D0196141

## CLASSIFICATIONS AND PROTOTYPE DRUGS

The classifications used in this book are based on the system used by the American Hospital Formulary Service (AHFS). This book further classifies drugs by therapeutic uses, enabling the nurse to identify drugs in the same class that have similar indications for use. Thus, the book provides a framework for understanding how drugs in a given class are used in clinical practice. The pharmacologic classification appears immediately after the **Classification** heading, followed by the **Therapeutic** classification. In general, all drugs in a class will have similar actions, uses, adverse effects, and nursing implications. Therefore, we have selected certain drugs that are representative of a classification or its subclassification— **prototype drugs** to aid the nurse in understanding the classification of drugs. Prototype drug monographs are identified with a small

icon. The user can refer to the prototype drug to develop a better understanding of drugs that belong within the same classification or subclassification. When a drug belongs to a classification that has a designated prototype drug, that prototype is identified directly below the therapeutic classification. The **Classifications Scheme** on pages xi–xviii identifies the drug prototype

considered to be representative of each class. All prototype drugs are highlighted in **bold** type in the index for quick identification. Some drugs have a unique mechanism of action or therapeutic effect. In these cases, there is no prototype drug to be identified.

## PREGNANCY CATEGORY

In December 2014, the FDA released a final rule replacing the historic "letter categories" with new detail subsections describing the risk of medication exposure in the real-world context of caring for pregnant patients. These changes will be implemented over the next several years; until that time, the historic "letter" categories will still be in use and therefore are included below for reference. Drugs may be described as **Pregnancy Category** A, B, C, D, or X according to the risk to the fetus, with A being the

---

**AMIODARONE HYDROCHLORIDE** ℗
(a-mee'oh-da-rone)
Cordarone, Nexterone, Pacerone
**Classification:** ANTIARRHYTHMIC, CLASS III
Therapeutic: CLASS III ANTIARRHYTHMIC; ANTIANGINAL

lowest and X the highest risk. Refer to Appendix C, *FDA Pregnancy Information*, for additional details.

## CONTROLLED SUBSTANCES

In the United States, **Controlled Substances** are classified as belonging to one of five schedules (I to V) according to abuse potential. Schedule I has the highest and Schedule V has the lowest potential for abuse. When a drug is a controlled substance, information about the schedule of the drug is found at the bottom of the yellow box. Refer to Appendix B, *U.S. Schedules of Controlled Substances*, for a complete description of each schedule.

## AVAILABILITY

Because drugs come in a variety of dosages and forms, the authors include a section devoted to **Availability** in each monograph. This section identifies the available dosage forms (e.g., tablets, capsules).

> **AVAILABILITY** Tablet; injection

## ACTION & *THERAPEUTIC EFFECT*

Each monograph describes the **Action** by which the specific drug produces physiologic and biochemic changes at the cellular, tissue, and organ levels. This information helps the user understand how the drug works in the body and makes it easier to learn its adverse reactions, and cautious uses. The *Therapeutic Effect,*

which is set in italics for clarity and ease of use is the reason why a drug is prescribed. Therapeutic effectiveness of the drug can be determined by monitoring improvement in the condition for which the drug is prescribed.

> **ACTION & *THERAPEUTIC EFFECT***
> Acts directly on all cardiac tissues by prolonging duration of action potential and refractory period. Slows conduction time through the AV node and can interrupt the reentry pathways through the AV node. *Effective in prevention or suppression of cardiac arrhythmias.*

## USES AND UNLABELED USES

The therapeutic applications of each drug are described in terms of approved (i.e., FDA-labeled) **Uses** and **Unlabeled Uses.** An unlabeled use is one that does not appear on the drug label or in the manufacturer's literature but is supported by medical literature or expert consensus.

> **USES** Prophylaxis and treatment of life-threatening ventricular arrhythmias and supraventricular arrhythmias, particularly with atrial fibrillation.
>
> **UNLABELED USES** Treatment of nonexertional angina, conversion of atrial fibrillation to normal sinus rhythm, paroxysmal supraventricular tachycardia, ventricular rate control due to accessory pathway conduction in pre-excited atrial arrhythmia, after defibrillation and epinephrine in cardiac arrest, AV nodal reentry tachycardia.

## CONTRAINDICATIONS AND CAUTIOUS USE

Many drugs have **Contraindications** and therefore should not be used in specific conditions, such as during pregnancy or pathologic disorders. In other cases, the drug requires **Cautious Use** because of a greater than average risk of untoward effects.

> **CONTRAINDICATIONS** Hypersensitivity to amiodarone, iodine, or benzyl alcohol; cardiogenic shock, severe sinus bradycardia, second- or third-degree AV block unless a pacemaker is available, severe sinus-node dysfunction or sick sinus syndrome, bradycardia causing syncopy (except in patients with functioning pacemaker); congenital or acquired QR prolongation syndromes, or history of torsades de pointes; pregnancy (category D); lactation.
>
> **CAUTIOUS USE** Severe hepatic disease, cirrhosis; Hashimoto's thyroiditis, goiter, thyrotoxicosis, or history of other thyroid dysfunction; severe hepatic impairment; CHF, older adults; Fabry disease especially with visual disturbances; electrolyte imbalance, hypokalemia, hypomagnesemia, hypovolemia; preexisting lung disease, COPD; open heart surgery.

## ROUTE & DOSAGE

The **Routes and Dosages** are highlighted in a blue box for easy access. Route of administration is specified as subcutaneous, IM, IV, PO, PR, nasal, ophthalmic, vaginal, topical, aural, intradermal, or intrathecal. Dosages are listed according to indication or FDA-approved labeled use(s). One of the hallmarks of this drug guide is the comprehensive dosage information it provides. The guide includes adult, geriatric, and pediatric dosages, as well as dosages for neonates and infants whenever applicable. This section also indicates dosage adjustments for renal impairment (based on creatinine clearance), hepatic impairment, patients undergoing hemodialysis, and obese patients (based on ideal body weight), as well as chemotherapeutic dosage adjustments based on these factors. Additionally, information about the need for dosage adjustments based on pharmacogenetic variables [e.g., cytochrome (CYP) system of enzymes] is provided as available.

> ## ROUTE & DOSAGE
>
> ### Arrhythmias
>
> *Adult:* **PO Loading Dose** 800–1600 mg/day in 1–2 doses for 1–3 wk **PO Maintenance Dose** 400–600 mg/day in 1–2 doses **IV Loading Dose** 150 mg over 10 min followed by 360 mg over next 6 h **IV Maintenance Dose** 540 mg over 18 h (0.5 mg/min), may continue at 0.5 mg/min **Convert IV to PO** Duration of infusion less than 1 wk use 800–1600 mg **PO,** 1–3 wk use 600–800 mg **PO,** greater than 3 wk use 400 mg **PO**
> *Child:* **IV** 5 mg/kg then repeat (max: 300 mg total)
> ***Hepatic Impairment Dosage Adjustment***
> Adjustment only suggested in severe hepatic impairment

## ADMINISTRATION

Drug administration is an important primary role for the nurse. Organized by different routes, the **Administration** section lists comprehensive instructions for administering, handling, and storing medications.

---

### ADMINISTRATION
- Note: Correct hypokalemia and hypomagnesemia prior to initiation of therapy.

### Oral
- Give consistently with respect to meals. Avoid grapefruit juice.
- Note: Only a prescriber experienced with the drug and treatment of life-threatening arrhythmias should give loading doses.
- Note: GI symptoms commonly occur during high-dose therapy, especially with loading doses. Symptoms usually respond to dose reduction or divided dose given with food, including milk.

---

## INTRAVENOUS DRUG ADMINISTRATION

Within the **Administration** section of appropriate monographs, the authors highlight intravenous drugs, indicated by a vertical color bar. This section provides users with comprehensive instructions on how to **Prepare** and **Administer** direct, intermittent, and continuous intravenous medications. When different from adults, intravenous administration and preparation for pediatric patients is provided. It also includes **Solution/Additive** and **Y-Site** incompatibility for every monograph, where appropriate, to indicate which drugs and solutions should not be mixed with the intravenous

drug. This is crucial information for drug administration. A chart for **Y-Site Compatibility** for common intravenous drugs is located inside the back cover of this drug guide. These enhancements eliminate the need for additional resources for intravenous administration.

---

### Intravenous

*PREPARE:* **IV Infusion: First rapid loading dose infusion:** Add 150 mg (3 mL) amiodarone to 100 mL D5W to yield 1.5 mg/mL. **Second infusion during first 24 h (slow loading dose and maintenance infusion):** Add 900 mg (18 mL) amiodarone to 500 mL D5W to yield 1.8 mg/mL. **Maintenance infusions after the first 24 h:** Prepare concentrations of 1–6 mg/mL amiodarone. Note: Use central line to give concentrations greater than 2 mg/mL.

*ADMINISTER:* **IV Infusion:** Initial infusion rate should not exceed 30 mg/min. Loading dose is usually given over 10 min in adults and 20–60 min in children. Note: See manufacturer's guidelines for **Nexterone** administration.

*INCOMPATIBILITIES:* **Solution/additive: Aminophylline, amoxicillin/clavulanic acid, cefazolin, floxacillin, furosemide, quinidine. Y-site: Acyclovir, allopurinol, amifostine, aminocaproic acid, aminophylline, amoxicillin, ampicillin, ampicillin/sulbactam, argatroban, atenolol, bivalirudin, cefamandole, cefazolin, cefotaxime, cefotetan, ceftazidime, ceftopribole, chloramphenicol, cytarabine, dantrolene, dexamethasone, diazepam, digoxin, doxorubicin, drotrecogin, ertapenem, fludarabine, fluorouracil, foscarnet, fosphenytoin, ganciclovir, gemtuzumab, heparin, hydrocortisone, imipenem/cilastatin, ketorolac, leucovorin, levofloxacin, magnesium sulfate, mechlorethamine, melphalan, meropenem, methotrexate,**

micafungin, mitomycin, paclitaxel, pentobarbital, phenytoin,
piperacillin, piperacillin/tazo-
bactam, potassium acetate, potassium phosphate, quinidine,
ranitidine, sodium bicarbonate,
sodium phosphate, SMZ/TMP,
thiopental, thiotepa, tigecycline,
verapamil.

## ADVERSE EFFECTS

Virtually all drugs have **Adverse
Effects** that may be bothersome to
some individuals but not to others.
Adverse effects with an incidence
of ≥2% are listed by body system
or organs. The most common adverse effects appear in *italic* type,
whereas those that are life-threatening are underlined. Users of the
drug guide will find a key at the
bottom of every page as a quick
reminder.

---

**ADVERSE EFFECTS** (≥1%) **CNS:**
Peripheral neuropathy (*muscle weakness*, wasting numbness, tingling),
*fatigue*, abnormal gait, dyskinesias,
*dizziness*, paresthesia, headache.
**CV:** Bradycardia, *hypotension* (IV),
sinus arrest, cardiogenic shock,
CHF, arrhythmias; AV block. **Special Senses:** *Corneal microdeposits*,
blurred vision, optic neuritis, optic
neuropathy, permanent blindness,
corneal degeneration, macular degeneration, photosensitivity. **GI:** *Anorexia, nausea, vomiting, constipation,*
hepatotoxicity. **Metabolic:** Hyperthyroidism or hypothyroidism; may cause
neonatal hypo- or hyperthyroidism if
taken during pregnancy. **Respiratory:**
(Pulmonary toxicity) Alveolitis, pneumonitis (fever, dry cough, dyspnea),
interstitial pulmonary fibrosis, fatal
gasping syndrome with IV in children.
**Skin:** Slate-blue pigmentation, *photosensitivity*, rash. **Other:** With chronic
use, angioedema.

---

## DIAGNOSTIC TEST INTERFERENCE

**Diagnostic Test Interference**
describes the effect of the drug on
various tests and alerts the nurse to
possible misinterpretations of test
results when applicable. The name
of the specific test altered is highlighted in **bold italic** type.

---

**DIAGNOSTIC TEST INTERFERENCE**
Ammonium chloride may increase
***blood ammonia*** and ***AST,*** decrease ***serum magnesium*** (by
increasing urinary magnesium
excretion), and decrease ***urine
urobilinogen.***

---

## INTERACTIONS

When applicable, this section lists
individual drugs, drug classes,
foods, and herbs that have relevant
interactions with the drug discussed in the monograph. Drugs
may interact to inhibit or enhance
one another. Thus, drug interactions may improve the therapeutic
response, lead to therapeutic failure, or produce specific adverse
reactions. Only drugs that have
been shown to cause clinically
significant and documented interactions with the drug discussed in
the monograph are identified. Note
that generic drugs appear in **bold**
type, and drug classes appear in
SMALL CAPS. Also listed are lab tests
that may have inaccurate results
due to effects of the drug.

---

**INTERACTIONS Drug:** Significantly increases **digoxin** levels;
enhances pharmacologic effects
and toxicities of **disopyramide,**

procainamide, quinidine, flecainide, lidocaine, lovastatin, simvastatin; anticoagulant effects of ORAL ANTICOAGULANTS enhanced; **verapamil, diltiazem,** BETA-ADRENERGIC BLOCKING AGENTS may potentiate sinus bradycardia, sinus arrest, or AV block; may increase **phenytoin** levels 2- to 3-fold; **cholestyramine** may decrease amiodarone levels; **fentanyl** may cause bradycardia, hypotension, or decreased output; may increase **cyclosporine** levels and toxicity; **cimetidine** may increase amiodarone levels; **ritonavir** may increase risk of amiodarone toxicity, including cardiotoxicity; **simvastatin** doses over 20 mg increase risk of rhabdomyolysis; **loratadine** use may increase risk of QT prolongation. **Food: Grapefruit juice** may increase amiodarone concentrations. **Herbal: Echinacea** may increase hepatotoxicity, **St. John's wort** may decrease efficacy. **Lab Test:** Affects thyroid function tests, causing an increase in serum $T_4$ and serum reverse $T_3$ levels, and a decline in serum $T_3$ levels.

**PHARMACOKINETICS** Absorption: 22–86% absorbed. **Onset (PO):** 2–3 days to 1–3 wk. **Peak:** 3–7 h. **Distribution:** Concentrates in adipose tissue, lungs, kidneys, spleen; crosses placenta; 96% protein bound. **Metabolism:** Extensively in liver; undergoes some enterohepatic cycling; via CYP2C8 and 3A4. **Elimination:** Excreted chiefly in bile and feces; also in breast milk. **Half-Life:** Biphasic, initial 2.5–10 days, terminal 40–55 days.

## PHARMACOKINETICS

This section identifies how the drug moves throughout the body. **Pharmacokinetics** lists the mechanisms of absorption, distribution, metabolism, elimination, and half-life when known. It also provides information about onset, peak, and duration of the drug action. Where appropriate, information appears for protein-binding and CYP450 impact.

## NURSING IMPLICATIONS

Under the headings **Black Box Warning, Assessment & Drug Effects,** and **Patient & Family Education,** the nurse can quickly and easily identify needed information and incorporate it into the appropriate steps of the nursing process. Before administering a drug, the nurse should read **Nursing Implications** to determine the assessments that should be made before and after administration of the drug, the indicators of drug effectiveness, laboratory tests recommended for individual drugs, and the essential patient and/or family education related to the drug.

## BLACK BOX WARNING

The U.S. Food and Drug Administration (FDA) can require a pharmaceutical company to place a warning in the literature describing potentially serious or life-threatening risks associated with a prescription drug. This type of warning is commonly referred to as a "black box warning" because it appears in the manufacturer's literature printed within a box outlined in black. If a drug has a black box warning, the warning will appear in each monograph directly under the **Nursing Implication** heading.

## NURSING IMPLICATIONS

### Black Box Warning

*Amiodarone has been associated with pulmonary toxicity (sometimes severe and potentially fatal), liver injury (ranging from mild to severe), and development of arrhythmias (heart block or sinus bradycardia).*

### Assessment & Drug Effects

- Monitor BP carefully during infusion and slow the infusion if significant hypotension occurs; bradycardia should be treated by slowing the infusion or discontinuing if necessary. Monitor heart rate and rhythm and BP until drug response has stabilized; report promptly symptomatic bradycardia. Sustained monitoring is essential because drug has an unusually long half-life.
- Monitor for S&S of: Adverse effects, particularly conduction disturbances and exacerbation of arrhythmias, in patients receiving other antiarrhythmic drugs; drug-induced hypothyroidism or hyperthyroidism (see Appendix F), especially during early treatment period; pulmonary toxicity (progressive dyspnea, fatigue, cough, pleuritic pain, fever) throughout therapy.
- Monitor for elevations of AST and ALT. If elevations persist or if they are 2–3 times above normal baseline readings, reduce dosage or withdraw drug promptly to prevent hepatotoxicity and liver damage.

- Auscultate chest periodically or when patient complains of respiratory symptoms. Check for diminished breath sounds, rales, pleuritic friction rub; observe breathing pattern. Drug-induced pulmonary function problems **must be** distinguished from CHF or pneumonia. Keep prescriber informed.
- Anticipate possible CNS symptoms within a week after amiodarone therapy begins. Proximal muscle weakness, a common side effect, intensified by tremors presents a great hazard to the ambulating patient. Assess severity of symptoms. Supervision of ambulation may be indicated.
- Monitor lab tests: Baseline and periodic serum electrolytes (i.e., potassium and magnesium); baseline and semiannual LFTs; baseline and periodic thyroid functions.

### Patient & Family Education

- Check pulse daily once stabilized, or as prescribed. Report a pulse less than 60.
- Take oral drug consistently with respect to meals. Do not drink grapefruit juice while taking this drug.
- Become familiar with potential adverse reactions and report those that are bothersome to the prescriber.
- Use dark glasses to ease photophobia; some patients may not be able to go outdoors in the daytime even with such protection.
- Follow recommendation for regular ophthalmic exams, including funduscopy and slit-lamp exam.
- Wear protective clothing and a barrier-type sunscreen that physically blocks penetration of skin by ultraviolet light to prevent a photosensitivity reaction (erythema, pruritus); avoid exposure to sun and sunlamps.

## THERAPEUTIC EFFECTIVENESS

Therapeutic effectiveness of a drug can be determined by monitoring improvement in the condition for which the drug is prescribed, and by using the **Assessment & Drug Effects** section. Drugs have multiple uses or indications. Therefore, it is important to know why a drug is being prescribed for a specific patient (**Uses** and **Unlabeled Uses**). In the italicized sentences at the end of the **Action & *Therapeutic Effect*** section in all monographs, specific indicators of the effectiveness of the drug are provided. Additionally, in the **Route & Dosage** table for each drug, the dosages are listed according to the indications for FDA-labeled use(s) of the drug. Furthermore, the **Therapeutic** classifications listed within the gold box at the beginning of the monograph provide the nurse with further assistance in determining and evaluating the therapeutic effectiveness of the drug.

# PEARSON
# NURSE'S
## DRUG GUIDE
# 2019

Kelly M. Shields, PharmD
Associate Dean and Professor of Pharmacy Practice
Raabe College of Pharmacy
Ohio Northern University
Ada, Ohio

Kami L. Fox, DNP, RN, APRN, CPNP-PC
Director/Chair and Associate Professor of Nursing
Ohio Northern University
Ada, Ohio

Christina Liebrecht, DNP, RN
Associate Professor of Nursing
Ohio Northern University
Ada, Ohio

 Pearson

330 Hudson Street, NY NY 10013

Copyright © 2019 by Pearson Education, Inc., Hoboken, NJ 07030

www.pearson.com

1    18

ISBN 0-13-520485-2/978-0-13-520485-6

PRINTED IN THE UNITED STATES OF AMERICA

# CONTENTS

To

*Rick, Kris, Leah, and Katelyn for*
*their willing sacrifice of time and their patience.*

◆

To

*Frostie, the first nurse that loved*
*and cared for me. My parents Karron, Marion,*
*and my family: Ken, Amelia, Nolan, and Sophia*
*for their unconditional love, support, and guiding*
*light that allow me to provide safe and*
*compassionate care to others.*

◆

*My family—Jay,*
*Amanda, Rachel, and Brie—Thank you for all of*
*your love, encouragement, laughter, and support.*
*And, my students, who soak up learning and*
*inspire me.*

◆

*And a special thank you to Billie Ann Wilson*
*and Margaret T. Shannon;*

*without whom this work would not have been possible*

# ABOUT THE AUTHORS

**Kelly M. Shields** is currently Associate Dean and Professor of Pharmacy Practice at Ohio Northern University's Raabe College of Pharmacy. She holds a Doctor of Pharmacy from Butler University and completed a fellowship in Natural Product Information and Research at University of Missouri-Kansas City. She has practiced pharmacy in retail, community, and academic settings and has worked as a freelance medical writer.

**Kami L. Fox** is the Director/Chair and Associate Professor of the Department of Nursing at Ohio Northern University. She holds a BS and MS in Nursing from Wright State University in Dayton, Ohio, and a DNP from the University of Toledo. She is a certified pediatric nurse practitioner in primary care.

**Christina M. Liebrecht** is Associate Professor of Nursing at Ohio Northern University. She holds a BS in Nursing from University of Toledo, an MS in Nursing from Walden University, and Doctorate in Nursing Practice from the University of Toledo. She has been in nursing education for the last 19 years with a focus on medical surgical nursing, fundamentals of nursing, and community health nursing as well as the use of simulation to support student learning and safe practice. She continues to practice as a medical surgical nurse in the acute care setting.

## ABOUT THE AUTHORS

### PHARMACY CONSULTANT

A special acknowledgment to **Zachary Woods, PharmD, RPh,** PGY1 Pharmacy Practice Resident, Ohio Northern University who is a tremendous addition to the author team as a contributor for the monographs of the new drugs in this edition. We are grateful for his expertise and for his valued input.

We wish to thank the following individuals for conducting thorough reviews of the drug information in this book for its accuracy, currency, relevance, presentation, accessibility, and use. Their feedback guided us in developing a better book for nurses.

**Nile Barnes, Pharm.D.**
The University of Texas at Austin
Austin, TX

**Karen Bastianelli, Pharm.D.**
University of Minnesota
Duluth, MN

**Kalin M. Clifford, Pharm.D.**
Texas Tech University Health Center
Dallas, TX

**Vinh N. Kieu, Pharm.D**
George Mason University
Fairfax, VA

# PREFACE

***Pearson Nurse's Drug Guide 2019*** is a current and reliable reference designed to provide comprehensive information needed to make appropriate decisions regarding drug administration. This new edition includes 18 new monographs for drugs recently approved by the Food and Drug Administration (FDA), and over 400 updates to drug indications, available dosage forms, adverse effects, dosages, and more. IV administration information has been updated regarding adults as well as children. There are subheadings for IV preparation and administration of IV medications for children (when available), which add to the ease of locating appropriate information by age.

Each drug monograph provides the necessary information for safe and effective drug administration. The user should read all the information provided. Occasionally, the user will be referred to Appendix F, *Glossary of Key Terms, Clinical Conditions, and Associated Signs and Symptoms*. This unique glossary provides valuable information regarding common assessment findings related to therapeutic effectiveness or ineffectiveness of specific drugs.

The authors recognize that the decision-making process related to drug administration is a cyclical one. For example, assessments are made both prior to and after drug administration. Thus, nursing diagnoses and interventions may change as a result of an *achieved therapeutic effect, therapeutic failure, manifestation of an adverse effect,* or *demonstration of a learning need*. The authors believe that the users of this drug reference will find that the clear and logical design of the drug monographs facilitates decision making and supports the nursing process.

Since physicians, advanced practice nurses, and other health professionals have prescriptive privileges, the term *prescriber* is used throughout this book.

## ORGANIZATION

The ***Pearson Nurse's Drug Guide 2019*** is user friendly. To help readers better understand how to use the drug guide, the authors illustrate and describe all the components of a drug monograph in the ***How to Use the Pearson Nurse's Drug Guide 2019,*** immediately after the front cover of the book.

In this drug guide, all drugs are listed alphabetically according to their generic names. Pharmacologic classifications are paired with therapeutic classifications for every drug monograph for ease of use by nurse clinicians and students alike. Each drug is indexed by both its generic and trade names in the back of the guide to make it easier for the user to locate individual drug monographs. Trade names followed by a maple leaf indicate that brand of the drug is available in Canada.

If a drug is not listed in the alphabetical section, it may be a combination drug, which is a drug made up of more than one generic component. Common combination drugs are listed under their trade names in the index and in Appendix E, *Prescription Combination Drugs*. The appendix identifies the generic components and the amount of each active ingredient contained in the combination. Users of this drug guide will find the page numbers for monographs of the component drugs in this appendix to make access to this information easier and faster.

## APPENDICES

Several helpful tables and charts in this drug guide include: Appendix A, *Ocular Medications, Low Molecular Weight Heparins, Inhaled Corticosteroids, Topical Corticosteroids*, and *Topical Antifungal Agents*; Appendix B, *U.S. Schedules of Controlled Substances*; Appendix C, *FDA Pregnancy Information*; Appendix D, *Oral Dosage Forms That Should Not Be Crushed*; Appendix E, *Prescription Combination Drugs*; Appendix F, *Glossary of Key Terms, Clinical Conditions, and Associated Signs and Symptoms*; Appendix G, *Abbreviations*; Appendix H, *Herbal and Dietary Supplement Table*; Appendix I, *Look-Alike, Sound-Alike Medications*, which highlights medications that are commonly involved in medication errors; Appendix J, *Vaccines*, which highlights vaccines commonly seen/administered in practice.

## INDEX

The index in the ***Pearson Nurse's Drug Guide 2019*** is perhaps the most often-used section in the entire book. All generic, trade, and combination drugs are listed in this index. Whenever a trade name is listed, the generic drug monograph is listed in parentheses. Additionally, classifications are listed and identified in SMALL CAPS, whereas all prototype drugs are highlighted in **bold** type. Drugs belonging to various classifications and subclassifications, including therapeutic classes, are also cross-referenced in this index. As a special feature, the index includes entries for combination drugs (e.g., Tylenol with Codeine) with index references to component drugs as well as the combination drug reference to Appendix E. Medications listed in Appendix A (*Ocular Medications, Low Molecular Weight Heparins, Inhaled Corticosteroids, Topical Corticosteroid, and Topical Antifungal Agents*) or Appendix J (*Vaccines*) are also cross-referenced in the index.

## ACKNOWLEDGMENTS

We wish to express our appreciation to our past and present students who have provided the inspiration for this work. It is for these individuals and all who strive for excellence in patient care that this work was undertaken.

**Kelly M. Shields, PharmD**
**Kami L. Fox, DNP, RN, APRN, CPNP-PC**
**Christina Liebrecht, DNP, RN**

# ABACAVIR SULFATE
(a-ba′ca-vir)

Ziagen

**Classifications:** ANTIRETROVIRAL; NUCLEOSIDE REVERSE TRANSCRIPTASE INHIBITOR (NRTI)
**Therapeutic:** ANTIRETROVIRAL (NRTI)
**Prototype:** Lamivudine

**AVAILABILITY** Tablet; oral solution

## ACTION & *THERAPEUTIC EFFECT*
Abacavir inhibits the activity of viral reverse transcriptase (RT) by competing with natural DNA nucleoside and by incorporation into viral DNA. Abacavir prevents viral DNA replication. *Viral load decreases as measured by an increased $CD_4$ lymphocyte cell count and suppression of HIV RNA, indicated by decreased HIV RNA copies, in HIV-positive individuals with little or no exposure to zidovudine (AZT).*

**USES** Treatment of HIV infection in combination with other antiretroviral agents.

**CONTRAINDICATIONS** Hypersensitivity to abacavir; serious and sometimes fatal hypersensitivity to abacavir have been reported; lactic acidosis; creatinine clearance of less than 50 mL/min; severe hepatomegaly with severe steatosis; moderate to severe hepatic impairment; lactation.

**CAUTIOUS USE** Patients with HLA-B*5701 allele (high risk for hypersensitivity reaction); prior resistance to another nucleoside reverse transcriptase inhibitor (NRTI); history of cardiac disease; hypertension, hyperlipidemia, DM, smoking; older adults; pregnancy (category C). Safe use in children younger than 3 mo has not been established.

## ROUTE & DOSAGE

### HIV Infection
*Adult:* **PO** 300 mg b.i.d. or 600 mg once daily
*Child (3 mo–16 y):* **PO** 8 mg/kg b.i.d. (max: 300 mg b.i.d.)
*Patients weighing 14 to less than 21 kg:* **PO** 150 mg twice daily; *21 to less than 30 kg:* **PO** 150 mg qam and 300 mg in the evening; *greater than 30 kg:* **PO** 300 mg twice daily

### Hepatic Impairment Dosage Adjustment
*Mild (Child-Pugh score 5–6):* 200 mg b.i.d.

## ADMINISTRATION
### Oral
- Tablets and oral solution are interchangeable on a mg-for-mg basis.
- Store tablets and liquid at 20°–25° C (68°–77° F). Liquid may be refrigerated.

**ADVERSE EFFECTS (≥1%) Body as a Whole:** Hypersensitivity reactions (including fever, skin rash, fatigue, nausea, vomiting, diarrhea, abdominal pain); malaise; lethargy; myalgia; arthralgia; paresthesia; edema; shortness of breath. **CNS:** Insomnia, *headache, fever.* **CV:** Hypotension (associated with hypersensitivity reaction), heart attack. **GI:** Hepatomegaly with steatosis, *nausea, vomiting, diarrhea, anorexia,* pancreatitis, increased GGT, increased liver function tests. **Skin:** *Rash.* **Other:** Lactic acidosis, renal insufficiency.

**INTERACTIONS Drug: Alcohol** may increase abacavir blood levels Use caution with **ribavirin.**

**PHARMACOKINETICS Absorption:** Rapidly absorbed, 83% bioavailable. **Distribution:** Distributes into

Common adverse effects in *italic;* life-threatening effects <u>underlined;</u> generic names in **bold;** classifications in SMALL CAPS; ♣ Canadian drug name; ● Prototype drug

1

extravascular space and erythrocytes; 50% protein bound. **Metabolism:** Metabolized by alcohol dehydrogenase and glucuronyl transferase to inactive metabolites. **Elimination:** 84% in urine, primarily as inactive metabolites; 16% in feces. **Half-Life:** 1.5 h.

## NURSING IMPLICATIONS

### Black Box Warning

*Abacavir has been associated with serious and sometimes fatal hypersensitivity reactions especially in those with the HLA-B\*5701 allele; and with lactic acidosis and severe hetatomegaly, sometimes fatal.*

### Assessment & Drug Effects

- Monitor for S&S of hypersensitivity: fever, skin rash, fatigue, GI distress (nausea, vomiting, diarrhea, abdominal pain). Withhold drug and immediately notify prescriber if hypersensitivity develops.
- Monitor for S&S of lactic acidosis [e.g., hyperventilation, lethargy, plasma pH less than 7.35 and lactate greater than 5–6 mol/L (mEq/L)], hepatomegaly, and renal insufficiency. Withhold drug and immediately notify prescriber for S&S of acidosis or hepatotoxicity.
- Monitor lab tests: Baseline screening for HLA-B\*5701; periodic LFTs, BUN and creatinine, CBC with differential, triglyceride levels, and blood glucose (especially in diabetics.)

### Patient & Family Education

- Take drug exactly as prescribed at indicated times. Missed dose: Take immediately, then resume dosing schedule. Do not double a dose.
- Withhold drug immediately and notify prescriber at first sign of hypersensitivity or liver damage (see Assessment & Drug Effects).

- Carry Warning Card provided with drug at all times.

# ABALOPARATIDE
(a-bal'oh-par'a-tide)

Tymlos

**Classifications:** PARATHYROID AGENTS
Therapeutic: PARATHYROID HORMONE ANALOG

**AVAILABILITY** Subcutaneous injection, multiuse pen

**ACTION & *THERAPEUTIC EFFECT***
Analog of human parathyroid hormone related peptide which acts as an agonist at the PTH1 receptor. *Results in stimulation of osteoblast function and increased bone mass.*

**USES** Osteoporosis in postmenopausal women, at high risk of fracture, who have failed or cannot tolerate other therapies.

**CAUTIOUS USE** Urolithiasis; pregnancy; lactation. Safety and efficacy in children not established.

## ROUTE & DOSAGE

### Osteoporosis
*Adult:* **Subcutaneous** 80 mcg daily

## ADMINISTRATION

### Subcutaneous
- Inject subcutaneously into the periumbilical region of the abdomen.
- Rotate sites each day and administer at approximately the same time each day.

**ADVERSE EFFECTS** (≥ 2%) **CNS:** *Dizziness, headache,* fatigue. **Endocrine and Metabolic:** *Increased uric acid,* hypercalcemia. **Urinary:** *Hypercalciuria.* **Integumentary:**

---

Common adverse effects in *italic;* life-threatening effects <u>underlined</u>; generic names in **bold;** classifications in SMALL CAPS; ◆ Canadian drug name; ◉ Prototype drug

*Erythema at injection site, swelling at injection site,* pain at injection site. **Cardiac:** Palpitations, orthostatic hypotension, tachycardia. **GI:** *Nausea,* upper abdominal pain. **Metabolic:** Hypercalcemia.

**PHARMACOKINETICS Absorption:** 36% bioavailability. **Distribution:** 70% protein bound. **Metabolism:** Proteolytic degradation into small peptide groups. **Elimination:** Urine. **Half-Life:** 1.7 h.

## NURSING IMPLICATIONS

### Black Box Warning

*Abaloparatide was associated with an increased risk of osteosarcoma in animal studies; avoid use in patients with increased risk for osteosarcoma at baseline.*

### Assessment & Drug Effects
• Monitor for and report orthostatic hypotension.
• Monitor serum calcium; bone mineral density (BMD) should be evaluated 1–2 y after initiating therapy and every 2 y thereafter.

### Patient & Family Education
• Notify prescriber immediately if you experience bone pain, pain anywhere that does not go away, a lump, or swelling under the skin that is tender.
• Notify prescriber if you have signs of high calcium levels such as weakness, confusion, feeling tired, headache, upset stomach, vomiting, constipation, or bone pain.
• Notify prescriber if you experience signs or symptoms of allergic reaction such as rash, hives, itching, shortness of breath, wheezing, cough, swelling of the face, lips, tongue, or throat; or any other signs.

• To lower the chance of feeling dizzy, change positions and sit and stand slowly. Be careful going up and down stairs.

## ABATACEPT
(a-ba-ta'sept)
Orencia
**Classifications:** BIOLOGIC AND IMMUNOLOGICAL; IMMUNOMODULATOR; DISEASE-MODIFYING ANTIRHEUMATIC DRUG (DMARD)
**Therapeutic:** ANTIRHEUMATIC (DMARD); ANTI-INFLAMMATORY

**AVAILABILITY** Lyophilized powder for injection; solution for injection

**ACTION & THERAPEUTIC EFFECT**
Inhibits T-cell (T-lymphocyte) activation by binding to CD80 and CD86, thereby blocking interaction with CD28 receptors on T-cells. Blocking this interaction inhibits a costimulatory signal necessary for full activation of T-lymphocytes. Activated T-lymphocytes are implicated in the pathogenesis of RA and are found in the synovium of patients with RA. *It relieves RA symptoms and slows progression of structural damage. It improves RA physical function in adults with active RA who have had an inadequate response to other drugs.*

**USES** Treatment of moderate to severe rheumatoid arthritis or juvenile rheumatoid arthritis.

**CONTRAINDICATIONS** Known hypersensitivity to abatacept, live vaccines; active infections; coadministration with anakinra, TNF antagonists, other biologic RA therapy; lactation.

Common adverse effects in *italic;* life-threatening effects underlined; generic names in **bold;** classifications in SMALL CAPS; ♣ Canadian drug name; ⊙ Prototype drug

3

CAUTIOUS USE COPD; malignancies; pregnancy (category C); children younger than 6 y.

## ROUTE & DOSAGE

### Rheumatoid Arthritis

*Adult (weight less than 60 kg):* **IV** Initial dose: 500 mg every 2 wk × 3 doses; *weight 60–100 kg:* 750 mg every 2 wk × 3 doses; *weight greater than 100 kg:* 1000 mg every 2 wk × 3 doses then every 4 wk; **Subcutaneous** 125 mg weekly

### Juvenile Idiopathic Arthritis

*Child (at least 6 y, weight less than 75 kg):* **IV** 10 mg/kg, repeat at wk 2 and 4, then monthly (max: 1000 mg); *weight 75–100 kg:* 750 mg at wk 2 and 4, then monthly; *weight at least 100 kg:* 1000 mg at wk 2 and 4, then monthly

## ADMINISTRATION

### Subcutaneous

- Abatacept for subcutaneous injection is supplied in a 125mg/mL prefilled syringe.
- Do not remove the small bubble of air in the syringe and do not pull back on the plunger head before injection.
- Ensure that the full contents of the syringe are injected. Rotate injection sites.
- Prefilled syringes must be stored at 2°–8° C (36°–46° F). Do not freeze.
- Allow prefilled syringe and autoinjector to warm to room temperature for 30–60 min prior to administration.

### Intravenous

- Note: The prefilled syringe is for subcutaneous injection only. Do not use for IV infusion.

*PREPARE:* **IV Infusion:** Use the supplied silicone-free disposable syringe with an 18–21 gauge needle to reconstitute the vial. ▪ Add 10 mL sterile water to each 250 mL to yield 25 mg/mL. ▪ To avoid foaming, gently swirl until completely dissolved. Do not shake or vigorously agitate. ▪ After dissolving, vent the vial with a needle to dissipate any foam. ▪ The reconstituted solution **must be** further diluted to a total of 100 mL as follows: From a 100 mL NS IV bag remove a volume equal to the total volume of abatacept in the reconstituted vials (e.g., for 2 vials, remove 20 mL). Using the supplied silicone-free syringe, slowly add the reconstituted abatacept to the IV bag and gently mix. ▪ The final concentration of the IV solution will be approximately 5, 7.5, or 10 mg/mL, depending on whether 2, 3, or 4 vials are used. ▪ Discard any unused abatacept.

*ADMINISTER:* **IV Infusion:** Use a 0.2–1.2 micron low-protein-binding filter. Infuse over 30 min.

*INCOMPATIBILITIES:* **Solution/additive:** Should not be infused in the same intravenous line with other agents. **Y-site:** Should not be infused in the same intravenous line with other agents.

- Store at 2°–8° C (36°–46° F). Protect from light.

## ADVERSE EFFECTS (≥1%) **Body as a Whole:** Infusion-related reactions, <u>malignancies</u>, *cough*, hypersensitivity reactions. **CNS:** *Headache*, dizziness. **CV:** Hypertension. **GI:** *Nausea*, dyspepsia. **Musculoskeletal:** Back pain, pain in extremity. **Respiratory:** *Upper respiratory tract infection, nasopharyngitis*, sinusitis, influenza, bronchitis. **Skin:** Rash. **Urogenital:** Urinary tract infection.

**INTERACTIONS Drug:** TNF ANTAG-ONISTS increase the risk of serious infections. Avoid use of LIVE VAC-CINES. Avoid use of **anakinra.**

**PHARMACOKINETICS Half-Life:** 13.1 days.

## NURSING IMPLICATIONS

### Assessment & Drug Effects
- Prior to initiating treatment with abatacept, screen for latent TB in-fection with a TB skin test.
- Monitor for S&S of hypersensi-tivity (e.g., hypotension, urticaria, and dyspnea); discontinue infu-sion and notify prescriber if any of these occur.
- Monitor for S&S of infection. Withhold drug and notify pre-scriber if patient develops a seri-ous infection.
- Monitor for deterioration of respira-tory status in patients with COPD.

### Patient & Family Education
- Report any of the following to a health care provider: Any type of infection, a positive TB skin test, a recent vaccination, a persistent cough, unexplained weight loss, fever, sore throat, or night sweats.
- Report S&S of an allergic reaction that may develop within 24 h of receiving abatacept (e.g., hives swollen face, eyelids, lips, tongue, throat, or trouble breathing).
- Do not accept immunizations with live vaccines while taking or within 3 mo of discontinuing abatacept.

## ABCIXIMAB ©

(ab-cix′i-mab)

ReoPro

**Classifications:** ANTIPLATELET; GLYCOPROTEIN IIB/IIIA INHIBITOR Therapeutic: PLATELET AGGREGATION INHIBITOR

**AVAILABILITY** Solution

## ACTION & *THERAPEUTIC EFFECT*
Abciximab is a human-murine mon-oclonal antibody Fab (fragment an-tigen binding) fragment that binds to the glycoprotein IIb/IIIa (GPIIb/IIIa) receptor sites of platelets. *Abciximab inhibits platelet aggre-gation by preventing fibrinogen, von Willebrand's factor, and other molecules from adhering to GPIIb/IIIa receptor sites of the platelets.*

**USES** Adjunct to aspirin and heparin for the prevention of acute cardiac ischemic complications in patients undergoing percutaneous translu-minal coronary angioplasty (PTCA).

**UNLABELED USES** Acute MI, Ka-wasaki disease.

**CONTRAINDICATIONS** Hypersen-sitivity to abciximab or to murine pro-teins; active internal bleeding; GI or GU bleeding within 6 wk; history of CVA within 2 y or a CVA with severe neurologic deficit; thrombocytopenia (less than 100,000 cells/mL); recent major surgery or trauma; intracranial neoplasm, aneurysm, severe hyper-tension; history of vasculitis; use of dextran before or during PTCA.

**CAUTIOUS USE** Patients weighing less than 75 kg; history of previous GI disease; recent thrombolytic therapy; PTCA within 12 h of MI; unsuccessful PTCA; PTCA procedure lasting longer than 70 min; older adults; pregnancy (category C); lactation. Safe use in children has not been established.

## ROUTE & DOSAGE

| PTCA |
| --- |
| *Adult:* **IV** 0.25 mg/kg bolus 10–60 min prior to angioplasty, followed by continuous infusion of 0.125 mcg/kg/min (up to 10 mcg/min) for next 12–24 h |

## ADMINISTRATION

### Intravenous

Do not shake vial. Discard if visible opaque particles are noted.
■ Use a nonpyrogenic low protein-binding 0.2- or 0.22-micron filter when withdrawing drug into a syringe from the 2 mg/mL vial and when infusing as continuous IV.

*PREPARE:* **Direct:** No dilution required. **Continuous:** Inject 5 mL of abciximab (10 mg) into 250 mL of NS or D5W.

*ADMINISTER:* **Direct:** Give undiluted bolus dose over 5 min. **Continuous:** Infuse at no more than 15 mL/h (10 mcg/min) via an infusion pump over 12 h to 24 h.

*INCOMPATIBILITIES:* **Solution/additive:** Infuse through ˙separate IV line. **Y-site:** Infuse through separate IV line.

■ Discard any unused drug at the end of the 12 h infusion as well as any unused portion left in vial. ■ Store vials at 2°–8° C (36°–46° F).

## ADVERSE EFFECTS (≥1%) **Hematologic:** *Bleeding*, including intracranial, retroperitoneal, and hematemesis; thrombocytopenia.

## INTERACTIONS **Drug:** ORAL ANTICOAGULANTS, NSAIDS, **dipyridamole, ticlopidine, dextran** may increase risk of bleeding. Herbal: Gingko can increase bleeding risk.

## PHARMACOKINETICS **Onset:** Greater than 90% inhibition of platelet aggregation within 2 h. **Duration:** Approximately 48 h. **Half-Life:** 30 min.

## NURSING IMPLICATIONS

### Assessment & Drug Effects

■ Monitor for S&S of: Bleeding at all potential sites (e.g., catheter insertion, needle puncture, or cutdown sites; GI, GU, or retroperitoneal sites); hypersensitivity that may occur any time during administration.
■ Avoid or minimize unnecessary invasive procedures and devices to reduce risk of bleeding.
■ Elevate head of bed 30° or less and keep limb straight when femoral artery access is used; following sheath removal, apply pressure for 30 min.
■ Stop infusion immediately and notify prescriber if bleeding or S&S of hypersensitivity occurs.
■ Monitor lab tests: Baseline platelet count, PT, aPTT, and ACT, then repeat every 2–4 h during first 24 h; aPTT or ACT prior to arterial sheath removal (do not remove unless aPTT is 50 sec or less or ACT is 75 sec or less).

### Patient & Family Education

■ Report any S&S of bleeding immediately.

## ABEMACICLIB

(uh-beh′muh-sy′klib)

Verzenio

**Classifications:** ANTINEOPLASTIC AGENT; CYCLIN-DEPENDENT KINASE INHIBITOR

Therapeutic: ANTINEOPLASTIC

## AVAILABILITY Tablet

## ACTION & *THERAPEUTIC EFFECT*

Potent small molecule cycline-dependent kinase inhibitor that blocks retinoblastoma tumor suppressor protein phosphoryulation and prevents progression through cell cycle resulting in arrest of the G1 phase. *Results in decreased tumor size.*

## USES Monotherapy in HR-positive, HER2-negative advanced or metastatic breast cancer in patients with disease progression following

endocrine therapy and prior chemotherapy in metastatic setting. Used in combination with fulvestrant for treatment of HR-positive, HER2-negative advanced or metastatic breast cancer in women with disease progression following endocrine therapy.

**CAUTIOUS USE** Hepatic impairment; pregnancy; lactation. Safety and efficacy in children not established.

## ROUTE & DOSAGE

**Breast Cancer**

*Adult:* **PO Monotherapy** 200 mg b.i.d. until disease progression or unacceptable toxicity; **PO Combination therapy** 150 mg b.i.d. (in combination with fulvestrant and potential gonadotropin releasing hormone agonist) until disease progression or unacceptable toxicity

*Toxicity Dosage Adjustment*

See package insert

## ADMINISTRATION

**Oral**

- Administer at approximately the same times each day.
- May be administered with or without food. Swallow whole, do not crush, chew, or split tablets.

**ADVERSE EFFECTS** (≥ 2%) **CNS:** *Dizziness, headache, fatigue.* **Integumentary:** *Alopecia.* **GI:** *Weight loss, nausea, decreased appetite, abdominal pain, vomiting, constipation, stomatitis, xerostomia, dysgeusia.* **Hematologic:** *Anemia, decreased lymphocyte count, neutropenia,* thrombocytopenia, leukopenia. **Hepatic:** *Increased serum ALT/AST.* **Muscular:** *Arthralgia.* **Renal:** *Increased serum*

*creatinine.* **Respiratory:** *Cough.* **Endocrine and Metabolic:** Dehydration. **Body as a Whole:** *Infection, fever,* venous thromboembolism.

**INTERACTIONS Drug:** Abemaciclib is a substrate of CYP3A4 (major); avoid combination with strong inducers (e.g., carbamazepine, phenytoin, rifampin. **Herbal:** St. John's wort.

**PHARMACOKINETICS Absorption:** 45% bioavailability (after single 200 mg oral dose). **Distribution:** 96% protein bound. **Metabolism:** Hepatic, CYP3A4, forms active metabolites. **Elimination:** 81% in feces, 3% in urine. **Half-Life:** 18.3 h; up to 55 h in patients with severe hepatic impairment.

## NURSING IMPLICATIONS

### Assessment & Drug Effects

- Monitor for and report S&S of severe diarrhea, dehydration, or infection
- Use effective form of birth control; notify doctor immediately if you become pregnant.
- Perform pregnancy testing prior to initiating treatment.
- Monitor lab tests: CBC with differential, platelet count, and LFTs at baseline, every 2 wk for the first 2 mo, then monthly for 2 mo.

### Patient & Family Education

- Notify prescriber if you experience signs or symptoms of allergic reaction such as rash, hives, itching, shortness of breath, wheezing, cough, swelling of the face, lips, tongue, or throat; or any other signs.
- Bleeding may occur with this medication. Be careful to avoid injury. Use a soft toothbrush and an electric razor.
- Notify prescriber right away if you have signs of a blood clot such as

Common adverse effects in *italic;* life-threatening effects <u>underlined</u>; generic names in **bold;** classifications in SMALL CAPS; ♣ Canadian drug name; ⊕ Prototype drug

7

chest pain or pressure; coughing up blood; shortness of breath; swelling, warmth, numbness, change of color, or pain in the leg or arm; or trouble speaking or swallowing.
- Use effective form of birth control while on this medication and for 3 wk after your last dose. Notify prescriber immediately if you become pregnant.

## ABIRATERONE ACETATE
(a'bir-a'ter-one as'e-tate)

Zytiga

**Classifications:** ANTINEOPLASTIC; ANTIANDROGEN; ANDROGEN BIOSYNTHESIS INHIBITOR
Therapeutic: ANTIANDROGEN

**AVAILABILITY** Tablet

## ACTION & *THERAPEUTIC EFFECT*
Inhibits the enzyme required for androgen biosynthesis in testicular, adrenal, and prostatic tumor tissues. Enzyme inhibition may also result in increased mineralocorticoid production in the adrenal glands. *Decreased levels of serum testosterone and other androgens slow the growth of androgen-sensitive carcinomas.*

**USES** Metastatic castration-resistant prostate cancer.

**CONTRAINDICATIONS** Severe hepatic impairment (Child-Pugh class C); pregnancy (category X).

**CAUTIOUS USE** History of CV disease (e.g., heart failure, hypertension, recent MI, ventricular arrhythmias); hypokalemia; fluid retention; concurrent steroid therapy, especially during dosage adjustment or with concurrent infection or stress; moderate hepatic impairment

(Child-Pugh class B). Abiratrone is not indicated for use in children.

## ROUTE & DOSAGE

**Metastatic Prostate Cancer**

*Adult:* **PO** 1000 mg once daily in combination with **PO** prednisone 5 mg b.i.d.

**Hepatic Impairment Dosage Adjustment**

*Moderate impairment (Child-Pugh class B score 7–9):* **PO** 250 mg once daily
*Severe impairment (Child-Pugh class C score greater than 10):* Do not use

## ADMINISTRATION
**Oral**
- Give on an empty stomach 2 h before or 1 h after food.
- Tablets should be swallowed whole with water.
- Women who are or may be pregnant must use gloves to handle abiraterone.
- Store at 15°–30° C (59°–86° F).

**ADVERSE EFFECTS** (≥1%) **CV:** *Arrhythmia*, <u>cardiac failure</u>, chest pain or discomfort, *hot flush, hypertension*. **GI:** *Diarrhea*, dyspepsia. **Metabolic:** *Edema*, elevated ALT and AST, elevated total bilirubin, elevated triglycerides, hypokalemia, hypophosphatemia. **Musculoskeletal:** *Joint discomfort and swelling, muscle discomfort*. **Respiratory:** *Cough*, upper respiratory tract infection. **Urogenital:** Nocturia, *urinary frequency, urinary tract infection*.

**INTERACTIONS Drug:** Abiraterone can increase the levels of drugs requiring CYP2D6 (e.g., **dextromethorphan, thioridazine**).

Strong inhibitors of CYP3A4 (e.g., **ketoconazole, itraconazole, clarithromycin, atazanavir, nefazodone, saquinavir, telithromycin, ritonavir, indinavir, nelfinavir, voriconazole**) increase abiraterone while inducers of CYP3A4 (e.g., **phenytoin, carbamazepine, rifampin, rifabutin, rifapentine, phenobarbital**) decrease levels of abiraterone. **Herbal: St. John's wort. Food:** Must be taken on an empty stomach.

**PHARMACOKINETICS:** 2 h. **Distribution:** Over 99% plasma protein bound. **Metabolism:** In the liver to an active metabolite. **Elimination:** Fecal (88%) and renal (5%). **Half-Life:** 7–17 h.

## NURSING IMPLICATIONS

### Assessment & Drug Effects

- Monitor BP and cardiac function especially with a history of CV disease.
- Monitor for and report signs of fluid retention (e.g., sudden weight gain, peripheral edema).
- Monitor for and report S&S of hypokalemia or hepatotoxicity (see Appendix F). Withhold drug and notify prescriber if AST/ALT is above 5 × ULN or bilirubin above 3 × ULN.
- Monitor lab tests: Baseline LFTs, then q2wk for first 3 mo, then monthly thereafter; periodic serum electrolytes (especially potassium).

### Patient & Family Education

- Do not take this drug within 2 h before or 1 h after consuming food.
- A condom should be used during sexual intercourse with a woman who is or could become pregnant.
- Report any of the following to a health care provider: Sudden weight gain, swelling of feet or legs, palpitations, unusual weakness, muscle pain, S&S of a urinary tract infection.

# ACAMPROSATE CALCIUM
(a-cam-pro'sate)
**Campral**

**Classifications:** SUBSTANCE ABUSE DETERRENT
**Therapeutic:** SUBSTANCE ABUSE INHIBITOR

**AVAILABILITY** Delayed release tablet

**ACTION & *THERAPEUTIC EFFECT***
Thought to interact with CNS glutamate and GABA neurotransmitter systems and help restore normal balance between neuronal excitation and inhibition. *Reduces craving for alcohol intake due to chronic use, but does not cause alcohol aversion or a disulfiram-like reaction as a result of ethanol ingestion.*

**USES** Maintenance of abstinence from alcohol in patients with alcoholism.

**CONTRAINDICATIONS** Hypersensitivity to acamprosate calcium or any of its components; suicidal ideation; severe renal impairment (CrCl less than 30 mL/min).

**CAUTIOUS USE** Moderate renal impairment; depression; pregnancy (category C); lactation. Safety and efficacy of acamprosate not established in adolescents or children younger than 18 y.

## ROUTE & DOSAGE

| Maintenance of Alcohol Abstinence |
| --- |
| *Adult:* **PO** Two 333 mg tablets t.i.d. |

Common adverse effects in *italic*; life-threatening effects underlined; generic names in **bold**; classifications in SMALL CAPS; ♥ Canadian drug name; ⓓ Prototype drug

9

### Renal Impairment Dosage Adjustment

*CrCl 30–50 mL/min:* 333 mg t.i.d.;
*less than 30 mL/min:* Do not use

## ADMINISTRATION

### Oral
▪ Ensure that the drug is not chewed or crushed. It **must be** swallowed whole.
▪ Store at 15°–30° C (59°–86° F).

## ADVERSE EFFECTS (≥1%) **Body as a Whole:** Flu syndrome, chills. **CNS:** Depression, anxiety, insomnia, asthenia, dizziness, paresthesia, headache, somnolence, decreased libido, amnesia, abnormal thinking, tremor. **CV:** Palpitation, syncope. **GI:** *Diarrhea,* nausea, vomiting, anorexia, flatulence, dry mouth, abdominal pain, dyspepsia, constipation, increased appetite. **Metabolic:** Peripheral edema, weight gain. **Musculoskeletal:** Musculoskeletal pain. **Respiratory:** Rhinitis, cough, dyspnea, pharyngitis, bronchitis. **Skin:** Pruritus, diaphoresis, rash. **Special Senses:** Abnormal vision, taste perversion. **Urogenital:** Impotence.

## PHARMACOKINETICS **Absorption:** 11% bioavailability. **Metabolism:** Not metabolized. **Elimination:** Renal. **Half-Life:** 20–33 h.

## NURSING IMPLICATIONS

### Assessment & Drug Effects
▪ Monitor for S&S of depression or suicidal thinking.
▪ Monitor for: Impaired judgment or thinking; dizziness or impaired motor skills. Take appropriate protective measures.

### Patient & Family Education
▪ Report any alcohol consumption while taking acamprosate.
▪ Report promptly any of the following: Unusual anxiousness

or nervousness; depression or suicidal thoughts; burning or tingling sensations in arms, legs, hands, or feet; chest pains or palpitations; difficulty urinating.
▪ Do not drive or engage in other hazardous activities until reaction to the drug is known.

## ACARBOSE ⓟ
(a-car′bose)
*Precose*
**Classifications:** ANTIDIABETIC; ALPHA-GLUCOSIDASE INHIBITOR
**Therapeutic:** ANTIDIABETIC

## AVAILABILITY Tablet

## ACTION & *THERAPEUTIC EFFECT*
Delays digestion of carbohydrates by inhibition of pancreatic amylase and intestinal hydrolase enzymes, resulting in slowed absorption of glucose molecules into the blood stream. *Causes slower and smaller rise in postprandial blood glucose.*

## USES In conjunction with diet and exercise for type 2 diabetes.

## UNLABELED USES Adjunctive treatment of type 1 diabetes.

## CONTRAINDICATIONS Inflammatory bowel disease, colon ulcers, partial bowel obstruction, predisposition for obstruction; lactation.

## CAUTIOUS USE GI distress or liver disorders, pregnancy (category B); children younger than 18 y.

## ROUTE & DOSAGE

### Type 2 Diabetes Mellitus
*Adult:* **PO** Start with 25 mg daily to t.i.d. with meals, titrate to individual response (max: 150 mg/day for 60 kg or less, 300 mg/day for greater than 60 kg)

## ADMINISTRATION

### Oral

- Remove drug from foil wrapper immediately before administration.
- Give drug with first bite at each of the three main meals.
- Do not store above 25° C (77° F). Keep tightly closed and protect from moisture.

## ADVERSE EFFECTS (≥1%) CNS:
Sleepiness, weakness, dizziness, headache, vertigo (may be due to poor diabetic control). **Endocrine:** Hypoglycemia (especially in combination with sulfonylureas and insulin). **GI:** *Diarrhea, flatulence, abdominal distention,* borborygmi, increased liver function tests. **Hematologic:** Anemia (especially iron deficiency). **Skin:** Erythema, exanthema, urticaria.

## INTERACTIONS Drug: SULFONY-
LUREAS may increase hypoglycemic effects. Drugs that induce hyperglycemia (e.g., THIAZIDES, CORTICOS-TEROIDS, PHENOTHIAZINES, ESTROGENS, **phenytoin, isoniazid**) may decrease effectiveness of acarbose. May decrease the effect of **digoxin. Herbal: Ginseng** may increase hypoglycemic effects.

## PHARMACOKINETICS Absorption:
0.5–2% is absorbed intact from GI tract. **Peak:** Peak blood glucose reduction approximately 70 min after dose. **Metabolism:** In GI tract by intestinal bacteria and digestive enzymes. **Elimination:** 35% in urine, 51% in feces, 5% in air as $CO_2$. **Half-Life:** 2 h.

## NURSING IMPLICATIONS

### Assessment & Drug Effects
- Treat hypoglycemia with dextrose; not with sucrose (table sugar).

- Monitor lab tests: Frequent blood glucose and periodic HbA1C; periodic LFTs; Hct and Hgb if anemia suspected.

### Patient & Family Education
- Note: Acarbose prevents the breakdown of table sugar. Have a source of dextrose, such as dextrose paste, available to treat low blood sugar.
- Monitor closely blood glucose, especially following dosage changes.
- Report abdominal distress; dietary adjustment or dosage reduction may be warranted.
- Monitor weight and report significant changes.

# ACEBUTOLOL HYDROCHLORIDE
(a-se-byoo-toe'lole)
Sectral

**Classifications:** BETA-ADRENERGIC ANTAGONIST; ANTIHYPERTENSIVE; CLASS II ANTIARRHYTHMIC
**Therapeutic:** ANTIHYPERTENSIVE; CLASS II ANTIARRHYTHMIC
**Prototype:** Propranolol

## AVAILABILITY Capsule

## ACTION & *THERAPEUTIC EFFECT*
Beta$_1$-selective adrenergic blocking agent with mild sympathomimetic activity (partial beta-agonist activity). Produces negative chronotropic and inotropic activity (i.e., decreases exercise-induced heart rate, inhibits reflex orthostatic tachycardia, and decreases cardiac output at rest and during exercise). *Decreases both systolic and diastolic BP at rest and during exercise. Exhibits antiarrhythmic activity (class II antiarrhythmic agent).*

## USES Treatment of mild to moderate
hypertension. Management of recurrent stable ventricular arrhythmias.

Common adverse effects in *italic;* life-threatening effects underlined; generic names in **bold;** classifications in SMALL CAPS; ♣ Canadian drug name; ⊙ Prototype drug

11

**UNLABELED USES** Supraventricular arrhythmias, chronic stable angina pectoris.

**CONTRAINDICATIONS** Overt CHF, second- or third-degree AV block, severe bradycardia, cardiogenic shock; acute bronchospasm, pulmonary edema; lactation.

**CAUTIOUS USE** Impaired cardiac function, well-compensated CHF, mesenteric or peripheral vascular disease; cerebrovascular disease; patients undergoing major surgery involving general anesthesia; renal or hepatic impairment; labile diabetes mellitus; hyperthyroidism; bronchospastic disease (asthma, emphysema); avoid abrupt withdrawal; pregnancy (category B); children younger than 12 y.

## ROUTE & DOSAGE

**Hypertension**

*Adult:* **PO** 400–800 mg/day in 1–2 divided doses (max: 1200 mg/day)
*Geriatric:* **PO** 200–400 mg/day (max: 800 mg/day)

**Ventricular Arrhythmias**

*Adult:* **PO** 200 mg b.i.d. increased to 600–1200 mg/day

**Renal Impairment Dosage Adjustment**

*CrCl less than 50 mL/min:* Reduce dose by 50%; *less than 25 mL/min:* Reduce dose by 75%; *Intermittent hemodialysis:* Reduce dose by 75%

## ADMINISTRATION

**Oral**
- Check BP and apical pulse before administration. If heart rate is less

than 60 bpm or other ordered parameter, consult prescriber.
- Drug is usually discontinued gradually over a period of 2 wk.
- Store at 15°–30° C (59°–86° F).

**ADVERSE EFFECTS** (≥1%) **Body as a Whole:** *Fatigue.* **CNS:** Dizziness, insomnia, drowsiness, confusion, fainting. **CV:** *Bradycardia,* hypotension, CHF. **GI:** Nausea, *diarrhea, constipation,* flatulence. **Hematologic:** Agranulocytosis, *antinuclear antibodies (ANA).* **Metabolic:** Hypoglycemia (may mask symptoms of a hypoglycemic reaction). **Respiratory:** Bronchospasm, pulmonary edema, dyspnea. **Urogenital:** Decreased libido; impotence.

**DIAGNOSTIC TEST INTERFERENCE** False-negative test results possible (see **propranolol**).

**INTERACTIONS Drug:** Other HYPOTENSIVE AGENTS, DIURETICS increase hypotensive effect; with **albuterol, metaproterenol, terbutaline,** or **pirbuterol,** there is mutual antagonism with acebutolol; NSAIDS blunt hypotensive effect; decreases hypoglycemic effect of **glyburide;** increases bradycardia and sinus arrest with **amiodarone.**

**PHARMACOKINETICS Absorption:** Average bioavailability of 40%. (In geriatric patients, bioavailability increases twofold.) **Peak:** 3 h. **Distribution:** Minimally into CSF; crosses placenta; is excreted in breast milk. **Metabolism:** In liver. **Elimination:** In urine, feces. **Half-Life:** 3–4 h.

## NURSING IMPLICATIONS

**Assessment & Drug Effects**
- Monitor BP and cardiac status throughout therapy. Observe for and report marked bradycardia or hypotension, especially when patient is also receiving a

catecholamine-depleting drug (e.g., reserpine).

- Monitor I&O ratio and pattern and report changes to prescriber (e.g., dysuria, nocturia, oliguria, weight change).
- Monitor for S&S of CHF, especially peripheral edema, dyspnea, activity intolerance.
- Monitor lab tests: Periodic tests for drug induced positive ANA titer during long-term therapy, especially in women and older adults; periodic CBC with long-term therapy.

**Patient & Family Education**

- Know parameters for withholding drug (e.g., pulse less than 60).
- Do not breast feed while taking this drug without consulting prescriber.
- Note: Common adverse effects include insomnia, drowsiness, and confusion.
- Do not drive or engage in potentially hazardous activities until response to drug is known.
- Do not increase, decrease, omit, or discontinue drug regimen without advice from the prescriber. Abrupt withdrawal may worsen angina or precipitate MI in patient with heart disease.
- Contact prescriber promptly at the first signs or symptoms of CHF (see Appendix F).
- Report muscle and joint pain to prescriber. Discontinuation of drug therapy usually reverses these adverse effects.
- Monitor for loss of glycemic control if diabetic.
- Note: Drug may mask symptoms of hypoglycemia (see Appendix F) and potentiate insulin-induced hypoglycemia in diabetics.
- Avoid use of OTC oral cold preparations and topical nasal decongestants unless approved by the prescriber.

# ACETAMINOPHEN, (PARACETAMOL) 

(a-seat-a-mee'noe-fen)

Abenol ◆, A'Cenol, Acephen, Anacin-3, Anuphen, APAP, Atasol ◆, Campain ◆, Dolanex, Exdol ◆, Halenol, Liquiprin, Ofirmev, Panadol, Pedric, Robigesic ◆, Rounox ◆, Tapar, Tempra, Tylenol, Tylenol Arthritis, Valadol

**Classifications:** NONNARCOTIC ANALGESIC, ANTIPYRETIC
Therapeutic: NONNARCOTIC ANALGESIC; ANTIPYRETIC

**AVAILABILITY** Suppository; tablet/caplet; extended release tablet/capsule; liquid; injection

**ACTION & THERAPEUTIC EFFECT** Produces analgesia by elevation of the pain threshold. Reduces fever by inhibiting the action of endogenous pyrogens on the heat-regulating centers in the brain by blocking the formation and release of prostaglandins in the CNS. *It provides temporary analgesia for mild to moderate pain. In addition, acetaminophen lowers body temperature in individuals with a fever.*

**USES** Fever reduction. Temporary relief of mild to moderate pain. Generally as substitute for aspirin when the latter is not tolerated or is contraindicated.

**CONTRAINDICATIONS** Hypersensitivity to acetaminophen or phenacetin. Acute liver failure has been associated with doses that exceed 4000 mg per day.

**CAUTIOUS USE** Repeated administration to patients with anemia, G6PD deficiency, renal or hepatic disease; arthritic or rheumatoid conditions affecting children

Common adverse effects in *italic;* life-threatening effects underlined; generic names in **bold;** classifications in SMALL CAPS; ◆ Canadian drug name; ⊙ Prototype drug

13

younger than 12 y; alcoholism; malnutrition; thrombocytopenia; bone marrow depression, immunosuppression; pregnancy (category C).

## ROUTE & DOSAGE

### Mild to Moderate Pain, Fever

Adult: **PO** 325–650 mg q4–6h (max: 4 g/day); **PR** 650 mg q4–6h (max: 4 g/day); **IV** 1000 mg q6h or 650 q4h prn
Child: **PO** 10–15 mg/kg q4–6h **PR** 2–5 y: 120 mg q4–6h (max: 720 mg/day); 6–12 y: 325 mg q4–6h (max: 2.6 g/day)
Child (2 yr or older): **IV** 15 mg/kg/dose q6h or 12.5 mg/kg/dose q4h prn
Neonate: **PO** 10–15 mg/kg q6–8h

## ADMINISTRATION

### Oral

- Ensure that extended release tablets are not crushed or chewed. These must be swallowed whole.
- Chewable tablets should be thoroughly chewed and wetted before they are swallowed.
- Do not coadminister with a high carbohydrate meal; absorption rate may be significantly retarded.
- Store in light-resistant containers at room temperature, preferably at 15°–30° C (59°–86° F).

### Rectal

- Insert suppositories beyond the rectal sphincter.

### Intravenous

**PREPARE: Intermittent:** For adults and adolescents weighing 50 kg (110 lb) or more, give without dilution by attaching a vented IV set directly to the 100 mL (1000 mg)

vial. For patients weighing less than 50 kg (110 lb), withdraw the needed dose from a sealed 1000 mg vial and place in an empty sterile container (e.g., plastic IV bag, syringe) for infusion.
**ADMINISTER: Intermittent:** Infuse over 15 min. For small volume pediatric doses up to 60 mL, use a syringe pump to administer over 15 min. Store at controlled temperature and use within 6 h after opening.

**ADVERSE EFFECTS** (≥1%) **Body as a Whole:** Negligible with recommended dosage; rash. **Acute poisoning:** Anorexia, nausea, vomiting, dizziness, lethargy, diaphoresis, chills, epigastric or abdominal pain, diarrhea; onset of hepatotoxicity: elevation of serum transaminases (ALT, AST) and bilirubin; hypoglycemia, hepatic coma, acute renal failure (rare). **Chronic ingestion:** Neutropenia, pancytopenia, leukopenia, thrombocytopenic purpura, hepatotoxicity in alcoholics, renal damage.

**DIAGNOSTIC TEST INTERFERENCE**
False increases in **urinary 5-HIAA** (5-hydroxyindoleacetic acid) byproduct of serotonin; false decreases in **blood glucose** (by **glucose oxidase–peroxidase procedure**); false increases in urinary glucose (with certain instruments in glucose analyses); and false increases in **serum uric acid** (with **phosphotungstate method**). High doses or long-term therapy: hepatic, renal, and hematopoietic function (periodically).

**INTERACTIONS Drug: Cholestyramine** may decrease acetaminophen absorption. With chronic coadministration, BARBITURATES, **carbamazepine, phenytoin,** and **rifampin** may increase potential for chronic

Common adverse effects in *italic;* life-threatening effects underlined; generic names in **bold;** classifications in SMALL CAPS; ♣ Canadian drug name; ⊘ Prototype drug

hepatotoxicity. Chronic, excessive ingestion of **alcohol** will increase risk of hepatotoxicity.

## PHARMACOKINETICS **Absorption:** Rapid and almost complete absorption (PO); less complete absorption from rectal suppository. **Peak:** 0.5–2 h. **Duration:** 3–4 h. **Distribution:** In all body fluids; crosses placenta. **Metabolism:** Extensively in liver. **Elimination:** 90–100% of drug excreted as metabolites in urine; excreted in breast milk. **Half-Life:** 1–3 h.

## NURSING IMPLICATIONS

### Black Box Warning

*Doses in excess of 4000 mg/day have been associated with acute liver failure.*

### Assessment & Drug Effects

▪ Monitor for S&S of: Hepatotoxicity, even with moderate acetaminophen doses, especially in individuals with poor nutrition or who have ingested alcohol (3 or more alcoholic drinks daily) over prolonged periods; poisoning, usually from accidental ingestion or suicide attempts; potential abuse from psychological dependence (withdrawal has been associated with restless and excited responses).

### Patient & Family Education

▪ Do not take other medications (e.g., cold preparations) containing acetaminophen without medical advice; overdosing and chronic use can cause liver damage and other toxic effects.
▪ Do not self-medicate adults for pain more than 10 days (5 days in children) without consulting a prescriber.
▪ Do not use this medication without medical direction for: Fever persisting longer than 3 days, fever over 39.5° C (103° F), or recurrent fever.
▪ Do not give children more than 5 doses in 24 h unless prescribed by prescriber.

## ACETAZOLAMIDE ⓟ
(a-set-a-zole'a-mide)
Acetazolam ◆, Apo-Acetazolamide ◆, Diamox Sequels
**Classifications:** CARBONIC ANHYDRASE INHIBITOR
Therapeutic: DIURETIC; ANTICONVULSANT; ANTIGLAUCOMA

**AVAILABILITY** Tablet; sustained release capsule; powder for injection

## ACTION & *THERAPEUTIC EFFECT*
A potent carbonic anhydrase inhibitor that decreases the secretion of aqueous humor in the eye, retards excessive abnormal discharges from CNS neurons, and increases renal loss of bicarbonate ions which carry out sodium, water, and potassium thus lowering intraocular pressure. *Reduces seizure activity and intraocular pressure. Additionally, it has a diuretic effect.*

**USES** Focal Absence seizures; reduction of intraocular pressure in open-angle glaucoma and secondary glaucoma; preoperative treatment of acute closed-angle glaucoma; edema.

**UNLABELED USES** Hydrocephalus; familial periodic paralysis, metabolic alkalosis, nystagmus, urinary alkalinization.

**CONTRAINDICATIONS** Hypersensitivity to carbonic anhydrase inhibitors, marked renal and hepatic disease; Addison's disease or other types of adrenocortical insufficiency; hyponatremia, hypokalemia,

---

Common adverse effects in *italic;* life-threatening effects underlined; generic names in **bold;** classifications in SMALL CAPS; ◆ Canadian drug name; ⓟ Prototype drug

15

# ACETAZOLAMIDE

hyperchloremic acidosis; prolonged administration to patients with hyphema; chronic noncongestive angle-closure glaucoma.

**CAUTIOUS USE** Hypersensitivity to sulfonamides and derivatives (e.g., thiazides), history of hypercalciuria; DM, renal impairment; gout, patients receiving digitalis, obstructive pulmonary disease, older adults; respiratory acidosis; pregnancy (category C).

## ROUTE & DOSAGE

### Glaucoma
*Adult:* **PO** 250 mg 1–4 × day; 500 mg sustained release b.i.d., up to 1 g/day; **IM/IV** 500 mg, may repeat in 2–4 h

### Absence Seizures
*Adult:* **PO/IV** 8–30 mg/kg/day in 1–4 doses

### Edema
*Adult:* **PO/IV** 250–375 mg every a.m. (5 mg/kg); may be given every other day if condition improves

### Altitude Sickness
*Adult:* **PO** 250 mg q6–12h or 500 mg sustained release q12–24h, starting 24–48 h before climb and continuing for 48 h at high altitude

### Renal Impairment Dosage Adjustment
*CrCl 10–50 mL/min:* Extend interval to q12h; *less than 10 mL/min:* Use not recommended

### Hemodialysis Dosage Adjusment
Administer post-dialysis

## ADMINISTRATION

### Oral
- Administer diuretic dose in the morning to avoid interrupted sleep.
- Give with food or meals to minimize GI upset.
- Note: If tablet(s) cannot be swallowed, soften tablet(s) (not sustained release form) in 2 tsp of hot water and add to 2 tsp of honey/syrup to disguise bitter taste; avoid syrups containing alcohol or glycerin, or crush tablet(s) and suspend in syrup (250–500 mg/5 mL syrup). Prepare just before administration. Drug does not dissolve in fruit juices.
- Store oral preparations at 15°–30° C (59°–86° F) unless otherwise directed.

### Intramuscular
- Reconstitute as for IV administration. See PREPARE Direct.
- Give IM for rapid lowering of intraocular pressure or in patients unable to take oral dosage.
- Note: The intramuscular dosage is not the route of choice because the alkalinity of the solution makes the injection painful.

### Intravenous

*PREPARE:* **Direct:** Reconstitute each 500 mg vial with at least 5 mL of sterile water for injection to yield approximately 100 mg/mL. ▪ May be used as prepared or further diluted. **IV Infusion:** Dilute reconstituted solution with D5W or NS. Use within 24 h of reconstitution.
*ADMINISTER:* **Direct:** Give at a rate of 500 mg or fraction thereof over 1 min. **IV Infusion:** Give as a continuous infusion over 4–8 h.
*INCOMPATIBILITIES:* **Solution/additive:** Amino acid, multivitamin **Y-site: Diltiazem, TPN.**

## ADVERSE EFFECTS (≥1%) CNS:
Paresthesias, sedation, malaise,

disorientation, depression, fatigue, muscle weakness, <u>flaccid paralysis</u>. **GI:** Anorexia, nausea, vomiting, weight loss, dry mouth, thirst, diarrhea. **Hematologic:** Bone marrow depression with <u>agranulocytosis, hemolytic anemia, aplastic anemia, leukopenia, pancytopenia</u>. **Metabolic:** Increased excretion of calcium, potassium, magnesium, and sodium, metabolic acidosis, hyperglycemia, hyperuricemia. **Ocular:** Transient myopia. **Urogenital:** Glycosuria, urinary frequency, polyuria, dysuria, hematuria, crystalluria. **Other:** Exacerbation of gout, hepatic dysfunction, <u>Stevens-Johnson syndrome</u>.

### DIAGNOSTIC TEST INTERFERENCE
Monitor for false-positive ***urinary protein*** determinations; falsely high values for ***urine urobilinogen;*** depressed ***iodine uptake*** values (exception: hypothyroidism).

### INTERACTIONS Drug: Renal excretion of AMPHETAMINES, **ephedrine, flecainide, quinidine, procainamide,** TRICYCLIC ANTIDEPRESSANTS may be decreased, thereby enhancing or prolonging their effects. Renal excretion of **lithium, phenobarbital** may be increased. **Amphotericin B** and CORTICOSTEROIDS may accelerate **potassium** loss. **Digoxin** may predispose persons with hypokalemia to **digitalis** toxicity; puts patients on high doses of SALICYLATES at high risk for SALICYLATE toxicity.

### PHARMACOKINETICS Absorption:
Well absorbed from GI tract. **Onset:** 1 h regular release; 2 h sustained release; 2 min IV. **Peak:** 2–4 h reg; 8–18 h sustained; 15 min IV. **Duration:** 8–12 h reg; 18–24 h sustained; 4–5 h IV. **Distribution:** Distributed throughout body; crosses placenta. **Elimination:** In urine. **Half-Life:** 2.4–5.8 h.

## NURSING IMPLICATIONS
### Assessment & Drug Effects
- Establish baseline weight before initial therapy and weigh daily thereafter when used to treat edema.
- Monitor for S&S of: Mild to severe metabolic acidosis; potassium loss which is greatest early in therapy (see hypokalemia in Appendix F).
- Monitor I&O especially when used with other diuretics.
- Monitor lab tests: Baseline serum pH, blood gases, urinalysis, CBC, and serum electrolytes and periodically during prolonged therapy or concomitant therapy with other diuretics or digitalis.

### Patient & Family Education
- Maintain adequate fluid intake (1.5–2.5 L/24 h; 1 liter is approximately equal to 1 quart) to reduce risk of kidney stones.
- Do not breast-feed while taking this drug without consulting prescriber.
- Report any of the following: Numbness, tingling, burning, drowsiness, and visual problems, sore throat or mouth, unusual bleeding, fever, skin or renal problems.
- Eat potassium-rich diet and take potassium supplement when taking this drug in high doses or for prolonged periods.
- Use caution when engaging in hazardous activities until reaction to drug is known.

## ACETYLCYSTEINE
(a-se-til-sis'tay-een)

Acetadote, N-Acetyl-cysteine, Mucomyst, Parvolex ◆

**Classifications:** MUCOLYTIC; ANTIDOTE

Therapeutic: MUCOLYTIC; ANTIDOTE

Common adverse effects in *italic*; life-threatening effects <u>underlined</u>; generic names in **bold**; classifications in SMALL CAPS; ◆ Canadian drug name; ⦿ Prototype drug

17

## ACETYLCYSTEINE

**AVAILABILITY** Solution for inhalation; solution for injection

**ACTION & *THERAPEUTIC EFFECT***
Probably acts by disrupting disulfide linkages of mucoproteins in purulent and nonpurulent bronchial secretions. In acetaminophen overdose, it helps to prevent hepatotoxicity by serving as a substrate for the toxic metabolites of acetaminophen. *Lowers viscosity and facilitates the removal of secretions. Removes the toxic metabolites of acetaminophen.*

**USES** Adjuvant therapy in patients with abnormal mucous secretions in acute and chronic bronchopulmonary diseases, and in pulmonary complications of cystic fibrosis and surgery, tracheostomy, and atelectasis. Also used in diagnostic bronchial studies and as an antidote for acute acetaminophen poisoning.

**UNLABELED USES** Meconium ileus; prevention of radiocontrast-induced renal dysfunction.

**CONTRAINDICATIONS** Hypersensitivity to acetylcysteine; patients at risk of gastric hemorrhage.

**CAUTIOUS USE** Patients with asthma, severe hepatic disease, esophageal varices, peptic ulcer disease; debilitated patients with severe respiratory insufficiency; older adults; pregnancy (category B); lactation.

## ROUTE & DOSAGE

**Mucolytic**

*Adult:* **Inhalation** 1–10 mL of 20% solution q4–6h or 2–20 mL of 10% solution q4–6h; **Direct Instillation** 1–2 mL of 10–20% solution q1–4h
*Child:* **Inhalation** 3–5 mL of 20% solution or 6–10 mL of 10% solution 3–4 × day

*Infant:* **Inhalation** 1–2 mL 20% solution or 2–4 mL of 10% solution 3–4 × day

**Acetaminophen Toxicity**

*Adult/Child:* **PO** 140 mg/kg followed by 70 mg/kg q4h for 17 doses (use a 5% solution)
*Adult/Adolescent/Child:* **IV** 150 mg/kg infused over 60 min, followed by 50 mg/kg over 4 h, then 100 mg/kg over 16 h; total dose 300 mg/kg over 21 h

## ADMINISTRATION

### Inhalation and Instillation
- Prepare dilution within 1 h of use; drug does not contain an antimicrobial agent. A light purple discoloration does not significantly impair drug's effectiveness.
- Dilute the 20% solution with NS or water for injection. The 10% solution may be used undiluted.
- Give by direct instillation into tracheostomy (1–2 mL of 10–20% solution).
- Instruct patient to clear airway, if possible, coughing productively prior to aerosol administration to ensure maximum effect.
- Store opened vial in refrigerator to retard oxidation; use within 96 h.
- Store unopened vial at 15°–30° C (59°–86° F), unless otherwise directed.

### Oral
- Dilute the 20% solution 1:3 with cola, orange juice, or other soft drink to make a 5% solution. If administered via a gastric tube, water may be used as the diluent.
- Freshly prepare all diluted solutions and use within 1 h of preparation.

### Intravenous

*PREPARE:* **IV Infusion:** Acetylcysteine reacts with certain metals and rubber; use IV equipment made of plastic or glass.

- Dilute all required doses in D5W as follows: For loading dose, add a dose equal to 150 mg/kg to 200 mL; for second dose, add a dose equal to 50 mg/kg to 500 mL; for third dose, add a dose equal to 100 mg/kg to 1000 mL. ■ Note: The total IV volume should be reduced for patients less than 40 kg and for those with fluid restriction. In small children, individualize the total IV volume to avoid water intoxication and hyponatremia.

*ADMINISTER:* **IV Infusion:** Give loading dose over 60 min, second dose 1 over 4 h, third dose 2 over 16 h. Complete all infusions over 21 h.

*INCOMPATIBILITIES:* **Y-site: Ceftazidime.**

- Store reconstituted solution for up to 24 h at 15°–30° C (59°–86° F).

## ADVERSE EFFECTS (≥1%) CNS:
Dizziness, drowsiness. **GI:** Nausea, *vomiting,* stomatitis, hepatotoxicity (urticaria). **Respiratory:** Bronchospasm, rhinorrhea, burning sensation in upper respiratory passages, epistaxis.

## PHARMACOKINETICS  Onset:
1 min. **Peak:** 5–10 min. **Metabolism:** Deacetylated in liver to cysteine.

## NURSING IMPLICATIONS
### Assessment & Drug Effects
- During IV infusion, carefully monitor for fluid overload and signs of hyponatremia (i.e., changes in mental status).
- Monitor for S&S of aspiration of excess secretions, and for bronchospasm (unpredictable); withhold drug and notify prescriber immediately if either occurs.

- Have suction apparatus immediately available. Increased volume of respiratory tract fluid may be liberated; suction or endotracheal aspiration may be necessary to establish and maintain an open airway. Older adults and debilitated patients are particularly at risk.
- Nausea and vomiting may occur, particularly when face mask is used, due to unpleasant odor of drug and excess volume of liquefied bronchial secretions.
- Monitor lab tests: ABGs, pulmonary functions and pulse oximetry as indicated; baseline serum acetaminophen level (for toxicity), LFTs, bilirubin, serum electrolytes, BUN, and plasma glucose.

### Patient & Family Education
- Report difficulty with clearing the airway or any other respiratory distress.
- Report nausea, as an antiemetic may be indicated.
- Note: Unpleasant odor of inhaled drug becomes less noticeable with continued use.

## ACITRETIN
(a ci tree'tin)

Soriatane

**Classifications:** RETINOID
**Therapeutic:** ANTIPSORIATIC
**Prototype:** Isotretinoin

## AVAILABILITY Capsule

## ACTION & *THERAPEUTIC EFFECT*
Binds to the retinoic acid receptors in the skin, thus modifying gene expression, epithelial cell growth, and cell differentiation. *Acitretin is a highly toxic metabolite of retinol (vitamin A).*

## USES Treatment of severe, recalcitrant psoriasis in adults.

---

Common adverse effects in *italic;* life-threatening effects <u>underlined</u>; generic names in **bold;** classifications in SMALL CAPS; ♣ Canadian drug name; ⊙ Prototype drug

**UNLABELED USES** Eczema, lichen planus.

**CONTRAINDICATIONS** Hypersensitivity to acitretin or sensitivity to parabens; hepatoxicity; hepatitis; severe renal impairment or renal failure, development of psychiatric symptoms (depression, etc); pregnancy (category X) for at least 3 y after use; lactation.

**CAUTIOUS USE** Patients with impaired hepatic function, history of mental illness; DM; obesity, history of pancreatitis, hypertriglyceridemia, hypercholesterolemia, coronary artery disease, retinal disease, degenerative joint disease.

## ROUTE & DOSAGE

### Psoriasis

*Adult:* **PO** 25–50 mg daily with main meal

## ADMINISTRATION

### Oral

- Administer as single dose with main meal because food enhances absorption.
- Store at 15°–25° C (59°–77° F) and protect from light. After opening, avoid exposure to high temperatures and humidity.

## ADVERSE EFFECTS (≥1%) **Body as a Whole:** *Hyperesthesia, paresthesias, arthralgia, progression of existing spinal hyperostosis, rigors,* back pain, hypertonia, myalgia, fatigue, hot flashes, increased appetite. **CNS:** Headache, depression, aggressive feelings and thoughts of self-harm, insomnia, somnolence. **CV:** Flushing, edema. **GI:** *Dry mouth, increased liver function tests, increased triglycerides and cholesterol,* hepatitis, gingival bleeding, gingivitis, increased saliva, stomatitis, thirst, ulcerative stomatitis, abdominal pain, diarrhea, nausea, tongue disorder. **Special Senses:** Blurred vision, blepharitis, conjunctivitis, decreased night vision/night blindness, eye pain, photophobia; earache, tinnitus; taste perversion. **Respiratory:** Sinusitis. **Skin:** *Alopecia, skin peeling, dry skin, nail disorders, pruritus, rash, cheilitis, skin atrophy, paronychia,* abnormal skin odor and hair texture, cold/clammy skin, increased sweating, purpura, seborrhea, skin ulceration, sunburn. **Other:** *Rhinitis, epistaxis, xerophthalmia.*

**INTERACTIONS Drug:** Use with **ethanol** causes longer half-life than acitretin; interferes with the contraceptive efficacy of **progestin**-only ORAL CONTRACEPTIVES. Use with **methotrexate** increases the risk of hepatitis. Do not use with **methotrexate** or TETRACYCLINES. **Food:** Avoid supplemental **vitamin A.**

**PHARMACOKINETICS Absorption:** Rapidly from GI tract, optimal absorption when taken with food. **Peak:** 2–5 h. **Distribution:** Crosses placenta, distributed into breast milk. **Metabolism:** Active metabolite, *cis*-acitretin. **Elimination:** In both urine and feces. **Half-Life:** 49 h acitretin, 63 h *cis*-acitretin.

## NURSING IMPLICATIONS

### Black Box Warning

*Severe birth defects and/or fetal death have occurred when either parent is/was treated with acitretin. Hepatotoxicity has occurred infrequently.*

## Assessment & Drug Effects

- Monitor for S&S of pancreatitis or loss of glycemic control in diabetics. Report either condition immediately to prescriber.
- Monitor lab tests: Baseline and q1–2wk (until response to drug is known) lipid profile and LFTs; periodic blood glucose and HbA1C.

## Patient & Family Education

- If either parent has been treated with acitretin, use two forms of effective contraception for 1 mo before and at least 3 y following therapy because of the serious risk of fetal deformities that could result from exposure to this medication.
- Do not breast-feed while taking this drug.
- Note: Transient worsening of psoriasis may occur during early therapy.
- Review common adverse effects of drug; lag time of 2–3 mo may be necessary before drug effect is evident.
- Discontinue drug and report immediately to prescriber if visual problems develop.
- Note: Dry eyes with decreased tolerance for contact lenses may occur.
- Do not drink alcohol while taking this drug; it increases risk of hepatotoxicity and hypertriglyceridemia; females should avoid alcohol during and for 2 mo following therapy.
- Avoid excessive amounts of vitamin A (consult prescriber).
- Do not donate blood for 3 y following therapy.
- Avoid excessive exposure to sunlight or UV light.

## ACLIDINIUM BROMIDE

(a-cli-di′ni-um bro′mide)

Tudorza Pressair

**Classification:** ANTICHOLINERGIC; ANTIMUSCARINIC; ANTISPASMODIC; BRONCHODILATOR

Therapeutic: BRONCHODILATOR

**Prototype:** Atropine

**AVAILABILITY** Powder for inhalation

## ACTION & *THERAPEUTIC EFFECT*

A long-acting antimuscarinic, anticholinergic agent that inhibits M3 receptors in bronchial smooth muscles. *Promotes bronchodilation and relieves bronchospasms associated with COPD.*

**USES** Treatment of bronchospasm associated with chronic obstructive pulmonary disease (COPD).

**CONTRAINDICATIONS** Hypersensitivity to aclidinium; acute or paradoxical episodes of bronchospasm.

**CAUTIOUS USE** Narrow angle glaucoma; urinary retention; hypersensitivity to milk proteins; pregnancy (category C); lactation. Safety and efficacy in children younger than 18 y not established.

## ROUTE & DOSAGE

**Chronic Obstructive Pulmonary Disorder**

*Adult:* **Oral Inhalation** 400 mcg b.i.d.

## ADMINISTRATION

### Inhalation

- Open pouch immediately before use.
- Ensure that powder does not contact eyes.
- Store inhaler inside the sealed pouch at 15°–30° C (59°–86° F).

**ADVERSE EFFECTS** (≥1%) **Body as a Whole:** Fall, hypersensitivity

Common adverse effects in *italic;* life-threatening effects underlined; generic names in **bold;** classifications in SMALL CAPS; ♣ Canadian drug name; ⊙ Prototype drug

21

reactions. **CNS:** Headache. **GI:** Diarrhea, toothache, vomiting. **Respiratory:** Cough, nasopharyngitis, rhinitis, sinusitis.

**INTERACTIONS Drug:** Additive anticholinergic effects if used in combination with another ANTICHOLINERGIC AGENT.

**PHARMACOKINETICS Absorption:** 6% bioavailability. **Onset:** 10 min. **Metabolism:** Broken down to inactive metabolites. **Elimination:** Renal (54–65%) and fecal (20–33%). **Half-Life:** 5–8 h.

**NURSING IMPLICATIONS**

**Assessment & Drug Effects**

- Monitor closely anyone with a history of hypersensitivity to atropine.
- Monitor I&O and assess for urinary retention.
- Monitor for and report promptly S&S of narrow-angle glaucoma (e.g., severe eye pain, eye edema and redness, often accompanied by nausea and vomiting).

**Patient & Family Education**

- Do not use as a rescue medication.
- Stop using aclidinium and report to prescriber if paradoxical bronchospasms occur.
- Report to prescriber if you experience painful urination or have difficulty passing urine (e.g., frequent urination, urination in weak stream or drips).
- Report promptly any of the following signs of acute narrow-angle glaucoma: Eye pain or discomfort, blurred vision, visual halos, colored images, or red eyes.

**ACRIVASTINE/ PSEUDOEPHEDRINE**

(a-cri-vas'teen)

**Semprex-D (combination with pseudoephedrine)**

**Classifications:** H$_1$-RECEPTOR ANTAGONIST; DECONGESTANT
**Therapeutic:** ANTIHISTAMINE; DECONGESTANT
**Prototype:** Diphenhydramine

**AVAILABILITY** Acrivastine 8 mg/ pseudoephedrine 60 mg capsules

**ACTION & THERAPEUTIC EFFECT**
An H$_1$-receptor histamine antagonist that controls histamine-mediated symptoms and acts on sympathetic nerve endings. It shrinks swollen nasal mucous membranes and reduces nasal congestion of the mucosa. *It is effective in allergic rhinitis by reducing nasal congestion and decreasing respiratory mucosa swelling.*

**USES** Seasonal and perennial allergic rhinitis with nasal congestion.

**CONTRAINDICATIONS** Hypersensitivity to acrivastine, triprolidine, pseudoephedrine, or ephedrine; severe hypertension or severe coronary artery disease; patients on MAO inhibitor drugs; uncontrolled hypertension; tachycardia, acute cardiac arrhythmias; closed-angle glaucoma.

**CAUTIOUS USE** Renal insufficiency, hypertension, DM, ischemic heart disease, increased intraocular pressure, hyperthyroidism, BPH, GI disorders, older adults, pregnancy (category B); lactation. Safety and efficacy in children younger than 12 y not established.

**ROUTE & DOSAGE**

| Allergic Rhinitis |
|---|
| *Adult:* **PO** 1 cap q4–6h |

### Renal Impairment Dosage Adjustment

CrCl less than 48 mL/min: Do not use

## ADMINISTRATION

### Oral

- Do not give to patients with a creatinine clearance of 48 mL/min or less.
- Store at 15°–25° C (59°–77° F); protect from light and moisture.

## ADVERSE EFFECTS (≥1%) CNS:
Headache, vertigo, dizziness, insomnia, jitteriness, *drowsiness*. GI: Nausea, diarrhea, dry mouth, dyspepsia.

## INTERACTIONS Drug: Alcohol
may increase psychomotor impairment.

## PHARMACOKINETICS Absorption:
Rapidly from GI tract. Onset: 1 h. Duration: Approximately 12 h. Metabolism: In liver. Elimination: Approximately 65% excreted unchanged in urine. Half-Life: 1.5 h.

## NURSING IMPLICATIONS

### Assessment & Drug Effects

- Monitor for dizziness, sedation, urinary obstruction, and hypotension, especially in older adults.
- Assess for significant drowsiness, which may necessitate drug discontinuation.
- Monitor lab tests: Periodic creatinine clearance.

### Patient & Family Education

- Do not use this drug in combination with other OTC antihistamines or decongestants.
- Do not drive or engage in potentially hazardous activities until response to drug is known.
- Do not take alcohol or other CNS depressants while taking this drug.

## ACYCLOVIR, ACYCLOVIR SODIUM ℗
(ay-sye′kloe-ver)
Zovirax

**Classifications:** ANTIVIRAL
Therapeutic: ANTIVIRAL; ANTIHERPES

## AVAILABILITY
Capsule; tablet; oral suspension; injection; ointment, cream

## ACTION & THERAPEUTIC EFFECT
It preferentially interferes with DNA synthesis of herpes simplex virus types 1 and 2 (HSV-1 and HSV-2) and varicella-zoster virus, thereby inhibiting viral replication. *Acyclovir reduces viral shedding and formation of new lesions and speeds healing time. It demonstrates antiviral activity against herpes virus simplex (B virus), Epstein-Barr (infectious mononucleosis), varicella-zoster and cyto-megalovirus, but does not eradicate the latent herpes virus.*

## USES
Parenterally for treatment of viral encephalitis, treatment of herpes simplex, and treatment of varicella-zoster virus (shingles/chickenpox). Used orally for treatment of herpes simplex treatment, and prophylaxis and treatment of varicella-zoster virus (shingles/chickenpox). Used topically for herpes labialis (cold sores), initial episodes of herpes genitalis and in non-life-threatening mucocutaneous herpes simplex virus infections in immunocompromised patients.

## UNLABELED USES
Treatment of eczema herpeticum caused by HSV localized and disseminated herpes zoster, CMV prophylaxis, pharyngitis, stomatitis, varicella prophylaxis.

## CONTRAINDICATIONS
Hypersensitivity to acyclovir and valacyclovir.

---

Common adverse effects in *italic*; life-threatening effects <u>underlined</u>; generic names in **bold**; classifications in SMALL CAPS; ♣ Canadian drug name; ℗ Prototype drug

**CAUTIOUS USE** Renal insufficiency, dehydration, seizure disorders, or neurologic disease; immunocompromised individuals; older adults; pregnancy (category B).

## ROUTE & DOSAGE

### Cold Sores

*Adult/Adolescents (12 y or older):* **Topical** Apply 5 × day for 4 days

### Genital Herpes Simplex

*Adult:* **PO** 400 mg t.i.d. for 5–14 day cycle; **IV** 5 mg/kg q8h × 7 days **Topical** Apply q3h 6 × day × 7 days

### Herpes Simplex Immunocompromised Patient

*Adult:* **IV** 5 mg/kg q8h × 7 days
*Child:* **IV** 10 mg/kg q8h × 7 days

### Prophylaxis for Genital Herpes Simplex

*Adult:* **PO** 400 mg b.i.d.

### Herpes Zoster

*Adult:* **PO** 800 mg q4h 5 × day × 7–10 days
*Child:* **PO** 80 mg/kg/day in 5 divided doses

### Herpes Zoster (in immunocompromised patients)

*Adult/Adolescent:* **IV** 10 mg/kg q8h × 7 days
*Child (less than 12 y):* **IV** 20 mg/kg q8h × 7–10 days

### Viral Encephalitis

*Adult:* **IV** 10 mg/kg q8h × 10 days
*Child (3 mo to less than 12 y):* **IV** 20 mg/kg q8h × 10 days
*Neonate (younger than 3 mo):* **IV** 10 mg/kg q8h × 10 days

### Varicella Zoster

*Child/Adolescent:* **PO** 20 mg/kg (max: 800 mg) q.i.d. for 5 day cycle initiated within 24 h of onset of rash
*Adult:* **IV** 10 mg/kg q8h × 7 days
*Child:* **IV** 20 mg/kg q8h × 7 days

### *Obesity Dosage Adjustment*

Patient dose should be calculated using IBW.

### *Renal Impairment Dosage Adjustment*

*CrCl 25–50 mL/min:* Standard dose q12h; *10–25 mL/min:* Standard dose q24h; *less than 10 mL/min:* Give half normal dose q24h (see package insert for neonatal renal impairment adjustment)

### *Hemodialysis Dosage Adjustment*

Administer dose after dialysis

## ADMINISTRATION

### Oral

- Shake suspension well prior to use.
- Store capsules in tight, light-resistant containers at 15°–30° C (59°–86° F) unless otherwise directed.

### Topical

- Wash hands thoroughly before and after treatment of lesions and after handling and disposition of secretions.
- Apply approximately ½ inch of cream or ointment ribbon for each 4 square inches of surface area. Use sufficient ointment or cream to completely cover lesions.
- Apply topical preparation with finger cot or surgical glove.
- Store at 15°–25° C (59°–78° F) unless otherwise directed.

### Intravenous

***PREPARE: Intermittent:*** Reconstitute by adding 10 mL sterile water for injection to 500-mg vial to yield 50 mg/mL. Note: Do not use bacteriostatic water for injection containing benzyl alcohol. Shake well. ▪ Further dilute to 7 mg/mL or less to reduce risk of renal injury and phlebitis. Example: Add 1 mL of reconstituted solution to 9 mL of diluent to yield 5 mg/mL. ▪ Use standard electrolyte and glucose solutions (e.g., NS, LR, D5W) for dilution.

*ADMINISTER:* **Intermittent:** Administer by constant infusion over at least 1 h to prevent renal tubular damage. Rapid or bolus IV administration **must be** avoided. ▪ Monitor IV flow rate carefully; infusion pump or microdrip infusion set preferred.

*INCOMPATIBILITIES:* **Solution/additive:** Bacteriostatic water for injection, **dobutamine, dopamine.** **Y-site: Amifostine, aminocaproic acid, amsacrine, amphotericin B, ampicillin/sulbactam, aztreonam, cefepime, chlorpromazine, ciprofloxacin, codeine, daptomycin, diazepam, dobutamine, dopamine, doxorubicin, epinephrine, epirubicin, eptifibatide, esmolol, fenoldopam, foscarnet, gemcitabine, gemtuzumab, haloperidol, hydralazine, hydroxyzine, idarubicin, irinotecan, ketamine, ketorolac, labetolol, levofloxacin, lidocaine, methyldopate, midazolam, mycophenolate, nitroprusside, ondansetron, palonosetron, pentamidine, phenylephrine, phenytoin, piperacillin/tazobactam, potassium phosphate, procainamide, prochlorperazine, promethazine, quinupristin/dalfopristin, sargramostim, streptozocin, tacrolimus, ticarcillin/clavulanate, TPN, vecuronium, verapamil, vinorelbine.**

▪ Refrigerated reconstituted solution may precipitate; however, crystals will redissolve at room temperature. ▪ Store acyclovir powder and reconstituted solutions at controlled room temperature, preferably at 15°–30° C (59°–86° F) unless otherwise directed by manufacturer. ▪ Use reconstituted solution within 12 h. Use diluted solution within 24 h.

**ADVERSE EFFECTS** (≥1%) **Body as a Whole:** Generally minimal and infrequent. **CNS:** *Headache,* lightheadedness, lethargy, fatigue, tremors, confusion, seizures, dizziness. **GI:** *Nausea, vomiting, diarrhea.* **Urogenital:** Glomerulonephritis, renal pain, renal tubular damage, acute renal failure. **Skin:** Rash, urticaria, pruritus, burning, stinging sensation, irritation, sensitization. **Other:** Inflammation or phlebitis at IV injection site, sloughing (with extravasation), thrombocytopenic purpura/hemolytic uremic syndrome.

**INTERACTIONS Drug: Probenecid** decreases acyclovir elimination; **zidovudine** may cause increased drowsiness and lethargy.

**PHARMACOKINETICS Absorption:** Oral dose is 15–30% absorbed. **Peak:** 1.5–2 h after oral dose. **Distribution:** Into most tissues with lower levels in the CNS; crosses placenta. **Metabolism:** Drug is primarily excreted unchanged. **Elimination:** Renally eliminated; also excreted in breast milk. **Half-Life:** 2.5–5 h.

## NURSING IMPLICATIONS

### Assessment & Drug Effects

▪ Observe infusion site during infusion and for a few days following infusion for signs of tissue damage.
▪ Monitor I&O and hydration status. Keep patient adequately hydrated

Common adverse effects in *italic;* life-threatening effects underlined; generic names in **bold;** classifications in SMALL CAPS; ♣ Canadian drug name; ⊙ Prototype drug

25

during first 2 h after infusion to maintain sufficient urinary flow and prevent formation of renal stones. Consult physician about amount and length of time oral fluids need to be pushed after IV drug treatment.

- Monitor for S&S of: Reinfection in pregnant patients; acyclovir-induced neurologic symptoms in patients with history of neurologic problems; drug resistance in immunocompromised patients receiving prolonged or repeated therapy; acute renal failure with concomitant use of other nephrotoxic drugs or preexisting renal disease.
- Monitor for adverse effects and viral resistance with long-term prophylactic use of the oral drug.
- Monitor lab tests: Baseline and periodic renal function tests, particularly with IV administration.

### Patient & Family Education

- Start therapy as soon as possible after onset of S&S for best results.
- Maintain a good fluid intake while receiving this drug.
- Do not exceed recommended dosage, frequency of drug administration, or specified duration of therapy. Contact prescriber if relief is not obtained or adverse effects appear.
- Cleanse affected areas with soap and water 3–4 × daily prior to topical application; dry well before application. With application to genitals, wear loose-fitting clothes over affected areas.
- Refrain from sexual intercourse while herpes lesions are present; neither topical nor systemic drug prevents transmission to other individuals.
- Avoid topical drug contact in or around eyes. Report unexplained eye symptoms to prescriber immediately (e.g., redness, pain);

untreated infection can lead to corneal keratitis and blindness.

## ADALIMUMAB

(a-da-lim'u-mab)

Humira

**Classifications:** BIOLOGICAL RESPONSE MODIFIER; IMMUNOMODULATOR; TUMOR NECROSIS FACTOR (TNF) MODIFIER; DISEASE-MODIFYING ANTIRHEUMATIC DRUG (DMARD)

Therapeutic: ANTIRHEUMATIC; DMARD; ANTI-INFLAMMATORY

**Prototype:** Etanercept

AVAILABILITY Solution for injection

ACTION & *THERAPEUTIC EFFECT*
A human recombinant IgG1 monoclonal antibody. It neutralizes the effects of tumor necrosis factor (TNF)-alpha by blocking its interaction with cell surface TNF receptors. This mechanism blocks the normal inflammatory and immune responses controlled by TNF-alpha. *Reduces the levels of acute phase inflammatory reactants (C-reactive protein, ESR, interleukin-6) thus decreasing overall joint inflammation; also reduces levels of enzymes that produce tissue remodeling responsible for cartilage destruction. In RA, it reduces the overproduction of TNF-alpha (principally by macrophages) in rheumatoid joints.*

USES Treatment of moderate to severe rheumatoid arthritis or psoriatic arthritis, polyarticular juvenile arthritis, ankylosing spondylitis, psoriasis, treatment of Crohn's disease, ulcerative colitis, uveitis.

CONTRAINDICATIONS Hypersensitivity to adalimumab or mannitol; serious infection including TB, sepsis; live vaccines; development of lupus-like syndrome while using adalimumab; neoplastic disease.

Common adverse effects in *italic;* life-threatening effects underlined; generic names in **bold;** classifications in SMALL CAPS; ♣ Canadian drug name; ◯ Prototype drug

**CAUTIOUS USE** History of recurrent infection or conditions predisposing to infection; recurrent history of sensitivity to monoclonal antibodies; CHF; neurologic disease; patients residing in areas with endemic TB or histoplasmosis; latent TB infection prior to therapy; history of or carriers of Hepatitis B; demyelinating disorders; Crohn's disease; ulcerative colitis; surgery; older adults; pregnancy (category B); lactation. Safe use in children younger than 4 y has not been established

## ROUTE & DOSAGE

### Rheumatoid Arthritis/Ankylosing Spondylitis

*Adult:* **Subcutaneous** 40 mg every other wk (may use 40 mg every wk if not on concomitant methotrexate)

### Polyarticular Juvenile Arthritis

*Adolescent/Child (2 y or older and 30 kg or more):* **Subcutaneous** 40 mg every other wk
*Adolescent/Child (2 y or older and 15–30 kg):* **Subcutaneous** 20 mg every other wk *Child (2 y or older and 10–15 kg):* **Subcutaneous** 10 mg every other wk

### Crohn's Disease /Moderate Ulcerative Colitis

*Adult/Adolescent/Child (6 y or older and over 40 kg):* **Subcutaneous** Initial dose of 160 mg (dose can be administered as 4 injections in 1 day or as 2 injections/day for 2 consecutive days), then 80 mg at wk 2, followed by 40 mg every other wk beginning at wk 4
*Child/Adolescent (6 y or older and 17–40 kg):* **Subcutaneous** 80 mg then 40 mg 2 wk later, followed by 20 mg every other wk starting at wk 4

### Plaque Psoriasis

*Adult:* **Subcutaneous** 80 mg then after 1 wk 40 mg every other wk

### Uveitis

*Adult:* **Subcutaneous** 30 mg, then 40 mg every other wk

## ADMINISTRATION

### Subcutaneous

- Do not administer to persons with active infections. Evaluate for latent TB with TB skin test prior to initiation of therapy.
- Leave at room temperature for 15 to 30 min prior to use.
- Inspect prefilled syringe for particulate matter and discoloration prior to subcutaneous injection.
- Rotate injection sites and do not inject into skin that is red, bruised, tender, or hard. After injecting the drug, do not rub the site. Inject in thigh or lower abdomen sites.
- Discard any remaining solution in prefilled syringe, as it contains no preservatives.
- Store in original carton at 2°–4° C (38°–48° F). Protect from light. Do not use beyond the expiration date.

**ADVERSE EFFECTS** (≥1%) **Body as a Whole:** *Infections* (especially reactivation of latent tuberculosis), sepsis, may see increase in malignancies (lymphoma), back pain, fever, allergic reactions (including anaphylactic shock), *flu-like symptoms, fatigue, sinusitis.* **CNS:** *Headache.* **CV:** Hypertension, increased serum alkaline phosphatase, arrhythmia exacerbation, cardiac arrest. **GI:** *Nausea, vomiting,* abdominal pain, GI perforation. **Hematologic:** *Development of ANA antibodies,* hematuria. **Respiratory:** *Upper respiratory infection, sinusitis* asthma, dyspnea. **Skin:** *Injection site reactions (erythema, itching, hemorrhage, pain,*

Common adverse effects in *italic;* life-threatening effects underlined; generic names in **bold;** classifications in SMALL CAPS; ✚ Canadian drug name; ⊕ Prototype drug

27

*swelling), rash,* urticaria, fixed drug reaction. **Urogenital:** Urinary tract infection, hematuria. **Neuromuscular and Skeletal:** Increased creatine phosphokinase.

**INTERACTIONS Drug:** Do not give live virus vaccines to patient on adalimumab; not recommended for use with other TNF BLOCKERS (**etanercept, infliximab, rilonacept, anakinra**). Do not use with **abatacept, tofacitinib,** or **rituximab.**

**PHARMACOKINETICS Absorption:** 64% absorbed from subcutaneous injection site. **Peak:** 131 h. **Distribution:** Minimal beyond vascular/synovial space. **Elimination:** Higher clearance in presence of anti-adalimumab antibodies, lower clearance with increasing age. **Half-Life:** 11.8 days (10–20 days).

## NURSING IMPLICATIONS

### Black Box Warning

*Adalimumab has been associated with increased risk of severe, potentially fatal, infections. Children and adolescents are at risk for development of malignancies.*

### Assessment & Drug Effects

- Monitor for and report lupus-like syndrome (e.g., joint pain, rash on cheeks or arms that is sensitive to sun).
- Monitor for and report promptly S&S of infection, including TB. Monitor known HBV carriers for signs of active HBV infection during therapy and for several months after therapy is discontinued.
- Monitor neurologic status closely. Report any change in status such as blurred vision or paresthesia.
- Monitor for signs or symptoms of liver dysfunction.

### Patient & Family Education

- Live vaccines should not be accepted by persons taking this drug.
- Report promptly any of the following to the prescriber: Unexplained joint pain, rash on cheeks or arms, fever, sore throat or other signs of infection, changes in vision, numbness or tingling in extremities.
- Severe and sometimes deadly infections have happened in patients who take this drug. Caution should be taken to minimize exposure to infectious agents.

## ADAPALENE
(a-da′pa-leen)
Differin
**Classifications:** ANTIACNE; RETINOID
Therapeutic: ANTIACNE
**Prototype:** Isotretinoin

**AVAILABILITY** Gel; cream; lotion

**ACTION & *THERAPEUTIC EFFECT*** A topical retinoid-like compound that modulates cellular differentiation, keratinization, and inflammatory processes related to the pathology of acne vulgaris. Topical adapalene may normalize the differentiation of epithelial follicular cells. *Adapalene decreases the inflammatory process and acne formation.*

**USES** Treatment of acne vulgaris.

**UNLABELED USES** Rosacea.

**CONTRAINDICATIONS** Hypersensitivity to adapalene or any of the components of the gel, irritating topical products, and sunburn; skin abrasion, eczema, seborrheic dermatitis.

**CAUTIOUS USE** Pregnancy (category C); lactation. Safety and efficacy in children younger than 12 y not established.

## ROUTE & DOSAGE

**Acne**

*Adult/Adolescent:* Apply once daily to affected areas in evening

## ADMINISTRATION

**Topical**

- Apply a thin film to clean skin, avoiding eyes, lips, mucous membranes, cuts, abrasions, eczematous or sunburned skin.
- Do not apply to skin recently treated with preparations containing sulfur, resorcinol, or salicylic acid.
- Store at 20°–25° C (68°–77° F).

## ADVERSE EFFECTS (≥1%) **Skin:**
*Erythema, scaling, dryness, pruritus, burning,* skin irritation, stinging, acne flares, sunburn.

## PHARMACOKINETICS **Absorption:** Minimal through intact skin. **Elimination:** Primarily in bile.

## NURSING IMPLICATIONS

**Assessment & Drug Effects**

- Monitor therapeutic effectiveness, which is indicated by improvement after 8–12 wk of treatment; early therapy may be marked by apparent worsening of acne.
- Note: Cutaneous reactions (e.g., erythema, scaling, pruritus) are common and normally diminish after first month of therapy.

**Patient & Family Education**

- Apply only as directed; excessive application will not result in faster healing but will cause marked redness, peeling, and discomfort.
- Minimize exposure to sunlight and sunlamps, and use sunscreen and protective clothing as needed.

## ADEFOVIR DIPIVOXIL
(a-de′fo-vir)

Hepsera

**Classifications:** ANTIVIRAL; NUCLEOTIDE ANALOG

**Therapeutic:** ANTIVIRAL

## AVAILABILITY Tablet

## ACTION & *THERAPEUTIC EFFECT*
Inhibits human hepatitis virus (HBV) DNA polymerase (reverse transcriptase) by competing with its DNA and by causing DNA chain termination after its incorporation into viral DNA. This results in inhibition of HBV DNA replication. *A nucleotide analog with activity against human hepatitis B virus (HBV).*

## USES Treatment of chronic hepatitis B.

## CONTRAINDICATIONS Hypersensitivity to adefovir; untreated or unknown human immunodeficiency virus (HIV); exacerbations of hepatitis B, especially in patients who have discontinued anti-hepatitis B therapy; lactation.

## CAUTIOUS USE Decreased cardiac function due to concomitant disease or other drug therapy; concomitant use of highly nephrotoxic drugs; renal dysfunction; coadministration with drugs that reduce renal function or compete for active tubular secretion; older adults; pregnancy (category C); children younger than 2 y. Appropriate infant immunizations should be used to prevent neonatal acquisition of the hepatitis B virus.

## ROUTE & DOSAGE

**Hepatitis B**

*Adult:* PO 10 mg daily

Common adverse effects in *italic;* life-threatening effects underlined; generic names in **bold;** classifications in SMALL CAPS; ♣ Canadian drug name; ⊙ Prototype drug

29

### Renal Impairment Dosage Adjustment

CrCl 20–49 mL/min: 10 mg q48h; 10–19 mL/min: 10 mg q72h

### Hemodialysis Dosage Adjustment

10 mg q7days following dialysis

## ADMINISTRATION

### Oral

- May be given without regard to food.
- Store in original container at 15°–30° C (59°–86° F).

## ADVERSE EFFECTS (≥1%) CNS:
*Asthenia,* headache. **GI:** Abdominal pain, nausea, flatulence, diarrhea, dyspepsia, exacerbation of hepatitis after discontinuation of therapy, hepatomegaly. **Metabolic:** *Increased ALT, AST,* increased creatine kinase, amylase, lactic acidosis. **Urogenital:** *Hematuria,* glycosuria, increased serum creatinine, nephrotoxicity. **Other:** HIV resistance in patient with unrecognized HIV, hematuria.

## INTERACTIONS **Drug:** Risk of lactic acidosis when used with NUCLEOSIDE ANALOGS. **Ibuprofen** increases bioavailability of adefovir.

## PHARMACOKINETICS **Absorption:** Adefovir dipivoxil is a prodrug. 59% of dose is absorbed as active drug. **Peak:** 1–4 h. **Distribution:** Minimal protein binding. **Metabolism:** Adefovir dipivoxil is rapidly converted to active adefovir. **Elimination:** Primarily in urine. **Half-Life:** 7.5 h.

## NURSING IMPLICATIONS

### Black Box Warning

*Adefovir has been associated with severe, acute exacerbations of hepatitis, nephrotoxicity, HIV resistance, lactic acidosis, and severe hepatomegaly with steatosis.*

### Assessment & Drug Effects

- Withhold drug and notify prescriber if lactic acidosis is suspected [e.g., hyperventilation, lethargy, plasma pH less than 7.35 and lactate greater than 5–6 mol/L (mEq/L)].
- Monitor for and promptly report S&S of hepatomegaly with steatosis, or other signs of liver injury.
- Monitor lab tests: Baseline and periodic renal function tests (monitor more often with preexisting impairment or other risk factors for renal impairment); periodic LFTs, creatinine kinase, serum amylase, and routine blood chemistries including serum electrolytes.

### Patient & Family Education

- Report any of the following to prescriber: Blood in urine, unexplained weakness, or exacerbation of S&S of hepatitis.
- Patients who discontinue adefovir should be monitored at repeated intervals over a period of time for hepatic function.

## ADENOSINE
(a-den'o-sin)

Adenocard, Adenoscan

**Classifications:** ANTIARRHYTHMIC
Therapeutic: ANTIARRHYTHMIC

## AVAILABILITY Injection

## ACTION & *THERAPEUTIC EFFECT*
Slows conduction through the atrioventricular (AV) and sinoatrial (SA) nodes. Can interrupt the reentry pathways through the AV node. *Restores normal sinus rhythm in patients with paroxysmal supraventricular tachycardia.*

**USES** Conversion to sinus rhythm of paroxysmal supraventricular tachycardia (PSVT) including PSVT associated with accessory bypass tracts (Wolff-Parkinson-White syndrome). "Chemical" thallium stress test.

**UNLABELED USES** Afterload-reducing agent in low-output states; to prevent graft occlusion following aortocoronary bypass surgery; to produce controlled hypotension during cerebral aneurysm surgery.

**CONTRAINDICATIONS** AV block, preexisting second- and third-degree heart block or sick sinus rhythm without pacemaker, since a heart block may result.

**CAUTIOUS USE** Asthmatics, unstable angina, stenotic valvular disease, hypovolemia; hepatic and renal failure; pregnancy (category C).

**ROUTE & DOSAGE**

**Supraventricular Tachycardia**

*Adult/Adolescent (weight 50 kg or more):* IV 6 mg bolus initially; after 1–2 min may give two additional 12 mg bolus doses for a total of 3 doses.
Do not exceed 12 mg in any one dose.
*Neonate/Infant/Child:* IV 0.05–1 mg/kg bolus; additional doses may be increased by 0.05–1 mg/kg q2min (max: 12 mg/dose)

**Stress Thallium Test**

*Adult:* IV 140 mcg/kg/min × 6 min (max: 0.84 mg/kg total dose)

**ADMINISTRATION**

**Intravenous**

Make sure solution is clear at time of use.

▪ Discard unused portion (contains no preservatives).

**PREPARE:** **Direct:** No dilution is required.
**ADMINISTER:** **Direct:** *Supraventricular Tachycardia:* Give rapid bolus over 1–2 sec. *Thallium Stress Test:* Give bolus over 6 min. ▪ If given by IV line, administer as proximally as possible, and follow with a rapid saline flush.

▪ Store at room temperature 15°–30° C (59°–86° F). Do not refrigerate, as crystallization may occur. If crystals do form, dissolve by warming to room temperature.

**ADVERSE EFFECTS** (≥1%) **CNS:** Headache, light-headedness, dizziness, tingling in arms (from IV infusion), apprehension, blurred vision, burning sensation (from IV infusion). **CV:** *Transient facial flushing,* sweating, palpitations, chest pain, atrial fibrillation or flutter. **Respiratory:** Shortness of breath, transient *dyspnea,* chest pressure. **GI:** Nausea, metallic taste, tightness in throat. **Other:** Irritability in children.

**INTERACTIONS** **Drug:** **Dipyridamole** can potentiate the effects of adenosine; **theophylline** will block the electrophysiologic effects of adenosine; **carbamazepine** may increase risk of heart block.

**PHARMACOKINETICS** **Absorption:** Rapid uptake by erythrocytes and vascular endothelial cells after IV administration. **Onset:** 20–30 sec. **Metabolism:** Rapid uptake into cells; degraded by deamination to inosine, hypoxanthine, and adenosine monophosphate. **Elimination:** Route unknown. **Half-Life:** 10 sec.

Common adverse effects in *italic;* life-threatening effects underlined; generic names in **bold;** classifications in SMALL CAPS; ♣ Canadian drug name; ⓖ Prototype drug

31

## NURSING IMPLICATIONS

### Assessment & Drug Effects

- Monitor for S&S of bronchospasm in asthma patients. Notify prescriber immediately.
- Use a hemodynamic monitoring system during administration; monitor BP and heart rate and rhythm continuously for several minutes after administration.
- Note: Adverse effects are generally self-limiting due to short half-life (10 sec).
- Note: At the time of conversion to normal sinus rhythm, PVCs, PACs, sinus bradycardia, and sinus tachycardia, as well as various degrees of AV block, are seen on the ECG. These usually last only a few seconds and resolve without intervention.

### Patient & Family Education

- Note: Flushing may occur along with a feeling of warmth as drug is injected.

## ADO-TRASTUZUMAB EMTANSINE

(A-doh-tras-too′zoo-mab em-tan′seen)

Kadcyla

**Classifications:** IMMUNOMODULATOR; MONOCLONAL ANTIBODY; ANTINEOPLASTIC; ANTI-HUMAN EPIDERMAL GROWTH FACTOR RECEPTOR (ANTI-HER)
Therapeutic: ANTINEOPLASTC; IMMUNOMODULATOR; ANTI-HER
**Prototype:** Trastuzumab

**AVAILABILITY** Powder for injection

**ACTION & *THERAPEUTIC EFFECT***
Binds to the HER2 receptors on the cell surface and is then brought into the cell where it is degraded into catabolites that disrupt the microtubule networks in the cell, resulting in cell cycle arrest and apoptotic cell death. *Causes death of HER2-positive breast cancer cells.*

**USES** Treatment of patients with HER2-positive, metastatic breast cancer who previously received trastuzumab and a taxane, separately or in combination.

**CONTRAINDICATIONS** Pregnancy (category D).

**CAUTIOUS USE** Interstitial lung disease or pneumonitis; hypersensitivity; thrombocytopenia; lactation.

## ROUTE & DOSAGE

**HER2-Positive, Metastatic Breast Cancer**

*Adult:* **IV** 3.6 mg/kg q 3wk
***Hepatic Impairment Dosage Adjustment***

*AST/ALT greater than 5 to less than or equal to 20 × ULN:* Withhold therapy; resume with dosage reduction when AST/ALT is less than or equal to 5 × ULN
*Total bilirubin greater than 3 to less than or equal to 10 × ULN:* Withhold therapy; resume with dosage reduction when total bilirubin less than or equal to 1.5 × ULN

Permanently discontinue use if AST/ALT is greater than 3 × ULN and total bilirubin is greater than 2 × ULN

**Thrombocytopenia**

*Platelet count 25,000/mm³ to less than 50,000 mm³:* Withhold therapy; resume at same dose when platelet count is greater than or equal to 75,500 m³
*Platelet count less than 25,000/mm³:* Withhold treat; resume with dosage reduction when platelet count is greater than or equal to 75,500 m³

***Recommended Dosage Reduction Schedule for Adverse Events***

*First reduction:* 3 mg/kg

Common adverse effects in *italic;* life-threatening effects underlined; generic names in **bold;** classifications in SMALL CAPS; ◆ Canadian drug name; ⊙ Prototype drug

*Second reduction:* 2.4 mg/kg
Discontinue if further reduction is required

## ADMINISTRATION

### Intravenous

Give antipyretics prior to infusion. **Do not** substitute adotrastuzumab emtansine (Kadcyla) for or with trastuzumab (Herceptin).

*PREPARE:* **IV Infusion:** Slowly inject 5 mL SW for injection or 8 mL SW for injection into the 100 mg or 160 mg vial, respectively, to yield 20 mg/mL. Swirl gently until dissolved but **do not shake.** Reconstituted solution will be clear to slightly opalescent. Should be used immediately.
From the 20 mg/mL reconstituted vial, withdraw the needed dose and add to 250 mL NS. Gently invert bag to dissolve. **Do not shake.**
*ADMINISTER:* **IV Infusion:** Infuse through a 0.22 micron in-line, non–protein filter. Give first infusion over 90 min; give subsequent infusions over 30 min if prior infusions well tolerated.
*INCOMPATIBILITIES:* **Solution/additive:** Do not mix with dextrose. **Y-site:** Do not mix or administer as an infusion with other medications.

- Store at 2°–8° C (36°–46° F) if not used immediately. Discard after 4 h.

## ADVERSE EFFECTS (≥1%) **Body as a Whole:** Asthenia, chills, *fatigue*, hypersensitivity reactions, infusion-related reaction, peripheral edema, peripheral neuropathy, pyrexia. **CNS:** Dizziness, *headache*, insomnia. **CV:** Hypertension, left ventricular dysfunction. **GI:** Abdominal pain, *constipation*, diarrhea, dry mouth, dyspepsia, *nausea*, stomatitis, vomiting. **Hematological:** Anemia, neutropenia, thrombocytopenia. **Metabolic:** AST/ALT increase, bilirubin increase, blood alkaline phoshatase increase, hemoglobin decrease, hypokalemia. **Musculoskeletal:** Arthralgia, *musculoskeletal pain*, myalgia. **Respiratory:** Cough, dyspnea, epistaxis, pneumonitis. **Skin:** Pruritus, rash. **Special Senses:** Blurred vision, conjunctivitis, dry eye, lacrimation. **Urogenital:** Urinary tract infection.

## INTERACTIONS **Drug:** Strong CYP3A4 inhibitors (e.g., **ketoconazole, itraconazole, clarithromycin, atazanavir, indinavir, nefazodone, nelfinavir, ritonavir, saquinavir, telithromycin, voriconazole**) may increase the levels of adotrastuzumab.

## PHARMACOKINETICS **Distribution:** 93% plasma protein bound. **Metabolism:** In liver to active and inactive compounds. **Half-Life:** 4 d.

## NURSING IMPLICATIONS

### Black Box Warning

*Adotrastuzumab emtansine has been associated with severe, potentially fatal, hepatotoxicity, and reduction in left ventricular ejection fraction. It can cause fetal harm and fetal death.*

### Assessment & Drug Effects

- Monitor for S&S of a hypersensitivity reaction during and for at least 90 min after IV infusion. Slow or stop infusion if a significant infusion-related or hypersensitivity reaction occurs.
- Monitor vital signs frequently during and after IV infusion.
- Monitor for S&S of neurotoxicity. Withhold dose and report to

Common adverse effects in *italic*; life-threatening effects <u>underlined</u>; generic names in **bold;** classifications in SMALL CAPS; ♣ Canadian drug name; ⓟ Prototype drug

33

prescriber if Grade 3 or 4 neuropathy develops.

- Monitor for and report promptly S&S of acute hepatitis and/or CHF.
- Monitor pulmonary status and report S&S of pulmonary toxicity (e.g., dyspnea, cough, fatigue, and pulmonary infiltrates).
- Monitor lab tests: Initial HERS2 testing to determine eligibility; prior to each dose, LFTs and platelet count.

**Patient & Family Education**
- Do not breast-feed while being treated with this drug.
- Use effective means of contraception during and for 6 mo after the last dose of this drug.
- Notify prescriber immediately if you suspect you are pregnant.
- Notify prescriber immediately if you experience S&S of liver damage (e.g., nausea, vomiting, right upper abdominal pain, jaundice, dark urine, generalized itching, anorexia), shortness of breath, cough, swelling of the ankles/ legs, palpitations, weight gain of more than 5 lbs in 24 h, dizziness or loss of consciousness.

# AFATINIB
(a-fa′ti-nib)
Gilotrif
**Classifications:** ANTINEOPLASTIC; KINASE INHIBITOR
Therapeutic: ANTINEOPLASTIC
**Prototype:** Erlotinib

**AVAILABILITY** Tablet

## ACTION & *THERAPEUTIC EFFECT*
Epidermal growth factor receptors (EGFR) are expressed or overexpressed in many cancers. EGFR expression is associated with poor prognosis (i.e., development of metastasis and resistance to chemotherapy, hormonal therapy, and radiation therapy). *Inhibits upregulation or overexpression of EGRF in cancer cells, thus diminishing their capacity for cell proliferation, cell survival, and decreasing their invasive capacity and metastases.*

**USES** First-line treatment of patients with metastatic non-small cell lung cancer (NSCLC) whose tumors have epidermal growth factor receptor (EGFR) exon 19 deletions or exon 21 (L858R) substitution mutations as detected by an FDA-approved test.

**CONTRAINDICATIONS** Lifethreatening bullous, blistering, or exfoliative skin lesions; confirmed interstitial lung disease (ILD); severe drug-induced hepatic impairment; persistent ulcerative keratitis; symptomatic left ventricular dysfunction; severe or intolerable adverse reaction occurring at a dose of 20 mg per day; pregnancy (category D); lactation.

**CAUTIOUS USE** Diarrhea, bullous and exfoliative skin disorders, keratitis; mild to moderate interstitial lung disease; metastatic breast cancer; mild to moderate hepatic impairment; patients with HER2-positive metastatic breast cancer. Safety and efficacy in children not established.

## ROUTE & DOSAGE

### Non-Small Cell Lung Cancer (NSCLC)
*Adult:* **PO** 40 once daily
***Toxicity Dosage Adjustment***
*Hold therapy for any of the following:*
National Cancer Institute Common Terminology Criteria for Adverse Effects (NCI CTCAE) Grade 3 or higher

Common adverse effects in *italic;* life-threatening effects underlined; generic names in **bold;** classifications in SMALL CAPS; ♣ Canadian drug name; ◯ Prototype drug

Diarrhea greater than or equal to Grade 2 persisting for 2 or more consecutive days while on anti-diarrheal medication

Grade 2 cutaneous reactions that are prolonged (greater than or equal to 7 days) or intolerable

**Hepatotoxicity Dosage Adjustment**

Grade 2 or higher renal toxicity

When toxicity resolves, resume therapy at 10mg/d less than dose that caused toxicity. Permanently discontinue if toxicity occurs at dose of 20 mg/day.

**Dosage Adjustment with Concomitant Use of P-gp Inhibitors or Inducers**

*P-gp inhibitor:* Reduce dose to 30 mg/day if not tolerated. If P-gp inhibitor is discontinued, resume previous dose.
*P-gp inducer:* Increase dose to 50mg/day as tolerated. If P-gp inducer is discontinued, wait 2–3 wk and resume previous dose.

## ADMINISTRATION

### Oral

- Give on an empty stomach at least 1 h before or 2 h after a meal.
- Store at 20°–25° C (68°–77° F).

### ADVERSE EFFECTS (≥10%) **Body as a Whole:** Cystitis, *paronychia*, pyrexia. **GI:** Cheilitis, *diarrhea, stomatitis*, nausea, vomiting, decreased appetite. **Metabolic:** ALT/AST increased, increased serum bilirubin, decreased appetite, decreased weight, *hypokalemia*. **Respiratory:** Epistaxis, rhinorrhea. **Skin:** *Dermatitis acneiform, dry skin*, pruritus, *rash*. **Special Senses:** Conjunctivitis.

## INTERACTIONS **Drug:** Inhibitors of P-gp (e.g., **amiodarone, azithromycin, cyclosporine A, diltiazem, erythromycin, itraconazole, ketoconazole, nelfinavir, quinidine, ritonavir, saquinavir, tacrolimus, verapamil**) can increase the levels of afatinib. Inducers of P-gp (e.g., **carbamazepine, phenobarbital, phenytoin, rifampin**) can decrease the levels of afatinib. **Herbal:** St. John's wort can decrease the levels of afatinib.

## PHARMACOKINETICS **Absorption:** 92% bioavailable. **Peak:** 2–5 h. **Distribution:** 95% plasma protein bound. **Metabolism:** Minimal metabolism in liver. **Elimination:** Primarily fecal (85%). **Half-Life:** 37 h.

## NURSING IMPLICATIONS

### Assessment & Drug Effects

- Monitor vital signs throughout the course of therapy.
- Monitor for diarrhea; withhold drug and notify prescriber if diarrhea lasts more than 48 h or if patient shows S&S of dehydration.
- Monitor for and report skin lesions (e.g., rash, erythema). Withhold drug and notify prescriber if blistering occurs.
- Monitor for and report eye inflammation, excessive lacrimation, light sensitivity, blurred vision, and eye pain.
- Monitor lab tests: Baseline and periodic LFTs; periodic serum electrolytes.

### Patient & Family Education

- Women should use highly effective means of birth control during and for at least 2 wk after termination of therapy. Notify prescriber immediately if a pregnancy occurs or is suspected.
- Promptly report if diarrhea develops; seek medical attention promptly for severe or persistent diarrhea.

Common adverse effects in *italic*; life-threatening effects underlined; generic names in **bold**; classifications in SMALL CAPS; ✚ Canadian drug name; ⊙ Prototype drug

35

- Minimize sun exposure with protective clothing and use of sunscreen.
- Report promptly new or worsening symptoms of adverse effects on the heart or lungs (e.g., trouble breathing, shortness of breath, cough, fever, exercise intolerance, fatigue, swelling of the ankles/legs, palpitations, or sudden weight gain).
- Report symptoms of liver damage (e.g., yellow skin or eyes, dark urine, right-sided abdominal pain, lethargy, easy bleeding or bruising).
- Report immediately eye pain, swelling, redness, blurred vision, or other vision changes.

# ALBENDAZOLE
(al-ben'da-zole)
Albenza
**Classifications:** ANTHELMINTIC
**Therapeutic:** ANTHELMINTIC
**Prototype:** Praziquantel

**AVAILABILITY** Tablet; chewable tablet

## ACTION & *THERAPEUTIC EFFECT*
A broad-spectrum oral anthelmintic agent. It is the only anthelmintic drug active against all stages of the helminth life cycle (ova, larvae, and adult worms). Its mechanism of action appears to cause selective degeneration of cytoplasmic microtubules in the intestinal cells of the helminths and larvae. *Albendazole ultimately causes decreased ATP production in the helminths, resulting in energy depletion, which kills the worms.*

**USES** Treatment of neurocysticercosis caused by pork tapeworm (*Taenia solium*), hydatid disease caused by the larval form of dog tapeworm (*Echinococcus granulosus*).

**UNLABELED USES** Giardiasis, pinworm infection, hookworm infection, microsporidosis.

**CONTRAINDICATIONS** Hypersensitivity to the benzimidazole class of compounds or any components of albendazole; hepatic enzymes twice the ULN; clinically significant decreases in blood cell counts.

**CAUTIOUS USE** Hepatic dysfunction; retinal lesions, pregnancy (category C); lactation; children younger than 6y.

## ROUTE & DOSAGE

**Neurocysticercosis**

*Adult/Adolescent/Child: (6 y or older, weight less than 60 kg):* **PO** 15 mg/kg/day divided b.i.d. for 8–30 day cycle (max: 800 mg/day); *weight 60 kg or more:* 400 mg b.i.d. for 8–30 days

**Hydatid Disease**

*Adult/Child: (6 y or older, weight less than 60 kg* (15 mg/kg/day divided b.i.d. × 28 days, then 14 days drug free and repeat for 2 more cycles (max: 800 mg/day); *weight 60 kg or more:* 400 mg b.i.d. for 28-day cycle (then 14 days without drug and repeat regimen for 3 cycles)

## ADMINISTRATION
Oral

- In young children, tablets should be crushed or chewed and swallowed with water.
- Give with meals. Absorption is significantly increased with a fatty meal.
- Do not exceed maximum total daily dose of 800 mg.
- Store at 20°–25° C (68°–77° F).

**ADVERSE EFFECTS** (≥1%) **Body as a Whole:** Hypersensitivity

Common adverse effects in *italic;* life-threatening effects <u>underlined;</u> generic names in **bold;** classifications in SMALL CAPS; ♣ Canadian drug name; ● Prototype drug

reactions. **CNS:** *Headache,* dizziness, vertigo, increased intracranial pressure, meningeal signs, fever. **GI:** *Abnormal liver function tests,* abdominal pain, nausea, *vomiting.* **Hematologic:** (Rare) Reversible <u>leukopenia</u>, granulocytopenia, pancytopenia, <u>agranulocytosis</u>. **Skin:** Rash, urticaria, reversible alopecia.

**INTERACTIONS Drug: Cimetidine, praziquantel, dexamethasone** increase levels. **Food:** Avoid **grapefruit juice.**

**PHARMACOKINETICS Absorption:** Poorly absorbed, absorption enhanced with a fatty meal. **Peak:** 2–5 h. **Distribution:** 70% protein bound; widely distributed, including cyst fluid and CSF; secreted into animal breast milk. **Metabolism:** In liver to active metabolite. **Elimination:** In bile. **Half-Life:** 9 h.

## NURSING IMPLICATIONS

### Assessment & Drug Effects

- Withhold drug and notify prescriber if WBC count falls below normal or liver enzymes are elevated.
- Note: Patients should be concurrently treated with appropriate steroid and anticonvulsant therapy.
- Monitor lab tests: Prior to each 28-day cycle and q2wk during cycle, WBC count, absolute neutrophil count, and LFTs.

### Patient & Family Education

- Take with meals (see ADMINISTRATION), but avoid grapefruit juice while taking this drug.
- Do not become pregnant during or for at least 1 mo after therapy.

## ALBIGLUTIDE

(al-bi-glu'tide)

Tanzeum

**Classifications:** ANTIDIABETIC; GLUCAGON-LIKE PEPTIDE-1 RECEPTOR AGONIST; INCRETIN MIMETIC
**Therapeutic:** ANTIDIABETIC
**Prototype:** Exenatide

**AVAILABILITY** Lyophilized powder for reconstitution

**ACTION & *THERAPEUTIC EFFECT***
An agonist of glucagon-like peptide-1 (GLP-1). Enhances glucose-dependent insulin secretion by the pancreas, suppresses glucagon secretion, and slows gastric emptying thereby decreasing glucagon stimulation of hepatic glucose output and insulin demand. *Improves glycemic control by reducing fasting and postprandial glucose concentrations in patients with type 2 diabetes.*

**USES** Type 2 diabetes mellitus in combination with diet and exercise.

**CONTRAINDICATIONS** Hypersensitivity to albiglutide; Type 1 diabetes; personal or family history of medullary thyroid carcinoma; history of Multiple Endocrine Neoplasia Syndrome type 2 (MEN2); pancreatitis; lactation.

**CAUTIOUS USE** History of pancreatitis; concurrent insulin secretagogues (e.g., sulfonylureas) or insulin; hypoglycemia; renal impairment; pregnancy (category C). Safety and efficacy in children younger than 18 y not established.

## ROUTE & DOSAGE

**Type 2 Diabetes Mellitus**
Adult: **Subcutaneous** 30 mg wk; may increase to 50 mg wk

## ADMINISTRATION

**Subcutaneous**
- Reconstitute powder with the diluent contained in the pen device.

Common adverse effects in *italic;* life-threatening effects <u>underlined</u>; generic names in **bold**; classifications in SMALL CAPS; ✦ Canadian drug name; ⊕ Prototype drug

37

Refer to manufacturer's product labeling for full reconstitution instructions. Administer within 8 h of reconstitution.

▪ Inject into the upper arm, thigh, or abdomen; use a different injection site each wk.

▪ Administer on the same day each wk, without regard to meals or time of day. The day may be changed, as long as the last dose was at least 4 days before.

▪ Store unused pens at 2°–8° C (36°–46° F); may be stored at room temperature (up to 30° C [86° F]) for up to 4 wk prior to use.

**ADVERSE EFFECTS** (≥ 1%) **Body as a Whole:** Influenza, angioedema, *injection site reaction.* **CV:** Atrial fibrillation, angioedema. **GI:** *Diarrhea*, gastroesophageal reflux disease, *nausea*, vomiting. **Metabolic:** Antibody development, *hypoglycemia*, increase gamma glutamyl transferase. **Musculoskeletal:** Arthralgia, back pain. **Respiratory:** Cough, pneumonia, *upper respiratory tract infection.* **Skin:** Rash at injection site.

**INTERACTIONS Drug:** Albiglutide causes a delay of gastric emptying, and may alter the absorption of concomitantly administered oral medications. May increase risk of hypoglycemia with **insulin detemir, pasireotide,** or **chloroquine**.

**PHARMACOKINETICS Onset:** 3–5 days **Metabolism:** Degradation to small peptides. **Half-Life:** 5 days.

## NURSING IMPLICATIONS

### Black Box Warning

*Albiglutide belongs to a class of drugs that has been associated with thyroid-C cell tumors.*

### Assessment & Drug Effects

▪ Monitor for S&S of pancreatitis (acute abdominal pain with/without vomiting). If pancreatitis is suspected, withhold drug and notify prescriber immediately.

▪ Monitor lab tests: Periodic HbA1C and renal function tests.

### Patient & Family Education

▪ Teach patient and caregivers proper preparation and administration of subcutaneous injection.

▪ If a dose is missed, inject as soon as possible within 3 days after the missed dose; then resume on the usual day.

▪ If more than 3 days have passed since the dose was missed, omit the missed dose and resume at the next regularly scheduled weekly dose. Report promptly symptoms of thyroid tumors (e.g., mass in the neck, difficulty swallowing or breathing, persistent hoarseness).

▪ Report promptly any of the following: Abdominal pain, severe dizziness, fainting, problems with urination, or signs of hypoglycemia.

▪ Women of childbearing age should consider stopping albiglutide at least 1 mo before a planned pregnancy.

▪ Do not breast-feed without consulting prescriber.

## ALBUTEROL ⊕

(al-byoo'ter-ole)

Accuneb, Novosalmol ◆ Pro-Air HFA, Proventil HFA, ReliOn Ventolin HFA, Ventolin HFA, VoSpire ER

**Classifications:** BRONCHODILATOR (RESPIRATORY SMOOTH MUSCLE RELAXANT); BETA-ADRENERGIC AGONIST
Therapeutic: BRONCHODILATOR

**AVAILABILITY** Tablet; extended release tablet; syrup; capsule for inhalation; solution for inhalation; actuation

## ACTION & *THERAPEUTIC EFFECT*
Moderately selective beta$_2$-adrenergic agonist that acts prominently on smooth muscles of trachea, bronchi, uterus, and vascular supply to skeletal muscles. Inhibits histamine release by mast cells. Produces bronchodilation by relaxing smooth muscles of bronchial tree. *Bronchodilation decreases airway resistance, facilitates mucous drainage, and increases vital capacity.*

## USES
To relieve bronchospasm associated with acute or chronic asthma, bronchitis, or other reversible obstructive airway diseases. Also used to prevent exercise-induced bronchospasm.

## CONTRAINDICATIONS
Albuterol or levalbuterol hypersensitivity; congenital long QT syndrome. Use of oral syrup in children younger than 2 y. Use of inhalator in children younger than 4 y.

## CAUTIOUS USE
Cardiovascular disease, renal impairment, hypertension, hyperthyroidism, diabetes mellitus, older adults; history of seizures; hypersensitivity to sympathomimetic amines or to fluorocarbon propellant used in inhalation aerosols; pregnancy (category C).

## ROUTE & DOSAGE

### Bronchospasm
*Adult:* **PO** 2–4 mg 3–4 × day; 4–8 mg sustained release 2 × day; **Inhaled** 1–2 inhalations q4–6h
*Child (2 to less than 6 y):* **PO** 0.1–0.2 mg/kg t.i.d. (max: 4 mg/dose); *6 to less than 12 y:* 2 mg 3–4 × day; **Inhaled** *4 to less than 12 y:* 1–2 inhalations q4–6h

### Prevention of Exercise-Induced Brochospasm
*Adult:* **Inhaled** 2 inhalations 30 min prior to exercise
*Child (4 y or older):* **Inhaled** 2 inhalations 30 min prior to exercise

## ADMINISTRATION

### Oral
- Do not crush extended release tablets. Scored tablets may be broken in half.
- Note: An initial dose of 2 mg t.i.d. or q.i.d. is recommended for older adult patients.
- Store tablets and syrup at 2°–25° C (36°–77° F) in tight, light-resistant container.

### Inhalation
- If ordered with beclomethasone, give 20–30 min before beclomethasone unless otherwise directed by prescriber.
- Administer albuterol inhalation aerosol canister only with the actuator provided.
- Store canisters at 15°–30° C (59°–86° F) away from heat and direct sunlight.

## ADVERSE EFFECTS (≥1%)
**Body as a Whole:** Hypersensitivity reaction. **CNS:** *Tremor,* anxiety, *nervousness,* restlessness, convulsions, weakness, headache, hallucinations. **CV:** Palpitation, chest pain, edema, hypertension, hypotension, bradycardia, reflex tachycardia. **Respiratory:** *Bronchospasm, rhinitis, URI.* **Special Senses:** Blurred vision, dilated pupils. **GI:** Nausea, vomiting. **Other:** Muscle cramps, hoarseness.

## DIAGNOSTIC TEST INTERFERENCE
Transient small increases in **plasma glucose** may occur.

Common adverse effects in *italic;* life-threatening effects <u>underlined</u>; generic names in **bold;** classifications in SMALL CAPS; ✚ Canadian drug name; ◐ Prototype drug

39

**INTERACTIONS Drug:** With **epinephrine,** other SYMPATHOMIMETIC BRONCHODILATORS, possible additive effects; MAO INHIBITORS, TRICYCLIC ANTIDEPRESSANTS potentiate action on vascular system; BETA-ADRENERGIC BLOCKERS antagonize the effects of both drugs.

**PHARMACOKINETICS Onset:** Inhaled: 5–15 min; PO: 30 min. **Peak:** Inhaled: 0.5–2 h; PO: 2.5 h. **Duration:** Inhaled: 3–6 h; PO: 4–6 h (8–12 h with sustained release). **Metabolism:** In liver by CYP3A4; may cross the placenta. **Elimination:** 76% of dose eliminated in urine in 3 days. **Half-Life:** 2.75 h.

## NURSING IMPLICATIONS

### Assessment & Drug Effects

- Monitor therapeutic effectiveness which is indicated by significant subjective improvement in pulmonary function within 60–90 min after drug administration.
- Monitor for: S&S of fine tremor in fingers, which may interfere with precision handwork; CNS stimulation, particularly in children 2–6 y (hyperactivity, excitement, nervousness, insomnia), tachycardia, GI symptoms. Report promptly to prescriber.
- Consult prescriber about giving last albuterol dose several hours before bedtime, if drug-induced insomnia is a problem.
- Monitor lab tests: Periodic ABGs, pulmonary functions, and pulse oximetry.

### Patient & Family Education

- Review directions for correct use of medication and inhaler (see ADMINISTRATION).
- Avoid contact of inhalation drug with eyes.

- Do not increase number or frequency of inhalations without advice of prescriber.
- Notify prescriber if albuterol fails to provide relief because this can signify worsening of pulmonary function and a reevaluation of condition/therapy may be indicated.
- Note: Albuterol can cause dizziness or vertigo; take necessary precautions.
- Do not use OTC drugs without prescriber approval. Many medications (e.g., cold remedies) contain drugs that may intensify albuterol action.

## ALCLOMETASONE DIPROPIONATE
(al-clo-met′a-sone)
Aclovate
**See Appendix A-4.**

## ALENDRONATE SODIUM
(a-len′dro-nate)
Binosto, Fosamax, Fosamax Plus D
**Classifications:** BISPHOSPHONATE; BONE METABOLISM REGULATOR
Therapeutic: BONE METABOLISM REGULATOR
**Prototype:** Etidronate

**AVAILABILITY** Tablet; effervescent tablet; oral solution

**ACTION & THERAPEUTIC EFFECT**
Inhibits osteoclast-mediated bone resorption. Antiresorption mechanism is thought to be localized to resorption sites of active bone turnover and to have minimal to no interference with bone mineralization. *Alendronate decreases bone resorption, thus minimizing loss of bone density.*

Common adverse effects in *italic;* life-threatening effects <u>underlined</u>; generic names in **bold;** classifications in SMALL CAPS; ♣ Canadian drug name; ✿ Prototype drug

**USES** Prevention and treatment of osteoporosis; Paget's disease. Treatment of glucocorticoid-induced osteoporosis.

**CONTRAINDICATIONS** Hypersensitivity to alendronate or other bisphosphonates; achalasia, esophageal stricture, severe renal impairment (CrCl less than 35 mL/min); hypocalcemia; inability to stand or sit upright for at least 30 min; invasive dental procedures.

**CAUTIOUS USE** Renal impairment, CHF, restricted sodium intake; hyperphosphatemia, liver disease, fever or infection, active upper GI problems; pregnancy (category C); lactation.

## ROUTE & DOSAGE

**Treatment of Osteoporosis**

*Adult:* **PO** 10 mg once/day (max: 40 mg/day) or 70 mg qwk

**Prevention of Osteoporosis**

*Adult:* **PO** 5 mg daily or 35 mg qwk

**Treatment of Steroid-Induced Osteoporosis**

*Adult:* **PO** 5 mg daily

**Treatment of Paget's Disease**

*Adult:* **PO** 40 mg once/day for 6 mo

*Renal Impairment Dosage Adjustment*

*CrCl less than 35 mL/min:* Use not recommended

## ADMINISTRATION

**Oral**

- Correct hypocalcemia before administering alendronate.
- Administer in the morning at least 30 min before the first food,

beverage, or medication. Do not administer within 2 h of calcium-containing foods, beverages, or medications. At least 30 min should elapse after alendronate dose before taking any other drugs.

- *Tablet:* Give with 8 oz of plain water.
- *Effervescent tablet:* Dissolve in 4 oz of plain water at room temp. Wait at least 5 min after effervescence stops. Stir the solution for approximately 10 seconds just before administration.
- *Oral solution:* Give with at least 2 oz of water.
- Keep patient sitting up or ambulating for 30 min after taking drug and until the first food of the day is eaten.
- Store according to manufacturer's directions.

**ADVERSE EFFECTS** (≥1%) **Endocrine:** Hypocalcemia, hypophosphatemia. **GI:** Esophageal irritation and *ulceration, nausea, vomiting, abdominal pain, dyspepsia,* diarrhea, constipation, flatulence. **Other:** Arthralgias, myalgias, headache, rash, alopecia.

**INTERACTIONS Drug: Ranitidine** increases alendronate availability. Aspirin increases risk of GI bleed. **Food: Calcium** and food (especially dairy products) reduce alendronate absorption.

**PHARMACOKINETICS Absorption:** 0.5–1% from GI tract (absorption significantly decreased by calcium and food). **Onset:** 3–6 wk. **Duration:** 12 wk after discontinuation. **Distribution:** Rapid skeletal uptake. **Metabolism:** Not metabolized. **Elimination:** Up to 50% excreted unchanged in urine. **Half-Life:** Up to 10 h.

---

Common adverse effects in *italic;* life-threatening effects underlined; generic names in **bold;** classifications in SMALL CAPS; ✤ Canadian drug name; ☻ Prototype drug

## NURSING IMPLICATIONS

### Assessment & Drug Effects
- Diagnostic test: Bone density scan every 12–18 mo.
- Discontinue drug if the CrCl less than 35 mL/min.
- Monitor lab tests: Baseline and periodic albumin-adjusted serum calcium, serum phosphate, serum alkaline phosphatase, fasting and 24 h urinary calcium, and serum electrolytes; periodic renal function tests and LFTs.

### Patient & Family Education
- Review directions for taking drug correctly (see ADMINISTRATION).
- Report fever, especially when accompanied by arthralgia and myalgia.

## ALFENTANIL HYDROCHLORIDE
(al-fen'ta-nill)

Alfenta

**Classifications:** NARCOTIC OPIATE AGONIST ANALGESIC; GENERAL ANESTHETIC
**Therapeutic** NARCOTIC ANALGESIC; GENERAL ANESTHETIC
**Prototype:** Morphine
**Controlled Substance:** Schedule II

### AVAILABILITY Injection

### ACTION & *THERAPEUTIC EFFECT*
A narcotic agonist analgesic with CNS effects that appear to be related to interaction of drug with opiate receptors. *Analgesia is mediated through changes in the perception of pain at the spinal cord and at higher levels in the CNS.*

### USES General anesthesia induction and maintenance, and sedation maintenance.

### UNLABELED USES Severe pain.

### CONTRAINDICATIONS Coagulation disorders, bacteremia, infection at injection site; lactation.

### CAUTIOUS USE Older adults, history of pulmonary disease; pregnancy (category C). Safety in children younger than 12 y is not established.

## ROUTE & DOSAGE

| Anesthesia |
| --- |
| *Adult:* **IV** induction 130–245 mcg/kg; maintenance 0.5–1.5 mcg/kg/min |
| **Conscious Sedation** |
| *Adult:* **IV** 3–8 mcg/kg then 3–5 mcg/kg q5–20 min or continuous infusion of 0.25–1 mcg/kg/min (total 3–40 mcg/kg) |
| *Obesity Dosage Adjustment* |
| Dose based on IBW |
| *Hepatic Impairment Dosage Adjustment* |
| Maintenance dosage adjustment recommended |

## ADMINISTRATION
Intravenous

*PREPARE:* **Direct or Continuous:** Alfentanil is available in a concentration of 500 mcg/mL. Small volumes may be given direct IV undiluted or diluted in 5 mL of NS. ▪ For IV infusion, add 20 mL of alfentanil to 230 mL of compatible IV solution to yield 40 mcg/mL. Compatible IV solutions include NS, D5/NS, D5W, and LR. ▪ Note: Alfentanil may be diluted to concentrations of 25–80 mcg/mL.
*ADMINISTER:* **Direct** Administer over at least 3 min. Do not administer more rapidly. **Continuous:** Administer at a rate of

0.25–1 mcg/kg/min. Note: Dose may be individualized.

***INCOMPATIBILITIES*: Y-site: Amphotericin B, amphotericin B (lipid), dantrolene, diazepam, diazoxide, lansoprazole, pantoprazole, phenytoin, sulfamethoxazole/trimethoprim.**

▪ Store at 15°–30° C (59°–86° F). Avoid freezing.

## ADVERSE EFFECTS (≥1%) Body as a Whole: Thoracic muscle rigidity, flushing, diaphoresis; extremities feel heavy and warm. **CNS:** Dizziness, euphoria, drowsiness. **CV:** Hypotension, hypertension, tachycardia, bradycardia. **GI:** *Nausea,* vomiting, anorexia, constipation, cramps. **Respiratory:** Apnea, respiratory depression, dyspnea.

## INTERACTIONS  Drug: BETA-ADRENERGIC BLOCKERS increase incidence of bradycardia; CNS DEPRESSANTS such as BARBITURATES, TRANQUILIZERS, NEUROMUSCULAR BLOCKING AGENTS, OPIATES, and INHALATION GENERAL ANESTHETICS may enhance the cardiovascular and CNS effects of alfentanil in both magnitude and duration; enhancement or prolongation of postoperative respiratory depression also may result from concomitant administration of any of these agents with alfentanil.

## PHARMACOKINETICS  Onset: 2 min. **Duration:** Injection 30 min; continuous infusion 45 min. **Distribution:** Crosses placenta. **Metabolism:** In liver by CYP3A4. **Elimination:** Excreted in breast milk. **Half-Life:** 46–111 min.

## NURSING IMPLICATIONS
### Assessment & Drug Effects
▪ Monitor for S&S of increased sympathetic stimulation (arrhythmias) and evidence of depressed

postoperative analgesia (tachycardia, pain, pupillary dilation, spontaneous muscle movement) if a narcotic antagonist has been administered to overcome residual effects of alfentanil.
▪ Evaluate adequacy of spontaneous ventilation carefully during postoperative period.
▪ Monitor vital signs carefully during postoperative period; check for bradycardia, especially if patient is also taking a beta-blocker.
▪ Note: Dizziness, sedation, nausea, and vomiting are common when drug is used as a postoperative analgesic.

### Patient & Family Education
▪ Report unpleasant adverse effects when drug is used for patient-controlled analgesia.

## ALFUZOSIN
(al-fuz'o-sin)
UroXatral, Xatral ◆
**Classifications:** ALPHA-ADRENERGIC ANTAGONIST
**Therapeutic:** GENITOURINARY SMOOTH MUSCLE RELAXER
**Prototype:** Tamsulosin

## AVAILABILITY Tablet

## ACTION & *THERAPEUTIC EFFECT*
A short-acting, selective antagonist at alpha-1 receptors with a low incidence of hypotension and sexual dysfunction. Alpha-1 receptors cause contraction of smooth muscle in the prostate, prostatic capsule, prostatic urethra, bladder base, and bladder neck. *Blockade of alpha-1 receptors by alfuzosin causes smooth muscles in the bladder neck and prostate to relax, thereby reducing pressure on the urethra and improving urine flow*

*rate. This results in a reduction in BPH symptoms.*

**USES** Treatment of symptomatic benign prostatic hypertrophy (BPH).

**CONTRAINDICATIONS** Hypersensitivity to alfuzosin; moderate or severe hepatic insufficiency; angina; QT prolongation; carcinoma of the prostate.

**CAUTIOUS USE** Coronary artery disease, cardiac arrhythmias; mild hepatic disease; severe renal impairment; dizziness, light-headedness, orthostatic hypotension; pregnancy (category B).

## ROUTE & DOSAGE

**Benign Prostatic Hypertrophy**
*Adult:* **PO** 10 mg daily

## ADMINISTRATION

**Oral**
- Give immediately after same meal each day.
- Ensure that extended release tablet is not crushed or chewed. It **must be** swallowed whole.
- Store at 15°–30° C (59°–86° F). Protect from light and moisture.

**ADVERSE EFFECTS** (≥1%) **Body as a Whole:** Fatigue, pain. **CNS:** Dizziness, headache. **GI:** Abdominal pain, dyspepsia, constipation, nausea. **CV:** Orthostatic hypotension thrombocytopenia. **Respiratory:** Upper respiratory infection, bronchitis, sinusitis, pharyngitis. **Urogenital:** Impotence, priapism.

**INTERACTIONS Drug:** Increased risk of hypotension with other ANTIHYPERTENSIVE AGENTS or PDE5 INHIBITORS **ketoconazole, itraconazole,** PROTEASE INHIBITORS may increase alfuzosin levels and toxicity. Contraindicated

with ANTIRETROVIRAL PROTEASE INHIBITORS or potent CYP3A4 inhibitors.

**PHARMACOKINETICS Absorption:** 80% protein bound **Peak:** 8 h. **Metabolism:** In liver by CYP3A4. **Elimination:** 69% in feces, 24% in urine. **Half-Life:** 10 h.

## NURSING IMPLICATIONS

### Assessment & Drug Effects
- Monitor CV status and BP, especially with concurrent antihypertensive drugs or inhibitors of CYP3A4. See INTERACTIONS.
- Check postural vital signs for orthostatic hypotension within a few hours following administration.
- Withhold drug and report new or worsening angina to prescriber.
- Monitor lab tests: Baseline and periodic LFTs.

### Patient & Family Education
- Inform prescriber about all other prescription, nonprescription, or herbal drugs being taken.
- Make position changes slowly to minimize dizziness.
- Do not drive or engage in other hazardous activities until reaction to drug is known.

## ALIROCUMAB
(a-lir-o-cu′mab)
Praluent

**Classifications:** MONOCLONAL ANTIBODY; PROPROTEIN CONVERTASE SUBTILISIN KEXIN TYPE 9 (PCSK9) INHIBITOR; ANTILIPIDEMIC; LIPID LOWERING
**Therapeutic:** ANTILIPIDEMIC

**AVAILABILITY** Pre-filled pens and solutions for injection

## ACTION & THERAPEUTIC EFFECT
Inhibits the binding of an enzyme

(proprotein convertase subtilisin kexin type 9 [PCSK9]) to LDL-C receptors in the liver, thus releasing the receptors to attach to LDL-C and clear LDL-C from the blood stream. *Lowers the level of LDL-C in the blood stream reducing the risk of CV disease.*

**USES** Adjunct treatment for adults with heterozygous familial hypercholesterolemia or clinical atherosclerotic cardiovascular disease who are receiving maximum tolerated statin therapy and require additional lowering of LDL-C.

**CONTRAINDICATIONS** Serious hypersensitivity to alirocmab or any component of the formulation.

**CAUTIOUS USE** Pregnancy; lactation. Safety and efficacy in children younger than 18 y not established.

## ROUTE & DOSAGE

**Heterozygous Familial Hypercholesterolemia**

*Adult:* Subcutaneous 75 mg q2wk; may increase to 150 mg q2wk

## ADMINISTRATION

### Subcutaneous

- Warm prefilled pen or syringe to room temperature for 30–40 min. Do not shake.
- Inject into the thigh, abdomen, or upper arm; rotate injection site with each injection. Do not coadminister with any other injectable drug.
- Store at 2°–8° C (36°–46° F) and protect from light. Do not leave unrefrigerated at 25° C (77° F) for more than 24 h.

**ADVERSE EFFECTS** (≥1%) **Body as a Whole:** Contusion, hypersensitivity reactions, influenza, injection site reactions. **Metabolic:** Elevated liver enzymes. **Musculoskeletal:** Musculoskeletal pain, muscle spasms, myalgia. **Respiratory:** Bronchitis, cough, *nasopharyngitis*, sinusitis. **Urogenital:** Urinary tract infection.

**PHARMACOKINETICS Peak:** 3–7 days. **Metabolism:** Peptide degradation. **Half-Life:** 17–20 days.

## NURSING IMPLICATIONS

### Assessment & Drug Effects

- Monitor for hypersensitivity reactions. Withhold drug and notify prescriber if hypersensitivity develops (e.g., hypersensitivity vasculitis, pruritus, rash, and urticaria).
- Monitor lab tests: Baseline LDL-C, repeat in 4–8 wk and after dose titrations, then periodically thereafter; periodic LFTs.

### Patient & Family Education

- Discontinue the drug and seek prompt medical attention if any signs or symptoms of serious allergic reactions occur (e.g., skin rash, itching, burning, pain).
- Prefilled syringes should not be reused.

## ALISKIREN

(a-lis'ki-ren)

Tekturna

**Classifications:** RENIN ANGIOTENSIN SYSTEM ANTAGONIST; ANTIHYPERTENSIVE

Therapeutic: DIRECT RENIN INHIBITOR; ANTIHYPERTENSIVE

**AVAILABILITY** Tablet

## ACTION & *THERAPEUTIC EFFECT*

A direct renin inhibitor that reduces plasma renin activity and inhibits the conversion of angiotensinogen to angiotensin I (ANG I) and subsequent production of angiotensin II (ANG II).

---

Common adverse effects in *italic;* life-threatening effects <u>underlined</u>; generic names in **bold**; classifications in SMALL CAPS; ♣ Canadian drug name; ⊙ Prototype drug

*Lowers blood pressure by decreasing vasoconstriction and aldosterone production, thus reducing sodium reabsorption and fluid retention.*

**USES** Treatment of hypertension.

**CONTRAINDICATIONS** Hypersensitivity to aliskiren; hyperkalemia; hypercalcemia; diabetics who are receiving ARBs or ACE inhibitors; dehydration, hypovolemia or salt depletion; pregnancy (category D second and third trimester); lactation; hypotension.

**CAUTIOUS USE** Patients with CrCl less than 30 mL/min; history of angioedema; respiratory disorders; history of airway surgery; DM; moderate renal impairment; renal stenosis, severe heart failure, post-MI; older adults; pregnancy (category C first trimester); children younger than 18 y.

## ROUTE & DOSAGE

**Hypertension**

*Adult:* **PO** 150 mg once daily (can increase to 300 mg once daily)

## ADMINISTRATION

**Oral**
- Give consistently at same time daily with or without meals.
- Store at 15°–30° C (59°–86° F) and protect from light.

**ADVERSE EFFECTS** (≥1%) **CNS:** *Headache, dizziness.* **GI:** *Diarrhea.* **Metabolic:** Hyperkalemia. **Skin:** Angioedema, rash. **Neuromuscular and Skeletal:** Increased creatine phosphokinase. **Renal:** Increased blood urea nitrogen, increased serum creatinine.

**INTERACTIONS Drug:** Enhances effects of other ANTIHYPERTENSIVE AGENTS. DIURETIC effect may be reduced. **Ketoconazole** increases the plasma level of aliskiren, while **irbesartan** decreases its plasma level.

**PHARMACOKINETICS Absorption:** 2.5%. **Peak:** 1–3 h; clinical effect seen in 2 wk. **Metabolism:** Less than 10% via liver. **Elimination:** Primarily in stool. **Half-Life:** 24 h.

## NURSING IMPLICATIONS

### Black Box Warning

*Aliskiren has been associated with fetal injury and/or death.*

**Assessment & Drug Effects**
- Monitor for hypotension at the initiation of therapy, following dosage change, and on a regular basis throughout.
- Monitor for angioedema, which may occur any time during treatment. Withhold drug and immediately report to prescriber.
- Monitor lab tests: Periodic serum electrolytes, especially with concurrent ACE inhibitor.
- Evaluate renal status prior to beginning therapy. Assess BUN, serum potassium, and serum creatinine.

**Patient & Family Education**
- Discontinue drug and notify health care provider immediately if pregnancy occurs.
- Full therapeutic effect is usually obtained by 2 wk of therapy.
- Report immediately any of the following: Swelling about the face, lips, tongue; difficulty breathing or swallowing; swelling of hands or feet.
- High fat meals interfere with the absorption of this drug. Do not take drug following a high fat meal.
- Do not use salt substitutes or potassium supplements without consulting prescriber.

- Monitor lab tests: Periodic serum potassium.

# ALITRETINOIN (9-*cis*-RETINOIC ACID)

(a-li-tre′ti-noyne)

Panretin

**Classifications:** ANTIACNE (RETINOID)
Therapeutic: ANTIACNE
**Prototype:** Isotretinoin

## AVAILABILITY Gel

## ACTION & *THERAPEUTIC EFFECT*

Naturally occurring retinoid that binds to and activates all known retinoid receptors in cells, which regulate cellular differentiation and proliferation in both healthy and neoplastic cells. *Inhibits the growth of Kaposi's sarcoma (KS) in HIV patients. It does not prevent the development of new KS lesions.*

## USES Treatment of cutaneous lesions of AIDS-related Kaposi's sarcoma.

## UNLABELED USES Cutaneous T-cell lymphomas.

## CONTRAINDICATIONS Hypersensitivity to alitretinoin or other retinoids including vitamin A; when systemic anti-KS therapy is required; pregnancy (category D), lactation.

## CAUTIOUS USE Cutaneous T-cell lymphoma. Safety and efficacy in children younger than 18 y, or adults 65 y or older, are unknown.

## ROUTE & DOSAGE

### Cutaneous Kaposi's Sarcoma

*Adult:* **Topical** Apply sufficient gel to cover lesions b.i.d., may increase application to 3–4 × daily if tolerated

## ADMINISTRATION

### Topical

- Apply gel liberally over lesions; avoid unaffected skin and mucous membranes.
- Dry 3–5 min before covering with clothes. Do not cover with occlusive dressing.
- Store at 15°–30° C (59°–86° F).

## ADVERSE EFFECTS (≥1%) **Skin:** Erythema, edema, vesiculation, *rash, burning pain,* pruritus, exfoliative dermatitis, excoriation, paresthesia.

## INTERACTIONS **Drug:** Increased toxicity with insect repellents containing DEET.

## PHARMACOKINETICS **Absorption:** Minimal.

## NURSING IMPLICATIONS

### Assessment & Drug Effects

- Monitor for S&S of dermal toxicity (e.g., erythema, edema, vesiculation).

### Patient & Family Education

- Allow up to 14 wk for therapeutic response.
- Discontinue drug immediately if pregnancy occurs.
- Avoid exposure of medicated skin to sunlight or sun lamps.
- Contact prescriber if inflammation, swelling, or blisters appear on medicated areas.

# ALLOPURINOL

(al-oh-pure′i-nole)

Aloprim, Apo-allopurinol-A ✦, Zyloprim

**Classifications:** ANTIGOUT
Therapeutic: ANTIGOUT

## AVAILABILITY Tablet; powder for injection

---

Common adverse effects in *italic*; life-threatening effects underlined; generic names in **bold**; classifications in SMALL CAPS; ✦ Canadian drug name; ⊙ Prototype drug

47

## ACTION & *THERAPEUTIC EFFECT*
Reduces endogenous uric acid by selectively inhibiting action of xanthine oxidase, the enzyme responsible for converting hypoxanthine to xanthine and xanthine to uric acid (end product of purine catabolism). *Urate pool is decreased by the lowering of both serum and urinary uric acid levels, and hyperuricemia is prevented.*

**USES** To control hyperuricemia, gout, nephrolithiasis, renal calculus, uric acid nephropathy.

**CONTRAINDICATIONS** Hypersensitivity to allopurinol; as initial treatment for acute gouty attacks; idiopathic hemochromatosis (or those with family history); HLA-B*5801 genotype (strongly associated with allopurinol induced severe cutaneous reactions).

**CAUTIOUS USE** Impaired hepatic or renal function, bone marrow suppression, pregnancy (category C). Use with caution when performing tasks which require mental alertness due to CNS effects.

## ROUTE & DOSAGE

### Treatment of Hyperuricemia
*Adult/Adolescent/Child (10 y and older):* **PO** 600–800 mg/day (in divided doses); **IV** 200–400 mg/m²/day (max: 600 mg/day) in 1–4 divided doses
*Child (less than 10 y):* **PO** 300 mg/day; *(less than 6 y):* **PO** 150 mg/day; **IV** 200 mg/m²/day in 1–4 divided doses

### Treatment of Recurrent Renal Calculi
*Adult:* **PO** 200–300 daily (may divide dose)

### Gout
*Adult:* **PO** 100 mg daily increase as needed for patient response (max: 800 mg/day)
**Renal Impairment Dosage Adjustment**
*CrCl 10–20 mL/min:* **PO** 200 mg/day; **IV** 100 mg; *3–9 mL/min:* 100 mg daily; *less than 3 mL/min:* 100 mg with extended interval between doses (24 h or more)
**Hemodialysis Dosage Adjustment**
See package insert

## ADMINISTRATION
### Oral
- Give after meals.
- Administer fluids for sufficient urine output.
- Store at 15°–30° C (59°–86° F) in a tightly closed container.

### Intravenous
*PREPARE:* **Intermittent:** Reconstitute a single dose vial (500 mg) with 25 mL of sterile water for injection to yield 20 mg/mL. ▪ **Must be** further diluted with NS or D5W to a concentration of 6 mg/mL or less. ▪ Note: Adding 2.3 mL of diluent yields 6 mg/mL.
*ADMINISTER:* **Intermittent** Usually administered over 30 min.
*INCOMPATIBILITIES:* Solution/additive: **Amikacin, amphotericin B, carmustine, cefotaxime, chlorpromazine, cimetidine, clindamycin, cytarabine, dacarbazine, daptomycin, daunorubicin, diltiazem, diphenhydramine, doxorubicin, doxycycline, droperidol, epirubicin, ertapenem, etoposide, floxuridine, gentamicin, haloperidol, hydroxyzine, idarubicin, imipenem-cilastatin,**

irinotecan, mechlorethamine, meperidine, methylpred-nisolone, metoclopramide, metoprolol, minocycline, myco-phenolate, nalbuphine, netil-micin, ondansetron, pa-lonosetron, pancuronium, potassium acetate, prochlor-perazine, promethazine, sodium bicarbonate, strepto-zocin, tacrolimus, tobramycin, vecuronium, vinorelbine.

## ADVERSE EFFECTS (≥1%) CNS:
Drowsiness, headache. GI: Nau-sea, vomiting, diarrhea, abdomi-nal discomfort. Hematologic: (Rare) <u>Agranulocytosis, aplastic anemia, bone marrow depres-sion, thrombocytopenia</u>. Skin: Urticaria or pruritus, rash, pruritic maculopapular rash, toxic. Other: <u>Hepatotoxicity</u>, increased liver enzymes, increased serum alka-line phosphatase, acute gout.

## DIAGNOSTIC TEST INTERFERENCE
Possibility of elevated blood lev-els of *alkaline phosphatase* and *serum transaminases (AST, ALT)*, and decreased blood *Hct, Hgb, leukocytes.*

## INTERACTIONS Drug: Alco-hol may inhibit renal excretion of uric acid; ampicillin, amoxi-cillin increase risk of skin rash; enhances anticoagulant effect of warfarin; toxicity from azathio-prine, mercaptopurine, cyclo-phosphamide, cyclosporin in-creased; increases hypoglycemic effects of chlorpropamide; THI-AZIDES increase risk of allopuri-nol toxicity and hypersensitivity (especially with impaired renal function); ACE INHIBITORS increase risk of hypersensitivity; high dose vitamin C increases risk of kid-ney stone formation. Do not use with didanosine or pegloticase.

## PHARMACOKINETICS Absorp-tion: 80–90% from GI tract. Onset: 24–48 h. Peak: 2–6 h. Metabolism: 75–80% to the active metabolite oxypurinol. Elimination: Slowly ex-creted in urine; excreted in breast milk. Half-Life: 1–3 h; oxypurinol, 18–30 h.

## NURSING IMPLICATIONS
### Assessment & Drug Effects
- Monitor for therapeutic effec-tiveness which is indicated by normal serum and urinary uric acid levels usually by 1–3 wk, gradual decrease in size of tophi, absence of new tophaceous deposits (after approximately 6 mo), with consequent relief of joint pain and increased joint mobility.
- Monitor for S&S of an acute gouty attack which is most likely to oc-cur during first 6 wk of therapy.
- Monitor patients with renal disor-ders more often; they tend to have a higher incidence of renal stones and drug toxicity problems.
- Report onset of rash or fever im-mediately to prescriber; withhold drug. Life-threatening toxicity syndrome can occur 2–4 wk af-ter initiation of therapy (more common with impaired renal function) and is generally ac-companied by malaise, fever, and aching, a diffuse erythematous, desquamating rash, hepatic dys-function, eosinophilia, and wors-ening of renal function.
- Monitor lab tests: Baseline then monthly CBC, LFTs, and kidney function tests; serum uric acid q1–2wk; periodic urine pH.

### Patient & Family Education
- Drink enough fluid to produce urinary output of at least 2000 mL/day (fluid intake of at least 3000 mL/day). (Note that 1000 mL is

Common adverse effects in *italic*; life-threatening effects <u>underlined</u>; generic names in **bold**; classifications in SMALL CAPS; ♣ Canadian drug name; ⊙ Prototype drug

49

approximately equal to 1 quart.) Report diminishing urinary output, cloudy urine, unusual color or odor to urine, pain or discomfort on urination.

- Report promptly the onset of itching or rash. Stop drug if a skin rash appears, and report to prescriber.
- Do not drive or engage in potentially hazardous activities until response to drug is known.

## ALMOTRIPTAN
(al-mo-trip′tan)
Axert
**Classifications:** SEROTONIN 5-HT$_1$ RECEPTOR AGONIST
Therapeutic: ANTIMIGRAINE
**Prototype:** Sumatriptan

**AVAILABILITY** Tablet

## ACTION & *THERAPEUTIC EFFECT*
Selective agonist that binds with high affinity to serotonin receptors found on extracerebral and intracranial blood vessels. Due primarily to its effects on 5-HT$_{1D}$ and 5-HT$_{1B}$ serotonin receptors on cranial blood vessels, it causes vasoconstriction and decreases inflammation and neurotransmission. *This results in constriction of cranial vessels that become dilated during a migraine attack and reduces signal transmission in the pain pathways.*

**USES** Treatment of migraine headache with or without aura.

**CONTRAINDICATIONS** Hypersensitivity to almotriptan malate; significant cardiovascular disease such as ischemic heart disease, coronary artery vasospasms, MI, angina, arteriosclerosis, cardiac arrhythmias, history of cerebrovascular events, or uncontrolled hypertension; stroke, Wolff-Parkinson-White syndrome, within 24 h of receiving another 5-HT$_1$ agonist or an ergotamine-containing or ergot-type drug; basilar or hemiplegic migraine.

**CAUTIOUS USE** Significant risk factors for coronary artery disease unless a cardiac evaluation has been done; hypertension; risk factors for cerebrovascular accident; diabetes; colitis; smoking; obesity; peripheral vascular disease, impaired liver or kidney function, Raynaud's disease, older adults; pregnancy (category C); lactation; children.

## ROUTE & DOSAGE

**Migraine Headache**
*Adult:* **PO** 6.25–12.5 mg; if headache returns, may repeat after at least 2 h (max: 2 tabs/24 h)

**Renal Impairment Dosage Adjustment**
*CrCl less than 10 mL/min:* 6.25 mg (max: 12.5 mg/day)

**Hepatic Impairment Dosage Adjustment**
6.25 mg (max: 12.5 mg/day)

## ADMINISTRATION
**Oral**
- Do not give within 24 h of an ergot-containing drug.
- Administer any time after symptoms of migraine appear.
- Do not administer a second dose without consulting the prescriber for any attack during which the FIRST dose did **not** work.
- Give a second dose if headache was relieved by first dose but symptoms return; however, wait at least 2 h after the first dose before giving a second dose.
- Do not give more than two doses in 24 h.
- Store at 15°–30° C (59°–86° F).

Common adverse effects in *italic;* life-threatening effects <u>underlined;</u> generic names in **bold;** classifications in SMALL CAPS; ♣ Canadian drug name; ⊘ Prototype drug

## ADVERSE EFFECTS (≥1%) Body as a Whole: Flushing. CNS: Drowsiness, headache, paresthesia. CV: Palpitations, tachycardia, serious cardiac events (including <u>MI</u>) have been reported within a few hours after administration. GI: Nausea, vomiting, dry mouth.

## INTERACTIONS Drug: **Dihydroergotamine, methysergide,** other 5-HT$_1$ AGONISTS may cause prolonged vasospastic reactions; SSRIS, **sibutramine** have rarely caused weakness, hyperreflexia, and incoordination; MAOIS should not be used with 5-HT$_1$ AGONISTS.

## PHARMACOKINETICS Absorption: Well absorbed, 70% reaches systemic circulation. Peak: 1–3 h. Distribution: 35% protein bound. Metabolism: 27% metabolized by monoamine oxidase. Elimination: 75% renally, 13% in feces. Half-Life: 3–4 h.

## NURSING IMPLICATIONS

### Assessment & Drug Effects

- Monitor cardiovascular status carefully following first dose in patients at relatively high risk for coronary artery disease (e.g., postmenopausal women, men over 40 years old, persons with known CAD risk factors) or who have coronary artery vasospasms.
- Report to prescriber immediately chest pain or tightness in chest or throat that is severe or does not quickly resolve following a dose of almotriptan.
- Pain relief usually begins within 10 min of ingestion, with complete relief in approximately 65% of all patients within 2 h.
- Monitor BP, especially in those being treated for hypertension.

### Patient & Family Education

- Notify prescriber immediately if symptoms of severe angina (e.g., severe or persistent pain or tightness in chest, back, neck, or throat) or hypersensitivity (e.g., wheezing, facial swelling, skin rash, or hives) occur.
- Do not take any other serotonin receptor agonist (e.g., Imitrex, Maxalt, Zomig, Amerge) within 24 h of taking almotriptan.
- Advise prescriber of any drugs taken within 1 wk of beginning almotriptan.
- Check with prescriber regarding drug interactions before taking any new OTC or prescription drugs.
- Report any other adverse effects (e.g., tingling, flushing, dizziness) at next prescriber visit.

# ALOGLIPTIN
(a-loh-grip'tin)
Nesina

**Classifications:** ANTIDIABETIC; INCRETIN MODIFIER; DIPEPTIDYL PEPTIDASE-4 (DPP-4) INHIBITOR
Therapeutic: ANTIDIABETIC; HORMONE MODIFIER; DPP-4 INHIBITOR
**Prototype:** Sitagliptin

## AVAILABILITY Tablet

## ACTION & *THERAPEUTIC EFFECT*
Slows inactivation of incretin hormones that are released by the intestine. As plasma glucose rises following food intake, incretin hormones stimulate release of insulin from the pancreas and lower glucagon secretion, resulting in reduced hepatic glucose production. *Sitagliptin lowers both fasting and postprandial plasma glucose levels.*

## USES Adjunct treatment of type 2 diabetes mellitus in combination with exercise and diet.

Common adverse effects in *italic;* life-threatening effects <u>underlined;</u> generic names in **bold;** classifications in SMALL CAPS; ♣ Canadian drug name; ⊙ Prototype drug

51

**CONTRAINDICATIONS** History of a serious hypersensitivity reaction (e.g., anaphylaxis, angioedema, or severe cutaneous reactions) to alogliptin-containing products; acute pancreatitis.

**CAUTIOUS USE** Hepatic dysfunction; concurrent use of insulin secretagogue (e.g., sulfonylurea) or insulin; renal impairment; older adults; heart failure; renal dysfunction; pregnancy (category B); lactation. Safety and efficacy in children not established.

## ROUTE & DOSAGE

**Type 2 Diabetes Mellitus**
*Adult:* **PO** 25 mg once daily
***Renal Impairment Dosage Adjustment***
*CrCl greater than or equal to 30 mL/min to 59 mL/min:* 12.5 mg once daily
*CrCl less than 30 mL/min:* 6.25 mg once daily

## ADMINISTRATION

**Oral**
- May be given without regard to meals.
- Note that dosage adjustment is recommended for moderate to severe renal impairment.
- Store at 20°–25° C (68°–77° F).

**ADVERSE EFFECTS** (≥1%) **CNS:** Headache. **Cardiac:** Heart failure. **Metabolic:** Hypoglycemia. **Respiratory:** Nasopharyngitis, upper respiratory infection. **Hepatic:** Increased serum ALT. **Renal:** Decreased GFR, impaired renal function.

**INTERACTIONS** May increase effect of SULONYLUREA or **insulin.** May cause hypoglycemia with other ANTIDIABETES drugs or **chloroquine.**

**PHARMACOKINETICS Absorption:** 100% bioavailable. **Peak:** 1–2 h. **Distribution:** 20% plasma protein bound. **Metabolism:** In liver. **Elimination:** Renal (76%) and fecal (13%). **Half-Life:** 21 h.

## NURSING IMPLICATIONS

### Assessment & Drug Effects
- Monitor for and report S&S of significant GI distress, including nausea, vomiting, and diarrhea.
- Monitor for S&S of hypoglycemia when used in combination with a sulfonylurea drug or insulin.
- Monitor lab tests: Baseline and periodic CrCl; baseline LFTs; periodic fasting and postprandial plasma glucose and HbA1C.

### Patient & Family Education
- Stop taking this drug and notify prescriber immediately if you have an allergic reaction (e.g., swelling of your face, lips, throat; difficulty swallowing or breathing; raised, red areas on your skin (hives); skin rash, itching, flaking, or peeling.
- Contact prescriber if you experience unexplained symptoms of liver problems (e.g., nausea or vomiting, abdominal pain, unusual tiredness, loss of appetite, dark urine, yellowing of your skin or the whites of your eyes).
- Taking this drug with another drug that can lower your blood sugar, such as a sulfonylurea or insulin, increases your risk of hypoglycemia.

## ALOSETRON
(a-lo'se-tron)
Lotronex
**Classifications:** SEROTONIN 5-HT$_3$ RECEPTOR ANTAGONIST
Therapeutic: GI

**AVAILABILITY** Tablet

---

Common adverse effects in *italic*; life-threatening effects underlined; generic names in **bold;** classifications in SMALL CAPS; ◆ Canadian drug name; ⊙ Prototype drug

## ACTION & *THERAPEUTIC EFFECT*

Potent and selective serotonin (5-HT$_3$) receptor antagonist. Serotonin 5-HT$_3$ receptors are extensively located on enteric neurons of the GI tract. Activation of these receptors affects amount of visceral pain experienced, transit time in the colon, and GI secretions. *Alosetron significantly controls GI pain, and severe diarrhea related to irritable bowel syndrome.*

## USES

Treatment of severe chronic irritable bowel syndrome (IBS) in women whose predominant symptom is diarrhea and whose symptoms have lasted longer than 6 mo and have failed to respond to conventional therapy.

## CONTRAINDICATIONS

Constipation, ischemic colitis, development of ischemic bowel symptoms such as sudden onset of rectal bleeding, bloody diarrhea, new or sudden worsening of abdominal pain; history of chronic or severe constipation, intestinal obstruction, toxic megacolon, GI adhesions, GI perforation, active diverticulitis, history of, or current Crohn's disease or ulcerative colitis; hypersensitivity to alosetron; thrombophlebitis, hypercoagulable state, inability to comply with Patient–Prescriber Agreement; severe hepatic impairment; lactation.

## CAUTIOUS USE

Hepatic insufficiency, renal impairment; older adults; pregnancy (category B). Safety and efficacy in children not established.

## ROUTE & DOSAGE

### Irritable Bowel Syndrome

*Adult:* **PO** Start with 0.5 mg b.i.d. for 4 wk, may increase to 1 mg b.i.d. if tolerated

## ADMINISTRATION

### Oral

- Ensure that the patient has signed the Patient–Prescriber Agreement prior to administering alosetron.
- Do not give this drug if the patient has constipation.
- Review the contraindications for this drug and ensure that the patient has none of the conditions for which the drug is contraindicated.
- Store at 25° C (77° F).

## ADVERSE EFFECTS (≥1%)

**Body as a Whole:** Malaise, fatigue, cramps, pain. **CNS:** Anxiety. **CV:** Tachyarrhythmias. **GI:** *Constipation,* abdominal pain, nausea, distention, reflux, hemorrhoids, hyposalivation, dyspepsia, ischemic colitis. **Skin:** Sweating, urticaria. **Urogenital:** Urinary frequency.

## INTERACTIONS

**Drug:** **Fluvoxamine** increases alosetron serum level.

## PHARMACOKINETICS

**Absorption:** Rapidly absorbed, average bioavailability of 50–60%. **Peak:** 1 h. **Distribution:** 82% protein bound. **Metabolism:** Extensively in liver by CYP2C9. **Elimination:** 73% in urine, 24% in feces. **Half-Life:** 1.5 h.

## NURSING IMPLICATIONS

### Black Box Warning

*Alosetron has been associated with infrequent, but serious and potentially fatal, GI adverse effects, including ischemic colitis and serious complications of constipation.*

### Assessment & Drug Effects

- Monitor for and report immediately signs of ischemic colitis such as new or worsening abdominal pain, bloody diarrhea, or blood in the stool.

- Withhold drug and notify prescriber if patient has not had adequate control of IBS symptoms after 4 wk of treatment with 1 mg twice a day.
- Monitor carefully patients who have decreased GI motility (e.g., older adults, persons receiving other drugs which may decrease GI motility) as they may be at greater risk of serious complications of constipation.
- Monitor carefully patients with any degree of hepatic insufficiency as they may be more susceptible to adverse drug effects.
- Monitor periodically for cardiac arrhythmias, especially with pre-existing cardiovascular disease.

### Patient & Family Education

- Read the Medication Guide before starting alosetron and each time you refill your prescription.
- Do not start taking alosetron if you are constipated.
- Discontinue alosetron immediately and contact your prescriber if you experience any of the following: Constipation, new or worsening abdominal pain, bloody diarrhea, or blood in the stool.
- Contact your prescriber immediately if constipation does not resolve after discontinuation of alosetron. Resume alosetron again only if constipation has resolved and your prescriber directs you to begin taking the medication again.
- Stop taking alosetron and contact your prescriber if IBS symptoms are not adequately controlled after 4 wk of taking 1 tablet twice a day.

## ALPRAZOLAM
(al-pray'zoe-lam)
Niravam, Xanax, Xanax XR

**Classifications:** ANXIOLYTIC; SEDATIVE-HYPNOTIC; BENZODIAZEPINE
**Therapeutic:** ANTIANXIETY; SEDATIVE-HYPNOTIC
**Prototype:** Lorazepam
**Controlled Substance:** Schedule IV

**AVAILABILITY** Tablet; sustained release tab; oral solution; orally disintegrating tab

### ACTION & THERAPEUTIC EFFECT
A CNS depressant that appears to act at the limbic, thalamic, and hypothalamic levels of the CNS. *Has antianxiety and sedative effects with addictive potential.*

**USES** Management of anxiety disorders or for short-term relief of anxiety symptoms. Also used as adjunct in management of anxiety associated with depression and agitation, and for panic disorders, such as agoraphobia.

**UNLABELED USES** Alcohol withdrawal.

### CONTRAINDICATIONS
Sensitivity to benzodiazepines; acute narrow angle glaucoma; pulmonary disease; use alone in primary depression or psychotic disorders, bipolar disorders, organic brain disorders; myasthenia gravis; pregnancy (category D); lactation.

### CAUTIOUS USE
Impaired hepatic function; history of alcoholism; renal impairment, hepatic disease; geriatric and debilitated patients; children younger than 18 y. Effectiveness for long-term treatment (greater than 4 mo) not established.

### ROUTE & DOSAGE

#### Anxiety Disorders
*Adult:* **PO** 0.25–0.5 mg t.i.d. (max: 4 mg/day)

Common adverse effects in *italic;* life-threatening effects underlined; generic names in **bold;** classifications in SMALL CAPS; ♣ Canadian drug name; ☻ Prototype drug

*Geriatric:* **PO** 0.125–0.25 mg b.i.d.

**Panic Attacks**

*Adult:* **PO** 1–2 mg t.i.d. (max: 8 mg/day); **Sustained release** Initiate with 0.5–1 mg once/day. Depending on the response, the dose may be increased at intervals of 3 to 4 days in increments of no more than 1 mg/day. Target range 3–6 mg/day (max: 10 mg/day).

**Hepatic Impairment Dosage Adjustment**

Reduce dose by 50% in hepatic impairment.
Do not discontinue abruptly.

## ADMINISTRATION

### Oral

- Reduce drug gradually when discontinuing drug.
- Store in light-resistant containers at 15°–30° C (59°–86° F), unless otherwise directed.

## ADVERSE EFFECTS (≥1%) CNS:
*Drowsiness, sedation,* lightheadedness, dizziness, syncope, depression, headache, confusion, insomnia, nervousness, fatigue, clumsiness, unsteadiness, rigidity, tremor, restlessness, paradoxical excitement, hallucinations. **CV:** Tachycardia, hypotension, ECG changes. **Special Senses:** Blurred vision. **Respiratory:** Dyspnea.

## INTERACTIONS Drug: Alcohol and other CNS DEPRESSANTS, ANTICONVULSANTS, ANTIHISTAMINES, BARBITURATES, NARCOTIC ANALGESICS, BENZODIAZEPINES compound CNS depressant effects; **cimetidine, disulfiram, fluoxetine,** TRICYCLIC ANTIDEPRESSANTS increase alprazolam levels (decreased metabolism); ORAL CONTRACEPTIVES may increase or decrease alprazolam effects. **Herbal: Kava, valerian** may potentiate sedation; **St. John's wort** decreases serum level of alprazolam.Cigarette smoking may decrease serum level of alprazolam by 50%.

## PHARMACOKINETICS Absorption: Rapidly absorbed. Peak: 1–2 h. Distribution: Crosses placenta. Metabolism: Oxidized in liver to inactive metabolites by CYP3A4. Elimination: Renal elimination. Half-Life: 12–15 h.

## NURSING IMPLICATIONS

### Assessment & Drug Effects

- Monitor for S&S of drowsiness and sedation, especially in older adults or the debilitated; they may require supervised ambulation and/or fall precautions.
- Monitor lab tests: Periodic blood counts, urinalyses, and blood chemistry studies during long-term therapy.

### Patient & Family Education

- Make position changes slowly and in stages to prevent dizziness.
- Do not use alcohol, other CNS depressants, or OTC medications containing antihistamines (e.g., sleep aids, cold, hay fever, or allergy remedies) without consulting prescriber.
- Do not drive or engage in potentially hazardous activities until response to drug is known.
- Taper dosage following continuous use; abrupt discontinuation of drug may cause withdrawal symptoms: Nausea, vomiting, abdominal and muscle cramps, sweating, confusion, tremors, convulsions.

---

Common adverse effects in *italic;* life-threatening effects <u>underlined</u>; generic names in **bold;** classifications in SMALL CAPS; ♣ Canadian drug name; ⊘ Prototype drug

# ALPROSTADIL (PGE₁)

(al-pross'ta-dil)
Caverject, Edex, Muse,
Prostin VR Pediatric
**Classification:** PROSTAGLANDIN
Therapeutic: PROSTAGLANDIN
**Prototype:** Epoprostenol

**AVAILABILITY** Injection; powder for injection; urethral suppository

## ACTION & THERAPEUTIC EFFECT

Preserves ductal patency by relaxing smooth muscle of ductus arteriosus. Alprostadil induces penile erection by relaxing the smooth muscles of the corpus cavernosum and dilating the cavernosal arteries and their penile arterioles. *Preserves ductal patency by relaxing smooth muscle of ductus arteriosus. It induces penile rigidity and erection by penile blood engorgement.*

## USES

Temporary measure to maintain patency of ductus arteriosus in infants with ductal-dependent congenital heart defects until corrective surgery can be performed. Also used in erectile dysfunction.

## CONTRAINDICATIONS

Ductus arteriosus respiratory distress syndrome (hyaline membrane disease); neonates with respiratory distress syndrome; hypersensitivity to alprostadil; patients with penile implants. **Muse, Edex:** Women, children, and newborns; lactation. **Muse:** Patients with urethral stricture, inflammation/infection of glans of penis, severe hypospadias, acute or chronic urethritis; sickle cell anemia or trait, thrombocytopenia, thrombocytosis; polycythemia, multiple myeloma.

**CAUTIOUS USE** Ductus arteriosus; bleeding tendencies; cardiovascular disease; erectile dysfunction; hypersensitivity to alprostadil; leukemia; penile anatomic deformations; patients on anticoagulants, vasoactive or antihypertensive drugs; pregnancy (category C).

## ROUTE & DOSAGE

### To Maintain Patency of Ductus Arteriosus

*Neonate:* **IV** 0.05–0.1 mcg/kg/min, may increase gradually (max: 0.4 mcg/kg/min)

### Erectile Dysfunction of Vasculogenic, Psychogenic, or Mixed Etiology

*Adult:* **Intracavernosal** Initiate with 2.5 mcg; if inadequate response, increase dose by 2.5 mcg. May then increase dose in 5 mcg increments until a suitable erection occurs, not exceeding 1 h in duration (max: 60 mcg).
*Adult:* **Intraurethral (Muse)** 125 mcg or 250 mcg; dose adjusted to patient satisfaction (max: 2 ×/24 h)

### Erectile Dysfunction of Pure Neurogenic Etiology

*Adult:* **Intracavernosal** Initiate with 1.25 mcg; if inadequate response, increase dose by 1.25 mcg, then increase by 2.5 mcg, may then increase dose in 5 mcg increments until a suitable erection occurs, not exceeding 1 h in duration; wait 24 h between doses (max: 60 mcg)

## ADMINISTRATION

### Intracavernosal Injection

- Administer only after proper training in the penile injection technique. Refer to information on administration provided to the patient by the manufacturer.
- Use reconstituted solutions immediately.
- Store dry powder at or below 25° C (77° F) for up to 3 mo. Do not freeze.

### Transurethral Insertion

- Refer to information on insertion of urethral suppository into the urethra provided to the patient by the manufacturer.

### Intravenous

**PREPARE: Continuous:** Dilute 500 mcg alprostadil with NS or D5W to volume appropriate for pump delivery system. ▪ Prepare fresh solution q24h. Discard unused portions. ▪ A 500 mcg ampule diluted in 250 mL yields a concentration of 2 mcg/mL.

**ADMINISTER: Continuous:** Infuse at rate of 0.05–0.1 mcg/kg/min up to a maximum of 0.4 mcg/kg/min. ▪ Reduce infusion rate immediately if arterial pressure drops significantly or if fever occurs. ▪ Discontinue promptly, if apnea or bradycardia occurs.

- Store at 2°–8° C (36°–46° F) unless otherwise directed by manufacturer. Protect from freezing.

## ADVERSE EFFECTS (≥1%) CNS:
*Fever,* seizures, lethargy. **CV:** *Flushing,* bradycardia, hypotension, syncope, tachycardia; CHF, ventricular fibrillation, shock. **GI:** Diarrhea, gastric regurgitation. **Hematologic:** Disseminated intravascular coagulation (DIC), thrombocytopenia. **Respiratory:** Apnea. **Urogenital:** Oliguria,

anuria. *Penile pain,* prolonged erection, priapism, penile fibrosis, injection site hematoma/ecchymosis, penile rash and edema, prostatitis, perineal pain. **Skin:** Rash on face and arms, alopecia. **Other:** Leg pain.

## INTERACTIONS Drug: May increase anticoagulant properties of **warfarin;** ANTIHYPERTENSIVE AGENTS increase risk of hypotension.

## PHARMACOKINETICS Onset: 15
min to 3 h. **Metabolism:** Rapidly in lungs. **Elimination:** Through kidneys. **Half-Life:** 5–10 min.

## NURSING IMPLICATIONS

### Black Box Warning

*Alprostadil has been associated with apnea in neonates.*

### Assessment & Drug Effects

#### Ductus Arteriosus

- Monitor for apnea especially during the first hour of infusion
- Monitor therapeutic effectiveness which is indicated by increased blood oxygenation (Po₂), usually evident within 30 min, in infants with cyanotic heart disease; increased pH in those with acidosis, increased systemic BP and urinary output, return of palpable pulses, and decreased ratio of pulmonary artery to aortic pressure in infants with restricted systemic blood flow.
- Monitor arterial pressure, ECG, heart rate, BP, respiratory rate, and temperature, throughout the infusion.
- Monitor lab tests: Arterial blood gases and blood pH throughout the infusion.

### Patient & Family Education

#### Erectile Dysfunction

- Follow carefully directions for penile injection provided by the manufacturer.

---

Common adverse effects in *italic;* life-threatening effects underlined; generic names in **bold;** classifications in SMALL CAPS; ♣ Canadian drug name; ⊙ Prototype drug

57

- Do not change dose without consulting the prescriber.
- Do not use intracavernosal injection more often than 3 × wk; allow at least 24 h between uses.
- Do not use more than 2 urethral suppository systems in a 24 h period.
- Report promptly any of the following: Nodules or hard tissue in penis; penile pain, redness, swelling, tenderness; or curvature of the erect penis.
- Seek immediate medical attention if an erection persists longer than 6 h.

## ALTEPLASE RECOMBINANT ℗

(al'te-plase)

Activase, Cathflo Activase

**Classification:** THROMBOLYTIC, TISSUE PLASMINOGEN ACTIVATOR
**Therapeutic:** THROMBOLYTIC ENZYME

## AVAILABILITY Injection

## ACTION & *THERAPEUTIC EFFECT*

A recombinant DNA-derived form of human tissue-type plasminogen activator that promotes thrombolysis by forming the active proteolytic enzyme, plasmin. *Plasmin is capable of degrading fibrin, fibrinogen, and factors V, VIII, and XII.*

## USES Acute MI management; acute ischemic stroke management; lysis of pulmonary embolism; reestablishing patency of occluded IV catheter.

## UNLABELED USES Lysis of arterial occlusions in peripheral and bypass vessels; DVT, intravascular catheter occlusion, parapneumonic pleural effusions.

## CONTRAINDICATIONS Hypersensitivity to alteplase; active internal bleeding, history of cerebrovascular accident (within 3 mo), aneurysm, recent (within 3 mo) intracranial or interspinal surgery or trauma, intracranial neoplasm, increased intracranial pressure; arteriovenous malformation, severe uncontrolled hypertension, likelihood of left heart thrombus, acute pericarditis, bacterial endocarditis, severe liver or renal dysfunction, septic thrombophlebitis; neurological deficit.

**CAUTIOUS USE** Recent major surgery (within 10 days), cerebral vascular disease, recent GI or GU bleeding, recent trauma, renal impairment, hypertension, hemorrhagic ophthalmic conditions; age greater than 75 y; children; pregnancy (category C); lactation.

## ROUTE & DOSAGE

### Acute MI

*Adult:* **IV** 60 mg over first hour, 20 mg/h over second hour, and 20 mg over third hour (for a total of 100 mg over 3 h. *Accelerated schedule with heparin and aspirin (weight greater than 67 kg):* 15 mg bolus, then 50 mg over next 30 min, then 35 mg over next 60 min. *Accelerated schedule with heparin and aspirin (weight 67 kg or less):* 15 mg bolus, then 0.75 mg/kg (not to exceed 50 mg) over next 30 min, then 0.5 mg/kg (not to exceed 35 mg) over next 60 min

### Acute Ischemic Stroke/ Thrombotic Stroke

*Adult:* **IV** 0.9 mg/kg over 60 min with 10% of dose as an initial bolus over 1 min (max: 90 mg)

**Pulmonary Embolism (Activase only)**

*Adult:* **IV** 100 mg infused over 2 h

**Reopen Occluded IV Catheter (Cathflo Activase only)**

*Adult/Child (greater than 30 kg):* **IV** Instill 2 mg/2 mL into dysfunctional catheter for 2 h. May repeat once if needed.

*Child (weight 10–29 kg):* **IV** Instill 110% of internal lumen volume (max: 2 mg in 2 mL). May repeat if function not restored within 2 h.

## ADMINISTRATION

### Intravenous

*PREPARE:* **IV Infusion:** Reconstitute the *50 mg vial* as follows: Do not use if vacuum in vial has been broken. Use a large-bore needle (e.g., 18 gauge) and do not prime needle with air. ▪ Dilute contents of vial with sterile water for injection supplied by manufacturer. ▪ Direct stream of sterile water into the lyophilized cake. Slight foaming is usual. Allow to stand until bubbles dissipate. Resulting concentration is 1 mg/mL. ▪ Reconstitute the *100-mg vial* using supplied transfer device for reconstitution. Follow manufacturer's directions.

*ADMINISTER:* **IV Infusion:** ▪ Start IV infusion as soon as possible after the thrombolytic event, preferably within 6 h. ▪ Administer drug as reconstituted (1 mg/mL) or further diluted with an equal volume of NS or D5W to yield 0.5 mg/mL. **Acute MI:** 3-h infusion: Administer 60% of total dose in the first hour for acute MI, with 6–10% given as a bolus dose over 1–2 min and remainder of first dose infused over hour 1. Follow with second dose (20% of total) over hour 2, and third dose (20% of total) over hour 3. ▪ For patients weighing less than 65 kg calculate dose using 1.25 mg/kg over 3 h. See accelerated schedule under Route & Dosage. **Pulmonary embolism:** Administer entire dose over a 2-h period. **Acute ischemic stroke:** Give 0.9 mg/kg (not to exceed 90 mg total dose) over 60 min with 10% of the total dose administered as an initial IV bolus over 1 min. ▪ Do not exceed a total dose of 100 mg. Higher doses have been associated with intracranial bleeding. ▪ Continue infusion of drug by flushing IV tubing with 30–50 mL of NS or D5W.

▪ Reconstituted drug is stable for 8 h in above solutions at room temperature (2°–30° C; 36°–86° F). Since there are no preservatives, discard any unused solution after that time.

*INCOMPATIBILITIES:* Solution/additive: **Dobutamine, dopamine, heparin.** Y-site: **Bivalirudin, dobutamine, dopamine, heparin, nitroglycerin.**

▪ Store above reconstituted solutions at room temperature 2°–30° C (36°–86° F) for no longer than 8 h. Discard any unused solution after that time.

## ADVERSE EFFECTS (≥1%) **Hematologic:** Internal and superficial bleeding (cerebral, retroperitoneal, GU, GI) stroke.

## PHARMACOKINETICS **Peak:** 5–10 min after infusion completed. **Duration:** Baseline values restored in 3 h. **Metabolism:** In liver. **Elimination:** In urine. **Half-Life:** 26.5 min.

## NURSING IMPLICATIONS

### Assessment & Drug Effects

- Monitor for S&S of excess bleeding q15min for the first hour of therapy, q30min for second to eighth hour, then q8h.
- Monitor neurologic checks throughout drug infusion q30min and qh for the first 8 h after infusion.
- Protect patient from invasive procedures because spontaneous bleeding occurs twice as often with alteplase as with heparin. IM injections are contraindicated. Minimize physical manipulation of patient during thrombolytic therapy to prevent bruising.
- Check vital signs frequently. Be alert to changes in cardiac rhythm.
- Report signs of bleeding: Gum bleeding, epistaxis, hematoma, spontaneous ecchymoses, oozing at catheter site, increased pain from internal bleeding. Stop the infusion, then resume when bleeding stops.
- Use the radial artery to draw ABGs. Pressure to puncture sites, if necessary, should be maintained for up to 30 min.
- Continue monitoring vital signs until laboratory reports confirm anticoagulant control; patient is at risk for postthrombolytic bleeding for 2–4 days after intracoronary alteplase treatment.
- Monitor lab tests: Baseline CBC, aPTT, PT, INR; Hct and Hgb, and platelet count as needed.

### Patient & Family Education

- Report promptly any of the following: Sudden severe headache, blood in urine, bloody or tarry stool, any sign of bleeding or oozing from injection/insertion sites.
- Remain quiet and on bedrest while receiving this medicine.

# ALTRETAMINE

(al-tre'ta-meen)

Hexalen

**Classifications:** ANTINEOPLASTIC; ALKYLATING

Therapeutic: ANTINEOPLASTIC

**Prototype:** Cyclophosphamide

**AVAILABILITY** Capsule

## ACTION & *THERAPEUTIC EFFECT*

A synthetic cytotoxic antineoplastic drug with an unknown mechanism of action. Its metabolites have cytotoxic properties. *Altretamine has demonstrated neoplastic activity in patients resistant to alkylating agents.*

**USES** Ovarian cancer.

**CONTRAINDICATIONS** Hypersensitivity to altretamine, severe bone marrow depression, neurologic toxicity, neurologic disease; pregnancy (category D); lactation.

**CAUTIOUS USE** Concerns related to bone marrow suppression, gastrointestinal toxicity, and neurotoxicity. Safety and efficacy in children not established.

## ROUTE & DOSAGE

### Ovarian Cancer

*Adult:* **PO** 260 mg/m²/day for 14 or 21 consecutive days in a 28-day cycle

## ADMINISTRATION

### Oral

- Give only under supervision of a qualified prescriber experienced in the use of antineoplastics.
- Give in 4 divided doses after meals and at bedtime.
- Hazardous agent; use appropriate precautions for handling and disposal.

- Altretamine is usually discontinued for 14 days or longer and restarted at 200 mg/m²/day if any of the following occur: Platelet count less than 0.075 mL; severe GI intolerance; WBC count less than 2000/mm³, granulocyte count less than 1000/mm³; or progressive neurotoxicity.
- Store at room temperature, 15°–30° C (59°–86° F).

## ADVERSE EFFECTS (≥1%) CNS:
*Paresthesias, peripheral numbness, ataxia.* GI: *Nausea, vomiting,* anorexia. **Hematologic:** Leukopenia, anemia, thrombocytopenia. **Hepatic:** Increased serum alkaline phosphatase. **Urogenital:** Increased blood urea nitrogen, increased serum creatinine. **Skin:** Alopecia, pruritus, skin rash.

## INTERACTIONS Drug:
Concomitant administration of TRICYCLIC ANTIDEPRESSANTS (**imipramine, amitriptyline**), MONOAMINE OXIDASE INHIBITORS, or **selegiline** result in orthostatic hypotension. Do not administer LIVE VACCINES. Avoid use with **sargramostim, filgramstim**. **Herbal:** Echinacea may reduce efficacy.

## PHARMACOKINETICS Absorption:
Rapidly from GI tract. Approximately 25% reaches systemic circulation. **Metabolism:** Rapidly demethylated in the liver. **Elimination:** 62% of the dose is excreted in the urine in 24 h. **Half-Life:** 4.7–10 h.

## NURSING IMPLICATIONS

### Black Box Warning

*Altretamine has been associated with severe neurotoxicity and bone marrow suppression.*

## Assessment & Drug Effects
- Perform a neurologic examination regularly; assess for the presence of paresthesias, peripheral numbness, ataxia, decreased sensations, and alterations in mood or consciousness.
- Withhold medication if neurologic symptoms fail to resolve with dose reduction. Notify prescriber.
- Monitor for nausea and vomiting, which are related to the cumulative dose of altretamine. After several weeks some patients develop tolerance to the GI effects. Antiemetics may be required to control GI distress.
- Use with caution in patients previously treated with **myelosuppressive** drugs or with pre-existing neurotoxicity.
- Monitor lab tests: Prior to each course of therapy and monthly, CBC with differential.

## Patient & Family Education
- Taking altretamine after meals or with food or milk may decrease nausea.
- Report symptoms indicative of neurotoxicity to prescriber (paresthesias, peripheral numbness, ataxia, decreased sensations, and alterations in mood or consciousness).

## ALUMINUM HYDROXIDE ⊕
(a-lu'mi-num)
ALternaGEL, Alu-Cap, Alugel, Alu-Tab, Amphojel, Dialume

## ALUMINUM CARBONATE, BASIC
Basaljel

## ALUMINUM PHOSPHATE
Phosphaljel

**Classifications:** ANTACID; ADSORBENT
**Therapeutic:** ANTACID

---

## AVAILABILITY
**Aluminum Hydroxide:** Tablet; capsule; suspension; **Aluminum Carbonate, Basic:** Tablet; capsule; suspension; **Aluminum Phosphate:** Tablet; capsule; suspension

## ACTION & *THERAPEUTIC EFFECT*
Nonsystemic antacid with moderate neutralizing action. Reduces acid concentration and pepsin activity by raising pH of gastric and intra-esophageal secretions. *Reduces gastric acidity by neutralizing the stomach acid content. Aluminum carbonate lowers serum phosphate by binding dietary phosphate to form insoluble aluminum phosphate, which is excreted in feces.*

## USES
Symptomatic relief of gastric hyperacidity associated with gastritis, esophageal reflux, and hiatal hernia; adjunct in treatment of gastric and duodenal ulcer. More commonly used in combination with other antacids. Aluminum carbonate is used primarily in conjunction with a low phosphate diet to reduce hyperphosphatemia in patients with renal insufficiency and for prophylaxis and treatment of phosphatic renal calculi.

## CONTRAINDICATIONS
Prolonged use of high doses in presence of low serum phosphate.

## CAUTIOUS USE
Renal impairment; gastric outlet obstruction; older adults; decreased bowel activity (e.g., patients receiving anticholinergic, antidiarrheal, or antispasmodic agents); patients who are dehydrated or on fluid restriction; pregnancy (category C).

## ROUTE & DOSAGE

### Antacid (Hydroxide and Phosphate)
*Adult:* **PO** 600 mg t.i.d. or q.i.d.

### Antacid (Carbonate)
*Adult:* **PO** 10–30 mL of regular suspension or 5–15 mL of extra strength suspension or 2 capsules or tablets q2h

### Phosphate Lowering (Carbonate)
*Adult:* **PO** 10–30 mL of regular suspension or 5–15 mL of extra strength suspension or 2–6 capsules or tablets 1 h p.c. and at bedtime

## ADMINISTRATION
### Oral
- Tablet **must be** chewed until it is thoroughly wetted before swallowing.
- Note for antacid use: Follow well-chewed tablet with one-half glass of water or milk; follow liquid preparation (suspension) with water to ensure passage into stomach. For phosphate lowering: Follow tablet, capsule, or suspension with full glass of water or fruit juice.
- Store at 15°–30° C (59°–86° F) in tightly closed container.

## ADVERSE EFFECTS (≥1%)
**GI:** *Constipation*, fecal impaction, intestinal obstruction. **CNS:** Dialysis dementia (thought to be due to aluminum intoxication). **Metabolic:** Hypophosphatemia, hypomagnesemia.

## INTERACTIONS
**Drug:** Aluminum will decrease absorption of **chloroquine, cimetidine, ciprofloxacin, digoxin, isoniazid,** IRON SALTS, NSAIDS, **norfloxacin, ofloxacin, phenytoin, phenothiazines, quinidine, tetracycline, thyroxine. Sodium polystyrene sulfonate** may cause systemic alkalosis.

## PHARMACOKINETICS
**Absorption:** Minimal absorption. **Peak:** Slow onset. **Duration:** 2 h when

taken with food; 3 h when taken 1 h after food. **Elimination:** In feces as insoluble phosphates.

## NURSING IMPLICATIONS

### Assessment & Drug Effects

- Note number and consistency of stools. Constipation is common and dose related. Intestinal obstruction from fecal concretions has been reported.
- Monitor lab tests: Periodic serum calcium and phosphorus levels with prolonged high-dose therapy or impaired renal function.

### Patient & Family Education

- Increase phosphorus in diet when taking large doses of these antacids for prolonged periods; hypophosphatemia can develop within 2 wk of continuous use of these antacids. The older adult in a poor nutritional state is at high risk.
- Antacid may cause stools to appear speckled or whitish.
- Report epigastric or abdominal pain; it is a clinical guide for adjusting dosage. Keep prescriber informed. Pain that persists beyond 72 h may signify serious complications.
- Seek medical help if indigestion is accompanied by shortness of breath, sweating, or chest pain, if stools are dark or tarry, or if symptoms are recurrent when taking this medication.
- Seek medical advice and supervision if self-prescribed antacid use exceeds 2 wk.

## ALVIMOPAN

(al-vi-mo′pan)

Entereg

**Classifications:** PERIPHERAL OPIOID RECEPTOR ANTAGONIST; GI MOTILITY STIMULANT

Therapeutic: GI MOTILITY STIMULANT

**AVAILABILITY** Capsule

## ACTION & *THERAPEUTIC EFFECT*

Morphine and other post-op analgesics are mu-opioid receptor agonists known to inhibit GI motility and prolong the duration of postoperative ileus. Alvimopan is a selective antagonist of mu-opioid receptors. *It competitively antagonizes the effect of morphine on contractility, shortening the duration of post-op ileus.*

**USES** To accelerate the time to upper and lower gastrointestinal recovery after partial large or small bowel resection surgery with primary anastomosis.

**UNLABELED USES** Constipation, opioid-induced constipation.

**CONTRAINDICATIONS** Therapeutic doses of opioids for greater than 7 consecutive days immediately pre-operative; end-stage renal disease; severe hepatic impairment (Child-Pugh class C).

**CAUTIOUS USE** Recent exposure to opioids; surgery for complete bowel obstruction; history of CAD or MI; pregnancy (category B); lactation. Safety and efficacy in children not established.

## ROUTE & DOSAGE

### Acceleration of Postoperative GI Recovery

*Adult:* **PO** 12 mg 0.5–5 h preoperative; then 12 mg b.i.d. up to 7 days

## ADMINISTRATION

### Oral

- Give pre-op dose 30 min–5 h before surgery.
- Do not exceed 15 doses (maximum allowed).

Common adverse effects in *italic;* life-threatening effects underlined; generic names in **bold;** classifications in SMALL CAPS; ♣ Canadian drug name; ⑩ Prototype drug

63

- Store at 15°–30° C (59°–86° F).
- Note: Hospitals **must be** registered in and have met all of the requirements for the **Enterag** Access Support and Education (E.A.S.E.) program in order to use alvimopan.

**ADVERSE EFFECTS** (≥3%) **GI:** Constipation, dyspepsia, flatulence. **Hematologic:** Anemia. **Metabolic:** Hypokalemia. **Musculoskeletal:** Back pain. **Urogenital:** Urinary retention.

**INTERACTIONS Food:** Decreased extent and rate of absorption if taken with a high fat meal.

**PHARMACOKINETICS Absorption:** Bioavailability 6%. **Peak:** 2 h. **Distribution:** 90–94% plasma protein bound. **Metabolism:** By intestinal flora. **Elimination:** Fecal (primary) and renal (35%). **Half-Life:** 10–18 h.

**NURSING IMPLICATIONS**
**Assessment & Drug Effects**
- Monitor frequently for return of bowel sounds and ability to pass flatus.
- Monitor closely patients with impaired renal function for adverse effects.
- Report to prescriber increasing abdominal pain, diarrhea, nausea and vomiting.
- Monitor lab tests: Serum potassium in those predisposed to hypokalemia.

**Patient & Family Education**
- Report promptly increasing abdominal pain and nausea.

---

**AMANTADINE HYDROCHLORIDE** 🅟
(a-man'ta-deen)
GOCOVRI, Symmetrel

**Classifications:** ANTIVIRAL; CENTRAL-ACTING CHOLINERGIC RECEPTOR ANTAGONIST; ANTIPARKINSON
**Therapeutic:** ANTIVIRAL; ANTIPARKINSON

**AVAILABILITY** Capsule; tablet; oral solution; extended release capsule

**ACTION & *THERAPEUTIC EFFECT***
Mechanism of action related to antiviral activity is poorly understood but may be due to prevention of release of viral nucleic acid into the host cell. Mechanism of action in parkinsonism may be related to release of dopamine from neuronal storage sites. *Active against several strains of influenza A virus. Effective in management of symptoms of parkinsonism when used in conjunction with other antiparkinson agents.*

**USES** Treatment of idiopathic parkinsonism or Parkinson's disease. Also used for prophylaxis and symptomatic treatment of influenza A infections.

**UNLABELED USES** Neuroleptic malignant syndrome (NMS), management of cocaine dependency, fatigue.

**CONTRAINDICATIONS** Hypersensitivity to amantadine or rimantadine, closed angle glaucoma; suicidal ideation; lactation.

**CAUTIOUS USE** History of epilepsy or other types of seizures; CHF, peripheral edema, orthostatic hypotension; recurrent eczematoid dermatitis; psychoses, severe psychoneuroses; hepatic disease; renal impairment; older adults, cerebral arteriosclerosis; pregnancy (category C). Safety in children younger than 1 y for Influenza A is not established.

## ROUTE & DOSAGE

### Influenza A Treatment

*Adult (younger than 65 y)/Child (9 y or older):* **PO** 200 mg once/day or 100 mg q12h
*Adult (65 y or older):* **PO** 100 mg once/day
*Child (1–8 y):* **PO** 4.4-8.8 mg/kg in 2 equal doses (max: 150 mg/day)

### Influenza A Prevention

*Adult (younger than 65 y):* **PO** 200 mg/day or 100 mg q12h; begin as soon as possible after initial exposure and continue for at least 10 days after exposure
*Adult (65 y or older):* **PO** 100 mg once daily
*HIV-Infected Adult/Adolescent/Child (10 y or older):* **PO** 100 mg twice daily
*Child (1–8 y):* **PO** 4.4-8.8 mg/kg/day (up to 150 mg/day) given in 2 divided doses (not more than 150 mg/day)

### Idiopathic Parkinsonism or Parkinson's Disease

*Adult:* **PO** 100 mg 1–2 × day, start with 100 mg/day if patient is on other antiparkinsonism medications

### Dyskinesia Associated with Parkinson's Disease

*Adult:*
**PO Extended release** 137 mg daily at bedtime, after 1 wk increase to 274 mg daily

### Drug-Induced Extrapyramidal Symptoms

*Adult:* **PO** 100 mg b.i.d. (max: 400 mg/day if needed)

### *Renal Impairment Dosage Adjustment*

*CrCl 30–50 mL/min:* **PO** 200 mg for 1st day, then 100 mg daily; *15–29 mL/min:* **PO** 100 mg for 1st day, then 100 mg on alternate days; *less than 15 mL/min:* 200 mg q7days

## ADMINISTRATION

### Oral

- Do not crush, chew, or divide capsules.
- Give with water, milk, or food.
- Use supplied calibrated device for measuring syrup formulation.
- Influenza prophylaxis: Drug should be initiated when exposure is anticipated and continued for at least 10 days.
- Used in conjunction with influenza A vaccine (generally in high-risk patients who have not been vaccinated previously) until protective antibodies develop (10–21 days) after vaccine administration.
- Schedule medication in the morning or, with q12h dosing, schedule 2nd dose several hours before bedtime. If insomnia is a problem, suggest patient limit number of daytime naps.
- Store in tightly closed container preferably at 15°–30° C (59°–86° F) unless otherwise directed by manufacturer. Avoid freezing.

## ADVERSE EFFECTS (≥1%) CNS:

*Dizziness, light-headedness,* headache, ataxia, irritability, anxiety, *nervousness, difficulty in concentrating,* mood or other mental changes, confusion, visual and auditory hallucinations, *insomnia,* nightmares, convulsions. **CV:** Orthostatic hypotension, peripheral edema, dyspnea. **Special Senses:** Blurring or loss of vision. **GI:** Anorexia, *nausea,* vomiting, dry mouth. **Hematologic:** Leukopenia, agranulocytosis.

Common adverse effects in *italic;* life-threatening effects underlined; generic names in **bold;** classifications in SMALL CAPS; ♣ Canadian drug name; ⊙ Prototype drug

65

**INTERACTIONS Drug: Alcohol** enhances CNS effects; may potentiate effects of ANTICHOLINERGICS. Use with **bupropion** can increase restlessness/agitation.

**PHARMACOKINETICS Absorption:** Almost completely absorbed from GI tract. **Onset:** Within 48 h. **Peak:** 1–4 h. **Distribution:** Through body fluids. **Metabolism:** Not metabolized. **Elimination:** 90% unchanged in urine. **Half-Life:** 9–37 h (prolonged in renal insufficiency).

## NURSING IMPLICATIONS
### Assessment & Drug Effects
- Monitor effectiveness. Note that with parkinsonism, maximum response occurs within 2 wk–3 mo. Effectiveness may wane after 6–8 wk of treatment; report change to prescriber.
- Monitor and report: Mental status changes; nervousness, difficulty concentrating, or insomnia; loss of seizure control; S&S of toxicity, especially with doses above 200 mg/day.
- Monitor for and report promptly suicidal ideation, especially in those with a history of psychiatric disorders.
- Establish a baseline profile of the patient's disabilities to accurately differentiate disease symptoms and drug-induced neuropsychiatric adverse reactions.
- Monitor vital signs for at least 3 or 4 days after increases in dosage; also monitor urinary output.
- Monitor for and report reduced salivation, increased akinesia or rigidity, and psychological disturbances that may develop within 4–48 h after initiation of therapy and after dosage increases with parkinsonism.

### Patient & Family Education
- Note: For influenza within 24 h but no later than 48 h after onset of symptoms.
- Make all position changes slowly, particularly from recumbent to upright position, in order to minimize dizziness.
- Report any of the following to prescriber: Shortness of breath, peripheral edema, significant weight gain, dizziness or lightheadedness, inability to concentrate, and other changes in mental status, suicidal ideation, difficulty urinating, and visual impairment.
- Do not drive and exercise caution with potentially hazardous activities until response to the drug is known.
- Note: People with Parkinson's disease should not discontinue therapy abruptly; doing so may precipitate a parkinsonian crisis with severe akinesia, rigidity, tremor, and psychic disturbances. Adhere to established dosage regimen.

## AMCINONIDE
(am-sin'oh-nide)
**See Appendix A-4.**

## AMIFOSTINE
(am-i-fos'teen)
Ethyol
**Classification:** CYTOPROTECTIVE
**Therapeutic:** CYTOPROTECTIVE

**AVAILABILITY** Solution for injection

**ACTION & THERAPEUTIC EFFECT**
Amifostine reduces cytotoxic damage induced by radiation or antineoplastic agents; this protective effect appears to be mediated by the formation of a metabolite of amifostine that removes free radicals from normal cells exposed to

cisplatin. *Amifostine is cytoprotective in the kidney, bone marrow, and GI mucosa, but not in the brain or spinal cord. The cytoprotection results in decreased myelosuppression and peripheral neuropathy.*

**USES** Reduction of the cumulative renal toxicity associated with cisplatin, xerostomia.

**UNLABELED USES** Reduction of paclitaxel toxicity, bone marrow suppression prophylaxis.

**CONTRAINDICATIONS** Sensitivity to aminothiol compounds or mannitol, patients with potentially curable malignancies, hypotensive patients or those who are dehydrated, exfoliated dermatitis; lactation.

**CAUTIOUS USE** Patients at risk for hypocalcemia, cardiovascular disease (i.e., arrhythmias, CHF, TIA, CVA); radiation therapy; renal disease; pregnancy (category C).

## ROUTE & DOSAGE

**Renal Protection**
Adult: IV 910 mg/m² once daily prior to chemotherapy

**Reduction of Xerostomia**
Adult: IV 200 mg/m² prior to radiation therapy

## ADMINISTRATION

**Intravenous**
Give antiemetics, adequately hydrate, and defer antihypertensives for 24 h prior to administration. Do not administer if patient is hypotensive or dehydrated. Consult prescriber.

*PREPARE:* **IV Infusion:** Reconstitute by adding 9.7 mL of NS injection to a single-dose vial to yield 50 mg/mL. ▪ May be further diluted with NS to a concentration as low as 5 mg/mL.

*ADMINISTER:* **IV Infusion:** Infuse over no more than 15 min, beginning 30 min before chemotherapy; place patient in supine position prior to and during infusion. ▪ For xerostomia, infuse over 3 min; begin 15–30 min before radiation.

*INCOMPATIBILITIES:* **Solution/additive:** Do not mix with any solutions other than NS. **Y-site:** Acyclovir, amphotericin B, amphotericin B lipid, cefoperazone, chlorpromazine, cisplatin, ganciclovir, hydroxyzine, minocycline, mycophenolate, prochlorperazine, quinupristin-dalfopristin.

▪ Store reconstituted solution at 15°–30° C (59°–86° F) for 5 h or refrigerate up to 24 h.

**ADVERSE EFFECTS** (≥1%) **CV:** *Transient reduction in blood pressure.* **GI:** *Nausea, vomiting.* **Other:** Infusion reactions (flushing, feeling of warmth or coldness, chills, dizziness, somnolence, hiccups, sneezing), hypocalcemia, hypersensitivity reactions.

**INTERACTIONS Drug:** ANTIHYPERTENSIVES could cause or potentiate hypotension.

**PHARMACOKINETICS Onset:** 5–8 min. **Metabolism:** In liver to active free thiol metabolite. **Elimination:** Renally excreted. **Half-Life:** 8 min.

## NURSING IMPLICATIONS
### Assessment & Drug Effects
▪ Monitor for S&S of hypocalcemia and fluid balance if vomiting is significant.

- Monitor BP every 5 min during infusion. Stop infusion if systolic BP drops significantly from baseline (e.g., 20% drop in systolic BP) and place patient flat with legs raised. Restart infusion if BP returns to normal in 5 min.

**Patient & Family Education**
- Know and understand adverse effects.

## AMIKACIN SULFATE

(am-i-kay'sin)

Amikin

**Classification:** AMINOGLYCOSIDE ANTIBIOTIC
**Therapeutic:** ANTIBIOTIC
**Prototype:** Gentamicin

**AVAILABILITY** Solution for injection

**ACTION & *THERAPEUTIC EFFECT***
Appears to inhibit protein synthesis in bacterial cells and is usually bactericidal. *Effective against a wide range of gram-negative bacteria, including many strains resistant to other aminoglycosides. Also effective against penicillinase- and non-penicillinase-producing* Staphylococcus.

**USES** Primarily for short-term treatment of serious infections of respiratory tract, bones, joints, skin, and soft tissue, CNS (including meningitis), peritonitis burns, recurrent urinary tract infections (UTIs).

**UNLABELED USES** Intrathecal or intraventricular administration, in conjunction with IM or IV dosage.

**CONTRAINDICATIONS** History of hypersensitivity or toxic reaction with an aminoglycoside antibiotic; lactation.

**CAUTIOUS USE** Impaired renal function; eighth cranial (auditory) nerve impairment; preexisting vertigo or dizziness, tinnitus, or dehydration; fever; myasthenia gravis; parkinsonism; hypocalcemia; older adults, premature infants, neonates and infants; pregnancy (category C).

## ROUTE & DOSAGE

**Moderate to Severe Infections**
*Adult:* **IV/IM** 5–7.5 mg/kg loading dose, then 7.5 mg/kg q12h (max: 15 mg/kg/day) for 7–10 days
*Child:* **IV/IM** 5–7.5 mg/kg loading dose, then 5 mg/kg q8h or 7.5 mg/kg q12h for 7–10 days (max: 1.5 g/day)
*Neonate:* **IV/IM** 10 mg/kg loading dose, then 7.5 mg/kg q12h for 7–10 days

**Uncomplicated UTI**
*Adult:* **IV/IM** 250 mg q12h

***Obesity Dosage Adjustment***
Calculate dose based on IBW

***Renal Impairment Dosage Adjustment***
*CrCl greater than 60 mL/min:* Normal dose q8h; *40–60 mL/min:* Normal dose q12h; *20–39 mL/min:* Half dose q24h; *less than 20 mL/min:* Administer loading dose then monitor closely

***Hemodialysis Dosage Adjustment***
Administer dose post-dialysis or give ⅔ dose as supplemental dose

## ADMINISTRATION

**Intramuscular**
- Use the 250 mg/mL vials for IM injection. Calculate the required dose and withdraw the equivalent number of mLs from the vial.

- Give deep IM into a large muscle.

**Intravenous**

Verify correct IV concentration and rate of infusion with prescriber for neonates, infants, and children.

*PREPARE:* **Intermittent:** Add contents of 500 mg vial to 100 or 200 mL D5W, NS injection, or other diluent recommended by manufacturer. ∎ For pediatric patients, volume of diluent depends on patient's fluid tolerance. ∎ Note: Color of solution may vary from colorless to light straw color or very pale yellow. Discard solutions that appear discolored or that contain particulate matter.

*ADMINISTER:* **Intermittent:** Give a single dose (including loading dose) over at least 30–60 min by IV infusion. ∎ Increase infusion time to 1–2 h for infants. ∎ Monitor infusion rate carefully. A rapid rise in serum amikacin level can cause respiratory depression (neuromuscular blockade) and other signs of toxicity.

*INCOMPATIBILITIES:* **Solution/additive: Aminophylline, amphotericin B, ampicillin,** CEPHALOSPORINS, **chlorothiazide, heparin,** PENICILLINS, **phenytoin, vitamin B complex with C. Y-site: Allopurinol, amphotericin B, azithromycin, hetastarch, propofol.**

- Store at 15°–30° C (59°–86° F) unless otherwise directed.

**ADVERSE EFFECTS** (≥1%) **CNS:** Neurotoxicity: Drowsiness, unsteady gait, weakness, clumsiness, paresthesias, tremors, convulsions, peripheral neuritis. **Special Senses:** *Auditory–ototoxicity,* high-frequency hearing loss, complete hearing loss (occasionally permanent); tinnitus; ringing or buzzing in ears; *Vestibular:*

Dizziness, ataxia. **GI:** Nausea, vomiting, hepatotoxicity. **Metabolic:** Hypokalemia, hypomagnesemia. **Skin:** Skin rash, urticaria, pruritus, redness. **Urogenital:** Oliguria, urinary frequency, hematuria, tubular necrosis, azotemia. **Other:** Superinfections.

**INTERACTIONS Drug:** ANESTHETICS, SKELETAL MUSCLE RELAXANTS have additive neuromuscular blocking effects; **acyclovir, amphotericin B, bacitracin, capreomycin, cephalosporins, colistin, cisplatin, carboplatin, methoxyflurane, polymyxin B, vancomycin, furosemide, ethacrynic acid** increase risk of ototoxicity and nephrotoxicity.

**PHARMACOKINETICS Peak:** 30 min IV; 45 min to 2 h IM. **Distribution:** Does not cross blood–brain barrier; crosses placenta; accumulates in renal cortex. **Elimination:** 94–98% renally in 24 h, remainder in 10–30 days. **Half-Life:** 2–3 h in adults, 4–8 h in neonates.

**NURSING IMPLICATIONS**

**Black Box Warning**

*Nephrotoxicity and ototoxicity (both vestibular and auditory) can occur especially with preexisting renal damage and/or high doses. Neuromuscular blockade and respiratory paralysis have been reported especially in those treated with anesthetics or neuromuscular blocking agents.*

**Assessment & Drug Effects**

- Baseline tests: Before initial dose, C&S; renal function and vestibulocochlear nerve function (and at regular intervals during therapy; closely monitor in the older adult, patients with documented ear problems, renal impairment, or during high dose or prolonged therapy).

- Monitor peak and trough amikacin blood levels: Draw blood 1 h after IM or immediately after completion of IV infusion; draw trough levels immediately before the next IM or IV dose.
- Monitor for and promptly report S&S of: Ototoxicity [primarily involves the cochlear (auditory) branch; high-frequency deafness usually appears first and can be detected only by audiometer]; indicators of declining renal function; respiratory tract infections and other symptoms indicative of superinfections.
- Monitor for and report auditory symptoms (tinnitus, roaring noises, sensation of fullness in ears, hearing loss) and vestibular disturbances (dizziness or vertigo, nystagmus, ataxia).
- Monitor and report any changes in I&O, oliguria, hematuria, or cloudy urine. Keeping patient well hydrated reduces risk of nephrotoxicity; consult prescriber regarding optimum fluid intake.
- Monitor respiratory status especially in those who have received anesthetics, neuromuscular blocking agents or multiple transfusions of citrated blood.
- Monitor lab tests: Baseline and frequent serum creatinine and BUN, complete urinalysis.

## Patient & Family Education

- Report immediately any changes in hearing or unexplained ringing/roaring noises or dizziness, and problems with balance or coordination.

# AMILORIDE HYDROCHLORIDE

(a-mill'oh-ride)

Midamor

**Classification:** DIURETIC, POTASSIUM-SPARING
**Therapeutic:** DIURETIC, POTASSIUM-SPARING; ANTIHYPERTENSIVE
**Prototype:** Spironolactone

## AVAILABILITY Tablet

## ACTION & *THERAPEUTIC EFFECT*

Induces urinary excretion of sodium and reduces excretion of potassium and hydrogen ions by direct action on distal renal tubules. *Lowers blood pressure by excretion of sodium ion and water from the kidney while sparing potassium excretion.*

## USES Adjunctive treatment of heart failure, hypertension.

## UNLABELED USES Ascites, hypokalemia.

## CONTRAINDICATIONS Hypersensitivity to amiloride; elevated serum potassium (greater than 5.5 mEq/L) anuria, acute or chronic renal insufficiency; evidence of diabetic nephropathy; type 1 diabetes mellitus; metabolic or respiratory acidosis.

## CAUTIOUS USE Debilitated patients; diet-controlled or uncontrolled diabetes mellitus; COPD; severe hepatic disease; older adult; pregnancy (category B); lactation. Safe use in children not established.

## ROUTE & DOSAGE

### HTN, HF, Hypokalemia
*Adult:* **PO** 5–10 mg/day, may increase up to 20 mg/day

### Renal Impairment Dosage Adjustment
*CrCl 10–50 mL/min:* Reduce dose by 50%

Common adverse effects in *italic;* life-threatening effects underlined; generic names in **bold;** classifications in SMALL CAPS; ♣ Canadian drug name; ⊙ Prototype drug

## ADMINISTRATION

### Oral

- Give once/day dose in the morning and schedule the second b.i.d. dose early to avoid interrupting sleep.
- Give with food to reduce possibility of gastric distress.
- Store at 15°–30° C (59°–86° F) in a tightly closed container unless otherwise directed.

### ADVERSE EFFECTS (≥1%) Body as a Whole: Generally well tolerated. CNS: *Headache,* dizziness, nervousness, confusion, paresthesias, drowsiness. CV: Cardiac arrhythmias. Metabolic: Hyperkalemia, hyponatremia, positive Coombs' test. Hematologic: Aplastic anemia. Special Senses: Tinnitus; nasal congestion. Visual disturbances, increased intraocular pressure. GI: *Diarrhea* or constipation, anorexia, *nausea,* vomiting, abdominal cramps, dry mouth, thirst. Urogenital: Polyuria, dysuria, bladder spasms, urinary frequency, impotence, decreased libido. Respiratory: Dyspnea, shortness of breath. Skin: Rash, pruritus, photosensitivity reactions. Other: Weakness, fatigue, muscle cramps.

### DIAGNOSTIC TEST INTERFERENCE

Discontinue at least 3 days before *Glucose Tolerance Test.*

### INTERACTIONS Drug: Blood from blood banks, ACE INHIBITORS (e.g., **captopril**), **spironolactone, triamterene,** POTASSIUM SUPPLEMENTS may cause hyperkalemia with cardiac arrhythmias; possibility of increased **lithium** toxicity (decreased renal elimination); possibility of altered **digoxin** response; NSAIDS may attenuate antihypertensive effects. Do not use with **eplerenone** or **quinidine. Food:** POTASSIUM-CONTAINING SALT SUBSTITUTES or foods high in **potassium** increase risk of hyperkalemia.

### PHARMACOKINETICS Absorption: 50% from GI tract. Onset: 2 h. Peak: 6–10 h. Duration: 24 h. Elimination: 20–50% unchanged in urine, 40% in feces. Half-Life: 6–9 h.

## NURSING IMPLICATIONS

### Black Box Warning

*Amiloride has been associated with severe, potentially fatal hyperkalemia especially in the elderly and those with renal impairment or diabetes.*

### Assessment & Drug Effects

- Monitor for S&S of hyperkalemia and hyponatremia (see Appendix F). Hyperkalemia occurs in about 10% of patients receiving amiloride and serum potassium can rise suddenly and without warning. It is more common in older adults and patients with diabetes or renal disease.
- Monitor ECG as warranted.
- Monitor lab tests: Serum potassium levels, particularly when therapy is initiated, whenever dosage adjustments are made, and during any illness that may affect kidney function; periodic BUN, creatinine, for patients with renal or hepatic dysfunction, diabetes mellitus, older adults, or the debilitated

### Patient & Family Education

- Learn S&S of hyperkalemia and hyponatremia (see Appendix F) and report to prescriber immediately.
- Do not take potassium supplements, salt substitutes, high intake of dietary potassium unless prescribed by prescriber.
- Do not drive or engage in potentially hazardous activities until response to drug is known.

## AMINOCAPROIC ACID

(a-mee-noe-ka-proe'ik)

---

Common adverse effects in *italic;* life-threatening effects underlined; generic names in **bold;** classifications in SMALL CAPS; ◆ Canadian drug name; ⓟ Prototype drug

71

Amicar

**Classifications:** COAGULATOR; SYSTEMIC HEMOSTATIC
**Therapeutic:** ANTIHEMORRHAGIC; ANTIFIBRINOLYTIC

**AVAILABILITY** Solution for injection; tablet; syrup

## ACTION & *THERAPEUTIC EFFECT*

Synthetic hemostatic agent with specific antifibrinolysis action. Inhibits plasminogen activator substance, and to a lesser degree plasmin (fibrinolysin), which is concerned with destruction of clots. *Acts as an inhibitor of fibrinolytic bleeding.*

**USES** To control excessive bleeding resulting from systemic hyperfibrinolysis; also used in urinary fibrinolysis associated with severe trauma, anoxia, shock, urologic surgery, and neoplastic diseases of GU tract.

**UNLABELED USES** To prevent hemorrhage in hemophiliacs undergoing dental extraction; as a specific antidote for streptokinase or urokinase toxicity; to prevent recurrence of subarachnoid hemorrhage, especially when surgery is delayed; for management of amegakaryocytic thrombocytopenia; and to prevent or abort hereditary angioedema episodes.

**CONTRAINDICATIONS** Severe renal impairment; active disseminated intravascular clotting (DIC); upper urinary tract bleeding (hematuria); hemophilia; benzyl alcohol hypersensitivity, especially in neonates; paraben hypersensitivity; lactation.

**CAUTIOUS USE** Cardiac, renal, or hepatic disease; renal impairment; history of pulmonary embolus or other thrombotic diseases; hypovolemia; pregnancy (category C).

## ROUTE & DOSAGE

**Hemostatic**

*Adult:* **PO/IV** 4–5 g during first hour, then 1–1.25 g qh for 8 h or until bleeding is controlled (max: 30 g/24h)

*Child:* **PO/IV** 100 mg/kg or 3 g/m² during first hour, then 33.3 mg²/kg qh (max: 18 g/m²/24 h)

**Renal Impairment Dosage Adjustment**

Reduce dose to 15–25% of normal dose

## ADMINISTRATION

### Oral

- Note: May need to give patient as many as 10 tablets or 4 tsp for a 5 g dose during the first hour of treatment.

### Intravenous

*PREPARE:* **IV Infusion:** Dilute parenteral aminocaproic acid before use. ■ Each 4 mL (1 g) is diluted with 50 mL of NS, D5W, or LR.
*ADMINISTER:* **IV Infusion:** Prescriber orders specific IV flow rate. ■ Usual rate is 5 g or a fraction thereof over first hour (5 g/250 mL). ■ Give each additional gram over 1 h. Avoid rapid infusion to prevent hypotension, faintness, and bradycardia or other arrhythmias.
*INCOMPATIBILITIES:* **Solution/additive: Fructose solution.**

- Store in tightly closed containers at 15°–30° C (59°–86° F) unless otherwise directed. Avoid freezing.

**ADVERSE EFFECTS** (≥1%) **CNS:** Dizziness, malaise, headache, seizures. **CV:** Faintness, orthostatic hypotension; dysrhythmias; thrombophlebitis, thromboses. **Special Senses:** Tinnitus, nasal congestion. Conjunctival

Common adverse effects in *italic;* life-threatening effects <u>underlined</u>; generic names in **bold;** classifications in SMALL CAPS; ✤ Canadian drug name; ◉ Prototype drug erythema. **GI:** Nausea, vomiting, cramps, diarrhea, anorexia. **Urogenital:** Diuresis, dysuria, urinary frequency, oliguria, reddish-brown urine (myoglobinuria), <u>acute renal failure</u>. Prolonged menstruation with cramping. **Skin:** Rash.

## DIAGNOSTIC TEST INTERFERENCE

***Serum potassium*** may be elevated (especially in patients with impaired renal function).

## INTERACTIONS **Drug:** ESTROGENS, ORAL CONTRACEPTIVES may cause hypercoagulation.

## PHARMACOKINETICS **Absorption:** Rapidly from GI tract. **Peak:** 2 h. **Distribution:** Readily penetrates RBCs and other body cells. **Elimination:** 80% as unmetabolized drug in 12 h.

## NURSING IMPLICATIONS

### Assessment & Drug Effects

- Check IV site at frequent intervals for extravasation.
- Observe for signs of thrombophlebitis. Change site immediately if extravasation or thrombophlebitis occurs (see Appendix F).
- Monitor and report S&S of myopathy: Muscle weakness, myalgia, diaphoresis, fever, reddish-brown urine (myoglobinuria), oliguria, as well as thrombotic complications: Arm or leg pain, tenderness or swelling, Homans' sign, prominence of superficial veins, chest pain, breathlessness, dyspnea. Drug should be discontinued promptly.
- Monitor vital signs and urine output.
- Monitor lab tests: With prolonged therapy, periodic creatine phosphokinase and urinalyses for early detection of myopathy.

### Patient & Family Education

- Report difficulty urinating or reddish-brown urine.
- Report arm or leg pain, chest pain, or difficulty breathing.

## AMINOPHYLLINE (THEOPHYLLINE ETHYLENEDIAMIDE)

(am-in-off'i-lin)

**Corophyllin ◆ , Paladron ◆**

**Classifications:** BRONCHODILATOR; RESPIRATORY SMOOTH MUSCLE RELAXANT; XANTHINE

**Therapeutic:** BRONCHODILATOR

**Prototype:** Theophylline

**AVAILABILITY** Solution for injection

## ACTION & *THERAPEUTIC EFFECT*

A xanthine derivative that relaxes smooth muscle in the airways of the lungs and suppresses the response of the airways to stimuli that constrict them. *It is a respiratory smooth muscle relaxant that results in bronchodilation.*

**USES** To prevent and relieve symptoms of acute bronchial asthma and treatment of bronchospasm associated with chronic bronchitis and emphysema.

**UNLABELED USES** As a respiratory stimulant in Cheyne-Stokes respiration; for treatment of apnea and bradycardia in premature infants; as cardiac stimulant and diuretic in treatment of CHF.

**CONTRAINDICATIONS** Hypersensitivity to xanthine derivatives or to ethylenediamine component; cardiac arrhythmias.

**CAUTIOUS USE** Severe hypertension, cardiac disease, arrhythmias; impaired hepatic function; diabetes mellitus; hyperthyroidism; glaucoma; prostatic hypertrophy; fibrocystic breast disease; history of peptic ulcer; neonates and young children, older adults; COPD, acute influenza or patients receiving influenza immunization; pregnancy (category C); lactation.

Common adverse effects in *italic;* life-threatening effects <u>underlined</u>; generic names in **bold;** classifications in SMALL CAPS; ◆ Canadian drug name; ⊙ Prototype drug

73

## ROUTE & DOSAGE

### Bronchospasm

*Adult:* **IV Loading Dose** 6 mg/kg over 30 min; **IV Maintenance Dose** *Nonsmoker:* 0.5 mg/kg/h; *smoker:* 0.8 mg/kg/h; *CHF or cirrhosis:* 0.1–0.2 mg/kg/h

*Child:* **IV Loading Dose** 6 mg/kg IV over 30 min; **IV Maintenance Dose** *1–9 y:* 1 mg/kg/h; *9 y or older:* 0.8 mg/kg/h; **IV** *6–11 mo:* 0.7 g/kg/h; *2 to less than 6 mo:* 0.5 mg/kg/h

### Neonatal Apnea

*Neonate:* **IV Loading Dose** 5 mg/kg

*Obesity Dosage Adjustment*
Calculate dose based on IBW

## ADMINISTRATION

### Intravenous

Verify correct IV concentration and rate of infusion with prescriber for neonates, infants, and children.

***PREPARE:*** **IV Infusion:** Dilute loading dose in 100–200 mL NS, D5W, D5/NS, or LR. For continuous or intermittent infusion dilute in 500–1000 mL. ▪ Do not use aminophylline solutions if discolored or if crystals are present.

***ADMINISTER:*** **IV Infusion:** Infuse at the ordered rate (mg/kg/h).

***INCOMPATIBILITIES:*** Solution/additive: **Amikacin, bleomycin,** CEPHALOSPORINS, **chlorpromazine, ciprofloxacin, clindamycin, dimenhydrinate, dobutamine, doxorubicin, epinephrine, hydralazine, hydroxyzine, insulin, isoproterenol, meperidine, methylprednisolone, morphine, nafcillin, norepineph-**rine, papaverine, penicillin G, pentazocine, procaine, prochlorperazine, promazine, promethazine, verapamil, vitamin B complex with C, zinc. Y-site: **Amiodarone, ampicillin, ascorbic acid, atracurium, azathioprine, buprenorphine, chlorpromazine, ciprofloxacin, clarithromycin, dantrolene, dexrazoxane, diazepam, diazoxide, dimendhyrinate, diphenhydramine, dobutamine, dolasetron, doxorubicin, epirubicin, fenoldopam, ganiciclovir, garenoxacin, gemtuzumab, haloperidol, hydralazine, idarubicin, lansoprazole, magnesium, midazolam, minocycline, mitomycin, moxifloxacin, mycophenolate, ondansetron, oritavancin, papervine, perfloxacin, pentamidine, pentazocin, phenytoin, prochlorperazine, promazine, quindine, quinupristin/dalfopristin, SMZ/TMP, thiamine, topotecan, TPN, vancomycin, verapamil, vinorelbine, warfarin.**

▪ Store at 15°–30° C (59°–86° F) in tightly closed containers unless otherwise directed.

## ADVERSE EFFECTS (≥1%) CNS:

*Nervousness,* restlessness, depression, insomnia, irritability, headache, dizziness, muscle hyperactivity, convulsions. **CV:** Cardiac arrhythmias, tachycardia (with rapid IV), hyperventilation, chest pain, <u>severe hypotension, cardiac arrest</u>. **GI:** *Nausea, vomiting, anorexia,* hematemesis, diarrhea, epigastric pain.

## INTERACTIONS Drug: Increas-

es **lithium** excretion, lowering **lithium** levels; **cimetidine,** high-dose **allopurinol** (600 mg/day), **ciprofloxacin, erythromycin,** troleandomycin can significantly increase theophylline levels. Herbal: St. John's wort may decrease effect.

## PHARMACOKINETICS Absorption: Most products are 100% absorbed from GI tract. Peak: IV 30 min; uncoated tablet 1 h; sustained release 4–6 h. Duration: 4–8 h; varies with age, smoking, and liver function. Distribution: Crosses placenta. Metabolism: Extensively in liver; by CYP1A2. Elimination: Parent drug and metabolites excreted by kidneys; excreted in breast milk. Half-Life: 3.7 h (child); 7.7 h (adult).

## NURSING IMPLICATIONS

### Assessment & Drug Effects

- Monitor for S&S of toxicity (generally related to theophylline serum levels over 20 mcg/mL). Observe patients receiving parenteral drug closely for signs of hypotension, arrhythmias, and convulsions until serum theophylline stabilizes within the therapeutic range.
- Monitor and record vital signs and I&O. A sudden, sharp, unexplained rise in heart rate may indicate toxicity.
- Note: Older adults, acutely ill, and patients with severe respiratory problems, liver dysfunction, or pulmonary edema are at greater risk of toxicity due to reduced drug clearance.
- Note: Children appear more susceptible to CNS stimulating effects of xanthines (nervousness, restlessness, insomnia, hyperactive reflexes, twitching, convulsions). Dosage reduction may be indicated.
- Monitor lab tests: Periodic serum theophylline levels.

### Patient & Family Education

- Note: Use of tobacco tends to increase elimination of this drug (shortens half-life), necessitating higher dosage or shorter intervals than in nonsmokers.
- Report excessive nervousness or insomnia. Dosage reduction may be indicated.
- Note: Dizziness is a relatively common side effect, particularly in older adults; take necessary safety precautions.
- Do not take OTC remedies for treatment of asthma or cough unless approved by prescriber.

## AMINOSALICYLIC ACID (*PARA*-AMINOSALICYLIC ACID)
(a-mee-noe-sal-i-sil'ik)
Paser

Classification: ANTITUBERCULOSIS
Therapeutic: ANTITUBERCULOSIS
Prototype: Isoniazid

**AVAILABILITY** Granule packets

## ACTION & *THERAPEUTIC EFFECT*
Suppresses growth and multiplication of *Mycobacterium tuberculosis* by preventing folic acid synthesis. Aminosalicylates reportedly have potent hypolipemic action. *Aminosalicylates are an effective antiinfective alone or in combined therapy and reduce serum cholesterol and triglycerides by lowering LDL and VLDL.*

**USES** Treat tuberculosis along with other medications.

## CONTRAINDICATIONS Hypersensitivity to aminosalicylates, salicylates, or to compounds containing *para*-aminophenyl groups (e.g., sulfonamides, certain hair dyes); G6PD deficiency, use of the sodium salt in patients on sodium restriction or CHF; lactation.

---

Common adverse effects in *italic;* life-threatening effects underlined; generic names in **bold;** classifications in SMALL CAPS; ♣ Canadian drug name; ⊘ Prototype drug

**CAUTIOUS USE** Impaired renal and hepatic function; blood dyscrasias; goiter; gastric ulcer; pregnancy (category C).

## ROUTE & DOSAGE

**Tuberculosis**

*Adult/Adolsecent/Child:* **PO** 4 g 3 × day (max: 12 g)

## ADMINISTRATION

### Oral

- Mix granules in apple sauce or yogurt, or suspend in an acidic drink such as fruit juice or tomato juice. Do not administer granules that have lost their tan color.
- Give with or immediately following meals to reduce irritative gastric effects.
- Store in tight, light-resistant containers in a cool, dry place, preferably at 15°–30° C (59°–86° F), unless otherwise directed.

**ADVERSE EFFECTS** (≥1%) **Body as a Whole:** Fever, chills, generalized malaise, joint pain, rash, fixed-drug eruptions, pruritus; vasculitis; Loeffler's syndrome. **CNS:** Psychotic reactions. **GI:** *Anorexia, nausea, vomiting, abdominal distress, diarrhea*, peptic ulceration, acute hepatitis, malabsorption. **Hematologic:** Leukopenia, agranulocytosis, eosinophilia, lymphocytosis, thrombocytopenia, hemolytic anemia; (G6PD deficiency); prothrombinemia. **Urogenital:** Renal (irritation), crystalluria. **Other:** With long-term administration, goiter.

**DIAGNOSTIC TEST INTERFERENCE** Aminosalicylates may interfere with urine **urobilinogen** determinations (using **Ehrlich's reagent**), and may cause false-positive **urinary protein** and **VMA** determinations

(with **diazoreagent**); false-positive **urine glucose** may result with **cupric sulfate tests** (e.g., **Benedict's solution**), but reportedly not with **glucose oxidase reagents** (e.g., **TesTape, Clinistix**). Reduces **serum cholesterol,** and possibly **serum potassium, serum PBI,** and 24-h **I-131 thyroidal uptake** (effect may last almost 14 days).

**INTERACTIONS Drug:** Increases hypoprothrombinemic effects of ORAL ANTICOAGULANTS; increased risk of crystalluria with **ammonium chloride, ascorbic acid;** decreased intestinal absorption of **cyanocobalamin, folic acid, digoxin;** ANTIHISTAMINES may inhibit PAS absorption; may increase or decrease **phenytoin** levels; **probenecid, sulfinpyrazone** decrease PAS elimination.

**PHARMACOKINETICS Absorption:** Almost completely from GI tract; sodium form more rapidly absorbed than the acid. **Peak:** 1.5–2 h. **Duration:** 4 h. **Distribution:** Well distributed to tissue and body fluids except CSF unless meninges are inflamed. **Metabolism:** In liver. **Elimination:** greater than 80% in urine in 7–10 h. **Half-Life:** 1 h.

## NURSING IMPLICATIONS

### Assessment & Drug Effects

- Monitor for abrupt onset of fever, particularly during the early weeks of therapy, and clinical picture resembling that of infectious mononucleosis (malaise, fatigue, generalized lymphadenopathy, splenomegaly, sore throat), as well as minor complaints of pruritus, joint pains, and headache, which strongly suggest hypersensitivity; report these symptoms promptly.
- Monitor I&O and encourage fluids. High concentrations of drug are excreted in urine, and this can cause crystalluria and hematuria.

### Patient & Family Education

- Note: Hypersensitivity reactions may occur after a few days, but most commonly in the fourth or fifth week; report promptly.
- Notify prescriber if sore throat or mouth, malaise, unusual fatigue, bleeding or bruising occurs.
- Note: Therapy generally lasts about 2 y. Adhere to the established drug regimen, and remain under close medical supervision to detect possible adverse drug effects during the treatment period. Resistant TB strains develop more rapidly when drug regimen is interrupted or is sporadic.
- Do not take aspirin or other OTC drugs without prescriber's approval.
- Discard drug if it discolors (brownish or purplish); this signifies decomposition.

## AMIODARONE HYDROCHLORIDE ℞

(a-mee'oh-da-rone)

Cordarone, Nexterone, Pacerone

**Classification:** ANTIARRHYTHMIC, CLASS III

**Therapeutic:** CLASS III ANTIARRHYTHMIC; ANTIANGINAL

### AVAILABILITY Tablet; injection

### ACTION & THERAPEUTIC EFFECT

Acts directly on all cardiac tissues by prolonging duration of action potential and refractory period. Slows conduction time through the AV node and can interrupt the reentry pathways through the AV node. *Effective in prevention or suppression of cardiac arrhythmias.*

### USES Prophylaxis and treatment of life-threatening ventricular arrhythmias and supraventricular arrhythmias, particularly with atrial fibrillation.

**UNLABELED USES** Treatment of nonexertional angina, conversion of atrial fibrillation to normal sinus rhythm, paroxysmal supraventricular tachycardia, ventricular rate control due to accessory pathway conduction in pre-excited atrial arrhythmia, after defibrillation and epinephrine in cardiac arrest, AV nodal reentry tachycardia.

**CONTRAINDICATIONS** Hypersensitivity to amiodarone, iodine, or benzyl alcohol; cardiogenic shock, severe sinus bradycardia, second- or third-degree AV block unless a pacemaker is available, severe sinus-node dysfunction or sick sinus syndrome, bradycardia causing syncopy (except in patients with functioning pacemaker); congenital or acquired QR prolongation syndromes, or history of torsades de pointes; pregnancy (category D); lactation.

**CAUTIOUS USE** Severe hepatic disease, cirrhosis; Hashimoto's thyroiditis, goiter, thyrotoxicosis, or history of other thyroid dysfunction; severe hepatic impairment; CHF, older adults; Fabry disease especially with visual disturbances; electrolyte imbalance, hypokalemia, hypomagnesemia, hypovolemia; preexisting lung disease, COPD; open heart surgery.

## ROUTE & DOSAGE

### Arrhythmias

*Adult:* **PO Loading Dose** 800–1600 mg/day in 1–2 doses for 1–3 wk; **PO Maintenance Dose** 400–600 mg/day in 1–2 doses; **IV Loading Dose** 150 mg over 10 min followed by 360 mg

Common adverse effects in *italic*; life-threatening effects underlined; generic names in **bold**; classifications in SMALL CAPS; ♣ Canadian drug name; ℗ Prototype drug

77

over next 6 h; **IV Maintenance Dose** 540 mg over 18 h (0.5 mg/min), may continue at 0.5 mg/min; **Convert IV to PO** Duration of infusion less than 1 wk use 800–1600 mg **PO**; 1–3 wk use 600–800 mg **PO**; greater than 3 wk use 400 mg **PO**
*Child:* **IV** 5 mg/kg then repeat (max: 300 mg total)

*Hepatic Impairment Dosage Adjustment*

Adjustment only suggested in severe hepatic impairment

## ADMINISTRATION

- Note: Correct hypokalemia and hypomagnesemia prior to initiation of therapy.

### Oral

- Give consistently with respect to meals. Avoid grapefruit juice.
- Note: Only a prescriber experienced with the drug and treatment of life-threatening arrhythmias should give loading doses.
- Note: GI symptoms commonly occur during high-dose therapy, especially with loading doses. Symptoms usually respond to dose reduction or divided dose given with food, including milk.

### Intravenous

*PREPARE:* **IV Infusion: First rapid loading dose infusion:** Add 150 mg (3 mL) amiodarone to 100 mL D5W to yield 1.5 mg/mL. **Second infusion during first 24 h (slow loading dose and maintenance infusion):** Add 900 mg (18 mL) amiodarone to 500 mL D5W to yield 1.8 mg/mL. **Maintenance infusions after the first 24 h:** Prepare concentrations of 1–6 mg/mL amiodarone. Note: Use central line to give concentrations greater than 2 mg/mL.

*ADMINISTER:* **IV Infusion:** Initial infusion rate should not exceed 30 mg/min. Loading dose is usually given over 10 min in adults and 20–60 min in children. Note: See manufacturer's guidelines for **Nexterone** administration.

*INCOMPATIBILITIES:* Solution/additive: **Aminophylline, amoxicillin/clavulanic acid, cefazolin, floxacillin, furosemide, quinidine.** Y-site: **Acyclovir, allopurinol, amifostine, aminocaproic acid, aminophylline, amoxicillin, ampicillin, ampicillin/sulbactam, argatroban, atenolol, bivalirudin, cefamandole, cefazolin, cefotaxime, cefotetan, ceftazidime, ceftopribole, chloramphenicol, cytarabine, dantrolene, dexamethasone, diazepam, digoxin, doxorubicin, drotrecogin, ertapenem, fludarabine, fluorouracil, foscarnet, fosphenytoin, ganciclovir, gemtuzumab, heparin, hydrocortisone, imipenem/cilastatin, ketorolac, leucovorin, levofloxacin, magnesium sulfate, mechlorethamine, melphalan, meropenem, methotrexate, micafungin, mitomycin, paclitaxel, pentobarbital, phenytoin, piperacillin, piperacillin/tazobactam, potassium acetate, potassium phosphate, quinidine, ranitidine, sodium bicarbonate, sodium phosphate, SMZ/TMP, thiopental, thiotepa, tigecycline, verapamil.**

- Store at 15°–30° C (59°–86° F) protected from light, unless otherwise directed.

## ADVERSE EFFECTS (≥1%) CNS:
Peripheral neuropathy (*muscle*

*weakness,* wasting numbness, tingling), *fatigue,* abnormal gait, dyskinesias, *dizziness,* paresthesia, headache. **CV:** Bradycardia, *hypotension* (IV), sinus arrest, cardiogenic shock, CHF, arrhythmias; AV block. **Special Senses:** *Corneal microdeposits,* blurred vision, optic neuritis, optic neuropathy, permanent blindness, corneal degeneration, macular degeneration, photosensitivity. **GI:** *Anorexia, nausea, vomiting, constipation,* hepatotoxicity. **Metabolic:** Hyperthyroidism or hypothyroidism; may cause neonatal hypo- or hyperthyroidism if taken during pregnancy. **Respiratory:** (Pulmonary toxicity) Alveolitis, pneumonitis (fever, dry cough, dyspnea), interstitial pulmonary fibrosis, *fatal gasping syndrome* with IV in children. **Skin:** Slate-blue pigmentation, *photosensitivity,* rash. **Other:** With chronic use, angioedema.

**INTERACTIONS Drug:** Significantly increases **digoxin** levels; enhances pharmacologic effects and toxicities of **disopyramide, procainamide, quinidine, flecainide, lidocaine, lovastatin, simvastatin;** anticoagulant effects of ORAL ANTICOAGULANTS enhanced; **verapamil, diltiazem,** BETA-ADRENERGIC BLOCKING AGENTS may potentiate sinus bradycardia, sinus arrest, or AV block; may increase **phenytoin** levels 2- to 3-fold; **cholestyramine** may decrease amiodarone levels; **fentanyl** may cause bradycardia, hypotension, or decreased output; may increase **cyclosporine** levels and toxicity; **cimetidine** may increase amiodarone levels; **ritonavir** may increase risk of amiodarone toxicity, including cardiotoxicity; **simvastatin** doses over 20 mg increase risk of rhabdomyolysis; **loratadine** use may increase risk of QT prolongation. **Food:** Grapefruit

**juice** may increase amidarone concentrations. **Herbal: Echinacea** may increase hepatotoxicity, **St. John's wort** may decrease efficacy. **Lab Test:** Affects thyroid function tests, causing an increase in serum $T_4$ and serum reverse $T_3$ levels, and a decline in serum $T_3$ levels.

**PHARMACOKINETICS Absorption:** 22–86% absorbed. **Onset (PO):** 2–3 days to 1–3 wk. **Peak:** 3–7 h. **Distribution:** Concentrates in adipose tissue, lungs, kidneys, spleen; crosses placenta; 96% protein bound. **Metabolism:** Extensively in liver; undergoes some enterohepatic cycling; via CYP2C8 and 3A4. **Elimination:** Excreted chiefly in bile and feces, also in breast milk **Half-Life:** Biphasic, initial 2.5–10 days, terminal 40–55 days.

## NURSING IMPLICATIONS

### Black Box Warning

*Amiodarone has been associated with pulmonary toxicity (sometimes severe and potentially fatal), liver injury (ranging from mild to severe), and development of arrhythmias (heart block or sinus bradycardia).*

### Assessment & Drug Effects

- Monitor BP carefully during infusion and slow the infusion if significant hypotension occurs; bradycardia should be treated by slowing the infusion or discontinuing if necessary. Monitor heart rate and rhythm and BP until drug response has stabilized; report promptly symptomatic bradycardia. Sustained monitoring is essential because drug has an unusually long half-life.
- Monitor for S&S of: Adverse effects, particularly conduction disturbances and exacerbation of arrhythmias, in patients receiving other

Common adverse effects in *italic;* life-threatening effects underlined; generic names in **bold;** classifications in SMALL CAPS; ♣ Canadian drug name; ◉ Prototype drug

79

antiarrhythmic drugs; drug-induced hypothyroidism or hyperthyroidism (see Appendix F), especially during early treatment period; pulmonary toxicity (progressive dyspnea, fatigue, cough, pleuritic pain, fever) throughout therapy.

- Monitor for elevations of AST and ALT. If elevations persist or if they are 2–3 times above normal baseline readings, reduce dosage or withdraw drug promptly to prevent hepatotoxicity and liver damage.
- Auscultate chest periodically or when patient complains of respiratory symptoms. Check for diminished breath sounds, rales, pleuritic friction rub; observe breathing pattern. Drug-induced pulmonary function problems **must be** distinguished from CHF or pneumonia. Keep prescriber informed.
- Anticipate possible CNS symptoms within a week after amiodarone therapy begins. Proximal muscle weakness, a common side effect, intensified by tremors presents a great hazard to the ambulating patient. Assess severity of symptoms. Supervision of ambulation may be indicated.
- Monitor lab tests: Baseline and periodic serum electrolytes (i.e., potassium and magnesium); baseline and semiannual LFTs; baseline and periodic thyroid functions.

### Patient & Family Education

- Check pulse daily once stabilized, or as prescribed. Report a pulse less than 60.
- Take oral drug consistently with respect to meals. Do not drink grapefruit juice while taking this drug.
- Become familiar with potential adverse reactions and report those that are bothersome to the prescriber.
- Use dark glasses to ease photophobia; some patients may not be able to go outdoors in the daytime even with such protection.
- Follow recommendation for regular ophthalmic exams, including funduscopy and slit-lamp exam.
- Wear protective clothing and a barrier-type sunscreen that physically blocks penetration of skin by ultraviolet light to prevent a photosensitivity reaction (erythema, pruritus); avoid exposure to sun and sunlamps.

# AMITRIPTYLINE HYDROCHLORIDE
(a-mee-trip'ti-leen)
Apo-Amitriptyline ✦, Levate ✦, Novotriptyn ✦
**Classification:** TRICYCLIC ANTIDEPRESSANT
Therapeutic: ANTIDEPRESSANT
**Prototype:** Imipramine

## AVAILABILITY Tablet

## ACTION & *THERAPEUTIC EFFECT*
Inhibits the reuptake of serotonin (5-HT) and norepinephrine from the synaptic gap; also inhibits norepinephrine reuptake to a moderate degree. Restoration of the levels of these neurotransmitters is a proposed mechanism of its antidepressant action. *Interference with the reuptake of serotonin and norepinephrine results in the antidepressant activity of amitriptyline.*

## USES Endogenous depression.

## UNLABELED USES Prophylaxis
for cluster, migraine, and chronic tension headaches; neuropathic pain, to increase muscle strength in myotonic dystrophy, enuresis, fibromyalgia, insomnia, panic disorder, social anxiety disorder, and as sedative for nondepressed patients.

Common adverse effects in *italic;* life-threatening effects <u>underlined;</u> generic names in **bold;** classifications in SMALL CAPS; ✦ Canadian drug name; ⊙ Prototype drug

**CONTRAINDICATIONS** TCA hypersensitivity; acute recovery period after MI, cardiac arrhythmias, AV block, long-QT prolongation; suicidal ideation; history of seizure disorders; lactation, children younger than 12 y.

**CAUTIOUS USE** Prostatic hypertrophy, history of urinary retention or obstruction; angle-closure glaucoma; diabetes mellitus; history of hematologic disorders; history of alcoholism; GERD, BPH; hyperthyroidism; patient with cardiovascular, hepatic, or renal dysfunction; patient with suicidal tendency, electroshock therapy; elective surgery; schizophrenia; respiratory disorders; Parkinson's disease; seizure disorders; older adults, adolescents; pregnancy (category C).

## ROUTE & DOSAGE

**Antidepressant**

*Adult:* **PO** / 5 mg/day in divided doses, may gradually increase to 150–300 mg/day
*Adolescent/Geriatric:* **PO** 10 mg t.i.d. with 20 mg at bedtime (max: 150–200 mg/day)

**Pharmacogenetic Dosage Adjustment**

*CYP2D6 poor metabolizers:* Dose at 60–75% of normal dose

## ADMINISTRATION

**Oral**

- Give with or immediately after food to reduce possibility of GI irritation. Tablet may be crushed if patient is unable to take it whole; administer with food or fluid.
- Give increased doses preferably in late afternoon or at bedtime due to sedative action that precedes antidepressant effect.

- Note that dose is usually tapered over 2 wk at discontinuation to prevent withdrawal symptoms (headache, nausea, malaise, musculoskeletal pain, panic attack, weakness).

**ADVERSE EFFECTS** (≥1%) **CNS:** *Drowsiness, sedation, dizziness,* nervousness, restlessness, fatigue, headache, insomnia, abnormal movements (extrapyramidal symptoms), seizures. **CV:** *Orthostatic hypotension,* tachycardia, palpitation, ECG changes. **Special Senses:** Blurred vision, mydriasis. **GI:** *Dry mouth,* increased appetite especially for sweets, *constipation,* weight gain, sour or metallic taste, nausea, vomiting. **Urogenital:** *Urinary retention.* **Skin:** Alopecia, urticaria. **Other:** (Rare) Bone marrow depression.

**INTERACTIONS** **Drug:** Avoid drugs affecting QT interval. CNS DEPRESSANTS, **alcohol,** HYPNOTICS, barbiturates, SEDATIVES potentiate CNS depression; ANTICOAGULANTS, ORAL, may increase hypoprothrombinemic effect; **levodopa,** SYMPATHOMIMETICS (e.g., **epinephrine, norepinephrine**), possibility of sympathetic hyperactivity with hypertension and hyperpyrexia; MAO INHIBITORS, possibility of severe reactions, toxic psychosis, cardiovascular instability; **methylphenidate** increases plasma TCA levels; THYROID DRUGS may increase possibility of arrhythmias; **cimetidine** may increase plasma TCA levels. **Herbal:** **St. John's wort** may cause serotonin syndrome.

**PHARMACOKINETICS** **Absorption:** Rapidly from GI tract. **Peak:** 2–12 h. **Distribution:** Crosses placenta. **Metabolism:** In liver (CYP2D6). **Elimination:** Primarily in urine; enters breast milk. **Half-Life:** 10–50 h.

---

Common adverse effects in *italic;* life-threatening effects underlined; generic names in **bold;** classifications in SMALL CAPS; ♣ Canadian drug name; ● Prototype drug

81

## NURSING IMPLICATIONS

### Black Box Warning

*Amitriptyline has been associated with increased risk of suicidal thinking and behavior in children and adolescents, especially during the first few months of treatment.*

### Assessment & Drug Effects

- Monitor for S&S of drowsiness and dizziness (initial stages of therapy); institute measures to prevent falling. Monitor for overdose or suicide ideation especially in children and adolescents and in patients who use excessive amounts of alcohol.
- Eye examinations (including glaucoma testing) are recommended particularly for older adults, adolescents, and patients receiving high doses/prolonged therapy.
- Monitor BP and pulse rate in patients with preexisting cardiovascular disease. Assess for orthostatic hypotension especially in older adults. Withhold drug if there is a rise or fall in systolic BP (by 10–20 mm Hg), or a sudden increase or a significant change in pulse rate or rhythm. Notify prescriber.
- Monitor I&O, including bowel elimination pattern.
- Monitor lab tests: Baseline and periodic amitriptyline level (level greater than 300 mg/mL associated with increased adverse effects); periodic blood glucose.

### Patient & Family Education

- Monitor weight; drug may increase appetite or a craving for sweets.
- Understand that tolerance/adaptation to anticholinergic actions (see Appendix F) usually develops with maintenance regimen. Keep prescriber informed.
- Relieve dry mouth by taking frequent sips of water and increasing total fluid intake.
- Make position change slowly and in stages to prevent dizziness.
- Do not drive or engage in potentially hazardous activities until response to drug is known.
- Do not use OTC drugs without consulting prescriber while on TCA therapy; many preparations contain sympathomimetic amines.
- Note: Amitriptyline may turn urine blue-green.

## AMLODIPINE

(am-lo'di-peen)

Norvasc

**Classifications:** CALCIUM CHANNEL BLOCKER; ANTIHYPERTENSIVE
Therapeutic: ANTIHYPERTENSIVE; ANTIANGINAL
**Prototype:** Nifedipine

### AVAILABILITY Tablet

### ACTION & *THERAPEUTIC EFFECT*

A calcium channel blocking agent that selectively blocks calcium influx across cell membranes of cardiac and vascular smooth muscle without changing serum calcium concentrations. It reduces coronary vascular resistance, increases coronary blood flow, decreases peripheral vascular resistance, increases oxygen delivery to myocardial tissue, and increases cardiac output. *Amlodipine reduces systolic, diastolic, and mean arterial blood pressure. It also decreases pain due to angina.*

### USES Treatment of mild to moderate hypertension and stable/variant angina.

Common adverse effects in *italic;* life-threatening effects <u>underlined</u>; generic names in **bold;** classifications in SMALL CAPS; ♣ Canadian drug name; ☻ Prototype drug

**CONTRAINDICATIONS** Hypersensitivity to amlodipine; hypotension; severe obstructive coronary artery disease; severe aortic stenosis; lactation.

**CAUTIOUS USE** Hepatic impairment; concomitant use with hypotension; CHF, severe obstructive CAD, ventricular dysfunction; older adults; GERD; hepatic disease; pregnancy (category C); children younger than 6 y.

## ROUTE & DOSAGE

**Hypertension**

*Adult:* PO 5–10 mg once daily
*Geriatric:* Start with 2.5 mg, adjust dose at intervals of not less than 2 wk
*Adolescent/Child (6 y or older):* PO 2.5–5 mg daily (max: 10 mg)

**Stable/Vasospastic Angina**

*Adult:* PO 5–10 mg daily (usually 10 mg)

**Hepatic Impairment Dosage Adjustment**

Start with 2.5 mg, adjust dose at intervals of not less than 2 wk

## ADMINISTRATION

**Oral**
- Give drug without regard to meals.
- Note: Doses are usually titrated upward over a period of 14 days or more rapidly if warranted.
- Store at 15°–30° C (59°–86° F).

**ADVERSE EFFECTS** (≥1%) **CV:** Palpitations, flushing tachycardia, *peripheral or facial edema*, bradycardia, chest pain, syncope, postural hypotension. **CNS:** Lightheadedness, fatigue, *headache*. **GI:** Abdominal pain, nausea, anorexia, constipation, dyspepsia, dysphagia, diarrhea, flatulence, vomiting. **Urogenital:** Sexual dysfunction, frequency, nocturia. **Respiratory:** Dyspnea. **Skin:** Flushing, rash. **Other:** Arthralgia, cramps, myalgia.

**INTERACTIONS Drug: Adenosine** may increase the risk of bradycardia; **bosentan** may decrease efficacy of amlodipine; additive hypotensive effects with other ANTIHYPERTENSIVE AGENTS; AZOLE ANTIFUNGALS (e.g., **fluconazole, itraconazole**) may inhibit metabolism of amlodipine; **itraconazole** may increase edema. Use caution with **ezetimibe** or **simvastatin** due to increased risk of myopathy. CYP3A4 inducers (**rifampin, rifabutin, carbamazepine, phenytoin**) may increase needed amlodipine dose. **Food: Grapefruit juice** may increase amlodipine levels. **Herbal: Ephedra, ma huang, melatonin** may antagonize antihypertensive effects. **St. John's wort** may reduce clinical efficacy.

**PHARMACOKINETICS Absorption:** Greater than 90% absorbed from GI tract. **Peak:** 6–9 h. **Duration:** 24 h. **Distribution:** Greater than 95% protein bound. **Metabolism:** In liver (CYP3A4) to inactive metabolites. **Elimination:** In urine (less than 5–10% excreted unchanged), 20–25% in feces. **Half-Life:** Less than 45 y: 28–69 h; greater than 60 y: 40–120 h.

## NURSING IMPLICATIONS

### Black Box Warning

*Amlodipine has been associated with fetal injury and death.*

**Assessment & Drug Effects**
- Monitor BP for therapeutic effectiveness. BP reduction is greatest

---

Common adverse effects in *italic;* life-threatening effects <u>underlined</u>; generic names in **bold;** classifications in SMALL CAPS; ♣ Canadian drug name; ○ Prototype drug

83

after peak levels of amlodipine are achieved 6–9 h following oral doses.

- Monitor for S&S of dose-related peripheral or facial edema that may not be accompanied by weight gain; rarely, severe edema may cause discontinuation of drug.
- Monitor BP with postural changes. Report postural hypotension. Monitor more frequently when additional antihypertensives or diuretics are added.
- Monitor heart rate; dose-related palpitations (more common in women) may occur.

### Patient & Family Education

- Discontinue drug immediately and report to prescriber if pregnancy is suspected.
- Do not breast-feed while taking this drug.
- Report significant swelling of face or extremities.
- Exercise caution when standing and walking due to possible dose-related light-headedness/dizziness.
- Report shortness of breath, palpitations, irregular heartbeat, nausea, or constipation to prescriber.

## AMMONIUM CHLORIDE
(ah-mo′ni-um)

**Classification:** ELECTROLYTIC BALANCE AGENT
Therapeutic: ACIDFIER; ELECTRO-LYTE REPLACEMENT

### AVAILABILITY Injection

### ACTION & *THERAPEUTIC EFFECT*

Acidifying property is due to conversion of ammonium ion ($NH_4^+$) to urea in liver with liberation of $H^+$ and $Cl^-$. Potassium excretion also increases acid, but to a lesser extent. *Effective as a systemic acidifier in metabolic alkalosis by releasing $H^+$ ions which lower pH.*

USES Treatment of hypochloremic states and metabolic alkalosis.

CONTRAINDICATIONS Severe renal or hepatic insufficiency; primary respiratory acidosis.

CAUTIOUS USE Cardiac edema, cardiac insufficiency, pulmonary insufficiency; pregnancy (category B); lactation.

### ROUTE & DOSAGE

**Metabolic Alkalosis and Hypochloremic States**

*Adult/Child:* IV Dose calculated on basis of $CO_2$ combining power or serum Cl deficit, 50% of calculated deficit is administered slowly

### ADMINISTRATION

**Intravenous**
Check with prescriber for slower rate for infants.

*PREPARE:* **Intermittent:** Dilute each 20 mL vial in 500–1000 mL NS. Do not exceed a concentration of 1–2%.
*ADMINISTER:* **Intermittent:** Give slowly to avoid serious adverse effects (ammonia toxicity) and local irritation and pain. ▪ Give at a rate not to exceed 5 mL/min.
*INCOMPATIBILITIES:* **Solution/additive: Dimenhydrinate. Y-site: Warfarin.**

- Avoid freezing. ▪ Concentrated solutions crystallize at low temperatures. ▪ Crystals can be dissolved by placing intact container in a warm water bath and warming to room temperature.

### ADVERSE EFFECTS (≥1%) **Body as a Whole:** Most secondary to ammonia toxicity. **CNS:** Headache, depression, drowsiness, twitching, excitability; EEG abnormalities. **CV:** Bradycardia and other arrhythmias.

**GI:** Gastric irritation, nausea, vomiting, anorexia. **Metabolic:** Metabolic acidosis, hyperammonia. **Respiratory:** Hyperventilation. **Skin:** Rash. **Urogenital:** Glycosuria. **Other:** Pain and irritation at IV site.

## DIAGNOSTIC TEST INTERFERENCE
Ammonium chloride may increase *blood ammonia* and *AST,* decrease *serum magnesium* (by increasing urinary magnesium excretion), and decrease *urine urobilinogen.*

## INTERACTIONS **Drug: Aminosalicylic acid** may cause crystalluria; increases urinary excretion of AMPHETAMINES, **flecainide, mexiletine, methadone, ephedrine, pseudoephedrine;** decreased urinary excretion of SULFONYLUREAS, SALICYLATES.

## PHARMACOKINETICS **Absorption:** Completely absorbed in 3–6 h. **Metabolism:** In liver to HCl and urea. **Elimination:** Primarily in urine.

## NURSING IMPLICATIONS
### Assessment & Drug Effects
- Assess IV infusion site frequently for signs of irritation. Change site as warranted.
- Monitor for S&S of the following: Metabolic acidosis (mental status changes including confusion, disorientation, coma, respiratory changes including increased respiratory rate and depth, exertional dyspnea); ammonium toxicity (cardiac arrhythmias including bradycardia, irregular respirations, twitching, seizures).
- Monitor I&O ratio and pattern. The diuretic effect of ammonium chloride is compensatory and lasts only 1–2 days.

- Monitor lab tests: Baseline and periodic $CO_2$ combining power, serum electrolytes, and urinary and arterial pH.

### Patient & Family Education
- Report pain at IV injection site.

## AMOXAPINE
(a-mox'a-peen)
**Classification:** TRICYCLIC ANTIDEPRESSANT
Therapeutic: ANTIDEPRESSANT
**Prototype:** Imipramine

## AVAILABILITY Tablet

## ACTION & *THERAPEUTIC EFFECT*
Antidepressant activity and mild sedation are thought to be due to reduced reuptake of norepinephrine and serotonin at the cell membrane of the neuron, thus increasing the level of both neurotransmitters. *Enhancement of neurotransmitters results in its antidepressant activity.*

## USES Depression accompanied by anxiety or aggression.

## CONTRAINDICATIONS Hypersensitivity to other tricyclic compounds; acute recovery period after MI; AV block; MAOI therapy; suicidal ideation; lactation.

## CAUTIOUS USE History of convulsive disorders, schizophrenia, manic depression, electroshock therapy; alcohol abuse; history of urinary retention, benign prostatic hypertrophy; angle-closure glaucoma or increased intraocular pressure; cardiovascular disorders; impaired renal or hepatic function; elective surgery; pregnancy (category C); children younger than 18 y.

---

## ROUTE & DOSAGE

### Antidepressant

*Adult:* **PO** Start at 50 mg b.i.d. or t.i.d., may increase on third day to 100 mg t.i.d. Maintenance doses less than 300 mg/day as single dose at bedtime.

## ADMINISTRATION

### Oral

- Give with or after food to reduce GI irritation; tablet may be crushed and taken with fluid or mixed with food.
- Give maintenance dose as a single dose at bedtime to minimize daytime sedation and other annoying drug adverse effects.
- Do not abruptly discontinue drug. Doses should be tapered over 2 wk.
- Store at 15°–30° C (59°–86° F) in tightly closed container unless otherwise directed.

## ADVERSE EFFECTS (≥1%) CNS:
*Drowsiness,* dizziness, headache, fatigue, *sedation,* lethargy; extrapyramidal effects (acute dystonic reactions, panic attacks, parkinsonism, tardive dyskinesia), neuroleptic malignancy syndrome (NMS); seizures (overdosage). **CV:** Orthostatic hypotension. **GI:** Constipation, diarrhea, flatulence, *dry mouth,* peculiar taste, nausea, heartburn. **Special Senses:** Blurred vision, dry eyes. **Urogenital:** Nephrotoxicity (overdosage).

## INTERACTIONS Drug: May decrease response to ANTIHYPERTENSIVES; CNS DEPRESSANTS, **alcohol,** HYPNOTICS, BARBITURATES, SEDATIVES potentiate CNS depression; may increase hypoprothrombinemic effect of ORAL ANTICOAGULANTS; **ethchlorvynol,** transient delirium; with **levodopa,** SYMPATHOMIMETICS (e.g., **epinephrine, norepinephrine**), possibility of sympathetic hyperactivity with hypertension and hyperpyrexia; with MAO INHIBITORS, possibility of severe reactions: toxic psychosis, cardiovascular instability; **methylphenidate** increases plasma TCA levels; thyroid drugs may increase possibility of arrhythmias; **cimetidine** may increase plasma TCA levels. **Herbal: Ginkgo** may decrease seizure threshold, **St. John's wort** may cause serotonin syndrome.

## PHARMACOKINETICS Absorption: Rapidly absorbed. **Peak:** 1–2 h. **Distribution:** Probably crosses placenta; distributed into breast milk. **Metabolism:** Via CYP2D6; active metabolite. **Elimination:** 60% in urine in 6 days; 7–18% in feces. **Half-Life:** 8 h parent drug, 30 h metabolite.

## NURSING IMPLICATIONS

### Black Box Warning

*Amoxapine has been associated with increased risk of suicidal thinking and behavior especially in children, adolescents, and young adults.*

### Assessment & Drug Effects

- Supervise patient closely during therapy for suicidal ideation, worsening of clinical condition, and other potential serious adverse effects.
- Monitor therapeutic effectiveness. Initial antidepressant effect (mild euphoria, increased energy) may occur within 4–7 days; however, in most patients clinical response does not occur until after 2–3 wk of drug therapy.
- Report immediately signs of neuroleptic malignant syndrome:

Common adverse effects in *italic;* life-threatening effects underlined; generic names in **bold;** classifications in SMALL CAPS; ♣ Canadian drug name; ◉ Prototype drug

Fever, sweating, rigidity (catatonia), unstable BP, rapid, irregular pulse; changes in level of consciousness, coma. Although rare, it can be life-threatening if drug is not stopped immediately. Death can result from acute respiratory, renal, or cardiovascular failure.

- Report immediately the onset of signs of tardive dyskinesia (see Appendix F); careful observation/reporting may prevent irreversibility.
- Monitor I&O ratio and bowel elimination pattern. Report continuing constipation.

### Patient & Family Education

- Report promptly suicidal ideation. Children, adolescents, and young adults may be especially vulnerable to suicidal thoughts.
- Do not abruptly discontinue drug. Dosage should be tapered over 2 wk. Maintain established dosage regimen. Do not skip, reduce, or double doses or change dose intervals.
- Minimize alcohol intake as it may potentiate drug effects, thus increasing the dangers of overdosage or suicidal ideation.
- Drink at least 2000 mL (approximately 2 qts) fluid daily and eat foods with high fiber content (if allowed) to provide needed roughage.
- Monitor weight at least weekly and report significant weight gain.
- Do not drive or engage in potentially hazardous tasks until response to drug is known.
- Rinse mouth frequently with clear water, especially after eating, to relieve mouth dryness.
- Do not take any prescription or OTC drugs without consulting prescriber.

## AMOXICILLIN
(a-mox-i-sill'in)

**Amoxil, Apo-Amoxi ♦, Moxatag**

**Classifications:** ANTIBIOTIC; AMINOPENICILLIN
Therapeutic: ANTIBIOTIC
**Prototype:** Ampicillin

**AVAILABILITY** Tablet; capsule; powder for suspension; extended release tab; chewable tablet

**ACTION & THERAPEUTIC EFFECT**
Broad-spectrum semisynthetic aminopenicillin and analog of ampicillin. Like other penicillins, amoxicillin inhibits the final stage of bacterial cell wall synthesis by binding to specific penicillin-binding proteins (PBPs) located inside the cell wall of rapidly multiplying bacteria. It results in bacterial cell lysis and death. *Active against both aerobic gram-positive and aerobic gram-negative bacteria.*

**USES** Infections of ear, nose, throat, GU tract, skin, and soft tissue caused by susceptible bacteria. Also used in uncomplicated gonorrhea.

**CONTRAINDICATIONS** Hypersensitivity to penicillins; infectious mononucleosis.

**CAUTIOUS USE** History of or suspected atopy or allergy (hives, eczema, hay fever, asthma); history of cephalosporin or carbapenem hypersensitivity; colitis, dialysis, diarrhea, GI disease; viral infection, syphilis, severe hepatic impairment; renal impairment or failure, diabetes mellitus, leukemia, pregnancy (category B); lactation.

Common adverse effects in *italic;* life-threatening effects underlined; generic names in **bold;** classifications in SMALL CAPS; ♦ Canadian drug name; ⊕ Prototype drug

87

## ROUTE & DOSAGE

### Mild to Moderate Infections

*Adult:* **PO** 250–500 mg q8h
*Child/Infant (3 mo or older):* **PO** 25–50 mg/kg/day (max: 60–80 mg/kg/day) divided q8h or 200–400 mg q12h
*Neonate/Infant (younger than 3 mo):* **PO** 20–30 mg/kg/day divided q12h

### Severe Infections

*Adult:* **PO** 875mg q12h or 500 mg q8h

### Gonorrhea

*Adult:* **PO** 3 g as single dose with 1 g probenecid
*Child (2 y or older):* **PO** 50 mg/kg as single dose with probenecid 25 mg/kg

### Tonsillitis/Pharyngitis

*Adult/Adolescent:* **PO Extended release** 775 mg daily × 10d

### Renal Impairment Dosage Adjustment

*CrCl 10–30 mL/min:* 250–500 mg q12h; *less than 10 mL/min:* 250–500 mg q24h

### Hemodialysis Dosage Adjustment

Administer extra dose after dialysis

## ADMINISTRATION

### Oral

- Ensure that chewable tablets are chewed or crushed before being swallowed with a liquid.
- Do not crush or chew extended release tablets.
- Place reconstituted pediatric drops directly on child's tongue or add to formula, milk, fruit juice, water, ginger ale, or other soft drink. Have child drink all the prepared dose promptly.
- Store in tightly covered containers at 15°–30° C (59°–86° F) unless otherwise directed. Reconstituted oral suspensions are stable for 7 days at room temperature.

## ADVERSE EFFECTS (≥1%) **Body as a Whole:** As with other penicillins. Hypersensitivity (rash, <u>anaphylaxis</u>), superinfections. **GI:** Diarrhea, nausea, vomiting, <u>pseudomembranous colitis</u> (rare). **Hematologic: Hemolytic anemia**, eosinophilia, <u>agranulocytosis</u> (rare). **Skin:** Pruritus, urticaria, or other skin eruptions. **Special Senses:** Conjunctival ecchymosis.

## DIAGNOSTIC TEST INTERFERENCE

False positive reactions may occur with **Clinitest, Benedict's solution** or **Fehling's solution.**

## INTERACTIONS **Probenecid** prolongs the activity of amoxicillin. ORAL CONTRACEPTIVE efficacy may be reduced. Levels of **methotrexate** may be increased. Increase monitoring in patients taking ANTICOAGULANTS.

## PHARMACOKINETICS **Absorption:** Nearly complete absorption. **Peak:** 1–2 h. **Distribution:** Diffuses into most tissues and body fluids, except synovial fluid and CSF (unless meninges are inflamed); crosses placenta; distributed into breast milk in small amounts. **Metabolism:** In liver. **Elimination:** 60% in urine. **Half-Life:** 1–1.3 h.

## NURSING IMPLICATIONS

### Assessment & Drug Effects

- Determine previous hypersensitivity reactions to penicillins, cephalosporins, and other allergens prior to therapy.
- Monitor for S&S of an urticarial rash (usually occurring within a few days after start of drug)

Common adverse effects in *italic;* life-threatening effects <u>underlined;</u> generic names in **bold;** classifications in SMALL CAPS; ♣ Canadian drug name; ⊘ Prototype drug

suggestive of a hypersensitivity reaction. If it occurs, look for other signs of hypersensitivity (fever, wheezing, generalized itching, dyspnea), and report to prescriber immediately.

- Report onset of generalized, erythematous, maculopapular rash (ampicillin rash) to prescriber. Ampicillin rash is not due to hypersensitivity; however, hypersensitivity should be ruled out.
- Monitor for and report diarrhea which may indicate pseudomembranous colitis.
- Monitor lab tests: Baseline C&S prior to initiation of therapy, periodic renal, hepatic, and hematologic functions with prolonged therapy.

**Patient & Family Education**

- Take drug around the clock, do not miss a dose, and continue therapy until all medication is taken, unless otherwise directed by prescriber.
- Report to prescriber onset of diarrhea and other possible symptoms of superinfection (see Appendix F).

# AMOXICILLIN AND CLAVULANATE POTASSIUM

(a-mox-i-sill'in)

Amoclan, Augmentin, Augmentin-ES600, Augmentin XR, Clavulin ◆

**Classifications:** BETA-LACTAM ANTIBIOTIC; AMINOPENICILLIN
Therapeutic: ANTIBIOTIC
**Prototype:** Ampicillin

**AVAILABILITY** Chewable tablet; oral suspension; 1000 mg amoxicillin/62.5 mg clavulanate sustained release tablet

**ACTION & THERAPEUTIC EFFECT**
As a beta-lactam antibiotic, amoxicillin is bactericidal. It inhibits the final stage of bacterial cell wall synthesis by binding with specific penicillin-binding proteins (PBPs) that are located inside the bacterial cell wall that leads to bacterial cell lysis and death. *Effectiveness of ampicillin is synergistic in combination with clavulanic acid. Clavulanic acid in combination with ampicillin inhibits enzyme (beta-lactamase) degradation of amoxicillin and by synergism extends both spectrum of activity and bactericidal effect of amoxicillin against many strains of beta-lactamase-producing bacteria resistant to amoxicillin alone.*

**USES** Infections caused by susceptible beta-lactamase-producing organisms: Lower respiratory tract infections, acute bacterial sinusitis, community acquired pneumonia, otitis media, sinusitis, skin and skin structure infections, and UTI.

**CONTRAINDICATIONS** Hypersensitivity to penicillins; infectious mononucleosis; patient with previous history of drug-induced cholestasis, jaundice, or other hepatic dysfunction.

**CAUTIOUS USE** Allergic disorders; cephalosporin hypersensitivity; GI disorders; colitis; hepatic or renal impairment; older adults; pregnancy (category B); lactation.

## ROUTE & DOSAGE

| Mild to Moderate Infections |
|---|
| *Adult:* **PO** 250 or 500 mg tablet (each with 125 mg clavulanic acid) q8–12h; Sustained release tabs: 2 tablets (2000 mg amoxicillin/125 mg clavulanate) q12h × 7–10 days |
| *Child (weight less than 40 kg):* **PO** 20–40 mg/kg/day (based on |

---

Common adverse effects in *italic;* life-threatening effects <u>underlined;</u> generic names in **bold;** classifications in SMALL CAPS; ◆ Canadian drug name; ⊙ Prototype drug

89

amoxicillin component) divided q8–12h; *3 mo or older:* 90 mg/kg/day of 600 ES divided q12h × 10 days

*Neonate: Infant (younger than 3 mo):* **PO** 30 mg/kg/day (amoxicillin) divided q12h

## ADMINISTRATION

### Oral

- Give at the start of a meal to minimize GI upset and enhance absorption.
- Reconstitute oral suspension by adding amount of water specified on container to provide a 5 mL suspension. Tap bottle before adding water to loosen powder, then add water in 2 portions, agitating suspension well before each addition.
- Agitate suspension well just before administration of each dose.
- Give dialysis patient an additional 2 doses on the day of dialysis; one dose during and another dose after dialysis.
- Store tablets in tight containers at less than 24° C (71° F). Reconstituted oral suspension should be refrigerated at 2°–8° C (36°–46° F), then discarded after 10 days.

## ADVERSE EFFECTS (≥1%) GI:
*Diarrhea,* nausea, vomiting. **Skin:** Rash, urticaria. **Other:** Candidal vaginitis; moderate increases in serum ALT, AST; hypersensitivity reactions, glomerulonephritis; agranulocytosis (rare).

## DIAGNOSTIC TEST INTERFERENCE

May interfere with **urinary glucose** determinations using **cupric sulfate, Benedict's solution, Clinitest;** does not affect **glucose oxidase methods** (e.g., **Clinistix, Tes-Tape**). Positive direct **antiglobulin (Coombs')** test results may be report-

ed, a reaction that could interfere with **hematologic studies** or with **transfusion cross-matching** procedures.

## INTERACTIONS Drug: Probene-
**cid** prolongs the activity of amoxicillin. Oral contraceptive efficacy may be reduced. Levels of **methotrexate** may be increased. Increase monitoring in patients taking anticoagulants.

## PHARMACOKINETICS Absorption: Nearly complete absorption. **Peak:** 1–2 h. **Distribution:** Diffuses into most tissues and body fluids, except synovial fluid and CSF (unless meninges are inflamed); crosses placenta; distributed into breast milk in very small amounts. **Metabolism:** In liver. **Elimination:** 50–73% of the amoxicillin and 25–45% of the clavulanate dose excreted in urine in 2 h. **Half-Life:** Amoxicillin 1–1.3 h, clavulanate 0.78–1.2 h.

## NURSING IMPLICATIONS

### Assessment & Drug Effects

- Determine previous hypersensitivity reactions to penicillins, cephalosporins, and other allergens prior to therapy.
- Monitor for S&S of an urticarial rash (usually occurring within a few days after start of drug) suggestive of a hypersensitivity reaction. If it occurs, look for other signs of hypersensitivity (fever, wheezing, generalized itching, dyspnea), and report to prescriber immediately.
- Monitor for and report diarrhea which may indicate pseudomembranous colitis.
- Monitor lab tests: Baseline C&S prior to initiation of therapy.

### Patient & Family Education

- Female patients should report onset of symptoms of *Candidal vaginitis* (e.g., moderate amount of white, cheesy, nonodorous vaginal discharge; vaginal inflammation and itching; vulvar excoriation, inflammation, burning, itching). Therapy may have to be discontinued.

- Report onset of diarrhea and other possible symptoms of superinfection to prescriber (see Appendix F).

## AMPHETAMINE SULFATE ℗
(am-fet′a-meen)
**Adderall, Adderall XR**
**Classification:** CEREBRAL STIMULANT; ANOREXIANT
**Therapeutic:** CEREBRAL STIMULANT
**Controlled Substance:** Schedule II

**AVAILABILITY** Tablet; **Adderall:** Tablet; sustained release capsules

## ACTION & *THERAPEUTIC EFFECT*
Marked stimulant effect on CNS thought to be due to action on cerebral cortex and possibly the reticular activating system. Acts indirectly on adrenergic receptors by increasing synaptic release of norepinephrine in the brain and by blocking reuptake of norepinephrine at presynaptic membranes. *CNS stimulation results in increased motor activity, diminished sense of fatigue, alertness, wakefulness, and mood elevation. Anorexigenic effect thought to result from direct inhibition of hypothalamic appetite center as well as mood elevation.*

## USES
Narcolepsy, attention deficit disorder in children and adults (hyperkinetic behavioral syndrome, minimal brain dysfunction). Use as short-term adjunct to control exogenous obesity not generally recommended because of its potential for abuse.

## CONTRAINDICATIONS
Hypersensitivity to sympathomimetic amines; history of drug abuse; severe agitation; hyperthyroidism; diabetes mellitus; moderate to severe hypertension, advanced arteriosclerosis, angina pectoris or other cardiovascular disorders; Gilles de la Tourette disorder; glaucoma; during or within 14 days after treatment with MAOIs; lactation.

## CAUTIOUS USE
Mild hypertension; pregnancy (category C); children younger than 3 y.

## ROUTE & DOSAGE

### Narcolepsy
*Adult:* **PO** 5–60 mg/day divided q4–6h in 2–3 doses
*Child (12 y or older):* **PO** 10 mg/day, may increase by 10 mg/day at weekly intervals; *6–12 y:* 5 mg/day, may increase by 5 mg at weekly intervals

### Attention Deficit Disorder
*Adult/Adolescent:* **PO Extended release** 10 mg once daily in a.m.; may increase by 5–10 mg at weekly intervals if needed (max: 30 mg/day)
*Child (6y):* **PO** 5 mg 1–2 × day, may increase by 5 mg at weekly intervals (max: 40 mg/day); *3–5 y:* 2.5 mg 1–2 × day, may increase by 2.5 mg at weekly intervals; **Extended release** 10 mg once daily in a.m.; may increase by 5–10 mg at weekly intervals if needed (max: 30 mg/day)

### Obesity Dosage Adjustment
*Adult:* **PO** 5–10 mg 1 h before meals

## ADMINISTRATION
### Oral
- Give first dose on awakening or early in a.m. when prescribed for narcolepsy.

---

Common adverse effects in *italic;* life-threatening effects underlined; generic names in **bold;** classifications in SMALL CAPS; ◆ Canadian drug name; ℗ Prototype drug

91

- Give last dose no later than 6 h before patient retires to avoid insomnia.
- Ensure that sustained release capsules are not crushed or chewed.
- Store at 15°–30° C (59°–86° F) unless otherwise directed.

**ADVERSE EFFECTS** (≥1%) **Body as a Whole:** Allergy, urticaria, <u>sudden death</u> (reported in children with structural cardiac abnormalities). **CNS:** *Irritability,* psychosis, *restlessness,* nervousness, headache, *insomnia,* weakness, *euphoria,* dysphoria, drowsiness, trembling, hyperactive reflexes. **CV:** *Palpitation,* elevated BP; tachycardia, vasculitis. **Urogenital:** Impotence and change in libido with high doses. **GI:** Dry mouth, anorexia, unusual weight loss, nausea, vomiting, diarrhea, or constipation.

**DIAGNOSTIC TEST INTERFERENCE** Elevations in **serum thyroxine (T$_4$)** levels with high amphetamine doses.

**INTERACTIONS Drug: Acetazolamide, sodium bicarbonate** decrease amphetamine elimination; **ammonium chloride, ascorbic acid** increase amphetamine elimination; effects of both amphetamine and BARBITURATES may be antagonized if given together; **furazolidone** may increase BP effects of amphetamines, and interaction may persist for several weeks after **furazolidone** is discontinued; **guanethidine** antagonizes antihypertensive effects; because MAO INHIBITORS, **selegiline** can precipitate hypertensive crisis (fatalities reported), do not administer amphetamines during or within 14 days of these drugs; PHENOTHIAZINES may inhibit mood elevating effects of amphetamines; TRICYCLIC ANTIDEPRESSANTS enhance amphetamine effects through increased **norepinephrine** release;

BETA AGONISTS increase cardiovascular adverse effects.

**PHARMACOKINETICS Absorption:** Rapid. **Peak effect:** 1–5 h. **Duration:** Up to 10 h. **Distribution:** All tissues, especially CNS. **Metabolism:** In liver. **Elimination:** Renal; excreted into breast milk. **Half-Life:** 10–30 h.

## NURSING IMPLICATIONS

### Black Box Warning

*Amphetamine has high abuse potential and misuse can cause severe cardiovascular adverse effects as well as sudden death.*

### Assessment & Drug Effects
- Monitor drug use and be alert for signs of misuse.
- Monitor for S&S of toxicity in children. Response to this drug is more variable in children than adults; acute toxicity has occurred over a wide dosage range.
- Monitor for S&S of insomnia or anorexia. Report complaints to prescriber. Dosage reduction may be required.
- Monitor BP and HR, especially in those with hypertension.
- Monitor diabetics closely for loss of glycemic control.
- Monitor growth in children; drug may be discontinued periodically to allow for normal growth.
- Note: Drug's excitatory and euphoric effects are associated with a high abuse potential.

### Patient & Family Education
- Keep prescriber informed of clinical response and persistent or bothersome adverse effects. This drug exerts a stimulating effect that masks fatigue; after exhilaration disappears, fatigue and depression are usually greater than before, and a longer period of rest is needed.

- Report insomnia or undesired weight loss.
- Do not drive or engage in potentially hazardous tasks until response to drug is known.
- Rinse mouth frequently with clear water, especially after eating, to relieve mouth dryness; increase fluid intake, if allowed; chew sugarless gum or sourballs.
- Note: Meticulous oral hygiene is required because decreaseds saliva encourages demineralization of tooth surfaces and mucosal erosion.
- Avoid caffeine-containing beverages because caffeine increases amphetamine effects.
- Note that drug is usually tapered gradually following prolonged administration of high doses. Abrupt withdrawal may result in lethargy, profound depression, or other psychotic manifestations that may persist for several weeks.

## AMPHOTERICIN B 💊

(am-foe-ter'i-sin)

Amphocin, Fungizone

**Classification:** ANTIFUNGAL
Therapeutic: ANTIFUNGAL

**AVAILABILITY** Powder for injection; suspension; cream, lotion, ointment

## ACTION & *THERAPEUTIC EFFECT*

Fungistatic antibiotic that exerts antifungal action on both resting and growing cells at least in part by selectively binding to sterols in fungus cell membrane resulting in cell death. *Fungicidal at higher concentrations, depending on sensitivity of fungus.*

**USES** Used Intravenously for a wide spectrum of potentially fatal systemic fungal (mycotic) infections. Has been used to potentiate antifungal effects of flucytosine (*Ancobon*) and

to provide anticandidal prophylaxis in certain susceptible patients receiving immunosuppressive therapy. Used topically for cutaneous and mucocutaneous infections caused by *Candida* (monilia).

**UNLABELED USES** Treatment of candiduria, fungal endocarditis, meningitis, septicemia; fungal infections of urinary bladder and urinary tract; amebic meningoencephalitis and paracoccidioidomycosis.

**CONTRAINDICATIONS** Hypersensitivity to amphotericin; lactation.

**CAUTIOUS USE** Severe bone marrow depression; renal function impairment; anemia; pregnancy (category B), oral supsension (category C).

## ROUTE & DOSAGE

### Systemic Infections (Amphocin, Fungizone)

*Adult:* **IV Test Dose** 1 mg dissolved in 20 mL of D5W by slow infusion (over 10–30 min); **IV Maintenance Dose** 0.25–0.3 mg/kg/day infused over 4–6 h, may gradually increase by 0.125–0.25 mg/kg/day up to 1–1.5 mg/kg/day (max dose: 1.5 mg/kg)

*Child:* **IV Test Dose** 0.1 mg/kg up to 1 mg dissolved in 20 mL of D5W by slow infusion (over 10–30 min); **IV Maintenance Dose** 0.4 mg/kg/day infused over 4–6 h, may increase by 0.25 mg/kg/day to target dose of 0.25–1 mg/kg/day infused over 2–6 h (max: 1.5 mg/kg)

### *Renal Impairment Dosage Adjustment*

The dose can be reduced or interval extended

Common adverse effects in *italic*; life-threatening effects <u>underlined</u>; generic names in **bold**; classifications in SMALL CAPS; ✦ Canadian drug name; 💊 Prototype drug

93

## ADMINISTRATION

### Intravenous

*PREPARE:* **Typically** prepared by pharmacy service due to complex technique required for IV solution preparation. Each brand of amphotericin is prepared differently according to manufacturer's directions. ▪ Refer to specific manufacturer's guidelines for preparation of IV solutions.

*ADMINISTER:* **Intermittent:** Use a 1-micron filter. ▪ Infuse total daily dose over 2–6 h. Use longer infusion time for better tolerance. ▪ Alert: Rapid infusion of any amphotericin can cause cardiovascular collapse. If hypotension or arrhythmias develop interrupt infusion and notify prescriber. ▪ Protect IV solution from light during administration. ▪ Note incompatibilities. When given through an existing IV line, flush before and after with D5W. ▪ Initiate therapy using the most distal vein possible and alternate sites with each dose if possible to reduce the risk of thrombophlebitis. ▪ Check IV site frequently for patency.

*INCOMPATIBILITIES:* **Solution/additive:** Any **saline**-containing solution (precipitate will form), PARENTERAL NUTRITION SOLUTIONS, **amikacin, calcium chloride, calcium gluconate, chlorpromazine, cimetidine, ciprofloxacin, diphenhydramine, dopamine, edetate calcium disodium, gentamicin, kanamycin, magnesium sulfate, meropenem, metaraminol, methyldopa, penicillin G, polymyxin, potassium chloride, prochlorperazine, ranitidine, streptomycin, verapamil. Y-site:** AMINOGLYCOSIDES, PENICILLINS, PHENOTHIAZINES, **allopurinol, amifostine, amsacrine, aztreonam, bivalirudin, cefepime, cefpirome, cisatracurium, dex-medetomidine, docetaxel, doxorubicin liposome, enalaprilat, etoposide, fenoldopam, filgrastim, fluconazole, foscarnet, gemcitabine, granisetron, heparin** (flush lines with **D5W**, not **NS**), **hetastarch, lansoprazole, linezolid, melphalan, meropenem, ondansetron, paclitaxel, pemetrexed, piperacillin/tazobactam, propofol, TPNs, vinorelbine.**

▪ Store according to manufacturer's recommendations for reconstituted and unopened vials.

## ADVERSE EFFECTS (≥1%) **Body as a Whole:** Hypersensitivity (pruritus, urticaria, skin rashes, fever, dyspnea, <u>anaphylaxis</u>); *fever, chills.* **CNS:** Headache, sedation, muscle pain, arthralgia, weakness. **CV:** Hypotension, <u>cardiac arrest</u>. **Special Senses:** Ototoxicity with tinnitus, vertigo, loss of hearing. **GI:** Nausea, vomiting, diarrhea, epigastric cramps, anorexia, weight loss. **Hematologic:** Anemia, <u>thrombocytopenia</u>. **Metabolic:** *Hypokalemia, hypomagnesemia.* **Urogenital:** <u>Nephrotoxicity</u>, urine with low specific gravity. **Skin:** Dry, erythema, pruritus, burning sensation; allergic contact dermatitis, exacerbation of lesions. **Other:** Pain; arthralgias, thrombophlebitis (IV site), superinfections.

## INTERACTIONS **Drug:** AMINOGLYCOSIDES, **capreomycin, cisplatin, carboplatin, colistin, cyclosporine, mechlorethamine, furosemide, vancomycin** increase the possibility of nephrotoxicity; CORTICOSTEROIDS potentiate hypokalemia; with DIGITALIS GLYCOSIDES, hypokalemia increases the risk of **digitalis** toxicity.

## PHARMACOKINETICS **Peak:** 1–2 h after IV infusion. **Duration:**

20 h. **Distribution:** Minimal amounts enter CNS, eye, bile, pleural, pericardial, synovial, or amniotic fluids; similar plasma and urine concentrations. **Elimination:** Excreted renally; can be detected in blood up to 4 wk and in urine for 4–8 wk after discontinuing therapy. **Half-Life:** 24–48 h.

## NURSING IMPLICATIONS

### Black Box Warning

*Amphotericin should be reserved for progressive and potentially fatal fungal infections.*

### Assessment & Drug Effects

- Monitor for S&S of local inflammatory reaction or thrombosis at injection site, particularly if extravasation occurs.
- Monitor cardiovascular and respiratory status and observe patient closely for adverse effects during initial IV therapy. If a test dose (1 mg over 20–30 min) is given, monitor vital signs every 30 min for at least 4 h. Febrile reactions (fever, chills, headache, nausea) occur in 20–90% of patients, usually 1–2 h after beginning infusion, and subside within 4 h after drug is discontinued. The severity of this reaction usually decreases with continued therapy. Keep prescriber informed.
- Monitor I&O and weight. Report immediately: Oliguria, any change in I&O ratio and pattern, or appearance of urine [e.g., sediment, pink or cloudy urine (hematuria)], abnormal renal function tests, unusual weight gain or loss. Generally, renal damage is reversible if drug is discontinued when first signs of renal dysfunction appear.
- Report to prescriber and withhold drug, if BUN exceeds 40 mg/dL or serum creatinine rises above 3 mg/dL. Dosage should be

reduced or drug discontinued until renal function improves.
- Consult prescriber for guidelines on adequate hydration and adjustment of daily dose as a possible means of avoiding or minimizing nephrotoxicity.
- Report promptly any evidence of hearing loss or complaints of tinnitus, vertigo, or unsteady gait. Tinnitus may not be a complaint in older adults or the very young. Other signs of ototoxicity (i.e., vertigo or hearing loss) are more reliable indicators of ototoxicity in these age groups.
- Baseline C&S prior to initiation of therapy; baseline and periodic BUN, serum creatinine, creatinine clearance; periodic CBC, serum electrolytes (especially $K^+$, $Mg^{++}$, $Na^+$, $Ca^{++}$), and LFTs.

### Patient & Family Education

- Maintain a high fluid intake of 2–3 L (approximately 2–3 qts) of fluid daily if not directed otherwise.
- Report promptly chills, fever, or unusual weakness.

## AMPHOTERICIN B LIPID-BASED

Abelcet, Amphotec, AmBisome

**Classification:** ANTIFUNGAL
**Therapeutic:** ANTIFUNGAL
**Prototype:** AMPHOTERICIN B

**AVAILABILITY Abelcet:** Suspension for injection; **Amphotec:** Powder for injection; **AmBisome:** Powder for injection

## ACTION & *THERAPEUTIC EFFECT*

Fungistatic antibiotic that exerts antifungal action on both resting and growing cells at least in part by selectively binding to sterols in fungus cell membrane. This results

Common adverse effects in *italic;* life-threatening effects <u>underlined</u>; generic names in **bold;** classifications in SMALL CAPS; ♥ Canadian drug name; ⊙ Prototype drug

95

in fungal cell death. *Fungicidal at higher concentrations, depending on sensitivity of fungus.*

**USES** Used Intravenously for a wide spectrum of potentially fatal systemic fungal (mycotic) infections.

**UNLABELED USES** Treatment of candiduria, fungal endocarditis, meningitis, septicemia; fungal infections of urinary bladder and urinary tract; amebic meningoencephalitis, and paracoccidioidomycosis.

**CONTRAINDICATIONS** Hypersensitivity to amphotericin; lactation.

**CAUTIOUS USE** Severe bone marrow depression; renal function impairment; anemia; pregnancy (category B).

## ROUTE & DOSAGE

**Systemic Infections (Abelcet)**
*Adult/Child:* **IV** 5 mg/kg/day

**(Amphotec)**
*Adult/Child:* **IV Test Dose** 10 mL (1.6–8.3 mg) of initial dose infused over 10–30 min; **IV Maintenance Dose** 3–4 mg/kg/day (max: 7.5 mg/kg/day) infused at 1 mg/kg/h

**(AmBisome)**
*Adult/Child:* **IV** 3–5 mg/kg/day infused over 1–2 h

**Cryptococcal Meningitis in HIV (AmBisome)**
*Adult:* **IV** 6 mg/kg/day infused over 2 h

**Leishmaniasis (AmBisome)**
*Adult (Immunocompetent):* **IV** 3 mg/kg/day on days 1–5, 14, and 21; may repeat if necessary.
*Immunocompromised:* 4 mg/kg/day on days 1–5, 10, 17, 24, 31, and 38

## ADMINISTRATION

### Intravenous

**PREPARE:** Each brand of amphotericin is prepared differently according to manufacturer's directions. ▪ Refer to specific manufacturer's guidelines for preparation of IV solutions.

**ADMINISTER: IV Infusion:** Flush existing line with D5W before infusion. Shake IV bag to ensure thorough mixing. Give at a rate of 2.5 mg/kg/h. Do not use an in-line filter. If the infusion exceeds 2 h, shake infusion bag q2h to mix.

**ALERT:** Rapid infusion of any amphotericin can cause cardiovascular collapse. If hypotension or arrhythmias develop interrupt infusion and notify prescriber. ▪ Protect IV solution from light during administration. ▪ Note incompatibilities. When given through an existing IV line, flush before and after with D5W. ▪ Initiate therapy using the most distal vein possible and alternate sites with each dose if possible to reduce the risk of thrombophlebitis. ▪ Check IV site frequently for patency.

**INCOMPATIBILITIES: Solution/additive:** Any **saline**-containing solution (precipitate will form), PARENTERAL NUTRITION SOLUTIONS. **Y-site:** AMINOGLYCOSIDES, PENICILLINS, PHENOTHIAZINES, **alfentanil, amikacin, ampicillin, ampicillin/sulbactam, atenolol, aztreonam, bretylium, buprenorphine, butorphanol, calcium salts, carboplatin, cefazolin, cefepime, ceftazidime, ceftriaxone, chlorpromazine, cimetidine, cisatracurium, cyclophosphamide, cyclosporine, cytarabine, diazepam, digoxin, diphenhydramine, dobutamine,**

Common adverse effects in *italic;* life-threatening effects underlined; generic names in **bold;** classifications in SMALL CAPS; ✤ Canadian drug name; ⊘ Prototype drug dopamine, doxorubicin, doxorubicin liposome, droperidol, enalaprilat, esmolol, etoposide, famotidine, fluconazole, fluorouracil, haloperidol, heparin (flush lines with **D5W**, not **NS**), heta-startch, hydromorphone, hydroxyzine, imipenem/cilastatin, labetalol, leucovorin, lidocaine, magnesium sulfate, meperidine, mesna, metoclopramide, midazolam, mitoxantrone, morphone, nalbuphine, naloxone, netilmicin, ofloxacin, ondansetron, paclitaxel, phenytoin, piperacillin, piperacillin/tazobactam, potassium chloride, prochlorperazine, promethazine, propranolol, ranitidine, remifentanil, sodium bicarbonate, ticarcillin/clavulanate, vecuronium, verapamil, vinorelbine.

- Do not mix **Abelcet** or **Amphotec** with any other drugs.

- Store according to manufacturer's recommendations for reconstituted and unopened vials.

## ADVERSE EFFECTS (≥1%) **Body as a Whole:** Hypersensitivity (pruritus, urticaria, skin rashes, fever, dyspnea, anaphylaxis); *fever, chills.* **CNS:** Headache, sedation, muscle pain, arthralgia, weakness. **CV:** Hypotension, cardiac arrest. **Special Senses:** Ototoxicity with tinnitus, vertigo, loss of hearing. **GI:** Nausea, vomiting, diarrhea, epigastric cramps, anorexia, weight loss. **Hematologic:** Anemia, thrombocytopenia. **Metabolic:** *Hypokalemia, hypomagnesemia.* **Urogenital:** Nephrotoxicity, urine with low specific gravity. **Skin:** Dry, erythema, pruritus, burning sensation; allergic contact dermatitis, exacerbation of lesions. **Other:** Pain; arthralgias, thrombophlebitis (IV site), superinfections.

## INTERACTIONS **Drug:** AMINOGLYCOSIDES, **capreomycin, cisplatin, carboplatin, colistin, cyclosporine, mechlorethamine, furosemide, vancomycin** increase the possibility of nephrotoxicity; CORTICOSTEROIDS potentiate hypokalemia; with DIGITALIS GLYCOSIDES, hypokalemia increases the risk of **digitalis** toxicity.

## PHARMACOKINETICS **Peak:** 1–2 h after IV infusion. **Duration:** 20 h. **Distribution:** Minimal amounts enter CNS, eye, bile, pleural, pericardial, synovial, or amniotic fluids; similar plasma and urine concentrations. **Elimination:** Excreted renally; can be detected in blood up to 4 wk and in urine for 4–8 wk after discontinuing therapy. **Half-Life:** 24–48 h.

## NURSING IMPLICATIONS
### Assessment & Drug Effects
- Monitor for S&S of local inflammatory reaction or thrombosis at injection site, particularly if extravasation occurs.
- Monitor cardiovascular and respiratory status and observe patient closely for adverse effects during initial IV therapy. If a test dose (1 mg over 20–30 min) is given, monitor vital signs every 30 min for at least 4 h. Febrile reactions (fever, chills, headache, nausea) occur in 20–90% of patients, usually 1–2 h after beginning infusion, and subside within 4 h after drug is discontinued. The severity of this reaction usually decreases with continued therapy. Keep prescriber informed.
- Monitor I&O and weight. Report immediately oliguria, any change in I&O ratio and pattern, or appearance of urine [e.g., sediment, pink or cloudy urine (hematuria)], abnormal renal function tests, unusual weight gain or loss. Generally,

renal damage is reversible if drug is discontinued when first signs of renal dysfunction appear.

- Report to prescriber and withhold drug if BUN exceeds 40 mg/dL or serum creatinine rises above 3 mg/dL. Dosage should be reduced or drug discontinued until renal function improves.
- Consult prescriber for guidelines on adequate hydration and adjustment of daily dose as a possible means of avoiding or minimizing nephrotoxicity.
- Report promptly any evidence of hearing loss or complaints of tinnitus, vertigo, or unsteady gait. Tinnitus may not be a complaint in older adults or the very young. Other signs of ototoxicity (i.e., vertigo or hearing loss) are more reliable indicators of ototoxicity in these age groups.
- Monitor lab tests: Baseline C&S prior to initiation of therapy; baseline and periodic renal function tests; periodic CBC, serum electrolytes (especially $K^+$, $Mg^{++}$, $Na^+$, $Ca^{++}$), and LFTs.

**Patient & Family Education**
- Maintain a high fluid intake of 2–3 L (approximately 2–3 qts) of fluid daily if not directed otherwise.
- Report promptly chills, fever, or unusual weakness.

## AMPICILLIN ⓟ
(am-pi-sill′in)
Novo-Ampicillin ♦

## AMPICILLIN SODIUM
Ampicin ♦, Penbritin ♦
**Classifications:** ANTIBIOTIC; AMINOPENICILLIN
**Therapeutic:** ANTIBIOTIC

**AVAILABILITY** Capsule; oral suspension; injection

## ACTION & *THERAPEUTIC EFFECT*
A broad-spectrum, semisynthetic aminopenicillin that is bactericidal but is inactivated by penicillinase (beta-lactamase). Like other penicillins, ampicillin inhibits the final stage of bacterial cell wall synthesis by binding to specific penicillin-binding proteins (PBPs) located inside the bacterial cell wall resulting in lysis and death of bacteria. *Effective against gram-positive bacteria as well as some gram-negative bacteria.*

**USES** Infections of GU, respiratory, and GI tracts and skin and soft tissues; also gonococcal infections, bacterial meningitis, otitis media, sinusitis, and septicemia and for prophylaxis of bacterial endocarditis. Used parenterally only for moderately severe to severe infections.

**CONTRAINDICATIONS** Hypersensitivity to ampicillin or other penicillins; infections caused by penicillinase-producing organisms; infectious mononucleosis.

**CAUTIOUS USE** History of hypersensitivity to cephalosporins; GI disorders; renal disease or impairment; pregnancy (category B); lactation.

## ROUTE & DOSAGE

**Systemic Infections**

*Adult:* **PO/IV/IM** 250–500 mg q6h
*Child (less than 40 kg):* **PO/IV** 25–50 mg/kg/day divided q6–8h
*Neonate:* **IV/IM** Younger than 7 days, weight 2000 g: 50 mg/kg/day divided q12h; Younger than 7 days, weight 2000 g or more: 75 mg/kg/day divided q8h; 7 days or older, weight 1200 g or more: 50 mg/kg/day

Common adverse effects in *italic;* life-threatening effects <u>underlined</u>; generic names in **bold**; classifications in SMALL CAPS; ♦ Canadian drug name; ⓟ Prototype drug

divided q12h; *7 days or older,*
*weight 1200–2000 g:* 75 mg/kg/
day divided q8h; *7 days or older,*
*weight greater than 2000 g:*
100 mg/kg/day divided q6h

**Meningitis**

*Adult/Child:* **IV** 150–200 mg/kg/
day divided q3–4h
*Neonate:* **IV/IM** *Younger than*
*7 days, weight less than 2000 g:*
100 mg/kg/day divided q12h;
*Younger than 7 days, weight*
*2000 g or more:* 150 mg/kg/day
divided q8h; *older than 7 days,*
*weight less than 1200 g:* 100 mg/
kg/day divided 2h; *older than 7*
*days, weight 1200–2000 g:* 150
mg/kg/day divided q8h; *older*
*than 7 days, weight greater than*
*2000 g:* 200 mg/kg/day divided
q6h

**Gonorrhea**

*Adult:* **PO** 3.5 g with 1 g
probenecid × 1; **IV/IM** 500 mg
q8–12h

**Bacterial Endocarditis**
**Prophylaxis**

*Adult:* **IV** 2 g 30 min before
procedure
*Child:* **IV** 50 mg/kg 30 min before
procedure (max: 2 g)

**Group B Strep Prophylaxis**

*Adult:* **IV** 2 g, then 1 g q4h until
delivery

***Renal Impairment Dosage***
***Adjustment***

*CrCl 10–30 mL/min:* Give
q6–12h; *less than 10 mL/min:*
Give q12h

***Hemodialysis Dosage Adjustment***

Dose should be given after dialysis

## ADMINISTRATION

### Oral

- Give with a full glass of water on
an empty stomach (at least 1 h
before or 2 h after meals) for
maximum absorption. Food
hampers rate and extent of oral
absorption.

### Intramuscular

- Reconstitute each vial by adding
the indicated amount of sterile water for injection or bacteriostatic
water for injection (1.2 mL to
125 mg; 1 mL to 250 mg; 1.8 mL to
500 mg; 3.5 mL to 1 g; 6.8 mL
to 2 g). All reconstituted vials yield
250 mg/mL except the 125 mg vial
which yields 125 mg/mL. Administer within 1 h of preparation.
- Withdraw the ordered dose and
inject deep IM into a large muscle.

### Intravenous

Verify correct IV concentration
and rate of infusion with prescriber for administration to neonates, infants, and children.

*PREPARE:* **Direct/Intermittent:** Reconstitute as follows with sterile
water for injection: Add 5 mL to
500 mg or fraction thereof; add
7.4 mL to 1 g; add 14.8 mL to 2 g
Final concentration **must be**
30 mg/mL or less; may be given
direct IV as prepared or further
diluted in 50 mL or more of NS,
D5W, D5/NS, D5W/0.45NaCl, or
LR. ■ Stability of solution varies
with diluent and concentration of
solution. Solutions in NS are stable for up to 8 h at room temperature; other solutions should be
infused within 2–4 h of preparation. Give direct IV within 1 h of
preparation. ■ Wear disposable
gloves when handling drug
repeatedly; contact dermatitis
occurs frequently in sensitized
individuals.

---

Common adverse effects in *italic;* life-threatening effects <u>underlined;</u> generic names
in **bold;** classifications in SMALL CAPS; ♣ Canadian drug name; ❷ Prototype drug

99

***ADMINISTER:*** **Direct/Intermittent:** Infuse 500 mg or less slowly over 3–5 min. Give 1–2 g over at least 15 min. ▪ With solutions of 100 mL or more, set rate according to amount of solution, but no faster than direct IV rate. ▪ Convulsions may be induced by too rapid administration.

***INCOMPATIBILITIES:*** **Solution/additive:** Do not add to a **dextrose**-containing solution unless entire dose is given within 1 h of preparation. **Aztreonam, cefepime, hydrocortisone, prochlorperazine.** **Y-site:** **Amphotericin B, epinephrine, fenoldopam, fluconazole, hydralazine, lansoprazole, midazolam, nicardipine, ondansetron, sargramostim, TPN, verapamil, vinorelbine.**

▪ Store capsules and unopened vials at 15°–30° C (59°–86° F) unless otherwise directed. Keep oral preparations tightly covered.

## ADVERSE EFFECTS (≥1%) **Body as a Whole:** Similar to those for penicillin G. Hypersensitivity (pruritus, urticaria, eosinophilia, hemolytic anemia, interstitial nephritis, <u>anaphylactoid reaction</u>); superinfections. **CNS:** Convulsive seizures with high doses. **GI:** *Diarrhea,* nausea, vomiting, <u>pseudomembranous colitis</u>. **Other:** Severe pain (following IM); phlebitis (following IV). **Skin:** *Rash.*

## DIAGNOSTIC TEST INTERFERENCE
Elevated ***CPK*** levels may result from local skeletal muscle injury following IM injection. ***Urine glucose:*** High urine drug concentrations can result in false-positive test results with ***Clinitest*** or ***Benedict's*** [enzymatic ***glucose oxidase methods*** (e.g., ***Clinistix, Diastix, TesTape***) are not affected].

***AST*** may be elevated (significance not known).

## INTERACTIONS **Drug: Allopurinol** increases incidence of rash. Effectiveness of the AMINOGLYCO-SIDES may be impaired in patients with severe end-stage renal disease. **Chloramphenicol, erythromycin,** and **tetracycline** may reduce bactericidal effects of ampicillin; this interaction is primarily significant when low doses of ampicillin are used. Ampicillin may interfere with the contraceptive action of oral contraceptives (**estrogens**). Female patients should be advised to consider nonhormonal contraception while on antibiotics. **Food:** Food may decrease absorption of ampicillin, so it should be taken 1 h before or 2 h after meals.

## PHARMACOKINETICS **Absorption:** Oral dose is 50% absorbed. Peak effect: 5 min IV, 1 h IM, 2 h PO. **Duration:** 6–8 h. **Distribution:** Most body tissues; high CNS concentrations only with inflamed meninges; crosses the placenta. **Metabolism:** Minimal hepatic metabolism. **Elimination:** 90% in urine; excreted into breast milk. **Half-Life:** 1–1.8 h.

## NURSING IMPLICATIONS
### Assessment & Drug Effects
▪ Determine previous hypersensitivity reactions to penicillins, cephalosporins, and other allergens prior to therapy. Monitor closely for signs of hypersensitivity during first 30 min after administration.
▪ Note: Sodium content of IV drug should be considered in patients on sodium restriction.
▪ Inspect skin daily and instruct patient to do the same. The appearance of a rash should be carefully evaluated to differentiate

a nonallergenic ampicillin rash from a hypersensitivity reaction. Report rash promptly to prescriber.
- Monitor for and report diarrhea which may indicate pseudomembranous colitis.
- Monitor lab tests: Baseline C&S prior to initiation of therapy; baseline and periodic renal, hepatic, and hematologic function tests, particularly during prolonged or high-dose therapy.

**Patient & Family Education**

- Report diarrhea to prescriber; do not self-medicate. Give a detailed report to the prescriber regarding onset, duration, character of stools, associated symptoms, temperature and weight loss to help rule out the possibility of drug-induced, potentially fatal pseudomembranous colitis (see Appendix F).
- Report S&S of superinfection (onset of black, hairy tongue; oral lesions or soreness; rectal or vaginal itching; vaginal discharge; loose, foul-smelling stools; or unusual odor to urine).
- Notify prescriber if no improvement is noted within a few days after therapy is started.
- Take medication around the clock; continue taking medication until it is all gone (usually 10 days) unless otherwise directed by prescriber or pharmacist.

# AMPICILLIN SODIUM AND SULBACTAM SODIUM

(am-pi-sill'in/sul-bak'tam)

Unasyn

**Classifications:** ANTIBIOTIC; AMINOPENICILLIN
Therapeutic: ANTIBIOTIC
**Prototype:** Ampicillin

**AVAILABILITY** Injection

## ACTION & *THERAPEUTIC EFFECT*

Ampicillin inhibits the final stage of bacterial cell wall synthesis by binding to specific penicillin-binding proteins (PBPs) located inside the bacterial cell wall, thus destroying the cell wall. Sulbactam inhibits beta-lactamases, most frequently responsible for transferred drug resistance. Thus the spectrum of drugs affected by the combination of the two is increased. *Effective against both gram-positive and gram-negative bacteria including those that produce beta-lactamase and nonbeta-lactamase producers. Ampicillin without sulbactam is not effective against beta-lactamase producing strains.*

**USES** Treatment of infections due to susceptible organisms in skin and skin structures, intra-abdominal infections, and gynecologic infections.

**CONTRAINDICATIONS** Hypersensitivity to ampicillin or other penicillins; mononucleosis; infections caused by penicillinase-producing organisms.

**CAUTIOUS USE** Hypersensitivity to cephalosporins; GI disorders; renal disease or impairment; pregnancy (category B) or lactation.

## ROUTE & DOSAGE

### Systemic Infections

*Adult/Adolescent/Child (weight greater than 40 kg):* **IV/IM** 1.5–3 g q6h (max: 4 g sulbactam/day) *Child (1 y or older, less than 40 kg):* **IV** 300 mg/kg/day (200 mg/kg ampicillin and 100 mg/kg sulbactam) divided q6h

### *Renal Impairment Dosage Adjustment*

*CrCl 15–29 mL/min:* Give q12h; *5–14 mL/min:* Give q24h *Dialysis:* Give dose after dialysis

---

Common adverse effects in *italic;* life-threatening effects underlined; generic names in **bold;** classifications in SMALL CAPS; ♣ Canadian drug name; ⊙ Prototype drug

## ADMINISTRATION

### Intramuscular

- Reconstitute solution with sterile water for injection by adding 6.4 mL diluent to a 3 g vial. Each mL contains 250 mg ampicillin and 125 mg sulbactam.
- Give deep IM into a large muscle. Rotate injection sites.

### Intravenous

*PREPARE:* **Direct/Intermittent:** Reconstitute each 1.5 g vial with 3.2 mL of sterile water for injection to yield 375 mg/mL (250 mg ampicillin/125 mg sulbactam); must further dilute with NS, D5W, D5/NS, D5W/0.45NS, or LR to a final concentration within the range of 3–45 mg/mL. *ADMINISTER:* **Direct:** Give slowly over at least 10–15 min. **Intermittent:** Infuse solutions of less than 50 mL over 10–15 min and solutions of 50–100 mL over 15–30 min. With solutions of 100 mL or more, set rate according to amount of solution but no faster than direct IV rate (e.g., 100 mL over 30 min). ▪ Convulsions may be induced by too rapid administration. ▪ Use only freshly prepared solution; administer within 1 h after preparation. *INCOMPATIBILITIES:* **Solution/additive:** Do not add to a **dextrose**-containing solution unless entire dose is given within 1 h of preparation. **Ciprofloxacin, tranexamic acid. Y-site:** Acyclovir, amiodarone, amphotericin B, azathioprine, caspofungin, chlorpromazine, ciprofloxacin, dacarbazine, dantrolene, danorubicin, diazepam, diazoxide, dobutamine, dolasetron, doxorubicin, doxycycline, epirubicin, ganciclovir, garenoxacin, hydralazine, hydrocortisone, hydroxyzine, idarubicin, lansoprazole, lorazepam, mechlorethamine, methylprednisolone, midazolam, minocycline, mitoxantrone, mycophenolate, nesiritide, nicardipine, ondansetron, papaverine, pentamidine, pentazocine, phenytoin, prochlorperazine, promethazine, protamine, quinidine, quinupristin/dalfopristin sargramostim, SMZ/TMP, topotecan, tranexamic, verapamil, vinorelbine.**

- Store powder for injection at 15°–30° C (59°–86° F) before reconstitution. Storage times and temperatures vary for different concentrations of reconstituted solutions; consult manufacturer's directions.

## ADVERSE EFFECTS (≥1%) **Body as a Whole:** Hypersensitivity (rash, itching, <u>anaphylactoid reaction</u>), fatigue, malaise, headache, chills, edema. **GI:** *Diarrhea, nausea,* vomiting, abdominal distention, candidiasis. **Hematologic:** Neutropenia, <u>thrombocytopenia</u>. **Urogenital:** Dysuria. **CNS:** Seizures. **Other:** Local pain at injection site; thrombophlebitis.

## INTERACTIONS **Drug: Allopurinol** increases incidence of rash; effectiveness of the AMINOGLYCOSIDES may be impaired in patients with severe end stage renal disease; **chloramphenicol, erythromycin, tetracycline** may reduce bactericidal effects of ampicillin—this interaction is primarily significant when low doses are used; ampicillin may interfere with the contraceptive action of ORAL CONTRACEPTIVES—female patients should be advised to consider nonhormonal contraception while on antibiotics.

Common adverse effects in *italic;* life-threatening effects <u>underlined;</u> generic names in **bold;** classifications in SMALL CAPS; ♣ Canadian drug name; ⓞ Prototype drug

## PHARMACOKINETICS Peak:
Immediate after IV. **Duration:** 6–8 h. **Distribution:** Most body tissues; high CNS concentrations only with inflamed meninges; crosses placenta; appears in breast milk. **Metabolism:** Minimal hepatic metabolism. **Elimination:** In urine. **Half-Life:** 1 h.

## NURSING IMPLICATIONS

### Assessment & Drug Effects
- Determine previous hypersensitivity reactions to penicillins, cephalosporins, and other allergens prior to therapy.
- Report promptly unexplained bleeding (e.g., epistaxis, purpura, ecchymoses).
- Monitor patient carefully during the first 30 min after initiation of IV therapy for signs of hypersensitivity and anaphylactoid reaction (see Appendix F). Serious anaphylactoid reactions require immediate use of emergency drugs and airway management.
- Monitor for and report diarrhea which may indicate pseudomembranous colitis. Observe for and report other S&S of superinfection.
- Monitor I&O ratio and pattern. Report dysuria, urine retention, and hematuria.
- Monitor lab tests: Baseline C&S prior to initiation of therapy; baseline and periodic renal, hepatic, and hematologic function tests, particularly during prolonged or high-dose therapy.

### Patient & Family Education
- Report chills, wheezing, pruritus (itching), respiratory distress, or palpitations to prescriber immediately.
- Report diarrhea to prescriber; do not self-medicate.

## ANAGRELIDE HYDROCHLORIDE
(a-na′gre-lyde)

Agrylin

**Classifications:** ANTICOAGULANT; ANTIPLATELET
Therapeutic: ANTIPLATELET; REDUCER OF PLATELET COUNT

## AVAILABILITY Capsule

## ACTION & THERAPEUTIC EFFECT
Causes dose-related reduction in platelet production. It inhibits platelet aggregation by affecting several aggregating agents (e.g., thrombin and arachidonic acid, ADP, and collagen). *Anagrelide is associated with significant decreases in platelet counts and is thought to prevent early changes in shape of platelets.*

## USES Essential thrombocythemia.

## UNLABELED USES Polycythemia vera, chronic myelogenous leukemia.

## CONTRAINDICATIONS Severe hepatic impairment; congenital QT prolongation; hypokalemia; lactation.

## CAUTIOUS USE Cardiovascular disease, history of acquired QT prolongation; mild and moderate hepatic impairment, renal impairment; pulmonary disease; jaundice; pregnancy (category C); children.

## ROUTE & DOSAGE

### Essential Thrombocythemia

*Adult (16 y or older):* **PO** Start with 0.5 mg q.i.d. or 1 mg b.i.d. × 1 wk, may increase by 0.5 mg/day qwk until platelet count is less than 600,000/mcL (max: 10 mg/day)

---

Common adverse effects in *italic*; life-threatening effects underlined; generic names in **bold**; classifications in SMALL CAPS; ♣ Canadian drug name; ⊘ Prototype drug

103

**Hepatic Impairment Dosage Adjustment**

0.5 mg daily for 1 wk

## ADMINISTRATION

### Oral

- Make sure dosage increments do not exceed 0.5 mg/day in any 1 wk.
- Store at 15°–25° C (59°–77° F) in a light-resistant container.

## ADVERSE EFFECTS (≥1%) **Body as a Whole:** *Asthenia, pain,* paresthesia, back pain, malaise, fever, chills, photosensitivity. **CNS:** *Headache, dizziness,* CVA, syncope, seizures. **CV:** *Palpitations,* chest pain, tachycardia, peripheral edema, *edema (general),* CHF, MI, cardiomyopathy, heart block, atrial fibrillation, pericarditis, arrhythmia, hemorrhage. **GI:** *Diarrhea, abdominal pain, nausea,* flatulence, vomiting, dyspepsia, anorexia, pancreatitis, constipation, GI hemorrhage, and ulceration. **Hematologic:** Anemia, thrombocytopenia, ecchymoses, lymphedema. **Respiratory:** *Dyspnea,* pulmonary infiltrates, pulmonary fibrosis, pulmonary hypertension. **Skin:** Rash, urticaria. **Other:** Dysuria.

## PHARMACOKINETICS **Absorption:** 70% from GI tract. Food reduces bioavailability. **Onset:** 7–14 days. **Duration:** Increased platelet counts were observed 4 days after discontinuing drug. **Metabolism:** Extensively metabolized. **Elimination:** Primarily in urine as metabolites. **Half-Life:** 1.3–1.8 h.

## NURSING IMPLICATIONS

### Assessment & Drug Effects

- Monitor for therapeutic effectiveness which is indicated by reduction of platelets for at least 4 wk to 600,000/mcL or less or 50% from baseline.
- Monitor for S&S of CHF or myocardial ischemia.
- Monitor for S&S of renal toxicity in patients with renal insufficiency (creatinine 2 mg/dL or more).
- Monitor for S&S of hepatic toxicity in patients with liver functions greater than 1.5 times upper limit of normal.
- Monitor lab tests: Platelet count q2days for first wk, weekly thereafter until maintenance dose reached; frequent Hgb, WBC count, LFTs, BUN, creatinine, and serum electrolytes while platelet count is being lowered.

### Patient & Family Education

- Contact prescriber if palpitations, fluid retention, breathing difficulty, or any other distressful symptoms develop.
- Avoid excessive exposure to sunlight or UV light.

## ANAKINRA

(an-a-kin′ra)

Kineret

**Classifications:** IMMUNOMODULATOR; INTERLEUKIN-1 RECEPTOR ANTAGONIST; DISEASE-MODIFYING ANTIRHEUMATIC DRUG (DMARD)

**Therapeutic:** ANTIRHEUMATIC; DMARD

## AVAILABILITY Solution for injection

## ACTION & *THERAPEUTIC EFFECT*

An interleukin-1 (IL-1) receptor antagonist that inhibits IL-1 binding to interleukin receptors present in both bone and cartilage (as well as other tissues). IL-1 is produced in response to inflammation and mediates various responses of tissues, including inflammatory and immunologic responses. *Anakinra competes with interleukin-1 (IL-1) by inhibiting it from binding to its receptor sites in tissues.*

**USES** Treatment of rheumatoid arthritis; neonatal-onset multisystem inflammatory disease (NOMID).

**CONTRAINDICATIONS** Hypersensitivity to anakinra, *E. coli*–derived products, latex; active infections; live vaccines.

**CAUTIOUS USE** Neutropenia, immunosuppressed patients, or patients with frequent, serious infections; asthmatics; older adults; renal impairment; pregnancy (category B), lactation; children.

## ROUTE & DOSAGE

**Rheumatoid Arthritis**

*Adult:* Subcutaneous 100 mg daily

**NOMID**

*Adult:* Subcutaneous 1–2 mg/kg daily, may taper up to max dose: 8 mg/kg/day

*Child:* Subcutaneous 1–2 mg/kg; may increase to 3–4mg/kg/day

## ADMINISTRATION

**Subcutaneous Only**

- Do not give anakinra if the patient has an active infection.
- Note that anakinra should not ordinarily be given with tumor necrosis factor (TNF) blocking agents.
- Discard any unused portions as the drug contains no preservative.
- Check expiration date and do not use if expired, discolored, or if an excessive number of translucent particles appears in the syringe.
- To decrease injection site reactions, apply a cold compress before/after injection and warm solution to room temperature 60–90 min before injection.
- Store in the refrigerator at 2°–8° C (36°–46° F). **Do not freeze or shake.** Protect from light.

**ADVERSE EFFECTS** (≥1%) **Body as a Whole:** *Bacterial infections (URI, sinusitis, flu, other), fever.* **CNS:** Headache. **GI:** Pharyngitis, nausea, vomiting, diarrhea, abdominal pain. **Hematologic:** Decreased neutrophil count, antibody formation. **Other:** *Fever, injection site reactions (erythema, ecchymosis, edema, inflammation, pain).*

**INTERACTIONS Drug:** Increased risk of infection with live virus vaccine, TUMOR NECROSIS FACTOR MODIFIERS. Increased risk of neutropenia as well as infection with **etanercept** and **infliximab.**

**PHARMACOKINETICS Absorption:** 95% absorbed subcutaneous site. **Peak:** 3–7 h. **Elimination:** In urine. **Half-Life:** 4–6 h.

## NURSING IMPLICATIONS

### Assessment & Drug Effects

- Monitor for S&S of infection (e.g., pneumonia or other URI, cellulitis). Withhold drug and notify prescriber if these appear.
- Monitor closely patients with impaired renal function for S&S of adverse drug reactions.
- Assess for injection site reactions manifested by erythema, ecchymosis, inflammation, and pain.
- Monitor lab tests: Absolute TB baseline test, absolute neutrophil count (ANC) prior to initiating anakinra, monthly for 3 mo, and q3mo thereafter for 1 y.

### Patient & Family Education

- Review carefully the "Information for Patients and Caregivers" leaflet for detailed instructions on handling and injecting anakinra.
- Give the injection at approximately the same time every day.

---

Common adverse effects in *italic*; life-threatening effects <u>underlined</u>; generic names in **bold**; classifications in SMALL CAPS; ♣Canadian drug name; ⊕ Prototype drug

- Administer only 1 dose (the entire contents of 1 prefilled glass syringe) per day. Discard any unused portions as the drug contains no preservative. Do not save unused drug.
- Do not permit vaccination with live vaccines while taking anakinra.
- Withhold drug and notify prescriber for S&S of upper respiratory, skin, or other infection(s).

# ANASTROZOLE ℗ᵣ

(a-nas'tro-zole)

Arimidex

**Classifications:** ANTINEOPLASTIC; NONSTEROIDAL AROMATASE INHIBITOR
Therapeutic: ANTINEOPLASTIC

## AVAILABILITY Tablet

## ACTION & THERAPEUTIC EFFECT

Anastrozole is a potent and selective nonsteroidal aromatase inhibitor that converts estrone to estradiol. It lowers serum estrogen levels in postmenopausal women without interfering with adrenal steroid synthesis. *Inhibiting the biosynthesis of estrogens is one way to deprive tumors of estrogens, and thus restrict tumor growth.*

## USES Early and advanced breast cancer with hormone receptor positive or hormone status unknown in postmenopausal women.

## CONTRAINDICATIONS Premenopausal women, postmenopausal hormone replacement therapy; severe hepatic disease, pregnancy (category D); lactation.

## CAUTIOUS USE Mild to moderate hepatic disease; older adults; children.

## ROUTE & DOSAGE

**Breast Cancer**
*Adult:* **PO** 1 mg once daily

## ADMINISTRATION

### Oral

- Give on an empty stomach, 1 h before or 2 h after meals, because food affects extent of absorption.
- Store at 20°–25° C (68°–77° F).

## ADVERSE EFFECTS (≥1%) CNS:
Asthenia, headache, hot flushes, pain, dizziness, depression, paresthesia, malaise, insomnia, confusion, anxiety, nervousness. **CV:** Chest pain, hypertension, thrombophlebitis, ischemic cardiac events, edema. **GI:** *Diarrhea,* nausea, vomiting, constipation, abdominal pain, anorexia, dry mouth, increased liver function tests (ALT, AST, GGT). **Respiratory:** Dyspnea, cough, pharyngitis, bronchitis, rhinitis, sinusitis. **Other:** Rash, peripheral edema, pelvic pain, flulike syndrome.

## PHARMACOKINETICS Absorption: Rapidly absorbed from GI tract. **Distribution:** 40% protein bound. **Metabolism:** 85% metabolized in liver to inactive metabolites. **Elimination:** 10% excreted unchanged; 60% as metabolites in urine. **Half-Life:** 50 h.

## NURSING IMPLICATIONS

### Assessment & Drug Effects

- Assess for hypertension, complications of edema, thrombotic events, and signs of liver toxicity.
- Monitor lab tests: Periodic total cholesterol and lipid profile.

### Patient & Family Education

- Recognize common adverse effects and seek information on measures to control discomfort.
- Seek medical attention if you experience chest pain, calf pain, or shortness of breath; unexplained loss of appetite or nausea; jaundice.

Common adverse effects in *italic;* life-threatening effects underlined; generic names in **bold;** classifications in SMALL CAPS; ♣ Canadian drug name; ℗ Prototype drug

# ANIDULAFUNGIN

(a-ni-dul'a-fun-gin)
Eraxis
**Classifications:** ECHINOCANDIN ANTIFUNGAL
Therapeutic: ANTIFUNGAL
**Prototype:** Caspofungin

**AVAILABILITY** Powder for injection

**ACTION & *THERAPEUTIC EFFECT***
Anidulafungin is a semisynthetic echinocandin that inhibits glucan synthase, an enzyme present in fungal cells. Glucan is an essential component of the fungal cell wall; therefore, anidulafungin causes fungal cell death. *Interferes with reproduction and growth of susceptible fungi.*

**USES** Treatment of candidemia and other *Candida* infections caused by *C. albicans, C. glabrata, C. parapsilosis,* and *C. tropicalis.* Treatment of esophageal candidiasis.

**UNLABELED USES** Fungal prophylaxis in immunocompromised children who are hospitalized with neutropenia.

**CONTRAINDICATIONS** Hypersensitivity to anidulafungin or another echinocandin antifungal; lactation.

**CAUTIOUS USE** Hepatic impairment; pregnancy (category C). Safety and efficacy in children not established.

## ROUTE & DOSAGE

### Candidemia and Other *Candida* Infections

*Adult:* **IV** 200 mg loading dose on day 1, then 100 mg IV daily for at least 14 days after last positive culture

### Esophageal Candidiasis

*Adult:* **IV** 100 mg loading dose on day 1, then 50 mg IV daily for at least 14 days (and for at least 7 days after resolution of symptoms)

## ADMINISTRATION

**Intravenous**

*PREPARE:* **IV Infusion:** The reconstituted solution must be further diluted in NS or D5W to a final concentration of 0.77 mg/mL as follows: Dilute a 50 mg dose in 50 mL IV fluid; dilute a 100 mg dose in 100 mL IV fluid; dilute a 200 mg dose in 200 mL IV fluid.
*ADMINISTER:* **IV Infusion:** Give at a rate **no greater** than 1.1 mg/min. **Do not** give a bolus dose.
*INCOMPATIBILITIES:* **Y-site: Amphotericin B, ertapenem, sodium bicarbonate.**

▪ Store unreconstituted vials, reconstituted vials, and companion diluent vials at 15°–30° C (59°–86° F). Reconstituted vials **must be** further diluted and administered within 24 h.

**ADVERSE EFFECTS** (≥1%) **Body as a Whole:** Hypersensitivity. **CNS:** Headache. **GI:** Diarrhea, nausea. **Hematologic:** Neutropenia. **Metabolic:** Increased alkaline phosphatase, increased ALT, increased gamma-glutamyl transferase, hypokalemia. **Skin:** Rash.

**INTERACTIONS Drug: Cyclosporin** increases overall systemic exposure (i.e., area under the curve, or AUC).

**PHARMACOKINETICS Distribution:** 84% protein bound. **Metabolism:** Nonhepatic degradation to inactive metabolites. **Elimination:** Fecal. **Half-Life:** 40–50 h.

## NURSING IMPLICATIONS

### Assessment & Drug Effects

- Prior to initiating therapy with anidulafungin, obtain specimen for fungal culture.
- Monitor for and report S&S of hypersensitivity (e.g., dyspnea, flushing, hypotension, swelling about the face, pruritus, rash, and urticaria), abnormal LFTs, or liver dysfunction (e.g., jaundice, clay-colored stools).
- Discontinue infusion if signs of hypersensitivity appear.
- Monitor cardiac status especially with a preexisting history of dysrhythmias.
- Monitor for S&S hypokalemia and hepatic toxicity (see Appendix F).
- Monitor diabetics for loss of glycemic control.
- Monitor lab tests: Baseline and periodic LFTs.

### Patient & Family Education

- Report any of the following immediately if experienced during or shortly after infusion: Difficulty breathing, swelling about the face, itching, rash.
- Report S&S of jaundice to the prescriber: Clay-colored stool, dark urine, yellow skin or sclera, unexplained abdominal pain, or fatigue.

## APIXABAN

(a-pix′a-ban)

Eliquis

**Classifications:** ANTICOAGULANT; ANTITHROMBOTIC; SELECTIVE FACTOR XA INHIBITOR

Therapeutic: ANTICOAGULANT; ANTITHROMBOTIC

**Prototype:** Rivaroxaban

**AVAILABILITY** Tablet

## ACTION & *THERAPEUTIC EFFECT*

A reversible, selective active site inhibitor of factor Xa that does not require antithrombin III for antithrombotic activity; indirectly inhibits platelet aggregation induced by thrombin. *By inhibiting FXa, apixaban decreases thrombin generation and clot development.*

**USES** Reduction of the risk of stroke and systemic embolism in patients with nonvalvular atrial fibrillation, DVT prophylaxis.

**CONTRAINDICATIONS** Severe hypersensitivity to apixaban; active pathological bleeding; 48 h before surgery; severe hepatic impairment; CrCl less than 25 mL/min; prosthetic heart valves or significant rheumatic heart disease; lactation.

**CAUTIOUS USE** Moderate hepatic or renal impairment; older adults; pregnancy (category B). Safety and efficacy in children not established.

## ROUTE & DOSAGE

### Reduction of Stroke and Systemic Embolism

*Adult:* **PO** 5 mg b.i.d.
*Adult with at least 2 of the following: 80 y or older, weight 60 kg or less, or serum creatinine 1.5 mg/dL or more:* **PO** 2.5 mg b.i.d.

### DVT Prophylaxis

*Adult:* **PO** 2.5 mg b.i.d. × 12 d (after knee replacement) or × 35 d (after hip replacement)

### DVT/PE Treatment

*Adult:* **PO** 10 mg b.i.d. × 7d then 5 mg bid

### *Dosage Adjustment if Coadministered with Dual CYP3A4 and P-gp Inhibitors*

Decrease dose to 2.5 mg b.i.d.

Common adverse effects in *italic;* life-threatening effects <u>underlined;</u> generic names in **bold;** classifications in SMALL CAPS; ♣ Canadian drug name; ⊘ Prototype drug

*Renal Impairment Dosage Adjustment (for patients with Nonvalvular Atrial Fibrillation)*

Adult 80 y or older and/or weighs 60 kg or less with serum creatinine 1.5 mg/dL or more: **PO** 2.5 mg twice daily

## ADMINISTRATION

### Oral

- May be given without regard to food.
- For patients that have difficulty swallowing, apixaban can be crushed and suspended in apple juice or applesauce for prompt administration. Alternatively, tablets can be crushed and suspended in 60 mL of water and promptly delivered through nasogastric tube.
- Store at 20°–25° C (68°–77° F).

## ADVERSE EFFECTS (≥ 1%) Hematological: *Increased bleeding risk*, anemia.

## INTERACTIONS Drug: Inhibitors of CYP3A4 and P-gp (e.g., **ketoconazole, itraconazole, ritonavir, clarithromycin**) may increase apixaban levels. Inducers of CYP3A4 and P-gp (e.g., **rifampin, carbamazepine, phenytoin, primidone**) may decrease apixaban levels. Use with POTASSIUM-SPARING DIURETICS may increase serum potassium. Avoid use with other ANTICOAGULANT agents. **Herbal: St. John's wort** may decrease apixaban levels.

## PHARMACOKINETICS Absorption: 50% bioavailable. Peak: 3–4 h. Distribution: 87% plasma protein bound. Metabolism: In liver (25%). Elimination: Renal (27%) and fecal (73%). Half-Life: 12 h.

## NURSING IMPLICATIONS

### Black Box Warning

*Discontinuing apixaba without replacement with another anticoagulant increases the risk of thrombotic events in patients with nonvalvular atrial fibrillation.*

### Assessment & Drug Effects

- Report promptly suspected or overt bleeding. Patients are at higher risk for bleeding with concomitant use of drugs such as aspirin, antiplatelet agents or anticoagulants agents, thrombolytic agents, SSRIs, SNRIs, or NSAIDs.
- Note: There is no established way to reverse anticoagulant effect of apixaban, which can persist for about 24 h after last dose.

### Patient & Family Education

- Do not stop taking this drug without consulting your prescriber.
- If you miss a dose, take it as soon as you remember but do not take more than one dose at the same time to make up for a missed dose.
- Do not take aspirin or other OTC pain relievers, such as NSAIDs, that could increase the risk of bleeding.
- Report promptly to prescriber if you experience any of the following: Unexpected, prolonged, or severe bleeding; red, pink, or brown urine; red or black tarry stools; coughing up blood; vomiting blood or your vomit looks like coffee grounds; unexpected pain, swelling, or joint pain; headaches, feeling dizzy or weak.
- Do not breast-feed while taking this drug.

## APOMORPHINE HYDROCHLORIDE

(a-po-mor'feen)

---

Common adverse effects in *italic*; life-threatening effects underlined; generic names in **bold**; classifications in SMALL CAPS; ◆Canadian drug name; ☺ Prototype drug

109

**Apokyn**
**Classifications:** ANTIPARKINSON;
DOPAMINE RECEPTOR AGONIST
**Therapeutic:** ANTIPARKINSON
**Prototype:** Levodopa

**AVAILABILITY** Injection

**ACTION & *THERAPEUTIC EFFECT***
A central dopamine receptor agonist that is thought to stimulate centrally located postsynaptic dopamine $D_2$-type receptors. *Diminishes hypomobility associated with "off" episodes ("end-of-dose wearing off" and unpredictable "on/off" episodes) in persons with advanced Parkinson's disease.*

**USES** Rescue of "off" episodes associated with advanced Parkinson's disease.

**CONTRAINDICATIONS** Hypersensitivity to the drug or its ingredients (i.e., sodium metabisulfite), benzyl alcohol hypersensitivity; renal failure; QT prolongation; heart failure, or shock; depression, suicidal ideation; decreased alertness, seizures, seizure disorder, unconscious state or coma, decreased alertness; lactation.

**CAUTIOUS USE** Hypersensitivity to sulfites; cardiovascular, cerebrovascular, respiratory, renal, or hepatic disease; CNS depression, history of (chronic) depression or suicidal ideation; hypotension; vomiting; bradycardia; hypokalemia and hypomagnesemia; older adult; pregnancy (category C).

**ROUTE & DOSAGE**

**"Off" Episodes of
Parkinson's Disease**

*Adult:* **Subcutaneous** Start with a test dose where BP can be closely monitored. Escalate test dose no sooner than 2 h after last dose until dose is not tolerated or patient has response. *If test dose of 0.2 mL (2 mg) is tolerated and has positive response:* Continue with 0.2 mL (2 mg); *if no response:* Use test dose of 0.4 mL (4 mg); *if tolerated and has a positive response:* Continue with 0.3 mL (3 mg); *if 0.4 mL test dose is not tolerated:* Try 0.3 mL (3 mg) test dose; *if 0.3 mL is tolerated:* Continue with 0.2 mL (2 mg). May increase by 1 mg every few days, generally should not exceed 0.4 mL (4 mg) as an outpatient (max: 0.6 mL as single injection and max 5 injections/day) *If therapy is interrupted for 1 wk:* Restart with 2 mg dose.

**ADMINISTRATION**

**Subcutaneous**
- Aspirate to avoid intravascular injection and ensure the injection is subcutaneous and not intradermal.
- Rotate subcutaneous sites to reduce skin reactions.
- If the patient has not received apomorphine in more than 1 wk, reinstitute it by starting with the initial test dose and titrating to the desired dose.
- Apomorphine causes nausea and vomiting; thus the recommendation is to give 300 mg of trimethobenzamide PO t.i.d., starting 3 days before the first injection and continued for at least the first 2 mo of treatment.
- Store at 15°–30° C (59°–86° F).

**ADVERSE EFFECTS** (≥1%) **Body as a Whole:** Weakness, yawning, tiredness. **CNS:** CNS depression, *dizziness, drowsiness,* headache, lightheadedness, euphoria, restlessness, tremor, depression, *dyskinesias, hallucinations.* **CV:** Acute circulatory failure, *angina,* bradycardia, hypertension, *orthostatic hypotension,* QT prolongation, vasovagal response, syncope. **GI:** *Nausea, vomiting,* hypersalivation, taste perversions. **Metabolic:** Peripheral edema. **Respiratory:** Respiratory depression, tachypnea, cough, pharyngitis, *rhinitis.* **Skin:** Contact dermatitis, *bruising,* granuloma, pruritus, sweating. **Urogenital:** *Frequent penile erections,* painful erections.

**INTERACTIONS Drug:** Alosetron, **dolasetron, granisetron, ondansetron, palonosetron** may cause severe hypotension and unconsciousness; **alfuzosin, amoxapine, bepridil, chloroquine, clozapine, cyclobenzaprine, droperidol, flecainide, halofantrine, halothane, levomethadyl,** LOCAL ANESTHETICS, MACROLIDES **(clarithromycin, erythromycin, troleandomycin), maprotiline, mefloquine, methadone, pentamidine,** PHENOTHIAZINES, **probucol, gatifloxacin, gemifloxacin, grepafloxacin, levofloxacin, moxifloxacin, sparfloxacin, tacrolimus,** TRICYCLIC ANTIDEPRESSANTS, **amiodarone, clozapine, disopyramide, dofetilide, dolasetron, haloperidol, ibutilide, mesoridazine, palonosetron, pimozide, procainamide, quinidine, thioridazine, sotalol, ziprasidone** may exacerbate QT$_c$ prolongation; may increase CNS depression with other CNS depressants, including TRICYCLIC ANTIDEPRESSANTS, ANXIOLYTICS, SEDATIVES, HYPNOTICS, **dronabinol,** GENERAL ANESTHETICS, **mirtazapine, nefazodone,** OPIATE AGONISTS, **pramipexole, ropinirole,** SKELETAL MUSCLE RELAXANTS, **tramadol, trazodone. Herbal: Kava** may increase the symptoms of Parkinson's disease.

**PHARMACOKINETICS Absorption:** Subcutaneous absorption dependent on site utilized—abdominal injection absorbed faster than thigh; lowering the temperature of the injection site slows absorption. **Onset:** 7–14 min. **Peak:** 40–60 min. **Duration:** Up to 2 h. **Distribution:** 85–90% protein bound. **Metabolism:** Metabolized by glucuronidation, sulfation, and N-demethylation. **Elimination:** Excreted by kidneys. **Half-Life:** 30–60 min

## NURSING IMPLICATIONS

### Assessment & Drug Effects
- Periodic ECG, especially in those with known CV disease.
- Withhold drug and notify prescriber for S&S of torsades de pointes (i.e., palpitations and syncope), especially in those with bradycardia or suspected hypokalemia or hypomagnesemia.
- Monitor closely for orthostatic hypotension, especially when doses are increased, and in patients taking antihypertensive medications and vasodilators (especially nitrates).
- Monitor orthostatic vital signs. Institute fall precautions, especially if orthostatic hypotension occurs.

### Patient & Family Education
- Avoid the use of alcohol while taking this drug.
- Report promptly any of the following: Irregular or fast, pounding heartbeat, or palpitations; dizziness, light-headedness, or fainting; unexplained weakness, tiredness, or sleepiness; confusion, hallucinations, or depression; unusual body movements; vomiting; or prolonged painful erections.
- Do not engage in potentially hazardous activities until reaction to drug is known.

Common adverse effects in *italic;* life-threatening effects underlined; generic names in **bold**; classifications in SMALL CAPS; ♣ Canadian drug name; ☯ Prototype drug

111

# APRACLONIDINE

(a-pra-clo'ni-deen)

Iopidine

See Appendix A-1.

# APREMILAST

(a-prem'i-last)

Otezla

**Classifications:** ANTIARTHRITIC; PHOSPHODIESTERASE 4 INHIBITOR

Therapeutic: ANTIARTHRITIC

**AVAILABILITY** Tablet

## ACTION & *THERAPEUTIC EFFECT*

Inhibits the enzyme, phosphodiesterase 4 (PDE4), specific for cAMP which results in increased intracellular cAMP levels and regulation of numerous inflammatory mediators (e.g., decreased expression of nitric oxide synthase, TNF-alpha, and IL 23). *Decrease pain and inflammation in affected joint and other tissues.*

**USES** Treatment of adult patients with active psoriatic arthritis.

**CONTRAINDICATIONS** Known hypersensitivity to apremilast or any components in the formulation; suicidal ideation; unexplained or clinically significant weight loss.

**CAUTIOUS USE** History of depression and/or suicidal thoughts; weight loss; severe renal impairment; pregnancy (category C); lactation. Safety and efficacy in children younger than 18 y not established.

## ROUTE & DOSAGE

### Psoriatic Arthritis

*Adult:* **PO** 30 mg b.i.d. following a 5 day titration: *Day 1:* 10 mg in a.m.; *Day 2:* 10 mg b.i.d.; *Day 3:* 10 mg a.m., 20 mg p.m.; *Day 4:* 20 mg b.i.d.; *Day 5:* 20 mg a.m., 30 mg p.m.

### *Renal Impairment Dosage Adjustment*

*CrCl less than 30 mL/min:* 30 mg once daily

## ADMINISTRATION

### Oral
- Administer without regard to food.
- Tablet **must not be** crushed, chewed, or divided.
- Store below 30° C (86° F).

**ADVERSE EFFECTS** (≥ 1%) **Body as a Whole:** Fatigue, folliculitis. **CNS:** Depression, *headache,* insomnia, sinus headache, tooth abcess. **GI:** *Diarrhea,* dyspepsia, *nausea,* vomiting. **Metabolic:** Decreased appetite, decreased weight. **Musculoskeletal:** Abdominal pain upper, back pain. **Respiratory:** Bronchitis, nasopharyngitis, upper respiratory tract infection.

**INTERACTIONS Drug:** Strong CYP450 inducers (i.e., **rifampin**) decrease the levels of apremilast. **Herbal: St. John's wort** may decrease the levels of apremilast.

**PHARMACOKINETICS Absorption:** 73% bioavailable. **Peak:** 2.5 h. **Distribution:** 68% plasma protein bound. **Metabolism:** Hepatic oxidation and conjugation. **Elimination:** Renal (58%) and fecal (39%). **Half-Life:** 6–9 h.

## NURSING IMPLICATIONS

### Assessment & Drug Effects
- Monitor weight regularly during therapy. Report significant weight loss.
- Monitor for and report promptly signs or symptoms of depression, suicidal thoughts, or other significant mood changes.

Common adverse effects in *italic;* life-threatening effects <u>underlined;</u> generic names in **bold;** classifications in SMALL CAPS; ✚ Canadian drug name; ◯ Prototype drug

- Monitor lab tests: Periodic renal function test.

**Patient & Family Education**

- Report promptly to prescriber if you experience any of the following: Excessive weight loss, suicidal thoughts, depression, anxiety, restlessness, irritability, panic attacks, or mood changes.

# APREPITANT ⊕
(a-pre'pi-tant)

# FOSAPREPITANT
(fos-a-pre'pi-tant)

Emend

**Classifications:** CENTRAL ACTING MISCELLANEOUS; ANTIEMETIC; SUBSTANCE P/NEUROKININ 1 (NK₁) RECEPTOR ANTAGONIST
Therapeutic: ANTIEMETIC

**AVAILABILITY** Capsule; powder for injection; oral suspension

**ACTION & THERAPEUTIC EFFECT**
Aprepitant is a selective substance P/neurokinin 1 (NK₁) receptor antagonist. Substance P and the NK-1 receptors are present in areas in the brain that control the emetic reflex. Aprepitant crosses the blood–brain barrier and occupies brain NK₁ receptors. Peripheral blockade by NK₁ receptor antagonists at receptors located in the GI is an additional hypothesized mechanism of action. *Aprepitant augments the antiemetic activity of the 5-HT₃-receptor antagonist, ondansetron, and inhibits both the acute and delayed phases of emesis induced by chemotherapy agents.*

**USES** Chemotherapy induced nausea/vomiting, postoperative nausea/vomiting.

**CONTRAINDICATIONS** Hypersensitivity to aprepitant; lactation.

**CAUTIOUS USE** Chemotherapeutic agents metabolized through CY-P3A4; severe hepatic impairment; severe renal impairment without dialysis; pregnancy (category B); children younger than 18 y.

## ROUTE & DOSAGE

**Chemotherapy-Induced Nausea and Vomiting**
*Adult:* **PO** 125 mg 1 h prior to chemotherapy, then 80 mg q a.m. for the next 2 days in conjunction with other antiemetics. **IV** 115 mg substituted for oral dose on day 1
**Postoperative Nausea/ Vomiting**
*Adult:* **PO** 40 mg within 3 h of anesthesia induction

## ADMINISTRATION

**Oral**
- Ensure that capsule is swallowed whole with a full glass of water. Do not crush or sprinkle the contents of the capsule.
- Give 1 h before start of chemotherapy.
- Store at 20°–25° C (68°–77° F). Keep the desiccant in the original bottle.

**Intravenous (Fosaprepitant)**

*PREPARE:* **Infusion:** Inject 5 mL NS onto the inside of the 150 mg vial to prevent foaming. Swirl gently to dissolve. Withdraw contents of the vial and add to 145 mL NS. *ADMINISTER:* **Infusion:** Infuse over 20–30 min. Longer infusion times may be used if patient complains of burning.

- Reconstituted drug is stable for 24 h at room temperature.

**ADVERSE EFFECTS** (≥1%) **Body as a Whole:** <u>Serious hypersensitivity reactions, serious infusion-related reactions including anaphylaxis</u>

---

Common adverse effects in *italic;* life-threatening effects <u>underlined;</u> generic names in **bold;** classifications in SMALL CAPS; ◆ Canadian drug name; ⊕ Prototype drug

and anaphylactic shock, *fatigue,* asthenia, malaise, dehydration, fever. **CV:** Bradycardia, hypotension, hypertension, tachycardia. **CNS:** Dizziness, insomnia, headache, peripheral neuropathy, confusion, depression. **GI:** *Constipation, diarrhea, anorexia, nausea,* hiccups, abdominal pain, gastritis, gastroesophageal reflux, abnormal or impaired taste (dysgeusia), dyspepsia, flatulence, hypersalivation, increased taste disturbance, increased AST and ALT. **Hematologic:** Neutropenia, anemia. **Musculoskeletal:** Pain, weakness, myalgia. **Respiratory:** Cough, dyspnea, upper or lower respiratory infection, pneumonitis, respiratory insufficiency. **Special Senses:** Tinnitus.

**INTERACTIONS Drug:** Increased risk of cardiovascular toxicity with **dofetilide, pimozide;** may decrease **warfarin** concentrations and INR; may decrease levels and effectiveness of ORAL CONTRACEPTIVES; **carbamazepine, griseofulvin, modafinil, rifabutin, rifapentine, phenobarbital, primidone** may decrease antiemetic efficacy; may increase levels of **dexamethasone.** Because aprepitant is a substrate of CYP3A4, many additional drug interactions are theoretically possible. Do not use with **eliglustat, flibanerin, lomitapide. Food: Grapefruit juice** may decrease effectiveness of aprepitant. **Herbal: St. John's wort** may decrease effectiveness of aprepitant.

**PHARMACOKINETICS Absorption:** 60–65% of oral dose reaches systemic circulation. **Peak:** 4 h. **Duration:** 95% protein bound; readily crosses the blood–brain barrier. **Metabolism:** In liver by CYP3A4. **Elimination:** Not renally excreted. **Half-Life:** 9–12 h.

## NURSING IMPLICATIONS

### Assessment & Drug Effects

- Monitor cardiac status especially with preexisting CV disease or concurrent use of any CYP3A4 substrate drug (e.g., ketoconazole, itraconazole, nefazodone, troleandomycin, clarithromycin).
- Monitor lab tests: PT/INR 7–10 days after 3-day regimen with concurrent warfarin use; phenytoin level with concurrent use; serum electrolytes, UA, and CBC.

### Patient & Family Education

- Report immediately to prescriber any of the following: Skin rash; difficulty breathing or shortness of breath; rapid, slow, or irregular heartbeat; changes in BP; dizziness or confusion; unexplained sharp or severe pain in leg or stomach; rectal bleeding. Inform prescriber of all other drugs or herbal products you are using. Do not take new drugs (prescription, OTC, herbal) without first consulting prescriber.
- Use barrier contraception in addition to oral contraceptives while taking drug and one mo after discontinuation of the drug.

## ARGATROBAN ℗

(ar-ga'tro-ban)

**Classifications:** ANTICOAGULANT; DIRECT THROMBIN INHIBITOR **Therapeutic:** ANTITHROMBOTIC; DIRECT THROMBIN INHIBITOR

**AVAILABILITY** Injection

## ACTION & *THERAPEUTIC EFFECT*

A direct thrombin inhibitor capable of inhibiting the action of both free and clot-bound thrombin. *Reversibly binds to the thrombin active site, thereby blocking clot-forming activity of thrombin.*

USES Prophylaxis or treatment of thrombosis in patients with heparin-induced thrombocytopenia (HIT); prophylaxis or treatment of coronary artery thrombosis during percutaneous coronary interventions (PCI) in patients at risk for HIT; treatment/prophylaxis of pulmonary embolism.

UNLABELED USES Treatment of disseminated intravascular coagulation (DIC).

CONTRAINDICATIONS Hypersensitivity to argatroban. Any bleeding including intracranial bleeding, GI bleeding, retroperitoneal bleeding; lactation.

CAUTIOUS USE Diseased states with increased risk of hemorrhaging; severe hypertension, GI ulcerations, hepatic impairment; spinal anesthesia, stroke, surgery, trauma; pregnancy (category B), children with HIT.

## ROUTE & DOSAGE

### Prevention & Treatment of Thrombosis

Adult: **IV** 2 mcg/kg/min, may be adjusted to maintain an aPTT of 1.5–3 × baseline (max: 10 mcg/kg/min)

### Hepatic Impairment Dosage Adjustment

0.5 mcg/kg/min, may be adjusted to maintain an aPTT of 1.5–3 × baseline (max: 10 mcg/kg/min)

### Prophylaxis or Treatment of Coronary Thrombosis during PCI

Adult: **IV** Initiate at 25 mcg/kg/min, then bolus of 350 mcg/kg administered via a large bore IV line over 3–5 min, then 25 mcg/kg/min by continuous infusion;

maintain activated clotting time (ACT) 300–450 sec; *if ACT below 300 sec:* Increase infusion to 30 mcg/kg/min; *if ACT over 450 sec:* Decrease infusion to 15 mcg/kg/min

## ADMINISTRATION

**Intravenous**

Note: Argatroban **must be** diluted to 1 mg/mL prior to infusion.

*PREPARE:* **Continuous:** Dilute each 2.5 mL vial by mixing with 250 mL of D5W, NS, or LR to yield 1 mg/mL. ▪ Mix by repeated inversion of the diluent bag for 1 min.

*ADMINISTER:* **Continuous for Heparin-Induced Thrombocytopenia (HIT/HITTS):** Before administration, discontinue heparin and obtain a baseline aPTT. ▪ Give at a rate of 2 mcg/kg/min, or as ordered. Lower initial doses are required with hepatic impairment. ▪ Check aPTT 2 h after initiation of therapy. After the initial dose, adjust dose (not to exceed 10 mcg/kg/min) until the steady-state aPTT is 1.5 to 3 × baseline (not to exceed 100 sec). **Continuous for Percutaneous Coronary Intervention:** Start an infusion at 25 mcg/kg/min and give a bolus of 350 mcg/kg, via a large bore IV line, over 3–5 min. ▪ Check ACT 5–10 min after the bolus dose. If the ACT is greater than 450 sec, decrease infusion rate to 15 mcg/kg/min. If ACT is less than 300 sec, give an additional bolus of 150 mcg/kg and increase infusion to 30 mcg/kg/min. ▪ Check ACT q5–10min to maintain an ACT level 300–450 sec.

▪ Diluted solutions are stable for 24 h at 25° C (77° F) in ambient indoor light. ▪ Protect from direct

Common adverse effects in *italic;* life-threatening effects <u>underlined;</u> generic names in **bold;** classifications in SMALL CAPS; ♣Canadian drug name; ⦿ Prototype drug

115

sunlight. Store solutions refrigerated at 2°–8° C (36°–46° F) in the dark.

**ADVERSE EFFECTS** (≥1%) **Body as a Whole:** Fever, sepsis, pain, allergic reactions (rare). **CV:** Hypotension, <u>cardiac arrest</u>, ventricular tachycardia. **GI:** Diarrhea, nausea, vomiting, coughing, abdominal pain. **Hematologic:** <u>Major GI bleed</u>, *minor GI bleeding, hematuria, decrease Hgb/Hct*, groin bleed, hemoptysis, brachial bleed. **Respiratory:** Dyspnea. **Urogenital:** UTI.

**INTERACTIONS Drug: Heparin** results in increased bleeding; may prolong PT with **warfarin;** may increase risk of bleeding with THROMBOLYTICS or NSAIDs. **Herbal: Feverfew, garlic, ginger, ginkgo** may increase potential for bleeding.

**PHARMACOKINETICS Peak:** 1–3 h. **Distribution:** In extracellular fluid; 54% protein bound. **Metabolism:** In liver by CYP3A4/5. **Elimination:** Primarily in bile (78%). **Half-Life:** 39–51 min.

**NURSING IMPLICATIONS**

**Assessment & Drug Effects**

- **Heparin-Induced Thrombocytopenia:** Monitor aPTT. Dose adjustment may be needed to reach the target aPTT. Check aPTT 2 h after initiation of therapy. After the initial dose, adjust dose (not to exceed 10 mcg/kg/min), until the steady-state aPTT is 1.5 to 3 × baseline (not to exceed 100 sec).
- Monitor cardiovascular status carefully during therapy.
- Monitor for and report S&S of bleeding: Ecchymosis, epistaxis, GI bleeding, hematuria, hemoptysis.
- Note: Patients with history of GI ulceration, hypertension, recent trauma, or surgery are at increased risk for bleeding.
- Monitor neurologic status and report immediately focal or generalized deficits.
- Monitor lab tests: Baseline and periodic ACT with PCI; baseline and periodic aPTT with heparin-induced thrombocytopenia, platelet count, Hgb and Hct; daily INR when argatroban and warfarin are co-administered.

**Patient & Family Education**

- Report immediately any of the following to prescriber: Unexplained back or stomach pain; black, tarry stools; blood in urine, coughing up blood; difficulty breathing; dizziness or fainting spells; heavy menstrual bleeding; nosebleeds; unusual bruising or bleeding at any site.

## ARIPIPRAZOLE

(a-rip′i-pra-zole)

Abilify, Abilify Discmelt, Abilify Maintena, Aristada

**Classifications:** ATYPICAL ANTIPSYCHOTIC; DOPAMINE SYSTEM STABILIZER
Therapeutic: ANTIPSYCHOTIC
**Prototype:** Clozapine

**AVAILABILITY** Tablet; disintegrating tablets; oral solution; injection; extended release injection

**ACTION & *THERAPEUTIC EFFECT*** Efficacy of aripiprazole may be mediated through a combination of partial agonist activity at $D_2$ and $5-HT_{1A}$ receptors and antagonist activity at $5-HT_{2A}$ receptors. *Partial dopaminergic agonist property of aripiprazole accounts for antipsychotic treatment of schizophrenic and bipolar individuals.*

**USES** Treatment of schizophrenia, bipolar mania, maintenance in bipolar 1 disorder, adjunct treatment in major depressive disorder, irritability associated with autism; Tourette's syndrome.

**UNLABELED USES** Restless leg syndrome, behavioral symptoms of dementia, acute psychosis, agitation.

**CONTRAINDICATIONS** Hypersensitivity to aripiprazole; dementia related psychosis in elderly due to increased mortality; QT prolongation; suicidal ideation; neuroleptic malignant syndrome (NMS); severe neutropenia; lactation.

**CAUTIOUS USE** History of seizures or conditions that lower seizure threshold (e.g., Alzheimer's dementia); history of suicides; suicidal tendencies, depression; increased risk of suicidality in children, adolescents and young adults; brain tumor; psychosis related to Alzheimer disease; patients driving or operating heavy machinery; DM; patients with known cardiovascular disease (history of MI or ischemic heart disease, heart failure, or conduction abnormalities), CVA, or conditions that predispose to hypotension (dehydration, hypovolemia, etc.); dysphagia; ethanol intoxication; hyperglycemia; DM; hypothermia; obesity; older adults; adults and children with severe depression, children younger than 10 y with bipolar mania or schizophrenia, children younger than 6 y with autistic disorder; pregnancy (category C).

## ROUTE & DOSAGE

### Schizophrenia
*Adult:* **PO** 10–15 mg once daily, may increase at 2-wk intervals (max: 30 mg/day); **IM Aristada** 441 mg, 662 mg, or 882 mg monthly or 882 mg q6w; or 1,064 mg q2mo

*Adolescent/Child (10 y or older):* **PO** 2 mg daily, increase to 5 mg after 2 days, increase to 10 mg after 2 more days. Can increase up to 30 mg.

### Bipolar Mania
*Adult:* **PO** 15–30 mg once daily; **IM Abilify Maintena** 400 mg monthly
*Adolescent/Child (10 y or older):* **PO** 2 mg daily, increase to 5 mg after 2 days, increase to 10 mg after 2 more days. Can increase up to 30 mg.

### Agitation Associated with Schizophrenia/Bipolar
*Adult:* **IM** 9.75 mg (range: 5.25–15 mg)

### Adjunct in Major Depression
*Adult:* **PO** 2–5 mg daily

### Irritability Associated with Autism
*Adolescent/Child (6 y or older):* **PO** 2 mg daily, increase as needed

### Tourette's Syndrome
*Child/Adolescent (6 y or older, weight over 50 kg):* **PO** 2 mg daily, after 2 days increase to 5 mg daily, then after 5 days increase to 10 mg daily

### Pharmacogentic Dosage Adjustment
*Reduced CYP2D6 expression (i.e., poor metabolizers):* Reduce to 50% of usual dose

## ADMINISTRATION

### Oral
- Remove tablet from blister pack immediately before administration. Do not push the tablet through the foil because this could damage the tablet.
- Administer with or without regard to food.

---

Common adverse effects in *italic*; life-threatening effects <u>underlined</u>; generic names in **bold**; classifications in SMALL CAPS; ♣ Canadian drug name; ● Prototype drug

- Orally disintegrating tablet should be given without water; however, if needed, liquid may be given. Do not split orally disintegrating tablet.
- Oral solution can be given up to 6 mo after opening, but should not exceed expiration date.
- Note that dose should be reduced by 50% with concurrent treatment with ketoconazole, quinidine, fluoxetine, or paroxetine.
- Store at 25° C (77° F). Excursions permitted to 15 °–30 ° C (59 °–86 ° F). Use within 6 mo of opening.

**Intramuscular**
- Inject slowly and deeply into a large muscle.
- Ensure that drug is not injected Intravenously or subcutaneously.
- Make sure to rotate between deltoid and gluteal injection sites.
- Store at 15°–30° C (59°–86° F).

**ADVERSE EFFECTS** (≥1%) **Body as a Whole:** *Headache,* asthenia, fever, flu-like symptoms, peripheral edema, chest pain, neck pain, neck rigidity. **CNS:** *Anxiety, agitation, insomnia, light-headedness, somnolence, akathisia, agitation, headache,* tremor, extrapyramidal symptoms, depression, drowsiness, nervousness, increased salivation, hostility, suicidal thought, manic reaction, abnormal gait, confusion, cogwheel rigidity. **CV:** Hypertension, tachycardia, hypotension, bradycardia. Risk of stroke in elderly with dementia-related psychosis. **GI:** *Nausea, vomiting, constipation,* anorexia, weight gain. **Hematologic:** Ecchymosis, anemia. **Metabolic:** Weight gain, weight loss, *hyperglycemia,* diabetes mellitus, increased creatine kinase, changes in cholesterol levels. **Musculoskeletal:** Muscle cramp. **Respiratory:** Rhinitis, cough. **Skin:** Rash. **Special Senses:** Blurred vision.

**INTERACTIONS Drug:** CYP3A4 inducers (**carbamazepine, phenytoin,** etc.) will decrease aripiprazole levels (may need to double aripiprazole dose); use with CYP2D6 or CYP3A4 inhibitors (**ketoconazole, quinidine, fluoxetine, paroxetine,** etc.) may increase aripiprazole levels (reduce dose by 50%); may cause additive sedation with other SEDATIVES (**alcohol, tramadol,** BARBITURATES, etc.); may enhance effects of ANTIHYPERTENSIVE AGENTS. Do not use with **fluconazole** or **dofetilide** due to risk of QT prolongation. **Herbal: St. John's wort** may decrease aripiprazole levels. **Food:** High fat meals may delay time to peak plasma levels.

**PHARMACOKINETICS Absorption:** 87% bioavailable. **Distribution:** Extensively protein bound. **Peak:** 3–5 h. **Metabolism:** In liver by CYP3A4 and 2D6. Major metabolite, has some activity. **Elimination:** 55% in feces, 25% in urine. **Half-Life:** 75 h (94 h for metabolite); 146 h (poor metabolizers).

## NURSING IMPLICATIONS

**Black Box Warning**

*Aripiprazole has been associated with increased mortality in the elderly with dementia-related psychosis, and suicidal thinking and behavior in children, adolescents, and young adults.*

**Assessment & Drug Effects**
- Monitor for and report immediately worsening depression or suicidal ideation, especially in children, adolescents, and young adults.
- Monitor cardiovascular status. Assess for and report orthostatic hypotension. Take BP supine then in sitting position. Report systolic

Common adverse effects in *italic;* life-threatening effects underlined; generic names in **bold;** classifications in SMALL CAPS; ♣ Canadian drug name; ⊕ Prototype drug

drop of greater than 15–20 mm Hg. Patients at increased risk are those who are dehydrated, hypovolemic, or receiving concurrent antihypertensive therapy.

- Monitor for S&S of infection especially in elderly patients with dementia.
- Monitor body temperature in situations likely to elevate core temperature (e.g., exercising strenuously, exposure to extreme heat, receiving drugs with anticholinergic activity, or being subject to dehydration).
- Monitor for and report signs of tardive dyskinesia.
- Monitor for and immediately report S&S of neuroleptic malignant syndrome (NMS) (see Appendix F). Withhold drug if NMS is suspected.
- Monitor diabetics for loss of glycemic control.
- Monitor weight and waist circumference at baseline and at 4, 8, and 12 wk, then quarterly.
- Monitor weight and waist circumference at baseline and at 4, 8, and 12 wk and then quarterly.
- Monitor lab tests: Periodic Hct, Hgb, and blood glucose; periodic CPK and myoglobinuria if NMS is suspected, frequent CBC with history of low WBC or drug-induced low WBC.

**Patient & Family Education**

- Report promptly deterioration of mental status or behavior (especially suicidal ideation).
- Carefully monitor blood glucose levels if diabetic.
- Do not drive or engage in other potentially hazardous activities until reaction to drug is known.
- Avoid situations where you are likely to become overheated or dehydrated.
- Notify prescriber if you become pregnant or intend to become pregnant while taking this drug.

## ASCORBIC ACID (VITAMIN C)
Apo-C ♦, Cecon, Cevalin, CeVi-Sol ♦, Flavorcee, Redoxon ♦, Vita-C

## ASCORBATE, SODIUM
(a-skor′bate)
Cenolate, Ortho-CS 250
**Classification:** VITAMIN
Therapeutic: VITAMIN SUPPLEMENT; URINARY ACIDIFIER

**AVAILABILITY** Tablet; injection

**ACTION & THERAPEUTIC EFFECT**
Water-soluble vitamin essential for synthesis and maintenance of collagen and intercellular ground substance of body tissue cells, blood vessels, cartilage, bones, teeth, skin, and tendons. Humans are unable to synthesize ascorbic acid in the body therefore, it **must be** consumed daily. *Increases protective mechanism of the immune system, thus supporting wound healing, and resistance to infection.*

**USES** Prophylaxis and treatment of scurvy and as a dietary supplement.

**UNLABELED USES** To acidify urine; to prevent and treat cancer; to treat idiopathic methemoglobinemia; as adjuvant during deferoxamine therapy for iron toxicity; in megadoses will possibly reduce severity and duration of common cold. Widely used as an antioxidant in formulations of parenteral tetracycline and other drugs.

**CONTRAINDICATIONS** Use of sodium ascorbate in patients on sodium restriction; use of calcium ascorbate in patients receiving digitalis.

---

**CAUTIOUS USE** Excessive doses in patients with G6PD deficiency; hemochromatosis, thalassemia, sideroblastic anemia, sickle cell anemia; patients prone to gout or renal calculi; pregnancy (category C).

## ROUTE & DOSAGE

**Vitamin C Deficiency**
*Adult:* **PO** 75–90 mg daily; **IV** 100–250 mg 1–2 × per day
*Child:* **PO/IV** 15–45 mg/day

## ADMINISTRATION

### Oral
- Give oral solutions mixed with food.
- Dissolve effervescent tablet in a glass of water immediately before ingestion.

### Intravenous
Verify correct IV concentration and rate of infusion for children with prescriber.

*PREPARE:* **Direct/Continuous/Intermittent:** Give diluted in solutions such as NS, D5W, D5/NS, LR. ▪ Be aware that parenteral vitamin C is incompatible with many drugs. ▪ Consult pharmacist for compatibility information.
*ADMINISTER:* **Direct:** Give slowly. Avoid rapid IV injection. **Continuous/Intermittent (preferred):** Give at ordered rate determined by volume of solution to be infused.
*INCOMPATIBILITIES:* **Solution/additive: Aminophylline, bleomycin, erythromycin, nafcillin, sodium bicarbonate, theophylline. Y-site: Aminophylline, azathioprine, ceftazidime, ceftriaxone, chloramphenicol, dantrolene, diazepam, diazoxide, erythromycin, etomidate, ganciclovir, hydralazine, hydroxocobalamine, iamrinone, midazolam, minocycline, nitrorusside, papaverine, pentamidine, penobarbital, phenytoin, propofol, sulfamethoxazole/trimethoprim.**

- Store in airtight, light-resistant, nonmetallic containers, away from heat and sunlight, preferably at 15°–30° C (59°–86° F), unless otherwise specified by manufacturer.

**ADVERSE EFFECTS** (≥1%) **GI:** Nausea, vomiting, heartburn, diarrhea, or abdominal cramps (high doses). **Hematologic:** Acute hemolytic anemia (patients with deficiency of G6PD); sickle cell crisis. **CNS:** Headache (high doses). **Urogenital:** Urethritis, dysuria, crystalluria, hyperoxaluria, or hyperuricemia (high doses). **Other:** Mild soreness at injection site; dizziness and temporary faintness with rapid IV administration.

## DIAGNOSTIC TEST INTERFERENCE

High doses of ascorbic acid can produce false-negative results for *urine glucose* with *glucose oxidase* methods (e.g., *Clinitest, TesTape, Diastix*); false-positive results with *copper reduction methods* (e.g., Benedict's solution, Clinitest). May produce false-negative tests for *occult blood* in stools if taken within 48–72 h of test.

**INTERACTIONS Drug:** Large doses may attenuate hypoprothrombinemic effects of ORAL ANTICOAGULANTS; SALICYLATES may inhibit ascorbic acid uptake by leukocytes and tissues, and ascorbic acid may decrease elimination of SALICYLATES; chronic high doses of ascorbic acid may diminish the effects of **disulfiram**. Avoid use with **deferoxamine.**

Common adverse effects in *italic*; life-threatening effects <u>underlined</u>; generic names in **bold**; classifications in SMALL CAPS; ♣ Canadian drug name; ⊘ Prototype drug

## PHARMACOKINETICS **Absorption:** Readily absorbed PO; however, absorption may be limited with large doses. **Distribution:** Widely distributed to body tissues; crosses placenta; distributed into breast milk. **Metabolism:** In liver. **Elimination:** Rapidly in urine when plasma level exceeds renal threshold of 1.4 mg/dL.

## NURSING IMPLICATIONS

### Assessment & Drug Effects
- Monitor for S&S of acute hemolytic anemia, sickle cell crisis.
- Monitor lab tests: Periodic Hct, Hgb, and serum electrolytes.

### Patient & Family Education
- High doses of vitamin C are not recommended during pregnancy.
- Take large doses of vitamin C in divided amounts because the body uses only what is needed at a particular time and excretes the rest in urine.
- Megadoses can interfere with absorption of vitamin $B_{12}$.
- Note: Vitamin C increases the absorption of iron when taken at the same time as iron-rich foods.

## ASENAPINE
(a-sin'a-peen)

Saphris

**Classification:** ATYPICAL ANTIPSYCHOTIC; SEROTONIN ANTAGONIST; ANTIDEPRESSANT
Therapeutic: ANTIPSYCHOTIC; ANTIMANIC; ANTIDEPRESSANT
**Prototype:** Clozapine

**AVAILABILITY** Sublingual tablet

## ACTION & *THERAPEUTIC EFFECT*
Mechanism of action thought to be related to antagonism of certain CNS dopamine ($D_2$) and serotonin ($5-HT_{2A}$) receptors. *Effect on serotonin and dopamine receptors may account for activity of asenapine against the negative symptoms of psychotic disorders.*

**USES** Acute treatment of schizophrenia; acute treatment of manic or mixed episodes associated with bipolar disorder (bipolar I disorder) with or without psychotic features.

**CONTRAINDICATIONS** Dementia-related psychosis; ketoacidosis; severe neutropenia (ANC less than 1000/mm³); patients with history of torsades de pointes related to drugs; suicidal ideation; severe hepatic impairment (Child-Pugh class C).

**CAUTIOUS USE** Tardive dyskinesia (especially women); cardiovascular disease (history of MI, ischemic heart disease, HF, conduction abnormalities, bradycardia), cerebrovascular disease, dehydration, hypovolemia, diabetes mellitus; history of seizures; Alzheimer's dementia; older adults; history of suicidal tendencies; pregnancy (category C); lactation. Use in children younger than 10 y of age not established.

## ROUTE & DOSAGE

### Schizophrenia
*Adult:* **SL** 5 mg b.i.d.; increase up to 10 mg b.i.d. as tolerated

### Bipolar Disorder
*Adult:* **SL** Start at 10 mg b.i.d., may decrease to 5 mg b.i.d. if higher dose not tolerated.
*Adolescent/Child (10 y or older):* **SL** 2.5 mg b.i.d. may increase after 3 days to 5 mg b.i.d.

## ADMINISTRATION
### Sublingual
- Tablet must be placed under tongue and allowed to dissolve completely.
- Ensure that tablet is not split, crushed, chewed, or swallowed.
- Eating and drinking should be avoided for 10 min after administration.
- Store at 15°–30° C (59°–86° F).

**ADVERSE EFFECTS** (≥1%) **Body as a Whole:** Fatigue, irritability, pain in extremities, suicidal thoughts. **CNS:** Agitation, akathisia, anxiety, *dizziness*, dysgeusia, *extrapyramidal symptoms, headache, insomnia, somnolence.* **CV:** Hypertension. **GI:** Constipation, dyspepsia, nausea, vomiting. **Metabolic:** Increased appetite, increased weight. **Musculoskeletal:** Arthralgia. **Respiratory:** Dry mouth, oral hypoesthesia, salivary hypersecretion.

**INTERACTIONS Drug: Fluvoxamine** and **imipramine** can increase asenapine levels. Do not use with **fluconazole, dofetilide,** or **itraconazole** due to risk of QT prolongation.

**PHARMACOKINETICS Absorption:** Bioavailability 35%. **Peak:** 0.5–1.5 h. **Distribution:** 95% plasma protein bound. **Metabolism:** In liver via CYP1A2. **Elimination:** 50% renal; 40% fecal. **Half-Life:** 24 h.

## NURSING IMPLICATIONS

### Black Box Warning

*Asenapine has been associated with increased mortality in the elderly with dementia-related psychosis.*

### Assessment & Drug Effects
- Monitor BP, HR, and weight. Monitor orthostatic vital signs with concurrent antihypertensive therapy or any condition that predisposes to hypotension (e.g., advanced age, dehydration).
- Monitor for orthostatic hypotension and syncope, especially early in therapy.
- Monitor for S&S of infection especially in elderly patients with dementia.
- Monitor diabetics or those at risk for diabetes for loss of glycemic control.
- Withhold drug and report promptly S&S of neuroleptic malignant syndrome (see Appendix F).
- Monitor lab tests: Baseline and periodic CBC.

### Patient & Family Education
- Be alert for and report worsening of condition, including ideas of suicide.
- Make position changes slowly, especially from lying or sitting to a standing position.
- If diabetic, monitor blood sugar closely for loss of control.
- Stop taking the drug and report immediately any of the following: High fever, muscle rigidity, altered mental status, or palpitations.
- Avoid engaging in hazardous activities until response to drug is known.
- Avoid alcohol while taking this drug.

# ASPIRIN (ACETYLSALICYLIC ACID) Ⓟ
(as′pe-ren)

Alka-Seltzer, A.S.A., Aspergum, Astrin ♦, Bayer, Bayer Children's, Cosprin, Easprin, Ecotrin, Empirin, Entrophen ♦, Halfprin, Measurin, Novasen ♦, St. Joseph Children's, Supasa ♦, Triaphen-10 ♦, ZORprin

Common adverse effects in *italic*; life-threatening effects <u>underlined</u>; generic names in **bold**; classifications in SMALL CAPS; ♦ Canadian drug name; Ⓟ Prototype drug

**Classifications:** NONNARCOTIC ANALGESIC, SALICYLATE; ANTIPYRETIC; ANTIPLATELET
Therapeutic: ANALGESIC; ANTIPYRETIC; ANTIPLATELET

## AVAILABILITY

Chewable tablet; tablet; enteric-coated tablet; sustained release tablet; suppository

## ACTION & *THERAPEUTIC EFFECT*

Major action is primarily due to inhibiting the formation of prostaglandins involved in the production of inflammation, pain, and fever. **Anti-Inflammatory Action:** Inhibits prostaglandin synthesis. As an anti-inflammatory agent, aspirin appears to be involved in enhancing antigen removal and in reducing the spread of inflammatory substances. **Analgesic Action:** Principally peripheral with limited action in the CNS in the hypothalamus; results in relief of mild to moderate pain. **Antipyretic Action:** Suppress the synthesis of prostaglandin in or near the hypothalamus. Aspirin also lowers body temperature by indirectly causing centrally mediated peripheral vasodilation and sweating. **Antiplatelet Action:** Aspirin powerfully inhibits platelet aggregation. *Reduces inflammation, pain, and fever. Also inhibits platelet aggregation, reducing ability of blood to clot.*

## USES

To relieve pain of low to moderate intensity. Also for various inflammatory conditions, such as acute rheumatic fever, systemic lupus, rheumatoid arthritis, osteoarthritis, bursitis, and calcific tendonitis, and to reduce fever in selected febrile conditions. Used to reduce recurrence of TIA due to fibrin platelet emboli and risk of stroke in men; to prevent recurrence of MI; as prophylaxis against MI in men with unstable angina.

**UNLABELED USES** As prophylactic against thromboembolism; to prevent cataract and progression of diabetic retinopathy; and to control symptoms related to gluten sensitivity.

## CONTRAINDICATIONS

History of hypersensitivity to salicylates including methyl salicylate (oil of wintergreen); patients with "aspirin triad" (aspirin sensitivity, nasal polyps, asthma); chronic rhinitis; acute bronchospasm; agranulocytosis; head trauma; increased intracranial pressure; intracranial bleeding; history of GI ulceration, bleeding, or other problems; hemophilia, or other bleeding disorders; severe renal or hepatic insufficiency; alcoholism; older adults; pregnancy (category D in third trimester); children with fever and children weighing less than 25 mg; lactation.

## CAUTIOUS USE

Otic diseases; gout; children with fever accompanied by dehydration; hyperthyroidism; immunosuppressed individuals; asthma; history of GI disease; history of gout; cardiac disease; G6PD deficiency; vitamin K deficiency; preoperatively; Hodgkin's disease; alcohol use; hypoprothrombinemia; vitamin K deficiency; pregnancy (category C in first and second trimester). Prematures, neonates, or children younger than 2 y, except under advice and supervision of prescriber; children or teenagers with chickenpox or influenza-like illnesses because of possible association with Reye's syndrome.

## ROUTE & DOSAGE

| Mild to Moderate Pain, Fever |
| --- |
| *Adult:* **PO/PR** 350–650 mg q4h (max: 4 g/day) |

---

*Child:* **PO/PR** 10–15 mg/kg in 4–6 h (max: 3.6 g/day)

**Arthritic Conditions**

*Adult:* **PO** 3.6–5.4 g/day in 4–6 divided doses
*Child:* **PO** 80–100 mg/kg/day in 4–6 divided doses (max: 130 mg/kg/day)

**Thromboembolic Disorders**

*Adult:* **PO** 81–325 mg daily

**TIA Prophylaxis**

*Adult:* **PO** 650 mg b.i.d.

**MI Prophylaxis**

*Adult:* **PO** 80–325 mg/day

## ADMINISTRATION

### Oral

- Give with a full glass of water (240 mL), milk, food, or antacid to minimize gastric irritation.
- Do not give to children or adolescents with chickenpox or flu-like symptoms.
- Enteric-coated tablets dissolve too quickly if administered with milk and should not be crushed or chewed.

### Rectal

- Ensure that suppository is inserted beyond the internal sphincter.
- Store at 15°–30° C (59°–86° F) in airtight container and dry environment unless otherwise directed by manufacturer. Store suppositories in a cool place or refrigerate but do not freeze.

## ADVERSE EFFECTS (≥1%) **Body as a Whole:** Hypersensitivity (urticaria, <u>bronchospasm, anaphylactic shock (laryngeal edema)</u>). **CNS:** Dizziness, confusion, drowsiness. **Special Senses:** Tinnitus, hearing loss. **GI:** *Nausea,* vomiting, diarrhea, anorexia, *heartburn, stomach pains,* *ulceration,* occult bleeding, GI bleeding. **Hematologic:** <u>Thrombocytopenia, hemolytic anemia</u>, prolonged bleeding time. **CV:** Edema, hypotension. **Skin:** Petechiae, easy bruising, rash. **Urogenital:** Impaired renal function. **Other:** Prolonged pregnancy and labor with increased bleeding.

## DIAGNOSTIC TEST INTERFERENCE

Bleeding time is prolonged 3–8 days (life of exposed platelets) following a single 325-mg (5 grains) dose of aspirin. Large doses of salicylates equivalent to 5 g or more of aspirin per day may cause prolonged *prothrombin time* by decreasing prothrombin production; interference with *pregnancy tests* (using mouse or rabbit); decreases in *serum cholesterol, potassium, PBI, T3* and *T4 concentrations,* and an increase in *T3 resin uptake. Serum uric acid* may increase when plasma salicylate levels are below 10 and decrease when above 15 mg/dL using colorimetric methods. *Urine 5-HIAA:* Aspirin may interfere with tests using fluorescent methods. *Urine ketones:* Salicylates interfere with Gerhardt test (reaction with ferric chloride produces a reddish color that persists after boiling). *Urine glucose:* Moderate to large doses of salicylates equivalent to an aspirin dosage 2.4 g/day or more may produce false-negative results with glucose oxidase methods (e.g., *Clinistix, TesTape*) and false-positive results with copper reduction methods *(Benedict's solution, Clinitest). Urinary PSP excretion* may be reduced by salicylates. Salicylates may cause *urine VMA* to be falsely elevated (by most tests), or reduced (by Pisano method). Salicylates may interfere with or cause false decreases in plasma theophylline levels using

Common adverse effects in *italic;* life-threatening effects <u>underlined;</u> generic names in **bold;** classifications in SMALL CAPS; ✤ Canadian drug name; ⊙ Prototype drug

Schack and Waxler method. High plasma salicylate levels may cause abnormalities in *liver function tests.*

## INTERACTIONS Drug: Amino-salicylic acid increases risk of SALICYLATE toxicity. Ammonium chloride and other ACIDIFYING AGENTS decrease renal elimination and increase risk of SALICYLATE toxicity. ANTICOAGULANTS increase risk of bleeding. ORAL HYPOGLYCEMIC AGENTS increase hypoglycemic activity with aspirin doses greater than 2 g/day. CARBONIC ANHYDRASE INHIBITORS enhance SALICYLATE toxicity. CORTICO-STEROIDS add to ulcerogenic effects. Methotrexate toxicity is increased. Low doses of SALICYLATES may antagonize uricosuric effects of probenecid and sulfinpyrazone. Herbal: Feverfew, garlic, ginger, ginkgo, evening primrose oil may increase bleeding potential.

## PHARMACOKINETICS Absorption: 80–100% absorbed (depending on formulation), primarily in stomach and upper small intestine. Peak levels: 15 min to 2 h. Distribution: Widely distributed in most body tissues; crosses placenta. Metabolism: Aspirin is hydrolyzed to salicylate in GI mucosa, plasma, and erythrocytes; salicylate is metabolized in liver. Elimination: 50% of dose is eliminated in the urine in 2–4 h (low doses) or 15–30 h (high doses). Excreted into breast milk. Half-Life: Aspirin 15–20 min; salicylate 2–18 h (dose dependent).

## NURSING IMPLICATIONS

### Assessment & Drug Effects

- Monitor for loss of tolerance to aspirin. Symptoms usually occur 15 min to 3 h after ingestion: Profuse rhinorrhea, erythema, nausea, vomiting, intestinal cramps, diarrhea.
- Monitor closely the diabetic child for need to adjust insulin dose. Children on high doses of aspirin are particularly prone to hypoglycemia (see Appendix F).
- Monitor for salicylate toxicity. In adults, a sensation of fullness in the ears, tinnitus, and decreased or muffled hearing are the most frequent symptoms.
- Monitor children for S&S of salicylate toxicity manifested by: hyperventilation, agitation, mental confusion, or other behavioral changes, drowsiness, lethargy, sweating, and constipation.

### Patient & Family Education

- Use enteric-coated tablets, extended release tablets, buffered aspirin, or aspirin administered with an antacid to reduce GI disturbances.
- Discontinue aspirin use with onset of ringing or buzzing in the ears, impaired hearing, dizziness, GI discomfort or bleeding, and report to prescriber.
- Do not use aspirin for self-medication of pain (adults) beyond 5 days without consulting a prescriber. Do not use aspirin longer than 3 days for fever (adults and children), never for fever over 38.9° C (102° F) in older adults or 39.5° C (103° F) in children and adults under 60 y or for recurrent fever without medical direction.
- Consult prescriber before using aspirin for any fever accompanied by rash, severe headache, stiff neck, marked irritability, or confusion (all possible symptoms of meningitis).
- Avoid alcohol when taking large doses of aspirin.
- Observe and report signs of bleeding (e.g., petechiae, ecchymoses, bleeding gums, bloody or black stools, cloudy or bloody urine).
- Maintain adequate fluid intake when taking repeated doses of aspirin.

---

## ATAZANAVIR
(a-ta-zan′a-vir)
*Reyataz*
**Classifications:** ANTIRETROVIRAL;
PROTEASE INHIBITOR
**Therapeutic:** PROTEASE INHIBITOR
**Prototype:** Saquinavir

**AVAILABILITY** Capsule; oral powder

**ACTION & *THERAPEUTIC EFFECT***
Selectively inhibits protease enzymes need for the replication of HIV and production of mature viruses; reduces the viral load and increases CD4+ cell count. *Protease inhibition renders the virus noninfectious. Because HIV protease inhibitors inhibit the HIV replication cycle midway in the process, they are active in acutely and chronically infected cells.*

**USES** Treatment of HIV infection in combination with other antiretroviral agents.

**CONTRAINDICATIONS** Previously demonstrated severe hypersentivity reaction to atazanavir; severe hepatic insufficiency; ESRD with hemodialysis; lactation.

**CAUTIOUS USE** Mild to moderate hepatic impairment, hepatitis B or C; elevated bilirubin; severe renal impairment; DM; diabetic ketoacidosis; hemophilia, hepatic disease; hepatitis; jaundice; cholelithiasis, hypercholesterolemia, hypertriglyceridemia; preexisting conduction system disease (e.g., marked first-degree AV block or second- or third-degree AV block); obesity; older adults; pregnancy (category B); infants younger than 3 mo or weighing less than or equal to 10 kg.

## ROUTE & DOSAGE

### HIV Infection
*Adult/Adolescent: Child (older than 6 y and weight greater than 39 kg):* **PO** 400 mg once/day with a light meal OR 300 mg once/day with 100 mg of ritonavir
*Adolescent/Child (6 y or older and weight 32 to less than 39 kg):* **PO** 250 mg plus ritonavir (100 mg) once daily
*Adolescent/Child (6 y or older and weight 25 to less than 32 kg):* **PO** 200 mg plus ritonavir (100 mg) once daily (i.e., 7 mg/kg plus ritonavir 4 mg/kg)
*Adolescent/Child (6 y or older and weight 20 to less than 25 kg):* **PO** 150 mg plus ritonavir (80 mg)
*Adolescent/Child (6 y or older and weight 15 to less than 20 kg):* **PO** 150 mg plus ritonavir (80 mg) once daily
*Infant/child (3 mo old and 10 to less than 15 kg):* **PO** 200 mg (plus ritonavir) daily kg
*Infant/child (3 mo or older and 15 kg to less than 25 kg:* **PO** 250 mg (plus ritonavir) daily

### Hepatic Impairment Dosage Adjustment
*Moderate impairment (Child-Pugh class B):* Reduce dose to 300 mg once a day. *Severe impairment:* Not recommended for use.

## ADMINISTRATION
### Oral
- Give with a light meal, not on an empty stomach.
- **Do not** open capsules, they must be given whole.
- May mix oral powder in one tablespoon of food such as

Common adverse effects in *italic;* life-threatening effects <u>underlined</u>; generic names in **bold;** classifications in SMALL CAPS; ♣ Canadian drug name; ● Prototype drug

applesauce or yogurt. May mix with a minimum of 30 mL of liquid for infants who can drink from a cup. For infants less than 6 mo, mix oral powder with infant formula and give using an oral dosing syringe. Administration using an infant bottle is not recommended because full dose may not be delivered.

- When co-administered with didanosine buffered formulations, give atazanavir (with food) 2 h before or 1 h after didanosine.
- Give 2 h before/1 h after antacids or buffered drugs.
- Store at 15°–30° C (59°–86° F).

**ADVERSE EFFECTS** (≥1%) **Body as a Whole:** *Peripheral neuropathy,* fever, pain, fatigue, allergic reaction, angioedema, asthenia, burning sensation, chest pain, edema, generalized edema, heat sensitivity, malaise, pallor, peripheral edema, photosensitivity, substernal chest pain, sweating. **CNS:** *Headache,* depression, insomnia, dizziness, abnormal dreams, agitation, amnesia, anxiety, confusion, decreased libido, emotional lability, hallucination, hostility, hyperkinesia, hypesthesia, psychosis, sleep disorder, somnolence, suicide attempt. **CV:** Cardiac arrest, heart block (PR prolongation), hypertension, myocarditis, palpitation, syncope, vasodilatation. **GI:** Hyperbilirubinemia, *jaundice, nausea, vomiting, diarrhea,* abdominal pain, anorexia, aphthous stomatitis, colitis, constipation, dental pain, dyspepsia, enlarged abdomen, esophageal ulcer, esophagitis, flatulence, gastritis, gastroenteritis, gastrointestinal disorder, hepatitis, hepatomegaly, hepatosplenomegaly, liver damage, liver fatty deposit, pancreatitis, peptic ulcer. **Endocrine:** Decreased male fertility. **Hematologic:** Ecchymosis, purpura. **Metabolic:** Lipodystrophy syndrome, hypercholesterolemia, hypertriglyceridemia. **Musculoskeletal:** Myalgia, arthralgia. **Respiratory:** *Cough,* dyspnea, hiccup. **Skin:** *Rash,* alopecia, cellulitis, dermatophytosis, dry skin, eczema, nail disorder, pruritus, seborrhea, urticaria, vesiculobullous rash. **Special Senses:** Otitis, taste perversion, tinnitus. **Urogenital:** Abnormal urine, amenorrhea, gynecomastia, hematuria, menstrual disorder, oliguria, pelvic pain, polyuria, proteinuria, urinary frequency, urinary tract infection.

**INTERACTIONS** **Drug:** There are extensive drug interactions reported; check the package insert for complete listing. May increase levels and toxicity of **cyclosporine,** systemic **lidocaine, sirolimus, tacrolimus, amiodarone, alfuzosin, dronedarone, eplerenone;** increase risk of myopathy and rhabdomyolysis with **atorvastatin, lovastatin, simvastatin;** may increase risk of heart block with **diltiazem;** ANTACIDS, H₂-RECEPTOR ANTAGONISTS, PROTON PUMP INHIBITORS may decrease absorption of atazanavir; may increase toxicity of **irinotecan;** increased risk of prolonged sedations with BENZODIAZEPINES; **indinavir** may increase risk of hyperbilirubinemia; **didanosine, efavirenz, rifampin** may decrease atazanavir levels; **ergotamine, dihydroergotamine, bepridil, pimozide** may cause serious adverse reactions; may increase risk of hypotension, visual changes, and priapism with **sildenafil, tadalafil, vardenafil.** Avoid use of **sildenafil, alfuzosin, salmeterol,**

and **bosentan. Herbal: St. John's wort, red yeast rice** may decrease atazanavir levels.

**PHARMACOKINETICS Absorption:** 68% into systemic circulation; taking with food enhances bioavailability. **Peak:** 2–2.5 h. **Metabolism:** In liver by CYP3A4. **Elimination:** 70% in feces, 13% in urine. **Half-Life:** 7 h.

## NURSING IMPLICATIONS

### Assessment & Drug Effects

- Monitor CV status and ECG closely, especially with concurrent treatment with other drugs known to prolong the PR interval.
- Monitor for and report promptly S&S of lactic acidosis (see metabolic acidosis, Appendix F).
- Monitor neonates and infants exposed to atazanavir in utero for severe hyperbilirubinemia during the first few days of life.
- Monitor lab tests: Baseline and periodic CD4+ cell count, HIV RNA viral load, and LFTs; total bilirubin if jaundiced; periodic PT/INR with concurrent warfarin therapy; frequent blood glucose, especially if diabetic.

### Patient & Family Education

- Do not alter the dose or discontinue therapy without consulting prescriber.
- Inform prescriber of all prescription, nonprescription, or herbal meds being used.
- Report promptly any of the following: Dizziness or light-headedness; muscle pain (especially with concurrent statin therapy); severe nausea, vomiting (especially if red or "coffee-ground" in appearance), stomach pain, black tarry stools; yellowing of skin or whites of eyes; skin rash or itchy skin; sore throat, fever, or other S&S of infection; unexplained tiredness or weakness.

- If taking both sildenafil and atazanavir, promptly report any of the following sildenafil-associated adverse effects: Hypotension, visual changes, or prolonged penile erection.

## ATENOLOL
(a-ten'oh-lole)
Apo-Atenolol ♦, Tenormin
**Classifications:** BETA-ADRENERGIC ANTAGONIST; ANTIHYPERTENSIVE
Therapeutic: ANTIHYPERTENSIVE; ANTIANGINAL
**Prototype:** Propranolol

**AVAILABILITY** Tablet

**ACTION & *THERAPEUTIC EFFECT***
Atenolol selectively blocks beta$_1$-adrenergic receptors located chiefly in cardiac muscle. Mechanisms for antihypertensive action include central effect leading to decreased sympathetic outflow to periphery, reduction in renin activity with consequent suppression of the renin–angiotensin–aldosterone system, and competitive inhibition of catecholamine binding at beta-adrenergic receptor sites. *Reduces rate and force of cardiac contractions (negative inotropic action); cardiac output is reduced as well as systolic and diastolic BP. Atenolol decreases peripheral vascular resistance both at rest and with exercise.*

**USES** Management of hypertension as a single agent or concomitantly with other antihypertensive agents, and in treatment of stable angina pectoris, MI. Reduction of cardiovascular mortality and MI prophylaxis.

**UNLABELED USES** Antiarrhythmic, mitral valve prolapse, tremor, and migraine prophylaxis.

**CONTRAINDICATIONS** Sinus bradycardia, greater than first-degree heart block, uncompensated heart failure, cardiogenic shock, abrupt discontinuation, untreated pheochromocytoma; pregnancy (category D); lactation.

**CAUTIOUS USE** Hypertensive patients with CHF controlled by digitalis and diuretics, vasospastic angina (Prinzmetal's angina); bronchospastic disease; asthma, bronchitis, emphysema, and COPD; major depression; diabetes mellitus; impaired renal function, dialysis; myasthenia gravis; pheochromocytoma, hyperthyroidism, thyrotoxicosis; older adults.

## ROUTE & DOSAGE

### Hypertension, Angina

*Adult:* PO 25–50 mg/day, may increase to 100 mg/day
*Child:* PO 0.8–1.5 mg/kg/day (max: 2 mg/kg/day)

### MI

*Adult:* PO Start 50 mg/day

### Reduction of CV Risk/MI

*Adult:* PO 100 mg/day in 1–2 divided doses

### Renal Impairment Dosage Adjustment

*CrCl 15–35 mL/min:* Max dose: 50 mg/day; *less than 15 mL/min:* Max dose: 25 mg/day

## ADMINISTRATION

### Oral

- Crush tablets, if necessary, before administration and give with fluid of patient's choice. Administration with orange juice may lower bioavailability more significantly than other foods.
- When drug is discontinued, it should be tapered and not stopped abruptly.

- Store in tightly closed, light-resistant container at 15°–30° C (59°–86° F) unless otherwise directed.

**ADVERSE EFFECTS** (≥1%) **CNS:** Dizziness, vertigo, light-headedness, syncope, fatigue or weakness, lethargy, drowsiness, insomnia, mental changes, depression. **CV:** *Bradycardia, hypotension, CHF,* cold extremities, leg pains, dysrhythmias. **GI:** Nausea, vomiting, diarrhea. **Respiratory:** Pulmonary edema, pulmonary embolism, dyspnea, <u>bronchospasm</u>. **Other:** May mask symptoms of hypoglycemia; sexual dysfunction (specifically, erectile dysfunction).

**INTERACTIONS** **Drug:** **Atropine** and other ANTICHOLINERGICS may increase atenolol absorption from GI tract; NSAIDS may decrease hypotensive effects; may mask symptoms of a hypoglycemic reaction induced by **insulin,** SULFONYLUREAS; may increase **lidocaine** levels and toxicity; pharmacologic and toxic effects of both atenolol and **verapamil** are increased. **Prazosin, terazosin** may increase severe hypotensive response to first dose of atenolol. May have additive electrophysiologic effects with **amiodarone.**

**PHARMACOKINETICS** **Absorption:** 50% of dose absorbed. **Peak:** 2–4 h. **Duration:** 24 h. **Distribution:** Does not readily cross blood–brain barrier. **Metabolism:** No hepatic metabolism. **Elimination:** 40–50% in urine; 50–60% in feces. **Half-Life:** 6–7 h.

## NURSING IMPLICATIONS

### Black Box Warning

*Abruptly stopping atenolol in patients with angina may cause*

Common adverse effects in *italic*; life-threatening effects <u>underlined</u>; generic names in **bold**; classifications in SMALL CAPS; ♣ Canadian drug name; ◉ Prototype drug

129

*severe exacerbation of angina, MI, and ventricular arrhythmias.*

### Assessment & Drug Effects
- Measure trough BP (just prior to scheduled dose) to determine efficacy.
- Check apical pulse before administration in patients receiving digitalis (both drugs slow AV conduction). If below 60 bpm (or other ordered parameter), withhold dose and consult prescriber.
- Monitor BP throughout dosage adjustment period. Consult prescriber for acceptable parameters.
- Monitor diabetics for loss of glycemic control.

### Patient & Family Education
- Do not abruptly discontinue this drug.
- Adhere closely to dose regimen. Sudden discontinuation of drug can exacerbate angina and precipitate tachycardia or MI in patients with coronary artery disease, and thyroid storm in patients with hyperthyroidism.
- Make position changes slowly and in stages, particularly from recumbent to upright posture.
- If diabetic, closely monitor blood glucose values.

## ATOMOXETINE
(a-to-mox'e-teen)
**Strattera**
**Classification:** MISCELLANEOUS PSYCHOTHERAPEUTIC
**Therapeutic:** ADHD AGENT

### AVAILABILITY Capsule

### ACTION & *THERAPEUTIC EFFECT*
Selective inhibition of the presynaptic norepinephrine transporter, resulting in norepinephrine reuptake inhibition. *Improved attentiveness,* *ability to follow through on tasks with less distraction and forgetfulness, and diminished hyperactivity.*

### USES
Acute and maintenance treatment of attention deficit/hyperactivity disorder (ADHD) in adults and children.

### CONTRAINDICATIONS
Hypersensitive to atomoxetine or any of its constituents; concomitant use or use within 2 wk of MAOIs; narrow angle glaucoma; structural cardiac abnormalities or other serious heart problems; pheochromocytoma or history of pheochromocytoma; jaundice or liver injury; suicidal ideation; major depressive disorder (MDD); lactation.

### CAUTIOUS USE
Severe liver injury may progress to liver failure or death in a small percentage of patients. History of hypertension, tachycardia, cardiovascular or cerebrovascular disease; any condition that predisposes to hypotension; urinary retention or urinary hesitancy; history of bipolar disorder; history of suicidal tendencies; increased risk of suicidal ideation in children and adolescents; pregnancy (category C).

### ROUTE & DOSAGE

**ADHD**

*Adult/Adolescent/Child (older than 6 y and weight greater than 70 kg):* **PO** Start with 40 mg in morning. May increase after 3 days to target dose of 80 mg/day q.a.m. or as divided dose. May increase (max: 100 mg/day if needed)

*Child/Adolescent (weight less than 70 kg):* **PO** Start with 0.5 mg/kg/day. May increase after 3 days to target dose of 1.2 mg/kg/day.

Administer q.a.m. or divided dose (max: 1.4 mg/kg or 100 mg, whichever is less)

**Hepatic Impairment Dosage Adjustment**

*Child-Pugh class B:* Initial and target doses should be reduced to 50% of the normal dose
*Child-Pugh class C:* Initial dose and target doses should be reduced to 25% of normal dose

**Pharmacogenetic Dosage Adjustment/Patients Receiving Concurrent CYP2D6 Inhibitors**

*CYP2D6 poor metabolizers: Children/adolescents (weight less than 70 kg):* Start at 0.5 mg/kg, adjust upward only after 4 wk if well tolerated; *adults/adolescents (weight greater than 70 kg).* Start at 40 mg/day, adjust upward only after 4 wk if well tolerated; do not exceed 80 mg

## ADMINISTRATION
**Oral**
- Note that total daily dose in children and adolescents is based on weight. Determine that ordered dose is appropriate for weight prior to administration of drug.
- Note manufacturer recommends dosage adjustments with concomitant administration of strong CYP2D6 inhibitors (e.g., paroxetine, fluoxetine, quinidine). Consult prescriber.
- Store at 15°–30° C (59°–86° F).

**ADVERSE EFFECTS** (≥1%) **Body as a Whole:** Flu-like syndrome, flushing, fatigue, fever, rigors. **CNS:** Dizziness, *headache,* somnolence, crying, tearfulness, irritability, mood swings, *insomnia,* depression, tremor, early morning awakenings, paresthesias, abnormal dreams, decreased libido, sleep disorder, <u>suicidal ideation</u>. **CV:** Increased blood pressure, sinus tachycardia, palpitations. **GI:** *Upper abdominal pain,* constipation, dyspepsia, *nausea, vomiting, decreased appetite,* anorexia, dry mouth, diarrhea, flatulence, <u>severe liver injury (rare)</u>. **Endocrine:** Hot flushes, sexual dysfunction. **Metabolic:** Weight loss. **Hepatic:** Hepatotoxicity. **Musculoskeletal:** Arthralgia, myalgia. **Respiratory:** *Cough,* rhinorrhea, nasal congestion, sinusitis. **Skin:** Dermatitis, pruritus, increased sweating. **Special Senses:** Mydriasis. **Urogenital:** Urinary hesitation/retention, dysmenorrhea, ejaculation dysfunction, impotence, delayed onset of menses, irregular menstruation, prostatitis; priapism, male pelvic pain.

**INTERACTIONS Drug: Albuterol** may potentiate cardiovascular effects of atomoxetine; CYP2D6 inhibitors (**fluoxetine, paroxetine, quinidine**) may increase atomoxetine levels and toxicity; MAOIS may precipitate a hypertensive crisis; may attenuate effects of ANTIHYPERTENSIVE AGENTS.

**PHARMACOKINETICS Absorption:** Well absorbed from GI tract. **Distribution:** 98% protein bound. **Peak:** 1–2 h. **Metabolism:** In liver by CYP2D6. **Elimination:** Primarily in urine. **Half-Life:** 5.2 h.

## NURSING IMPLICATIONS

**Black Box Warning**

*Atomoxetine has been associated with increased suicidal thinking and behavior in children and adolescents.*

### Assessment & Drug Effects

- Evaluate for continuing therapeutic effectiveness especially with long-term use.
- Report increased aggression and irritability as these may indicate a need to discontinue the drug.
- Monitor children and adolescents for behavior changes that may indicate suicidal ideation, including aggression and anxiety that may be precursors of it.
- Monitor cardiovascular status especially with preexisting hypertension.
- Monitor HR and BP at baseline, following a dose increase, and periodically while on therapy.
- Monitor lab tests: Periodic LFTs.

### Patient & Family Education

- Instruct patients on S&S of liver toxicity.
- Report any of the following to the prescriber: Indicators of suicidal ideation in children and adolescents; chest pains or palpitations, urinary retention or difficulty initiating voiding urine, appetite loss and weight loss, or insomnia.
- Make position changes slowly if you experience dizziness with arising from a lying or sitting position.
- Do not drive or engage in potentially hazardous activities until reaction to the drug is known.

## ATORVASTATIN CALCIUM

(a-tor-va'sta-tin)

Lipitor

**Classifications:** ANTILIPEMIC; HMG-COA; REDUCTASE INHIBITOR (STATIN)
**Therapeutic:** ANTILIPEMIC; STATIN
**Prototype:** Lovastatin

**AVAILABILITY** Tablet

## ACTION & *THERAPEUTIC EFFECT*

An inhibitor of HMG-CoA, an enzyme essential to hepatic production of cholesterol; increases the number of hepatic LDL receptors, thus increasing LDL uptake and catabolism. *Atorvastatin reduces LDL and total triglyceride (TG) production as well as increases the plasma level of high-density lipids (HDL).*

**USES** Adjunct to diet for the reduction of LDL cholesterol and triglycerides in patients with primary hypercholesterolemia and mixed dyslipidemia, prevention of cardiovascular disease in patients with multiple risk factors.

**CONTRAINDICATIONS** Hypersensitivity to atorvastatin, myopathy, active liver disease, unexplained persistent transaminase elevations, hepatic encephalopathy, hepatitis, active hepatic disease; jaundice, rhabdomyolysis; uncontrolled seizure disorders; pregnancy (category X); lactation.

**CAUTIOUS USE** Hypersensitivity to other HMG-CoA reductase inhibitors, history of liver disease, older adults; renal impairment; patients who consume substantial quantities of alcohol; surgery. Safety and efficacy in children younger than 10 y not established.

## ROUTE & DOSAGE

**Hypercholesterolemia/ Prevention of Cardiovascular Disease**

*Adult:* **PO** Start with 10–40 mg daily, may increase up to 80 mg/day

*Child/Adolescent (10 to less than 17 y):* **PO** Start with 10 mg daily, may increase up to 20 mg/day

Common adverse effects in *italic;* life-threatening effects underlined; generic names in **bold;** classifications in SMALL CAPS; ✦ Canadian drug name; ⊙ Prototype drug

## ADMINISTRATION

### Oral
- May be given at any time of day.
- Store at 20°–25° C (68°–77° F).

## ADVERSE EFFECTS (≥1%) **Body as a Whole:** Back pain, asthenia, hypersensitivity reaction, myalgia, rhabdomyolysis. **CNS:** Headache, insomnia. **GI:** Abdominal pain, constipation, diarrhea, dyspepsia, flatulence, increased liver function tests. **Respiratory:** Sinusitis, pharyngitis. **Skin:** Rash. **GU:** Urinary tract infection.

## INTERACTIONS **Drug:** May increase **digoxin** levels 20%, increases levels of **norethindrone**; **erythromycin** may increase atorvastatin levels 40%; MACROLIDE ANTIBIOTICS, **cyclosporine, delavirdine, gemfibrozil, niacin, clofibrate,** AZOLE ANTIFUNGALS (**ketoconazole, itraconazole**) may increase risk of rhabdomyolysis; **nelfinavir** may increase atorvastatin levels. Concurrent use of **lopinavir** or **ritonavir** requires decrease of dose of **atorvastatin. Food: Grapefruit juice** (greater than 1 qt/day) may increase risk of myopathy and rhabdomyolysis. Fiber may decrease effect, separate doses. **Lab Test:** May increase fasting glucose and HgA1C.

## PHARMACOKINETICS **Absorption:** Rapidly from GI tract. 30% reaches the systemic circulation. **Onset:** Cholesterol reduction—2 wk. **Peak:** Plasma concentration, 1–2 h; effect 2–4 wk. **Distribution:** 98% or greater protein bound. Crosses placenta, distributed into breast milk of animals. **Metabolism:** In the liver by CYP3A4 to active metabolites. **Elimination:** Primarily in bile; less than 2% in urine. **Half-Life:** 14 h; 20–30 h for active metabolites.

## NURSING IMPLICATIONS

### Assessment & Drug Effects
- Monitor for therapeutic effectiveness which is indicated by reduction in the level of LDL-C. Monitor diabetics for loss of glycemic control.
- Assess for muscle pain, tenderness, or weakness; and, if present, monitor CPK level (discontinue drug with marked elevations of CPK or if myopathy is suspected).
- Monitor carefully for digoxin toxicity with concurrent digoxin use.
- Monitor prediabetics and diabetics for loss of glycemic control.
- Monitor lab tests: Lipid levels within 2–4 wk after initiation of therapy or upon change in dosage; LFTs at 6 and 12 wk after initiation or elevation of dose, and periodically thereafter; periodic HbgA1c.

### Patient & Family Education
- Report promptly any of the following: Unexplained muscle pain, tenderness, or weakness, especially with fever or malaise; yellowing of skin or eyes; stomach pain with nausea, vomiting, or loss of appetite; skin rash or hives.
- Do not take drug during pregnancy because it may cause birth defects. Immediately inform prescriber of a suspected or known pregnancy.
- Inform prescriber regarding concurrent use of any of the following drugs: Erythromycin, niacin, antifungals, or birth control pills.
- Minimize alcohol intake while taking this drug.

## ATOVAQUONE
(a-to′va-quone)

**Mepron**

**Classification:** ANTIPROTOZOAL
**Therapeutic:** ANTIPROTOZOAL
**Prototype:** Metronidazole

## AVAILABILITY Oral suspension

Common adverse effects in *italic;* life-threatening effects underlined; generic names in **bold;** classifications in SMALL CAPS; ◆ Canadian drug name; ⊘ Prototype drug

133

## ACTION & *THERAPEUTIC EFFECT*

Atovaquone is an antiprotozoal with antipneumocystic activity, including *Pneumocystis carinii* (PCP) and the *Plasmodium* species. The site of action in PCP is linked to inhibition of the electron transport system in the mitochondria. This results in the inhibition of nucleic acid and ATP synthesis. *Effective against* P. carinii *and the* Plasmodium *species, as well as other protozoans.*

## USES

Second-line oral therapy of mild to moderate *P. carinii* pneumonia (PCP) in immunocompromised patients intolerant of co-trimoxazole.

## UNLABELED USES

May be effective in the treatment of cerebral toxoplasmosis.

## CONTRAINDICATIONS

History of potential life-threatening allergies to atovaquone.

## CAUTIOUS USE

Severe PCP, concurrent pulmonary diseases, older adults, impaired hepatic function; pregnancy (category C); lactation; neonates and infants.

## ROUTE & DOSAGE

**Mild to Moderate *Pneumocystis Carinii* Pneumonia (PCP)**

*Adult:* **PO** 750 mg (5 mL) suspension b.i.d. for 21 days

## ADMINISTRATION

**Oral**

- Give with meals because food significantly enhances absorption.
- Store at room temperature 15°–30° C (59°–86° F) unless otherwise directed by the manufacturer.

## ADVERSE EFFECTS (≥1%)

**Body as a Whole:** *Fever.* **CV:** Hypotension. **CNS:** *Headache, insomnia, dizziness, strange or vivid dreams, anxiety, depression.* **Hematologic:** Anemia, neutropenia. **Metabolic:** Hyponatremia, hypoglycemia. **GI:** *Nausea, diarrhea, vomiting,* abdominal pain, anorexia, dyspepsia, oral candidiasis, oral ulcers. **Skin:** *Rash,* pruritus, erythema multiforme. **Respiratory:** Cough, sinusitis.

## DIAGNOSTIC TEST INTERFERENCE

May cause increase in **amylase** and other **liver function tests.**

## INTERACTIONS

**Drug:** **Zidovudine** may increase risk of bone marrow toxicity. **Food:** Oral absorption is increased 3- to 4-fold when administered with food, especially with fatty foods.

## PHARMACOKINETICS

**Absorption:** Poor, absorption improved when taken with a fatty meal. **Duration:** 6–23 wk after a 3-wk course of therapy. **Distribution:** Penetrates poorly into cerebrospinal fluid; greater than 99.9% protein bound. **Metabolism:** Not metabolized. **Elimination:** Greater than 94% in feces over 21 days (enterohepatically cycled). **Half-Life:** 2–3 days.

## NURSING IMPLICATIONS

### Assessment & Drug Effects

- Assess for therapeutic failure in patients with GI disorders that may limit absorption of drug.
- Monitor lab tests: Periodic CBC with differential, blood glucose, serum sodium, creatinine, BUN, and serum amylase.

### Patient & Family Education

- Note: It is necessary to take this drug exactly as prescribed because it is slowly eliminated from the body.

# ATOVAQUONE/PROGUANIL HYDROCHLORIDE

(a-to'va-quone/pro'gua-nil)

Malarone, Malarone Pediatric

**Classification:** ANTIMALARIAL
**Therapeutic:** ANTIMALARIAL
**Prototype:** Chloroquine HCl and Metronidazole

**AVAILABILITY** Atovaquone 250 mg/proguanil HCl 100 mg (adult dose), atovaquone 62.5 mg/proguanil HCl 25 mg (pediatric dose) tablets

**ACTION & *THERAPEUTIC EFFECT***
Combination of two antimalarial drugs. Atovaquone inhibits electron transport system in mitochondria of the malaria parasite, thus interfering with nucleic acid and ATP synthesis of the parasite. Proguanil interferes with DNA synthesis of the malaria parasite. *This drug combination has synergistic activity toward malarial treatment because each component has a different mode of action.*

**USES** Prevention and treatment of malaria due to *P. falciparum,* even in chloroquine-resistant areas.

**CONTRAINDICATIONS** Known hypersensitivity to atovaquone or proguanil; severe malaria.

**CAUTIOUS USE** Cerebral malaria, complicated malaria, pulmonary edema; renal failure, renal impairment; hepatic disease; lactation; older adults; African Americans, Chinese, Japanese; diarrhea, emesis, GI disease; hepatic disease, infection, sunlight (UV) exposure; pregnancy (category C).

## ROUTE & DOSAGE

### Prevention of Malaria

*Adult:* **PO** 1 tablet daily with food starting 1–2 days before travel to malarial area and continuing for 7 days after return

*Child (weight 11–20 kg):* **PO** 1 pediatric tablet daily; *weight 21–30 kg:* 2 pediatric tablets daily; *weight 31–40 kg:* 3 pediatric tablets daily; *weight greater than 40 kg:* 1 adult tablet daily with food starting 1–2 days before travel to malarial area and continuing for 7 days after return

### Treatment of Malaria

*Adult:* **PO** 4 tablets as a single daily dose for 3 days
*Child (weight 5–8 kg):* **PO** 2 pediatric tablets; *weight 9–10 kg:* 3 pediatric tablets; *weight 11–20 kg:* 1 adult tablet; *weight 21–30 kg:* 2 adult tablets; *weight 31–40 kg:* 3 adult tablets; *weight greater than 40 kg:* 4 adult tablets as a single daily dose for 3 days

## ADMINISTRATION

### Oral

- Give at the same time each day with food or a drink containing milk.
- Give a repeat dose if vomiting occurs within 1 h after dosing.

**ADVERSE EFFECTS** (≥1%) **Body as a Whole:** Fever, *myalgia,* back pain, asthenia, anorexia. **Digestive:** *Nausea, abdominal pain, diarrhea,* dyspepsia. **CNS:** *Headache.* **Respiratory:** Cough. **Skin:** Pruritus. **Other:** Anaphylactic reaction.

**INTERACTIONS Drug: Rifampin, rifabutin, tetracycline** may

Common adverse effects in *italic;* life-threatening effects underlined; generic names in **bold;** classifications in SMALL CAPS; ✦Canadian drug name; ● Prototype drug

135

decrease serum levels; **metoclopramide** may decrease absorption.

## PHARMACOKINETICS Absorption: Atovaquone (A), Poor, absorption improved when taken with a fatty meal; **Proguanil (P),** Extensively absorbed. **Duration: A,** 6–23 wk after a 3-wk course of therapy. **Distribution: A,** Penetrates poorly into cerebrospinal fluid; greater than 99.9% protein bound; **P,** 75% protein bound. **Metabolism: A,** Not metabolized; **P,** Metabolized by CYP2C19 to cycloguanil. **Elimination: A,** Greater than 94% in feces over 21 days (enterohepatically cycled); **P,** Primarily in urine. **Half-Life: A,** 2–3 days; **P,** 12–21 h.

## NURSING IMPLICATIONS

### Assessment & Drug Effects

- Monitor for S&S of parasitemia in patients receiving tetracycline and in those experiencing diarrhea or vomiting.
- Note: Only use metoclopramide to control vomiting if other antiemetics are not available.
- Monitor lab tests: Periodic AST and ALT, especially with long-term therapy.

### Patient & Family Education

- Take this drug at the same time each day for maximum effectiveness.
- Note: Absorption of this drug may be reduced with diarrhea and vomiting. Consult prescriber if either of these occurs.

## ATRACURIUM BESYLATE ℞

(a-tra-kyoor'ee-um)

**Classifications:** NONPOLARIZING SKELETAL MUSCLE RELAXANT; NEUROMUSCULAR ANTAGONIST

Therapeutic: SKELETAL MUSCLE RELAXANT

**AVAILABILITY** Solution for injection

## ACTION & *THERAPEUTIC EFFECT*
Inhibits neuromuscular transmission by binding competitively with acetylcholine at muscle end plate receptors. *Synthetic skeletal muscle relaxant that produces short duration of neuromuscular blockade, exhibits minimal direct effects on cardiovascular system, and has less histamine-releasing action.*

**USES** Adjunct for general anesthesia to produce skeletal muscle relaxation during surgery; to facilitate endotracheal intubation. Especially useful for patients with severe renal or hepatic disease, limited cardiac reserve, and in patients with low or atypical pseudocholinesterase levels.

**CONTRAINDICATIONS** Myasthenia gravis.

**CAUTIOUS USE** When appreciable histamine release would be hazardous (as in asthma or anaphylactoid reactions, significant cardiovascular disease), neuromuscular disease (e.g., Eaton–Lambert syndrome), carcinomatosis, electrolyte or acid–base imbalances, dehydration, impaired pulmonary function; pregnancy (category C); lactation; children younger than 1 mo.

## ROUTE & DOSAGE

### Skeletal Muscle Relaxation

*Adult/Child (2 y or older):* **IV** 0.4–0.5 mg/kg initial dose, then 0.08–0.1 mg/kg bolus 20–45 min after the first dose and q15–25 min thereafter; reduce doses if used with general anesthetics
*Child (1 mo to less than 2 y):* **IV** 0.3–0.4 mg/kg

### Mechanical Ventilation

*Adult:* **IV** 5–9 mcg/kg/min by continuous infusion

Common adverse effects in *italic;* life-threatening effects underlined; generic names in **bold;** classifications in SMALL CAPS; ♣ Canadian drug name; ℞ Prototype drug

## ADMINISTRATION

- Verify correct concentration and rate of infusion for infants and children with prescriber.

### Intravenous

*PREPARE:* **Direct:** Give initial bolus dose undiluted. **Continuous:** Maintenance dose **must be** diluted with NS, D5W or D5/NS. Maximum concentration should be 0.5 mg/mL. Do not mix in same syringe or administer through same needle as used for alkaline solutions [incompatible with alkaline solutions (e.g., barbiturates)].

*ADMINISTER:* **Direct:** Give as bolus dose over 30–60 sec. **Continuous:** Give infusion at rate required to maintain desired effect.

*INCOMPATIBILITIES:* **Solution/additive: Lactated Ringer's, aminophylline, cefazolin, heparin, nitroprusside quinidine, ranitidine, sodium nitroprusside. Y-site: Aminophylline, amphotericin B, cefonicid, cefoperazone, cefoxitin, ceftazidime, dantrolene, diazepam, diazoxide, furosemide, ganciclovir, indomethacin, pantoprazole, pentobarbital, phenobarbital, phenytoin, propofol, sodium bicarbonate.**

- Store at 2°–8° C (36°–46° F) to preserve potency unless otherwise directed. Avoid freezing.

## ADVERSE EFFECTS (≥1%) **CV:** Bradycardia, tachycardia. **Respiratory:** Respiratory depression. **Other:** Increased salivation, anaphylaxis.

## INTERACTIONS **Drug:** GENERAL ANESTHETICS increase magnitude and duration of neuromuscular blocking action; AMINOGLYCOSIDES, **bacitracin, polymyxin B, clindamycin, lidocaine, parenteral magnesium, quinidine, quinine, trimethaphan, verapamil** increase neuromuscular blockade; DIURETICS may increase or decrease neuromuscular blockade; **lithium** prolongs duration of neuromuscular blockade; NARCOTIC ANALGESICS present possibility of additive respiratory depression; **succinylcholine** increases onset and depth of neuromuscular blockade; **phenytoin** may cause resistance to or reversal of neuromuscular blockade.

## PHARMACOKINETICS **Onset:** 2 min. **Peak:** 3–5 min. **Duration:** 60–70 min. **Distribution:** Well distributed to tissues and extracellular fluids; crosses placenta; distribution into breast milk unknown. **Metabolism:** Rapid nonenzymatic degradation in bloodstream. **Elimination:** 70–90% in urine in 5–7 h. **Half-Life:** 20 min.

## NURSING IMPLICATIONS

### Assessment & Drug Effects

- Note: Personnel and equipment required for endotracheal intubation, administration of oxygen under positive pressure, artificial respiration, and assisted or controlled ventilation **must be** immediately available.
- Evaluate degree of neuromuscular blockade and muscle paralysis to avoid risk of overdosage by qualified individual using peripheral nerve stimulator.
- Monitor BP, pulse, and respirations and evaluate patient's recovery from neuromuscular blocking (curare-like) effect as evidenced by ability to breathe naturally or to take deep breaths and cough, keep eyes open, lift head keeping mouth closed, adequacy

Common adverse effects in *italic*; life-threatening effects underlined; generic names in **bold**; classifications in SMALL CAPS; ♣ Canadian drug name; ⊘ Prototype drug

137

of hand-grip strength. Notify prescriber if recovery is delayed.

- Note: Recovery from neuromuscular blockade usually begins 35–45 min after drug administration and is almost complete in about 1 h. Recovery time may be delayed in patients with cardiovascular disease, edematous states, and in older adults.

- Monitor lab tests: Baseline serum electrolytes, acid–base balance, and renal function tests.

## ATROPINE SULFATE ℗
(a'troe-peen)

Atropair ◆

**Classifications:** ANTICHOLINERGIC; ANTIMUSCARINIC; ANTIARRHYTHMIC

Therapeutic: ANTISECRETORY; ANTIARRHYTHMIC; BRONCHODILATOR

**AVAILABILITY** Solution for injection, ophthalmic ointment, ophthalmic drops

## ACTION & *THERAPEUTIC EFFECT*
Acts by selectively blocking all muscarinic responses to acetylcholine (ACh). Antisecretory action (vagolytic effect) suppresses sweating, lacrimation, salivation, and secretions from nose, mouth, pharynx, and bronchi. Blocks vagal impulses to heart causing decreased AV conduction time, increased HR and cardiac output, and shortened PR interval. *Potent bronchodilator when bronchoconstriction has been induced by parasympathomimetics, and decreases bronchial secretions. Decreases GI spasm. Produces mydriasis and cycloplegia by blocking responses of iris sphincter muscle and ciliary muscle of lens to cholinergic stimulation. Increases heart rate and cardiac output.*

**USES** Adjunct in symptomatic treatment of GI disorders (e.g., peptic ulcer, pylorospasm, GI hypermotility, irritable bowel syndrome) and spastic disorders of biliary tract. Relaxes upper GI tract and colon during hypotonic radiography. **Ophthalmic Use:** To produce mydriasis and cycloplegia before refraction and for treatment of anterior uveitis and iritis. **Preoperative Use:** To suppress salivation, perspiration, and respiratory tract secretions; to reduce incidence of laryngospasm, reflex bradycardia arrhythmia, and hypotension during general anesthesia. **Cardiac Uses:** For sinus bradycardia or asystole during CPR or that is induced by drugs or toxic substances (e.g., pilocarpine, beta-adrenergic blockers, organophosphate pesticides, and *Amanita* mushroom poisoning); for management of selected patients with symptomatic sinus bradycardia and associated hypotension and ventricular irritability; for diagnosis of sinus node dysfunction and in evaluation of coronary artery disease during atrial pacing; for management of chronic symptomatic sinus node dysfunction. **Other Uses:** Oral inhalation for short-term treatment and prevention of bronchospasms associated with asthma, bronchitis, and COPD and as drying agent in upper respiratory infection. Adjunctive therapy for hypermotility of GI tract.

## CONTRAINDICATIONS Hypersensitivity to belladonna alkaloids; asthma, angle-closure glaucoma; parotitis; intestinal atony, paralytic ileus, achalasia, pyloric

stenosis, obstructive diseases of GI tract, severe ulcerative colitis, toxic megacolon; tachycardia; acute hemorrhage; myasthenia gravis.

**CAUTIOUS USE** Myocardial infarction, hypertension, hypotension; coronary artery disease, CHF, tachy-arrhythmias; gastric ulcer, hiatal hernia with reflux esophagitis; hyperthyroidism; COPD; autonomic neuropathy; hepatic or renal disease; debilitated patients; Down syndrome; autonomic neuropathy, spastic paralysis, brain damage in children; patients exposed to high environmental temperatures; patients with fever; BPH; older adults; pregnancy (category C); lactation; infants.

## ROUTE & DOSAGE

### Preanesthesia

*Adult:* **IV/IM/Subcutaneous** 0.4–0.6 mg 30–60 min before surgery
*Child (weight less than 5 kg):* **IV/IM/Subcutaneous** 0.04 mg/kg; *5 kg and greater:* 0.03 mg/kg 30–60 min before surgery (max: 0.4 mg)

### Bradyarrhythmias

*Adult:* **IV/IM** 1 mg q2–3min (max: 3 mg)
*Child:* **IV/IM** 0.01–0.03 mg/kg for 1–2 doses

### Organophosphate Antidote

*Adult:* **IV/IM** 1–2 mg q5–60min until muscarinic signs and symptoms subside (may need up to 50 mg)
*Child:* **IV/IM** 0.05 mg/kg q10–30min until muscarinic signs and symptoms subside

### COPD

*Adult:* **Inhalation** 0.025 mg/kg diluted with 3–5 mL saline, via nebulizer 3–4 × daily (max: 2.5 mg/day)
*Child:* **Inhalation** 0.03–0.05 mg/kg diluted with 3–5 mL saline, via nebulizer 3–4 × daily

### Uveitis

*Adult/Child:* **Ophthalmic** 1–2 drops of solution or small amount of ointment in eye up to t.i.d.

### Cycloplegia

*Adult:* **Ophthalmic** 1 drop of solution or small amount of ointment in eye 1 h before the procedure
*Child:* **Ophthalmic** 1–2 drops in eye b.i.d. for 1–3 days prior to procedure or a small amount of ointment in conjunctival sac t.i.d. for 1–3 days prior to procedure with last dose applied several hours before the procedure

## ADMINISTRATION

### Ocular

- Use a gloved finger to compress the lacrimal sac for 2–3 min after instillation to prevent excessive systemic absorption.

### Subcutaneous/Intramuscular

- Inject undiluted. When using AtroPen, inject into the outer thigh at a 90 degree angle.

### Intravenous

**PREPARE: Direct:** Give undiluted or diluted in up to 10 mL of sterile water.
**ADMINISTER: Direct:** Give 1 mg or fraction thereof over 1 min directly into a Y-site.
**INCOMPATIBILITIES: Solution/additive: Pantoprazole. Y-site: Amphotericin B (conven-**

tional), **dantrolene, diaze-pam, diazoxide, pantopra-zole, phenytoin, SMZ/TMP, thiopental.**

▪ Store at room temperature 15°–30° C (59°–86° F) in protected airtight, light-resistant containers unless otherwise directed by manufacturer.

## ADVERSE EFFECTS (≥1%) CNS:
Headache, ataxia, dizziness, excitement, irritability, convulsions, drowsiness, fatigue, weakness; mental depression, confusion, disorientation, hallucinations. **CV:** Hypertension or hypotension, ventricular tachycardia, palpitation, paradoxical bradycardia, AV dissociation, atrial or <u>ventricular fibrillation</u>. **GI:** Dry mouth with thirst, dysphagia, loss of taste; nausea, vomiting, constipation, delayed gastric emptying, antral stasis, paralytic ileus. **Urogenital:** Urinary hesitancy and retention, dysuria, impotence. **Skin:** Flushed, dry skin; anhidrosis, rash, urticaria, contact dermatitis, allergic conjunctivitis, fixed-drug eruption. **Special Senses:** Mydriasis, blurred vision, photophobia, increased intraocular pressure, cycloplegia, eye dryness, local redness.

## DIAGNOSTIC TEST INTERFERENCE
**Upper GI series:** Findings may require qualification because of anticholinergic effects of atropine (reduced gastric motility and delayed gastric emptying). **PSP excretion test:** Atropine may decrease urinary excretion of PSP (phenolsul-fonphthalein).

## INTERACTIONS Drug: Aman-tadine, ANTIHISTAMINES, TRICYCLIC ANTIDEPRESSANTS, quinidine, dis-opyramide, procainamide add to anticholinergic effects. Levo-

**dopa** effects decreased. **Methotrimeprazine** may precipitate extrapyramidal effects. Antipsychotic effects of PHENOTHIAZINES are decreased due to decreased absorption.

## PHARMACOKINETICS Absorption: Well absorbed from all administration sites. Peak effect: 30 min IM, 2–4 min IV, 1–2 h subcutaneous, 1.5–4 h inhalation, 30–40 min topical. **Duration:** Inhibition of salivation 4 h; mydriasis 7–14 days. **Distribution:** In most body tissues; crosses blood–brain barrier and placenta. **Metabolism:** In liver. **Elimination:** 77–94% in urine in 24 h. **Half-Life:** 2–3 h.

## NURSING IMPLICATIONS
### Assessment & Drug Effects
▪ Monitor vital signs. HR is a sensitive indicator of patient's response to atropine. Be alert to changes in quality, rate, and rhythm of HR and respiration and to changes in BP and temperature.
▪ Initial paradoxical bradycardia following IV atropine usually lasts only 1–2 min; it most likely occurs when IV is administered slowly (more than 1 min) or when small doses (less than 0.5 mg) are used. Postural hypotension occurs when patient ambulates too soon after parenteral administration.
▪ Note: Frequent and continued use of eye preparations, as well as overdosage, can have systemic effects. Some atropine deaths have resulted from systemic absorption following ocular administration in infants and children.
▪ Monitor I&O, especially in older adults and patients who have had surgery (drug may contribute to urinary retention).
▪ Monitor CNS status. Older adults and debilitated patients some-

times manifest drowsiness or CNS stimulation (excitement, agitation, confusion) with usual doses of drug or other belladonna alkaloids. Supervision of ambulation may be indicated.
- Monitor infants, small children, and older adults for "atropine fever" (hyperpyrexia due to suppression of perspiration and heat loss), which increases the risk of heatstroke.
- Patients receiving atropine via inhalation sometimes manifest mild CNS stimulation with doses in excess of 5 mg and mental depression and other mental disturbances with larger doses.

**Patient & Family Education**
- Follow measures to relieve dry mouth: Adequate hydration; small, frequent mouth rinses with tepid water; meticulous mouth and dental hygiene; gum chewing or sucking sugarless sourballs.
- Note: Drug causes drowsiness, sensitivity to light, blurring of near vision, and temporarily impairs ability to judge distance. Avoid driving and other activities requiring visual acuity and mental alertness.
- Discontinue ophthalmic preparations and notify prescriber if eye pain, conjunctivitis, palpitation, rapid pulse, or dizziness occurs.

## AURANOFIN ℗

(au-rane'eh-fin)

Ridaura

**Classifications:** GOLD COMPOUND; IMMUNOLOGIC; ANTI-INFLAMMATORY; ANTI-RHEUMATIC
Therapeutic: ANTI-INFLAMMATORY; ANTIRHEUMATIC

**AVAILABILITY** Capsule

**ACTION & *THERAPEUTIC EFFECT***
Strongly lipophilic and almost neutral in solution, properties that may facilitate transport across cell membranes. Has immunomodulatory and anti-inflammatory effects, although mechanism of action is not understood. Gold is taken up by macrophages possibly causing inhibition of phagocytosis and lysosomal enzyme release resulting in an anti-inflammatory effect. Gold also causes decreased serum immunoglobulin concentrations and rheumatoid factor titers resulting in immunomodulatory effect. *Auranofin is immunomodulatory and anti-inflammatory.*

**USES** Management of rheumatoid arthritis.

**CONTRAINDICATIONS** History of gold-induced necrotizing enterocolitis, renal disease, exfoliative dermatitis or bone marrow aplasia, recent radiation therapy, history of severe toxicity from previous exposure to gold or other heavy metals; uncontrolled CHF; marked hypertension; SLE; lactation.

**CAUTIOUS USE** Inflammatory bowel disease, rash, liver disease, renal disease; history of bone marrow depression; older adults; DM; CHF; pregnancy (category C).

## ROUTE & DOSAGE

**Rheumatoid Arthritis**
*Adult:* **PO** 6 mg/day in 1–2 divided doses, may increase to

6–9 mg/day in 3 divided doses after 6 mo (max: 9 mg/day)

*hematuria, pruritus, rash, stomatitis, and persistent diarrhea may occur.*

## ADMINISTRATION

### Oral

- Give capsule with food or fluid of patient's choice.
- Store at 15°–30° C (59°–86° F); protect from light and moisture.
- Note: Expiration date is 4 y after date of manufacture.

## ADVERSE EFFECTS (≥1%) GI: *Diarrhea, abdominal cramping* and pain; *nausea,* vomiting, anorexia, dysphagia; *stomatitis,* glossitis, metallic taste; flatulence, constipation, GI bleeding, melena. **Hematologic:** Thrombocytopenia, leukopenia, eosinophilia, agranulocytosis, aplastic anemia. **Urogenital:** Proteinuria, hematuria, renal failure. **Skin:** *Rash, pruritus,* dermatitis, urticaria.

## INTERACTIONS Drug: May increase phenytoin levels.

## DIAGNOSTIC TEST INTERFERENCE

Auranofin may enhance response to a *tuberculin skin test.*

## PHARMACOKINETICS Absorption: 20% from small intestine. Peak: 2 h. **Distribution:** Highest concentrations in kidneys, spleen, lungs, adrenals, and liver; unknown if crosses placenta; small amounts distributed into breast milk. **Elimination:** 60% of absorbed gold eliminated in urine, remainder in feces. **Half-Life:** 11–23 days.

## NURSING IMPLICATIONS

### Black Box Warning

*Gold toxicity, manifested by bone marrow suppression, proteinuria,*

### Assessment & Drug Effects

- Monitor for therapeutic effectiveness which develops slowly and is not usually apparent for 3–4 mo.
- Report any of the following S&S promptly: Unexplained bleeding or bruising, metallic taste, sore mouth; pruritus, rash; diarrhea and melena; yellow skin and sclera; unexplained cough or dyspnea.
- Monitor lab tests: Periodic CBC with differential and platelet count; periodic LFTs and renal function tests.

### Patient & Family Education

- Report adverse effects of therapy, especially abdominal cramping and pain; discontinuance of therapy may be necessary.
- Report metallic taste and pruritus with or without rash. These are among earliest symptoms of impending gold toxicity.
- Do not change dosage (dose or dose interval) by omission, increase, or decrease without first consulting prescriber.
- Use antidiarrheal OTC drug and high-fiber diet for drug-induced diarrhea.
- Avoid exposure to sunlight or to artificial ultraviolet light to prevent photosensitivity reaction.
- Rinse mouth with water frequently for symptomatic treatment of mild stomatitis. Avoid commercial mouth rinses; clean teeth with soft tooth brush and gentle brushing to avoid gingival trauma. Floss at least once daily.

Common adverse effects in *italic;* life-threatening effects underlined; generic names in **bold;** classifications in SMALL CAPS; ♣ Canadian drug name; ⊙ Prototype drug

# AVANAFIL

(a-van'a-fil)

Stendra

**Classification:** PHOSPHODIESTERASE (PDE) INHIBITOR; IMPOTENCE AGENT
Therapeutic: IMPOTENCE AGENT
**Prototype:** Sildenafil

## AVAILABILITY Tablet

## ACTION & *THERAPEUTIC EFFECT*

Enhances the effect of nitric oxide (NO) release in the corpus cavernosum during sexual stimulation. NO causes increased levels of cGMP, producing smooth muscle relaxation in the corpus cavernosum and allowing inflow of blood into the penis. NO inhibits PDE5, an enzyme responsible for degrading cGMP in the corpus cavernosum. *Promotes sustained erection only in the presence of sexual stimulation.*

## USES Treatment of erectile dysfunction.

## CONTRAINDICATIONS Hypersensitivity to avanafil; severe hepatic impairment (Child Pugh class C); severe renal impairment (CrCl less than 30 mL/min).

## CAUTIOUS USE Preexisting cardiovascular disease; bleeding disorders; active peptic ulcer disease; mild-to-moderate renal or hepatic impairment; alcohol consumption; concurrent antihypertensive drugs; pregnancy (category C). Safety and efficacy in children younger than 18 y not established.

## ROUTE & DOSAGE

### Erectile Dysfunction
*Adult:* **PO** 50–100 mg 30 min prior to sexual activity (max: 200 mg once daily) *Concurrent moderate CYP34A inhibitor:* Max dose: 50 mg/24 h

## ADMINISTRATION

### Oral
- May be given without regard to food.
- Should be taken only once daily.
- Store at 20°–30° C (77°–86° F).

**ADVERSE EFFECTS** (≥1%) **Body as a Whole:** Back pain, flushing, influenza, rash. **CNS:** Dizziness, headache. **CV:** Abnormal electrocardiogram, hypertension **GI:** Constipation, diarrhea, dyspepsia, nausea. **Musculoskeletal:** Arthralgia, back pain. **Respiratory:** Bronchitis, nasal congestion, nasopharyngitis, sinus congestion, sinusitis, upper respiratory tract infection.

**INTERACTIONS Drug:** Coadministration with **alcohol,** ALPHA₁ ANTAGONISTS (i.e., **doxazosin, terazosin**), ANTIHYPERTENSIVE AGENTS (i.e., **amlodipine, enalapril**), **sodium nitroprusside** or ORGANIC NITRATES (i.e., **isosorbide mononitrate, nitroglycerin**) may cause an excessive decrease in blood pressure. Strong (i.e., **atazanavir, clarithromycin, indinavir, itraconazole, ketoconazole, nefazodone, nelfinavir, ritonavir, saquinavir, telithromycin**) and moderate (i.e., **aprepitant, diltiazem, erythromycin, fluconazole, fosamprenavir, verapamil**) inhibitors of CYP3A4 can increase the levels of avanafil. **Food: Grapefruit juice** may increase the levels of avanafil.

---

Common adverse effects in *italic;* life-threatening effects <u>underlined;</u> generic names in **bold;** classifications in SMALL CAPS; ♣ Canadian drug name; ⊘ Prototype drug

143

## PHARMACOKINETICS  Onset:
30–45 min. **Distribution:** 99% plasma protein bound. **Metabolism:** Hepatic transformation to active and inactive compounds. **Elimination:** Fecal (62%) and renal (21%). **Half-Life:** 5 h.

## NURSING IMPLICATIONS

### Assessment & Drug Effects
- Monitor cardiac response to drug, including changes in BP and HR.
- Assess for and report promptly sudden loss of vision, decrease or loss of hearing, or tinnitus.

### Patient & Family Education
- Take no more than once daily.
- Ensure that prescriber has a complete list of all other concurrent medications.
- Report promptly painful erections or prolonged erections lasting 4 h or longer.
- Stop taking drug and seek immediate medical attention for any of the following: Sudden decrease or loss of hearing, with or without tinnitus and dizziness; sudden loss of vision.
- Reduce or eliminate alcohol consumption when using this drug.

# AXITINIB
(ax-i'ti-nib)

Inlyta

**Classification:** ANTINEOPLASTIC; KINASE INHIBITOR
**Therapeutic:** ANTINEOPLASTIC
**Prototype:** Erlotinib

## AVAILABILITY Tablet

## ACTION & THERAPEUTIC EFFECT
Inhibits receptor tyrosine kinases, including vascular endothelial growth factor receptors. These receptors are implicated in pathologic angiogenesis and tumor growth. Thought to inhibit renal tumor growth and cancer progression.

## USES Treatment of advanced renal cell carcinoma.

## CONTRAINDICATIONS  Hypertensive crisis; active brain hemorrhage; recent GI bleeding or perforation; within 24 h of elective surgery; reversible posterior leukoencephalopahy syndrome (RPLS); pregnancy (category D); lactation.

## CAUTIOUS USE Hypertension; hepatic impairment; renal impairment; mild-to-moderate proteinuria; history of CVA, TIA, MI, or retinal artery occlusion; history of Grade 3 or 4 venous thrombosis; history of GI bleeding. Safety and efficacy in children younger than 18 y not established.

## ROUTE & DOSAGE

### Renal Cell Carcinoma
*Adult:* **PO** 5 mg b.i.d.; can titrate up to 10 mg b.i.d. or down to 2 mg b.i.d.

### Hepatic Impairment Dosage Adjustment
*Moderate impairment (Child Pugh Class B):* Reduce starting dose to approximately half

## ADMINISTRATION

### Oral
- May be given without regard to food.
- Ensure that tablets are swallowed whole with sufficient water.
- Do not re-administer if patient vomits; wait until next scheduled dose.
- Store at 20°–25° C (68°–77° F).

## ADVERSE EFFECTS (≥1%) Body as a Whole:
Dehydration, epistaxis, hematuria, hemoptysis, mucosal inflammation, *palmar-plantar erythrodysesthesia (hand-foot) syndrome*, proteinuria, upper abdominal pain. **CNS:** *Asthenia*, dizziness, *fatigue*, headache. **CV:** <u>Deep vein thrombosis</u>, *hypertension*, <u>transient ischemic attack</u>. **GI:** Abdominal pain, *constipation, decreased appetite, diarrhea*, dyspepsia, hemorrhoids, *nausea*, rectal hemorrhage, stomatitis, *vomiting*. **Hematological:** anemia, bicarbonate decreased, creatinine increased, hemoglobin decreased, hyperkalemia, hypoalbuminemia, hypocalcemia, hypophosphatemia, hypothyroidism, lipase increased, *weight loss*; lymphocytes decreased, platelets decreased, polycythemia, white blood cells decreased. **Metabolic:** ALT and AST increased, alteration of glucose and sodium levels, amylase increased. **Musculoskeletal:** Arthralgia, myalgia, pain in extremity. **Respiratory:** Cough, dyspnea, pulmonary embolism. **Skin:** Alopecia, dry skin, erythema, pruritus, rash. **Special Senses:** Dysgeusia, *dysphonia*, retinal-vein occlusion/thrombosis, tinnitus.

## INTERACTIONS Drug:
Strong CYP3A4/5 inhibitors (i.e., **atazanavir, clarithromycin, indinavir, itraconazole, ketoconazole, nefazodone, nelfinavir, ritonavir, saquinavir, telithromycin**) may increase the levels of axitinib. Strong (i.e., **carbamazepine, dexamethasone, phenobarbital, phenytoin, rifabutin, rifampin, rifapentine**) and moderate (i.e., **bosentan, efavirenz, etravirine, modafinil, nafcillin**) CYP3A4/5 inducers may decrease the levels of axitinib. **Food:** Grapefruit or grapefruit juice may increase the levels of axitinib.

**Herbal: St. John's wort** may decrease the levels of axitinib.

## PHARMACOKINETICS Absorption:
58% bioavailability. **Peak:** 2.5–4.1 h. **Distribution:** 99% plasma protein bound. **Metabolism:** Extensive hepatic metabolism. **Elimination:** Fecal (41%) and renal (23%). **Half-Life:** 2.5–6.1 h.

## NURSING IMPLICATIONS

### Assessment & Drug Effects
- Monitor BP at baseline and frequently throughout therapy.
- Assess for and report promptly S&S suggestive of thromboembolic events (e.g., DVT, TIA, chest pain).
- Monitor for and report promptly S&S of hemorrhage, GI perforation, or fistula formation.
- Monitor lab tests: Baseline and periodic thyroid function tests, LFTs, CBC with differential, serum electrolytes, serum glucose, and urinalysis for proteinuria.

### Patient & Family Education
- Frequent monitoring of BP is recommended throughout therapy.
- Exercise caution with activities that could result in bleeding.
- Report promptly any of the following: Unexplained bleeding episodes; persistent or severe abdominal pain; any neurologic deficit (e.g., seizure, confusion, visual disturbances, frequent or severe headaches).
- Men and women should use effective means of birth control during therapy.
- Contact your prescriber immediately if you or your partner becomes pregnant during treatment.
- Do not breastfeed while receiving this drug.

Common adverse effects in *italic;* life-threatening effects <u>underlined</u>; generic names in **bold;** classifications in SMALL CAPS; ✚ Canadian drug name; ⊙ Prototype drug

145

# AZACITIDINE

(a-za-ci'ti-deen)

Vidaza

**Classifications:** ANTINEOPLASTIC; ANTIMETABOLITE (PYRIMIDINE)

Therapeutic: ANTINEOPLASTIC

**Prototype:** Fluorouracil

**AVAILABILITY** Powder for injection

## ACTION & *THERAPEUTIC EFFECT*

Causes changes in DNA in abnormal blood-forming cells in the bone marrow, resulting in restoration of normal function to tumor-suppressor genes that are responsible for regulating cell differentiation and growth. *Cytotoxic effects of azacitidine cause the death of rapidly dividing cancer cells that are no longer responsive to normal growth control mechanisms.*

**USES** Treatment of myelodysplastic syndrome, specifically refractory anemia.

**UNLABELED USES** Refractory acute and chronic myelogenous leukemia.

**CONTRAINDICATIONS** Hypersensitivity to azacitidine or mannitol; advanced malignant hepatic tumors, myelodysplastic syndrome with hepatic impairment; hepatotoxicity; vaccination; active infection; dental work; intramuscular injections, if platelets are less than 50,000 mm³; pregnancy (category D); lactation.

**CAUTIOUS USE** Hypoalbuminemia (less than 3 g/dL); hepatic disease; bone marrow depression; dental disease; history of varicella zoster or other herpes infections; renal impairment, renal failure; older adults. Safety and efficacy in children not established.

## ROUTE & DOSAGE

### Myelodysplastic Syndrome

*Adult:* **Subcutaneous** 75 mg/m² once daily for 7 days every 4 wk; may increase to 100 mg/m² if no beneficial response is seen after 2 treatment cycles and no toxicity other than nausea and vomiting has occurred

### *Renal Impairment Dosage Adjustment*

If unexplained elevations of BUN or creatinine occur, the next cycle should be delayed until the values return to normal or baseline, and the dose should be reduced by 50% in the next course

## ADMINISTRATION

### Subcutaneous

- Reconstitute by slowly injecting 4 mL of sterile water for injection into 100 mg vial to yield 25 mg/mL. Invert 2–3 times and gently rotate until a uniform suspension is achieved. The suspension will be cloudy. If not used immediately, see directions for storage.
- Doses greater than 4 mL should be divided equally into 2 syringes and injected into 2 separate sites. Rotate sites for each injection (thigh, abdomen, or upper arm). Give subsequent injections at least 1 in from an old site and never into areas where the site is tender, bruised, red, or hard.
- Storage: Reconstituted suspension may be kept in the vial or syringe. May refrigerate for up to 8 h. Before use, suspension may be kept at room temperature for up to 30 min. Resuspend by inverting the syringe 2–3 times and gently roll between the palms for 30 sec immediately before administration.

Common adverse effects in *italic;* life-threatening effects underlined; generic names in **bold;** classifications in SMALL CAPS; ♣ Canadian drug name; ⦿ Prototype drug

**ADVERSE EFFECTS** (≥1%) **Body as a Whole:** *Fever, fatigue, malaise, weakness, asthenia, limb pain, back pain,* lymphadenopathy, hematoma, night sweats, cellulitis, lethargy. **CNS:** *Dizziness, headache, depression,* syncope. **CV:** *Chest pain,* cardiac murmur, tachycardia, hypotension. **GI:** *Nausea, vomiting, diarrhea, constipation, anorexia, weight loss, abdominal pain,* stomatitis, dyspepsia. **Hematologic:** *Anemia,* thrombocytopenia, leukopenia, neutropenia, *ecchymosis, febrile neutropenia.* **Metabolic:** *Peripheral edema.* **Musculoskeletal:** *Myalgia, arthralgia,* muscle cramps. **Respiratory:** *Cough, dyspnea, pharyngitis, nasopharyngitis, pneumonia,* wheezing, pleural effusion, rhonchi. **Skin:** *Injection site erythema, injection site reactions, rash, pruritus, sweating,* urticaria. **Urogenital:** *Dysuria,* urinary tract infection

**INTERACTIONS Drug:** ANTICOAGU-LANTS, NSAIDS, ANTIPLATELET AGENTS may increase risk of bleeding; **filgrastim, sargramostim** may interfere with the efficacy of azacitidine if given within 24 h of azacitidine dose.

**PHARMACOKINETICS Peak:** 30 min. **Metabolism:** In liver. **Elimination:** By kidneys. **Half-Life:** 4 h.

## NURSING IMPLICATIONS

### Assessment & Drug Effects

- Monitor for S&S of drug toxicity in those with renal insufficiency.
- Withhold drug and notify prescriber for any of the following: S&S of hepatic or renal insufficiency; lab values that indicate leukopenia, neutropenia, thrombocytopenia, or hepatic or renal insufficiency; or serum bicarbonate levels less than 20 mEq/L.

- Monitor lab tests: Baseline LFTs and serum creatinine; baseline and periodic CBC with differential.

### Patient & Family Education

- Promptly report S&S of infection or indication of unusual bleeding tendencies (e.g., dark, tarry stools and easy bruising).
- Women should avoid becoming pregnant and men should not father a child while taking this drug.

## AZATHIOPRINE

(ay-za-thye'oh-preen)

**Azasan, Imuran**

**Classifications:** IMMUNOSUPPRESSANT; DISEASE-MODIFYING RHEUMATIC DRUG (DMARD)
**Therapeutic:** IMMUNOSUPPRESSANT; ANTI-INFLAMMATORY; ANTIRHEUMATIC; DMARD
**Prototype:** Cyclosporine

**AVAILABILITY** Tablet; powder for injection

## ACTION & *THERAPEUTIC EFFECT*

Antagonizes purine metabolism and appears to inhibit DNA, RNA, and normal protein synthesis in rapidly growing cells. *Suppresses T cell effects before transplant rejection. Has immunosuppressant and anti-inflammatory properties.*

**USES** Adjunctive agent to prevent rejection of kidney allografts. Also used in patients with active rheumatoid arthritis.

**UNLABELED USES** SLE, lupus nephritis, psoriatic arthritis; ulcerative colitis, pemphigus, nephrotic syndrome, and other inflammatory and immunologic diseases.

Common adverse effects in *italic;* life-threatening effects underlined; generic names in **bold**; classifications in SMALL CAPS; ◆ Canadian drug name; ⊘ Prototype drug

147

**CONTRAINDICATIONS** Hypersensitivity to azathioprine or mercaptopurine; clinically active infection, immunization of patient or close family members with live virus vaccines; anuria; pancreatitis; patients previously treated with alkylating agents (increased risk of neoplasms), concurrent radiation therapy; development of GI toxicity to drug; pregnancy (category D); lactation.

**CAUTIOUS USE** Impaired kidney and liver function; MG; serious infections. Safety and efficacy in children not established.

## ROUTE & DOSAGE

### Kidney Transplant Rejection
Adult: **PO** 3–5 mg/kg/day initially, may be able to reduce to 1–3 mg/kg/day; **IV** 3–5 mg/kg/day initially, may be able to reduce to 1–3 mg/kg/day; switch to **PO**

### Rheumatoid Arthritis
Adult: **PO** 1 mg/kg/day initially, may be increased by 0.5 mg/kg/day a 6 wk intervals if needed up to 2.5 mg/kg/day

### Obesity Dosage Adjustment
Doses calculated on IBW

## ADMINISTRATION

### Oral
- Give oral drug in divided doses (as prescribed) with food or immediately after meals to minimize gastric disturbances.

### Intravenous

*PREPARE:* **Direct/Intermittent:** Reconstitute by adding 10 mL sterile water for injection into vial; swirl until dissolved. May be given as prepared or further diluted with 50 mL NS, D5W, or D5/NS. ▪ Reconstituted solution may be stored at room temperature but **must be** used within 24 h after reconstitution (contains no preservatives).

*ADMINISTER:* **Direct/Intermittent:** May infuse over 30 min to 8 h. Typical infusion time is 30–60 min or longer. ▪ If longer infusion time is ordered, the final volume of the IV solution is increased appropriately. Check with prescriber.

*INCOMPATIBILITIES:* **Y-site: amikacin, ampicillin/sulbactam, ascorbic acid, aztreonam, bumetanide, buprenorphine, zutophanol, calcium chloride, CEPHALOSPORINS, chloramphenicol, chlorpromazine, cimetidine, clindamycin, dantrolene, diazepam, diazoxide, diphenydramine, dobutamine, dopamine, doxycycline, ephedrine, epinephrine, esmolol, famotidine, ganciclovir, gentamicin, haloperidol, hydralazine, hydrocortisone, hydroxyzine, imipenem/cilastin, isoproterenol, ketorolac, labetolol, lidocaine, magnesium sulfate, meperidine, methyldopate, miconazole, midazolam, milrinone acetate, minocycline, morphine, nafcillin, nalbuphine, nitroprusside, norepinephrine, ondansetron, papaverine, pentazocine, phenylephrine, phenytoin, piperacillin, procainamide, prochlorperazine, promethazine, pyridoxine, quinidine, ritodrine, rocuronium, sodium bicarbonate, streptokinase, succinylcholine, sulfamethaxazole/rimethoprim, tacrolimus, thiamine, ticarcillin, tobramycin, tolazoline, vancomycin, verapamil**

Common adverse effects in *italic;* life-threatening effects underlined; generic names in **bold;** classifications in SMALL CAPS; ✚ Canadian drug name; ◓ Prototype drug

- Store at 15°–30° C (59°–86° F) in tightly closed, light-resistant containers unless otherwise directed.

## ADVERSE EFFECTS (≥1%) Body as a Whole: Hypersensitivity (skin eruptions, rash, arthralgia). GI: Nausea, vomiting, anorexia, esophagitis, diarrhea, steatorrhea. Hepatic: Hepatic toxicity, hepatitis with elevations in bilirubin, alkaline phosphatase, AST, ALT, biliary stasis, toxic hepatitis. Hematologic: <u>Bone marrow depression</u>, <u>thrombocytopenia</u>, <u>leukopenia</u>, anemia, <u>agranulocytosis</u>, pancytopenia. Other: *Secondary infection (immunosuppression);* dysarthria, alopecia; carcinogenic and teratogenic potential reported.

## DIAGNOSTIC TEST INTERFERENCE
Azathioprine may decrease plasma and urinary *uric acid* in patients with gout; may falsely increase *serum creatinine* values.

## INTERACTIONS Drug: Allopurinol increases effects and toxicity of azathioprine by reducing metabolism of the active metabolite; **allopurinol** doses should be decreased by one third or one fourth; **tubocurarine** and other NONDEPOLARIZING SKELETAL MUSCLE RELAXANTS may reverse or inhibit neuromuscular blocking effects. **Ribavirin** or **peginterferon alfa-2A** increase risk of pancytopenia.

## PHARMACOKINETICS Absorption: Readily from GI tract. Distribution: Crosses placenta. Metabolism: Extensively in liver to active metabolite mercaptopurine. Elimination: In urine. Half-Life: 3 h.

## NURSING IMPLICATIONS

### Black Box Warning

*Chronic use of azathioprine has been associated with development of lymphoma.*

### Assessment & Drug Effects
- Monitor therapeutic efficacy which usually requires 6–8 wk of therapy for patients with rheumatoid arthritis (improvement in morning stiffness and grip strength). If no improvement has occurred after 12-wk trial period, drug is generally discontinued.
- Monitor for toxicity. Drug has a high toxic potential. Because it may have delayed action, dosage should be reduced or drug withdrawn at the first indication of an abnormally large or persistent decrease in leukocyte or platelet count.
- Monitor vital signs. Report signs of infection.
- Monitor I&O ratio; note color, character, and specific gravity of urine. Report an abrupt decrease in urinary output or any change in I&O ratio.
- Monitor for signs of abnormal bleeding [easy bruising, bleeding gums, petechiae, purpura, melena, epistaxis, dark urine (hematuria), hemoptysis, hematemesis]. If thrombocytopenia occurs, invasive procedures should be withheld, if possible.
- Monitor lab tests: Baseline CBC with differential and platelet count, then weekly during 1st mo, and twice during both 2nd and 3rd mo, or more frequently if indicated (e.g., by dosage or therapy changes); periodic LFTs and renal function tests throughout therapy.

### Patient & Family Education
- Chronic use of this drug has been associated with development of blood cancers in patients with inflammatory bowel disease.
- Avoid contact with anyone who has a cold or other infection and report signs of impending infection. Exercise scrupulous personal

hygiene because infection is a constant hazard of immunosuppressive therapy.

▪ Practice birth control during therapy and for 4 mo after drug is discontinued. This drug is associated with potential hazards in pregnancy.

▪ Do not receive/take vaccinations or other immunity-conferring agents during therapy because they may precipitate unusually severe reactions due to the immunosuppressive effects of the drug.

## AZELAIC ACID
(a'ze-laic)
Azelex, Finacea
**Classification:** ANTIACNE
Therapeutic: ANTIACNE
**Prototype:** Isotretinoin

### AVAILABILITY Cream; gel

### ACTION & *THERAPEUTIC EFFECT*
Azelaic acid is a naturally occurring dicarboxylic acid. Antimicrobial action is attributable to inhibition of microbial cellular protein synthesis. A normalization of keratinization of the follicle occurs and it reduces the number of acne lesions. *Reduces the number of inflammatory pustules and papules.*

### USES Mild to moderate inflammatory acne vulgaris, mild to moderate rosacea.

### CONTRAINDICATIONS Hypersensitivity to any component in the drug.

### CAUTIOUS USE Dark complexion, pregnancy (category B); lactation. Safety and efficacy in children younger than 12 y not established.

## ROUTE & DOSAGE

**Acne Vulgaris, Rosacea**
*Adult/Child (12 y and older):*
**Topical** Apply thin film to clean and dry area b.i.d.

## ADMINISTRATION
**Topical**
▪ Wash and dry skin thoroughly prior to application of drug.
▪ Apply by thoroughly massaging a thin film of the cream or gel into the affected area. Avoid occlusive dressing.
▪ Wash hands before and after application of cream or gel.
▪ Store at 15°–30° C (59°–86° F).

### ADVERSE EFFECTS (≥1%) **Skin:**
Pruritus, burning, stinging, tingling, erythema, dryness, rash, peeling, irritation, contact dermatitis, vitiligo depigmentation, hypertrichosis. **Other:** Worsening of asthma.

### PHARMACOKINETICS **Absorption:** Approximately 4% absorbed through the skin. **Onset:** 4–8 wk. **Distribution:** Into all tissues. **Metabolism:** Partially by beta oxidation in liver. **Elimination:** Primarily in urine. **Half-Life:** 12 h.

## NURSING IMPLICATIONS
### Assessment & Drug Effects
▪ Assess for signs of hypopigmentation and report immediately.
▪ Monitor for sensitivity or severe irritation, which may warrant drug dosage reduction or discontinuation.

### Patient & Family Education
▪ Learn proper application of cream or gel and avoid contact with eyes or mucous membranes.
▪ Wash eyes with copious amounts of water if contact with medication occurs.

Common adverse effects in *italic;* life-threatening effects <u>underlined;</u> generic names in **bold;** classifications in SMALL CAPS; ♣ Canadian drug name; ◐ Prototype drug

- Note: Transient pruritus, burning, and stinging are common; however, severe skin irritation or hypopigmentation should be reported.

## AZELASTINE HYDROCHLORIDE
(a-ze-las'teen)

Astelin, Astepro, Optivar

**Classifications:** ANTIHISTAMINE; $H_1$-RECEPTOR ANTAGONIST; NASAL AND OCULAR ANTIHISTAMINE
Therapeutic: ANTIHISTAMINE
**Prototype:** Diphenhydramine

**AVAILABILITY** Nasal spray; ophthalmic solution

**ACTION & *THERAPEUTIC EFFECT***
Potent histamine $H_1$ receptor antagonist and inhibitor of mast cell release of histamine. *Effective in the symptomatic treatment of seasonal allergic rhinitis and as a nasal decongestant.*

**USES** Allergic conjunctivitis, allergic rhinitis, ocular pruritus, vasomotor rhinitis

**CONTRAINDICATIONS** Hypersensitivity to azelastine; pregnancy (category C). Safety and efficacy in children younger than 5 y nasal spray use not established.

**CAUTIOUS USE** Hepatic or renal disease; asthmatics; older adults; lactation. **Astepro** nasal spray in children younger than 5 y.

## ROUTE & DOSAGE

### Allergic Rhinitis
*Adult/Adolescent:* **Intranasal**
1–2 sprays/nostril b.i.d.
*Child (5–11 y):* **Intranasal**
1 spray/nostril b.i.d.

### Perennial Allergic Rhinitis (Astepro only)
*Adult/Adolescent:* **Intranasal**
2 sprays/nostril b.i.d.

**Ocular Pruritus**
See Appendix A-1.

## ADMINISTRATION

**Intranasal**
- Prime delivery unit before first use (see manufacturer's instructions).
- Instruct patient to clear nasal passages prior to drug installation; then tilt head forward slightly and sniff gently when drug is sprayed into each nostril.
- Store the bottle upright at room temperature, 15°–30° C (59°–86° F).

**ADVERSE EFFECTS (≥1%) Body as a Whole:** Fatigue, dizziness. **GI:** Dry mouth, nausea. **Metabolic:** Weight gain. **CNS:** *Headache, somnolence.* **Respiratory:** Pharyngitis, *rhinitis,* paroxysmal sneezing, *cough,* asthma. **Special Senses:** *Bitter taste, nasal burning,* epistaxis, conjunctivitis.

**INTERACTIONS Drug: Alcohol** and CNS DEPRESSANTS, sedating ANTIHISTAMINES may cause reduced alertness.

**PHARMACOKINETICS Absorption:** 40% from nasal inhalation. **Peak:** 2–3 h. **Metabolism:** Active metabolites. **Elimination:** Primarily in feces. **Half-Life:** 22 h.

## NURSING IMPLICATIONS

**Assessment & Drug Effects**
- Monitor level of alertness especially in older adults and with concurrent use of other CNS depressants.

---

Common adverse effects in *italic;* life-threatening effects underlined; generic names in **bold;** classifications in SMALL CAPS; ♣ Canadian drug name; ⊙ Prototype drug

151

## Patient & Family Education

- Follow manufacturer's directions for priming the metered dose spray unit before first use and after storage of greater than 3 days.
- Tilt head forward while instilling spray. Avoid getting spray in eyes.
- Do not drive or engage in potentially hazardous activities until response to drug is known.
- Avoid concurrent use of CNS depressants, such as alcohol, while taking this drug.
- Discard spray unit and dispensing package bottle after 3 mo.

## AZILSARTAN MEDOXOMIL

(ay'-zil-sar'-tan me-dox'-oh-mil)

Edarbi

**Classifications:** ANGIOTENSIN II RECEPTOR ANTAGONIST; ANTIHYPERTENSIVE
**Therapeutic:** ANTIHYPERTENSIVE
**Prototype:** Losartan

### AVAILABILITY Tablet

### ACTION & *THERAPEUTIC EFFECT*

An angiotensin II receptor blocker (ARB) that prevents binding of angiotension II to $AT_1$ receptors in vascular smooth muscle and other tissues. *Lowers blood pressure thus reducing the risk for fatal and nonfatal cardiovascular events (e.g., stroke and myocardial infarction).*

### USES Hypertension, either alone or in combination with other agents.

### CONTRAINDICATIONS Pregnancy D; lactation.

### CAUTIOUS USE Severe CHF, renal artery stenosis, volume depletion, and renal impairment; older adults; women of childbearing age. Safety and efficacy in children younger than 18 y not established.

## ROUTE & DOSAGE

### Hypertension

*Adult:* **PO** 80 mg once daily; consider 40 mg once daily if on high-dose diuretic

## ADMINISTRATION

### Oral

- May be given without regard to meals.
- Store at 15°–30° C (59°–86° F), and protect from light and moisture.

### ADVERSE EFFECTS (≥1%) CNS:
Dizziness, fatigue. **CV:** Hypotension. **GI:** Diarrhea. **Metabolic:** Hyperkalemia. **Skin:** Rash.

### INTERACTIONS Drug: Concurrent use of azilsartan with NSAIDs may cause deterioration of renal function in patients who are older adults, volume-depleted, on diuretic therapy, or have compromised renal function.

### PHARMACOKINETICS Absorption: 60% bioavailability. Distribution: Greater than 99% plasma protein bound. **Metabolism:** In the liver to pharmacologically inactive metabolites. **Elimination:** Fecal (55%) and renal (42%). **Half-Life:** 11 h.

## NURSING IMPLICATIONS

### Assessment & Drug Effects

### Black Box Warning

*Azilsartan has been associated with fetal injury and fetal death. It **must not** be used by pregnant women.*

- Monitor HR and BP at regular intervals.
- Monitor for and report S&S of orthostatic hypotension, especially with volume depletion or with concurrent diuretic use.

Common adverse effects in *italic;* life-threatening effects <u>underlined;</u> generic names in **bold;** classifications in SMALL CAPS; ♣ Canadian drug name; ⊙ Prototype drug

- Monitor lab tests: Periodic CBC especially with those at risk for anemia; periodic serum creatinine, especially with preexisting renal impairment.

**Patient & Family Education**
- Report to prescriber if you become or plan to become pregnant.
- Stop taking the drug and immediately report to prescriber if you suspect that you are pregnant.
- Make position changes slowly, especially from lying or sitting to standing.
- Report promptly to prescriber if you experience faintness or dizziness or if you develop a rash.

# AZITHROMYCIN

(a-zi-thro-mye'sin)

AzaSite, Zithromax, Zmax

**Classification:** MACROLIDE ANTIBIOTIC
**Therapeutic:** ANTIBIOTIC
**Prototype:** Erythromycin

**AVAILABILITY** Tablet; oral suspension; solution for injection; ophthalmic drops; extended release oral suspension

**ACTION & THERAPEUTIC EFFECT**
A macrolide antibiotic that reversibly binds to the 50S ribosomal subunit of susceptible organisms and consequently inhibits protein synthesis. *Effective for treatment of mild to moderate infections caused by pyogenic organisms.*

**USES** Pneumonia, respiratory tract infections, pharyngitis/tonsillitis, gonorrhea, nongonococcal urethritis, skin and skin structure infections due to susceptible organisms, otitis media, *Mycobacterium avium–intracellulare* complex infections, acute bacterial sinusitis; pelvic inflammatory disease.

**Zmax:** Acute bacterial sinusitis and community acquired pneumonia. **AzaSite:** Bacterial conjunctivitis.

**UNLABELED USES** Bronchitis, *Helicobacter pylori* gastritis, Lyme disease, prostatitis, cystic fibrosis, typhoid fever, dental infection.

**CONTRAINDICATIONS** Hypersensitivity to azithromycin, erythromycin, or any of the macrolide or ketolide antibiotics, history of cholestatic jaundice/hepatic dysfunction associated with prior use of azithromycin; hepatitis.

**CAUTIOUS USE** Hepatic or renal impairment; GI disease; altered cardiac conduction, ventricular arrhythmias, bradyarrhythmias, QT prolongation; history of torsade de pointes; MG; superinfection; older adults or debilitated persons; GFR less than 10 mL/min; pregnancy (category B); lactation; children younger than 6 mo.

## ROUTE & DOSAGE

**Bacterial Infections** (see package insert for dosing on specific causative agent)

*Adult:* **PO** 500 mg on day 1, then 250 mg q24h for 4 more days; **IV** 500 mg daily for at least 2 days, administer 1 mg/mL over 3 h or 2 mg/mL over 1 h
*Child (6 mo and older):* **PO** 10 mg/kg on day 1, then 5 mg/kg for 4 more days (max: 250 mg/day)

**Acute Bacterial Sinusitis**

*Adult:* **PO** 500 mg once daily × 3 days. **Zmax:** Single one-time dose of 2 g
*Child (6 mo or older):* **PO** 10 mg/kg once daily × 3 days

**Otitis Media**

*Child (6 mo and older):* **PO** 30 mg/kg as a single dose or 10 mg/kg once daily (not to exceed 500 mg/day) for

---

Common adverse effects in *italic;* life-threatening effects <u>underlined</u>; generic names in **bold;** classifications in SMALL CAPS; ♦ Canadian drug name; ⊙ Prototype drug

153

3 days or 10 mg/kg as a single dose on day 1 followed by 5 mg/kg/day on days 2–5

**Gonorrhea**

*Adult:* **PO** 2 g as a single dose

**Chancroid**

*Adult:* **PO** 1 g as a single dose
*Child:* **PO** 20 mg/kg as single dose (max: 1 g)

**Pelvic Inflammatory Disease**

*Adult/Adolescent:* **IV** 500 mg × 1–2 days then **PO** 250 mg daily to complete 7 day course

**Bacterial Conjunctivitis**

*Adult:* Ophthalmic 1 drop b.i.d. × 2 days then daily × 5 days

***Renal Impairment Dosage Adjustment***

*CrCl less than 10 mL/min:* Use with caution

## ADMINISTRATION

### Oral

- Give extended-release oral suspension (Zmax) at least 1 h before or 2 h after a meal. Tablets may be taken without regard to food.
- Suspension should be taken within 12 h of reconstitution.

### Intravenous

***PREPARE: Intermittent:*** Reconstitute 500-mg vial with 4.8 mL of sterile water for injection and shake until dissolved. ▪ Final concentration is 100 mg/mL. ▪ Solution **must be** further diluted to 1 or 2 mg/mL by adding 5 mL of the 100-mg/mL solution to 500 mL or 250 mL, respectively, of D5W, D5/NS, 0.45NaCl, or other compatible solution.

***ADMINISTER: Intermittent:*** Administer 1 mg/mL over 3 h. Infuse 2 mg/mL over 1 h. ▪ Note: Do not give a bolus dose.

***INCOMPATIBILITIES:* Solution/additive: Ciprofloxacin. Y-site:** Amikacin, amiodarone, amphotericin B, aztreonam, cefotaxime, ceftazidime, ceftriaxone, cefuroxime, chlorpromazine, ciprofloxacin, clindamycin, diazepam, doxorubicin, epirubicin, famotidine, fentanyl, furosemide, garenoxacin, gemtuzumab, gentamicin, imipenem/cilastatin, ketorolac, levofloxacin, midazolam, mitoxantrone, morphine, mycophenolate, nicardipine, ondansetron, pentamidine, phenytoin, piperacillin/tazobactam, potassium, quinupristin/dalfopristin, thiopental, ticarcillin/clavulanate, tobramycin.

- Store drug when diluted as directed for 24 h at or below 30° C (86° F) or for 7 days under 5° C (41° F).

## ADVERSE EFFECTS (≥1%) CNS:
Headache, dizziness, drowsiness, fatigue, vertigo. **GI:** *Nausea, vomiting, diarrhea,* abdominal pain; mild elevations in liver function tests. **Dermatologic:** *pruritus, rash.* **Genitourinary:** vaginitis. **CV:** Arrythmia, chest pain. **General:** Pain at injection site, local inflammation.

## DIAGNOSTIC TEST INTERFERENCE
Liver function tests: Reversible, asymptomatic elevations in *liver enzymes (AST, ALT, gamma glutamyl transferase, alkaline phosphatase)* have been reported in some patients treated with azithromycin.

## INTERACTIONS Drug: ANTACIDS may
decrease peak level of azithromycin; may increase toxicity of **digoxin, cyclosporine, phenytoin, dihydroergotamine. Nelfinavir** may increase side effects of azithromycin.

Common adverse effects in *italic;* life-threatening effects <u>underlined</u>; generic names in **bold;** classifications in SMALL CAPS; ✤ Canadian drug name; ⊙ Prototype drug

Use with **dronedarone** may increase QT interval. Effects of **warfarin** may be potentiated. Do not use with **amiodarone, dofetilide, ivermectin, mifepristone, saquinavir, ziprasidone. Food:** Food will decrease the amount of azithromycin absorbed by 50%.

## PHARMACOKINETICS Absorption:
37% of dose reaches the systemic circulation. **Onset:** 48 h. **Peak:** 2–3 h (immediate release) 3–5 h (extended release). **Distribution:** Extensively into tissues including sputum, blister, and vaginal secretions; tissue concentrations are often higher than serum concentrations. **Metabolism:** In liver. **Elimination:** 5–12% of dose in urine. **Half-Life:** 60–70 h.

## NURSING IMPLICATIONS

### Assessment & Drug Effects
- Monitor for and report loose stools or diarrhea, since pseudomembranous colitis (see Appendix F) **must be** ruled out.
- Report immediately any S&S of hypersensitivity; though rare, these reactions can be serious.
- Monitor closely for and report promptly any of the following: Prolonged QT interval, bradyarrhythmias.
- Assess results of culture and sensitivity tests and allergies prior to beginning therapy.
- Monitor lab tests: Frequent PT and INR with concurrent warfarin use.

### Patient & Family Education
- Direct sunlight (UV) exposure should be minimized during therapy with drug.
- Report onset of loose stools or diarrhea.
- If being used to treat STD, use protection against transmission.

# AZTREONAM
(az-tree'oh-nam)
Azactam, Cayston
**Classifications:** ANTIBIOTIC; MONOBACTAM ANTIBIOTIC
Therapeutic: ANTIBIOTIC
**Prototype:** Imipenem-cilastatin

## AVAILABILITY Vial

## ACTION & *THERAPEUTIC EFFECT*
Acts by inhibiting synthesis of bacterial cell wall by preferentially binding to specific penicillin-binding proteins (PBP) in the bacterial cell wall. *Highly resistant to beta-lactamases and does not readily induce their formation. Spectrum of activity limited to aerobic, gram-negative bacteria.*

**USES** Gram-negative infections of urinary tract, lower respiratory tract, skin and skin structures; and for intra-abdominal and gynecologic infections, septicemia, and as adjunctive therapy for surgical infections, community acquired pneumonia. Inhalation form for cystic fibrosis.

**CONTRAINDICATIONS** Hypersensitivity to aztreonam; viral infections.

**CAUTIOUS USE** History of hypersensitivity reaction to penicillin, cephalosporins, or to other drugs; impaired renal or hepatic function, older adults; pregnancy (category B); lactation. For **Cayston** inhalation only: Safety and efficacy not established in pediatric patients younger than 7 y; patients with FEV$_1$ less than 25% or greater than 75% predicted, or colonized with *Burkholderia cepacia*.

## ROUTE & DOSAGE

**Urinary Tract Infection**
*Adult/Adolescent:* **IV/IM** 0.5–1 g q8–12h

Common adverse effects in *italic;* life-threatening effects underlined; generic names in **bold;** classifications in SMALL CAPS; ♣ Canadian drug name; ⊘ Prototype drug

155

*Child/Infant (9 mo or older):* **IV** 30 mg/kg q6–8h

**Moderate to Severe Infections**

*Adult:* **IV/IM** 1–2 g q8–12h (max: 8 g/24 h)

*Child:* **IV** 30 mg/kg/day q6–8h

**Community-Acquired Pneumonia**

*Adult:* **IV** 1–2 g q8–12h or 2 g q6–8h

**Cystic Fibrosis Improvement in Respiratory Symptoms**

*Adult/Adolescent/Child (7 y or older):* **Inhaled** 75 mg t.i.d. × 28 days

*Renal Impairment Dosage Adjustment*

*CrCl 10–30 mL/min:* Reduce dose 50%; *less than 10 mL/min:* Reduce dose by 75%

*Hemodialysis Dosage Adjustment*

Reduce dose to 12.5% and give after hemodialysis

## ADMINISTRATION

### Inhalation

- Administer immediately after reconstitution.
- Administer only via an Altera Nebulizer System after patient has used a bronchodilator. Short-acting bronchodilators can be taken 15 min–4 h before Cayston. Long-acting bronchodilators can be taken 30 min–12 h before Cayston.

### Intramuscular

- Reconstitute with at least 3 mL of diluent/gram of drug for IM injection. Immediately and vigorously shake vial to dissolve. Suitable diluents include sterile water for injection; bacteriostatic water for injection (with benzyl alcohol and propyl parabens); NS 0.9% for injection.
- Give IM injections deeply into large muscle mass such as the upper outer quadrant of the gluteus maximus or lateral thigh. Rotate injection sites.

### Intravenous

Verify correct IV concentration and rate of infusion/injection with prescriber before giving to neonates, infants, and children.

*PREPARE:* **Direct** Reconstitute a single dose with 6–10 mL of sterile water for injection. ▪ Immediately shake vial until solution is dissolved. May be given direct IV as prepared or further diluted for IV infusion. ▪ Reconstituted solutions are colorless to light straw yellow and turn slightly pink on standing. **For intermittent infusion:** Each gram of reconstituted aztreonam **must be** further diluted in at least 50 mL of D5W, NS, or other solution approved by manufacturer to yield a concentration not to exceed 20 mg/mL.

*ADMINISTER:* **Direct:** Give over 3–5 min. **Intermittent:** Give over 20–60 min through Y-site.

*INCOMPATIBILITIES:* **Solution/additive: Ampicillin, metronidazole, nafcillin. Y-site: Acyclovir, alatrofloxacin, amphotericin B, amphotericin B cholesteryl complex, amsacrine, azathioprine, azithromycin, chlorpromazine, dantrolene, daunorubicin, erythromycin, ganciclovir, milrinone acetate, indomethacin, lansoprazole, lorazepam, metronidazole, mitomycin, mitoxantrone, mycophenolate, oritavancin, pantoprazole, papaverine, pentamidine, pentazocine, pentobarbital, phenytoin, prochlorperazine, quinidine, streptozocin, trastuzumab.**

## ADVERSE EFFECTS (≥1%) Body as a Whole: Hypersensitivity (urticaria, eosinophilia, <u>anaphylaxis</u>). CNS:

Headache, dizziness, confusion, paresthesias, insomnia, seizures. **GI:** Nausea, *diarrhea,* vomiting, elevated liver function tests. **Hematologic:** Eosinophilia. **Special Senses:** Tinnitus, nasal congestion, sneezing, diplopia. **Skin:** Rash, purpura, erythema multiforme, exfoliative dermatitis, diaphoresis; petechiae, pruritus. **Other:** Local reactions (phlebitis, thrombophlebitis (following IV), pain at injection sites), superinfections (gram-positive cocci), vaginal candidiasis.

## DIAGNOSTIC TEST INTERFERENCE

Aztreonam may cause transient elevations of *liver function tests,* increases in *PT* and *PTT,* minor changes in *Hgb,* and positive *Coombs' test.*

## INTERACTIONS Drug: **Imipenem-cilastatin, cefoxitin** may be antagonistic.

## PHARMACOKINETICS Peak: 1 h

IM. **Distribution:** Widely distributed including synovial and blister fluid, bile, bronchial secretions, prostate, bone, and CSF; crosses placenta; distributed into breast milk in small amounts. **Metabolism:** Not extensively metabolized. **Elimination:** 60–70% in urine within 24 h. **Half-Life:** 1.6–2.1 h.

## NURSING IMPLICATIONS

### Assessment & Drug Effects

- Inspect IV injection sites daily for signs of inflammation. Pain and phlebitis occur in a significant number of patients.
- Monitor for and report loose stools or diarrhea, since pseudomembranous colitis (see Appendix F) **must be** ruled out.
- Monitor for S&S of opportunistic infections (rectal or vaginal itching or discharge, fever, cough) and promptly report onset to prescriber. Overgrowth of nonsusceptible

organisms, particularly *staphylococci, streptococci,* and fungi, is a threat, especially in patients receiving prolonged or repeated therapy.
- Monitor lab tests: Baseline C&S prior to initiation of therapy. Baseline and periodic renal function tests, particularly in older adults and in those with history of renal impairment.

### Patient & Family Education

- Determine previous hypersensitivity reactions to penicillins, cephalosporins, and other allergens prior to therapy.
- Report promptly any of the following: Unexplained diarrhea or loose stools, any sign of allergic reaction, any worsening symptoms.
- Note: IV therapy may cause a change in taste sensation. Report interference with eating.

## BACITRACIN
(bass-i-tray'sin)
Baci-IM
**Classification:** ANTIBIOTIC
**Therapeutic:** ANTIBIOTIC

## AVAILABILITY Vial; ophthalmic ointment

## ACTION & THERAPEUTIC EFFECT

Interferes with the bacterial cell membrane by inhibiting cell wall synthesis. *Spectrum of antibacterial activity similar to that of penicillin. Active against many gram-positive organisms. Ineffective against most other gram-negative organisms.*

## USES Parenteral therapy restricted to infants with staphylococcal pneumonia and empyema where adequate laboratory facilities and constant supervision are available. Used topically in treatment of superficial infections of skin.

Common adverse effects in *italic;* life-threatening effects underlined; generic names in **bold;** classifications in SMALL CAPS; ♣ Canadian drug name; ⊘ Prototype drug

157

**B**

**UNLABELED USES** Orally for treatment of antibiotic-associated colitis.

**CONTRAINDICATIONS** Toxic reaction or renal dysfunction associated with bacitracin; pulmonary disease; atopic individuals.

**CAUTIOUS USE** Hypersensitivity to neomycin; myasthenia gravis or other neuromuscular disease; renal impairment; pregnancy (category C); lactation.

## ROUTE & DOSAGE

**Systemic Infections**

*Infant (weight less than 2.5 kg):* **IM** Up to 900 units/kg/24 h divided q8–12h; *weight greater than 2.5 kg:* Up to 1000 units/kg/24h divided q8–12h

**Skin Infections**

*Adult:* **Topical** Apply thin layer of ointment b.i.d., t.i.d., as solution of 250–1000 units/mL in wet dressing

## ADMINISTRATION

**Intramuscular**

- Reconstitute with NS containing 2% procaine hydrochloride (prescribed). Do not reconstitute with diluents containing parabens because solution may precipitate or become cloudy.
- Alternate injection sites since injections are painful.
- Powder vials should be stored in refrigerator at 2°–8° C (36°–46° F). Store solution for a maximum of 1 wk if refrigerated. Inactivation occurs at room temperature.

**Topical**

- Clean affected area prior to application. May be covered with a sterile bandage.

- Store ointments in tightly closed containers at 15°–30° C (59°–86° F) unless otherwise directed.

**ADVERSE EFFECTS (≥1%) GI:** Anorexia, nausea, vomiting, diarrhea, rectal itching and burning. **Hematologic:** Systemic use: Bone marrow depression, blood dyscrasias; eosinophilia. **Body as a Whole:** Hypersensitivity (erythema, <u>anaphylaxis</u>). **Urogenital:** <u>Nephrotoxicity</u>; dose related: Increased BUN, uremia, <u>renal tubular and glomerular necrosis</u> (IM route). **Special Senses:** Tinnitus. **Other:** Pain and inflammation at injection site, fever, superinfection, neuromuscular blockade <u>with respiratory depression</u>.

**INTERACTIONS Drug:** With AMINO-GLYCOSIDES, possibility of additive nephrotoxic and neuromuscular blocking effects; with **tubocurarine** and other NONDEPOLARIZING SKELETAL MUSCLE RELAXANTS, possibility of additive neuromuscular blocking effects.

**PHARMACOKINETICS Absorption:** Poorly absorbed from intact or denuded skin or mucous membranes. **Peak:** 1–2 h IM. **Duration:** 6–8 h. **Distribution:** Widely distributed including peritoneal and ascitic fluids. **Elimination:** Slow renal excretion (10–40% in 24 h).

## NURSING IMPLICATIONS

**Black Box Warning**

*Parenteral form of bacitracin has been associated with nephrotoxicity, especially with concurrent use of other nephrotoxic drugs.*

#### Assessment & Drug Effects

- Monitor I&O during parenteral therapy. Adequate hydration and urinary output are important to reduce possibility of renal toxicity.
- Inspect urine for turbidity and hematuria, and watch for other S&S of urinary tract dysfunction. Report any changes in urination pattern (e.g., oliguria, urinary frequency, nocturia).
- Note: Prolonged use may result in overgrowth of nonsusceptible organisms, especially *Candida albicans*.
- Monitor lab tests: Baseline C&S prior to initiation of therapy, baseline and periodic kidney function tests.

#### Patient & Family Education

- Report local allergic reactions with topical applications (e.g., itching, burning, redness).

## BACLOFEN

(bak'loe-fen)

**Lioresal**

**Classifications:** CENTRAL ACTING SKELETAL MUSCLE RELAXANT; GABA AGONIST

**Therapeutic:** SKELETAL MUSCLE RELAXANT

**Prototype:** Cyclobenzaprine

**AVAILABILITY** Tablet; orally disintegrating tablet; ampule

## ACTION & *THERAPEUTIC EFFECT*

Centrally acting skeletal muscle relaxant that depresses monosynaptic and polysynaptic afferent reflex activity at spinal cord level. Baclofen stimulates the GABA receptors, which results in decreased excitatory input into alpha-motor neurons. *Reduces skeletal muscle spasm caused by upper motor neuron lesions.*

**USES** Symptomatic relief of painful spasms in multiple sclerosis and in the management of detrusor

sphincter dyssynergia in spinal cord injury or disease.

**UNLABELED USES** Treatment of trigeminal neuralgia and of tardive dystonia associated with antipsychotic medications, chronic pain.

**CONTRAINDICATIONS** Coagulopathy, bacteremia, intramuscular or intrathecal administration; lactation.

**CAUTIOUS USE** Impaired renal and hepatic function; bipolar disorder, psychosis, schizophrenia, seizure disorders, seizures, stroke, cerebral palsy, depression, DM, dialysis, head trauma, PKU, epilepsy; thrombocytopenia; psychiatric or brain disorders; older adults, pregnancy (category C); children younger than 2 y.

## ROUTE & DOSAGE

### Muscle Spasm

*Adult:* **PO** 5 mg t.i.d., may increase by 5 mg/dose q3days prn (max: 80 mg/day)
*Child (2–7 y):* **PO** 10–15 mg/day divided q8h, may increase by 5–15 mg/day q3days (max: 40 mg/day); *8 y or older:* 10–15 mg/day divided q8h, may increase by 5–15 mg/day q3days (max: 60 mg/day)
*Adult:* **Intrathecal** Prior to infusion pump implantation, initiate trial dose of 50 mcg/mL bolus administered in intrathecal space by barbotage over 1 min or less. Observe patient over next 4–8 h for significant decrease in muscle spasm. If response is less than desired, administer second bolus of 75 mcg/1.5 mL and observe 4–8 h. May repeat in 24 h with a 100 mcg/2-mL bolus if necessary.
*Post-implant titration:* Use screening dose if response lasted longer than

Common adverse effects in *italic;* life-threatening effects underlined; generic names in **bold**; classifications in SMALL CAPS; ♣ Canadian drug name; ⊙ Prototype drug

159

12 h or double screening dose if response lasted less than 12 h and administer over 24 h. After first 24 h, decrease dose by 10–30% q24h until desired response achieved. Maintenance doses range from 12–1500 mcg/day, with most patients maintained on 300–800 mcg/day.

## ADMINISTRATION

### Oral
- Give with food or milk to avoid GI distress.

### Intrathecal
- Give by direct intrathecal injection (via lumbar puncture or catheter) over at least 1 min or longer.
- Dilute *only* with sterile, preservative-free NS injection. Baclofen **must be** diluted to a concentration of 50 mcg/mL when preparing test doses.
- Intrathecal infusion pump: Do not abruptly discontinue as serious adverse effects may develop.
- Store at 15°–30° C (59°–86° F) in tightly closed container unless otherwise directed.

## ADVERSE EFFECTS (≥1%) CNS:
*Transient drowsiness,* vertigo, dizziness, weakness, fatigue, headache, confusion, insomnia; ataxia, loss of seizure control in epileptic patients; abrupt discontinuation of intrathecal administration may result in high fever, altered mental status, exaggerated rebound spasticity, and muscle rigidity, that in rare cases has advanced to rhabdomyolysis, <u>multiple organ-system failure, and death.</u> **CV:** Hypotension. **Special Senses:** Tinnitus, nasal congestion; blurred vision, mydriasis, nystagmus, diplopia, strabismus, miosis. **GI:** Nausea, constipation, vomiting; mild increases in AST, and alkaline phosphatase, jaundice. **Urogenital:** Urinary frequency.

## DIAGNOSTIC TEST INTERFERENCE
Possibility of increases in *blood-glucose,* serum *alkaline phosphatase,* and *AST levels.*

## INTERACTIONS Drug: Alcohol,
CNS DEPRESSANTS, MAO INHIBITORS, ANTIHISTAMINES compound CNS depression; baclofen may increase blood **glucose** levels, making it necessary to increase dosage of SULFONYLUREAS, **insulin.**

## PHARMACOKINETICS Absorption:
Readily from GI tract. **Peak:** 2–3 h. **Duration:** 8 h. **Distribution:** Minimal amounts cross blood–brain barrier; crosses placenta; distribution into breast milk unknown. **Metabolism:** 15% in liver. **Elimination:** 70–85% in urine within 72 h; some elimination in feces. **Half-Life:** 3–4 h.

## NURSING IMPLICATIONS

### Black Box Warning

*Abrupt discontinuation of intrathecal baclofen has resulted in severe adverse reactions including high fever, altered mental status, exaggerated spasticity and muscle rigidity; rarely, rhabdomyolysis, multiple organ-system failure, and death have occurred.*

### Assessment & Drug Effects
- Supervise ambulation. Initially, the loss of spasticity induced by baclofen may affect patient's ability to stand or walk.
- Monitor for orthostatic hypotension. Fall precautions may be necessary.
- Observe carefully for CNS side effects: Mental confusion, depression, hallucinations. Older adults are especially sensitive to this drug.
- Monitor patients with epilepsy for possible loss of seizure control.
- Monitor lab tests: Baseline and periodic blood sugar and LFTs.

Common adverse effects in *italic;* life-threatening effects <u>underlined;</u> generic names in **bold;** classifications in SMALL CAPS; ♣ Canadian drug name; ⊙ Prototype drug

**Patient & Family Education**

- Do not stop this drug unless directed to do so by prescriber. Drug withdrawal needs to be accomplished gradually over a period of 2 wk or more. Abrupt withdrawal following prolonged administration may cause anxiety, agitated behavior, auditory and visual hallucinations, severe tachycardia, acute exacerbation of spasticity, and seizures.
- Note: CNS depressant effects will be additive to other CNS depressants, including alcohol.
- Monitor blood glucose for loss of glycemic control if diabetic.
- Do not drive or engage in other potentially hazardous activities until the response to drug is known.
- Do not self-dose with OTC drugs without prescriber's approval.

## BALSALAZIDE
(bal-sal'a-zide)

Colazal, Giazo

**Classifications:** MUCOUS MEMBRANE AGENT; ANTI-INFLAMMATORY
**Therapeutic:** ANTI-INFLAMMATORY
**Prototype:** Mesalamine (5-ASA)

**AVAILABILITY** Capsule; tablet

## ACTION & *THERAPEUTIC EFFECT*
A prodrug of mesalamine that remains intact until it reaches the lumen of the colon. Thought to decrease inflammation of the mucous lining of the colon by blocking cyclooxygenase and inhibiting prostaglandin synthesis in the lining of the colon. *An anti-inflammatory agent and a prodrug of 5-ASA.*

**USES** Treatment of mild to moderate active ulcerative colitis.

**CONTRAINDICATIONS** Prior hypersensitivity to salicylates, balsalazide.

**CAUTIOUS USE** Hypersensitivity to mesalamine, sulfasalazine, olsalazine, salicylate. Allergic response to any medications; hepatic or renal impairment; pyloric stenosis; older adults; pregnancy (category B); lactation; children younger than 5 y.

## ROUTE & DOSAGE

**Ulcerative Colitis**

*Adult:* **PO** 3 capsules t.i.d. for 8–12 wk OR 3 tablets b.i.d.
*Adolescent/Child (5 y or older):* 2250 mg (1–3 caps) t.i.d. for up to 8 wk

## ADMINISTRATION
**Oral**
- Give in a consistent manner with respect to food intake (i.e., either always with or always without food).
- Capsules may be opened and sprinkled on applesauce for ease of swallowing.
- Store at room temperature, preferably at 15°–30° C (59°–86° F).

**ADVERSE EFFECTS** (≥1%) **Body as a Whole:** Arthralgia, fatigue, fever, pain, back pain. **CNS:** Headache, insomnia. **GI:** Abdominal pain, nausea, diarrhea, vomiting, rectal bleeding, flatulence, dyspepsia, coughing, anorexia. **Respiratory:** Rhinitis, pharyngitis.

**INTERACTIONS** Avoid for 6 wk after VARICELLA VACCINE.

**PHARMACOKINETICS Absorption:** Low and variable absorption from the colon. **Distribution:** 99%

Common adverse effects in *italic;* life-threatening effects <u>underlined</u>; generic names in **bold;** classifications in SMALL CAPS; ♣ Canadian drug name; ⊚ Prototype drug

161

protein bound. **Metabolism:** Metabolized in colon to release 5-aminosalicylic acid. **Elimination:** Feces.

## NURSING IMPLICATIONS

### Assessment & Drug Effects

- Monitor for S&S of myelosuppression in patients also receiving azathioprine. Monitor S&S of colitis, including rectal bleeding and frequent stools. Report worsening symptoms.
- Monitor lab tests: Baseline and periodic renal function tests; periodic CBC especially in older adults; periodic LFTS with liver disease.

### Patient & Family Education

- Report worsening of S&S of colitis to prescriber (e.g., diarrhea, abdominal pain, fever, rectal bleeding).

## BASILIXIMAB ℗

(bas-i-lix'i-mab)

Simulect

**Classifications:** IMMUNOSUPPRESSANT; MONOCLONAL ANTIBODY; INTERLEUKIN-2 RECEPTOR ANTAGONIST

Therapeutic: IMMUNOSUPPRESSANT

**AVAILABILITY** Powder for injection

## ACTION & *THERAPEUTIC EFFECT*

Immunosuppressant agent that is an interleukin-2 (IL-2) receptor monoclonal antibody produced by recombinant DNA technology. Binds to and blocks the interleukin-2R-alpha chain (CD-25 antibodies) on surface of activated T lymphocytes. *Binding to CD-25 antibodies inhibits a critical pathway in the immune response of the lymphocytes involved in allograft rejection.*

**USES** Prophylaxis of acute renal transplant rejection.

**UNLABELED USE** Liver transplant rejection prophylaxis.

**CONTRAINDICATIONS** Hypersensitivity to mannitol or murine protein; serious infection or exposure to viral infections (e.g., chickenpox, herpes zoster); lactation.

**CAUTIOUS USE** History of untoward reactions to dacliximab or other monoclonal antibodies; pregnancy (category B).

## ROUTE & DOSAGE

### Transplant Rejection Prophylaxis

*Adult/Child (weight greater than 35 kg):* **IV** 20 mg within 2 h prior to surgery then 20 mg 4 days post-transplant
*Child (weight less than 35 kg, 2–15 y):* **IV** 10 mg within 2 h prior to surgery then 10 mg 4 days post-transplant

## ADMINISTRATION

### Intravenous

*PREPARE:* **Direct/IV infusion:** Add 2.5 mL or 5 mL sterile water for injection to the 10 mg or 20 mg vial, respectively. Rock vial gently to dissolve. ■ May be given as prepared direct IV as a bolus dose or further diluted in an infusion bag to a volume of 50 mL in NS or D5W. The resulting solution has a concentration of 2.5 mg/mL. ■ Invert IV bag to dissolve but do not shake. ■ Discard if diluted solution is colored or has particulate matter. ■ Use IV solution immediately.
*ADMINISTER:* **Direct:** Give bolus over 20–30 min. **IV Infusion:** Infuse the ordered dose of diluted drug over 20–30 min.

▪ If necessary, the diluted solution may be stored at room temperature for 4 h or at 2°–8° C (36°–46° F) for 24 h. Discard after 24 h. ▪ Store undiluted drug at 2°–8° C (36°–46° F).

**ADVERSE EFFECTS** (≥1%) **Body as a Whole:** Pain, peripheral edema, edema, fever, viral infection, asthenia, arthralgia, acute hypersensitivity reactions with any dose. **CNS:** *Headache, tremor,* dizziness, *insomnia,* paresthesias, agitation, depression. **CV:** *Hypertension,* chest pain, hypotension, arrhythmias. **GI:** *Constipation, nausea, diarrhea, abdominal pain,* vomiting, dyspepsia, moniliasis, flatulence, GI hemorrhage, melena, esophagitis, erosive stomatitis. **Hematologic:** *Anemia,* thrombocytopenia, thrombosis, polycythemia, hematoma, hemorrhage, hypoproteinemia, leukopenia, purpura. **Respiratory:** Dyspnea, URI, cough, rhinitis, pharyngitis, bronchospasm. **Skin:** Poor wound healing, *acne.* **Urogenital:** Dysuria, UTI, albuminuria, hematuria, oliguria, frequency, renal tubular necrosis, urinary retention, genital edema (male), impotence. **Other:** Cataract, conjunctivitis. **Metabolic:** *Hyperkalemia,* hypokalemia, hyperglycemia, hyperuricemia, hypophosphatemia, hypocalcemia, increased weight, hyper-cholesterolemia, acidosis. **Neuromuscular:** Tremor.

**INTERACTIONS Drug:** Do not use with **alefacpet** or LIVE VACCINES. Use with **gefinitib** can increase risk of adverse reactions. **Herbal:** Do not use with **echinacea.**

**PHARMACOKINETICS Distribution:** Binds to interleukin-2R-alpha sites on lymphocytes. **Half-Life:** 7.2 ± 3.2 days in adults, 11.5 ± 6.3 days in children.

**NURSING IMPLICATIONS**

**Assessment & Drug Effects**

▪ Monitor carefully for and immediately report S&S of opportunistic infection or anaphylactic reaction (see Appendix F).
▪ Monitor CV status with periodic BP measurements.
▪ Monitor lab tests: Periodic serum electrolytes, lipid profile, and uric acid.

**Patient & Family Education**

▪ Report any distressing adverse effects.
▪ Avoid vaccination for 2 wk following last dose of drug.

## BCG (BACILLUS CALMETTE-GUÉRIN) VACCINE

(ba-cil'lus cal'met-te guer'in)

Tice, TheraCys

**Classifications:** BIOLOGIC RESPONSE MODIFIER; VACCINE; IMMUNOMODULATOR
**Therapeutic:** ANTINEOPLASTIC; IMMUNOMODULATOR

**AVAILABILITY** Powder for suspension

**ACTION & THERAPEUTIC EFFECT**
BCG vaccine is an attenuated, live bacterial culture of the Bacillus of Calmette and Guérin (BCG) strain of *Mycobacterium bovis* and induces active immunity against *Mycobacterium tuberculosis.* BCG live is thought to cause a local, chronic inflammatory response involving macrophage and leukocyte infiltration of the bladder. This leads to destruction of superficial tumor cells. *BCG vaccine is an immunization agent for tuberculosis (TB). BCG is active immunotherapy that stimulates the immune mechanism to reject the tumor. It enhances the cytotoxicity of macrophages.*

Common adverse effects in *italic;* life-threatening effects underlined; generic names in **bold;** classifications in SMALL CAPS; ♣ Canadian drug name; ⦿ Prototype drug

163

*BCG live is used intravesically as a biological response modifier for bladder cancer in situ.*

**USES** Carcinoma in situ of the bladder.

**UNLABELED USES** Malignant melanoma.

**CONTRAINDICATIONS** Impaired immune responses, immunosuppressive corticosteroid therapy, active TB, concurrent infections; recent TURP, severe hematuria; positive HIV serology; fever; UTI; angioedema; bone marrow suppression; chemotherapy; infection; mycobacterial infection; radiation therapy; tuberculosis; lactation.

**CAUTIOUS USE** Hypersensitivity to BCG; high risk for HIV; bladder irritation; pregnancy (category C).

## ROUTE & DOSAGE

### Carcinoma of the Bladder

*Adult:* **Intravesical** 1 vial **TheraCys** into bladder weekly × 6 wk then 1 vial at 3, 6, 12, 18, and 24 mo following the initial dose; 1 vial of **Tice** weekly × 6 wk then monthly × 6–12 mo

### Prevention of Tuberculosis (Tice Only)

Apply vaccine with syringe and needle by dropping onto 1 to 2 inch area of horizontally positioned surface of cleansed dry skin in the deltoid region of the arm

See Appendix J.

## ADMINISTRATION

### Intravesical Instillation

- **TheraCys:** Dilute 3 vials of **TheraCys** in 50 mL of sterile preservative free NS and instill into bladder slowly by gravity flow via urethral catheter. Patient retains suspension for 2 h and then voids.
- **Important:** Exercise care when handling BCG vaccine to avoid contact with the product. BCG is a biohazardous material.
- Store dry BCG powder, reconstituted vaccine, and diluent refrigerated at 2°–8° C (35°–46° F). Use reconstituted solution within 2 h.

### Percutaneous Application

- Apply vaccine with syringe and needle by dropping onto 1 to 2 inch area of horizontally positioned surface of cleansed dry skin in the deltoid region of the arm.
- Pull skin taut and puncture skin with multiple puncture device centered over the vaccine. Apply pressure for 5 seconds.
- Spread vaccine evenly over puncture area.
- Apply loose covering and keep area dry for 24 h.

**ADVERSE EFFECTS** (≥1%) **CNS:** Intravesical administration: *Malaise,* dizziness, headache, weakness. **Endocrine:** Hyperpyrexia. **GI:** Abdominal pain, anorexia, constipation, nausea, vomiting, diarrhea; hepatic dysfunction following intratumor injection, granulomatous hepatitis. **Urogenital:** Intravesical administration: Bladder spasms, clot retention, decreased bladder capacity, decreased urine flow, *dysuria, hematuria,* incontinence, nocturia, UTI, cystitis, hemorrhagic cystitis, penile pain, prostatism, urinary frequency. **Hematologic:** Thrombocytopenia, eosinophilia, *anemia,* leukopenia, disseminated intravascular coagulation. **Respiratory:** Cough (rare), pulmonary granulomas, pulmonary infection. **Skin:** Abscess with

Common adverse effects in *italic;* life-threatening effects underlined; generic names in **bold;** classifications in SMALL CAPS; ♣ Canadian drug name; ⊙ Prototype drug

recurrent discharge, red papule that scales or ulcerates in about 5–6 wk, dermatomyositis, granulomas at injection site 4–6 wk after inoculation, keloid formation, lupus vulgaris. **Body as a Whole:** Systemic BCG infection, *chills, flulike syndrome,* anaphylaxis (rare), allergic reactions, lymphadenitis, fever.

## DIAGNOSTIC TEST INTERFERENCE
Prior BCG vaccination may result in false-positive *tuberculin skin test (PPD).* Following BCG vaccination, tuberculin sensitivity may persist for months to years.

## INTERACTIONS **Drug:** Concurrent antibiotic therapy may diminish therapeutic effect. **Cyclosporine** may reduce the immunologic response to BCG vaccine. Avoid IMMUNOSUPPRESSANT and MYELOSUPPRESSIVE agents. Avoid LIVE VACCINES.

## NURSING IMPLICATIONS

### Black Box Warning

*BCG is a biohazardous material. Accidental exposure has resulted in serious, and sometimes fatal, infections.*

### Assessment & Drug Effects
- Monitor for S&S of systemic BCG infection: Fever, chills, severe malaise, or cough.
- Assess for regional lymph node enlargement and report fistula formation.
- Monitor lab tests: Culture blood and urine if systemic infection is suspected.

### Patient & Family Education
- Report promptly S&S of infections including fever, chills, or unexplained fatigue and weakness.

- Retain instillation in bladder for as long as possible (up to 2 h) before voiding.
- Unless instructed otherwise, increase fluid intake to flush bladder after first voiding.
- Disinfect voided urine with bleach for 15 min before flushing.

# BECAPLERMIN
(be-cap'ler-min)
Regranex
**Classification:** PLATELET-DERIVED GROWTH FACTOR (PDGF)
Therapeutic: GROWTH FACTOR

## AVAILABILITY Gel

## ACTION & *THERAPEUTIC EFFECT*
It induces fibroblast proliferation in new granulation tissue. *It is effective against diabetic neuropathic ulcers that involve subcutaneous or deeper tissue, and also have an adequate blood supply. Hence it promotes wound healing of diabetic ulcers.*

## USES Lower-extremity diabetic neuropathic ulcers, wound management.

## CONTRAINDICATIONS Hypersensitivity to becaplermin; cresol or paraben hypersensitivity; neoplasms at site of application; wounds that close by primary intention; increased risk of death in patients with DM.

## CAUTIOUS USE Systemic infection; peripheral vascular disease; ulcer wounds related to arterial or venous insufficiency; thermal, electrical, or radiation burns at wound site; malignancy; older adults; pregnancy (category C); lactation; children younger than 16 y.

Common adverse effects in *italic;* life-threatening effects underlined; generic names in **bold;** classifications in SMALL CAPS; ♣ Canadian drug name; ❿ Prototype drug

165

## ROUTE & DOSAGE

### Diabetic Neuropathic Ulcers

*Adult/Adolescent (16 y or older):*
**Topical** Calculate the length of gel based on ulcer size and apply once/day until healed; reassess if ulcer not completely healed in 20 wk

## ADMINISTRATION

**Topical**
- Squeeze calculated length of gel onto clean, firm, nonabsorbable surface.
- Apply even layer to ulcer area with clean tongue depressor or cotton swab and cover with saline-moistened dressing. After 12 h, remove dressing, clean ulcer by rinsing with water or saline to remove residual gel, and apply new saline-moistened dressing without becaplermin for next 12 h. Repeat cycle.
- Apply only to ulcers with good blood supply.
- Dosage calculation: Measure greatest length ($L$) and greatest width ($W$) of ulcer in inches or centimeters; using 15-g tube multiply $(L \times W) \times 0.6$ for dose in inches or $(L \times W)/4$ for dose in cm; using 2-g tube multiply $(L \times W) \times 1.3$ for dose in inches or $(L \times W)/2$ for dose in cm.
- Store at 2°–8° C (36°–46° F). Do not freeze and do not use beyond expiration date.

**ADVERSE EFFECTS** (≥1%) **Skin:** Erythematous rash.

**PHARMACOKINETICS Absorption:** Less than 3% absorbed into systemic circulation.

## NURSING IMPLICATIONS

**Assessment & Drug Effects**
- Therapeutic efficacy: 30% decrease in ulcer size after 10 wk or complete healing after 20 wk.
- Monitor for and report appearance of erythematous rash.

**Patient & Family Education**
- Consult wound care provider who typically recalculates dosage weekly/biweekly.
- Follow directions for application carefully. Gel may be measured out on waxed paper.
- Wash hands prior to application and do not allow tip of tube to contact ulcer or any surface.
- Report worsening ulceration or development of skin rash.

## BECLOMETHASONE DIPROPIONATE

(be-kloe-meth'a-sone)

Beconase AQ, QVAR, Vancenase AQ

**See Appendix A-3.**

## BEDAQUILINE

(bed-ak'wi-leen)

Sirturo

**Classifications:** ANTI-INFECTIVE; ANTITUBERCULOSIS; INHIBITOR OF MYCOBACTERIAL ATP SYNTHETASE
**Therapeutic:** ANTITUBERCULOSIS

**AVAILABILITY** Tablet

**ACTION & *THERAPEUTIC EFFECT***
Bedaquiline inhibits mycobacterial ATP synthase, an enzyme essential for the generation of energy in Mycobacterium tuberculosis. *Bedaquiline is bactericidal, thus it causes Mycobacterium tuberculosis cell death.*

**USES** Combination therapy in adults (18 y or older) with pulmonary multi-drug resistant tuberculosis (MDR-TB) when other effective treatment regimens are not available.

Common adverse effects in *italic;* life-threatening effects <u>underlined;</u> generic names in **bold;** classifications in SMALL CAPS; ♣ Canadian drug name; ⊙ Prototype drug

166

**CONTRAINDICATIONS** Significant ventricular irregularities; QTcF interval of greater than 500 msec (confirmed by repeat ECG); recent MI; lactation.

**CAUTIOUS USE** Concurrent use with drugs that prolong the QT segment; severe renal or hepatic impairment; HIV-TB co-infected patients; patients with TB other than in the lungs; older adults; pregnancy (category B). Safety and efficacy in children younger than 18 y not established.

## ROUTE & DOSAGE

### Treatment of MDR Tuberculosis

*Adult:* **PO** 400 mg once daily for 2 wk; reduce to 200 mg 3 × wk with at least 48 h between doses for wk 3–24.

## ADMINISTRATION

### Oral

- Give with food. Note that bedaquiline should only be used in combination with other drugs to which the patient's TB has been, or is likely to be susceptible.
- Tablets should be swallowed whole and should not be crushed or chewed.
- Store in a tight, light-resistant container at 15°–30° C (59°–86° F).

**ADVERSE EFFECTS** (>1%) **Body as a Whole:** Anorexia, *hemoptysis*. **CNS:** *Headache.* **CV:** *Chest pain,* QT prolongation. **GI:** *Nausea.* **Metabolic:** ALT/AST increase, blood amylase increase. **Musculoskeletal:** *Arthralgia.* **Skin:** Rash.

**INTERACTIONS Drug:** Inhibitors of CYP3A4 (e.g., **itraconazole, ketoconazole, lopoinavir, ritonavir**) may increase the levels of bedaquiline. Inducers of CYP3A4 (e.g., RIFAMYCINS) may decrease the levels of bedaquiline. Coadministration with other QT prolonging drugs (FLUOROQUINOLONES, MACROLIDES, **clofazimine**) may increase the risk QT prolongation. **Herbal: St. John's wort** may decrease bedaquiline levels.

**PHARMACOKINETICS Peak:** 5 h. **Distribution:** Greater than 99.9% plasma protein bound. **Metabolism:** In liver. **Elimination:** Primarily fecal. **Half-Life:** 5.5 mo (slow release from peripheral tissues).

## NURSING IMPLICATIONS

### Black Box Warning

*Bedaquiline has been associated with an increased risk of death and should be used ONLY when required to provide an effective treatment regimen. QT prolongation can occur with bedaquiline.*

### Assessment & Drug Effects

- Monitor heart rate and rhythm with periodic ECG. Report promptly rapid rate or irregular beat.
- Monitor for and report promptly S&S of hepatoxicity.
- Monitor lab tests: Baseline and periodic sputum cultures and LFTs.

### Patient & Family Education

- During wk 1 and 2, bedaquiline is taken daily.
- During wk 3–24, take no more 600 mg in a 7 day period (e.g., 200 mg M–W–F).
- Always take bedaquiline with other medicines prescribed for you to treat TB.
- Report promptly to prescriber if you experience any of the following: Irregular or rapid heart beat; unexplained nausea or vomiting, stomach pain, fever, weakness,

Common adverse effects in *italic;* life-threatening effects underlined; generic names in **bold;** classifications in SMALL CAPS; ♣ Canadian drug name; ● Prototype drug

167

itching, unusual tiredness, loss of appetite, light colored stool, dark urine, yellowing of your skin or the white of your eyes.
- Do not breast-feed while taking this drug.

# BELIMUMAB

(be-lim'ue-mab)

Benlysta

**Classifications:** BIOLOGICAL RESPONSE MODIFIER; MONOCLONAL ANTIBODY; IMMUNOLOGIC AGENT

Therapeutic: IMMUNOSUPPRESSANT

**Prototype:** Basiliximab

## AVAILABILITY Powder for injection

## ACTION & *THERAPEUTIC EFFECT*

A monoclonal antibody that inhibits the survival of B cells, including autoreactive B cells, and reduces the differentiation of B cells into immunoglobulin-producing plasma cells. *Helps control lupus erythematosus by decreasing the level of a specific immunoglobulin G responsible for the damaging effects of lupus.*

## USES Treatment of active, autoantibody-positive systemic lupus erythematosis (SLE) in adults who are receiving standard therapy.

## CONTRAINDICATIONS Previous hypersensitivity to belimumab; development of progressive multifocal leukoencephalopathy due to belimumab.

## CAUTIOUS USE New onset or chronic infection; psychiatric disorders; depression or suicidal behavior; black patients due to low response rate; pregnancy (category C); lactation. Safety and efficacy not established in children.

## ROUTE & DOSAGE

### Systemic Lupus Erythematosis
*Adult:* **IV** 10 mg/kg q2wk for 3 doses, then q4wk

## ADMINISTRATION

### Intravenous
- Use only in a setting capable of managing hypersensitivity reactions.

*PREPARE:* **IV Infusion:** Place vial at room temperature for 10–15 min. Reconstitute with sterile water for injection by adding 1.5 mL or 4.8 mL to the 120 mg or 400 mg vial, respectively, to yield 80 mg/mL. Minimize foaming by directing stream to side of vial, then swirl gently for 60 sec. Keep at room temperature, swirling for 60 sec q5min until dissolved. Withdraw the required dose of belimumab, then remove from 250 mL of NS a volume equal to the volume of the dose. Add belimumab to the NS and invert to mix.

*ADMINISTER:* **IV Infusion: Do not** give IV push or bolus. Infuse over 1 h through a dedicated IV line. Do not mix with other solutions or drugs. ▪ Monitor closely for S&S of an infusion reaction. Stop infusion, institute supportive measures and notify prescriber if an infusion reaction (or hypersensitivity) is suspected.

*INCOMPATIBILITIES:* **Solution/additive: Dextrose** solutions.

- May store reconstituted solution for up to 7 h at 2°–8° C (36°–46° F). Protect from light. Total time from reconstitution to completion of infusion should not exceed 8 h.

**ADVERSE EFFECTS** (≥1%) **Body as a Whole:** Cystitis, pain in the extremities, *pyrexia,* infection. **CNS:** Depression, insomnia, migraine headache. **GI:** *Diarrhea,* gastroenteritis, *nausea.* **Hematological:** Leukopenia. **Respiratory:** Bronchitis, *nasopharyngitis,* pharyngitis.

**PHARMACOKINETICS Half-Life:** 19.4 days.

## NURSING IMPLICATIONS

### Assessment & Drug Effects

- Monitor vital signs often during and after infusion.
- Monitor closely for S&S of infusion reaction or hypersensitivity. Stop the infusion and notify prescriber if any of these occur.
- Monitor closely if a new infection develops.
- Assess for depression, anxiety, or other manifestations of psychiatric problems. Report immediately suicidal ideation.

### Patient & Family Education

- Report immediately any of the following: Difficulty breathing, wheezing, rash, itching, swelling of the face or tongue, chest pain, or other discomfort during drug infusion.
- Inform prescriber immediately of new or worsening mental health problems such as anxiety, depression, or thoughts of suicide.
- Live vaccines received within 30 days of beginning or concurrently with belimumab therapy may not be effective. Seek advice of prescriber.
- Do not breast-feed while taking this drug without consulting prescriber.
- Women should use effective means of contraception during and for at least 4 mo following termination of treatment.

## BELINOSTAT
(be-lin'o-stat)
Beleodaq

**Classifications:** ANTINEOPLASTIC; HISTONE DEACETYLASE INHIBITOR
**Therapeutic:** ANTINEOPLASTIC

**AVAILABILITY** Lyophilized powder for reconstitution

## ACTION & *THERAPEUTIC EFFECT*
Inhibits the enzyme, histone deacetylase, resulting in accumulation of acetyl groups in cells, leading to cell cycle arrest and apoptosis of tumor cells; drug has preferential cytotoxicity toward tumor cells versus normal cells. *Inhibits proliferation of peripheral T-cell lymphoma cells.*

**USES** Treatment of patients with relapsed or refractory peripheral T-cell lymphoma (PTCL).

**CONTRAINDICATIONS** Tumor lysis syndrome due to belinostat; pregnancy (category D); lactation.

**CAUTIOUS USE** Anemia; neutropenia; thrombocytopenia; hepatic impairment; renal impairment. Safety and efficacy in children younger than 18 y not established.

## ROUTE & DOSAGE

| Peripheral T-Cell Lymphoma |
| --- |
| *Adult:* **IV** 1000 mg/m² on days 1–5 of a 21-day cycle; can repeat every 21 days |
| **Hematologic Toxicity Dosage Adjustment** |
| *ANC less than 0.5 × 10⁹/L (any platelet count):* Reduce dose to 750 mg/m² |
| *Platelet count less than 25 × 10⁹/L (any nadir ANC):* Reduce to 750 mg/m² |

Common adverse effects in *italic;* life-threatening effects underlined; generic names in **bold;** classifications in SMALL CAPS; ♣ Canadian drug name; ⊘ Prototype drug

169

### Nonhematologic Toxicity Dosage Adjustment

*Any CTCAE Grade 3 or 4 adverse reaction (except nausea, vomiting, and diarrhea):* Reduce to 750 mg/m²
*Recurrence of CTCAE Grade 3 or 4 adverse reactions after two dosage reductions:* Discontinue therapy
*Grade 3 or 4 nausea, vomiting, or diarrhea:* Reduce dose only if the duration is greater than 7 days with supportive management

### Patients with Reduced UGT1A1 Activity Dosage Adjustment

*Patients homozygous for the UGT1A1\*28 allele:* Reduce initial dose to 750 mg/m²

## ADMINISTRATION

### Intravenous

This drug is a cytotoxic agent and caution should be used to prevent any contact with the drug. Follow institutional or standard guidelines for preparation, handling, and disposal of cytotoxic agents.
*PREPARE:* **IV Infusion:** Reconstitute 500 mg vial with 9 mL SW to yield 50 mg/mL. Swirl vial until dissolved. Further dilute required dose in 250 mL NS.
*ADMINISTER:* **IV Infusion:** Give over 30 min through a 0.22-micron inline filter; if infusion site pain occurs, increase infusion time to 45 min.

- Store drug vials at 15°–30° C (59°–86° F). May store reconstituted solution up to 12 h and solutions diluted for infusion up to 36 h (including infusion time) at 15°–30° C (59°–86° F).

## ADVERSE EFFECTS (≥ 2%) **Body as a Whole:** *Fever*, infection, injection site pain, <u>multi-organ failure</u>. **CNS:** Chills, dizziness, *fatigue*, headache. **CV:** Hypotension, *peripheral edema*, phlebitis, <u>QT prolongation</u>. **GI:** Abdominal pain, constipation, decreased appetite, diarrhea, *nausea, vomiting*. **Hematological:** *Anemia*, <u>thrombocytopenia</u>. **Metabolic:** Hypokalemia, increased lactate dehydrogenase, increase serum creatinine. **Respiratory:** *Cough*, dyspnea, pneumonia. **Skin:** Pruritus, *skin rash*.

## INTERACTIONS **Drug:** Strong inhibitors of UGT1A1 will increase belinostat levels, and concomitant administration is contraindicated.

## PHARMACOKINETICS **Distribution:** 93–96% plasma protein bound. **Metabolism:** In liver by UGT1A1. **Elimination:** Primarily renal. **Half-Life:** 1.1 h.

## NURSING IMPLICATIONS

### Assessment & Drug Effects

- Monitor for and report S&S of GI toxicity (e.g., nausea, vomiting, diarrhea), hepatic dysfunction, infection, or tumor lysis syndrome (e.g., weakness or lethargy, edema, cardiac symptoms, shortness of breath, muscle cramp).
- Withhold drug and notify prescriber if an infection is suspected.
- Monitor lab tests: Baseline and weekly CBC with platelets and differential; renal function tests and LFTs at baseline and before each cycle; periodic serum electrolytes.

### Patient & Family Education

- Report promptly to prescriber if you experience any of the following: Signs of infection, unexplained bleeding, severe dizziness, fainting, irregular heart rate, shortness of breath, or swelling extremities.

- Report promptly signs of liver toxicity such as yellowing of the skin or the white part of eyes (jaundice), dark urine, itching, or pain in the right upper stomach area.
- GI distress is common but report to prescriber significant anorexia, nausea, or diarrhea.
- Women of reproductive age should avoid pregnancy during treatment with this drug.
- Do not breast-feed while taking this drug.

## BENAZEPRIL HYDROCHLORIDE
(ben-a'ze-pril)

Lotensin

**Classifications:** ANTIHYPERTENSIVE; RENIN ANGIOTENSIN SYSTEM ANTAGONIST
**Therapeutic:** ANTIHYPERTENSIVE, ACE INHIBITOR
**Prototype:** Enalapril

### AVAILABILITY Tablet

### ACTION & *THERAPEUTIC EFFECT*
Lowers blood pressure by specific inhibition of the angiotensin converting enzyme (ACE) and thus by decreasing angiotensin II (a potent vasoconstrictor) and aldosterone secretion. *Achieves an antihypertensive effect by suppression of the renin-angiotensin-aldosterone system.*

### USES Treatment of mild to moderate hypertension.

### UNLABELED USES CHF, renoprotective agent, diabetic nephropathy.

### CONTRAINDICATIONS Hypersensitivity to benazepril or another ACE inhibitor; history of angioedema; coadministration with aliskiren in patients with DM; development of jaundice or elevated hepatic enzymes while taking benazepril; pregnancy (category D); lactation; children with a CrCl less than 30 mL/h.

### CAUTIOUS USE Renal impairment, renal-artery stenosis; patients with hypovolemia, receiving diuretics, undergoing dialysis; patients in whom excessive hypotension would present a hazard (e.g., cerebrovascular insufficiency; CHF; hepatic impairment; women of childbearing age; DM; older adults; children younger than 6 y.

## ROUTE & DOSAGE

### Hypertension

*Adult/Adolescent:* **PO** 10–40 mg/day in 1–2 divided doses (max: 80 mg/day)
*Child (6 y or older):* **PO** 0.2–0.6 mg/kg daily (max: 40 mg/day)

### Renal Impairment Dosage Adjustment

*CrCl less than 30 mL/min:* Use 5 mg starting dose.

## ADMINISTRATION
### Oral
- Consult prescriber about initial dose if patient is also receiving diuretics. Typically an initial dose of 5 mg is used to minimize the risk of hypotension.
- Store at room temperature, but not above 30° C (86° F).

---

Common adverse effects in *italic;* life-threatening effects <u>underlined;</u> generic names in **bold;** classifications in SMALL CAPS; ♣ Canadian drug name; ⊙ Prototype drug

**B**

## ADVERSE EFFECTS (≥1%) CV: Hypotension. CNS: *Headache,* dizziness, fatigue, weakness. Endocrine: Hyperkalemia (at higher doses). GI: Nausea, diarrhea or constipation, gastritis. Urogenital: Azotemia, oliguria, renal failure in patients with CHF. Respiratory: Cough, rhinitis, bronchitis. Other: Back pain.

## DIAGNOSTIC TEST INTERFERENCE

Elevations in *serum bilirubin* have been observed after benazepril administration. Benazepril inhibits *aldosterone* secretion, which causes an increase in *serum potassium.*

## INTERACTIONS Drug: POTASSIUM-SPARING DIURETICS may increase the risk of hyperkalemia. Benazepril may increase **lithium** toxicity. Use with **azathioprine** increases risk of myelosuppression. Use with **pregabalin** can increase angioedema risk. Contraindicated with **sacubitril/valsartan.**

## PHARMACOKINETICS Absorption: Readily from GI tract; 37% reaches the systemic circulation. Peak: 2–6 h. Duration: 20–24 h. Distribution: Small amounts cross the blood–brain barrier; crosses placenta; small amount excreted in breast milk. Metabolism: In liver to active metabolite, benazeprilat. Elimination: Benazeprilat is primarily excreted in urine. Half-Life: Benazepril 0.6 h; benazeprilat 22 h.

## NURSING IMPLICATIONS

### Black Box Warning

*Benazepril may cause fetal injury and death.*

### Assessment & Drug Effects

- Assess for hypotension, especially in patients who may be volume depleted (e.g., prolonged diuretic therapy, recent vomiting or diarrhea, salt restriction) or who have CHF.
- Monitor lab tests: Periodic renal function tests during first few weeks of therapy.

### Patient & Family Education

- Discontinue drug and report to prescriber if pregnancy is suspected or detected.
- Do not use salt substitutes unless recommended by prescriber.
- Report swelling of face, eyes, lips, or tongue or difficulty breathing immediately to prescriber.

## BENDAMUSTINE

(ben-da-mus'teen)

Bendeka, Treanda

Classifications: ANTINEOPLASTIC; ALKYLATING AGENT

Therapeutic: ANTINEOPLASTIC

Prototype: Cyclophosphamide

## AVAILABILITY Powder for injection

## ACTION & *THERAPEUTIC EFFECT*

Alkylating agent that causes the formation of intrastrand and interstrand crosslinks between DNA molecules, thus resulting in inhibition of DNA replication, repair and transcription. *Active against both dividing and resting neoplastic lymphocytes.*

## USES Treatment of chronic lymphocytic leukemia (CLL), indolent B cell non-Hodgkin's lymphoma (NHL).

## UNLABELED USES Treatment of mantle cell lymphoma.

## CONTRAINDICATIONS Known hypersensitivity (e.g., anaphylaxic reaction) to bendmustine or mannitol); infusion reaction; pregnancy (category D); lactation.

Common adverse effects in *italic;* life-threatening effects <u>underlined</u>; generic names in **bold;** classifications in SMALL CAPS; ♣ Canadian drug name; ● Prototype drug

**CAUTIOUS USE** Myelosuppression; mild hepatic or mild-to-moderate renal impairment; grade 3 or 4 infusion reaction; infection; dermatologic toxicity; extravasation; gastrointestinal toxicities; hypokalemia; infection; malignancies; tumor lysis syndrome; children younger than 6 y.

## ROUTE & DOSAGE

### Chronic Lymphocytic Leukemia

*Adult:* **IV** 100 mg/m² on days 1 and 2 of a 28-day cycle, up to 6 cycles

### Hematologic Toxicity Dosage Adjustment

*Grade 3 or higher:* Reduce dose to 50 mg/m² on days 1 and 2 of each cycle; *if grade 3 or higher toxicity recurs:* Reduce the dose to 25 mg/m² on days 1 and 2 of each cycle.

*Grade 4 hematologic toxicity:* Hold dose until neutrophil above 1000 and platelets above 75,000.

### Non-Hodgkin's Lymphoma

*Adult:* **IV** 120 mg/m² on days 1 and 2 q21days; up to 8 cycles

### Toxicity Dosage Adjustment

- *For grade 3 or greater non-hematologic toxicity or grade 4 hematologic toxicity:* Reduce dose to 90 mg/m²
- *For recurrent grade 3 or greater non-hematologic toxicity or recurrent grade 4 hematologic toxicity:* Reduce dose to 60 mg/m²

## ADMINISTRATION

### Intravenous

Exercise caution in handling and disposal. Avoid contact with skin. Wash immediately with soap and water if contact occurs.

*PREPARE:* **IV Infusion:** Reconstitute with sterile water for injection; add 5 mL to the 25 mg vial or 20 mL to the 100 mg vial to yield 5 mg/mL; should dissolve completely in 5 min. ▪ Withdraw required dose within 30 min of reconstitution and immediately add to 500 mL of NS.
*ADMINISTER:* **IV Infusion:** Infuse over 30 min for CLL and 60 min for NHL.

## ADVERSE EFFECTS (≥5%) **Body as a Whole:** Hypersensitivity, infection, *pyrexia.* **CNS:** Headache, dizziness, insomnia, chills, fatigue. **GI:** Diarrhea, *nausea, vomiting,* anorexia, stomatitis, abdominal pain, decreased appetite, dyspepsia. **Hematologic:** *Anemia,* leukopenia, lymphocytopenia, bone marrow depression, *neutropenia,* thrombocytopenia, dehydration. **Metabolic:** Hyperuricemia, weight loss. **Respiratory:** Cough, nasopharyngitis. **Skin:** Pruritus, rash. **Cardiovascular:** Peripheral edema. **Hepatic:** Increased serum bilirubin.

## INTERACTIONS **Drug:** Compounds that inhibit CYP1A2 (**atazanavir, cimetidine, ciprofloxacin, fluvoxamine, omeprazole, zileuton**) will increase levels of bendamustine but decrease levels of its active metabolite. Avoid **clozapine** due to additive bone marrow suppression. Use with NSAIDs may cause thrombocytopenia.

## PHARMACOKINETICS **Distribution:** 95% protein bound. **Metabolism:** Hepatic oxidation by CYP1A2. **Elimination:** Primarily fecal (90%). **Half-Life:** 40 min.

---

Common adverse effects in *italic;* life-threatening effects underlined; generic names in **bold;** classifications in SMALL CAPS; ♣ Canadian drug name; ◐ Prototype drug

173

**B**

## NURSING IMPLICATIONS

### Assessment & Drug Effects

- Monitor closely for infusion reactions (i.e., chills, fever, pruritus, rash) and signs of anaphylaxis. Reactions are more likely with the second and subsequent cycles. Discontinue infusion immediately and notify prescriber for severe reactions.
- Maintain adequate hydration status to minimize risk of tumor lysis syndrome.
- Monitor for and report S&S of infection.
- If extravasation occurs, stop infusion immediately and disconnect tubing from IV cannula. Gently aspirate extravasated solution and remove cannula. Apply dry, cold compress for 20 min 4 × daily.
- Monitor lab tests: Baseline and weekly Hgb, WBC with differential, and platelet count; frequent serum potassium and uric acid; frequent renal function tests with preexisting renal impairment.

### Patient & Family Education

- Men and women should use reliable contraception to avoid pregnancy during and for 3 mo after bendamustine therapy is completed.
- Do not drive or engage in other dangerous activities until reaction to drug is known.
- Report promptly any of the following: Signs of infection, nausea, vomiting, diarrhea, worsening rash, itching, shortness of breath. cough, or swelling of face, lips, tongue, or throat.

## BENZALKONIUM CHLORIDE

(benz-al-koe′nee-um)

Benza, Benzalchlor-50, Germicin, Pharmatex ♣, Sabol, Zephiran

**Classification:** TOPICAL ANTIBIOTIC
**Therapeutic:** ANTIBIOTIC

**AVAILABILITY** Concentrate, solution, tincture/tincture spray

**ACTION & *THERAPEUTIC EFFECT***
Bactericidal or bacteriostatic action (depending on concentration), probably due to inactivation of bacterial enzyme. *Effective against bacteria, some fungi (including yeasts) and certain protozoa. Generally not effective against spore-forming organisms.*

**USES** Antisepsis of intact skin, mucous membranes, superficial injuries, and infected wounds; also for irrigations of the eye and body cavities and for vaginal douching. A component of several contact lens wetting and cushioning solutions, and a preservative for ophthalmic solutions.

**CONTRAINDICATIONS** Casts, occlusive dressings, anal or vaginal packs, lactation.

**CAUTIOUS USE** Irrigation of body cavities; pregnancy (category C).

**ROUTE & DOSAGE**

**Minor Wounds or Preoperative Disinfection**
*Adult:* **Topical** 1:750 tincture or spray

**Preoperative Disinfection of Denuded Skin and Mucous Membranes**
*Adult:* **Topical** 1:10,000–1:2000 solution

**Wet Dressings**
*Adult:* **Topical** 1:5000 solution

Common adverse effects in *italic*; life-threatening effects underlined; generic names in **bold**; classifications in SMALL CAPS; ♣ Canadian drug name; ⊙ Prototype drug

**Urinary Bladder Irrigation**

*Adult:* **Topical** 1:20,000–1:5000 solution

**Urinary Bladder Instillation**

*Adult:* **Topical** 1:40,000–1:20,000 solution

**Irrigation of Deep Infected Wounds**

*Adult:* **Topical** 1:20,000–1:3000 solution

**Vaginal Irrigation**

*Adult:* **Topical** 1:5000–1:2000 solution

**Sterile Storage of Instruments, Thermometers, Ampules**

*Adult:* **Topical** 1:750 solution

## ADMINISTRATION
### Topical
- Use sterile water for injection as diluent for aqueous solutions to be instilled in wounds or body cavities. For other uses, fresh sterile distilled water is used.
- Irrigate eyes immediately and repeatedly with water if medication solution stronger than 1:5000 enters eyes; see a prescriber promptly.
- Rinse first with water, then with 70% alcohol, before applying benzalkonium for preoperative skin preparation.
- Consult prescriber about proper dilution of solutions used on denuded skin or inflamed or irritated tissues.
- Store at room temperature, preferably at 15°–30° C (59°–86° F) in airtight container, protected from light.

## ADVERSE EFFECTS (≥1%) Body as a Whole: Few or no toxic effects

in recommended dilutions. **Skin:** Erythema, local burning, hypersensitivity reactions.

## NURSING IMPLICATIONS
### Assessment & Drug Effects
- Monitor wounds carefully. Report increasing signs of infection or lack of healing.

## BENZOCAINE
(ben'zoe caine)

Anesthetic Lubricant, Anbesol Cold Sore Therapy, Chigger-Tox, Dermoplast, Foille, Hurricaine, Orabase with Benzocaine, Orajel, Solar-caine, T-Caine

**Classifications:** LOCAL ANESTHETIC (ESTER TYPE); ANTIPRURITIC
**Therapeutic:** LOCAL ANESTHETIC; ANTIPRURITIC
**Prototype:** Procaine

**AVAILABILITY** Spray; cream; ointment; lotion; gel; liquid; otic solution

## ACTION & THERAPEUTIC EFFECT
Produces surface anesthesia by inhibiting conduction of nerve impulses from sensory nerve endings. Almost identical to procaine in chemical structure, but has prolonged duration of anesthetic action. *Temporary relief of pain and discomfort.*

**USES** Temporary relief of pain and discomfort in pruritic skin problems, minor burns and sunburn, minor wounds, and insect bites. Preparations are also available for toothache, minor sore throat pain, canker sores, hemorrhoids, rectal fissures, pruritus ani or vulvae, and for use as anesthetic-lubricant for passage of catheters and endoscopic tubes.

Common adverse effects in *italic;* life-threatening effects underlined; generic names in **bold;** classifications in SMALL CAPS; ♣ Canadian drug name; ☯ Prototype drug

175

## CONTRAINDICATIONS

Hypersensitivity to benzocaine or other PABA derivatives (e.g., sunscreen preparations), or to any of the components in the formulation; use of ear preparation in patients with perforated eardrum or ear discharge; applications to large areas. **Dental Use:** Children younger than 2 y. **Anesthetic Lubricant:** Infants younger than 1 y.

## CAUTIOUS USE

History of drug sensitivity; denuded skin or severely traumatized mucosa; lactation; pregnancy (category C).

## ROUTE & DOSAGE

**Anesthetic**

*Adult:* **Topical** Lowest effective dose (usually 3–4 × per day)
*Child:* **Topical** Lower strengths

## ADMINISTRATION

**Topical**

- Avoid contact of all preparations with eyes and be careful not to inhale mist when spray form is used.
- Do not use spray near open flame or cautery and do not expose to high temperatures. Hold can at least 12 inches (30 cm) away from affected area when spraying.
- Store at 15°–30° C (59°–86° F) in tight, light-resistant containers unless otherwise specified.

## ADVERSE EFFECTS (≥1%)

**Body as a Whole:** Low toxicity; sensitization in susceptible individuals; allergic reactions, anaphylaxis. **Hematologic:** Methemoglobinemia reported in infants. **Dermatologic:** Contact dermatitis, localized erythema, burning, stinging.

## INTERACTIONS

**Drug:** Benzocaine may antagonize antibacterial activity of SULFONAMIDES.

## PHARMACOKINETICS

**Absorption:** Poorly absorbed through intact skin; readily absorbed from mucous membranes. **Peak:** 1 min. **Duration:** 15–30 min. **Metabolism:** By plasma cholinesterases and to a lesser extent by hepatic cholinesterases. **Elimination:** In urine.

## NURSING IMPLICATIONS

### Assessment & Drug Effects

- Assess swallowing when used on oral mucosa, as benzocaine may interfere with second (pharyngeal) stage of swallowing; hold food and liquids accordingly.
- Assess for sensitivity. Local anesthetics are potentially sensitizing to susceptible individuals when applied repeatedly or over extensive areas.

### Patient & Family Education

- Use specific benzocaine preparation ONLY as prescribed or recommended by manufacturer.
- Discontinue medication if the condition persists, worsens, or if signs of sensitivity, irritation, or infection occur.

## BENZONATATE ⓟ

(ben-zoe'na-tate)

Tessalon Perles, Zonatuss

**Classification:** ANTITUSSIVE
**Therapeutic:** COUGH SUPPRESSANT

## AVAILABILITY Capsule

## ACTION & *THERAPEUTIC EFFECT*

Nonnarcotic antitussive activity that acts periperally by anesthetizing the receptors in the respiratory bronchi, lungs, and pleura, thus reducing the cough reflex. *Decreases frequency and intensity of nonproductive cough.*

## USES Symptomatic treatment of cough.

Common adverse effects in *italic;* life-threatening effects underlined; generic names in **bold;** classifications in SMALL CAPS; ♣ Canadian drug name; ⓟ Prototype drug

**UNLABELED USES** Hiccups.

**CONTRAINDICATIONS** Hypersensitivity to benzonatate.

**CAUTIOUS USE** Pregnancy (category C); lactation; children younger than 10 y.

## ROUTE & DOSAGE

**Antitussive**

*Adult/Child (10 y or older):* **PO** 100 mg t.i.d. (max: 600 mg/day)

## ADMINISTRATION

**Oral**
- Ensure that soft capsules called perles are swallowed whole.
- Store in airtight containers protected from light.

**ADVERSE EFFECTS** (≥1%) **CNS:** Drowsiness, sedation, headache, mild dizziness. **GI:** Constipation, nausea. **Skin:** Rash, pruritus. **Respiratory:** Hypersensitivity reaction (bronchospasm, laryngospasm, anaphylaxis).

**INTERACTIONS** Use with MAO INHIBITORS may increase risk of hypotension.

**PHARMACOKINETICS Onset:** 15–20 min. **Duration:** 3–8 h.

## NURSING IMPLICATIONS

**Assessment & Drug Effects**
- Auscultate lungs anteriorly and posteriorly at scheduled intervals.
- Observe character and frequency of coughing and volume and quality of sputum. Keep prescriber informed.

**Patient & Family Education**
- Do not chew or allow perle to dissolve in mouth; swallow whole. If perle dissolves in mouth, the mouth, tongue, and pharynx will be anesthetized. Also, it is unpleasant to taste.

- Use with caution while driving or operating machinery.

# BENZPHETAMINE HYDROCHLORIDE
(benz-fet'a-meen)

**Classifications:** CEREBRAL STIMULANT; ANOREXIANT
**Therapeutic:** ANOREXIANT
**Prototype:** Amphetamine
**Controlled Substance:** Schedule III

**AVAILABILITY** Tablet

## ACTION & *THERAPEUTIC EFFECT*

Indirect-acting sympathomimetic amine with amphetamine-like actions but with fewer side effects than amphetamine. Anorexiant effect thought to be secondary to stimulation of hypothalamus releasing stored catecholamines in the CNS. *Effective as an appetite suppressant.*

**USES** Short-term management of exogenous obesity.

**CONTRAINDICATIONS** Known hypersensitivity to sympathomimetic amines; angle closure glaucoma; advanced arteriosclerosis, angina pectoris, severe cardiovascular disease, moderate to severe hypertension; hyperthyroidism, agitated states; history of drug abuse; lactation; pregnancy (category X).

**CAUTIOUS USE** Diabetes mellitus; older adults; psychosis; mild hypertension; children younger than 12 y.

## ROUTE & DOSAGE

**Obesity**

*Adult/Adolescent:* **PO** 25–50 mg 1–3 × day

Common adverse effects in *italic;* life-threatening effects underlined; generic names in **bold**; classifications in SMALL CAPS; ♦ Canadian drug name; ⊕ Prototype drug

177

## ADMINISTRATION

### Oral

- Give as a single daily dose, preferably midmorning or midafternoon, according to patient's eating habits.
- Schedule daily dose no later than 6 h before patient retires to avoid insomnia.
- Store in tight, light-resistant containers at 15°–30° C (59°–86° F) unless otherwise directed.

## ADVERSE EFFECTS (≥1%) CNS:

Euphoria, irritability, hyperactivity, nervousness, *restlessness, insomnia,* tremor, headache, light-headedness, dizziness, depression following stimulant effects. Marked insomnia, irritability, hyperactivity, personality changes, psychosis, dermatoses. **CV:** *Palpitation,* tachycardia, elevated BP, irregular heartbeat. **GI:** Xerostomia, nausea, vomiting, diarrhea or constipation, abdominal cramps.

## INTERACTIONS Drug: **Acetazolamide, sodium bicarbonate**

decrease AMPHETAMINE elimination; **ammonium chloride, ascorbic acid** increase AMPHETAMINE elimination; BARBITURATES may antagonize the effects of both drugs; **furazolidone** may increase BP effects of AMPHETAMINES, and interaction may persist for several weeks after discontinuation of **furazolidone; guanethidine** antagonizes antihypertensive effects; because MAO INHIBITORS, **selegiline** can cause hypertensive crisis (fatalities reported); do not administer AMPHETAMINES during or within 14 days of these drugs; PHENOTHIAZINES may inhibit mood-elevating effects of AMPHETAMINES; BETA AGONISTS increase AMPHETAMINE's adverse cardiovascular effects. Do not use with **meperidine.** Do not use with other ANORECTIC AGENTS. **Herbal:** Do not use with **melatonin.**

## PHARMACOKINETICS Absorption: Readily absorbed from GI tract. **Duration:** 4 h. **Metabolism:** Via CYP3A4. **Elimination:** Renal elimination.

## NURSING IMPLICATIONS

### Assessment & Drug Effects

- Assess for signs of excessive CNS stimulation: Insomnia, restlessness, tremor, palpitations. These may indicate need for dosage adjustment.
- Monitor vital signs; report elevated BP, tachycardia, and irregular heart rhythm.
- Monitor diabetics for loss of glycemic control.

### Patient & Family Education

- Note: Anorexiant effects are temporary and tolerance may occur; long-term use is not indicated.
- Do not drive or engage in potentially hazardous activities until response to drug is known.
- Do not terminate high dosage therapy abruptly; GI distress, stomach cramps, trembling, unusual tiredness, weakness, and mental depression may result.

## BENZTROPINE MESYLATE ℗

(benz′troe-peen)

Apo-Benztropine ◆, Cogentin, PMS Benztropine ◆

**Classifications:** CENTRALLY ACTING CHOLINERGIC RECEPTOR ANTAGONIST; ANTIPARKINSON
Therapeutic: ANTIPARKINSON

## AVAILABILITY Tablet, injectable solution

## ACTION & *THERAPEUTIC EFFECT*

Synthetic centrally acting anticholinergic agent that acts by diminishing excess cholinergic effect associated with dopamine deficiency. *Suppresses tremor and rigidity; does not alleviate tardive dyskinesia.*

Common adverse effects in *italic;* life-threatening effects underlined; generic names in **bold;** classifications in SMALL CAPS; ◆ Canadian drug name; ℗ Prototype drug

**USES** Parkinson's disease or Parkinsonism, drug-induced extrapyramidal symptoms.

**CONTRAINDICATIONS** Narrow-angle glaucoma; myasthenia gravis; obstructive diseases of GU and GI tracts; tendency to tachycardia; tardive dyskinesia achalasia, myasthenia gravis; megacolon; children younger than 3 y.

**CAUTIOUS USE** Older adults or debilitated patients, patients with poor mental outlook, mental disorders; tachycardia; autonomic neuropathy; enlarged prostate; hypertension; history of renal or hepatic disease; pregnancy (category C); lactation; children older than 3 y.

## ROUTE & DOSAGE

### Parkinsonism
*Adult:* **PO/IM** 0.5–1 mg/day, may gradually increase if needed up to 6 mg/day

### Extrapyramidal Reactions
*Adult:* **PO/IM/IV** 1–4 mg once or twice daily
*Child (3 y or older):* **PO/IM/IV** 0.02–0.05 mg/kg/dose once or twice daily

### Acute Dystonia
*Adult:* **IV** 1–2 mg daily

## ADMINISTRATION

### Oral
- Give immediately after meals or with food to prevent gastric irritation. Tablet can be crushed and sprinkled on or mixed with food.
- Initiate and withdraw drug therapy gradually; effects are cumulative.
- Store in tightly covered, light-resistant container at 15°–30° C (59°–86° F) unless otherwise directed.

### Intramuscular
- Inject undiluted solution deeply into a large muscle.

### Intravenous
IV administration to infants and children: Verify correct IV concentration with prescriber.

*PREPARE:* **Direct:** Give undiluted.
*ADMINISTER:* **Direct:** Give 1 mg or a fraction thereof over 1 min.

**ADVERSE EFFECTS** (≥1%) **CNS:** *Sedation, drowsiness, dizziness, paresthesias; agitation, irritability, restlessness, nervousness, insomnia, hallucinations, delirium, mental confusion, toxic psychosis, muscular weakness, ataxia, inability to move certain muscle groups.* **CV:** Palpitation, tachycardia, flushing. **Special Senses:** Blurred vision, mydriasis, photophobia. **GI:** Nausea, vomiting, *constipation, dry mouth,* distention, paralytic ileus. **Urogenital:** Dysuria, urinary retention. **Body as a Whole:** hyperthermia, fever.

**INTERACTIONS Drug: Amantadine,** TRICYCLIC ANTIDEPRESSANTS, MAO INHIBITORS, PHENOTHIAZINES, **procainamide, quinidine** have additive anticholinergic effects and cause confusion, hallucinations, paralytic ileus. **Nifedipine** extended release increases the risk of GI obstruction.

**PHARMACOKINETICS Onset:** 15 min IM/IV; 1 h PO. **Duration:** 6–10 h.

## NURSING IMPLICATIONS

### Assessment & Drug Effects
- Monitor I&O ratio and pattern. Advise patient to report difficulty in urination or infrequent voiding. Dosage reduction may be indicated.
- Closely monitor for appearance of S&S of onset of paralytic ileus including intermittent constipation,

Common adverse effects in *italic;* life-threatening effects underlined; generic names in **bold;** classifications in SMALL CAPS; ♣ Canadian drug name; ● Prototype drug

179

**B**

abdominal pain, diminution of bowel sounds on auscultation, and distention.

- Monitor HR especially in patients with a tendency toward tachycardia.
- Monitor for and report muscle weakness or inability to move certain muscle groups. Dosage reduction may be needed.
- Supervise ambulation and use protective measures as necessary.
- Report immediately S&S of CNS depression or stimulation. These usually require interruption of drug therapy.

### Patient & Family Education

- Do not drive or engage in potentially hazardous activities until response to drug is known. Seek help walking as necessary.
- Avoid alcohol and other CNS depressants because they may cause additive drowsiness. Do not take OTC cold, cough, or hay fever remedies unless approved by prescriber.
- Sugarless gum, hard candy, and rinsing mouth with tepid water will help dry mouth.
- Avoid strenuous exercise in hot weather; diminished sweating may require dose adjustments because of possibility of heat stroke.

## BETAMETHASONE

(bay-ta-meth'a-sone)

## BETAMETHASONE BENZOATE

## BETAMETHASONE DIPROPIONATE

AlphaTrex, Diprolene, Sernivo

## BETAMETHASONE VALERATE

Betaderm ♦, Betnovate ♦, Luxiq

**Classifications:** ADRENAL CORTICOSTEROID; GLUCOCORTICOID; ANTI-INFLAMMATORY
Therapeutic: ANTI-INFLAMMATORY; ADRENAL CORTICOSTEROID
**Prototype:** Hydrocortisone

**AVAILABILITY** **Betamethasone Acetate and Betamethasone Sodium:** 3 mg acetate, 3 mg sodium phosphate/mL suspension; **Betamethasone Benzoate and Betamethasone Dipropionate:** Injection; **Betamethasone Valerate:** Ointment; cream; lotion; foam.

## ACTION & *THERAPEUTIC EFFECT*

Synthetic, long-acting glucocorticoid with minor mineralocorticoid properties but strong immunosuppressive, anti-inflammatory, and metabolic actions. *Relieves anti-inflammatory manifestations and is an immunosuppressive agent.*

**USES** Reduces serum calcium in hypercalcemia, suppresses undesirable inflammatory or immune responses, produces temporary remission in nonadrenal disease, and blocks ACTH production in diagnostic tests. Topical use provides relief of inflammatory manifestations of corticosteroid-responsive dermatoses.

**UNLABELED USES** Prevention of neonatal respiratory distress syndrome (hyaline membrane disease).

**CONTRAINDICATIONS** Corticosteroid hypersensitivity; idiopathic thrombocytopenic purpura (ITP).

**CAUTIOUS USE** Fungal infection; acne vulgaris, acne rosacea;

Cushing's syndrome; vaccination; ocular herpes simplex; osteoporosis; diverticulitis, nonspecific ulcerative colitis, abscess or other pyrogenic infection, peptic ulcer disease; asthmatics; DM; hypertension; renal insufficiency; MG; pregnancy (category C); lactation; children.

## ROUTE & DOSAGE

### Anti-Inflammatory Agent

*Adult:* **IM/IV** Up to 9 mg/day as sodium phosphate

*Child:* **IM** 0.0175–0.125 mg/kg/day or 0.5–0.75 mg/m²/day divided q6–8h

### Topical
See Appendix A-4.

### Respiratory Distress Syndrome

*Adult:* **IM** 2 mL of sodium phosphate to mother once daily, 2–3 days before delivery

## ADMINISTRATION

### Intramuscular

- Use Celestone Soluspan for intra-articular, IM, and intralesional injection. The preparation is not intended for IV use. Do not mix with diluents containing preservatives (e.g., parabens, phenol).
- Use 1% or 2% lidocaine hydrochloride if prescribed. Withdraw betamethasone mixture first, then lidocaine; shake syringe briefly.

### Intravenous

*PREPARE:* **Direct/IV Infusion:** Give by direct IV undiluted or further diluted for infusion in D5W or NS.
*ADMINISTER:* **Direct:** Give over one min. **Infusion:** Give at a rate

determined by the total amount of IV fluid.
*INCOMPATIBILITIES:* **Solution/additive** and **Y-site:** Do not infuse with other drugs.

## ADVERSE EFFECTS (≥1%) **Body as a Whole:** Hypersensitivity or anaphylactoid reactions; aggravation or masking of infections; malaise, weight gain, obesity. Most adverse effects are dose and treatment duration dependent. **CNS:** Vertigo, headache, nystagmus, ataxia (rare), increased intracranial pressure with papilledema (usually after discontinuation of medication), mental disturbances, aggravation of pre-existing psychiatric conditions, insomnia. **CV:** Hypertension; syncopal episodes, thrombophlebitis, thromboembolism or fat embolism, palpitation, tachycardia, necrotizing angitis, CHF. **Endocrine:** Suppressed linear growth in children, decreased glucose tolerance, hyperglycemia, manifestations of latent diabetes mellitus; hypocorticism; amenorrhea and other menstrual difficulties. **Special Senses:** Posterior subcapsular cataracts (especially in children), glaucoma, exophthalmos, increased intraocular pressure with optic nerve damage, perforation of the globe, fungal infection of the cornea, decreased or blurred vision. **Metabolic:** Hypocalcemia; *sodium and fluid retention;* hypokalemia and hypokalemic alkalosis; negative nitrogen balance. **GI:** *Nausea,* increased appetite, ulcerative esophagitis, pancreatitis, abdominal distention, peptic ulcer with perforation and hemorrhage, melena; decreased serum concentration of vitamins A and C. **Hematologic:** Thrombocytopenia. **Musculoskeletal:** Osteoporosis, compression fractures, muscle wasting and weakness, tendon rupture, aseptic

---

Common adverse effects in *italic;* life-threatening effects underlined; generic names in **bold;** classifications in SMALL CAPS; ♣ Canadian drug name; ⊙ Prototype drug

necrosis of femoral and humeral heads (all resulting from long-term use). **Skin:** Skin thinning and atrophy, *acne, impaired wound healing;* petechiae, ecchymosis, easy bruising; suppression of skin test reaction; hypopigmentation or hyperpigmentation, hirsutism, acneiform eruptions, subcutaneous fat atrophy; allergic dermatitis, urticaria, angioneurotic edema, increased sweating. **Urogenital:** Increased or decreased motility and number of sperm; urinary frequency and urgency, enuresis. **With Parenteral Therapy, IV Site:** Pain, irritation, necrosis, atrophy, sterile abscess; Charcot-like arthropathy following intra-articular use; burning and tingling in perineal area (after IV injection).

## DIAGNOSTIC TEST INTERFERENCE

May increase *serum cholesterol, blood glucose, serum sodium, uric acid* (in acute leukemia) and *calcium* (in bone metastasis). It may decrease *serum calcium, potassium, PBI, thyroxin (T₄), triiodothyronine (T₃) and reduce thyroid I 131* uptake. It increases *urine glucose* level and *calcium* excretion; decreases *urine 17-OHCS* and *17-KS* levels. May produce false-negative results with *nitroblue tetrazolium test* for systemic bacterial infection and may suppress reactions to skin tests.

## INTERACTIONS Drug: BARBITU-
RATES, **phenytoin, rifampin** may reduce pharmacologic effect of betamethasone by increasing its metabolism. Use with caution in patients taking **amiodarone.**

## PHARMACOKINETICS Peak: 1–2 h
**Half-Life:** 35–54 h.

## NURSING IMPLICATIONS
### Assessment & Drug Effects
- Assess therapeutic efficacy. Response following intra-articular, intralesional, or intrasynovial administration occurs within a few hours and persists for 1–4 wk. Following IM administration response occurs in 2–3 h and persists for 3–7 days.

### Patient & Family Education
- Monitor weight at least weekly.
- Discontinue slowly after systemic use of 1 wk or longer. Abrupt withdrawal, especially following high doses or prolonged use, can cause dizziness, nausea, vomiting, fever, muscle and joint pain, weakness.

## BETAXOLOL HYDROCHLORIDE
(be-tax'oh-lol)
Betoptic, Betoptic-S, Kerlone
**Classifications:** EYE PREPARATION; MIOTIC (ANTIGLAUCOMA); BETA-ADRENERGIC ANTAGONIST; ANTIHYPERTENSIVE
Therapeutic: ANTIGLAUCOMA (MIOTIC); ANTIHYPERTENSIVE
**Prototype:** Propranolol

## AVAILABILITY Tablet; ophthalmic solution; opthalmic suspension

## ACTION & THERAPEUTIC EFFECT
Acts as a beta₁-selective adrenergic receptor blocking agent, especially at the cardioselective beta₁ receptors. Its antihypertensive effect is thought to be due to: (1) decreasing cardiac output, (2) reducing sympathetic nervous system outflow to the periphery resulting in vasodilatation, and (3) suppression of renin activity in the kidney. It reduces intraocular pressure within the eye by

Common adverse effects in *italic;* life-threatening effects <u>underlined</u>; generic names in **bold;** classifications in SMALL CAPS; ♣ Canadian drug name; ⊕ Prototype drug

decreasing the production of aqueous humor. *It has antihypertensive and antiglaucoma effects.*

**USES** Hypertension. Ocular use for intraocular hypertension, chronic open angle glaucoma (see Appendix A-1).

**CONTRAINDICATIONS** Hypersensitivity to beta-blockers; sinus bradycardia, AV block greater than first degree, cardiogenic shock, overt cardiac failure; lactation.

**CAUTIOUS USE** History of CHF, angina; renal impairment, hyperthyroidism or thyroid disease; DM; bronchiospastic diseases; evidence of airflow obstruction or reactive airway disease, depression; cardiovascular insufficiency; peripheral vascular disease; older adults; pregnancy (category C); children younger than 18 y.

## ROUTE & DOSAGE

**Hypertension**

*Adult:* **PO** 10–20 mg daily (no benefit above 20 mg/day)
*Elderly:* **PO** Start with 5 mg/day and taper up

**Renal Impairment Dosage Adjustment**

*CrCl less than 60 mL/min:*
Administer 50% of dose (max: 20 mg/day)

**Chronic Open-Angle Glaucoma/ Ocular Hypertension**

See Appendix A-1.

## ADMINISTRATION

**Oral**

▪ Check pulse before administering betaxolol, oral or ophthalmic. If there are extremes (rate or rhythm), withhold medication and notify prescriber.

**Opthalmic**

▪ Shake opthalmic suspension before use.
▪ After instillation of drops, instruct patient to close eyes to distribute medication.
▪ Apply finger pressure to lacrimal sac for 1–2 min following application.
▪ Wait 5 min before administering any other opthalmic drug product.

**ADVERSE EFFECTS** (≥1%) **CV:** Bradycardia, hypotension, arrhythmia, AV block. **CNS:** Depression, dizziness, headache. **Respiratory:** Increased airway resistance. **Special Senses:** With ophthalmic solution, *mild ocular stinging* and discomfort, tearing.

**INTERACTIONS Drug: Reserpine** and other CATECHOLAMINE-DEPLETING AGENTS, **amiodarone, bretylium** may cause additive hypotensive effects or bradycardia. **Verapamil** may cause additive heart block.

**PHARMACOKINETICS Absorption:** 90% bioavailable. **Onset:** 0.5–1 h. **Peak:** 2 h. **Duration:** Greater than 12 h. **Metabolism:** In liver. **Elimination:** 30–40% in urine, 50–60% in bile and feces. **Half-Life:** 12–22 h.

## NURSING IMPLICATIONS

**Assessment & Drug Effects**

▪ Monitor pulse rate and BP at regular intervals in patients with known heart disease.
▪ Report promptly onset of bradycardia or signs of CHF.
▪ Monitor therapeutic efficacy. Some patients develop tolerance during long-term therapy.
▪ Taper dosage slowly when discontinuing.

Common adverse effects in *italic*; life-threatening effects <u>underlined</u>; generic names in **bold;** classifications in SMALL CAPS; ♣ Canadian drug name; ⊙ Prototype drug

183

**B**

**Patient & Family Education**

- Report unusual pulse rate or significant changes to prescriber according to parameters provided.
- Adhere to regimen EXACTLY as prescribed. Do not stop drug abruptly; angina may be exacerbated; dosage is reduced over a period of 1–2 wk.
- Report difficulty in breathing promptly to prescriber. Drug withdrawal may be indicated.

# BETHANECHOL CHLORIDE ℞

(be-than'e-kole)

Urecholine

**Classification:** DIRECT-ACTING CHOLINERGIC
**Therapeutic:** CHOLINERGIC

## AVAILABILITY Tablet

## ACTION & *THERAPEUTIC EFFECT*

Synthetic choline ester with effects similar to those of acetylcholine (ACh). Acts directly on postsynaptic receptors, and since it is not hydrolyzed by cholinesterase, its actions are more prolonged than those of ACh. Produces muscarinic effects primarily on GI tract and urinary bladder. Increases tone and peristaltic activity of esophagus, stomach, and intestine; contracts detrusor muscle of urinary bladder, usually enough to initiate micturition. *Bethanechol is indicated for the treatment of urinary retention associated with neurogenic bladder.*

## USES Acute postoperative and postpartum nonobstructive (functional) urinary retention, and for neurogenic atony of urinary bladder with retention.

## UNLABELED USES Anticholinergic syndrome, GERD, ileus.

## CONTRAINDICATIONS COPD; latent or active bronchial asthma; hyperthyroidism; recent urinary bladder surgery, cystitis, bacteriuria, urinary bladder neck or intestinal obstruction, peptic ulcer, recent GI surgery, peritonitis; marked vagotonia, pronounced vasomotor instability, AV conduction defects, severe bradycardia, hypotension or hypertension, coronary artery disease, recent MI; epilepsy, parkinsonism; lactation, children younger than 8 y.

## CAUTIOUS USE Urinary retention; bacteriemia; patients at risk for syncopy; pregnancy (category C).

## ROUTE & DOSAGE

**Urinary Retention**

*Adult:* **PO** 5–10 mg hourly until goals attained (max: 50 mg dose), usually 10–50 mg 3–4 × daily

## ADMINISTRATION

**Oral**

- Give on an empty stomach (1 h before or 2 h after meals) to lessen possibility of nausea and vomiting, unless otherwise advised by prescriber.

## ADVERSE EFFECTS (≥1%) **Body as a Whole:** (Dose-related) Increased sweating, malaise, headache, substernal pain or pressure, hypothermia. **CV:** Hypotension with dizziness, faintness, flushing, orthostatic hypotension (large doses); mild reflex tachycardia, atrial fibrillation (hyperthyroid patients), <u>transient complete heart block</u>. **Special Senses:** Blurred vision, miosis, lacrimation. **GI:** Nausea, vomiting, abdominal cramps, diarrhea, borborygmi, belching, salivation, fecal incontinence (large doses), urge to defecate (or urinate).

**Respiratory:** Acute asthmatic attack, dyspnea (large doses).

## DIAGNOSTIC TEST INTERFERENCE

Bethanechol may cause increases in *serum amylase* and *serum lipase,* by stimulating pancreatic secretions, and may increase *AST, serum bilirubin,* and *BSP retention* by causing spasms in sphincter of Oddi.

## INTERACTIONS Drug: Amoxapine, ANTIMUSCARINICS, **maprotiline,** TRICYCLIC ANTIDEPRESSANTS **may decrease the effect of bethanechol. Neostigmine,** other CHOLINESTERASE INHIBITORS compound cholinergic effects and toxicity; **procainamide, quinidine, atropine, epinephrine** antagonize effects of bethanechol.

## PHARMACOKINETICS Absorption: Poorly absorbed. Onset: 30 min. Duration: 1 h. Metabolism: Unknown. Elimination: Unknown

## NURSING IMPLICATIONS

### Assessment & Drug Effects

- Monitor BP and pulse. Report early signs of overdosage: Salivation, sweating, flushing, abdominal cramps, nausea.
- Monitor I&O. Observe and record patient's response to bethanechol.
- Monitor respiratory status. Promptly report dyspnea or any other indication of respiratory distress.
- Supervise ambulation as indicated by patient response to drug.

### Patient & Family Education

- Make position changes slowly and in stages, particularly from lying down to standing.
- Do not stand still for prolonged periods; sit or lie down at first indication of faintness.

- Do not drive or engage in potentially hazardous activities until response to drug is known.
- Note: Drug may cause blurred vision; take appropriate precautions.

## BETRIXABAN
(be-trix'a-ban)
Bevyxxa

**Classifications:** ANTICOAGULANT; ANTITHROMBOTIC; DIRECT ORAL ANTICOAGULANT; FACTOR XA INHIBITOR
Therapeutic: ANTICOAGULANT; ANTITHROMBOTIC
*[antithrombotic]*

## AVAILABILITY Capsule

## ACTION & *THERAPEUTIC EFFECT*

Inhibits fibrin clot formation via inhibition of factor Xa which catalyzes the conversion of prothrombin to thrombin. *Reduces venous thromboembolism (VTE) risk.*

## USES Venous thromboembolism prophylaxis in hospitalized adults.

## CONTRAINDICATIONS Hypersensitivity to betrixaban or components of the capsule, active pathological bleeding.

## CAUTIOUS USE Severe hypersensitivity to betrixaban, active pathological bleeding; hepatic impairment; renal impairment; pregnancy; lactation. Safety and efficacy in patients younger than 18 y not established.

## ROUTE & DOSAGE

### VTE Prophylaxis

*Adult:* **PO** 160 mg on day one, then 80 mg daily for 35–42 days

### Renal Impairment Dosage Adjustment

Common adverse effects in *italic;* life-threatening effects underlined; generic names in **bold;** classifications in SMALL CAPS; ♣ Canadian drug name; ● Prototype drug

185

CrCL 15-30 mL/min: 80 mg on day one, then 40 mg daily for 35–42 days

## ADMINISTRATION

### Oral
- Give with food at the same time each day.

## ADVERSE EFFECTS (≥ 2%) **Cardiac:** Hypertension. **CNS:** Headache. **Endocrine and Metabolic:** Hypokalemia. **Urinary:** UTI, hematuria. **GI:** Nausea, constipation, diarrhea. **Hematologic:** Hemorrhage. **Respiratory:** Epistaxis.

## INTERACTIONS **Drug:** Decrease dose by 50% for patients on P-GLYCOPROTEIN INHIBITORS (e.g., **amiodarone, azithromycin, clarithromycin, ketoconazole, verapamil**).

## PHARMACOKINETICS **Absorption:** 34% bioavailability. **Onset:** Peak effect in 3–4 h. **Metabolism:** Minimal via CYP-independent hydrolysis. **Elimination:** 85% in feces, 11% in urine. **Half-Life:** 19–27 h.

## NURSING IMPLICATIONS

### Black Box Warning

*Betrixaban may be associated with epidural or spinal hematomas in those receiving neuraxial anesthesia or undergoing spinal puncture.*

### Assessment & Drug Effects
- Monitor for and report S&S of bleeding.
- Routine monitoring of coagulation tests is not required; anti-FXa assay may be helpful in guiding clinical decisions.

### Patient & Family Education
- Notify provider if you use this drug before you have a spinal or epidural procedure.
- Notify prescriber if you experience signs or symptoms of allergic reaction such as rash, hives, itching, shortness of breath, wheezing, cough, swelling of the face, lips, tongue, or throat; or any other signs.
- Notify prescriber immediately if you have signs of bleeding such as throwing up blood or coffeeground appearing vomit; coughing up blood; blood in the urine; black, red, or tarry stools; bleeding from the gums; vaginal bleeding that is not normal; bruises without a reason or that get bigger; or any bleeding that is very bad or can't be stopped.
- You may bleed more easily. Be careful and avoid injury. Use a soft toothbrush and and elecric razor.

## BEVACIZUMAB
(be-va-ci-zu′mab)
*Avastin*

**Classifications:** ANTINEOPLASTIC; BIOLOGICAL RESPONSE MODIFIER; MONOCLONAL ANTIBODY
**Therapeutic:** ANTINEOPLASTIC

## AVAILABILITY Injection

## ACTION & *THERAPEUTIC EFFECT*
Binds to vascular endothelial growth factor (VEGF) and prevents the interaction of VEGF with its receptors on the surface of endothelial cells. This blocks endothelial cell proliferation and new blood vessel formation in tumor cells. *Believed to cause reduction of microvascularization in the tumor inhibiting the progression of metastatic disease.*

## USES Metastatic colorectal cancer, non–small-cell lung cancer, malignant

Common adverse effects in *italic*; life-threatening effects underlined; generic names in **bold**; classifications in SMALL CAPS; ♣ Canadian drug name; ⊕ Prototype drug

glioblastoma, metastic renal cell carcinoma.

**UNLABELED USES** Age-related macular degeneration.

**CONTRAINDICATIONS** Nephrotic syndrome; hemorrhage; recent hemoptysis; GI perforation; nephritic syndrome; leucopenia; surgery within 28 days; dental work within 20 days; necrotizing fasciitis; severe arterial thromboembolic event due to drug; hypertensive crisis; pulmonary embolism; posterior reversible encephalopathy syndrome (PRES); nephrotic syndrome due to drug; lactation.

**CAUTIOUS USE** Hypersensitivity to bevacizumab; renal insufficiency; hypertension, history of arterial thromboembolic, cardiovascular, or cerebrovascular disease; CHF; history of GI bleeding, older adults; pregnancy (category C). Safety and efficacy in children and infants not established.

## ROUTE & DOSAGE

**Metastatic Colorectal Cancer**
*Adult:* **IV** 5–10 mg/kg q14days until disease progression; in conjunction with other chemotherapy

**Non–Small-Cell Lung Cancer**
*Adult:* **IV** 15 mg/kg q3wk

**Glioblastoma/Metastatic Renal Cell Carcinoma**
*Adult:* **IV** 10 mg/kg q14days in 28-day cycle

## ADMINISTRATION

**Intravenous**

*PREPARE:* **IV Infusion:** Withdraw the desired dose of 5 mg/kg and

dilute in 100 mL of NS injection.
- Do not shake and do **not** mix or administer with dextrose solutions. Discard any unused portion.
*ADMINISTER:* **IV Infusion: Do not** administer IV push or bolus.
- Infuse first dose over 90 min; if well tolerated, infuse second dose over 60 min; if well tolerated, infuse all subsequent doses over 30 min.
*INCOMPATIBILITIES:* **Solution/additive: Dextrose**-containing solutions. **Y-site: Dextrose**-containing solutions.

- Store diluted solution at 2°–8° C (36°–46° F) for up to 8 h. Store vials at 2°–8° C (36°–46° F); do not freeze and protect from light.

**ADVERSE EFFECTS** (≥1%) **Body as a Whole:** *Asthenia,* pain, wound dehiscence, tracheoesophageal (TE) fistula formation. **CNS:** Syncope, *headache,* anxiety, dizziness, confusion, abnormal gait, leukoencephalopathy. **CV:** DVT, *hypertension,* heart failure, hypotension, intra-abdominal thrombosis, cerebrovascular events. **GI:** *Abdominal pain, diarrhea,* constipation, nausea, vomiting, anorexia, stomatitis, dyspepsia, weight loss, flatulence, dry mouth, colitis, gastrointestinal perforation. **Hematologic:** Leukopenia, *neutropenia,* thrombocytopenia, hemorrhage, *thromboembolism.* **Metabolic:** Hypokalemia, hyperbilirubinemia, hyperglycemia, hypoalbuminemia, hypomagnesemia, ovarian failure, weight loss. **Musculoskeletal:** Myalgia. **Respiratory:** Upper respiratory infection, epistaxis, dyspnea, hemoptysis. **Skin:** Exfoliative dermatitis, alopecia. **Special Senses:** Taste disorder, increased tearing. **Urogenital:** *Proteinuria,* urinary frequency/urgency.

Common adverse effects in *italic;* life-threatening effects underlined; generic names in **bold;** classifications in SMALL CAPS; ♣ Canadian drug name; ☺ Prototype drug

187

**PHARMACOKINETICS  Half-Life:** 20 days (11–50 days).

## NURSING IMPLICATIONS

### Black Box Warning

*Bevacizumab has been associated with increased risk of potentially fatal GI perforation, wound healing complications, and hemorrhage.*

### Assessment & Drug Effects

- Monitor for S&S of an infusion reaction (hypersensitivity); infusion should be interrupted in all patients with severe infusion reactions and appropriate therapy instituted.
- Withhold drug and promptly notify prescriber for S&S of CHF, hemorrhage (e.g., epistaxis, hemoptysis, or GI bleeding), or unexplained abdominal pain.
- Monitor BP at least every 2–3 wk; if hypertension develops, monitor more frequently, even after discontinuation of bevacizumab.
- Monitor for dizziness, lightheadedness, or loss of balance. Take appropriate safety measures.
- Monitor lab tests: Urinalysis for proteinuria and 24 h urine if protein 2+ or greater.

### Patient & Family Education

- Report any of the following to the prescriber: Bloody or black, tarry stool; changes in patterns of urination; swelling of legs or ankles; increased shortness of breath; severe abdominal pain; change in mental awareness, inability to talk or move one side of the body.

## BEXAROTENE
(bex-a-ro'teen)

Targretin

**Classifications:** RETINOID; ANTINEOPLASTIC
**Therapeutic:** ANTINEOPLASTIC
**Prototype:** Isotretinoin

**AVAILABILITY** Capsule; gel

**ACTION & *THERAPEUTIC EFFECT***
Selectively binds to retinoid X receptors (RXR). Activation of the RXR pathway leads to cell death by interfering with cellular differentiation and proliferation of cells. *Inhibits the growth of tumor cells of squamous (skin) cell origin inducing tumor regression.*

**USES** Treatment of cutaneous manifestations of cutaneous T-cell lymphoma, mycosis fungoides.

**CONTRAINDICATIONS** Hypersensitivity to bexarotene; pregnancy (category X); lactation.

**CAUTIOUS USE** Hypersensitivity to retinoid agents; CAD; DM; alcoholism, history of pancreatitis, hepatitis; lipid abnormalities; hepatic impairment; thyroid disease; women of childbearing age. Safety and efficacy in children not established.

**ROUTE & DOSAGE**

### T-Cell Lymphoma

*Adult:* **PO** 300 mg/m²/day as a single dose if no response after 8 wk, may increase to 400 mg/m²/day. Adjust dose downward in 100 mg/m²/day increments if toxicity occurs. **Topical** Apply once every other day × 1 wk increase frequency at weekly intervals to once/day, b.i.d., t.i.d., and q.i.d.

## ADMINISTRATION

### Oral

- Give drug with or immediately following a meal. Ensure that capsules are swallowed whole.
- Do not initiate therapy in a woman of childbearing age until the possibility of pregnancy has been completely ruled out.

### Topical

- Apply a generous coating only to skin lesions; avoid normal skin.
- Do not cover with clothing until gel dries.
- Store capsules and gel at 20°–25° C (36°–77° F). Protect from light and avoid high temperatures and humidity after bottle or tube is opened.

### ADVERSE EFFECTS (≥1%) Body as a Whole: *Headache, asthenia, infection,* chills, fever, flu-like syndrome, back pain, bacterial infection. CNS: Insomnia, depression, agitation. CV: *Peripheral edema,* hypertension, angina, syncope. GI: *Abdominal pain, nausea,* diarrhea, vomiting, anorexia. Endocrine: *Hyperthyroidism.* Hematologic: Leukopenia, anemia, hypochromic anemia. Metabolic: *Hyperlipidemia, hypercholesterolemia,* increased LDH. Skin: *Rash, dry skin,* exfoliative dermatitis, alopecia, photosensitivity.

### PHARMACOKINETICS Absorption: Best with a fat-containing meal. Peak: 2 h. Distribution: Greater than 99% protein bound. Metabolism: Metabolized by CYP3A4. Elimination: Primarily in bile. Half-Life: 7 h.

## NURSING IMPLICATIONS

### Black Box Warning

*The oral form of bexarotene has been associated with serious birth defects.*

### Assessment & Drug Effects

- Monitor (with oral dose) for S&S of: Hypothyroidism, hypertriglyceridemia, hypercholesterolemia, and pancreatitis.
- Lab tests (with oral dose): Baseline blood lipids, then weekly for 2–4 wk, and every 8 wk thereafter; baseline LFTs then repeat at 1, 2, 4 wk, and every 8 wk thereafter; baseline WBC and thyroid function tests, then repeat periodically thereafter; periodic serum calcium; for females, pregnancy test monthly throughout therapy.
- Withhold oral drug and notify prescriber if triglycerides greater than 400 mg/dL or AST, ALT, or bilirubin greater than 3 × upper limit of normal.

### Patient & Family Education

- Use effective methods of contraception (both men and women) while taking/using this drug and for at least 1 mo after the last dose of the drug.
- Do not take this drug if you are or could be pregnant.
- Report immediately any of the following: Swelling in the face, lips, or wheezing; persistent bloating, constipation, diarrhea, vomiting, or stomach pain; persistent headache, severe drowsiness or weakness.
- Report changes in vision to the prescriber. An ophthalmologic evaluation may be needed.
- Limit exposure to sunlight or sun lamps and wear sunscreen.
- Report significant skin irritation.

## BEZLOTOXUMAB
(bez-loe-tox′ue-mab)
Zinplava
**Classifications:** ANTITOXIN; MONOCLONAL ANTIBODY
**Therapeutic:** ANTITOXIN

Common adverse effects in *italic;* life-threatening effects underlined; generic names in **bold;** classifications in SMALL CAPS; ◆ Canadian drug name; ⊘ Prototype drug

189

**AVAILABILITY** Solution for injection

**ACTION & *THERAPEUTIC EFFECT***
A human monoclonal antibody
that binds to *Clostridium difficile*
toxin B and neutralizes it. *Bezlo-
toxumab binds to a specific epitope
on toxin B that is conserved across
reported strains of Clostridium difficile. It does not have antibacterial
activity nor does it bind to Clostridium difficile toxin A.*

**USES** In combination with antibacterial therapy to reduce the
recurrence of *Clostridium difficile*
infection in patients 18 y or older
who are at high risk for recurrence.

**CAUTIOUS USE** Heart failure,
pregnancy, lactation.

**ROUTE & DOSAGE**

**Clostridium Difficile**
*Adult:* **IV** 10 mg/kg single dose
over 60 min

**ADMINISTRATION**

**Intravenous**

***PREPARE:*** **IV Infusion:** Do not
shake the vial. Withdraw the required volume from the vial and
transfer into an intravenous bag
of either 0.9% sodium chloride or
5% dextrose to prepare a diluted
solution with a final concentration of 1–10 mg/mL. Mix the
diluted solution by gentle inversion; do not shake.
***ADMINISTER:*** **IV Infusion:** Infuse
over 60 min using a sterile, non-
pyrogenic, low-protein binding
0.2–0.5 micron in-line or add-on
filter.

▪ Do not administer IV push.
▪ Store at room temperature for
16 h or under refrigeration for up

to 24 h. If refrigerated, allow solution to come to room temperature
before administering.

**ADVERSE EFFECTS** (>1%) **Body
as a Whole:** Fatigue, *infusion related reactions*, pyrexia. **CNS:** Dizziness, headache. **CV:** Heart failure,
hypertension. **GI:** Nausea. **Respiratory:** Dyspnea.

**INTERACTIONS** Due to metabolic
catabolism, none are expected.

**PHARMACOKINETICS Metabo-
lism:** Metabolic catabolism. **Half-
Life:** 19 days.

**NURSING IMPLICATIONS**

**Assessment & Drug Effects**
▪ Monitor for signs or symptoms of
an infusion-related reaction.
▪ Monitor for elevated BP or signs
or symptoms of heart failure.

**Patient & Family Education**
▪ This medication is used to lower
the chance of a bacterial infection
called *Clostridium difficile (C diff)*
from coming back.
▪ Notify health care provider if you
are breast-feeding or if you are
pregnant or planning to become
pregnant.

**BICALUTAMIDE**
(bi-ca-lu′ta-mide)
Casodex
**Classifications:** ANTINEOPLASTIC;
HORMONE
Therapeutic: ANTINEOPLASTIC;
NON-STEROIDAL ANTIANDROGEN
**Prototype:** Flutamide

**AVAILABILITY** Tablet

**ACTION & *THERAPEUTIC EFFECT***
Inhibits the pharmacologic effects
of androgen by binding to androgen

receptors in target tissue. *Prostatic carcinoma is androgen sensitive; it responds to removal of the source of androgen or treatment that counteracts the effects of androgen.*

**USES** In combination with a luteinizing hormone-releasing hormone (LHRH) analog for advanced prostate cancer.

**UNLABELED USES** Prevention of recurrent priapism.

**CONTRAINDICATIONS** Hypersensitivity to bicalutamide, pregnancy (category X), hepatic failure; lactation.

**CAUTIOUS USE** Moderate to severe hepatic impairment; glucose intolerance; diabetes mellitus. Safety and efficacy in children not established.

## ROUTE & DOSAGE

**Advanced Prostate Cancer**
*Adult:* PO 50 mg once/day

## ADMINISTRATION

**Oral**
- Give drug at the same time each day.
- Start treatment with bicalutamide at the same time as treatment with a luteinizing hormone-releasing hormone (LHRH) analog.
- Store at 15°–30° C (59°–86° F).

## ADVERSE EFFECTS (≥1%) CNS:
Dizziness, paresthesia, insomnia, anxiety, decreased libido, confusion, neuropathy, somnolence, nervousness, headache. **CV:** *Hot flashes,* hypertension, chest pain, CHF. **GI:** *Constipation, nausea, diarrhea,* vomiting, increased liver function tests, abdominal pain, anorexia, dyspepsia, dry mouth, melena. **Urogenital:** Nocturia, hematuria, UTI,

impotence, gynecomastia, incontinence, frequency, dysuria, urinary retention, urgency. **Metabolic:** Peripheral edema, hyperglycemia, weight loss, weight gain, gout. **Musculoskeletal:** Myasthenia, arthritis, myalgia, leg cramps, pathologic fractures. **Skin:** Rash, sweating, dry skin, pruritus, alopecia. **Body as a Whole:** Flu syndrome, bone pain, infection, anemia.

**INTERACTIONS Drug:** May increase effects of ORAL ANTICOAGULANTS. Bicalutamide concentrations may be increased by PROTEASE INHIBITORS, **fluoxetine, fluvoxamine, erythromycin** and other CYP3A4 inhibitors. Efficacy of bicalutamide may be decreased by **bosentan, carbamazapine,** BARBITURATES, and other CYP3A4 inducers.

**PHARMACOKINETICS Absorption:** Readily from GI tract. **Metabolism:** In liver. **Elimination:** In urine and feces. **Half-Life:** 5.8 days.

## NURSING IMPLICATIONS

**Assessment & Drug Effects**
- Monitor for S&S of disease progression.
- Monitor lab tests: Baseline LFTs, then regularly during first 4 mo of treatment and periodically thereafter; periodic PSA; with concurrent warfarin therapy, frequent PT and INR.

**Patient & Family Education**
- Report jaundice or any other troubling adverse effects immediately.

## BIMATOPROST
(bi-mat'o-prost)
**Lumigan**
**See Appendix A-1.**

---

Common adverse effects in *italic;* life-threatening effects <u>underlined</u>; generic names in **bold;** classifications in SMALL CAPS; ◆ Canadian drug name; ⊕ Prototype drug

191

B

# BISACODYL ⊕
(bis-a-koe'dill)

Apo-Bisacodyl ✦, Bisacolax, BiscoLax ✦, Dacodyl, Deficol, Doxidan, Dulcolax, Fleet Bisacodyl, Laxit ✦, Theralax

**Classification:** STIMULANT LAXATIVE
Therapeutic: LAXATIVE

**AVAILABILITY** Tablet, enteric coated; delayed release tablet; suppository; enema

**ACTION & *THERAPEUTIC EFFECT***
Expands intestinal fluid volume by increasing epithelial permeability. *Induces peristaltic contractions by direct stimulation of sensory nerve endings in the colonic wall.*

**USES** Temporary relief of acute constipation and for evacuation of colon before GI procedures.

**CONTRAINDICATIONS** Acute surgical abdomen, nausea, vomiting, abdominal cramps, intestinal obstruction, fecal impaction; use of rectal suppository in presence of anal or rectal fissures, ulcerated hemorrhoids, proctitis, bowel obstruction or perforation, ileus.

**CAUTIOUS USE** Pregnancy (category C); lactation.

## ROUTE & DOSAGE

**Laxative**

*Adult:* **PO** 5–15 mg prn (max: 30 mg for special procedures); **PR** 10 mg prn
*Child (6 y or older):* **PO** 5–10 mg prn; *2 y or older:* **PR** 10 mg; *younger than 2 y:* **PR** 5 mg

## ADMINISTRATION
### Oral
- Give in the evening or before breakfast because of action time required.
- Ensure that enteric-coated tablets are swallowed whole; they should not be crushed or chewed. Do not give within 1 h of antacids or milk.
- Store tablets in tightly closed containers at temperatures not exceeding 30° C (86° F).

### Rectal
- Suppository may be inserted at the time bowel movement is desired.
- Storage is same as tablets.

**ADVERSE EFFECTS** (≥1%) Systemic effects not reported. Mild cramping, nausea, diarrhea, fluid and electrolyte disturbances (especially potassium and calcium).

**INTERACTIONS Drug:** ANTACIDS will cause early dissolution of enteric-coated tablets, resulting in abdominal cramping.

**PHARMACOKINETICS Absorption:** 5–15% from GI tract. **Onset:** 6–8 h PO; 15–60 min PR. **Metabolism:** In liver. **Elimination:** In urine, bile, and breast milk.

## NURSING IMPLICATIONS
### Assessment & Drug Effects
- Evaluate periodically patient's need for continued use of drug; bisacodyl usually produces 1 or 2 soft-formed stools daily.
- Monitor patients receiving concomitant anticoagulants. Indiscriminate use of laxatives results in decreased absorption of vitamin K.

### Patient & Family Education
- Add high-fiber foods slowly to regular diet to avoid gas and

diarrhea. Adequate fluid intake includes at least 6–8 glasses/day.

# BISMUTH SUBSALICYLATE ⊕
(bis'muth)

Pepto-Bismol

**Classifications:** ANTIDIARRHEAL; SALICYLATE

Therapeutic: ANTIDIARRHEAL

**AVAILABILITY** Tablet/capsule; liquid

## ACTION & *THERAPEUTIC EFFECT*

Hydrolyzed in GI tract to salicylate, which is believed to inhibit synthesis of prostaglandins responsible for GI hypermotility and inflammation. *It acts as a direct mucosal protective agent. Efficacy as an antidiarrheal appears to be due to direct antimicrobial action and to an antisecretory effect on intestinal secretions exposed to toxins.*

**USES** Prophylaxis and treatment of traveler's diarrhea (turista) and for temporary relief of indigestion.

**UNLABELED USES** *Helicobacter pylori* associated with peptic ulcer disease.

**CONTRAINDICATIONS** Hypersensitivity to aspirin or other salicylates; coagulopathy; severe hepatic impairment; use for more than 2 days in presence of high fever or in children younger than 3 y unless prescribed by prescriber; chickenpox or flu; dysentery.

**CAUTIOUS USE** Diabetes and gout; alcoholism; renal impairment; older adults; smoking; pregnancy (category C); lactation.

## ROUTE & DOSAGE

### Diarrhea

*Adult:* **PO** 30 mL or 2 tab q30–60min prn (max: 8 doses/day)
*Child (3 to less than 6 y):* **PO** 5 mL or 1/2 tab q30–60min prn (max: 8 doses/day); *6 y to less than 9 y:* 2/3 tab or 10 mL q30–60min prn (max: 8 doses/day); *9–12 y:* 15 mL or 1 tab q30–60min prn (max: 8 doses/day)

### Traveler's Diarrhea

*Adult:* **PO** 2–4 tab or 15–30 mL q.i.d. for 3 wk

### Peptic Ulcer Disease

*Adult:* **PO** 2 tablets q.i.d. with 2 additional antibiotics for 10–14 days
*Child (younger than 10 y):* **PO** 15 mL q.i.d. × 6 wk

## ADMINISTRATION

### Oral

- Ensure chewable tablets are chewed or crushed before being swallowed and followed with at least 8 oz water or other liquid.
- Store at 15°–30° C (59°–86° F) unless otherwise directed.

**ADVERSE EFFECTS** (≥1%) **GI:** Temporary *darkening of stool* and tongue, metallic taste, bluish gum line; bleeding tendencies. With high doses: Fecal impaction. **CNS:** Encephalopathy (disorientation, muscle twitching). **Hematologic:** Bleeding tendency. **Special Senses:** Tinnitus, hearing loss.

**DIAGNOSTIC TEST INTERFERENCE** Because bismuth subsalicylate is radiopaque, it may interfere with *radiographic studies* of GI tract.

---

Common adverse effects in *italic*; life-threatening effects underlined; generic names in **bold**; classifications in SMALL CAPS; ♣ Canadian drug name; ⊕ Prototype drug

193

**INTERACTIONS Drug:** Bismuth may decrease the absorption of TETRACYCLINES, QUINOLONES (**ciprofloxacin, norfloxacin, ofloxacin**). May increase level of **aspirin.**

**PHARMACOKINETICS Absorption:** Undergoes chemical dissociation in GI tract to bismuth subcarbonate and sodium salicylate; bismuth is minimally absorbed, but the salicylate is readily absorbed.

## NURSING IMPLICATIONS

### Assessment & Drug Effects

- Monitor bowel function; note that stools may darken and tongue may appear black. These are temporary effects and will disappear without treatment.
- Monitor lab tests: *H. pylori* breath test when used for peptic ulcers.

### Patient & Family Education

- Note: Bismuth contains salicylate. Use caution when taking aspirin and other salicylates. Many OTC medications for colds, fever, and pain contain salicylates.
- Consult prescriber if diarrhea is accompanied by fever or continues for more than 2 days.
- Note: Temporary grayish black discoloration of tongue and stool may occur.

## BISOPROLOL FUMARATE

(bis-o-pro'lol fum'a-rate)

Zebeta

**Classifications:** BETA-ADRENERGIC ANTAGONIST; ANTIHYPERTENSIVE
**Therapeutic:** ANTIHYPERTENSIVE
**Prototype:** Propranolol

## AVAILABILITY Tablet

## ACTION & *THERAPEUTIC EFFECT*

Long-acting cardioselective (beta-$_1$) adrenoreceptor blocking agent that decreases HR, BP, contractile force, and cardiac workload, thus reducing myocardial oxygen consumption and increasing blood flow to the myocardium. *Bisoprolol has antianginal properties, especially improving exercise tolerance. It reduces both systolic and diastolic blood pressure at rest and with exercise.*

**USES** Hypertension.

**UNLABELED USES** Angina, heart failure, atrial flutter.

**CONTRAINDICATIONS** History of hypersensitivity to bisoprolol, severe sinus bradycardia, second- and third-degree AV block, overt cardiac failure, cardiogenic shock; pulmonary edema; lactation.

**CAUTIOUS USE** Asthma or COPD bronchospastic disease; PVD; DM; Prinzmetal's angina; hyperthyroidism; renal or hepatic insufficiency, CVA; stroke; pregnancy (category C); lactation. Safety and efficacy in children not established.

## ROUTE & DOSAGE

### Hypertension

*Adult:* **PO** 5 mg once daily, may increase to 20 mg/day if necessary

### Hepatic Impairment Dosage Adjustment
Start with 2.5 mg daily

### Renal Impairment Dosage Adjustment
*CrCl less than 40 mL/min:* Start with 2.5 mg daily

## ADMINISTRATION

### Oral

- Note: The half-life of the drug is increased in those with significant liver dysfunction; usual initial dose is 2.5 mg and may be carefully titrated upward if necessary.

▪ Discontinue drug gradually over a period of 1–2 wk to avoid rebound, withdrawal angina, or hypertension.

▪ Store at room temperature, 15°–30° C (59°–86° F).

## ADVERSE EFFECTS (≥1%) CNS:
Dizziness, fatigue, vertigo, anxiety, headache, sleep disturbances. CV: Bradycardia, ortho-static hypotension, rebound/withdrawal angina or hypertension following abrupt discontinuation, may exacerbate intermittent claudication. Endocrine: Increases serum levels of VLDL-C and decreases levels of HDL-C lipoproteins, may cause slight rise in serum potassium. GI: Abdominal pain, dyspepsia, nausea, vomiting, constipation, diarrhea. Respiratory: Asthma, bronchospasm, cough, dyspnea, pharyngitis, sinusitis. Skin: Rash, acne, pruritus, eczema. Other: Arthralgia.

## INTERACTIONS Drug: Amiodarone
may cause significant bradycardia; BETA-BLOCKERS may reduce glucose tolerance, inhibit insulin secretion, alter rate of recovery from hypoglycemia, reduce peripheral circulation, and suppress hypoglycemic symptoms; rifampin decreases bisoprolol blood levels.

## PHARMACOKINETICS Absorption:
Readily from GI tract; 82–94% reaches systemic circulation. Peak: Therapeutic effect 2–4 wk. Duration: 24 h. Distribution: Some CNS penetration. Metabolism: 50% in liver by CYP3A4. Elimination: 50–60% unchanged in urine. Half-Life: 10–12.4 h.

## NURSING IMPLICATIONS
### Assessment & Drug Effects
▪ Monitor BP frequently during periods of dose adjustment or drug withdrawal. Monitor postural vital signs for orthostatic hypotension.

▪ Monitor for activity-induced angina both during therapy and following discontinuation of drug.

▪ Monitor for and report severe hypotension and bradycardia. Dosage adjustment may be required.

▪ Monitor for bronchospasms in patients with a history of asthma or COPD.

▪ Monitor diabetics for loss of glycemic control.

▪ Monitor lab tests: Periodic CBC, electrolytes, renal function, LFTs lipid profile.

### Patient & Family Education
▪ Report orthostatic hypotension and dizziness to prescriber.

▪ Do not discontinue drug abruptly unless specifically instructed to do so.

▪ Note: Drug-induced nightmares and unpleasant dreams are possible when taking this drug.

▪ Monitor blood glucose for loss of glycemic control if diabetic.

## BIVALIRUDIN
(bi-val'i-ru-den)
Angiomax
Classifications: ANTICOAGULANT; DIRECT THROMBIN INHIBITOR
Therapeutic: ANTITHROMBOTIC
Prototype: Argatroban

## AVAILABILITY Vial

## ACTION & THERAPEUTIC EFFECT
Inhibits thrombin by specifically binding to (and thus inhibiting) cell

Common adverse effects in *italic;* life-threatening effects underlined; generic names in **bold;** classifications in SMALL CAPS; ♣ Canadian drug name; ⊕ Prototype drug

195

sites required to cleave fibrinogen into fibrin. *Reversibly binds to the thrombin active site, thereby blocking the thrombogenic activity of thrombin.*

**USES** Used with aspirin as an anticoagulant in patients undergoing PTCA or PCR, patients at risk for HIT undergoing PCI, heparin-induced thrombocytopenia.

**UNLABELED USES** DVT prevention, unstable angina/non-ST-evaluation myocardial infarction.

**CONTRAINDICATIONS** Hypersensitivity to bivalirudin; cerebral aneurysm, intracranial hemorrhage; patients with increased risk of bleeding (e.g., recent surgery, trauma, CVA, hepatic disease); coagulopathy; lactation.

**CAUTIOUS USE** Asthma or allergies; blood dyscrasia or thrombocytopenia; GI ulceration, serious hepatic disease; hypertension, renal impairment, pregnancy (category B). Safety and efficacy in children not established.

## ROUTE & DOSAGE

**Anticoagulation**

*Adult:* **IV** 0.75 mg/kg bolus (5 min after the bolus, ACT should be performed and 0.3 mg/kg given if needed) followed by 1.75 mg/kg/h for the duration of the procedure, may continue at 0.2 mg/kg/h up to 20 h if needed; intended for use with aspirin 300–325 mg

**Heparin Induced Thrombocytopenia**

*Adult:* **IV** 0.75 mg/kg bolus then 1.75 mg/kg/hr

**Renal Impairment Dosage Adjustment**

*CrCl less than 30 mL/min:* Give maintenance dose of 1 mg/kg/h

**Hemodialysis Dosage Adjustment**

Give 0.25 mg/kg/h maintenance dose

## ADMINISTRATION
**Intravenous**

*PREPARE:* **Direct/Continuous:** Direct IV bolus dose and initial 4-h continuous infusion: Reconstitute each 250 mg vial with 5 mL of sterile water for injection; gently swirl until dissolved. ▪ Must further dilute each reconstituted vial in 50 mL of D5W or NS to yield 5 mg/mL. **Continuous:** Subsequent low-dose, continuous infusions: Reconstitute each 250 mg vial as above. ▪ Further dilute each reconstituted vial in 500 mL of D5W or NS to yield 0.50 mg/mL.

*ADMINISTER:* **Direct:** Give bolus dose over 3–5 sec. **Continuous:** Give 1.75 mg/kg/h for the duration of the PTCA procedure. ▪ Subsequent doses, give 0.2 mg/kg/h for up to 20 h as ordered.

*INCOMPATIBILITIES:* **Y-site:** **Alte-plase, amiodarone, ampho-tericin B, caspofungin, chlorpromazine, dantrolene, diazepam, dobutamine, lansoprazole, pentamidine, pentazocine, phenytoin, prochlorperazine, quinidine, quinupristine/dalfopristin, reteplase, streptokinase, vancomycin.**

▪ Store reconstituted vials refrigerated at 2°–8° C (35.6°–46.4° F) for up to 24 h. Store diluted concentrations between 0.5 mg/mL and 5 mg/mL at room temperature, 15°–30° C (59°–86° F), for up to 24 h.

**ADVERSE EFFECTS** (≥1%) **Body as a Whole:** *Back pain,* pain, fever.

Common adverse effects in *italic;* life-threatening effects <u>underlined;</u> generic names in **bold;** classifications in SMALL CAPS; ♣ Canadian drug name; ⊙ Prototype drug

**CV:** *Hypotension,* hypertension, bradycardia. **GI:** *Nausea,* vomiting, dyspepsia, abdominal pain. **Hematologic:** Bleeding. **CNS:** *Headache,* anxiety, nervousness. **Urogenital:** Urinary retention, pelvic pain. **Other:** Injection site pain.

**INTERACTIONS** ANTICOAGULANTS may increase risk of bleeding.

**PHARMACOKINETICS Duration:** 1 h. **Distribution:** No protein binding. **Metabolism:** Proteolytic cleavage and renal metabolism. **Elimination:** Renal. **Half-Life:** 25 min.

## NURSING IMPLICATIONS

### Assessment & Drug Effects

- Monitor cardiovascular status carefully during therapy.
- Monitor for and report S&S of bleeding: Ecchymosis, epistaxis, GI bleeding, hematuria, hemoptysis.
- Patients with history of GI ulceration, hypertension, recent trauma or surgery are at increased risk for bleeding.
- Monitor neurologic status and report immediately: Focal or generalized deficits.
- Monitor lab tests: Baseline and periodic ACT, aPTT, PT, platelet count, Hgb and Hct; periodic serum creatinine, stool for occult blood, urinalysis.

### Patient & Family Education

- Report any of the following immediately: Unexplained back or stomach pain; black, tarry stools; blood in urine, coughing up blood; difficulty breathing; dizziness or fainting spells; heavy menstrual bleeding; nosebleeds; unusual bruising or bleeding at any site.

## BLEOMYCIN SULFATE
(blee-oh-mye'sin)

**Classifications:** ANTINEOPLASTIC; ANTIBIOTIC
**Therapeutic:** ANTINEOPLASTIC
**Prototype:** Doxorubicin

**AVAILABILITY** Powder for injection

## ACTION & *THERAPEUTIC EFFECT*
By unclear mechanism, blocks DNA, RNA, and protein synthesis. A cell cycle-phase nonspecific agent widely used in combination with other chemotherapeutic agents because it lacks significant myelosuppressive activity. *This mixture of cytotoxic antibiotics from a strain of* Streptomyces *verticillus has strong affinity for skin and lung tumor cells, in contrast to its low affinity for cells in hematopoietic tissue.*

**USES** As single agent or in combination with other agents, as adjunct to surgery and radiation therapy. Squamous cell carcinomas of head, neck, penis, testicles, cervix, and vulva; lymphomas (including reticular cell sarcoma, lymphosarcoma, Hodgkin's); malignant pleural effusions.

**UNLABELED USES** *Mycosis fungoides* and *Verruca vulgaris* (common warts), AIDS-related Kaposi's sarcoma.

**CONTRAINDICATIONS** History of hypersensitivity or idiosyncrasy to bleomycin; pulmonary infection; concurrent radiation therapy; women of childbearing age, pregnancy (category D); lactation.

**CAUTIOUS USE** Compromised hepatic, renal, or pulmonary function; peripheral vascular disease; history of tobacco use; previous cytotoxic drug or radiation therapy.

Common adverse effects in *italic;* life-threatening effects underlined; generic names in **bold;** classifications in SMALL CAPS; ✦ Canadian drug name; ⊘ Prototype drug

197

## ROUTE & DOSAGE

### Squamous Cell Carcinoma, Testicular Carcinoma

*Adult/Child:* **Subcutaneous/IM/ IV** 10–20 units/m$^2$ or 0.25–0.5 units/kg 1–2 × wk (max: 300–400 units)

### Lymphomas

*Adult/Adolescent:* **Subcutaneous/IM/ IV** 10–20 units/m$^2$ 1–2 × wk after a 1–2 units test dose × 2 doses

### Malignant Pleural Effusion

*Adult:* **Intrapleural** 60 units single dose

### Cervical, Penile, Vuvlvar, Head-Neck Cancer

*Adult:* **IV/IM/Subcutaneous** 5–20 units/m$^2$ (0.25–0.5 units/kg)

### Renal Impairment Dosage Adjustment

*CrCl 40–50 mL/min:* Reduce dose 30%; *CrCl 30–39 mL/min:* Reduce dose 40%; *CrCl 20–29 mL/min:* Reduce dose 45%; *CrCl 10–19 mL/min:* Reduce dose 55%; *CrCl 5–10 mL/min:* Reduce dose 60%

## ADMINISTRATION

Note: Due to risk of anaphylactoid reaction, give lymphoma patients 2 units or less for first two doses. If no reaction, follow regular dosage schedule.

### Subcutaneous/Intramuscular

- Reconstitute with sterile water, NS, or bacteriostatic water by adding 1–5 mL to the 15 units vial or 2–10 mL to the 30 units vial. Amount of diluent is determined by the total volume of solution that will be injected.

- Inject IM deeply into upper outer quadrant of buttock; change sites with each injection.

### Intravenous

IV administration to infants and children: Verify correct IV concentration and rate of infusion with prescriber.

*PREPARE:* **Intermittent:** Dilute each 15 units with at least 5 mL of sterile water or NS. ▪ May be further diluted in 50–100 mL of the chosen diluent. ▪ Do not dilute with any solution containing D5W.

*ADMINISTER:* **Intermittent:** Give each 15 units or fraction thereof over 10 min through Y-tube of free-flowing IV.

*INCOMPATIBILITIES:* **Solution/additive: Aminophylline, ascorbic acid, cefazolin, diazepam, hydrocortisone, methotrexate, mitomycin, nafcillin, penicillin G, terbutaline Y-site: amphotericin B, dantrolene, diazepam, phenytoin, tigecycline.**

- Store unopened ampules at 15°–30° C (59°–86° F) unless otherwise specified by manufacturer.

## ADVERSE EFFECTS (≥1%) **Body as a Whole:** Hypersensitivity (anaphylactoid reaction); *mild febrile reaction.* **CNS:** Headache, mental confusion. **GI:** Stomatitis, ulcerations of tongue and lips, anorexia, nausea, vomiting, diarrhea, weight loss. **Hematologic:** Thrombocytopenia, leukopenia, (rare). **Respiratory:** Pulmonary toxicity (dose and age-related); interstitial pneumonitis, pneumonia, or fibrosis. **Skin:** Diffuse alopecia (reversible), *hyperpigmentation, pruritic erythema,* vesiculation, acne, thickening of skin and nail beds, *patchy hyperkeratosis,* striae, peeling, bleeding. **Other:** Pain at tumor site; phlebitis; necrosis at injection site, shivering.

Common adverse effects in *italic;* life-threatening effects underlined; generic names in **bold;** classifications in SMALL CAPS; ♣ Canadian drug name; ⦿ Prototype drug

**INTERACTIONS Drug:** Other ANTI-NEOPLASTIC AGENTS increase bone marrow toxicity; decreases effects of **digoxin, phenytoin,** avoid use with LIVE VACCINES.

**PHARMACOKINETICS Distribution:** Concentrates mainly in skin, lungs, kidneys, lymphocytes, and peritoneum. **Metabolism:** Unknown. **Elimination:** 60–70% recovered in urine as parent compound. **Half-Life:** 2 h.

## NURSING IMPLICATIONS

### Black Box Warning

*Bleomycin has been associated with severe hypersensitivity reactions and severe pulmonary, renal, and hepatic toxicity.*

### Assessment & Drug Effects

- Monitor closely for an acute reaction (hypotension, hyperpyrexia, chills, confusion, wheezing, cardiopulmonary collapse). Anaphylactoid reaction can be fatal (see Appendix F). It may occur immediately or several hours after first or second dose, especially in lymphoma patients.
- Monitor temperature. Febrile reaction (mild chills and fever) is relatively common and usually occurs within the first few hours after administration of a large single dose and lasts about 4–12 h. Reaction tends to become less frequent with continued drug administration, but can recur at any time.
- Monitor respiratory status and report promptly any of the following: SOB, cough, fatigue, loss of appetite, and weight loss.
- Monitor for and report any of the following: Unexplained bleeding or bruising; evidence of deterioration of renal function (changed

I&O ratio and pattern, decreasing creatinine clearance, weight gain or edema); evidence of pulmonary toxicity (nonproductive cough, chest pain, dyspnea).
- Check weight at regular intervals under standard conditions. Weight loss and anorexia may persist a long time after therapy has been discontinued.
- Report promptly symptoms of skin toxicity (hypoesthesia, urticaria, tender swollen hands) that may develop in second or third week of treatment and after 150–200 units of bleomycin have been administered. Therapy may be discontinued.

### Patient & Family Education

- Avoid OTC drugs during antineoplastic treatment period unless approved by prescriber.
- Report skin irritation which may not develop for several weeks after therapy begins.
- Hyperpigmentation may occur in areas subject to friction and pressure, skin folds, nail cuticles, scars, and intramuscular sites.

## BLINATUMOMAB

(bli-na-tu′mo-mab)

Blincyto

**Classifications:** ANTINEOPLASTIC; IMMUNOMODULATOR; MONOCLONAL ANTIBODY

**Therapeutic:** ANTINEOPLASTIC

**Prototype:** Basiliximab

**AVAILABILITY** Lyophilized powder for reconstitution and injection

### ACTION & THERAPEUTIC EFFECT

Binds to CD19 on B-cells and CD3 on T-cells. It activates T cells by connecting CD3 on the T-cell with CD19 on B-cells (malignant and benign), thus forming a connection between a

Common adverse effects in *italic;* life-threatening effects underlined; generic names in **bold;** classifications in SMALL CAPS; ♣ Canadian drug name; ⊙ Prototype drug

199

cytotoxic T-cell and the cancer target B-cell. It mediates the production of cytolytic proteins, release of inflammatory cytokines, and proliferation of T cells, which result in lysis of CD19-positive cancer cells.

**USES** Treatment of Philadelphia chromosome-negative relapsed or refractory B-cell precursor acute lymphoblastic leukemia (ALL).

**CONTRAINDICATIONS** Known hypersensitivity to blinatumomab; cytokine release syndrome (CRS); tumor lysis syndrome; lactation.

**CAUTIOUS USE** History of hypersensitivity reactions; infection; increased AST, ALT, and GGT; increased bilirubin; neurologic toxicity; neutropenia and febrile neutropenia; pregnancy (category C).

## ROUTE & DOSAGE

### Acute Lymphocytic Leukemia (ALL)

*Adult (45 kg or greater):* **IV** Cycle 1: 9 mcg/day on days 1–7 and 28 mcg/day on days 8–28; cycles 2–5: 28 mcg/day on days 1–28

### Dosing Adjustments Based on Toxicities

*Cytokine Release Syndrome (CRS)*

*Grade 3:* Withhold until resolved, then restart at 9 mcg/day, and increase to 28 mcg/day after 7 days if the toxicity does not recur
*Grade 4:* Discontinue permanently

*Neurological Toxicity*

*Grade 3:* Withhold until Grade 1 or less for at least 3 days, then restart at 9 mcg/day, and increase to 28 mcg/day after 7 days; if toxicity reoccurs at 9 mcg/day, or does not resolve in 7 days, discontinue permanently

*Grade 4 or if more than one seizure occurs:* Discontinue permanently

*Other Clinically Relevant Adverse Reactions*

*Grade 3:* Withhold until toxicity level is Grade 1 or less, then restart at 9 mcg/day, and increase to 28 mcg/day after 7 days if the toxicity does not recur. If toxicity does not resolve in 14 days, discontinue permanently
*Grade 4:* Consider discontinuing permanently

## ADMINISTRATION

- This drug is a cytotoxic agent and caution should be used to prevent any contact with the drug. Follow institutional or standard guidelines for preparation, handling, and disposal of cytotoxic agents.
- Premedicate with dexamethasone 20 mg IV 1 h before first dose of each cycle, prior to a step dose (such as cycle 1 day 8), or when restarting infusion after interruption of 4 or more h.

**Intravenous**

*PREPARE:* **IV Continuous:** Preparation must be done in a pharmacy in a laminar flow hood.

*ADMINISTER:* **IV Continuous:** Infuse through a dedicated line with a non-pyrogenic, low protein-binding, 0.2 micron in-line filter at a rate of 10 mL/h for 24 h or 5 mL/h for 48 h. Prime the IV line only with the prepared solution for infusion. Do not prime with NS. Use programmable, lockable, non-elastomeric infusion pump with an alarm to give at a constant flow rate. **Important Note:** Do not flush the infusion line, especially when changing infusion bags. Flushing when changing bags or at completion of infusion can result in excess dosage.

- Store: Solutions for infusion are stable for up to 48 h at 23°–27° C (73°–81° F) or up to 8 days at 2°–8° C (36°–46° F).

**ADVERSE EFFECTS** (>1%) **Body as a Whole:** Chest pain, *chills,* confusion, cytokine release syndrome, disorientation, edema, *fatigue, pathogenic infections, peripheral edema, pyrexia.* **CNS:** Aphasia, cognitive disorder, convulsion, dizziness, encephalopathy, *headache, insomnia,* memory impairment, paresthesia, *tremor.* **CV:** Alterations in blood pressure, tachycardia. **GI:** Abdominal pain, *constipation, diarrhea, nausea,* vomiting. **Hematological:** *Anemia, febrile neutropenia,* leukocytosis, leukopenia, lymphopenia, *neutropenia,* sepsis, thrombocytopenia. **Metabolic:** Decreased appetite, decreased immunoglobulins, hyperglycemia, hypoalbuminemia, *hypokalemia,* hypomagnesemia, *hypophosphatemia,* increased ALT/AST, increased blood bilirubin, increased gamma-glutamyltransferase, increased weight, tumor lysis syndrome. **Musculoskeletal:** Arthralgia, back pain, bone pain, pain in extremity. **Respiratory:** *Cough, dyspnea,* pneumonia. **Skin:** Rash.

**PHARMACOKINETICS Metabolism:** Protein degradation. **Half-Life:** 2.1 h.

## NURSING IMPLICATIONS

### Black Box Warning

*Blinatumomab has been associated with potentially life-threatening cytokine release syndrome, and severe, potentially life-threatening neurological toxicities.*

### Assessment & Drug Effects

- Monitor for neurotoxicity (e.g., confusion, lack of coordination or

balance, speech disorders); if suspected, stop infusion and notify prescriber immediately.
- Monitor for S&S of cytokine release syndrome (e.g., pyrexia, headache, nausea, weakness, hypotension, increased transaminases, and elevated total bilirubin); if suspected, stop infusion and notify prescriber immediately.
- Monitor for S&S of hypokalemia (see Appendix F) or infection, and report if either is suspected.
- Monitor lab tests: Baseline and periodic CBC with differential and LFTs; periodic serum electrolytes.

### Patient & Family Education

- Report promptly to prescriber any of the following: Fever, persistent headache, weakness, dizziness, lack of coordination, confusion or disorientation, problems with speech, swelling of extremities.
- Refrain from driving or engaging in hazardous occupations or activities while receiving this drug.
- Women should use reliable means of contraception while receiving this drug.
- Do not breast-feed while receiving this drug.
- If diabetic, monitor for loss of glycemic control.

## BOCEPREVIR ⓟ

(boe-se′pre-vir)

Victelis

**Classifications:** ANTIVIRAL; VIRAL PROTEIN INHIBITOR; PROTEASE INHIBITOR; DIRECT-ACTING ANTIVIRUS; ANTIHEPATITIS
**Therapeutic:** ANTIHEPATITIS

**AVAILABILITY** Capsule

## ACTION & *THERAPEUTIC EFFECT*

A direct-acting antiviral that inhibits an HCV protease enzyme needed

Common adverse effects in *italic;* life-threatening effects underlined; generic names in **bold;** classifications in SMALL CAPS; ◆ Canadian drug name; ⓟ Prototype drug

201

for replication of HCV in the host cells. *Effective in treatment of hepatitis C genotype 1.*

**USES** Treatment of chronic hepatitis C virus (HCV) genotype 1 infection in adult patients with compensated liver disease.

**CONTRAINDICATIONS** Hypersensitivity to boceprevir; men whose female partners are pregnant; coadministration with drugs that are highly dependent on CYP3A4/5 for clearance or are potent CYP3A4/5 inducers (see drug interactions); older adults; pregnancy (category X in combination with ribavirin and peginterferon alfa); lactation.

**CAUTIOUS USE** Anemia, neutropenia, and thromboembolic events; older adults; pregnancy (category B when used alone). Safety and efficacy in children not established.

**ROUTE & DOSAGE**

**Chronic Hepatitis C Infection**

*Adult:* **PO** 800 mg t.i.d. begin treatment 4 wk after initiating therapy with ribavirin and peginterferon alfa. Therapy duration varies based on HCV RNA concentrations; see package insert for duration.

**ADMINISTRATION**

**Oral**
- Give with a meal or light snack.
- Doses should be given approximately q7–9 h.
- Boceprevir **must be** given in combination with peginterferon alfa and ribavirin (started 4 wk prior to adding boceprevir).

- Store 2°–8° C (36°–46° F). Can be stored at room temperature up to 25° C (77° F) for 3 mo. Avoid excessive heat.

**ADVERSE EFFECTS** (≥1%) **Body as a Whole:** Arthralgia, chills, decreased appetite, dyspnea on exertion. **CNS:** Asthenia, dizziness, *fatigue, headache,* insomnia, irritability. **GI:** Diarrhea, dry mouth, *dysgeusia, nausea,* vomiting. **Hematological:** *Anemia,* neutropenia. **Metabolic:** Decreased hemoglobin, neutropenia. **Skin:** Alopecia, dry skin, rash.

**INTERACTIONS Drug:** Strong CYP3A4 inhibitors (e.g., **ketoconazole, itraconazole, voriconazole, clarithromycin, nefazodone, ritonavir, saquinavir, nelfinavir, indinavir, atazanavir,** and **telithromycin**) can increase boceprevir levels, while potent CYP3A4 inducers (e.g., **rifampin, dexamethasone, phenytoin, carbamazepine,** and **phenobarbital**) can decrease boceprevir levels. Due to its ability to inhibit CYP3A4/5, boceprevir can increase plasma levels of other compounds requiring CYP3A4/5 (e.g., **ketoconazole, itraconazole, voriconazole, posiconazole, budesonide, fluticasone,** ri-**fampin** and other RIFAMYCINS, **alfuzosin,** ERGOT ALKALOIDS, HMG CoA REDUCTASE INHIBITORS). Boceprevir can increase adverse effects of **desipramine** and **trazodone.** Use of BENZODIAZEPINES with boceprevir may increase the risk of respiratory depression. Boceprevir increases the cardiovascular effects of **salmeterol.** Combination use with **colchicine** increases the risk of colchicine toxicity. Boceprevir increases the risk of hyperkalemia if used with **drospirenone.** Boceprevir can increase **digoxin** levels. Boceprevir may alter the levels of **warfarin.**

Use caution with concurrent ESTRO-GEN use. **Food:** Co-administration with food enhances bioavailability. **Herbal: St. John's wort** may decrease the levels of boceprevir.

## PHARMACOKINETICS **Peak:** 2 h. **Distribution:** Approximately 75% plasma protein bound. **Metabolism:** Hepatic metabolism to inactive compounds. **Elimination:** Fecal (79%) and renal (9%). **Half-Life:** 3.4 h.

## NURSING IMPLICATIONS
### Assessment & Drug Effects
- Monitor for and report S&S of anemia or infection.
- Compile a complete list of all drugs, vitamins, herbals, etc. used by the patient.
- Withhold drug and notify prescriber if pregnancy is suspected.
- Monitor lab tests: CBC with differential at baseline and wk 4, 8, 12; HCV-RNA levels at wk 4, 8, 12, 24, end of treatment, and periodically thereafter; monthly pregnancy tests during treatment and for 6 mo thereafter.

### Patient & Family Education
- Women who are pregnant or men whose female partners are pregnant should not take boceprevir. Notify prescriber immediately if a pregnancy develops.
- Use at least two forms of effective birth control during and for 6 mo after completion of therapy. Systemic hormonal contraceptives may not be effective while taking boceprevir.
- If a dose is missed and it is less than 2 h before next dose is due, skip the missed dose; if it is 2 h or more before the next dose is due, take the missed dose and resume dosing schedule.
- Boceprevir interacts with a large number of drugs. Inform prescriber

about any prescription and nonprescription medicines, vitamins, and herbal supplements you are taking.
- Do not breast-feed while taking this drug without consulting prescriber.

## BORTEZOMIB ⊘
(bor-te-zo′mib)
Velcade
**Classifications:** ANTINEOPLASTIC; BIOLOGICAL RESPONSE MODIFIER; PROTEOSOME INHIBITOR
**Therapeutic:** ANTINEOPLASTIC; SIGNAL TRANSDUCTION INHIBITOR (STI)

**AVAILABILITY** Powder for injection

## ACTION & *THERAPEUTIC EFFECT*
An inhibitor of proteasome, which is responsible for regulation of protein expression and degradation of damaged or obsolete proteins within the cell; its activity is critical to activation or suppression of cellular functions including the cell cycle, oncogene expression, and apoptosis. *Proteasome inhibition may reverse some of the changes that allow proliferation of malignant cells and suppress apoptosis (programmed cell death) in malignant cells.*

**USES** Treatment of relapsed or refractory multiple myeloma or mantle cell lymphoma.

**UNLABELED USES** Myelomatous pleural effusion, non-Hodgkin's lymphoma.

**CONTRAINDICATIONS** Hypersensitivity to bortezomib, boron, or mannitol; acute diffuse infiltrative pulmonary disease due to drug; posterior reversible encephalopathy

Common adverse effects in *italic;* life-threatening effects underlined; generic names in **bold;** classifications in SMALL CAPS; ♣ Canadian drug name; ⊘ Prototype drug

203

syndrome (PRES); pregnancy (category D); lactation.

**CAUTIOUS USE** Peripheral neuropathy; history of syncope, dehydration, hypotension; history of allergies, asthma; preexisting electrolyte or acid-base disturbances, especially hypokalemia or hyponatremia; diabetic mellitus; liver disease; myelosuppression, renal impairment; risk factors for cardiac disease; history of peripheral neuropathy or other neurologic disorders; risk factors for pulmonary disorders; GI toxicities. Safety and efficacy in children not established.

## ROUTE & DOSAGE

### Multiple Myeloma/Mantle Cell Lymphoma (failed previous therapy)

*Adult:* **IV** 1.3 mg/m² days 1, 4, 8, and 11 followed by a 10-day rest period; at least 72 h should elapse between consecutive doses; 3 wk period is a treatment cycle

### Previously Untreated Multiple Myeloma

*Adult:* **IV** 1.3 mg/m²/dose on days 1, 4, 8, and 11 followed by a 10-day rest period (days 12–21) then on days 22, 25, 29, and 32 followed by a 10-day rest period; 6 wk is one course

### *Toxicity Dosage Adjustment*

Withhold dose with grade 3 or 4 hematologic toxicity, when symptoms resolve dose may be reduced 25% and restarted.

### *Hemodialysis Dosage Adjustment*

Administer after hemodialysis

### *Hepatic Impairment Dosage Adjustment*

Moderate/severe impairment (bilirubin above 1.5 × ULN) reduce dose to 0.7 mg/m²

## ADMINISTRATION

### Intravenous

Wear protective gloves and prevent contact with skin.

***PREPARE: Direct:*** Reconstitute 3.5 mg vial with 3.5 mL of NS for injection to yield 1 mg/mL. ▪ Discard if not clear and colorless. Label reconstituted drug for IV use. Give within 8 h of reconstitution.

***ADMINISTER: Direct:*** Give as a bolus dose over 3–5 sec. Flush before/after with NS.

***INCOMPATIBILITIES: Solution/additive:*** Do not recommend mixing or injecting with any other drugs.

### Subcutaneous

▪ Reconstitute 3.5 mg vial with 1.4 mL of NS to yield 2.5 mg/mL. Label reconstituted drug for subcutaneous use.
▪ Inject into thigh or abdomen. Rotate injection sites. New injections sites should be at least one inch from old sites.
▪ If local site reaction occurs, the less concentrated form (1 mg/mL) for IV bolus injection may be given subcutaneously.
▪ Store unopened vials at 15°–30° C (59°–86° F). Protect from light.
▪ Store reconstituted vials at 15°–30° C (59°–86° F). ▪ Give within 8 h of reconstitution. May store up to 3 h in a syringe; however, total storage time must not exceed 8 h when exposed to normal indoor lighting.

## ADVERSE EFFECTS (≥1%) **Body as a Whole:** *Asthenia, weakness,*

*fatigue, malaise, fever, dehydration, peripheral neuropathy, rigors, herpes zoster.* **CNS:** *Insomnia, headache, paresthesia, dizziness, anxiety.* **CV:** *Edema,* hypotension, *orthostatic hypotension.* **GI:** *Nausea, vomiting, diarrhea, anorexia, abdominal pain, constipation, dyspepsia, dysphagia.* **Hematologic:** Thrombocytopenia, leukopenia, *neutropenia, anemia.* **Musculoskeletal:** *Arthralgia, musculoskeletal pain, bone pain, myalgia, back pain, muscle cramps.* **Respiratory:** *Dyspnea, cough, upper respiratory infection.* **Skin:** *Rash, pruritus.* **Special Senses:** *Blurred vision, diplopia.*

## INTERACTIONS **Drug:** Hypoglycemia and hyperglycemia have been reported with ANTIDIABETIC AGENTS; ANTIHYPERTENSIVE AGENTS may exacerbate hypotension; ANTICOAGULANTS, **antithymocyte globulin,** NSAIDS, PLATELET INHIBITORS, **aspirin,** THROMBOLYTIC AGENTS may increase risk of bleeding. **Food: Grapefruit juice** may increase drug levels.

## PHARMACOKINETICS **Distribution:** 85% protein bound. **Metabolism:** In the liver (CYP3A4, CYP2C19, CYP1A2). **Half-Life:** 9–15 h.

## NURSING IMPLICATIONS

### Assessment & Drug Effects
- Monitor for and report S&S of neuropathy (e.g., hyperesthesia, hypoesthesia, paresthesia, discomfort or neuropathic pain).
- Monitor diabetics for loss of glycemic control.
- Monitor postural vital signs for orthostatic hypotension.
- Monitor for S&S of developing a pulmonary disorder.

- Monitor I&O and assess for S&S of dehydration or electrolyte imbalance if vomiting and/or diarrhea develop.
- Monitor for exacerbation of CHF, or acute onset of CHF.
- Monitor lab tests: CBC with platelet count prior to each dose; baseline and periodic LFTs; frequent blood glucose in diabetics.

### Patient & Family Education
- Report promptly any of the following: Dizziness, light-headedness or fainting spells; numbness, tingling, or other unusual sensations; signs of infection (e.g., fever, chills, cough, sore throat); bruising, pinpoint red spots on the skin; black, tarry stools, nosebleeds, or any other sign of bleeding.
- Monitor closely blood glucose level if diabetic.
- Report increased S&S of CHF, or acute onset of these S&S.
- Do not drive or engage in other hazardous activities until reaction to drug is known.
- Report any S&S of respiratory difficulty.
- Females should use reliable methods of contraception to avoid pregnancy while on this drug.

## BOSUTINIB
(bo-su'ti-nib)
Bosulif
**Classification:** ANTINEOPLASTIC; KINASE INHIBITOR
Therapeutic: ANTINEOPLASTIC
**Prototype:** Erlotinib

## AVAILABILITY Tablet

## ACTION & *THERAPEUTIC EFFECT*
A tyrosine kinase inhibitor that blocks certain enzymes (e.g., Bcr-Abl

Common adverse effects in *italic;* life-threatening effects underlined; generic names in **bold;** classifications in SMALL CAPS; ♣ Canadian drug name; ☺ Prototype drug

205

kinase) which promote CML. *Slows progression of CML.*

**USES** Treatment of chronic phase, accelerated phase, or blast phase Philadelphia chromosome-positive chronic myelogenous leukemia (CML) in adults who are resistant or intolerant to prior therapy.

**CONTRAINDICATIONS** Hypersensitivity to bosutinib; pregnancy (category D); lactation.

**CAUTIOUS USE** Diarrhea; myelosuppression; renal impairment; hepatic impairment; bone density changes; bone marrow suppression; fluid retention; gastrointestinal toxicity; hemorrhage; pancreatitis; QT prolongation; older adults. Safety and efficacy in children younger than 18 y not established.

## ROUTE & DOSAGE

### Chronic Myelogenous Leukemia (CML)

*Adult:* **PO** 500 mg once daily until disease progression or drug intolerance. May escalate to 600 mg daily if target response levels are not reached and adverse reactions are less than Grade 3.

### Hepatic Impairment Dosage Adjustment

*For elevation of ALT/AST levels greater than or equal to 5 × the upper limit of normal (ULN):* Withhold until ALT/AST levels are less than or equal to 2.5 × ULN and reduce dose to 400 mg once daily. *If levels are not less than or equal to 2.5 ULN after 4 wk:* Discontinue bosutinib.

*If ALT/AST levels are greater than or equal to 3 × ULN and bilirubin levels are greater than 2 × ULN and alkaline phosphatase levels are less than 2 × ULN:* Discontinue bosutinib.

### Treatment-Related Toxicity Dosage Adjustments

### Hematologic Toxicity Dosage Adjustment

*If ANC is less than 1000 × 10⁶/L or platelet count is less than 50,000 × 10⁶/L:* Hold bosutinib. *If ANC is greater than or equal to 1000 × 10⁶/L and platelet count is greater than or equal to 50,000 × 10⁶/L within 2 wk:* Resume bosutinib at normal dose. *If recovery takes longer than 2 wks:* Reduce dose by 100 mg/day.

### Diarrhea Dosage Adjustment

*Grade 3 or 4 diarrhea:* Hold bosutinib until recovery to Grade 1 toxicity or lower; resume therapy at 400 mg/day

## ADMINISTRATION

### Oral
- Give with food.
- Tablets should be swallowed whole and not crushed, cut, or chewed.
- Follow proper handling and disposal precautions for anticancer drugs.
- Avoid exposure to crushed or broken tablets.
- Store at 15°–30° C (59°–86° F).

**ADVERSE EFFECTS** (≥1%) **Body as a Whole:** *Abdominal pain,* anaphylactic shock, anemia, chest pain, edema, *fatigue,* hepatotoxicity, hypersensitivity, influenza, malaise, pain, *pyrexia.* **CNS:** Headache, dizziness, dysgeusia. **CV:** Pericardial effusion, pericarditis, prolonged

QT interval, edema. **GI:** Acute pancreatitis, *diarrhea*, gastritis, GI hemorrhage, *nausea*, *vomiting*. **Hematological:** *Anemia*, neutropenia, *thrombocytopenia*. **Metabolic:** Hypophosphatemia, hypokalemia. **Musculoskeletal:** Arthralgia, back pain, myalgia. **Respiratory:** Bronchitis, cough, dyspnea, nasopharyngitis, pleural effusion, pneumonia, pulmonary edema, pulmonary hypertension, respiratory failure, respiratory tract infection. **Skin:** Acne, drug eruption, erythema multiforme, exfoliative rash, pruritus, *rash*, urticaria. **Special Senses:** Tinnitus. **Urogenital:** Renal failure.

**INTERACTIONS Drug:** Strong or moderate inhibitors of CYP3A (e.g., **ketoconazole**) and/or P-glycoprotein may increase the levels of bosutinib. Strong or moderate inducers (e.g., **rifampin**) of CYP3A may decrease the levels of bosutinib. PROTON PUMP INHIBITORS (e.g., **lansoprazole, omeprazole**) can decrease the absorption of bosutinib. **Food:** Grapefruit or grapefruit juice may increase the levels of bosutinib. **Herbal:** St. John's wort may decrease the levels of bosutinib.

**PHARMACOKINETICS Peak:** 4–6 h. **Distribution:** 94% plasma protein bound. **Metabolism:** Hepatic oxidation. **Elimination:** Fecal (91%) and renal (3%). **Half-Life:** 22.5 h.

## NURSING IMPLICATIONS

### Assessment & Drug Effects
- Monitor closely for GI toxicity.
- Monitor vital signs and assess for fluid retention (e.g., peripheral edema, pleural effusion, pulmonary edema).
- Monitor for S&S of hepatotoxicity (See Appendix F).
- Monitor lab tests: CBC with differential weekly for 1 mo and monthly thereafter; monthly LFTs for 3 mo or more often if indicated, then periodically thereafter.

### Patient & Family Education
- If a dose is missed beyond 12 h, do not take until next scheduled dose.
- Report promptly any of the following: Jaundice; S&S of infection; unusual bruising or bleeding; sudden weight gain or extremity swelling; shortness of breath.
- Women should use effective means of birth control during therapy and for at least 30 days following completion of therapy.
- Contact your prescriber immediately if you become pregnant during treatment.
- Do not breast-feed while receiving this drug.

# BOTULINUM TOXIN TYPE A
(bo'tul-i-num)
Botox, BOTOX Cosmetic

# ONABOTULINUM A

**Classifications:** SKELETAL MUSCLE RELAXANT; ANTISPASMODIC
**Therapeutic:** MUSCLE RELAXANT; ANTISPASMODIC

**AVAILABILITY** Powder for injection

## ACTION & *THERAPEUTIC EFFECT*
Blocks neuromuscular transmission by binding to receptor sites on motor nerve terminals, entering the nerve terminals, and inhibiting the release of acetylcholine. *When*

Common adverse effects in *italic;* life-threatening effects underlined; generic names in **bold;** classifications in SMALL CAPS; ♣ Canadian drug name; ⊙ Prototype drug

207

*injected intramuscularly at therapeutic doses, botulinum toxin type A produces partial chemical denervation of the muscle resulting in a localized reduction in muscle activity.*

**USES** Treatment of blepharospasm, cervical dystonia, strabismus, facial wrinkles, severe axillary hyperhidrosis, spasticity, urinary incontinence, chronic migraine.

**UNLABELED USES** Achalasia.

**CONTRAINDICATIONS** Presence of infection at the proposed injection site(s); hypersensitivity to Botox. Patients with dysphagia or respiratory compromise.

**CAUTIOUS USE** Hypersensitivity to albumin; individuals with peripheral motor neuropathic diseases (e.g., amyotrophic lateral sclerosis, or motor neuropathy), or neuromuscular junctional disorders (e.g., myasthenia gravis or Lambert-Eaton syndrome); neuromuscular disorders; ocular disease; cardiovascular disease; elderly; inflammation at the proposed injection site; weakness in the target muscle(s); pregnancy (category C); lactation; children.

## ROUTE & DOSAGE

**Blepharospasm**

*Adult/Child (12 y or older):*
**Intradermal** 1.25–2.5 units injected at each site, may repeat in 3 mo if needed; cumulative dose should not exceed 200 units in a 30-day period

**Cervical Dystonia**

*Adult/Adolescent (16 y or older):*
**IM** 198–300 units divided among affected muscles

**Facial Wrinkles**

*Adult:* **IM** 20 units divided among affected muscles in 5 step doses, may repeat in 3–4 mo if needed

**Spasticity**

*Adult:* **IM**, Initiate with lowest dose 75–360 units divided among muscles

*Child (2–18 y):* **IM** 4 units/kg (max: 200 units/treatment) q3mo

**Axillary Hyperhidrosis**

*Adult:* **IM** 50 units/site

**Migraine Prophylaxis**

*Adult:* **IM** 155U/treatment across 31 sites (see prescribing information)

**Overactive Bladder**

*Adult:* **IM** 100 units/treatment

## ADMINISTRATION

**Intramuscular, Intradermal**

- Slowly inject required amount of nonpreserved NS (see dilution calculation) into vial. Discard vial if a vacuum does not pull diluent into vial. Gently rotate to mix. Discard if not clear, colorless, and free of particulate matter. Dilution calculation: Add 1, 2, 4, or 6 mL of NS to yield, respectively, 10 units/0.1 mL, 5 units/0.1 mL, 2.5 units/0.1 mL, 1.25 units/0.1 mL.
- Store at 2°–8° C (36°–46° F) (refrigerated). Administer within 4 h of reconstitution.

**INCOMPATIBILITIES:** Do not mix with other solutions/additives.

Common adverse effects in *italic;* life-threatening effects <u>underlined;</u> generic names in **bold;** classifications in SMALL CAPS; ♣ Canadian drug name; ● Prototype drug

**ADVERSE EFFECTS** (≥1%) **Body as a Whole:** Injection site reactions (localized pain, tenderness, bruising), neck pain, flu-like symptoms, hypertonia, asthenia, fever. **CNS:** *Headache.* **GI:** *Dysphagia,* dry mouth, fever, nausea. **Hematologic:** Ecchymosis. **Musculoskeletal:** Local muscle weakness, dysarthria. **Respiratory:** Rhinitis, upper respiratory infection. **Special Senses:** *Ptosis,* superficial punctate keratitis, dry eyes, ocular irritation, lacrimation, photophobia, keratitis, diplopia.

**INTERACTIONS Drug:** AMINOGLYCOSIDES, NEUROMUSCULAR BLOCKING AGENTS may potentiate neuromuscular blockade; **chloroquine** may antagonize blocking effects.

## NURSING IMPLICATIONS

### Assessment & Drug Effects

- Evaluate for therapeutic efficacy, maximal at about 1–2 wk (lasting 3–4 mo).

### Patient & Family Education

- Inform prescriber about all prescription, nonprescription, and herbal drugs being taken.
- Report immediately any of the following: Difficulty breathing or swallowing, problem with speech; unusual bleeding, bruising, or swelling around injection site.
- Note: Effects of the injection generally last 3–4 mo and then repeat treatments may be given.

## BRENTUXIMAB

(bren-tuk'see-mab)

Adcetris

**Classifications:** BIOLOGICAL RESPONSE MODIFIER; MONOCLONAL ANTIBODY; CD-30

SPECIFIC ANTIBODY; ANTINEOPLASTIC
**Therapeutic:** ANTINEOPLASTIC
**Prototype:** Basiliximab

**AVAILABILITY** Lyophilized powder for injection

## ACTION & *THERAPEUTIC EFFECT*

An antibody-drug complex that binds to a protein (CD 30) on the surface of lymphoma cells and is internalized into these cells where it releases a microtubule disrupting agent. *Causes cell cycle arrest and apoptosis of lymphoma cells.*

**USES** Treatment of Hodgkin lymphoma in patients non-responsive to autologous stem cell transplant (ASCT) or non-Hodgkin's lymphoma.

**CONTRAINDICATIONS** Development of Progressive Multifocal Leukoencephalopathy (PML) or Stevens–Johnson syndrome; concurrent use with bleomycin; pregnancy (category D); lactation.

**CAUTIOUS USE** Hypersensitivity to brentuximab due to infusion reaction; bone marrow depression; renal and hepatic impairment; history of peripheral neuropathy; history of pulmonary disease; older adults. Safety and efficacy in children not established.

## ROUTE & DOSAGE

**Hodgkin Lymphoma or Systemic Anaplastic Large Cell Lymphoma**

*Adult:* **IV** 1.8 mg/kg q3wk for maximum of 16 cycles

**Peripheral Neuropathy Dosage Adjustment**

*Grade 2/3 peripheral neuropathy:* Stop treatment until toxicity

Common adverse effects in *italic*; life-threatening effects underlined; generic names in **bold**; classifications in SMALL CAPS; ♣ Canadian drug name; ⊘ Prototype drug

209

resolves to grade 1 or better. Reduce dosage to 1.2 mg/kg q3wk

*For Grade 4 peripheral neuropathy:* Discontinue treatment

**Neutropenia Dosage Adjustment**

*Grade 3/4 neutropenia:* Stop treatment until toxicity resolves to baseline or grade 2 or better. Consider the use of growth factors (CSFs) for subsequent cycles

*Grade 4 neutropenia (despite the use of growth factors):* Discontinue treatment or reduce dosage to 1.2 mg/kg IV q3wk

## ADMINISTRATION

**Intravenous**

▪ Premedication with acetaminophen, an antihistamine and a corticosteroid are recommended for prior infusion reactions.

*PREPARE:* **IV Infusion:** Reconstitute each 50 mg vial with 10.5 mL sterile water (SW) for injection to yield 5 mg/mL. Direct the stream of SW on to side of vial and not into powder. Swirl gently to dissolve. Do not shake. Immediately withdraw the required volume of reconstituted solution and add to a minimum of 100 mL of NS, D5W, or LR to produce a final concentration of 0.4–1.8 mg/mL. Invert bag gently to mix.

*ADMINISTER:* **IV Infusion:** Give over 30 min. Do not give IV push or bolus.

*INCOMPATIBILITIES:* **Solution/additive:** Do not mix or administer as an IV infusion with any other medicinal products.

▪ Store refrigerated, if necessary, at 2°–8° C (36°–46° F). Should be used immediately after preparation

but no later than 24 h following reconstitution.

**ADVERSE EFFECTS** (≥10%) **Body as a Whole:** Chills, *fatigue*, pain, peripheral edema, *pyrexia*. **CNS:** Anxiety, dizziness, headache, insomnia, *peripheral neuropathy*. **GI:** *Abdominal pain*, constipation, *diarrhea, nausea, vomiting*. **Hematological:** *Anemia*, lymphadenopathy, *neutropenia, thrombocytopenia*. **Metabolic:** Decreased appetite, weight loss. **Musculoskeletal:** Arthralgia, back pain, muscle spasms, myalgia, pain in extremity. **Respiratory:** *Cough*, dyspnea, oropharyngeal pain, *upper respiratory tract infection*. **Skin:** Alopecia, dry skin, night sweats, pruritus, *rash*.

**INTERACTIONS Drug:** Monomethyl auristatin E (MMAE), one of the components of brentuximab is primarily metabolized by CYP3A4. Strong inhibitors of CYP3A4 (e.g., **ketoconazole, delavirdine, indinavir, itraconazole**) may increase the levels of brentuximab. Strong inducers of CYP3A4 (i.e., **phenobarbital, rifampin** may decrease the levels of brentuximab. **Herbal:** **St. John's wort** and **Hypericum perforatum** may reduce the levels of brentuximab.

**PHARMACOKINETICS Peak:** 1–3 d. **Distribution:** 68–82% plasma protein bound. **Metabolism:** Oxidative metabolism. **Elimination:** Primarily fecal. **Half-Life:** 4–6 d.

## NURSING IMPLICATIONS

**Assessment & Drug Effects**

### Black Box Warning

*Brentuximab has been associated with progressive JC virus infection resulting in progressive multifocal leukoencephalopathy (PML) and death.*

- Discontinue infusion immediately and institute supportive measures if hypersensitivity (see Appendix F) is suspected.
- Monitor closely for and report promptly S&S of an infusion reaction (e.g., chills, nausea, dyspnea, pruritus, fever, cough).
- Monitor cardiac status throughout infusion and during the immediate period thereafter.
- Monitor closely for a report S&S of peripheral neuropathy (e.g., hypo/hyperesthesia, paresthesia, burning sensation, nerve pain, weakness). Withhold drug and notify prescriber for new or worsening grade 2 or 3 neuropathy.
- Monitor lab tests: Baseline and prior to each dose, CBC with differential.

**Patient and Family Education**

- Report any of the following to prescriber: Chills, rash, or difficulty breathing within 24 h of infusion; numbness or tingling of hands or feet; muscle weakness; fever of 100.5° F or greater; unexplained cough; or pain on urination.
- Women should use effective means of contraception and avoid breast-feeding while being treated with brentuximab.

# BREXPIPRAZOLE

(brex-pi-pra'zole)

Rexulti

**Classifications:** ATYPICAL ANTIPSYCHOTIC; ANTIDEPRESSANT
Therapeutic: ANTIPSYCHOTIC; ANTIDEPRESSANT
**Prototype:** Clozapine

**AVAILABILITY** Tablets

## ACTION & THERAPEUTIC EFFECT

Exhibits partial agonist activity for 5-HT$_{1A}$ and D$_2$ receptors and antagonist activity for 5-HT$_{2A}$ receptors.

*May improve mood and affect in major depressive disorder, and may improve overall functional capability in schizophrenia.*

**USES** Adjunctive treatment of major depressive disorder (MDD) and treatment of schizophrenia.

**CONTRAINDICATIONS** Hypersensitivity to brexpiprazole or any component of the formulation; dementia related psychosis; suicidal ideation.

**CAUTIOUS USE** History of suicidal thoughts; extrapyramidal symptoms; hyperglycemia; DM; obesity; orthostatic hypotension; dyslipidemia; seizures, impaired core body temperature regulation; esophageal dysmotility; pregnancy (third trimester); lactation. Safety and efficacy in people younger than 18 y not established.

## ROUTE & DOSAGE

| Major Depressive Disorder (MDD) |
| --- |
| *Adult:* **PO** 0.5 to 1 mg once daily; titrate weekly to max of 3 mg |
| **Schizophrenia** |
| *Adult:* **PO** 1 mg once daily on days 1–4; titrate to 2 mg once daily on days 5–7, then to 4 mg on day 8 |
| ***Hepatic Impairment Dosage Adjustment*** |
| *Severe hepatic impairment (Child-Pugh score 7 or greater):* Max daily doses: 2 mg (MDD) and 3 mg (schizophrenia) |
| ***Renal Impairment Dosage Adjustment*** |
| *Moderate, severe, or end-stage renal impairment (CrCl less than 60 mL/min):* Max daily doses: 2 mg (MDD) and 3 mg (schizophrenia) |

Common adverse effects in *italic;* life-threatening effects underlined; generic names in **bold;** classifications in SMALL CAPS; ♣ Canadian drug name; ☻ Prototype drug

211

**B**

### Pharmacogenetic Dosage Adjustment/Concomitant CYP Inducers or Inhibitors

*CYP2D6 poor metabolizers, or taking concomitant strong CYP2D6 or strong CYP3A4 inhibitors:* Half of usual dose
*CYP2D6 poor metabolizers taking concomitant strong/moderate CYP3A4 inhibitors, or taking concomitant strong/moderate CYP2D6 inhibitors with strong/moderate CYP3A4 inhibitors:* One quarter of usual dose
*Taking concomitant strong CYP3A4 inducers:* Double usual dose over 1–2 wk

## ADMINISTRATION

### Oral

- May give without regard to food.
- Store at 15°–30° C (59°–86° F).

## ADVERSE EFFECTS (>1%) **Body as a Whole:** Anxiety, dystonia, extrapyramidal symptoms, fatigue, increased risk of death, restlessness. **CNS:** Abnormal dreams, akathisia, dizziness, headache, insomnia, seizures, somnolence, tremor. **CV:** Orthostatic hypotension, stroke. **GI:** Abdominal pain, constipation, diarrhea, dry mouth, dyspepsia, flatulence, nausea, salivary hypersecretion. **Hematological:** Agranulocytosis, leukopenia, neuroleptic malignant syndrome, neutropenia. **Metabolic:** Decreased blood cortisol, hyperglycemia, increased appetite, increased blood creatine phosphate, increased blood prolactin, increased triglycerides, increased weight. **Musculoskeletal:** Myalgia. **Respiratory:** Nasopharyngitis. **Skin:** Hyperhidrosis. **Special Senses:** Blurred vision. **Urogenital:** Urinary tract infection.

## INTERACTIONS **Drug:** Concomitant use with strong CYP3A4 inhibitors (e.g., **clarithromycin, itraconazole, ketoconazole**) and/or strong CYP2D6 inhibitors (e.g., **fluoxetine, paroxetine, quinidine**) will increase the blood levels of brexpiprazole. Concomitant use with strong CYP3A4 inducers (e.g., **rifampin**) will decrease the blood levels of brexpiprazole. **Herbal: St. John's wort** will decrease the levels of brexpiprazole.

## PHARMACOKINETICS **Absorption:** 95% bioavailable. **Peak:** 4 h. **Distribution:** 99% plasma protein bound. **Metabolism:** Hepatic oxidation. **Elimination:** Renal (25%) and fecal (46%). **Half-Life:** 91 h.

## NURSING IMPLICATIONS

### Black Box Warning

*Brexpiprazole has been associated with increased mortality in elderly patients with dementia-related psychosis, and increased risk of suicidal thoughts and behavior in those 24 y and younger.*

### Assessment & Drug Effects

- Monitor mental status; report worsening of clinical S&S and emergence of suicidal thoughts and behaviors.
- Monitor for extrapyramidal symptoms (EPS) such as tardive dyskinesia (see Appendix F). Withhold drug and notify prescriber if EPS develop.
- Monitor BP at baseline, repeat 3 mo after therapy initiated, then yearly thereafter.
- Monitor closely those at risk for aspiration as esophageal dysmotility and dysphagia may occur.
- Monitor weight, BMI, waist circumference at baseline; repeat at

Common adverse effects in *italic;* life-threatening effects underlined; generic names in **bold;** classifications in SMALL CAPS; ♣ Canadian drug name; ◉ Prototype drug

212

4, 8, and 12 wk or after changing therapy, then q3mo thereafter; report weight gain of 5% or more of initial weight.
- Monitor lab tests: Periodic CBC with differential, fasting blood glucose, lipid profile.

**Patient & Family Education**
- Report new or worsening depression symptoms, especially sudden changes in mood, behaviors, thoughts, or feelings.
- Report promptly suicidal thoughts or actions.
- Avoid drinking alcohol while taking this drug.
- Report promptly any of the following: Restlessness, uncontrolled movement on your face, tongue or other body parts; difficulty swallowing; weight gain; excessive urination or thirst; lightheadedness upon arising.
- Avoid becoming overheated and maintain adequate hydration with liquids.
- Women should use effective means of contraception while taking this drug.
- Do not breast-feed while taking this drug without consulting the prescriber.

# BRIMONIDINE TARTRATE
(bry-mon'i-deen)
Alphagan P
**See Appendix A-1.**

# BRINZOLAMIDE
(brin-zol'a-mide)
Azopt
**See Appendix A-1.**

# BRIVARACETAM
(briv'a-ra'se-tam

Brivact
**Classifications:** ANTICONVULSANT
Therapeutic: ANTICONVULSANT

**AVAILABILITY** Tablet; oral solution; solution for injection

**ACTION & *THERAPEUTIC EFFECT***
Exact mechanism has not been determined; however, brivaracetam is highly selective for synaptic vesicle protein 2A (SV2A) in the brain. *This is thought to contribute to the anticonvulsant effect.*

**USES** Adjunctive therapy in the treatment of partial-onset seizures in patients 16 y or older with epilepsy.

**CONTRAINDICATIONS** Hypersensitivity to brivaracetam.

**CAUTIOUS USE** Abrupt discontinuation, depression, driving or operating machinery, geriatric, hepatic disease, suicidal ideation, pregnancy, lactation.

**ROUTE & DOSAGE**

**Epilepsy**
*Adult:* **PO** or **IV** 50 mg b.i.d.; may adjust to 25 mg b.i.d. or 100 mg b.i.d.

***Hepatic Impairment Dosage Adjustment***
Initial dose of 25 mg b.i.d. (max dose: 75 mg b.i.d.)

**ADMINISTRATION**
Oral
- May be administered without regard to meals.
- Swallow tablets whole; do not crush or chew tablets.
- Oral solution does not need to be diluted.

---

Common adverse effects in *italic;* life-threatening effects <u>underlined;</u> generic names in **bold;** classifications in SMALL CAPS; ♣ Canadian drug name; ☻ Prototype drug

213

▪ Discard unused oral solution after 5 mo of first opening the bottle.

### Intravenous

*PREPARE:* **IV Infusion:** No need to dilute but can be diluted in 0.9% sodium chloride, LR, or 5% dextrose.
*ADMINISTER:* **IV Infusion:** May be given intravenously over 2–15 min.

▪ Store after dilution for no more than 4 h at room temperature.

### ADVERSE EFFECTS (>1%) **Body as a Whole:** Asthenia, lethargy, malaise. **CNS:** Ataxia, balance disorder, coordination abnormal, dizziness, fatigue, hypersomnia, irritability, nystagmus, psychiatric events, sedation, suicidal thoughts and behavior. **GI:** Constipation, nausea, vomitting. **Hematologic:** Decreased white blood cell levels.

### INTERACTIONS **Drug:** **Rifampin** increases the levels of brivaracetam. Brivaracetam may increase the levels of **phenytoin** and **carbamazepine.**

### PHARMACOKINETICS **Peak:** 1 h. **Distribution:** Less than 20% plasma protein bound. **Metabolism:** Hepatic to inactive metabolites. **Elimination:** Primarily renal (greater than 95%). **Half-Life:** 9 h.

### NURSING IMPLICATIONS

#### Assessment & Drug Effects

▪ Assess other medications that patient is taking, alternative therapies, or dosage adjustments that might be needed.
▪ Monitor for signs or symptoms of depression or suicidal ideation.
▪ Monitor lab tests: Obtain CBC with differential, LFTs, and renal function tests.

#### Patient & Family Education

▪ Notify your health care provider if you are breast-feeding or if you are pregnant or planning to become pregnant.
▪ Upon starting this medication, avoid driving or performing other tasks which require you to be alert.
▪ Call your health care provider right away if you feel sad or depressed, nervous, restless, grouchy, panicky; have a change in mood; or have suicidal thoughts.

## BRODALUMAB
(broe-dalu′mab)
Siliq
**Classifications:** MONOCLONAL ANTIBODY; ANTIPSORIATIC AGENT; ANTI-INTERLEUKIN 17-RECEPTOR ANTIBODY
Therapeutic: ANTIPSORIATIC

### AVAILABILITY Subcutaneous injection, prefilled syringe

### ACTION & *THERAPEUTIC EFFECT* Human monoclonal IgG2 antibody that antagonizes the interleukin-17 receptor, a pathway to block cytokine-induced inflammatory response. *Reduces inflammatory response in moderate to severe plaque psoriasis.*

### USES Treatment of plaque psoriasis in patients who have not responded, or stopped responding, to other systemic treatments.

### CONTRAINDICATIONS Crohn's disease.

### CAUTIOUS USE Crohn's disease; pregnancy; lactation. Safety and efficacy in children not established.

### ROUTE & DOSAGE

| Psoriasis |
|---|
| *Adult:* **Subcutaneous** 210 mg once a wk for 3 wk, then 210 mg |

Common adverse effects in *italic;* life-threatening effects <u>underlined;</u> generic names in **bold;** classifications in SMALL CAPS; ◆ Canadian drug name; ⊕ Prototype drug

every 2 wk; discontinue if response not seen after 12–16 wk

## ADMINISTRATION

### Subcutaneous

- Allow prefilled syringe to reach room temperature for approx 30 min prior to injecting; do not use if solution is not clear, or discolored.
- Administer subcutaneously into the thigh, abdomen more than 2 in from umbilicus, or outer upper arm.
- Do not inject into tissue that is tender, bruised, red, hard, scaly, or affected by psoriasis.

## ADVERSE EFFECTS (≥ 2%) Body as a Whole: *Infection.* CNS: *Fatigue.* GI: *Nausea, diarrhea.* Hematologic: Neutropenia, antibody development. Integumentary: *Tinea, injection site reaction.* Muscular: *Arthralgia, myalgia.* Respiratory: *Oropharyngeal pain.*

## INTERACTIONS Avoid use with live vaccines; unknown influence on CYP450 enzymes, consider monitoring effect of medications with narrow therapeutic index.

## PHARMACOKINETICS Absorption: 55% bioavailability. Distribution: Follows nonlinear pharmacokinetics. Onset: Peak effect in 3 days. Metabolism: Similar to endogenous IgG.

## NURSING IMPLICATIONS

### Black Box Warning

*Brodalumab use is associated with an increased risk of suicidal ideation and behavior; advise patients to seek medical attention if symptoms develop while on treatment with brodalumab. Only available through a REMS program.*

### Assessment & Drug Effects

- Evaluate for tuberculosis infection prior to treatment.
- Monitor for signs of suicidal ideation or behavior.
- Monitor for signs of infection including active tuberculosis.
- Routine monitoring of coagulation tests is not required; anti-FXa assay may be helpful in guiding clinical decisions.

### Patient & Family Education

- Notify prescriber if you have suidical thoughts or behaviors.
- Notify prescriber if you experience signs or symptoms of allergic reaction such as rash, hives, itching, shortness of breath, wheezing, cough, swelling of the face, lips, tongue, or throat; or any other signs.
- Prior to initiating treatment, notify prescriber if you have been diagnosed with Crohn's disease or have active TB.

---

## BROMFENAC
(brom'fen-ac)
Xibrom
**See Appendix A-1.**

---

## BROMOCRIPTINE MESYLATE
(broe-moe-krip'teen)
Cycloset, Parlodel

**Classifications:** ERGOT ALKALOID; DOPAMINE RECEPTOR AGONIST; ANTIPARKINSON
**Therapeutic:** ERGOT REPLACEMENT; ANTIDYSKINETIC; ANTIPARKINSON; GLYCEMIC CONTROL AGENT
**Prototype:** Ergotamine

## AVAILABILITY Tablet; capsule

## ACTION & *THERAPEUTIC EFFECT*
Reduces elevated serum prolactin levels in men and women by acti-

Common adverse effects in *italic*; life-threatening effects underlined; generic names in **bold**; classifications in SMALL CAPS; ♣ Canadian drug name; ☺ Prototype drug

215

vating postsynaptic dopaminergic receptors in hypothalamus to stimulate release of prolactin-inhibiting factor. Activates dopaminergic receptors ($D_2$ receptors) in neostriatum of CNS, which may explain action in parkinsonism. *Restores ovulation and ovarian function in amenorrheic women, thus correcting female infertility secondary to elevated prolactin levels. Activates dopaminergic receptors in CNS resulting in antiparkinsonism effect. Improves glycemic control in Type 2 diabetics.*

**USES** Acromegaly, hyperprolactinemia, infertility, Parkinson's disease, pituitary adenoma. As adjunct to diet and exercise in Type 2 diabetes.

**UNLABELED USES** To prevent postpartum lactation, to relieve premenstrual symptoms, mastalgia, and cocaine withdrawal.

**CONTRAINDICATIONS** Hypersensitivity to ergot alkaloids; uncontrolled hypertension; severe ischemic heart disease or peripheral vascular disease; pituitary tumor; lactation. **Cycloset:** Type 1 diabetes mellitus or diabetic ketoacidosis; synopal migraine due to hypertensive episodes. **Parlodel:** Uncontrolled hypertension; postpartum period in women with history of CAD, or severe cardiovascular conditions; normal prolactin levels, preeclampsia, eclampsia.

**CAUTIOUS USE** Hepatic and renal dysfunction; history of psychiatric disorder; history of GI bleeding or peptic ulcer; history of MI with residual arrhythmia; pregnancy (category C); children.

## ROUTE & DOSAGE

**Amenorrhea or Galactorrhea, Female Infertility**

*Adult:* **PO** 1.25–2.5 mg/day (max: 2.5 mg 2–3 × day)

**Parkinson's Disease**

*Adult:* **PO** 1.25 day (increase by 2.5 mg q14–28 days)

**Acromegaly**

*Adult:* **PO** 1.25–2.5 mg/day for 3 days, then increase by 1.25–2.5 mg q3–7days until desired effect is achieved, usually 30–60 mg/day in divided doses

**Adjunct in Type 2 Diabetes (Cycloset)**

*Adult:* **PO** 0.8 mg daily in the a.m., titrate up (max: 1.6–4.8 mg)

## ADMINISTRATION

### Oral

- Give with meals, milk, or other food to reduce incidence of GI side effects.
- Have patient in supine position before receiving first dose because dizziness and fainting may occur. For this reason, initial dose is usually prescribed for evening administration.
- Store in tightly closed, light-resistant containers, preferably at 15°–30° C (59°–86° F) unless otherwise directed.

**ADVERSE EFFECTS** (≥1%) **Body as a Whole:** Mostly dose related. **CNS:** Headache, dizziness, vertigo, lightheadedness, fainting, sedation, nightmares, insomnia, dyskinesia, ataxia; mania, nervousness, anxiety, depression. **CV:** *Orthostatic hypotension,* <u>shock</u>, postpartum hypertension, palpitation, extra-systoles, Raynaud's phenomenon, red, tender, hot, edematous extremities (erythromelalgia), exacerbation of angina, arrhythmias, acute MI. **Special Senses:** Blurred vision, burning sensation in eyes, blepharospasm, diplopia. **GI:** *Nausea,* vomiting, abdominal cramps, epigastric pain, constipation (long-term use) or diarrhea; metallic taste, dry mouth, dysphagia, anorexia, peptic ulcers **Skin:** Urticaria, rash, mottling, livedo reticularis. **Other:** Fatigue, nasal congestion, asthenia.

**INTERACTIONS Drug:** Possibility of decreased tolerance to **alcohol;** ANTIHYPERTENSIVE AGENTS add to hypotensive effects; ORAL CONTRACEPTIVES, **estrogen, progestins** may interfere with effect of bromocriptine by causing amenorrhea and galactorrhea; PHENOTHIAZINES, TRICYCLIC ANTIDEPRESSANTS, **methyldopa, reserpine** can cause an increase in **prolactin,** which may interfere with bromocriptine activity.

**PHARMACOKINETICS Absorption:** 28% from GI tract. **Peak:** 1–2 h. **Duration:** 4–8 h. **Metabolism:** In liver by CYP3A4. **Elimination:** 85% in feces in 5 days; 3–6% in urine. **Half-Life:** 50 h.

## NURSING IMPLICATIONS

### Assessment & Drug Effects

- Monitor vital signs closely during the first few days and periodically throughout therapy.
- Monitor for and report psychotic symptoms and other adverse reactions in Parkinson's patients.
- Improvement in Parkinson's disease may be noted in 30–90 min following administration of

bromocriptine, with maximum effect in 2 h.
- Monitor lab tests: Periodic CBC, LFTs and renal functions with prolonged therapy.

### Patient & Family Education

- Make position changes slowly and in stages, especially from lying down to standing, and to dangle legs over bed for a few minutes before walking. Lie down immediately if light-headedness or dizziness occurs.
- Do not drive or engage in other potentially hazardous activities until response to drug is known.
- Avoid exposure to cold and report the onset of pallor of fingers or toes.
- Note: Use barrier-type contraceptive measures until normal ovulating cycle is restored. Oral contraceptives are contraindicated.

## BROMPHENIRAMINE MALEATE

(brome-fen-ir′a-meen)

Veltane

**Classification:** ANTIHISTAMINE; H₁-RECEPTOR ANTAGONIST
**Therapeutic:** ANTIHISTAMINE
**Prototype:** Diphenhydramine

**AVAILABILITY** Injection; elixir; tablet; ingredient in many oral combination products containing a decongestant, expectorant, and/or analgesic

## ACTION & *THERAPEUTIC EFFECT*

Antihistamine that competes with histamine for H₁-receptor sites on effector cells in the bronchi and bronchioles, thus blocking histamine-mediated responses.

Common adverse effects in *italic;* life-threatening effects underlined; generic names in **bold;** classifications in SMALL CAPS; ♣ Canadian drug name; ⊘ Prototype drug

217

*Effective against upper respiratory symptoms and allergic manifestations.*

**USES** Symptomatic treatment of allergic manifestations. Also used in various cough mixtures and antihistamine-decongestant cold formulations.

**CONTRAINDICATIONS** Hypersensitivity to antihistamines; acute asthma; newborns.

**CAUTIOUS USE** Older adults; prostatic hypertrophy; GI obstruction; asthma; narrow-angle glaucoma; COPD, cardiovascular or renal disease; seizure disorders; hyperthyroidism; pregnancy (category C); lactation.

## ROUTE & DOSAGE

**Allergy**

*Adult:* **PO** 4–8 mg t.i.d. or q.i.d. or 8–12 mg of sustained release b.i.d. or t.i.d.
*Geriatric:* **PO** 4 mg 1–2 × day
*Child (6 y or older):* **PO** 2–4 mg t.i.d. or q.i.d. or 8–12 mg of sustained release b.i.d. (max: 12 mg/24 h); *younger than 6 y:* 0.5 mg/kg in 3–4 divided doses

## ADMINISTRATION

**Oral**

▪ Give with meals or a snack to prevent gastric irritation.

▪ Store in tightly covered container at 15°–30° C (59°–86° F) unless otherwise directed. Elixir should be protected from light. Avoid freezing.

**ADVERSE EFFECTS** (≥1%) **Body as a Whole:** Hypersensitivity reaction (urticaria, increased sweating, agranulocytosis). **CNS:** *Sedation,* drowsiness, dizziness, headache, disturbed coordination. **GI:** Dry mouth, throat, and nose, stomach upset, constipation. **Special Senses:** Ringing or buzzing in ears. **Skin:** Rash, photosensitivity.

## DIAGNOSTIC TEST INTERFERENCE
May cause false-negative **allergy skin tests.**

**INTERACTIONS Drug: Alcohol** and other CNS DEPRESSANTS add to sedation.

**PHARMACOKINETICS Peak:** 3–9 h. **Duration:** Up to 48 h. **Distribution:** Crosses placenta. **Elimination:** 40% in urine within 72 h; 2% in feces. **Half-Life:** 12–34 h.

## NURSING IMPLICATIONS
**Assessment & Drug Effects**

▪ Drowsiness, sweating, transient hypotension, and syncope may follow IV administration; reaction to drug should be evaluated. Keep prescriber informed.
▪ Note: Older adults tend to be particularly susceptible to drug's sedative effect, dizziness, and hypotension. Most symptoms respond to reduction in dosage.
▪ Monitor lab tests: Periodic CBC with long-term therapy.

**Patient & Family Education**

▪ Acute hypersensitivity reaction can occur within minutes to hours after drug ingestion. Reaction is manifested by high fever, chills, and possible development of ulcerations of mouth and throat, pneumonia, and prostration. Patient should seek medical attention immediately.
▪ Sugarless gum, lemon drops, or frequent rinses with warm water may relieve dry mouth.

- Do not drive or perform other potentially hazardous activities until response to drug is known.
- Do not take alcoholic beverages or other CNS depressants (e.g., tranquilizers, sedatives, pain or sleeping medicines) without consulting prescriber.

## BUDESONIDE

(bu-des'o-nide)

Entocort EC, Pulmicort, Rhinocort Aqua, UCERIS

**Classifications:** ADRENAL CORTICOSTEROID GLUCOCORTICOID; ANTI-INFLAMMATORY

Therapeutic: RESPIRATORY INHALANT; ANTI-INFLAMMATORY; ADRENAL CORTICOSTEROID

**Prototype:** Hydrocortisone

**AVAILABILITY** Inhalation powder, nasal spray, nebulizer solution, oral capsule, extended release tablet

### ACTION & *THERAPEUTIC EFFECT*
Its anti-inflammatory action on nasal mucosa is thought to be a result of decreased IgE synthesis and decreased arachidonic acid metabolism. *Glucocorticoids have a wide range of inhibitory activities against multiple cell types (e.g., neutrophils, macrophages) and mediators (e.g., histamine, cytokines) involved in allergic and nonallergic/irritant-mediated inflammation.*

**USES** Treatment of allergic and perennial rhinitis, maintain remission in mild to moderate Crohn's disease or ulcerative colitis; prophylaxis for asthma.

**CONTRAINDICATIONS** Hypersensitivity to budesonide; status asthmaticus, acute bronchospasms; peptic ulcer disease; lactation (**oral**).

**CAUTIOUS USE** Active or quiescent tuberculosis; infections of respiratory tract; in sun-treated fungal, bacterial, or systemic viral infections or ocular herpes simplex; recent nasal septal ulcers; recurrent epistaxis; nasal surgery or trauma; psychosis; myasthenia gravis; diabetes mellitus; seizure disorders; hepatic impairment. **Oral:** Pregnancy (category C). **Nasal:** Pregnancy (category B); lactation.

## ROUTE & DOSAGE

**Crohn's Disease**

*Adult:* **PO** 9 mg once daily for up to 8 wk, may taper to 6 mg daily for 2 wk prior to discontinuing. May repeat 8-wk course for recurring episodes of active Crohn's disease.

**Ulcerative Colitis**

*Adult:* **PO** 9 mg daily for up to 8 wk

**Asthma Prophylaxis, Rhinitis**

See Appendix A-3.

## ADMINISTRATION

**Oral**

- Ensure that capsules and extended release formulations are swallowed whole and not chewed.
- Give only in the morning.
- Patients with moderate to severe liver disease should be monitored for increased signs and/or symptoms of hypercorticism. Reducing the dose of Entocort EC capsules should be considered in these patients.

---

Common adverse effects in *italic;* life-threatening effects underlined; generic names in **bold;** classifications in SMALL CAPS; ◆ Canadian drug name; ◎ Prototype drug

- Store at 25° C (77° F); excursions permitted to 15°–30° C (59°–86° F).

## ADVERSE EFFECTS (≥1%) Body as a Whole: Arthralgia, fatigue, fever, hyperkinesis, myalgia, asthenia, paresthesia, tremor. CNS: Dizziness, emotional lability, facial edema, nervousness, *headache,* agitation, confusion, insomnia, drowsiness. CV: Chest pain, hypertension, palpitations, sinus tachycardia. GI: Abdominal pain, dyspepsia, gastroenteritis, oral candidiasis, xerostomia, diarrhea, nausea, vomiting, cramps. Hematologic: Epistaxis. Metabolic: Hypokalemia, weight gain. Respiratory: Bronchospasms, *infections,* cough, rhinitis, sinusitis, dyspnea, hoarseness, wheezing. Skin: Eczema, pruritus, purpura, rash, alopecia. Special Senses: Contact dermatitis, reduced sense of smell, nasal pain. Urogenital: Intermenstrual bleeding, dysuria.

## INTERACTIONS Drug: Ketoconazole may increase oral budesonide concentrations and toxicity; toxicity may also occur with **anastrozole** (high doses only), **clarithromycin, cyclosporine, danazol, delavir-dine, diltiazem, erythromycin, fluconazole, fluoxetine, fluvoxamine, indinavir, isoniazid, INH, itraconazole, mibefradil, nefazodone, nelfinavir, nicardipine, norfloxacin, oxiconazole, quinidine, quinine, ritonavir, saquinavir, troleandomycin, verapamil,** and **zafirlukast. Food: Grapefruit juice** will significantly increase bioavailability of oral budesonide.

## PHARMACOKINETICS Absorption: 20% (nasal) dose, 6–13% of (orally inhaled) dose, 9% PO dose reaches systemic circulation; PO form is absorbed from duodenum at pH greater than 5.5; oral bioavailability increases 2.5 × in hepatic cirrhosis. Onset: 8–12 in inhaled, 2 wk oral. Peak: 2 wk inhaled, 8 wk oral delayed by high-fat meal. Distribution: 90% protein bound. Metabolism: 85% of absorbed dose undergoes first pass metabolism by CYP3A4. Elimination: 60% in urine, 40% in feces. Half-Life: 2–3.6 h.

## NURSING IMPLICATIONS

### Assessment & Drug Effects

- Monitor closely for S&S of hypercorticism if concomitant doses of ketoconazole or other CYP3A4 inhibitors (see Drug Interactions) are being given.
- Monitor patients with moderate to severe liver disease for increased S&S of hypercorticism.
- Monitor lab tests: Periodic serum potassium.

### Patient & Family Education

- Notify the prescriber immediately for any of the following: Itching, skin rash, fever, swelling of face and neck, difficulty breathing, or if you develop S&S of infection.
- Do not drink grapefruit juice or eat grapefruit regularly.
- Avoid people with infections, especially those with chickenpox or measles if you have never had these conditions.

## BUMETANIDE
(byoo-met′a-nide)
Bumex
**Classifications:** FLUID AND WATER BALANCE AGENT; LOOP DIURETIC

Common adverse effects in *italic;* life-threatening effects <u>underlined;</u> generic names in **bold;** classifications in SMALL CAPS; ♣ Canadian drug name; ⊙ Prototype drug

Therapeutic: DIURETIC; ANTIHYPER-
TENSIVE
**Prototype:** Furosemide

## AVAILABILITY Tablet; injection

## ACTION & *THERAPEUTIC EFFECT*
Sulfonamide derivative that causes
both potassium and magnesium
loss. Inhibits sodium and chloride
reabsorption by direct action on
proximal ascending limb of the
loop of Henle. Also appears to inhibit phosphate and bicarbonate
reabsorption. *Produces only mild
hypotensive effects at usual diuretic
doses. Controls formation of edema.*

## USES Edema, heart failure.

## UNLABELED USES Ascites, hyper-
calcemia, hypertension.

## CONTRAINDICATIONS Hyper-
sensitivity to bumetanide or to other sulfonamides; anuria, markedly
elevated BUN; hepatic coma;
ventricular arrhythmias; severe
electrolyte deficiency; lactation.

## CAUTIOUS USE Hepatic cirrho-
sis; renal impairment; severe renal
disease; history of gout; history of
pancreatitis; history of hypersensitivity to furosemide; diabetes mellitus;
acute MI; older adults; pregnancy
(category C).

## ROUTE & DOSAGE

### Edema
*Adult:* **PO** 0.5–2 mg once/day,
may repeat at 4–5 h intervals if
needed (max: 10 mg/day); **IV/
IM** 0.5–1 mg over 1–2 min,
repeated q2–3h prn (max:
10 mg/day)

## ADMINISTRATION

### Oral
- Give with food or milk to reduce
  risk of gastrointestinal irritation.
- Administered in the morning as a
  single dose, either daily or by intermittent schedule.

### Intramuscular
- Use undiluted solution for injection.

### Intravenous

*PREPARE:* **Direct/Continuous:** Give
direct IV undiluted (typical) or
diluted for infusion with D5W,
NS, LR.
*ADMINISTER:* **Direct:** Give IV push
at a rate of a single dose over 1–2
min. **Continuous:** Give diluted
solution over 1–2 min or at prescribed rate.
*INCOMPATIBILITIES:* Solution/ad-
ditive: **Dobutamine. Y-site:
Amphotericin B, azathio-
prine, chlorpromazine, dantrolene, diazepam, diazoxide,
fenoldopam, ganciclovir, gemtuzumab, haloperidol, midazolam, minocycline, ofloxacin,
oritavancin, papaverine, phenytoin, quinupristin/dalfo-
pristin, sulfamethoxazole/tri-
methoprim.**
- Diluted infusion should be used
  within 24 h after preparation.

- Store in tight, light-resistant container at 15°–30° C (59°–86° F) unless otherwise directed.

## ADVERSE EFFECTS (≥1%) **Body
as a Whole:** Sweating, hyperventilation, glycosuria. **CNS:** Dizziness, headache, weakness, fatigue. **CV:** Hypotension, ECG
changes, chest pain, *hypovolemia*. **GI:** Nausea, vomiting, abdominal or stomach pain, GI distress, diarrhea, dry mouth.

Common adverse effects in *italic;* life-threatening effects underlined; generic names
in **bold;** classifications in SMALL CAPS; ♣ Canadian drug name; ⊘ Prototype drug

221

**B**

**Metabolic:** *Hypokalemia,* hyponatremia, hyperuricemia, hyperglycemia; *hypomagnesemia;* decreased calcium, chloride. **Musculoskeletal:** Muscle cramps, muscle pain, stiffness or tenderness; arthritic pain. **Special Senses:** Ear discomfort, ringing or buzzing in ears, impaired hearing.

**INTERACTIONS Drug:** AMINOGLYCOSIDES, **cisplatin** increase risk of ototoxicity; bumetanide increases risk of hypokalemia-induced **digoxin** toxicity; NONSTEROIDAL ANTI-INFLAMMATORY DRUGS (NSAIDS) may attenuate diuretic and hypotensive response; **probenecid** may antagonize diuretic activity; bumetanide may decrease renal elimination of **lithium; sotalol** may increase risk of cardiotoxicity.

**PHARMACOKINETICS Absorption:** Readily from GI tract. **Onset:** 30–60 min PO; 40 min IV. **Peak:** 0.5–2 h. **Duration:** 4–6 h. **Distribution:** Distributed into breast milk. **Metabolism:** In liver. **Elimination:** 80% in urine in 48 h, 10–20% in feces. **Half-Life:** 60–90 min.

## NURSING IMPLICATIONS

### Black Box Warning

*Bumetanide has been associated with profound diuresis resulting in serious fluid and electrolyte imbalances.*

### Assessment & Drug Effects

- Monitor I&O and report onset of oliguria or other changes in I&O ratio and pattern promptly.

- Monitor weight, BP, and pulse rate. Assess for hypovolemia by taking BP and pulse rate while patient is lying, sitting, and standing. Older adults are particularly at risk for hypovolemia with resulting thrombi and emboli.
- Monitor for S&S of hypomagnesemia and hypokalemia (see Appendix F) especially in those receiving digitalis or who have CHF, hepatic cirrhosis, ascites, diarrhea, or potassium-depleting nephropathy.
- Monitor for hearing difficulty or ear discomfort. Patients at risk of ototoxic effects include those receiving the drug IV, especially at high doses, those with severely impaired renal function, and those receiving other potentially ototoxic or nephrotoxic drugs (see Appendix F).
- Monitor diabetics for loss of glycemic control.
- Monitor lab tests: Baseline and periodic serum electrolytes, blood studies (for dyscrasias), LFTs and kidney function tests, uric acid (particularly patients with history of gout), and blood glucose.

### Patient & Family Education

- Report promptly to prescriber symptoms of electrolyte imbalance (e.g., weakness, dizziness, fatigue, faintness, confusion, muscle cramps, headache, paresthesias).
- Eat potassium-rich foods such as fruit juices, potatoes, cereals, skim milk, and bananas while taking bumetanide.
- Report S&S of ototoxicity promptly to prescriber (see Appendix F).
- Monitor blood glucose for loss of glycemic control if diabetic.

# BUPRENORPHINE HYDROCHLORIDE

(byoo-pre-nor′feen)

Buprenex, Butrans, Suboxone

**Classifications:** ANALGESIC; NARCOTIC (OPIATE AGONIST–ANTAGONIST)
Therapeutic: NARCOTIC ANALGESIC
**Prototype:** Pentazocine
**Controlled Substance:** Schedule III

**AVAILABILITY** Injection; sublingual tablet; transdermal patch

## ACTION & *THERAPEUTIC EFFECT*

Opiate agonist antagonist with agonist activity approximately 30 × that of morphine and antagonist activity equal to or up to 3 × that of naloxone. Respiratory depression occurs infrequently, probably due to drug's opiate antagonist activity. *Dose-related analgesia results from a high affinity of buprenorphine for mu-opioid receptors and as an antagonist at the kappa-opiate receptors in the CNS. Naloxone is an antagonist at the mu-opioid receptor.*

**USES** *Injectable* used for moderate to severe pain. *Sublingual tablets* used for treatment of opioid dependence.

**UNLABELED USES** *Injectable* to reverse fentanyl-induced anesthesia. *Sublingual tablets* may be used to ease cocaine withdrawal.

**CONTRAINDICATIONS** Hypersensitivity to buprenorphine; significant respiratory depression; acute or severe bronchial asthma without resuscitative equipment; paralytic ileus; severe hepatic impairment; lactation.

**CAUTIOUS USE** Patient with history of opiate use or substance abuse; family or personal history of alcohol dependency or mental illness; unstable cardiac status; personal or family history of QT prolongation; compromised respiratory function [e.g., COPD, cor pulmonale, decreased respiratory reserve, hypoxia, hypercapnia, or preexisting respiratory depression]; hypothyroidism, myxedema, adenal insufficient including Addison's disease; severe renal impairment; mild to moderate hepatic impairment; geriatric or debilitated patients; acute alcoholism, delirium tremens; hypovolemia; cardiovascular disease including acute MI, prostatic hypertrophy, urethral stricture; comatose patient; patients with CNS depression, head injury, or intracranial lesion; history of seizures, biliary tract dysfunction; old er or debilitated adults; pregnancy (category C). Safety and efficacy in children not established.

## ROUTE & DOSAGE

### Postoperative Pain

*Adult/Adolescent (13 y or older):*
**IV/IM** 0.3 mg q6h up to 0.6 mg q4h or 25–50 mcg/h by IV infusion
*Geriatric:* **IV/IM** 0.15 mg q6h
*Child (2–12 y):* **IV/IM** 2–6 mcg/kg q4–6h prn

### Opioid Dependence/Cocaine Withdrawal

*Adult/Adolescent:* **SL** Initiate with 8 mg daily on day 1 at

Common adverse effects in *italic;* life-threatening effects underlined; generic names in **bold;** classifications in SMALL CAPS; ♣ Canadian drug name; ⊙ Prototype drug

223

least 4 h after last opioid dose, 16 mg daily on day 2, then switch to maintenance therapy at the same buprenorphine dose as day 2 (e.g., 16 mg daily). Adjust dose daily until opiate withdrawal effects are suppressed. Maintenance dose range 4–24 mg/day buprenorphine.

**Moderate to Severe Pain**

*Adult:* **Topical** One 5 mcg/h patch q7days (titrate at minimum interval of 72 h)

## ADMINISTRATION

### Sublingual

- Place sublingual tablets under tongue until dissolved. For doses requiring more than two tablets, place all tablets at once under tongue, or if patient cannot accommodate all tablets, place two tablets at a time under tongue.
- Instruct to hold the tablets under tongue until dissolved; advise not to swallow.

### Transdermal

- Apply only to intact, hairless or nearly hairless skin. If needed, clip (but do not shave) hair from skin. Prior to application, clean site with clear water and allow to dry completely; do not use soaps, alcohol, oils, or lotions on application site.
- Each system is worn for 7 days. May apply to upper outer arm, upper chest, upper back, or the side of the chest. Tape edges in place if needed.
- Rotate sites. Must wait at least 21 days before reusing a skin site.

### Intramuscular

- Give undiluted, deep IM into a large muscle.

### Intravenous

*PREPARE:* **Direct/IV Infusion:** May be given undiluted direct IV or further dilute each 1 mL (0.3 mg) ampule in 50 mL of D5W, NS, D5NS, or LR to yield 6 mcg/mL for infusion. • Do not use if discolored or contains particulate matter.

*ADMINISTER:* **Direct:** Give slowly at a rate of 0.3 mg over 2 min to a patient in a recumbent position. **IV Infusion:** Give by slow infusion over 3 min or longer depending on volume of IV solution.

*INCOMPATIBILITIES:* **Solution/additive: Diltiazem, floxacillin, furosemide, lorazepam. Y-site: Alemtuzumab, aminophylline, amphotericin B cholesteryl sulfate complex, ampicillin, azathioprine, dantrolene, diazepam, diazoxide, doxorubicin liposome, fluorouracil, gemtuzumab, indomethacin, lansoprazole pantoprazole, pentobarbital, phenobarbital, phenytoin, sodium bicarbonate, SMZ/TMP.**

- Store at 15°–30° C (59°–86° F); avoid freezing.

## ADVERSE EFFECTS (≥1%) CNS:
*Sedation, drowsiness,* dizziness, vertigo, *headache,* amnesia, euphoria, asthenia, *insomnia, pain* (when used for withdrawal), *withdrawal symptoms.* **CV:** Hypotension, vasodilation. **Special Senses:** Miosis. **GI:** *Nausea,* vomiting, diarrhea, *constipation.* **Respiratory:** Respiratory depression, hyperventilation. **Skin:** Pruritus, injection site reactions, *sweating.*

**INTERACTIONS Drug: Alcohol,** OPIATES, other CNS DEPRESSANTS, BENZODIAZEPINES augment CNS depression; **diazepam** may cause respiratory or cardiovascular collapse; AZOLE ANTIFUNGALS (e.g., **fluconazole**), MACROLIDE ANTIBIOTICS (e.g., **erythromycin**), and PROTEASE INHIBITORS (e.g., **saquinavir**) may increase buprenorphine levels.

**PHARMACOKINETICS Absorption:** Widely variable sublingual absorption. **Onset:** 10–30 min IM/IV. **Peak:** 1 h IM/IV; 2–6 h SL. **Duration:** 6–10 h. **Metabolism:** Extensively in liver by CYP3A4 to active metabolite norbuprenorphine. **Elimination:** 70% in feces, 30% in urine in 7 days. **Half-Life:** 2.2 h IM/IV; 37 h SL.

## NURSING IMPLICATIONS

### Black Box Warning

*Buprenorphine has been associated with severe, potentially fatal respiratory depression; it also has a high potential for abuse. Prolonged use during pregnancy can cause life-threatening neonatal withdrawal syndrome.*

### Assessment & Drug Effects

- Monitor respiratory status during therapy. Buprenorphine-induced respiratory depression is about equal to that produced by 10 mg morphine, but onset is slower, and if it occurs, it lasts longer.
- Monitor I&O ratio and pattern: Urinary retention is a potential adverse effect.
- Supervise ambulation; drowsiness occurs in 66% of patients taking this drug.

- Monitor lab tests: Baseline LFTs and renal function tests.

### Patient & Family Education

- Do not drive or engage in other potentially hazardous activities until response to drug is known.
- Do not use alcohol or other CNS depressing drugs without consulting prescriber. An additive effect exists between buprenorphine hydrochloride and other CNS depressants including alcohol.

## BUPROPION HYDROCHLORIDE
(byoo-pro'pi-on)

Budeprion XL, Forfivo XL, Wellbutrin, Wellbutrin SR, Wellbutrin XL, Zyban

## BUPROPION HYDROBROMIDE
Aplenzin

**Classification:** ANTIDEPRESSANT
**Therapeutic:** ANTIDEPRESSANT

**AVAILABILITY** Tablet; sustained release tablet; extended release tablet; hydrobromide form

## ACTION & *THERAPEUTIC EFFECT*
The neurochemical mechanism of bupropion is not fully understood. It selectively inhibits the neuronal reuptake of dopamine and norepinephrine, but does not inhibit monoamine oxidase or reuptake serotonin. The primary action is thought to be dopaminergic and/or noradrenergic. *Its antidepressive effect is related to dopaminergic or noradrenergic properties.*

**USES** Depression, smoking cessation, seasonal affective disorder.

Common adverse effects in *italic;* life-threatening effects underlined; generic names in **bold;** classifications in SMALL CAPS; ✤ Canadian drug name; ● Prototype drug

225

**UNLABELED USES** Neuropathic pain, ADHD.

**CONTRAINDICATIONS** Hypersensitivity to bupropion; seizure disorder; current or prior diagnosis of bulimia or anorexia nervosa; suicidal ideation; concurrent 14 days of MAO inhibitor use; head trauma; CNS tumor; recent MI; abrupt discontinuation, lactation.

**CAUTIOUS USE** Renal or hepatic function impairment; drug abuse or dependence; hypertension, CHF, MI, renal impairment; severe hepatic impairment, hepatic disease, biliary cirrhosis; suicidal tendencies; major depressive disorders (MDD); bipolar disorder, mania, psychosis, schizophrenia; DM; ethanol intoxication, tics, Tourette's syndrome; older adults; pregnancy (category C); children younger than 18 y.

## ROUTE & DOSAGE

**Depression/Seasonal Affective Disorder**

*Adult:* **PO Immediate release** 100 mg b.i.d. then titrate to 100 mg t.i.d.; **Sustained release** 150 mg daily then titrate to 150 mg b.i.d. (or 300 mg daily Wellbutrin SR); **Aplenzin:** 174 mg daily can increase to 348 mg daily (max: 522 mg/day)
*Geriatric:* **PO** May require reduced initial dose

**Smoking Cessation**

*Adult:* **PO** Start with 150 mg once daily × 3 days, then increase to 150 mg b.i.d. (max: 300 mg/day) for 7–12 wk

**Hepatic Impairment Dosage Adjustment**

Start at lower dose, decrease dose or dosage frequency

## ADMINISTRATION
**Oral**
- Administer as a single dose in the morning. May be given with or without food.
- Immediate release tablets should be given at approximately 6-h intervals, or longer as directed.
- Ensure that extended release and sustained release tablets are not chewed or crushed. They **must be** swallowed whole.
- Store away from heat, direct light, and moisture.

**ADVERSE EFFECTS (≥1%) Body as a Whole:** Weight loss, weight gain. **CNS:** Seizures. The risk of seizure appears to be strongly associated with dose (especially greater than 450 mg/day) *agitation, insomnia, dry mouth, blurred vision, headache, dizziness, tremor.* **GI:** *Nausea, vomiting, constipation.* **CV:** Tachycardia. **Respiratory:** Pharyngitis. **Skin:** Rash, diaphoresis.

**INTERACTIONS Drug:** May increase metabolism of **carbamazepine, cimetidine, phenytoin, phenobarbital,** decreasing their effect; may increase incidence of adverse effects of **levodopa,** contraindicated with MAO INHIBITORS.

**PHARMACOKINETICS Absorption:** Readily from GI tract. **Onset:** 3–4 wk. **Peak:** 1–3 h. **Metabolism:** In liver to active metabolites by CYP2B6; may inhibit CYP2D6. **Elimination:** 80% in urine. **Half-Life:** 8–24 h.

## NURSING IMPLICATIONS

### Black Box Warning

*Bupropion has been associated with increased risk of suicidal thoughts and behavior in children, adolescents, and young adults. Serious neuropsychiatric events have occurred in patients during use and during treatment discontinuation.*

### Assessment & Drug Effects

- Monitor for therapeutic effectiveness. The full antidepressant effect of drug may not be realized for 4 or more weeks
- Monitor for and report promptly worsening of depression or suicidal ideation.
- Monitor respiratory status and report promptly S&S of respiratory depression.
- Monitor blood pressure prior to initiation of treatment and periodically.
- Use extreme caution when administering drug to patient with history of seizures, cranial trauma, or other factors predisposing to seizures; during sudden and large increments in dose, seizure potential is increased.
- Report significant restlessness, agitation, anxiety, and insomnia. Symptoms may require treatment or discontinuation of drug.
- Monitor for and report delusions, hallucinations, psychotic episodes, confusion, and paranoia.
- Monitor lab tests: Periodic renal function tests and LFTs.

### Patient & Family Education

- Monitor weight at least weekly. Report significant changes in weight (±5 lb) to prescriber.
- Minimize or avoid alcohol because it increases the risk of seizures.

- Report promptly suicidal thoughts, especially when treated for depression.
- Do not drive or engage in potentially hazardous activities until response to drug is known because judgment or motor and cognitive skills may be impaired.
- Do not abruptly discontinue drug. Gradual dosage reduction may be necessary to prevent adverse effects.
- Do not take any OTC drugs without consulting prescriber.

## BUSPIRONE HYDROCHLORIDE

(byoo-spye'rone)

BuSpar

**Classification:** ANXIOLYTIC
**Therapeutic:** ANTIANXIETY
**Prototype:** Lorazepam

**AVAILABILITY** Tablet

**ACTION & *THERAPEUTIC EFFECT***
An anxiolytic with agonist effects on presynaptic dopamine receptors and also a high affinity for serotonin (5-HT$_{1A}$) receptors. *Antianxiety effect is due to serotonin reuptake inhibition and agonist effects on dopamine receptors of the brain.*

**USES** Management of anxiety disorders and for short-term treatment of generalized anxiety.

**UNLABELED USES** Adjuvant for nicotine withdrawal, premenstrual syndrome.

**CONTRAINDICATIONS** Concomitant use of MAOI therapy; lactation.

**CAUTIOUS USE** Moderate to severe renal or hepatic impairment, pregnancy (category B); children less than 18 y.

Common adverse effects in *italic;* life-threatening effects underlined; generic names in **bold;** classifications in SMALL CAPS; ♣ Canadian drug name; ☻ Prototype drug

227

## ROUTE & DOSAGE

### Anxiety

*Adult:* **PO** 7.5–15 mg/day in divided doses, may increase by 5 mg/day q2–3days as needed (max: 60 mg/day)
*Geriatric:* **PO** 5 mg b.i.d., may increase dose (max: 60 mg/day)

## ADMINISTRATION

### Oral

- Give with food to decrease nausea.
- Store at 15°–30° C (59°–86° F) in tightly closed container unless otherwise directed.

## ADVERSE EFFECTS (≥1%) **CNS:**
Numbness, paresthesia, tremors, *dizziness, headache,* nervousness, *drowsiness,* lightheadedness, dream disturbances, decreased concentration, excitement, mood changes. **CV:** Tachycardia, palpitation. **Special Senses:** Blurred vision. **GI:** *Nausea,* vomiting, dry mouth, abdominal/gastric distress, diarrhea, constipation. **Urogenital:** Urinary frequency, hesitancy. **Musculoskeletal:** Arthralgias. **Respiratory:** Hyperventilation, shortness of breath. **Skin:** Rash, edema, pruritus, flushing, easy bruising, hair loss, dry skin. **Other:** Fatigue, weakness.

## DIAGNOSTIC TEST INTERFERENCE
Buspirone may increase serum concentrations of *hepatic aminotransferases (ALT, AST).*

## INTERACTIONS **Drug:** May cause hypertension with MAO INHIBITORS, **trazodone,** possible increase in liver transaminases; increased **haloperidol** serum levels. **Food: Grapefruit juice** may increase drug levels. **Herbal: St. John's wort** may increase drug levels.

## PHARMACOKINETICS **Absorption:** Readily from GI tract, undergoes first pass metabolism. **Onset:** 5–7 days. **Peak:** 1 h. **Metabolism:** In liver. **Elimination:** 30–63% in urine as metabolites within 24 h. **Half-Life:** 2–4 h.

## NURSING IMPLICATIONS

### Assessment & Drug Effects

- Monitor for therapeutic effectiveness. Desired response may begin within 7–10 days; however, optimal results take 3–4 wk. Reinforce the importance of continuing treatment to patient.
- Monitor for and report dystonia, motor restlessness, and involuntary repetitious movement of facial or cervical muscle.
- Observe for and report swollen ankles, decreased urinary output, changes in voiding pattern, jaundice, itching, nausea, or vomiting.

### Patient & Family Education

- Report any of the following immediately: Involuntary, repetitive movements of face or neck; weakness, nervousness, nightmares, headache, or blurred vision; depression or thoughts of suicide.
- Do not use OTC drugs without advice of the prescriber while taking buspirone.
- Do not drive or engage in other potentially hazardous activities until response to drug is known.
- Discuss limits of alcohol intake with prescriber; cautious use is generally advised.

## BUSULFAN
(byoo-sul'fan)
Busulfex, Myleran
**Classifications:** ANTINEOPLASTIC; ALKYLATING AGENT
Therapeutic: ANTINEOPLASTIC
**Prototype:** Cyclophosphamide

**AVAILABILITY** Tablet; injection

**ACTION & *THERAPEUTIC EFFECT***
Potent cytotoxic alkylating agent thought to bring about changes in DNA that block replication and cause its cytotoxic effects. *Causes cell death in slowly proliferating stem cells.*

**USES** Chronic myelogenous leukemia, stem cell transplant preparation.

**CONTRAINDICATIONS** Therapy-resistant chronic lymphocytic leukemia; lymphoblastic crisis of chronic myelogenous leukemia; bone marrow depression, immunizations (patient and household members), chickenpox (including recent exposure), herpetic infections; pregnancy (category D); lactation.

**CAUTIOUS USE** Men and women in childbearing years; hepatic disease; history of gout or urate renal stones; prior irradiation or chemotherapy.

**ROUTE & DOSAGE**

**Chronic Myelogenous Leukemia**
*Adult:* **PO** 4–8 mg/day or 1.8–4 mg/m² daily until maximal clinical and hematologic improvement, may use 1–4 mg/day if remission is shorter than 3 mo
*Child:* **PO** 0.06–0.12 mg/kg/day or 1.8–4.6 mg/m² as a daily dose

**Stem Cell Transplant Preparation**
*Adult:* **IV** (used with cyclophosphamide) 0.8 mg/kg IBW or ABW (whichever is lower) q6h × 4 days

*Obesity Dosage Adjustment*
In obese patients, use adjusted ideal body weight = IBW + 0.25 × (actual weight − IBW)

**ADMINISTRATION**
**Oral**
- Hazardous agent; NIOSH recommends single gloving for administration of intact tablets. If manipulation of tablets is necessary (e.g., to prepare in an oral solution) double glove, wear protective gown, and prepare in controlled device.
- Give at same time each day.
- Give on an empty stomach to minimize nausea and vomiting.
- Store in tightly capped, light-resistant container at 15°–30° C (59°–86° F), unless otherwise specified.

**Intravenous**
***PREPARE: Intermittent:*** Prepare a volume of NS or D5W IV solution that is 10 × the volume of busulfan needed. ▪ Using a 5 micron nylon filter (supplied), withdraw the needed dose of busulfan. Remove needle and filter and use a new, nonfiltered needle to add busulfan to the IV fluid. (Always add busulfan to IV fluid rather than IV fluid to busulfan.) ▪ Mix by inverting the IV bag several times.
***ADMINISTER: Intermittent:*** Infuse via a central venous catheter over 2 h. ▪ Flush line before/after infusion with at least 5 mL D5W or NS.

**ADVERSE EFFECTS** (≥1%) **Hematologic:** Major toxic effects are related to bone marrow failure; agranulocytosis (rare), pancytopenia, thrombocytopenia, leukopenia, *anemia.* **Urogenital:** Flank pain, renal calculi, uric acid nephropathy, acute

Common adverse effects in *italic;* life-threatening effects underlined; generic names in **bold;** classifications in SMALL CAPS; ♣ Canadian drug name; ⊙ Prototype drug

229

renal failure, gynecomastia, testicular atrophy, azoospermia, impotence, sterility in males, ovarian suppression, menstrual changes, amenorrhea (potentially irreversible), menopausal symptoms. **Respiratory:** Irreversible pulmonary fibrosis ("busulfan lung"). **Gastrointestinal:** *Vomiting, nausea, mucositis, stomatitis, anorexia.* **Skin:** Alopecia, hyperpigmentation. **Other:** Endocardial fibrosis, dizziness, cholestatic jaundice, infections.

## DIAGNOSTIC TEST INTERFERENCE
Busulfan may decrease *urinary 17-OHCS* excretion, and may increase *blood and urine uric acid* levels.

## INTERACTIONS
**Drug: Probenecid, sulfinpyrazone** may increase uric acid levels. Do not administer LIVE VACCINES. **Herbal:** Do not use with echinacea.

## PHARMACOKINETICS
**Absorption:** Readily from GI tract. **Peak:** 4 h. **Duration:** 4 h. **Metabolism:** In liver by CYP3A4. **Elimination:** 10–50% in urine within 48 h.

## NURSING IMPLICATIONS

### Black Box Warning

*Busulfan can cause severe bone marrow hypoplasia. Malignant tumors and acute leukemias have been associated with this drug.*

### Assessment & Drug Effects
- Withhold drug and notify prescriber immediately at the first sign of abnormal decrease in any of the formed elements of the blood.
- Monitor the following: Vital signs, weight, I&O ratio and pattern. Urge patient to increase fluid intake to 10–12 (8 oz) glasses daily

(if allowed) to assure adequate urinary output.
- Monitor for and report symptoms suggestive of superinfection (see Appendix F), particularly when patient develops leukopenia.
- Avoid invasive procedures during periods of platelet count depression.
- Monitor lab tests: Baseline and weekly Hgb, Hct, WBC with differential, platelet count; LFTs, kidney function, serum uric acid as needed, serum bilirubin (total and direct).

### Patient & Family Education
- Report to prescriber any of the following: Easy bruising or bleeding, cloudy or pink urine, dark or black stools; sore mouth or throat, unusual fatigue, blurred vision, flank or joint pain, swelling of lower legs and feet; yellowing white of eye, dark urine, light-colored stools, abdominal discomfort, or itching (hepatotoxicity).
- Use contraceptive measures during busulfan therapy and for at least 3 mo after drug is withdrawn.

## BUTABARBITAL SODIUM
(byoo-ta-bar'bi-tal)

Butisol Sodium

**Classifications:** BARBITURATE; ANXIOLYTIC; SEDATIVE-HYPNOTIC
Therapeutic: ANTIANXIETY; SEDATIVE-HYPNOTIC
**Prototype:** Phenobarbital
**Controlled Substance:** Schedule III

## AVAILABILITY
Tablet

## ACTION & THERAPEUTIC EFFECT
Intermediate-acting barbiturate that appears to act at thalamus level of the brain, where it interferes with transmission of impulses to the cerebral cortex. *Preoperative sedative agent that also is an effective antianxiety agent.*

Common adverse effects in *italic;* life-threatening effects underlined; generic names in **bold;** classifications in SMALL CAPS; ♣ Canadian drug name; ◉ Prototype drug

**USES** Sedation induction and maintenance.

**CONTRAINDICATIONS** Hypersensitivity to barbituates, history of or latent porphyria; uncontrolled pain; severe respiratory disease; history of addiction; lactation.

**CAUTIOUS USE** Severe renal or hepatic impairment; acute abdominal conditions; head trauma, history of seizures; history of suicide or depression; history of herpes infection; older adults or debilitated patients; pregnancy (category C).

## ROUTE & DOSAGE

**Daytime Sedation**
Adult: **PO** 15–30 mg t.i.d. or q.i.d.

**Preoperative Sedation**
Adult: **PO** 50–100 mg 60–90 min before surgery
Child: **PO** 2–6 mg/kg/dose (max: 100 mg)

## ADMINISTRATION
Oral
- Take on an empty stomach (i.e., 1 h before or 2 h after a meal).
- Schedule slow withdrawal following long-term use to avoid precipitating withdrawal symptoms.
- Store at 20°–25° C (68°–77° F).

**ADVERSE EFFECTS** (≥1%) **CNS:** Drowsiness, *residual sedation* ("hangover"), headache.

**INTERACTIONS Drug: Alcohol** and other CNS DEPRESSANTS add to CNS and respiratory depression; butabarbital increases the metabolism of ORAL ANTICOAGULANTS, BETA-BLOCKERS, CORTICOSTEROIDS, **doxycycline, griseofulvin, quinidine,** THEOPHYLLINES, ORAL CONTRACEPTIVES, decreasing their effectiveness. **Herbal: Kava, valerian** may potentiate sedation.

**PHARMACOKINETICS Absorption:** Readily from GI tract. **Onset:** 40–60 min. **Peak:** 3–4 h. **Duration:** 6–8 h. **Distribution:** Crosses placenta; distributed into breast milk. **Metabolism:** In liver. **Elimination:** In urine primarily as metabolites. **Half-Life:** Average 100 h.

## NURSING IMPLICATIONS
### Assessment & Drug Effects
- Assess for adverse effects. Older adults and debilitated patients sometimes manifest excitement, confusion, or depression. Children also may react with paradoxical excitement. Side rails may be advisable. Report these reactions to prescriber.

### Patient & Family Education
- Do not drive or engage in other potentially hazardous activities until response to drug is known.
- Do not drink alcoholic beverages while taking this drug. Other CNS depressants may produce additive drowsiness; do not take without approval of prescriber.

## BUTENAFINE HYDROCHLORIDE
(bu-ten'a-feen)
Lotrimin Ultra, Mentax
**Classification:** ANTIFUNGAL ANTIBIOTIC
**Therapeutic:** ANTIFUNGAL
**Prototype:** Terbinafine

**AVAILABILITY** Cream

## ACTION & THERAPEUTIC EFFECT
Exerts antifungal action by inhibiting fungal sterol synthesis that is needed in formation of the fungal cell membrane. *Antifungal effectiveness against interdigital tinea pedis (athlete's foot), tinea corporis (ringworm), and tinea cruris (jock itch).*

Common adverse effects in *italic;* life-threatening effects underlined; generic names in **bold;** classifications in SMALL CAPS; ✦ Canadian drug name; ⊙ Prototype drug

231

**USES** Treatment of tinea pedis, tinea corporis, and tinea cruris.

**CONTRAINDICATIONS** Hypersensitivity to butenafine; ophthalmic or vaginal administration.

**CAUTIOUS USE** Hypersensitivity to naftifine or tolnaftate; pregnancy (category B); lactation; children younger than 12 y.

## ROUTE & DOSAGE

**Tinea Pedis**

*Adult/Child (12 y or older):*
**Topical** Apply to affected area and surrounding skin b.i.d. × 7 days or daily × 4 wk

**Tinea Corporis, Tinea Cruris**

*Adult/Child (younger than 12 y):*
**Topical** Apply to affected area and surrounding skin once daily

## ADMINISTRATION

**Topical**
- Apply sufficient cream to cover affected skin and surrounding areas.
- Do not use occlusive dressing unless specifically directed to do so.
- Store at 5°–30° C (41°–86° F).

**ADVERSE EFFECTS** (≥1%) **Skin:** Burning/stinging at application site, contact dermatitis, erythema, irritation, itching.

## NURSING IMPLICATIONS

**Assessment & Drug Effects**
- Note: 2–4 wk of therapy are usually required for effective treatment.

**Patient & Family Education**
- Discontinue medication and notify prescriber if irritation or sensitivity develops.
- Avoid contact with mucous membranes.
- Wash hands thoroughly before and after application of cream.

# BUTOCONAZOLE NITRATE

(byoo-toe-koe′na-zole)

Femstat 3, Gynazole 1

**Classification:** AZOLE ANTIFUNGAL ANTIBIOTIC

Therapeutic: ANTIFUNGAL

**Prototype:** Fluconazole

## AVAILABILITY Cream

## ACTION & *THERAPEUTIC EFFECT*

Imidazole derivative with antifungal activity. Alters fungal cell membrane permeability, permitting loss of essential intra-cellular constituents with consequent loss of ability to replicate. *Has fungicidal effect as well as effectiveness against some gram-positive bacteria.*

**USES** Local treatment of vulvovaginal candidiasis.

**CAUTIOUS USE** Hypersensitivity to azole antifungals; HIV patients; diabetes mellitus; pregnancy (category C); lactation; children less than 12 y.

## ROUTE & DOSAGE

**Vulvovaginal Candidiasis**

*Adult:* **Topical** 1 applicator full intravaginally at bedtime for 3 days, may be extended another 3 days if needed

*Pregnant women:* **Topical** 1 applicator full intravaginally at bedtime for 6 days

## ADMINISTRATION

**Topical Intravaginal**
- Continue treatment even during menstruation.
- Store medication at 15°–30° C (59°–86° F); avoid extreme temperature and freezing.

Common adverse effects in *italic;* life-threatening effects underlined; generic names in **bold;** classifications in SMALL CAPS; ♣ Canadian drug name; ☻ Prototype drug

**ADVERSE EFFECTS** (≥1%) **Urogenital:** Vulvar or vaginal burning, vulvar itching, discharge, soreness, swelling; urinary frequency and burning. **Skin:** Itching of fingers. **CNS:** Headache.

**PHARMACOKINETICS Absorption:** Small amount absorbed systemically from intravaginal administration. **Distribution:** Crosses placenta in animals. **Metabolism:** In liver. **Elimination:** In both urine and feces within 4–7 days. **Half-Life:** 21–24 h.

## NURSING IMPLICATIONS

### Assessment & Drug Effects
- Monitor for therapeutic effectiveness. Candidiasis in nonpregnant women is usually controlled in 3 days.

### Patient & Family Education
- Take medication exactly as prescribed; do not increase or decrease dosage or discontinue or extend treatment period. Contact prescriber if symptoms (vaginal burning, discharge, or itching) persist; drug may be discontinued if acute irritation occurs.
- Patient's sexual partner should wear a condom during intercourse.

## BUTORPHANOL TARTRATE
(byoo-tor'fa-nole)

Stadol, Stadol NS

**Classifications:** ANALGESIC; NARCOTIC (OPIATE AGONIST-ANTAGONIST)
**Therapeutic:** NARCOTIC ANALGESIC
**Prototype:** PENTAZOCINE
**Controlled Substance:** Schedule IV

**AVAILABILITY** Solution for injection; spray

## ACTION & *THERAPEUTIC EFFECT*
Synthetic, centrally acting analgesic that acts as agonist on one type of opioid receptor and as a competitive antagonist at others. Site of analgesic action believed to be subcortical, possibly in the limbic system of the brain. Respiratory depression does not increase appreciably with higher doses, as it does with morphine, but duration of action increases. *Narcotic analgesic that relieves moderate to severe pain.*

**USES** Relief of moderate to severe pain, preoperative or preanesthetic sedation and analgesia, obstetric analgesia during labor, cancer pain, renal colic, burns.

**UNLABELED USES** Musculoskeletal and post-episiotomy pain.

**CONTRAINDICATIONS** Narcotic-dependent patients; opiate agonist hypersensitivity.

**CAUTIOUS USE** History of drug abuse or dependence; emotionally unstable individuals; head injury, increased intracranial pressure; acute MI, ventricular dysfunction, coronary insufficiency, hypertension; patients undergoing biliary tract surgery; respiratory depression, bronchial asthma, obstructive respiratory disease; and renal or hepatic dysfunction; prior to labor, pregnancy (category C). Safe use in children under 18 y not established.

## ROUTE & DOSAGE

| Pain Relief |
|---|
| *Adult:* **IM** 1–4 mg q3–4h as needed (max: 4 mg/dose); **IV** 0.5–2 mg q3–4h as needed |

Common adverse effects in *italic;* life-threatening effects underlined; generic names in **bold;** classifications in SMALL CAPS; ♣ Canadian drug name; ⊘ Prototype drug

233

**B**

*Geriatric:* **IM/IV** 0.25–1 mg q6–8h; **Intranasal** 1 mg (1 spray) in one nostril, may repeat in 90 sec, then may repeat these 2 doses q3–4h prn

**Adjunct to Balanced Anesthesia**

*Adult:* **IV** 2 mg before induction or 0.5–1 mg in increments during anesthesia

**Labor**

*Adult:* **IV/IM** 1–2 mg may repeat in 4 h

*Renal Impairment Dosage Adjustment*

*GFR less than 10 mL/min:* Use 50% of dose

*Hepatic Impairment Dosage Adjustment*

Use half normal dose and at least 6 h interval

## ADMINISTRATION

**Intranasal**
- Give 1 spray into one nostril only. One spray provides a 1 mg dose.

**Intramuscular**
- Give preoperative IM injection 60–90 min before surgery.

**Intravenous**

**PREPARE: Direct:** Give undiluted.
**ADMINISTER: Direct:** Give at a rate of 2 mg over 3–5 min.
**INCOMPATIBILITIES: Y-site: Amphotericin B cholesteryl, lansoprazole, midazolam.**

- Store at 15°–30° C (59°–86° F) unless otherwise directed. Protect from light.

## ADVERSE EFFECTS (≥1%) CNS:
Drowsiness, *sedation*, headache, vertigo, dizziness, floating feeling, weakness, lethargy, confusion, light-headedness, insomnia, nervousness, <u>respiratory depression</u>. **CV:** Palpitation, bradycardia. **GI:** Nausea. **Skin:** Clammy skin, tingling sensation, flushing and warmth, cyanosis of extremities, diaphoresis, sensitivity to cold, urticaria, pruritus. **Genitourinary:** Difficulty in urinating, biliary spasm.

**INTERACTIONS Drug: Alcohol** and other CNS DEPRESSANTS augment CNS and respiratory depression.

**PHARMACOKINETICS Onset:** 10–30 min IM; 1 min IV. **Peak:** 0.5–1 h IM; 4–5 min IV. **Duration:** 3–4 h IM; 2–4 h IV. **Distribution:** Crosses placenta; distributed into breast milk. **Metabolism:** In liver in inactive metabolites. **Elimination:** Primarily in urine. **Half-Life:** 3–4 h.

## NURSING IMPLICATIONS

### Assessment & Drug Effects
- Monitor for respiratory depression. Do not administer drug if respiratory rate is less than 12 breaths/min.
- Monitor vital signs. Report marked changes in BP or bradycardia.
- Note: If used during labor or delivery, observe neonate for signs of respiratory depression.
- Note: Drug can induce acute withdrawal symptoms in opiate-dependent patients.
- Drug is usually withdrawn gradually following chronic administration. Abrupt withdrawal may produce vomiting, loss of appetite, restlessness, abdominal cramps, increase in BP and temperature, mydriasis, faintness. Withdrawal symptoms peak 48 h after discontinuation of drug.

### Patient & Family Education
- Lie down to control drug-induced nausea.
- Do not take alcohol or other CNS depressants with this drug without consulting prescriber because of possible additive effects.

- Do not drive or engage in other potentially hazardous activities until response to drug is known.

# CABAZITAXEL
(ka-baz'i tax-el)

Jevtana

**Classifications:** ANTINEOPLASTIC; TAXANE; MICROTUBULE INHIBITOR
**Therapeutic:** ANTINEOPLASTIC; ANTIMICROTUBULE
**Prototype:** Paclitaxel

**AVAILABILITY** Solution for injection

**ACTIONS & THERAPEUTIC EFFECT**
Cabazitaxel binds to the microtubule network essential for interphase and mitosis of the cell cycle stabilizing the microtubules involved in cell division and preventing their normal functioning. *This antimicrotubular effect results in inhibition of mitosis in cancer cells.*

**USES** Treatment of prostate cancer.

**CONTRAINDICATIONS** Neutrophil count of 1500/mm³ or less; severe hypersensitivity to cabazitaxel or drugs formulated with polysorbate 80; severe hepatic impairment (total bilirubin more than 3 × ULN); pregnancy (category D); lactation.

**CAUTIOUS USE** Neutropenia; history of hypersensitivity reactions; GI distress (nausea, vomiting, diarrhea); renal or hepatic impairment; patients 65 y or greater. Safety and efficacy in children not established.

# ROUTE & DOSAGE

**Prostate Cancer**
*Adult:* **IV** 25 mg/m² over 1 h, repeat q3wk (max: 10 cycles)

## Toxicity Dosage Adjustment

*Grade 3 or greater neutropenia:* Delay treatment until ANC greater than 1500/mm³. Reduce dose to 20 mg/m². Use G-CSF for secondary prophylaxis.

*Patients who develop febrile neutropenia:* Delay treatment until improvement, and until ANC is greater than 1500/mm³. Reduce dose to 20 mg/m². Use G-CSF for secondary prophylaxis.

*Grade 3 or greater diarrhea or persisting diarrhea:* Delay treatment until improvement or resolution. Reduce dose to 20 mg/m². Discontinue cabazitaxel if toxicity persists with 20 mg/m² dose.

**Hepatic Impairment Dosage Adjustment**

*Total bilirubin 1–1.5 × ULN:* Reduce dose to 20 mg/m²

*Total bilirubin 1.5–3 × ULN:* Reduce dose to 15 mg/m²

*Total bilirubin more than 3 × ULN:* Should not be given to patients

# ADMINISTRATION

**Intravenous**
- Premedicate at least 30 min prior to each dose to avoid severe hypersensitivity: Dexamethasone 8 mg (or equivalent), dexchlorpheniramine 5 mg or diphenhydramine 25 mg, and ranitidine 50 mg (or equivalent). • This drug is a cytotoxic agent and caution should be used to prevent any contact with the drug. Follow institutional or standard guidelines for preparation, handling, and disposal of cytotoxic agents.

Common adverse effects in *italic;* life-threatening effects underlined; generic names in **bold;** classifications in SMALL CAPS; ✦ Canadian drug name; ☻ Prototype drug

235

**C**

*PREPARE:* **Continuous:** Prepare under aseptic conditions. **Do not** use infusion containers or equipment made with PVC or polyurethane. *First dilution:* Add all of the supplied diluent to the 60 mg vial of cabazitaxel. ▪ Direct flow of diluent onto inside wall of the cabazitaxel vial; inject slowly to limit foaming then invert vial gently for 45 sec to mix. ▪ Allow vial to stand until foam dissipates then inspect to ensure there are no visible particles. ▪ The resulting solution (10 mg/mL of cabazitaxel) should be further diluted within 30 min. *Second dilution:* Withdraw required dose and dilute in 250 mL or more of NS or D5W to yield a concentration no greater than 0.26 mg/mL. Solution should be clear without precipitate. ▪ Use immediately.
*ADMINISTER:* **Continuous:** Infuse over 1 h through a 0.22 micron in-line filter. **Do not** use tubing containing PVC or polyurethane. ▪ Monitor closely during infusion for S&S of hypersensitivity. Stop infusion immediately and institute supportive care should a hypersensitivity reaction occur.
*INCOMPATIBILITIES:* **Solution/additive:** Unknown. **Y-site:** Unknown.

▪ Store undiluted at 15°–30° C (59°–86° F). First dilution should be used immediately. Second dilution may be stored for 8 h at room temperature (including 1 h infusion time) or for a total of 24 h if refrigerated (including 1 h infusion time).

**ADVERSE EFFECTS** (≥5%) **Body as a Whole:** *Alopecia,* mucosal inflammation, pain, peripheral edema, *pyrexia.* **CNS:** *Asthenia,* dizziness, *dysgeusia, fatigue,* headache, *periphery neuropathy.* **CV:** Arrhythmia, hypotension. **GI:** *Abdominal pain,* *constipation, diarrhea,* dyspepsia, *nausea, vomiting.* **Hematological:** *Anemia,* febrile neutropenia, *leukopenia, neutropenia, thrombocytopenia.* **Metabolic:** *Anorexia,* dehydration, weight loss. **Musculoskeletal:** *Arthralgia, back pain,* muscle spasms. **Respiratory:** *Cough, dyspnea.* **Urogenital:** Dysuria, *hematuria,* urinary tract infections.

**INTERACTIONS Drug:** Coadministration of CYP3A4 inducers (e.g., **carbamazepine, phenobarbital, phenytoin, rifabutin, rifampin, rifapentine**) can decrease the levels of cabazitaxel. Coadministration of strong CYP3A4 inhibitors (e.g., **atazanavir, clarithromycin, indinavir, itraconazole, ketoconazole, nefazodone, nelfinavir, ritonavir, saquinavir, telithromycin, voriconazole**) can increase the levels of cabazitaxel. **Food:** Grapefruit juice can increase the levels of cabazitaxel. **Herbal:** St. John's wort can decrease the levels of cabazitaxel.

**PHARMACOKINETICS Distribution:** 89–92% plasma protein bound. **Metabolism:** Extensively metabolized in the liver. **Elimination:** Primarily fecal elimination. **Half-Life:** 95 h.

## NURSING IMPLICATIONS

### Black Box Warning

*Cabazitaxel has been associated with deaths from complications of severe neutropenia. Severe hypersensitivity reactions have also occurred.*

### Assessment & Drug Effects

▪ Monitor for hypersensitivity reactions especially during cycles 1 and 2. S&S requiring treatment and discontinuation of the drug include: Hypotension, bronchospasm, and generalized rash/erythema. Discontinue immediately and manage symptoms aggressively.

Common adverse effects in *italic;* life-threatening effects <u>underlined</u>; generic names in **bold;** classifications in SMALL CAPS; ♣ Canadian drug name; ● Prototype drug

- Monitor vital signs frequently, especially during the first hour of infusion. Cardiac monitoring may be indicated for those with conduction abnormalities.
- Monitor for S&S of infection. Withhold drug and notify prescriber immediately if oral temperature reaches 101° F or is sustained at 100.4° F or higher over a 1 h period.
- Monitor for and report promptly severe or persistent diarrhea as it may cause dehydration and electrolyte imbalances.
- Monitor lab tests: Weekly CBC with differential during cycle 1 and prior to each cycle thereafter; baseline and periodic LFTs and kidney function tests; periodic serum electrolytes, especially if diarrhea occurs.

**Patient & Family Education**

- Report immediately to prescriber S&S of hypersensitivity during drug infusion: Rash or itching, skin redness, difficulty breathing, chest pain or throat tightness, swelling of face, or feeling faint.
- Report severe or persistent diarrhea or vomiting as additional medications may be required.
- Avoid aspirin, NSAIDs, or alcohol to minimize GI distress.
- Do not drink grapefruit juice while taking this drug.
- Report unusual bruising or bleeding (e.g., blood in urine, or dark tarry stools).
- Use caution with exposure to potential sources of infection during periods when your blood count is low.

# CABERGOLINE
(ka-ber'go-leen)
Dostinex
**Classifications:** ERGOT ALKALOID; DOPAMINE RECEPTOR AGONIST

**Therapeutic:** DOPAMINE RECEPTOR AGONIST; ANTI-PARKINSON
**Prototype:** Ergotamine

**AVAILABILITY** Tablet

## ACTION & THERAPEUTIC EFFECT
Cabergoline is a synthetic ergot derivative, long-acting dopamine receptor agonist with a high affinity for $D_2$ receptors in the anterior pituitary. It also suppresses prolactin secretion. *Cabergoline inhibits both puerperal lactation and pathologic hyperprolactinemia. Exhibits antiparkinsonism effects due to increased levels of dopamine.*

**USES** Treatment of hyperprolactinemia.

**UNLABELED USES** Parkinson's disease, restless leg syndrome.

**CONTRAINDICATIONS** Uncontrolled hypertension and hypersensitivity to ergot derivatives; pregnancy-induced hypertension, preeclampsia, eclampsia, lactation.

**CAUTIOUS USE** Hepatic function impairment; older adults; psychosis; pregnancy (category B). Safety and efficacy in pediatric patients are unknown.

## ROUTE & DOSAGE

**Hyperprolactinemia**
*Adult:* **PO** Start with 0.25 mg 2 × wk, may increase by 0.25 mg 2 × wk (max: 1 mg 2 × wk)

## ADMINISTRATION
Oral
- Give on same days each week.

**ADVERSE EFFECTS** (≥1%) **Body as a Whole:** Asthenia, fatigue, hot flashes. **CV:** Postural hypotension.

Common adverse effects in *italic;* life-threatening effects <u>underlined;</u> generic names in **bold;** classifications in SMALL CAPS; ♣ Canadian drug name; ☯ Prototype drug

237

C

**GI:** *Nausea, constipation,* abdominal pain, dyspepsia, vomiting, dry mouth, diarrhea, flatulence. **Endocrine:** Breast pain, dysmenorrhea. **CNS:** *Headache, dizziness,* paresthesia, somnolence, depression, nervousness.

**INTERACTIONS Drug:** Concurrent use with PHENOTHIAZINES, BUTYROPH-ENONES, THIOXANTHINES, and **meto-clopramide** decreases therapeutic effects of both drugs.

**PHARMACOKINETICS Absorption:** Rapidly absorbed in GI tract, undergoes first-pass metabolism. **Peak:** 2–3 h. **Distribution:** 40–42% protein bound. Crosses placenta. **Metabolism:** Extensively metabolized. **Elimination:** Approximately 22% in urine, 60% in feces. **Half-Life:** 63–69 h.

## NURSING IMPLICATIONS

### Assessment & Drug Effects

- Monitor for hypotension, especially when given with other drugs known to lower BP.
- Monitor lab tests: Periodic serum prolactin level.

### Patient & Family Education

- Discontinue this drug once prescriber advises that serum prolactin level has been maintained for 6 mo.

## CABOZANTINIB

(ka′- boe-zan′- ti-nib)

Cometriq

**Classifications:** ANTINEOPLASTIC; KINASE INHIBITOR
Therapeutic: ANTINEOPLASTIC
**Prototype:** Erlotinib

**AVAILABILITY** Gelatin capsule

## ACTION & *THERAPEUTIC EFFECT*

Cabazantinib inhibits tyrosine kinases which are enzymes required for cancer cell formation (oncogenesis), metastasis, tumor angiogenesis, and maintenance of the tumor microenvironment. *Slows development of progressive, metastatic medullary thyroid cancer.*

**USES** Treatment of patients with progressive, metastatic medullary thyroid cancer (MTC).

**CONTRAINDICATIONS** GI perforation or fistula; severe hemorrhage; MI, cerebral infarction, serious arterial thromboembolic events; wound dehiscence; hypertensive crisis or uncontrollable hypertenstion; osteonecrosis of the jaw; nephrotic syndrome; reversible posterior leukoencephalopathy syndrome (RPLS); within 28 days of dental procedures; moderate or severe hepatic impairment; pregnancy (category D); lactation.

**CAUTIOUS USE** Hypertension; mild hepatic impairment; coadministration of strong CYP3A4 inducers/inhibitors.

## ROUTE & DOSAGE

### Metastatic Medullary Thyroid Cancer

*Adult:* **PO** 140 mg once daily until disease progression or unacceptable toxicity occurs.

### *Hepatic Impairment Dosage Adjustment*

*Moderate and severe impairment:* Not recommended

### *Toxicity Dosage Adjustment*

*Grade 4 hematologic toxicity, grade 3 or higher non-hematologic toxicity, or intolerable grade 2 toxicity:* Hold therapy until resolution/improvement (i.e., return to baseline or resolution to grade 1); then reduce daily dose by 40 mg. If patient previously receiving cabozantinib 60 mg/day, resume this dosage if tolerated, otherwise discontinue therapy.

**Dosage Adjustment If Coadministered with a Strong CYP3A4 Inhibitor or Inducer**

*Strong CYP3A4 Inhibitor:* Decrease dose by 40 mg; resume previous dose 2–3 days after discontinuing the strong inhibitor *Strong CYP3A4 Inducer:* Increase dose by 40 mg (max: 180 mg); resume previous dose 2–3 days after discontinuing strong inducer

## ADMINISTRATION

### Oral

- Give with at least 240 mL (8 oz) of water on an empty stomach (at least 2 h before/1 h after eating).
- Capsules must be swallowed whole. They should not be opened or crushed.
- Store at 15°–30° C (59°–86° F).

## ADVERSE EFFECTS (≥1%) Body

**as a Whole:** Asthenia, *fatigue,* osteonecrosis of the jaw. **CNS:** Anxiety, dizziness, dysgeusia, headache, paresthesia, peripheral neuropathy, peripheral sensory neuropathy. **CV:** Hypertension, hypotension. **GI:** Abdominal pain, *burning mouth syndrome,* constipation, *diarrhea,* dyspepsia, dysphagia, GI perforation and fistula, glossitis, *glossodynia,* hemorrhoids, *nausea, oral pain, oropharyngeal pain, stomatitis,* vomiting. **Hematological:** Hemorrhage, lymphopenia, neutropenia, thromboembolism, thrombocytopenia. **Metabolic:** ALT/AST increase, ALP increase, *decreased appetite, decreased weight,* dehydration, hyperbilirubinemia, hypocalcemia, hypokalemia, hypomagnesemia, hyponatremia. **Musculoskeletal:**

Arthralgia, muscle spasms, musculoskeletal chest pain. **Respiratory:** Dysphonia. **Skin:** Alopecia, depigmentation, dry skin, erythema, graying, hair color changes, hyperkeratosis, *palmar-plantar erythrodysesthesia syndrome (PPES).*

## INTERACTIONS Drug: Strong in-

hibitors of CYP3A4 (e.g., **atazanavir, clarithromycin, indinavir, itraconazole, ketoconazole, nefazodone, nelfinavir, ritonavir, saquinavir, telithromycin, voriconazole**) can increase the levels of cabozantinib. Strong inducers of CYP3A4 (e.g., **carbamazepine, dexamethasone, phenobarbital, phenytoin, rifampin, rifabutin, rifapentine**) may decrease the levels of cabozantinib. **Herbal: St. John's wort** may decrease the levels of cabozantinib.

## PHARMACOKINETICS Peak: 2–5 h.

**Distribution:** Greater than 99.7% plasma protein bound. **Metabolism:** In liver. **Elimination:** Fecal (54%) and renal (27%). **Half-Life:** 55 h.

## NURSING IMPLICATIONS

### Black Box Warning

*Cabozantinib has been associated with GI perforation and fistula formation, and severe, potentially fatal, hemorrhage*

### Assessment & Drug Effects

- Monitor BP at baseline and periodically thereafter.
- Monitor for S&S of thrombotic events (e.g., MI, PE).
- Monitor for S&S of GI perforation and fistula formation (e.g., blood in stool, hematemesis, abdominal pain).
- Assess for development of hand–foot syndrome (e.g., redness,

---

Common adverse effects in *italic;* life-threatening effects underlined; generic names in **bold;** classifications in SMALL CAPS; ✦ Canadian drug name; ⊕ Prototype drug

C

swelling, blisters, pain in hands and feet).
- Report immediately to prescriber if patient presents with seizures, headache, visual disturbances, confusion or altered mental function.
- Monitor lab tests: Periodic urinalysis for protein.

**Patient & Family Education**
- Practice good oral hygiene while taking this drug.
- Contact your prescriber immediately if you experience signs of bleeding (e.g., coughing up blood or blood clots, vomiting blood or vomit looks like coffee-grounds, red or black tarry stools, heavy menstrual bleeding).
- Contact prescriber immediately for any of the following: Progressive rash, painful sores in mouth, significant weight loss, or severe diarrhea.
- Do not consume grapefruit or grapefruit juice while taking this drug.
- Men and women should use effective contraception during therapy and for at least 4 mo after last dose.
- Do not breast-feed while taking this drug.

# CAFFEINE ℗

(kaf-een')
Caffedrine, Dexitac, NoDoz, Quick Pep, S-250, Tirend, Vivarin

## CAFFEINE AND SODIUM BENZOATE

## CITRATED CAFFEINE
Cafcit

**Classifications:** RESPIRATORY AND CEREBRAL STIMULANT; XANTHINE
Therapeutic: RESPIRATORY AND CEREBRAL STIMULANT

**AVAILABILITY** Tablet; capsule; caffeine citrate oral solution; caffeine citrate injection

## ACTION & *THERAPEUTIC EFFECT*
Caffeine is structurally similar to adenosine, and is capable of binding to adenosine receptors on the surface of cells without activating them, thereby acting as a competitive inhibitor. Antagonism of adenosine receptors stimulates: The vagal nucleus, reducing heart rate; the vasomotor center, constricting blood vessels; and the respiratory center, increasing respiratory rate. It also promotes release of the neurotransmitters (i.e., monoamines and acetylcholine) which causes stimulant effects. *Effective in managing neonatal apnea, and as an adjuvant for pain control in headaches and following dural puncture. Relief of headache is perhaps due to mild cerebral vasoconstriction action and increased vascular tone.*

**USES** Orally as a mild CNS stimulant to aid in staying awake and restoring mental alertness, and as an adjunct in narcotic and nonnarcotic analgesia. Used parenterally as an emergency stimulant in acute circulatory failure, as a diuretic, and for neonatal apnea.

**UNLABELED USES** Topical treatment of atopic dermatitis; to relieve spinal puncture headache.

**CONTRAINDICATIONS** Acute MI, symptomatic cardiac arrhythmias, palpitations; peptic ulcer; pulmonary disease; insomnia, panic attacks.

**CAUTIOUS USE** Diabetes mellitus; hiatal hernia; psychotic disorders; dementia; depressive disorders; hepatic disease; hypertension with heart disease; pregnancy (category C); lactation.

Common adverse effects in *italic;* life-threatening effects underlined; generic names in **bold;** classifications in SMALL CAPS; ♣ Canadian drug name; ℗ Prototype drug

## ROUTE & DOSAGE

**Mental Stimulant**
*Adult:* **PO** 100–200 mg q3–4h prn

**Circulatory Stimulant**
*Adult:* **IM** 200–500 mg prn

**Apnea of Prematurity (Caffeine Citrate Only)**
*Neonate (28–33 wk gestation):* **PO/IV** 20 mg/kg (loading dose); then, after 24 h, 5 mg/kg/day

## ADMINISTRATION

### Oral
- Powdered form may be dissolved in the patient's liquid of choice.

### Intramuscular
- Give deep IM into a large muscle.

### Intravenous
Note: IV route reserved for emergency situations only.

*PREPARE:* **IV Infusion:** May be diluted for infusion in D5W.
*ADMINISTER:* **IV Infusion:** A syringe infusion pump is recommended. • Give loading dose over 30 min and maintenance dose over at least 10 min.
*INCOMPATIBILITIES:* **Y-site:** Acyclovir, furosemide, lorazepam, nitroglycerin, oxacillin, pantoprazole.

## ADVERSE EFFECTS (≥1%) **CV:**
Tingling of face, flushing, palpitation, tachycardia, arrhythmia, angina, ventricular ectopic beats. **GI:** Nausea, vomiting; epigastric discomfort, gastric irritation (oral form), diarrhea, hematemesis, kernicterus (neonates). **CNS:** *Nervousness, insomnia,* restlessness, irritability, confusion, agitation, fasciculations, delirium, twitching, tremors, clonic convulsions. **Respiratory:** Tachypnea. **Special Senses:** Scintillating scotomas, tinnitus. **Urogenital:** Increased urination, diuresis.

## DIAGNOSTIC TEST INTERFERENCE
Caffeine reportedly may interfere with diagnosis of pheochromocytoma or neuroblastoma by increasing urinary excretion of *catecholamines,* *VMA,* and *5-HIAA* and may cause false positive increases in *serum urate* (by *Bittner method*).

## INTERACTIONS **Drug:** Increases effects of **cimetidine;** increases cardiovascular stimulating effects of BETA-ADRENERGIC AGONISTS; possibly increases **theophylline** toxicity.

## PHARMACOKINETICS **Absorption:** Rapid. **Peak:** 15–45 min. **Distribution:** Widely throughout body; crosses blood–brain barrier and placenta. **Metabolism:** In liver. **Elimination:** In urine as metabolites; excreted in breast milk in small amounts. **Half-Life:** 3–5 h in adults, 36–144 h in neonates.

## NURSING IMPLICATIONS

### Assessment & Drug Effects
- Monitor vital signs closely as large doses may cause intensification rather than reversal of severe drug-induced depressions.
- Observe children closely following administration as they are more susceptible than adults to the CNS effects of caffeine.
- Monitor lab tests: Frequent blood glucose and periodic HbA1C levels in diabetics.

### Patient & Family Education
- Caffeine in large amounts may impair glucose tolerance in diabetics.

Common adverse effects in *italic;* life-threatening effects underlined; generic names in **bold;** classifications in SMALL CAPS; ✦ Canadian drug name; ☺ Prototype drug

241

- Do not consume large amounts of caffeine as headache, dizziness, anxiety, irritability, nervousness, and muscle tension may result from excessive use, as well as from abrupt withdrawal of coffee (or oral caffeine). Withdrawal symptoms usually occur 12–18 h following last coffee intake.

# CALCIPOTRIENE

(cal-ci′po-tri-een)

Dovonex, Sorilux

**Classification:** VITAMIN D ANALOG
Therapeutic: VITAMIN D ANALOG
**Prototype:** Calcitriol

**AVAILABILITY** Ointment; foam; cream; scalp solution

## ACTION & *THERAPEUTIC EFFECT*

Calcipotriene is a synthetic vitamin $D_3$ analog for the treatment of moderate plaque psoriasis. *Calcipotriene controls psoriasis by inhibiting proliferation of psoriatic skin, reducing the number of polymorphonuclear leukocytes (PMNs) in the skin cells, and decreasing the number of epithelial cells.*

**USES** Treatment of psoriasis.

## CONTRAINDICATIONS
Hypersensitivity to calcipotriene, hypercalcemia or vitamin D toxicity, lactation.

## CAUTIOUS USE
History of nephrolithiasis; dermatoses other than psoriasis; older adults; pregnancy (category C). Safety and efficacy in children not established.

## ROUTE & DOSAGE

*Adult:* **Topical** Apply a thin layer to affected area once or twice daily

## ADMINISTRATION

### Topical
- A thin layer should be applied to the affected skin and rubbed in gently and completely.
- Calcipotriene should not be applied to the face.
- Wash hands before and after application of medication.

**ADVERSE EFFECTS** (≥1%) **Skin:** Facial dermatitis, burning, stinging, erythema, folliculitis, mild transient itching.

**PHARMACOKINETICS Absorption:** 6% absorbed systemically. **Onset:** 1 wk. **Peak:** 8 wk. **Duration:** 4 wk. **Metabolism:** Recycled via liver. **Elimination:** In bile.

## NURSING IMPLICATIONS

### Assessment & Drug Effects
- Observe reductions in scaling, erythema, and lesion thickness indicating a positive therapeutic response.
- Significant reduction in psoriatic lesions usually occurs following 1 wk of treatment. Marked improvement is generally noted by the 8th wk of treatment.
- Monitor lab tests: Periodic serum calcium, phosphate, and calcitriol levels during long-term therapy.

### Patient & Family Education
- Treatment with calcipotriene may be indefinite, as reappearance of psoriatic lesions is common following discontinuation of the drug.
- Adverse effects may include burning and stinging with drug application; these are usually transient.
- Do not mix calcipotriene with any other topical medicine.

Common adverse effects in *italic;* life-threatening effects <u>underlined;</u> generic names in **bold;** classifications in SMALL CAPS; ♣ Canadian drug name; ⦾ Prototype drug

▪ Report appearance of facial dermatitis (redness and scaling around mouth and nose).

# CALCITONIN (SALMON)
Fortical, Miacalcin

**Classification:** BONE METABOLISM REGULATOR
Therapeutic: BONE METABOLISM REGULATOR

**AVAILABILITY** Solution for injection; spray

## ACTION & THERAPEUTIC EFFECT
Calcitonin opposes the effects of parathyroid hormone on bone and kidneys, reduces serum calcium by binding to a specific receptor site on osteoclast cell membrane, and alters transmembrane passage of calcium and phosphorus. Promotes renal excretion of calcium and phosphorus. *Effective in osteoporosis due to inhibition of bone resorption. Effective in symptomatic hypercalcemia by rapidly lowering serum calcium.*

**USES** Symptomatic Paget's disease of bone (osteitis deformans), postmenopausal osteoporosis. Orphan drug approval (calcitonin human): Short-term adjunctive treatment of severe hypercalcemic emergencies.

**UNLABELED USES** Diagnosis and management of medullary carcinoma of thyroid; treatment of osteogenesis imperfecta.

**CONTRAINDICATIONS** Hypersensitivity to fish proteins or to calcitonin; hypocalcemia.

**CAUTIOUS USE** Renal impairment; osteoporosis; pernicious anemia; Zollinger–Ellison syndrome; older

adults; pregnancy (category C); lactation. Safe use in children younger than 12 y not established.

## ROUTE & DOSAGE

**Paget's Disease**
*Adult:* **Subcutaneous/IM** 100 international units/day, may decrease to 50–100 international units/day or every other day

**Hypercalcemia**
*Adult:* **Subcutaneous/IM** 4 international units/kg q12h, may increase to 8 international units/kg q6h if needed

**Postmenopausal Osteoporosis**
*Adult:* **Subcutaneous/IM** 100 international units/day; **Intranasal** 1 spray (200 international units) daily, alternate nostrils

## ADMINISTRATION
**Allergy Test Dose**
▪ An allergy skin test is usually done prior to initiation of therapy. The appearance of more than mild erythema or wheal 15 min after intracutaneous injection indicates that the drug should not be given.

**Intranasal**
▪ Activate the pump prior to first use; hold bottle upright and depress white side arms 6 times.
▪ The nasal spray is administered in one nostril daily; alternate nostrils.

**Subcutaneous**
▪ Calcitonin human is administered only by subcutaneous injection; calcitonin salmon may be administered by subcutaneous or IM injection.

**Intramuscular**
▪ Use IM route when the volume to be injected is greater than 2 mL.
▪ Rotate injection sites.

---

Common adverse effects in *italic;* life-threatening effects <u>underlined</u>; generic names in **bold;** classifications in SMALL CAPS; ♣ Canadian drug name; ⊘ Prototype drug

- Store calcitonin (human) at or below 25° C (77° F), protected from light, unless otherwise specified by manufacturer.
- Store calcitonin (salmon) in refrigerator, preferably at 2°–8° C (36°–46° F) unless otherwise directed.

**ADVERSE EFFECTS** (≥1%) **Body as a Whole:** Headache, eye pain, feverish sensation, hypersensitivity reactions, <u>anaphylaxis</u>, tremor. Reported for Cibacalcin only: Urinary frequency, chills, chest pressure, weakness, paresthesias, tender palms and soles, dizziness, nasal congestion, shortness of breath. **GI:** *Transient nausea*, vomiting, anorexia, unusual taste sensation, abdominal pain, diarrhea. **Skin:** Inflammatory reactions at injection site, flushing of face or hands, pruritus of earlobes, edema of feet, skin rashes. **Urogenital:** Nocturia, diuresis, abnormal urine sediment.

**INTERACTIONS Drug:** May decrease serum **lithium** levels.

**PHARMACOKINETICS Onset:** 15 min. **Peak:** 4 h. **Duration:** 8–24 h. **Distribution:** Does not cross placenta; distribution into breast milk unknown. **Metabolism:** In kidneys. **Elimination:** In urine. **Half-Life:** 1.25 h.

## NURSING IMPLICATIONS

### Assessment & Drug Effects

- Have readily available parenteral calcium, particularly during early therapy. Hypocalcemic tetany is a theoretical possibility.
- Examine urine specimens periodically for sediment with long-term therapy.
- Examine nasal passages prior to treatment with the nasal spray and anytime nasal irritation occurs.
- Nasal ulceration or heavy bleeding are indications for drug discontinuation.

- Monitor for hypocalcemia (see Signs & Symptoms, Appendix F). Theoretically, calcitonin can lead to hypocalcemic tetany. Latent tetany may be demonstrated by Chvostek's or Trousseau's signs and by serum calcium values: 7–8 mg/dL (latent tetany); below 7 mg/dL (manifest tetany).
- Monitor lab tests: Baseline and periodic serum calcium.

### Patient & Family Education

- Watch for redness, warmth, or swelling at injection site and report to prescriber, as these may indicate an inflammatory reaction. The transient flushing that commonly occurs following injection of calcitonin, particularly during early therapy, may be minimized by administering the drug at bedtime. Consult prescriber.
- Maintain your drug regimen to prevent early relapses even though symptoms have improved.
- Ensure that you feel comfortable using the nasal pump properly. Notify prescriber if significant nasal irritation occurs.
- Consult prescriber before using OTC preparations. Some supervitamins, hematinics, and antacids contain calcium and vitamin D (vitamin may antagonize calcitonin effects).

## CALCITRIOL ⊕

(kal-si-trye'ole)

**Calcijex, Rocaltrol, Vectical**

**Classification:** VITAMIN D ANALOG
Therapeutic: VITAMIN D ANALOG

**AVAILABILITY** Capsule; oral solution; solution for injection; ointment

## ACTION & *THERAPEUTIC EFFECT*

Synthetic form of an active metabolite of ergocalciferol (vitamin $D_2$). In the liver, cholecalciferol (vitamin $D_3$) and ergocalciferol

Common adverse effects in *italic;* life-threatening effects <u>underlined</u>; generic names in **bold**; classifications in SMALL CAPS; ♣ Canadian drug name; ⊕ Prototype drug (vitamin $D_2$) are enzymatically metabolized to calcifediol, an activated form of vitamin $D_3$ in the kidney. Patients with non-functioning kidneys are unable to synthesize sufficient calcitriol. *By promoting intestinal absorption and renal retention of calcium, calcitriol elevates serum calcium levels, decreases elevated blood levels of phosphate and parathyroid hormone. Thus it decreases subperiosteal bone resorption and mineralization defects.*

**USES** Management of hypocalcemia in patients undergoing chronic renal dialysis and in patients with hypoparathyroidism or pseudohypoparathyroidism. Patients with hyperparathyroidism in moderate to severe chronic renal failure not on dialysis; psoriasis; renal osteodystrophy.

**UNLABELED USES** Selected patients with vitamin D-dependent rickets, familial hypophosphatemia; osteopetrosis; osteoporosis.

**CONTRAINDICATIONS** Hypersensitivity to calcitriol; hypercalcemia or vitamin D toxicity.

**CAUTIOUS USE** Hyperphosphatemia, renal failure; sarcoidosis; patients receiving digitalis glycosides; older adults; pregnancy (category C).

## ROUTE & DOSAGE

### Hypocalcemia

*Adult:* **PO** 0.25 mcg/day, may be increased by 0.25 mcg/day q4–8wk for dialysis patients or q2–4wk for hypoparathyroid patients if necessary; **IV** 1–2 mcg 3 × wk at the end of dialysis, may need up to 3 mcg 3 × wk
*Child:* **PO** *On hemodialysis:* 0.25–2 mcg/day

### Renal Osteodystrophy (Stage 3 or 4 Chronic Kidney Disease)

*Adult/Adolescent/Child (3 y or older):* **PO** 0.25 mcg/day may increase; monitor closely and adjust as needed
*Child (younger than 3 y):* **PO** 0.01–0.015 mcg/kg/day. Monitor closely and adjust as needed

## ADMINISTRATION

### Oral

- Oral dose can be taken either with food or milk or on an empty stomach. Discuss with prescriber.
- When given for hypoparathyroidism, the dose is given in the morning.
- Capsules should be protected from heat, light, and moisture. Store in tightly closed container.
- Store at 15°–30° C (59°–87° F). Do not refrigerate.

### Intravenous

*PREPARE:* **Direct:** Give undiluted.
*ADMINISTER.* **Direct:** Give IV push over 30–60 sec

**ADVERSE EFFECTS** (≥1%) **Body as a Whole:** Muscle or bone pain. **CV:** Palpitation. **GI:** Anorexia, nausea, vomiting, dry mouth, thirst, constipation, abdominal cramps, metallic taste. **Metabolic:** Vitamin D intoxication, hypercalcemia, hypercalciuria, hyperphosphatemia. **CNS:** Headache, weakness. **Special Senses:** Blurred vision, photophobia. **Urogenital:** Increased urination.

**INTERACTIONS Drug:** THIAZIDE DIURETICS may cause hypercalcemia; calcifediol-induced hypercalcemia may precipitate digitalis arrhythmias in patients receiving DIGITALIS GLYCOSIDES.

Common adverse effects in *italic;* life-threatening effects <u>underlined;</u> generic names in **bold;** classifications in SMALL CAPS; ✦ Canadian drug name; ⊙ Prototype drug

245

## PHARMACOKINETICS Absorption:
Readily absorbed from GI tract. **Onset:** 2–6 h. **Peak:** 10–12 h. **Duration:** 3–5 days. **Metabolism:** In liver. **Elimination:** Mainly in feces. **Half-Life:** 3–6 h.

## NURSING IMPLICATIONS

### Assessment & Drug Effects

- Effectiveness of therapy depends on an adequate daily intake of calcium and phosphate. The prescriber may prescribe a calcium supplement on an as-needed basis.
- Monitor for hypercalcemia (see Signs & Symptoms, Appendix F). During dosage adjustment period, monitor serum calcium levels particularly twice weekly to avoid hypercalcemia.
- If hypercalcemia develops, withhold calcitriol and calcium supplements and notify prescriber. Drugs may be reinitiated when serum calcium returns to normal.
- Monitor lab tests: Baseline and periodic serum calcium, phosphorus, magnesium, alkaline phosphatase, creatinine; urinary calcium and phosphorus levels q24h.

### Patient & Family Education

- Oral/IV: Discontinue the drug if experiencing any symptoms of hypercalcemia (see Appendix F) and contact prescriber.
- Oral/IV: Do not use any other source of vitamin D during therapy, since calcitriol is the most potent form of vitamin $D_3$. This will avoid the possibility of hypercalcemia.
- Oral/IV: Consult prescriber before taking an OTC medication. (Many products contain calcium, vitamin D, phosphates, or magnesium, which can increase adverse effects of calcitriol.)

- Oral/IV: Maintain an adequate daily fluid intake unless you have kidney problems, in which case consult your prescriber about fluids.
- Stop using ointment and contact physician if severe irritation occurs.
- Avoid natural or artificial sunlight when using ointment.
- Limit ointment use to no more than 2 tubes/wk.

## CALCIUM CARBONATE
Apo-Cal ♦, BioCal, Calcite-500, Calsan ♦, Cal-Sup, Caltrate ♦, Chooz, Dicarbosil, Equilet, Mallamint, Mega-Cal, Nu-Cal, Os-Cal, Oystercal, Titralac, Tums

## CALCIUM ACETATE
PhosLo

## CALCIUM CITRATE
Citracal

## CALCIUM PHOSPHATE TRIBASIC (TRICALCIUM PHOSPHATE)

## CALCIUM LACTATE
Cal-Lac

**Classifications:** FLUID AND ELECTROLYTIC REPLACEMENT SOLUTION; ANTACID
**Therapeutic:** NUTRITIONAL SUPPLEMENT; ANTACID
**Prototype:** Calcium gluconate

**AVAILABILITY Calcium carbonate:** Tablet. **Calcium acetate:** Tablet. **Calcium citrate:** Tablet. **Calcium phosphate tribasic:** Tablet

## ACTION & *THERAPEUTIC EFFECT*
Calcium carbonate is a rapid-acting antacid with high neutralizing

Common adverse effects in *italic;* life-threatening effects <u>underlined</u>; generic names in **bold;** classifications in SMALL CAPS; ♣ Canadian drug name; ⊙ Prototype drug

capacity and relatively prolonged duration of action. Decreases gastric acidity, thereby inhibiting proteolytic action of pepsin on gastric mucosa. All forms of calcium salts are used for calcium replacement therapy. *Effectively relieves symptoms of acid indigestion and useful as a calcium supplement.*

**USES** Relief of transient symptoms of hyperacidity as in acid indigestion, heartburn, peptic esophagitis, and hiatal hernia. Also as calcium supplement in treatment of mild calcium deficiency states. Control of hyperphosphatemia in chronic renal failure (calcium acetate).

**UNLABELED USES** For treatment of hyperphosphatemia in patients with chronic renal failure and to lower BP in selected patients with hypertension.

**CONTRAINDICATIONS** Hypercalcemia and hypercalciuria (e.g., hyperparathyroidism, vitamin D overdosage, decalcifying tumors, bone metastases), calcium loss due to immobilization, severe renal failure, renal calculi, GI hemorrhage or obstruction, dehydration, digitalis toxicity; hypochloremic alkalosis, ventricular fibrillation, cardiac disease.

**CAUTIOUS USE** Decreased bowel motility (e.g., with anticholinergics, antidiarrheals, antispasmodics), older adults; **Calcium acetate:** Pregnancy (category B); children.

## ROUTE & DOSAGE

All doses are in terms of *elemental calcium:*

- 1 g calcium carbonate = 400 mg (20 mEq, 40%) elemental calcium
- 1 g calcium acetate = 250 mg (12.6 mEq, 25%) elemental

calcium; 1 g calcium citrate = 210 mg (12 mEq, 21%) elemental calcium
- 1 g tricalcium phosphate = 390 mg (19.3 mEq, 39%) elemental calcium; calcium lactate = 130 mg (6.5 mEq, 13%) elemental calcium

**Supplement for Osteoporosis**

*Adult:* **PO** 1–2 g b.i.d. or t.i.d.

**Antacid**

*Adult:* **PO** 0.5–2 g 4–6 × day

**Hyperphosphatemia**

*Adult:* **PO** Calcium acetate 2–4 tablets with each meal

**Supplement for Mild Hypercalcemia**

*Child:* **PO** 500 mg/kg/day in divided doses (lactate)

## ADMINISTRATION

**Oral**

- When used as antacid, give 1 h after meals and at bedtime. When used as calcium supplement, give 1–1½ h after meals, unless otherwise directed by prescriber.
- Chewable tablet should be chewed well before swallowing or allowed to dissolve completely in mouth, followed with water. Powder form may be mixed with water.
- Ensure that sustained release form of drug is not chewed or crushed. It **must be** swallowed whole.

**ADVERSE EFFECTS** (≥1%) **GI:** *Constipation* or laxative effect, acid rebound, nausea, eructation, *flatulence,* vomiting, fecal concretions. **Metabolic:** Hypercalcemia with alkalosis, metastatic calcinosis, hypercalciuria, hypomagnesemia, hypophosphatemia (when phosphate intake is low). **CNS:** Mood and mental changes. **Urogenital:** Polyuria, renal calculi.

Common adverse effects in *italic;* life-threatening effects underlined; generic names in **bold;** classifications in SMALL CAPS; ✤ Canadian drug name; ⊕ Prototype drug

247

**INTERACTIONS Drug:** May enhance inotropic and toxic effects of **digoxin; magnesium** may compete for GI absorption; decreases absorption of TETRACYCLINES, QUINOLONES **(ciprofloxacin).**

**PHARMACOKINETICS Absorption:** Approximately ⅓ of dose absorbed from small intestine. **Distribution:** Crosses placenta. **Elimination:** Primarily in feces; small amounts in urine, pancreatic juice, saliva, breast milk.

## NURSING IMPLICATIONS

### Assessment & Drug Effects

- Note number and consistency of stools. If constipation is a problem, prescriber may prescribe alternate or combination therapy with a magnesium antacid or advise patient to take a laxative or stool softener as necessary.
- Record amelioration of symptoms of hypocalcemia (see Signs & Symptoms, Appendix F).
- Observe for S&S of hypercalcemia in patients receiving frequent or high doses, or who have impaired renal function (see Appendix F).
- Monitor lab tests: Weekly serum and urine calcium with prolonged therapy and in those with renal dysfunction.

### Patient & Family Education

- Do not continue this medication beyond 1–2 wk, since it may cause acid rebound, which generally occurs after repeated use for 1 or 2 wk and leads to chronic use. It is potentially dangerous to self-medicate. Do not take antacids longer than 2 wk without medical supervision.
- Avoid taking calcium carbonate with cereals or other foods high in oxalates. Oxalates combine with calcium carbonate to form insoluble, nonabsorbable compounds.
- Do not use calcium carbonate repeatedly with foods high in

vitamin D (such as milk) or sodium bicarbonate, as it may cause milk-alkali syndrome: hypercalcemia, distaste for food, headache, confusion, nausea, vomiting, abdominal pain, metabolic alkalosis, hypercalciuria, polyuria, soft tissue calcification (calcinosis), hyperphosphatemia, and renal insufficiency. Predisposing factors include renal dysfunction, dehydration, electrolyte imbalance, and hypertension.

## CALCIUM CHLORIDE

**Classification:** FLUID AND ELECTROLYTIC REPLACEMENT SOLUTION
**Therapeutic:** FLUID AND ELECTROLYTE REPLACEMENT
**Prototype:** Calcium gluconate

**AVAILABILITY** Solution for injection

## ACTION & *THERAPEUTIC EFFECT*

Ionizes readily and provides excess chloride ions that promote acidosis and temporary (1–2 days) diuresis secondary to excretion of sodium. *Rapidly and effectively restores serum calcium levels in acute hypocalcemia of various origins and an effective cardiac stabilizer under conditions of hyperkalemia or resuscitation.*

**USES** Treatment of cardiac resuscitation when epinephrine fails to improve myocardial contractions; for treatment of acute hypocalcemia (as in tetany due to parathyroid deficiency, vitamin D deficiency, alkalosis, insect bites or stings, and during exchange transfusions), for treatment of hypermagnesemia, and for cardiac disturbances of hyperkalemia.

Common adverse effects in *italic*; life-threatening effects underlined; generic names in **bold**; classifications in SMALL CAPS; ♣ Canadian drug name; ⊘ Prototype drug

**CONTRAINDICATIONS** Ventricular fibrillation, hypercalcemia, digitalis toxicity, injection into myocardium or other tissue.

**CAUTIOUS USE** Digitalized patients; sarcoidosis, renal insufficiency, history of renal stone formation; cardiac arrhythmias; dehydration; diarrhea; cor pulmonale, respiratory acidosis, respiratory failure; pregnancy (category A, category C in high doses).

## ROUTE & DOSAGE

**All doses are in terms of elemental calcium:**

- 1 g calcium chloride = 272 mg (13.6 mEq) elemental calcium

**Hypocalcemia**

*Adult:* IV 0.5–1 g (7–14 mEq) at 1–3 day intervals as determined by patient response and serum calcium levels
*Child:* IV 2.7–5 mg/kg administered slowly

**Hypocalcemic Tetany**

*Adult:* IV 4.5–16 mEq prn
*Child:* IV 0.5–0.7 mEq/kg t.i.d. or q.i.d.
*Neonate:* IV 2.4 mEq/kg/day in divided doses

**CPR**

*Adult:* IV 2–4 mg/kg, may repeat in 10 min
*Child:* IV 20 mg/kg, may repeat in 10 min

## ADMINISTRATION

**Intravenous**

*IV administration to neonates, infants, and children:* Verify correct IV concentration and rate of infusion with prescriber.

*PREPARE:* **Direct:** May be given undiluted or diluted (preferred) with an equal volume of NS for injection. ▪ Solution should be warmed to body temperature before administration.

*ADMINISTER:* **Direct:** Give at 0.5–1 mL/min or more slowly if irritation develops. Avoid rapid administration. ▪ Use a small-bore needle and inject into a large vein to minimize venous irritation and undesirable reactions. ▪ Do not use scalp veins for injection in children. ▪ Following injection, keep recumbent for a short time.

*INCOMPATIBILITIES:* **Solution/additive: Amphotericin B, chlorpheniramine, dobutamine,** concentration-dependent incompatibility with other ELECTROLYTES. **Y-site: Amphotericin B cholesteryl complex, propofol, sodium bicarbonate.**

**ADVERSE EFFECTS** (≥1%) **Body as a Whole:** Tingling sensation. With rapid IV, sensations of heat waves (peripheral vasodilation), fainting. **CV:** (With rapid infusion) hypotension, bradycardia, cardiac arrhythmias, <u>cardiac arrest</u>. **Skin:** Pain and burning at IV site, severe venous thrombosis, necrosis and sloughing (with extravasation).

**INTERACTIONS Drug:** May enhance inotropic and toxic effects of **digoxin;** antagonizes the effects of **verapamil** and possibly other CALCIUM CHANNEL BLOCKERS.

**PHARMACOKINETICS Distribution:** Crosses placenta. **Elimination:** Primarily in feces; small amounts in urine, pancreatic juice, saliva, and breast milk.

## NURSING IMPLICATIONS
**Assessment & Drug Effects**
- Monitor ECG and BP and observe patient closely during

Common adverse effects in *italic;* life-threatening effects <u>underlined</u>; generic names in **bold;** classifications in SMALL CAPS; ✦ Canadian drug name; ◍ Prototype drug

249

administration. IV injection may be accompanied by cutaneous burning sensation and peripheral vasodilation, with moderate fall in BP.

- Advise ambulatory patient to remain in bed for 15–30 min or more depending on response following injection.
- Observe digitalized patients closely since an increase in serum calcium increases risk of digitalis toxicity.
- Monitor lab tests: Frequent serum pH and serum calcium.

### Patient & Family Education

- Remain in bed for 15–30 min or more following injection and depending on response.
- Symptoms of mild hypercalcemia, such as loss of appetite, nausea, vomiting, or constipation may occur. If hypercalcemia becomes severe, call health care provider if feeling confused or extremely excited.
- Do not use other calcium supplements or eat foods high in calcium, like milk, cheese, yogurt, eggs, meats, and some cereals, during therapy.

## CALCIUM GLUCONATE ℗

(gloo'koe-nate)

**Classification:** ELECTROLYTE AND WATER BALANCE
Therapeutic: ELECTROLYTE REPLACEMENT SOLUTION

**AVAILABILITY** Tablet; intravenous solution; capsule

## ACTION & *THERAPEUTIC EFFECT*

Calcium gluconate acts like digitalis on the heart, increasing cardiac muscle tone and force of systolic contractions (positive inotropic effect). *Rapidly and effectively restores serum calcium levels in acute hypocalcemia of various origins;* *also effective as a cardiac stabilizer under conditions of hyperkalemia or resuscitation.*

**USES** Treatment of acute symptomatic hypocalcemia. Also as antidote for magnesium sulfate, for acute symptoms of lead colic, to decrease capillary permeability in sensitivity reactions, and to relieve muscle cramps from insect bites or stings. Oral calcium may be used to maintain normal calcium balance and to prevent primary osteoporosis. Also in osteoporosis, osteomalacia, chronic hypoparathyroidism, rickets, and as adjunct in treatment of myasthenia gravis and Eaton–Lambert syndrome.

**UNLABELED USES** To antagonize aminoglycoside-induced neuromuscular blockage, and as "calcium challenge" to diagnose Zollinger–Ellison syndrome and medullary thyroid carcinoma, management of severe hypermagnesemia.

**CONTRAINDICATIONS** Ventricular fibrillation, metastatic bone disease, injection into myocardium; renal calculi, hypercalcemia, predisposition to hypercalcemia (hyperparathyroidism, certain malignancies); digitalis toxicity.

**CAUTIOUS USE** Digitalized patients, renal or cardiac insufficiency, arrhythmias; dehydration; diarrhea; hyperphosphatemia; sarcoidosis, history of lithiasis, immobilized patients; pregnancy (category C). The amount of calcium in breast milk is homeostatically regulated and not altered by maternal calcium intake. Decision to continue or discontinue lactation during therapy should take into account risk of the infant exposure, the benefits of breast-feeding to the infant, and benefits of treatment for the mother.

Common adverse effects in *italic;* life-threatening effects underlined; generic names in **bold;** classifications in SMALL CAPS; ◆ Canadian drug name; ℗ Prototype drug

## ROUTE & DOSAGE

**All doses are in terms of elemental calcium:**

- 1 g calcium gluconate = 90 mg (4.5 mEq, 9.3%) elemental calcium

**Supplement for Osteoporosis**
*Adult:* **PO** 1–2 g b.i.d. to q.i.d.
*Child:* **PO** 45–65 mg/kg/day in divided doses
*Neonate:* **PO** 50–130 mg/kg/day (max: 1 g)

**Hypocalcemia**
*Adult:* **IV** 1–4 g over 2–4 h then reassess calcium measurement
*Child:* **IV** 200–500 mg/kg/day (max: 2–3 g/dose)

**Hypocalcemic Tetany**
*Adult:* **IV** 2–3 g prn
*Child:* **IV** 100–500 mg/kg/dose, may repeat q6–8h
*Neonate:* **IV** 200 mg followed by 500 mg/kg/day infusion

**CPR**
*Adult:* **IV** 1.5–3 grams over 2–5 min

**Hyperkalemia with Cardiac Toxicity**
*Adult:* **IV** 500–800 mg (max: 3 g)

## ADMINISTRATION

**Oral**
- Ensure that chewable tablets are chewed or crushed before being swallowed with a liquid. Powder, take with food or liquid.
- Give with meals to enhance absorption.

**Intravenous**

*PREPARE:* **Direct:** May be given undiluted. **Intermittent/Continuous:** May be diluted in 1000 mL of NS.

*ADMINISTER:* **Direct/Intermittent/Continuous:** Due to the risk of particulates, American Regent, Inc. recommends the use of a 0.22 micron inline filter for IV administration (1.2 micron filter if admixture contains lipids). ▪ Give slowly, not to exceed 200 mg/min for adults or 100 mg/min for children. Use a small-bore needle into a large vein to avoid possibility of extravasation and resultant necrosis. ▪ With children, scalp veins should be avoided. Avoid rapid infusion. ▪ High concentrations of calcium suddenly reaching the heart can cause fatal cardiac arrest.

*INCOMPATIBILITIES:* **Solution/additive: Amphotericin B, cefamandole, dobutamine, methylprednisolone, metoclopramide,** concentration-dependent incompatibility with other ELECTROLYTES. **Y-site: Amphotericin B cholesteryl complex, cangrelor, ceftobiprole medocaril, ceftriaxone sodium, dantrolene sodium, diazepam, diazoxide, fluconazole, foscarnet sodium, fosphenytoin sodium, gemtuzumab ozogamicin, inamirone lactate, indomethacin, lansoprazole, meropenem pantoprazole, methylprednisolone sodium succinate, minocycline hydrochloride, mycophenolate mofetil hydrochloride, oxacillin sodium, pemetrexed, phenytoin sodium, potassium phosphates, quinupristin-dalfopristin, sodium bicarbonate, sodium phosphates, sulfamethoxazole-trimethoprim, tedizolid phosphate, topotecan hydrochloride.**
- Injection should be stopped if patient complains of any discomfort. ▪ If extravasation

Common adverse effects in *italic*; life-threatening effects <u>underlined</u>; generic names in **bold**; classifications in SMALL CAPS; ✤ Canadian drug name; ⊙ Prototype drug

251

occurs, stop the infusion, disconnect (leave needle/cannula in place); gently aspirate extravasated solution (**do not** flush the line). ▪ Patient should be advised to remain in bed for 15–30 min or more following injection, depending on response.

▪ Store intact IV vials at 20°–25 ° C (68°–77° F). Do not freeze. Discard unused portion within 4 h after initial puncture. Store oral at room temperature.

**ADVERSE EFFECTS** (≥1%) **Body as a Whole:** Tingling sensation. With rapid IV, sensations of heat waves (peripheral vasodilation), fainting. **GI:** PO preparation: Chalky taste, constipation, increased gastric acid secretion. **CV:** (With rapid infusion) hypotension, bradycardia, cardiac arrhythmias, cardiac arrest. **Skin:** Pain and burning at IV site, severe venous thrombosis, necrosis and sloughing (with extravasation).

**DIAGNOSTIC TEST INTERFERENCE** IV calcium may cause false decreases in *serum and urine magnesium* (by *Titan yellow method*) and transient elevations of *plasma 11-OHCS* levels by *Glenn–Nelson technique.* Values usually return to control levels after 60 min; *urinary steroid values (17-OHCS)* may be decreased.

**INTERACTIONS Drug:** May enhance inotropic and toxic effects of **digoxin; magnesium** may compete for GI absorption; decreases absorption of TETRACYCLINES, QUINOLONES **(ciprofloxacin);** antagonizes the effects of **verapamil** and possibly other CALCIUM CHANNEL BLOCKERS (IV administration).

**PHARMACOKINETICS Absorption:** 30% from small intestine.

**Onset:** Immediately after IV. **Distribution:** Crosses placenta. **Elimination:** Primarily in feces; small amounts in urine, pancreatic juice, saliva, and breast milk.

## NURSING IMPLICATIONS
### Assessment & Drug Effects
▪ Assess for cutaneous burning sensations and peripheral vasodilation, with moderate fall in BP, during direct IV injection.
▪ Monitor ECG during IV administration to detect evidence of hypercalcemia: Decreased QT interval associated with inverted T wave.
▪ Observe IV site closely. Extravasation may result in tissue irritation and necrosis.
▪ Monitor for hypocalcemia and hypercalcemia (see Signs & Symptoms, Appendix F).
▪ Monitor lab tests: Frequent serum calcium, phosphorus, albumin, and magnesium during sustained therapy.

### Patient & Family Education
▪ Report S&S of hypercalcemia (see Appendix F) promptly to your care provider.
▪ Milk and milk products are the best sources of calcium (and phosphorus). Other good sources include dark green vegetables, soy beans, tofu, and canned fish with bones.
▪ Calcium absorption can be inhibited by zinc-rich foods: Nuts, seeds, sprouts, legumes, soy products (tofu).
▪ Check with prescriber before self-medicating with a calcium supplement.

## CALCIUM POLYCARBOPHIL
(pol-ee-kar′boe-fil)
FiberCon, FiberGen

Common adverse effects in *italic;* life-threatening effects underlined; generic names in **bold**; classifications in SMALL CAPS; ◆ Canadian drug name; ⊙ Prototype drug

**Classifications:** BULK LAXATIVE; ANTIDIARRHEAL
Therapeutic: BULK LAXATIVE; ANTIDIARRHEAL
**Prototype:** Psyllium hydrophilic mucilloid

## AVAILABILITY Tablet

## ACTION & *THERAPEUTIC EFFECT*

Hydrophilic, bulk-producing laxative that restores normal moisture level and bulk content of intestinal tract. In constipation, retains free water in intestinal lumen, thereby indirectly opposing dehydrating forces of the bowel; in diarrhea, when intestinal mucosa is incapable of absorbing fluid, drug absorbs fecal fluid to form a gel. *Relieves constipation or diarrhea associated with bowel disorders and acute nonspecific diarrhea.*

## USES Treatment and prevention of constipation; treatment of IBS.

## CONTRAINDICATIONS GI obstruction.

## CAUTIOUS USE Pregnancy (category A; category C in high doses); lactation; children younger than 6 y.

## ROUTE & DOSAGE

### Constipation

*Adult:* **PO** 1 g 1–4 × day or as needed (max: 6 g/24 h)
*Child (6–12 y):* **PO** 500 mg 1–4 × day (max: 3 g/24 h); *3 to less than 6 y:* 500 mg 1–2 × day (max: 1.5 g/24 h)

## ADMINISTRATION

### Oral

▪ Administer with at least 180–240 mL (6–8 oz) water or other fluid

of patient's choice when used as a laxative and with at least 60–90 mL (2–3 oz) of fluid when used as an antidiarrheal. Chewed tablets should not be swallowed dry.
▪ If diarrhea is severe, dose can be repeated every half hour up to maximum daily dose.

## ADVERSE EFFECTS (≥1%) GI:
*Flatulence,* abdominal fullness, intestinal obstruction; laxative dependence (long-term use).

## PHARMACOKINETICS Absorption: Not absorbed from the intestine. Bowel movement usually occurs within 12–72 h. Elimination: In feces.

## NURSING IMPLICATIONS

### Assessment & Drug Effects

▪ Evaluate effectiveness of medication. If it is ineffective as an antidiarrheal, report to prescriber.
▪ Report promptly rectal bleeding, very dark stools, or abdominal pain.

### Patient & Family Education

▪ You will likely have a bowel movement within 12–72 h.
▪ This is an OTC product. Take this drug exactly as ordered. Do not increase the dose if response is inadequate. Consult prescriber. Do not use other laxatives while you are taking calcium polycarbophil.

## CANAGLIFLOZIN 🅟

(kan'a-gli-floe'zin)
Invokana

**Classifications:** ANTIDIABETIC; SODIUM-GLUCOSE CO-TRANSPORTER 2 (SGLT2) INHIBITOR
Therapeutic: ANTIDIABETIC; SGLT2 INHIBITOR

## AVAILABILITY Tablet

## ACTION & *THERAPEUTIC EFFECT*

Inhibits the sodium-glucose cotransporter 2 (SGLT2) in the

Common adverse effects in *italic;* life-threatening effects underlined; generic names in **bold;** classifications in SMALL CAPS; ♣ Canadian drug name; 🅟 Prototype drug

253

proximal renal tubules that is responsible for the majority of the reabsorption of filtered glucose in the kidney. *Canagliflozin inhibits SGLT2 thus allowing more glucose to be removed from the blood stream and excreted by the kidney.*

**USES** Adjunct therapy for the treatment of type 2 diabetes mellitus in combination with diet and exercise.

**CONTRAINDICATIONS** History of serious hypersensitivity reaction to canagliflozin; Type 1 DM; severe renal impairment (eGFR of 30 mL/min/l.73m²), ESRD, or on dialysis; severe hepatic impairment; lactation.

**CAUTIOUS USE** Hypotension; cardiovascular disease; diabetic ketoacidosis; renal impairment; low systolic blood pressure; increases in low density cholesterol; moderate hepatic impairment; renal insufficiency, reduced intravascular volume; history of genital mycotic infections especially in uncircumcised men; older adults; pregnancy (category C). Safety and efficacy in children younger than 18 y not established.

## ROUTE & DOSAGE

**Type 2 Diabetes Mellitus**
*Adult:* **PO** 100 mg once daily; can increase up to 300 mg once daily

**Hepatic Impairment Dosage Adjustment**
*Severe Impairment:* Not recommended

**Renal Impairment Dosage Adjustment**
*eGFR 45–59 mL/min/1.73m²:* Do not exceed 100 mg daily.
*eGFR less than 45 mL/min/1.73m²:* Not recommended

## ADMINISTRATION

**Oral**
▪ Give before the first meal of the day.
▪ Store at 15°–30° C (59°–86° F).

**ADVERSE EFFECTS** (≥1%) **Body as a Whole:** Dehydration, dry mouth, polydipsia, syncope, thirst. **CNS:** Asthenia, fatigue. **CV:** Hypotension, intravascular volume depletion, orthostatic hypotension. **GI:** Abdominal pain, constipation, nausea. **Endocrine:** Hypoglycemia. **Metabolic:** Increased LDL, increased phosphate, hyperkalemia, *hypermagnesemia*, increased serum creatinine, pancreatitis. **Hematologic:** *Hyperkalemia, hypermagnesemia,* hypoglycemia, increased hemaglobin, increased LDL, *increased phosphate.* **Musculoskeletal:** Bone fractures. **Skin:** Angioedema, erythema, pruritus, rash. **Urogenital:** *Candidiasis, vaginitis,* increase urination, urinary tract infections.

**INTERACTIONS Drug: Rifampin** and other inducers of UGT enzymes (e.g., **phenobarbital, phenytoin, ritonavir, carbamazepine, efavirenz, fosphenytoin**) can decrease the levels of canagliflozin. Canagliflozin can increase the levels of **digoxin.** LOOP DIURETICS increase risk of hypotension.

**PHARMACOKINETICS Absorption:** 65% bioavailable. **Peak:** 1–2 h. **Distribution:** 99% plasma protein bound. **Metabolism:**

Common adverse effects in *italic;* life-threatening effects underlined; generic names in **bold;** classifications in SMALL CAPS; ♣ Canadian drug name; ● Prototype drug

Glucuronidation by UGT. **Elimination:** Renal (30%) and fecal (52%). **Half-Life:** 10.6–13.1 h.

## NURSING IMPLICATIONS

### Black Box Warning

*Lower limb amputation. An approximate two-fold increased risk of lower limb amputations associated in two large randomized, placebo controlled trials in patients with cardiovascular disease (CVD) or were at risk for CVD. Amputations of the toe and midfoot were most frequent.*

### Assessment & Drug Effects

- Monitor BP throughout therapy as drug causes intravascular volume depletion.
- Monitor for symptomatic hypotension especially at the initiation of therapy and in the older adult or those taking other drugs that lower BP.
- Monitor for S&S of genital fungal infections.
- Monitor for lower limb and feet ulcerations, sores, or infections.
- Monitor lab tests: Baseline and periodic kidney function tests; periodic HbA1C, serum potassium (in those predisposed to hyperkalemia), magnesium, phosphate, and lipid profile.

### Patient & Family Education

- Monitor blood sugar as directed by prescriber. Note that this drug will cause sugar to appear in your urine.
- Report to prescriber if you experience S&S of hypoglycemia (see Appendix F).
- Report to prescriber any S&S of an allergic reaction (e.g., rash, hives).
- Maintain adequate fluid intake as drug can cause dehydration. Inform prescriber if you experience dizziness upon standing.

- Yeast infections of the vagina and penis (especially in uncircumcised men) may occur. Report promptly for treatment.
- Report to prescriber if a pregnancy is suspected.
- Discontinue breast-feeding while taking this drug.

## CANDESARTAN CILEXETIL

(can-de-sar'tan ci-lex'e-til)

*Atacand*

**Classification:** ANGIOTENSIN II RECEPTOR ANTAGONIST, ANTIHYPERTENSIVE

*Therapeutic:* ANTIHYPERTENSIVE
**Prototype:** Losartan

### AVAILABILITY Tablet

### ACTION & *THERAPEUTIC EFFECT*

Angiotensin II receptor (type $AT_1$) antagonist. Angiotensin II is a potent vasoconstrictor and primary vasoactive hormone of the renin–angiotensin–aldosterone system. Candesartan selectively blocks binding of angiotensin II to the $AT_1$ receptors found in many tissues (e.g., vascular smooth muscle, adrenal glands). *Results in blocking the vasoconstricting and aldosterone-secreting effects of angiotensin II, resulting in an antihypertensive effect. Effectively lowers BP from hypertensive to normotensive range.*

### USES Hypertension, heart failure.

### CONTRAINDICATIONS Known

sensitivity to candesartan or any other angiotensin II ($AT_1$) receptor antagonist (e.g., losartan, valsartan); primary hyperaldosteronism; bilateral renal artery stenosis; pregnancy (category D second and third trimesters); lactation; children

---

Common adverse effects in *italic;* life-threatening effects <u>underlined</u>; generic names in **bold**; classifications in SMALL CAPS; ✦ Canadian drug name; ⊘ Prototype drug

C

younger than 1 y for hypertension, or children with GFR less than 30 mL/min/1.73 m$^2$.

**CAUTIOUS USE** Unilateral renal artery stenosis; aortic or mitral valve stenosis; hypertrophic cardiomyopathy; CHF; DM; moderate hepatic or renal impairment, significant renal failure; children; pregnancy (category C first trimester); lactation.

## ROUTE & DOSAGE

### Hypertension

*Adult:* **PO** Start at 16 mg daily (range 8–32 mg divided once or twice daily)
*Adolescent/Child: (6 y or older weighing more than 50 kg):* **PO** 8–16 mg given in single or divided doses; adjust based on response; *6 y or older weighing less than 50 kg:* 4–8 mg given in single or divided doses; adjust based on response
*Child (1 to younger than 6 y):* **PO** 0.2 mg/kg/day; adjust based on response

### Heart Failure

*Adult:* **PO** Start at 4 mcg once daily, double the dose at 2 wk intervals as tolerated by the patient until a dose of 32 mg is reached

### *Hepatic Impairment Dosage Adjustment*

*Moderate hepatic impairment:* Initiate therapy at lower dose

## ADMINISTRATION

### Oral

- Volume depletion should be corrected prior to initiation of therapy to prevent hypotension.
- Dose is individualized and may be given once or twice daily. The daily dose may be titrated up to 32 mg; larger doses are not likely to provide additional benefit.

**ADVERSE EFFECTS** (≥1%) **Body as a Whole:** Fatigue, peripheral edema, back pain, arthralgia. **CV:** Chest pain. **GI:** Nausea, abdominal pain, diarrhea, vomiting. **CNS:** Headache, dizziness. **Respiratory:** Cough, sinusitis, upper respiratory infection, pharyngitis, rhinitis. **Urogenital:** Albuminuria.

**INTERACTIONS Drug:** May increase risk of **lithium** toxicity.

**PHARMACOKINETICS Absorption:** 15% reaches systemic circulation. **Peak:** Serum concentration, 3–4 h; therapeutic effect, 2–4 wk. **Duration:** 24 h. **Distribution:** Greater than 99% protein bound; crosses placenta; distributed into breast milk. **Metabolism:** Minimally in liver. **Elimination:** Primarily in bile (67%) and urine (33%). **Half-Life:** 9–12 h.

## NURSING IMPLICATIONS

### Black Box Warning

*Candesartan cilexetil has been associated with fetal injury and death.*

### Assessment & Drug Effects

- Monitor BP as therapeutic effectiveness is indicated by decreases in systolic and diastolic BP within 2 wk with maximal effect at 4–6 wk.
- Monitor for transient hypotension in volume/salt-depleted patients; if hypotension occurs, place in supine position and notify prescriber.
- Monitor BP periodically; trough readings, just prior to the next scheduled dose, should be made when possible.

- Monitor lab tests: Periodic BUN and creatinine, serum potassium, LFTs, and CBC with differential.

**Patient & Family Education**
- Stop taking this drug and inform your prescriber immediately if you become pregnant.
- You may not notice maximum pressure-lowering effect for 6 wk.
- Report episodes of dizziness especially when making position changes.

## CAPECITABINE
(cap-e-si'ta-been)
Xeloda
**Classifications:** ANTINEOPLASTIC; ANTIMETABOLITE, PYRIMIDINE
**Therapeutic:** ANTINEOPLASTIC
**Prototype:** 5-Fluorouracil (5-FU)

**AVAILABILITY** Tablet

## ACTION & *THERAPEUTIC EFFECT*
Pyrimidine antagonist and cell cycle specific antimetabolite. Prodrug of 5-FU. Blocks actions of enzymes essential to normal DNA and RNA synthesis. May become incorporated into RNA molecules of tumor cells, thereby interfering with RNA and protein synthesis. *Reduces or stabilizes tumor size in metastatic breast cancer and colorectal cancer.*

**USES** Metastatic breast cancer and colorectal cancer.

**UNLABELED USES** Ovarian cancer.

**CONTRAINDICATIONS** Hypersensitivity to capecitabine, doxifluridine, 5-FU; myelosuppression; dihydropyrimidine dehydrogenase (DPD) deficiency; females of childbearing age; active infection; jaundice; severe renal failure (less than 30 mL/min); pregnancy (category D); lactation.

**CAUTIOUS USE** Mild to moderate renal or hepatic dysfunction; bacterial or viral infection; coronary artery disease, angina, cardiac arrhythmias; history of varicella zoster or other herpes infections; older adults; children younger than 18 y.

## ROUTE & DOSAGE

**Breast Cancer, Colorectal Cancer**
Adult: **PO** 1250 mg/m$^2$ b.i.d. × 2 wk (timing of second cycle differs based on other medications used)

**Renal Impairment Dosage Adjustment**
CrCl 30–50 mL/min: Reduce dose by 25%; less than 30 mL/min: Do not use

**Toxicity Dosage Adjustment**
See package insert

## ADMINISTRATION
**Oral**
- Hazardous agent: NIOSH recommends single gloving for administration of intact tablets. If it is necessary to manipulate the tablets (e.g., to prepare an oral solution), it is recommended to double glove, and prepare in a controlled device.
- Morning and evening doses (about 12 h apart) should be given within 30 min after the meal. Water is the preferred liquid for taking this drug.

**ADVERSE EFFECTS** (≥1%) **Body as a Whole:** *Fatigue,* pyrexia, pain, myalgia. **CV:** Edema. **GI:** *Severe diarrhea, nausea, vomiting, stomatitis,* abdominal pain, constipation, dyspepsia, *anorexia.* **Hematologic:**

Common adverse effects in *italic;* life-threatening effects underlined; generic names in **bold;** classifications in SMALL CAPS; ♣ Canadian drug name; ❼ Prototype drug

257

Neutropenia, thrombocytopenia, anemia, lymphopenia. **Metabolic:** Dehydration, hyperbilirubinemia. **CNS:** Paresthesias, headache, dizziness, insomnia. **Skin:** Hand-and-foot syndrome, *dermatitis,* nail disorder. **Special Senses:** Eye irritation.

**INTERACTIONS Drug: Leucovorin** increases concentration and toxicity of **5-FU,** altered coagulation and/or bleeding reported with **warfarin** and **NSAIDs.** Avoid or monitor closely with other agents that may cause neutropenia (**deferiprone, clozapine**). **Food:** Food decreases extent of absorption.

**PHARMACOKINETICS Absorption:** Absorption significantly reduced by food. **Peak:** 1.5–2 h. **Distribution:** Approx 35% protein bound. **Metabolism:** Extensively metabolized to 5-FU. **Elimination:** In urine. **Half-Life:** 45 min.

## NURSING IMPLICATIONS

### Black Box Warning

*When capecitabine is given to patients using oral coumarin-derivative anticoagulants (e.g., warfarin), there is increased risk of bleeding and death from hemorrhage. These adverse effects may occur as late as several months after starting capecitabine or even after stopping capecitabine.*

### Assessment & Drug Effects
- Monitor carefully for S&S of grade 2 or greater toxicity: Diarrhea greater than 4 BMs/day or at night; vomiting greater than 1 time/24 h; significant loss of appetite or anorexia; stomatitis; hand-and-foot syndrome (pain, swelling, erythema, desquamation, blistering); temperature = 100.5° F; and S&S of infection.

- Withhold drug and immediately report S&S of grade 2 or greater toxicity.
- Withhold drug and notify prescriber if PT and INR are prolonged beyond the normal range in those with concurrent warfarin therapy.
- Monitor for dehydration and replace fluids as needed.
- Monitor carefully patients with coronary artery disease for S&S of cardiotoxicity (e.g., increasing angina).
- Monitor lab tests: Periodic CBC with differential and LFTs. Frequent PT and INR with concurrent warfarin therapy. Serum bilirubin, serum creatinine, and serum alkaline phosphatase.

### Patient & Family Education
- Report immediately significant nausea, loss of appetite, diarrhea, soreness of tongue, fever of 100.5° F or more, or signs of infection. Review patient drug package insert carefully for more detail.
- For female patients, it is a necessity to use contraceptive methods. Inform prescriber immediately if you become pregnant.

## CAPREOMYCIN
(kap-ree-oh-mye′sin)
**Capastat**
**Classifications:** ANTIBIOTIC; ANTITUBERCULOSIS
**Therapeutic:** ANTITUBERCULOSIS
**Prototype:** Isoniazid

**AVAILABILITY** Powder for injection

## ACTION & *THERAPEUTIC EFFECT*
Polypeptide antibiotic that is bactericidal against strains of Mycobacterium tuberculosis. The exact action is not fully known. Should not be

used alone. *Effective second-line antimycobacterial in conjunction with other antitubercular drugs.*

**USES** Treatment of active tuberculosis when primary agents cannot be tolerated or when causative organism has become resistant.

**CONTRAINDICATIONS** Lactation.

**CAUTIOUS USE** Hypersensitivity to antibiotics, including capreomycin, or to other drugs; renal insufficiency (extreme caution); acoustic nerve impairment; history of allergies (especially to drugs); preexisting liver disease; myasthenia gravis; parkinsonism; pregnancy (category C). Safe use in children not established.

## ROUTE & DOSAGE

**Tuberculosis**

*Adult:* **IM/IV** 1 g/day (not to exceed 20 mg/kg/day) for 60–120 days, then 1 g 2–3 × wk × 18–24 mo

**Renal Impairment Dosage Adjustment**

*CrCl 25–50 mL/min:* Reduce dose by 50%; *10–24 mL/min:* Reduce dose by 50% and give q48h; *less than 10 mL/min:* Reduce dose by 50% and give twice weekly

## ADMINISTRATION

**Intramuscular**

- Reconstitute by adding 2 mL of NS injection or sterile water for injection to each 1 g vial. Allow 2–3 min for drug to dissolve completely.
- Make IM injections deep into large muscle mass. Superficial injections are more painful and are associated with sterile abscess. Rotate injection sites.

- Solution may become pale straw color and darken with time, but this does not indicate loss of potency.
- After reconstitution, solution may be stored for use within 24 h.

**Intravenous**

**PREPARE: IV Infusion:** Reconstitute by adding 2 mL of NS or sterile water to each 1 g to yield 370 mg/mL. ▪ Allow 2–3 min to dissolve, then add required dose to 100 mL of NS.
**ADMINISTER: IV Infusion:** Give over 60 min. Avoid rapid infusion.

**ADVERSE EFFECTS** (≥1%) **Skin:** Urticaria, maculopapular rash, photosensitivity. **Hematologic:** Leukocytosis, <u>leukopenia</u>, *eosinophilia*. **CNS:** Neuromuscular blockage (large doses: Skeletal muscle weakness, respiratory depression or arrest). **Urogenital:** Nephrotoxicity (long-term therapy), tubular necrosis. **Special Senses:** *Ototoxicity,* eighth nerve (auditory and vestibular) damage. **Metabolic:** Hypokalemia, and other electrolyte imbalances. **Other:** Impaired hepatic function (decreased BSP excretion); IM site reactions: Pain, induration, excessive bleeding, sterile abscesses.

## DIAGNOSTIC TEST INTERFERENCE

**BSP** and **PSP** excretion tests may be decreased.

**INTERACTIONS Drug:** Increased risk of nephrotoxicity and ototoxicity with AMINOGLYCOSIDES, **amphotericin B, colistin, polymyxin B, cisplatin, vancomycin.**

**PHARMACOKINETICS Peak:** 1–2 h. **Distribution:** Does not cross blood–brain barrier; crosses placenta. **Elimination:** 52% in urine

Common adverse effects in *italic;* life-threatening effects <u>underlined</u>; generic names in **bold**; classifications in SMALL CAPS; ♣ Canadian drug name; ⊘ Prototype drug

259

unchanged in 12 h; small amount in bile. **Half-Life:** 4–6 h.

## NURSING IMPLICATIONS

### Black Box Warning

*Capreomycin has been associated with VIII cranial nerve impairment and renal injury.*

### Assessment & Drug Effects

- Observe injection sites for signs of excessive bleeding and inflammation.
- Dosage of capreomycin is typically reduced in patients with impaired renal function, as it is cumulative. Follow renal function tests closely.
- Monitor closely for vestibular and/or auditory nerve impairment especially in those with preexisting renal insufficiency.
- Monitor I&O rates and pattern: Report immediately any change in output or I&O ratio, any unusual appearance of urine, or elevation of BUN above 30 mg/dL.
- Evaluate hearing and balance by audiometric measurements (twice weekly or weekly) and tests of vestibular function (periodically).
- Monitor lab tests: Baseline C&S prior to therapy; baseline and weekly renal function tests; baseline and frequent serum electrolytes and LFTs.

### Patient & Family Education

- Report any change in hearing or disturbance of balance. These effects are sometimes reversible if drug is withdrawn promptly when first symptoms appear.
- Ensure that you know about adverse reactions and what to do about them. Report immediately the appearance of any unusual symptom, regardless of how vague it may seem.

## CAPSAICIN

(cap-say'i-sin)

Axsain, Capsaicin, Capsin, Capzasin-P, Dolorac, Qutenza, Trixaicin, Zostrix, Zostrix-HP

**Classification:** TOPICAL ANALGESIC
Therapeutic: TOPICAL ANALGESIC

**AVAILABILITY** Lotion cream; gel, topical patch

**ACTION & THERAPEUTIC EFFECT** Capsaicin depletes and prevents reaccumulation of Substance P, the primary chemical mediator of pain impulses from the periphery to the CNS. *Renders skin and joints insensitive to pain; therefore, it serves as an effective peripheral analgesic.*

**USES** Temporary relief of pain from arthritis, neuralgias, diabetic neuropathy, and herpes zoster.

**UNLABELED USES** Phantom limb pain, psoriasis, intractable pruritus.

**CONTRAINDICATIONS** Hypersensitivity to capsaicin or any ingredient in the cream.

**CAUTIOUS USE** Patients on ACE inhibitors. Safety and efficacy in children younger than 2 y not established.

## ROUTE & DOSAGE

### Analgesia

*Adult/Child (2 y or older):* **Topical** Apply to affected area not more than 3–4 × day

## ADMINISTRATION
### Topical
- Apply to affected areas only and avoid contact with eyes or broken or irritated skin.

- If applied with bare hand, wash immediately following application.
- Use only nitrile gloves when handling a capsaicin patch.
- Avoid tight bandages over areas of application of the cream.
- If necessary for adherence, clip hair (do not shave) on skin where patch will be applied.
- Patch may be cut (before removing protective liner) to match size and shape of treatment area.
- Leave patch on for 60 min. To ensure contact, a dressing may be applied.
- Following patch removal, apply cleansing gel to treatment area and leave on for at least 1 min.

## ADVERSE EFFECTS (≥1%) CNS:
Concentration greater than 1%: Neurotoxicity, hyperalgesia. **Skin:** *Burning, stinging, redness,* itching. **Other:** Cough.

## INTERACTIONS Drug:
May increase incidence of cough with ACE INHIBITORS.

## PHARMACOKINETICS Onset:
Postherpetic neuralgia: 2–6 wk.

## NURSING IMPLICATIONS
### Assessment & Drug Effects
- Monitor for significant pain relief, which may require 4–6 wk of application 3 or 4 × daily.
- Monitor for and report signs of skin breakdown as these generally indicate need for drug discontinuation.

### Patient & Family Education
- Report local discomfort at site of application if discomfort is distressing or persists beyond the first 3–4 days of use.
- Use caution in handling contact lenses following application of cream. Wash hands thoroughly before touching lenses.
- Notify prescriber if symptoms do not improve or condition worsens within 14–28 days.

## CAPTOPRIL
(kap'toe-pril)
**Classifications:** RENIN ANGIOTENSIN SYSTEM ANTAGONIST; ANTIHYPERTENSIVE
**Therapeutic:** ANTIHYPERTENSIVE; ACE INHIBITOR
**Prototype:** Enalapril

## AVAILABILITY Tablet

## ACTION & THERAPEUTIC EFFECT
Lowers blood pressure by specific inhibition of the angiotensin-converting enzyme (ACE) utilized by renin in the formation of angiotensin II, a potent vasoconstrictor. ACE inhibition alters hemodynamics without compensatory changes in cardiac output (except in patients with CHF). Inhibition of ACE also leads to decreased circulating aldosterone. *Effective in management of hypertension, and in congestive heart failure with resulting decreases in dyspnea and improved exercise tolerance.*

## USES
Hypertension; heart failure, diabetic nephropathy, left ventricular dysfunction post MI; proteinuria.

## UNLABELED USES
Idiopathic edema; hypertensive emergency, scleroderma renal crisis.

## CONTRAINDICATIONS
History of angioedema, hypersensitivity to captopril or ACE inhibitors; coadministration with alskiren in patients with DM; hypotension; jaundice, or marked elevations of hepatic enzymes; pregnancy (category D); lactation.

Common adverse effects in *italic;* life-threatening effects underlined; generic names in **bold;** classifications in SMALL CAPS; ♣ Canadian drug name; ⊘ Prototype drug

261

**CAUTIOUS USE** Impaired renal function, patient with solitary kidney; collagen-vascular diseases (scleroderma, SLE); autoimmune disease, bone marrow suppression, coronary or cerebrovascular disease; black patients; surgery; cardiomyopathy, aortic stenosis; severe salt/volume depletion; heart failure, hyperkalemia, older adults, children.

## ROUTE & DOSAGE

### Hypertension
*Adult/Adolescent:* **PO** 12.5–25 mg b.i.d. or t.i.d., may increase to 50 mg t.i.d. (max: 450 mg/day)

### Heart Failure
*Adult:* **PO** 25 mg b.i.d.; may increase to 50 mg t.i.d. if needed (max: 450 mg/day)

### Proteinuria with Diabetic Nephropathy
*Adult:* **PO** 25 mg t.i.d.

### Left Ventricular Function Post MI
*Adult:* **PO** 6.25–12.5 mg t.i.d.

### Renal Insufficiency Dosage Adjustment
*CrCl 10–50 mL/min:* 75% of dose; *less than 10 mL/min:* 50% of dose

## ADMINISTRATION

### Oral
- Give captopril 1 h before meals. Food reduces absorption by 30–40%.
- Store in light-resistant containers at no more than 30° C (86° F) unless otherwise directed.

## ADVERSE EFFECTS (≥1%) **Body as a Whole:** Hypersensitivity reactions, serum sickness-like reaction, arthralgia, skin eruptions. **CV:** Tachycardia, first dose hypotension, dizziness, fainting. **GI:** Altered taste sensation (loss of taste perception, persistent salt or metallic taste); weight loss, intestinal angioedema. **Hematologic:** Hyperkalemia, neutropenia, agranulocytosis (rare). **Respiratory:** *Cough.* **Skin:** *Maculopapular rash,* urticaria, pruritus, angioedema, photosensitivity. **Urogenital:** Azotemia, impaired renal function, nephrotic syndrome, membranous glomerulonephritis. **Other:** Positive antinuclear antibody (ANA) titers.

## DIAGNOSTIC TEST INTERFERENCE
False-positive *urine acetone* (using *sodium nitroprusside reagent*). Captopril may decrease *fasting blood sugar.*

## INTERACTIONS **Drug:** NITRATES, DIURETICS, and ANTIHYPERTENSIVES enhance hypotensive effects. POTASSIUM-SPARING DIURETICS **(spironolactone, amiloride)** increase potassium levels. May increase risk of angioedema when used with **pregabalin;** increased risk of hyperkalemia with **aliskiren.** ANTACIDS may decrease absorption. Use with **digoxin** (though common) requires reduction in digoxin dose. **Food:** Decreases absorption; take 30–60 min before meals.

## PHARMACOKINETICS **Absorption:** 60–75% absorbed; food may decrease absorption 25–40%. **Onset:** 15 min. **Peak:** 1–2 h. **Duration:** 6–12 h. **Distribution:** To all tissues except CNS; crosses placenta. **Metabolism:** Some liver metabolism. **Elimination:** Primarily in urine; excreted in breast milk.

## NURSING IMPLICATIONS

### Black Box Warning

*Captopril has been associated with fetal injury and death.*

Common adverse effects in *italic;* life-threatening effects underlined; generic names in **bold;** classifications in SMALL CAPS; ✚ Canadian drug name; Ⓟ Prototype drug

## Assessment & Drug Effects

- Monitor BP closely following the first dose. A sudden exaggerated hypotensive response may occur within 1–3 h of first dose, especially in those with high BP or on a diuretic and restricted salt intake.
- Monitor therapeutic effectiveness. At least 2 wk of therapy may be required before full therapeutic effects are achieved.
- Monitor lab tests: Baseline urine protein levels and monthly for the first 8 mo of treatment and then periodically thereafter, WBC and differential before therapy is begun and at approximately 2-wk intervals for the first 3 mo of therapy and then periodically thereafter.

## Patient & Family Education

- Report to prescriber without delay the onset of unexplained fever, unusual fatigue, sore mouth or throat, easy bruising or bleeding. Mild skin eruptions are most likely to appear during the first 4 wk of therapy and may be accompanied by fever and eosinophilia.
- Taste impairment occurs in 5–10% of patients and generally reverses in 2–3 mo even with continued therapy.
- Notify prescriber if you become or suspect you are pregnant.
- Use OTC medications only with approval of the prescriber.

## CARBACHOL INTRAOCULAR
(kar'ba-kole)

Miostat

**See Appendix A-1.**

## CARBAMAZEPINE ⓟ
(kar-ba-maz'e-peen)

Apo-Carbamazepine ♦, Carbatrol, Epitol, Equetro, Mazepine ♦, PMS-Carbamazepine ♦, Tegretol, Tegretol XR

**Classification:** ANTICONVULSANT; TRICYCLIC
**Therapeutic:** ANTICONVULSANT; ANTIMANIA

**AVAILABILITY** Tablet; extended release tablet; extended release capsule; oral suspension

## ACTION & *THERAPEUTIC EFFECT*
Inhibits sustained repetitive impulses and reduces post-tetanic synaptic transmission in the spinal cord. It limits the spread of seizure activity. Provides relief in trigeminal neuralgia by reducing synaptic transmission within trigeminal nucleus. Unknown mechanism in regard to bipolar disorder. *Effective anticonvulsant for a range of seizure disorders and as an adjuvant reduces depressive signs and symptoms and stabilizes mood. It is effective for pain and other symptoms associated with neurologic disorders.*

**USES** Partial seizures, bipolar disorder, mania, neuropathic pain, tonic-clonic seizures, trigeminal neuralgia.

**UNLABELED USES** Diabetic neuropathy, agitation, postherpetic neuralgia, hiccups.

**CONTRAINDICATIONS** Hypersensitivity to carbamazepine and to TCAs or MAOI therapy; history of myelosuppression or hematologic reaction to other drugs; leukopenia; bone marrow depression; within 14 d use of MAOI drugs; increased IOP; SLE; hepatic, or renal failure; hyponatremia; coronary artery disease;

**C**

hypertension; petit mal (absent) seizures, atonic or myoclonic seizures; suicidal ideation; acute intermediate porphyria; presence of HLA-B*1502 gene increases risk of Stevens–Johnson syndrome or toxic epidermal necrolysis especially common in Asian ancestry; pregnancy (category D).

**CAUTIOUS USE** The older adult; history of cardiac disease or impairment, alcoholism; history of suicidal thoughts; hepatic disease or impairment; cardiac arrhythmias; mixed seizure disorder including atypical absence seizures; children younger than 6 y.

## ROUTE & DOSAGE

**Seizures**

*Adult:* PO 200 mg b.i.d., gradually increased to 800–1200 mg/day in 3–4 divided doses. **Tegretol XR** dosed b.i.d.
*Child: (Younger than 6 y):* PO 10–20 mg/kg/day, may gradually increase weekly (recommended max: 35 mg/kg/day in 3–4 divided doses); *6–12 y:* 100 mg b.i.d., gradually increased to 400–800 mg/day in 3–4 divided doses (max: 1 g/day); *younger than 6 y:* 20–30 mg/kg/day in 3–4 divided doses

**Trigeminal Neuralgia**

*Adult:* PO 100 mg b.i.d., gradually increased by 100 mg increments q12h until relief; usual dose 200–800 mg/day in 3–4 divided doses (max: 1.2 g/day). **Tegretol XR** dosed b.i.d.

**Bipolar Disorder (Equetro)**

*Adult:* PO 200 mg b.i.d.

## ADMINISTRATION

**Oral**

- Do not administer within 14 days of patient receiving a MAO inhibitor.
- Give with a meal to increase absorption.
- Ensure that chewable tablets are chewed or crushed before being swallowed with a liquid.
- Ensure that sustained release form of drug is not chewed or crushed. It **must be** swallowed whole.
- Do not administer carbamazepine suspension simultaneously with other liquid medications: A precipitate may form in the stomach.

**ADVERSE EFFECTS** (≥1%) **Body as a Whole:** Myalgia, arthralgia, leg cramps, carbamazepine-induced SLE. **CV:** Edema, syncope, arrhythmias, heart block. **GI:** Nausea, vomiting, anorexia, abdominal pain, diarrhea, constipation, dry mouth and pharynx, abnormal liver function tests, hepatitis, cholestatic and hepatocellular jaundice, pancreatitis. **Endocrine:** Hypothyroidism, SIADH. **Hematologic:** Aplastic anemia, *leukopenia* (transient), leukocytosis, agranulocytosis, eosinophilia, thrombocytopenia. **CNS:** Dizziness, vertigo, drowsiness, disturbances of coordination, ataxia, confusion, headache, fatigue, listlessness, speech difficulty, development of minor motor seizures, hyperreflexia, akathisia, involuntary movements, tremors, visual hallucinations, activation of latent psychosis, aggression; agitation, respiratory depression. **Skin:** Skin rashes, urticaria, petechiae, erythema multiforme, Stevens–Johnson syndrome, photosensitivity reactions, altered skin pigmentation, exfoliative dermatitis, alopecia. **Special Senses:** Abnormal hearing acuity, scotomas, conjunctivitis, blurred

Common adverse effects in *italic*; life-threatening effects underlined; generic names in **bold**; classifications in SMALL CAPS; ✦ Canadian drug name; ⊕ Prototype drug vision, transient diplopia, oculomotor disturbances, oscillopsia, nystagmus. **Urogenital:** Urinary frequency or retention, oliguria, impotence.

## DIAGNOSTIC TEST INTERFERENCE

May cause false positive *TCA screen;* may interact with pregnancy tests.

## INTERACTIONS **Drug:** Serum
concentrations of other ANTICONVULSANTS or **ranolazine** may decrease because of increased metabolism; **verapamil, erythromycin, ketoconazole, nefazodone, voriconazole,** may increase carbamazepine levels; decreases hypoprothrombinemic effects of ORAL ANTICOAGULANTS; increases metabolism of ESTROGENS, thus decreasing effectiveness of ORAL CONTRACEPTIVES. Reduces concentration of **delavirdine, etravirine. Food:** Grapefruit juice may increase drug levels. **Herbal:** Ginkgo may decrease anticonvulsant effectiveness.

## PHARMACOKINETICS **Absorption:** Slowly from GI tract. **Peak:** 2–8 h. **Distribution:** Widely distributed; high concentrations in CSF; crosses placenta; distributed into breast milk. **Metabolism:** In liver by CYP3A4; can induce liver microsomal enzymes. **Elimination:** In urine and feces. **Half-Life:** Variable due to autoinduction: 25–65 h then 14–16 h (with repeated use).

## NURSING IMPLICATIONS

### Black Box Warning

*Serious and sometime fatal dermatologic reactions have occurred with carbamazepine in those who carry the HLA-B\*1502 allele (e.g., persons of Asian ancestry). Carbamazepine has been associated with development of aplastic anemia and agranulocytosis.*

### Assessment & Drug Effects

- Monitor for therapeutic effectiveness and loss of seizure control. Some patients develop tolerance to the effects of carbamazepine.
- Monitor for the following reactions, which commonly occur during early therapy: Drowsiness, dizziness, light-headedness, ataxia, gastric upset.
- Monitor for and report promptly skin rash or any other sign of dermatologic toxicity.
- Withhold drug and notify prescriber if the following signs occur: RBC less than 4 million/mm³, Hct less than 32%, Hgb less than 11 g/dL, WBC less than 4000/mm³, platelet count less than 100,000/mm³, reticulocyte count less than 20,000/mm³, serum iron greater than 150 mg/dL.
- Monitor for toxicity, which can develop when serum concentrations are even slightly above the therapeutic range.
- Monitor I&O ratio and vital signs during period of dosage adjustment. Report oliguria, signs of fluid retention, changes in I&O ratio, and changes in BP or pulse patterns.
- Doses higher than 600 mg/day may precipitate arrhythmias in patients with heart disease.
- Confusion and agitation may be aggravated in the older adult.
- Monitor lab tests: Prior to initiation of therapy HLA-B\*1502 testing is recommended; baseline and periodic CBC with differential, platelet count, LFTs, and kidney function tests; periodic lipid profile and serum calcium.

### Patient & Family Education

- Discontinue drug and notify prescriber immediately if early signs of toxicity or a possible

Common adverse effects in *italic;* life-threatening effects underlined; generic names in **bold;** classifications in SMALL CAPS; ♣ Canadian drug name; ● Prototype drug

265

hematologic problem appear, (e.g., skin rash, anorexia, fever, sore throat or mouth, malaise, unusual fatigue, tendency to bruise or bleed, petechiae, ecchymoses, bleeding gums, nose bleeds).

- Avoid hazardous tasks requiring mental alertness and physical coordination until reaction to drug is known, since dizziness, drowsiness, and ataxia are common adverse effects.
- Report promptly to prescriber development of an unexplained skin reaction.
- Avoid excessive sunlight, as photosensitivity reactions have been reported. Apply a sunscreen (if allowed) with SPF of 12 or above.
- Carbamazepine may cause breakthrough bleeding and may also affect the reliability of oral contraceptives.
- Be aware that abrupt withdrawal of any anticonvulsant drug may precipitate seizures or even status epilepticus.

# CARBIDOPA-LEVODOPA ℗

(kar-bi-doe'pa)
Sinemet, Sinemet-CR, Parcopa

# CARBIDOPA

Lodosyn

**Classifications:** DOPAMINE RECEPTOR AGONIST; ANTIPARKINSON
Therapeutic: ANTIPARKINSON

**AVAILABILITY Carbidopa:** Tablet. **Carbidopa/Levodopa:** Tablet; sustained release tablet; orally disintegrating tablet

## ACTION & THERAPEUTIC EFFECT

Carbidopa prevents peripheral metabolism of levodopa and thereby makes more levodopa available for transport to the brain. Carbidopa does not cross blood–brain barrier and therefore does not affect metabolism of levodopa within the brain. *Effective in management of symptoms of Parkinson's disease and parkinsonism of secondary origin while improving life expectancy and quality of life.*

**USES** Symptomatic treatment of idiopathic Parkinson's disease (paralysis agitans), postencephalitic parkinsonism, and parkinsonism following carbon dioxide and manganese intoxication. Carbidopa is available alone from manufacturer, on request by prescriber, for use with levodopa when separate titration of each agent is indicated, and for investigational purposes.

**CONTRAINDICATIONS** Hypersensitivity to carbidopa or levodopa; narrow-angle glaucoma; history of or suspected melanoma; lactation.

**CAUTIOUS USE** Cardiovascular, hepatic, pulmonary, or renal disorders; history of MI; urinary retention; history of peptic ulcer; psychiatric states; endocrine disease; chronic wide-angle glaucoma; seizure disorders; pregnancy (category C). Safe use in children younger than 18 y is not established. Safe use in women of childbearing potential is not established.

## ROUTE & DOSAGE

**Parkinson's Disease in Patients Not Currently Receiving Levodopa**

*Adult:* **PO** 1 tablet containing 10 mg carbidopa/100 mg levodopa *or* 25 mg carbidopa/100 mg levodopa t.i.d., increased by 1 tablet daily or every other day up to 6 tablets/day

Common adverse effects in *italic;* life-threatening effects underlined; generic names in **bold;** classifications in SMALL CAPS; ♣ Canadian drug name; ℗ Prototype drug

**Patients Receiving Levodopa**

*Adult:* **PO** 1 tablet of the 25/250 mixture t.i.d. or q.i.d., adjusted by ½–1 tablet as needed up to 8 tablets/day (start at 20–25% of initial dose of levodopa)

## ADMINISTRATION

### Oral

- Ensure that sustained release form of drug (Sinemet CR) is not chewed or crushed. It may be broken in half but otherwise swallowed whole.
- Give consistently with respect to food. High protein meals may interfere with absorption of levodopa.
- When patient has been taking levodopa alone, carbidopa-levodopa is usually initiated with a morning dose after patient has been without levodopa for at least 8 h.
- Store in tight, light-resistant containers.

## ADVERSE EFFECTS (≥1%) **Body as a Whole:** Hoarseness, unusual breathing patterns, neuroleptic malignant syndrome. **CV:** Orthostatic hypotension, irregular heartbeat, palpitation, arrhythmias, phlebitis, edema. **GI:** Nausea, anorexia, dry mouth, bruxism, vomiting, excess salivation. **Hematologic:** Hemolytic and nonhemolytic anemia, thrombocytopenia, agranulocytosis. **Metabolic:** Abnormal liver function tests, abnormal BUN. **CNS:** *Involuntary movements (dyskinetic, dystonic, choreiform),* ataxia, muscle twitching, increase in hand tremor, numbness, headache, dizziness, euphoria, fatigue, confusion, insomnia, nightmares, mental disturbances, anxiety, depression with suicidal tendencies, delirium, seizures. **Skin:** Body odor, skin rash, dark sweat, loss of hair. **Special Senses:** Blepharospasm, mydriasis, miosis, blurred vision, diplopia, oculogyric crisis. **Urogenital:** Dark urine, priapism, urinary frequency, retention, incontinence.

## DIAGNOSTIC TEST INTERFERENCE

**Urine glucose:** False-negative tests may result with use of *glucose oxidase methods* (e.g., *Clinistix, TesTape*) and false-positive results with *copper reduction methods* (e.g., *Benedict's, Clinitest*), especially in patients receiving large doses. It is reported that *Clinistix* and *TesTape* may be used if reading is taken at margin of wet and dry tape. There is also the possibility of false-positive tests for *urinary ketones* by *dipstick tests* [e.g., *Acetest* (equivocal), *Ketostix, Labstix*] false elevation of *serum* and *urinary uric acid* levels by *colorimetric methods* (*not* with *uricase*); and interference with *urine PKU test* results.

## INTERACTIONS Drug: MAO INHIBITORS may precipitate hypertensive crisis; TRICYCLIC ANTIDEPRESSANTS potentiate postural hypotension; ANTICHOLINERGIC AGENTS may enhance levodopa effects but can exacerbate involuntary movements; **methyldopa, guanethidine** increase hypotensive and CNS effects; PHENOTHIAZINES, haloperidol, **phenytoin, papaverine** may interfere with levodopa effects.

## PHARMACOKINETICS Absorption: 40–70% of carbidopa absorbed after PO dose; carbidopa may enhance absorption of levodopa. **Distribution:** Widely distributed in most body tissues except CNS; crosses placenta; excreted in breast milk. **Elimination:** In urine. **Half-Life:** 2 h.

---

Common adverse effects in *italic;* life-threatening effects underlined; generic names in **bold;** classifications in SMALL CAPS; ♣ Canadian drug name; ✪ Prototype drug

267

## NURSING IMPLICATIONS
### Assessment & Drug Effects

- Make accurate observations and report promptly adverse reactions and therapeutic effects. Rate of dosage increase is determined primarily by patient's tolerance and response to levodopa.
- Monitor vital signs, particularly during period of dosage adjustment. Report alterations in BP, pulse, and respiratory rate and rhythm.
- Monitor all patients closely for behavior changes. Patients in depression should be closely observed for suicidal tendencies.
- Monitor for changes in intraocular pressure in patients with chronic wide-angle glaucoma.
- Monitor patients with diabetes carefully for alterations in diabetes control. Frequent monitoring of blood sugar is advised.
- Report promptly abnormal involuntary movement such as facial grimacing, exaggerated chewing, protrusion of tongue, rhythmic opening and closing of mouth, bobbing of head, jerky arm and leg movements, and exaggerated respiration.
- Assess for "on-off" phenomenon: Sudden, unpredictable loss of drug effectiveness ("off" effect), which lasts 1 min–1 h. This is followed by an equally abrupt return of function ("on" effect). Sometimes symptoms can be controlled by increasing number of doses/day.
- Monitor therapeutic effects. Some patients manifest increase in bradykinesia ("leg freezing" or slow body movement). The patient is unable to start walking and frequently falls. Reduction of dosage may be indicated in these patients.
- Patients who require more frequent drug administration are most likely to manifest gradual return of parkinsonian symptoms toward the end of a dose period.
- Monitor lab tests: Periodic blood glucose, LFTs, renal function tests, CBC with differential, Hgb and Hct.

### Patient & Family Education

- Follow prescriber's directions regarding continuation or discontinuation of levodopa. Both adverse reactions and therapeutic effects occur more rapidly with carbidopa–levodopa combination than with levodopa alone.
- Make positional changes slowly and in stages, particularly from recumbent to upright position, dangle your legs a few minutes before standing, and walk in place before ambulating, as some patients experience weakness, dizziness, and faintness. Tolerance to this effect usually develops within a few months of therapy. Support stockings may help. Consult prescriber.
- Report muscle twitching and spasmodic winking promptly, as these may be early signs of overdosage.
- You may notice elevation of mood and sense of well-being before any objective improvement. Resume activities gradually and observe safety precautions to avoid injury.
- Maintain your prescribed drug regimen. Abrupt withdrawal can lead to parkinsonian crisis with return of marked muscle rigidity, akinesia, tremor, hyperpyrexia, mental changes.
- Avoid driving or other hazardous activities until reaction to drug is determined.
- Levodopa may cause urine to darken on standing and may also cause sweat to be dark-colored. This effect is not clinically significant.

Common adverse effects in *italic*; life-threatening effects underlined; generic names in **bold**; classifications in SMALL CAPS; ✦ Canadian drug name; ⊙ Prototype drug

- Wear medical identification. Inform all health care providers that you are taking carbidopa-levodopa.

## CARBINOXAMINE
(car-bi-nox'a-meen)
Karbinal ER
**Classification:** ANTIHISTAMINE;
$H_1$-RECEPTOR ANTAGONIST
**Therapeutic:** ANTIHISTAMINE;
SEDATING $H_1$-ANTAGONIST
**Prototype:** Diphenhydramine

**AVAILABILITY** Oral suspension; oral solution; tablet

## ACTION & THERAPEUTIC EFFECT
Carbinoxamine competes for $H_1$-receptor sites on effector cells thus blocking histamine release. *Has antihistaminic, anticholinergic (drying), antitussive, and sedative properties.*

**USES** Allergic conjunctivitis, allergic rhinitis, rhinorrhea, pruritus, sneezing, urticaria.

**CONTRAINDICATIONS** Hypersensitivity to carbinoxamine; lower respiratory tract symptoms (including acute asthma); MAOI therapy, MAOI coadministration; lactation; children younger than 2 y.

**CAUTIOUS USE** Hypersensitivity to antihistamines of similar structure; history of asthma; COPD; convulsive disorders; increased IOP; hyperthyroidism; hypertension, cardiovascular disease; hepatic disease; diabetes mellitus, prostatic hyperplasia/urinary obstruction, pyloroduodenal obstruction, older adults; pregnancy (category C); young children.

## ROUTE & DOSAGE

**Allergic Conjunctivitis, Allergic Rhinitis, Rhinorrhea, Pruritus, Sneezing, Urticaria**
*Adult/Adolescent:* **PO** 4–8 mg q6–8h (max: 32 mg/day)
*Child ( 2 to younger than 6 y):* **PO** 0.2–0.4 mg/kg/day divided into 3–4 doses; *6 y or older:* 2–4 mg q6–8h

## ADMINISTRATION

**Oral**
- Administer on an empty stomach with water. Shake suspension well before administering.
- Store a 15°–30° C (59°–86° F). Protect from light.

**ADVERSE EFFECTS** (≥1%) **Body as a Whole:** <u>Anaphylactic shock</u>, chills, excessive perspiration, polyuria, photosensitivity, weakness. **CNS:** Acute labyrinthitis, blurred vision, confusion, convulsions, diplopia, disturbed coordination, dizziness, euphoria, excitation, fatigue, headache, hysteria, insomnia, irritability, nervousness, neuritis, paresthesia, restlessness, *sedation*, tinnitus, tremor, vertigo. **CV:** Extrasystoles, headache, hypotension, palpitations, tachycardia, chest tightness. **GI:** Anorexia, constipation, diarrhea, epigastric distress, heartburn, nausea, vomiting. **Hematological:** <u>Agranulocytosis</u>, hemolytic anemia, <u>thrombocytopenia</u>. **Otic:** Labyrinthitis, tinnitus **Respiratory:** Dryness of mouth, nose and throat, nasal stuffiness, thickening of bronchial secretions. **Skin:** Drug rash, photosensitivity, urticaria. **Urogenital:** Difficult urination, increased urinary

Common adverse effects in *italic;* life-threatening effects <u>underlined</u>; generic names in **bold**; classifications in SMALL CAPS; ♣ Canadian drug name; ☯ Prototype drug

269

frequency, urinary retention, early menses.

**INTERACTIONS Drug:** MAO INHIBITORS may prolong and intensify the anticholinergic effects of carbinoxamine. Carbinoxamine may enhance the effects of TRICYCLIC ANTIDEPRESSANTS, BARBITURATES, **alcohol,** and other CNS DEPRESSANTS.

**PHARMACOKINETICS Onset:** 15–30 m. **Peak:** 1 h. **Metabolism:** Extensive hepatic metabolism to inactive compounds. **Elimination:** Primarily renal. **Half-Life:** 10–20 h.

**NURSING IMPLICATIONS**

**Assessment & Drug Effects**

▪ Monitor CV status especially with preexisting cardiovascular disease.
▪ Monitor for adverse effects especially in young children and older adults.
▪ Supervise ambulation and institute fall precautions as necessary.

**Patient & Family Education**

▪ Do not use alcohol and other CNS depressants because of the possible additive CNS depressant effects.
▪ Do not drive or engage in other potentially hazardous activities until the response to drug is known.
▪ Increase fluid intake, if not contraindicated; drug has a drying effect (thickens bronchial secretions) that may make expectoration difficult.

**CARBOPLATIN**

(car-bo-pla'tin)

**Classifications:** ANTINEOPLASTIC; ALKYLATING AGENT

**Therapeutic:** ANTINEOPLASTIC
**Prototype:** Cyclophosphamide

**AVAILABILITY** Solution for injection

**ACTION & *THERAPEUTIC EFFECT***
It produces interstrand DNA crosslinkages, thus interfering with DNA, RNA, and protein synthesis. Carboplatin is cell-cycle nonspecific and induces programmed cell death. *Full or partial activity against a variety of cancers resulting in reduction or stabilization of tumor size. Useful in patients with impaired renal function, patients unable to accommodate high-volume hydration, or patients at high risk for neurotoxicity and/or ototoxicity.*

**USES** Ovarian cancer.

**UNLABELED USES** Combination therapy for breast, cervical, colon, endometrial, head and neck, and lung cancer; leukemia, lymphoma, and melanoma.

**CONTRAINDICATIONS** History of severe reactions to carboplatin or other platinum compounds, severe bone marrow depression; significant bleeding; impaired renal function; pregnancy (category D); lactation.

**CAUTIOUS USE** Use with other nephrotoxic drugs; coagulopathy; previous radiation therapy; renal impairment.

**ROUTE & DOSAGE**

**Ovarian Cancer**

*Adult:* **IV** 360 mg/m² once q4wk. May be repeated when neutrophil count is at least 2000 mm³ and platelet count is at least 100,000 mm³. If neutrophil and platelet

Common adverse effects in *italic;* life-threatening effects underlined; generic names in **bold**; classifications in SMALL CAPS; ✤ Canadian drug name; ⦿ Prototype drug counts are lower, dose of carboplatin should be reduced by 50–75% of initial dose. Alternatively, 400 mg/m² as a 24-h infusion for 2 consecutive days can be used.

**Renal Impairment Dosage Adjustment**

CrCl 41–59 mL/min: Dose 250 mg/m²; 16–40 mL/min: Dose 200 mg/m²

**Hemodialysis Dosage Adjustment**
Initial dose not to exceed 150 mg/m²

## ADMINISTRATION
**Intravenous**

*PREPARE:* **IV Infusion:** Do not use needles or IV sets containing aluminum. ▪ Immediately before use, reconstitute with either sterile water for injection or D5W or NS as follows: 50-mg vial plus 5 mL diluent; 150-mg vial plus 15 mL diluent; 450-mg vial plus 45 mL diluent. All dilutions yield 10 mg/mL. ▪ May be further diluted for infusion with D5W or NS to concentrations as low as 0.5 mg/mL.
*ADMINISTER:* **IV Infusion:** Give IV solution over 15 min or longer, depending on total amount of solution and patient tolerance. ▪ Lengthening duration of administration may decrease nausea and vomiting. ▪ Premedication with a parenteral antiemetic 30 min before and on a scheduled basis thereafter is normally used. ▪ Do not repeat doses until the neutrophil count is at least 2000/mm³ and platelet count at least 100,000/mm³.
*INCOMPATIBILITIES:* Solution/additive: **Sodium bicarbonate, fluorouracil, mesna.** Y-site: **Amphotericin B cholesteryl complex, lansoprazole.**

▪ Protect from light. Reconstituted solutions are stable for 8 h at room temperature; discard solutions 8 h after dilution.

## ADVERSE EFFECTS (≥1%) Body as a
**Whole:** Hypersensitivity reactions. **GI:** *Mild to moderate nausea and vomiting,* anorexia, hypogeusia, dysgeusia, mucositis, diarrhea, constipation, elevated liver enzymes. **Hematologic:** <u>Thrombocytopenia, leukopenia, neutropenia, anemia.</u> **Metabolic:** *Mild hyponatremia, hypomagnesemia, hypocalcemia, and hypokalemia.* **CNS:** Peripheral neuropathy. **Skin:** Rash, alopecia. **Special Senses:** Tinnitus. **Urogenital:** Nephrotoxicity.

## DIAGNOSTIC TEST INTERFERENCE
Decreased *calcium levels;* mild increases in *liver function tests;* decreased levels of *magnesium, potassium,* and *sodium.*

## INTERACTIONS Drug: AMINOGLY-
COSIDES may increase the risk of ototoxicity and nephrotoxicity. May decrease **phenytoin** levels.

## PHARMACOKINETICS Onset: 8 wk
(2 cycles). **Duration:** 2–16 mo. **Distribution:** Highest concentration in the liver, lung, kidney, skin, and tumors. Not bound to plasma proteins. **Metabolism:** Hydrolyzed in the serum. **Elimination:** Primarily by the kidneys; 60–80% excreted in urine within 24 h. **Half-Life:** 3 h.

## NURSING IMPLICATIONS

### Black Box Warning

*Carboplatin has been associated with severe bone marrow suppression. Anaphylactic-type reactions have occurred within minutes of administration.*

---

**C**

## Assessment & Drug Effects

- Monitor closely during first 15 min of infusion, since severe allergic reactions have occurred within minutes of carboplatin administration.
- Monitor results of peripheral blood counts. Leukopenia, neutropenia, and thrombocytopenia are dose related and may produce dose-limiting toxicity.
- Monitor for peripheral neuropathy (e.g., paresthesias), ototoxicity, and visual disturbances.
- Monitor serum electrolyte studies, because carboplatin has been associated with decreases in sodium, potassium, calcium, and magnesium. Special precautions may be warranted for patients on diuretic therapy.
- Monitor lab tests: Baseline and periodic CBC with differential, platelet count, Hgb and Hct; baseline kidney function tests and prior to each infusion; periodic serum electrolytes.

## Patient & Family Education

- Learn about the range of potential adverse effects. Strategies for nausea prevention should receive special attention.
- During therapy you are at risk for infection and hemorrhagic complications related to bone marrow suppression. Avoid unnecessary exposure to crowds or infected persons during the nadir period.
- Report paresthesias (numbness, tingling), visual disturbances, or symptoms of ototoxicity (hearing loss and/or tinnitus).

## CARBOPROST TROMETHAMINE ℗℞

(kar'boe-prost)

**Hemabate**

**Classifications:** PROSTAGLANDIN; OXYTOCIC
**Therapeutic:** OXYTOCIC

**AVAILABILITY** Solution for injection

## ACTION & *THERAPEUTIC EFFECT*

Synthetic analog of naturally occurring prostaglandin $F_2$ alpha with longer duration of biological activity. Stimulates myometrial contractions of gravid uterus at term labor. Mean time to abortion 16 h; mean dose required 2.6 mL. *Effectively stimulates uterine contraction and is used to induce abortion. Useful in treatment of postpartum hemorrhage due to uterine atony unresponsive to usual measures.*

**USES** Pregnancy termination. Also for refractory postpartum bleeding.

**UNLABELED USES** To reduce blood loss secondary to uterine atony; to induce labor in intrauterine fetal death and hydatidiform mole.

**CONTRAINDICATIONS** Acute pelvic inflammatory disease; active cardiac, pulmonary, renal, or hepatic disease; pregnancy (category D); lactation.

**CAUTIOUS USE** History of asthma; adrenal disease; anemia; hypotension; hypertension; diabetes mellitus; epilepsy; history of uterine surgery; cervical stenosis; fibroids.

## ROUTE & DOSAGE

**Abortion, Postpartum Bleeding**

*Adult:* **IM** Initial: 250 mcg (1 mL) repeated at 1.5–3.5-h intervals if indicated by uterine response. Dosage may be increased to 500

Common adverse effects in *italic;* life-threatening effects <u>underlined;</u> generic names in **bold;** classifications in SMALL CAPS; ♣ Canadian drug name; ℗ Prototype drug

mcg (2 mL) if uterine contractility is inadequate after several doses of 250 mcg (1 mL), not to exceed total dose of 12 mg or continuous administration for more than 2 days.

## ADMINISTRATION

### Intramuscular

▪ Give deep IM into a large muscle. Aspirate carefully before injecting drug to avoid inadvertent entry into blood vessel which can result in bronchospasm, tetanic contractions, and shock. Do not use same site for subsequent doses.

▪ Store drug in refrigerator at 2°–4° C (36°–39° F) unless otherwise specified.

### ADVERSE EFFECTS (≥1%) Body as a Whole: Fever, flushing, chills, cough, headache, pain (muscles, joints, lower abdomen, eyes), hiccups, breast tenderness. GI: *Nausea, diarrhea, vomiting.*

### PHARMACOKINETICS Peak: 30–90 min. Elimination: Renal within 24 h.

## NURSING IMPLICATIONS

### Assessment & Drug Effects

▪ Monitor uterine contractions and observe and report excessive vaginal bleeding and cramping pain. Save all clots and tissue for prescriber inspection and laboratory analysis.

▪ Check vital signs at regular intervals. Carboprost-induced febrile reaction occurs in more than 10% of patients and **must be** differentiated from endometritis, which occurs around third day after abortion.

### Patient & Family Education

▪ Report promptly onset of bleeding, foul-smelling discharge, abdominal pain, or fever.

▪ Since ovulation may reoccur as early as 2 wk post-abortion, consider appropriate contraception.

## CARFILZOMIB
(car-fil-zo′mib)
Kyprolis
**Classification:** ANTINEOPLASTIC; PROTEOSOME INHIBITOR; SIGNAL TRANSDUCTION INHIBITOR
Therapeutic: ANTINEOPLASTIC
**Prototype:** Bortezomib

**AVAILABILITY** Sterile lyophilized powder

### ACTION & *THERAPEUTIC EFFECT*
Plays a regulatory role in cell proliferation by destroying proteins that trigger cell-cycle progression and cell survival pathways in certain cancers; produces antiproliferative and proapoptotic effects leading to cell death in solid and hematologic tumor cells. *Delays tumor growth in multiple myeloma and other hematologic tumors and solid tumors.*

**USES** Relapsed or refractory multiple myeloma.

**CONTRAINDICATIONS** Pregnancy (category D); lactation.

**CAUTIOUS USE** Cardiac and pulmonary disease; CHF; MI within 6 mo; thrombocytopenia; hepatic disease. Avoid oral contraceptives or other hormonal contraceptives with increased risk of thrombosis. Safety and efficacy in children younger than 18 y not established.

---

## ROUTE & DOSAGE

### Multiple Myeloma

*Adult:* **IV** 20 mg/m² on days 1, 2, 8, 9, 15, 16 of 28 d cycle. Increase to 27 mg/m² on subsequent 28 d cycles if tolerated.

### Hepatic Impairment Dosage Adjustment

*Grade 3 or 4 liver toxicity:* Hold therapy until resolved or return to baseline; may restart at a reduced level (from 27 to 20 mg/m² or from 20 to 15 mg/m²); doses may be re-escalated if tolerated.

### Renal Impairment Dosage Adustment

*Serum creatinine greater than or equal to 2 × baseline:* Hold therapy until return to Grade 1 or baseline; may restart at a reduced level (from 27 to 20 mg/m² or from 20 to 15 mg/m²); doses may be re-escalated if tolerated.

### Dose Modifications Due to Other Toxicities

*Grade 3 or 4 toxicities:* Hold therapy until resolution or a return to baseline; consider reducing the dose one level (27 to 20 mg/m² or 20 to 15 mg/m²); doses may be re-escalated if tolerated. Refer to manufacturer's guidelines for specifics.

## ADMINISTRATION

### Intravenous

▪ Hazardous agent. Single glove during receiving and unpacking. For administration: double gloving, protective gown. Premedication: Give 4 mg dexamethasone prior to all doses during cycle 1, during the first cycle of dose escalation to 27 mg/m², and if infusion reaction symptoms appear during subsequent cycles. ▪ Hydration: Prior to each dose in cycle 1, give 250–500 mL of IV, NS, or other IV fluid. Give an additional 250–500 mL of IV fluids as needed. Continue IV hydration, as needed, in all subsequent cycles.

*PREPARE:* **IV Infusion:** Hazardous agent: Double glove and follow appropriate precautions for handling and disposal. Remove vial from refrigeration just prior to use. Reconstitute 60 mg vial with 29 mL sterile water for injection to yield 2 mg/mL. Direct stream against side of vial to prevent foaming. Swirl gently for 1 min or until completely dissolved. Do not shake. If foam appears, allow to stand until foam dissipates. Withdraw required dose and dilute in 50 mL or 100 mL D5W.

*ADMINISTER:* **IV Infusion:** Infuse over 10–30 min. **Do not** give as bolus dose. Flush IV line before/after with D5W.

*INCOMPATIBILITIES:* **Solution/additive:** Do not mix with other solutions or medications. **Y-site:** Do not mix with other solutions or medications.

▪ May store reconstituted drug up to 24 h refrigerated and up to 4 h at room temperature. Protect from light.

## ADVERSE EFFECTS (≥1%) **Body as a Whole:** Asthenia, chills, pain, peripheral edema, pyrexia, tumor lysis syndrome. **CNS:** Dizziness, *fatigue*, headache, hypoesthesia, intercranial hemorrhage, insomnia. **CV:** Chest wall pain, cardiac arrest, congestive heart failure, anemia, hypertension. **GI:** Anorexia, constipation, *diarrhea*, abdominal pain, *nausea*, vomiting,

gastrointestinal hemorrhage. **Hematological:** *Anemia*, leukopenia, lymphopenia, neutropenia, *thrombocyopenia*. **Metabolic:** AST increased, hypercalcemia, hyperglycemia, hypokalemia, hypomagnesemia, hyponatremia, hypophosphatemia. **Musculoskeletal:** Arthralgia, *back pain*, muscle spasms, pain in extremity. **Respiratory:** Cough, *dyspnea*, pneumonia, upper respiratory tract infection. **Urogenital:** Acute renal failure.

**INTERACTIONS** Consider increasing ANC monitoring if used with **clozapine**.

**PHARMACOKINETICS** **Distribution:** 97% plasma protein bound. **Metabolism:** Extensive hydrolytic metabolism. **Half-Life:** 1 h.

### NURSING IMPLICATIONS

#### Assessment & Drug Effects

- Check for pregnancy status
- Maintain adequate fluid volume status throughout treatment; closely monitor for fluid overload.
- Monitor cardiac and respiratory status closely during drug administration period.
- Monitor for evidence of tumor lysis syndrome (TLS). Signs of TLS include nausea and vomiting, dyspnea, irregular HR, cloudy urine, lethargy, and/or joint discomfort.
- Immediately stop infusion if dyspnea occurs. Do not resume infusion until symptoms return to baseline. Consult prescriber.
- Monitor for peripheral neuropathy.
- Monitor lab tests: Baseline and frequent CBC with differential and platelet count, serum electrolytes, LFTs, and renal function tests.

#### Patient & Family Education

- Report promptly any of the following: Chest pain, shortness of breath, chills, cough, fever, or swelling of the feet or legs.
- Maintain adequate hydration especially when experiencing diarrhea or vomiting. Seek guidance from prescriber if experiencing dizziness, light-headedness, or fainting.
- Do not drive or engage in other potentially dangerous activities until reaction to drug is known.
- Women should use effective means of birth control during therapy.
- Contact your prescriber immediately if you become pregnant during treatment.
- Do not breast-feed while receiving this drug.

## CARIPRAZINE
(car-i-pra′zine)
Vraylar

**Classifications:** ATYPICAL ANTIPSYCHOTIC; MOOD STABILIZER
**Therapeutic:** ANTIPSYCHOTIC; ANTIMANIC; ANTIDEPRESSANT
**Prototype:** Clozapine

**AVAILABILITY** Capsules

**ACTION & THERAPEUTIC EFFECT** The mechanism of action is unknown, but may be mediated by partial agonist activity at central dopamine $D_2$ and serotonin 5-HT$_{1A}$ receptors and antagonist activity at serotonin 5-HT$_{2A}$ receptors. *Stabilizes mood and improves ability to perform activities of daily living.*

**USES** Treatment of schizophrenia and acute treatment of manic or mixed episodes associated with bipolar I disease.

**CONTRAINDICATIONS** Known hypersensitivity to cariprazine and any component in the formulation; neuroleptic malignant syndrome (NMS).

**CAUTIOUS USE** Commitment use of a strong CYP3A4 inhibitor or

Common adverse effects in *italic;* life-threatening effects underlined; generic names in **bold;** classifications in SMALL CAPS; ♣ Canadian drug name; ✪ Prototype drug

275

**C**

inducer; tardive dyskinesia; hyperglycemia and DM; dyslipidemia; weight gain; esophageal motility disorder; orthostatic hypotension.

## ROUTE & DOSAGE

### Schizophrenia or Bipolar I Disease

*Adult:* **PO** Initial dose of 1.5 mg once daily; can increase to 3 mg once daily on day 2, then titrate up to maximum of 6 mg once daily

### Hepatic Impairment Dosage Adjustment

*Severe Impairment:* Not recommended

### Renal Impairment Dosage Adjustment

*Severe Impairment (CrCL < 30 mL/min):* Not recommended

### Concomitant CYP3A4 Inhibitors and Inducers Dosage Adjustments

*Strong CYP3A4 inhibitor:* Reduce usual dose by half
*Strong CYP3A4 inducer:* Not recommended

## ADMINISTRATION

### Oral

- May be given without regard to food.
- Store at 15°–30° C (59°–86° F) and protect from light.

**ADVERSE EFFECTS (≥1%) Body as a Whole:** Agitation, anxiety, fatigue, insomnia, pyrexia, restlessness. **CNS:** *Akathisia,* dizziness, *extrapyramidal symptoms, headache,* somnolence. **CV:** Hypertension, tachycardia. **GI:** Abdominal pain, constipation, diarrhea, dry mouth, dyspepsia, nausea, toothache, *vomiting.* **Metabolic:** Decreased appetite, increased blood creatine phosphokinase, increased hepatic enzymes, weight gain. **Musculoskeletal:** Arthalgia, back pain, dystonia, pain in extremity. **Respiratory:** Cough, nasopharyngitis, oropharyngeal pain. **Special Senses:** Blurred vision. **Urogenital:** Urinary tract infection.

**INTERACTIONS Drug:** Concomitant use with strong CYP3A4 inhibitors (e.g., **itraconazole, ketoconazole**) increases the levels of cariprazine; concomitant use with strong CYP3A4 inducers (e.g., **rifampin, carbamazepine**) decreases the levels of cariprazine. **Herbal:** St. John's wort decreases the levels of cariprazine.

**PHARMACOKINETICS Peak:** 3–6 h. **Distribution:** 91–97% plasma protein bound. **Metabolism:** Hepatic metabolism to both active and inactive metabolites. **Elimination:** Renal. **Half-Life:** 2–4 days.

## NURSING IMPLICATIONS

### Black Box Warning

*Cariprazine has been associated with increased mortality in elderly patients with dementia-related psychosis.*

### Assessment & Drug Effects

- Monitor for orthostatic hypotension, especially early in treatment.
- Monitor closely those at risk for aspiration as esophageal dysmotility and dysphagia may occur.
- Monitor for a report promptly S&S of tardive dyskinesia and neuroleptic malignant syndrome (see Appendix F).
- Monitor weight and report excessive increases in weight gain, BMI, and waist circumference.
- Monitor diabetics for loss of glycemic control.

---

Common adverse effects in *italic*; life-threatening effects <u>underlined</u>; generic names in **bold**; classifications in SMALL CAPS; ♣ Canadian drug name; ⦾ Prototype drug

- Monitor lab tests: Baseline and periodic CBC with differential, blood glucose, and lipid profile.

**Patient & Family Education**

- Use caution with activities requiring mental alertness until response to drug is known.
- Use caution when arising from a supine or sitting position as dizziness or fainting may occur.
- Report promptly any of the following: Restlessness; uncontrolled movement of the face, tongue or other body parts; weight gain; excessive urination or thirst; lightheadedness upon arising.
- Avoid overheating and maintain adequate hydration with liquids.
- Monitor blood glucose closely if diabetic.
- Notify prescriber of any other prescription or nonprescription drugs taken as significant drug interactions may occur and dosage adjustments may be warranted.
- Women should use effective means of birth control while taking this drug. Report promptly to prescriber if a pregnancy is suspected.

# CARISOPRODOL

(kar-eye-soe-proe'dole)

**Soma**

**Classification:** CENTRALLY-ACTING SKELETAL MUSCLE RELAXANT
**Therapeutic:** SKELETAL MUSCLE RELAXANT
**Prototype:** Cyclobenzaprine
**Controlled Substance:** Schedule IV

## AVAILABILITY Tablet

## ACTION & *THERAPEUTIC EFFECT*

Centrally acting skeletal muscle relaxant that appears to cause slight reduction in muscle tone leading to relief of pain and discomfort of muscle spasm. *Effective spasmolytic while reducing pain associated with acute musculoskeletal disorders*.

**USES** Acute treatment of musculoskeletal pain.

**CONTRAINDICATIONS** Hypersensitivity to carisoprodol and related compounds (e.g., meprobamate, carbamate); acute intermittent porphyria.

**CAUTIOUS USE** Impaired liver or kidney function, addiction-prone individuals; seizure disorder; pregnancy (category C); lactation; children younger than 16 y.

## ROUTE & DOSAGE

**Muscle Spasm**
*Adult/Adolescent:* PO 250–350 mg t.i.d.

## ADMINISTRATION

**Oral**

- Give with food, as needed, to reduce GI symptoms. Last dose should be taken at bedtime.
- Store in tightly closed container.

**ADVERSE EFFECTS (≥1%) Body as a Whole:** Eosinophilia, asthma, fever, <u>anaphylactic shock</u>. **CV:** Tachycardia, postural hypotension, facial flushing. **GI:** Nausea, vomiting, hiccups. **CNS:** *Drowsiness, dizziness,* vertigo, ataxia, tremor, headache, irritability, depressive reactions, syncope, insomnia. **Skin:** Skin rash, erythema multiforme, pruritus.

**INTERACTIONS Drug: Alcohol,** CNS DEPRESSANTS potentiate CNS effects. Do not use with **meprobamate.**

**PHARMACOKINETICS Onset:** 30 min. **Duration:** 4–6 h. **Distribution:** Crosses placenta. **Metabolism:** In liver by CYP2C19. **Elimination:** By kidneys; excreted in breast milk (2–4 × the plasma concentrations). **Half-Life:** 8 h.

Common adverse effects in *italic;* life-threatening effects <u>underlined</u>; generic names in **bold;** classifications in SMALL CAPS; ♣ Canadian drug name; ⊕ Prototype drug

277

## NURSING IMPLICATIONS

### Assessment & Drug Effects

- Monitor for allergic or idiosyncratic reactions that generally occur from the first to the fourth dose in patients taking the drug for the first time. Symptoms usually subside after several hours; they are treated by supportive and symptomatic measures.
- Abuse potential is high. Monitor use.

### Patient & Family Education

- Avoid driving and other potentially hazardous activities until response to the drug has been evaluated. Drowsiness is a common side effect and may require reduction in dosage.
- Report to prescriber if symptoms of dizziness and faintness persist. Symptoms may be controlled by making position changes slowly and in stages.
- Do not take alcohol or other CNS depressants (effects may be additive) unless otherwise directed by prescriber.
- Discontinue drug and notify prescriber if skin rash, diplopia, dizziness, or other unusual signs or symptoms appear.

## CARMUSTINE
(kar-mus'teen)
BiCNU, Gliadel
**Classifications:** ANTINEOPLASTIC; ALKYLATING
Therapeutic: ANTINEOPLASTIC
**Prototype:** Cyclophosphamide

**AVAILABILITY** Solution for injection; wafer

## ACTION & *THERAPEUTIC EFFECT*

Highly lipid-soluble compound with cell-cycle-nonspecific activity against rapidly proliferating cells. Produces cross-linkage of DNA strands, thereby blocking DNA, RNA, and protein synthesis in tumor cells. *Drug metabolites are thought to be responsible for antineoplastic activities. Full or partial activity against a variety of cancers results in reduction or stabilization of tumor size and increased survival rates.*

**USES** As single agent or with other antineoplastics in treatment of Hodgkin's disease and other lymphomas, melanoma, primary and metastatic tumors of brain, and GI tract malignancies.

**UNLABELED USES** Treatment of carcinomas of breast and lungs, Ewing's sarcoma, Burkitt's tumor, malignant melanoma, and topically for mycosis fungoides.

**CONTRAINDICATIONS** History of pulmonary function impairment; recent illness with or exposure to chickenpox or herpes zoster; infection; severe bone marrow depression, decreased circulating platelets, leukocytes, or erythrocytes; pregnancy (category D); lactation.

**CAUTIOUS USE** Hepatic and renal insufficiency; Patient with bone marrow suppression, patients with nausea and vomiting, patient with previous cytotoxic medication, or radiation therapy; history of herpes infections.

## ROUTE & DOSAGE

| Previously Untreated Patients — Carcinoma |
|---|
| *Adult:* **IV** 150–200 mg/m² q6wk in one dose *or* given over 2 days; adjust for hematologic toxicity |
| **Glioblastoma Multiforme (recurrent)** |
| *Adult:* **Implantation (wafer)** 8 wafers (7.7 mg each) implanted intracranially into in the resection cavity |

## ADMINISTRATION

### Topical
- Follow application directions provided by prescriber.

### Intravenous

*PREPARE:* **IV Infusion:** Wear disposable gloves and protective gown. Hazardous agent. Contact of drug with skin can cause burning, dermatitis, and hyperpigmentation. ▪ Add supplied diluent to the 100 mg vial. Further dilute with 27 mL of sterile water for injection to yield a concentration of 3.3 mg/mL. ▪ Each dose is then added to 100–500 mL of D5W or NS. ▪ Avoid using PVC IV tubing and bags. ▪ Protect from light. Reconstituted solution is stable for 24 h refrigerated to 2°–8° C; (36°–46° F) in a glass container. Must use within 8 h at room temperature if protected from light.

*ADMINISTER:* **IV Infusion:** Infuse a single dose over at least 2 h. Adequate dilution will reduce pain of administration. ▪ Avoid starting infusion into dorsum of hand, wrist, or the antecubital veins; extravasation in these areas can damage underlying tendons and nerves leading to loss of mobility of entire limb. Frequently check rate of flow and blood return during infusion; monitor injection site for extravasation.
- If there is any question about patency, line should be restarted.

*INCOMPATIBILITIES:* **Solution/additive: Dextrose 5%, sodium bicarbonate. Y-site: Allopurinol.**

- Reconstituted solutions of carmustine are clear and colorless and may be stored at 2°–8° C (36°–46° F) for 8 h protected from light.
- Store unopened vials at 2°–8° C (36°–46° F), protected from light, unless otherwise directed by manufacturer. ▪ Signs of decomposition of carmustine in unopened vial: Liquefaction and appearance of oil film at bottom of vial. Discard drug in this condition.

## ADVERSE EFFECTS (≥1%) **Hematologic:** Delayed myelosuppression (dose-related); thrombocytopenia. **CNS:** Dizziness, confusion, ataxia, headache, *seizures.* **Respiratory:** Pulmonary infiltration or fibrosis. **Skin:** Skin flushing and burning pain at injection site, hyperpigmentation of skin (from contact), alopecia. **Special Senses:** (With high doses) Eye infarctions, retinal hemorrhage, suffusion of conjunctiva. **GI:** Stomatitis, constipation, *nausea, vomiting, diarrhea.* **Urogenital:** Renal failure, gynecomastia.

## INTERACTIONS Drug: **Cimetidine** may potentiate neutropenia and thrombocytopenia.

## PHARMACOKINETICS **Distribution:** Readily crosses blood–brain barrier, CSF concentrations 15–70% of plasma concentrations. **Metabolism:** Rapidly metabolized. **Elimination:** 60–70% in urine in 96 h; 6% via lungs, 1% in feces; excreted in breast milk.

## NURSING IMPLICATIONS

### Black Box Warning

*Carmustine has been associated with severe, delayed bone marrow depression leading to hemorrhage and/or severe infection. Pulmonary toxicity may occur even years after termination of treatment.*

### Assessment & Drug Effects
- Monitor for nausea and vomiting (dose related), which may occur

Common adverse effects in *italic*; life-threatening effects underlined; generic names in **bold**; classifications in SMALL CAPS; ♣ Canadian drug name; ● Prototype drug

279

within 2 h after drug administration and persist for up to 6 h.

- Monitor vital signs throughout infusion.
- Monitor blood pressure closely during high dose BMT infusion; supine positions (Trandelenburg position may be necessary), fluid support and vasopressor support should be available.
- Report symptoms of lung toxicity (cough, shortness of breath, fever) to the prescriber immediately.
- Be alert to signs of hepatic toxicity (jaundice, dark urine, pruritus, light-colored stools) and renal insufficiency (dysuria, oliguria, hematuria, swelling of lower legs and feet).
- Monitor lab tests: Baseline CBC with differential and platelet count, repeat following infusion at weekly intervals for at least 6 wk; baseline and periodic LFTs and renal function tests.

### Patient & Family Education

- Report burning sensation immediately, as carmustine can cause burning discomfort even in the absence of extravasation. Infusion will be discontinued and restarted in another site. Ice application over the area may decrease the discomfort.
- Intense flushing of skin may occur during IV infusion. This usually disappears in 2–4 h.
- You will be highly susceptible to infection and to hemorrhagic disorders. Be alert to hazardous periods that occur 4–6 wk after a dose of carmustine. If possible, avoid invasive procedures (e.g., IM injections, enemas, rectal temperatures) during this period.
- Report promptly the onset of sore throat, weakness, fever, chills, infection of any kind, or abnormal bleeding (ecchymosis, petechiae, epistaxis, bleeding gums, hematemesis, melena).

# CARTEOLOL HYDROCHLORIDE

(car'tee-oh-lole)

Ocupress

**Classifications:** BETA-ADRENERGIC ANTAGONIST; ANTIHYPERTENSIVE

Therapeutic: ANTIHYPERTENSIVE; BETA-ADRENERGIC BLOCKER

**Prototype:** Propranolol

## AVAILABILITY Solution

## ACTION & *THERAPEUTIC EFFECT*

Carteolol is a beta-adrenergic blocking agent (antagonist) that competes for available beta receptor sites. It inhibits both beta$_1$ receptors (chiefly in cardiac muscle) and beta$_2$ receptors (chiefly in the bronchial and vascular musculature). *It interferes with production and outflow of aqueous humor.*

## USES Chronic open-angle glaucoma.

## CONTRAINDICATIONS Sinus bradycardia, severe CHF; greater than first-degree heart block, cardiogenic shock, CHF secondary to tachycardia treatable with beta-blockers, overt cardiac failure, hypersensitivity to beta-blocking agents, persistent severe bradycardia, bronchial asthma or bronchospasm, and severe COPD; pulmonary edema.

## CAUTIOUS USE CHF patients treated with digitalis and diuretics, peripheral vascular disease; diabetes, hypoglycemia, thyrotoxicosis; renal disease; CVA; pregnancy (category C); lactation.

## ROUTE & DOSAGE

### Open-Angle Glaucoma

*Adult:* **Ophthalmic** 1 drop in affected eye b.i.d.

Common adverse effects in *italic;* life-threatening effects underlined; generic names in **bold;** classifications in SMALL CAPS; ♣ Canadian drug name; ◯ Prototype drug

## ADMINISTRATION

### Conjunctival

- For topical use only. Wash hands before use. To avoid contamination, do not touch dropper tip to eyelids or other surfaces.
- Remove contact lenses prior to administration; wait 15 min before reinserting if using products containing benzalkoniumchloride.

## ADVERSE EFFECTS (≥1%) Special

**Senses:** Conjunctival hyperemia, lacrimation, and ocular irritation.

## INTERACTIONS Drug: DIURETICS

and other HYPOTENSIVE AGENTS increase hypotensive effect.

## PHARMACOKINETICS Absorption: 25% reaches systemic circulation. **Metabolism:** In liver to active metabolite. **Elimination:** Primarily in urine.

## NURSING IMPLICATIONS

### Assessment & Drug Effects

- Assess conjunctiva and corneal surfaces for any edema or discoloration.
- Contact prescriber with patient complaints of eye pain or any disturbances in vision (blurry, cloudy, double vision, or decreased night vision).

### Patient & Family Education

- Make sure that dropper does not touch the eye during administration.
- Report to prescriber any drooping of the eyelid, drainage from the eye, changes in vision (blurry, cloudy, double vision, unable to tolerate light, or decreased night vision).
- Do not discontinue medication abruptly, since sudden withdrawal may precipitate or exacerbate angina.
- Report slow pulse rate, confusion or depression, dizziness or lightheadedness, skin rash, fever, sore throat, or unusual bleeding or bruising.

- Be cautious while driving or performing other hazardous activities until response to drug is known.
- Take your pulse before and after taking the medication. If it is much slower than normal rate (or less than 50 bpm), check with your prescriber.

## CARVEDILOL

(car-ve-di'lol)

Coreg, Coreg CR ♦

**Classifications:** ALPHA- and BETA-ADRENERGIC ANTAGONIST; ANTIHYPERTENSIVE

**Therapeutic:** ANTIHYPERTENSIVE; ADRENERGIC BLOCKER

**Prototype:** Propanolol HCl

## AVAILABILITY Tablet; extended release capsule

## ACTION & *THERAPEUTIC EFFECT*

Adrenergic receptor blocking agent that contributes to blood pressure reduction. Peripheral vasodilatation and, therefore, decreased peripheral resistance results from alpha₁-blocking activity. *An effective antihypertensive agent reducing BP to normotensive range and useful in managing some angina, dysrhythmias, and CHF by decreasing myocardial oxygen demand and lowering cardiac workload.*

## USES Management of essential hypertension, CHF, left ventricular dysfunction post MI, cardiomyopathy.

## UNLABELED USES Angina, atrial fibrillation, gastroesophageal varices.

## CONTRAINDICATIONS Patients with class IV decompensated

C

cardiac failure, abrupt cessation in CAD patients; hypersensitivity to any component of the formulation, possibility of cross-reactivity with other alpha/beta adrenergic blocking agents; bronchial asthma, or related bronchospastic conditions (e.g., chronic bronchitis and emphysema), pulmonary edema; second- and third-degree AV block, sick sinus syndrome, cardiogenic shock or severe bradycardia, lactation.

**CAUTIOUS USE** Patients on MAOI agents, DM; hypoglycemia; patients at high risk for anaphylactic reaction, PVD; cerebrovascular insufficiencies, major depression, hepatic or renal impairment; older adults; pregnancy (category C); children younger than 18 y.

## ROUTE & DOSAGE

### Heart Failure

*Adult (weight less than 85 kg):* **PO Immediate release** Start with 3.125 mg b.i.d. × 2 wk, may double dose q2wk as tolerated up to 25 mg b.i.d.; *weight greater than 85 kg:* 50 mg b.i.d.; **Extended release** 10 mg qd × 2 wk may increase up to 80 mg

### Left Ventricular Dysfunction Post MI

*Adult:* **PO Immediate release** 3.125–6.25 mg b.i.d., can double every 3–10 days as tolerated; **Extended release** 10–20 mg daily

### Hypertension

*Adult:* **PO Immediate release** Start with 6.25 mg b.i.d., may increase by 6.25 mg b.i.d. (max: 25 mg b.i.d.); **Extended release** 20 mg daily, may increase to 40 mg daily

## ADMINISTRATION

### Oral

- Take baseline blood pressure and pulse rate prior to and following first dose.
- Give with food to slow absorption and minimize risk of orthostatic hypotension.
- Extended release capsules should not be crushed, chewed or divided. Capsules may be opened and sprinkled on applesauce for immediate use.
- Dose increments should be made at 7- to 14-day intervals.
- Store at less than 30° C (less than 86° F). Protect from light and moisture.

**ADVERSE EFFECTS** (≥1%) **Body as a Whole:** Increased sweating, *fatigue*, chest pain, pain, arthralgia, weight gain. **CV:** Bradycardia, *hypotension*, syncope, hypertension, AV block, angina edema. **GI:** Diarrhea, nausea, abdominal pain, vomiting. **Respiratory:** Sinusitis, dyspnea, bronchitis, cough. **Hematologic:** Thrombocytopenia. **Metabolic:** Hyperglycemia, weight increase, gout. **CNS:** *Dizziness,* headache, paresthesias.

**INTERACTIONS Drug:** **Rifampin** significantly decreases **carvedilol** levels; **cimetidine** may increase **carvedilol** levels; **clonidine, reserpine,** MAO INHIBITORS may cause hypotension or bradycardia; **carvedilol** may increase **digoxin** levels and may enhance hypoglycemic effects of **insulin** and oral HYPOGLYCEMIC AGENTS, may enhance the effects of ANTIHYPERTENSIVES. **Amiodarone** and **fluconazole** increase side effects.

**PHARMACOKINETICS Absorption:** Rapidly from GI tract, 25–35% reaches the systemic circulation.

Common adverse effects in *italic*; life-threatening effects <u>underlined</u>; generic names in **bold**; classifications in SMALL CAPS; ✦ Canadian drug name; ❂ Prototype drug

**Peak:** Antihypertensive effect 7–14 days. **Distribution:** Greater than 98% protein bound. **Metabolism:** In the liver by CYP2D6 and CYP2C9. **Elimination:** Primarily through feces. **Half-Life:** 7–10 h.

## NURSING IMPLICATIONS

### Assessment & Drug Effects

- Monitor for therapeutic effectiveness which is indicated by lessening of S&S of CHF and improved BP control.
- Monitor for worsening of symptoms in patients with PVD.
- Withhold drug and notify prescriber at the first sign of hepatic toxicity (see Appendix F).
- Monitor digoxin levels with concurrent use; plasma digoxin concentration may increase.
- Monitor lab tests: Periodic LFTs.

### Patient & Family Education

- Do not abruptly discontinue taking this drug.
- Make position changes slowly due to the risk of orthostatic hypotension.
- Do not engage in hazardous activities while experiencing dizziness.
- If you have diabetes, the drug may increase effects of hypoglycemic drugs and mask S&S of hypoglycemia.

## CASPOFUNGIN ℗

(cas-po-fun'gin)

Cancidas

**Classifications:** ANTIBIOTIC; ECHINOCANDIN ANTIFUNGAL

Therapeutic: ANTIFUNGAL

**AVAILABILITY** Powder for injection

## ACTION & *THERAPEUTIC EFFECT*

Caspofungin is an antifungal agent that inhibits the synthesis of an integral component of the fungal cell wall of susceptible species. *Interferes with reproduction and growth of susceptible fungi.*

**USES** Treatment of invasive aspergillosis in those refractory to or intolerant of other antifungal therapies; empirical therapy for presumed fungal infection with febrile neutropenia; treatment of candidemia and intra-abdominal abscesses, peritonitis, and pleural space infections due to *Candida*.

**UNLABELED USES** Treatment of esophageal candidiasis with or without oropharyngeal candidiasis (thrush).

**CONTRAINDICATIONS** Hypersensitivity (e.g., anaphylaxis) to any component of this product; mannitol; not studied in patients with ESRF.

**CAUTIOUS USE** Patients with moderate hepatic insufficiency; cholestasis; older adults; pregnancy (category C); lactation; children younger than 18 y. Not recommended for adults with severe hepatic impairment and children 3 mo to younger than 18 y with any degree of hepatic impairment.

## ROUTE & DOSAGE

### Invasive *Aspergillosis*, Empirical Therapy, *Candida*

Adult: **IV** 70 mg on day 1, then 50 mg daily thereafter

## ADMINISTRATION

### Intravenous

Allow vial to come to room temperature.

***PREPARE: IV Infusion:*** Reconstitute a 50 or 70-mg vial with 10.5 mL of NS, sterile water for injection, or bacteriostatic water for injection to yield 5 mg/mL and

Common adverse effects in *italic;* life-threatening effects underlined; generic names in **bold;** classifications in SMALL CAPS; ♣ Canadian drug name; ℗ Prototype drug

283

7 mg/mL, respectively. Mix gently until clear. ▪ Withdraw the required dose of reconstituted solution and add to 250 mL of NS, 1/2NS, or 1/4NaCl, or LR. **Do not** use diluents or IV solutions containing dextrose.

*ADMINISTER:* **IV Infusion:** Give slowly over at least 1 h. Do not coinfuse with any other medication.

*INCOMPATIBILITIES:* **Solution/additive:** Any **dextrose**-containing solution. Do not mix or co-infuse with any other medications. **Y site: Aminocaproic acid, amphotercin B, ampicillin, atenolol, bivalirudin, cefazolin, cefepime, cefoperazone, cefotaxime, cefotetan, cefoxitin, ceftaroline, ceftazidime, ceftobiprole, ceftriaxone, cefuroxime, chloramphenicol, clindamycin, dantrolene, dexamethasone, diazepam, digoxin, doxacurium, enalaprilat, ephedrine, ertapenem, fluorouracil, foscarnet, fosphenytoin, furosemide, gemtuzumab, heparin, ketorolac, lansoprazole, lidocaine, methotrexate, methylprednisolone, mivacurium, nafcilln, nitroprusside, pamidronate, pancuronium, pemetrexed, pentobarbital, phenobarbital, phenytoin, piperacillin/ tazobactam, ranitidine.**

▪ Reconstituted solution should be stored at or below 25° C (77° F) for 1 h prior to preparing the IV solution for infusion. ▪ Store IV solution for up to 24 h at or below 25° C (77° F) or 48 h at 2°–8° C (36°–46° F).

**ADVERSE EFFECTS** (≥1%) **Body as a Whole:** Anaphylaxis, chills, *injection site reaction,* sensation of warmth, fever, chills. **CNS:** Headache. **CV:** Sinus tachycardia, *hypotension,* edema. **GI:** *Nausea, vomiting,* diarrhea, *hypotension edema* abdominal pain. **Hematologic/ Lymphatic:** *Phlebitis, thrombophlebitis,* vasculitis, *anemia.* **Hepatic:** *Elevated liver enzymes.* **Metabolic:** Anorexia, *hypokalemia.* **Musculoskeletal:** Pain, myalgia. **Respiratory:** Acute respiratory distress syndrome, dyspnea. **Skin:** Rash, facial swelling, pruritus.

**INTERACTIONS Drug:** **Cyclosporine** increases overall systematic exposure to caspofungin; inducers of drug clearance or mixed inducer/ inhibitors (e.g., **carbamazepine, dexamethasone, efavirenz, nelfinavir, nevirapine, phenytoin, rifampin**) can decrease caspofungin levels; caspofungin decreases the overall systematic exposure to **tacrolimus.**

**PHARMACOKINETICS Distribution:** 97% protein bound. **Metabolism:** Liver and plasma to inactive metabolites. **Elimination:** Both in urine and feces. **Half-Life:** 9–11 h.

**NURSING IMPLICATIONS**

**Assessment & Drug Effects**
▪ Monitor for S&S of hypersensitivity during IV infusion; frequently monitor IV site for thrombophlebitis.
▪ Monitor for and report S&S of fluid retention (e.g., weight gain, swelling, peripheral edema), especially with known cardiovascular disease.
▪ Monitor blood levels of tacrolimus with concurrent therapy.
▪ Monitor lab tests: Baseline and periodic LFTs; periodic kidney function tests, serum electrolytes, CBC with differential, and platelet count.

**Patient & Family Education**
▪ Report immediately any of the following: Facial swelling, wheezing, difficulty breathing or swallowing, tightness in chest, rash, hives, itching, or sensation of warmth.

Common adverse effects in *italic;* life-threatening effects underlined; generic names in **bold;** classifications in SMALL CAPS; ✢ Canadian drug name; ⊕ Prototype drug

# CEFACLOR ⊕℗

(sef'a-klor)

Ceclor ✦

**Classifications:** ANTIBIOTIC;
SECOND-GENERATION CEPHALOSPORIN

Therapeutic: ANTIBIOTIC

**AVAILABILITY** Capsule; sustained release tablet suspension

## ACTION & THERAPEUTIC EFFECT

Preferentially binds to one or more of the penicillin-binding proteins (PBPs) located on cell walls of susceptible organisms. This inhibits third and final stages of bacterial cell wall synthesis, thus killing bacterium. *Effective in treating acute otitis media and acute sinusitis where causative agent is resistant to other antibiotics. Useful in treating respiratory and urinary tract infections.*

**USES** Treatment of otitis media and infections of upper and lower respiratory tract, urinary tract, and skin and skin structures caused by ampicillin-resistant *H. influenzae;* acute uncomplicated UTI.

**CONTRAINDICATIONS** Hypersensitivity to cephalosporins and related antibiotics.

**CAUTIOUS USE** History of sensitivity to penicillins or other drug allergies; GI disease, colitis; markedly impaired renal function; older adults; coagulopathy; pregnancy (category B); lactation.

## ROUTE & DOSAGE

**Mild to Moderate Infections**

*Adult:* **PO** 250–500 mg q8h, or Ceclor CD 250–500 mg/q12h

*Child (1 mo or older):* **PO** 20–40 mg/kg/day divided q8h (max: 2 g/day)

## ADMINISTRATION

**Oral**

- Give sustained release tablets with food to enhance absorption. Food does not affect absorption of capsules.
- Ensure that sustained release tablets are not chewed or crushed. They **must be** swallowed whole.
- After stock oral suspension is prepared, it should be kept refrigerated. Expiration date should appear on label. Discard unused portion after 14 days. Shake well before pouring.
- Store pulvules in tightly closed container unless otherwise directed.

**ADVERSE EFFECTS** (≥1%) **Body as a Whole:** Serum sickness-like reaction, eosinophilia, joint pain or swelling, fever, superinfections. **GI:** *Diarrhea,* nausea, vomiting, anorexia, pseudomembranous <u>colitis</u> (rare). **Skin:** Urticaria, pruritus, morbilliform eruptions.

**DIAGNOSTIC TEST INTERFERENCE** May produce positive *direct Coombs' test.* False-positive *urine glucose* determinations may result with use of *copper sulfate reduction methods* (e.g., *Clinitest* or *Benedict's reagent*) but not with *glucose oxidase* (enzymatic) *tests* such as *Clinistix, Diastix, TesTape.*

**INTERACTIONS Drug:** Avoid live vaccines.

**PHARMACOKINETICS Absorption:** Well absorbed; acid stable. **Peak:** 30–60 min. **Elimination:** 60% of dose eliminated renally in 8 h; crosses placenta; excreted in breast milk. **Half-Life:** 0.5–1 h.

---

Common adverse effects in *italic;* life-threatening effects <u>underlined</u>; generic names in **bold**; classifications in SMALL CAPS; ✦ Canadian drug name; ℗ Prototype drug

## NURSING IMPLICATIONS

### Assessment & Drug Effects

- Determine previous hypersensitivity to cephalosporins, penicillins, and other drug allergies before therapy is initiated.
- Report persistent diarrhea, as interruption of therapy may be necessary.
- Monitor for manifestations of drug hypersensitivity (see Appendix F). Discontinue drug and promptly report them if they appear.
- Monitor for manifestations of superinfection (see Appendix F). Promptly report their appearance.
- Monitor lab tests: Baseline C&S prior to initiation of therapy.

### Patient & Family Education

- Report promptly any signs or symptoms of superinfection (see Appendix F).
- Yogurt or buttermilk (if allowed) may serve as a prophylactic against intestinal superinfections by helping to maintain normal intestinal flora.

## CEFADROXIL

(sef-a-drox'ill)

**Classifications:** ANTIBIOTIC; FIRST-GENERATION CEPHALOSPORIN
Therapeutic: ANTIBIOTIC
**Prototype:** Cefazolin

**AVAILABILITY** Capsule; tablet; oral suspension

## ACTION & *THERAPEUTIC EFFECT*

Drug penetrates bacterial cell wall, resists beta-lactamases, and inactivates enzymes essential to cell wall synthesis thus killing the bacterium. *Active against organisms that liberate cephalosporinase and penicillinase (beta-lactamases).*

*Effective in reducing signs and symptoms of urinary tract infections, bone and joint infections, skin and soft tissue infections, and pharyngitis.*

**USES** Urinary tract infections, infections of skin and skin structures, pharyngitis and tonsillitis.

**UNLABELED USES** Endocarditis prophylaxis, rheumatic fever prophylaxis.

**CONTRAINDICATIONS** Hypersensitivity to cephalosporins; drug induced seizure activity.

**CAUTIOUS USE** Sensitivity to penicillins or other drug allergies; markedly impaired renal function, older adults; GI disease, history of GI disease particularly colitis, coagulopathy; pregnancy (category B); lactation; children less than 2 y.

## ROUTE & DOSAGE

**Uncomplicated Urinary Tract Infection**

*Adult:* **PO** 1–2 g/day in 1–2 divided doses
*Child:* **PO** 30 mg/kg/day in 2 divided doses

**Skin and Skin Structure Infections, Streptococcal Pharyngitis, or Tonsillitis**

*Adult:* **PO** 1 g/day in 1–2 divided doses
*Child:* **PO** 30 mg/kg/day in 2 divided doses

***Renal Impairment Dosage Adjustment***

*CrCl less than 25 mL/min:*
*Adult:* **PO** 1 g q24h
*Child:* **PO** 15 mg/kg q24h

---

Common adverse effects in *italic;* life-threatening effects <u>underlined</u>; generic names in **bold;** classifications in SMALL CAPS; ♣ Canadian drug name; ⊘ Prototype drug

## ADMINISTRATION

### Oral

- Give with food or milk to reduce nausea. If nausea persists, termination of therapy may be necessary.
- Follow directions for mixing oral suspension found on drug label. Reconstituted suspension contains 125 or 250 mg cefadroxil/5 mL.
- Shake suspension well before use; discard after 14 days.
- Store in tight container unless otherwise directed. Oral suspensions are stable for 14 days under refrigeration at 2°–8° C (36° 46° F). Avoid freezing. Note expiration date on label.

## ADVERSE EFFECTS (≥1%) Body as a Whole: Hypersensitivity [rash, swollen eyelids (angioedema), pruritus, chills], superinfections. GI: Nausea, *diarrhea,* vomiting, heartburn, gastritis, bloating, abdominal cramps.

## DIAGNOSTIC TEST INTERFERENCE

False-positive *urine glucose* determinations using *copper sulfate reduction reagents,* such as *Clinitest* or *Benedict's reagent, Positive direct Coombs' test* may interfere with *cross-matching procedures* and *hematologic studies.* False-positive **serum/urine creatine** with **Jaffe** reaction.

## INTERACTIONS Drug: Probenecid decreases renal excretion of cefadroxil. Do not use with **BCG.**

## PHARMACOKINETICS Absorption: Acid stable; rapidly absorbed from GI tract. Peak: 1 h. Elimination: 90% unchanged in urine within 8 h; bacterial inhibitory levels persist 20–22 h; crosses placenta; excreted in breast milk. Half-Life: 1–12 h.

## NURSING IMPLICATIONS

### Assessment & Drug Effects

- Determine previous hypersensitivity to cephalosporins, penicillins, and other drug allergies, before therapy is initiated.
- Monitor for manifestations of drug hypersensitivity (see Signs & Symptoms, Appendix F). Discontinue drug and promptly report them if they appear.
- Monitor for manifestations of superinfection (see Signs & Symptoms, Appendix F). Promptly report their appearance.
- Monitor I&O ratio and pattern.
- Monitor lab tests: Baseline C&S prior to initiation of therapy; baseline and periodic renal function studies in patients with renal function impairment.

### Patient & Family Education

- Report promptly the onset of rash, urticaria, pruritus, or fever, as the possibility of an allergic reaction is high, if you are allergic to penicillin.
- Take medication for the full course of therapy as directed by your prescriber.
- Report promptly S&S of superinfections (see Appendix F).

## CEFAZOLIN SODIUM 🅟

(sef-a'zoe-lin)

Ancef

**Classifications:** ANTIBIOTIC; FIRST-GENERATION CEPHALOSPORIN
Therapeutic: ANTIBIOTIC

## AVAILABILITY Solution for injection

## ACTION & *THERAPEUTIC EFFECT*

Preferentially binds to one or more of the penicillin-binding proteins (PBP) located on cell walls of

Common adverse effects in *italic;* life-threatening effects underlined; generic names in **bold;** classifications in SMALL CAPS; ♣ Canadian drug name; 🅟 Prototype drug

287

susceptible organisms. This inhibits third and final stages of bacterial cell wall synthesis, thus killing
the bacterium. *Effective treatment
for bone and joint infections, biliary tract infections, endocarditis
prophylaxis and treatment, respiratory tract and genital tract infections, septicemia and skin infections,
and surgical prophylaxis.*

**USES** Severe infections of urinary
and biliary tracts, skin, soft tissue,
and bone, and for bacteremia and
endocarditis caused by susceptible
organisms; also perioperative prophylaxis in patients undergoing procedures associated with high risk of
infection (e.g., open heart surgery).

**CONTRAINDICATIONS** Hypersensitivity to any cephalosporin
and related antibiotics.

**CAUTIOUS USE** History of penicillin sensitivity, impaired renal
function, patients on sodium restriction; seizure disorders; coagulopathy; GI disease, colitis; pregnancy (category B).

## ROUTE & DOSAGE

### Moderate to Severe Infections

*Adult:* **IV/IM** 250 mg–2 g q8h,
up to 2 g q4h (max: 12 g/day)
*Child:* **IV/IM** 25–100 mg/kg/day in
3–4 divided doses, up to 100 mg/
kg/day (not to exceed adult doses)
*Neonate (Younger than 7 days):*
**IV** 40 mg/kg/day divided q12h;
*7 days or older:* 40–60 mg/kg/
day divided q8–12h

### Surgical Prophylaxis

*Adult:* **IV/IM** 1–2 g 30–60 min
before surgery, then 0.5–1 g q8h
*Child:* **IV/IM** 25–50 mg/kg
30–60 min before surgery, then
q8h for 24 h

### Renal Impairment Dosage Adjustment

*CrCl less than 35 mL/min:* Dose
q12h; *10 mL/min:* Dose q24h

## ADMINISTRATION

### Intramuscular

- Preparation of IM solution: Reconstitute with sterile water for
injection, bacteriostatic water for
injection, or 0.9% sodium chloride injection.
- Reconstituted solutions are stable
for 24 h at room temperature and
for 96 h refrigerated.
- IM injections should be made
deep into large muscle mass. Pain
on injection is usually minimal.
Rotate injection sites.

### Intravenous

*IV administration to neonates,
infants, and children:* Verify
correct IV concentration and rate
of infusion with prescriber.

*PREPARE:* **Direct:** Add 2 mL sterile
water for injection to the 500 mg
vial to yield 225 mg/mL, or add
2.5 mL to the 1 g vial to yield 330
mg/mL. Shake well to dissolve.
- Further dilute with 5 mL sterile
water for injection. **Intermittent:**
After initial vial reconstitution,
add required dose to 50–100 mL
of NS or D5W.

*ADMINISTER:* **Direct/Intermittent:**
Infuse 1 g over 5 min or longer as
determined by the amount of solution. - The risk of IV site reactions may be reduced by proper
dilution of IV solution, use of
small bore IV needle in a large
vein, and by rotating injection
sites.

*INCOMPATIBILITIES:* Solution/ad-
ditive: AMINOGLYCOSIDES, **atracurium, bleomycin, cimetidine,
clindamycin, lidocaine, raniti-**

Common adverse effects in *italic;* life-threatening effects <u>underlined</u>; generic names
in **bold;** classifications in SMALL CAPS; ♣ Canadian drug name; ⊘ Prototype drug

dine. Y-site: **Amiodarone**, AMINOGLYCOSIDES, **amphotericin B cholesteryl complex, azathioprine, calcium chloride, caspofungin, cefotaxime, chlorpromazine, cisatracurium, dacarbazine, dantrolene, danorubicin, diazepam, diazoxide, diphenhydramine, dobutamine, dolasetron, dopamine, doxorubicin, doxycycline, erythromycin, ganciclovir, garenoxacin, gemtuzumab, haloperidol, hydralazine, hydromorphone, hydroxyzine, idarubicin, inamrinone, lansoprazole, levofloxacin, minocycline, mitomycin, mitoxantrone, mivacurium, mycophenolate, netlimicin, papaverine, pemetrexed, pentamidine, pentazocine, pentobarbital, pentamidine, phentolamine, phenytoin, prochlorperazine, protamine, pyridoxine, quinidine, quinprustin/ dalfopristin, sodium citrate, SM7/TMP, tobramycin,** high dose **vancomycin, vinorelbine.**

## ADVERSE EFFECTS (≥1%) Body as a Whole: Anaphylaxis, fever, eosinophilia, superinfections, seizure (high doses in patients with renal insufficiency). **GI:** *Diarrhea,* anorexia, abdominal cramps. **Skin:** Maculopapular rash, urticaria.

## DIAGNOSTIC TEST INTERFERENCE
Because of cefazolin effect on the *direct Coombs' test,* transfusion *cross-matching procedures* and *hematologic studies* may be complicated. False-positive *urine glucose* determinations are possible with use of *copper sulfate tests* (e.g., *Clinitest* or *Benedict's reagent*) but not with *glucose oxidase tests* such as *TesTape, Diastix,* or *Clinistix.*

## INTERACTIONS Drug: Probenecid decreases renal elimination of cefazolin.

## PHARMACOKINETICS Peak: 1–2 h after IM; 5 min after IV. **Distribution:** Poor CNS penetration even with inflamed meninges; high concentrations in bile and in diseased bone; crosses placenta. **Elimination:** 70% unchanged in urine in 6 h; small amount excreted in breast milk. **Half-Life:** 90–130 min.

## NURSING IMPLICATIONS
### Assessment & Drug Effects
- Determine history of hypersensitivity to cephalosporins, penicillins, and other drugs, before therapy is initiated.
- Monitor I&O rates and pattern: Be alert to changes in BUN, serum creatinine.
- Prompt attention should be given to onset of signs of hypersensitivity (see Appendix F).
- Promptly report the onset of diarrhea. Pseudomembranous colitis, a potentially life-threatening condition, starts with diarrhea.
- Monitor lab tests: Baseline C&S prior to initiation of therapy.

### Patient & Family Education
- Report promptly any signs or symptoms of superinfection (see Appendix F).
- Report signs of coagulation problems such as easy bruising and nosebleeds.

## CEFDINIR
(cef'di-nir)
Omnicef
**Classifications:** ANTIBIOTIC; THIRD–GENERATION CEPHALOSPORIN
Therapeutic: ANTIBIOTIC
**Prototype:** Cefotaxime sodium

---

C

**AVAILABILITY** Capsule; suspension

## ACTION & *THERAPEUTIC EFFECT*

Has bactericidal activity resulting from the inhibition of cell wall synthesis through an affinity for penicillin binding proteins (PBPs). Stable in the presence of a variety of bacterial beta-lactamase enzymes. *Effective against a wide variety of gram-positive and gram-negative bacteria.*

**USES** Community-acquired pneumonia, acute exacerbations of chronic bronchitis, acute maxillary sinusitis, pharyngitis, tonsillitis, uncomplicated skin infections, bacterial otitis media.

**CONTRAINDICATIONS** Hypersensitivity to cefdinir and other cephalosporins.

**CAUTIOUS USE** Hypersensitivity to penicillins, penicillin derivatives; renal impairment; ulcerative colitis or antibiotic-induced colitis; bleeding disorders; GI disorders; liver or kidney disease; pregnancy (category B); lactation. Safety and efficacy in neonates and infants younger than 6 mo old not established.

## ROUTE & DOSAGE

**Community-Acquired Pneumonia, Skin Infections**
*Adult:* **PO** 300 mg q12h × 10 days
*Child/Infant (6 mo–12 y):* **PO** 7 mg/kg q12h × 10 days

**Chronic Bronchitis, Maxillary Sinusitis, Pharyngitis, Tonsillitis**
*Adult/Adolescent:* **PO** 600 mg q24h × 10 d or 300 mg q12h × 5–10 days
*Child/Infant (6 mo–12 y):* **PO** 14 mg/kg q24h × 10 d or 7 mg/kg q12h × 5–10 days

**Renal Impairment Dosage Adjustment**
*Adult: CrCl less than 10 mL/min:* 300 mg daily
*Child:* 7 mg/kg daily

**Hemodialysis Dosage Adjustment**
300 mg or 7 mg/kg dose PO every other day; dose given at the end of each session

## ADMINISTRATION

**Oral**
- Do not give within 2 h of aluminum- or magnesium-containing antacids or iron supplements.
- Reconstitute oral suspension to 125 mg/mL by adding water (38 to 60 mL bottle or 63 to 100 mL bottle). Shake well before each use.
- Store in tightly closed container. Discard after 10 days.

**ADVERSE EFFECTS** (≥1%) **GI:** *Diarrhea*, nausea, abdominal pain. **Metabolic:** Increased GGT, increased urine protein, hematuria. **CNS:** Headache. **Skin:** Rash, cutaneous moniliasis. **Urogenital:** Vaginal moniliasis, vaginitis.

**DIAGNOSTIC TEST INTERFERENCE**
False positive for *ketones* or *glucose* in urine using *nitroprusside* or *Clinitest;* may cause false positive *Direct Coomb's test.*

**INTERACTIONS Drug:** ANTACIDS should be taken at least 2 h before or after cefdinir; **probenecid** prolongs cefdinir elimination; **iron** decreases absorption.

**PHARMACOKINETICS Absorption:** 16–25% bioavailability. **Peak:** 2–4 h. **Distribution:** 60–70% protein bound; penetrates sinus tissue,

Common adverse effects in *italic*; life-threatening effects <u>underlined</u>; generic names in **bold**; classifications in SMALL CAPS; ♣ Canadian drug name; ⊘ Prototype drug

blister fluid, lung tissue, middle ear fluid. **Metabolism:** Hepatic. **Elimination:** In urine. **Half-Life:** 1.6 h.

## NURSING IMPLICATIONS

### Assessment & Drug Effects

- Determine previous hypersensitivity to cephalosporins, penicillins, and other drug allergies before therapy is initiated.
- Carefully monitor for and immediately report S&S of: Hypersensitivity, superinfection, or pseudomembranous colitis (see Appendix F).
- Discontinue drug and notify prescriber if seizures associated with drug therapy occur.

### Patient & Family Education

- Allow a minimum of 2 h between cefdinir and antacids containing aluminum or magnesium, or drugs containing iron.
- Immediately contact prescriber if a rash, diarrhea, or new infection (e.g., yeast infection) develops.

## CEFDITOREN PIVOXIL

(cef-di-tor'en)

Spectracef

**Classifications:** ANTIBIOTIC; THIRD-GENERATION CEPHALOSPORIN

**Therapeutic:** ANTIBIOTIC

**Prototype:** Cefotaxime sodium

## AVAILABILITY Tablet

## ACTION & *THERAPEUTIC EFFECT*

Has bactericidal activity resulting from the inhibition of cell wall synthesis through an affinity for penicillin-binding proteins (PBPs). Stable in the presence of a variety of bacterial beta-lactamase enzymes, including penicillinases and some cephalosporinases. *Antibacterial activity is effective against both aerobic gram-positive and aerobic gram-negative bacteria.*

**USES** Acute exacerbation of bacterial chronic bronchitis, pharyngitis, tonsillitis, pneumonia, uncomplicated skin and skin-structure infections.

**CONTRAINDICATIONS** Known allergy to cephalosporins or cefditoren; carnitine deficiency; milk protein hypersensitivity (not lactose intolerance).

**CAUTIOUS USE** History of hypersensitivity to penicillin; renal or hepatic impairment; poor nutritional status; coagulopathy; diabetes mellitus; colitis, GI disease; older adults; concurrent anticoagulant therapy; pregnancy (category B); lactation. Safety and efficacy in children younger than 12 y not established.

## ROUTE & DOSAGE

**Chronic Bronchitis/Pneumonia**

*Adult/Adolescent:* **PO** 400 mg b.i.d. × 10–14 days

**Pharyngitis, Tonsillitis, Skin Infections, Uncomplicated Skin/Soft Tissue Infections**

*Adult:* **PO** 200 mg b.i.d. × 10 days

**Renal Impairment Dosage Adjustment**

*CrCl 30–49 mL/min:* **200 mg b.i.d.;** *less than 30 mL/min:* **200 mg daily**

## ADMINISTRATION

### Oral

- Give with food to enhance absorption.
- Do not give within 2 h of an antacid or $H_2$-receptor antagonist (such as cimetidine).

---

Common adverse effects in *italic;* life-threatening effects <u>underlined</u>; generic names in **bold;** classifications in SMALL CAPS; ♣ Canadian drug name; ⊙ Prototype drug

291

■ Store at 15°–30° C (58°–86° F). Protect from light and moisture.

## ADVERSE EFFECTS (≥1%) GI: *Diarrhea*, nausea, abdominal pain, dyspepsia, vomiting. **Hematologic:** Anemia, leukocytosis. **CNS:** Headache. **Urogenital:** Vaginal moniliasis, hematuria. **Endocrine:** Increased glucose.

## DIAGNOSTIC TEST INTERFERENCE
May cause false negative *ferricynaide test,* may induce positive *Direct Coomb's test.*

## INTERACTIONS Drug: ANTACIDS, H₂-RECEPTOR ANTAGONISTS may decrease absorption; **probenecid** will decrease elimination.

## PHARMACOKINETICS Absorption: 14% reaches systemic circulation. **Distribution:** 88% protein bound, distributes into blister fluid, tonsils. **Metabolism:** Hydrolyzed. **Elimination:** Primarily in urine. **Half-Life:** 1.6 h.

## NURSING IMPLICATIONS
### Assessment & Drug Effects
■ Obtain history of hypersensitivity to cephalosporins, penicillins, and other drug allergies.
■ Monitor for manifestations of drug hypersensitivity (see Appendix F). Withhold drug and report promptly to prescriber if they appear.
■ Monitor for and report promptly manifestations of superinfection (see Appendix F), especially diarrhea. Diarrhea may indicate a change in intestinal flora and development of enterocolitis.
■ Monitor for and report immediately signs of seizure activity or loss of seizure control.
■ Monitor lab tests: Baseline C&S prior to initiating therapy. Baseline and periodic renal function tests; frequent PT in those at risk for increased prothrombin time; as indicated, Hct and Hgb, CBC with differential, urinalysis, serum electrolytes, and LFTs.

### Patient & Family Education
■ Do not take within 2 h of antacids or other drugs used to reduce stomach acids.
■ Discontinue drug and report to prescriber signs of an allergic reaction (e.g., rash, urticaria, pruritus, fever).
■ Report promptly S&S of superinfection (see Appendix F), especially unexplained diarrhea. Antibiotic-associated colitis is a superinfection that may occur in 4–9 days or as long as 6 wk after drug is discontinued.
■ Use daily yogurt or buttermilk (if allowed) as a prophylactic against intestinal superinfections.

## CEFEPIME HYDROCHLORIDE
(cef'e-peem)
**Classifications:** ANTIBIOTIC; FOURTH-GENERATION CEPHALOSPORIN
**Therapeutic:** ANTIBIOTIC; CEPHALOSPORIN
**Prototype:** Cefotaxime sodium

## AVAILABILITY Solution for injection

## ACTION & *THERAPEUTIC EFFECT*
Cefepime preferentially binds to one or more of the penicillin-binding proteins (PBPs) located on cell walls of susceptible organisms. This inhibits the third and final stages of bacterial cell wall synthesis, thus killing the bacteria (bactericidal). *Cefepime is similar to third-generation cephalosporins with respect to broad*

Common adverse effects in *italic;* life-threatening effects underlined; generic names in **bold;** classifications in SMALL CAPS; ♣ Canadian drug name; ⊘ Prototype drug

*gram-negative coverage; however, cefepime has broader gram-positive coverage than third-generation cephalosporins.*

**USES** Uncomplicated and complicated UTI, skin and soft tissue infections, pneumonia. Empiric monotherapy for febrile neutropenic patients.

**CONTRAINDICATIONS** Hypersensitivity to cefepime, other cephalosporins, severe reaction to penicillins, or other beta-lactam antibiotics; hypersensitivity to corn products (solutions containing dextrose only); development of neurotoxicity from use of drug.

**CAUTIOUS USE** Patients with history of GI disease, particularly colitis; renal insufficiency; CrCl of 60 mL/min or less; diabetics; older adults; pregnancy (category B); lactation.

## ROUTE & DOSAGE

#### Mild to Moderate UTI
*Adult:* **IV/IM** 0.5–1 g q12h for 7–10 days

#### Moderate to Severe UTI
*Adult/Adolescent/Child (greater than 40 kg):* **IV** 2g q12h for 10 days
*Child (40 kg or lighter)/Infant (older than 2 mo):* **IV** 50 mg/kg q12h for 10 days

#### Febrile Neutropenia
*Adult/Adolescent/Child (greater than 40 kg):* **IV** 2 g q8h for 7 days or until resolution of neutropenia
*Child (lighter than 40 kg)/Infant (older than 2 mo):* **IV** 50 mg/kg q8h until resolution of neutropenia

#### Community-Acquired Pneumonia
*Adult:* **IV** 1–2g q8h

#### Intraabdominal Infections/ Skin Infection
*Adult:* **IV** 2 g q12h × 7–10 days

#### Renal Impairment Dosage Adjustment
*CrCl 30–60 mL/min:* Dose q24h; *11–29 mL/min:* Give 50% of normal dose q24h for maintenance doses; *less than 10 mL/min:* Reduce the maintenance dose by 50% and extend the interval to q24h

#### Hemodialysis Dosage Adjustment
Administer dose after dialysis

## ADMINISTRATION

#### Intramuscular
- Reconstitute the 1 g vial with 2.4 mL of one of the following: Sterile water for injection, 0.9% NaCl injection, bacteriostatic water for injection with parabens or benzyl alcohol, or other compatible solution to yield 280 mg/mL.

#### Intravenous
*PREPARE:* **Intermittent:** Dilute 1 or 2 g vial with 10 mL of a compatible diluent to yield 100 mg/mL for 1 g vial and 160 mg/mL for 2 g vial. Further dilute in one of the following: NS, D5W, D5/NS or other compatible solution.
*ADMINISTER:* **Intermittent:** Infuse over 30 min; with Y-type administration set, discontinue other compatible solutions while infusing cefepime.
*INCOMPATIBILITIES:* Solution/additive: AMINOGLYCOSIDES, **aminophylline, metronidazole.** Y-site: **Acetylcysteine, acyclovir,**

Common adverse effects in *italic;* life-threatening effects underlined; generic names in **bold;** classifications in SMALL CAPS; ♣ Canadian drug name; ✪ Prototype drug

293

alemtuzumab, amphotericin B, amphotericin B cholesteryl complex, amphotericin B liposomal, argatroban, asparginase, caspofungin, chlordiazepoxide, chlorpromazine, cimetidine, ciprofloxacin, cisplatin, dacarbazine, daunorubicin, dexrazoxane, diazepam, diltiazem, diphenhydramine, dobutamine, dolasetron, dopamine, doxorubicin, droperidol, enalaprilat, epirubicin, erythromycin, etoposide, famotidine, filgrastim, floxuridine, gallium, ganciclovir, gemcitabine, haloperidol, hydroxyzine, idarubicin, ifosfamide, irinotecan, lansoprazole, magnesium sulfate, mannitol, mechlorethamine, meperidine, metoclopramide, midazolam, mitomycin, mitoxantrone, morphine, nalbuphine, nesiritide, nicardipine, ofloxacin, ondansetron, oxaliplatin, pantoprazole, premetrexed, phenytoin, piritramide, plicamycin, prochlorperazine, promethazine, quinupristin-dalfopristin, streptozocin, tacrolimus, temocillin, theophylline, topotecan, vancomycin, vecuronium, vinblastine, vincristine, voriconazole.

• Store reconstituted solution at 20°–25° C (68°–77° F) for 24 h or in refrigerator at 2°–8° C (36°–46° F) for 7 days. Protect from light.

**ADVERSE EFFECTS** (≥1%) **Body as a Whole:** Eosinophilia. **GI:** Antibiotic-associated colitis, diarrhea, nausea, oral moniliasis, vomiting, elevated liver function tests (ALT, AST). **CNS:** Headache, fever. **Skin:** Phlebitis, pain, inflammation, rash, pruritus, urticaria. **Urogenital:** Vaginitis.

## DIAGNOSTIC TEST INTERFERENCE
Positive **Coombs' test** without hemolysis. May cause false-positive **urine glucose test** with **Clinitest.**

## INTERACTIONS Drug: AMINOGLYCOSIDES may increase risk of nephrotoxicity and have additive/synergistic effects. May decrease efficacy of ORAL CONTRACEPTIVES. **Probenecid** may increase levels.

## PHARMACOKINETICS Absorption: Well absorbed after IM administration; serum levels significantly lower than after equivalent IV dose. **Distribution:** Widely distributed, may cross inflamed meninges; crosses placenta, secreted into breast milk. **Metabolism:** In liver. **Elimination:** In urine. **Half-Life:** 2 h.

## NURSING IMPLICATIONS
### Assessment & Drug Effects
• Determine history of hypersensitivity reactions to cephalosporins, penicillins, or other drugs before therapy is initiated.
• Monitor for S&S of hypersensitivity (see Appendix F). Report their appearance promptly and discontinue drug.
• Monitor for S&S of superinfection or pseudomembranous colitis (see Appendix F); immediately report either to prescriber.
• With concurrent high-dose aminoglycoside therapy, closely monitor for nephrotoxicity and ototoxicity.
• Monitor lab tests: Baseline C&S before initiation of therapy; frequent renal function tests, especially with known renal impairment.

### Patient & Family Education
• Promptly report S&S of hypersensitivity (e.g., rash) or superinfection, especially unexplained diarrhea (see Appendix F).

Common adverse effects in *italic;* life-threatening effects underlined; generic names in **bold;** classifications in SMALL CAPS; ♣ Canadian drug name; ● Prototype drug

# CEFIXIME
(ce-fix'ime)

**Suprax**

**Classifications:** BETA-LACTAM ANTIBIOTIC; THIRD-GENERATION CEPHALOSPORIN

**Therapeutic:** ANTIBIOTIC

**Prototype:** Cefotaxime sodium

**AVAILABILITY** Liquid suspension; tablet; capsule

**ACTION & THERAPEUTIC EFFECT** It inhibits the third and final stages of bacterial cell wall synthesis by preferentially binding to specific penicillin-binding proteins (PBPs) located inside the bacterial cell wall. *Cefixime is highly stable in the presence of beta-lactamases (penicillinases and cephalosporinases) and therefore has excellent activity against a wide range of gramnegative bacteria. It is bactericidal against susceptible bacteria.*

**USES** Uncomplicated UTI, otitis media, pharyngitis, tonsillitis, and bronchitis.

**CONTRAINDICATIONS** Patients with known allergy to the cephalosporin group of antibiotics, severe reaction to penicillin.

**CAUTIOUS USE** Allergy to penicillin, history of colitis, renal insufficiency, seizure disorders; GI disease, coagulopathy, pregnancy (category B), children; lactation.

## ROUTE & DOSAGE

### Infection

*Adult/Adolescent/Child (greater than 45kg):* **PO** 400 mg/day in 1–2 divided doses

*Child:* **PO** 8 mg/kg/day in 1–2 divided doses

### Renal Impairment Dosage Adjustment

*CrCl 21–60 mL/min:* Give 65% of dose; *less than 20 mL/min:* Give 50% of dose

## ADMINISTRATION

### Oral

- Do not substitute tablets for liquid in treatment of otitis media because of lack of bioequivalence.
- Ensure that chewable tablets are chewed or crushed before swallowing.
- After reconstitution, suspension may be kept for 14 days at room temperature or refrigerated. Store away from heat and light. Keep tightly closed and shake well before using.

**ADVERSE EFFECTS** (≥1%) **GI:** *Diarrhea,* loose stools, nausea, vomiting, dyspepsia, flatulence. **CNS:** Drug fever, headache, dizziness. **Skin:** Rash, pruritus. **Urogenital:** Vaginitis, genital pruritus.

**INTERACTIONS Drug.** AMINOGLYCOSIDES may increase risk of nephrotoxicity and have additive/synergistic effects. May decrease efficacy of ORAL CONTRACEPTIVES. **Probenecid** may increase levels.

**PHARMACOKINETICS Absorption:** 40–50% from GI tract. **Peak:** 2–6 h. **Distribution:** Into breast milk. **Elimination:** 50% in urine, 50% in bile. **Half-Life:** 3–4 h.

## NURSING IMPLICATIONS

### Assessment & Drug Effects

- Determine previous hypersensitivity reactions to cephalosporins, penicillins, and history of other allergies, particularly to drugs prior to initiation of therapy.

Common adverse effects in *italic*; life-threatening effects underlined; generic names in **bold**; classifications in SMALL CAPS; ♣ Canadian drug name; ⊙ Prototype drug

295

C

- Monitor for superinfections (see Appendix F) caused by overgrowth of nonsusceptible organisms, particularly during prolonged use.
- Monitor I&O rates and pattern: Nephrotoxicity occurs more frequently in patients older than 50 y, with impaired renal function, in the debilitated, and in patients receiving high doses or other nephrotoxic drugs.
- Carefully monitor anyone with a history of allergies. Report manifestations of hypersensitivity (see Appendix F).
- Promptly report loose stools or diarrhea, which may indicate pseudomembranous colitis (see Appendix F). Discontinuation of drug may be necessary.
- Monitor lab tests: Baseline C&S prior to initiation of therapy.

### Patient & Family Education

- Report loose stools or diarrhea during drug therapy and for several weeks after. Older adult patients are especially susceptible to pseudomembranous colitis.

---

## CEFOTAXIME SODIUM ⊙

(sef-oh-taks′eem)

Claforan

**Classifications:** BETA-LACTAM ANTIBIOTIC; THIRD-GENERATION CEPHALOSPORIN

Therapeutic: ANTIBIOTIC

**AVAILABILITY** Solution for injection

## ACTION & *THERAPEUTIC EFFECT*

Preferentially binds to one or more of the penicillin-binding proteins (PBP) located on cell walls of susceptible organisms. This inhibits third and final stages of bacterial cell wall synthesis, thus killing the bacteria. *Generally active against a wide variety of gram-negative bacteria including*

*most of the Enterobacteriaceae. Also active against some organisms resistant to first- and second-generation cephalosporins, and aminoglycoside antibiotics and penicillins.*

**USES** Serious infections of lower respiratory tract, skin and skin structures, bones and joints, CNS (including meningitis and ventriculitis), gynecologic and GU tract infections, including uncomplicated gonococcal infections caused by penicillinase-producing *Neisseria gonorrhoeae* (PPNG). Also used to treat bacteremia or septicemia, intra-abdominal infections, and for perioperative prophylaxis.

**UNLABELED USES** Treatment of disseminated gonococcal infections (gonococcal arthritis-dermatitis syndrome) Lyme disease, typhoid fever.

**CONTRAINDICATIONS** Hypersensitivity to cefotaxime, or cephalosporins antibiotics.

**CAUTIOUS USE** History of Type I hypersensitivity reactions to penicillin; history of allergy to other beta-lactam antibiotics; coagulopathy; renal impairment; older adults; history of colitis or other GI disease; pregnancy (category B).

## ROUTE & DOSAGE

### Moderate to Severe Infections

*Adult:* **IV/IM** 1–2 g q8–12h, up to 2 g q4h (max: 12 g/day)
*Child (1 wk or younger):* **IV/IM** 50 mg/kg q12h; *1–4 wk:* 50 g/kg/q8h; *1 mo–12 y:* 50–180 mg/kg/day divided q6–8h (max: 12 g/24 h)

### Uncomplicated Gonorrhea

*Adult/Adolescent/Child (greater than 45 kg):* **IM** 500 mg as single dose

**Surgical Prophylaxis**
*Adult:* **IV/IM** 1 g 30–90 min before surgery

**Renal Impairment Dosage Adjustment**
*CrCl less than 20 mL/min:* Reduce dose by 50%

**Hemodialysis Dosage Adjustment**
Supplemental dose may be needed

## ADMINISTRATION

### Intramuscular

- Dilute with SW for injection as follows: 2 mL for the 500 mg vial to yield 230 mg/mL; 3 mL for the 1 g vial to yield 300 mg/mL; 5 mL for the 2 g vial to yield 330 mg/mL.
- Administer IM injection deeply into large muscle mass (e.g., upper outer quadrant of gluteus maximus). Aspirate to avoid inadvertent injection into blood vessel. If IM dose is 2 g, divide dose and administer into 2 different sites.

### Intravenous

*IV administration to neonates, infants, and children:* Verify correct IV concentration and rate of infusion with prescriber.

- Do not admix cefotaxime with sodium bicarbonate or any fluid with a pH greater than 7.5. ▪Risk of phlebitis may be reduced by use of a small needle in a large vein.

*PREPARE:* **Direct:** Add 10 mL diluent to vial with 1 or 2 g drug providing a solution containing 95 or 180 mg/mL, respectively. **Intermittent:** To 1 or 2 g drug add 50 or 100 mL D5W, NS, D5/NS, D5/.45% NaCl, LR, or other compatible diluent. **Continuous:** Dilute in 500–1000 mL compatible IV solution.

*ADMINISTER:* **Direct:** Give over 3–5 min. **Intermittent:** Give over 15–30 min, preferably via butterfly or scalp vein-type needles. **Continuous:** Infuse over 6–24 h.

*INCOMPATIBILITIES:* Solution/additive: AMINOGLYCOSIDES, **aminophylline. Y-site: Alemtuzumab, allopurinol, amiodarone, amphotericin B liposome, azathioprine, azithromycin, capsofungin, cefazolin, ceftazidime, ceftizoxime, chloramphenicol, chlorpromazine, cisatracurium, dacarbazine, dantrolene, danorubicin, diazepam, diazoxide, diphenhydramine, dobutamine, dolasetron, doxorubicin, filgrastim, fluconazole, ganciclovir, gemcitabine, gemtuzumab, hetastarch, hydroxyzine, idarubicin, irinotecan, methylprednisolone, minocycline, mitoxantrone, mycophenolate, pantoprazole, papaverine, pemetrexed, pentamidine, pentazocine, phenytoin, prochlorperazine, promethazine, protamine, quinidine, quinupristin/dalfopristin, sodium bicarbonate, sulfamethoxazole/trimethoprim, trastuzumab, vancomycin, vecuronium.**

- Protect from excessive light. Reconstituted solutions may be stored in original containers for 24 h at room temperature; for 10 days under refrigeration at or below 5° C (41° F); or for at least 13 wk in frozen state.

## ADVERSE EFFECTS (≥1%) **Body as a Whole:** Fever, nocturnal perspiration, inflammatory reaction at IV site, phlebitis, thrombophlebitis; pain, induration, and tenderness at IM site, superinfections. **GI:** Nausea, vomiting, *diarrhea,* abdominal pain, colitis, pseudomembranous colitis, anorexia. **Metabolic:** Transient increases

Common adverse effects in *italic;* life-threatening effects underlined; generic names in **bold;** classifications in SMALL CAPS; ♣ Canadian drug name; ☻ Prototype drug

297

C

in serum AST, ALT, LDH, bilirubin, alkaline phosphatase concentrations. **Skin:** Rash, pruritus.

## DIAGNOSTIC TEST INTERFERENCE

May cause falsely elevated **serum** or **urine creatinine** values **(Jaffe reaction).** Positive **direct antiglobulin (Coombs') test;** false positive urinary glucose test using cupric sulfate.

## INTERACTIONS Drug: **Probenecid** decreases renal elimination.

## PHARMACOKINETICS Peak:

30 min after IM; 5 min after IV. **Distribution:** CNS penetration except with inflamed meninges; also penetrates aqueous humor, ascitic and prostatic fluids; crosses placenta. **Metabolism:** In liver to active metabolites. **Elimination:** 50–60% unchanged in urine in 24 h; small amount excreted in breast milk. **Half-Life:** 1 h.

## NURSING IMPLICATIONS

### Assessment & Drug Effects

- Determine previous hypersensitivity reactions to cephalosporins and penicillins, and history of other allergies, particularly to drugs, before therapy is initiated.
- Monitor I&O rates and patterns, especially with higher doses or concurrent aminoglycoside therapy. Report significant changes in I&O.
- Superinfection due to overgrowth of nonsusceptible organisms may occur, particularly with prolonged therapy.
- Report onset of diarrhea promptly. Check for fever. If diarrhea is mild, discontinuation of cefotaxime may be sufficient.
- If diarrhea is severe, suspect antibiotic-associated pseudomembranous colitis, a life-threatening superinfection (may occur in 4–9 days or as long as 6 wk after cephalosporin therapy is discontinued).
- Monitor lab tests: Baseline C&S before initiation of therapy; periodic renal function tests; periodic CBC with differential with high doses or prolonged therapy.

### Patient & Family Education

- Report any early signs or symptoms of superinfection promptly. Superinfections caused by overgrowth of nonsusceptible organisms may occur, particularly during prolonged use.
- Yogurt or buttermilk, 120 mL (4 oz) of either (if allowed), may serve as a prophylactic against intestinal superinfection by helping to maintain normal intestinal flora.
- Report loose stools or diarrhea.

## CEFOTETAN DISODIUM
(se-fo-tee′tan)
Cefotan

**Classifications:** ANTIBIOTIC; SECOND-GENERATION CEPHALOSPORIN
Therapeutic: ANTIBIOTIC
**Prototype:** Cefotaxime sodium

## AVAILABILITY Solution for injection

## ACTION & *THERAPEUTIC EFFECT*

Preferentially binds to one or more of the penicillin-binding proteins (PBP) located on cell walls of susceptible organisms. This inhibits third and final stages of bacterial cell wall synthesis, thus killing the bacterium. *Generally less active against susceptible Staphylococci than first-generation cephalosporins, but has broad spectrum of activity against gram-negative bacteria when compared to first- and second-generation cephalosporins. It also*

Common adverse effects in *italic*; life-threatening effects underlined; generic names in **bold;** classifications in SMALL CAPS; ♣ Canadian drug name; ⊘ Prototype drug *shows moderate activity against gram-positive organisms. It is active against the Enterobacteriaceae and anaerobes.*

**USES** Infections caused by susceptible organisms in urinary tract, lower respiratory tract, skin and skin structures, bones and joints, gynecologic tract; also intra-abdominal infections, bacteremia, and perioperative prophylaxis.

**CONTRAINDICATIONS** Known allergy to cephalosporins and individuals who have experienced a cephalosporin-associated hemolytic anemia; pseudomembranous colitis.

**CAUTIOUS USE** Hypersensitivity to cefotetan, penicillins, or other drugs; preexisting coagulopathy; colitis, GI disease; renal impairment; cancer patients; patients in debilitated state; older adults; pregnancy (category B); lactation. Safety and efficacy in children not established.

## ROUTE & DOSAGE

**Moderate to Severe Infections**
*Adult:* **IV/IM** 1–2 g q12h

**UTI**
*Adult:* **IV** 500 mg q12h or 1–4 g/day

**Surgical Prophylaxis**
*Adult/Adolescent:* **IV/IM** 1–2 g 30–60 min before surgery

**Renal Impairment Dosage Adjustment**
*CrCl greater than 30 mL/min:* Regular dose q12h; *10–30 mL/min:* Regular dose q24h; *less than 10 mL/min:* Regular dose q48h

**Hemodialysis Dosage Adjustment**
Give ¼ dose q24h on days between sessions, ½ dose on day of dialysis

## ADMINISTRATION

### Intramuscular
- For IM reconstitution (follow manufacturer's directions for selection of diluent), add 2 mL diluent to 1 g vial or 3 mL to the 2 g vial; yields approximately 400 or 500 mg/mL, respectively.
- For IM administration, inject well into body of large muscle such as upper outer quadrant of buttock (gluteus maximus).

### Intravenous
IV administration to infants and children: Verify correct IV concentration and rate of infusion with prescriber.

*PREPARE:* **Direct:** Dilute each 1 g with 10 mL of sterile water for injection. **Intermittent:** Dilute each 1 g with 50–100 mL of D5W or NS.
*ADMINISTER:* **Direct:** Give over 3–5 min. **Intermittent:** Give a single dose over 30 min. ▪ For IV infusion, solution may be given for longer period of time through tubing system through which other IV solutions are being given.
*INCOMPATIBILITIES:* **Solution/additive:** AMINOGLYCOSIDES, **heparin, promethazine,** TETRACYCLINES. **Y-site:** AMINOGLYCOSIDES, **cistracurium, lansoprazole, pemetrexed, promethazine, vancomycin, vinorelbine.**

- Protect sterile powder from light; store at or below 22° C (71.6° F); remains stable 24 mo after date of manufacture. May darken with age, but potency is unaffected. ▪ Reconstituted solutions: Stable for 24 h at 25° C (77° F); 96 h when refrigerated at 5° C (41° F); or at least 1 wk when frozen at –20° C (–4° F).

**ADVERSE EFFECTS** (≥1%) **Body as a Whole:** Fever, chills, injection site pain, inflammation, disulfiram-like reaction.

Common adverse effects in *italic;* life-threatening effects <u>underlined;</u> generic names in **bold;** classifications in SMALL CAPS; ♣ Canadian drug name; ⊘ Prototype drug

299

**GI:** Nausea, vomiting, *diarrhea,* abdominal pain, antibiotic-associated colitis. **Hematologic:** Thrombocytopenia, prolongation of bleeding time or prothrombin time. **Skin:** Rash, pruritus.

## DIAGNOSTIC TEST INTERFERENCE

May cause falsely elevated *serum* or *urine creatinine* values *(Jaffe reaction).* False-positive reactions for *urine glucose* have not been reported using *copper sulfate reduction methods* (e.g., *Benedict's, Clinitest*); however, since it has occurred with other cephalosporins, it may be advisable to use *glucose oxidase tests (Clinistix, TesTape, Diastix).* Positive *direct antiglobulin (Coombs') test* results may interfere with *hematologic studies* and *cross-matching* procedures.

## INTERACTIONS **Drug: Probenecid** decreases renal elimination of cefotetan; **alcohol** produces disulfiram reaction; **chloramphenicol** may effect therapeutic activity.

## PHARMACOKINETICS **Peak:** 1.5–3 h after IM. **Distribution:** Poor CNS penetration; widely distributed to body tissues and fluids, including bile, sputum, prostatic and peritoneal fluids; crosses placenta. **Elimination:** 51–81% unchanged in urine; 20% in bile; small amount in breast milk. **Half-Life:** 180–270 min.

## NURSING IMPLICATIONS

### Assessment & Drug Effects

- Determine history of hypersensitivity to cephalosporins and penicillins, and other drug allergies, before therapy begins.
- Report onset of loose stools or diarrhea. If diarrhea is severe, suspect pseudomembranous colitis (see

Appendix F) caused by *Clostridium difficile.* Check temperature. Report fever and severe diarrhea to prescriber; drug should be discontinued.
- Monitor lab tests: Baseline C&S before initiation of therapy. Periodic hematologic studies and renal function tests, especially if cefotetan dose is high or if therapy is prolonged.

### Patient & Family Education

- Report promptly S&S of superinfection (see Appendix F).
- Report loose stools or diarrhea.

## CEFOXITIN SODIUM

(se-fox'i-tin)

**Classifications:** ANTIBIOTIC; SECOND-GENERATION CEPHALOSPORIN
**Therapeutic:** ANTIBIOTIC
**Prototype:** Cefaclor

## AVAILABILITY Solution for injection

## ACTION & *THERAPEUTIC EFFECT*

Preferentially binds to one or more of the penicillin-binding proteins (PBP) located on cell walls of susceptible organisms, thus making it bactericidal. *It shows enhanced activity against a wide variety of gram-negative organisms and is effective for mixed aerobic-anaerobic infections.*

## USES Infections caused by susceptible organisms in the lower respiratory tract, urinary tract, skin and skin structures, bones and joints; also intra-abdominal endocarditis, gynecologic infections, septicemia, uncomplicated gonorrhea, and perioperative prophylaxis in prosthetic arthroplasty or cardiovascular surgery.

## CONTRAINDICATIONS Known hypersensitivity to cefoxitin or cephalosporins.

CAUTIOUS USE History of sensitivity to penicillin, or other drugs; impaired renal function; coagulopathy; GI disease, colitis; seizure disorders; patients with overt or subclinical diabetes; older adults; pregnancy (category B); children younger than 3 mo.

## ROUTE & DOSAGE

### Moderate to Severe Infections

*Adult:* **IV/IM** 1 g every 4 h or 2 g q6-8h up to 12 g/day
*Child (3 mo or older):* **IV/IM** 80–160 mg/kg/day in 4–6 divided doses (max: 12 g/day)

### Surgical Prophylaxis

*Adult:* **IV/IM** 2 g 30–60 min before surgery, then 2 g q6h for 24 h
*Child:* **IV/IM** 30–40 mg/kg 30–60 min before surgery, then 30–40 mg q6h for 24 h

### Pelvic Inflammatory Disease

*Adult/Adolescent:* **IV** 2 g q6h (with **doxycylcine**)

### Cesarean Surgery

*Adult:* **IV/IM** 2 g after clamping umbilical cord

### Renal Impairment Dosage Adjustment

*CrCl 30–50 mL/min:* 1–2 g q8–12h; *10–29 mL/min:* 1–2 g q12–24h; *5–9 mL/min:* 0.5–1 g q12–24h; *greater than 5 mL/min:* 0.5–1 g q24–48h

### Hemodialysis Dosage Adjustment

Dose of 1–2 g post dialysis

## ADMINISTRATION

### Intramuscular

- Reconstitute each 1 g with 2 mL sterile water for injection or 0.5 or 1% lidocaine hydrochloride (without epinephrine), used to reduce discomfort of IM injection. After reconstitution for IM use, shake vial and allow solution to stand until it becomes clear.
- Administer IM injections deep into large muscle mass such as upper outer quadrant of gluteus maximus. Aspirate before injecting drug. Rotate injection sites.

### Intravenous

IV administration to neonates, infants and children: Verify correct IV concentration and rate of infusion/injection with prescriber.

*PREPARE:* **Direct:** Reconstitute each 1 g with 10 mL sterile water, D5W, or NS. **Intermittent:** Following reconstitution, dilute 1–2 g in 50–100 mL of D5W or NS. **Continuous:** Dilute large doses in 1000 mL of D5W, D10W or NS.
*ADMINISTER:* **Direct:** Give over 3–5 min. **Intermittent:** Give over 10–60 min. **Continuous:** Give at a rate determined by the volume of solution. ▪ Reconstituted solution may become discolored (usually light yellow to amber) if exposed to high temperatures; however, potency is not affected. ▪ Solution may be cloudy immediately after reconstitution; let stand and it will clear.
*INCOMPATIBILITIES:* **Solution/additive:** AMINOGLYCOSIDES, **ranitidine. Y-site: Alemtuzumab, ampicillin/sulbactam,** AMINOGLYCOSIDES, **azathioprine, caspofungin, ceftizoxime, chloramphenicol, cisatracurium, dantrolene, danorubicin, diazepam, diazoxide, diphenhydramine, dobutamine, dolasetron, doxorubicin, doxycycline, epirubicin, erythromycin, fenoldopam, filgrastim, ganciclovir, garenoxacin, gatifloxacin, gembtuzumab, haloperidol,**

Common adverse effects in *italic;* life-threatening effects <u>underlined</u>; generic names in **bold;** classifications in SMALL CAPS; ♣ Canadian drug name; ⊙ Prototype drug

301

**C**

hetastarch, hydroxyzine, ida-rubicin, inamrinone, insulin, labetalol, lansoprazole, levo-floxacin, methylprednisolone, minocycline, mitoxantrone, mycophenolate, papaverine, pemetrexed, pentamidine, pentazocine, pentobarbital, phenobarbital, phentolamine, polymixin, prochlorperazine, promethazine, protamine, qui-nidine, quinupristine/dalfo-pristin, sodium bicarbonate, SMZ/TMP, trastuzumab, van-comycin, vinorelbine.

▪ After reconstitution, solution is stable for 24 h at 25° C (77° F); 7 days when refrigerated at 4° C (39° F), or 30 wk when frozen at –20° C (–4° F).

**ADVERSE EFFECTS** (≥1%) **Body as a Whole:** Drug fever, eosinophilia, superinfections, local reactions: pain, tenderness, and induration (IM site), thrombophlebitis (IV site). **GI:** *Diarrhea,* pseudomembranous colitis. **Skin:** Rash, exfoliative dermatitis, pruritus, urticaria. **Metabolic:** Increased hepatic enzymes, thrombocytopenia. **Urogenital:** Nephrotoxicity, interstitial nephritis.

**DIAGNOSTIC TEST INTERFERENCE**
Cefoxitin causes false-positive (black-brown or green-brown color) *urine glucose* reaction with *copper reduction reagents* such as *Benedict's* or *Clinitest,* but not with *enzymatic glucose oxidase reagents (Clinistix, TesTape).* With high doses, falsely elevated *serum and urine creatinine* (with *Jaffe reaction*) reported. False-positive *direct Coombs' test* (may interfere with *cross-matching procedures* and *hematologic studies*) has also been reported.

**INTERACTIONS Drug: Probene-cid** decreases renal elimination of cefoxitin.

**PHARMACOKINETICS Peak:** 20–30 min after IM; 5 min after IV. **Distribution:** Poor CNS penetration even with inflamed meninges; widely distributed in body tissues including pleural, synovial, and ascitic fluid and bile; crosses placenta. **Elimination:** 85% unchanged in urine in 6 h, small amount in breast milk. **Half-Life:** 45–60 min.

**NURSING IMPLICATIONS**
**Assessment & Drug Effects**
▪ Determine previous hypersensitivity to cephalosporins, penicillins, and other drug allergies before therapy is initiated.
▪ Inspect injection sites regularly. Report evidence of inflammation and patient's complaint of pain.
▪ Monitor I&O rates and pattern: Nephrotoxicity occurs most frequently in patients older than 50 y, in patients with impaired renal function, the debilitated, and in patients receiving high doses or other nephrotoxic drugs.
▪ Be alert to S&S of superinfections (see Appendix F). This condition is most apt to occur in older adult patients, especially when drug has been used for prolonged period.
▪ Report onset of diarrhea (may be dose related). If severe, pseudomembranous colitis (see Signs & Symptoms, Appendix F) **must be** ruled out. Older adult patients are especially susceptible.
▪ Monitor lab tests: Baseline C&S prior to therapy; CBC with differential, periodic renal function tests, test for *clostridium difficile* if patient develops diarrhea.

### Patient & Family Education

- Report promptly S&S of superinfection (see Appendix F).
- Report watery or bloody loose stools or severe diarrhea.
- Report severe vomiting or stomach pain.
- Report infusion site swelling, pain, or redness.

## CEFPODOXIME
(cef-po-dox'eem)

Vantin

**Classifications:** ANTIBIOTIC; THIRD-GENERATION CEPHALOSPORIN
**Therapeutic:** ANTIBIOTIC
**Prototype:** Cefotaxime sodium

**AVAILABILITY** Tablet; liquid suspension

## ACTION & THERAPEUTIC EFFECT
Inhibits the final stage of bacterial cell wall synthesis by preferentially binding to specific penicillin-binding proteins (PBPs) within the bacterial cell wall. *Highly active against gram-negative bacteria*.

## USES
Gonorrhea, otitis media, lower and upper respiratory tract infections, urinary tract infections.

## UNLABELED USES
Skin and soft tissue infections.

## CONTRAINDICATIONS
Known hypersensitivity to cephalosporins.

## CAUTIOUS USE
History of Type I hypersensitivity reactions to penicillins; renal impairment; coagulopathy; history of colitis or other GI disease; pregnancy (category B); lactation; children.

## ROUTE & DOSAGE

**Respiratory Tract, Skin, and Soft Tissue Infections**
*Adult:* **PO** 200 mg q12h for 10 days

*Child:* **PO** 10 mg/kg/day divided q12h

**Urinary Tract Infections**
*Adult:* **PO** 100 mg q12h

**Gonorrhea**
*Adult:* **PO** 200 mg as single dose

**Otitis Media**
*Child (5 mo–12 y):* **PO** 10 mg/kg/day divided q12–24h

## ADMINISTRATION

### Oral
- Give with food to enhance absorption.
- Give 1 h before or 2 h after an antacid.
- Consult prescriber regarding patients with renal impairment (i.e., creatinine clearance less than 30 mL/min); dosage intervals should be every 12 h.
- Preparation of suspension: To either the 50 mg/5 mL strength or the 100 mg/5 mL strength, add 25 mL of distilled water, then shake vigorously for 15 seconds. Next, to the 50 mg/5 mL strength add 33 mL, or to the 100 mg/5 mL strength add 32 mL, of distilled water, and shake for at least 3 minutes.
- Store suspension for up to 14 days in a refrigerator [2°–8° C (36°–46° F)]. Shake well before using.

## ADVERSE EFFECTS (≥1%)
**Body as a Whole:** Eye itching, cough, epistaxis, fever, decreased appetite, malaise. **GI:** Diarrhea, nausea, vomiting, abdominal pain, soft stools, flatulence, <u>pseudomembranous colitis</u> (rare). **CNS:** Rare: Headache, asthenia, dizziness, fatigue, anxiety, insomnia, flushing, nightmares, weakness. **Urogenital:** Vaginal candidiasis. **Skin:** Urticaria, rash, scaling, peeling.

---

Common adverse effects in *italic;* life-threatening effects <u>underlined</u>; generic names in **bold**; classifications in SMALL CAPS; ♣ Canadian drug name; ⊙ Prototype drug

**C**

**INTERACTIONS Drug:** ANTACIDS, **ranitidine** may decrease absorption. **Food:** Food may increase the absorption.

**PHARMACOKINETICS Absorption:** 40–50% absorbed from GI tract. **Onset:** Therapeutic effect in 3 days. **Distribution:** Distributes well into inflammatory, pulmonary, and pleural fluid, and tonsils. Some distribution into prostate. 40% bound to plasma proteins. Distributed into breast milk. **Elimination:** 80% in urine. **Half-Life:** 2–3 h.

## NURSING IMPLICATIONS

### Assessment & Drug Effects

- Determine history of hypersensitivity reactions to cephalosporins and penicillins, and history of allergies, particularly to drugs, before therapy is initiated.
- Report onset of loose stools or diarrhea. Although pseudomembranous enterocolitis (see Appendix F) rarely occurs, this potentially life-threatening complication should be ruled out.
- Monitor for manifestations of hypersensitivity (see Appendix F). Discontinue drug and report S&S of hypersensitivity promptly.
- Monitor I&O (especially with high doses). Report significant changes.
- Monitor lab tests: Baseline C&S before initiation of therapy.

### Patient & Family Education

- Report any signs or symptoms of hypersensitivity immediately.
- Report loose stools or diarrhea.

## CEFPROZIL

(cef'pro-zil)

**Classifications:** ANTIBIOTIC; SECOND-GENERATION CEPHALOSPORIN

**Therapeutic** ANTIBIOTIC
**Prototype:** Cefaclor

**AVAILABILITY** Tablet; liquid; suspension

## ACTION & *THERAPEUTIC EFFECT*

Generally resistant to hydrolysis by beta-lactamases. Preferentially binds to proteins in cell walls of susceptible organisms, thus killing the bacteria. *Third-generation cephalosporins are more active and have a broader spectrum against gram-negative bacteria than first- or second-generation of cephalosporins.*

**USES** Upper and lower respiratory tract infections, otitis media, skin infections.

**CONTRAINDICATIONS** Known hypersensitivity to cephalosporin.

**CAUTIOUS USE** Hypersensitivity to penicillins, or other drugs; coagulopathy; renal impairment, renal disease; GI disease, especially colitis; pregnancy (category B); infants.

## ROUTE & DOSAGE

**Pharyngitis/Tonsillitis/Acute Sinusitus/Lower RTI**
*Adult:* **PO** 250–500 mg q12–24h for 10–14 days

**Otitis Media**
*Child (6 mo to 12 y):* **PO** 15 mg/kg q12h

**Skin Infection**
*Adult:* **PO** 250–500 q12h or 500 q24h
*Child (2–12 y):* **PO** 20 mg/kg q24h

Common adverse effects in *italic;* life-threatening effects underlined; generic names in **bold;** classifications in SMALL CAPS; ✦ Canadian drug name; ⊘ Prototype drug

### Renal Impairment Dosage Adjustment

*CrCl less than 29 mL/min:* Reduce dose 50%

## ADMINISTRATION

### Oral

- Drug may be given without regard to meals.
- Consult prescriber for patients with impaired renal function. Dose is reduced by 50% when creatinine clearance is 0–29 mL/min.
- Administer after hemodialysis since drug is partially removed by dialysis.
- After reconstitution, oral suspension is refrigerated. Discard unused portion after 14 days.

## ADVERSE EFFECTS (≥1%) Body as a Whole: Hypersensitivity reactions, superinfections. GI: Nausea, vomiting, diarrhea, abdominal pain. Hematologic: Eosinophilia. CNS: Headache. Skin: Rash, diaper rash. Urogenital: Genital pruritus, vaginal candidiasis

## DIAGNOSTIC TEST INTERFERENCE

May cause a positive *direct Coombs' test;* false-positive reactions for *urine glucose* with *copper reduction tests* such as *Benedict's* or *Fehling's solution* or *Clinitest tablets.*

## INTERACTIONS Drug: Probenecid prolongs the elimination of cefprozil.

## PHARMACOKINETICS Absorption: Readily from GI tract. Peak: 1–2 h. Distribution: Distributes into blister fluid at 50% of the serum level. Elimination: Primarily by kidneys. Half-Life: 1–2 h.

## NURSING IMPLICATIONS

### Assessment & Drug Effects

- Determine previous hypersensitivity to cephalosporins or penicillins before treatment.
- Withhold drug and notify prescriber if hypersensitivity occurs (e.g., rash, urticaria).
- Monitor for and report diarrhea, as pseudomembranous colitis is a potential adverse effect.
- Monitor for and report signs of superinfection (see Appendix F)
- When given concurrently with other cephalosporins or aminoglycosides, monitor for signs of nephrotoxicity.
- Monitor lab tests: Baseline C&S before therapy.

### Patient & Family Education

- Report rash or other signs of hypersensitivity immediately.
- Report signs of superinfection (see Appendix F).
- Report loose stools and diarrhea even after completion of drug therapy.

## CEFTAROLINE

(cef tar'o-line)

Teflaro

**Classifications:** BETA-LACTAM ANTIBIOTIC; THIRD-GENERATION CEPHALOSPORIN
**Therapeutic:** ANTIBIOTIC
**Prototype:** Cefotaxime

## AVAILABILITY Powder for injection

## ACTION & *THERAPEUTIC EFFECT*

It preferentially binds to one or more of the penicillin-binding proteins (PBP) located on the cell walls of susceptible organisms. This inhibits the third and final stages of cell wall

Common adverse effects in *italic;* life-threatening effects <u>underlined</u>; generic names in **bold;** classifications in SMALL CAPS; ♣ Canadian drug name; ⊕ Prototype drug

305

synthesis, thus destroying the bacterium. *Effective against certain gram-positive and gram-negative bacteria responsible for complicated, acute skin infections and community-acquired pneumonia.*

**USES** Treatment of acute bacterial skin and skin structure infections (ABSSSI) and community-acquired bacterial pneumonia (CABP) caused by susceptible microorganisms: *Haemophilus influenzae.*

**CONTRAINDICATIONS** Known hypersensitivity to ceftaroline or other cephalosporins; *C. difficile*-associated diarrhea.

**CAUTIOUS USE** Previous hypersensitivity to penicillins or carbapenems; renal impairment; direct Coombs' test seroconversion; pregnancy (category B); lactation. Safety and efficacy in children not established.

## ROUTE & DOSAGE

**Acute Bacterial Skin and Skin Structure Infections (ABSSSI) or Community-Acquired Bacterial Pneumonia (CABP)**

*Adult:* **IV** 600 mg infused over 1 h q12h for 5–14 days

***Renal Impairment Dosage Adjustment***

*CrCl greater than 30 to 50 mL/ min:* 400 mg over 1 h q12h; *15–30 mL/min:* 300 mg over 1 h q12h; *less than 15 mL/min:* 200 mg over 1 h q12h

***Hemodialysis Dosage Adjustment***

Administer dose after hemodialysis

## ADMINISTRATION
Intravenous

*PREPARE:* **Intermittent:** Reconstitute the 400 or 600 mg vial with 20 mL of sterile water to yield 20 or 30 mg/mL, respectively. ▪ Mix gently then withdraw the required dose and add to at least 250 mL of NS, D5W, 2.5% DW, 0.45% NaCl, or LR. ▪ Do not mix with or add to solutions containing other drugs.

*ADMINISTER:* **Intermittent:** Give at a constant rate over 1 h. ▪ Monitor closely for S&S of hypersensitivity (see Appendix F). If suspected, stop infusion and notify prescriber immediately.

*INCOMPATIBILITIES:* **Solution/additive:** Do not mix with another drug. **Y-site:** Do not mix with another drug. ▪ Use within 6 h when stored at room temperature or within 24 h if refrigerated.

**ADVERSE EFFECTS** (≥2%) **Body as a Whole:** Phlebitis. **GI:** Constipation, *diarrhea, nausea, vomiting.* **Metabolic:** Elevated ALT and AST levels, hypokalemia. **Skin:** Rash.

**DIAGNOSTIC TEST INTERFERENCE** Ceftaroline can cause false positive results for a ***Direct Coombs' Test***.

**INTERACTIONS Drug: Probenecid** may decrease the renal excretion of ceftaroline.

**PHARMACOKINETICS Peak:** 1 h. **Distribution:** Approximately 20% plasma protein bound. **Metabolism:** Dephosphorylated to active metabolite; hydrolyzed to inactive metabolite. **Elimination:** Primarily renal (88%) with minor fecal (6%). **Half-Life:** 1.6 h.

Common adverse effects in *italic;* life-threatening effects underlined; generic names in **bold;** classifications in SMALL CAPS; ♣ Canadian drug name; ⊙ Prototype drug

## NURSING IMPLICATIONS

### Assessment & Drug Effects

- Determine previous hypersensitivity reactions to cephalosporins and penicillins, and history of other allergies, particularly to drugs, before therapy is initiated.
- Monitor closely for S&S of hypersensitivity (see Appendix F).
- Monitor I&O rates and patterns, especially with concurrent aminoglycoside therapy. Report significant changes in I&O.
- Report promptly onset of diarrhea. If fever is present and diarrhea is severe, suspect antibiotic-associated pseudomembranous colitis (may occur during therapy or following discontinuation of ceftaroline).
- Monitor lab tests: Baseline C&S before initiation of therapy; baseline and periodic kidney function tests, especially in the older adult; periodic serum electrolytes, CBC with differential, platelet count, and LFTs.

### Patient & Family Education

- Report promptly frequent watery stools or bloody diarrhea.
- Yogurt or buttermilk may serve as a prophylactic against mild forms of diarrhea.
- Report any signs of hypersensitivity (see Appendix F).

## CEFTAZIDIME

(sef'taz-i-deem)

Fortaz, Tazicef

**Classifications:** ANTIBIOTIC; THIRD-GENERATION CEPHALOSPORIN

Therapeutic: ANTIBIOTIC

**Prototype:** Cefotaxime sodium

**AVAILABILITY** Solution for injection; powder for solution for injection

## ACTION & THERAPEUTIC EFFECT

Preferentially binds to one or more of the penicillin-binding proteins (PBP) located on cell walls of susceptible microbes; this inhibits the final stage of bacterial cell wall synthesis, leading to cell death of the bacterium. *More active and has a broader spectrum against aerobic gram-negative bacteria than do either first- or second-generation agents.*

**USES** To treat infections of lower respiratory tract, skin and skin structures, urinary tract, bones, and joints; also used to treat bacteremia, gynecologic, intra-abdominal, and CNS infections (including meningitis).

**UNLABELED USES** Surgical prophylaxis.

**CONTRAINDICATIONS** Hypersensitivity to ceftazidime or cephalosporins; viral disease.

**CAUTIOUS USE** Hypersensitivity to penicillins, or other drugs, coagulopathy, renal disease, renal impairment; GI disease; colitis; older adults; pregnancy (category B); lactation.

## ROUTE & DOSAGE

### Moderate to Severe Infections

*Adult:* **IV/IM** 1–2 g q8–12h, up to 2 g q6h
*Geriatric:* **IV/IM** 1–2 g q12h
*Child:* **IV/IM** 90–150 mg/kg/day divided q8h (max: 2 g/dose)
*Neonate (4 wk or younger):* **IV** 50 mg/kg q8–12h

### Very Severe Infection

*Adult:* **IV** 2 g q8h

---

Common adverse effects in *italic;* life-threatening effects <u>underlined</u>; generic names in **bold;** classifications in SMALL CAPS; ◆ Canadian drug name; ◯ Prototype drug

**C**

### Renal Impairment Dosage Adjustment

Adult: **IV/IM**
CrCl 31–50 mL/min: 1 g q12h;
CrCl 16–30 mL/min: 1 g q24h;
CrCl 6–15 mL/min: 1 g then 500 mg q24h; CrCl less than 5 mL/min: 1 g then 500 mg q48h

## ADMINISTRATION

### Intramuscular

- Reconstitute by adding 3 mL sterile water or bacteriostatic water for injection or 0.5% or 1% lidocaine HCl injection to 1 g vial to yield 280 mg/mL.
- Inject into large muscle mass (e.g., upper outer quadrant of gluteus maximus or lateral part of thigh).

### Intravenous

**PREPARE:** **Direct:** Using SW for injection: Add 5.3 mL to 500 mg vial then withdraw 5 mL for a 500 mg dose; or add 10 mL to 1 g vial then withdraw 10 mL for a 1 g dose; or add 56 mL to a 6 g vial then withdraw 10 mL for a 1 g dose. **Intermittent:** Prepare as for direct injection then further dilute with 50–100 mL of D5W, NS, or LR. **ADMINISTER:** **Direct:** Give over 3–5 min. **Intermittent:** Give over 15–30 min. ▪ If given through a Y-type set, discontinue other solutions during infusion of ceftazidime. **INCOMPATIBILITIES:** **Solution/additive:** AMINOGLYCOSIDES, **amikacin, aminophylline, ciprofloxacin, ranitidine, sodium bicarbonate, teicoplanin.** Y-site: **Acetylcysteine, alatrofloxacin, amiodarone,** AMINOGLYCOSIDES, **amphotericin B cholesteryl complex, amsacrine, ascorbic acid, atracurium, azathioprine, azithromycin, calcium chloride, caspofungin, cefotaxime, chloramphenicol, chlorprom-**azine, clarithromycin, dantrolene, danorubicin, diazepman, diazoxide, diphenhydramine, doxorubicin liposome, doxycycline, epirubic, erythromycin, fluconazole, ganciclovir, gemtuzumab, haloperidol, hydroxyzine, idarubicin, lansoprazole, midazolam, minocycline, mitxantrone, mycophenolate, nicardipine, nitroprusside, ondansetron, pantoprazole, papaverine, pemetrexed, pentamidine, pentazocine, pentobarbital, phenytoin, piritamide, prochlorperzaine, promethazine, propofol, protamine, quinidine, quinupristin/dalfopristin, sargramostim, sulfamethoxazole/trimethoprim, temocillin, theophylline, thiamine, ticarcillin, vancomycin, verapamil, warfarin.**

- Protect sterile powder from light. Reconstituted solution is stable 7 days when refrigerated at 4°–5° C (39°–41° F); for 18–24 h when stored at 15°–30° C (59°–86° F).

## ADVERSE EFFECTS (≥1%) **Body as a Whole:** Fever, phlebitis, pain or inflammation at injection site, superinfections. **GI:** Nausea, vomiting, *diarrhea*, abdominal pain, metallic taste, drug-associated <u>pseudomembranous colitis</u>. **Skin:** Pruritus, rash, urticaria. **Urogenital:** Vaginitis, candidiasis.

## DIAGNOSTIC TEST INTERFERENCE

False-positive reactions for *urine glucose* have been reported using *copper sulfate* (e.g., *Benedict's solution, Clinitest*). *Glucose oxidase tests (Clinistix, TesTape)* are unaffected. May cause positive *direct antiglobulin (Coombs') test* results, which can interfere with *hematologic studies* and *transfusion cross-matching procedures*.

**INTERACTIONS Drug: Probenecid** decreases renal elimination of ceftazidine. May reduce efficacy of bowel preparation kits. May impact efficacy of ORAL CONTRACEPTIVES. May increase bleeding risk with **warfarin**.

**PHARMACOKINETICS Peak:** 1 h. **Distribution:** CNS penetration with inflamed meninges; also penetrates bone, gallbladder, bile, endometrium, heart, skin, and ascitic and pleural fluids; crosses placenta. **Metabolism:** Not metabolized. **Elimination:** 80–90% unchanged in urine in 24 h; small amount in breast milk. **Half-Life:** 1.5–2 h.

**NURSING IMPLICATIONS**

**Assessment & Drug Effects**

▪ Determine history of hypersensitivity to cephalosporins and penicillins, and other drug allergies, before therapy begins.
▪ If administered concomitantly with another antibiotic, monitor renal function and report it symptoms of dysfunction appear (e.g., changes in I&O ratio and pattern, dysuria).
▪ Be alert to onset of rash, itching, and dyspnea. Check patient's temperature. If it is elevated, suspect onset of hypersensitivity reaction (see Appendix F).
▪ Monitor for superinfection. (See Appendix F.)
▪ If diarrhea occurs and is severe, suspect pseudomembranous colitis (caused by *Clostridium difficile*). Report severe diarrhea to prescriber.
▪ Monitor lab tests: Baseline C&S before initiation of therapy; serum BUN/creatinine.

**Patient & Family Education**

▪ Report loose stools or diarrhea promptly.

▪ Report any signs or symptoms of superinfection promptly (see Appendix F).

**CEFTAZIDIME AND AVIBACTAM**
(cef-ta-zi'deem and a-vi-bac'tam)
Avicaz

**Classifications:** THIRD GENERATION CEPHALOSPORIN (ceftazidime); NON-BETA-LACTAM BETA LACTAMASE INHIBITOR (avibactam)
**Therapeutic:** ANTIBIOTIC

**AVAILABILITY** Sterile powder for reconstitution and injection

**ACTION & THERAPEUTIC EFFECT**
Bactericidal action of **ceftazidime** is mediated through binding to essential penicillin-binding proteins (PBPs); **avibactam** inactivates some beta-lactamases and protects **ceftazidime** from degradation by certain beta-lactamases. *Drug has antibacterial activity against certain gram-negative and gram-positive bacteria.*

**USES** In combination with metronidazole for the treatment of complicated intra-abdominal infections (cIAI) caused by the following susceptible microorganisms: *Escherichia coli, Klebsiella pneumoniae, Proteus mirabilis, Providencia stuartii, Enterobacter cloacae, Klebsiella oxytoca,* and *Pseudomonas aeruginosa* in patients 18 y or older; as a single combination agent for the treatment of complicated urinary tract infections (cUTI) including pyelonephritis caused by the following susceptible microorganisms: *Escherichia coli, Klebsiella pneumoniae, Citrobacter koseri, Enterobacter aerogenes, Enterobacter cloacae, Citrobacter freundii, Proteus* spp., and *Pseudomonas aeruginosa* in patients 18 y or older.

Common adverse effects in *italic;* life-threatening effects underlined; generic names in **bold;** classifications in SMALL CAPS; ♣ Canadian drug name; ☺ Prototype drug

309

**C**

## CONTRAINDICATIONS Known
serious hypersensitivity to ceftazidime, avibactam, or other members of the cephalosporin class.

## CAUTIOUS USE History of penicillin
allergy; renal impairment; seizures or other neurologic events. Safety and efficacy in children younger than 18 y not established.

## ROUTE & DOSAGE

### Complicated Infections
*Adult:* **IV** 2.5g q8h for 5–14 days

### Renal Impairment Dosage Adjustment
*CrCL 31–50 mL/min:* 1.25g q8h
*CrCL 16–30 mL/min:* 0.94g q12h
*CrCL 6–15 mL/min:* 0.94g q24h
*CrCL less than 6 mL/min:* 0.94g q48h

## ADMINISTRATION
### Intravenous

**PREPARE:** **Intermittent:** Reconstitute with 10 mL of one of the following: SW, NS, D5W, LR. Mix gently to yield ceftazidime 0.167 g/mL and avibactam 0.042 g/mL. Further dilute in NS, D5W, or LR to a total volume of 50–250 mL.
**ADMINISTER:** **Intermittent:** Infuse over 2 h. Monitor closely for anaphylaxis during the first dose.

- Store at room temperature for up to 12 h and refrigerated for up to 24 h.

## ADVERSE EFFECTS (≥1%) CNS:
Dizziness. **CV:** Anxiety. **GI:** *Abdominal pain*, constipation, *nausea*, *vomiting*. **Hematological:** Eosinophilia, thrombocytopenia. **Metabolic:** Hypokalemia, *increased ALT, increased blood alkaline phosphatase*, increased gamma-glutamyl transferase, prolonged prothrombin time. **Skin:** Rash. **Urogenital:** <u>Acute renal failure</u>, renal impairment

## DIAGNOSTIC TEST INTERFERENCE
Ceftazidime may cause a false-positive reaction for ***glucose tests*** in the urine.

## INTERACTIONS Drug: Probenecid decreases the elimination of avibactam.

## PHARMACOKINETICS Distribution: Minimal plasma protein binding. **Metabolism:** Minimal. **Elimination:** Renal excretion. **Half-Life:** 2.2 h (avibactam) and 3.3 h (ceftazidime).

## NURSING IMPLICATIONS
### Assessment & Drug Effects
- Monitor for and report promptly signs of hypersensitivity, including skin reactions. Stop infusion and contact prescriber if a hypersensitivity reaction is suspected.
- Report promptly the onset of diarrhea. Check for fever and monitor fluid and electrolyte balance.
- Monitor for and report promptly signs of adverse nervous system reactions (i.e., confusion, hallucinations, stupor, seizures, impaired motor activity).
- Monitor lab test: Baseline renal function tests, and repeat daily with renal impairment.

### Patient & Family Education
- Report immediately if watery or bloody diarrhea develop up to 2 mo after treatment.
- Report immediately the following: Muscle rigidity, tremors, or difficulty with motor activity.
- Do not breast-feed while taking this drug without consulting a prescriber.

# CEFTIBUTEN

(sef-ti-bu'ten)

Cedax

**Classifications:** BETA-LACTAM ANTIBIOTIC; THIRD-GENERATION CEPHALOSPORIN

Therapeutic: ANTIBIOTIC

**Prototype:** Cefotaxime sodium

**AVAILABILITY** Capsule; liquid suspension

## ACTION & *THERAPEUTIC EFFECT*

Ceftibuten preferentially binds to one or more of the penicillin-binding proteins located in the cell wall of susceptible organisms. This inhibits the final stage of bacterial cell wall synthesis, killing the bacterium. *It has antibacterial activity against both gram-negative and gram-positive bacteria.*

**USES** Acute bacterial exacerbations of chronic bronchitis; acute bacterial otitis media; pharyngitis or tonsillitis.

**CONTRAINDICATIONS** Known hypersensitivity to ceftibuten or cephalosporins.

**CAUTIOUS USE** Hypersensitivity to cephalosporins or penicillin or other drugs; history of colitis or diabetes; renal impairment; GI disease; coagulopathy; renal impairment; older adults; pregnancy (category B); lactation. Safety and efficacy in infants younger than 6 mo not established.

## ROUTE & DOSAGE

**Mild to Moderate Infections**

*Adult:* **PO** 400 mg once daily for 10 days

*Renal Impairment Dosage Adjustment*

*CrCl 30–49 mL/min:* 200 mg q24h; *less than 30 mL/min:* 100 mg q24h

*Child (6 mo–12 y):* **PO** 9 mg/kg once daily (max: 400 mg) for 10 days

*Renal Impairment Dosage Adjustment*

*CrCl 30–49 mL/min:* 4.5 mg/kg q24h; *less than 30 mL/min:* 2.25 mg/kg q24h

## ADMINISTRATION

### Oral

- Give oral suspension 1 h before or 2 h after a meal.
- Children weighing more than 45 kg may receive maximum daily dose.
- Hemodialysis patients should receive drug at the end of dialysis.
- Store capsules at 2°–25° C (36°–77° F); keep container tightly closed. Reconstituted oral suspension is stable for 14 days under refrigeration at 2°–8° C (36°–46° F).

**ADVERSE EFFECTS** (≥1%) **Body as a Whole:** Dyspnea, dysuria, fatigue, vaginitis, moniliasis, urticaria, pruritus, rash, paresthesia, taste perversion. **GI:** Nausea, vomiting, diarrhea, dyspepsia, abdominal pain, anorexia, constipation, dry mouth, eructation, flatulence. **CNS:** Headache, dizziness, nasal congestion, somnolence.

**INTERACTIONS Drug:** AMINOGLYCOSIDES may increase risk of nephrotoxicity and have additive/synergistic effects. May decrease efficacy of ORAL CONTRACEPTIVES. **Probenecid** may increase levels.

**PHARMACOKINETICS Absorption:** Rapidly from GI tract. **Peak:** Approx 2–3 h. **Distribution:** Bronchial mucosa levels are approx 37%

Common adverse effects in *italic;* life-threatening effects <u>underlined</u>; generic names in **bold;** classifications in SMALL CAPS; ♣ Canadian drug name; ● Prototype drug

311

of plasma levels, middle ear levels approx 50% of plasma levels. **Elimination:** Primarily in urine. **Half-Life:** 1.5–2.5 h.

## NURSING IMPLICATIONS

### Assessment & Drug Effects

- Determine history of hypersensitivity reactions to cephalosporins, penicillins, or other drugs, before therapy is initiated. Monitor for S&S of hypersensitivity (see Appendix F); report their appearance promptly and discontinue drug.
- Monitor for S&S of superinfection or pseudomembranous colitis (see Appendix F); immediately report either to prescriber.
- Closely monitor patients with renal impairment; if seizures develop, discontinue drug and notify prescriber.
- Monitor lab tests: Baseline C&S before initiation of therapy.

### Patient & Family Education

- If on dialysis treatment, take this drug after dialysis.
- Report any S&S of hypersensitivity, superinfection, and pseudomembranous colitis promptly.

## CEFTRIAXONE SODIUM

(sef-try-ax'one)

Rocephin

**Classifications:** ANTIBIOTIC; THIRD-GENERATION CEPHALOSPORIN
Therapeutic: ANTIBIOTIC
**Prototype:** Cefotaxime sodium

**AVAILABILITY** Solution for injection

## ACTION & THERAPEUTIC EFFECT

Preferentially binds to one or more of the penicillin-binding proteins (PBP) located on cell walls of susceptible organisms. This inhibits third and final stages of bacterial cell wall synthesis, thus killing the bacterium. *Similar to other third-generation cephalosporins, ceftriaxone is effective against serious gram-negative organisms and also penetrates the CSF in concentrations useful in treatment of meningitis.*

**USES** Infections caused by susceptible organisms in lower respiratory tract, skin and skin structures, urinary tract, bones and joints; also intra-abdominal infections, pelvic inflammatory disease, uncomplicated gonorrhea, meningitis, and surgical prophylaxis.

**CONTRAINDICATIONS** Known hypersensitivity to cephalosporins; viral infections; neonates with hyperbilirubinemia 28 days or younger; neonates with calcium-containing infusions; signs and symptoms of gallbladder disease.

**CAUTIOUS USE** Hypersensitivity to penicillin or other drugs; impaired vitamin K synthesis; coagulopathy; hepatic or renal disease; history of GI disease, colitis; older adults; pregnancy (category B).

## ROUTE & DOSAGE

### Moderate to Severe Infections, CAP, UTI

*Adult:* **IV/IM** 1–2 g q12–24h × 4–14 days (max: 4 g/day)
*Child:* **IV/IM** 50–75 mg/kg/day in 2 divided doses × 4–14 days (max: 2 g/day)

### Bacterial Otitis Media

*Child:* **IM** 50 mg/kg (max: 1 g)

### Meningitis

*Adult:* **IV/IM** 2 g q12h
*Child:* **IV/IM** 100 mg/kg/day in 2 divided doses (max: 4 g/day)

### Surgical Prophylaxis
*Adult:* **IV/IM** 1 g 30–120 min before surgery

### Uncomplicated Gonorrhea
*Adult:* **IM** 250 mg as single dose
*Child:* **IM** 125 mg as single dose

## ADMINISTRATION

### Intramuscular
- Reconstitute the 1 or 2 g vial by adding 2.1 or 4.2 mL, respectively, of sterile water for injection. Yields 350 mg/mL. See manufacturer's directions for other dilutions.
- Give deep IM into a large muscle.

### Intravenous
IV administration to infants and children: Verify correct IV concentration and rate of infusion with prescriber.

*PREPARE:* **Intermittent:** Reconstitute each 250 mg with 2.4 mL of sterile water, D5W, NS, or D5/NS to yield 100 mg/mL. • Further dilute with 50–100 mL of the selected IV solution.

*ADMINISTER:* **Intermittent:** Give over 30 min. Do not administer simultaneously with calcium-containing IV solutions, including infusions via a Y-site. In patients other than neonates (28 days and younger), ceftriaxone- and calcium-containing solutions may be administered sequentially if infusion lines are thoroughly flushed between infusions with a compatible fluid.

*INCOMPATIBILITIES:* **Solution/additive:** AMINOGLYCOSIDES, **aminophylline, clindamycin, lido-caine, linezolid, metronidazole, theophylline, calcium**-containing products such as parenteral nutrition. **Y-site: Alatrofloxacin, alemtuzumab,** AMINOGLYCOSIDES, **amphotericin B cholesteryl complex, amsacrine, ascorbic acid, azathioprine, azithromycin, calcium**-containing products, **capreomycin, caspofungin, chloramphenicol, chlor-pro-mazine, clindamycin, dantro-lene, danorubicin, diazepam, diazoxide, diphenhy-dra-mine, dobutamine, dolasetron, doxorubicin, epirubicin, filgrastim, fluconazole, ganciclovir, garenoxacin, gemtuzumab, haloperidol, hydralazine, hydroxyzine, idarubicin, imipenem-cilastin, irinotecan, labetalol, leucovorin, magnesium sulfate, minocycline, mitoxantrone, mycophenolate, papaverine, pentamidine, pentazocine, pentobarbital, phenytoin, pro-chlorperazine, promethazine, protamine, quin-idine, quinupristin/dalfopristin, SMZ/TMP, tobramycin, vancomycin, vinorelbine.**

- Protect sterile powder from light. Store at 15°–25° C (59°–77° F). • Reconstituted solutions: Diluent, concentration of solutions are determinants of stability. See manufacturer's instructions for storage.

## ADVERSE EFFECTS (≥1%) **Body as a Whole:** Pruritus, fever, chills, pain, induration at IM injection site; phlebitis (IV site). **GI:** *Diarrhea,* abdominal cramps, pseudomembranous colitis, biliary sludge. **Urogenital:** Genital pruritus; moniliasis.

## DIAGNOSTIC TEST INTERFERENCE
Causes prolonged *PT/INR* during therapy.

## INTERACTIONS Drug: **Probenecid** decreases renal elimination of

Common adverse effects in *italic;* life-threatening effects <u>underlined</u>; generic names in **bold**; classifications in SMALL CAPS; ✦ Canadian drug name; ● Prototype drug

313

C

ceftriaxone; **alcohol** produces disulfiram reaction; effect of **warfarin** may be increased.

## PHARMACOKINETICS  **Peak:**
1.5–4 h after IM; immediately after IV. **Distribution:** Widely in body tissues and fluids; good CNS penetration; crosses placenta. **Metabolism:** Not metabolized. **Elimination:** 33–65% unchanged in urine; also in bile and breast milk. **Half-Life:** 5–10 h.

## NURSING IMPLICATIONS
### Assessment & Drug Effects
- Determine history of hypersensitivity reactions to cephalosporins and penicillins and history of other allergies, particularly to drugs, before therapy is initiated.
- Inspect injection sites for induration and inflammation. Rotate sites. Note IV injection sites for signs of phlebitis (redness, swelling, pain).
- Monitor for manifestations of hypersensitivity (see Appendix F). Report promptly.
- Watch for and report: Petechiae, ecchymotic areas, epistaxis, or any unexplained bleeding. Ceftriaxone appears to alter vitamin K–producing gut bacteria; therefore, hypoprothrombinemic bleeding may occur.
- Report promptly development of diarrhea. The incidence of antibiotic-produced pseudomembranous colitis (see Appendix F) is higher than with most cephalosporins.
- Monitor lab tests: Baseline C&S before initiation of therapy. PT and INR with concurrent warfarin.

### Patient & Family Education
- Report any signs of bleeding.
- Report loose stools or diarrhea promptly.

## CEFUROXIME SODIUM
(se-fyoor-ox'eem)
Zinacef

## CEFUROXIME AXETIL
Ceftin
**Classifications:** ANTIBIOTIC; SECOND-GENERATION CEPHALOSPORIN
Therapeutic: ANTIBIOTIC
**Prototype:** Cefaclor

**AVAILABILITY** Tablet; liquid suspension; solution for injection

## ACTION & *THERAPEUTIC EFFECT*
Preferentially binds to one or more of the penicillin-binding proteins (PBP) located on cell walls of susceptible organisms. This inhibits third and final stages of bacterial cell wall synthesis, thus killing the bacterium. *Similar to other second-generation cephalosporins, cefuroxime is more active against gram-negative bacteria than are first-generation cephalosporins but not as active as third-generation cephalosporins.*

**USES** Infections caused by susceptible organisms in the lower respiratory tract, urinary tract, skin, and skin structures; also used for treatment of meningitis, gonorrhea, and otitis media and for perioperative prophylaxis (e.g., open-heart surgery), early Lyme disease.

**CONTRAINDICATIONS** Known hypersensitivity to cephalosporins; viral infections.

**CAUTIOUS USE** History of allergy, particularly to drugs; penicillin sensitivity; renal insufficiency; history of seizures; history of colitis or

Common adverse effects in *italic;* life-threatening effects <u>underlined</u>; generic names in **bold;** classifications in SMALL CAPS; ♣ Canadian drug name; ⊙ Prototype drug

other GI disease; pregnancy (category B); lactation.

## ROUTE & DOSAGE

### Moderate to Severe Infections

*Adult:* **PO** 250–500 mg q12h; **IV/ IM** 750 mg–1.5 g q6–8h
*Child (3 mo–12 y):* **PO** 10–15 mg/kg (125–250 mg) q12h; **IV/ IM** 50–100 mg/kg/day divided q8h (max: 6 g/day)

### Pneumonia

*Adult:* **IV/IM** 0.75-1.5 g q8h

### Bacterial Meningitis

*Adult:* **IV/IM** 1.5–3 g q8h
*Child/Infant (3 mo and older):* **IV/IM** 200–240 mg/kg/day divided q6–8h; reduced to 100 mg/kg/day upon improvement

### Surgical Prophylaxis

*Adult/Adolescent:* **IV/IM** 1.5 g 30–60 min before surgery, then 750 mg q8h for 24 h

### Renal Impairment Dosage Adjustment

*CrCl 10–20 mL/min:* Give q12h; *less than 10 mL/min:* Give q24h

### Hemodialysis Dosage Adjustment

Give supplemental dose

## ADMINISTRATION

### Oral

- Cefuroxime tablets and oral suspension are not substitutable on a mg-for-mg basis.
- The oral suspension is for infants and children 3 mo to 12 y. Each teaspoon (5 mL) contains the equivalent of 125 mg cefuroxime. Shake oral suspension well before each use.

### Intramuscular

- Shake IM suspension gently before administration. IM injections should be made deeply into large muscle mass. Rotate injection sites.

### Intravenous

*IV administration to neonates, infants and children:* Verify correct IV concentration and rate of infusion/injection with prescriber.

*PREPARE:* **Direct:** Dilute each 750 mg with 8 mL sterile water, D5W, or NS. **Intermittent:** Further dilute in 50–100 mL of compatible solution. **Continuous:** May be added to 1000 mL of IV compatible solution. *ADMINISTER:* **Direct:** Give slowly over 3–5 min. **Intermittent:** Give over 30 min. **Continuous:** Give over 6–24 h.

*INCOMPATIBILITIES:* **Solution/additive:** AMINOGLYCOSIDES, **ciprofloxacin, ranitidine. Y-site: Alemtuzumab,** AMINOGLYCOSIDES, **azathioprine, azithromycin, calcium chloride, caspofungin, chlorpromazine, cisatracurium, clarithromycin, dantrolene, daunorubicin, dexamethasone, diazepam, diazoxide, diphenhydramine, dobutamine, dolasetron, doxorubicin, doxycycline, epirubicin, filgrastim, fluconazole, ganciclovir, garenoxacin, haloperidol, hydralazine, hydroxyzine, idarubicin, inamrinone, labetalol, magnesium, midazolam, minocycline, mitomycin, mitoxantrone, mycophenolate, nicardipine, papaverine, pentamidine, pentazocine, pentobabital, phenobarbital, phentolamine, phenytoin, polymyxin B, prochlorperazine, promethazine, protamine, quinidine, quinupristin/dalfopristin, SMZ/TMP, vancomycin, vinorelbine.**

---

Common adverse effects in *italic;* life-threatening effects <u>underlined</u>; generic names in **bold;** classifications in SMALL CAPS; ✦ Canadian drug name; ❶ Prototype drug

315

C

• Store powder protected from light unless otherwise directed. After reconstitution, store suspension at 2°–30° C (36°–86° F). Discard after 10 days.

## ADVERSE EFFECTS (≥1%) **Body as a Whole:** Thrombophlebitis (IV site); pain, burning, cellulitis (IM site); superinfections, positive Coombs' test. **GI:** *Diarrhea*, nausea, antibiotic-associated colitis. **Skin:** Rash, pruritus, urticaria. **Urogenital:** Increased serum creatinine and BUN, decreased creatinine clearance.

## DIAGNOSTIC TEST INTERFERENCE
Cefuroxime causes false-positive (black-brown or green-brown color) *urine glucose* reaction with *copper reduction reagents* (e.g., *Benedict's* or *Clinitest*) but not with *enzymatic glucose oxidase reagents* (e.g., *Clinistix, TesTape*). False-positive *direct Coombs' test* (may interfere with *cross-matching procedures* and *hematologic studies*) has been reported.

## INTERACTIONS **Drug: Probenecid** decreases renal elimination of cefuroxime, thus prolonging its action.

## PHARMACOKINETICS **Absorption:** Well absorbed from GI tract; hydrolyzed to active drug in GI mucosa. **Peak:** PO 2 h; IM 30 min. **Distribution:** Widely distributed in body tissues and fluids; adequate CNS penetration with inflamed meninges; crosses placenta. **Elimination:** 66–100% in 24 h; in breast milk. **Half-Life:** 1–2 h.

## NURSING IMPLICATIONS
### Assessment & Drug Effects
• Determine history of hypersensitivity reactions to cephalosporins, penicillins, and history of aller-

gies, particularly to drugs, before therapy is initiated.
• Report onset of loose stools or diarrhea. Pseudomembranous colitis (see Signs & Symptoms, Appendix F) should be ruled out as the cause of diarrhea during and after antibiotic therapy.
• Monitor for manifestations of hypersensitivity (see Appendix F). Discontinue drug and report their appearance promptly.
• Monitor lab tests: Baseline C&S before initiation of therapy. Periodic renal function tests.

### Patient & Family Education
• Report loose stools or diarrhea promptly.
• Report any signs or symptoms of hypersensitivity (see Appendix F).

## CELECOXIB ℗
(cel-e-cox'ib)
Celebrex
**Classifications:** ANALGESIC, NONSTEROIDAL ANTI-INFLAMMATORY DRUG (NSAID); CYCLOOXYGENASE-2 (COX-2) INHIBITOR; ANTI-INFLAMMATORY
**Therapeutic:** ANALGESIC, NSAID; COX-2 INHIBITOR; ANTIINFLAMMATORY; ANTIRHEUMATIC

## AVAILABILITY Capsule

## ACTION & *THERAPEUTIC EFFECT*
Inhibits prostaglandin synthesis by inhibiting cyclooxygenase-2 (COX-2), but does not inhibit cyclooxygenase-1 (COX-1). *Exhibits anti-inflammatory, analgesic, and antipyretic activities. Reduces or eliminates the pain of rheumatoid and osteoarthritis.*

## USES Relief of S&S of osteoarthritis and rheumatoid arthritis. Treatment

Common adverse effects in *italic;* life-threatening effects <u>underlined</u>; generic names in **bold;** classifications in SMALL CAPS; ♣ Canadian drug name; ℗ Prototype drug

of acute pain and primary dysmenorrhea; ankylosing spondylitis, juvenile rheumatoid arthritis.

**CONTRAINDICATIONS** Hypersensitivity to celecoxib, salicylate, or sulfonamide; asthmatic patients with aspirin triad; GI bleeding; advanced renal disease; development of S&S of renal impairment due to drug; severe hepatic impairment; development of S&S of hepatic impairment due to drug; anemia; pain from CABG surgery; pregnancy (category D third trimester); lactation.

**CAUTIOUS USE** Patients who are CYP2C9 poor metabolizers; patients who weigh less than 50 kg; mild or moderate hepatic impairment; elevated LTFs; renal insufficiency; prior history of GI bleeding or peptic ulcer disease; alcoholics; asthmatics; bone marrow suppression; CVA; PVD; fluid retention and/or HF; known risks for cardiovascular disease; kidney disease; hypertension; fluid retention; older adults; pregnancy (category C first and second trimester); children with systemic-onset juvenile rheumatoid arthritis younger than 2 y.

## ROUTE & DOSAGE

### Osteoarthritis/Arthritis/Ankylosing Spondylitis
*Adult:* **PO** 100 mg b.i.d. or 200 mg daily

### Rheumatoid Arthritis
*Adult:* **PO** 100–200 mg b.i.d.

### Acute Pain, Dysmenorrhea
*Adult:* **PO** 400 mg 1st dose, then 200 mg same day if needed, then 200 mg b.i.d. prn

### FAP
*Adult:* **PO** 400 mg b.i.d.

### Juvenile Rheumatoid Arthritis
*Adolescent/Child (2 y or older, weight greater than 25 kg):* **PO** 100 mg b.i.d.
*Child (2 y or older, weight 10–25 kg):* **PO** 50 mg b.i.d.

### Hepatic Dosage Adjustment
*Child-Pugh class B:* Reduce dose by 50%

### Pharmacogenetic Dosage Adjustment
*Poor CYP2C9 metabolizers:* Start with ½ normal dose

## ADMINISTRATION

### Oral
- Give 2 h before/after magnesium- or aluminum-containing antacids.
- Store in tightly closed container and protect from light.

**ADVERSE EFFECTS** (≥1%) **Body as a Whole:** Back pain, peripheral edema. Increased risk of cardiovascular events. **GI:** Abdominal pain, diarrhea, dyspepsia, flatulence, nausea. **CNS:** Dizziness, headache, insomnia. **Respiratory:** Pharyngitis, rhinitis, sinusitis, URI. **Skin:** Rash. **CV:** Stroke, MI.

**INTERACTIONS Drug:** May diminish effectiveness of ACE INHIBITORS; **fluconazole** increases celecoxib concentrations; may increase **lithium** concentrations; may increase INR in older patients on **warfarin.**

**PHARMACOKINETICS Peak:** 3 h. **Distribution:** 97% protein bound; crosses placenta. **Metabolism:** In liver by CYP2C9. **Elimination:** Primarily in feces (57%), 27% in urine. **Half-Life:** 11.2 h.

---

Common adverse effects in *italic*; life-threatening effects <u>underlined</u>; generic names in **bold**; classifications in SMALL CAPS; ♣ Canadian drug name; ⊙ Prototype drug

317

## NURSING IMPLICATIONS

### Black Box Warning

*Celecoxib may increase the risk of serious, potentially fatal thrombosis (e.g., MI and stroke) and GI adverse events (e.g., bleeding, ulceration, and perforation).*

### Assessment & Drug Effects

- Monitor for S&S of GI bleeding that may occur suddenly and without warning, especially in older patients.
- Monitor for development of thrombotic events even in those with no prior history of cardiovascular problems.
- Monitor closely lithium levels when the two drugs are given concurrently.
- Monitor closely PT/INR when used concurrently with warfarin.
- Monitor for fluid retention and edema especially in those with a history of hypertension or CHF.
- Monitor lab tests: Periodic Hct and Hgb, LFTs, renal function tests, and serum electrolytes.

### Patient & Family Education

- Seek immediate medical attention for any of the following: Chest pain, shortness of breath, sudden weakness, slurring of speech, or other S&S of a stroke.
- Promptly report any of the following: Unexplained weight gain, edema, skin rash.
- Stop taking celecoxib and promptly report to prescriber if any of the following occurs: S&S of liver dysfunction including nausea, fatigue, lethargy, itching, jaundice, abdominal pain, and flu-like symptoms; S&S of GI ulceration including black, tarry stools and upper GI distress.

- Avoid using celecoxib during the third trimester of pregnancy.

# CEPHALEXIN
(sef-a-lex'in)
Keflex
**Classifications:** BETA-LACTAM ANTIBIOTIC; FIRST-GENERATION CEPHALOSPORIN
Therapeutic: ANTIBIOTIC
**Prototype:** Cefazolin

**AVAILABILITY** Capsule; oral suspension

**ACTION & *THERAPEUTIC EFFECT*** Preferentially binds to one or more of the penicillin-binding proteins (PBP) located on cell walls of susceptible organisms. This inhibits third and final stages of bacterial cell wall synthesis, thus killing the bacterium. *Broad-spectrum, first-generation cephalosporin active against many gram-positive aerobic cocci and much less active against gram-negative bacteria or anaerobic organisms.*

**USES** To treat infections caused by susceptible pathogens in respiratory and urinary tracts, middle ear, skin, soft tissue, and bone.

**CONTRAINDICATIONS** Known hypersensitivity to cephalosporin antibiotics; viral infections; prophylactic use.

**CAUTIOUS USE** History of hypersensitivity to penicillin or other drug allergy; severely impaired renal function; GI disease, colitis; hepatic disease; coagulopathy; pregnancy (category B); lactation. Safe use in younger than 2 y not established.

Common adverse effects in *italic;* life-threatening effects underlined; generic names in **bold;** classifications in SMALL CAPS; ♣ Canadian drug name; ⦿ Prototype drug

## ROUTE & DOSAGE

**Mild to Moderate Infection**

*Adult:* **PO** 250–500 mg q6h
*Child:* **PO** 25–100 mg/kg/day in 4 divided doses

**Skin and Skin Structure Infections**

*Adult:* **PO** 500 mg q12h
*Adolescent/Child:* **PO** 25–50 mg/kg/day q12h

**Otitis Media**

*Child:* **PO** 75–100 mg/kg/day in 4 divided doses

## ADMINISTRATION

### Oral

- Cephalexin oral suspension should be refrigerated; discard unused portions 14 days after preparation. Label should indicate expiration date. Keep tightly covered. Shake suspension well before pouring.

## ADVERSE EFFECTS (≥1%) **Body as a Whole:** Angioedema, anaphylaxis, superinfections. **GI:** *Diarrhea* (generally mild), nausea, vomiting, anorexia, abdominal pain. **CNS:** Dizziness, headache, fatigue. **Skin:** Rash, urticaria.

## DIAGNOSTIC TEST INTERFERENCE

False-positive *urine glucose* determinations using *copper sulfate reagents* (e.g., *Clinitest, Benedict's reagent*). Positive *direct Coombs' test* may complicate transfusion *cross-matching procedures* and *hematologic studies.*

## INTERACTIONS **Drug:** Probenecid decreases renal elimination of cephalexin. **Metformin** can decrease absorption of cephalexin.

## PHARMACOKINETICS **Absorption:** Rapidly from GI tract; stable in stomach acid. **Peak:** 1 h. **Distribution:** Widely distributed in body fluids with highest concentration in kidney; crosses placenta. **Elimination:** 80–100% unchanged in urine in 8 h; excreted in breast milk. **Half-Life:** 38–70 min.

## NURSING IMPLICATIONS

### Assessment & Drug Effects

- Determine history of hypersensitivity reactions to cephalosporins and penicillin and history of other drug allergies before therapy is initiated.
- Monitor for manifestations of hypersensitivity (see Signs & Symptoms, Appendix F). Discontinue drug and report their appearance promptly.
- Monitor lab tests: Periodic renal function tests and LFTs with prolonged therapy.

### Patient & Family Education

- Keep prescriber informed if adverse reactions appear.
- Be alert to S&S of superinfections (see Appendix F). These symptoms should be reported promptly and appropriate therapy instituted.

## CERITINIB

(ce-ri'ti-nib)

Zykadia

**Classifications:** ANTINEOPLASTIC; KINASE INHIBITOR
**Therapeutic:** ANTINEOPLASTIC
**Prototype:** Erlotinib

## AVAILABILITY Capsule

## ACTION & *THERAPEUTIC EFFECT*

Potent inhibitor of anaplastic lymphoma kinase (ALK), an en-

Common adverse effects in *italic*; life-threatening effects underlined; generic names in **bold**; classifications in SMALL CAPS; ♣ Canadian drug name; ⊕ Prototype drug

319

zyme involved in the pathogenesis of non-small-cell lung cancer. ALK gene mutations may result in expression of oncogenic fusion proteins that increase cellular proliferation and survival of tumor cells which express these fusion proteins. *ALK inhibition reduces proliferation of lung cancer cells expressing the genetic alteration.*

**USES** Treatment of anaplastic lymphoma kinase (ALK) positive metastatic non-small-cell lung cancer (NSCLC) in patients who have progressed on or are intolerant to crizotinib.

**CONTRAINDICATIONS** Severe hepatotoxicity, severe QTc prolongation, or Interstitial Lung Disease (ILD)/Pneumonitis due to drug use; pregnancy (category D); lactation.

**CAUTIOUS USE** GI, hepatic, or pulmonary toxicity; QTc prolongation; CHF; bradycardia; DM, hyperglycemia. Safety and efficacy in children younger than 18 y not established.

**ROUTE & DOSAGE**

**Non-Small Cell Lung Cancer (NSCLC)**
*Adult:* **PO** 750 mg daily

*Concomitant Use of Strong CYP3A4 Inducers/Inhibitors Dosage Adjustment*

Reduce dose by approximately one-third, rounded to nearest 150 mg dosage strength if taken with a strong CYP3A4 inhibitor. If strong CYP3A4 inhibitor is discontinued, resume previous dose. Avoid concomitant use with strong CYP3A4 inducers

*Hepatic Impairment Dosage Adjustment*

*ALT or AST elevation greater than 5 × ULN with total bilirubin 2 × ULN or less:* Withhold until recovery or 3 × ULN or less, resume with 150 mg dose reduction
*ALT or AST elevation greater than 3 × ULN with total bilirubin 2 × ULN or greater in the absence of cholestasis or hemolysis:* Permanently discontinue

*Treatment-Related Toxicity Dosage Adjustment*

*Any grade interstitial lung disease (ILD) or pneumonitis:* Permanently discontinued
*Cardiac (QT prolongation, bradycardia), metabolic (hyperglycemia) and GI toxicities:* See manufacturer's guidelines.

**ADMINISTRATION**
**Oral**
- Give on an empty stomach at least 2 h before/after a meal.
- Store at 15°–30° C (59°–86° F).

**ADVERSE EFFECTS** (≥ 1%) **Body as a Whole:** Fatigue, neuropathy. **CV:** <u>Bradycardia, prolonged QT interval.</u> **GI:** Abdominal pain, constipation, decreased appetite, *diarrhea*, dyspepsia, dysphagia, gastroesophageal reflux disease, *nausea, vomiting.* **Hematological:** Decreased hemoglobin. **Metabolic:** Decreased serum phosphate, hyperglycemia, *increased serum ALT and AST*, increased serum bilirubin, increased serum creatinine, increased serum lipase. **Respiratory:** <u>Interstitial pulmonary disease.</u>

Common adverse effects in *italic;* life-threatening effects <u>underlined;</u> generic names in **bold;** classifications in SMALL CAPS; ✦ Canadian drug name; ◎ Prototype drug

**Skin:** Acneiform dermatitis, maculopapular rash. **Special Senses:** Visual disturbances.

**INTERACTIONS Drug:** Strong CYP3A4 inhibitors (e.g., **ketoconazole**, MACROLIDE ANTIBIOTICS, **nefazodone**, **ritonavir**) increase the levels of ceritinib. Strong CYP3A4 inducers (e.g., **carbamazepine, phenytoin, rifampin**) decrease the levels of ceritinib. **Food:** Grapefruit and grapefruit juice may increase the levels of ceritinib. **Herbal: St. John's wort** decreases the levels of ceritinib.

**PHARMACOKINETICS Peak:** 4–6 h. **Distribution:** 97% plasma protein bound. **Metabolism:** Hepatic oxidation. **Elimination:** Primarily fecal (92%). **Half-Life:** 41 h.

## NURSING IMPLICATIONS

### Assessment & Drug Effects

- Monitor diabetics or those with glucose intolerance for loss of glycemic control (i.e., hyperglycemia).
- Monitor for and report promptly S&S of GI or hepatic toxicity, pneumonitis (e.g., shortness of breath, chest pain, cough with/without mucus), or cardiac arrhythmias (e.g., QTc prolongation and bradycardia with heart rate less than 50).
- Monitor lab tests: Baseline and periodic CBC with differential, LFTs, renal function tests, and blood glucose.

### Patient & Family Education

- Do not drink grapefruit juice or eat grapefruit during treatment.
- Report promptly to prescriber if you experience any of the following: Severe or persistent GI distress or signs of liver toxicity (e.g., excessive fatigue, jaundice, loss of appetite, itchy skin, nausea and vomiting, abdominal pain); shortness of breath or chest pain; abnormal heart beats (palpitations), lightheadedness, or dizziness.
- Tell prescriber if you are taking any OTC drugs for reflux or acid stomach.
- Women of reproductive age should avoid pregnancy during treatment with this drug.
- Do not breast-feed while taking this drug.

# CERTOLIZUMAB PEGOL
(cer-to'li-zu-mab)
Cimzia

**Classifications:** BIOLOGIC RESPONSE MODIFIER; IMMUNOMODULATOR; TUMOR NECROSIS FACTOR (TNF) MODIFIER
**Therapeutic:** TNF MODIFIER; IMMUNOLOGIC; ANTIRHEUMATIC
**Prototype:** Etanercept

**AVAILABILITY** Powder for injection; solution for injection

## ACTION & *THERAPEUTIC EFFECT*
A fragment of an antibody Fab fragment with specificity for tumor necrosis factor (TNF)-alpha. This causes a reduction in the production of proinflammatory cytokines including interleukin-1 beta as well as TNF-alpha. Increased levels of TNF-alpha are found in the bowel wall areas that are affected by Crohn's disease and RA. *Reduces inflammatory cytokine production in Crohn's disease. It also decreases the serum level of C-reactive protein, a direct measure of the inflammatory process related to Crohn's disease. Effective for treatment of adults with moderately to severely active rheumatoid arthritis.*

**USES** Reduction of signs and symptoms, as well as maintenance of clinical response, in patients with moderately to severely active Crohn's

Common adverse effects in *italic*; life-threatening effects underlined; generic names in **bold**; classifications in SMALL CAPS; ◆ Canadian drug name; ⊕ Prototype drug

321

C

disease. For treatment of moderate to severely active rheumatoid arthritis.

**UNLABELED USES** Psoriasis.

**CONTRAINDICATIONS** Active chronic or localized infections (e.g., TB, histoplasmosis, other fungal infections); HBV reactivation; lupus-like syndrome.

**CAUTIOUS USE** History of recurrent infection; concurrent immunosuppressive therapy; past/current residence in region where TB and histoplasmosis are endemic; CNS demyelinating disease; neurologic disorders, including seizure disorder, optic neuritis, peripheral neuropathy; recurrent/previous hematologic disorders; heart failure; hypersensitivity response to other TNF blocker(s); older adults; pregnancy (category B); lactation. Safety and efficacy in children not established.

## ROUTE & DOSAGE

**Crohn's Disease**

*Adult:* **Subcutaneous** 400 mg (two 200 mg injections) at wk 0, 2, and 4, then 400 mg q4wk if clinical response occurs

**Rheumatoid Arthritis**

*Adult:* **Subcutaneous** Two 200 mg injections, at wk 0, 2, and 4, then 200 mg every other week

## ADMINISTRATION

**Subcutaneous**

- Reconstitute two 200 mg vials by adding 1 mL sterile water to each using a 20-gauge needle. Swirl gently then allow to sit to dissolve (may require up to 30 min); yields 200 mg/mL. Use within 2 h of reconstitution.

- Use two separate syringes with 20-gauge needles; withdraw 1 mL from each vial. Change to 23-gauge needles and inject into two separate sites on the abdomen or thigh.
- Store reconstituted solution. May be kept at room temperature for no longer than 2 h and refrigerated for up to 24 h.

**ADVERSE EFFECTS** (≥1%) **Body as a Whole:** *Rash*, erythema nodosum, injection-site pain, pain in extremity, peripheral edema, pneumonia, *increased risk of serious infections (bacterial, mycobacterial, fungal, viral)* **GI:** Abdominal pain. **Musculoskeletal:** *Arthralgia.* **Urogenital:** Pyelonephritis.

**DIAGNOSTIC TEST INTERFERENCE** Certolizumab may cause erroneously elevated **activated partial thromboplastin time (aPTT)** assay results.

**INTERACTIONS Drug:** Coadministration of **anakinra, abatacept** may cause increased risks of serious infections and neutropenia. Do not use with TNF ALPHA BLOCKERS.

**PHARMACOKINETICS Absorption:** 80% bioavailable. **Peak:** 54–171 h. **Half-Life:** 14 days.

## NURSING IMPLICATIONS

### Black Box Warning

*Certolizumab has been associated with serious, potentially fatal, infections.*

**Assessment & Drug Effects**

- Prior to initiating therapy, patient should be evaluated for TB risk factors and latent TB. Monitor for S&S of TB throughout therapy.

- Report promptly any S&S of infection or hypersensitivity reaction. (See Appendix F for S&S.)
- Monitor closely carriers of HBV for signs of active infection. If suspected, withhold injection and notify prescriber.
- Monitor closely patients with heart failure for worsening cardiac status.
- Monitor for and report promptly any abnormal neurologic finding or unexplained bruising or bleeding.
- Monitor lab tests. Baseline TB test; periodic CBC with platelet count.

**Patient & Family Education**
- Report promptly any of the following: S&S of infections, such as persistent fever; signs of an allergic reaction (e.g., hives, itching, swelling); unexplained bleeding or bruising.
- Do not accept vaccination with live (or attenuated) vaccines while on certolizumab.

## CETIRIZINE
(ce-tir′i-zeen)
Reactine ♦, Zyrtec

## LEVOCETIRIZINE
(lev-o-ce-tir′i-zeen)
Xyzal

**Classifications:** ANTIHISTAMINE; H₁-RECEPTOR ANTAGONIST; NON-SEDATING
Therapeutic: ANTIHISTAMINE, NON-SEDATING
**Prototype:** Loratadine

**AVAILABILITY** Tablet; chewable tablet; syrup. **Levocetirizine:** Syrup; tablet

## ACTION & *THERAPEUTIC EFFECT*
A potent H₁-receptor antagonist and an antihistamine without significant anticholinergic or CNS activity. Low lipophilicity combined with its H₁-receptor selectivity probably accounts for its relative lack of anticholinergic and sedative properties. *Effectively treats allergic rhinitis and chronic urticaria by eliminating or reducing the local and systemic effects of histamine release.*

**USES** Seasonal and perennial allergic rhinitis and chronic idiopathic urticaria.

**CONTRAINDICATIONS** Hypersensitivity to H₁-receptor antihistamines or hydroxyzine; lactation.

**CAUTIOUS USE** Moderate to severe renal impairment, hepatic impairment, pregnancy (category B), children.

## ROUTE & DOSAGE

**Allergic Rhinitis**
*Adult:* PO 5–10 mg once/day
*Child (2 to younger than 6 y):* PO 2.5 mg daily (max: 5 mg/day); 6 y or older: 5–10 mg daily

**Allergic Rhinitis (Levocetirizine)**
*Adult/Adolescent/Child (6 y or older):* PO 2.5–5 mg once/day
*Child (2 to younger than 6 y:)* PO 1.25 mg each evening

**Chronic Urticaria**
*Adult:* PO 10 mg daily or b.i.d.

**Chronic Urticaria (Levocetirizine)**
*Adult/Adolescent/Child (6 y or older):* PO 2.5–5 mg each evening
*Child (6 mo to younger than 6 y):* PO 1.25 mg each evening

---

Common adverse effects in *italic;* life-threatening effects underlined; generic names in **bold;** classifications in SMALL CAPS; ♣ Canadian drug name; ⦿ Prototype drug

323

**C**

***Renal Impairment Dosage Adjustment (Levocetirizine)***
*CrCl 51–80 mL/min:* **2.5 mg daily;** *30–50 mL/min:* **2.5 mg every other day;** *10–29 mL/min:* **2.5 mg twice a week;** *less than 10 mL/min:* **Do not use**

## ADMINISTRATION
### Oral
- May be administered with or without food.
- Consult prescriber about dosage if significant adverse effects appear. As elimination half-life is prolonged in the older adult, dosage adjustments may be warranted.
- Store at 20°–25° C (68°–77° F); excursions at 15°–30° C (59°–86° F).

## ADVERSE EFFECTS (≥1%) GI:
Constipation, diarrhea, dry mouth. **CNS:** *Drowsiness, sedation, headache,* depression. **CV:** Syncope.

## INTERACTIONS Drug: **Theophylline** may decrease cetirizine clearance leading to toxicity. Use with **scopolamine** or **atropine** may cause anticholinergic effects. Alcohol may enhance the CNS depressant effect. May enhance the depressant effect of CNS depressants.

## PHARMACOKINETICS Absorption: Readily from GI tract. **Peak:** 1 h. **Distribution:** 93% protein bound; minimal CNS concentrations. **Metabolism:** Minimal (by CYP3A4). **Elimination:** 60% unchanged in urine within 24 h, 5% in feces. **Half-Life:** 7.4 h (cetirizine), 8–9 h (levocetirizine).

## NURSING IMPLICATIONS
### Assessment & Drug Effects
- Monitor for drug interactions. As the drug is highly protein bound, the potential for interactions with other protein-bound drugs exists.
- Monitor for sedation, especially the older adult.

### Patient & Family Education
- Do not use in combination with OTC antihistamines.
- Do not engage in driving or other hazardous activities, before experiencing your responses to the drug.

## CETRORELIX
(ce-tro-re′lix)
**Cetrotide**
**Classification:** GONADOTROPIN-RELEASING HORMONE (GnRH) ANTAGONIST
**Therapeutic:** LUTEINIZING HORMONE-RELEASING HORMONE RECEPTOR ANTAGONIST

## AVAILABILITY Solution for injection

## ACTION & THERAPEUTIC EFFECT
Competes with natural GnRH for binding to membrane receptors on pituitary cells and thus controls the release of LH and FSH. *Prevents premature LH surges in patients undergoing controlled ovarian hyperstimulation for assisted reproduction.*

## USES Treatment of infertility as part of an assisted reproduction program.

## UNLABELED USES BPH, endometriosis.

## CONTRAINDICATIONS Hypersensitivity to cetrorelix, extrinsic peptide hormones, mannitol, gonadotropin-releasing hormone analogs; primary ovarian failure; renal

failure; pregnancy (category X); known or suspected pregnancy; lactation.

**CAUTIOUS USE** Hepatic insufficiency; polycystic ovary syndrome.

## ROUTE & DOSAGE

**Infertility**

*Adult:* **Subcutaneous** 0.25 mg/ days during early to mid follicular phase of the cycle (stimulation day 5 or 6) following the initiation of FSH or 3 mg as a single dose is administered when the serum estradiol level is indicative of an appropriate stimulation response, usually on FSH stimulation day 7 (range day 5–9). If HCG has not been administered within 4 days after the injection of 3 mg, then 0.25 mg should be administered once daily until HCG administration.

## ADMINISTRATION

**Subcutaneous**

- Reconstitute the 0.25 or 3 mL vial with 1 or 3 mL, respectively, of sterile water for injection.
- Inject into lower abdominal wall following reconstitution. Rotate injection sites.
- Store the 3 mg dose at room temperature, 15°–30° C (59°–86° F). Store the 0.25 mg dose in the refrigerator.

## ADVERSE EFFECTS (≥1%) CNS:
Headache. **GI:** Nausea, vomiting, abdominal pain. **Endocrine:** Hot flashes. **Skin:** Pruritus at injection

site. **Urogenital:** Ovarian enlargement, ovarian hyperstimulation syndrome, pelvic pain.

**INTERACTIONS Drug: Cimetidine, methyldopa, metoclopramide, reserpine,** PHENOTHIAZINES may interfere with fertility efforts. **Herbal: Black cohosh, DHEA** may antagonize fertility efforts.

**PHARMACOKINETICS Absorption:** 85% absorbed from subcutaneous injection site. **Peak:** 1–2 h. **Metabolism:** Metabolized by peptidases. **Elimination:** 2–4% in urine, 5–10% in bile. **Half-Life:** 62 h after single dose, 20 h after multiple doses.

## NURSING IMPLICATIONS

### Assessment & Drug Effects
- Monitor weight and report development of edema and/or shortness of breath.
- Monitor lab tests: Routine blood chemistries.

### Patient & Family Education
- Contact prescriber immediately for any of the following: Abdominal or stomach pain, persistent or severe nausea, vomiting or diarrhea; decreased urination; pelvic pain; moderate to severe bloating, rapid weight gain; shortness of breath; swelling of lower legs.

## CETUXIMAB
(ce-tux'i-mab)
**Erbitux**
**Classifications:** ANTINEOPLASTIC; MONOCLONAL ANTIBODY; EPIDERMAL GROWTH FACTOR RECEPTOR (EGFR) INHIBITOR
**Therapeutic:** ANTINEOPLASTIC
**Prototype:** Erlotinib

Common adverse effects in *italic;* life-threatening effects <u>underlined</u>; generic names in **bold;** classifications in SMALL CAPS; ♣ Canadian drug name; ☻ Prototype drug

325

C

**AVAILABILITY** Solution for injection

## ACTION & *THERAPEUTIC EFFECT*

Cetuximab is a recombinant, monoclonal antibody that binds specifically to the epidermal growth factor receptor (EGFR, HER1, c-ErbB-1) on both normal and tumor cells. Binding to the EGFR results in inhibition of cell growth, induction of apoptosis, and decreased vascular endothelial growth factor production. *Overexpression of EGFR is detected in many human cancers, including those of the colon and rectum. Cetuximab inhibits the growth and survival of tumor cells that overexpress the EGFR.*

**USES** Metastatic colorectal cancer, squamous cancer of head and neck.

**CONTRAINDICATIONS** Lactation within 60 days of using cetuximab; worsening of preexisting pulmonary edema or interstitial lung disease; serious infusion reaction to drug.

**CAUTIOUS USE** Infusion reaction, especially with first-time users; history of hypersensitivity to murine proteins or cetuximab; cardiac disease, coronary artery disease, CHF, arrhythmias; pulmonary disease, pulmonary fibrosis; UV exposure, radiation therapy; older adults; pregnancy (category C). Safety in children not established.

## ROUTE & DOSAGE

**Colorectal Cancer/Head and Neck Cancer**

*Adult:* IV Start with 400 mg/m$^2$ over 2 h; continue with 250 mg/m$^2$ over 1 h weekly

## ADMINISTRATION

**Intravenous**

Administer with full resuscitation equipment available and under the supervision of a prescriber experienced with chemotherapy. ▪ Premedication with an H$_1$-receptor antagonist (e.g., diphenhydramine 50 mg IV) is recommended. ▪ Monitor for an infusion reaction for at least 1 h following completion of infusion.

*PREPARE:* **IV Infusion:** ▪ Do not shake or further dilute vial. Do not mix with other medication. ▪ Inject cetuximab solution into a sterile, evacuated container or bag (i.e., glass, polyolefin, ethylene vinyl acetate, DEHP plasticized PVC, or PVC); repeat until needed dose has been added to container, using a new needle for each vial. ▪ Attach to infusion set with a low-protein-binding 0.22-micron filter and prime line with cetuximab. May also administer by syringe and syringe pump; use a new needle and filter for each vial.

*ADMINISTER:* **IV Infusion: Do not** administer a bolus dose. ▪ Give IV infusion via an infusion pump or syringe pump; use a low-protein binding 0.22 micron in-line filter. Give initial infusion over 120 min and subsequent infusions over 60 min. Do not exceed 10 mg/min. ▪ Flush line with NS after infusion.

*INCOMPATIBILITIES:* **Solution/additive:** Do not mix with other additives.

▪ Store unopened vials at 2°–8° C (36°–46° F). Note: Vials may contain a small amount of easily visible, white particles. ▪ Cetuximab in IV bag is stable for up to 12 h refrigerated and up to 8 h at 20°–25° C (68°–77° F).

---

Common adverse effects in *italic;* life-threatening effects <u>underlined</u>; generic names in **bold;** classifications in SMALL CAPS; ♣ Canadian drug name; ● Prototype drug

326

**ADVERSE EFFECTS (≥1%) Body as a Whole:** Infusion reactions (allergic reaction, anaphylactoid reaction, fever, chills, dyspnea, bronchospasm stridor, hoarseness, urticaria, hypotension), *fever,* sepsis, *asthenia, malaise,* pain, infection. **CNS:** *Headache,* insomnia, depression, fatigue. **CV:** Cardiopulmonary arrest. **GI:** *Nausea, vomiting, diarrhea, abdominal pain, constipation,* stomatitis, dyspepsia. **Hematologic:** Leukopenia, anemia, neutropenia. **Metabolic:** Weight loss, peripheral edema, dehydration, hypomagnesemia, hypokalemia. **Respiratory:** Pulmonary embolism, pulmonary fibrosis (rare), *dyspnea,* cough. **Skin:** *Rash,* alopecia, pruritus, desquamation, radiodermatitis, changes in nails, acne vulgaris. **Urogenital:** Kidney failure. **Hepatic:** Increased AST, ALT, ASP.

**INTERACTIONS** Do not use with **penicillamine**.

**PHARMACOKINETICS Half-Life:** 114 h (75–188 h).

## NURSING IMPLICATIONS

### Black Box Warning

*Cetuximab has been associated with severe, potentially fatal, infusion reactions, and with cardiopulmonary arrest.*

### Assessment & Drug Effects
- Monitor throughout infusion and for 1 h after completion of infusion for development of an infusion reaction.
- Discontinue infusion immediately and notify prescriber for S&S of a severe infusion reaction: Chills, fever, bronchospasm, stridor, hoarseness, urticaria, and/or hypotension. Carefully monitor until complete resolution of all S&S.

- Monitor pulmonary status and report onset of acute or worsening pulmonary symptoms.
- Premedication with antihistamines is recommended.
- Monitor lab tests: Periodic serum magnesium, calcium, and potassium over 8 wk.

### Patient & Family Education
- Report immediately: Difficulty breathing, wheezing, shortness of breath, hives, faintness and/or dizziness anytime during IV infusion.
- Report promptly any of the following: Eye inflammation, mouth sores, skin rash, redness, or severe dry skin.
- Wear sunscreen and a hat and limit sun exposure while being treated with this drug.

## CEVIMELINE HYDROCHLORIDE
(cev-i-may'leen)

Evoxac

**Classifications:** CHOLINERGIC AGONIST; CHOLINERGIC ENHANCER
**Therapeutic:** CHOLINERGIC RECEPTOR ENHANCER

**AVAILABILITY** Capsule

**ACTION & THERAPEUTIC EFFECT** Cholinergic agent that binds to muscarinic receptors. *Increases secretion of exocrine glands, such as salivary and sweat glands. It relieves severe dry mouth.*

**USES** Treatment of dry mouth in patients with Sjögren's syndrome.

**CONTRAINDICATIONS** Hypersensitivity to cevimeline; uncontrolled asthma; acute iritis; narrow-angle glaucoma; lactation.

Common adverse effects in *italic;* life-threatening effects underlined; generic names in **bold;** classifications in SMALL CAPS; ◆ Canadian drug name; ● Prototype drug

327

**CAUTIOUS USE** Controlled asthma; chronic bronchitis, COPD; cardiac disease, cardiac arrhythmias, myocardial infarction; history of nephrolithiasis or cholelithiasis; older adults; pregnancy (category C). Safety and efficacy in children not established.

## ROUTE & DOSAGE

**Dry Mouth**
*Adult:* **PO** 30 mg t.i.d.

## ADMINISTRATION

**Oral**
▪ May be administered with food to decrease GI upset.
▪ Store refrigerated at 2°–8° C (35.6°–46.4° F) with occasional fluctuations at 15°–30° C (59°–86° F).

**ADVERSE EFFECTS** (≥1%) **Body as a Whole:** *Excessive sweating, headache,* back pain, dizziness, fatigue, pain, hot flushes, rigors, tremor, hypertonia, myalgia, fever, eye pain, earache, flu-like symptoms. **CNS:** Insomnia, anxiety, vertigo, depression, hyporeflexia. **CV:** Peripheral edema, chest pain, palpitations. **GI:** *Nausea, diarrhea,* excessive salivation, dyspepsia, abdominal pain, coughing, vomiting, constipation, anorexia, dry mouth, hiccup. **Respiratory:** *Rhinitis, sinusitis, upper respiratory tract infection,* pharyngitis, bronchitis. **Skin:** Rash, conjunctivitis, pruritus. **Special Senses:** Abnormal vision. **Urogenital:** Urinary tract infection.

**INTERACTIONS Drug:** BETA-ADRENERGIC AGONISTS may cause conduction disturbances; PARASYMPATHOMIMETIC DRUGS may have additive effects.

**PHARMACOKINETICS Absorption:** Rapidly absorbed. **Peak:** 1.5–2 h. **Distribution:** Less than 20% protein bound. **Metabolism:** In liver by CYP2D6 and 3A3/4. **Elimination:** Primarily in urine. **Half-Life:** 5 h.

## NURSING IMPLICATIONS

**Assessment & Drug Effects**
▪ Monitor for S&S of increased airway resistance, especially in patient with asthma, bronchitis, emphysema, or COPD.
▪ Report S&S of excess cholinergic activity (e.g., diaphoresis, frequent urge to urinate, nausea and/or diarrhea).
▪ Monitor lab tests: Routine blood chemistry during long-term therapy.

**Patient & Family Education**
▪ Do not drive or engage in potentially hazardous activities until response to drug is known.
▪ Consult prescriber if confusion, dizziness, or faintness occur.
▪ Report diminished night vision or depth perception.
▪ Drink fluids liberally (2000–3000 mL/day) in the event of excessive sweating.

## CHARCOAL, ACTIVATED (LIQUID ANTIDOTE)

Actidose, CharcoAid, Charcocaps, Charcodote, Insta-Char

**Classifications:** ANTIDOTE; ADSORBENT
Therapeutic: ANTIDOTE

**AVAILABILITY** Liquid suspension

**ACTION & THERAPEUTIC EFFECT**
Acts by binding (adsorbing) toxic substances, thereby inhibiting their

Common adverse effects in *italic;* life-threatening effects <u>underlined;</u> generic names in **bold;** classifications in SMALL CAPS; ♣ Canadian drug name; ❹ Prototype drug

GI absorption, enterohepatic circulation, and thus bioavailability. *Action appears to result from drug diffusion from plasma into GI tract where it is adsorbed by activated charcoal. Effectively adsorbs toxins in the gut preventing their systemic absorption and impact.*

**USES** General purpose emergency antidote in the treatment of poisonings by most drugs and chemicals. Gastric dialysis (repetitive doses) in uremia to adsorb various waste products from GI tract; severe acute poisoning. Has been used to adsorb intestinal gases in treatment of dyspepsia, flatulence, and distention (value in these conditions not established). Sometimes used topically as a deodorant for foul-smelling wounds and ulcers.

**CONTRAINDICATIONS** Reportedly not effective for poisonings by cyanide, mineral acids, caustic alkalis, organic solvents, iron, ethanol, methanol; gag reflex depression, coma; GI obstruction; quinidine or quinine hypersensitivity.

**CAUTIOUS USE** Pregnancy (category C); lactation.

## ROUTE & DOSAGE

**Acute Poisonings**
*Adult:* **PO** 30–100 g in at least 180–240 mL (6–8 oz) of water or 1 g/kg
*Child (1–12 y):* **PO** 1–2 g/kg or 15–30 g in at least 6–8 oz of water
*Infant (younger than 1 y):* **PO** 1 g/kg

**Gastric Dialysis**
*Adult:* **PO** 20–40 g q6h for 1 or 2 days

**GI Disturbances**
*Adult:* **PO** 520–975 mg p.c. up to 5 g/day

## ADMINISTRATION
**Oral**
- In an emergency, dose may be approximated by stirring sufficient activated charcoal into tap water to make a slurry the consistency of soup (about 20–30 g in at least 240 mL of water).
- Activated charcoal can be swallowed or given through a nasogastric tube. If administered too rapidly, patient may vomit.
- Store in tightly covered container.

**ADVERSE EFFECTS** (>1%) **GI:** Vomiting (rapid ingestion of high doses), constipation, diarrhea (from sorbitol).

**INTERACTIONS Drug:** May decrease absorption of all other oral medications—administer at least 2 h apart.

**PHARMACOKINETICS Absorption:** Not absorbed. **Elimination:** In feces.

## NURSING IMPLICATIONS
**Assessment & Drug Effects**
- Record appearance, color, consistency, frequency, and relative amount of stools. Inform patient that activated charcoal will color feces black.

## CHLORAMBUCIL
(klor-am'byoo-sil)
Leukeran
**Classifications:** ANTINEOPLASTIC; ALKYLATING AGENT
**Therapeutic:** ANTINEOPLASTIC; NITROGEN MUSTARD
**Prototype:** Cyclophosphamide

**AVAILABILITY** Tablets

## ACTION & THERAPEUTIC EFFECT
Potent aromatic derivative of the alkylating agent nitrogen mustard

Common adverse effects in *italic;* life-threatening effects underlined; generic names in **bold;** classifications in SMALL CAPS; ♣ Canadian drug name; ⊘ Prototype drug

329

C

which is slowest acting and least toxic of the nitrogen mustards. A cell-cycle nonspecific drug (kills both resting and dividing cells), it causes cytotoxic cross linkage in DNA, thus preventing synthesis of DNA, RNA, and proteins. *Lymphocytic effect is marked; thus it is effective in treatment of various lymphomas.*

**USES** As single agent or with other antineoplastics in treatment of chronic lymphocytic leukemia, non-Hodgkin's lymphoma, Hodgkin's disease.

**UNLABELED USES** Nonneoplastic conditions: Vasculitis complicating rheumatoid arthritis, autoimmune hemolytic anemias associated with cold agglutinins, lupus glomerulonephritis, idiopathic nephrotic syndrome, polycythemia vera, macroglobulinemia.

**CONTRAINDICATIONS** Hypersensitivity to chlorambucil or to other alkylating agents; administration within 4 wk of a full course of radiation or chemotherapy; full dosage if bone marrow is infiltrated with lymphomatous tissue or is hypoplastic; smallpox and other vaccines; pregnancy (category D); lactation.

**CAUTIOUS USE** Excessive or prolonged dosage, pneumococcus vaccination, history of seizures or head trauma.

## ROUTE & DOSAGE

### Palliative Treatment of CLL
*Adult:* **PO** 0.1–0.2 mg/kg/day (usual dose 4–10 mg/day)

### Hodgkin's Disease
*Adult/Adolescent/Child:* **PO** 0.2 mg/kg/day

### Non-Hodgkin's Lymphoma
*Adult/Adolescent/Child:* **PO** 0.1–0.2 mg/kg/day × 3–6 wk

## ADMINISTRATION

### Oral
- Control nausea and vomiting by giving entire daily dose at one time, 1 h before breakfast or 2 h after evening meal, or at bedtime. Consult prescriber.
- Store in tightly closed, light-resistant container.

**ADVERSE EFFECTS** (≥1%) **Body as a Whole:** Drug fever, skin rashes, papilledema, alopecia, peripheral neuropathy, sterile cystitis, pulmonary complications, seizures (high doses). **GI:** Low incidence of gastric discomfort, hepatotoxicity. **Hematologic:** Bone marrow depression: *Leukopenia*, thrombocytopenia, anemia. **Metabolic:** Sterility, hyperuricemia.

**INTERACTIONS Drug:** May have to adjust dose of **allopurinol, colchicine** because of chlorambucil-associated hyperuricemia.

**PHARMACOKINETICS Absorption:** Rapidly and completely from GI tract. **Peak:** 1 h. **Distribution:** Extensively bound to plasma and tissue proteins; crosses placenta. **Metabolism:** In liver. **Elimination:** 60% in urine as metabolites within 24 h. **Half-Life:** 1.5–2.5 h.

## NURSING IMPLICATIONS

### Black Box Warning

*Chlorambucil has been associated with severe bone marrow suppression, and with infertility and severe fetal abnormalities.*

Common adverse effects in *italic;* life-threatening effects underlined; generic names in **bold;** classifications in SMALL CAPS; ♣ Canadian drug name; ⊙ Prototype drug

### Assessment & Drug Effects

- Leukopenia usually develops after the third week of treatment; it may continue for up to 10 days after last dose, then rapidly return to normal.
- Avoid or reduce to minimum injections and other invasive procedures (e.g., rectal temperatures, enemas) when platelet count is low.
- Monitor lab tests: Baseline and weekly CBC, Hgb, WBC total and differential counts, and serum uric acid.

### Patient & Family Education

- Do not take chlorambucil if you are or suspect you are pregnant.
- Notify prescriber if the following symptoms occur: Unusual bleeding or bruising, sores on lips or in mouth; flank, stomach, or joint pain; fever, chills, or other signs of infection, sore throat, cough, dyspnea.
- Report immediately the onset of a skin reaction.
- Drink at least 10–12 glasses [240 mL (8 oz) each] of fluid/day, if not contraindicated.

# CHLORAMPHENICOL SODIUM SUCCINATE

(klor-am-fen′i-kole)

**Classification:** ANTIBIOTIC
**Therapeutic:** BROAD-SPECTRUM ANTIBIOTIC

**AVAILABILITY** Solution for injection

## ACTION & *THERAPEUTIC EFFECT*

Synthetic broad-spectrum antibiotic believed to act by binding to the 50S ribosome of bacteria and thus interfering with protein synthesis. *Effective against a wide variety of gram-negative and gram-positive bacteria and most anaerobic microorganisms.*

**USES** Severe infections when other antibiotics are ineffective or are contraindicated.

**CONTRAINDICATIONS** History of hypersensitivity or toxic reaction to chloramphenicol; influenza; treatment of minor infections, prophylactic use; typhoid carrier state, history or family history of drug-induced bone marrow depression lactation.

**CAUTIOUS USE** Impaired hepatic or renal function, premature and full-term infants, children; intermittent porphyria; patients with G6PD deficiency; patient or family history of drug-induced bone marrow depression; pregnancy (category C).

## ROUTE & DOSAGE

**Serious Infections**

*Adult:* **IV** 50–100 mg/kg/day in 4 divided doses
*Adolescent/Child/Infant:* **IV** 50 mg/ kg/day in 4 divided doses

## ADMINISTRATION

**Intravenous**

IV administration to neonates, infants, children: Verify correct IV concentration and rate of infusion with prescriber.

*PREPARE:* **Direct:** Dilute each 1 g with 10 mL of sterile water or D5W.
*ADMINISTER:* **Direct:** Give slowly over a period of at least 1 min.
*INCOMPATIBILITIES:* **Solution/additive: Chlorpromazine, erythromycin, hydroxyzine, metronidazole, glycopyrrolate, polymyxin B, prochlorperazine, promethazine, vancomycin. Y-site: Ascorbic acid, azathioprine, benzotropine,**

butorphanol, casopfungin, cefotaxime, ceftazidime, ceftizosime, ceftriaxone, chlorpromazine, cimetidine, dantrolene, diazepam, diazoxide, diltiazem, diphenydramine, dobutamine, dopamine, doxycycline, erythromycin, esmolol, famotidine, fluconazole, ganciclovir, gatifloxacin, gemcitabine, gentamicin, haloperidol, hydralazine, hydroxyzine, idarubicin, irinotecan, labetalol, mechlorethamine, meperidine, metaraminol, methyldopate, midazolam, minocycline, mycophenolate, nafcillin, nalbupine, ondansetron, pantoprazole, papaverine, pemetrexed, pentamidine, pentazocine, phentolamine, phenytoin, polymyxin B, procainamide, prochlorperazine, promethazine, protamine, pyridoxine, quinidine, sulfamethoxazole/trimethoprim, thiamine, tigecycline, tolaxoline, vancomycin, vecuronium, verapamil, vinorelbine.

▪ Solution for infusion may form crystals or a second layer when stored at low temperatures. Solution can be clarified by shaking vial. ▪ Do not use cloudy solutions.

## ADVERSE EFFECTS (≥1%) Body as a Whole: Hypersensitivity, angioedema, dyspnea, fever, anaphylaxis, superinfections, Gray syndrome. GI: Nausea, vomiting, diarrhea, perianal irritation, enterocolitis, glossitis, stomatitis, unpleasant taste, xerostomia. Hematologic: Bone marrow depression (dose-related and reversible): Reticulocytosis, leukopenia, granulocytopenia, thrombocytopenia, increased plasma iron, reduced Hgb, hypoplastic anemia, hypoprothrombinemia.

Non-dose-related and irreversible pancytopenia, agranulocytosis, aplastic anemia, paroxysmal nocturnal hemoglobinuria, leukemia. CNS: Neurotoxicity: Headache, mental depression, confusion, delirium, digital paresthesias, peripheral neuritis. Skin: Urticaria, contact dermatitis, maculopapular and vesicular rashes, fixed-drug eruptions. Special Senses: Visual disturbances, optic neuritis, optic nerve atrophy, contact conjunctivitis.

## DIAGNOSTIC TEST INTERFERENCE
Possibility of false-positive results for *urine glucose* by *copper reduction methods* (e.g., *Benedict's solution, Clinitest*).

## INTERACTIONS Drug: The metabolism of chlorpropamide, dicumarol, phenytoin, tolbutamide may be decreased, prolonging their activity. Phenobarbital decreases chloramphenicol levels. The response to iron preparations, folic acid, and vitamin B_{12} may be delayed. Do not use with ranolazine. Monitor INR when using with warfarin. Do not use with LIVE VACCINES. Avoid use with deferiprone.

## PHARMACOKINETICS Peak: 1 h. Distribution: Widely distributed to most body tissues; concentrates in liver and kidneys; penetrates CNS; crosses placenta. Metabolism: Inactivated in liver. Elimination: Much longer in neonates; metabolite and free drug excreted in urine; excreted in breast milk. Half-Life: 1.5–4.1 h.

## NURSING IMPLICATIONS

### Black Box Warning

*Chloramphenicol has been associated with serious and potentially fatal blood dyscrasias.*

Common adverse effects in *italic;* life-threatening effects underlined; generic names in **bold;** classifications in SMALL CAPS; ♣ Canadian drug name; ⊕ Prototype drug

## Assessment & Drug Effects

- Check temperature at least q4h. Usually chloramphenicol is discontinued if temperature remains normal for 48 h.
- Monitor I&O ratio or pattern: Report any appreciable change.
- Withhold drug and notify prescriber if lab values indicate bone marrow suppression.
- Monitor for S&S of gray syndrome, which has occurred 2–9 days after initiation of high dose chloramphenicol therapy in premature infants and neonates and in children 2 y or younger. Report early signs: Abdominal distention, failure to feed, pallor, changes in vital signs.
- Monitor lab tests: Baseline C&S, CBC, platelets, serum iron, and reticulocyte cell counts q48h during therapy, and periodically thereafter. Weekly chloramphenicol blood levels or more frequently with hepatic dysfunction and in patients receiving therapy for longer than 2 wk.

## Patient & Family Education

- A bitter taste may occur 15–20 sec after IV injection; it usually lasts only 2–3 min.
- Report immediately sore throat, fever, fatigue, petechiae, nose bleeds, bleeding gums, or other unusual bleeding or bruising, or any other suspicious sign or symptom.
- Watch for S&S of superinfection (see Appendix F).
- Notify prescriber immediately if signs of hypersensitivity reaction (see Appendix F), irritation, superinfection, or other adverse reactions appear.

# CHLORDIAZEPOXIDE HYDROCHLORIDE

(klor-dye-az-e-pox'ide)

**Librium, Solium ♦**

**Classifications:** ANXIOLYTIC; SEDATIVE-HYPNOTIC; BENZODIAZEPINE
**Therapeutic:** ANTIANXIETY; SEDATIVE-HYPNOTIC
**Prototype:** Lorazepam
**Controlled Substance:** Schedule IV

**AVAILABILITY** Capsule

## ACTION & *THERAPEUTIC EFFECT*

Benzodiazepine derivative that acts on the limbic, thalamic, and hypothalamic areas of the CNS. Has long-acting hypnotic properties. Causes mild suppression of REM sleep and of deeper phases, particularly stage 4, while increasing total sleep time. *Produces mild anxiolytic (reduces anxiety), sedative, anticonvulsant, and skeletal muscle relaxant effects.*

**USES** Relief of various anxiety and tension states, preoperative apprehension and anxiety, and for management of alcohol withdrawal.

**UNLABELED USES** Essential, familial, and senile action tremors.

**CONTRAINDICATIONS** Hypersensitivity to chlordiazepoxide and other benzodiazepines; narrow-angle glaucoma, prostatic hypertrophy, shock, comatose states, primary depressive disorder or psychoses, acute alcohol intoxication; pregnancy (category D); lactation.

**CAUTIOUS USE** Anxiety states associated with impending depression, history of impaired hepatic or renal function; addiction-prone individuals, blood dyscrasias; in the older adult, debilitated patients, children; aggressive or hyperactive children; hyperkinesis; children younger than 6 y.

---

Common adverse effects in *italic;* life-threatening effects <u>underlined</u>; generic names in **bold;** classifications in SMALL CAPS; ♦ Canadian drug name; ⊙ Prototype drug

C

## ROUTE & DOSAGE

### Mild Anxiety, Preoperative Anxiety

*Adult:* **PO** 5–10 mg t.i.d. or q.i.d.
*Geriatric:* **PO** 5 mg b.i.d. to q.i.d.
*Child:* **PO** 5 mg b.i.d. to q.i.d.;
may be increased to 10 mg t.i.d.

### Severe Anxiety and Tension

*Adult:* **PO** 20–25 mg t.i.d. or q.i.d.

### Alcohol Withdrawal Syndrome

*Adult:* **PO** 50–100 mg prn up to 300 mg/day

## ADMINISTRATION

### Oral

▪ Give with or immediately after meals or with milk to reduce GI distress. If an antacid is prescribed, it should be taken at least 1 h before or after chlordiazepoxide to prevent delay in drug absorption.
▪ Store in tight, light-resistant containers at room temperature unless otherwise specified by manufacturer.

## ADVERSE EFFECTS (≥1%) **Body as a Whole:** Edema, pain in injection site, jaundice, hiccups, <u>respiratory depression</u>. **CV:** Orthostatic hypotension, tachycardia, changes in ECG patterns seen with rapid IV administration. **GI:** Nausea, dry mouth, vomiting, constipation, increased appetite. **CNS:** *Drowsiness,* dizziness, *lethargy,* changes in EEG pattern; vivid dreams, nightmares, headache, vertigo, syncope, tinnitus, confusion, hallucinations, parodoxic rage, depression, delirium, ataxia. **Skin:** Photosensitivity, skin rash. **Urogenital:** Urinary frequency.

## DIAGNOSTIC TEST INTERFERENCE

Chlordiazepoxide increases ***serum bilirubin, AST*** and ***ALT;*** decreases ***radioactive iodine uptake;*** and may falsely increase readings for ***urinary 17-OHCS*** (modified ***Glenn-Nelson*** technique).

## INTERACTIONS **Drug: Alcohol,** CNS DEPRESSANTS, ANTICONVULSANTS potentiate CNS depression; **cimetidine** increases **chlordiazepoxide** plasma levels, thus increasing toxicity; may decrease antiparkinson effects of **levodopa;** may increase **phenytoin** levels; smoking decreases sedative and antianxiety effects. **Herbal: Kava, valerian** may potentiate sedation.

## PHARMACOKINETICS **Absorption:** Well absorbed from GI tract. **Peak:** 1–4 h. **Distribution:** Widely distributed throughout body; crosses placenta. **Metabolism:** In liver via CYP3A4 to long-acting active metabolite. **Elimination:** Slowly excreted in urine (may last several days); excreted in breast milk. **Half-Life:** 5–30 h.

## NURSING IMPLICATIONS

### Assessment & Drug Effects

▪ Monitor for S&S of orthostatic hypotension and tachycardia; observe closely and monitor vital signs.
▪ Check BP and pulse before giving benzodiazepine in early part of therapy. If blood pressure falls 20 mm Hg or more or if pulse rate is above 120 bpm, notify prescriber.
▪ Monitor I&O until drug dosage is stabilized. Report changes in I&O ratio and dysuria to prescriber.
▪ Monitor for S&S of paradoxic reactions—excitement, stimulation, disturbed sleep patterns, acute rage—which may occur during first few weeks of therapy in psychiatric patients and in hyperactive and aggressive children receiving

chlordiazepoxide. Withhold drug and report to prescriber.

- Assess patient's sleep pattern. If dreams or nightmares interfere with rest, notify prescriber.
- Supervise ambulation, especially with older adults & debilitated patients.
- Monitor lab tests: Periodic CBC and LFTs during prolonged therapy.

**Patient & Family Education**

- Abrupt discontinuation of drug in patients receiving high doses for long periods (4 mo or longer) has precipitated withdrawal symptoms, but not for at least 5–7 days because of slow elimination.
- Long-term use of this drug may cause mouth soreness. Good oral hygiene can alleviate the discomfort.
- Avoid activities requiring mental alertness until reaction to the drug has been evaluated.
- Avoid drinking alcoholic beverages. When combined with chlordiazepoxide, effects of both are potentiated.
- Avoid excessive sunlight. Use sun screen lotion (SPF 12 or above) if allowed.

# CHLOROQUINE PHOSPHATE ⊕

(klor'oh-kwin)

Aralen

**Classification:** ANTIMALARIAL
Therapeutic: ANTIMALARIAL; AMEBICIDE

**AVAILABILITY** Tablet

**ACTION & *THERAPEUTIC EFFECT***

Antimalarial activity is believed to be based on its ability to form complexes with DNA of parasite, thereby inhibiting replication and transcription to RNA and nucleic acid synthesis. *Acts as a suppressive agent in patient with* P. vivax *or* P. malariae *malaria; terminates acute attacks and increases intervals between treatment and relapse of malaria. Abolishes the acute attack of* P. falciparum *malaria but does not prevent the infection.*

**USES** Treatment and prophylaxis of malaria, amebiasis.

**UNLABELED USES** Discoid and systemic lupus erythematosus, porphyria cutanea tarda, solar urticaria, polymorphous light eruptions, and in rheumatoid arthritis.

**CONTRAINDICATIONS** Hypersensitivity to 4-aminoquinolines, psoriasis; ocular disease, porphyria, renal disease, 4-aminoquinoline-induced retinal or visual field changes.

**CAUTIOUS USE** Impaired hepatic function, alcoholism, eczema, patients with G6PD deficiency, infants and children, hematologic, GI, cardiac disease, diabetes, and neurologic disorders; pregnancy (category C); children. Safe use in women of childbearing potential not established.

**ROUTE & DOSAGE**

| Doses are expressed in terms of chloroquine base |
| --- |
| **Acute Malaria** |
| *Adult (weight 60 kg or more):* **PO** 600 mg base followed by 300 mg base at 6, 24, and 48 h |
| *Adult (less than 60 kg)/Child:* **PO** 10 mg base/kg, then 5 mg base/kg at 6, 24, and 48 h |

Common adverse effects in *italic;* life-threatening effects <u>underlined</u>; generic names in **bold**; classifications in SMALL CAPS; ✦Canadian drug name; ⊕ Prototype drug

335

**C**

## Malaria Suppression

*Adult:* **PO** 300 mg base the same day each week starting 2 wk before exposure and continuing for 4–6 wk after leaving the area of exposure (max: 300 mg base/wk)
*Child:* **PO** 5 mg base/kg the same day each week starting 2 wk before exposure and continuing for 4–6 wk after leaving the area of exposure (max: 300 mg base/wk)

## Extraintestinal Amebiasis

*Adult:* **PO** 600 mg base/day for 2 days, then 300 mg base/day for 2–3 wk
*Child:* **PO** 10 mg base/kg/day for 2–3 wk

## ADMINISTRATION

### Oral

- Give immediately before or after meals to minimize GI distress.
- Monitor child's dose closely. Children are extremely susceptible to overdosage.

## ADVERSE EFFECTS (≥1%) **Body as a Whole:** Slight weight loss, myalgia, lymphedema of upper limbs. **CV:** Hypotension; ECG changes. **GI:** *Diarrhea,* abdominal cramps, *nausea,* vomiting, anorexia. **Hematologic:** Hemolytic anemia in patients with G6PD deficiency. **Metabolic:** Hypoglycemia. **CNS:** Mild transient headache, fatigue, irritability, confusion, nightmares, skeletal muscle weakness, paresthesias, reduced reflexes, vertigo, <u>suicidal ideation</u>. **Skin:** Bleaching of scalp, eyebrows, body hair, and freckles, pruritus, patchy alopecia (reversible). **Special Senses:** (Usually reversible): Blurred vision, disturbances of accommodation, night blindness, scotomas, visual field defects, photophobia, corneal edema, opacity or deposits, ototoxicity (rare).

## INTERACTIONS **Drug: Aluminum-** and **magnesium-**containing ANTACIDS and LAXATIVES decrease chloroquine absorption, so separate administration by at least 4 h; chloroquine may interfere with response to **rabies vaccine.** Use caution with ANTIDIABETES medications due to increased risk of hypoglycemia. Do not use with **posaconazole** or **fluconazole** due to risk of torsades de pointes. **Food:** Taking **lemon juice** decreases therapeutic effect.

## PHARMACOKINETICS **Absorption:** Rapidly and almost completely absorbed. **Peak:** 1–2 h. **Distribution:** Widely distributed; concentrates in lungs, liver, erythrocytes, eyes, skin, and kidneys; crosses placenta. **Metabolism:** Partially in liver to active metabolites. **Elimination:** In urine; excreted in breast milk. **Half-Life:** 70–120 h.

## NURSING IMPLICATIONS

### Assessment & Drug Effects

- Monitor for changes in ECG, especially with a preexisting cardiac condition.
- Obtain baseline opthalmologic exam and monitor for changes in vision. Retinopathy (generally irreversible) can be progressive even after termination of therapy. Patient may be asymptomatic or complain of night blindness, scotomas, visual field changes, blurred vision, or difficulty in focusing. Withhold drug and report immediately to prescriber.
- Monitor lab tests: Baseline CBC before initiation of therapy and periodically in patients on long-term therapy.

Common adverse effects in *italic;* life-threatening effects <u>underlined</u>; generic names in **bold;** classifications in SMALL CAPS; ♣ Canadian drug name; ⦿ Prototype drug

### Patient & Family Education

- Report promptly visual or hearing disturbances, muscle weakness, or loss of balance, symptoms of blood dyscrasia (fever, sore mouth or throat, unexplained fatigue, easy bruising or bleeding).
- Use of dark glasses in sunlight or bright light may provide comfort (because of photophobia) and reduce risk of ocular damage.
- Avoid driving or other potentially hazardous activities until reaction to drug is known.
- May cause rusty yellow or brown discoloration of urine.
- Do not drink lemon juice along with chloroquine. It decreases the drug's effectiveness.

---

# CHLOROTHIAZIDE
(klor-oh-thye'a-zide)

# CHLOROTHIAZIDE SODIUM
Diuril

**Classifications:** ELECTROLYTE AND WATER BALANCE AGENT; THIAZIDE DIURETIC; ANTIHYPERTENSIVE
**Therapeutic:** THIAZIDE DIURETIC; ANTIHYPERTENSIVE
**Prototype:** Hydrochlorothiazide

**AVAILABILITY** Oral suspension; tablet; solution for injection

## ACTION & *THERAPEUTIC EFFECT*

Produces diuresis by direct action on the distal convoluted tubules. Inhibits reabsorption of sodium, potassium, and chloride ions. *Promotes renal excretion of sodium (and water), bicarbonate, and potassium. Antihypertensive mechanism is due to decreased peripheral resistance and reduced blood pressure.*

**USES** Edema associated with CHF, renal dysfunction ascites, hypertension.

**UNLABELED USES** Hypercalciuria.

**CONTRAINDICATIONS** Hypersensitivity to thiazide or sulfonamides; anuria; hypokalemia; hyponatremia; hypercalcemia; renal failure; jaundiced neonates.

**CAUTIOUS USE** History of sulfa allergy; impaired renal or hepatic function or gout; SLE; diabetes mellitus, older adult or debilitated patients, pancreatitis, sympathectomy; pregnancy (category C).

## ROUTE & DOSAGE

| Hypertension, Edema |
| --- |
| *Adult:* **PO** 500 mg–1 g/day in 1–2 divided doses; **IV** 500 mg–1 g/day in 1–2 divided doses |
| *Child (6 mo or older):* **PO** 10–20 mg/kg/day in 1–2 doses (max: 375 mg) |
| *Infant (younger than 6 mo):* **PO** 10–20 mg/kg/day divided in 2 doses |

## ADMINISTRATION

### Oral
- Give with or after food to prevent gastric irritation. Extent of absorption appears to be increased by taking it with food.
- Schedule daily doses to avoid nocturia and interrupted sleep.

### Intravenous
- Reserve for emergency or when patient unable to take oral medication. ■ IV administration to infants and children: Verify correct IV concentration and rate of infusion with prescriber.

**PREPARE: Intermittent** Reconstitute the 500-mg vial with at least 18 mL sterile water for injection. ■ May be further diluted with D5W or NS. **Must be** prepared immediately before use.

---

Common adverse effects in *italic*; life-threatening effects <u>underlined</u>; generic names in **bold**; classifications in SMALL CAPS; ♣ Canadian drug name; ⓟ Prototype drug

*ADMINISTER:* **Intermittent:** Give at a rate of 500 mg over 5 min. ▪ Thiazide preparations are extremely irritating to the tissues, and great care **must be** taken to avoid extravasation. ▪ If infiltration occurs, stop medication, remove needle, and apply ice if area is small.

*INCOMPATIBILITIES:* **Solution/additive:** Amikacin, chlorpromazine, hydralazine, insulin, levorphanol, methadone, morphine, norepinephrine, pentobarbital, polymyxin B, procaine, prochlorperazine, promazine, promethazine, streptomycin, trifluromazine, vancomycin, vitamin B complex with C, warfarin. **Y-site:** Chlorpromazine, codeine, hydralazine, prochlorperazine, promazine, promethazine, tacrolimus, TPN.

▪ Store tablets, PO solutions, and parenteral dosage forms at 15°–30° C (59°–86° F) unless otherwise directed by manufacturer. ▪ Unused reconstituted IV solutions may be stored at room temperature up to 24 h. Use only clear solutions.

## ADVERSE EFFECTS (≥1%) **Body as a Whole:** Fever, respiratory distress, anaphylactic reaction. **CV:** Irregular heart beat, weak pulse, orthostatic hypotension. **GI:** Vomiting, acute pancreatitis, diarrhea abdominal pain, constipation. **Hematologic:** Agranulocytosis (rare), aplastic anemia (rare), asymptomatic hyperuricemia, hyperglycemia, glycosuria, SIADH secretion. **Metabolic:** *Hypokalemia,* hypercalcemia, hyponatremia, hypochloremic alkalosis, elevated cholesterol and triglyceride levels. **CNS:** Unusual fatigue, dizziness, mental changes, vertigo, headache. **Skin:** Urticaria, photosensitivity, skin rash.

## DIAGNOSTIC TEST INTERFERENCE
May interfere with *parathyroid function tests.*

## INTERACTIONS **Drug:** CORTICOSTEROIDS, **topiramate** increase hypokalemic effects of chlorothiazide; the hypoglycemic effects of SULFONYLUREAS and **insulin** may be antagonized; intensifies hypoglycemic and hypotensive effects of **diazoxide;** increased potassium and magnesium loss may cause **digoxin** toxicity; decreases **lithium** excretion, increasing its toxicity; increases risk of NSAID-induced renal failure and may attenuate diuresis. Use with **amifostine** may have increased risk of **hypotension.**

## PHARMACOKINETICS **Absorption:** Incompletely absorbed PO. **Onset:** 2 h PO; 15 min IV. **Peak:** 3–6 h PO; 30 min IV. **Duration:** 6–12 h PO; 2 h IV. **Distribution:** Throughout extracellular tissue; concentrates in kidney; crosses placenta. **Metabolism:** Does not appear to be metabolized. **Elimination:** In urine and breast milk. **Half-Life:** 45–120 min.

## NURSING IMPLICATIONS
### Assessment & Drug Effects
▪ Monitor for therapeutic effect. Antihypertensive action of a thiazide diuretic requires several days before effects are observed; usually optimum therapeutic effect is not established for 3–4 wk.
▪ Monitor for hyperglycemia. Thiazide therapy can cause hyperglycemia (see Appendix F) and glycosuria in diabetic and diabetic-prone individuals.
▪ Monitor patients with gout. Asymptomatic hyperuricemia can be produced because of interference with uric acid excretion.
▪ Establish baseline weight before initiation of therapy. Weigh patient

Common adverse effects in *italic;* life-threatening effects underlined; generic names in **bold;** classifications in SMALL CAPS; ♣ Canadian drug name; ⊙ Prototype drug

at the same time each a.m. under standard conditions. A gain of more than 1 kg (2.2) within 2 or 3 days and a gradual weight gain over the week's period is reportable.

- Monitor BP closely during early drug therapy.
- Inspect skin and mucous membranes daily for evidence of petechiae in patients receiving large doses and those on prolonged therapy.
- Monitor I&O rates and patterns: Excessive diuresis may cause electrolyte imbalance and necessitate prompt dosage adjustment.
- Monitor patients on digitalis therapy for S&S of hypokalemia (see Appendix G), which can precipitate digitalis intoxication.
- Monitor lab tests: Baseline and periodic blood count, serum electrolytes, $CO_2$, kidney function tests, uric acid, and blood glucose.

### Patient & Family Education

- Urination will occur in greater amounts and with more frequency than usual, and there will be an unusual sense of tiredness. With continued therapy, diuretic action decreases; BP lowering effects usually are maintained, and sense of tiredness diminishes.
- Make position changes slowly to minimize risks associated with orthostatic hypotension.
- Report to prescriber any illness accompanied by prolonged vomiting or diarrhea
- Avoid drinking large quantities of coffee or other caffeine drinks. Caffeine has a diuretic effect.
- Report S&S of hypokalemia, hypercalcemia, or hyperglycemia (see Appendix F).
- Hypokalemia may be prevented if the daily diet contains potassium-rich foods. Eat a banana and drink at least 6 oz orange juice every day.

- Report photosensitivity reaction to prescriber. Photosensitivity may occur 1½–2 wk after initial sun exposure.

## CHLORPHENIRAMINE MALEATE
(klor-fen-eer'a-meen)

Aller-Chlor, Chlo-Amine, Chlor-Trimeton, Chlor-Tripolon ♦, Novopheniram ♦, Phenetron, Telachlor, Teldrin, Trymegan

**Classification:** ANTIHISTAMINE ($H_1$-RECEPTOR ANTAGONIST)
Therapeutic: ANTIHISTAMINE
**Prototype:** Diphenhydramine

**AVAILABILITY** Tablet; sustained release tablet; syrup

## ACTION & *THERAPEUTIC EFFECT*
Competes with histamine for $H_1$-receptor sites on effector cells; thus it promotes capillary permeability and edema formation and constrictive action on respiratory, gastrointestinal, and vascular smooth muscles. *Has effective antihistamine reaction resulting in decreasing allergic symptomatology.*

**USES** Symptomatic relief of various uncomplicated allergic conditions; to prevent transfusion and drug reactions in susceptible patients, and as adjunct to epinephrine and other standard measures in anaphylactic reactions.

**CONTRAINDICATIONS** Hypersensitivity to antihistamines of similar structure; lower respiratory tract symptoms, narrow-angle glaucoma, obstructive prostatic hypertrophy or other bladder neck

---

Common adverse effects in *italic*; life-threatening effects underlined; generic names in **bold**; classifications in SMALL CAPS; ♦ Canadian drug name; ✪ Prototype drug obstruction, GI obstruction or stenosis; premature and newborn infants; during or within 14 days of MAO INHIBITOR therapy.

**CAUTIOUS USE** Convulsive disorders, increased intraocular pressure, hyperthyroidism, cardiovascular disease, hepatic disease; BPH; GI obstruction; hypertension, diabetes mellitus, history of bronchial asthma, COPD, older adult patients, patients with G6PD deficiency; pregnancy (category C), lactation.

## ROUTE & DOSAGE

### Symptomatic Allergy Relief

*Adult:* **PO** 2–4 mg t.i.d. or q.i.d. *or* 8–12 mg b.i.d. or t.i.d. (max: 24 mg/day)
*Geriatric:* **PO** 4 mg daily or b.i.d. *or* 8 mg sustained release at bedtime
*Child (6–12 y):* **PO** 2 mg q4–6h (max: 12 mg/day); *2 to younger than 6 y:* 1 mg q4–6h

## ADMINISTRATION

### Oral

- Give on an empty stomach for fastest response.
- Sustained release tablets should be swallowed whole and not crushed or chewed.
- Ensure that chewable tablets are chewed or crushed before being swallowed with a liquid.

**ADVERSE EFFECTS** (≥1%) **Body as a Whole:** Sensation of chest tightness. **CV:** Palpitation, tachycardia, mild hypotension or hypertension. **GI:** Epigastric distress, anorexia, nausea, vomiting, constipation, or diarrhea. **CNS:** *Drowsiness,* sedation, headache, dizziness, vertigo, fatigue, disturbed coordination, tremors, euphoria, nervousness, restlessness, insomnia. **Special Senses:** *Dryness of mouth,* nose, and throat, tinnitus, vertigo, acute labyrinthitis, thickened bronchial secretions, blurred vision, diplopia. **Urogenital:** Urinary frequency or retention, dysuria.

## DIAGNOSTIC TEST INTERFERENCE

Antihistamines should be discontinued 4 days before **skin testing** procedures for allergy because they may obscure otherwise positive reactions.

## INTERACTIONS **Drug: Alcohol (ethanol)** and other CNS DEPRESSANTS produce additive sedation and CNS depression.

## PHARMACOKINETICS **Absorption:** Well absorbed from GI tract; about 45% of dose reaches systemic circulation intact. **Onset:** Within 6 h. **Peak:** 2–6 h. **Distribution:** Highest concentrations in lung, heart, kidney, brain, small intestine, and spleen. **Metabolism:** By CYP3A4. **Half-Life:** 12–43 h.

## NURSING IMPLICATIONS

### Assessment & Drug Effects

- Monitor for CNS depression and sedation, especially when chlorpheniramine is given in combination with other CNS depressants.
- Monitor BP in hypertensive patients since chlorpheniramine may elevate BP.

### Patient & Family Education

- Avoid driving a car and other potentially hazardous activities until drug response has been determined.
- Avoid or minimize alcohol intake. Antihistamines have additive effects with alcohol.
- Report any of the following: Tinnitus or palpitations.
- Consult prescriber before taking additional OTC drugs for allergy relief.

# CHLORPROMAZINE ⊕

(klor-proe'ma-zeen)

## CHLORPROMAZINE HYDROCHLORIDE

Sonazine, Thorazine

**Classifications:** ANTIPSYCHOTIC, PHENOTHIAZINE; ANTIEMETIC
Therapeutic: ANTIPSYCHOTIC; ANTIEMETIC

**AVAILABILITY** Tablet; sustained release capsule; syrup; oral concentrate; solution for injection

## ACTION & *THERAPEUTIC EFFECT*

Phenothiazine derivative with actions at all levels of CNS with a mechanism that produces strong antipsychotic effects. Antiemetic effect due to suppression of the chemoreceptor trigger zone (CTZ). Mechanism thought to be related to blockade of postsynaptic dopamine receptors in the brain. *Effective in decreasing psychotic symptoms. Also has antiemetic effects due to its action on the CTZ.*

**USES** To control manic phase of manic-depressive illness, for symptomatic management of psychotic disorders, including schizophrenia, in management of severe nausea and vomiting, to control excessive anxiety and agitation before surgery, and for treatment of severe behavior problems in children (e.g., attention deficit disorder). Also used for treatment of acute intermittent porphyria, intractable hiccups, and as adjunct in treatment of tetanus.

**CONTRAINDICATIONS** Hypersensitivity to phenothiazine derivatives, sulfite, or benzyl alcohol; withdrawal states from alcohol; CNS depression; comatose states, brain damage, bone marrow depression, Reye's syndrome; lactation.

**CAUTIOUS USE** Agitated states accompanied by depression, seizure disorders, dementia-related psychosis in the older adult, respiratory impairment due to infection or COPD; glaucoma, diabetes, hypertensive disease, peptic ulcer, prostatic hypertrophy; thyroid, cardiovascular, and hepatic disorders; patients exposed to extreme heat or organophosphate insecticides; previously detected breast cancer; pregnancy (category C); children younger than 6 mo.

## ROUTE & DOSAGE

### Psychotic Disorders, Agitation

*Adult:* **PO** 25–100 mg t.i.d. or q.i.d., may need up to 1000 mg/day; **IM/IV** 25–50 mg up to 600 mg q4–6h
*Child (6 mo or older):* **PO** 0.55 mg/kg q4–6h prn up to 500 mg/day; *6 mo or older* **IM/IV** 0.5–1 mg/kg q6–8h

### Nausea and Vomiting

*Adult:* **PO** 10–25 mg q4–6h prn; **IM/IV** 25–50 mg q4–6h prn
*Child (6 mo or older):* **PO** 0.55 mg/kg q4–6h prn up to 500 mg/day; **IM/IV** 0.55 mg/kg q6–8h

### Dementia

*Geriatric:* **PO** Initial 10–25 mg 1–2 × day, may increase q4–7days by 10–25 mg/day (max: 800 mg/day)

### Intractable Hiccups

*Adult:* **PO/IM** 25–50 mg t.i.d. or q.i.d.

### Tetanus

*Adult:* **IM/IV** 25–50 mg q6–8h
*Child:* **IM/IV** 0.5 mg/kg q6–8h

Common adverse effects in *italic*; life-threatening effects underlined; generic names in **bold;** classifications in SMALL CAPS; ♣Canadian drug name; ⊕ Prototype drug

341

**C**

### Nausea and Vomiting during Surgery

*Adult/Adolescent:* **IV** 2 mg q2min prn (max total: 25 mg)
*Child/Infant 6 mo or older:* **IV** 1 mg q2min prn (max total: 0.25 mg/kg)

### Intractable Hiccups

*Adult/Adolescent:* **IV** 25–50 mg in 500–1000 mL NS, not to exceed 1 mg/min

## ADMINISTRATION

### Oral

- Give with food or a full glass of fluid to minimize GI distress.
- Mix chlorpromazine concentrate just before administration in at least ½ glass juice, milk, water, coffee, tea, carbonated beverage, or with semisolid food.
- Ensure that sustained release form of drug is not chewed or crushed. It **must be** swallowed whole.

### Intramuscular/Intravenous

- Avoid parenteral drug contact with skin, eyes, and clothing because of its potential for causing contact dermatitis.
- Keep patient recumbent for at least 30 min after parenteral administration. Observe closely. Report hypotensive reactions.

### Intramuscular

- Inject IM preparations slowly and deep into upper outer quadrant of buttock. If irritation is a problem, consult prescriber about diluting medication with normal saline or 2% procaine. Rotate injection sites.

### Intravenous

*PREPARE:* **Direct:** Dilute 25 mg with 24 mL of NS to yield 1 mg/mL. **Continuous:** May be further diluted in up to 1000 mL of NS.

*ADMINISTER:* **Direct:** Administer 1 mg or fraction thereof over 1 min for adults and over 2 min for children. **Continuous:** Give slowly at a rate not to exceed 1 mg/min.

- Lemon yellow color of parenteral preparation does not alter potency; if otherwise colored or markedly discolored, solution should be discarded.

*INCOMPATIBILITIES:* **Solution/additive: Aminophylline, amphotericin B, ampicillin, chloramphenicol, chlorothiazide, methohexital, penicillin G, pentobarbital, phenobarbital. Y-site: Allopurinol, amifostine, amphotericin B cholesteryl complex, aztreonam, bivalirudin, cefepime, etoposide, furosemide, lansoprazole, linezolid, melphalan, methotrexate, paclitaxel, piperacillin/tazobactam, remifentanil, sargramostim.**

- All forms are stored preferably at 15°–30° C (59°–86° F) protected from light, unless otherwise specified by the manufacturer. Avoid freezing.

## ADVERSE EFFECTS (≥1%) **Body as a Whole:** Idiopathic edema, muscle necrosis (following IM), SLE-like syndrome, sudden unexplained death. **CV:** Orthostatic hypotension, palpitation, tachycardia, ECG changes (usually reversible): Prolonged QT and PR intervals, blunting of T waves, ST depression. **GI:** Dry mouth; constipation, adynamic ileus, cholestatic jaundice, aggravation of peptic ulcer, dyspepsia, increased appetite. **Hematologic:** Agranulocytosis, thrombocytopenic purpura, pancytopenia (rare). **Metabolic:** Weight gain, hypoglycemia, hyperglycemia, glycosuria (high doses), enlargement of parotid glands. **CNS:** *Sedation,*

Common adverse effects in *italic;* life-threatening effects <u>underlined</u>; generic names in **bold;** classifications in SMALL CAPS; ♣ Canadian drug name; ● Prototype drug

342

*drowsiness,* dizziness, restlessness, <u>neuroleptic malignant syndrome</u>, tardive dyskinesias, tumor, syncope, headache, weakness, insomnia, reduced REM sleep, bizarre dreams, cerebral edema, <u>convulsive seizures</u>, <u>hypothermia</u>, inability to sweat, depressed cough reflex, *extrapyramidal symptoms,* EEG changes. **Respiratory:** <u>Laryngospasm</u>. **Skin:** Fixed-drug eruption, urticaria, reduced perspiration, contact dermatitis, exfoliative dermatitis, photosensitivity, eczema, anaphylactoid reactions, hypersensitivity vasculitis; hirsutism (long-term therapy). **Special Senses:** Blurred vision, lenticular opacities, mydriasis, photophobia. **Urogenital:** Anovulation, infertility, pseudopregnancy, menstrual irregularity, gynecomastia, galactorrhea, priapism, inhibition of ejaculation, reduced libido, urinary retention and frequency.

## DIAGNOSTIC TEST INTERFERENCE

Chlorpromazine (phenothiazines) may increase *cephalin flocculation,* and possibly other *liver function tests;* also may increase *PBI.* False-positive result may occur for *amylase, 5-hydroxyindole acetic acid, phenylketonuria, porphobilinogens, urobilinogen (Ehrlich's reagent),* and *urine bilirubin (Bili-Labstix).* False-positive or false-negative *pregnancy test* results possibly caused by a metabolite of phenothiazines, which discolors urine depending on test used.

## INTERACTIONS **Drug:** Alcohol,

CNS DEPRESSANTS increase CNS depression; ANTACIDS, ANTIDIARRHEALS decrease absorption—space administration 2 h before or after administration of chlorpromazine; could increase the risk of QT prolongation when used with other agents that also have this effect (e.g., **amiodarone**); **phenobarbital** increases metabolism of phenothiazine; GENERAL ANESTHETICS increase excitation and hypotension; antagonizes antihypertensive action of **guanethidine; phenylpropanolamine** poses possibility of sudden death; TRICYCLIC ANTIDEPRESSANTS intensify hypotensive and anticholinergic effects; ANTICONVULSANTS decrease seizure threshold—may need to increase anticonvulsant dose. **Herbal: Kava** increases risk and severity of dystonic reaction.

## PHARMACOKINETICS **Absorption:** Rapid absorption with considerable first pass metabolism in liver; rapid absorption after IM. **Onset:** 30–60 min. **Peak:** 2–4 h PO; 15–20 min IM. **Duration:** 4–6 h. **Distribution:** Widely distributed; accumulates in brain; crosses placenta. **Metabolism:** In liver by CYP2D6. **Elimination:** In urine as metabolites; excreted in breast milk. **Half-Life:** Biphasic 2 and 30 h.

## NURSING IMPLICATIONS

### Black Box Warning

*Chlorpromazine has been associated with increased mortality in the older adult with dementia-related psychosis.*

### Assessment & Drug Effects

- Note that this drug is not approved for use in older adults with dementia-related psychosis.
- Establish baseline BP (in standing and recumbent positions), and pulse, before initiating treatment.
- Monitor BP frequently. Hypotensive reactions, dizziness, and sedation are common during early therapy, particularly in patients on high doses and in the older adult receiving parenteral doses.

Common adverse effects in *italic;* life-threatening effects <u>underlined</u>; generic names in **bold;** classifications in SMALL CAPS; ♣ Canadian drug name; ⊙ Prototype drug

343

- Monitor cardiac status with baseline ECG in patients with preexisting cardiovascular disease.
- Be alert for signs of neuroleptic malignant syndrome (see Appendix G). Report immediately.
- Report extrapyramidal symptoms that occur most often in patients on high dosage, the pediatric patient with severe dehydration and acute infection, the older adult, and women. Reduce smoking, if possible.
- Monitor I&O ratio and pattern: Urinary retention due to mental depression and compromised renal function may occur.
- Be alert to complaints of diminished visual acuity, reduced night vision, photophobia, and a perceived brownish discoloration of objects. Patient may be more comfortable with dark glasses.
- Monitor diabetics or prediabetics on long-term, high-dose therapy for reduced glucose tolerance and loss of diabetes control.
- Ocular examinations, and EEG (in patients older than 50 y) are recommended before and periodically during prolonged therapy.
- Monitor lab tests: Periodic CBC with differential, LFTs, and blood glucose.

### Patient & Family Education

- Take medication as prescribed and keep appointments for follow-up evaluation of dosage regimen. Improvement may not be experienced until 7 or 8 wk into therapy.
- May cause pink to red-brown discoloration of urine.
- Wear protective clothing and sunscreen lotion with SPF above 12 when outdoors, even on dark days. Photosensitivity causes exposed skin areas to have appearance of an exaggerated sunburn.

If reaction occurs, report to prescriber.
- Practice meticulous oral hygiene. Oral candidiasis occurs frequently in patients receiving phenothiazines.
- Avoid driving a car or undertaking activities requiring precision and mental alertness until drug response is known.
- Do not abruptly stop this drug. Abrupt withdrawal of drug or deliberate dose skipping, especially after prolonged therapy with large doses, can cause onset of extrapyramidal symptoms (see Appendix F) and severe GI disturbances. When drug is to be discontinued, dosage **must be** tapered off gradually over a period of several weeks.

## CHLORPROPAMIDE
(klor-proe′pa-mide)
Novopropamide ◆
**Classifications:** ANTIDIABETIC; SULFONYLUREA
Therapeutic: ANTIDIABETIC
**Prototype:** Glyburide

**AVAILABILITY** Tablet

**ACTION & *THERAPEUTIC EFFECT***
Lowers blood glucose by stimulating beta cells in pancreas to synthesize and release endogenous insulin. *Antidiabetic effect is due to the ability of the drug to stimulate beta cells of the pancreas to manufacture and release insulin. Therapeutic effectiveness is indicated by HbA1C level in normal range.*

**USES** Type 2 diabetes mellitus.

**UNLABELED USES** Neurogenic diabetes insipidus.

CHLORPROPAMIDE

**CONTRAINDICATIONS** Known hypersensitivity to sulfonylureas and sulfonamides; diabetes complicated by severe infection; acidosis; severe renal, hepatic, or thyroid insufficiency; lactation.

**CAUTIOUS USE** Older adult patients, Addison's disease, CHF, and hepatic porphyria; pregnancy (category C). Safe use in children not established.

### ROUTE & DOSAGE

**Antidiabetic**

*Adult:* **PO** Initial: 250 mg/day with breakfast, adjust by 50–125 mg/day q3–5days until glycemic control is achieved, up to 750 mg/day

### ADMINISTRATION
**Oral**
- Give as a single morning dose with breakfast or 3 doses and taken with meals.
- Store at 15°–30° C (59°–86° F) in a tightly closed container, unless otherwise directed.

**ADVERSE EFFECTS** (≥1%) **Body as a Whole:** Flushing, photosensitivity, alcohol intolerance. **GI:** GI distress, anorexia, nausea, diarrhea, constipation, cholestatic jaundice. **Hematologic:** Leukopenia, thrombocytopenia, agranulocytosis. **Metabolic:** Hypoglycemia, antidiuretic effect (SIADH), dilutional hyponatremia, water intoxication. **CNS:** Drowsiness, muscle cramps, weakness, paresthesias. **Skin:** Rash, pruritus.

**INTERACTIONS Drug:** Adverse effects of ORAL ANTICOAGULANTS, **phenytoin,** SALICYLATES, NSAIDS may be increased along with those of chlorpropamide; THIAZIDE DIURETICS may increase blood sugar; **alcohol** produces disulfiram reaction; **probenecid,** MAO INHIBITORS may increase hypoglycemic effects. **Herbal: Garlic, ginseng** may increase hypoglycemic effects.

**PHARMACOKINETICS Absorption:** Readily from GI tract. **Onset:** 1 h. **Peak:** 3–6 h. **Distribution:** Highly protein bound; distributed into breast milk. **Metabolism:** In liver. **Elimination:** 80–90% in urine in 96 h. **Half-Life:** 36 h.

### NURSING IMPLICATIONS
**Assessment & Drug Effects**
- Report dizziness, shortness of breath, malaise, fatigue.
- Monitor for S&S of hypoglycemia (see Appendix F)
- Monitor I&O ratio and pattern: Infrequently, chlorpropamide produces an antidiuretic effect, with resulting severe hyponatremia, edema, and water intoxication. If fluid intake far exceeds output and edema develops (weight gain), report to the prescriber.
- Monitor lab tests: Periodic fasting and postprandial blood glucose; HbA1C every 3 mo; baseline and periodic hematologic tests and LFTs, particularly in patients receiving high doses.

**Patient & Family Education**
- Report hypoglycemic episodes to prescriber. Because chlorpropamide has a long half-life, hypoglycemia can be severe.
- Report any of the following immediately to prescriber: Skin eruptions, malaise, fever, or photosensitivity. A change to another hypoglycemic agent may be indicated.

Common adverse effects in *italic;* life-threatening effects underlined; generic names in **bold;** classifications in SMALL CAPS; ♣ Canadian drug name; ⊙ Prototype drug

345

# CHLORTHALIDONE

(klor-thal′i-done)

**Classifications:** ELECTROLYTE & WATER BALANCE AGENT; DIURETIC; ANTIHYPERTENSIVE

**Therapeutic:** DIURETIC; ANTIHYPERTENSIVE

**Prototype:** Hydrochlorothiazide

## AVAILABILITY Tablet

## ACTION & *THERAPEUTIC EFFECT*

Sulfonamide derivative that increases excretion of sodium and chloride by inhibiting their reabsorption in the cortical diluting segment of the ascending loop of Henle. *Antihypertensive effect is correlated to the decrease in extracellular and intracellular volumes. Decreased volume results in reduced cardiac output with subsequent decrease in peripheral resistance.*

**USES** Hypertension, adjunctive therapy in edema.

**CONTRAINDICATIONS** Hypersensitivity to sulfonamide or thiazide derivatives; anuria, hypokalemia; toxemia; hyperparathroidism; lactation; neonates with jaundice.

**CAUTIOUS USE** History of renal and hepatic disease, hyponatremia, hypochloremia; gout, SLE, diabetes mellitus; history of allergy or bronchial asthma; pregnancy (category B).

## ROUTE & DOSAGE

### Hypertension

*Adult:* **PO** 15–25 mg/day, may be increased to 100 mg/day if needed
*Child:* **PO** 2 mg/kg 3 × wk

### Edema

*Adult:* **PO** 50–100 mg/day, may be increased to 200 mg/day if needed
*Child:* **PO** 2 mg/kg 3 × wk (adjust to response)

## ADMINISTRATION

### Oral

- Administer as single dose in a.m. to reduce potential for interrupted sleep because of diuresis.
- Consult prescriber when chlorthalidone is used as a diuretic; an intermittent dose schedule may reduce incidence of adverse reactions.
- Store tablets in tightly closed container at 15°–30° C (59°–86° F) unless otherwise advised.

**ADVERSE EFFECTS** (≥1%) **CV:** Orthostatic hypotension. **GI:** Anorexia, nausea, vomiting, diarrhea, constipation, cramping, jaundice. **Hematologic:** Agranulocytosis, thrombocytopenia, aplastic anemia. **CNS:** Dizziness, vertigo, paresthesias, headache. **Metabolic:** *Hypokalemia,* hyponatremia, hypochloremia, hypercalcemia, glycosuria, hyperglycemia, exacerbation of gout. **Skin:** Rash, urticaria, photosensitivity, vasculitis. **Urogenital:** Impotence.

**INTERACTIONS Drug:** Increased risk of **digoxin** toxicity because of hypokalemia; CORTICOSTEROIDS, **amphotericin B** increases hypokalemia; decreases **lithium** elimination; **dofetilide** may increase potential for arrythmia; may antagonize the hypoglycemic effects of SULFONYLUREAS; NSAIDS may attenuate diuretic effects; **cholestyramine** decreases thiazide absorption.

**PHARMACOKINETICS Absorption:** Readily from GI tract. **Onset:**

---

2 h. **Peak:** 3–6 h. **Duration:** 24–72 h. **Distribution:** Crosses placenta; appears in breast milk. **Elimination:** 30–60% in urine in 24 h. **Half-Life:** 54 h.

## NURSING IMPLICATIONS
### Assessment & Drug Effects
- Establish baseline BP measurements and check at regular intervals during period of dosage adjustment when chlorthalidone is used for hypertension.
- Be alert to signs of hypokalemia (see Appendix F). Older adult patients are more sensitive to adverse effects of drug-induced diuresis because of age-related changes in the cardiovascular and renal systems.
- Monitor lithium and digoxin levels closely when either of these drugs is used concurrently.
- Monitor lab tests: Baseline and periodic serum electrolytes, kidney function tests, uric acid, and blood glucose (especially in patients with diabetes).

### Patient & Family Education
- Maintain adequate potassium intake, monitor weight, and make a daily estimate of I&O ratio.

## CHLORZOXAZONE
(klor-zox′a-zone)
**Classification:** CENTRALLY ACTING SKELETAL MUSCLE RELAXANT
**Therapeutic:** SKELETAL MUSCLE RELAXER; ANTISPASMODIC
**Prototype:** Cyclobenzaprine

## AVAILABILITY Tablet

## ACTION & THERAPEUTIC EFFECT
Centrally acting skeletal muscle relaxant that acts indirectly by depressing nerve transmission through polysynaptic pathways in spinal cord, subcortical centers, and brain stem; also possibly has a sedative effect. *Effectively controls muscle spasms and pain associated with musculoskeletal conditions.*

## USES
Symptomatic treatment of muscle spasm and pain associated with various musculoskeletal conditions.

## CONTRAINDICATIONS
Impaired liver function; alcoholism; hepatic disease, jaundice; lactation.

## CAUTIOUS USE
Patients with known allergies or history of drug allergies; renal impairment or failure; CNS depression; older adult patients; pregnancy (category C).

## ROUTE & DOSAGE

**Skeletal Muscle Relaxant**

*Adult:* PO 250–500 mg t.i.d. or q.i.d. (max: 3 g/day)
*Child:* PO 20 mg/kg/day in 3–4 divided doses

## ADMINISTRATION
### Oral
- Give with food or meals to prevent gastric distress. If necessary, tablet may be crushed and mixed with food or liquid (e.g., milk, fruit juice).
- Store in tight container at 15°–30° C (59°–86° F) unless otherwise directed.

## ADVERSE EFFECTS (≥1%) GI:
Anorexia, heartburn, nausea, vomiting, constipation, diarrhea, abdominal pain, hepatotoxicity: Jaundice, liver damage. **CNS:** *Drowsiness, dizziness,* light-headedness, headache, malaise, overstimulation. **Skin:** Erythema, rash, pruritus, urticaria, petechiae, ecchymoses.

## INTERACTIONS Drug:
Alcohol, CNS DEPRESSANTS add to CNS depression.

Common adverse effects in *italic;* life-threatening effects underlined; generic names in **bold;** classifications in SMALL CAPS; ♣ Canadian drug name; ☻ Prototype drug

347

**C**

## PHARMACOKINETICS Absorption: Readily absorbed from GI tract. **Onset:** 1 h. **Peak:** 1–4 h. **Duration:** 3–4 h. **Distribution:** Not known if crosses placenta or distributed into breast milk. **Metabolism:** In liver. **Elimination:** In urine. **Half-Life:** 66 min.

## NURSING IMPLICATIONS

### Assessment & Drug Effects

- Monitor ambulation during early drug therapy; some patients may require supervision.
- Note: Since chlorzoxazone metabolite may discolor urine, dark urine cannot be a reliable sign of a hepatotoxic reaction.
- Monitor lab tests: Periodic LFTs in patients receiving long-term therapy.

### Patient & Family Education

- Avoid activities requiring mental alertness, judgment, and physical coordination until reaction to drug is known, since sedation, drowsiness, and dizziness may occur.
- Drug may discolor urine orange to purplish red, but this is of no clinical significance.
- Discontinue drug and notify prescriber if signs of hypersensitivity (see Appendix F) or of liver dysfunction appear (abdominal discomfort, yellow sclerae or skin, pruritus, malaise, nausea, vomiting).
- Check with prescriber before taking an OTC depressant (e.g., antihistamine, sedative, alcohol) since effects may be additive.

## CHOLESTYRAMINE RESIN ℗

(koe-less-tear′a-meen)

LoCHOLEST, Questran, Questran Light, Prevalite

**Classifications:** ANTILIPEMIC; BILE ACID SEQUESTRANT

**Therapeutic:** CHOLESTEROL-LOWERING

## AVAILABILITY Powder for suspension; tablet

## ACTION & *THERAPEUTIC EFFECT*
Adsorbs and combines with intestinal bile acids in exchange for chloride ions to form an insoluble, nonabsorbable complex that is excreted in the feces. As a result, bile salts are continually (but not entirely) prevented from reentry into the enterohepatic circulation, thus increasing fecal loss of bile acids. *The resin anion-exchange agent increases fecal loss of bile acids, which leads to lowered serum total cholesterol by decreasing (LDL) cholesterol, and reducing bile acid deposit in dermal tissues (decreasing pruritus). Serum triglyceride levels may increase or remain unchanged.*

## USES As adjunct to diet therapy in management of patients with primary hypercholesterolemia (type IIa hyperlipidemia) with a significant risk of atherosclerotic heart disease and MI; for relief of pruritus secondary to partial biliary stasis.

## UNLABELED USES To control diarrhea caused by excess bile acids in colon; for hyperoxaluria.

## CONTRAINDICATIONS Complete biliary obstruction or biliary cirrhosis, cholelithiasis; GI obstruction; hypersensitivity to bile acid sequestrants; coagulopathy; lactation.

## CAUTIOUS USE Bleeding disorders; hemorrhoids; impaired GI function, decreased GI motility; peptic ulcer, malabsorption states (e.g., steatorrhea); phenylketonuria

**(Questran Light** only); renal disease; pregnancy (category C). Safe use in children 6 y or younger not established.

## ROUTE & DOSAGE

### Hypercholesterolemia
*Adult:* **PO** 4 g b.i.d. to q.i.d. a.c. and at bedtime, may need up to 24 g/day
*Child:* **PO** 240 mg/kg/day in 3 divided doses

### Hyperlipoproteinemia
*Adult:* **PO** 4–8 g b.i.d. to q.i.d. a.c. and at bedtime (32 g/day or less)

### Pruritus
*Adult:* **PO** 4 g b.i.d. to q.i.d. a.c. and at bedtime (16 g/day or less)

## ADMINISTRATION

### Oral
- Place contents of one packet or one level scoopful on surface of at least 120 to 180 mL (4–6 oz) of water or other preferred liquid. Permit drug to hydrate by standing without stirring 1–2 min, twirling glass occasionally, then stir until suspension is uniform. Rinse glass with small amount of liquid and have patient drink remainder to ensure entire dose is taken. Administer before meals.
- Store in tightly closed container at 15°–30° C (59°–86° F) unless otherwise specified.

## ADVERSE EFFECTS (≥1%) **GI:**
*Constipation,* fecal impaction, hemorrhoids, abdominal pain and distension, flatulence, bloating sensation, belching, nausea, vomiting, heartburn, anorexia, diarrhea, steatorrhea. **Endocrine:** Increased libido. **Metabolic:** Weight loss or gain, iron, calcium, vitamin A, D, and K deficiencies (from poor absorp-

tion); hypoprothrombinemia, hyperchloremic acidosis, decreased erythrocyte folate levels. **Skin:** Rash, irritations of skin, tongue, and perianal areas. **Special Senses:** Arcus juvenilis, uveitis.

## DIAGNOSTIC TEST INTERFERENCE
Cholestyramine therapy may be accompanied by increased *serum AST, phosphorus, chloride,* and *alkaline phosphatase* levels; decreased *serum calcium, sodium,* and *potassium* levels.

## INTERACTIONS **Drug:** Decreases the absorption of ORAL ANTICOAGULANTS, **digoxin,** TETRACYCLINES, **penicillins, phenobarbital,** THYROID HORMONES, THIAZIDE DIURETICS, IRON SALTS, FAT-SOLUBLE VITAMINS (A, D, E, K) from the GI tract administer cholestyramine 4 h before or 2 h after these drugs. Can bind to and affect absorption of any drug.

## PHARMACOKINETICS **Absorption:** Not absorbed from GI tract. **Elimination:** Excreted in feces as insoluble complex.

## NURSING IMPLICATIONS

### Assessment & Drug Effects
- Be alert to early symptoms of hypoprothrombinemia (petechiae, ecchymoses, abnormal bleeding from mucous membranes, tarry stools) and report their occurrence promptly. Long-term use of cholestyramine resin can increase bleeding tendency.
- Monitor bowel function. Preexisting constipation may be worsened in the older adult and women.
- Consult prescriber regarding supplemental vitamins A and D and folic acid that may be required by patient on long-term therapy.

---

Common adverse effects in *italic;* life-threatening effects <u>underlined;</u> generic names in **bold;** classifications in SMALL CAPS; ♣Canadian drug name; ⓟ Prototype drug

C

- Monitor lab tests: Periodic CBC, platelet count, serum electrolytes, and lipid profile.

**Patient & Family Education**

- Report constipation to prescriber. High-bulk diet with adequate fluid intake is an essential adjunct to cholestyramine treatment and generally resolves the problems of constipation and bloating sensation.
- Do not omit doses. Sudden withdrawal can promote uninhibited absorption of other drugs taken concomitantly, leading to toxicity or overdosage.
- GI adverse effects usually subside after the first month of drug therapy.
- The following symptoms may be drug-induced and should be reported promptly: Severe gastric distress with nausea and vomiting, unusual weight loss, black stools, severe hemorrhoids (GI bleeding), sudden back pain.

# CHOLINE MAGNESIUM TRISALICYLATE

(cho'leen mag-ne'si-um tri-sal'i-ci-late)

**Classifications:** ANALGESIC (SALICYLATE), NONSTEROIDAL ANTI-INFLAMMATORY DRUG (NSAID); ANTIPYRETIC
Therapeutic: ANALGESIC, NSAID
**Prototype:** Aspirin

**AVAILABILITY** Tablet; liquid

**ACTION & *THERAPEUTIC EFFECT***
Inhibits prostaglandin synthesis by reversibly inhibiting cyclooxygenase (both COX-1 and COX-2), resulting in its anti-inflammatory properties as well as its analgesic property. *Has anti-inflammatory, analgesic, and antipyretic action.*

**USES** Osteoarthritis, rheumatoid arthritis, and other arthrides.

**CONTRAINDICATIONS** Hypersensitivity to nonacetylated salicylates; children and teenagers with chickenpox, influenza, or flu symptoms because of the potential for Reye's syndrome; coagulopathy, anticoagulant therapy, G6PD deficiency; pregnancy (category D third trimester); contraindicated in late pregnancy, near term, or in labor and delivery; children younger than 6 y.

**CAUTIOUS USE** Chronic renal and hepatic failure, history of GI disease, peptic ulcer; patients on coumadin or heparin, anemia; hypovolemic states; older adults; pregnancy (category C first and second trimester); lactation.

## ROUTE & DOSAGE

| Arthritis |
|---|
| *Adult:* **PO** 1–2.5 g/day in 1–3 divided doses (max: 4.5 g/day) |

## ADMINISTRATION

**Oral**

- Give with food to reduce gastric upset. Do not give with antacids.
- Store at 15°–30° C (59°–86° F).

**ADVERSE EFFECTS** (≥1%) **GI:** Vomiting, diarrhea. **CNS:** Headache, vertigo, confusion, drowsiness. **Special Senses:** Tinnitus.

**INTERACTIONS Drug: Aminosalicylic acid** increases risk of salicylate toxicity; **ammonium chloride** and other **acidifying agents** decrease its renal elimination, increasing risk of salicylate toxicity; ANTICOAGULANTS increase risk of bleeding; CARBONIC

Common adverse effects in *italic;* life-threatening effects <u>underlined</u>; generic names in **bold;** classifications in SMALL CAPS; ✦ Canadian drug name; ⊙ Prototype drug

ANHYDRASE INHIBITORS enhance salicylate toxicity; CORTICOSTEROIDS compound ulcerogenic effects; increases **methotrexate** toxicity; low doses of salicylates may antagonize uricosuric effects of **probenecid, sulfinpyrazone.**

## PHARMACOKINETICS **Absorption:** Readily absorbed from small intestine. **Onset:** 30 min. **Peak:** 1–3 h. **Metabolism:** In liver. **Elimination:** In urine. **Half-Life:** 2–3 h.

## NURSING IMPLICATIONS

### Assessment & Drug Effects
- As with other NSAIDS, the antipyretic and anti inflammatory effects may mask usual S&S of infection or other diseases
- Assess for GI discomfort; nausea, gastric irritation, indigestion, diarrhea, and constipation are frequent complaints.
- Monitor for S&S of bleeding. Closely monitor PT if used concurrently with warfarin.

### Patient & Family Education
- Avoid taking aspirin, NSAIDS, or acetaminophen concurrently with drug.
- Avoid dangerous activities until reaction to drug is determined, due to possible CNS effects (e.g., vertigo, drowsiness).
- Report tinnitus or persistent gastric irritation and epigastric pain.
- Report any unexplained bruising or bleeding to prescriber.
- Hypoglycemic effects may be enhanced for those with type 2 diabetes taking an oral hypoglycemic agent (OHA).
- Do not give to children or teenagers with chickenpox, influenza, or flu symptoms because of association with Reye's syndrome.

# CHORIONIC GONADOTROPIN
(go-nad'oh-troe-pin)
**Pregnyl**
**Classification:** HUMAN CHORIONIC GONADOTROPIN (HCG) HORMONE
**Therapeutic:** HCG HORMONE

## AVAILABILITY Solution for injection

## ACTION & *THERAPEUTIC EFFECT*
Promotes production of gonadal steroid hormones by stimulating interstitial cells of the testes to produce androgen and the corpus luteum of the ovary to produce progesterone. *Administration of HCG to women of childbearing age with normal functioning ovaries causes maturation of the ovarian follicle and triggers ovulation.*

## USES Prepubertal cryptorchidism not due to anatomic obstruction and male hypogonadism secondary to pituitary deficiency. Also used in conjunction with menotropins to induce ovulation and pregnancy in infertile women in whom the cause of anovulation is secondary; ovulation usually occurs within 18 h. To stimulate spermatogenesis in males with hypogonadism.

## UNLABELED USES Corpus luteum dysfunction.

## CONTRAINDICATIONS Known hypersensitivity to HCG, hypogonadism of testicular origin, hamster protein hypersensitivity; hypertrophy or tumor of pituitary, prostatic carcinoma or other androgen-dependent neoplasms, precocious puberty; ovarian failure; dysfunctional uterine bleeding; adrenal insufficiency; uncontrolled thyroid disease; pregnancy (category X).

Common adverse effects in *italic;* life-threatening effects underlined; generic names in **bold;** classifications in SMALL CAPS; ♣ Canadian drug name; ☻ Prototype drug

351

**CAUTIOUS USE** Epilepsy, migraine, asthma, cardiac or renal disease; endometriosis; thrombophlebitis; lactation. Safe use in children younger than 4 y has not been established.

## ROUTE & DOSAGE

### Prepubertal Cryptorchidism

*Child:* **IM** 4000 units 3 × wk for 3 wk, *or* 5000 units every other day for 4 doses, *or* 500–1000 units 3 × wk for 4–6 wk

### Hypogonadotropic Hypogonadism

*Adult:* **IM** 500–1000 units 3 × wk for 3 wk, then 2 × wk for 3 wk *or* 4000 units 3 × wk for 6–9 mo followed by 2000 units 3 × wk for 3 mo

### Stimulation of Spermatogenesis

*Adult:* **IM** 5000 units 3 × wk until normal testosterone levels are achieved (4–6 mo), then 2000 units 2 × wk with menotropins for 4 mo

### Induction of Ovulation

*Adult:* **IM** 500–1000 units 1 day following last dose of menotropins

## ADMINISTRATION

### Intramuscular

- Reconstitute only with diluent supplied by manufacturer.
- Following reconstitution solution is stable for 30–90 day, depending on manufacturer, when refrigerated; thereafter potency decreases.
- Give IM into a large muscle.
- Store powder for injection at 15°–30° C (59°–86° F) unless otherwise directed.

**ADVERSE EFFECTS** (≥1%) **Body as a Whole:** Edema, pain at injection site, <u>arterial thromboembolism</u>. **Endocrine:** Gynecomastia, precocious puberty, increased urinary steroid excretion, ectopic pregnancy (incidence low). When used with menotropins (human menopausal gonadotropin): Ovarian hyperstimulation (ascites with or without pain, pleural effusion, ruptured ovarian cysts with resultant hemoperitoneum, multiple births). **CNS:** Headache, irritability, restlessness, depression, fatigue.

**DIAGNOSTIC TEST INTERFERENCE** *Pregnancy tests:* Possibility of false results.

**INTERACTIONS Herbal: Black cohosh** may antagonize fertility effects.

**PHARMACOKINETICS Onset:** 2 h. **Peak:** 6 h. **Distribution:** Testes in males, ovaries in females. **Elimination:** 10–12% in urine within 24 h. **Half-Life:** 23 h.

## NURSING IMPLICATIONS

### Assessment & Drug Effects

- Assess prepubescent males for development of secondary sex characteristics.
- Assess females for and report excessive menstrual bleeding, irregular menstrual cycles, and abdominal/pelvic distention or pain.

### Patient & Family Education

- Report promptly onset of abdominal pain and distension (ovarian hyperstimulation syndrome).
- Report to prescriber if the following appear: Axillary, facial, pubic hair; penile growth; acne; deepening of voice. Induction of androgen secretion by HCG may induce precocious puberty in patient treated for cryptorchidism.
- Observe for signs of fluid retention. A weight chart should be maintained for a biweekly record. Report to prescriber if weight gain is associated with edema.

# CICLESONIDE
(ci-cle-so'nide)
Alvesco, Omnaris, Zetonna
**See Appendix A-3.**

# CICLOPIROXOLAMINE
(sye-kloe-peer'ox)
Loprox, Penlac Nail Lacquer
**Classification:** ANTIFUNGAL
ANTIBIOTIC
Therapeutic: ANTIFUNGAL
ANTIBIOTIC

**AVAILABILITY** Cream; ointment; nail
lacquer; shampoo

## ACTION & *THERAPEUTIC EFFECT*
Inhibits transport of amino acids
within fungal cell, thereby interfering with synthesis of fungal protein,
RNA, and DNA. *Effective against the
following organisms: Dermatophytes,
yeasts, some species of* Mycoplasma
*and* Trichomonas vaginalis, *and
certain strains of gram-positive and
gram-negative bacteria.*

**USES** Topically for treatment of
tinea cruris and tinea corporis
(ringworm) due to *Trichophyton
rubrum, Trichophyton mentagrophytes, Epidermophyton floccosum,*
and *Microsporum canis,* and for
tinea (pityriasis) versicolor due to
*M. furfur;* also cutaneous candidiasis (moniliasis) caused by *Candida
albicans.* Nail lacquer indicated for
onychomycosis of fingernails and
toenails due to *T. rubrum;* seborrheic dermatitis of the scalp.

**CONTRAINDICATIONS** Hypersensitivity to ciclopiroxolamine or to
any component in the formulation.

**CAUTIOUS USE** Type 1 diabetic
patient; history of seizure disorder;
immunosuppression; pregnancy
(category B); lactation. Safe use in
children younger than 10 y not established.

## ROUTE & DOSAGE

### Tinea
*Adult:* **Topical** Massage cream into
affected area and surrounding skin
twice daily, morning and evening

### Onychomycosis
*Adult:* **Topical** Paint affected
nail(s) under the surface of the nail
and on the nail bed once daily at
bedtime (at least 8 h before
washing). After 7 days, remove
lacquer with alcohol and remove
or trim away unattached nail.
Continue up to 48 wk.

### Seborrheic Dermatitis
*Adult:* **Topical** Wet hair and apply
approximately 1 tsp (5 mL) to the
scalp (may use up to 10 mL for
long hair), leave on scalp for
3 min, then rinse. Repeat
treatment twice/wk × 4 wk, with
a minimum of 3 days between
applications.

## ADMINISTRATION
### Topical
- Wash hands thoroughly before
  and after treatments.
- Consult with prescriber about
  specific procedure for cleansing
  the skin before medication is applied. Regardless of method used,
  dry skin thoroughly before drug
  application.
- Avoid occlusive dressing, wrapping, or clothing over site where
  cream is applied.
- Store at 15°–30° C (59°–86° F) unless otherwise directed.

---

Common adverse effects in *italic;* life-threatening effects underlined; generic names
in **bold;** classifications in SMALL CAPS; ♣ Canadian drug name; ● Prototype drug

**C**

**ADVERSE EFFECTS** (≥1%) **Skin:** Irritation, pruritus, burning, worsening of clinical condition.

**PHARMACOKINETICS Absorption:** 1.3% absorbed through intact skin. **Distribution:** Distributed to epidermis, corium (dermis), including hair and hair follicles and sebaceous glands; not known if crosses placenta or is distributed into breast milk. **Elimination:** Excreted primarily by kidneys. **Half-Life:** 1.7 h.

## NURSING IMPLICATIONS

### Assessment & Drug Effects

▪ Monitor for therapeutic effectiveness. Tinea versicolor generally responds to drug treatment in about 2 wk. Tinea pedis ("athlete's foot"), tinea corporis (ringworm), tinea cruris ("jock itch"), and candidiasis (moniliasis) require about 4 wk of therapy.

### Patient & Family Education

▪ Use medication for the prescribed time even though symptoms improve.

▪ Report skin irritation or other possible signs of sensitization. A reaction suggestive of sensitization warrants drug discontinuation.

▪ Do not use occlusive dressings or wrappings.

▪ Avoid contact of drug in or near the eyes.

▪ Wear light clothing and footwear that will allow ventilation. Loose-fitting cotton underwear or socks are preferred.

## CIDOFOVIR
(cye-do'fo-ver)
Vistide
**Classification:** ANTIVIRAL
Therapeutic: ANTIVIRAL
**Prototype:** Acyclovir

**AVAILABILITY** Solution for injection

## ACTION & *THERAPEUTIC EFFECT*
Cidofovir, a nucleotide analog, suppresses cytomegalovirus (CMV) replication by inhibiting CMV DNA polymerase. Cidofovir reduces the rate of viral DNA synthesis of CMV. *It is limited for use in treating CMV retinitis in patients with AIDS. Also effective against herpes viruses and other viruses.*

**USES** Treatment/prophylaxis of CMV retinitis in patients with AIDS.

**CONTRAINDICATIONS** Hypersensitivity to cidofovir, history of severe hypersensitivity to probenecid or other sulfa-containing medications; childbearing women and men without barrier contraception; acute renal failure; serum creatinine more than 1.5 mg/dL, creatinine clearance 55 mL/min or less, or urine protein 100 mg/dL or more; lactation.

**CAUTIOUS USE** Renal function impairment, DM, myelosuppression, previous hypersensitivity to other nucleoside analogs; older adults; pregnancy (category C). Safety and efficacy in children not established.

## ROUTE & DOSAGE

### CMV Retinitis: Induction and Maintenance

*Adult:* **IV** 5 mg/kg once weekly for 2 wk. Also give 2 g probenecid 3 h prior to infusion and 1 g 8 h after infusion (4 g total). Continue every 2 wk.

### Renal Impairment Dosage Adjustment

If serum Cr increases by 0.3–0.4, lower dose to 3 mg/kg

## ADMINISTRATION

- Pretreatment: Prehydrate with IV of 1 L NS infused over 1–2 h immediately before cidofovir infusion. If able to tolerate fluid load, infuse second liter over 1–3 h starting at beginning (or end) of cidofovir infusion.

### Intravenous

*PREPARE:* **IV Infusion:** Dilute the calculated dose in 100 mL of NS. *ADMINISTER:* **IV Infusion:** Give over 1 h at constant rate. ▪ Do not coadminister with other agents with significant nephrotoxic potential.

- Store vials at 20°–25° C (68°–77° F); may store diluted IV solution at 2°–8° C (36°–46° F) for up to 24 h.

### ADVERSE EFFECTS (≥1%) **Body as a Whole:** Infection, allergic reactions. **GI:** Nausea, vomiting, diarrhea. **Metabolic:** Metabolic acidosis. **Hematologic:** Neutropenia. **CNS:** *Fever, headache,* asthenia. **Respiratory:** Dyspnea, pneumonia. **Special Senses:** Ocular hypotony. **Urogenital:** *Nephrotoxicity, proteinuria.*

### INTERACTIONS **Drug:** AMINOGLYCOSIDES, **amphotericin B, foscarnet, pentamidine** can increase risk of nephrotoxicity.

### PHARMACOKINETICS **Duration:** Probenecid increases serum levels and area under concentration–time curve. **Elimination:** 80–100% in urine; probenecid delays urinary excretion.

## NURSING IMPLICATIONS

### Black Box Warning

*Cidofovir has been associated with severe renal impairment and neutropenia.*

### Assessment & Drug Effects

- Periodic visual acuity tests and measurement of intraocular pressure are recommended.
- Note that probenecid is typically given concurrently to minimize potential nephrotoxicity. Potential adverse effects of probenecid include headache, nausea, vomiting, hypersensitivity reactions.
- Monitor for S&S of hypersensitivity (see Appendix F). Report their appearance promptly.
- Monitor lab tests: Serum creatinine and urine protein within 48 h prior to each dose. WBC with differential prior to each dose.

### Patient & Family Education

- Initiate or continue regular ophthalmologic exams.
- Be alert to potential adverse reactions caused by probenecid (e.g., headache, nausea, vomiting, hypersensitivity reactions) and cidofovir.

## CILOSTAZOL
(sil-os'tah-zol)

**Classifications:** ANTIPLATELET; PHOSPHODIESTERASE INHIBITOR

**Therapeutic:** PERIPHERAL VASODILATOR; PLATELET AGGREGATION INHIBITOR

### AVAILABILITY Tablet

### ACTION & *THERAPEUTIC EFFECT*
Mechanism of action in intermittent claudication not completely understood. Known to suppress degradation of cAMP with resultant vasodilation and inhibition of platelet aggregation. *Increases the skin temperature of the extremities and improves claudication. Effectiveness is indicated by increased ability to walk further without claudication.*

### USES Intermittent claudication.

### CONTRAINDICATIONS CHF of any severity; hypersensitivity to

Common adverse effects in *italic;* life-threatening effects underlined; generic names in **bold;** classifications in SMALL CAPS; ♣Canadian drug name; ● Prototype drug

355

cilostazol; acute MI; hemostatic disorders or pathologic bleeding; lactation.

**CAUTIOUS USE** Cardiac arrhythmias, MI within 6 mo; valvular heart disease; peptic ulcer disease; renal failure; hepatic impairment; pregnancy (category C). Safety and efficacy in children younger than 18 y not established.

## ROUTE & DOSAGE

**Intermittent Claudication**

*Adult:* **PO** 100 mg b.i.d., may need to reduce to 50 mg b.i.d. with concomitant CYP3A4 or CYP2C19 inhibitors

## ADMINISTRATION

**Oral**

- Give at least 30 min before or 2 h after a meal. Do not give with grapefruit juice.
- Store at 20°–25° C (68°–77° F).

**ADVERSE EFFECTS** (≥1%) **Body as a Whole:** Back pain, *headache,* infection, myalgia. **CNS:** Dizziness, vertigo. **CV:** Palpitations, tachycardia. **GI:** Abdominal pain, *abnormal stools, diarrhea,* dyspepsia, flatulence, nausea. **Respiratory:** Cough, pharyngitis, rhinitis.

**INTERACTIONS Drug: Diltiazem, erythromycin, fluconazole, fluvoxamine, fluoxetine, ketoconazole, itraconazole,** MACROLIDE ANTIBIOTICS, **nefazodone, omeprazole, sertraline,** PROTEASE INHIBITORS may increase cilostazol levels and adverse effects. Do not use with **defibrotide. Herbal: Evening primrose oil** may increase bleeding risk. **Food:** High fat meals may increase peak concentrations. **Grapefruit juice** may increase concentration.

**PHARMACOKINETICS Onset:** 2–4 wk. **Distribution:** 95–98% protein bound. May be excreted in breast milk. **Metabolism:** Metabolized by CYP3A4 to active metabolites. **Elimination:** Metabolites primarily excreted in urine and feces. **Half-Life:** 11–13 h.

## NURSING IMPLICATIONS

**Assessment & Drug Effects**

- Monitor therapeutic effectiveness indicated by ability to walk farther without leg pain.
- Monitor for S&S of CHF. Do not give cilostazol to patients with preexisting CHF.

**Patient & Family Education**

- Avoid grapefruit or grapefruit juice while taking cilostazol.
- Allow 2–12 wk for therapeutic response.
- Monitor for signs of abnormal bleeding.

## CIMETIDINE ⓟ

(sye-met'i-deen)

Tagamet HB

**Classification:** ANTISECRETORY (H$_2$-RECEPTOR ANTAGONIST)

Therapeutic: ANTISECRETORY

**AVAILABILITY** Tablet; oral solution

## ACTION & *THERAPEUTIC EFFECT*

Has high selectivity for inhibition of histamine H$_2$-receptors on parietal cells of the stomach, thus suppressing all phases of daytime and nocturnal basal gastric acid secretion in the stomach. Indirectly reduces pepsin secretion. *Blocks the H$_2$-receptors on the parietal cells of the stomach, thus decreasing gastric acid secretion; raises the pH of the stomach and thereby reduces pepsin secretion.*

**USES** Short-term treatment of active duodenal ulcer and prevention of ulcer recurrence (at reduced dosage) after it is healed. Also used for short-term treatment of active benign gastric ulcer, pathologic hypersecretory conditions such as Zollinger-Ellison syndrome, and heartburn.

**UNLABELED USES** Prophylaxis of stress-induced ulcers, upper GI bleeding, and aspiration pneumonitis; gastroesophageal reflux; chronic urticaria; acetaminophen toxicity.

**CONTRAINDICATIONS** Known hypersensitivity to cimetidine or other H$_2$-receptor antagonists.

**CAUTIOUS USE** Older adults or critically ill patients; impaired renal or hepatic function; organic brain syndrome; gastric ulcers; immunocompromised patients, pregnancy (category B); children younger than 12 y.

## ROUTE & DOSAGE

**GERD**

*Adult/Adolescent:* **PO** 800 mg b.i.d. or 400 mg q.i.d. × 12 w
*Child:* **PO** 20–40 mg/kg/day in divided doses

**Duodenal Ulcer, Acute Treatment**

*Adult/Adolescent:* **PO** 300 mg q.i.d. *or* 400 mg b.i.d. *or* 800 mg × 12 w
*Child:* **PO** 20–40 mg/kg/day in 4 divided doses

**Duodenal Ulcer, Maintenance Therapy**

*Adult/Adolescent:* **PO** 400 mg at bedtime

**Heartburn**

*Adult:* **PO** 200 mg 2–4 × day

**Pathologic Hypersecretory Disease**

*Adult:* **PO** 300 mg q.i.d. (max: 2400 mg/day)

**Renal Impairment Dosage Adjustment**

*CrCl less than 30 mL/min:* Reduce daily dose by 50%

**Hemodialysis Dosage Adjustment**
Give scheduled dose after dialysis

## ADMINISTRATION

**Oral**
- If an antacid is being used, give 1 h before or 2 h after the antacid.

**ADVERSE EFFECTS** (>1%) **Body as a Whole:** Fever. **CV (rare):** Cardiac arrhythmias and cardiac arrest after rapid IV bolus dose. **GI:** Mild transient diarrhea; severe diarrhea, constipation, abdominal discomfort. **Hematologic:** Increased prothrombin time; neutropenia (rare), thrombocytopenia (rare), aplastic anemia. **Metabolic:** Slight increase in serum uric acid, BUN, creatinine; transient pain at IM site; hypospermia. **Musculoskeletal:** Exacerbation of joint symptoms in patients with preexisting arthritis. **CNS:** Drowsiness, dizziness, light-headedness, depression, headache, reversible confusional states, paranoid psychosis. **Skin:** Rash, Stevens–Johnson syndrome, reversible alopecia. **Urogenital:** Gynecomastia and breast soreness, galactorrhea, reversible impotence.

## DIAGNOSTIC TEST INTERFERENCE
Cimetidine may cause false-positive *Hemoccult test for gastric bleeding* if test is performed within 15 min of oral cimetidine administration.

**INTERACTIONS Drug:** Cimetidine decreases the hepatic metabolism of **warfarin, phenobarbital, phenytoin, diazepam,**

Common adverse effects in *italic;* life-threatening effects underlined; generic names in **bold;** classifications in SMALL CAPS; ♣ Canadian drug name; ⊙ Prototype drug

357

**propranolol, lidocaine, theophylline,** thus increasing their activity and toxicity; ANTACIDS may decrease absorption of cimetidine.

## PHARMACOKINETICS Absorption: 70% from GI tract. **Peak:** 1–1.5 h. **Distribution:** Widely distributed; crosses blood–brain barrier and placenta. **Metabolism:** In liver by CYP1A2 and 3A4. **Elimination:** Most of drug excreted in urine in 24 h; excreted in breast milk. **Half-Life:** 2 h.

## NURSING IMPLICATIONS

### Assessment & Drug Effects
- Monitor pulse of patient during first few days of drug regimen. Bradycardia should be reported. Pulse usually returns to normal within 24 h after drug discontinuation.
- Monitor I&O ratio and pattern: Particularly in the older adult, severely ill, and in patients with impaired renal function.
- Be alert to onset of confusional states, particularly in the older adult or severely ill patient. Symptoms occur within 2–3 days after first dose; report immediately. Symptoms usually resolve within 3–4 days after therapy is discontinued.
- Check BP and report an elevation to the prescriber, if patient complains of severe headache.
- Monitor lab tests: Periodic CBC, renal function tests, and LFTs during long-term therapy.

### Patient & Family Education
- Seek advice about self-medication with any OTC drug.
- Report breast tenderness or enlargement. Mild bilateral gynecomastia and breast soreness may occur after 1 mo or more of therapy. It may disappear spontaneously or remain throughout therapy.

- Report recurrence of gastric pain or bleeding (black, tarry stools or "coffee ground" vomitus) immediately, and notify prescriber if diarrhea continues more than 1 day.
- Avoid driving and other potentially hazardous activities until reaction to drug is known.
- Duodenal or gastric ulcer is a chronic, recurrent condition that requires long-term maintenance drug therapy.

# CINACALCET HYDROCHLORIDE
(sin-a-kal'set)

Sensipar

**Classifications:** PARATHYROID HORMONE; CALCIUM RECEPTOR AGONIST
Therapeutic: PARATHYROID HORMONE

## AVAILABILITY Tablet

## ACTION & *THERAPEUTIC EFFECT*
Directly lowers parathyroid hormone (PTH) levels by increasing sensitivity of calcium-sensing receptors on parathyroid gland to extracellular calcium. This causes decreased calcium and phosphate adsorption from bone, and thus decreased serum calcium and phosphate levels. *Lowers PTH production; this also decreases rate of bone turnover and bone fibrosis in chronic renal failure disease (CRFD).*

## USES Primary or secondary hyperparathyroidism; hypercalcemia in patients with parathyroid cancer.

## CONTRAINDICATIONS Hypersensitivity to cinacalcet; hypocalcemia or lower limit of normal serum calcium; chronic kidney disease patients not on dialysis; lactation.

## CAUTIOUS USE Moderate and severe hepatic impairment, history of seizures; hypotension; heart failure;

history of QT prolongation; history of arrhythmias; pregnancy (category C); children younger than 18 y.

## ROUTE & DOSAGE

### Hyperparathyroidism
Adult: PO Start with 30 mg once daily; may increase q2–4wk until target iPTH of 150–300 pg/mL (max: 300 mg/day)

### Hypercalcemia
Adult: PO 30 mg twice daily; titrate q2–4wk as 60 mg b.i.d., 90 mg b.i.d., then 90 mg 3–4 × daily as needed to normalize calcium concentrations

## ADMINISTRATION
### Oral
- Give with food or shortly after a meal.
- Tablets should be swallowed whole and not divided, crushed, or chewed.
- Do not give to patient with hypocalcemia.
- Store at 15°–30° C (59°–86° F).

**ADVERSE EFFECTS** (≥1%) **Body as a Whole:** Dizziness, asthenia, noncardiac chest pain, dialysis access infection. **CV:** Hypertension. **GI:** *Nausea, vomiting, diarrhea,* anorexia, constipation. **Metabolic:** Hypocalcemia. **Musculoskeletal:** *Myalgia,* adynamic bone disease (renal osteodystrophy).

**INTERACTIONS Drug:** May increase **amoxapine, atomoxetine, carvedilol, clozapine, codeine, cyclobenzaprine, dexfenfluramine, dextromethorphan, donepezil, fenfluramine, flecainide, fluoxetine, haloperidol, hydrocodone, maprotiline, meperidine, methadone, methamphetamine,**

**metoprolol, mexiletine, morphine, oxycodone, paroxetine, perphenazine, propafenone, propranolol, risperidone, thioridazine** (use may be contraindicated with cinacalcet), **timolol, tramadol, trazodone,** TRICYCLIC ANTIDEPRESSANTS, **venlafaxine, zolpidem** levels; cinacalcet levels may be increased by strong CYP3A4 inhibitors such as **amiodarone, aprepitant, clarithromycin, dalfopristin, diltiazem, erythromycin, fluconazole, fluvoxamine, itraconazole, ketoconazole, miconazole, nefazodone, quinupristin, troleandomycin, verapamil, voriconazole. Food: Grapefruit juice** may increase cinacalcet levels.

**PHARMACOKINETICS Peak:** 2–6 h. **Distribution:** 93–97% protein bound. **Metabolism:** In liver by CYP3A4. **Elimination:** 80% by kidneys, 15% in feces. **Half-Life:** 30–40 h.

## NURSING IMPLICATIONS
### Assessment & Drug Effects
- Monitor for S&S of hypocalcemia (e.g., paresthesias, myalgias, cramping, tetany, convulsions).
- Withhold drug and notify prescriber for serum calcium less than 7.5 mg/dL or symptoms of hypocalcemia. Drug should not be resumed until serum calcium levels reach 8 mg/dL, and/or symptoms of hypocalcemia resolve.
- Closely monitor iPTH and serum calcium with concurrent administration of a strong CYP3A4 (e.g., ketoconazole, erythromycin, itraconazole).
- Monitor lab tests: Baseline serum calcium, repeat within a week of initiation or dosage adjustment, and iPTH 1–4 wk after initiation of drug or dose adjustment; thereafter, monthly serum calcium and

Common adverse effects in *italic*; life-threatening effects underlined; generic names in **bold**; classifications in SMALL CAPS; ♣Canadian drug name; ☺ Prototype drug

359

phosphorus (more often with a history of a seizure disorder), and iPTH every 1–3 mo.

**Patient & Family Education**

- Report promptly any of the following: Seizure or convulsion; muscle spasms or cramping of the abdomen, back, legs, face; burning, numbness, pricking, tickling, or tingling of the face, lips, tongue, hands, or feet; changes in mental status.

# CIPROFLOXACIN HYDROCHLORIDE ⊙

(ci-pro-flox′a-cin)

Cetraxal, Cipro, Cipro XR, OTIPRIO

# CIPROFLOXACIN OPHTHALMIC

Ciloxan

**Classification:** QUINOLONE ANTIBIOTIC

**Therapeutic:** ANTIBIOTIC

**AVAILABILITY** Tablet; extended release tablet; suspension; solution for injection; ophthalmic solution; otic drops

## ACTION & *THERAPEUTIC EFFECT*

Inhibits DNA-gyrase, an enzyme necessary for bacterial DNA replication and some aspects of transcription, repair, recombination, and transposition. *Effective against many gram-positive and aerobic gram-negative organisms.*

**USES** UTIs, lower respiratory tract infections, skin and skin structure infections, bone and joint infections, GI infection or infectious diarrhea, chronic bacterial prostatitis, gonorrhea, urethritis, nosocomial pneumonia, acute sinusitis. Post-exposure prophylaxis for anthrax. **Ophthalmic:** Corneal ulcers, bacterial conjunctivitis caused by *Staphylococci, Streptococci,* and *Pseudomonas aeruginosa.* **Otic:** Otitis externa.

**CONTRAINDICATIONS** Known hypersensitivity to ciprofloxacin or other quinolones, concurrent administration of tizanidine, syphilis, viral infection; history of myasthenia gravis; peripheral neuropathy; tendon inflammation or tendon pain; lactation.

**CAUTIOUS USE** Known or suspected CNS disorders (i.e., severe cerebral arteriosclerosis or seizure disorders); myocardial ischemia, atrial fibrillation, QT prolongation, CHF; GI disease, colitis; CVA; uncorrected hypokalemia; severe renal impairment and crystalluria during ciprofloxacin therapy; pregnancy (category C); children.

## ROUTE & DOSAGE

**Uncomplicated UTI**

*Adult:* **PO** 250 mg q12h or 500 mg XR daily × 3 days; **IV** 200 mg q12h × 7–14 days

**Complicated UTI**

*Adult:* **PO** 250–500 mg q12h or 1000 mg XR daily × 7–14 days; **IV** 200–400 mg q12h × 7–14 days

**Respiratory Tract Infections**

*Adult:* **IV** 400 mg q8–12h × 7–14 days; **PO** 500–750 q12h × 7–14 days

**Pneumonia**

*Adult:* **IV** 400 mg q8–12h × 10–14days

**Acute Sinusitis**

*Adult:* **PO** 500 mg b.i.d. × 10 days

**Moderate to Severe Systemic Infection**

*Adult:* **PO** 500–750 mg q12h; **IV** 200–400 mg q8–12h

### Skin/Skin Structure Infection

*Adult:* **PO** 500–750 mg q12h × 7–14 days; **IV** 400 mg q8–12h × 7–14 days

### Renal Impairment Dosage Adjustment

*Adult (CrCl 30–50 mL/min):* **PO** 250–500 mg q12h; **IV** No change in dose; *less than 30 mL/min:* **PO** 250–500 mg q18h; **IV** 200–400 mg q18–24h

### Bacterial Conjunctivwitis

*Adult:* **Ophthalmic** 1–2 drops in conjunctival sac q2h while awake for 2 days, then 1–2 drops q4h while awake for the next 5 days
**Ointment** ½-inch ribbon into conjunctival sac t.i.d. × 2 days, then b.i.d. × 5 days

### Corneal Ulcers

*Adult:* **Ophthalmic** 2 drops q15min for 6 h, 2 drops q30min for the next 18 h, then 2 drops q1h for 24 h, then 2 drops q4h for 14 days

### Otitis Externa

*Adult/Adolescent/Child (1 y or older):* 0.25 mL into affected ears q12h × 7 days

## ADMINISTRATION

▪ For patients with renal impairment, oral and IV doses are lowered according to creatinine clearance.

### Ophthalmic

▪ Apply ointment or solution directly into the conjunctival sac when treating conjunctivitis.

### Oral

▪ Do not give an antacid within 4 h of the oral ciprofloxacin dose. May administer with food to minimize GI upset.

▪ Swallow whole; do not split, crush, or chew.

### Otic

▪ Warm solution by holding container in hands for at least 1 min to minimize dizziness.
▪ Patient should lie on opposite side and remain for 1 min after instillation.

### Intravenous

*PREPARE:* **Intermittent:** Dilute in NS or D5W to a final concentration of 0.5–2 mg/mL. ▪ Typical dilutions are 200 mg in 100–250 mL and 400 mg in 250–500 mL.

*ADMINISTER:* **Intermittent:** Give slowly over 60 min. Avoid rapid infusion and use of a small vein.

*INCOMPATIBILITIES:* Solution/additive: **Aminophylline, amoxicillin, amoxicillin/clavulanate potassium, amphotericin B, ampicillin/sulbactam, ceftazidime, cefuroxime, clindamycin, heparin, metronidazole, piperacillin, sodium bicarbonate, ticarcillin.** Y-site: **Aminophylline, ampicillin, ampicillin/sulbactam, azithromycin, cefepime, dexamethasone, drotrecogin alfa, furosemide, heparin, hydrocortisone, lansoprazole, phenytoin, propofol, sodium bicarbonate, theophylline, TPN, warfarin.**

▪ Discontinue other IV infusion while infusing ciprofloxacin or infuse through another site.
▪ Reconstituted IV solution is stable for 14 days refrigerated.

## ADVERSE EFFECTS (≥1%) GI:

Nausea, vomiting, diarrhea, cramps, gas, pseudomembranous colitis. **Metabolic:** Transient increases in liver transaminases, alkaline phosphatase, lactic dehydrogenase, and eosinophilia count. **Musculoskeletal:** Tendon rupture, cartilage erosion. **CNS:** Headache, vertigo,

Common adverse effects in *italic;* life-threatening effects <u>underlined</u>; generic names in **bold;** classifications in SMALL CAPS; ♣Canadian drug name; ☻ Prototype drug

361

malaise, peripheral neuropathy, nervousness, insomnia seizures (especially with rapid IV infusion). **Skin:** Rash, phlebitis, pain, burning, pruritus, and erythema at infusion site; photosensitivity. **Special Senses:** *Local burning and discomfort, crystalline precipitate on superficial portion of cornea,* lid margin crusting, scales, foreign body sensation, itching, and conjunctival hyperemia. **Respiratory:** Rhinitis, pharyngitis.

**DIAGNOSTIC TEST INTERFERENCE**
May cause false positive on *opiate screening tests.*

**INTERACTIONS Drug:** May increase **theophylline** levels 15–30%; ANTACIDS, **sulcralfate, iron** decrease absorption of ciprofloxacin; may increase PT for patients on **warfarin.** Do not use with **dofetilide, dronderarone, ziprasidone** due to risk of increased QT prolongation. Do not use with **tizanidine.** Avoid use with **zolpidem** due to increased exposure. **Food: Calcium** decreases the levels of ciprofloxacin.

**PHARMACOKINETICS Absorption:** 60–80% from GI tract; opthalmic: Minimal absorption through cornea or conjunctiva. **Onset:** Topical 0.5–2 h. **Duration:** Topical 12 h. **Peak:** Immediate release: 0.5–2 h; Cipro XR: 1–2.5 h; Proquin XR: 3.5–8.7 h. **Distribution:** Widely distributed including prostate, lung, and bone; crosses placenta; distributed into breast milk. **Elimination:** Primarily in urine with some biliary excretion. **Half-Life:** 3.5–4 h.

**NURSING IMPLICATIONS**

### Black Box Warning

*Ciprofloxacin (oral and IV) has been associated with increased risk of tendinitis and tendon rupture, and with exacerbations of muscle weakness in persons with myasthenia gravis.*

### Assessment & Drug Effects

- Report tendon inflammation or pain. Drug should be discontinued.
- Monitor I&O ratio and patterns: Patients should be well hydrated; assess for S&S of crystalluria.
- Monitor persons with myasthenia gravis for exacerbations of muscle weakness.
- Monitor plasma theophylline concentrations with concurrent use, since drug may interfere with half-life.
- Administration with theophylline derivatives or caffeine can cause CNS stimulation.
- Assess for S&S of GI irritation (e.g., nausea, diarrhea, vomiting, abdominal discomfort) in clients receiving high dosages and in older adults.
- Monitor PT and INR in patients receiving coumarin therapy.
- Assess for S&S of superinfections (see Appendix F).
- Monitor lab tests: Baseline C&S, periodic LFTs, renal function tests, and CBC with differential with prolonged therapy.

### Patient & Family Education

- Immediately report tendon inflammation or pain. Drug should be discontinued.
- Fluid intake of 2–3 L/day is advised, if not contraindicated.
- Report sudden, unexplained joint pain.
- Restrict caffeine due to the following effects: Nervousness, insomnia, anxiety, tachycardia.
- Use sunscreen and avoid overexposure to sunlight.
- Report nausea, diarrhea, vomiting, and abdominal pain or discomfort.
- Use caution with hazardous activities until reaction to drug is known. Drug may cause light-headedness.

Common adverse effects in *italic*; life-threatening effects <u>underlined</u>; generic names in **bold**; classifications in SMALL CAPS; ♣ Canadian drug name; ⦿ Prototype drug

# CISATRACURIUM BESYLATE

(cis-a-tra-kyoo-ri'um)

Nimbex

**Classifications:** NONDEPOLAR-
IZING SKELETAL MUSCLE RELAXANT;
NEUROMUSCULAR BLOCKER
Therapeutic: SKELETAL MUSCLE
RELAXANT
**Prototype:** Atracurium

**AVAILABILITY** Solution for injection

## ACTION & *THERAPEUTIC EFFECT*

It binds competitively to cholinergic receptors on the motor endplate of neurons, antagonizing
the action of acetylcholine. *Blocks*
*neuromuscular transmission of*
*nerve impulses.*

**USES** Adjunct to general anesthesia to facilitate tracheal intubation
and provide skeletal muscle relaxation during surgery or mechanical
ventilation.

**CONTRAINDICATIONS** Hyper
sensitivity to cisatracurium or other
related agents; rapid-sequence en
dotracheal intubation.

**CAUTIOUS USE** History of hemiparesis, electrolyte imbalances,
burn patients, pulmonary disease,
COPD; neuromuscular diseases
(e.g., myasthenia gravis), older
adults, renal function impairment,
pregnancy (category B), lactation.
Safe use in children younger than
1 mo not established.

## ROUTE & DOSAGE

### Intubation

*Adult:* **IV** 0.15 or 0.20 mg/kg
*Child (2–12 y):* **IV** 0.1–0.15 mg/kg
*Infant (1 mo or older):* **IV**
0.15 mg/kg

### Maintenance

*Adult:* **IV** 0.03 mg/kg q20min prn
or 1–2 mcg/kg/min
*Child (2 y or older):* **IV** 1–2 mcg/
kg/min

### Mechanical Ventilation in ICU

*Adult:* **IV** 3 mcg/kg/min (can range
from 0.5 to 10.2 mcg/kg/min)

## ADMINISTRATION

- Administer carefully adjusted,
individualized doses using a
peripheral nerve stimulator to
evaluate neuromuscular function.
- Given only by or under supervision of expert clinician familiar
with the drug's actions and potential complications.
- Have immediately available personnel and facilities for resuscitation and life support and an antagonist of cisatracurium.
- Note that 10-mL multiple-dose vials
contain benzyl alcohol and should
not be used with neonates.

### Intravenous

*PREPARE:* **Direct:** Give undiluted.
**IV Infusion:** Dilute 10 mg in 95 mL
or 40 mg in 80 mL of compatible
IV fluid to prepare 0.1 mg/mL or
0.4 mg/mL, respectively, IV solution. • Compatible IV fluids include D5W, NS, D5/NS, D5/LR.
**ICU IV Infusion (Mechanical Ven-
tilation):** Dilute the contents of
the 200 mg vial (i.e., 10 mg/mL)
in 1000 mL or 500 mL of compatible
IV fluid to prepare 0.2 mg/mL or
0.4 g/mL, respectively, IV solutions.
*ADMINISTER:* **Direct:** Give a single
dose over 5–10 sec. **IV Infusion:** Adjust the rate based on patient's weight.
*INCOMPATIBILITIES:* Solution/ad-
ditive: Ketorolac, propofol (dose
dependent). Y-site: Amphotericin B, amphotericin B cholesteryl complex, ampicillin,

Common adverse effects in *italic*; life-threatening effects <u>underlined</u>; generic names
in **bold**; classifications in SMALL CAPS; ✦Canadian drug name; ◐ Prototype drug

363

C

**cefazolin, cefotaxime, cefotetan, cefuroxime, diazepam, furosemide, ganciclovir, heparin, methylprednisolone, sodium bicarbonate, trimethoprim/sulfamethoxazole.**

▪ Refrigerate vials at 2°–8° C (36°–46° F). Protect from light. Diluted solutions may be stored refrigerated or at room temperature for 24 h.

**ADVERSE EFFECTS** (≥1%) **CV:** Bradycardia, hypotension, flushing. **Respiratory:** Bronchospasm. **Skin:** Rash.

**PHARMACOKINETICS Onset:** Varies from 1.5 to 3.3 min (higher dose has faster onset). **Peak:** Varies from 1.5 to 3.3 min (higher dose has faster peak). **Duration:** Varies with dose from 46 to 121 min (higher dose, longer recovery time). **Metabolism:** Undergoes Hoffman elimination (pH- and temperature-dependent degradation) and hydrolysis by plasma esterases. **Elimination:** In urine. **Half-Life:** 22 min.

**NURSING IMPLICATIONS**

**Assessment & Drug Effects**

▪ Time-to-maximum neuromuscular block is ≈1 min slower in the older adult.
▪ Monitor for bradycardia, hypotension, and bronchospasms; monitor ICU patients for spontaneous seizures.

# CISPLATIN (cis-DDP, cis-PLATINUM II)

(sis'pla-tin)

Abiplatin ✦, Platinol

**Classifications:** ANTINEOPLASTIC; ALKYLATING AGENT
**Therapeutic:** ANTINEOPLASTIC
**Prototype:** Cyclophosphamide

**AVAILABILITY** Solution for injection

**ACTION & *THERAPEUTIC EFFECT*** A heavy metal complex that produces cross linkage in DNA of rapidly dividing cells, thus preventing DNA, RNA, and protein synthesis. *Cell cycle-nonspecific (i.e., effective throughout the entire cell life cycle).*

**USES** Established combination therapy (cisplatin, vinblastine, bleomycin) in patient with metastatic testicular tumors and with doxorubicin for metastatic ovarian tumors following appropriate surgical or radiation therapy.

**UNLABELED USES** Carcinoma of endometrium, bladder, head, and neck.

**CONTRAINDICATIONS** History of hypersensitivity to cisplatin or other platinum-containing compounds; impaired renal function of CrCl below 30 mL/min; severe myelosuppression; impaired hearing; active infection; history of gout and urate renal stones, renal failure; hypomagnesia; Raynaud syndrome; pregnancy (category D).

**CAUTIOUS USE** Previous cytotoxic drug or radiation therapy with other ototoxic and nephrotoxic drugs; peripheral neuropathy; hyperuricemia; electrolyte imbalances, moderate renal impairment; hepatic impairment; history of circulatory disorders. Safe use in children not established.

**ROUTE & DOSAGE**

**Testicular Neoplasms**

*Adult:* **IV** 20 mg/m²/day for 5 days q3–4wk for 3 courses

**Ovarian Neoplasms**

*Adult (with cyclophosphamide):* **IV** 75–100 mg/m² once q4wk; *single agent:* 100 mg/m² once q4wk

### Advanced Bladder Cancer
*Adult:* **IV** 50–75 mg/m$^2$ q3–4 wk

## ADMINISTRATION

- Usually a parenteral antiemetic agent is administered 30 min before cisplatin therapy is instituted and given on a scheduled basis throughout day and night as long as necessary.
- Before the initial dose is given, hydration is started with 1–2 L IV infusion fluid to reduce risk of nephrotoxicity and ototoxicity.

### Intravenous

*PREPARE:* **IV Infusion:** Use disposable gloves when preparing cisplatin solutions. If drug accidentally contacts skin or mucosa, wash immediately and thoroughly with soap and water. ▪ Do not use any equipment containing aluminum. ▪ Withdraw required dose and dilute in 2 L D5W 5% dextrose in ½ or ⅓ normal saline containing 37.5 g mannitol.
*ADMINISTER:* **IV Infusion:** Give 2 L over 6–8 h.
*INCOMPATIBILITIES:* **Solution/additive: 5% dextrose, fluorouracil, mesna, metoclopramide, sodium bicarbonate, thiotepa. Y-site: Amifostine, amphotericin B, cholesteryl, cefepime, lansoprazole, piperacillin/ tazobactam, thiotepa, TPN.**

- Hydration and forced diuresis are continued for at least 24 h after drug administration to ensure adequate urinary output.

- Store at 15°–30° C (59°–86° F). Do not refrigerate. Protect from light. Once vial is opened, solution is stable for 28 days protected from light or 7 days in fluorescent light.

## ADVERSE EFFECTS (≥1%) **Body as a Whole:** Anaphylactic-like reactions. **CV:** Cardiac abnormalities. **GI:** *Marked nausea, vomiting,* anorexia, stomatitis, xerostomia, diarrhea, constipation. **Hematologic:** Myelosuppression (25–30% patients): Leukopenia, thrombocytopenia; hemolytic anemia, hemolysis. **Metabolic:** Hypocalcemia, *hypomagnesemia,* hyperuricemia, elevated AST, SIADH. **CNS:** Seizures, headache; peripheral neuropathies (may be irreversible): Paresthesia, unsteady gait, clumsiness of hands and feet, exacerbation of neuropathy with exercise, loss of taste. **Special Senses:** Ototoxicity (may be irreversible): Tinnitus, hearing loss, deafness, vertigo, blurred vision, changes in ability to see colors (optic neuritis, papilledema). **Urogenital:** Nephrotoxicity.

## INTERACTIONS **Drug:** AMINOGLYCOSIDES, **amphotericin B, vancomycin,** other **nephrotoxic drugs** increase nephrotoxicity and acute renal failure—try to separate by at least 1–2 wk; AMINOGLYCOSIDES, **furosemide** increase risk of ototoxicity.

## PHARMACOKINETICS **Peak:** Immediately after infusion. **Distribution:** Widely distributed in body fluids and tissues; concentrated in kidneys, liver, and prostate; accumulated in tissues. **Metabolism:** Not known. **Elimination:** 15–50% in urine within 24–48 h. **Half-Life:** 73–290 h.

## NURSING IMPLICATIONS

### Black Box Warning

*Cisplatin has been associated with severe renal toxicity, ototoxicity, and anaphylactic reactions.*

### Assessment & Drug Effects
- Obtain baseline ECG and cardiac monitoring during induction

Common adverse effects in *italic;* life-threatening effects underlined; generic names in **bold;** classifications in SMALL CAPS; ✦ Canadian drug name; ⊙ Prototype drug

365

therapy because of possible myocarditis or focal irritability.

- Monitor for anaphylactoid reactions (particularly in patient previously exposed to cisplatin), which may occur within minutes of drug administration.
- Audiometric testing should be performed before the first dose and before each subsequent dose. Ototoxicity (reported in 31% of patients) may occur after a single dose of 50 mg/m². Children who receive repeated doses are especially susceptible.
- Monitor closely for dose-related adverse reactions. Drug action is cumulative; therefore severity of most adverse effects (such as neurotoxicity) increases with repeated doses.
- Suspect ototoxicity if patient manifests tinnitus or difficulty hearing in the high frequency range.
- Monitor and report abnormal bowel elimination; diarrhea is a possible response to GI irritation.
- Inspect oral membranes for xerostomia (white patches and ulcerations) and tongue for signs of fungal overgrowth (black, furry appearance).
- Monitor lab tests: Baseline and before each cycle, renal function tests and serum electrolytes; weekly CBC with differential and platelet count; periodic LFTs.

### Patient & Family Education

- Continue maintenance of adequate hydration (at least 3000 mL/24 h oral fluid if prescriber agrees) and report promptly: Reduced urinary output, flank pain, anorexia, nausea, vomiting, dry mucosae, itching skin, urine odor on breath, fluid retention, and weight gain.
- Avoid rapid changes in position to minimize risk of dizziness or falling.
- Tingling, numbness, and tremors of extremities, loss of vision, sense, and taste, and constipation are

early signs of neurotoxicity. Report their occurrence promptly to prevent irreversibility.

- Report tinnitus or any hearing impairment.
- Report promptly evidence of unexplained bleeding and easy bruising.
- Report unusual fatigue, fever, sore mouth and throat, abnormal body discharges.

# CITALOPRAM HYDROBROMIDE

(cit-a-lo′pram)

Celexa

**Classification:** SELECTIVE SEROTONIN-REUPTAKE INHIBITOR (SSRI)
**Therapeutic:** ANTIDEPRESSANT
**Prototype:** Fluoxetine

**AVAILABILITY** Tablet; oral solution

**ACTION & *THERAPEUTIC EFFECT***
Selective serotonin reuptake inhibitor (SSRI) with an antidepressant effect presumed to be linked to its inhibition of CNS presynaptic neuronal uptake of serotonin. *Selective serotonin reuptake inhibition mechanism results in the antidepressant activity of citalopram.*

**USES** Depression.

**UNLABELED USES** Anxiety, hot flashes, obsessive-compulsive disorder, post-traumatic stress disorder, panic disorder.

**CONTRAINDICATIONS** Hypersensitivity to citalopram; unstable heart disease, congenital QT prolongation, recent MI; concurrent use of MAOIs or use within 14 days of discontinuing MAOIs; mania; volume depleted, hyponatremia; bipolar depression; suicidal ideation.

**CAUTIOUS USE** Hypersensitivity to other SSRIs; hepatic insufficiency; history of potential suicide; dehydration; severe renal impairment or renal failure; cardiovascular disease (e.g., dysrhythmias, conduction defects, myocardial ischemia); history of QT prolongation; history of drug abuse; history of seizure disorders or suicidal tendencies; history of mania; ECT treatments; narrow angle glaucoma; older adults; pregnancy (category C); lactation; children younger than 18 y.

## ROUTE & DOSAGE

**Depression**

*Adult:* **PO** Start at 20 mg daily, may increase to 40 mg daily if needed
*Geriatric:* **PO** 20 mg daily

## ADMINISTRATION

**Oral**

- Do not begin this drug within 14 days of stopping an MAOI.
- Reduced doses are advised for the older adult and those with hepatic or renal impairment.
- Dose increments should be separated by at least 1 wk.
- Store at 15°–30° C (59°–86° F) in a tightly closed container and protect from light.

**ADVERSE EFFECTS** (≥1%) **Body as a Whole:** Asthenia, fatigue, fever, arthralgia, myalgia, hyperhidrosis. **CV:** Tachycardia, postural hypotension, hypotension. **GI:** *Nausea,* vomiting, diarrhea, dyspepsia, abdominal pain, *dry mouth,* anorexia, flatulence. **CNS:** Dizziness, *insomnia, somnolence,* agitation, tremor, anxiety, paresthesia, migraine, neuromalignant syndrome. **Respiratory:** URI, rhinitis, sinusitis. **Skin:** Increased sweating. **Urogenital:** Dysmenorrhea, decreased libido, ejaculation disorder, impotence.

**INTERACTIONS Drug:** Combination with MAOIS could result in hypertensive crisis, hyperthermia, rigidity, myoclonus, autonomic instability; **cimetidine** may increase citalopram levels; **linezolid** may cause serotonin syndrome. Do not use with **bretylium**. **Herbal: St. John's wort** may cause serotonin syndrome.

**PHARMACOKINETICS Absorption:** Rapidly absorbed from GI tract; approximately 80% reaches systemic circulation. **Peak:** Steady-state serum concentrations in 1 wk; peak blood levels at 4 h. **Distribution:** 80% protein bound; crosses placenta; distributed into breast milk. **Metabolism:** In liver by CYP3A4 and CYP2C9 enzymes. **Elimination:** 20% in urine, 80% in bile. **Half-Life:** 35 h.

## NURSING IMPLICATIONS

**Black Box Warning**

*Citalopram has been associated with increased suicidal thinking and behavior especially in children, adolescents, and young adults.*

**Assessment & Drug Effects**

- Watch closely for worsening of depression or emergence of suicidal ideations.
- Monitor for therapeutic effectiveness: Indicated by elevation of mood; 1–4 wk may be needed before improvement is noted.
- Monitor periodically HR and BP, and carefully monitor complete cardiac status in person with known or suspected cardiac disease.

- Monitor closely older adult patients for adverse effects especially with doses greater than 20 mg/day.
- Monitor lab tests: Periodic LFTs, CBC, serum sodium; lithium levels when the two drugs are given concurrently.

**Patient & Family Education**

- Report immediately worsening of clinical condition, including suicidal ideation or other unusual changes in behavior.
- Do not engage in hazardous activities until reaction to this drug is known.
- Do not abruptly stop taking this drug. It should be gradually tapered to minimize withdrawal symptoms.
- Avoid using alcohol while taking citalopram.
- Report distressing adverse effects including any changes in sexual functioning or response.
- Periodic ophthalmology exams are advised with long-term treatment.

# CLADRIBINE
(cla'dri-been)
**Classifications:** ANTINEOPLASTIC; ANTIMETABOLITE, PURINE ANTAGONIST
Therapeutic: ANTINEOPLASTIC; ANTI-METABOLITE
**Prototype:** 6-Mercaptopurine

**AVAILABILITY** Solution for injection

## ACTION & *THERAPEUTIC EFFECT*
Cladribine is a synthetic antineoplastic agent with selective toxicity toward certain normal and malignant lymphocytes and monocytes. It accumulates intracellularly, preventing repair of single-stranded DNA breaks and ultimately interfering with cellular metabolism and DNA synthesis. *Cladribine is cytotoxic to both actively dividing and quiescent lymphocytes and monocytes, inhibiting both DNA synthesis and repair.*

**USES** Treatment of hairy cell leukemia.

**UNLABELED USES** Advanced cutaneous T-cell lymphomas, acute myeloid leukemia, autoimmune hemolytic anemia, mycosis fungoides, chronic lymphotic leukemia, non-Hodgkin's lymphomas.

**CONTRAINDICATIONS** Hypersensitivity to cladribine; severe bone marrow suppression; severe neurologic toxicity; acute nephrotoxicity; pregnancy (category D); lactation.

**CAUTIOUS USE** Hepatic or renal impairment; previous radiation therapy or chemotherapy; bone marrow depression. Safety and efficacy in children not established.

## ROUTE & DOSAGE

**Hairy Cell Leukemia**
*Adult:* **IV** 0.09–0.1 mg/kg/day by 7 days continuous infusion

## ADMINISTRATION
- Use disposable gloves and protective clothing when handling the drug.
- Wash immediately if skin contact occurs.

**Intravewnous**

*PREPARE:* **IV Infusion reservoir usually prepared by pharmacists as follows:** Add the calculated dose of cladribine through a sterile 0.22 micron disposable hydrophilic syringe filter to an infusion bag containing 500 mL of NS.

***ADMINISTER:*** **IV Infusion:** Give through a central line and control by a pump device.
***INCOMPATIBILITIES:*** **Solution/additive:** Do not mix with any other diluents or drugs.

▪ Diluted solutions of cladribine may be stored refrigerated for up to 8 h prior to administration. ▪ Store unopened vials in refrigerator [2°–8° C (36°–46° F)], and protect from light.

## ADVERSE EFFECTS (≥1%) CNS:
Headache, dizziness. **GI:** Nausea, diarrhea. **Hematologic:** *Myelosuppression (neutropenia), anemia, thrombocytopenia.* **Metabolic:** *Fever.* **CNS:** Headache, dizziness. **Urogenital:** Elevated serum creatinine. **Body as a Whole:** *infection, rash, fatigue.*

## INTERACTIONS Drug: Additive risk
of bleeding with ANTICOAGULANTS, NSAIDS, PLATELET INHIBITORS, SALICYLATES.

## PHARMACOKINETICS Onset:
Therapeutic effect 10 days to 4 mo. **Duration:** 7–25+ mo. **Distribution:** Crosses placenta; distributed into breast milk. **Metabolism:** In malignant leukocytes, cladribine is phosphorylated to active forms, which are subsequently incorporated into cellular DNA. **Half-Life:** Initial 35 min, terminal 6.7 h.

## NURSING IMPLICATIONS

### Black Box Warning

*Cladribine has been associated with severe bone marrow suppression and acute nephrotoxicity.*

### Assessment & Drug Effects
▪ Monitor vital signs during and after drug infusion. Fever (above 100° F) is common during the 5th to 7th day in patients with hairy cell leukemia, and severe fever (above 104° F) may develop within the first month of therapy.
▪ Closely monitor hematologic status; myelosuppression is common during the first month after starting therapy.
▪ Monitor for and report S&S of infection. Note that within the first month, fever may occur in the absence of infection.
▪ With high doses of cladribine, monitor for neurologic toxicity and acute nephrotoxicity.
▪ Monitor lab tests: Frequent hematologic studies; periodic serum creatinine and LFTs.

### Patient & Family Education
▪ Be fully informed regarding adverse responses to the drug.
▪ Understand the need for close follow-up during and after treatment with the drug.

## CLARITHROMYCIN
(clar′i-thro-my-sin)
**Biaxin, Biaxin XL**
**Classification:** MACROLIDE ANTIBIOTIC
**Therapeutic:** ANTIBIOTIC
**Prototype:** Erythromycin

## AVAILABILITY Tablet; sustained release tablet; oral suspension

## ACTION & *THERAPEUTIC EFFECT*
A semisynthetic macrolide antibiotic that binds to the 50S ribosomal subunit of susceptible bacterial organisms and, thereby, blocks RNA-mediated bacterial protein synthesis of bacteria. *It is active against both aerobic and anaerobic gram-positive and gram-negative organisms.*

## USES Treatment of upper respiratory,
lower respiratory infections; community-acquired pneumonia; acute maxil-

C

lary sinusitis; otitis media; and skin and soft tissue infections. Prevention and treatment of *Mycobacterium avium* complex (MAC) infections in patients with HIV. Used in combination for *Helicobacter pylori*.

## CONTRAINDICATIONS Hypersensitivity to clarithromycin, erythromycin, or any other macrolide antibiotics; history of cholestatic jaundice/hepatic dysfunction with previous use of clarithromycin; S&S of hepatitis; acute porphyria; congenital QT prolongation or history of QT prolongation; ventricular cardiac arrhythmia including torsades de pointes; viral infections.

## CAUTIOUS USE Renal impairment, older adults, GI disease, colitis; myasthenia gravis; pregnancy (category C); lactation. Safety and efficacy in infants younger than 6 mo not established.

## ROUTE & DOSAGE

### Mild to Moderate Infections

*Adult:* **PO** 250–500 mg b.i.d. × 7–14 days or 1000 mg XL daily for 7–14 days
*Child:* **PO** 7.5 mg/kg q12h

### MAC Infections (with Other Agents)

*Adult:* **PO** 500 mg q12h
*Child /Adolescent/Infant (6 mo or older):* **PO** 7.5 mg/kg q12h

### H. pylori Infections (with other medications)

*Adult:* **PO** 500 mg b.i.d.

### Renal Impairment Dosage Adjustment

*CrCl less than 30 mL/min:* Decrease dose by 50%

## ADMINISTRATION

### Oral

- Ensure that sustained release form of drug is not chewed or crushed. It **must be** swallowed whole.
- Shake suspension well before use.
- Store at 15°–30° C (59°–86° F).

## ADVERSE EFFECTS (≥1%) GI: Diarrhea, abdominal discomfort, nausea, abnormal taste, dyspepsia. **Hematologic:** Eosinophilia. **CNS:** Headache. **Skin:** Rash, urticaria.

## DIAGNOSTIC TEST INTERFERENCE May increase *serum AST* and *ALT levels.*

## INTERACTIONS Drug: May increase **theophylline** levels; drugs known to interact with **erythromycin** (i.e., **digoxin, carbamazepine, triazolam, warfarin, ergotamine, dihydroergotamine**) should be monitored carefully for increased levels and toxicity; **pimozide** may increase risk of arrhythmias. **Food: Grapefruit juice** increases risk of adverse effects.

## PHARMACOKINETICS Absorption: Readily from GI tract; 50% reaches the systemic circulation. **Peak:** 2–4 h. **Distribution:** Into most body tissue (excluding CNS); high pulmonary tissue concentrations. **Metabolism:** Partially in the liver; active 14-OH metabolite acts synergistically with the parent compound against *H. influenzae.* **Elimination:** 20% unchanged in urine; 10–15% of 14-OH metabolite excreted in urine. **Half-Life:** 3–5 h.

## NURSING IMPLICATIONS

### Assessment & Drug Effects

- Inquire about previous hypersensitivity to other macrolides (e.g., erythromycin) before treatment.
- Withhold drug and notify prescriber, if hypersensitivity occurs (e.g., rash, urticaria).

---

Common adverse effects in *italic;* life-threatening effects <u>underlined;</u> generic names in **bold;** classifications in SMALL CAPS; ♣ Canadian drug name; ⦿ Prototype drug

- Monitor for and report loose stools or diarrhea, since pseudomembranous colitis **must be** ruled out.
- When clarithromycin is given concurrently with anticoagulants, digoxin, or theophylline, blood levels of these drugs may be elevated. Monitor appropriate serum levels and assess for S&S of drug toxicity.

### Patient & Family Education
- Complete prescribed course of therapy.
- Report rash or other signs of hypersensitivity immediately.
- Report loose stools or diarrhea even after completion of drug therapy.

## CLEMASTINE FUMARATE

(klem'as-teen)

Tavist-1

**Classification:** ANTIHISTAMINE ($H_1$-RECEPTOR ANTAGONIST)
**Therapeutic:** ANTIHISTAMINE
**Prototype:** Diphenhydramine

**AVAILABILITY** Tablet; syrup

### ACTION & THERAPEUTIC EFFECT
An antihistamine ($H_1$-receptor antagonist) that competes for $H_1$-receptor sites on cells, thus blocking histamine effectiveness. Has greater selectivity for peripheral $H_1$-receptors and, consequently, it produces little sedation. Has prominent antipruritic activity and low incidence of unpleasant adverse effects. *Effective in controlling various allergic reactions (e.g., nasal congestion, sneezing, itching).*

**USES** Symptomatic relief of allergic rhinitis and mild uncomplicated allergic skin manifestations such as urticaria and angioedema.

**CONTRAINDICATIONS** Hypersensitivity to clemastine or to other antihistamines of similar chemical structure; lower respiratory tract symptoms, including acute asthma; concomitant MAOI therapy; closed-angle glaucoma; lactation.

**CAUTIOUS USE** History of bronchial asthma, COPD; increased intraocular pressure; GI or GU obstruction; hyperthyroidism; hepatic disease; cardiovascular disease, hypertension, older adults; pregnancy (category B). Safety and efficacy in children younger than 5 y not established.

## ROUTE & DOSAGE

### Allergic Rhinitis
*Adult:* **PO** 1.34 mg b.i.d., may increase up to 8.04 mg/day
*Child (6 y or older):* **PO** 0.67 mg b.i.d., may increase up to 4.02 mg/day; *younger than 6 y:* 0.335–0.67 mg/kg/day in 2 divided doses (max: 1.34 mg/day)

### Allergic Urticaria
*Adult:* **PO** 2.68 mg b.i.d. or t.i.d., may increase up to 8.04 mg/day
*Child:* **PO** 1.34 mg b.i.d., may increase up to 4.02 mg/day

## ADMINISTRATION

### Oral
- Drug may be administered with food, water, or milk to reduce possibility of gastric irritation.
- Older adult patients usually require less than average adult dose.
- Store at 15°–30° C (59°–86° F) unless otherwise directed.

**ADVERSE EFFECTS** (≥1%) **Body as a Whole:** <u>Anaphylaxis</u>, excess perspiration, chills. **CV:** Hypotension, palpitation, tachycardia, extrasystoles. **GI:** *Dry mouth,* epigastric distress, anorexia, nausea,

Common adverse effects in *italic;* life-threatening effects <u>underlined;</u> generic names in **bold;** classifications in SMALL CAPS; ♣ Canadian drug name; ⊘ Prototype drug

371

vomiting, diarrhea, constipation. **Hematologic:** Hemolytic anemia, thrombocytopenia, agranulocytosis. **CNS:** Sedation, *transient drowsiness,* dry nose and throat, headache, dizziness, weakness, fatigue, disturbed coordination; confusion, restlessness, nervousness, hysteria, convulsions, tremors, irritability, euphoria, insomnia, paresthesias, neuritis. **Respiratory:** Dry nose and throat, thickening of bronchial secretions, tightness of chest, wheezing, nasal stuffiness. **Skin:** Urticaria, rash, photosensitivity. **Special Senses:** Vertigo, tinnitus, acute labyrinthitis, blurred vision, diplopia. **Urogenital:** Difficult urination, urinary retention, early menses.

**INTERACTIONS Drug: Alcohol** and other CNS DEPRESSANTS increase sedation; MAO INHIBITORS may prolong and intensify anticholinergic effects.

**PHARMACOKINETICS Absorption:** Readily from GI tract. **Peak:** 5–7 h. **Duration:** 10–12 h. **Distribution:** Into breast milk. **Metabolism:** In liver. **Elimination:** In urine.

## NURSING IMPLICATIONS

### Assessment & Drug Effects

- Monitor for drowsiness, poor coordination, or dizziness, especially in the older adult or debilitated. Supervision of ambulation may be warranted.
- Assess for symptomatic relief with use of the medication.
- Monitor lab tests: Periodic hematologic studies with long-term use.

### Patient & Family Education

- Check with prescriber before taking alcohol or other CNS depressants, since effects may be additive.
- Clemastine may cause lethargy and drowsiness; therefore, necessary safety precautions should be taken.

- Older adults should make position changes slowly and in stages, particularly from recumbent to upright posture, as dizziness and hypotension occur more frequently than in younger patients.
- Avoid driving and other potentially hazardous activities until response to the drug has been established.

# CLEVIDIPINE BUTYRATE
(cle-vi-di′peen bu-ti′rate)
Cleviprex
**Classifications:** CALCIUM CHANNEL BLOCKER; ANTIHYPERTENSIVE
**Therapeutic:** ANTIHYPERTENSIVE
**Prototype:** Nifedipine

**AVAILABILITY** Emulsion for injection

**ACTION & *THERAPEUTIC EFFECT*** A calcium channel blocker that interferes with the influx of calcium during depolarization of arterial smooth muscle. Decreases systemic vascular resistance, thus lowering mean arterial pressure. *Decreases blood pressure.*

**USES** Treatment of hypertension, hypertensive emergency/urgency when oral administration is neither feasible nor desired.

**CONTRAINDICATIONS** Hypersensitivity to soybeans, soy products, eggs/egg products; defective lipid metabolism (e.g., pathologic hyperlipidemia, lipid nephrosis, acute pancreatitis); severe aortic stenosis.

**CAUTIOUS USE** Reflex tachycardia, hypotension, heart failure; lipid intake restriction; rebound hypertension following drug discontinuation; elderly; pregnancy (category C); lactation. Safety and efficacy in children not established.

Common adverse effects in *italic;* life-threatening effects underlined; generic names in **bold;** classifications in SMALL CAPS; ◆ Canadian drug name; ⊙ Prototype drug

## ROUTE & DOSAGE

### Hypertension

*Adult:* **IV** Initial dose of 1–2 mg/h. Titrate dose to desired BP: May initially double dose every 90 sec; as BP approaches goal, decrease dose increments to less than double the previous dose and lengthen time intervals between doses to q5–10min.

## ADMINISTRATION

**Intravenous**

*PREPARE:* **IV Infusion:** Supplied premixed, ready to use. Invert vial gently to produce a uniform emulsion.

*ADMINISTER:* **IV Infusion:** Use infusion device that permits calibrated rates. ▪ May infuse through a central or peripheral line using NS, D5W, D5W/NS, D5W/LR, LR, or 10% amino acid solution. ▪ Complete infusion within 12 h of entering vial.

*INCOMPATIBILITIES:* **Solution/additive:** Do not dilute in any IV solution. **Y-site:** Unknown; do not mix.

▪ Store refrigerated at 2°–8° C (36°–46° F). Do not return unopened vials to refrigeration once they have reached room temperature.

## ADVERSE EFFECTS (≥1%) CNS:
Headache. **CV:** Hypotension, reflex tachycardia. **GI:** Nausea, vomiting. **Other:** <u>Acute renal failure</u>.

## PHARMACOKINETICS Distribution: 99.5% plasma protein bound. **Metabolism:** In the plasma. **Elimination:** Renal (63–74%) and fecal (7–22%). **Half-Life:** 15 min.

## NURSING IMPLICATIONS

### Assessment & Drug Effects
▪ Monitor HR and BP continuously during infusion. Increases in HR

is a normal response to vasodilation and rebound hypertension may occur for at least 8 h after infusion is stopped.
▪ Monitor cardiac status continuously during infusion, especially with preexisting HF. Clevidipine may have a negative inotropic effect and exacerbate HF.

### Patient & Family Education
▪ Report promptly any of the following: Signs of heart failure; visual changes, weakness, or other signs of neurologic impairment.

## CLINDAMYCIN HYDROCHLORIDE ℗
(klin-da-mye'sin)
Cleocin, Dalacin C ♦

## CLINDAMYCIN PALMITATE HYDROCHLORIDE
Cleocin Pediatric

## CLINDAMYCIN PHOSPHATE
Cleocin Phosphate, Cleocin T, Dalacin C, Evoclin, Cleocin Vaginal Ovules or Cream

**Classification:** LINCOSAMIDE ANTIBIOTIC
**Therapeutic:** ANTIBIOTIC

**AVAILABILITY** Capsule; oral suspension; solution for injection; vaginal cream; suppository; gel, lotion; foam

## ACTION & *THERAPEUTIC EFFECT*
Suppresses protein synthesis by preventing peptide bond formation in bacterial ribosomes. *Particularly effective against susceptible strains of anaerobic streptococci as well as aerobic gram-positive cocci.*

**USES** Serious infections when less toxic alternatives are inappropriate. Topical applications are used

---

Common adverse effects in *italic;* life-threatening effects <u>underlined</u>; generic names in **bold;** classifications in SMALL CAPS; ♦ Canadian drug name; ℗ Prototype drug

**373**

in treatment of acne vulgaris. Vaginal applications are used in treatment of bacterial vaginosis in nonpregnant women.

**UNLABELED USES** In combination with pyrimethamine for toxoplasmosis in patients with AIDS.

**CONTRAINDICATIONS** History of hypersensitivity to clindamycin or lincomycin; meningitis; history of ulcerative colitis, or antibiotic-associated colitis; viral infection; UGI infections due to nonbacterial infections.

**CAUTIOUS USE** History of GI disease, severe hepatic disease; atopic individuals (history of eczema, asthma, hay fever); older adults; pregnancy (category B); lactation; children.

## ROUTE & DOSAGE

### Moderate to Severe Infections

*Adult:* **PO** 150–450 mg q6h; **IM/IV** 600–1200 mg/day in divided doses (max: 2700 mg/day)
*Child:* **PO** 8–20 mg/kg/day q6–8h; **IM/IV** 20–40 mg/kg/day in divided doses
*Neonate (7 days or younger, weight 2000 g or less):* **IM/IV** 10 mg/kg/day q12h; *7 days or younger, weight greater than 2000 g:* 15 mg/kg/day q8h; *7 days or older, weight less than 1200 g:* 10 mg/kg/day q12h; *7 days or older, weight 1200 g–2000 g:* 15 mg/kg/day q8h; *7 days or older, weight greater than 2000 g:* 20 mg/kg/day q6–8h

### Acne Vulgaris

*Adult:* **Topical** Apply to affected areas b.i.d.; 1% foam used for once daily application

### Bacterial Vaginosis

*Adult:* **Topical** Insert 1 suppository intravaginally at bedtime × 3 days, or insert 1 applicator full of cream intravaginally at bedtime × 7 days

## ADMINISTRATION

### Oral
- Administer clindamycin capsules with a full [240 mL (8 oz)] glass of water to prevent esophagitis. May administer with or without food.
- Note expiration date of oral solution; retains potency for 14 days at room temperature. Do not refrigerate, as chilling causes thickening and thus makes pouring it difficult.

### Topical
- Gel (except Clindagel), lotion, pledget, solution: Apply thin film twice daily to affected area. More than 1 pledget may be used.
- Clindagel, foam: Apply once daily to affected area.

### Intramuscular
- Deep IM injection is recommended. Rotate injection sites and observe daily for evidence of inflammatory reaction. Single IM doses should not exceed 600 mg.

### Intravenous
IV administration to neonates, infants, and children: Verify correct IV concentration and rate of infusion with prescriber.

*PREPARE:* **Intermittent: ADD-Vantage System:** Clindamycin may be reconstituted in 50 or 100 mL, respectively, of D5W or NS in the ADD diluent container. Refer to manufacturer's instructions for the ADD-Vantage system guidelines.
*ADMINISTER:* **Intermittent:** Never give a bolus dose. ▪ Do not give more than 1200 mg in a single

1-h infusion. ▪ Infusion rate should not exceed 30 mg/min.

**INCOMPATIBILITIES:** Solution/additive: **Aminophylline,** BARBITURATES, **calcium gluconate, ceftriaxone, ciprofloxacin, gentamicin, magnesium sulfate, ranitidine.** Y-site: **Allopurinol, amphotericin B, azathioprine, azithromycin, caspofungin, ceftriaxone, chlorpromazine, dantrolene, daunorubicin, diazepam, diazoxide, doxapram, filgrastim, fluconazole, ganciclovir, haloperidol, hydroxyzine, idarubicin, lansoprazole, minocycline, mitomycin, mitoxantrone, mycophenolate, oritavancin, papaverine, pentamidine, pentobarbital, phentolamine, phenytoin, prochlorperazine, promethazine, quinidine, quinupristin/dalfopristin, SMZ/TMP, temocillin.**

▪ Store in tight containers at 15° 30° C (59°–86° F) unless otherwise directed.

## ADVERSE EFFECTS (≥1%) Body as a Whole:

Fever, serum sickness, sensitization, swelling of face (following topical use), generalized myalgia, superinfections, proctitis, vaginitis, pain, induration, sterile abscess (following IM injections); thrombophlebitis (IV infusion). **CV:** Hypotension (following IM), <u>cardiac arrest</u> (rapid IV). **GI:** *Diarrhea,* abdominal pain, flatulence, bloating, *nausea, vomiting,* <u>pseudomembranous colitis;</u> esophageal irritation, loss of taste, medicinal taste (high IV doses), jaundice, abnormal liver function tests. **Hematologic:** <u>Leukopenia,</u> eosinophilia, <u>agranulocytosis, thrombocytopenia.</u> **Skin:** *Skin rashes,* urticaria, pruritus, dryness, contact dermatitis, gram-negative folliculitis, irritation, oily skin.

## DIAGNOSTIC TEST INTERFERENCE

Clindamycin may cause increases in *serum alkaline phosphatase, bilirubin, creatine phosphokinase (CPK)* from muscle irritation following IM injection; *AST, ALT.*

## INTERACTIONS Drug:

**Chloramphenicol, erythromycin** possibly are mutually antagonistic to clindamycin; neuromuscular blocking action enhanced by NEUROMUSCULAR BLOCKING AGENTS (**atracurium, tubocurarine, pancuronium**).

## PHARMACOKINETICS Absorption:

Approximately 90% absorbed from GI tract; 10% of topical application is absorbed through skin. **Peak:** 45–60 min PO; 3 h IM. **Duration:** 6 h PO; 8–12 h IM. **Distribution:** Widely distributed except for CNS; crosses placenta; distributed into breast milk. **Metabolism:** In liver. **Elimination:** In urine and feces. **Half-Life:** 2–3 h.

## NURSING IMPLICATIONS

### Black Box Warning

*Clindamycin has been associated with severe, potentially fatal, Clostridium difficile-associated diarrhea (CDAD)*

### Assessment & Drug Effects

▪ Monitor BP and pulse in patients receiving drug parenterally. Hypotension has occurred following IM injection. Advise patient to remain recumbent following drug administration until BP has stabilized.

▪ Severe diarrhea and colitis, including pseudomembranous colitis (i.e., *Clostridium difficile*-associated diarrhea or CDAD), have been associated with oral (highest incidence), parenteral, and topical clindamycin. Report immediately the onset of watery diarrhea, with or without fever. Symptoms may appear within a few days to

2 wk after therapy is begun or up to several weeks following cessation of therapy.

- Be alert to signs of superinfection (see Appendix F).
- Be alert for signs of anaphylactoid reactions (see Appendix F), which require immediate attention.
- Monitor lab tests: Baseline C&S; periodic CBC with differential, LFTs, and renal function tests.

**Patient & Family Education**

- Report loose stools or diarrhea promptly.
- Stop drug therapy if significant diarrhea develops (more than 5 loose stools daily) and notify prescriber.
- Do not self-medicate with antidiarrheal preparations. Antiperistaltic agents may prolong and worsen diarrhea by delaying removal of toxins from colon.

## CLOBETASOL PROPIONATE

(cloe-bay'ta-sol)

Clobex, Temovate, Embeline gel; Olux Foam

**See Appendix A-4.**

## CLOBAZAM

(kloe' ba zam)

Onfi

**Classifications:** BENZODIAZEPINE; ANTICONVULSANT
**Therapeutic:** ANTICONVULSANT
**Prototype:** Diazepam
**Controlled Substance:** Schedule IV

**AVAILABILITY** Tablet; oral suspension

## ACTION & *THERAPEUTIC EFFECT*

Mechanism of action believed to involve potentiation of GABAergic neurotransmission resulting from binding at the benzodiazepine site of the GABA$_A$ receptor. *Helps inhibit development of seizures associated with Lennox-Gastaut syndrome.*

**USES** Adjunctive treatment of seizures associated with Lennox-Gastaut syndrome (LGS)

**CONTRAINDICATIONS** Hypersensitivity to clobazam; severe hepatic impairment; signs and symptoms of Stevens–Johnson syndrome; suicidal ideation; lactation.

**CAUTIOUS USE** Hepatic impairment; severe renal impairment; history of substance abuse; history of suicidal thoughts or behaviors; pregnancy (category C); depression; drug withdrawal; older adults. Safety and efficacy in patients younger than 2 y not established.

## ROUTE & DOSAGE

**Adjunctive Treatment of Seizures**

*Adult and Children (2 y or older, weight over 30 kg):* **PO** 5 mg b.i.d., increase to 10 mg b.i.d. on day 7, then increase to 20 mg b.i.d. on day 14.; *weight 30 kg or less:* 5 mg once daily, increase to 5 mg b.i.d., on day 7, then increase to 10 mg b.i.d. on day 14

*Geriatric Patients (weight greater than 30 kg):* Use normal dose regimen; may increase to 20 mg b.i.d. on day 21; *weight 30 kg or less:* Initial dose of 5 mg once daily, increase to 5 mg b.i.d. on day 14, then increase to 10 mg b.i.d.

***Pharmacogenetic Dosage Adjustment***

*Poor CYP2C19 metabolizers:* Starting dose should be 5 mg/day; dose titration should proceed slowly according to weight, but to half the normal dose regimen. If necessary, additional titration to the 20 mg/day or 40 mg/day (depending on weight) may be started on day 21.

**Hepatic Impairment Dosage Adjustment**

*Mild to moderate impairment (Child-Pugh score 5 to 9):* Use geriatric dosing regimen

*Severe impairment:* Not recommended

## ADMINISTRATION

### Oral

- May give tablet whole or crushed and mixed in applesauce.
- Oral suspension: Insert provided adapter firmly into neck of bottle before first use and keep in place throughout use. Shake bottle well before every use. Use only the dosing syringe provided to measure dose.
- Give without regard to timing of meals.
- Abrupt discontinuation of this drug should be avoided. Drug should be tapered off by decreasing the daily dose every week by 5 to 10 mg.
- Store at 20° –25° C (68° – 77° F).

**ADVERSE EFFECTS** (≥5%) **Body as a Whole:** Fatigue, irritability, *pyrexia*. **CNS:** Aggresion, ataxia, drooling, dysarthria, insomnia, *lethargy*, psychomotor hyperactivity, sedation, *somnolence*. **GI:** Constipation, anorexia, dysphagia, *vomiting*. **Metabolic:** Alterations in appetite. **Respiratory:** Bronchitis, cough, pneumonia, upper respiratory tract infection. **Urogenital:** Urinary tract infection.

**INTERACTIONS Drug:** Clobazam may decrease the effectiveness of ORAL CONTRACEPTIVES and other drugs requiring CYP2D6 (e.g., **metoprolol, propranolol, aripiprazole, clozapine**). Strong and moderate inhibitors of CYP2C19 (e.g., **fluconazole, fluvoxamine, ticlopidine, omeprazole**) may result in increased levels of the active metabolite of clobazam. **Ethanol** increases the maximum plasma exposure of clobazam by 50%.

**PHARMACOKINETICS Absorption:** Approximately 100% bioavailable. **Peak:** 0.5–4 h. **Distribution:** 80–90% plasma protein bound. **Metabolism:** Extensive hepatic oxidation to active and inactive metabolites. **Elimination:** Renal (82%) and fecal (11%). **Half-Life:** 36–42 h.

## NURSING IMPLICATIONS

### Assessment & Drug Effects

- Monitor for adverse CNS effects (e.g., somnolence, sedation, new or worsening depression, impaired judgment, impaired motor skills), especially when used concurrently with other CNS depressants.
- Monitor for and report promptly suicidal thoughts or behaviors, or thoughts of self-harm.
- Monitor lab tests: Baseline and periodic LFTs.

### Patient & Family Education

- Promptly notify prescriber of suicidal ideation or thoughts of self-harm.
- Avoid potentially hazardous tasks, such as driving, until response to the drug is known.
- Do not drink alcohol while taking colbazam.
- Abruptly stopping colbazam may increase the risk of seizure activity.
- Women of childbearing age who use hormonal contraceptives should use alternative non-hormonal methods during and for 28 days after discontinuing colbazam.

---

Common adverse effects in *italic*; life-threatening effects underlined; generic names in **bold**; classifications in SMALL CAPS; ♣Canadian drug name; ⊕ Prototype drug

- Notify prescriber immediately if you become pregnant or intend to become pregnant, or if you are breast-feeding or intend to breast feed.

## CLOCORTOLONE PIVALATE
(kloe-kor'toe-lone)

Cloderm

**See Appendix A-4.**

## CLOFARABINE
(clo-fa-ra'been)

Clolar

**Classifications:** ANTINEOPLASTIC; PURINE ANTIMETABOLITE
Therapeutic: ANTINEOPLASTIC
**Prototype:** 6-Mercaptopurine

**AVAILABILITY** Solution for injection

**ACTION & *THERAPEUTIC EFFECT***
Clofarabine inhibits DNA repair within cancer cells, thus interfering with mitosis; it also disrupts the mitochondrial membrane, leading to cancer cell death. *Cytotoxic to rapidly proliferating and quiescent cancer cells.*

**USES** Relapsed or refractory acute lymphocytic leukemia (ALL) after at least 2 prior regimens.

**CONTRAINDICATIONS** Severe bone marrow suppression; active infection; venous occlusive liver disease; severe hepatotoxicity; pregnancy (category D); lactation.

**CAUTIOUS USE** Renal or hepatic function impairment; thrombocytopenia; neutropenia; previous chemotherapy or radiation therapy; history of viral infections such as herpes; history of cardiac disease or hypotension; females of childbearing age; older adults.

## ROUTE & DOSAGE

**Acute Lymphocytic Leukemia**
*Adolescent/Child:* **IV** 52 mg/m²/day for 5 days q2-6w

**Renal Impairment Dosage Adjustment**
*CrCl 30–60 mL/min:* Reduce dose by 50%

**Toxicity Dosage Adjustment**
*Grade 4 neutropenia lasting at least 4 wk:* Reduce dose by 50%

## ADMINISTRATION

- Do not give drugs with known renal toxicity during the 5 days of clofarabine administration.

**Intravenous**

***PREPARE:* IV Infusion:** Withdraw required dose from vial using a 0.2 micron filter syringe. ▪ Further dilute in 100 mL or more of D5W or NS prior to infusion to a final concentration between 0.15 and 0.4 mg/mL.
***ADMINISTER:* IV Infusion:** Give over 2 h.

- Store diluted solution at room temperature. Use within 24 h of mixing.

**ADVERSE EFFECTS** (≥1%) **CNS:** Anxiety, depression, dizziness, headache, irritability, somnolence. **CV:** *Tachycardia,* pericardial infusion, left ventricular systolic dysfunction (LSVT). **GI:** *Vomiting, nausea,* and *diarrhea,* abdominal pain, constipation. **Hematologic/Lymphatic:** *Anemia, leukopenia, thrombocytopenia,* neutropenia, febrile neutropenia. **Hepatic:** Jaundice, hepatomegaly. **Metabolic:** Anorexia, decreased appetite, edema, decreased weight. **Muscu-**

---

Common adverse effects in *italic;* life-threatening effects <u>underlined;</u> generic names in **bold;** classifications in SMALL CAPS; ♣ Canadian drug name; ❷ Prototype drug

**loskeletal:** Arthralgia, back pain, myalgia. **Respiratory:** Cough, dyspnea, epistaxis, pleural effusion, respiratory distress. **Skin:** Dermatitis, contusion, dry skin, erythema, palmar-plantar erythrodysesthesia syndrome, pruritus. **Body as a Whole:** Increased risk of infection.

## PHARMACOKINETICS
**Distribution:** 47% protein bound. **Metabolism:** Negligible. **Elimination:** Primarily unchanged in the urine. **Half-Life:** 5.2 h.

## NURSING IMPLICATIONS

### Assessment & Drug Effects
- Monitor vital signs frequently during infusion of clofarabine
- Monitor closely for S&S of capillary leak syndrome or systemic inflammatory response syndrome (e.g., tachypnea, tachycardia, hypotension, pulmonary edema). If either is suspected, immediately DC IV, institute supportive measures and notify prescriber.
- Monitor I&O rates and pattern and watch for S&S of dehydration, including dizziness, lightheadedness, fainting spells, or decreased urine output.
- Withhold drug and notify prescriber if hypotension develops for any reason during 5-day period of drug administration.
- Monitor lab tests. Baseline and periodic CBC and platelet counts; frequent LFTs and renal function tests during therapy.

### Patient & Family Education
- Report any distressing adverse effect of therapy to prescriber.
- Use effective measures to avoid pregnancy while taking this drug.

## CLOMIPHENE CITRATE
(kloe'mi-feen)

Clomid, Milophene, Serophene

**Classifications:** OVULATION STIMULANT; NONSTEROID SELECTIVE ESTROGEN RECEPTOR MODULATOR (SERM)
**Therapeutic:** OVULATION STIMULANT; ANTIESTROGENIC

**AVAILABILITY** Tablet

## ACTION & THERAPEUTIC EFFECT
Induces ovulation in selected infrequently ovulating or anovulatory women, blocking the normal negative feedback of circulating estradiol on the hypothalamus, thus preventing estrogen from lowering the output of gonadotropin releasing hormone (GnRH). *Stimulates pituitary release of luteinizing hormone (LH), follicle-stimulating hormone (FSH) and gonadotropins, leading to ovarian stimulation.*

**USES** Infertility in appropriately selected women desiring pregnancy whose partners are fertile and potent.

**UNLABELED USES** Male infertility, menstrual abnormalities, gynecomastia, fibrocystic breast disease, regulation of cycles in patients using rhythm method of contraception, endometrial hyperplasia, persistent lactation.

**CONTRAINDICATIONS** Neoplastic lesions, ovarian cyst; hepatic disease or dysfunction; abnormal uterine bleeding; endometriosis; primary ovarian failure; men with testicular failure; untreated thyroid disease; visual abnormalities; major depression or psychosis; thrombophlebitis; pregnancy (category X); lactation.

**CAUTIOUS USE** Polycystic ovarian enlargement, pelvic discomfort, sensitivity to pituitary gonadotropins.

Common adverse effects in *italic;* life-threatening effects underlined; generic names in **bold;** classifications in SMALL CAPS; ♣ Canadian drug name; ⊘ Prototype drug

379

C

## ROUTE & DOSAGE

### Infertility

Adult: **PO** First course: 50 mg/day for 5 days; start on 5th day of cycle following start of spontaneous or induced bleeding (with progestin) or at any time in the patient who has had no recent uterine bleeding Second course if ovulation: Repeat first course until conception or for 3 cycles Second course if no ovulation: 100 mg/day for 5 days as above (max: 100 mg/day)

## ADMINISTRATION

### Oral

- Each course of therapy should start on or about the 5th cycle day once ovulation has been established.
- Store at 15°–30° C (59°–86° F) in tightly capped, light-resistant container.

## ADVERSE EFFECTS (≥1%) **Body as a Whole:** *Vasomotor flushes,* breast discomfort, abdominal pain, heavy menses, exacerbation of endometriosis; mental depression, headache, fatigue, insomnia, dizziness, vertigo. **GI:** Nausea, vomiting, increased appetite with weight gain, constipation, bloating. **Endocrine:** Spontaneous abortion, multiple ovulations, ovarian failure, *ovarian hyperstimulation syndrome, enlarged ovaries with multiple follicular cysts.* **Special Senses:** Transient blurring, diplopia, scotomas, photophobia, floaters, prolonged after-images. **Urogenital:** Urinary frequency, polyuria.

## DIAGNOSTIC TEST INTERFERENCE

Clomiphene may increase BSP retention; **plasma transcortin, thyroxine** and **sex hormone binding globulin** levels. Also increases **follicle-stimulating** and **luteinizing hormone** secretion in most patients.

## INTERACTIONS **Herbal:** **Black cohosh** may antagonize infertility treatments.

## PHARMACOKINETICS **Absorption:** Readily absorbed from GI tract. **Metabolism:** In liver. **Elimination:** Primarily in feces in 5 days; the remainder is excreted slowly from enterohepatic pool or is stored in body fat for later release. **Half-Life:** 5 days.

## NURSING IMPLICATIONS

### Assessment & Drug Effects

- Monitor for abnormal bleeding. Report it immediately.
- Monitor for visual disturbances. Their occurrence indicates the need for a complete ophthalmologic evaluation. Drug will be stopped until symptoms subside.
- Pelvic pain indicates the need for immediate pelvic examination for diagnostic purposes.

### Patient & Family Education

- Take the medicine at same time every day to maintain drug levels and prevent forgetting a dose.
- Missed dose: Take drug as soon as possible. If not remembered until time for next dose, double the dose, then resume regular dosing schedule. If more than one dose is missed, check with prescriber.
- Report these symptoms: Hot flushes resembling those associated with menopause; nausea, vomiting, headache.
- Report promptly yellowing of eyes, light-colored stools, yellow, itchy skin, and fever symptomatic of jaundice.
- Stop taking clomiphene if pregnancy is suspected.
- Because of the possibility of lightheadedness, dizziness, and visual disturbances, do not perform

Common adverse effects in *italic*; life-threatening effects <u>underlined</u>; generic names in **bold**; classifications in SMALL CAPS; ✦ Canadian drug name; ⊕ Prototype drug hazardous tasks requiring skill and coordination in an environment with variable lighting.

- Report promptly excessive weight gain, signs of edema, bloating, decreased urinary output.
- If clomiphene is continued more than 1 y, patient should have an ophthalmologic examination at regular intervals.

# CLOMIPRAMINE HYDROCHLORIDE

(clo-mi'pra-meen)

Anafranil

**Classification:** TRICYCLIC ANTIDEPRESSANT
Therapeutic: ANTIPSYCHOTIC
**Prototype:** Imipramine

**AVAILABILITY** Capsule

**ACTION & THERAPEUTIC EFFECT** Inhibits reuptake of norepinephrine and serotonin at the presynaptic neuron. *The basis of its antidepressant effects is thought to be due to the elevated serum levels of norepinephrine and serotonin.*

**USES** Obsessive-compulsive disorder (OCD).

**UNLABELED USES** Panic disorder, autism, agoraphobia, depression.

**CONTRAINDICATIONS** Hypersensitivity to other tricyclic compounds and carbamazepine; MAOI therapy; acute recovery period after MI, QT elongation, cardiac arrhythmias (AV block, bundle-branch block); suicidal ideation.

**CAUTIOUS USE** History of convulsive disorders, prostatic hypertrophy, urinary retention, cardiovascular, hepatic, GI, or blood disorders; history

of seizure disorder; respiratory depression; diabetes mellitus; GERD; Parkinson's disease; closed-angle glaucoma; asthma; bipolar disorder; history of suicidal tendencies; older adults; pregnancy (category C); lactation; children younger than 10 y.

## ROUTE & DOSAGE

### Obsessive-Compulsive Disorder

*Adult:* **PO** 25 mg daily, gradually increase to 100 mg daily as tolerated over 2 wk, (max: 250 mg/day)
*Adolescent/Child (10 y or older):* **PO** 25 mg daily, gradually increase to 100 mg daily or 3 mg/kg (whichever is less) in divided doses as tolerated over 2 wk, then up to 200 mg or 3 mg/kg daily (whichever is less)

### *Pharmacogenetic Dosage Adjustment*

Poor CYP2D6 metabolizers should receive 60% of normal dose

## ADMINISTRATION

### Oral

- Give with meals to reduce GI adverse effects.
- Following titration to the full dose, drug may be given as a single dose at bedtime to reduce daytime sedation.
- Store at 15°–30° C (59°–86° F).

**ADVERSE EFFECTS** (≥1%) **Body as a Whole:** Diaphoresis. **CV:** Hypotension, tachycardia. **GI:** Constipation, *dry mouth*. **Endocrine:** Galactorrhea, hyperprolactinemia, amenorrhea, *weight gain,* change in libido. **Hematologic:** Leukopenia, agranulocytosis, thrombocytopenia, anemia. **CNS:** Mania, *tremor,* drowsiness, headache, insomnia,

Common adverse effects in *italic;* life-threatening effects underlined; generic names in **bold;** classifications in SMALL CAPS; ◆Canadian drug name; ⊕ Prototype drug

381

fatigue, dizziness, hyperthermia, neuroleptic malignant syndrome, seizures (especially with abrupt withdrawal). **Urogenital:** Delayed ejaculation, anorgasmia. **Respiratory:** Pharyngitis, rhinitis.

## DIAGNOSTIC TEST INTERFERENCE

Increased glucose may interfere with urine detection of **methadone.**

## INTERACTIONS Drug: MAO INHIBITORS

may precipitate hyperpyrexic crisis, tachycardia, or seizures; ANTIHYPERTENSIVE AGENTS potentiate orthostatic hypotension; CNS DEPRESSANTS, **alcohol** add to CNS depression; **norepinephrine** and other SYMPATHOMIMETICS may increase cardiac toxicity; **cimetidine** decreases hepatic metabolism, thus increasing imipramine levels; **methylphenidate** inhibits metabolism of **imipramine** and thus may increase its toxicity; **amoxapine** may increase risk of side effects. Do not use with **doeftilide, dronedarone,** or **ziprasidone** due to increased risk of QT prolongation. **Herbal: Ginkgo** may decrease seizure threshold; **St. John's wort** may cause serotonin syndrome.

## PHARMACOKINETICS Absorption:

Rapidly from GI tract; 20–78% reaches systemic circulation. **Onset:** Approx 4–10 wk. **Peak:** 2–6 h. **Distribution:** Widely distributed including the CSF; crosses placenta. **Metabolism:** Extensive first-pass metabolism in the liver; active metabolite is desmethylclomipramine. **Elimination:** 50–60% in urine, 24–32% in feces. **Half-Life:** 36 h.

## NURSING IMPLICATIONS

### Black Box Warning

*Clomipramine has been associated with increased suicidal thinking and behavior especially in children, adolescents, and young adults.*

### Assessment & Drug Effects

- Monitor for and report promptly suicidal thinking and behavior.
- Monitor for seizures, especially in those with predisposing factors or concurrent therapy with other drugs that lower seizure threshold.
- Monitor for and report signs of neuroleptic malignant syndrome (see Appendix F).
- Monitor for sedation and vertigo, especially at the beginning of therapy and following dosage increases. Supervision of ambulation may be indicated.
- Notify prescriber of fever and complaints of sore throat since these may indicate need to rule out adverse hematologic changes.
- Taper dosage slowly when discontinuing.
- Monitor lab tests: Periodic CBC with differential, platelet count, and Hct and Hgb. Periodic LFTs, especially with long-term therapy.

### Patient & Family Education

- Discontinue drug and report promptly to prescriber if suicidal ideation or behavior occurs.
- Do not take nonprescribed drugs or discontinue therapy without consent of prescriber. Abrupt discontinuation may cause nausea, headache, malaise, or seizures.
- Men should understand that the drug may cause impotence or ejaculation failure.
- Report promptly a sore throat accompanied by fever.
- Use caution with ambulation until response to drug is known.
- Moderate alcohol intake since it may potentiate adverse drug effects.

C

# CLONAZEPAM

(kloe-na'zi-pam)

Klonopin, Klonopin Wafers,
Rivotril ✦

**Classifications:** ANTICONVULSANT;
BENZODIAZEPINE
Therapeutic: ANTICONVULSANT;
ANTIANXIETY
**Prototype:** Diazepam
**Controlled Substance:** Schedule IV

**AVAILABILITY** Tablet; orally disintegrating wafer

## ACTION & *THERAPEUTIC EFFECT*

Benzodiazepine derivative with strong anticonvulsant activity that prevents seizures by potentiating the effects of GABA, an inhibitory neurotransmitter. Suppresses spread of seizure activity in the cortex, thalamus, and limbic regions of the brain. *Suppresses spike and wave discharge in absence seizures (petit mal) and decreases amplitude, frequency, duration, and spread of discharge in minor motor seizures.*

**USES** Alone or with other drugs in absence, myoclonic, and akinetic seizures, Lennox-Gastaut syndrome, absence seizures, panic disorder.

**UNLABELED USES** Insomnia, nystagmus, restless leg syndrome, complex partial seizure pattern, and generalized tonic-clonic convulsions.

**CONTRAINDICATIONS** Hypersensitivity to benzodiazepines; significant liver disease; acute narrow-angle glaucoma; pulmonary disease; coma or CNS depression; suicidal ideation; pregnancy (category D).

**CAUTIOUS USE** Renal or hepatic impairment; COPD; drug-controlled open-angle glaucoma; bipolar disorder, preexisting depression; history of suicidal thoughts; addiction-prone individuals; neuromuscular disease; mixed seizure disorders; debilitated individuals; older adults; children younger than 10 y; lactation.

## ROUTE & DOSAGE

### Seizures

*Adult/Adolescent (weight greater than 30 kg):* **PO** 1.5 mg/day in 3 divided doses, increased by 0.5–1 mg q3days until seizures are controlled or until intolerable adverse effects (max recommended dose: 20 mg/day)
*Child (younger than 10 y, weight 30 kg or less):* **PO** 0.01–0.03 mg/kg/day (not to exceed 0.05 mg/kg/day) in 3 divided doses; may increase by 0.25–0.5 mg q3days until seizures are controlled or until intolerable adverse effects (max recommended dose: 0.2 mg/kg/day)

### Panic Disorders

*Adult,* **PO** 0.25 mg b.i.d. initially, increase to 1 mg/day (max: 4 mg/day)

## ADMINISTRATION

### Oral

- Give largest dose at bedtime if daily dose cannot be equally divided.
- Place wafer form on tongue to dissolve.
- May be swallowed with or without water.
- Store in tightly closed container protected from light at 15°–30° C (59°–86° F) unless otherwise specified.

## ADVERSE EFFECTS (≥1%) CV:
Palpitations. **GI:** Dry mouth, sore gums, anorexia, coated tongue, increased salivation, increased

---

Common adverse effects in *italic;* life-threatening effects underlined; generic names in **bold;** classifications in SMALL CAPS; ✦Canadian drug name; ⓟ Prototype drug appetite, nausea, constipation, diarrhea. **Hematologic:** Anemia, leukopenia, thrombocytopenia, eosinophilia. **CNS:** *Drowsiness, sedation, ataxia,* insomnia, aphonia, choreiform movements, coma, dysarthria, "glassy-eyed" appearance, headache, hemiparesis, hypotonia, slurred speech, tremor, vertigo, confusion, depression, hallucinations, aggressive behavior problems, hysteria, suicide attempt. **Respiratory:** Chest congestion, respiratory depression, rhinorrhea, dyspnea, hypersecretion in upper respiratory passages. **Skin:** Hirsutism, hair loss, skin rash, ankle and facial edema. **Special Senses:** Diplopia, nystagmus, abnormal eye movements. **Urogenital:** Decreased libido, dysuria, enuresis, nocturia, urinary retention.

## DIAGNOSTIC TEST INTERFERENCE

Clonazepam causes transient elevations of *serum transaminase* and *alkaline phosphatase.*

## INTERACTIONS **Drug: Alcohol**

and other CNS DEPRESSANTS increase sedation and CNS depression; may increase **phenytoin** levels. CYP34A inhibitors may increase risk of toxicity. **Herbal: Kava, valerian** may potentiate sedation. Avoid use with marijuana due to exaggerated sedation.

## PHARMACOKINETICS **Absorption:** Readily absorbed from GI tract. **Onset:** 60 min. **Peak:** 1–2 h. **Duration:** Up to 12 h in adults; 6–8 h in children. **Distribution:** Crosses placenta; distributed into breast milk. **Metabolism:** In liver. **Elimination:** In urine primarily as metabolites. **Half-Life:** 18–40 h.

## NURSING IMPLICATIONS
### Assessment & Drug Effects
- Monitor for signs of suicidal ideation in depressive individuals.
- Both psychological and physical dependence may occur in the patient on long-term, high-dose therapy.
- Monitor for S&S of overdose, including somnolence, confusion, irritability, sweating, muscle and abdominal cramps, diminished reflexes, coma.
- Monitor lab tests: Periodic LFTs, platelet count, blood count, and renal function tests.

### Patient & Family Education
- Report loss of seizure control promptly. Anticonvulsant activity is often lost after 3 mo of therapy; dosage adjustment may reestablish efficacy.
- Do not abruptly discontinue this drug. Abrupt withdrawal can precipitate seizures. Other withdrawal symptoms include convulsion, tremor, abdominal and muscle cramps, vomiting, sweating.
- Do not drive a car or engage in other activities requiring mental alertness and physical coordination until reaction to the drug is known. Drowsiness occurs in approximately 50% of patients.

## CLONIDINE HYDROCHLORIDE
(kloe′ni-deen)

Catapres, Catapres-TTS, Dixaril ◆, Duraclon, Kapvay

**Classifications:** ANTIADRENERGIC; CENTRAL-ACTING ANTIHYPERTENSIVE; ANALGESIC
Therapeutic: ANTIHYPERTENSIVE; ANALGESIC
**Prototype:** Methyldopa

**AVAILABILITY** Tablet; transdermal patch; solution for injection; extended release tablet

## ACTION & *THERAPEUTIC EFFECT*

Centrally acting receptor agonist that stimulates alpha$_2$-adrenergic receptors in CNS to inhibit sympathetic cardioaccelerator and vasomotor centers. Central actions reduce plasma concentrations of norepinephrine. It decreases systolic and diastolic BP and heart rate. *Decreases systolic and diastolic BP and heart rate. Reportedly minimizes or eliminates many of the common clinical S&S associated with withdrawal of heroin, methadone, or other opiates.*

**USES** Hypertension, treatment of severe pain, ADHD.

**UNLABELED USES** Prophylaxis for migraine; treatment of dysmenorrhea, menopausal flushing, diarrhea, paroxysmal localized hyperhidroses; neuropathic pain; alcohol, smoking, opiate, and benzodiazepine withdrawal; Tourette's syndrome.

**CONTRAINDICATIONS** Hypersensitivity to clonidine; first line treatment of hypertension; coagulopathy. **Extended release:** Children younger than 6 y. **Patch:** Polyarteritis nodosa, scleroderma, SLE on affected areas. **Epidural:** Severe cardiovascular disease, or those who are hemodynamically unstable; infection at injection site; obstetric, postpartum, perioperative pain management; use above the C$_4$ dermatome.

**CAUTIOUS USE** Severe coronary insufficiency, recent MI, sinus node dysfunction, cerebrovascular disease; diabetes mellitus; renal impairment; chronic renal failure; Raynaud's disease, thromboangiitis obliterans; history of hypotension, heart block, bradycardia, or CVD; history of syncope; history of depression; addictive disorders; older adults; pregnancy (category C); lactation; children younger than 12 y. **Extended release:** children younger than 18 y and over 6 y. Adult use in ADHD of **Clonidine ER** has not been studied.

## ROUTE & DOSAGE

### Hypertension

*Adult:* **PO** 0.1 mg b.i.d., may increase by 0.1–0.2 mg/day until desired response is achieved (max: 2.4 mg/day); **Transdermal** 0.1 mg patch once q7days, may increase by 0.1 mg q1–2wk; **Extended release** 0.1 mg daily
*Geriatric:* **PO** Start with 0.1 mg once daily
*Child (12 years or older):* **PO** 0.2–0.6 mg/day in divided doses

### Severe Pain

*Adult:* **Epidural** Start infusion at 30 mcg/h and titrate to response. Use rates greater than 40 mcg/h with caution
*Child:* **Epidural** Start infusion at 0.5 mcg/kg/h and titrate to response.

### ADHD

*Adolescent/Child (6 y or older):* **PO Extended release** 0.1 mg qhs increase weekly to desired response

## ADMINISTRATION

### Oral

- Ensure that extended release tablets are swallowed whole. They should not be crushed or chewed.
- Give last PO dose immediately before patient retires to ensure overnight BP control and to minimize daytime drowsiness.
- Oral dosage is increased gradually over a period of weeks so as not

Common adverse effects in *italic;* life-threatening effects underlined; generic names in **bold;** classifications in SMALL CAPS; ♣Canadian drug name; ⦿ Prototype drug

385

to lower BP abruptly (especially important in the older adult).

- During change from PO clonidine to transdermal system, PO clonidine should be maintained for at least 24 h after patch is applied. Consult prescriber.

- Do not abruptly discontinue drug. It should be withdrawn over a period of 2–4 days. Abrupt withdrawal may result in a hypertensive crisis within 8–18 h.

- Store in tightly closed container at 15°–30° C (59°–86° F) unless otherwise directed.

### Transdermal

- Apply transdermal patch to dry skin, free of hair and rash. Avoid irritated, abraded, or scarred skin. Recommended areas for applying transdermal patch are upper outer arm and anterior chest. Rotate application sites and keep a record.

## ADVERSE EFFECTS (≥1%) CV: *Hypotension (epidural)*, postural hypotension (mild), peripheral edema, ECG changes, tachycardia, bradycardia, flushing, rapid increase in BP with abrupt withdrawal. GI: *Dry mouth, constipation,* abdominal pain, pseudo-obstruction of large bowel, altered taste, nausea, vomiting, hepatitis, hyperbilirubinemia, weight gain (sodium retention). CNS: *Drowsiness, sedation, dizziness,* headache, fatigue, weakness, sluggishness, dyspnea, vivid dreams, nightmares, insomnia, behavior changes, agitation, hallucination, nervousness, restlessness, anxiety, mental depression. Skin: Rash, pruritus, thinning of hair, exacerbation of psoriasis; with transdermal patch: Hyperpigmentation, recurrent herpes simplex, skin irritation, contact dermatitis, mild erythema. Special Senses: Dry eyes. Urogenital: Impotence, loss of libido.

## DIAGNOSTIC TEST INTERFERENCE
Avoid use of transdermal patch during **MRI**. Possibility of decreased urinary excretion of *aldosterone, catecholamines,* and *VMA* (however, sudden withdrawal of clonidine may cause increases in these values); transient increases in *blood glucose;* weakly positive *direct antiglobulin (Coombs') tests.*

## INTERACTIONS Drug: Alcohol
and other CNS DEPRESSANTS add to CNS depression; TRICYCLIC ANTIDEPRESSANTS may reduce antihypertensive effects. OPIATE ANALGESICS increase hypotension with epidural clonidine. Increased risk of bradycardia or AV block when epidural clonidine is used with **digoxin,** CALCIUM CHANNEL BLOCKERS, or BETA BLOCKERS. Use with other ANTIHYPERTENSIVES can have added effect. Avoid with MAO INHIBITORS and **guanethidine.** Mirtazapine may antagonize antihypertensive effects.

## PHARMACOKINETICS Absorption: Readily from GI tract. Onset: 30–60 min PO; 1–3 days transdermal. Peak: 2–4 h PO; 2–3 days transdermal. Duration: 8 h PO; 7 days transdermal. Distribution: Widely distributed; crosses blood–brain barrier; not known if crosses placenta or distributed into breast milk. Metabolism: In liver. Elimination: 80% in urine, 20% in feces. Half-Life: 6–20 h.

## NURSING IMPLICATIONS
### Assessment & Drug Effects
- Monitor BP closely. Determine positional changes (supine, sitting, standing).
- With epidural administration, frequently monitor BP and HR. Hypotension is a common side effect that may require intervention.

Common adverse effects in *italic;* life-threatening effects <u>underlined</u>; generic names in **bold;** classifications in SMALL CAPS; ✦ Canadian drug name; ◯ Prototype drug

- Monitor BP closely whenever a drug is added to or withdrawn from therapeutic regimen.
- Monitor I&O during period of dosage adjustment. Report change in I&O ratio or change in voiding pattern.
- Determine weight daily. Patients not receiving a concomitant diuretic agent may gain weight, particularly during first 3 or 4 days of therapy, because of marked sodium and water retention.
- Supervise closely patients with history of mental depression, as they may be subject to further depressive episodes.

**Patient & Family Education**
- Although postural hypotension occurs infrequently, make position changes slowly, and in stages, particularly from recumbent to upright position, and dangle and move legs a few minutes before standing. Lie down immediately if faintness or dizziness occurs.
- Avoid potentially hazardous activities until reaction to drug has been determined due to possible sedative effects.
- Do not omit doses or stop the drug without consulting the prescriber.
- Do not take OTC medications, alcohol, or other CNS depressants without prior discussion with prescriber.
- Avoid becoming overheated or dehydrated.
- Examine site when transdermal patch is removed and report to prescriber if erythema, rash, irritation, or hyperpigmentation occurs.
- If transdermal patch loosens, tape it in place with adhesive. The patch should never be cut or trimmed.

## CLOPIDOGREL BISULFATE ℗
(clo-pi'do-grel)
Plavix
**Classification:** ANTIPLATELET
Therapeutic: PLATELET AGGREGATION
INHIBITOR; ANTITHROMBOTIC

**AVAILABILITY** Tablet

## ACTION & *THERAPEUTIC EFFECT*
Inhibits platelet aggregation by selectively preventing the binding of adenosine diphosphate to its platelet receptor. The drug's effect on the adenosine diphosphate receptor of a platelet is irreversible. *Clopidogrel prolongs bleeding time, thereby reducing atherosclerotic events in high-risk patients.*

**USES** Acute coronary syndrome (ST or non-ST elevations). Secondary prevention of MI, stroke, and vascular death.

**UNLABELED USES** Reduction of restenosis after stent placement.

**CONTRAINDICATIONS** Hypersensitivity to clopidogrel; intracranial hemorrhage, peptic ulcer, or any other active pathologic bleeding; lactation. Discontinue clopidogrel 5 days before elective surgery including CABG. Discontinue for at least 24 h for emergency on pump CABG.

**CAUTIOUS USE** GI bleeding, peptic ulcer disease; patients at risk for increased bleeding; hepatic impairment; renal impairment; pregnancy (category B) Safety and efficacy not established in children.

## ROUTE & DOSAGE

**Secondary Prevention**
*Adult:* **PO** 75 mg daily

Common adverse effects in *italic;* life-threatening effects underlined; generic names in **bold;** classifications in SMALL CAPS; ◆Canadian drug name; ℗ Prototype drug

387

**Secondary Prevention in Patients with STEMI (ST segment Elevated MI)**

*Adult:* **PO** 75 mg daily with aspirin

**Acute Coronary Syndrome (Non-ST Elevation)**

*Adult:* **PO** 300 mg loading dose then 75 mg daily (use with aspirin)

*Phamacogenetic Dosage Adjustment*

*Poor CYP2C19 metabolizers:* May need a higher initial dose or another treatment strategy.

## ADMINISTRATION

### Oral

- Do not administer to persons with active pathologic bleeding.
- Discontinue drug 7 days prior to surgery.
- Store at 15°–30° C (59°–86° F) in tightly closed container and protect from light.

## ADVERSE EFFECTS (≥1%) **Body as a Whole:** Flu-like syndrome, fatigue, pain, arthralgia, back pain. **CV:** Chest pain, edema, hypertension, thrombocytopenic purpura. **GI:** Abdominal pain, dyspepsia, diarrhea, nausea, hypercholesterolemia. **Hematologic:** Thrombotic thrombocytopenic purpura, epistaxis. **CNS:** Headache, dizziness, depression. **Respiratory:** URI, dyspnea, rhinitis, bronchitis, cough. **Skin:** Rash, pruritus.

## INTERACTIONS **Drug:** NSAIDS may increase risk of bleeding events. PROTON PUMP INHIBITORS may decrease effectiveness. **Fluoxetine, citalopram,** or **fluvosamine** may decrease effectiveness. **Herbal: Garlic, ginger, ginkgo, evening primrose oil** may increase risk of bleeding.

## PHARMACOKINETICS **Absorption:** Rapidly from GI tract. **Onset:** 2 h; reaches steady state in 3–7 days. **Distribution:** 94–98% protein bound. **Metabolism:** via CYP2C19. **Elimination:** 50% in urine and 50% in feces. **Half-Life:** 8 h.

## NURSING IMPLICATIONS

### Black Box Warning

*Clopidogrel has diminished efficacy in patients who are CYP2C19 poor metabolizers.*

### Assessment & Drug Effects

- Carefully monitor for and immediately report S&S of GI bleeding, especially when coadministered with NSAIDS, aspirin, heparin, or warfarin.
- Evaluate patients with unexplained fever or infection for myelotoxicity.
- Monitor lab tests: Baseline test for CYP2C19 genotype; periodic platelet count and lipid profile.

### Patient & Family Education

- Report promptly any unusual bleeding (e.g., black, tarry stools).
- Avoid omeprazole, esomeprazole, or other over-the-counter acid-reducing drugs; do not take aspirin or NSAID use unless approved by prescriber.

## CLORAZEPATE DIPOTASSIUM
(klor-az'e-pate)

Tranxene

**Classifications:** ANXIOLYTIC; ANTICONVULSANT; BENZODIAZEPINE
**Therapeutic** ANTIANXIETY; ANTICONVULSANT
**Prototype:** Lorazepam
**Controlled Substance:** Schedule IV

## AVAILABILITY Capsule; tablet

## ACTION & *THERAPEUTIC EFFECT*

Exerts its effects through enhancement of GABA-benzodiazepine receptor complex, an inhibitory neurotransmitter. Clorazepate has depressant effects on the CNS, thus controlling anxiety associated with stress and also resulting in sedative effects. *Effective in controlling anxiety and withdrawal symptoms of alcohol.*

**USES** Management of anxiety disorders, short-term relief of anxiety symptoms, as adjunct in management of partial seizures, and symptomatic relief of acute alcohol withdrawal.

**CONTRAINDICATIONS** Hypersensitivity to clorazepate; acute narrow-angle glaucoma; depressive neuroses; pulmonary disease, COPD; psychotic reactions, drug abusers. Safe use during pregnancy (category D); lactation.

**CAUTIOUS USE** Hypersensitivity to other benzodiazepines; older adults; debilitated patients; hepatic disease; kidney disease; Parkinson's disease; neuromuscular disease; seizure disorders; bipolar disorder, mania, history of suicidal tendencies. Safe use in children younger than 9 y not established.

## ROUTE & DOSAGE

**Anxiety**
*Adult:* **PO** 15–30 mg daily may increase to 60 mg/day in divided doses (max: 60 mg/day)

**Acute Alcohol Withdrawal**
*Adult:* **PO** 30 mg followed by 30–60 mg in divided doses (max: 90 mg/day), taper by 15 mg/day over 4 days to 15–30 mg/day then gradually reduce to 7.5–15 mg/day until patient is stable

**Partial Seizures (Adjunctive)**
*Adult:* **PO** 7.5 mg t.i.d.
*Child (9–12 y):* **PO** 3.75–7.5 mg b.i.d., may increase by no more than 3.75 mg/wk (max: 60 mg/day)

## ADMINISTRATION

**Oral**
- Give with food to minimize gastric distress.
- Ensure that sustained-release form of drug is not chewed or crushed. It **must be** swallowed whole.
- Taper drug dose gradually over several days when drug is to be discontinued
- Store in a light-resistant container at 15°–30° C (59°–86° F) unless otherwise specified.

**ADVERSE EFFECTS** (≥1%) **Body as a Whole:** Allergic reactions, physiological and psychological dependence. **CV:** Hypotension. **GI:** GI disturbances, abnormal liver function tests, xerostomia. **Hematologic:** Decreased Hct, blood dyscrasias. **CNS:** *Drowsiness,* ataxia, dizziness, headache, paradoxical excitement, mental confusion, insomnia, suicidal ideation. **Special Senses:** Diplopia, blurred vision.

**INTERACTIONS Drug: Alcohol** and other CNS DEPRESSANTS compound CNS depression; clorazepate increases effects of **cimetidine, disulfiram,** causing excessive sedation; avoid **olanzapine** due to additive adverse effects. **Herbal: Ginkgo** may decrease anticonvulsant effectiveness.

**PHARMACOKINETICS Absorption:** Decarboxylated in stomach; absorbed as active metabolite, desmethyldiazepam. **Peak:** 1 h. **Duration:** 24 h. **Distribution:** Crosses

Common adverse effects in *italic*; life-threatening effects underlined; generic names in **bold**; classifications in SMALL CAPS; ♣ Canadian drug name; ⊕ Prototype drug

389

**C**

placenta; distributed into breast milk. **Metabolism:** In liver to oxazepam by CYP2C19 and CYP3A4. **Elimination:** Primarily in urine. **Half-Life:** 30–200 h.

## NURSING IMPLICATIONS

### Assessment & Drug Effects

- Drowsiness, a common side effect, is more likely to occur at initiation of therapy and with dose increments on successive days.
- Monitor patient with history of cardiovascular disease in early therapy for drug-induced responses. If systolic BP drops more than 20 mm Hg or if there is a sudden increase in pulse rate, withhold drug and notify prescriber.
- Monitor lab tests: Periodic blood count and LFTs throughout therapy.

### Patient & Family Education

- Take drug as prescribed and do not change dose or abruptly stop taking the drug without prescriber's approval.
- Do not self-dose with OTC drugs (cold remedies, sleep medications, antacids) without consulting prescriber.
- Avoid driving and other potentially hazardous activities until reaction to drug is known.
- Do not use alcohol and other CNS depressants while on clorazepate therapy.
- If a woman becomes pregnant during therapy or intends to become pregnant, communicate with prescriber about the desirability of discontinuing the drug.

## CLOTRIMAZOLE
(kloe-trim'a-zole)
Canesten ♦, Gyne-
Lotrimin, Gyne-
Lotrimin-3, Lotrimin,
Mycelex, Mycelex-G

**Classifications:** ANTIBIOTIC; AZOLE ANTIFUNGAL
Therapeutic: ANTIFUNGAL
**Prototype:** Fluconazole

**AVAILABILITY** Cream; solution; lotion; troches; vaginal tablet; vaginal cream

## ACTION & *THERAPEUTIC EFFECT*
Acts by altering fungal cell membrane permeability, permitting loss of phosphorous compounds, potassium, and other essential intracellular constituents with consequent loss of ability to replicate. *Has broad-spectrum fungicidal activity. Active against a wide variety of fungi, yeast, dermatophytes and certain gram-positive bacteria.*

**USES** Dermal infections including tinea pedis, tinea cruris, tinea corporis, tinea versicolor; also vulvovaginal and oropharyngeal candidiasis.

**UNLABELED USES** Trichomoniasis.

**CONTRAINDICATIONS** Ophthalmic uses; systemic mycoses.

**CAUTIOUS USE** Hyersensitivity to other azole antifungals; hepatic impairment, diabetes mellitus; HIV; recurrent infections; pregnancy (category C for oral troches; category B for topical use); lactation. **Troches:** Safe use in children younger than 12 y has not been established. **Oral:** Safe use in children younger than 3 y not established. **Topical:** Cautious use in children younger than 2 y.

## ROUTE & DOSAGE

### Dermal Infections
*Adult:* **Topical** Apply small amount onto affected areas b.i.d. a.m. and p.m.

Common adverse effects in *italic;* life-threatening effects <u>underlined;</u> generic names in **bold;** classifications in SMALL CAPS; ♣ Canadian drug name; ⊙ Prototype drug

### Vulvovaginal Infections

*Adult:* **Intravaginal** Insert 1 applicator full or one 100 mg vaginal tablet into vagina at bedtime for 7 days, or one 500 mg vaginal tablet at bedtime for 1 dose

### Oropharyngeal Candidiasis

*Adult/Child (older than 3 y):* **PO** 1 troche (lozenge) 4–5 × day q3h for 14 days

## ADMINISTRATION

### Oral

- Instruct patient taking the oral lozenge to allow it to dissolve slowly in mouth over 15–30 min for maximum effectiveness.

### Topical

- Apply skin cream and solution preparations sparingly. Protect hands with latex gloves when applying medication.
- Avoid contact of clotrimazole preparations with the eyes.
- Do not use occlusive dressings unless directed by prescriber to do so.
- Consult prescriber about skin cleansing procedure before applying medication. Regardless of procedure used, dry skin thoroughly.

### Vaginal

- Apply small amount of cream to irritated area of vulva for relief of external vulvar itching associated with vaginal yeast infection.
- Store cream and solution formulations at 15°–30° C (59°–86° F); do not store troches or vaginal tablets above 35° C (95° F) unless otherwise directed.

## ADVERSE EFFECTS (≥1%) **GI:** Abnormal liver function tests; occasional nausea and vomiting (with oral troche). **Skin:** Stinging, erythema, edema, vesication, desquamation, pruritus, urticaria, skin fissures. **Urogenital:** Mild burning sensation, lower abdominal cramps, bloating, cystitis, urethritis, mild urinary frequency, vulval erythema and itching, pain and vaginal soreness during intercourse.

**INTERACTIONS Drug:** Intravaginal preparations may inactivate SPERMICIDES.

**PHARMACOKINETICS Absorption:** Minimal systemic absorption; minimally absorbed topically. **Peak:** High saliva concentrations less than 3 h; high vaginal concentrations in 8–24 h. **Metabolism:** In liver. **Elimination:** Eliminated as metabolite in bile.

## NURSING IMPLICATIONS

### Assessment & Drug Effects

- Evaluate effectiveness of treatment. Report any signs of skin irritation with dermal preparations.
- Anticipate signs of clinical improvement within the first week of drug use.

### Patient & Family Education

- Use clotrimazole as directed and for the length of time prescribed by prescriber.
- Generally, clinical improvement is apparent during first week of therapy. Report to prescriber if condition worsens or if signs of irritation or sensitivity develop, or if no improvement is noted after 4 wk of therapy.
- If receiving the drug vaginally, your sexual partner may experience burning and irritation of penis or urethritis; refrain from sexual intercourse during therapy or have sexual partner wear a condom.

Common adverse effects in *italic;* life-threatening effects underlined; generic names in **bold;** classifications in SMALL CAPS; ♣ Canadian drug name; ⊙ Prototype drug

391

# CLOZAPINE ⊘
(clo'za-pin)

Clozaril, Fazaclo, Versacloz

**Classification:** ATYPICAL ANTIPSYCHOTIC
**Therapeutic:** ANTIPSYCHOTIC

**AVAILABILITY** Tablet; orally disintegrating tablet; oral suspension

**ACTION & THERAPEUTIC EFFECT**
Interferes with the binding of dopamine type 2 ($D_2$) and the serotonin type 2A ($5\text{-}HT_{2A}$) receptors; also acts as an antagonist at adrenergic, cholinergic, histaminergic and other dopaminergic and serotonergic receptors. *Improves symptoms in patients with treatment-resistant schizophrenia.*

**USES** Management of schizophrenia and schizoaffective disorder.

**UNLABELED USES** Bipolar disorder, dementia-related behavioral disorders, tremor.

**CONTRAINDICATIONS** Hypersensitivity to clozapine; history of clozapine-induced agranulocytosis or severe granulocytopenia; severe CNS depression, blood dyscrasia, patients with myeloproliferative disorders, uncontrolled epilepsy; chemotherapy, coma, leukemia, leukopenia, neutropenia, myocarditis; renal failure, dialysis, hepatitis, jaundice; suicidal ideation; dementia related psychosis; neuroleptic malignant syndrome (NMS); infants; lactation. Discontinue clozapine if QTc interval is more than 500 msec.

**CAUTIOUS USE** Arrhythmias, GI disorders, history of bone marrow depression; narrow-angle glaucoma, hepatic and renal impairment, prostatic hypertrophy, history of seizures; DM; patients at risk for diabetes; cardiovascular and/or pulmonary disease; cerebrovascular disease, cardiac arrhythmias, tachycardia, dehydration, neurologic disease, tardive dyskinesia, patients at risk for aspiration pneumonia due to drug-induced esophageal dysmotility; history of suicidal thoughts; history of seizures or predisposition for seizures; previous history of agranulocytosis; surgery, glaucoma, infection, older adults; pregnancy (category B). Safety and efficacy in children younger than 16 y not established.

## ROUTE & DOSAGE

### Schizophrenia

*Adult (16 y or older):* **PO** Initiate at 12.5 mg daily or b.i.d., then increase by 25–50 mg/day and titrate to a target dose of 350–450 mg/day in 3 divided doses, further increases (not more than twice weekly) can be made if necessary (max: 900 mg/day)

## ADMINISTRATION

### Oral

- Drug is usually withdrawn gradually over 1–2 wk if therapy must be discontinued.
- Store the drug away from heat or light.

**ADVERSE EFFECTS** (≥1%) **CV:** Orthostatic hypotension, *tachycardia,* ECG changes, increased risk of myocarditis especially during first month of therapy, pericarditis, pericardial effusion, cardiomyopathy, heart failure, MI, mitral insufficiency. **GI:** Nausea, dry mouth, constipation, hypersalivation. **Hematologic:** Agranulocytosis. **CNS:** Seizures,

Common adverse effects in *italic;* life-threatening effects underlined; generic names in **bold;** classifications in SMALL CAPS; ♣ Canadian drug name; ⊘ Prototype drug

*transient fever,* sedation, neuro-leptic malignant syndrome (rare), dystonic reactions (rare). **Metabolic:** Hyperglycemia, diabetes mellitus. **Urogenital:** Urinary retention. **Other:** Increased mortality from severe hematologic, cardiovascular, and respiratory adverse effects.

## INTERACTIONS Drug: Alcohol

and other CNS DEPRESSANTS compound depressant effects; ANTICHOLINERGIC AGENTS potentiate anticholinergic effects; ANTIHYPERTENSIVE AGENTS may potentiate hypotension; ANTINEOPLASTIC AGENTS may potentiate bone marrow suppression. **Herbal: St. John's wort** and **kava** may increase sedation.

## PHARMACOKINETICS Absorption: 

Readily absorbed from GI tract. **Onset:** 2–4 wk. **Peak:** 2.5 h. **Distribution:** Possibly distributed into breast milk. **Metabolism:** In liver. **Elimination:** 50% in urine, 30% in feces. **Half-Life:** 8–12 h.

## NURSING IMPLICATIONS

### Black Box Warning

*Clozapine has been associated with a significant risk of agranulocytosis, seizures (especially at higher doses), potentially fatal myocarditis (especially during, but not limited to, the first month of therapy, and orthostatic hypotension (especially during initial titration with dose acceleration).*

### Assessment & Drug Effects

- Monitor cardiovascular and respiratory status, especially during the first month of therapy. Report promptly S&S of potential cardiac problems.
- Monitor for development of tachycardia or hypotension, which may pose a serious risk for patients with compromised cardiovascular function.
- Monitor diabetics for loss of glycemic control.
- Monitor for seizure activity; seizure potential increases at the higher dose level.
- Monitor for S&S of NMS (see Appendix F) and tardive dyskinesia.
- Closely monitor for recurrence of psychotic symptoms if the drug is being discontinued.
- Monitor lab tests: Baseline WBC and absolute neutrophil count, then qwk × 6 mo, then q2wk for next 6 mo, then q4wk throughout therapy, and after drug discontinued, qwk × 4 wk; periodic blood glucose.

### Patient & Family Education

- Carefully monitor blood glucose levels if diabetic.
- Do not engage in any hazardous activity until response to the drug is known. Drowsiness and sedation are common adverse effects.
- Due to the risk of agranulocytosis (see Appendix F) it is important to comply with blood test regimen. Report flu-like symptoms, fever, sore throat, lethargy, malaise, or other signs of infection.
- Rise slowly to avoid orthostatic hypotension.
- Report immediately any of the following: Unexplained fatigue, especially with activity; shortness of breath, sudden weight gain or edema of the lower extremities.
- Take drug exactly as ordered.
- Do not use OTC drugs or alcohol without permission of prescriber.

## CODEINE
(koe'deen)

Common adverse effects in *italic;* life-threatening effects underlined; generic names in **bold;** classifications in SMALL CAPS; ◆Canadian drug name; ⊘ Prototype drug

393

# CODEINE SULFATE

**Classifications:** NARCOTIC (OPIATE AGONIST) ANALGESIC; ANTITUSSIVE
Therapeutic: NARCOTIC ANALGESIC; ANTITUSSIVE
**Prototype:** Morphine
**Controlled Substance:** Schedule II

**AVAILABILITY** Tablet; oral solution

## ACTION & *THERAPEUTIC EFFECT*

Opium agonist in the CNS. Analgesia is mediated through changes in the perception of pain at the spinal cord and higher levels in the CNS. The antitussive effects are mediated through direct action on receptors in the cough center of the medulla. *Analgesic potency is about one-sixth that of morphine; antitussive activity is also a little less than that of morphine.*

**USES** Symptomatic relief of mild to moderately severe pain when control cannot be obtained by nonnarcotic analgesics and to suppress hyperactive or nonproductive cough.

**CONTRAINDICATIONS** Hypersensitivity to codeine or other morphine derivatives; increased intracranial pressure, head injury, acute alcoholism; use during labor.

**CAUTIOUS USE** Prostatic hypertrophy, G6PD deficiency; GI disease; COPD, acute asthma; hepatic or renal disease; hepatitis; immunosuppression; hypothyroidism; debilitated patients, very young and very old patients; history of drug abuse; pregnancy (category C); lactation; children/adolescent.

## ROUTE & DOSAGE

### Analgesic

*Adult:* **PO** 15–60 mg q.i.d.
*Child:* 0.5–1 mg/kg q4–6h prn
(max: 60 mg/dose)

### Antitussive

*Adult:* **PO** 10–20 mg q4–6h prn
(max: 120 mg/24 h)
*Child (6–12 y):* **PO** 5–10 mg
q4–6h (max: 60 mg/24 h);
*2 to younger than 6 y:* 2.5–5 mg
q4–6h (max: 30 mg/24 h)

## ADMINISTRATION

### Oral

- Administer codeine with milk or other food to reduce possibility of GI distress.

**ADVERSE EFFECTS** (≥1%) **Body as a Whole:** Shortness of breath, anaphylactoid reaction. **CV:** Palpitation, hypotension, orthostatic hypotension, bradycardia, tachycardia, circulatory collapse. **GI:** *Nausea,* vomiting, *constipation.* **CNS:** *Dizziness,* light-headedness, *drowsiness,* sedation, lethargy, euphoria, agitation; restlessness, exhilaration, convulsions, narcosis, respiratory depression. **Skin:** Diffuse erythema, rash, urticaria, *pruritus,* excessive perspiration, facial flushing, fixed-drug eruption. **Special Senses:** Miosis. **Urogenital:** Urinary retention.

**INTERACTIONS Drug: Alcohol** and other CNS DEPRESSANTS augment CNS depressant effects. **Herbal: St. John's wort** may cause increased sedation.

**PHARMACOKINETICS Absorption:** Readily from GI tract. **Onset:** 15–30 min. **Peak:** 1–1.5 h. **Duration:** 4–6 h. **Distribution:** Crosses placenta; distributed into breast milk. **Metabolism:** In liver. **Elimination:** In urine. **Half-Life:** 2.5–4 h.

Common adverse effects in *italic*; life-threatening effects <u>underlined</u>; generic names in **bold**; classifications in SMALL CAPS; ♣ Canadian drug name; ⊙ Prototype drug

## NURSING IMPLICATIONS

### Black Box Warning

*Codeine has been associated with respiratory depression and death in children who are ultra-rapid metabolizers of codeine when used following tonsillectomy or adenoidectomy.*

### Assessment & Drug Effects

- Monitor closely for signs of respiratory depression. Withhold drug and notify prescriber if respiratory depression develops.
- Record relief of pain and duration of analgesia.
- Evaluate effectiveness as cough suppressant. Treatment of cough is directed toward decreasing frequency and intensity of cough without abolishing cough reflex, need to remove bronchial secretions.
- Supervise ambulation and use other safety precautions as warranted since drug may cause dizziness and light-headedness.
- Monitor for nausea, a common side effect. Report nausea accompanied by vomiting. Change to another analgesic may be warranted.

### Patient & Family Education

- Make position changes slowly and in stages, particularly from recumbent to upright posture. Lie down immediately if light-headedness or dizziness occurs.
- Lie down when feeling nauseated and notify prescriber if this symptom persists. Nausea appears to be aggravated by ambulation.
- Avoid driving and other potentially hazardous activities until reaction to drug is known. Codeine may impair ability to perform tasks requiring mental alertness.

- Do not take alcohol or other CNS depressants unless approved by prescriber.

## COLCHICINE

(kol'chi-seen)

Colcrys, Novocolchine ♦

**Classification:** ANTIGOUT
**Therapeutic:** ANTIGOUT

**AVAILABILITY** Tablet

### ACTION & *THERAPEUTIC EFFECT*

In gout anti-inflammatory action may involve a reduction in lactic acid production by leukocytes resulting in decreased uric acid deposition and a reduction in phagocytosis. Effect on fever may be due to preventing activation of neutrophils and monocytes. *Inhibition of inflammation and reduction of pain and swelling, which occurs in gouty arthritis. Colchicine is nonanalgesic and nonuricosuric.*

**USES** Prophylactically for recurrent gouty arthritis or for acute gout, treatment or prevention of Mediterranean fever.

**UNLABELED USES** Sarcoid arthritis, chondrocalcinosis (pseudogout), arthritis associated with erythema nodosum, leukemia, adenocarcinoma, acute calcific tendonitis, multiple sclerosis, primary biliary cirrhosis, mycosis fungoides, and Paget's disease.

**CONTRAINDICATIONS** Hypersensitivity to the drug; blood dyscrasias; severe GI, renal, hepatic, or cardiac disease.

**CAUTIOUS USE** Early manifestations of GI, renal, hepatic, or cardiac disease; hemotologic disorders; debilitated patients and older

Common adverse effects in *italic;* life-threatening effects <u>underlined;</u> generic names in **bold;** classifications in SMALL CAPS; ♣ Canadian drug name; ⊙ Prototype drug

395

adults; pregnancy (category C). Safe use in children not established.

## ROUTE & DOSAGE

### Acute Gouty Flare
*Adult:* PO 1.2 mg followed by 0.6 mg one hour later (max: 1.8 mg in one hour).

### Prophylaxis
*Adult:* PO 0.6 mg once or twice daily. Adult with concurrent CYP3A4 inhibitor use PO 0.3 mg every day or every other day

### Familial Mediterranean Fever
*Adult:* PO 1.2–2.4 mg in 1 or 2 doses.

### *Renal Impairment Dosage Adjustment*
*CrCl 30 mL/min:* Use 50% of normal dose

## ADMINISTRATION
### Oral
- Administer oral drug with milk or food to reduce possibility of GI upset.
- Preserve in tight, light-resistant containers preferably at 15°–30° C (59°–86° F), unless otherwise directed by manufacturer.

## ADVERSE EFFECTS (≥1%) GI:
*Nausea, vomiting, diarrhea, abdominal pain,* anorexia, hemorrhagic gastroenteritis, steatorrhea, hepatotoxicity, pancreatitis. **Hematologic:** Neutropenia, bone marrow depression, thrombocytopenia, agranulocytosis, aplastic anemia. **CNS:** Mental confusion, peripheral neuritis, syndrome of muscle weakness (accompanied by elevated serum creatine kinase). **Skin:** Severe irritation and tissue damage if IV administration leaks around injec-

tion site. **Urogenital:** Azotemia, proteinuria, hematuria, oliguria.

## DIAGNOSTIC TEST INTERFERENCE
False-positive *urine tests for RBCs and Hgb* reported.

## INTERACTIONS Drug: May decrease intestinal absorption of vitamin $B_{12}$. Do not use with PROTEASE INHIBITORS. Avoid CYP3A4 inhibitors. **Food: Grapefruit juice** may increase adverse effects.

## PHARMACOKINETICS Absorption: Rapidly from GI tract. Peak: 0.5–2 h; multiple peaks because of enterohepatic cycling. **Distribution:** Widely distributed; concentrates in leukocytes, kidney, liver, spleen, and intestinal tract. **Metabolism:** by P-glycoprotein and CYP3A4. **Elimination:** Primarily in feces.

## NURSING IMPLICATIONS
### Assessment & Drug Effects
- Monitor for dose-related adverse effects; they are most likely to occur during the initial course of treatment.
- Monitor for early signs of colchicine toxicity including weakness, abdominal discomfort, anorexia, nausea, vomiting, and diarrhea. Report to prescriber. To avoid more serious toxicity, drug should be discontinued promptly until symptoms subside.
- Monitor I&O ratio and pattern (during acute gouty attack): High fluid intake promotes excretion and reduces danger of crystal formation in kidneys and ureters.
- Monitor lab tests: Baseline and periodic serum uric acid and creatinine, CBC, platelet count, serum electrolytes, and urinalysis.

### Patient & Family Education
- Withhold drug and report to the prescriber the onset of GI symptoms or signs of bone marrow

depression (nausea, sore throat, bleeding gums, sore mouth, fever, fatigue, malaise, unusual bleeding or bruising).
- Avoid fermented beverages such as beer, ale, and wine as they may precipitate gouty attack.

# COLESEVELAM HYDROCHLORIDE

(co-less'e-ve-lam)

Welchol

**Classifications:** ANTIHYPERLIPIDEMIC; BILE ACID SEQUESTRANT
Therapeutic: CHOLESTEROL-LOWERING; BILE ACID SEQUESTRANT
**Prototype:** Cholestyramine resin

**AVAILABILITY** Tablet; powder for suspension

**ACTION & THERAPEUTIC EFFECT**
Binds with bile salts in the intestinal tract to form an insoluble complex that is excreted in the feces, thus reducing circulating cholesterol and increasing serum LDL removal rate. Serum triglyceride levels may increase slightly. *Decreases serum LDL and total cholesterol level. Removes bile salts from the intestine.*

**USES** Hypercholesterolemia, hyperlipoproteinemia, type 2 diabetes.

**CONTRAINDICATIONS** Hypersensitivity to colesevelam; complete biliary obstruction; history of hypertriglyceridemia-induced pancreatitis; serum triglyceride concentrations greater than 500 mg/dL; bowel obstruction.

**CAUTIOUS USE** Preexisting GI disorders or bowel disease, primary biliary cirrhosis, partial biliary obstruction, biliary atresia; diabetes mellitus; hypertriglyceridemia; older adults, malabsorption states; bleeding disorders; pregnancy (category B).

## ROUTE & DOSAGE

**Hypercholesterolemia**
*Adult:* **PO** 3 tablets b.i.d. with meals or 6 tablets daily with a meal, may be increased to 7 tablets/day or 1.875 gram packet b.i.d.

**Type 2 Diabetes**
*Adult:* **PO** 3 tablets b.i.d. or 6 tablets daily or 1.875 gram packet b.i.d.

## ADMINISTRATION

**Oral**
- Give with meals (mandatory) and adequate liquid (e.g., 8 oz).
- Administer concurrently ordered drugs at least 4 h prior to colesevelam.
- Store at 15°–30° C (59°–86° F) with occasional fluctuations to 40° C (90° F); protect from moisture.

**ADVERSE EFFECTS** (≥1%) **Body as a Whole:** Infection, pain, flu-like syndrome, asthenia, myalgia. **CNS:** Headache. **GI:** Abdominal pain, *flatulence, constipation,* diarrhea, nausea, dyspepsia. **Respiratory:** Sinusitis, rhinitis, cough, pharyngitis.

**INTERACTIONS Drug:** May decrease absorption of **verapamil.** Can bind and affect absorption of any drug.

**PHARMACOKINETICS Absorption:** Not absorbed. **Metabolism:** Not metabolized. **Elimination:** 0.05% in urine.

## NURSING IMPLICATIONS

**Assessment & Drug Effects**
- Withhold drug and notify prescriber for triglycerides greater than 300 mg/dL.
- Monitor lab tests: Baseline lipid profile, repeat at 3 mo, then q6–12 mo thereafter.

---

Common adverse effects in *italic;* life-threatening effects underlined; generic names in **bold;** classifications in SMALL CAPS; ✦Canadian drug name; ⑩ Prototype drug

**Patient & Family Education**
- Report S&S of GI distress (see Appendix F), especially constipation.

# COLESTIPOL HYDROCHLORIDE
(koe-les'ti-pole)
Cholestabyl ✦ , Colestid, Lestid ✦

**Classifications:** ANTIHYPERLIPIDEMIC; BILE ACID SEQUESTRANT
Therapeutic: CHOLESTEROL-LOWERING AGENT; BILE ACID SEQUESTRANT
**Prototype:** Cholestyramine

**AVAILABILITY** Tablet; powder for suspension

## ACTION & *THERAPEUTIC EFFECT*
Adsorbs and combines with intestinal bile acids in exchange for chloride ions to form an insoluble, nonabsorbable complex that is excreted in the feces. *Reduces circulating cholesterol and increases serum LDL removal rate. Serum triglycerides are not affected or are minimally increased.*

## USES
Pruritus associated with partial biliary obstruction; biliary cirrhosis; also as adjunct to diet therapy of patient with primary hypercholesterolemia (type IIa hyperlipoproteinemia) or with coronary artery disease unresponsive to diet or other measures alone.

## UNLABELED USES
Digitoxin overdose and hyperoxaluria and to control postoperative diarrhea caused by excess bile acids in colon.

## CONTRAINDICATIONS
Complete biliary obstruction, biliary cirrhosis; hypersensitivity to bile acid sequestrants; renal disease.

## CAUTIOUS USE
Hemorrhoids; bleeding disorders; malabsorption states; GI motility disorders, dysphagia; older adult; pregnancy (category C). Safe use in children not established.

## ROUTE & DOSAGE

| Hypercholesterolemia |
| --- |
| *Adult:* **PO** 15–30 g/day in 2–4 doses a.c. and at bedtime, or 1–2 tabs 1–2 × day |
| **Digitalis Toxicity** |
| *Adult:* **PO** 10 g followed by 5 g q6–8h as needed |

## ADMINISTRATION
**Oral**
- Give 30 min before a meal when ordered a.c.
- Ensure that tablets are not chewed or crushed. They **must be** swallowed whole.
- Always mix granule form with liquids, juices, soups, cereals, or pulpy fruits. Add powder to at least 90 mL fluid. When carbonated drink is used, slowly stir in a large glass because excess foaming may occur. Rinse glass with small amount extra fluid to be sure all the drug is taken.
- Drugs given concomitantly should be scheduled at least 1 h before or 4 h after ingestion of colestipol to reduce interference with their absorption (see drug interactions).
- Store at 15°–30° C (59°–86° F) in tightly closed container unless otherwise instructed.

## ADVERSE EFFECTS (≥1%) **Body as a Whole:** Joint and muscle pain, arthritis, shortness of breath. **GI:**

Common adverse effects in *italic;* life-threatening effects <u>underlined;</u> generic names in **bold;** classifications in SMALL CAPS; ✦ Canadian drug name; ⊘ Prototype drug

*Constipation,* abdominal pain or distention, belching, flatulence, nausea, vomiting, diarrhea. **Metabolic:** Transient increases in liver enzyme tests, serum phosphorus and chloride; decreases in serum sodium and potassium. **Skin:** Dermatitis, urticaria.

## INTERACTIONS **Drug:** Because it decreases the absorption from the GI tract of ORAL ANTICOAGULANTS, **digoxin,** TETRACYCLINES, PENICILLINS, **phenobarbital,** THYROID HORMONES, THIAZIDE DIURETICS, IRON SALTS, FAT-SOLUBLE VITAMINS (A, D, E, K), administer cholestyramine 4 h before or 2 h after these drugs. Can bind and affect absorption of any drug.

## PHARMACOKINETICS **Absorption:** Not absorbed from GI tract. **Elimination:** In feces as insoluble complex.

## NURSING IMPLICATIONS

### Assessment & Drug Effects

- Watch for changes in bowel elimination pattern. Constipation should not be allowed to persist without medical attention.
- Monitor lab tests: Baseline lipid profile, repeat at 3 mo, then q6–12 mo thereafter.

### Patient & Family Education

- To prevent drug interactions, it is important to keep to established schedule for taking colestipol and other drugs. See Drug Interactions.
- If receiving prolonged therapy, report unusual bleeding (vitamin K deficiency). Colestipol prevents absorption of fat-soluble vitamins (A, D, E, K).

# COLISTIMETHATE SODIUM
(koe-lis-ti-meth'ate)
Coly-Mycin M

**Classifications:** URINARY TRACT ANTIINFECTIVE; ANTIBIOTIC
**Therapeutic:** URINARY TRACT ANTIINFECTIVE
**Prototype:** Trimethoprim

**AVAILABILITY** Solution for injection

## ACTION & *THERAPEUTIC EFFECT*
Acts by affecting phospholipid component in bacterial cytoplasmic membranes with resulting damage and leakage of essential intracellular components. *Bactericidal against most gram-negative organisms, but not effective against* Proteus *or* Neisseria *species.*

**USES** Severe, acute, and chronic UTIs caused by organisms resistant to other antibiotics.

**CONTRAINDICATIONS** Hypersensitivity to polypeptide antibiotics; concurrent use of nephrotoxic and ototoxic drugs.

**CAUTIOUS USE** Impaired renal function; myasthenia gravis; older adult patients; pregnancy (category C); lactation; infants.

## ROUTE & DOSAGE

| Urinary Tract Infections |
| --- |
| *Adult/Child:* **IM/IV** 2.5–5 mg/kg/day divided in 2–4 doses (max: 5 mg/kg/day) |

---

Common adverse effects in *italic;* life-threatening effects <u>underlined;</u> generic names in **bold;** classifications in SMALL CAPS; ♣ Canadian drug name; ⊙ Prototype drug

### Renal Impairment Dosage Adjustment

*CrCl 50–79 mL/min:* Colistimethate sodium equivalent to 2.5–3.8 mg/kg/day of colistin base divided in 2 doses

*CrCl 30–49 mL/min:* Colistimethate sodium equivalent to 2.5 mg/kg/day of colistin base in 1–2 divided doses

*CrCl 10–29 mL/min:* Colistimethate sodium equivalent to 1.5 mg/kg of colistin base every 36 h

## ADMINISTRATION

### Intramuscular

- Reconstitute each 150-mg vial with 2 mL of sterile water for injection to yield a concentration of 75 mg/mL. Swirl vial gently during reconstitution to avoid bubble formation.
- IM injection should be made deep into upper outer quadrant of buttock.
- Patients commonly experience pain at injection site. Rotate sites.

### Intravenous

*PREPARE:* **Direct/Intermittent:** Prepare first half of total daily dose as directed for IM then further dilute with 20 mL sterile water for injection. ▪ Prepare second half of total daily dose by diluting further in 50 mL or more of D5W, NS, D5/NS, LR, or other compatible solution. ▪ IV infusion solution should be freshly prepared and used within 24 h.

*ADMINISTER:* **Direct/Intermittent:** First half of total daily dose: Give slowly over 3–5 min. ▪ Second half of total daily dose: Starting 1–2 h after the first half dose has been given, infuse the second half dose over the next 22–23 h.

*INCOMPATIBILITIES:* **Solution/additive: Cefazolin, cephapirin, erythromycin, hydrocortisone, hydroxyzine, kanamycin, linomycin.**

▪ Reconstituted solution may be stored in refrigerator at 2°–8° C (36°–46° F) or at controlled room temperature of 15°–30° C (59°–86° F). Use within 7 days. ▪ Store unopened vials at controlled room temperature.

## ADVERSE EFFECTS (≥1%) **Body as a Whole:** Drug fever, pain at IM site. **GI:** GI disturbances. **CNS:** Circumoral, lingual, and peripheral paresthesias; visual and speech disturbances, neuromuscular blockade (generalized muscle weakness, dyspnea, respiratory depression or paralysis), seizures, psychosis. **Respiratory:** Respiratory arrest after IM injection. **Skin:** Pruritus, urticaria, dermatoses. **Special Senses:** Ototoxicity. **Urogenital:** Nephrotoxicity.

## INTERACTIONS **Drug: Tubocurarine, pancuronium, atracurium,** AMINOGLYCOSIDES may compound and prolong respiratory depression; AMINOGLYCOSIDES, **amphotericin B, vancomycin** augment nephrotoxicity.

## PHARMACOKINETICS **Peak:** 1–2 h IM. **Duration:** 8–12 h. **Distribution:** Widely distributed in most tissues except CNS; crosses placenta; distributed into breast milk in low concentrations. **Metabolism:** In liver. **Elimination:**

66–75% in urine within 24 h.
**Half-Life:** 2–3 h.

## NURSING IMPLICATIONS
### Assessment & Drug Effects

- Report restlessness or dyspnea promptly. Respiratory arrest has been reported after IM administration.
- Monitor I&O ratio and patterns: Decrease in urine output or change in I&O ratio and rising BUN, serum creatinine, and serum drug levels (without dosage increase) are indications of renal toxicity. If they occur, withhold drug and report to prescriber.
- Be alert to neurologic symptoms: Changes in speech and hearing, visual changes, drowsiness, dizziness, ataxia, and transient paresthesias, and keep prescriber informed.
- Monitor closely postoperative patients who have received curariform muscle relaxants, ether, or sodium citrate for signs of neuromuscular blockade (delayed recovery, muscle weakness, depressed respiration).
- Monitor lab tests: Baseline C&S; periodic renal function tests and urine drug levels.

### Patient & Family Education

- Avoid operating a vehicle or other potentially hazardous activities while on drug therapy because of the possibility of transient neurologic disturbances.

## CONIVAPTAN HYDROCHLORIDE ℗+
(con-i-vap'tin)
Vaprisol

**Classifications:** ELECTROLYTIC & WATER BALANCE AGENT; DIURETIC; VASOPRESSIN ANTAGONIST
Therapeutic: VASOPRESSIN ANTAGONIST; DIURETIC

**AVAILABILITY** Solution for injection

## ACTION & *THERAPEUTIC EFFECT*
Conivaptan is a vasopressin receptor (V2) antagonist that reduces the effect of vasopressin in the kidney, thus increasing the excretion of free water into the renal collecting ducts. *Conivaptan increases urine output and decreases urine osmolality in patients with euvolemic hyponatremia, thus restoring serum sodium balance.*

**USES** Treatment of euvolemic and hypervolemic hyponatremia in hospitalized patients.

**CONTRAINDICATIONS** Hypersensitivity to conivaptan; CHF; hyponatremia associated with hypovolemia; hypotension, syncope; lactation.

**CAUTIOUS USE** Renal or hepatic function impairment; pregnancy (category C). Safety and efficacy in children not established.

## ROUTE & DOSAGE

### Hyponatremia
*Adult:* **IV** 20 mg loading dose followed by 20 mg IV over 24 h. May repeat 20 mg/day dose for 1–3 days, or may titrate up to 40 mg/day based on response. Total duration of infusion should not exceed 4 days.

Common adverse effects in *italic;* life-threatening effects underlined; generic names in **bold;** classifications in SMALL CAPS; ♣Canadian drug name; ℗ Prototype drug

401

## ADMINISTRATION

### Intravenous

*PREPARE:* **IV Infusion:** Packaged as 20 mg/100 mL IV solution. No further preparation is necessary.

*ADMINISTER:* **IV Infusion:** Give via a large vein and change infusion site every 24 h. *Loading dose:* Give over 30 min. *Maintenance dose:* Give over 24 h. ▪ Frequently monitor the serum sodium level. A reduction in dose or discontinuation of infusion may be required if the serum sodium rises too rapidly. Discontinue infusion immediately and notify prescriber of a rise in serum sodium greater than 12 mEq/L/24 h. **Do not** resume infusion if serum sodium continues to rise. ▪ Infusion may be resumed ONLY if hyponatremia persists or reoccurs and patient demonstrates no indication of neurologic impairment. If the serum sodium rises too slowly, the dose may be titrated up to 40 mg over 24 h.

*INCOMPATIBILITIES:* Solution/additive: **Lactated Ringer's solution, sodium chloride 0.9%.**

▪ Store vials at 25° C (77° F). Ampules should be stored in the original container and protected from light until ready for use. ▪ After diluting with D5W, the solution should be used immediately, with infusion completed within 24 h of mixing.

## ADVERSE EFFECTS (≥1%) **Body as a Whole:** Cannula-site reaction, *infusion-site reaction,* pain, peripheral edema, pyrexia, *thirst.*

**CNS:** Confusional state, *headache,* insomnia. **CV:** <u>Atrial fibrillation</u>, hypertension, hypotension, orthostatic hypotension, phlebitis. **GI:** Constipation, diarrhea, dry mouth, nausea, vomiting. **Hematologic:** Anemia. **Metabolic:** Dehydration, hyperglycemia, hypoglycemia, *hypokalemia,* hypomagnesemia, hyponatremia. **Respiratory:** Pneumonia. **Skin:** Erythema. **Special Senses:** Oral candidiasis.

## INTERACTIONS **Drug:** Compounds that inhibit CYP3A4 (e.g., **ketoconazole, itraconazole, clarithromycin, ritonavir, indinavir**) can increase conivaptan levels. Conivaptan can increase the levels of **digoxin** and drugs that require CYP3A4 for metabolism (e.g., **midazolam,** HMG COA REDUCTASE INHIBITORS, **amlodipine**). **Food: Grapefruit juice** may increase the level of conivaptan. **Herbal: St. John's wort** may decrease the level of conivaptan.

## PHARMACOKINETICS **Distribution:** 99% protein bound. **Metabolism:** Extensive hepatic metabolism. **Elimination:** Primarily fecal elimination (83%) with minor renal elimination. **Half-Life:** 5 h.

## NURSING IMPLICATIONS

### Assessment & Drug Effects

▪ Monitor infusion site for erythema, phlebitis, or other site reaction.
▪ Monitor vital signs and neurologic status frequently; report immediately S&S of hypernatremia (see Appendix F).
▪ Monitor digoxin blood levels with concurrent therapy and assess for S&S of digoxin toxicity.

Common adverse effects in *italic;* life-threatening effects <u>underlined</u>; generic names in **bold;** classifications in SMALL CAPS; ♣ Canadian drug name; ☯ Prototype drug

- Monitor I&O closely. Effective treatment is accompanied by increased urine output, whereas decreasing urine output and oliguria may indicate developing hypernatremia.
- Monitor lab tests: Baseline and frequent serum sodium, serum potassium, and urine osmolality.

**Patient & Family Education**

- Report any of the following to a health care provider: Pain at the infusion site, dizziness, confusion, palpitations, swelling of hands or feet.

## CORTISONE ACETATE
(kor'ti-sone)

Cortistan, Cortone

**Classifications:** ADRENOCORTICAL STEROID; ANTI-INFLAMMATORY

**Therapeutic:** ANTI-INFLAMMATORY; GLUCOCORTICOID REPLACEMENT; IMMUNOSUPPRESSANT

**Prototype:** Prednisone

**AVAILABILITY** Solution for injection

## ACTION & *THERAPEUTIC EFFECT*

Short-acting synthetic steroid with prominent glucocorticoid activity and minimal mineralocorticoid effects. Cortisone is converted in the body to cortisol, resulting in metabolic effects including promotion of protein, carbohydrate, and fat metabolism and interference with linear growth in children. *Has anti-inflammatory and immunosuppressive actions. Suppresses inflammation caused by radiant, mechanical, chemical, and infectious stimuli. Also suppress immune responses in diseases, such as in asthma, urticaria, or renal allograft.*

**USES** Replacement therapy for primary or secondary adrenocortical insufficiency and inflammatory and allergic disorders.

**CONTRAINDICATIONS** Hypersensitivity to glucocorticoids; psychoses; viral, fungal, or bacterial diseases of skin; Cushing's syndrome; immunologic procedures; pregnancy (category D); lactation.

**CAUTIOUS USE** Diabetes mellitus; hypertension, CHF; older adults; active or arrested tuberculosis; coagulopathy; hepatic disease; psychosis, emotional instability; renal disease, seizure disorders; active or latent peptic ulcer.

## ROUTE & DOSAGE

**Replacement or Inflammatory Disorders**

*Adult:* **PO/IM** 20–300 mg/day in 1 or more divided doses, try to reduce periodically by 10–25 mg/day to lowest effective dose
*Child:* **PO** 2.5–10 mg/kg/day divided q6–8h; **IM** 1–5 mg/kg/day divided q12–24h

## ADMINISTRATION

**Oral**

- Administer cortisone (usually in a.m.) with food or fluid of patient's choice to reduce gastric irritation.
- Sodium chloride and a mineralocorticoid are usually given with cortisone as part of replacement therapy.

**Intramuscular**

- Shake bottle well before withdrawing dose.
- Give deep IM into a large muscle.
- Drug **must be** gradually tapered rather than withdrawn abruptly.
- Store at 15°–30° C (59°–86° F) in tightly closed container unless

Common adverse effects in *italic;* life-threatening effects <u>underlined</u>; generic names in **bold;** classifications in SMALL CAPS; ♣ Canadian drug name; ⊘ Prototype drug

403

**C**

otherwise directed by manufacturer. Protect from heat and freezing.

## ADVERSE EFFECTS (≥1%) CV:
CHF, hypertension, *edema*. GI: *Nausea*, peptic ulcer, pancreatitis. **Endocrine:** Hyperglycemia. **Hematologic:** Thrombocytopenia. **Musculoskeletal:** *Compression fracture,* osteoporosis, muscle weakness. **CNS:** Euphoria, insomnia, vertigo, nystagmus. **Skin:** Impaired wound healing, petechiae, ecchymosis, acne. **Special Senses:** *Cataracts,* glaucoma, blurred vision.

## INTERACTIONS Drug: BARBITU-
RATES, **phenytoin, rifampin** decrease effects of cortisone.

## PHARMACOKINETICS Absorption:
Readily absorbed from GI tract. **Onset:** Rapid PO; 24–48 h IM. **Peak:** 2 h PO; 24–48 h IM. **Duration:** 1.25–1.5 days. **Distribution:** Concentrated in many tissues; crosses placenta; distributed in breast milk. **Metabolism:** In liver. **Elimination:** In urine. **Half-Life:** 0.5 h; HPA suppression: 8–12 h.

## NURSING IMPLICATIONS

### Assessment & Drug Effects

- Monitor for S&S of Cushing's syndrome (see Appendix F), especially in patients on long-term therapy.
- Cortisone may mask some signs of infection, and new infections may appear.
- Be alert to clinical indications of infection: Malaise, anorexia, depression, and evidence of delayed healing. (Classic signs of inflammation are suppressed by cortisone.)
- Report ecchymotic areas, unexplained bleeding, and easy bruising.

- Monitor lab tests: Periodic blood glucose and CBC with platelet count.

### Patient & Family Education

- Take drug exactly as prescribed. Do not alter dose intervals or stop therapy abruptly.
- Monitor weight and report a steady gain especially if it is accompanied by signs of fluid retention (e.g., edema of ankles or hands).
- Report changes in visual acuity, including blurring, promptly.
- Inform prescriber or dentist that cortisone is being taken.

## CROFELEMER
(kroe-fel′e-mer)

Fulyzaq

**Classifications:** ANTIDIARRHEAL; CHLORIDE ION CHANNEL BLOCKER
Therapeutic: ANTIDIARRHEAL

## AVAILABILITY    Delayed-release tablet

## ACTION & *THERAPEUTIC EFFECT*
Crofelemer blocks chloride ion secretion in the intestine and accompanying high volume water loss in diarrhea, normalizing the flow of chloride ions and water in the GI tract. *By decreasing water loss via the GI tract, diarrhea is substantially diminished.*

## USES Symptomatic relief of noninfectious diarrhea in patients with HIV/AIDS on anti-retroviral therapy.

## CONTRAINDICATIONS Diarrhea caused by infection; lactation.

## CAUTIOUS USE Pregnancy (category C); older adults. Safety and efficacy in children younger than 18 y not established.

## ROUTE & DOSAGE

**Diarrhea**
*Adult:* **PO** 125 mg b.i.d.

## ADMINISTRATION

**Oral**
▪ May be given without regard to food.
▪ Tablets must be swallowed whole. They should not be crushed or chewed.
▪ Store at 15°–30° C (59°–86° F).

## ADVERSE EFFECTS (≥1%) **Body as a Whole:** Abdominal distension, abdominal pain, acne, *cough, flatulence,* giardiasis, herpes zoster infection, pain in extremity, procedural pain, seasonal allergy. **CNS:** Depression. **CV:** Dizziness. **GI:** Constipation, dry mouth, dyspepsia, gastroenteritis, hemorrhoids, nausea. **Metabolic:** Decreased white blood cell count, increased ALT/AST, *increased bilirubin.* **Musculoskeletal:** Arthralgia, back pain, musculoskeletal pain. **Respiratory:** *Bronchitis,* nasopharyngitis, sinusitis, *upper respiratory tract infection.* **Skin:** Dermatitis. **Urogenital:** Nephrolithiasis, pollakiuria, urinary tract infection.

## INTERACTIONS **Drug:** Crofelemer may have additive effects with other antidiarrheal agents or those who produce constipation (i.e., OPIOIDS). Constipation and bowel obstruction have been reported in IBS patients taking **alosetron** in combination with other agents to control diarrhea.

## PHARMACOKINETICS **Absorption:** Minimal oral absorption. **Metabolism:** Not metabolized. **Elimination:** Not identified.

## NURSING IMPLICATIONS
### Assessment & Drug Effects
▪ Monitor bowel elimination. Report to prescriber if the number of daily episodes of watery diarrhea does not diminish.
▪ Note that infectious diarrhea will not respond to this therapy.

### Patient & Family Education
▪ Contact prescriber if diarrhea does not substantially diminish.

## CROMOLYN SODIUM ⊕
(kroe′moe-lin)
Crolom, Fivent ♦, Gastrocrom, Intal, Opticrom, Rynacrom ♦, Vistacrom ♦
**Classifications:** RESPIRATORY AGENT; MAST CELL STABILIZER; ANTI-INFLAMMATORY; ANTIASTHMATIC
Therapeutic: ANTIASTHMATIC; ANTI-INFLAMMATORY

**AVAILABILITY** Solution for nebulization; spray; nasal solution; ophthalmic solution; oral concentrate

## ACTION & *THERAPEUTIC EFFECT*
Inhibits release of bronchoconstrictors, histamine and slow-reacting substance of anaphylaxis, from sensitized pulmonary mast cells, thereby suppressing an allergic response. Additionally, cromolyn may also reduce the release of inflammatory leukotrienes. *Particularly effective for IgE-mediated or "extrinsic asthma" precipitated by exposure to specific allergen (e.g., pollens, dust, animal dander), by inhibiting the release of bronchoconstrictors.*

**USES** Primarily for prophylaxis of mild to moderate seasonal and

Common adverse effects in *italic*; life-threatening effects <u>underlined</u>; generic names in **bold**; classifications in SMALL CAPS; ♦ Canadian drug name; ⊕ Prototype drug

405

C

perennial bronchial asthma and allergic rhinitis. Also used for prevention of exercise-related bronchospasm, prevention of acute bronchospasm induced by known pollutants or antigens, and for prevention and treatment of allergic rhinitis. Orally for systemic mastocytosis. **Ophthalmic:** Allergic ocular disorders, conjunctivitis, vernal keratoconjunctivitis.

**UNLABELED USES** Orally for prophylaxis of GI and systemic reactions to food allergy.

**CONTRAINDICATIONS** Use of aerosol (because of fluorocarbon propellants) in patients with coronary artery disease or history of arrhythmias; dyspnea, acute asthma, status asthmaticus, or acute bronchospasm; patients unable to coordinate actions or follow instructions.

**CAUTIOUS USE** Renal or hepatic dysfunction; pregnancy (category B); lactation. **Inhalation and nasal spray:** Safe use in children younger than 6 y not established. Safe use in children under 6 y not established. **Ophthalmic:** Safe use under 2 y not established.

## ROUTE & DOSAGE

### Allergies

*Adult:* **Inhalation** Metered dose inhaler or capsule: 1 spray or 1 capsule inhaled q.i.d.; nasal solution: 1 spray in each nostril 3–6 × day at regular intervals
*Child (6y or older):* **Inhalation** Metered dose inhaler or capsule, same as for adult; *6 y or older:* Nasal solution, same as for adult

### Conjunctivitis

*Adult:* **PO** 2 ampules q.i.d. 30 min a.c. and at bedtime
*Child (2–12 y):* **PO** 1 ampule q.i.d. 30 min a.c. and at bedtime

### Mastocytosis

See Appendix A-1.

## ADMINISTRATION

### Oral
▪ Give at least 30 min before meals.

### Inhalation
▪ Patients should receive detailed instructions for each inhalation device. See manufacturer's instructions. Therapeutic effect is dependent on proper inhalation technique.
▪ Advise patient to clear as much mucus as possible before inhalation treatments.
▪ Instruct patient to exhale as completely as possible before placing inhaler mouthpiece between lips, tilt head backward and inhale rapidly and deeply with steady, even breaths. Remove inhaler from mouth, hold breath for a few seconds, then exhale into the air. Repeat until entire dose is taken.
▪ Protect cromolyn from moisture and heat. Store in tightly closed, light-resistant container at 15°–30° C (59°–86° F) unless otherwise directed.

## ADVERSE EFFECTS (≥1%) **Body as a Whole:** Peripheral eosinophilia, angioedema, bronchospasm, anaphylaxis (rare). **GI:** Swelling of parotid glands, dry mouth, slightly bitter aftertaste, *nausea,* vomiting, esophagitis. **CNS:** Headache, dizziness, peripheral neuritis. **Skin:** Erythema, urticaria, rash, contact dermatitis. **Special Senses:** *Sneezing, nasal stinging and burning,* dryness and *irritation of throat and trachea; cough;* nasal congestion, itchy, puffy eyes, lacrimation, *transient ocular burning, stinging.*

Common adverse effects in *italic*; life-threatening effects underlined; generic names in **bold;** classifications in SMALL CAPS; ✦ Canadian drug name; ⊙ Prototype drug

## PHARMACOKINETICS Absorption:
Approximately 8% of dose absorbed from lungs. **Onset:** 1 wk with regular use. **Peak:** 15 min. **Duration:** 4–6 h; may last as long as 2–3 wk. **Elimination:** In bile and urine in equal amounts. **Half-Life:** 80 min.

## NURSING IMPLICATIONS

### Assessment & Drug Effects

- Withhold drug and notify prescriber if any of the following occur; angioedema or bronchospasm.
- Monitor for exacerbation of asthmatic symptoms including breathlessness and cough that may occur in patients receiving cromolyn during corticosteroid withdrawal.
- For patients with asthma, therapeutic effects may be noted within a few days but generally not until after 1–2 wk of therapy.

### Patient & Family Education

- Throat irritation, cough, and hoarseness can be minimized by gargling with water, drinking a few swallows of water, or by sucking on a lozenge after each treatment.
- Talk to your prescriber about what to do in the event of an acute asthmatic attack. Cromolyn is of no value in acute asthma.
- Cromolyn does not eliminate the continued need for therapy with bronchodilators, expectorants, antibiotics, or corticosteroids, but the amount and frequency of use of these medications may be appreciably reduced.
- Report any unusual signs or symptoms. Hypersensitivity reactions (see Signs & Symptoms, Appendix F) can be severe and life-threatening. Drug should be discontinued if an allergic reaction occurs.

# CROTAMITON
(kroe-tam'i-ton)
Eurax

**Classifications:** SCABICIDE; ANTIPRURITIC
**Therapeutic:** SCABICIDE; ANTIPRURITIC
**Prototype:** Lindane

## AVAILABILITY Cream; lotion

## ACTION & THERAPEUTIC EFFECT
By unknown mechanisms, drug eradicates *Sarcoptes scabiei* and *effectively relieves itching.*

## USES Treatment of scabies and for symptomatic treatment of pruritus.

## CONTRAINDICATIONS Application to acutely inflamed skin, raw or weeping surfaces, eyes, or mouth; history of previous sensitivity to crotamiton.

## CAUTIOUS USE Pregnancy (category C), children.

## ROUTE & DOSAGE

### Scabies/Pruritus

*Adult:* **Topical** Apply a thin layer of cream from neck to toes; apply a second layer 24 h later; bathe 48 h after last application to remove drug

## ADMINISTRATION

### Topical

- Shake container well before use of solution.
- The skin **must be** thoroughly dry before applying medication.
- If drug accidentally contacts eyes, thoroughly flush out medication with water.

---

Common adverse effects in *italic*; life-threatening effects underlined; generic names in **bold**; classifications in SMALL CAPS; ◆ Canadian drug name; ⊘ Prototype drug

- Pruritus treatment: Massage medication gently into affected areas until it is completely absorbed. Repeat as needed (usually effective for 6–10 h).
- Store in tightly closed containers at 15°–30° C (59°–86° F). Do not freeze.

## ADVERSE EFFECTS (≥1%) Skin:
Skin irritation (particularly with prolonged use), rash, erythema, sensation of cooling, allergic sensitization.

## NURSING IMPLICATIONS
### Assessment & Drug Effects
- Monitor for and report significant skin irritation or allergic sensitization.

### Patient & Family Education
- Review package insert before treatment begins.
- Discontinue medication and report to prescriber if irritation or sensitization develops.

## CYANOCOBALAMIN
(sye-an-oh-koe-bal'a-min)
Anacobin ♦, Bedoz ♦,
Nascobal, Rubion ♦
**Classification:** VITAMIN B$_{12}$
Therapeutic: VITAMIN B$_{12}$

**AVAILABILITY** Tablet; nasal gel; nasal spray

## ACTION & THERAPEUTIC EFFECT
Vitamin B$_{12}$ is a cobalt-containing B complex vitamin essential for normal growth, cell reproduction, maturation of RBCs, nucleoprotein synthesis, maintenance of nervous system (myelin synthesis), and believed to be involved in protein and carbohydrate metabolism. *Therapeutically effective for treatment of vitamin B$_{12}$ deficiency and pernicious anemia.*

**USES** Vitamin B$_{12}$ deficiency due to malabsorption syndrome as in pernicious (Addison's) anemia, sprue; GI pathology, dysfunction, or surgery; fish tapeworm infestation, and gluten enteropathy. Also used in B$_{12}$ deficiency caused by increased physiologic requirements or inadequate dietary intake, and in vitamin B$_{12}$ absorption (Schilling) test.

**UNLABELED USES** To prevent and treat toxicity associated with sodium nitroprusside.

**CONTRAINDICATIONS** History of sensitivity to vitamin B$_{12}$, other cobalamins, or cobalt; early Leber's disease (hereditary optic nerve atrophy), indiscriminate use in folic acid deficiency.

**CAUTIOUS USE** Heart disease, anemia, pulmonary disease; pregnancy (category A for **PO** or **nasal route,** and category C for **parenteral**).

## ROUTE & DOSAGE

### Vitamin B$_{12}$ Deficiency
*Adult:* **IM/Deep Subcutaneous** 30 mcg/day for 5–10 days, then 100–200 mcg/mo
*Child:* **IM/Deep Subcutaneous** 100 mcg doses to a total of 1–5 mg over 2 wk, then 60 mcg/mo

### Pernicious Anemia
*Adult:* **IM/Deep Subcutaneous** 100–1000 mcg/day for 2–3 wk, then 100–1000 mcg q2–4wk

**Intranasal** one pump in one nostril once weekly
*Child:* **IM** 30–50 mcg/day × 2 wk to total of 1000 mcg, then 100 mcg/mo
*Infant:* **IM** 1000 mcg/day × at least 2 wk, then 50 mcg/mo

**Diagnosis of Megaloblastic Anemia**
*Adult:* **IM/Deep Subcutaneous** 1 mcg/day for 10 days while maintaining a low folate and vitamin B₁₂ diet

**Schilling Test**
*Adult:* **IM/Deep Subcutaneous** 1000 mcg × 1 dose

**Nutritional Supplement**
*Adult:* **PO** 1–25 mcg/day
*Child (younger than 1 y):* **PO** 0.3 mcg/day; *1 y or older:* 1 mcg/day

## ADMINISTRATION
### Oral
- PO preparations may be mixed with fruit juices. However, administer promptly since ascorbic acid affects the stability of vitamin B₁₂.
- Administration of oral vitamin B₁₂ with meals increases its absorption.

### Subcutaneous/Intramuscular
- Give deep subcutaneous by slightly tenting the skin at the injection site.
- IM may be given into any normal IM injection site.
- Preserved in light-resistant containers at room temperature preferably at 15°–30° C (59°–86° F) unless otherwise directed by manufacturer.

**ADVERSE EFFECTS** (≥1%) **Body as a Whole:** Feeling of swelling of body, <u>anaphylactic shock, sudden death</u>. **CV:** Peripheral vascular thrombosis, pulmonary edema, CHF. **GI:** Mild transient diarrhea. **Hematologic:** Unmasking of polycythemia vera (with correction of vitamin B₁₂ deficiency). **Metabolic:** Hypokalemia. **Skin:** Itching, rash, flushing. **Special Senses:** Severe optic nerve atrophy (patients with Leber's disease).

**DIAGNOSTIC TEST INTERFERENCE** Most antibiotics, methotrexate, and pyrimethamine may produce invalid diagnostic *blood assays for vitamin B₁₂*. Possibility of false-positive test for *intrinsic factor antibodies*.

**INTERACTIONS Drug:** Alcohol, **aminosalicylic acid, neomycin, colchicine** may decrease absorption of oral cyanocobalamin; **chloramphenicol** may interfere with therapeutic response to cyanocobalamin.

**PHARMACOKINETICS Absorption:** Intestinal absorption requires presence of intrinsic factor in terminal ileum. **Distribution:** Widely distributed; principally stored in liver, kidneys, and adrenals; crosses placenta, excreted in breast milk. **Metabolism:** Converted in tissues to active coenzymes; enterohepatically cycled. **Elimination:** 50–95% of doses 100 mcg or more are excreted in urine in 48 h. **Half-Life:** 6 days (400 days in liver).

## NURSING IMPLICATIONS
### Assessment & Drug Effects
- Obtain a careful history of sensitivities. Sensitization to cyanocobalamin can take as long as 8 y to develop.

---

Common adverse effects in *italic;* life-threatening effects <u>underlined</u>; generic names in **bold;** classifications in SMALL CAPS; ♣ Canadian drug name; ⦿ Prototype drug

409

**C**

- Monitor vital signs in patients with cardiac disease and in those receiving parenteral cyanocobalamin, and be alert to symptoms of pulmonary edema, which generally occur early in therapy.
- Characteristically, reticulocyte concentration rises in 3–4 days, peaks in 5–8 days, and then gradually declines as erythrocyte count and Hgb rise to normal levels (in 4–6 wk).
- Obtain a complete diet and drug history and inquire into alcohol drinking patterns for all patients receiving cyanocobalamin to identify and correct poor habits.
- Monitor lab tests: Baseline reticulocyte and erythrocyte counts, Hgb, Hct, vitamin $B_{12}$, and serum folate levels; then repeated between 5 and 7 days after start of therapy and at regular intervals during therapy. Monitor potassium levels during the first 48 h.

### Patient & Family Education

- Notify prescriber of any intercurrent disease or infection. Increased dosage may be required.
- To prevent irreversible neurologic damage resulting from pernicious anemia, drug therapy **must be** continued throughout life.
- Rich food sources of $B_{12}$ are nutrient-added breakfast cereals, vitamin $B_{12}$-fortified soy milk, organ meats, clams, oysters, egg yolk, crab, salmon, sardines, muscle meat, milk, and dairy products.

## CYCLOBENZAPRINE HYDROCHLORIDE ℞

(sye-kloe-ben′za-preen)
Amrix, Flexeril, Flexmid

**Classification:** CENTRAL ACTING SKELETAL MUSCLE RELAXANT
Therapeutic: SKELETAL MUSCLE RELAXANT; ANTISPASMODIC

**AVAILABILITY** Tablet; extended release capsule

## ACTION & *THERAPEUTIC EFFECT*

Relieves skeletal muscle spasm of local origin without interfering with muscle function. Believed to act primarily within CNS at brain stem. Depresses tonic somatic motor activity, although both gamma and alpha motor neurons are affected. *Relieves muscle spasm associated with acute, painful musculoskeletal conditions.*

**USES** Short-term adjunct to rest and physical therapy for relief of muscle spasm associated with acute musculoskeletal conditions. Not effective in treatment of spasticity associated with cerebral palsy or cerebral or cord disease.

**UNLABELED USES** Fibromyalgia.

**CONTRAINDICATIONS** Acute recovery phase of MI, cardiac arrhythmias, heart block or conduction disturbances, QT prolongation; CHF, hyperthyroidism; moderate or severe hepatic impairment; MAOI therapy within 14 days of use; cerebral palsy. **Extended release:** Do not use capsule for older adults.

**CAUTIOUS USE** Prostatic hypertrophy, history of urinary retention, seizures; cardiovascular disease; mild hepatic impairment; closed angle glaucoma; increased intraocular pressure; older adults, debilitated patients; history of psychiatric illness; pregnancy (category B); lactation. Safe use in children younger than 15 y not established.

## ROUTE & DOSAGE

### Muscle Spasm

*Adult/Adolescent (15 y or older):*
**PO** 5–10 mg t.i.d. (max: 30 mg/day); **Extended release** 15–30 mg daily
*Geriatric:* Start with 5 mg, adjust dose slowly

### Hepatic Impairment Dosage Adjustment

*Mild:* Start with 5 mg
*Moderate to Severe:* Not recommended

## ADMINISTRATION

### Oral

- Do not administer drug if patient is receiving an MAO inhibitor (e.g., furazolidone, isocarboxazid, pargyline, tranylcypromine).
- Do not open extended release capsules. They **must be** swallowed whole.
- Cyclobenzaprine is intended for short-term (2 or 3 wk) use.
- Store in tightly closed container, preferably at 15°–30° C (59°–86° F) unless otherwise directed by manufacturer.

## ADVERSE EFFECTS (≥1%) **Body as a Whole:** Edema of tongue and face, sweating, myalgia, hepatitis, alopecia. Shares toxic potential of tricyclic antidepressants. **CV:** Tachycardia, syncope, palpitation, vasodilation, chest pain, orthostatic hypotension, dyspnea; with high doses, possibility of severe arrhythmias. **GI:** *Dry mouth,* indigestion, unpleasant taste, coated tongue, tongue discoloration, vomiting, anorexia, abdominal pain, flatulence, diarrhea, paralytic ileus. **CNS:** *Drowsiness, dizziness,* weakness, fatigue, asthenia, paresthesias, tremors, muscle twitching, insomnia, euphoria, disorientation, mania, ataxia. **Skin:** Pruritus, urticaria, skin rash. **Urogenital:** Increased or decreased libido, impotence.

## INTERACTIONS **Drug:** **Alcohol,** BARBITURATES, other CNS DEPRESSANTS enhance CNS depression; potentiates anticholinergic effects of **phenothiazine** and other ANTICHOLINERGICS; MAO INHIBITORS may precipitate hypertensive crisis—use with extreme caution.

## PHARMACOKINETICS **Absorption:** Well absorbed from GI tract with some first-pass elimination in liver. **Onset:** 1 h. **Peak:** 3–8 h. **Duration:** 12–24 h. **Distribution:** 93% protein bound. **Metabolism:** In liver to inactive metabolites. **Elimination:** Slowly in urine with some elimination in feces; may be excreted in breast milk. **Half-Life:** 1–3 days.

## NURSING IMPLICATIONS

### Assessment & Drug Effects

- Supervision of ambulation may be indicated, especially in the older adult because of risk of drowsiness and dizziness.
- Withhold drug and notify prescriber if signs of hypersensitivity (e.g., pruritus, urticaria, rash) appear.

### Patient & Family Education

- Avoid driving and other potentially hazardous activities until reaction to drug is known. Adverse effects include drowsiness and dizziness.
- Avoid alcohol and other CNS depressants (unless otherwise directed by prescriber) because cyclobenzaprine enhances their effects.
- Dry mouth may be relieved by increasing total fluid intake (if not contraindicated).
- Keep prescriber informed of therapeutic effectiveness. Spasmolytic

effect usually begins within 1 or 2 days and may be manifested by lessening of pain and tenderness, increase in range of motion, and ability to perform ADL.

# CYCLOPHOSPHAMIDE ⓟ

(sye-kloe-foss'fa-mide)

Procytox ♦

**Classifications:** ANTINEOPLASTIC; NITROGEN MUSTARD; ALKYLATING AGENT

Therapeutic: ANTINEOPLASTIC

**AVAILABILITY** Tablet; solution for injection

## ACTION & *THERAPEUTIC EFFECT*

Cell-cycle–nonspecific alkylating agent that causes cross-linkage of DNA strands, thereby blocking synthesis of DNA, RNA, and protein. *Has pronounced antineoplastic effects and immunosuppressive activity.*

## USES

In treatment of malignant lymphoma, multiple myeloma, leukemias, mycosis fungoides (advanced disease), neuroblastoma, adenocarcinoma of ovary, carcinoma of breast, or malignant neoplasms of lung.

## UNLABELED USES

To prevent rejection in homotransplantation; to treat severe rheumatoid arthritis, multiple sclerosis, systemic lupus erythematosus, Wegener's granulomatosis, nephrotic syndrome.

## CONTRAINDICATIONS

Absolute contraindication with bladder or urinary tract obstruction. Hypersensitivity to cyclophosphamide; serious infections (including chickenpox, herpes zoster); live virus vaccines; severe myelosuppression; dehydration; severe hemorrhagic cystitis; pregnancy (category D); lactation.

## CAUTIOUS USE

History of radiation or cytotoxic drug therapy; hepatic and renal impairment, elderly; recent history of steroid therapy; history of cardiac disease or arrhythmias, bone marrow infiltration with tumor cells; history of urate calculi and gout; patients with leukopenia, thrombocytopenia; men and women of childbearing age.

## ROUTE & DOSAGE

### Neoplasm

*Adult:* **PO Initial** 1–5 mg/kg/day; **Maintenance** 1–5 mg/kg q7–10 days **IV** dose varies based on concurrent antineoplastic agents, see package insert for specific dosing
*Child:* **PO Initial** 2–8 mg/kg or 60–250 mg/m² ; **Maintenance** 2–5 mg/kg or 50–150 mg/m² twice weekly; **IV Initial** 2–8 mg/ kg or 60–250 mg/m²

### Renal Impairment Dosage Adjustment

*CrCl less than 10 mL/min:* Give 50% of dose; administer post-dialysis, give supplemental dose of 35%

## ADMINISTRATION

### Oral

- Administer in the morning PO drug on empty stomach. Do not cut, crush or chew tablets. Wash hands immediately if contact with broken tablet occurs. If nausea and vomiting are severe, however, it may be taken with food. An antiemetic medication may be prescribed to be given before the drug.
- Store cyclophosphamide PO solution in refrigerator at 2°–8° C (36°–46° F) and use within 14 days.

### Intravenous

*PREPARE:* **Direct:** Add 5 mL NS for each 100 mg and shake gently to dissolve. **Do not** reconstitute with sterile water for injection if giving direct IV. **Intermittent:** May be further diluted for infusion with 100–250 mL D5W, D5/NS, or 0.45% NaCl.

*ADMINISTER:* **Direct/Intermittent:** Give each 100 mg or fraction thereof over 10–15 min.

*INCOMPATIBILITIES:* **Y-site: Amphotericin B cholesteryl complex, amphotericin B colloidal, asparaginase, diazepam, gemtuzumab, lansoprazole, phenytoin.**

▪ If mixed with 5% dextrose or 5% dextrose and 0.9% sodium chloride for injection, store at room temperature for up to 24 h and refrigerated for up to 36 h.

## ADVERSE EFFECTS (≥1%) **Body as a Whole:** Transient dizziness, fatigue, facial flushing, diaphoresis, drug fever, anaphylaxis, secondary neoplasia. **GI:** *Nausea, vomiting,* mucositis, *anorexia,* hepatotoxicity, diarrhea. **Hematologic:** Leukopenia, *neutropenia,* acute myeloid leukemia, anemia, thrombophlebitis, interference with normal healing. **Metabolic:** Severe hyperkalemia, SIADH, hyponatremia, weight gain (but without edema) or weight loss, hyperuricemia. **Respiratory:** Pulmonary emboli and edema, pneumonitis, interstitial pulmonary fibrosis. **Skin:** *Alopecia* (reversible), transverse ridging of nails, pigmentation of nail beds and skin (reversible), nonspecific dermatitis, toxic epidermal necrolysis, Stevens–Johnson syndrome. **Urogenital:** Sterile hemorrhagic and nonhemorrhagic cystitis, bladder fibrosis, nephrotoxicity.

## DIAGNOSTIC TEST INTERFERENCE
Cyclophosphamide suppresses positive reactions to **Candida, *mumps, trichophytons,*** and ***tuberculin PPD skin tests. Papanicolaou (PAP)*** smear may be falsely positive.

## INTERACTIONS **Drug: Succinylcholine,** prolonged neuromuscular blocking activity; **doxorubicin** may increase cardiac toxicity.

## PHARMACOKINETICS **Absorption:** Readily from GI tract. **Peak:** 1 h PO. **Distribution:** Widely distributed, including brain, breast milk; crosses placenta. **Metabolism:** In liver by CYP3A4. **Elimination:** In urine as active metabolites and unchanged drug. **Half-Life:** 4–6 h.

## NURSING IMPLICATIONS
### Assessment & Drug Effects
▪ Assess for signs of unexplained bleeding or easy bruising which could indicate thrombocytopenia.

▪ Marked leukopenia is the most serious side effect. It can be fatal. Nadir may occur in 2–8 days after first dose but may be as late as 1 mo after a series of several daily doses. Leukopenia usually reverses 7–10 days after therapy is discontinued.

▪ During severe leukopenic period, protect patient from infection and trauma and from visitors and medical personnel who have colds or other infections.

▪ Report onset of unexplained chills, sore throat, tachycardia. Monitor temperature carefully and report an elevation immediately. The development of fever in a neutropenic patient (granulocyte count less than 1000) is a medical emergency because sepsis can develop quickly in these patients.

▪ Observe and report character of wound drainage. During period of neutropenia, purulent drainage may become serosanguineous because there are not enough WBC to create pus. Because of suppressed immune mechanisms,

Common adverse effects in *italic;* life-threatening effects underlined; generic names in **bold;** classifications in SMALL CAPS; ♣ Canadian drug name; ⊙ Prototype drug

413

wound healing may be prolonged or incomplete.

▪ Monitor I&O ratio and patterns: Since the drug is a chemical irritant, PO and IV fluid intake is generally increased to help prevent renal irritation and hemorrhagic cystitis. Have patient void frequently, especially after each dose and just before retiring to bed.

▪ Watch for symptoms of water intoxication or dilutional hyponatremia; patients are usually well hydrated as part of the therapy.

▪ Promptly report hematuria or dysuria. Drug schedule is usually interrupted and fluids are forced.

▪ Record body weight at least twice weekly (basis for dose determination). Alert prescriber to sudden change or slow, steady weight gain or loss over a period of time that appears inconsistent with caloric intake.

▪ Diarrhea may signal onset of hyperkalemia, particularly if accompanied by colicky pain, nausea, bradycardia, and skeletal muscle weakness. These symptoms warrant prompt reporting to prescriber.

▪ Monitor for hyperuricemia, which occurs commonly during early treatment period in patients with leukemias or lymphoma. Report edema of lower legs and feet; joint, flank, or stomach pain.

▪ Protect patient from potential sources of infection. Cyclophosphamide makes the patient particularly susceptible to varicellazoster infections (chickenpox, herpes zoster).

▪ Report any sign of overgrowth with opportunistic organisms, especially in patient receiving corticosteroids or who has recently been on steroid therapy.

▪ Report fever, dyspnea, and nonproductive cough. Pulmonary toxicity is not common, but the already debilitated patient is particularly susceptible.

▪ Monitor lab tests: Baseline total and differential leukocyte count, platelet count, and Hct, and repeat at least 2 × wk during maintenance period. Baseline and periodic LFTs, renal function, and serum electrolytes.

**Patient & Family Education**

▪ Adhere to dosage regimen and do not omit, increase, decrease, or delay doses. If for any reason drug cannot be taken, notify prescriber.

▪ Alopecia occurs in about 33% of patients on cyclophosphamide therapy. Hair loss may be noted 3 wk after therapy begins; regrowth (often differs in texture and color) usually starts 5–6 wk after drug is withdrawn and may occur while on maintenance doses.

▪ Use adequate means of contraception during and for at least 4 mo after termination of drug treatment. Breast-feeding should be discontinued before cyclophosphamide therapy is initiated.

▪ Amenorrhea may last up to 1 y after cessation of therapy in 10–30% of women.

# CYCLOSERINE
(sye-kloe-ser′een)
Seromycin
**Classification:** ANTITUBERCULOSIS
Therapeutic: ANTITUBERCULOSIS

**AVAILABILITY** Capsule

**ACTION & THERAPEUTIC EFFECT**
Inhibits cell wall synthesis in susceptible strains of bacteria. It competitively

Common adverse effects in *italic*; life-threatening effects <u>underlined</u>; generic names in **bold;** classifications in SMALL CAPS; ✦ Canadian drug name; ❷ Prototype drug interferes with the incorporation of D-alanine into the bacterial cell wall, resulting in cell death. *Effective against gram-positive and gram-negative bacteria and* Mycobacterium tuberculosis.

**USES** Treatment of tuberculosis, urinary tract infections.

**UNLABELED USES** Treatment of MAC.

**CONTRAINDICATIONS** Uncontrolled epilepsy; depression, severe anxiety, history of psychoses; severe renal insufficiency.

**CAUTIOUS USE** Renal impairment, anemia; chronic alcoholism; pregnancy (category C); lactation. Safe use in children not established.

### ROUTE & DOSAGE

**Tuberculosis**
*Adult:* **PO** 250 mg q12h for 2 wk, may increase to 250 q6–8h OR 15–20 mg/kg/day (max: 1 g/day)
**Urinary Tract Infection**
*Adult:* **PO** 250 mg q12h for 2 wk

### ADMINISTRATION

**Oral**
- Pyridoxine 200–300 mg/day may be ordered concurrently to prevent neurotoxic effects of cycloserine.
- Store in tightly closed container at 15°–30° C (59°–86° F) unless otherwise directed.

**ADVERSE EFFECTS** (≥1%) **CV:** Arrhythmias, CHF. **Hematologic:** Vitamin $B_{12}$ and folic acid deficiency, megaloblastic or sideroblastic anemia. **CNS:** *Drowsiness,* anxiety, *headache,* tremors, myoclonic jerking, convulsions, vertigo, visual disturbances, speech difficulties

(dysarthria), lethargy, depression, disorientation with loss of memory, confusion, nervousness, psychoses, tic episodes, character changes, hyperirritability, aggression, hyperreflexia, peripheral neuropathy, paresthesias, paresis, dyskinesias. **Skin:** Dermatitis, photosensitivity. **Special Senses:** Eye pain (optic neuritis), photophobia.

**INTERACTIONS Drug: Alcohol** increases risk of seizures; **ethionamide, isoniazid** potentiate neurotoxic effects; may inhibit **phenytoin** metabolism, increasing its toxicity.

**PHARMACOKINETICS Absorption:** 70–90% from GI tract. **Peak:** 3–4 h. **Distribution:** Distributed to lung, ascitic, pleural and synovial fluids, and CSF; crosses placenta; distributed into breast milk. **Metabolism:** Not metabolized. **Elimination:** 60–70% in urine within 72 h; small amount in feces. **Half-Life:** 10 h.

### NURSING IMPLICATIONS

**Assessment & Drug Effects**
- Maintenance of blood drug level below 30 mg/mL considerably reduces incidence of neurotoxicity. Possibility of neurotoxicity increases when dose is 500 mg or more or when renal clearance is inadequate.
- Observe patient carefully for signs of hypersensitivity and neurologic effects. Neurotoxicity generally appears within first 2 wk of therapy and disappears after drug is discontinued.
- Drug should be withheld and prescriber notified or dosage reduced if symptoms of CNS toxicity or hypersensitivity reaction (see Appendix F) develop.
- Monitor lab tests: Baseline C&S; weekly plasma drug levels; hematologic, renal function studies at regular intervals.

Common adverse effects in *italic;* life-threatening effects <u>underlined;</u> generic names in **bold;** classifications in SMALL CAPS; ♣ Canadian drug name; ☉ Prototype drug

415

C

## Patient & Family Education

- Take cycloserine after meals to prevent GI irritation.
- Notify prescriber immediately of the onset of skin rash and early signs of CNS toxicity (see Appendix F).
- Avoid potentially hazardous tasks such as driving until reaction to cycloserine has been determined.
- Take drug precisely as prescribed and to keep follow-up appointments. Continuous therapy may extend into months or years.

# CYCLOSPORINE ℗

(sye'kloe-spor-een)

Gengraf, Neoral, Restasis, Sandimmune

**Classifications:** BIOLOGIC RESPONSE MODIFIER; IMMUNOSUPPRESSANT

Therapeutic: IMMUNOSUPPRESSANT; ANTIRHEUMATIC; ANTIPSORIATIC

## AVAILABILITY Gengraf: Capsule. Neoral: Capsule; oral solution; solution for injection. Restasis: Ophthalmic emulsion. Sandimmune: Capsule; oral solution; injectable.

## ACTION & THERAPEUTIC EFFECT

Suppresses certain humoral immunity reactions (i.e., antigen-antibody reactions) and, to a greater extent, cell-mediated immune reactions. T-lymphocytes are preferentially inhibited (the T-helper cell is the main target, although the T-suppressor cell also may be suppressed). *Prevents allograft rejection in transplant patients. Additionally, it is a disease-modifying antirheumatic drug (DMARD) in RA patients that have not responded on methotrexate alone.*

## USES In conjunction with adrenal corticosteroids to prevent organ rejection after kidney, liver, and heart transplants (allografts). Also used for treatment of chronic transplant rejection in patients previously treated with other immunosuppressants; rheumatoid arthritis, severe psoriasis. Ophthalmic emulsion for the treatment of xerophthalmia.

**UNLABELED USES** Sjögren's syndrome, to prevent rejection of heart-lung and pancreatic transplants, ulcerative colitis.

**CONTRAINDICATIONS** Hypersensitivity to cyclosporine; recent contact with or bout of chickenpox, herpes zoster; administration of live virus vaccines to patient or family members; **Gengraf** and **Neoral** in psoriasis or RA patients with abnormal renal function, uncontrolled hypertension, or malignancies; ocular infection. **PO form:** Lactation.

**CAUTIOUS USE** Renal, hepatic, pancreatic, or bowel dysfunction; biliary tract disease, jaundice, hyperkalemia; electrolyte imbalance, hyperuricemia, hypertension; infection; radiation therapy, older adults, encephalopathy, fungal or viral infection, gout, herpes infection, lymphoma; neoplastic disease, malabsorption problems (e.g., liver transplant patients); older adults; females of childbearing age, pregnancy (category C).

## ROUTE & DOSAGE

### Prevention of Organ Rejection

*Can vary depending on transplanted organ and concurrent immunosuppresive use:* See package insert for details

*Adult/Child:* **PO** 14–18 mg/kg beginning 4–12 h before transplantation and continued for 1–2 wk after surgery, then gradual reduction by 5%/wk (max dose of microemulsion: 10 mg/kg/day)

**Maintenance** 5–10 mg/kg/day **IV** 5–6 mg/kg beginning 4–12 h before transplantation and continued after surgery until patient can take orally

**Rheumatoid Arthritis (Neoral)**

*Adult:* **PO** 2.5 mg/kg/day divided into 2 doses. May increase by 0.5–0.75 mg/kg/day q4wk to (max: 4 mg/kg/day)

**Severe Psoriasis (Neoral)**

*Adult:* **PO** 1.25 mg/kg b.i.d. If significant improvement has not occurred after 4 wk, may increase dose by 0.5 mg/kg/day every 2 wk (max: 4 mg/kg/day)

**Keratoconjunctivitis Sicca**

*Adult:* **Ophthalmic** 1 drop in affected eye(s) twice daily approximately 12 h apart

## ADMINISTRATION

### Oral

- Do not dilute oral solution with grapefruit juice. Dilute with orange or apple juice, stir well, then administer immediately.
- The various product brands may not be bioequivalent on a mg for mg basis. Do not interchange without prescriber supervision.

### Intravenous

*PREPARE:* **IV Infusion:** Dilute each 1 mL immediately before administration in 20–100 mL of D5W or NS. *ADMINISTER:* **IV Infusion:** Give by slow infusion over approximately 2–6 h. ▪Rapid IV can result in nephrotoxicity.

*INCOMPATIBILITIES:* Solution/additive: **Magnesium sulfate.** Y-site: **Amphotericin B cholesteryl complex, TPN.**

- Store preferably at 15°–30° C (59°–86° F) in well-closed containers. Do not refrigerate. ▪ Protect ampules from light.

## ADVERSE EFFECTS (≥1%) Body as a Whole: Lymphoma, gynecomastia, chest pain, leg cramps, edema, fever, chills, weight loss, increased risk of skin malignancies in psoriasis patients previously treated with methotrexate, psoralens, or UV light therapy. **CV:** *Hypertension,* MI (rare). **GI:** Gingival hyperplasia, diarrhea, nausea, *vomiting,* abdominal discomfort, anorexia, gastritis, constipation. **Hematologic:** Leukopenia, anemia, thrombocytopenia, *hypermagnesemia, hyperkalemia,* hyperuricemia, *decreased serum bicarbonate,* hyperglycemia. **CNS:** *Tremor,* convulsions, headache, paresthesias, hyperesthesia, flushing, night sweats, insomnia, visual hallucinations, confusion, anxiety, flat affect, depression, lethargy, weakness, paraparesis, ataxia, amnesia. **Skin:** *Hirsutism,* acne, oily skin, flushing. **Special Senses:** Sinusitis, tinnitus, hearing loss, sore throat. **Urogenital:** Urinary retention, frequency, *nephrotoxicity (oliguria).*

## DIAGNOSTIC TEST INTERFERENCE

*Hyperlipidemia* and abnormalities in *electrophoresis* reported; believed to be due to polyoxyl 35 castor oil **(Cremophor)** in IV cyclosporine.

## INTERACTIONS Drug: AMINOGLYCOSIDES, **danazol, diltiazem, doxycycline, erythromycin, ketoconazole, methylprednisolone, metoclopramide, nicardipine,** NSAIDS, **prednisolone, verapamil** may increase cyclosporine levels; **carbamazepine, isoniazid, octreotide, phenobarbital, phenytoin, rifampin** may decrease cyclosporine

Common adverse effects in *italic;* life-threatening effects <u>underlined;</u> generic names in **bold;** classifications in SMALL CAPS; ◆ Canadian drug name; ⊘ Prototype drug

417

C

levels; **acyclovir,** AMINOGLYCOSIDES, **amphotericin B, cidofovir, cimetidine, erythromycin, ketoconazole, melphalan, ranitidine, cotrimoxazole, trimethoprim** may increase risk of nephrotoxicity; POTASSIUM-SPARING DIURETICS, ACE INHIBITORS **(captopril, enalapril)** may potentiate hyperkalemia. **Food: Grapefruit juice** may increase concentration. **Herbal: St. John's wort** may decrease cyclosporine levels; **berberine** may increase toxicities.

## PHARMACOKINETICS **Absorption:** Variably and incompletely absorbed (30%). Microemulsion formulation (**Gengraf/Neoral**) has less variability and may produce significantly higher serum levels compared with the standard formulation. **Peak:** 3–4 h. **Distribution:** Widely distributed; 33–47% distributed to plasma; 41–50% to RBCs; crosses placenta; distributed into breast milk. **Metabolism:** In liver by CYP3A4, including significant first pass metabolism; considerable enterohepatic circulation. **Elimination:** Primarily in bile and feces; 6% in urine. **Half-Life:** 19–27 h.

## NURSING IMPLICATIONS
### Assessment & Drug Effects
- Observe patients receiving the drug parenterally for at least 30 min continuously after start of IV infusion, and at frequent intervals thereafter to detect allergic or other adverse reactions.
- Monitor I&O ratio and pattern: Nephrotoxicity has been reported in about one-third of transplant patients. It has occurred in mild forms as late as 2–3 mo after transplantation. In severe form, it can be irreversible, and therefore early recognition is critical.
- Monitor vital signs. Be alert to indicators of local or systemic infection

that can be fungal, viral, or bacterial. Also report significant rise in BP.
- Periodic tests should be made of neurologic function. Neurotoxic effects generally occur over 13–195 days after initiation of cyclosporine therapy. Signs and symptoms are reportedly fully reversible with dosage reduction or discontinuation of drug.
- Monitor blood or plasma drug concentrations at regular intervals, particularly in patients receiving the drug orally for prolonged periods, as drug absorption is erratic.
- Monitor lab tests: Baseline and periodic renal function, LFTs, and serum potassium. In psoriasis patients, CBC, BUN, uric acid, potassium, lipids, and magnesium biweekly during first 3 mo.

### Patient & Family Education
- Take medication with meals to reduce nausea or GI irritation.
- Enhance palatability of oral solution by mixing it with milk, chocolate milk, or orange juice, preferably at room temperature. Mix in a glass rather than a plastic container. Stir well, drink immediately, and rinse glass with small quantity of diluent to assure getting entire dose.
- Take medication at same time each day to maintain therapeutic blood levels.
- Practice good oral hygiene. Inspect mouth daily for white patches, sores, swollen gums.
- Hirsutism is reversible with discontinuation of drug.

## CYPROHEPTADINE HYDROCHLORIDE
(si-proe-hep′ta-deen)
Periactin, Vimicon ✦

Common adverse effects in *italic*; life-threatening effects <u>underlined</u>; generic names in **bold**; classifications in SMALL CAPS; ✦ Canadian drug name; 🅟 Prototype drug

**Classifications:** ANTIHISTAMINE; ANTIPRURITIC
**Therapeutic:** ANTIHISTAMINE
**Prototype:** Diphenhydramine

**AVAILABILITY** Tablet

## ACTION & *THERAPEUTIC EFFECT*

Competes with histamine for serotonin and $H_1$-receptor sites, thus preventing histamine-mediated responses. *Has significant antipruritic, local anesthetic, and antiserotonin activity.*

**USES** Symptomatic relief of various allergic conditions.

**UNLABELED USES** Cushing's disease, carcinoid syndrome, vascular headaches, appetite stimulant.

**CONTRAINDICATIONS** Hypersensitivity to cyproheptadine; MAOI therapy within 14 days; angle-closure glaucoma; stenosing peptic ulcer, symptomatic BPH, bladder neck obstruction, pyloroduodenal obstruction; older adults, debilitated patients; acute asthma attack; newborns, premature infants; lactation.

**CAUTIOUS USE** Patients predisposed to urinary retention; glaucoma; asthma; COPD; increased intraocular pressure; hyperthyroidism; cardiovascular or hepatic disease; hypertension; children with a family history of SIDS; pregnancy (category B), children. Safe use in children younger than 2 y not established.

## ROUTE & DOSAGE

**Allergies**
*Adult:* **PO** 4 mg t.i.d. or q.i.d. (4–20 mg/day), max: 0.5 mg/kg/day

*Geriatric:* **PO** Start with 4 mg b.i.d.
*Child:* **PO** 0.25 mg/kg/day in 3–4 divided doses (max: *2 to younger than 6 y:* 12 mg/day; *6–12 y:* 16 mg/day)

## ADMINISTRATION

**Oral**
- GI adverse effects may be minimized by administering drug with food or milk.
- Store in tightly covered container at 15°–30° C (59°–86° F) unless otherwise directed.

**ADVERSE EFFECTS** (≥1%) **GI:** *Dry mouth,* nausea, vomiting, epigastric distress, appetite stimulation, weight gain, transient decrease in fasting blood sugar level, increased serum amylase level, cholestatic jaundice. **CNS:** *Drowsiness,* dizziness, faintness, headache, tremulousness, fatigue, disturbed coordination. **Respiratory:** Thickened bronchial secretions. **Skin:** Skin rash. **Special Senses:** Dry nose and throat **Urogenital:** Urinary frequency, retention, and difficult urination.

**INTERACTIONS Drug:** **Alcohol** and CNS DEPRESSANTS add to CNS depression; TRICYCLIC ANTIDEPRESSANTS and other ANTICHOLINERGICS have additive anticholinergic effects; may inhibit pressor effects of **epinephrine.**

**PHARMACOKINETICS Absorption:** Readily absorbed from GI tract. **Duration:** 6–9 h. **Distribution:** Distribution into breast milk not known. **Metabolism:** In liver. **Elimination:** In urine.

## NURSING IMPLICATIONS

**Assessment & Drug Effects**
- Monitor level of alertness. In some patients, the sedative effect

Common adverse effects in *italic;* life-threatening effects underlined; generic names in **bold;** classifications in SMALL CAPS; ♣ Canadian drug name; ⊙ Prototype drug

419

disappears spontaneously after 3–4 days of drug administration.

- Since drug may cause dizziness, supervision of ambulation and other safety precautions may be warranted.

**Patient & Family Education**

- Avoid activities requiring mental alertness and physical coordination, such as driving a car, until reaction to the drug is known.
- Drug causes sedation, dizziness, and hypotension in older adults. Report these symptoms. Children are more apt to manifest CNS stimulation (e.g., confusion, agitation, tremors, hallucinations). Reduction in dosage may be indicated.
- Cyproheptadine may increase and prolong the effects of alcohol, barbiturates, narcotic analgesics, and other CNS depressants.
- Maintain sufficient fluid intake to help to relieve dry mouth and also reduce risk of cholestatic jaundice.

# CYTARABINE

(sye-tare'a-been)

**Classifications:** ANTINEOPLASTIC; ANTIMETABOLITE, PURINE ANTAGONIST

Therapeutic: ANTINEOPLASTIC

**Prototype:** 6-Mercaptopurine

**AVAILABILITY** Liposomal; powder for injection

## ACTION & *THERAPEUTIC EFFECT*

Although the mechanism of action is not completely understood, it appears to act through the inhibition of DNA polymerase thus blocking progression of certain cancer cells from the $G_1$ phase to the S-phase of the cell cycle. *Antineoplastic agent which has strong myelosuppressant activity.*

*Immunosuppressant properties are exhibited by obliterated cell-mediated immune responses, such as delayed hypersensitivity skin reactions.*

**USES** To induce and maintain remission in acute myelocytic leukemia, acute lymphocytic leukemia, and meningeal leukemia and for treatment of lymphomas. Used in combination with other antineoplastics in established chemotherapeutic protocols.

**CONTRAINDICATIONS** History of drug-induced myelosuppression; immunization procedures; active meningeal infection (**liposomal cytarabine**); pregnancy (category D) particularly during first trimester; lactation.

**CAUTIOUS USE** Impaired renal or hepatic function, elderly; neurologic disease; gout, drug-induced myelosuppression. Safe use in infants not established.

## ROUTE & DOSAGE

**Leukemias**

*Adult/Child:* **IV** 100–200 mg/m$^2$/ day by continuous infusion over 24 h; **Subcutaneous** 1 mg/kg 1–2 × wk; **Intrathecal** 5–75 mg once q4days or once/day for 4 days

**Renal Impairment Dosage Adjustment**

*Serum Cr of 1.5–1.9 mg/dL (or from baseline of 0.5–1.2 mg/dL):* Reduce to 1 g/m$^2$/dose.
*Serum Cr of 2 or more (or greater than 1.2 mg/dL change):* Do not exceed 100 mg/m$^2$/day.

## ADMINISTRATION

**Intrathecal**

- For intrathecal injection, reconstitute with an isotonic, buffered diluent without preservatives. Follow manufacturer's recommendations.

**Subcutaneous**

- Reconstitute sterile powder with bacteriostatic water for injection with benzyl alcohol (**without** benzyl alcohol for neonates).

**Intravenous**

*PREPARE:* **Direct:** Reconstitute with bacteriostatic water for injection (without benzyl alcohol for neonates) as follows: Add 5 mL to the 100-mg vial to yield 20 mg/mL; add 10 mL to the 500 mg vial to yield 50 mg/mL. Further dilute with 100 mL or more of D5W or NS. *ADMINISTER:* **Continuous:** Give over 24 h.

*INCOMPATIBILITIES:* Solution/additive: **Fluorouracil, gentamicin, heparin, hydrocortisone, insulin, nafcillin, oxacillin, penicillin G.** Y-site: **Allopurinol, amphotericin B cholesteryl sulfate complex, gallium, ganciclovir, lansoprazole, TPN.**

- Store cytarabine in refrigerator until reconstituted. • Reconstituted solutions may be stored at 15°–30° C (59°–86° F) for 48 h. Discard solutions with a slight haze.

**ADVERSE EFFECTS** (≥1%) **Body as a Whole:** Weight loss, sore throat, fever, thrombophlebitis and pain at injection site; pericarditis, bleeding (any site), pneumonia. Potentially carcinogenic and mutagenic. **GI:** *Nausea, vomiting,* diarrhea, stomatitis, oral or anal inflammation or ulceration, esophagitis, anorexia, hemorrhage, hepatotoxicity, jaundice. **Hematologic:** *Leukopenia, thrombocytopenia,* anemia, megaloblastosis, myelosuppression (reversible); transient hyperuricemia. **CNS:** Headache, neurotoxicity; peripheral neuropathy, brachial plexus neuropathy, personality change, neuritis, vertigo, lethargy, somnolence, confusion. **Skin:** Rash, erythema, freckling, cellulitis, skin ulcerations, pruritus, urticaria, bulla formation, desquamation. **Special Senses:** Conjunctivitis, keratitis, photophobia. **Urogenital:** Renal dysfunction, urinary retention.

**INTERACTIONS Drug:** GI toxicity may decrease **digoxin** absorption; decreases AMINOGLYCOSIDES activity against *Klebsiella pneumoniae*

**PHARMACOKINETICS Peak:** 20–60 min subcutaneous. **Distribution:** Crosses blood–brain barrier and placenta. **Metabolism:** In liver. **Elimination:** 80% in urine in 24 h. **Half-Life:** 1–3 h.

**NURSING IMPLICATIONS**

**Assessment & Drug Effects**

- Inspect patient's mouth before the administration of each dose. Toxicity necessitating dosage alterations almost always occurs. Report adverse reactions immediately.
- Hyperuricemia due to rapid destruction of neoplastic cells may accompany cytarabine therapy. A regimen that includes a uricosuric agent such as allopurinol, urine alkalinization, and adequate hydration may be started. To reduce potential for urate stone formation, fluids are forced in excess of 2 L, if tolerated. Consult prescriber.
- Monitor I&O ratio and pattern.
- Monitor body temperature. Be alert to the most subtle signs of infection, especially low-grade fever, and report promptly.
- When platelet count falls below 50,000/mm³ and polymorphonuclear leukocytes to below 1000/mm³, therapy may be suspended. WBC nadir is usually reached in

Common adverse effects in *italic*; life-threatening effects underlined; generic names in **bold**; classifications in SMALL CAPS; ♣ Canadian drug name; ⊚ Prototype drug

421

C

5–7 days after therapy has been stopped. Therapy is restarted with appearance of bone marrow recovery and when preceding cell counts are reached.
- Provide good oral hygiene to diminish adverse effects and chance of superinfection. Stomatitis and cheilosis usually appear 5–10 days into the therapy.
- Monitor lab tests: Periodic LFTs, CBC with differential, platelet count, serum creatinine, BUN, serum uric acid.

### Patient & Family Education
- Report promptly protracted vomiting or signs of nephrotoxicity (see Appendix F).
- Flu-like syndrome occurs usually within 6–12 wk after drug administration and may recur with successive therapy. Report chills, fever, achy joints and muscles.
- Practice good oral hygiene to minimize discomfort from stomatitis.
- Report any S&S of superinfection (see Appendix F).

## CYTOMEGALOVIRUS IMMUNE GLOBULIN (CMVIG, CMV-IVIG)
(cy-to-meg'a-lo-vi-rus)
CytoGam
**Classifications:** BIOLOGICAL RESPONSE MODIFIER; IMMUNOGLOBULIN
Therapeutic: IMMUNOGLOBULIN
**Prototype:** Peginterferon alfa-2a

**AVAILABILITY** Solution for injection

## ACTION & *THERAPEUTIC EFFECT*
Cytomegalovirus immune globulin (CMVIG) is a preparation of immunoglobulin G (IgG) antibodies with high concentrations of antibodies directed against cytomegalovirus (CMV). *The CMV antibodies attenuate or reduce the incidence of serious CMV disease, such as CMV-associated pneumonia, CMV-associated hepatitis, and concomitant fungi and parasitic superinfections.*

## USES
Attenuation of primary cytomegalovirus (CMV) disease associated with kidney transplantation.

## UNLABELED USES
Prevention of CMV disease in other organ transplants (especially heart) when the recipient is seronegative for CMV and the donor is seropositive.

## CONTRAINDICATIONS
History of previous severe reactions associated with CMVIG or other human immunoglobulin preparations, selective immunoglobulin A (IgA) deficiency.

## CAUTIOUS USE
Myelosuppression, maltose or sucrose hypersensitivity; renal insufficiency; DM; older adults; volume depletion; sepsis; paraproteinemia; cardiac disease; pregnancy (category C); lactation.

## ROUTE & DOSAGE

### Prevention of CMV Disease
*Adult:* **IV** 150 mg/kg within 72 h of transplantation, then 100 mg/kg 2, 4, 6, and 8 wk post-transplant, then 50 mg/kg 12 and 16 wk post-transplant

## ADMINISTRATION
### Intravenous
CMVIG should be administered through a separate IV line using an infusion pump. See manufacturer's directions if this is not possible.

Common adverse effects in *italic;* life-threatening effects <u>underlined;</u> generic names in **bold;** classifications in SMALL CAPS; ✣ Canadian drug name; ☻ Prototype drug

**PREPARE: IV Infusion:** Do not shake vial; avoid foaming. Predilution of CMV-IgIV (human) before infusion is not recommended. ▪ **Must be** completely infused within 12 h of entering the vial since solution contains no preservative.

**ADMINISTER: IV Infusion:** Use a constant infusion pump and give at rate of 15, 30, 60 mg/kg/h over first 30 min, second 30 min, third 30 min, respectively. Monitor closely during and after each rate change. ▪ If flushing, nausea, back pain, fever, or chills develops, slow or temporarily discontinue infusion. ▪ If BP begins to decrease, stop infusion and institute emergency measures. **Infusion of Subsequent IV Doses:** The intervals for increasing the dose from 15 to 30 to 60 mg may be shortened from 30 to 15 min. ▪ Never infuse more than 75 mL/h of CMVIG.

**ADVERSE EFFECTS** (≥1%) **Body as a Whole:** Muscle aches, back pain, anaphylaxis (rare), fever and chills during infusion. **CV:** Hypotension, palpitations. **GI:** Nausea, vomiting, metallic taste. **CNS:** Headache, anxiety. **Respiratory:** Shortness of breath, wheezing. **Skin:** Flushing.

**INTERACTIONS Drug:** May interfere with the immune response to LIVE VIRUS VACCINES **(BCG, measles/mumps/rubella, live polio),** defer vaccination with live viral vaccines for approximately 3 mo after administration of CMVIG; revaccination may be necessary if these vaccines were given shortly after CMVIG.

## NURSING IMPLICATIONS

### Assessment & Drug Effects
▪ Monitor vital signs preinfusion, before increases in infusion rate,

periodically during infusion, and postinfusion.
▪ Notify prescriber immediately if any of the following occur: Flushing, nausea, back pain, fall in BP, other signs of anaphylaxis.
▪ Emergency drugs should be available for treatment of acute anaphylactic reactions.
▪ Monitor for CMV-associated syndromes (e.g., leukopenia, thrombocytopenia, hepatitis, pneumonia) and for superinfections.

### Patient & Family Education
▪ Familiarize yourself with potential adverse effects and know which to report to prescriber.
▪ Defer vaccination with live viral vaccines for 3 mo after administration of CMVIG.

---

# DABIGATRAN ETEXILATE
(dab-i-ga′tran e-tex′i-late)
Pradaxa

**Classification:** ANTICOAGULANT; DIRECT THROMBIN INHIBITOR
**Therapeutic:** ANTITHROMBOTIC; THROMBIN INHIBITOR
**Prototype:** Argatroban

**AVAILABILITY** Capsule

## ACTION & THERAPEUTIC EFFECT
A direct inhibitor of thrombin which prevents thrombin-induced platelet aggregation and conversion of fibrinogen into fibrin during the coagulation cascade. *It prolongs the aPTT and TT, and it prevents development of a thrombus.*

**USES** Reduction of the risk of stroke, DVT and systemic embolism in patients with nonvalvular atrial fibrillation.

**CONTRAINDICATIONS** History of serious hypersensitivity to dabigatran etexilate; active pathological

Common adverse effects in *italic;* life-threatening effects underlined; generic names in **bold;** classifications in SMALL CAPS; ◆ Canadian drug name; ● Prototype drug

423

bleeding mechanical prosthetic heart valve; acute renal failure; CrCl less than 15 mL/min; lactation.

**CAUTIOUS USE** Medications or conditions (e.g., labor and delivery, chronic NSAID use, use of antiplatelet agents) that predispose to bleeding; severe renal impairment; spinal procedures; older adults; pregnancy (category C). Safety and efficacy in children not established.

## ROUTE & DOSAGE

### Risk of Stroke/DVT or Systemic Embolism Reduction
*Adult:* **PO** 150 mg b.i.d.

### VTE Prophylaxis in Patients Undergoing Hip Replacement
*Adult:* **PO** 110 mg × 1 day then 220 mg daily × 28–35 days

### Renal Impairment Dosage Adjustment
*CrCl greater than or equal to 15 to less than or equal to 30 mL/ min:* 75 mg b.i.d.; *CrCl less than 15 mL/min:* Not recommended

### Conversion from Dabigatran to Warfarin
*CrCl greater than 50 mL/min:* Start warfarin 3 d before discontinuing dabigatran; *CrCl 31–50 mL/min:* Start warfarin 2 d before discontinuing dabigatran; *CrCl 15–30 mL/min:* Start warfarin 1 d before discontinuing dabigatran; *CrCl less than 15 mL/min:* Not recommended

## ADMINISTRATION
### Oral
- Ensure that capsule is swallowed whole. It should not be opened or chewed and should be swallowed with a full glass of water.
- Converting from a parenteral anticoagulant: Start dabigatran up to 2 h before the next dose of parenteral drug was due or at time of discontinuation of an IV anticoagulant.
- Withhold drug and report to prescriber if active bleeding is suspected.
- Store at 15–30° C (59–86° F). Store in original package to protect from moisture. Once bottle is opened, use contents within 4 mo of opening.

**ADVERSE EFFECTS** (≥1%) **GI:** Abdominal pain or discomfort, diarrhea, epigastric discomfort, erosive gastritis, esophagitis, gastric hemorrhage, gastroesophogeal reflux disorder, gastrointestinal ulcer, hemorrhagic gastritis, hemorrhagic erosive gastritis, nausea. **Hematological:** *Increased risk of bleeding.*

**INTERACTIONS Drug:** Concomitant use with P-GLYCOPROTEIN INDUCERS (**rifampin, carbamazepine, phenobarbital, tipranaive**) reduces the levels of dabigatran. **Ketoconazole** increases levels and subsequent bleeding risk. Monitor when starting SSRI. Do not use with **apixaban** or **defibrotide** due to increased bleeding risk.

**PHARMACOKINETICS Absorption:** 3–7% bioavailable. **Peak:** 1 h. **Distribution:** 35% plasma protein bound. **Metabolism:** Esterase hydrolysis and glucuronide conjugation to active metabolites. **Elimination:** Primarily renal; unabsorbed drug excreted in feces. **Half-Life:** 12–17 h.

## NURSING IMPLICATIONS

### Black Box Warning

*Discontinuation of dabigatran without coverage with another*

Common adverse effects in *italic;* life-threatening effects underlined; generic names in **bold;** classifications in SMALL CAPS; ♣ Canadian drug name; ⊘ Prototype drug

*anticoagulant poses a risk of thrombotic events. Concomitant epidural/ spinal anesthesia or puncture may cause epidural or spinal hematoma, which may result in long-term or permanent paralysis.*

## Assessment & Drug Effects

- Monitor for and promptly report S&S of active bleeding.
- Monitor for and report promptly adverse GI effects including: Epigastric pain or discomfort, GERD, or abdominal pain or discomfort.
- Monitor lab tests: Periodic aPTT and PT; baseline and periodic renal function; CBC with differential as needed.

## Patient & Family Education

- Seek emergency care for any of the following: Unusual bruising; pink or brown urine; red or black, tarry stools; coughing up blood; vomiting blood, or vomit that looks like coffee grounds.
- Report promptly to prescriber any of the following: Pain, swelling or discomfort in a joint; nose bleeds or bleeding from gums; headaches, dizziness, or weakness; menstrual bleeding or vaginal bleeding that is heavier than normal; indigestion, gastric reflux, or nausea.
- Alert all health care providers that you are taking dabigatran before any invasive procedure, including dental procedures.

# DABRAFENIB MESYLATE

(da-braf'-e-nib)

Tafinlar

**Classifications:** ANTINEOPLASTIC; KINASE INHIBITOR
**Therapeutic:** ANTINEOPLASTIC
**Prototype:** Erlotinib

## AVAILABILITY Capsule

## ACTION & *THERAPEUTIC EFFECT*

Dabrafenib inhibits tyrosine kinases which are enzymes required for cancer cell formation (oncogenesis), metastasis, tumor angiogenesis, and maintenance of the tumor microenvironment. *Slows BRAF V600 mutation–positive melanoma cell growth resulting in decreased tumor cell growth.*

**USES** Treatment of patients with unresectable or metastatic melanoma with BRAF V600E mutation as detected by an FDA-approved test; non-small-cell lung cancer.

**CONTRAINDICATIONS** Wild-type BRAF melanoma; serious fever reactions to dabrafenib (104° or greater); palmar-plantar erythrodysesthesia syndrome (PPES); pregnancy (category D), lactation.

**CAUTIOUS USE** DM; history of hyperglycemia; G6PD deficiency. Safety and efficacy in children not established.

## ROUTE & DOSAGE

**Metastatic Melanoma**
*Adult:* **PO** 150 mg every 12 h
**Non-Small-Cell Lung Cancer**
*Adult:* **PO** 150 mg q12h in combination with **trametinib** 2mg daily

*Toxicity Dosage Adjustment*

*Fever of 101.3° F to 104° F:* Withhold until fever resolves; resume at same or reduced dose
*Fever higher than 104° F or complicated by rigors, hypotension, dehydration, or renal failure:* Permanently discontinue or resume at a reduced dose level once fever resolves

**D**

*Intolerable grade 2 toxicity or any grade 3 toxicity:* Withhold until toxicity resolves to grade 1 or less; resume at a reduced dose level
*Grade 4 toxicity, first occurrence:* Permanently discontinue or withhold therapy until toxicity resolves to grade 1 or less; resume at a reduced dose level
*Recurrent grade 4 toxicity:* Permanently discontinue therapy

**Recommended Dosage Reductions**

*First reduction:* 100 mg every 12 h
*Second reduction:* 75 mg every 12 h
*Third reduction:* 50 mg every 12 h
*Permanently discontinue:* Patient is unable to tolerate 50 mg every 12 h

## ADMINISTRATION

### Oral

- Give 1 h before or at least 2 h after a meal.
- Capsules must be swallowed whole. They must not be opened or crushed.
- Store at 15°–30° C (59°–86° F).

## ADVERSE EFFECTS ((≥1%)) **Body as a Whole:** *Alopecia,* chills, fatigue, hypersensitivity reactions, insomnia, *papilloma, pyrexia.* **CNS:** *Headache.* **CV:** Dizziness, anemia. **GI:** Constipation, *diarrhea,* abdominal pain, *anorexia,* vomiting, pancreatitis. **Metabolic:** *Hyperglycemia,* hyponatremia, *hypophosphatemia,* hypoalbuminemia, hypokalemia, hyperkalemia, *increased alkaline phosphatase.* **Musculoskeletal:** *Arthralgia,* back pain, myalgia, muscle spasms. **Respiratory:** Cough, nasopharyngitis. **Skin:** Cutaneous squamous cell carcinoma, *hyperkeratosis, palmar-plantar erythrodysesthesia syndrome (PPES),* rash. **Urogenital:** Interstitial nephritis.

## INTERACTIONS **Drug:** Strong inhibitors of CYP3A4 or CYP2C8 (e.g., **clarithromycin, gemfibrozil, ketoconazole, nefazodone**) may increase the levels of dabrafenib. Strong inducers of CYP3A4 or CYP2C8 (e.g., **carbamazepine, phenobarbital, phenytoin, rifampin**) may decrease the levels of dabrafenib. **Herbal: St. John's wort** may decrease the levels of dabrafenib.

## PHARMACOKINETICS **Absorption:** 95% bioavailable. **Peak:** 2 h. **Distribution:** 99.7% plasma protein bound. **Metabolism:** Hepatic oxidation. **Elimination:** Fecal (71%) and renal (23%). **Half-Life:** 8 h.

## NURSING IMPLICATIONS

### Assessment & Drug Effects

- Monitor existing melanoma lesions; report new lesions or changes in existing lesions.
- Monitor for and report S&S of uvitis (e.g., change in vision, photophobia, eye pain).
- Monitor diabetics for loss of glycemic control.
- Monitor lab tests: Periodic blood glucose with preexisting diabetes, LFTs.

### Patient & Family Education

- Report to prescriber: Changes in vision or eye pain; symptoms of severe hyperglycemia (e.g., excessive thirst, increase in volume or frequency of urination).
- Diabetics should monitor blood glucose frequently for loss of glycemic control.
- Women should use highly effective means of nonhormonal contraception during and for 4 wk after treatment.
- Do not breast-feed while taking this drug.

# DACARBAZINE
(da-kar'ba-zeen)

DTIC-Dome

**Classifications:** ANTINEOPLASTIC;
ALKYLATING AGENT
Therapeutic: ANTINEOPLASTIC
**Prototype:** Cyclophosphamide

**AVAILABILITY** Solution for injection

**ACTION & *THERAPEUTIC EFFECT***
Although exact mechanism of
action is unknown, it may have
alkylating properties and may
inhibit DNA synthesis by acting as
a purine analog. It is cell-cycle nonspecific. Either mechanism would
interfere with DNA replication,
RNA transcription, and protein synthesis in rapidly proliferating cells.
*Has carcinogenic, mutagenic, and
teratogenic effects.*

**USES** As single agent or in combination with other antineoplastics in
treatment of metastatic malignant
melanoma, refractory Hodgkin's
disease.

**UNLABELED USES** Various sarcomas and malignant glucagonoma.

**CONTRAINDICATIONS** Hypersensitivity to dacarbazine; severe
bone marrow suppression; active
infection; live vaccine; lactation.

**CAUTIOUS USE** Hepatic or renal
impairment; previous radiation
or chemotherapy; pregnancy
(category C).

## ROUTE & DOSAGE

### Neoplasms
*Adult:* **IV** 2–4.5 mg/kg/day for
10 days repeated at 4-wk
intervals or 250 mg/m²/day for
5 days repeated at 3-wk
intervals

### Hodgkin's Disease
*Adult:* **IV** 150 mg/m²/day ×
5 days; repeat at 4-wk intervals

## ADMINISTRATION

### Intravenous

*IV ADMINISTRATION TO INFANTS AND
CHILDREN:* Verify correct IV concentration and rate of infusion
with prescriber.
▪ Wear gloves when handling this
drug. If solution gets into the
eyes, wash them with soap and
water immediately, then irrigate
with water or isotonic saline.

*PREPARE:* **Direct:** Reconstitute drug
with sterile water for injection
to make a solution containing
10 mg/mL dacarbazine (pH 3.0–4.0)
by adding 9.9 mL to 100 mg or 19.7
mL to 200 mg. **IV Infusion:** Further
dilute reconstituted solution in
50–250 mL of D5W or NS.
*ADMINISTER:* **Direct:** Give by direct IV into a freely running IV
over 5 min. **IV Infusion** *(preferred):* Infuse IV over 30–60
min. ▪ If possible, avoid using antecubital vein or veins on dorsum of hand or wrist where ex
travasation could lead to loss of
mobility of entire limb. ▪ Avoid
veins in extremity with compromised venous or lymphatic drainage and veins near joint spaces.
*INCOMPATIBILITIES:* **Solution/ad-
ditive: Allopurinol, heparin,
hydrocortisone. Y-site: Allopurinol, cefepime, heparin,
piperacillin/tazobactam.**
▪ Administer dacarbazine only to
patients under close supervision
because close observation and
frequent laboratory studies are
required during and after therapy. ▪ **IV Extravasation:** Monitor
injection site frequently (instruct
patient to do so, if able). Give

Common adverse effects in *italic;* life-threatening effects underlined; generic names
in **bold;** classifications in SMALL CAPS; ✦ Canadian drug name; ☺ Prototype drug

427

prompt attention to patient's complaint of swelling, stinging, and burning sensation around injection site. ▪ Extravasation can occur painlessly and without visual signs. Danger areas for extravasation are dorsum of hand or ankle (especially if peripheral arteriosclerosis is present), joint spaces, and previously irradiated areas. ▪ If extravasation is suspected, infusion should be stopped immediately and restarted in another vein. Report to the prescriber. Prompt institution of local treatment is IMPERATIVE.

▪ Store reconstituted solution up to 72 h at 4° C (39° F) or at room temperature 15°–30° C (59°–86° F) for up to 8 h. ▪ Store diluted reconstituted solution for 24 h at 4° C (39° F) or at room temperature for up to 8 h. Protect from light.

**ADVERSE EFFECTS** (≥1%) **Body as a Whole:** Hypersensitivity (erythematosus, urticarial rashes, hepatotoxicity, photosensitivity); facial paresthesia and flushing, flu-like syndrome, myalgia, malaise, anaphylaxis. **CNS:** Confusion, headache, seizures, blurred vision. **GI:** *Anorexia, nausea, vomiting.* **Hematologic:** <u>Severe leukopenia and thrombocytopenia</u>, mild anemia. **Skin:** Alopecia. **Other:** *Pain along injected vein.*

**PHARMACOKINETICS Distribution:** Localizes primarily in liver. **Metabolism:** In liver by CYP1A2. **Elimination:** 35–50% in urine in 6 h. **Half-Life:** 5 h.

## NURSING IMPLICATIONS

### Black Box Warning

*Dacarbazine has been associated with hemopoietic depression and hepatic necrosis.*

### Assessment & Drug Effects

▪ Monitor IV site carefully for extravasation; if suspected, discontinue IV immediately and notify prescriber.
▪ Note: Skin damage by dacarbazine can lead to deep necrosis requiring surgical debridement, skin grafting, and even amputation. Older adults, the very young, comatose, and debilitated patients are especially at risk. Other risk factors include establishing an IV line in a vein previously punctured several times and the use of nonplastic catheters.
▪ Avoid, if possible, all tests and treatments during platelet nadir requiring needle punctures (e.g., IM). Observe carefully and report evidence of unexplained bleeding.
▪ Monitor for severe nausea and vomiting (greater than 90% of patients) that begin within 1 h after drug administration and may last for as long as 12 h.
▪ Check patient's mouth for ulcerative stomatitis prior to the administration of each dose.
▪ Monitor I&O ratio and pattern and daily temperature. Renal impairment extends the half-life and increases danger of toxicity. Report symptoms of renal dysfunction and even a slight elevation of temperature.
▪ Monitor lab tests: Baseline and periodic CBC with differential and Hct and Hgb.

### Patient & Family Education

▪ Learn about all potential adverse drug effects.
▪ Report flu-like syndrome that may occur during or even a week after treatment is terminated and last 7–21 days. Symptoms frequently recur with successive treatments.
▪ Avoid prolonged exposure to sunlight or to ultraviolet light during treatment period and for at least 2 wk after last dose. Protect exposed

Common adverse effects in *italic;* life-threatening effects <u>underlined;</u> generic names in **bold;** classifications in SMALL CAPS; ✤ Canadian drug name; ⊙ Prototype drug

skin with sunscreen lotion (SPF 15) and avoid exposure in midday.
- Report promptly the onset of blurred vision or paresthesia.

# DACLATASVIR
(da-cla-tas'vir)
Daklinza

**Classifications:** ANTIVIRAL; DIRECT-ACTING ANTIVIRAL; VIRAL PROTEIN INHIBITOR ANTIHEPATITIS
Therapeutic: ANTIHEPATITIS
**Prototype:** Boceprevir

## AVAILABILITY Tablets

## ACTION & THERAPEUTIC EFFECT
A direct-acting antiviral agent (DAA) that inhibits a nonstructural protein (i.e., NS5A) encoded by HCV. *Inhibits both viral RNA replication and virion assembly.*

## USES
In combination with sofosbuvir for the treatment of patients with chronic hepatitis C virus (HCV) genotype 3 infection.

## CONTRAINDICATIONS
Concurrent use with drugs that strongly induce CYP3A (e.g., phenytoin, carbamazepine, rifampin, St. John's wort).

## CAUTIOUS USE
Cardiac morbidities or advanced hepatic disease and concomitant use of amiodarone; pregnancy; lactation. Safety and efficacy in children not established.

## ROUTE & DOSAGE

**Hepatitis C Infection**

*Adult:* **PO** 60 mg once daily in combination with sofosbuvir for 12 wk

**Concomitant CYP3A4 Inhibitors and Inducers Dosage Adjustment**

*Strong CYP3A4 inhibitor:* Reduce to 30 mg once daily

*Moderate CYP3A inducer:* Increase to 90 mg once daily

## ADMINISTRATION
**Oral**
- May be given without regard to food.
- Store at 15°–30° C (59°–86° F).

## ADVERSE EFFECTS (>2%)
**Body as a Whole:** *Fatigue.* **CNS:** *Headache.* **GI:** Nausea, vomiting. **Metabolic:** Elevated lipase enzymes.

## INTERACTIONS
**Drug:** Strong and moderate inducers of CYP3A4 (e.g., **bosentan, dexamethasone, efavirenz, etravirine, modafinil, nafcillin, rifapentine**) may decrease the levels of daclatasvir. Strong inhibitors of CYP3A4 (e.g., **atazanavir, clarithromycin, indinavir, itraconazole, ketoconazole, nefazodone, nelfinavir, posaconazole, ritonavir, saquinavir, telithromycin, voriconazole**) may increase the levels of daclatasvir. Daclatasvir may increase the levels of **dabigatran, digoxin,** and HMG-COA REDUCTASE INHIBITORS. Daclatasvir may increase the levels of other drugs that are substrates of P-glycoprotein transporter (P-gp), organic anion transporting polypeptide (OATP), and/or breast cancer resistance protein (BCRP). **Herbal: St. John's wort** may decrease the levels of daclatasvir.

## PHARMACOKINETICS
**Absorption:** 67% bioavailable. **Peak:** 2 h. **Distribution:** 99% plasma protein bound. **Metabolism:** Hepatic oxidation. **Elimination:** Fecal (88%) and renal (6.6%). **Half-Life:** 12–15 h.

## NURSING IMPLICATIONS
**Assessment & Drug Effects**
- Monitor cardiac status with ECG during first 48 h if coadminis-

tered with sofosbuvir or amiodarone, or if amiodarone discontinued just prior to initiation of therapy with daclatasvir. Report immediately development of bradycardia.
- Ensure that all medications (prescription and OTC) the patient is taking are known to prescriber.
- Monitor lab tests: Baseline and periodic LFTs and serum creatinine.

**Patient & Family Education**
- Inform prescriber of all prescription and non-prescription drugs being taken. Potentially serious drug interaction may require dosage adjustments.
- If taking either sofosbuvir or amiodarone, monitor heart rate daily for the first 2 wk of therapy. If a slow heart rate develops, seek medical evaluation immediately. Symptoms may include near-fainting or fainting, dizziness or lightheadedness, weakness, excessive tiredness, shortness of breath, chest pain, confusion, or memory problems.
- Take appropriate precautions to prevent transmission of the hepatitis C virus during treatment because effect of treatment on transmission of the virus is unknown.

# DACTINOMYCIN
(dak-ti-noe-mye'sin)
Cosmegen
**Classifications:** ANTINEOPLASTIC; ANTHRACYCLINE (ANTIBIOTIC)
Therapeutic: ANTINEOPLASTIC
**Prototype:** Doxorubicin

**AVAILABILITY** Solution for injection

**ACTION & THERAPEUTIC EFFECT**
Complexes with DNA, thereby inhibiting DNA, RNA, and protein synthesis in actively proliferating cells. Potentiates effects of x-ray therapy and the converse also appears likely. *Has antineoplastic properties that result from inhibiting DNA and RNA synthesis.*

**USES** To treat Wilms' tumor, rhabdomyosarcoma, carcinoma of testes and uterus, Ewing's sarcoma, solid malignancies, gestational trophoblastic neoplasia, and sarcoma botryoides.

**UNLABELED USES** Malignant melanoma, Kaposi's sarcoma, osteogenic sarcoma, among others.

**CONTRAINDICATIONS** Acute infection; pregnancy (category D); lactation.

**CAUTIOUS USE** Previous therapy with antineoplastics or radiation within 3–6 wk, bone marrow depression; infections; history of gout; impairment of kidney or liver function; obesity; chickenpox, herpes zoster, and other viral infections. Safe use in infants younger than 6 mo is not known.

## ROUTE & DOSAGE

**Neoplasms**

*Adult/Adolescent/Child/Infant (6 mo or older):* IV 500 mcg/day for 5 days max, may repeat at 2–4 wk intervals if tolerated (if patient is obese or edematous, give 400–600 mcg/m²/day to relate dosage to lean body mass); monitor for symptoms of toxicity from overdosage

**Wilms' Tumor, Childhood Rhabdomyosarcoma, Ewing's Sarcoma, Nephroblastoma**

*Adult/Child:* IV 15 mcg/kg/day × 5 days with other agents

## Gestational Trophoblastic Neoplasia

*Adult:* **IV** 12 mcg/kg/day × 5 days or 500 mcg × 2 days with other agents

## Solid Tumor

*Adult/Adolescent/Child/Infant (6 mo or older):* **IV** 50 mcg/kg (lower extremity) or 35 mcg/kg (upper extremity)

## ADMINISTRATION

**Intravenous**

Use gloves and eye shield when preparing solution. If skin is contaminated, rinse with running water for 10 min; then rinse with buffered phosphate solution. ▪ If solution gets into the eyes, wash with water immediately; then irrigate with water or isotonic saline for 10 min.

*PREPARE:* **Direct:** Reconstitute 0.5 mg vial by adding 1.1 mL sterile water (without preservative) for injection; the resulting solution will contain approximately 0.5 mg/mL. **IV Infusion:** Further dilute reconstituted solution in 50 mL of D5W or NS for infusion.
*ADMINISTER:* **Direct:** Use two-needle technique for direct IV: Withdraw calculated dose from vial with one needle, change to new needle to give directly into vein without using an infusion. Give over 2–3 min. ▪ Or give directly into an infusing solution of D5W or NS, or into tubing or side arm of a running IV infusion. **IV Infusion:** Give diluted solution as a single dose over 15–30 min.
*INCOMPATIBILITIES:* **Y-site: Filgrastim.**

▪ Store drug at 15°–30° C (59°–86° F) unless otherwise directed. Protect from heat and light.

## ADVERSE EFFECTS (≥1%) GI: *Nausea, vomiting,* anorexia, abdominal pain, diarrhea, proctitis, GI ulceration, *stomatitis,* cheilitis, glossitis, dysphagia, hepatitis. **Hematologic:** Anemia (including aplastic anemia), agranulocytosis, *leukopenia, thrombocytopenia,* pancytopenia, reticulopenia. **Skin:** Acne, desquamation, hyperpigmentation and reactivation of erythema especially over previously irradiated areas, *alopecia* (reversible). **Other:** Malaise, fatigue, lethargy, fever, myalgia, anaphylaxis, gonadal suppression, hypocalcemia, hyperuricemia, thrombophlebitis; *necrosis, sloughing, and contractures at site of extravasation;* hepatitis, hepatomegaly.

## INTERACTIONS Drug: Elevated **uric acid** level produced by dactinomycin may necessitate dose adjustment of ANTIGOUT AGENTS; effects of both dactinomycin and other MYELOSUPPRESSANTS are potentiated; effects of both **radiation** and dactinomycin are potentiated, and dactinomycin may reactivate erythema from previous radiation therapy; **vitamin K** effects (antihemorrhagic) decreased, leading to prolonged clotting time and potential hemorrhage.

## PHARMACOKINETICS Distribution: Concentrated in liver, spleen, kidneys, and bone marrow; does not cross blood–brain barrier; crosses placenta. **Elimination:** 50% unchanged in bile and 10% in urine; only 30% in urine over 9 days. **Half-Life:** 36 h.

## NURSING IMPLICATIONS

### Black Box Warning

*Dactinomycin is highly toxic and extremely corrosive to soft tissue.*

---

Common adverse effects in *italic;* life-threatening effects underlined; generic names in **bold**; classifications in SMALL CAPS; ✢ Canadian drug name; ⊘ Prototype drug

**D**

*Extravasation will cause severe tissue damage.*

### Assessment & Drug Effects

- Observe injection site frequently; if extravasation occurs, stop infusion immediately. Restart infusion in another vein. Report to prescriber. Institute prompt local treatment to prevent thrombophlebitis and necrosis.
- Monitor for severe toxic effects that occur with high frequency. Effects usually appear 2–4 days after a course of therapy is stopped and may reach maximal severity 1–2 wk following discontinuation of therapy.
- Use antiemetic drugs to control nausea and vomiting, which often occur a few hours after drug administration. Vomiting may be severe enough to require intermittent therapy. Observe patient daily for signs of drug toxicity.
- Monitor temperature and inspect oral membranes daily for stomatitis.
- Monitor for stomatitis, diarrhea, and severe hematopoietic depression. These may require prompt interruption of therapy until drug toxicity subsides.
- Report onset of unexplained bleeding, jaundice, and wheezing. Also, be alert to signs of agranulocytosis (see Appendix F). Report to prescriber. Antibiotic therapy, protective isolation, and discontinuation of the antineoplastic are indicated.
- Observe and report symptoms of hyperuricemia (see Appendix F). Urge patient to increase fluid intake up to 3000 mL/day if allowed.
- Monitor lab tests: Frequent renal, hepatic, and bone marrow function tests. Frequent WBC counts, and platelet counts.

### Patient & Family Education

- Note: Infertility is a possible, irreversible adverse effect of this drug.
- Learn preventative measures to minimize nausea and vomiting.
- Note: Alopecia (hair loss) is an anticipated reversible adverse effect of this drug. Seek appropriate supportive guidance.

## DALBAVANCIN HYDROCHLORIDE

(dal-ba′van-sin)

Dalvance

**Classifications:** ANTIBIOTIC; GLYCOPROTEIN

Therapeutic: ANTIBIOTIC

**Prototype:** Vancomycin

**AVAILABILITY** Single-use vials containing sterile powder

**ACTION & *THERAPEUTIC EFFECT***
Binds to components required for the bacterial cell wall preventing cell wall synthesis. *It is bactericidal against* Staphylococcus aureus *and* Streptococcus pyogenes.

**USES** Parenterally for the treatment of acute bacterial skin and skin structure infections (ABSSSI) caused by designated susceptible strains of gram-positive microorganisms.

**CONTRAINDICATIONS** Hypersensitivity to dalbavancin or to any component of the formulation; pseudomembranous colitis due to drug.

**CAUTIOUS USE** Known hypersensitivity to other glycopeptide antibiotics; moderate to severe hepatic impairment; severe renal impairment; colitis; pregnancy (category C); lactation. Safety and efficacy in children younger than 18 y not established.

Common adverse effects in *italic;* life-threatening effects <u>underlined</u>; generic names in **bold;** classifications in SMALL CAPS; ✦ Canadian drug name; ⑳ Prototype drug

## ROUTE & DOSAGE

**Acute Bacterial Skin and Skin Structure Infection**

*Adult:* **IV** 1000 mg followed by 500 mg one wk later

**Renal Impairment Dosage Adjustment**

*CrCl less than 30 mL/min in patients not on hemodialysis:* Reduce to 750 mg initially and follow with 375mg

## ADMINISTRATION

**Intravenous**

*PREPARE:* **IV Infusion:** Reconstitute with 25 mL of SW for each 500 mg vial to yield 20 mg/mL. Swirl gently and invert vial several times until completely dissolved. Do not shake. Further dilute in D5W to a final concentration of 1–5 mg/mL.

*ADMINISTER:* **IV Infusion:** Infuse over 30 min. If using IV line for other drugs, flush before/after with D5W.

*INCOMPATIBILITIES:* **Solution/additive:** Normal saline. **Y-site:** Flush before/after infusion.

▪ Store vials at 15° C–30°C (59° F–86° F). Store reconstituted vial or IV solution up to 48 h at room temperature or under refrigeration.

## ADVERSE EFFECTS (≥ 1%)

**Body as a Whole:** Flushing, hypersensitivity, infusion site reactions, phlebitis. **CNS:** Dizziness, *headache.* **GI:** Abdominal pain, *Clostridium difficile*-associated diarrhea, *diarrhea,* GI hemorrhage, hematochezia, melena, *nausea,* oral candidiasis, pseudomembranous colitis, vomiting. **Hematological:** Anemia, eosinophilia, hematoma, hepatotoxicity,

increased INR, increased serum alkaline phosphatase, increased serum transaminases, leukopenia, neutropenia, petechia, thrombocythemia, thrombocytopenia, wound hemmorrhage. **Metabolic:** Hypoglycemia. **Respiratory:** Bronchospasm. **Skin:** Pruritus, skin rash, urticarial. **Urogenital:** Vulvovaginal infection.

## PHARMACOKINETICS

**Distribution:** 93% plasma protein bound. **Metabolism:** Minor. **Elimination:** Renal (45%) and fecal (20%). **Half-Life:** 8.5 days.

## NURSING IMPLICATIONS

### Assessment & Drug Effects

▪ Monitor patients for any infusion-related reactions.
▪ Monitor for S&S of superinfection, including *C. difficile*-associated diarrhea (CDAD) and pseudomembranous colitis, that may develop within days or up to several months after completion of therapy.
▪ If superinfection is suspected, withhold drug and contact prescriber.
▪ Monitor lab tests: Baseline serum urea nitrogen, serum creatinine, and LFTs.

### Patient & Family Education

▪ Report promptly to prescriber if you develop frequent watery or bloody diarrhea.
▪ Consult with prescriber if you are a female who is or plans to become pregnant.
▪ Do not breast-feed without consulting prescriber.

## DALFAMPRIDINE

(dal-fam'pri-deen)

Ampyra

**Classification:** NEUROLOGIC; POTASSIUM CHANNEL BLOCKER
**Therapeutic:** NEUROLOGIC

Common adverse effects in *italic;* life-threatening effects underlined; generic names in **bold;** classifications in SMALL CAPS; ◆ Canadian drug name; ⊕ Prototype drug

433

**AVAILABILITY** Extended release tablet

**ACTION & *THERAPEUTIC EFFECT*** The mechanism by which it exerts its therapeutic effect is not fully understood. *Improves walking speed in persons with multiple sclerosis.*

**USES** To improve walking speed in patients with multiple sclerosis.

**CONTRAINDICATIONS** History of seizures; moderate or severe renal impairment; concurrent use of other forms of 4-aminopyridine (4-AP, fampridine); lactation.

**CAUTIOUS USE** Mild renal impairment; urinary tract infections. Safe use in children younger than 18 y is not established.

## ROUTE & DOSAGE

**Multiple Sclerosis**
*Adult:* **PO** 10 mg q12h

***Renal Impairment Dosage Adjustment***
*CrCl 50 mL/min or less:*
Dalfampridine is contraindicated

## ADMINISTRATION

**Oral**
- Ensure that extended release tablet is swallowed whole. It should not be crushed or chewed.
- Store at 15°–30° C (59°–86° F).

**ADVERSE EFFECTS** (≥2%) **CNS:** Asthenia, balance disorder, dizziness, headache, *insomnia*, MS relapse, paresthesia. **GI:** Constipation, dyspepsia, nausea. **Musculoskeletal:** Back pain. **Respiratory:** Nasopharyngitis, pharyngolaryngeal pain. **Urogenital:** *Urinary tract infection.*

**PHARMACOKINETICS Absorption:** 96% bioavailability. **Peak:** 3–4 h.

**Metabolism:** Minimal. **Elimination:** Renal as unchanged drug. **Half-Life:** 5.2–6.5 h.

## NURSING IMPLICATIONS

### Assessment & Drug Effects
- Monitor closely for signs of seizure activity. Withhold drug and notify prescriber if a seizure occurs.
- Monitor for and report signs of urinary tract infection.
- Monitor I&O and report significant changes in output.
- Monitor lab tests: Baseline and periodic renal function tests.

### Patient & Family Education
- Stop taking drug and notify prescriber immediately if a seizure occurs.
- Tablets must be taken whole. Breaking the tablet may allow too much medication to be released too quickly increasing the risk of a seizure.
- Do not take more than 2 tablets in a 24 h period and maintain an approximate 12 h interval between doses.
- If you take too much dalfampridine, immediately call your prescriber or go to the nearest emergency room.

## DALTEPARIN SODIUM
(dal-tep-a'rin)
Fragmin
**See Appendix A-2**.

## DANAZOL
(da'na-zole)
Cyclomen ✦
**Classification:** ANDROGEN/ANABOLIC STEROID
Therapeutic: ANABOLIC STEROID
**Prototype:** Testosterone

**AVAILABILITY** Capsule

## ACTION & *THERAPEUTIC EFFECT*.
Suppresses pituitary output of FSH and LH, resulting in anovulation and associated amenorrhea. Has mild androgenic effects. *Interrupts progress and pain of endometriosis by causing atrophy and involution of both normal and ectopic endometrial tissue.*

## USES
Palliative treatment of endometriosis. Also used to treat fibrocystic breast disease and hereditary angioedema.

## UNLABELED USES
To treat precocious puberty, gynecomastia, menorrhagia, premenstrual syndrome (PMS), chronic immune thrombocytopenic purpura (ITP), autoimmune hemolytic anemia, hemophilia A and B.

## CONTRAINDICATIONS
Undiagnosed abnormal genital bleeding; porphyria, markedly impaired hepatic, renal, or cardiac function; peripheral neuropathy; vaginal bleeding; pregnancy (category X); lactation.

## CAUTIOUS USE
Migraine headache, epilepsy; seizure disorders; renal impairment; history of strokes; history of thrombotic disorders, CAD atherosclerosis; fibrocytic disease; older adults.

## ROUTE & DOSAGE

**Endometriosis**
*Adult:* PO 200–400 mg b.i.d. for 3–6 mo

**Fibrocystic Breast Disease**
*Adult:* PO 100–400 mg in 2 divided doses

**Hereditary Angioedema**
*Adult:* PO 200 mg b.i.d. or t.i.d., may decrease by 50% at intervals of 1–3 mo or longer

## ADMINISTRATION
**Oral**
- Start therapy during menstruation, or after a negative pregnancy test.
- Store capsules at 15°–30° C (59°–86° F) in a tightly closed container.

## ADVERSE EFFECTS (≥1%)
**Body as a Whole:** Hypersensitivity (skin rashes, nasal congestion). **Endocrine:** Androgenic effects (acne, mild hirsutism, deepening of voice, oily skin and hair, hair loss, edema, weight gain, pitch breaks, voice weakness, decrease in breast size); hypoestrogenic effects (*hot flashes;* sweating; emotional lability; nervousness; vaginitis with itching, drying, burning, or bleeding; *amenorrhea, irregular menstrual patterns*); impairment in glucose tolerance, rare splenic peliosis. **CNS:** Dizziness, sleep disorders, fatigue, tremor, irritability. **Special Senses:** Conjunctival edema. **CV:** Elevated BP. **GI:** Gastroenteritis, hepatic damage (rare), increased LDL, decreased HDL. **Urogenital:** Decreased libido. **Musculoskeletal:** Joint lock-up, joint swelling.

## INTERACTIONS
**Herbal:** **Echinacea** possibility of increased hepatotoxicity.

## PHARMACOKINETICS
**Elimination:** Other pharmacokinetic information is not known. **Half-Life:** 4.5 h.

## NURSING IMPLICATIONS

### Black Box Warning

*Danazol may cause fetal harm and should never be given to a pregnant woman. Danazol has been associated with thrombobosis, emboli, phlebitis, potentially fatal strokes, and benign intracranial hypertension.*

---

Common adverse effects in *italic;* life-threatening effects underlined; generic names in **bold;** classifications in SMALL CAPS; ♣ Canadian drug name; ⊘ Prototype drug

435

D

## Assessment & Drug Effects

- Routine breast examinations should be carried out during therapy. Carcinoma of the breast should be ruled out prior to start of therapy for fibrocystic breast disease. Advise patient to report to prescriber if any nodule enlarges or becomes tender or hard during therapy.
- Because danazol may cause fluid retention, patients with cardiac or renal dysfunction, epilepsy, or migraine should be observed closely during therapy, as these problems could worsen. Monitor weight.
- Drug-induced edema may compress the median nerve, producing symptoms of carpal tunnel syndrome. If patient complains of wrist pain that worsens at night, paresthesias in radial palmar aspect of the hand and fingers, consult prescriber.
- Monitor diabetics for loss of glycemic control.
- Monitor lab tests: Baseline and periodic LFTs. Patients with diabetes should be monitored for loss of glycemic control.

## Patient & Family Education

- Note: Pain and discomfort of endometriosis are usually relieved in 2 or 3 mo; the nodularity in 4–6 mo. Menses may be regular or irregular in pattern during therapy.
- Note: Drug-induced amenorrhea is reversible. Ovulation and cyclic bleeding usually return within 60–90 days after therapeutic regimen is discontinued as well as the potential for conception.
- Use a reliable nonhormonal contraceptive during treatment because ovulation may not be suppressed until 6–8 wk after therapy is begun. If pregnancy occurs while taking this drug, contact prescriber immediately.
- Report voice changes or other masculinizing effects promptly. Virilizing adverse effects may persist even after drug therapy is terminated.

# DANTROLENE SODIUM
(dan'troe-leen)

Dantrium, Revonto, Ryanodex

**Classification:** DIRECT-ACTING SKELETAL MUSCLE RELAXANT
**Therapeutic:** SKELETAL MUSCLE RELAXANT; ANTISPASMODIC

**AVAILABILITY** Capsule; solution for injection

## ACTION & *THERAPEUTIC EFFECT*
Hydantoin derivative with peripheral skeletal muscle relaxant action. Directly relaxes spastic muscle by interfering with calcium ion release from sarcoplasmic reticulum within skeletal muscle. *Relief of muscle spasticity, however, may be accompanied by muscle weakness sufficient to affect overall functional capacity of the patient. Dantrolene also can attenuate or prevent development of malignant hyperthermia.*

**USES** Orally for spasticity. Used intravenously for the management of malignant hyperthermia.

**UNLABELED USES** Neuroleptic malignant syndrome, exercise-induced muscle pain, and flexor spasms.

**CONTRAINDICATIONS** Active hepatic disease such as hepatitis and cirrhosis; drug-induced hepatitis; when spasticity is necessary to sustain upright posture and balance in locomotion or to maintain increased body function; spasticity due to rheumatic disorders; lactation.

**CAUTIOUS USE** Impaired cardiac or pulmonary function, muscular sclerosis; neuromuscular disease; myopathy; history of liver disease or dysfunction; patients older than

Common adverse effects in *italic;* life-threatening effects <u>underlined;</u> generic names in **bold;** classifications in SMALL CAPS; ◆ Canadian drug name; ⊕ Prototype drug

35 y, especially women; pregnancy (category C); long-time use in children. Safe use in children younger than 5 y is not established.

## ROUTE & DOSAGE

### Relief of Spasticity

*Adult:* **PO** 25 mg once/day, increase to 25 mg b.i.d. to q.i.d., may increase q7days up to 100 mg b.i.d. to q.i.d.

*Child (5 y or older):* **PO** 0.5 mg/ kg b.i.d., increase to 0.5 mg/kg t.i d. or q.i.d., may increase by 0.5 mg/kg up to 3 mg/kg b.i.d. to q.i.d. (max: 100 mg q.i.d.)

### Malignant Hyperthermia Treatment

*Adult/Child:* **IV** 1 mg/kg rapid direct IV push repeated prn up to a total of 10 mg/kg; **PO** May be necessary to continue orally with 1–2 mg/kg q.i.d. for 1–3 days to prevent recurrence

### Malignant Hyperthermia Preoperatively

*Adult:* **IV** 2.5 mg/kg infusion over 1 h may be repeated

*Adult/Child (5 y or older):* **PO** 4–8 mg/kg/day in divided doses for 1–2 days prior to surgery

### Hepatic Impairment Dosage Adjustment

Do not use in active liver disease

## ADMINISTRATION

### Oral

- Prepare oral suspension for a single dose, when necessary, by emptying contents of capsule(s) into fruit juice or other liquid. Shake suspension well before pouring.
- Avoid contamination, keep refrigerated, and use within several days, since it does not contain a preservative.

### Intravenous

*PREPARE:* **Direct:** Dilute each 20 mg with 60 mL sterile water without preservatives. Shake until clear. **Infusion:** Large volume used for prophylaxis may be transferred to plastic (not glass) infusion bags. *ADMINISTER:* **Direct:** Give by rapid direct IV push. Avoid extravasation; solution has a high pH and therefore is extremely irritating to tissue. ▪ Ensure IV patency prior to giving drug direct IV. **Infusion:** Give over 1 h.
*INCOMPATIBILITIES:* **Y-site:** Do not administer with other medications.

- Store capsules in tightly closed, light-resistant container. Contents of vial (for IV use) **must be** protected from direct light and used within 6 h after reconstitution, since it does not contain a preservative. ▪ Store both PO and parenteral forms at 15°–30° C (59°–86° F) unless otherwise directed.

## ADVERSE EFFECTS (≥1%) **Body as a Whole:** Hypersensitivity (pruritus, urticaria, eczematoid skin eruption, photosensitivity, eosinophilic pleural effusion). **CNS:** Drowsiness, *muscle weakness,* dizziness, light-headedness, unusual fatigue, speech disturbances, headache, confusion, nervousness, mental depression, insomnia, euphoria, seizures. **CV:** Tachycardia, erratic BP. **Special Senses:** Blurred vision, diplopia, photophobia. **GI:** *Diarrhea,* constipation, nausea, vomiting, anorexia, swallowing difficulty, alterations of taste, gastric irritation, abdominal cramps, GI bleeding; hepatitis, jaundice, hepatomegaly, hepatic necrosis (all related to prolonged use of high doses). **Urogeni-**

**D**

**tal:** Crystalluria with pain or burning with urination, urinary frequency, urinary retention, nocturia, enuresis, difficult erection.

**INTERACTIONS Drug: Alcohol** and other CNS DEPRESSANTS compound CNS depression; **estrogens** increase risk of hepatotoxicity in women older than 35 y; **verapamil** and other CALCIUM CHANNEL BLOCKERS increase risk of ventricular fibrillation and cardiovascular collapse with IV dantrolene.

**PHARMACOKINETICS Absorption:** Incompletely absorbed from GI tract. **Peak:** 5 h. **Distribution:** Crosses placenta. **Metabolism:** In liver. **Elimination:** In urine chiefly as metabolites. **Half-Life:** 8.7 h.

## NURSING IMPLICATIONS

### Black Box Warning

*Dantrolene has been associated with severe hepatic damage.*

### Assessment & Drug Effects

- Monitor for and report promptly S&S of hepatotoxicity (see Appendix F) that are more common in females and in those older than 35 y.
- Monitor vital signs during IV infusion. Also monitor ECG, CVP, and serum potassium.
- Supervise ambulation until patient's reaction to drug is known. Relief of spasticity may be accompanied by some loss of strength.
- Monitor patients with impaired cardiac or pulmonary function closely for cardiovascular or respiratory symptoms such as tachycardia, BP changes, feeling of suffocation.
- Monitor for and report symptoms of allergy and allergic pleural ef-

fusion: Shortness of breath, pleuritic pain, dry cough.
- Alert prescriber if improvement is not evident within 45 days. Drug may be discontinued because of the possibility of hepatotoxicity (see Appendix F).
- Monitor bowel function. Persistent diarrhea may necessitate drug withdrawal. Severe constipation with abdominal distention and signs of intestinal obstruction have been reported.
- Monitor lab tests: Baseline and periodic LFTs, blood cell counts, and renal function tests.

### Patient & Family Education

- Report promptly the onset of jaundice: Yellow skin or sclerae; dark urine, clay-colored stools, itching, abdominal discomfort. Hepatotoxicity frequently occurs between the 3rd and 12th mo of therapy.
- Do not drive or engage in other potentially hazardous activities until response to drug is known.
- Do not use OTC medications, alcoholic beverages, or other CNS depressants unless otherwise advised by prescriber. Liver toxicity occurs more commonly when other drugs are taken concurrently.

## DAPAGLIFLOZIN

(dap-a-gli-flo′sin)

Farxiga

**Classifications:** ANTIDIABETIC; SODIUM-GLUCOSE CO-TRANSPORTER 2 (SGLT2) INHIBITOR
**Therapeutic:** ANTIDIABETIC
**Prototype:** Canagliflozin

**AVAILABILITY** Tablets

## ACTION & *THERAPEUTIC EFFECT*

Inhibits the sodium-glucose cotransporter 2 (SGLT2) in the

proximal renal tubules that is responsible for the majority of the reabsorption of filtered glucose in the kidney. *Dapagliflozin inhibits SGLT2 thus allowing more glucose to be removed from the blood stream and excreted by the kidney.*

**USES** An adjunct to diet and exercise to improve glycemic control in adults with type 2 diabetes mellitus.

**CONTRAINDICATIONS** History of serious hypersensitivity reaction to dapagliflozin; severe renal impairment, end-stage renal disease, or dialysis; active bladder cancer, lactation.

**CAUTIOUS USE** Risk factors for hypotension; impaired renal function; hypoglycemia; ketoacidosis; genital mycotic infections; increased LDL C; history of bladder cancer; DM; older adults; pregnancy (category C). Safety and efficacy in children younger than 18 y not established.

## ROUTE & DOSAGE

**Type 2 Diabetes Mellitus**
*Adult:* PO 5 mg once daily; may increase to 10 mg

**Renal Impairment Dosage Adjustment**
*GFR less than 60 mL/min/ 1.73 m²:* Do not initiate
*GFR consistently falls to less than 60 mL/min/1.73 m²:* Discontinue

## ADMINISTRATION
**Oral**
- Give in the morning with/without food.
- Store at 15° C–30° C (59°F–86° F)

**ADVERSE EFFECTS** (≥ 1%) **Body as a Whole:** Influenza, pain in extremity. **CV:** Hypotension. **GI:** Constipation, nausea. **Metabolic:** Dyslipidemia, hypoglycemia, ketoacidosis. **Musculoskeletal:** Back pain, bone fracture. **Respiratory:** Nasopharyngitis. **Urogenital:** *Genital mycotic infection,* increased urination, urinary discomfort, urinary tract infection.

**INTERACTIONS Drug:** May potentiate the hypoglycemia effect of **insulin** and INSULIN SECRETAGOGUES. Monitor blood sugar closely if used with **rifampin** or **phenobarbital**.

**PHARMACOKINETICS Absorption:** 78% bioavailable after oral dose **Peak:** 2 h. **Distribution:** 9 1% plasma protein bound. **Metabolism:** In liver. **Elimination:** Renal (75%) and fecal (2 1%). **Half-Life:** 12.9 h.

## NURSING IMPLICATIONS
### Assessment & Drug Effects
- Monitor blood sugars (hypo/hyper glycemia).
- Monitor BP throughout therapy as drug causes intravascular volume depletion.
- Monitor for symptomatic hypotension especially at the initiation of therapy and in the older adult or those taking other drugs that lower BP.
- Monitor for S&S of genital fungal infections.
- Monitor lab tests: Baseline and periodic renal function tests; periodic HbA1C; periodic lipid profile.

### Patient & Family Education
- Monitor blood sugar as directed by prescriber. Note that this drug will cause sugar to appear in your urine.
- Report to prescriber if you experience S&S of hypoglycemia (see Appendix F).
- Report to prescriber any S&S of an allergic reaction (e.g., rash, hives).
- Maintain adequate fluid intake as drug can cause dehydration. Inform prescriber if you experience dizziness upon standing.

Common adverse effects in *italic;* life-threatening effects underlined; generic names in **bold;** classifications in SMALL CAPS; ♣ Canadian drug name; ⊕ Prototype drug

439

D

- Yeast infections of the vagina and penis (especially in uncircumcised men) may occur. Report promptly for treatment.
- Report to prescriber if a pregnancy is suspected.
- Discontinue breast-feeding while taking this drug.

## DAPSONE ℗

(dap'sone)

Aczone, Avlosulfon ◆

**Classification:** ANTILEPROSY (SULFONE)

Therapeutic: ANTILEPROSY

**AVAILABILITY** Tablet; gel

## ACTION & *THERAPEUTIC EFFECT*

Has bacteriostatic and bactericidal activity. Interferes with bacterial cell growth by competitive inhibition of folic acid synthesis by susceptible organisms. It also interferes with alternative pathways of complement system. *Effective against dapsone-sensitive multibacillary (borderline, borderline lepromatous, or lepromatous) leprosy, and dapsone-sensitive paucibacillary (indeterminate, tuberculoid, or borderline tuberculoid) leprosy. Gel form is effective against acne vulgaris.*

**USES** All forms of leprosy. Used in dapsone-sensitive multibacillary leprosy (with clofazimine and rifampin) and in dapsone-sensitive paucibacillary leprosy (with rifampin, clofazimine, or ethionamide). Also used prophylactically in contacts of patients with all forms of leprosy except tuberculoid and indeterminate leprosy. Used for treatment of dermatitis herpetiformis. **Gel** used for acne vulgaris.

**UNLABELED USES** Chemoprophylaxis of malaria (with pyrimethamine), systemic and discoid lupus erythematosus, pemphigus vulgaris, dermatosis (especially those associated with bullous eruptions, mucocutaneous lesions, inflammation or pustules); rheumatoid arthritis, allergic vasculitis; treatment of initial episodes of *P. carinii* pneumonia (with trimethoprim) in limited number of adults with AIDS.

**CONTRAINDICATIONS** Hypersensitivity to sulfones or its derivatives; advanced renal amyloidosis, anemia, methemoglobin reductase deficiency.

**CAUTIOUS USE** Sulfonamide hypersensitivity; chronic renal, hepatic, pulmonary, or cardiovascular disease, refractory anemias, albuminuria, G6PD deficiency; pregnancy (category C); lactation.

## ROUTE & DOSAGE

**Tuberculoid and Indeterminate-Type Leprosy**

*Adult:* **PO** 100 mg/day (with 6 mo of rifampin 600 mg/day) for a minimum of 3 y

**Lepromatous and Borderline Lepromatous Leprosy**

*Adult:* **PO** 100 mg/day for 10 y or more

*Child:* **PO** 1–2 mg/kg/day once daily in combination therapy (max: 100 mg/day)

**Dermatitis Herpetiformis**

*Adult:* **PO** 50 mg/day, may be increased to 300 mg/day if necessary (max: 500 mg/day)

**Prophylaxis for Close Contacts of Patient with Multibacillary Leprosy**

*Adult:* **PO** 50 mg/day

*Child (younger than 6 mo):* **PO** 6 mg 3 × wk; *6–23 mo:* 12 mg 3 × wk; *2–5 y:* 25 mg 3 × wk; *6–12 y:* 25 mg/day

Common adverse effects in *italic;* life-threatening effects underlined; generic names in **bold;** classifications in SMALL CAPS; ◆ Canadian drug name; ℗ Prototype drug

### *P. carinii* Pneumonia Prophylaxis

*Adult:* **PO** 50 mg b.i.d. or 100 mg daily
*Child:* **PO** 2 mg/kg once daily (max: 100 mg/day)

### Acne

**Topical** Apply pea-sized amount of gel to affected area b.i.d.

## ADMINISTRATION

### Oral

- Give with food to reduce possibility of GI distress.
- Store in tightly covered, light-resistant containers at 15°–30° C (59°–86° F). Drug discoloration apparently does not indicate a chemical change.

### Topical

- Clean skin with soap and water before application.

## ADVERSE EFFECTS (≥1%) Body as a Whole:

Hypersensitivity (cutaneous reactions); erythema multiforme, exfoliative dermatitis, toxic epidermal necrolysis (rare), allergic rhinitis, urticaria, fever, infectious mononucleosis-like syndrome. **CNS:** Headache, nervousness, insomnia, vertigo; paresthesia, *muscle weakness*. **CV:** Tachycardia. **GI:** Anorexia, nausea, vomiting, abdominal pain; toxic hepatitis, cholestatic jaundice (reversible with discontinuation of drug therapy); increased ALT, AST, LDH; hyperbilirubinemia. **Hematologic:** In patient with or without G6PD deficiency; *dose-related hemolysis,* Heinz body formation, *methemoglobinemia with cyanosis,* hemolytic anemia; aplastic anemia (rare), agranulocytosis. **Skin:** Drug-induced lupus erythematosus, phototoxicity. **Special Senses:** Blurred vision, tinnitus. **Other:** Male infertility; sulfone syndrome (fever, malaise, exfoliative dermatitis, hepatic necrosis with jaundice, lymphadenopathy, methemoglobinemia, anemia).

## INTERACTIONS Drug: Activated charcoal

decreases dapsone absorption and enterohepatic circulation; **pyrimethamine, trimethoprim** increase risk of adverse hematologic reactions; **rifampin** decreases dapsone levels 7–10 fold.

## PHARMACOKINETICS

**Absorption:** Rapidly and nearly completely absorbed from GI tract. **Peak:** 2–8 h. **Distribution:** Distributed to all body tissues; high concentrations in kidney, liver, muscle, and skin; crosses placenta; distributed into breast milk. **Metabolism:** In liver by CYP3A4. **Elimination:** 70–85% in urine; remainder in feces; traces of drug may be found in body for 3 wk after repeated doses. **Half-Life:** 20–30 h.

## NURSING IMPLICATIONS

### Assessment & Drug Effects

- Monitor for therapeutic effectiveness that may not appear for leprosy until after 3–6 mo of therapy.
- Determine periodic dapsone blood levels.
- Perform liver function tests in patients who complain of malaise, fever, chills, anorexia, nausea, vomiting, and have jaundice.
- Monitor severity of anemia. Nearly all patients demonstrate hemolysis.
- Monitor temperature during first few weeks of therapy. If fever is frequent or severe, leprosy reactional state should be ruled out.
- Monitor lab tests: Baseline then weekly CBC during the first month of therapy, at monthly intervals for at least 6 mo, and semiannually thereafter.

### Patient & Family Education

- Report symptoms of leprosy that do not improve within 3 mo or that get worse to prescriber.

---

Common adverse effects in *italic;* life-threatening effects underlined; generic names in **bold;** classifications in SMALL CAPS; ♣ Canadian drug name; ☺ Prototype drug

- Report the appearance of a rash with bullous lesions around elbows and other joints promptly. Drug-induced or worsening skin lesions require withdrawal of dapsone.
- Report symptoms of peripheral neuropathy with motor loss (muscle weakness) promptly.

# DAPTOMYCIN
(dap-to-my'sin)
Cubicin
**Classifications:** ANTIBIOTIC;
LIPOPEPTIDE
Therapeutic: ANTIBIOTIC

**AVAILABILITY** Solution for injection

**ACTION & THERAPEUTIC EFFECT**
It binds to bacterial membranes of gram-positive bacteria causing rapid depolarization of the membrane potential leading to inhibition of protein, DNA, and RNA synthesis and bacterial cell death. *Daptomycin is effective against a broad spectrum of gram-positive organisms, including both susceptible and resistant strains of* S. aureus.

**USES** Complicated skin and skin structure infections, bacteremia, endocarditis.

**UNLABELED USES** Vancomycin-resistant enterococci, MRSA-associated bone/joint infections, febrile neutropenia.

**CONTRAINDICATIONS** Hypersensitive reaction to daptomycin; pseudomembranous colitis; myopathy; eosinophilic pneumonia; nonbacterial infection.

**CAUTIOUS USE** Severe renal or hepatic impairment, end-stage renal failure; peripheral neuropathy; GI disease; history of rhabdomyolysis, or myopathy; older adults; pregnancy (category B); lactation. Safe use in infants is not established.

## ROUTE & DOSAGE

**Skin Infections**
*Adult:* **IV** 4 mg/kg q24h × 7–14 days
*Adolescent:* **IV** 5 mg/kg q24h × 14 d
*Children (7-11 y):* **IV** 7 mg/kg q24h x 14 d; *(2-6 y):* 9 mg/kg q24h x14d; *(1-2 y):* 10 mg/kg q24h x14 d

**Bacteremia (S. aureus)**
*Adult:* **IV** 6 mg/kg daily × 2–6 wk
*Adolescent:* **IV** 7 mg/kg every 24 h
*Children (7-11 y):* **IV** 9 mg/kg every 24 h; *(1–6 y):* 12 mg/kg every 24 h

**Endocarditis**
*Adult:* **IV** 6 mg/kg q24h x 2-6 wk

**Renal Impairment Dosage Adjustment**
*CrCl less than 30 mL/min:* administer q48h

**Hemodialyis Dosage Adjustment**
Dose by CrCl, administer after dialysis

## ADMINISTRATION
Intravenous

**PREPARE: IV Direct:** Note: Double check manufacturer's guidelines for reconstitution, not all recommend normal saline—varies by product. Slowly add 10 mL of NS to the 500 mg vial, pointing needle toward the wall of the vial. Gently rotate vial to wet the powder, then allow to

Common adverse effects in *italic;* life-threatening effects <u>underlined;</u> generic names in **bold;** classifications in SMALL CAPS; ✦ Canadian drug name; ⊙ Prototype drug

stand for 10 min. Gently rotate vial to completely dissolve. Yields 50 mg/mL. **IV Infusion:** Further dilute the 50 mg/mL solution in 50 mL of NS.
*ADMINISTER:* **Direct:** Inject over 2 min. **IV Infusion:** Infuse over 30 min; if same IV line is used for infusion of other drugs, flush line before/after with NS.
*INCOMPATIBILITIES:* **Solution/additive:** **Dextrose**-containing solutions. **Y-site: Acyclovir, alemtuzumab, allopurinol, amphotericin B, amphotericin B liposomal, blinatumomab, cytarabine, dantrolene, gemcitabine, gemtuzumab, imipenem/cilastin, methotrexate, metronidazole, minocycline, mitomycin, nesiritide, nitroglycerin, pantoprazole, pentazocine, pentobarbital, phenytoin, quinidine, remifentanil, streptozocin, sulfentanil, thiopental, vancomycin.**

■ Store unopened vials in 2°–8° C (36°–46° F). Avoid excessive heat. ■ Refer to manufacturer's labeling for specific storage and reconstitution guidelines— varies by product.

## ADVERSE EFFECTS (≥1%) **Body as a Whole:** Injection site reactions, fever, fungal infections. **CNS:** Headache, anxiety, *insomnia*, dizziness. **CV:** Hypotension, hypertension, peripheral edema, chest pain, atrial fibrillation. **GI:** Nausea, vomiting, diarrhea, abdominal pain, abnormal liver function tests. **Hematologic:** Anemia, eosinophilia, leukocytosis, thrombocytopenia. **Metabolic:** Elevated CPK, hypokalemia, elevated hepatic enzymes. **Musculoskeletal:** Limb pain, arthralgia, uncontrolled muscle movement. **Otic:** tinnitus. **Respiratory:** Dyspnea, pharyngolaryngeal pain. **Skin:** Rash, diaphoresis, ery-

thema, pruritus, hyperhidrosis. **Urogenital:** UTIs, renal failure.

## INTERACTIONS Do not use with bowel preparation kits. Use caution when also administering **tobramycin**.

## PHARMACOKINETICS **Elimination:** Primarily renal. **Distribution:** 90% protein bound. **Half-Life:** 8 h.

## NURSING IMPLICATIONS

### Assessment & Drug Effects
■ Monitor for and report: Muscle pain or weakness, especially with concurrent therapy with HMG-CoA reductase inhibitors (statin drugs); S&S of peripheral neuropathy, superinfection such as candidiasis, irregular pulse.
■ Withhold drug and notify prescriber if S&S of myopathy develop with CPK elevation greater than 1000 units/L (~5 × ULN), or if CPK level is 10 × ULN or greater.
■ Monitor lab tests: Baseline C&S and renal function tests.

### Patient & Family Education
■ Report any of the following to the prescriber: Muscle pain, weakness or unusual tiredness; numbness or tingling; difficulty breathing or shortness of breath; severe diarrhea or vomiting; skin rash or itching, dark urine, jaundice.

## DARBEPOETIN ALFA
(dar-be-po-e'tin)
Aranesp
**Classifications:** BLOOD FORMER; ERYTHROPOIESIS-STIMULATING AGENT
Therapeutic: ANTIANEMIC
**Prototype:** Epoetin alfa

AVAILABILITY Solution for injection

Common adverse effects in *italic*; life-threatening effects underlined; generic names in **bold;** classifications in SMALL CAPS; ♣ Canadian drug name; ⊘ Prototype drug

443

D

## ACTION & *THERAPEUTIC EFFECT*
An erythropoiesis-stimulating protein that stimulates red blood cell production in the bone marrow in response to hypoxia. *Darbepoetin stimulates release of reticulocytes from the bone marrow into the blood stream where they mature into RBCs.*

## USES
Treatment of anemia in patients with chronic renal failure or chemotherapy-associated anemia, treatment of chemotherapy-induced anemia in nonmyeloid malignancies.

## CONTRAINDICATIONS
Patients with uncontrolled hypertension; serious hypersensitivity to darbepoetin or human albumin; antibody-mediated anemia due to anti-erythropoietin antibodies; pure red cell aplasia that begins after treatment with darbepoetin alfa or other related drugs.

## CAUTIOUS USE
Controlled hypertension, elevated hemoglobin, folic acid or vitamin $B_{12}$ deficiencies, hematologic diseases; infections, inflammatory or malignant processes, osteofibrosis, occult blood loss, hemolysis, severe aluminum toxicity, bone marrow fibrosis, chronic renal failure patients not on dialysis; pregnancy (category C); lactation.

## ROUTE & DOSAGE

### Anemia
*Adult:* **IV/Subcutaneous** Initially, 0.45 mcg/kg once/wk. Reduce dose by 25% if there is a rapid increase (i.e., more than 1 g/dL in any 2-wk period) in Hgb or if the Hgb is approaching 12 g/dL. If the Hgb does not increase by 1 g/dL after 4 wk of therapy and iron stores are adequate, increase the dose by 25%. Maintenance dose is 0.26–0.65 mcg/kg once/wk.

### Converting Epoetin Alfa to Darbepoetin
*Adults:* **IV/Subcutaneous** Estimate the starting dose of darbepoetin alfa based on the total weekly dose of epoetin alfa at the time of conversion. If the patient was receiving epoetin alfa 2–3 × wk, administer darbepoetin alfa once/wk; if the patient was receiving epoetin alfa once/wk, administer darbepoetin alfa once every 2 wk. The route of administration (i.e., subcutaneous or IV) should be maintained. Note: The following darbepoetin alfa dosage recommendations are estimates based on total amount of epoetin alfa administered/wk. Because of individual variability, titrate doses to maintain the target Hgb.

### Estimated Starting Dose (titrate to maintain target Hgb)

### Previous Weekly Dose of Epoetin Alfa
- *1500–2499 units/wk:* Darbepoetin dose: 6.25 mcg/wk
- *2500–4999 units/wk:* Darbepoetin dose: 10–12.5 mcg/wk
- *5000–10,999 units/wk:* Darbepoetin dose: 20–25 mcg/wk
- *11,000–17,999 units/wk:* Darbepoetin dose: 40 mcg/wk
- *18,000–33,999 units/wk:* Darbepoetin dose: 60 mcg/wk
- *34,000–89,999 units/wk:* Darbepoetin dose: 100 mcg/wk
- *Greater than 90,000 units/wk:* Darbepoetin dose: 200 mcg/wk

**D**

## ADMINISTRATION

### All Routes

- Correct deficiencies of folic acid or vitamin $B_{12}$ prior to initiation of therapy.

### Subcutaneous

- Do not shake solution. Shaking may denature the darbepoetin, rendering it biologically inactive.
- Inspect solution for particulate matter prior to use. Do not use if solution is discolored or if it contains particulate matter.
- Use only one dose per vial, and do not reenter vial.
- Do not give with any other drug solution.

### Intravenous

*PREPARE:* **Direct:** Do not shake or dilute vials or prefilled syringes. Do not use vials or prefilled syringes that have been shaken.
*ADMINISTER:* **Direct:** Give direct IV as a bolus dose over 1 min.
- Discard any unused portion of the vial or syringe. It contains no preservatives.

## ADVERSE EFFECTS (≥1%) **Body as a Whole:** Injection site pain, *peripheral edema,* fatigue, fever, death, chest pain, fluid overload, access infection, access hemorrhage, flu-like symptoms, asthenia, *infection.* **CNS:** *Headache,* dizziness. **CV:** *Hypertension, hypotension, arrhythmias,* cardiac arrest, angina, chest pain, vascular access thrombosis, CHF, red cell aplasia. **GI:** *Nausea, vomiting, diarrhea,* constipation. **Musculoskeletal:** *Myalgia, arthralgia,* limb pain, back pain. **Respiratory:** *Upper respiratory infection, dyspnea, cough,* bronchitis. **Skin:** Pruritus. **Other:** Increased risk of thrombotic events and mortality in cancer patients.

## PHARMACOKINETICS **Absorption:** 37% absorbed from subcutaneous site. **Peak:** 24–72 h subcutaneous. **Distribution:** Distribution confined primarily to intravascular space. **Elimination:** 10% in urine. **Half-Life:** 21 h IV, 49 h subcutaneous.

## NURSING IMPLICATIONS

### Black Box Warning

*Darbepoetin has been associated with increased risk of MI, stroke, venous thromboembolism, thrombosis of vascular access, and tumor progression or recurrence.*

### Assessment & Drug Effects

- Control BP adequately prior to initiation of therapy and closely monitor and control during therapy. Report immediately S&S of CHF, cardiac arrhythmias, or sepsis. Note that hypertension is an adverse effect that **must be** controlled.
- Notify prescriber of a rapid rise in Hgb as dosage will need to be reduced because of risk of serious hypertension and other adverse events. Note that BP may rise during early therapy as Hgb increases.
- Monitor for premonitory neurologic symptoms (i.e., aura, and report their appearance promptly). The potential for seizures exists during periods of rapid Hgb increase (e.g., greater than 1.0 g/dL in any 2-wk period).
- Monitor closely and report immediately S&S of thrombotic events (e.g., MI, CVA, TIA), especially for patients with CRF.
- Monitor lab tests: Baseline and periodic transferrin and serum ferritin; Hgb twice weekly until stabi-

Common adverse effects in *italic;* life-threatening effects underlined; generic names in **bold;** classifications in SMALL CAPS; ♣ Canadian drug name; ⊙ Prototype drug

445

lized and maintenance dose is established, then weekly for at least 4 wk, and at regular intervals thereafter; periodic CBC with differential and platelet count; periodic BUN, creatinine, serum phosphorus, and serum potassium.

### Patient & Family Education
- Adhere closely to antihypertensive drug regimen and dietary restrictions.
- Monitor BP as directed by prescriber.
- Do not drive or engage in other potentially hazardous activity during the first 90 days of therapy because of possible seizure activity.
- Report any of the following to the prescriber: Chest pain, difficulty breathing, shortness of breath, severe or persistent headache, fever, muscle aches and pains, or nausea.

---

## DARIFENACIN HYDROBROMIDE

(dar-i-fen'a-sin)

Enablex

**Classifications:** ANTICHOLINERGIC; MUSCARINIC RECEPTOR ANTAGONIST; BLADDER ANTISPASMODIC
**Therapeutic:** BLADDER ANTISPASMODIC
**Prototype:** Oxybutin

**AVAILABILITY** Extended release tablet

### ACTION & *THERAPEUTIC EFFECT*

Darifenacin is a selective $M_3$ muscarinic receptor antagonist. Muscarinic $M_3$ receptors play an important role in contraction of the urinary bladder smooth muscle and stimulation of salivary secretion. *Control of urinary incontinence due to urgency and frequency.*

**USES** Treatment of overactive bladder with symptoms of urge urinary incontinence, urgency, and frequency.

**CONTRAINDICATIONS** Hypersensitivity to darifenacin; angioedema; severe hepatic impairment (Child-Pugh C class); patients at risk of urinary retention, gastric retention; pyloric stenosis, ileus; urinary retention; uncontrolled narrow-angle glaucoma.

**CAUTIOUS USE** Risk of urinary retention, clinically significant bladder outflow obstruction, renal disease; mild to moderate hepatic impairment; decreased GI motility, GERD, severe constipation, ulcerative colitis; myasthenia gravis; controlled narrow-angle glaucoma; pregnancy (category C); lactation. Safety and efficacy in patients with severe hepatic impairment is unknown.

### ROUTE & DOSAGE

| Overactive Bladder |
| --- |
| *Adult:* **PO** 7.5–15 mg daily |
| **Moderate Hepatic Impairment Dosage Adjustment** |
| *Child-Pugh B Class:* Max: 7.5 mg daily |

### ADMINISTRATION

**Oral**
- Ensure that the drug is not chewed or crushed. It **must be** swallowed whole.
- Note: Dosage should not exceed 7.5 mg daily with moderate hepatic impairment (i.e., Child-Pugh B class) or concurrent therapy

with potent inhibitors of CYP3A4 (e.g., itraconazole, clarithromycin, nefazodone, nelfinavir, ritonavir).
- Store 15°–30° C (59°–86° F). Protect from light.

## ADVERSE EFFECTS (≥1%) Body as a Whole:
Flu-like symptoms, urinary tract infection, angioedema **CNS:** *Headache,* asthenia, dizziness. **GI:** *Constipation, dry mouth, dyspepsia, nausea,* abdominal pain, diarrhea. **Opthalmic:** Dry eye syndrome, visual disturbances.

## INTERACTIONS Drug:
Potent inhibitors of CYP3A4 (e.g., **clarithromycin, erythromycin, itraconazole, ketoconazole, nefazodone, nelfinavir,** and **ritonavir**) increase darifenacin levels. Darifenacin will cause additive anticholinergic effects with other ANTICHOLINERGIC drugs. Darifenacin can increase **digoxin** concentrations. DIURETICS can increase bladder symptoms. **Food: Grapefruit juice** may increase darifenacin levels.

## PHARMACOKINETICS Absorption:
15–19% bioavailability. **Peak:** 7 h. **Distribution:** 98% protein bound. **Metabolism:** Extensive hepatic metabolism. **Elimination:** Renal and fecal. **Half-Life:** 13–19 h.

## NURSING IMPLICATIONS
### Assessment & Drug Effects
- Monitor for adverse effects of concurrently used drugs that have a narrow therapeutic window and are metabolized by CYP26D (e.g., flecainide, thioridazine, or TRICYCLIC ANTIDEPRESSANTS).
- Signs of toxicity: headache, confusion, hallucinations, and somnolence.
- Monitor lab tests: Frequent digoxin levels with concurrent therapy.

### Patient & Family Education
- Do not drive or engage in potentially hazardous activities until response to drug is known.
- Use caution in hot environments to minimize the risk of heat prostration.
- Report any of the following to a health care provider: Difficulty passing urine, unexplained nausea, or persistent constipation.

## DARUNAVIR
(da-run′a-ver)
Prezista
**Classifications:** ANTIRETROVIRAL; PROTEASE INHIBITOR
**Therapeutic:** HIV PROTEASE INHIBITOR
**Prototype:** Saquinavir

**AVAILABILITY** Tablet, oral suspension

## ACTION & THERAPEUTIC EFFECT
Darunavir is an inhibitor of HIV-1 protease that selectively inhibits the cleavage of HIV polyproteins in infected cells, thereby preventing the maturation of virus particles. *Darunavir reduces viral load (decreases the number of RNA copies) and increases the number of T helper CD4 cells.*

**USES** Treatment of HIV infection with other antiretroviral agents.

**UNLABELED USES** HIV prophylaxis.

## CONTRAINDICATIONS
Hypersensitivity to darunavir or protease inhibitors, ritonavir; severe hepatic impairment; pancreatitis; lactation.

## CAUTIOUS USE
Hypersensitivity to sulfa drugs; hepatic function impairment, hepatitis B or C; patients at risk for pancreatitis; severe renal

Common adverse effects in *italic;* life-threatening effects underlined; generic names in **bold;** classifications in SMALL CAPS; ◆ Canadian drug name; ⊙ Prototype drug

447

impairment, chronic renal failure; hemophilia A or B; concurrent autoimmune disease; sulfonamide allergy; DM; diabetes ketoacidosis; hyperglycemia; older adults; pregnancy (category C); children.

## ROUTE & DOSAGE

### HIV Infection, Treatment Naive
*Adult:* **PO** 800 mg daily with 100 mg ritonavir PO

### HIV Infection, Treatment Experienced
*Adult:* **PO** 600 mg b.i.d. with 100 mg ritonavir PO (Genetic screening to determine if 800 mg daily is needed.)
*Adolescent/Child:* Weight, genetic screen and previous drug exposure all affect dose; see package insert for dosing table.

*Pregnanacy Dosage Adjustment*
Decrease to 600 mg b.i.d.

## ADMINISTRATION

### Oral
- Give with food and coadminister with 100 mg ritonavir (adult dose).
- Tablets **must be** swallowed whole.
- Store at 15°–30° C (59°–86° F). Protect from light and moisture.

## ADVERSE EFFECTS (≥1%) CNS:
*Headache,* fatigue. **GI:** Abdominal pain, constipation, *diarrhea, vomiting.* **Skin:** Stevens–Johnson syndrome, rash, pruritus. **Hepatic:** Acute hepatitis. **Metabolic:** Hypercholesterolemia, increased LDL.

## INTERACTIONS Drug: AZOLE ANTIFUNGALS and **indinavir** increase the levels of darunavir. Coadministration of other inhibitors of

CYP3A4 may also increase darunavir. ANTICONVULSANTS (e.g., **carbamazepine, phenobarbital, phenytoin**), CORTICOSTEROIDS (e.g., **dexamethasone**), **efavirenz,** RIFAMYCINS (e.g., **rifampin, rifabutin**), and **saquinavir** may decrease darunavir levels. Darunavir may increase the levels of AZOLE ANTIFUNGALS, CORTICOSTEROIDS, **efavirenz, indinavir,** RIFAMYCINS, **amiodarone, bepridil, lidocaine, quinidine,** CALCIUM CHANNEL BLOCKERS (e.g., **nifedipine, nicardipine, felodipine**), **clarithromycin,** IMMUNOSUPPRESSANTS (e.g., **cyclosporine, sirolimus, tacrolimus**), PHOSPHODIESTERASE TYPE 5 INHIBITORS (e.g., **sildenafil, tadalafil, vardenafil**), and trazodone, due in part to its ability to inhibit CYP3A4. Darunavir decreases the levels of the **lopinavir/ritonavir** combination, ORAL CONTRACEPTIVES (e.g., **norethindrone**), **methadone,** SELECTIVE SEROTONIN REUPTAKE INHIBITORS [SSRIS (e.g., **paroxetine, sertraline**)], and **warfarin.** Use of BENZODIAZEPINES (e.g., **midazolam, triazolam**) increases the risk of prolonged or increased sedation or respiratory depression. Use of ERGOT ALKALOIDS may increase ergot toxicity. Coadministration with HMG COA REDUCTASE INHIBITORS increases the risk of myopathy. Combination use with **pimozide** increases the risk of cardiac arrhythmias. **Food:** Food enhances the bioavailability of darunavir. **Herbal:** St. John's wort decreases the level of darunavir.

## PHARMACOKINETICS Absorption: 82% absorbed (in combination with ritonavir). **Peak:** 2.5–4 h. **Distribution:** 95% protein bound. **Metabolism:** In the liver. **Elimination:** Primarily fecal (80%) with minor elimination in urine. **Half-Life:** 15 h.

## NURSING IMPLICATIONS

### Assessment & Drug Effects

- Monitor for and report S&S of pancreatitis, as this may be an indication for discontinuation of darunavir.
- Monitor for S&S of skin rash. Notify prescriber immediately if a severe rash appears.
- Monitor diabetics for loss of glycemic control.
- Increase monitoring of INR with concurrent warfarin therapy.
- Monitor for adverse effects or loss of efficacy of concurrent medications, as many drug interactions occur with darunavir.
- Monitor lab tests: Periodic CD4+ cell count, plasma HIV-RNA, lipid profile, LFTs, and plasma glucose.

### Patient & Family Education

- Follow directions for taking the drug (see Administration). If a dose is missed by more than 6 h, wait until the next regularly scheduled dose. If a dose is missed by less than 6 h, take a dose and continue with the next regularly scheduled dose.
- Ensure that you know which medicines should **not** be taken with darunavir, as serious consequences could occur.
- Report any of the following to a health care provider: Blistering, redness, or peeling skin or mucous membranes; severe skin rash.
- Use or add a barrier contraceptive if using an estrogen-containing oral contraceptive if you wish to prevent pregnancy.

## DASATINIB
(das-a'ti-nib)
Sprycel

**Classifications:** ANTINEOPLASTIC BIOLOGIC RESPONSE MODIFIER; KINASE INHIBITOR

**Therapeutic** ANTINEOPLASTIC
**Prototype:** Erlotinib

## AVAILABILITY Tablet

## ACTION & *THERAPEUTIC EFFECT*

Dasatinib is a BCR-ABL tyrosine kinase inhibitor. BCR-ABL tyrosine kinase is an enzyme produced by a chromosomal translocation associated with chronic myeloid leukemia (CML) and certain types of acute lymphocytic leukemias (Ph+ ALL). *Dasatinib inhibits the growth of CML and ALL cell lines overexpressing BCR-ABL kinase.*

## USES Treatment of chronic, accelerated, or myeloid or lymphoid blast phase chronic myelogenous leukemia (CML). Treatment of Philadelphia chromosome–positive (Ph+) acute lymphocytic leukemia (ALL) in adults.

## CONTRAINDICATIONS Hypersensitivity to dasatinib; active bleeding; pulmonary arterial hypertension; hypokalemia; hypomagnesemia; pregnancy (category D); lactation.

## CAUTIOUS USE Hepatic impairment; bacterial or viral infection; history of GI bleeding; interstitial pneumonia; pleural effusion; patients at risk for QT prolongation including patients with long QT syndrome; older adults. Safe use in children younger than 18 y not established.

## ROUTE & DOSAGE

### CML and Philadelphia Chromosome-Positive ALL

*Adult:* **PO** 140 mg once daily; may increase dose to 180 mg once daily.

Common adverse effects in *italic;* life-threatening effects underlined; generic names in **bold;** classifications in SMALL CAPS; ♣ Canadian drug name; ◑ Prototype drug

449

### Chronic Phase CML
*Adult:* **PO** 100 mg daily

### Dosage Adjustments for Neutropenia and Thrombocytopenia

**Chronic phase CML where absolute neutrophil count (ANC) less than 500/m³ and/or platelets less than 50,000/mm³**

*Step 1:* DC dasatinib until the ANC 1000/mm³ or more and platelets 50,000/mm³ or more

*Step 2:* If cell recovery occurs in 7 days or less, restart at original dose

*Step 3:* If platelets less than 25,000 mm³ and/or recurrence of ANC less than 500/mm³, resume at dose of 80 mg daily

**Accelerated phase CML, blast phase CML, and Ph⁺ ALL where ANC less than 500/mm³ and/or platelets less than 10,000/mm³**

*Step 1:* Assure that cytopenia is unrelated to the underlying leukemia. If so, DC until ANC 1000/mm³ or more and platelets 20,000/mm³ or more.

*Step 2:* Resume at starting dose

*Step 3:* If cytopenia recurs, repeat step 1 and resume at 50 mg b.i.d. (second episode) or 40 mg b.i.d. (third episode)

*Step 4:* If cytopenia is related to the underlying leukemia, may increase to 180 mg daily

## ADMINISTRATION
### Oral
▪ Do not crush or break tablets. They should be swallowed whole.

▪ Ensure that hypokalemia and hypomagnesemia are corrected prior to administering dasatinib.
▪ Store at 15°–30° C (59°–86° F).

## ADVERSE EFFECTS (≥1%) Body as a Whole: Chills, contusion, *febrile* neutropenia, *hemorrhage, infection,* malaise, *pain, pyrexia,* tumor lysis syndrome, weight gain or weight loss. **CNS:** *Asthenia,* anxiety, confusional state, CNS bleeding, depression, dizziness, dysgeusia, *fatigue, headache,* insomnia, neuropathy, somnolence, syncope, tremor, vertigo. **CV:** Arrhythmia, chest pain, angina, <u>congestive heart failure,</u> pericardial effusion, cardiomegaly, hypertension, hypotension, <u>myocardial infarction,</u> palpitations. **GI:** *Abdominal distention and pain,* anal fissure, *anorexia,* ascites, colitis, constipation, *diarrhea,* dysphagia, gastritis, *GI bleeding, nausea,* oral soft tissue disorder, *vomiting, mucosal inflammation.* **Hematologic:** *Anemia, neutropenia,* pancytopenia, <u>thrombocytopenia,</u> elevated ALT and AST, hypocalcemia, hypophosphatemia. **Metabolic:** Appetite disturbances, *fluid retention, edema,* hyperuricemia. **Musculoskeletal:** *Arthralgia, musculoskeletal pain,* muscle inflammation, myalgia, musculoskeletal stiffness. **Respiratory:** Asthma, *cough, dyspnea,* lung infiltration, *plural effusion,* pneumonia, pulmonary edema, pulmonary hypertension, *upper respiratory tract infection.* **Skin:** Acne, alopecia, dermatitis, dry skin, hyperhidrosis, nail disorder, photosensitivity reaction, pigmentation disorder, pruritus, *skin rash.* **Special Senses:** Conjunctivitis, dry eye, tinnitus. **Urogenital:** Gynecomastia, renal failure, urinary frequency.

Common adverse effects in *italic;* life-threatening effects <u>underlined</u>; generic names in **bold;** classifications in SMALL CAPS; ✿ Canadian drug name; ⊙ Prototype drug

## INTERACTIONS

**Drug:** **Aluminum-** and **magnesium**-based ANTACIDS decrease dasatinib absorption. AZOLE ANTIFUNGAL AGENTS (e.g., **ketoconazole, itraconazole**), MACROLIDE ANTIBIOTICS (e.g., **clarithromycin, erythromycin, telithromycin**), HIV PROTEASE INHIBITORS (e.g., **indinavir, nelfinavir, ritonavir, saquinavir**), **nefazodone,** and other inhibitors of CYP3A4 may increase dasatinib levels. Compounds that induce CYP3A4 (e.g., **carbamazepine, dexamethasone, phenobarbital, phenytoin, rifampin**) may decrease dasatinib levels. PROTON PUMP INHIBITORS and H₂ ANTAGONISTS may reduce the absorption of dasatinib due to long-term suppression of gastric acid secretion. Dasatinib may alter the plasma concentrations of other drugs that require CYP3A4 and have a narrow therapeutic window (e.g., **cyclosporine**, ERGOT ALKALOIDS). Dasatinib increases the levels of **simvastatin**. **Food:** Food enhances the bioavailability of dasatinib. **Herbal: St. John's wort** may decrease the level of dasatinib.

## PHARMACOKINETICS

**Peak:** 0.5–6 h. **Distribution:** 93–96% protein bound. **Metabolism:** Extensive hepatic metabolism. **Elimination:** Fecal. **Half-Life:** 3–5 h.

## NURSING IMPLICATIONS

### Assessment & Drug Effects

- Monitor for and report S&S of fluid retention (e.g., pleural or pericardial effusion, peripheral or pulmonary edema, ascites).
- Monitor for S&S of cardiac dysfunction (e.g., heart failure, arrhythmias). ECG monitoring may be needed to evaluate potential QT interval prolongation.
- Monitor for numerous adverse side effects of dasatinib. Immediately report suspected bleeding or infection.
- Monitor lab tests: Baseline and periodic serum potassium and magnesium; baseline CBC with differential (including ANC and platelet count), then weekly for first 2 mo, then monthly; periodic LFTs.

### Patient & Family Education

- Take antacids (if needed for GI distress) 2 h before or after dasatinib.
- Do not use OTC medications for heartburn (other than antacids) without consulting prescriber.
- Women should use effective means of contraception to avoid pregnancy during treatment.
- Inform your prescriber if you are pregnant or planning to become pregnant, as dasatinib may harm the fetus.
- Discontinue breast-feeding as it is not know if drug is excreted in breast milk.
- Report immediately to your health care provider any of the following: Bleeding (including wine- or coke-colored urine, or black tarry stools) or easy bruising, fever or other signs of an infection, severe lethargy or weakness.

---

# DAUNORUBICIN HYDROCHLORIDE

(daw-noe-roo'bi-sin)

Cerubidine

# DAUNORUBICIN CITRATED LIPOSOMAL

DaunoXome

**Classifications:** ANTINEOPLASTIC; ANTHRACYCLINE (ANTIBIOTIC)
**Therapeutic:** ANTINEOPLASTIC
**Prototype:** Doxorubicin HCl

---

Common adverse effects in *italic*; life-threatening effects underlined; generic names in **bold**; classifications in SMALL CAPS; ◆ Canadian drug name; ⊙ Prototype drug

451

**D**

**AVAILABILITY** **Daunorubicin HCl:** Solution for injection. **Daunorubicin Citrated Liposomal:** Solution for injection

## ACTION & *THERAPEUTIC EFFECT*
Cytotoxic and antimitotic anthracycline antibiotic that is cell-cycle specific for S-phase of cell division. Has rapid interaction with the DNA molecule changing its shape, thus resulting in inhibition of DNA, RNA, and protein synthesis. *Antineoplastic effects against acute leukemias with decreased incidence of cardiotoxicity than doxorubicin.*

**USES** To induce remission in acute nonlymphocytic/lymphocytic leukemia, advanced HIV-associated Kaposi's sarcoma.

**UNLABELED USES** Non-Hodgkin's lymphoma.

**CONTRAINDICATIONS** Severe myelosuppression; immunizations (patient, family), and preexisting cardiac disease unless risk-benefit is evaluated; uncontrolled systemic infection; pregnancy (category D); lactation.

**CAUTIOUS USE** History of gout, urate calculi, hepatic or renal function impairment; older adults with inadequate bone reserve due to age or previous cytotoxic drug therapy, radiation therapy, tumor cell infiltration of bone marrow, patient who has received potentially cardiotoxic drugs or related antineoplastics; children.

## ROUTE & DOSAGE

**Neoplasms**
*Adult (younger than 60 y):* **IV** 45 mg/m²/day on days 1, 2, and 3 of first course then days 1 and 2 of subsequent courses (max total cumulative dose: 500–600 mg/m²); *60 y or older:* 30 mg/m²/day on days 1, 2, and 3 of first course then days 1 and 2 of subsequent courses
*Child (2 y or older):* **IV** As combination therapy, 25 mg/m² weekly; *younger than 2 y:* 1 mg/kg

**Kaposi's Sarcoma (DaunoXome)**
*Adult:* **IV** 40 mg/m² over 1 h, repeat q2wk (withhold therapy if granulocyte count less than 750 cells/mm³)

***Renal Impairment Dosage Adjustment***
*If serum Cr greater than 3 mg/dL, give 50% of dose*

***Hepatic Impairment Dosage Adjustment***
*Total bilirubin 1.2–3 mg/dL:* Give 50% of dose
*Greater than 3–5 mg/dL:* Give 25% of dose
*Greater than 5 mg/dL:* Omit dose

## ADMINISTRATION

**Intravenous**
Hazardous Agent: Use double gloves and gown during preparation and administration for infusion to prevent skin contact with this drug. If contact occurs, decontaminate skin with copious amounts of water with soap.

**Daunorubicin HCl**
*PREPARE:* **Direct:** Reconstitute 20 mg vial with 4 mL sterile water for injection. The concentration of the solution will be 5 mg/mL.

- Withdraw dose into syringe containing 10–15 mL normal saline. **IV Infusion:** Dilute further in 100 mL NS or D5W as required.
*ADMINISTER:* **Direct:** Inject over approximately 3 min into the tubing or side arm of a rapidly flowing IV infusion of D5W or NS. **Infusion:** Give a single dose over 30–45 min.

### DaunoXome

*PREPARE:* **IV Infusion:** Each vial of **DaunoXome** contains the equivalent of 50 mg daunorubicin base. Dilute with enough D5W to produce a concentration of 1 mg/1 mL.
*ADMINISTER:* **IV Infusion:** Give **DaunoXome** over 60 min. Do not use a filter with **DaunoXome**.
*INCOMPATIBILITIES:* **Solution/additive:** Dexamethasone, heparin. **Y-site:** Acyclovir, allopurinol, aminophylline, amphotericin B, ampicillin, aztreonam, cefazolin sodium, cefepime, cefoperazone, cefotaxime, cefotetan disodium, cefoxitin, ceftazidime, ceftriaxone, cefuroxime, chloramphenicol, dantrolene, dexamethosone, diazepam, ertapenem sodium, fludarabine phosphate, foscarnet sodium, fosphenytoin sodium, furosemide, gallium nitrate, ganciclovir, sodium, heparin sodium, indomethacin sodium, ketorolac tromethamine, lansoprazole, levofloxacin, methohexital sodium, methylprednisolone sodium succinate, mitoxantrone hydrochloride,, nafcillin sodium, nitroprusside sodium, pantoprazole sodium, pemetrexed disodium, pentobarbital sodium, phenobarbital sodium, piperacillin/tazobactam, sulfamethoxazole-trimethoprim, thiopental sodium.

- Avoid extravasation because it can cause severe tissue necrosis.

- Store reconstituted solution at room temperature (15°–30° C; 59°–86° F) for 24 h and under refrigeration at 2°–8° C (36°–46° F) for 48 h. Protect from light.

### ADVERSE EFFECTS (≥1%) **Body as a Whole:** Fever. **CNS:** Amnesia, anxiety, ataxia, confusion, hallucinations, emotional lability, tremors. **CV:** Pericarditis, myocarditis, arrhythmias, chest pain, EKG abnormality, <u>cardiac arrest</u>, peripheral edema, CHF, hypertension, tachycardia. **GI:** *Acute nausea and vomiting* (mild), anorexia, *stomatitis*, mucositis, discoloration of saliva, diarrhea (occasionally) hemorrhage. **Urogenital:** Dysuria, red urine discoloration, nocturia, polyuria, dry skin. **Hematologic:** <u>Bone marrow depression thrombocytopenia, leukopenia,</u> anemia. **Skin:** Generalized *alopecia* (reversible), transverse pigmentation of nails, discoloration of sweat and tears, severe cellulitis or tissue necrosis at site of drug extravasation. **Endocrine:** Hyperuricemia, gonadal suppression.

### PHARMACOKINETICS **Distribution:** Highest concentrations in spleen, kidneys, liver, lungs, and heart; does not cross blood–brain barrier; crosses placenta. **Metabolism:** In liver to active metabolite. **Elimination:** 25% in urine, 40% in bile. **Half-Life:** 18.5–26.7 h.

Common adverse effects in *italic;* life-threatening effects <u>underlined;</u> generic names in **bold;** classifications in SMALL CAPS; ♣ Canadian drug name; ⓟ Prototype drug

453

## NURSING IMPLICATIONS

### Black Box Warning

*Daunorubicin has been associated with cardiac toxicity and CHF, severe local tissue necrosis, bone marrow suppression, dosages reduced with impaired renal or hepatic function.*

### Assessment & Drug Effects

- Monitor infusion site closely. With daunorubicin hydrochloride severe local tissue necrosis will result if extravasation occurs. In the event of extravasation, stop the infusion and do not flush. Leave the catheter or needle in place. Note that liposomal daunorubicin is not known to cause tissue damage with extravasation.
- Monitor during infusion of liposomal daunorubicin for back pain, flushing, and chest tightness. These symptoms may occur during the first 5 min of infusion. They subside when infusion is stopped and typically do not return if infusion resumed at a slower rate.
- Monitor serum bilirubin; drug dose needs to be reduced when bilirubin is greater than 1.2 mg/dL.
- Monitor BP, temperature, pulse, and respiratory function during treatment.
- Monitor for S&S of acute CHF. It can occur suddenly or in patients with compromised heart function because of previous radiation therapy to heart area.
- Report immediately: Breathlessness, orthopnea, change in pulse and BP parameters. Early clinical diagnosis of drug-induced CHF is essential for successful treatment.
- Report promptly S&S of superinfections including elevation of temperature, chills, upper respiratory tract infection, tachycardia, overgrowth with opportunistic organisms because myelosuppression imposes risk of superimposed infection (see Appendix F).
- Control nausea and vomiting (usually mild) by antiemetic therapy.
- Inspect oral membranes. Mucositis may occur 3–7 days after drug is administered.
- Monitor lab tests: Baseline and periodic Hct, platelet count, total and differential leukocyte count, serum uric acid, LFTs, and renal function tests.

### Patient & Family Education

- Avoid contact with persons with infections. The most hazardous period is when the WBC count is most suppressed.
- Use barrier contraceptives during treatment because this drug is teratogenic. Tell your prescriber immediately if you become pregnant during therapy.
- Note: A transient effect of the drug is to turn urine red on the day of infusion.

## DECITABINE

(de-sit′a-bine)

Dacogen

**Classifications:** ANTINEOPLASTIC; ANTIMETABOLITE; PYRIMIDINE

Therapeutic: ANTINEOPLASTIC

**Prototype:** 5-Fluorouracil

**AVAILABILITY** Lyophilized powder for injection

## ACTION & THERAPEUTIC EFFECT

An antimetabolite that exerts antineoplastic effects after its direct incorporation into DNA and inhibition of DNA transferase, causing loss of cell differentiation and cell death. Nonproliferating cells are resistant to the effects of decitabine. *Decitabine-induced changes in neoplastic cells may restore normal function to genes that are critical for control of cellular differentiation and proliferation.*

**USES** Treatment of patients with myelodysplastic syndrome (MDS).

**UNLABELED USES** Treatment of chronic myelogenous leukemia (CML).

**CONTRAINDICATIONS** Pregnancy (category D); lactation.

**CAUTIOUS USE** Moderate to severe renal failure; hepatic impairment, older adults. Safety and efficacy in children not established.

## ROUTE & DOSAGE

**Myelodysplastic Syndrome**

*Adult:* **IV** 15 mg/m² q8h × 3 days; repeat q6w for at least 4 cycles; or 20 mg/m2 × 5 days q4w.

## ADMINISTRATION

**Intravenous**

*PREPARE:* **IV Infusion:** Caution should be exercised when handling and preparing decitabine. Procedures for proper handling and disposal of antineoplastic drugs should be applied. ▪ Reconstitute each vial with 10 mL sterile water for injection to yield approximately 5 mg/mL at pH 6.7–7.3. Immediately after reconstitution, further dilute with NS, D5W, or LR to a final drug concentration of 0.1–1 mg/mL. ▪ Use within 15 min of reconstitution (see Storage).

*ADMINISTER:* **IV infusion:** Premedicate with standard antiemetic therapy. Give 15 mg/m² dose over 3 h and 20 mg/m² dose over 1 h.

▪ Store vials at 15°–30° C (59°–86° F). Unless used within 15 min of reconstitution, the diluted solution **must be** prepared using cold (2°–8° C) infusion fluids and stored at 2°–8° C (36°–46° F) for up to a maximum of 7 h until administration.

**ADVERSE EFFECTS** (≥5%) **Body as a Whole:** *Fatigue, pyrexia,* Mycobacterium avium complex infection, peripheral edema, bacteremia, candidal infection, cellulitis, injection site reactions, rigors, tenderness, transfusion reaction, sinusitis, staphylococcal infection. **CNS:** Intracranial hemorrhage, anxiety, confusion, dizziness, headache, hypesthesia, insomnia, pyrexia. **CV:** Cardiorespiratory arrest, cardiac murmur, hypotension. **GI:** *Nausea, vomiting, constipation, diarrhea,* abdominal distention and discomfort, anorexia, dyspepsia, gastroesophageal reflux disease, glossodynia, gingival bleeding, hemorrhoids, lip ulceration, stomatitis, tongue ulceration. **Hematologic:** *Anemia, neutropenia,* thrombocytopenia, hematoma, leukopenia, lymphadenopathy, thrombocythemia. **Metabolic:** *Hyperglycemia,* increased AST,

Common adverse effects in *italic*; life-threatening effects underlined; generic names in **bold**; classifications in SMALL CAPS; ✛ Canadian drug name; ⓟ Prototype drug

455

**D**

decreased blood albumin, increased blood alkaline phosphatase, altered blood bicarbonate, decreased blood bilirubin, decreased blood chloride, increased blood lactate dehydrogenase, increased blood urea, decreased total protein, dehydration, hyperbilirubinemia, altered potassium levels, hypoalbuminemia, hypomagnesemia, hyponatremia. **Musculoskeletal:** Arthralgia, back pain, chest wall pain, musculoskeletal discomfort, myalgia, pain in limb. **Respiratory:** *Cough,* lung crackles, hypoxia, pharyngitis, pneumonia, pulmonary edema, rales. **Skin:** Alopecia, ecchymosis, erythema, pallor, *petechiae,* pruritus, rash, skin lesion, swelling face, urticaria. **Special Senses:** Blurred vision. **Urogenital:** Dysuria, urinary frequency, urinary tract infection.

## PHARMACOKINETICS **Distribution:** Negligible plasma protein binding. **Half-Life:** 0.2–0.8 h.

## NURSING IMPLICATIONS

### Assessment & Drug Effects

- Withhold dose and notify prescriber of any of the following: Absolute neutrophil count (ANC) less than 1000/mcL; platelet count less than 50,000/mcL; serum creatinine at 2 mg/dL or higher; ALT, total bilirubin 2 × ULN or more; or an active or uncontrolled infection.
- Monitor for and report S&S of pulmonary or peripheral edema, cardiac arrhythmias, new-onset depression, or infection.
- Avoid IM injections with platelet counts less than 50,000/mcL.
- Monitor diabetics for loss of glycemic control.

- Monitor lab tests: CBC with differentials and platelet count prior to each chemotherapy cycle; baseline and periodic LFTs and serum creatinine.

### Patient & Family Education

- Do not accept vaccinations during treatment with decitabine.
- Avoid contact with anyone who recently received the oral poliovirus vaccine.
- Women of childbearing age should avoid becoming pregnant while receiving decitabine.
- Men should not father a child while receiving decitabine and for 2 mo after the end of therapy.
- Report any of the following to a health care provider: Signs of infection such as fever, chills, sore throat; signs of bleeding such as easy bruising, black, tarry stools, blood in the urine; irregular heart rate; significant tiredness or weakness.

## DEFEROXAMINE MESYLATE
(de-fer-ox′a-meen)

Desferal

**Classifications:** CHELATING AGENT; ANTIDOTE

Therapeutic: ANTIDOTE

**AVAILABILITY** Powder for injection

## ACTION & *THERAPEUTIC EFFECT*
Chelating agent with specific affinity for ferric ion and low affinity for calcium. Binds ferric ions to form a stable water soluble chelate readily excreted by kidneys. *Main effect is removal of iron from ferritin, hemosiderin, and transferrin in iron toxicity.*

**USES** Adjunct in treatment of acute iron intoxication or iron overload.

**UNLABELED USES** Aluminum toxicity.

**CONTRAINDICATIONS** Severe renal disease, anuria, pyelonephritis; primary hemochromatosis; acute infection.

**CAUTIOUS USE** History of pyelonephritis; cardiac dysfunction; aluminum overload; older adults; pregnancy (category C); lactation; infants and children younger than 3 y.

## ROUTE & DOSAGE

**Acute Iron Intoxication**

*Adult:* **IM/IV** 1 g followed by 500 mg at 4 h intervals for 2 doses, subsequent doses of 500 mg q4–12h may be given if necessary (max: 6 g/24 h), infuse at 15 mg/kg/h or less
*Child (3 y or older):* **IV** 15 mg/kg/h (max: 6 g/24 h); **IM** 40–90 mg/kg (up to 1 g) q4–8h

**Chronic Iron Overload**

*Adult:* **IM** 500 mg–1 g/day; **Subcutaneous** 1–2 g/day (20–40 mg/kg/day) infused over 8–24 h
*Child (3 y or older):* **IM** 500 mg–1 g/day; **Subcutaneous** 20–40 mg/kg/day over 8–12 h

## ADMINISTRATION

**Subcutaneous**

▪ Reconstitute by adding 5 mL sterile water for injection to each 500 mg vial or 20 mL to each 2 gram vial to yield 100 mg/mL. Dissolve completely.
▪ Give subcutaneously over 8–24 h using a portable minipump device.

**Intramuscular**

▪ Reconstitute by adding 2 mL sterile water for injection to 500

mg vial or 8 mL to the 2 g vial to yield 250 mg/mL. Dissolve completely.
▪ Use IM route for all patients not in shock; preferred route for acute intoxication.

**Intravenous**

For infants and children: Verify correct IV concentration and rate with prescriber.

*PREPARE:* **IV Infusion:** Reconstitute by adding 5 mL sterile water for injection to 500 mg vial to yield 100 mg/mL. ▪ After drug is completely dissolved, withdraw prescribed amount from vial and add to NS, D5W, or LR solution.

*ADMINISTER:* **IV Infusion:** *Adult:* Give initial dose at a rate not to exceed 15 mg/kg/h; give two subsequent 500 mg dose at 125 mg/h; give any additional doses over 4–12 h. *Child:* Give at 15 mg/kg/h. ▪ Do not infuse IV rapidly; such infusion is associated with the occurrence of more adverse effects.

*INCOMPATIBILITIES:* Solution/additive: **Iron dextran.**

▪ Store at room temperature 15°–30° C (59°–86° F) for not longer than 1 wk. Protect from light.

## ADVERSE EFFECTS (≥1%) Body as a Whole: Hypersensitivity (generalized itching, cutaneous wheal formation, rash, fever, <u>anaphylactoid reaction</u>). **CV:** Hypotension, tachycardia. **Special Senses:** Decreased hearing; blurred vision, decreased visual acuity and visual fields, color vision abnormalities, night blindness, retinal pigmentary degeneration. **GI:** Abdominal discomfort, diarrhea. **Urogenital:** Dysuria, exacerbation of pyelonephritis, orange-rose discoloration

Common adverse effects in *italic;* life-threatening effects <u>underlined;</u> generic names in **bold;** classifications in SMALL CAPS; ♣ Canadian drug name; ⊘ Prototype drug

457

**D**

of urine. **Other:** *Pain and induration at injection site.*

**INTERACTIONS Drug:** Use with
**ascorbic acid** increases cardiac
risk, **prochlorperazine** may cause
loss of consciousness.

**PHARMACOKINETICS Distribu-
tion:** Widely distributed in body
tissues. **Metabolism:** Forms nontoxic complex with iron. **Elimination:** Primarily in urine; some in
feces.

## NURSING IMPLICATIONS

### Black Box Warning

*Deferoxamine has been associat-
ed with potentially fatal acute renal failure, hepatic failure, and GI
hemorrhage.*

### Assessment & Drug Effects

- Monitor injection site. If pain and
  induration occur, move infusion
  to another site.
- Monitor I&O ratio and pattern.
  Report any change. Observe
  stools for blood (iron intoxication
  frequently causes necrosis of
  GI tract).
- Monitor for S&S of GI bleeding
  and/or ulceration; older adults
  are especially at risk when they
  have conditions causing low
  platelet counts.
- Note: Periodic ophthalmoscopic
  (slit lamp) examinations and au-
  diometry are advised for patients
  on prolonged or high-dose therapy for chronic iron overload.
- Monitor lab tests: Baseline and
  periodic renal function tests.

### Patient & Family Education

- Deferoxamine chelate makes
  urine turn a reddish color.

- Report promptly signs of GI
  bleeding.
- Consult prescriber if you are concurrently taking drugs than can
  cause GI bleeding such as NSAIDs,
  corticosteroids, oral osteoporosis
  drugs, or anticoagulants.
- Report blurred vision or any other
  visual abnormality.

## DEGARELIX ACETATE

(de-ga're-lix)

Firmagon

**Classification:** GONADOTROPIN-
RELEASING HORMONE (GNRH)
ANTAGONIST
Therapeutic: GNRH ANTAGONIST
**Prototype:** Ganirelix acetate

**AVAILABILITY** Powder for injection

## ACTION & *THERAPEUTIC EFFECT*

It binds reversibly to pituitary GnRH
receptors, reducing release of gonadotropins and, consequently, testosterone. *Testosterone suppression
slows growth of androgen-sensitive
prostate cancer cells as indicated by
decrease in PSA values.*

**USES** Treatment of advanced prostate cancer.

**CONTRAINDICATIONS** Hypersensitivity to degarelix; women
who are or may become pregnant
(category X); lactation.

**CAUTIOUS USE** Congenital long
QT syndrome; electrolyte abnormalities; CHF; older adults. Safety and efficacy in children not
established.

## ROUTE & DOSAGE

### Prostate Cancer

*Adult:* **Subcutaneous** Initial dose
of 240 mg in two 120 mg

injections, followed by 80 mg
q28days

## ADMINISTRATION
### Subcutaneous
- Glove should be worn for reconstitution. Follow carefully manufacturer's guidelines for reconstitution of the powder vial.
- Administer into the abdominal area within 1 h of reconstitution.
- Initial dose: Give as 2 subcutaneous injections of 120 mg each (at a concentration of 40 mg/mL).
- Maintenance dose: Give 1 subcutaneous injection of 80 mg (at a concentration of 20 mg/mL).
- Store at 25° C (77° F), excursions permitted at 15°–30° C (59°–86° F).

## ADVERSE EFFECTS (≥1%) Body as a Whole: *Injection-site reactions*, night sweats. **CNS:** Asthenia, chills, dizziness, fatigue, fever, headache, insomnia. **CV:** *Hot flashes*, hypertension. **GI:** Constipation, nausea, diarrhea. **Metabolic:** Increases in ALT, AST, and GGT, *weight gain*. **Musculoskeletal:** Arthralgia, back pain. **Urogenital:** Erectile dysfunction, gynecomastia, testicular atrophy, urinary tract infections.

## INTERACTIONS Drug: Degarelix may cause an additive effect with other drugs that prolong the QT interval prolongation (e.g., ANTIARRHYTHMIC AGENTS, **chlorpromazine, dolasetron, droperidol, mefloquine, mesoridazine, moxifloxacin, pentamidine, pimozide, tacrolimus, thioridazine, ziprasidone**).

## PHARMACOKINETICS Peak: 2 days. **Distribution:** 90% plasma protein bound. **Metabolism:** Hepatobiliary. **Elimination:** Biliary excretion 70–80%; urinary excretion 20–30%. **Half-Life:** 53 days.

## NURSING IMPLICATIONS
### Assessment & Drug Effects
- Monitor ECG and QT interval, especially with electrolyte imbalances, a history of CHF, and concurrent Class IA (e.g., quinidine) or III (e.g., amiodarone) antiarrhythmics.
- Monitor lab tests: Baseline and periodic PSA and serum testosterone; periodic LFTs.

### Patient & Family Education
- Hot flashes are a common side effect that usually subside spontaneously.
- Degarelix can decrease bone density leading to osteoporosis. With long-term therapy, bone density tests are advisable and supplemental calcium and vitamin D may reduce the risk of osteoporosis.

## DELAFLOXACIN
(del-a-floks'a-sin)
Baxdela
**Classifications:** QUINOLONE ANTIBIOTIC; ANTIBIOTIC
Therapeutic: ANTIBIOTIC
**Prototype:** Ciprofloxacin

## AVAILABILITY Tablet; powder for injection

## ACTION & THERAPEUTIC EFFECT
Inhibits DNA gyrase and topoisomerase enzymes which are required for bacterial DNA replication, transcription, repair, and recombination. *Used to treat acute bacterial skin infections.*

## USES Treatment of bacterial skin and skin structure infections.

Common adverse effects in *italic;* life-threatening effects underlined; generic names in **bold;** classifications in SMALL CAPS; ♣ Canadian drug name; ⊙ Prototype drug

459

**CONTRAINDICATIONS** Hypersensitivity to delafloxacin, quinolone antibiotics, or components of the tablet or powdered injection.

**CAUTIOUS USE** Hypersensitivity to delafloxacin, other fluoroquinolones, or any component of the formulation; myasthenia gravis; renal impairment; elderly; pregnancy; lactation. Safety and efficacy in patients younger than 18 y not established.

## ROUTE & DOSAGE

### Infection

*Adult:* **PO** 450 mg b.i.d. for 5–14 days; **IV** 300 mg b.i.d. for 5–14 days

### Renal Impairment Dosage Adjustment

*CrCL 15–29 mL/min:* **IV** 200 mg b.i.d.; **PO** No adjustment

*CrCL less than 15 mL/min:* **IV** Do not use; **PO** No adjustment

## ADMINISTRATION

### Oral

- Administer with or without food at least 2 h before or 6 h after antacids containing magnesium or aluminum, sucralfate, metal cations, or multivitamins containing zinc or iron.

### Intravenous

*PREPARE:* **IV Infusion:** Reconstitute 300 mg vials with 10.5 mL of D5W or NS, and shake vigorously until completely dissolved. Then dilute to a total volume of 250 mL with NS or D5W.

*ADMINISTER:* Administer intravenously over 60 min. Do not administer with any solution containing multivalent cations (calcium or magnesium) through the same IV line. Do not infuse with other medications.

*INCOMPATIBILITIES:* Not compatible with solutions containing multivalent cations (e.g., calcium or magnesium).

**ADVERSE EFFECTS** (≥ 2%) **CNS:** Headache. **GI:** *Nausea, diarrhea.* **Hepatic:** Increased serum transaminase.

**INTERACTIONS DRUG: Magnesium** or **aluminum**–containing antacids, **sucralfate, iron, calcium, zinc** may decrease absorption of delafloxacin. NSAIDS may increase risk of CNS reactions, including seizures; may cause hyper- or hypoglycemia in patients on ORAL HYPOGLYCEMIC AGENTS. Do not use with agents known to prolong QT interval **(bepridil, doeftilide, dronedarone, thioridazine, ziprasidone).**

**PHARMACOKINETICS Absorption: PO** 59% bioavailability, unaffected by food. **Distribution:** 84% protein (albumin) bound. **Metabolism:** Glucuronidation through $UGT_1A_1$, $UGT_1A_3$, and $UGT_2B_{15}$. **Elimination: PO** 50% in urine, 48% in feces; **IV** 65% in urine, 28% in feces. **Half-Life: PO** 4–8 h (multiple dose); **IV** 4 h.

## NURSING IMPLICATIONS

### Black Box Warning

*Quinolone antibiotics have been associated with tendinitis and tendon rupture; drug may exacerbate muscle weakness in those with MG. Quinolone antibiotics are also associated with peripheral neuropathy and central nervous system effects.*

### Assessment & Drug Effects
- Monitor for signs of infection.
- Routine monitoring of WBC and serum creatinine.

### Patient & Family Education
- Notify prescriber if you have symptoms of irritated or torn tendons or nerve problems in the arms, hands, legs, or feet.
- Notify prescriber if you experience signs or symptoms of allergic reaction such as rash, hives, itching, shortness of breath, wheezing, cough, swelling of the face, lips, tongue, or throat; or any other signs.

## DELAVIRDINE MESYLATE
(del-a-vir′deen)
Rescriptor
**Classifications:** ANTIVIRAL; NONNUCLEOSIDE REVERSE TRANSCRIPTASE INHIBITOR (NNRTI)
**Therapeutic:** ANTIVIRAL; NNRTI
**Prototype:** Efavirenz

### AVAILABILITY Tablet

### ACTION & THERAPEUTIC EFFECT
Nonnucleoside reverse transcriptase inhibitor (NNRTI) of HIV-1 binds directly to reverse transcriptase (RT) and disrupts RNA- and DNA-dependent DNA polymerase activities. *Prevents replication of the HIV-1 virus; resistant strains appear rapidly.*

### USES Treatment of HIV infection in combination with other antiretroviral agents.

### UNLABELED USES HIV prophylaxis.

### CONTRAINDICATIONS Hypersensitivity to delavirdine; lactation.

### CAUTIOUS USE Impaired liver function; older adults; achlorhydria;

pregnancy (category C). Safety and efficacy in combination with other anitretroviral agents not established in children younger than 16 y.

## ROUTE & DOSAGE

### HIV Infection
*Adult/Adolescent:* **PO** 400 mg t.i.d.

## ADMINISTRATION
### Oral
- Disperse in water by adding a single dose to at least 3 oz of water, let it stand for a few minutes, then stir to create a uniform suspension just prior to administration.
- Give drug to patients with achlorhydria with an acid beverage such as orange or cranberry juice.
- Store at 20°–25° C (68°–77° F) and protect from high humidity in a tightly closed container.

### ADVERSE EFFECTS (≥1%) **Body as a Whole:** Headache, fatigue, allergic reaction, chills, edema, arthralgia. **CNS:** Abnormal coordination, agitation, amnesia, anxiety, confusion, dizziness. **CV:** Chest pain, bradycardia, palpitations, postural hypotension, tachycardia. **GI:** Nausea, vomiting, diarrhea, increased LFTs, abdominal cramps, anorexia, aphthous stomatitis. **Hematologic:** Neutropenia. **Respiratory:** Bronchitis, cough, dyspnea. **Skin:** *Rash,* pruritus.

### INTERACTIONS **Drug:** ANTACIDS, H$_2$-RECEPTOR ANTAGONISTS decrease absorption; **didanosine** and **delavirdine** should be taken 1 h apart to avoid decreased delavirdine levels; **clarithromycin, fluoxetine, ketoconazole** may increase delavirdine levels; **carbamazepine, phenobarbital,**

Common adverse effects in *italic;* life-threatening effects underlined; generic names in **bold;** classifications in SMALL CAPS; ♣ Canadian drug name; ⓟ Prototype drug

461

**phenytoin, rifabutin, rifampin** may decrease delavirdine levels; delavirdine may increase levels of **clarithromycin, indinavir, saquinavir, dapsone, rifabutin, alprazolam, midazolam, triazolam,** DIHYDROPYRIDINE, CALCIUM CHANNEL BLOCKERS (e.g., **nifedipine, nicardipine,** etc.), **quinidine, warfarin.** Use with HMG-COA REDUCTASE INHIBITORS may increase the risk of rhabdomyolysis. Use with **pimozide** may cause cardiac arrhythmias. Use with **trazodone** may increase **trazodone** levels. Use with inhaled **fluticasone** may increase **fluticasone** levels. Use with HYPNOTICS, **alprazolam, midazolam, triazolam** can cause respiratory depression. **Herbal: St. John's wort** may decrease antiretroviral activity.

## PHARMACOKINETICS **Absorption:** Rapidly from GI tract, 80% reaches systemic circulation. **Peak:** 1 h. **Distribution:** 98% protein bound. **Metabolism:** In the liver by CYP3A4. **Elimination:** Half in urine, 44% in feces. **Half-Life:** 2–11 h.

## NURSING IMPLICATIONS

### Assessment & Drug Effects
▪ Therapeutic effectiveness: Indicated by decreased viral load.
▪ Monitor for and immediately report appearance of a rash, generally within 1–3 wk of starting therapy; rash is usually diffuse, maculopapular, erythematous, and pruritic.

### Patient & Family Education
▪ Take this drug exactly as prescribed. Missed doses increase risk of drug resistance.
▪ Do not take antacids and delavirdine at the same time; separate by at least 1 h.

▪ Report all prescription and nonprescription drugs used to prescriber because of multiple drug interactions.
▪ Discontinue medication and notify prescriber if rash is accompanied by any of the following: Fever, blistering, oral lesions, conjunctivitis, swelling, muscle or joint pain.

---

## DEMECLOCYCLINE HYDROCHLORIDE
(dem-e-kloe-sye'kleen)
Declomycin
**Classifications:** ANTIBIOTIC; TETRACYCLINE
Therapeutic: ANTIBIOTIC
**Prototype:** Tetracycline

---

**AVAILABILITY** Capsule; tablet

**ACTION & *THERAPEUTIC EFFECT***
Demeclocycline blocks the binding of transfer RNA (tRNA) to messenger RNA (mRNA) of bacteria. Therefore, bacterial protein synthesis is inhibited and bacterial cells are destroyed. *Effective against both gram-positive and gram-negative bacteria.*

**USES** Similar to those of tetracycline.

**UNLABELED USES** Treatment of chronic SIADH (syndrome of inappropriate antidiuretic hormone) secretion.

**CONTRAINDICATIONS** Hypersensitivity to any of the tetracyclines; severe renal or hepatic disease; cirrhosis, common bile duct obstruction; period of tooth development in fetus; pregnancy (category D); lactation; children younger than 8 y (causes permanent yellow discoloration of teeth, enamel hypoplasia, and retarded bone growth).

---

Common adverse effects in *italic;* life-threatening effects underlined; generic names in **bold;** classifications in SMALL CAPS; ♦ Canadian drug name; ⊘ Prototype drug

**CAUTIOUS USE** Mild or moderate impaired renal or hepatic function; nephrogenic diabetes insipidus.

## ROUTE & DOSAGE

**Anti-Infective**
Adult: **PO** 150 mg q6h or 300 mg q12h (max: 2.4 g/day)
Child (8 y or older): **PO** 8–12 mg/kg/day divided q8–12h

**Gonorrhea**
Adult: **PO** 600 mg followed by 300 mg q12h for 4 days

**SIADH**
Adult: **PO** 600–1200 mg/day in 3–4 divided doses

## ADMINISTRATION

### Oral

- Give not less than 1 h before or 2 h after meals. Foods rich in iron (e.g., red meat or dark green vegetables) or calcium (e.g., milk products) impair absorption.
- Concomitant therapy: Do not give antacids with tetracyclines.
- Check expiration date before giving drug. Renal damage and death have resulted from use of outdated tetracyclines.
- Store in tight, light-resistant containers, preferably at 15°–30° C (59°–86° F) unless otherwise directed. Tetracyclines form toxic products when outdated or exposed to light, heat, or humidity.

## ADVERSE EFFECTS (≥1%) **Body as a Whole:** Hypersensitivity [*photosensitivity,* pericarditis, anaphylaxis (rare)]. **GI:** *Nausea,* vomiting, *diarrhea,* esophageal irritation or ulceration, enterocolitis, abdominal cramps, anorexia. **Urogenital:** Diabetes insipidus, azotemia, hyperphosphatemia.

**Skin:** Pruritus, erythematous eruptions, exfoliative dermatitis.

## DIAGNOSTIC TEST INTERFERENCE

Like other tetracyclines, demeclocycline may cause false increases in **urine catecholamines** (**fluorometric** methods); false decreases in **urine urobilinogen;** and false-negative **urine glucose** with **glucose oxidase** methods (e.g., **Clinistix, TesTape**).

## INTERACTIONS **Drug:** ANTACIDS, IRON PREPARATION, **calcium, magnesium, zinc, kaolinpectin, sodium bicarbonate** can significantly decrease demeclocycline absorption; effects of **desmopressin** and demeclocycline antagonized; increases **digoxin** absorption, increasing risk of **digoxin** toxicity; **methoxyflurane** increases risk of renal failure. **Food: Dairy** products significantly decrease demeclocycline absorption; food may decrease drug absorption also.

## PHARMACOKINETICS **Absorption:** 60–80% absorbed from GI tract. **Peak:** 3–4 h. **Distribution:** Concentrated in liver; crosses placenta; distributed into breast milk. **Metabolism:** In liver; enterohepatic circulation. **Elimination:** 40–50% excreted in urine and 31% in feces in 48 h. **Half-Life:** 10–17 h.

## NURSING IMPLICATIONS

### Assessment & Drug Effects

- Monitor I&O ratio and pattern and record weights in patients with impaired kidney or liver function, or on prolonged or high dose therapy.
- Monitor lab tests: Baseline C&S and, with prolonged therapy, periodic serum electrolytes, kidney function, and LFTs.

---

Common adverse effects in *italic;* life-threatening effects underlined; generic names in **bold;** classifications in SMALL CAPS; ♣ Canadian drug name; ⊘ Prototype drug

**Patient & Family Education**

- Do not use antacids while taking this drug.
- Take drug on an empty stomach to enhance absorption. Because esophageal irritation and ulceration have been reported, take each dose with a full glass (240 mL) of water; remain upright for at least 90 sec after taking medication; and avoid taking drug within 1 h of lying down or bedtime.
- Notify prescriber if gastric distress is a problem; a snack or light meal free of dairy products may be added to the regimen.
- Report symptoms of superinfections (see Appendix F).
- Demeclocycline-induced phototoxic reaction can be unusually severe. Avoid sunlight as much as possible and use sunscreen.

# DENOSUMAB
(den-o' su-mab)
Prolia, Xgeva
**Classification:** MONOCLONAL ANTIBODY; RANK LIGAND INHIBITOR; BONE RESORPTION INHIBITOR
**Therapeutic:** MONOCLONAL ANTIBODY; BONE RESORPTION INHIBITOR

AVAILABILITY Solution for injection

ACTION & *THERAPEUTIC EFFECT*
Denosumab prevents RANKL (receptor activator of nuclear factor κB ligand, a protein essential for survival of osteoclasts) from activating its receptor, RANK, on the surface of osteoclasts. Prevention of the RANKL/RANK interaction inhibits osteoclast formation, function, and survival. *Decreases bone resorption and increases bone mass and strength.*

USES Treatment of osteoporosis; prevention of bone loss in patients with prostate or breast cancer, giant cell tumor of bone, hypercalcemia.

CONTRAINDICATIONS Preexisting hypocalcemia; lactation; pregnancy (category X) for **Prolia** and pregnancy (category D) for **Xgeva.**

CAUTIOUS USE Predisposition to hypocalcemia and electrolyte imbalance (e.g., history of hypoparathyroidism, thyroid or parathyroid surgery, malabsorption syndromes, removal of small intestine, severe renal impairment [(creatinine clearance less than 30 mL/min) or on dialysis]; dental work such as tooth extraction and/or infection; poor dental hygiene, or use of a dental appliance; any serous infection; older adults; presence of bone fractures. Safety and efficacy in children younger than 18 y not established. **Xgeva** has been used in children older than 13 y with skeletally mature status.

## ROUTE & DOSAGE

| Osteoporosis, Bone Loss in Cancer Patients |
|---|
| *Adult:* **Subcutaneous** 60 mg every 6 m |
| **Hypercalcemia of Malignancy/ Giant Cell Tumor** |
| *Adult:* **Subcutaneous** 120 mg every 4 wk (additional 120 mg on day 8 and 15 in first mo) |

## ADMINISTRATION
**Subcutaneous**
- Ensure that hypocalcemia is corrected prior to initiation of therapy.
- Bring syringe to room temperature by removing from refrigeration 15–30 min prior to injection. Do not warm any other way.
- Inject into upper arm, upper thigh, or abdomen.
- Store refrigerated.

Common adverse effects in *italic;* life-threatening effects <u>underlined;</u> generic names in **bold;** classifications in SMALL CAPS; ♣ Canadian drug name; ◯ Prototype drug

**ADVERSE EFFECTS** (≥2%) **Body as a Whole:** Cystitis, herpes zoster infection, hypercholesterolemia, peripheral edema, pharyngitis. **CNS:** Asthenia, insomnia, sciatica, vertigo, *fatigue, headache.* **CV:** Anginal pectoris, atrial fibrillation, hypertension. **GI:** Flatuence, gastroesophageal reflux disease, upper abdominal pain, diarrhea, nausea. **Hematological:** Anemia. **Musculoskeletal:** *Back pain,* bone pain, musculoskeletal pain, myalgia, *pain in extremity,* spinal osteoarthritis. **Metabolic:** Hypophosphatemia, chills. **Respiratory:** Pneumonia, upper respiratory tract infection, cough, dyspnea. **Skin:** Pruritus, rash.

**INTERACTIONS** Do not use with MONOCLONAL ANTIBODIES as that can increase toxic effect.

**PHARMACOKINETICS Peak:** 10 d. **Half-Life:** 25.4 d.

## NURSING IMPLICATIONS

### Assessment & Drug Effects

- Monitor for S&S of hypocalcemia (see Appendix F) and report immediately if any of these appear.
- Monitor for and report promptly any of the following: S&S of infection; skin reaction such as dermatitis, eczema, rash; or jaw pain.
- Monitor lab tests: Baseline and periodic serum calcium, phosphorus, and magnesium.

### Patient & Family Education

- Ensure that calcium and vitamin D supplements (usually 1000 mg calcium and at least 400 IU vitamin D daily) are taken exactly as ordered.
- Notify your prescriber immediately if you develop any of the following: S&S of low calcium (e.g., spasms, twitches, cramps; numbness or tingling in your fingers,

toes, or around your mouth); S&S of infection (e.g., fever or chills; skin that is red, hot, or swollen; abdominal pain; frequency, urgency, or burning with urination); signs of skin irritation (e.g., rash, itching, peeling); jaw pain.
- Practice meticulous oral hygiene while you are taking this drug.
- Inform prescriber if you become pregnant while taking this drug,

## DESIPRAMINE HYDROCHLORIDE
(dess-ip'ra-meen)
Norpramin

**Classification:** TRICYCLIC ANTIDEPRESSANT
**Therapeutic:** TRICYCLIC ANTIDEPRESSANT
**Prototype:** Imipramine

**AVAILABILITY** Tablets

## ACTION & *THERAPEUTIC EFFECT*
Antidepressant activity appears to be related to blocking reuptake of norepinephrine and serotonin in the CNS, thus increasing their levels. *Has antidepressant activity.*

**USES** Endogenous depression.

**UNLABELED USES** Attention deficit disorder, bulimia, diabetic neuropathy, panic disorder, postherpetic neuralgia.

**CONTRAINDICATIONS** Hypersensitivity to tricyclic compounds; recent MI, QT prolongation, cardiac arrhythmias, AV block, bundle branch block; concurrent use of MAOI therapy; suicidal ideation; lactation.

**CAUTIOUS USE** Urinary retention, prostatic hypertrophy; narrow-angle glaucoma; epilepsy; alcoholism; adolescents, older adults;

Common adverse effects in *italic;* life-threatening effects underlined; generic names in **bold;** classifications in SMALL CAPS; ♣ Canadian drug name; ⊙ Prototype drug

465

bipolar disease; thyroid; cardiovascular, renal, and hepatic disease; suicidal tendency; ECT; elective surgery; pregnancy (category C). Safe use in children younger than 6 y is not established.

## ROUTE & DOSAGE

### Antidepressant

*Adult:* PO 75–100 mg/day at bedtime or in divided doses, may gradually increase to 150–300 mg/day (use lower doses in older adult patients)
*Adolescent:* PO 25–50 mg/day in divided doses (max: 100 mg/day)
*Child (6–12 y):* PO 1–3 mg/kg/day in divided doses (max: 5 mg/kg/day)

### Pharmacogenetic Dosage Adjustment

*CYP2D6 poor metabolizers:* Start with 40% of normal dose

## ADMINISTRATION

### Oral

- Give drug with or immediately after food to reduce possibility of gastric irritation.
- Give maintenance dose at bedtime to minimize daytime sedation.
- Store drug in tightly closed container at 15°–30° C (59°–86° F) unless otherwise specified.

## ADVERSE EFFECTS (≥1%) **Body as a Whole:** Hypersensitivity (rash, urticaria, photosensitivity). **CNS:** *Drowsiness,* dizziness, weakness, fatigue, headache, insomnia, confusional states, depressive reaction, paresthesias, ataxia. **CV:** *Postural hypotension,* hypotension, palpitation, tachycardia, ECG changes, flushing, <u>heart block</u>. **Special Senses:** Tinnitus, parotid swelling; blurred vision, disturbances in accommodation, mydriasis, increased IOP. **GI:** *Dry mouth, constipation,* bad taste, diarrhea, nausea. **Urogenital:** *Urinary retention,* frequency, delayed micturition, nocturia; impaired sexual function, galactorrhea. **Hematologic:** <u>Bone marrow depression</u> and <u>agranulocytosis</u> (rare). **Other:** Sweating, craving for sweets, weight gain or loss, SIADH secretion, hyperpyrexia, eosinophilic pneumonia.

## INTERACTIONS **Drug:** May somewhat decrease response to ANTIHYPERTENSIVES; CNS DEPRESSANTS, **alcohol,** HYPNOTICS, BARBITURATES, SEDATIVES potentiate CNS depression; may increase hypoprothrombinemic effect of ORAL ANTICOAGULANTS; **ethchlorvynol** may cause transient delirium; **levodopa,** SYMPATHOMIMETICS (e.g., **epinephrine, norepinephrine**) pose possibility of sympathetic hyperactivity with hypertension and hyperpyrexia; MAO INHIBITORS pose possibility of severe reactions, toxic psychosis, cardiovascular instability; **methylphenidate** increases plasma TCA levels; THYROID AGENTS may increase possibility of arrhythmias; **cimetidine** may increase plasma TCA levels. **Herbal: Ginkgo** may decrease seizure threshold; **St. John's wort** may cause **serotonin** syndrome.

## PHARMACOKINETICS **Absorption:** Rapidly from GI tract and injection sites. **Peak:** 4–6 h. **Distribution:** Crosses placenta. **Metabolism:** In liver. **Elimination:** Primarily in urine. **Half-Life:** 7–60 h.

## NURSING IMPLICATIONS

### Black Box Warning

*Desipramine has been associated with suicidal thinking and behavior in children, adolescents, and young adults.*

### Assessment & Drug Effects

- Monitor children, adolescents, and young adults for signs of suicidal ideation and behavior.
- Monitor for therapeutic effectiveness: Usually not realized until after at least 2 wk of therapy.
- Monitor BP and pulse rate during early phase of therapy, particularly in older adult, debilitated, or cardiovascular patients. If BP rises or falls more than 20 mm Hg or if there is a sudden increase in pulse rate or change in rhythm, withhold drug and inform prescriber.
- Note: Drowsiness, dizziness, and orthostatic hypotension are signs of impending toxicity in patient on long-term, high dosage therapy. Prolonged QT or QRS intervals indicate possible toxicity. Report to prescriber.
- Observe patient with history of glaucoma. Report symptoms that may signal acute attack: Severe headache, eye pain, dilated pupils, halos of light, nausea, vomiting.
- Monitor bowel elimination pattern and I&O ratio. Severe constipation and urinary retention are potential problems of TCA therapy.

### Patient & Family Education

- Be alert for and promptly report unusual changes in behavior (e.g., anxiety, agitation, panic attacks, insomnia, irritability, hostility, aggressiveness), worsening of depression, or suicidal ideation.
- Make all position changes slowly and in stages, particularly from recumbent to standing position.
- Do not drive or engage in other potentially hazardous activities until reaction to drug is known.
- Take medication exactly as prescribed; do not change dose or dose intervals.
- Note: Patients who receive high doses for prolonged periods may experience withdrawal symptoms including headache, nausea, musculoskeletal pain, and weakness if drug is discontinued abruptly.
- Do not take OTC drugs unless prescriber has approved their use.
- Stop, or at least limit, smoking because it may increase the metabolism of desipramine, thereby diminishing its therapeutic action.

## DESLORATADINE

(des-lor-a-ta'deen)

Clarinex, Clarinex Reditabs

**Classifications:** NONSEDATING ANTIHISTAMINE, H₁-RECEPTOR ANTAGONIST
**Therapeutic:** ANTIHISTAMINE; ANTIALLERGIC
**Prototype:** Loratadine

**AVAILABILITY** Tablet; orally dissolving tablet; syrup

### ACTION & THERAPEUTIC EFFECT

A long-acting, nonsedating antihistamine with selective H₁-receptor antagonist properties. Reduces human mast cell release of inflammatory cytokines. Therefore, it also exhibits antiallergic effects. *Desloratadine is effective in controlling allergic rhinitis and inhibiting histamine-induced wheals and flare (hives).*

**USES** Treatment of seasonal or perennial allergic rhinitis and idiopathic urticaria.

**CONTRAINDICATIONS** Hypersensitivity to desloratadine or loratadine; neonates; infants.

**CAUTIOUS USE** Renal and hepatic insufficiencies; bladder neck obstruction or urinary retention; prostatic hypertrophy; asthma; glaucoma; pregnancy (category C); lactation. Safety and efficacy in children younger than 12 y not established.

Common adverse effects in *italic*; life-threatening effects underlined; generic names in **bold**; classifications in SMALL CAPS; ♦ Canadian drug name; ⊘ Prototype drug

467

D

## ROUTE & DOSAGE

### Allergic Rhinitis, Idiopathic Urticaria

*Adult:* **PO** 5 mg daily

### Renal Impairment Dosage Adjustment

*CrCl less than 50 mL/min:* 5 mg every other day

### Hepatic Impairment Dosage Adjustment

5 mg every other day

## ADMINISTRATION

### Oral

- Note that drug should be given every other day to patients with significant renal or hepatic impairment.
- Store at 2°–25° C (36°–77° F).

## ADVERSE EFFECTS (≥1%) **Body as a Whole:** Pharyngitis, fatigue, flu-like symptoms, myalgia. **CNS:** Somnolence, dizziness. **GI:** Dry mouth, nausea, dry throat. **Urogenital:** Dysmenorrhea.

## PHARMACOKINETICS **Absorption:** Well absorbed. **Peak:** 3 h. **Distribution:** 85–89% protein bound. **Metabolism:** Extensively metabolized in liver to 3-hydroxydesloratadine, an active metabolite. **Elimination:** Equally in urine and feces. **Half-Life:** 27 h.

## NURSING IMPLICATIONS

### Assessment & Drug Effects

- Monitor cardiovascular status and report significant changes in BP and palpitations or tachycardia.
- Concurrent drugs: Monitor ECG when used in combination with any other drug that can produce an additive effect causing QT interval prolongation.
- Monitor lab tests: Periodic renal function and LFTs.

### Patient & Family Education

- Drug may cause significant drowsiness in older adult patients and those with liver or kidney impairment.
- Note: Concurrent use of alcohol and other CNS depressants may have an additive effect.
- Do not take this drug more often than every other day if you have renal impairment.

## DESMOPRESSIN ACETATE

(des-moe-pres'sin)

**DDAVP, Noctiva, Stimate**

**Classification:** POSTERIOR PITUITARY HORMONE
**Therapeutic:** ANTIDIURETIC HORMONE (ADH); ANTIHEMOPHILIC FACTOR
**Prototype:** Vasopressin

**AVAILABILITY** Tablet; nasal spray; solution for injection

## ACTION & *THERAPEUTIC EFFECT*

Synthetic analog of natural posterior pituitary (antidiuretic) hormone, vasopressin. Reduces urine volume and osmolality of serum in patients with central diabetes insipidus by increasing reabsorption of water by kidney collecting tubules. Produces a dose-related increase in factor VIII (antihemophilic factor) and von Willebrand's factor. *Desmopressin is an effective replacement for antidiuretic hormone. It also can shorten or normalize bleeding time, and correct platelet adhesion abnormalities in certain patients with bleeding disorders.*

**USES** To control and prevent symptoms and complications of central (neurohypophyseal) diabetes insipidus, and to relieve temporary polyuria and polydipsia associated with trauma or surgery in the pituitary region; bleeding prophylaxis, enuresis.

**UNLABELED USES** To increase factor VIII activity in selected patients with mild to moderate hemophilia A and in type I von Willebrand's disease or uremia, and to control enuresis in children.

**CONTRAINDICATIONS** Nephrogenic diabetes insipidus, type II B von Willebrand's disease; CrCl less than 50 mL/min; hyponatremia, moderate to severe renal impairment. **PO form:** Patients with fluid and electrolyte imbalance.

**CAUTIOUS USE** Coronary artery insufficiency, hypertensive cardiovascular disease; psychogenic polydipsia; severe CHF; older adults; history of thromboembolic disease; diarrhea, electrolyte imbalance, nasal trauma; pregnancy (category B). **PO:** Children younger than 6 y. **Intranasal:** Children 3 mo and older.

## ROUTE & DOSAGE

**Diabetes Insipidus**

*Adult/Adolescent:* **Intranasal** 0.1–0.4 mL (10–40 mcg) in 1–3 divided doses; **IV/Subcutaneous** 2–4 mcg in 2 divided doses; **PO** 0.05 mg b.i.d. titrate to response
*Child (3 mo–12y):* **Intranasal** 0.05–0.3 mL in 1–2 divided doses; **IV/Subcutaneous** 0.3 mcg/kg infused over 1.5–30 min; *younger than 4 y:* **PO** 0.05 mg titrated to response

**Enuresis**

*Adult/Adolescent/Child (6 y or older):* **PO** 0.2 mg at bedtime, may titrate up to 0.6 mg at bedtime

**Nocturia**

*Adults (50–64 y):* **Intranasal** 1 spray (use 0.83 mcg strength in those at high risk for hyponatremia) in either nostril 30 min before bedtime

**Bleeding Prophylaxis in Patients with Von Willebrand's Disease**

*Adult/Child (3 mo or older):* **IV/Subcutaneous** 0.3 mcg/kg

30 min preoperative, may repeat in 48 h if needed
*Adult (over 50 kg):* **Intranasal** 1 spray each nostril, repeat in 8–24 h if needed
*Adult (50 kg or below)/Adolscent/Child:* **Intranasal** 1 spray, may repeat in 8–24 h if needed

**Renal Impairment Dosage Adjustment**

*CrCl less than 50 mL/min:* Do not use

## ADMINISTRATION

### Oral

- Note that 0.2 mg PO is equivalent to 10 mcg (0.1 mL) intranasal. May administer with or without food.

### Intranasal

- Follow manufacturer's instructions for proper technique with nasal spray.
- Give initial dose in the evening, and observe antidiuretic effect. Dose is increased each evening until uninterrupted sleep is obtained. If daily urine volume is more than 2 L after nocturia is controlled, morning dose is started and adjusted daily until urine volume does not exceed 1.5–2 L/24 h.

### Subcutaneous

- Give undiluted as direct injection.

### Intravenous

**PREPARE: Direct:** Give undiluted for diabetes insipidus. **IV Infusion:** Dilute 0.3 mcg/kg in 10 mL of NS (children weighing 10 kg or less) or 50 mL of NS (children greater than 10 kg and adults) for von Willebrand's disease (type I).
**ADMINISTER: Direct:** Give direct IV over 30 s for diabetes insipidus. **IV Infusion:** Give over 15–30 min for von Willebrand's disease (type I).

---

Common adverse effects in *italic*; life-threatening effects underlined; generic names in **bold**; classifications in SMALL CAPS; ♣ Canadian drug name; ⊕ Prototype drug

**D**

• Store parenteral and nasal solution in refrigerator preferably at 4° C (39.2° F) unless otherwise directed. Avoid freezing. • Nasal spray can be stored at room temperature. • Discard solutions that are discolored or contain particulate matter.

**ADVERSE EFFECTS** (≥1%) **All:** Dose related. **CNS:** Transient headache, drowsiness, dizziness, listlessness. **Special Senses:** Nasal congestion, rhinitis, nasal irritation. **GI:** Nausea, heartburn, mild abdominal cramps. **CV:** Hypertension. **Cardiac:** Hypertension. **Other:** Vulval pain, shortness of breath, facial flushing, pain and swelling at injection site, *hyponatremia.*

**INTERACTIONS Drug: Demeclocycline, lithium,** other VASO-PRESSORS may decrease antidiuretic response; **carbamazepine, chlorpropamide, clofibrate** may prolong antidiuretic response. NSAIDS or CORTICOSTEROIDS may increase risk of hyponatremia.

**PHARMACOKINETICS Absorption:** 10–20% through nasal mucosa. **Onset:** 15–60 min. **Peak:** 1–5 h. **Duration:** 5–21 h. **Distribution:** Small amount crosses blood–brain barrier; distributed into breast milk. **Half-Life:** 76 min.

**NURSING IMPLICATIONS**

**Assessment & Drug Effects**
• Monitor I&O ratio and pattern (intervals). Fluid intake **must be** carefully controlled, particularly in older adults and the very young to avoid water retention and sodium depletion.
• Weigh patient daily and observe for edema. Severe water retention may require reduction in dosage and use of a diuretic.
• Monitor BP during dosage-regulating period and whenever drug is administered parenterally.

• Monitor lab tests: Baseline and periodic urine and plasma osmolality.

**Patient & Family Education**
• Report upper respiratory tract infection or nasal congestion.
• Follow manufacturer's instructions for insertion to ensure delivery of drug high into nasal cavity and not down throat. A flexible calibrated plastic tube is provided.

**DESONIDE**

(dess'oh-nide)

DesOwen, Tridesilon

See Appendix A-4.

**DESOXIMETASONE**

(des-ox-i-met'a-sone)

Topicort

See Appendix A-4.

**DESVENLAFAXINE**

(des-ven-la-fax'een)

Pristiq

See Venlafaxime

**DEXAMETHASONE**

(dex-a-meth'a-sone)

Maxidex

**DEXAMETHASONE SODIUM PHOSPHATE**

**Classifications:** ADRENAL CORTICOSTEROID; GLUCOCORTICOID
Therapeutic: ADRENOCORTICAL STEROID; ANTI-INFLAMMATORY
**Prototype:** Prednisone

**AVAILABILITY Dexamethasone:** Tablet; oral solution. **Dexamethasone sodium phosphate:** Solution for injection; cream; ophthalmic solution; suspension

## ACTION & *THERAPEUTIC EFFECT*

Long-acting synthetic adrenocorticoid with intense anti-inflammatory (glucocorticoid) activity and minimal mineralocorticoid activity. **Anti-inflammatory action:** Prevents accumulation of inflammatory cells at sites of infection; inhibits phagocytosis, lysosomal enzyme release, and synthesis of potent mediators of inflammation, prostaglandins, and leukotrienes; reduces capillary dilation and permeability. **Immunosuppression:** Probably due to prevention or suppression of delayed hypersensitivity immune reaction. *Has anti inflammatory and immunosuppression properties.*

**USES** Adrenal insufficiency concomitantly with a mineralocorticoid; inflammatory conditions, allergic states, collagen diseases, hematologic disorders, cerebral edema, and addisonian shock. Also palliative treatment of neoplastic disease, as adjunctive short-term therapy in acute rheumatic disorders and GI diseases, and as a diagnostic test for Cushing's syndrome and for differential diagnosis of adrenal hyperplasia and adrenal adenoma.

**UNLABELED USES** As an antiemetic in cancer chemotherapy; as a diagnostic test for endogenous depression; and to prevent hyaline membrane disease in premature infants.

**CONTRAINDICATIONS** Hypersensitivity to any component of formulation, including sulfites; fungal infections; cerebral malaria; acute infections, active or resting tuberculosis, vaccinia, varicella, administration of live virus vaccines (to patient, family members), latent or active amebiasis; Cushing's syndrome; Kaposi sarcoma; rupture of posterior ocular lens capsule; neonates or infants weighing less than 1300 g;

lactation. **Topical use:** Rosacea, perioral dermatitis; venous stasis ulcers. **Ophthalmic use:** Primary open-angle glaucoma, eye infections, superficial ocular herpes simplex, keratitis, and tuberculosis of eye.

**CAUTIOUS USE** Hypersensitivity to corticosteroids; stromal herpes simplex, keratitis, GI disease; renal disease, DM; hypothyroidism, acute MI; myasthenia gravis, CHF, cirrhosis, psychiatric disorders; ocular disease such as cataracts, glaucoma, increased intraocular pressure, open-angle glaucoma; seizures; coagulopathy; older adults; pregnancy (category C); children.

## ROUTE & DOSAGE

| Allergies, Inflammation, Neoplasias (Note: Dosages are very individualized based on patient response) |
| --- |
| *Adult:* **PO** 0.25–4 mg b.i.d. to q.i.d.; **IM** 8–16 mg q1–3wk or 0.8–1.6 mg intralesional q1–3wk; **IV** 0.75–0.9 mg/kg/day divided q6–12h |
| *Child:* **PO/IV/IM** 0.08–0.3 mg/kg/day divided q6–12h |

| Adrenocorticol Function Abnormalities |
| --- |
| *Adult:* **PO/IV** 0.75–9 mg/day in divided doses, adjust to patient response |
| *Child:* **PO/IV** 0.03–0.3 mg/kg/day in divided doses, adjust to patient response |

| Cerebral Edema |
| --- |
| *Adult:* **IV** 10 mg followed by 4 mg q6h, reduce dose after 2–4 days then taper over 5–7 days |
| *Child:* **PO/IV/IM** 1–2 mg/kg loading dose, then 1–1.5 mg/kg/day divided q4–6h × 5 days (max: 16 mg/day) |

Common adverse effects in *italic;* life-threatening effects underlined; generic names in **bold;** classifications in SMALL CAPS; ♣ Canadian drug name; ⊙ Prototype drug

471

D

**Shock**

*Adult:* **IV** 1–6 mg/kg as a single dose or 40 mg repeated q2–6h if needed or 20 mg bolus then 3 mg/kg/day

**Dexamethasone Suppression Test**

*Adult:* **PO** 0.5 mg q6h for 48 h

**Test for Cushing's Syndrome**

*Adult:* **PO** 2 mg q6h × 48h

**Inflammation**

*Adult/Child:* **Ophthalmic/Topical/Inhalation/Intranasal** See Appendix A.

## ADMINISTRATION

### Oral

- Give the once-daily dose in the a.m. with food or liquid of patient's choice.
- Taper dosage over a period of time before discontinuing because adrenal suppression can occur with prolonged use.
- Do not store or expose aerosol to temperature above 48.9° C (120° F); do not puncture or discard into a fire or an incinerator.

### Intramuscular

- Give IM injection deep into a large muscle mass (e.g., gluteus maximus). Avoid subcutaneous injection: Atrophy and sterile abscesses may occur.
- Use repository form, dexamethasone acetate, for IM or local injection only. The white suspension settles on standing; mild shaking will resuspend drug.

### Intravenous

*PREPARE:* **Direct:** Give undiluted. **Intermittent:** Dilute in D5W or NS for infusion.

*ADMINISTER:* **Direct:** Give direct IV push over 1 min or less. **Intermittent:** Set rate as prescribed or

according to amount of solution to infuse.

*INCOMPATIBILITIES:* **Solution/additive:** Daunorubicin, diphenhydramine, doxorubicin, doxapram, glycopyrrolate, metaraminol, phenobarbital, vancomycin. **Y-site:** Ciprofloxacin, fenoldopam, idarubicin, midazolam, topotecan.

- Store at 15°–30° C (59°–86° F) unless otherwise directed.

## ADVERSE EFFECTS (≥1%) Aerosol Therapy: *Nasal irritation,* dryness, epistaxis, rebound congestion, bronchial asthma, anosmia, perforation of nasal septum. *Systemic Absorption*—**CNS:** Euphoria, insomnia, convulsions, increased ICP, vertigo, headache, ptosis, psychic disturbances. **CV:** CHF, hypertension, *edema.* **Endocrine:** Menstrual irregularities, *hyperglycemia;* cushingoid state; growth suppression in children; hirsutism. **Special Senses:** *Posterior subcapsular cataract,* increased IOP, glaucoma, exophthalmos, ocular hemorrhage. **GI:** Peptic ulcer with possible perforation, abdominal distension, nausea, increased appetite, heartburn, dyspepsia, pancreatitis, <u>bowel perforation</u>, *oral candidiasis.* **Musculoskeletal:** Muscle weakness, loss of muscle mass, <u>vertebral compression fracture</u>, pathologic fracture of long bones, tendon rupture. **Skin:** Acne, *impaired wound healing,* petechiae, ecchymoses, diaphoresis, allergic dermatitis, hypo- or hyperpigmentation, subcutaneous and cutaneous atrophy, burning and tingling in perineal area (following IV injection).

## DIAGNOSTIC TEST INTERFERENCE

*Dexamethasone suppression test for endogenous depression:* False positive results may be caused by

Common adverse effects in *italic;* life-threatening effects <u>underlined</u>; generic names in **bold;** classifications in SMALL CAPS; ♣ Canadian drug name; ⊙ Prototype drug

alcohol, **glutethimide, meproba-mate;** false-negative results may be caused by high doses of benzodiazepines (e.g., **chlordiazepoxide** and **cyproheptadine**), long-term glucocorticoid treatment, **indomethacin, ephedrine,** estrogens or hepatic enzyme-inducing agents **(phenytoin)** may also cause false-positive results in *test for Cushing's syndrome.*

**INTERACTIONS Drug:** BARBITURATES, **phenytoin, rifampin** increase steroid metabolism—dosage of dexamethasone may need to be increased; **amphotericin B,** DIURETICS compound potassium loss; **neostigmine, pyridostigmine** may cause severe muscle weakness in patients with myasthenia gravis; may inhibit antibody response to VACCINES, TOXOIDS. Do not use with **dasabuvir, ritonavir, emtricitabine, tenofovir.**

**PHARMACOKINETICS Absorption:** Readily from GI tract. **Onset:** Rapid. **Peak:** 1–2 h PO; 8 h IM. **Duration:** 2.75 days PO; 6 days IM; 1–3 wk intra lesional, intraarticular. **Distribution:** Crosses placenta; distributed into breast milk. **Metabolism:** Induces CYP3A4. **Elimination:** Hypothalamus-pituitary axis suppression: 36–54 h. **Half-life:** 3–4.5 h.

## NURSING IMPLICATIONS

### Assessment & Drug Effects

- Monitor and report S&S of Cushing's syndrome (see Appendix F) or other systemic adverse effects.
- Monitor neonates born to a mother who has been receiving a corticosteroid during pregnancy for symptoms of hypoadrenocorticism.
- Monitor for S&S of a hypersensitivity reaction (see Appendix F). The acetate and sodium phosphate formulations may contain bisulfites, parabens, or both; these inactive ingredients are allergenic to some individuals.

### Patient & Family Education

- Take drug exactly as prescribed.
- Report lack of response to medication or malaise, orthostatic hypotension, muscular weakness and pain, nausea, vomiting, anorexia, hypoglycemic reactions (see Appendix F), ocular changes, or mental depression to prescriber.
- Report changes in appearance and easy bruising to prescriber.
- Add potassium-rich foods to diet; report signs of hypokalemia (see Appendix F). Concomitant potassium-depleting diuretic can enhance dexamethasone-induced potassium loss.
- Note: Dexamethasone dose regimen may need to be altered during stress (e.g., surgery, infections, emotional stress, illness, acute bronchial attacks, trauma). Consult prescriber if change in living or working environment is anticipated.
- Discontinue drug gradually under the guidance of the prescriber.
- Note: It is important to prevent exposure to infection, trauma, and sudden changes in environmental factors, as much as possible, because drug is an immunosuppressor.

## DEXMEDETOMIDINE HYDROCHLORIDE ℗

(dex-med-e-to'mi-deen)

Precedex

**Classifications:** ALPHA₂-ADRENERGIC AGONIST; NONBARBITURATE SEDATIVE-HYPNOTIC
**Therapeutic:** SEDATIVE-HYPNOTIC

**AVAILABILITY** Solution for injection

## ACTION & THERAPEUTIC EFFECT

Stimulates alpha₂-adrenergic receptors in the CNS (primarily in

Common adverse effects in *italic;* life-threatening effects underlined; generic names in **bold;** classifications in SMALL CAPS; ◆ Canadian drug name; ℗ Prototype drug

473

**D**

the medulla oblongata) causing inhibition of the sympathetic vasomotor center of the brain resulting in sedative effects. *Sedative properties utilized in intubating patients and for initially maintaining them on a mechanical ventilator.*

**USES** Sedation of initially intubated or mechanically ventilated patients.

**CONTRAINDICATIONS** Hypersensitivity to dexmedetomidine.

**CAUTIOUS USE** Cardiac arrhythmias or cardiovascular disease, uncontrolled hypertension; hypotension; cerebrovascular disease; renal or hepatic insufficiency; signs of light anesthesia; older adults; pregnancy (category C); lactation. Safety and efficacy in children younger than 18 y not established.

## ROUTE & DOSAGE

### Sedation

*Adult:* **IV** 1 mcg/kg loading dose infused over 10 min, then continue with infusion of 0.2–0.7 mcg/kg/h for up to 24 h adjusted to maintain sedation

### Hepatic Impairment Dosage Adjustment

Reduce initial dosage

### Renal Impairment Dosage Adjustment

*CrCl less than 30 mL/min:* Reduce initial dose

## ADMINISTRATION

### Intravenous

**PREPARE: Continuous:** Withdraw 2 mL of dexmedetomidine and add to 48 mL of NS to yield 4 mcg/mL. Shake gently to mix.

**ADMINISTER: Continuous:** Administer using a controlled infusion device. ▪ A loading dose of 1 mcg/kg is infused over 10 min followed by the ordered maintenance dose. **Do not** use administration set containing natural rubber. **Do not** infuse longer than 24 h.
**INCOMPATIBILITIES: Y-site: Amphotericin B, diazepam, garenoxacin, gemtuzumab, irinotecan, pantoprazole, phenytoin.**

▪ Store at 15°–30° C (59°–86° F).

**ADVERSE EFFECTS** (≥1%) **Body as a Whole:** Pain, infection. **CV:** *Hypotension,* bradycardia, tachycardia, atrial fibrillation. **GI:** *Nausea,* constipation, thirst. **Respiratory:** Hypoxia, pleural effusion, pulmonary edema. **CNS:** Agitation. **Hematologic:** Anemia, leukocytosis. **Urogenital:** Oliguria.

**INTERACTIONS Drug:** BARBITURATES, BENZODIAZEPINES, GENERAL ANESTHETICS, OPIATE AGONISTS, ANXIOLYTICS, SEDATIVES/HYPNOTICS, **ethanol,** TRICYCLIC ANTIDEPRESSANTS, **tramadol,** PHENOTHIAZINES, SKELETAL MUSCLE RELAXANTS, **azatadine, brompheniramine, carbinoxamine, chlorpheniramine, clemastine, cyproheptadine, dexchlorpheniramine, dimenhydrinate, diphenhydramine, doxylamine, hydroxyzine, methdilazine, phenindamine, promethazine, tripelennamine** enhance CNS depression possibly prolong recovery from anesthesia.

**PHARMACOKINETICS Metabolism:** Extensively in liver (CYP2A6). **Elimination:** Primarily in urine. **Half-Life:** 2 h.

## NURSING IMPLICATIONS

### Assessment & Drug Effects

▪ Monitor for hypertension during loading dose; reduction of loading dose may be required.

Common adverse effects in *italic;* life-threatening effects <u>underlined</u>; generic names in **bold**; classifications in SMALL CAPS; ✣ Canadian drug name; ⊙ Prototype drug

- Monitor cardiovascular status continuously; notify prescriber immediately if hypotension or bradycardia occurs.

## DEXMETHYLPHENIDATE

(dex-meth-ill-fen'i-date)

Focalin, Focalin XR

**Classification:** CEREBRAL STIMULANT
**Therapeutic:** CEREBRAL STIMULANT
**Prototype:** Amphetamine
**Controlled Substance:** Schedule II

**AVAILABILITY** Tablet; extended release capsule

## ACTION & *THERAPEUTIC EFFECT*

Thought to block reuptake of norepinephrine and dopamine into presynaptic neurons and, thereby increases release of these substances into the synapse. *Is effective in controlling ADHD syndrome in conjunction with other measures (psychological, educational, and social).*

**USES** Attention deficit hyperactivity disorder (ADHD).

## CONTRAINDICATIONS

Hypersensitivity to methylphenidate; known structural cardiac abnormalities in children or adults, cardiomyopathy, congenital heart disease; coronary heart disease; severe agitation, marked anxiety, or tension; psychotic symptomatology; glaucoma; motor tics; family history of or diagnosis of Tourette's syndrome; concurrent MAOI therapy or within 14 days of discontinuation; occurrence of seizures without a history.

**CAUTIOUS USE** Moderate to severe hepatic insufficiency; depression; preexisting pyschosis; emotional instability, bipolar disorder, history of suicides; alcoholism or drug dependence; history of seizure disorders; hypertension, CHF, cardiac arrhythmias; hyperthyroidism; older adults; pregnancy (category C); lactation. Safe use in children younger than 6 y is not established.

## ROUTE & DOSAGE

**Attention Deficit Hyperactivity Disorder**

*Adult:* **PO** 2.5 mg b.i.d., may increase by 2.5–5 mg/day at weekly intervals (max: 20 mg/day). If converting from methylphenidate, start with ½ of methylphonidate dose. **Extended release** 10 mg daily, may increase by 5 mg at weekly intervals (max: 40 mg/day)

*Child (6 y or older):* **PO** 2.5 mg b.i.d., may increase by 2.5–5 mg/day at weekly intervals (max: 20 mg/day). If converting from methylphenidate, start with ½ of methylphenidate dose. **Extended release** 5 mg daily, may increase by 5 mg at weekly intervals (max: 20 mg/day)

## ADMINISTRATION

Oral

- Do not administer with or within 14 days following discontinuation of an MAO inhibitor.
- Give sustained release capsules whole. They should not be crushed or chewed.
- Give b.i.d. doses at least 4 h apart.
- Store at 15°–30° C (59°–86° F).

**ADVERSE EFFECTS** (≥1%) **Body as a Whole:** Fever, allergic reactions. **CNS:** Dizziness, insomnia, nervousness, tics, abnormal thinking,

D

hallucinations, emotional lability, CNS overstimulation or sympathomimetic effects (angina, anxiety, agitation, biting, blurred vision, delirium, diaphoresis, flushing or pallor, hallucinations, hyperthermia, labile blood pressure and heart rate (hypotension or hypertension), mydriasis, palpitations, paranoia, purposeless movements, psychosis, sinus tachycardia, tachypnea, or tremor]. **CV:** Hypertension, tachycardia. **GI:** *Abdominal pain,* anorexia, nausea, vomiting.

**INTERACTIONS Drug:** Additive stimulant effects with other STIMULANTS (including **amphetamine, caffeine**); increased vasopressor effects with **dopamine, epinephrine, norepinephrine, phenylpropanolamine, pseudoephedrine;** MAO INHIBITORS may cause hypertensive crisis; antagonizes hypotensive effects of **guanethidine,** may inhibit metabolism and increase serum levels of **fosphenytoin, phenytoin, phenobarbital,** and **primidone, warfarin,** TRICYCLIC ANTIDEPRESSANTS.

**PHARMACOKINETICS Absorption:** Well absorbed. **Peak:** 1–1.5 h. **Metabolism:** De-esterified in liver. No interaction with CYP450 system. **Elimination:** Primarily in urine. **Half-Life:** 2.2 h.

## NURSING IMPLICATIONS

### Black Box Warning

*Use dexmethylphenidate with extreme caution in those with a history of drug dependence or alcoholism.*

### Assessment & Drug Effects

- Monitor for potential abuse and dependence on this drug. Careful supervision is needed during drug withdrawal since severe depression may occur.
- Withhold drug and notify prescriber if patient has a seizure. Monitor

closely for loss of seizure control with a prior history of seizures.
- Monitor BP in all patients receiving this drug. Monitor cardiac status and report palpitations or other signs of arrhythmias.
- Monitor for signs of aggression or psychotic behavior in adolescents and children.
- Concurrent drugs: Monitor patients on BP-lowering drugs for loss of BP control. Monitor plasma levels of oral anticoagulants and anticonvulsants; doses of these drugs may need to be decreased.
- Monitor lab tests: Periodic CBC with differential and platelet count, and LFTs during prolonged therapy.

### Patient & Family Education

- Withhold drug and report immediately any of the following signs of overdose: Vomiting, agitation, tremors, muscle twitching, convulsions, confusion, hallucinations, delirium, sweating, flushing, headache, or high temperature.
- Note that drug is usually discontinued if improvement is not observed after appropriate dosage adjustment over 1 mo.

## DEXRAZOXANE
(dex-ra-zox'ane)
Totect, Zinecard
**Classifications:** ANTINEOPLASTIC; CYTOPROTECTIVE AGENT; CARDIOPROTECTIVE
**Therapeutic:** CARDIOPROTECTIVE FOR DOXORUBICIN

**AVAILABILITY** Solution for injection

## ACTION & *THERAPEUTIC EFFECT*

A derivative of EDTA that readily penetrates cell membranes. Dexrazoxane is converted intracellularly to a chelating agent that interferes with iron-mediated free radical generation thought to be partially responsible for one form of cardiomyopathy. *Cardioprotective effect is related to its chelating activity.*

**USES** Reduction of cardiomyopathy associated with a cumulative doxorubicin dose of 300 mg/m$^2$; extravasation due to anthracycline therapy.

**CONTRAINDICATIONS** Zinecard, generic products; use with chemotherapy regimens that do not contain an anthracycline; pregnancy (category D); lactation.

**CAUTIOUS USE** Myelosuppression, prior radiation or chemotherapy; renal failure or moderate to severe renal impairment; hepatic or cardiac impairment; older adults. Safety and efficacy in children not established.

## ROUTE & DOSAGE

### Cardiomyopathy

*Adult:* IV 10:1 ratio of dexrazoxane to doxorubicin

### Extravasation (Totect)

*Adult:* IV 1000mg/m$^2$ on day one and day two, then 500 mg/m$^2$ on day 3

### Renal Impairment Dosage Adjustment

*CrCl less than 40 mL/min:* Reduce dose by 50%

## ADMINISTRATION

### Intravenous

Wear gloves when handling dexrazoxane. Immediately wash with soap and water if drug contacts skin or mucosa.

■ Doxorubicin dose **must be** started within 30 min of beginning dexrazoxane.

*PREPARE:* **Direct:** Reconstitute by adding 25 or 50 mL of 0.167 M sodium lactate injection (provided by manufacturer) to the 250- or 500-mg vial, respectively, to produce a 10-mg/mL solution. **IV Infusion:** Further dilute reconstituted solution with NS or D5W to a concentration of 1.3–5 mg/mL for infusion.
*ADMINISTER:* **Direct:** Give bolus dose slowly. **IV Infusion:** Give over 10–15 min.
*INCOMPATIBILITIES:* **Y site: Acyclovir, allopurinol, aminophylline, amphotericin B, cefepime, dantrolene, diazepam, dobutamine, furosemide, ganciclovir, gemtuzumab, methotrexate, methylprednisolone, mitomycin, nafcillin, pantoprazole, pentobarbital, phenytoin, sodium phosphate, SMZ/TMP, thiopental, zidovudine.**

■ Store reconstituted solutions for 6 h at 15° 30° C (59°–86° F).

**ADVERSE EFFECTS** (≥1%) **All:** Adverse effects of dexrazoxane are difficult to distinguish from those of the chemotherapeutic agents but are dose related and include pain at injection site, <u>leukopenia, granulocytopenia, and thrombocytopenia</u>. **General:** Fatigue, neurotoxicity, fever, infection, sepsis, bone marrow depression. **CV:** Phlebitis. **Integumentary:** Erythema.

**PHARMACOKINETICS Distribution:** Not protein bound. **Metabolism:** In liver. **Elimination:** 42% in urine. **Half-Life:** 2–4 h.

## NURSING IMPLICATIONS

### Assessment & Drug Effects

■ Monitor cardiac function. Drug does not eliminate risk of doxorubicin cardiotoxicity.

Common adverse effects in *italic;* life-threatening effects <u>underlined;</u> generic names in **bold;** classifications in SMALL CAPS; ✦ Canadian drug name; ☺ Prototype drug

477

D

- Note: Adverse effects are likely due to concurrent cytotoxic drugs rather than dexrazoxane.
- Assess infusion site frequently; avoid extravasation.
- Monitor lab tests: Baseline and periodic blood cell counts; periodic LFTs and renal function tests.

**Patient & Family Education**
- Report any of the following to prescriber: Worsening shortness of breath, swelling extremities, or chest pains.

## DEXTRAN 40
(dex'tran)

Gentran 40, 10% LMD, Rheomacrodex

**Classification:** PLASMA VOLUME EXPANDER
Therapeutic: PLASMA VOLUME EXPANDER
**Prototype:** Albumin

**AVAILABILITY** Solution for injection

### ACTION & *THERAPEUTIC EFFECT*
A hypertonic colloidal solution that produces immediate and short-lived expansion of plasma volume by increasing colloidal osmotic pressure and drawing fluid from interstitial to intravascular space. *Cardiovascular response to volume expansion includes increased BP, pulse pressure, CVP, cardiac output, venous return to heart, and urinary output.*

**USES** Adjunctively to expand plasma volume and provide fluid replacement in treatment of shock or impending shock. Also used in prophylaxis and therapy of venous thrombosis and pulmonary embolism. Used as priming fluid or as additive to other primers during extracorporeal circulation.

**CONTRAINDICATIONS** Hypersensitivity to dextrans, severe renal failure, hypervolemic conditions, severe CHF, significant anemia, hypofibrinogenemia or other marked hemostatic defects including those caused by drugs, (e.g., heparin, warfarin); lactation.

**CAUTIOUS USE** Active hemorrhage; severe dehydration; chronic liver disease; impaired renal function; thrombocytopenia; patients susceptible to pulmonary edema or CHF; pregnancy (category C).

### ROUTE & DOSAGE

**Shock**

*Adult/Adolescent/Child:* **IV** Up to 20 mL/kg in the first 24 h (doses up to 10 mL/kg/day may be given for a maximum of 4 additional days if needed)

**Prophylaxis for Thromboembolic Complications**

*Adult:* **IV** 500–1000 mL (10 mL/kg) on the day of operation followed by 500 mL/day for 2–3 days, may continue with 500 mL q2–3days for up to 2 wk if necessary

**Priming for Extracorporeal Circulation**

*Adult:* **IV** 10–20 mL/kg added to perfusion circuit

### ADMINISTRATION

**Intravenous**
If blood is to be administered, draw a cross-match specimen before dextran infusion.

*PREPARE:* **IV Infusion:** Use only if seal is intact, vacuum is detectable, and solution is absolutely clear. ▪ No dilution required.
*ADMINISTER:* **IV Infusion:** Specific flow rate should be prescribed

---

Common adverse effects in *italic;* life-threatening effects <u>underlined</u>; generic names in **bold;** classifications in SMALL CAPS; ♣ Canadian drug name; ☯ Prototype drug

by prescriber. ▪ For emergency treatment of shock in adults give first 500 mL rapidly (e.g., 20–40 mL/min); give remaining portion of the daily dose over 8–24 h or at the rate prescribed.
*INCOMPATIBILITIES:* Solution/additive: **Amoxicillin, ampicillin, oxacillin, penicillin.**

▪ Store at a constant temperature, preferably 25° C (77° F). Once opened, discard unused portion because dextran contains no preservative.

## ADVERSE EFFECTS (≥1%) **Body as a Whole:** Hypersensitivity (mild to generalized urticaria, pruritus, ana-phylactic shock (rare), angioedema, dyspnea). **Other:** Renal tubular vacuolization (osmotic nephrosis), stasis and blocking oliguria, renal failure; increased AST and ALT, interference with platelet function, prolonged bleeding and coagulation times.

## DIAGNOSTIC TEST INTERFERENCE
When blood samples are drawn for study, notify laboratory that patient has received dextran. *Blood glucose:* False increases (utilizing *ortho-toluidine methods* or *sulfuric* or *acetic acid* hydrolysis). *Urinary protein:* False increases (utilizing *Lowry method*). *Bilirubin assays:* False increases when alcohol is used. *Total protein assays:* False increases using *biuret reagent. Rh testing, blood typing* and *cross-matching* procedures: Dextran may interfere with results (by inducing rouleaux formation) when *proteolytic enzyme techniques* are used (*saline agglutination* and *indirect antiglobulin methods* reportedly not affected).

## INTERACTIONS Drug: May potentiate **abciximab** anticoagulant effects.

## PHARMACOKINETICS Onset: Volume expansion within minutes of infusion. **Duration:** 12 h. **Metabolism:** Degraded to glucose and metabolized to $CO_2$ and water over a period of a few weeks. **Elimination:** 75% excreted in urine within 24 h; small amount excreted in feces.

## NURSING IMPLICATIONS
### Assessment & Drug Effects
▪ Evaluate patient's state of hydration before dextran therapy begins. Administration to severely dehydrated patients can result in renal failure.
▪ Monitor vital signs and observe patient closely for at least the first 30 min of infusion. Hypersensitivity reaction is most likely to occur during the first few minutes of administration. Terminate therapy at the first sign of a hypersensitivity reaction (see Appendix F).
▪ Monitor CVP as an estimate of blood volume status and a guide for determining dosage. Normal CVP: 5–10 cm $H_2O$.
▪ Observe for S&S of circulatory overload (see Appendix F).
▪ Note: When sodium restriction is indicated, know that 500 mL of dextran 40 in 0.9% normal saline contains 77 mEq of both sodium and chloride.
▪ Monitor I&O ratio and check urine specific gravity at regular intervals. Low urine specific gravity may signify failure of renal dextran clearance and is an indication to discontinue therapy.
▪ Report oliguria, anuria, or lack of improvement in urinary output (dextran usually causes an increase in urinary output). Discontinue dextran at first sign of renal dysfunction.

---

Common adverse effects in *italic;* life-threatening effects underlined; generic names in **bold;** classifications in SMALL CAPS; ♣ Canadian drug name; ⊘ Prototype drug

- High doses are associated with transient prolongation of bleeding time and interference with normal blood coagulation.
- Monitor lab tests: Baseline Hct and repeat Hct as needed.

**Patient & Family Education**
- Report immediately S&S of bleeding: Easy bruising, blood in urine, or dark tarry stool.

## DEXTROAMPHETAMINE SULFATE

(dex-troe-am-fet′a-meen)

Dexampex, Dexedrine, Oxydess II ◆, Spancap No. 1

**Classifications:** RESPIRATORY AND CEREBRAL STIMULANT; AMPHETAMINE; ANOREXIANT
Therapeutic: AMPHETAMINE; ANOREXIANT
**Prototype:** Amphetamine
**Controlled Substance:** Schedule II

**AVAILABILITY** Tablet; sustained release capsule

**ACTION & *THERAPEUTIC EFFECT***
A CNS stimulant that may cause diminished appetite through loss of acuity of smell and taste. *Is a more potent appetite suppressant than amphetamine. In hyperkinetic children, amphetamines reduce motor restlessness by an unknown mechanism.*

**USES** Adjunct in short-term treatment of exogenous obesity, narcolepsy, and attention deficit disorder with hyperactivity in children (also called minimal brain dysfunction or hyperkinetic syndrome).

**UNLABELED USES** Adjunct in epilepsy to control ataxia and drowsiness induced by barbiturates; to combat sedative effects of trimethadione in absence seizures.

**CONTRAINDICATIONS** Hypersensitivity to sympathomimetic amines, closed-angle glaucoma, agitated states, psychoses (especially in children), structural cardiac abnormalities, valvular heart disease; congenital heart disease, coronary heart disease, advanced arteriosclerosis, symptomatic heart disease, moderate to severe hypertension, hyperthyroidism, history of drug abuse, during or within 14 days of MAOI therapy; children younger than 3 y; lactation.

**CAUTIOUS USE** Bipolar disease; salicylate hypersensitivity; seizure disorders; suicidal ideation, depression; salicylate hypersensitivity; pregnancy (category C). Safety and efficacy in children younger than 6 y for narcolepsy and younger than 3 y for attention deficit disorder not established.

## ROUTE & DOSAGE

**Narcolepsy**

*Adult:* **PO** 5–20 mg 1–3 × day at 4–6 h intervals
*Child (6 to younger than 12 y):* **PO** 5 mg/day, may increase by 5 mg at weekly intervals; *12 y or older:* 10 mg/day, may increase by 10 mg at weekly intervals

**Attention Deficit Disorder**

*Child (3–5 y):* **PO** 2.5 mg 1–2 × day, may increase by 2.5 mg at weekly intervals; *6 y or older:* 5 mg 1–2 × day, may increase by 5 mg at weekly intervals (max: 40 mg/day)

**Obesity**

*Adult:* **PO** 5–10 mg 1–3 × day or 10–15 mg of sustained release once/day 30–60 min a.c.

Common adverse effects in *italic;* life-threatening effects <u>underlined;</u> generic names in **bold;** classifications in SMALL CAPS; ◆ Canadian drug name; ❷ Prototype drug

**D**

## ADMINISTRATION
### Oral

- Ensure that sustained release capsule is not chewed or crushed. It **must be** swallowed whole.
- Give 30–60 min before meals for treatment of obesity. Give long-acting form in the morning.
- Give last dose no later than 6 h before patient retires (10–14 h before bedtime for sustained release form) to avoid insomnia.
- Store in tightly closed containers at 15°–30° C (59°–86° F) unless otherwise directed.

## ADVERSE EFFECTS (≥1%) CNS:
Nervousness, *restlessness,* hyperactivity, *insomnia,* euphoria, dizziness, headache; *with prolonged use:* Severe depression, psychotic reactions. **CV:** Palpitations, tachycardia, elevated BP. **GI:** Dry mouth, unpleasant taste, anorexia, weight loss, diarrhea, constipation, abdominal pain. **Other:** Impotence, changes in libido, unusual fatigue, increased intraocular pressure, marked dystonia of head, neck, and extremities; sweating.

## DIAGNOSTIC TEST INTERFERENCE
Dextroamphetamine may cause significant elevations in *plasma corticosteroids* (evening levels are highest) and increases in *urinary epinephrine* excretion (during first 3 h after drug administration).

## INTERACTIONS Drug: Acetazolamide, sodium bicarbonate decrease dextroamphetamine elimination; **ammonium chloride, ascorbic acid** increase dextroamphetamine elimination; effects of both BARBITURATES and dextroamphetamine may be antagonized; **furazolidone** may increase BP effects of AMPHETAMINES—interaction may persist for several weeks after discontinuing **furazolidone;** antagonizes antihypertensive effects of **guanethidine;** MAO INHIBITORS, **selegiline** can cause—hypertensive crisis (fatalities reported)—do not administer AMPHETAMINES during or within 14 days of these drugs; PHENOTHIAZINES may inhibit mood-elevating effects of AMPHETAMINES; TRICYCLIC ANTIDEPRESSANTS enhance dextroamphetamine effects because of increased **norepinephrine** release; BETA-ADRENERGIC AGONISTS increase cardiovascular adverse effects.

## PHARMACOKINETICS Absorption:
Rapid. **Peak:** 1–5 h. **Duration:** Up to 10 h. **Distribution:** All tissues, especially the CNS. **Metabolism:** In liver. **Elimination:** Renal elimination; excreted in breast milk. **Half-Life:** 10–30 h.

## NURSING IMPLICATIONS

### Black Box Warning

*Dextroamphetamine has been associated with fatal respiratory depression in children younger than 2 y (do not use in this age group). Children older than 2 y may experience serious adverse effects.*

### Assessment & Drug Effects
- Monitor children, adolescents, and adults for signs and symptoms of respiratory depression and adverse cardiac reactions (e.g., arrhythmias).
- Monitor growth rate closely in children.
- Monitor children and adolescents for development of aggressive or abnormal behaviors.
- Note: Tolerance to anorexiant effects may develop after a few weeks, however, tolerance does not appear to develop when dextroamphetamine is used to treat narcolepsy.

### Patient & Family Education
- Swallow sustained release capsule whole with a liquid; do not chew or crush.

Common adverse effects in *italic;* life-threatening effects underlined; generic names in **bold;** classifications in SMALL CAPS; ♣ Canadian drug name; ⊘ Prototype drug

481

**D**

- Do not drive or engage in other potentially hazardous activities until response to drug is known.
- Drug is usually tapered off gradually following long-term use to avoid extreme fatigue, mental depression, and prolonged sleep pattern.

## DEXTROMETHORPHAN HYDROBROMIDE

(dex-troe-meth-or'fan)

Balminil DM ♣, Benylin DM, Cremacoat 1, Delsym, DM Cough, Hold, Koffex ♣, Mediquell, Neo-DM ♣, Ornex DM ♣, Pedia Care, Pertussin 8 Hour Cough Formula, Robidex ♣, Robitussin DM, Romilar CF, Romilar Children's Cough, Sedatuss ♣, Sucrets Cough Control

**Classification:** ANTITUSSIVE
**Therapeutic:** ANTITUSSIVE
**Prototype:** Benzonatate

**AVAILABILITY** Capsule; liquid; syrup

**ACTION & *THERAPEUTIC EFFECT***
Chemically related to morphine but without central hypnotic or analgesic effect. Controls cough spasms by depressing the cough center in medulla. Antitussive activity comparable to that of codeine. *Temporarily relieves coughing spasm.*

**USES** Temporary relief of cough spasms in nonproductive coughs.

**CONTRAINDICATIONS** Asthma, COPD, productive cough, persistent or chronic cough; severe hepatic function impairment. Concurrent administration with or within 2 wk of discontinuing an MAO inhibitor.

**CAUTIOUS USE** Chronic pulmonary disease; enlarged prostate; mild or moderate hepatic impairment; pregnancy (category C); lactation. Safe use in children younger than 2 y not established.

## ROUTE & DOSAGE

**Cough**

*Adult:/Adolescent:* **PO** 10–20 mg q4h or
30 mg q6–8h (max: 120 mg/day) or 60 mg of sustained action liquid b.i.d.
*Child (2 to younger than 6 y):*
**PO** 2.5–5 mg q4h or 7.5 mg q6–8h (max: 30 mg/day) or 15 mg sustained action liquid b.i.d.;
*6–11 y:* 5–10 mg q4h or 15 mg q6–8h (max: 60 mg/day) or 30 mg sustained action liquid b.i.d.

## ADMINISTRATION

**Oral**

- Do not give lozenges to children younger than 6 y.
- Ensure that extended release form of drug is not chewed or crushed. It **must be** swallowed whole.
- Note: Although soothing local effect of the syrup may be enhanced if given undiluted, depression of cough center depends only on systemic absorption of drug.

**ADVERSE EFFECTS** (≥1%) **CNS:** Dizziness, drowsiness, CNS depression with very large doses; excitability, especially in children. **GI:** GI upset, constipation, abdominal discomfort.

**INTERACTIONS Drug:** High risk of excitation, hypotension, and hyperpyrexia with MAO INHIBITORS. Due to potential of serotonin syndrome use caution with SSRIs.

**PHARMACOKINETICS Absorption:** Readily from GI tract. **Onset:** 15–30 min. **Duration:** 3–6 h. **Metabolism:** In liver. **Elimination:** In urine.

## NURSING IMPLICATIONS

### Black Box Warning

*Do not use in children younger than 2 y due to risk of fatal respiratory depression.*

### Assessment & Drug Effects

- Monitor for dizziness and drowsiness, especially when concurrent therapy with CNS depressant is used.

### Patient & Family Education

- Note: Treatment aims to decrease the frequency and intensity of cough without completely eliminating protective cough reflex.
- While dextromethorphan is available OTC, any cough persisting longer than 1 wk–10 days needs to be medically diagnosed.

## DIAZEPAM ⊕

(dye-az′e-pam)

Diastat, Diazemuls ◆, Valium

**Classifications:** BENZODIAZEPINE ANTICONVULSANT; ANXIOLYTIC
**Therapeutic:** ANTICONVULSANT; ANTIANXIETY
**Controlled Substance:** Schedule IV

**AVAILABILITY** Tablet; oral solution; solution for injection; rectal gel

## ACTION & *THERAPEUTIC EFFECT*

Acts at the limbic, thalamic, and hypothalamic regions of the CNS and produces CNS depression resulting in sedation, hypnosis, skeletal muscle relaxation, and anticonvulsant activity dependent on the dosage. *Has antianxiety, anticonvulsant, and skeletal muscle relaxation properties.*

**USES** Drug of choice for status epilepticus. Management of anxiety disorders, for short-term relief of anxiety symptoms, to allay anxiety and tension prior to surgery, cardioversion and endoscopic procedures, as an amnesic, and treatment for restless legs. Also used to alleviate acute withdrawal symptoms of alcoholism, voiding problems in older adults, and adjunctively for relief of skeletal muscle spasm associated with cerebral palsy, paraplegia, athetosis, stiffman syndrome, tetanus.

**CONTRAINDICATIONS** Acute narrow-angle glaucoma, untreated open-angle glaucoma, during or within 14 days of MAOI therapy; pregnancy (category D); lactation. **Injectable form:** Shock, coma, acute alcohol intoxication, depressed vital signs, obstetric patients.

**CAUTIOUS USE** Epilepsy, psychoses, mental depression; myasthenia gravis; impaired hepatic or renal function; neuromuscular disease; bipolar disorder, dementia, Parkinson's disease; organic brain syndrome, psychosis, suicidal ideation; drug abuse, addiction-prone individuals. **Injectable form:** Extreme caution in older adults, the very ill, and patients with COPD, or asthma; infant

## ROUTE & DOSAGE

| Status Epilepticus |
|---|
| *Adult:* **IV/IM** 5–10 mg, repeat if needed at 10–15 min intervals up to 30 mg, then repeat if needed q2–4h |
| *Child (5 y or older):* **IV** 1 mg/kg q2–5min (max: 10 mg), may repeat in 2–4 h |
| *Child/Infant (1 mo to younger than 5 y):* **IV** 0.2–0.5 mg slowly q2–5min up to 5 mg |
| *Neonate:* **IV** 0.1–0.3 mg/kg q15–30min (max total dose: 2 mg) |

| Muscle Spasm |
|---|
| *Adult/Adolescent/Child (5 y or older):* **IV** 5–10 mg q3–4h prn |

Common adverse effects in *italic;* life-threatening effects <u>underlined</u>; generic names in **bold;** classifications in SMALL CAPS; ◆ Canadian drug name; ⊕ Prototype drug

483

**D**

(larger dose for tetanus); **PO**
2–10 mg 3–4 × day
*Child/Infant (1 mo–5 y):* **IV**
1–2 mg q3–4h prn

**Anxiety**

*Adult/Adolescent:* **IV** 2–10 mg,
repeat if needed in 3–4 h; **PO**
2–10 mg 2–4 × day
*Child/Infant (6 mo or older):* **IV**
0.04–0.3 mg q2–4h (max:
0.6 mg/kg/8 h)

**Alcohol Withdrawal**

*Adult:* **IV** 10 mg then 5–10 mg in
3–4 h; **PO** 10 mg 3 or 4 × on day
1 then 5 mg 3–4 × day PRN

**Preoperative**

*Adult:* **IV** 5–15 mg 5–10 min
before procedure

## ADMINISTRATION

### Oral

- Ensure that sustained release
  form is not chewed or crushed. It
  **must be** swallowed whole. Give
  other tablets crushed with fluid or
  mixed with food if necessary.
- Supervise oral ingestion to ensure
  drug is swallowed.
- Avoid abrupt discontinuation of
  diazepam. Taper doses to termination.

### Intramuscular

- Give deep into large muscle mass.
  Inject slowly. Rotate injection sites.

### Intravenous

*PREPARE:* **Direct:** Do not dilute or
mix with any other drug.
*ADMINISTER:* **Direct:** Give direct
IV by injecting drug slowly, taking at least 1 min for each 5 mg
(1 mL) given to adults and taking
at least 3 min to inject 0.25 mg/
kg body weight of children. ▪ If
injection cannot be made

directly into vein, inject slowly
through infusion tubing as close
as possible to vein insertion.
▪ The emulsion form is incompatible with PVC infusion sets.
▪ Avoid small veins and take extreme care to avoid intra-arterial
administration or extravasation.
*INCOMPATIBILITIES:* Solution/ad-
ditive: **Bleomycin, dobutamine,
doxorubicin, epinephrine,
fluorouracil, furosemide, glycopyrrolate, nalbuphine, sodium bicarbonate.** Emulsion also
incompatible with **morphine.**
Y-site: **Amphotericin B cholesteryl complex, atracu-
rium, bivalirudin, cefepime,
dexmedetomidine, diltiazem,
fenoldopam, fluconazole, foscarnet, furosemide, heparin,
hetastarch, lansoprazole, linezolid, meropenem, oxaliplatin, pancuronium, potassium chloride, propofol,
remifentanil, tirofiban, vecuronium, vitamin B com-
plex with C.** Do not mix emulsion with any other drugs. Do not
administer through **polyvinyl
chloride (PVC)** infusion sets.

- Store in tight, light-resistant containers at 15°–30° C (59°–86° F),
  unless otherwise specified by
  manufacturer.

## ADVERSE EFFECTS (≥1%) **Body
as a Whole:** Throat and chest pain.
**CNS:** *Drowsiness,* fatigue, ataxia,
confusion, paradoxic rage, dizziness, vertigo, amnesia, vivid dreams,
headache, slurred speech, tremor;
EEG changes, tardive dyskinesia.
**CV:** Hypotension, tachycardia, edema, cardiovascular collapse. **Special
Senses:** Blurred vision, diplopia,
nystagmus. **GI:** Xerostomia, nausea,
constipation, hepatic dysfunction.
**Urogenital:** Incontinence, urinary
retention, gynecomastia (prolonged

use), menstrual irregularities, ovulation failure. **Respiratory:** Hiccups, coughing, <u>laryngospasm</u>. **Other:** Pain, venous thrombosis, phlebitis at injection site.

**INTERACTIONS Drug: Alcohol,** CNS DEPRESSANTS, ANTICONVULSANTS potentiate CNS depression; **cimetidine** increases diazepam plasma levels, increases toxicity; may decrease antiparkinson effects of **levodopa;** may increase **phenytoin** levels; smoking decreases sedative and antianxiety effects. **Herbal: Kava, valerian** may potentiate sedation.

**PHARMACOKINETICS Absorption:** Readily from GI tract; erratic IM absorption. **Onset:** 30–60 min PO; 15–30 min IM; 1–5 min IV. **Peak:** 1–2 h PO. **Duration:** 15 min–1 h IV; up to 3 h PO. **Distribution:** Crosses blood–brain barrier and placenta; distributed into breast milk. **Metabolism:** In liver to active metabolites. **Elimination:** Primarily in urine. **Half-Life:** 20–50 h.

**NURSING IMPLICATIONS**

**Assessment & Drug Effects**

- Monitor for adverse reactions. Most are dose related.
- Monitor for therapeutic effectiveness. Maximum effect may require 1–2 wk; patient tolerance to therapeutic effects may develop after 4 wk of treatment.
- Monitor for and report promptly signs of suicidal ideation especially in those treated for anxiety states accompanied by depression.
- Observe patient closely and monitor vital signs when diazepam is given parenterally; hypotension, muscular weakness, tachycardia, and respiratory depression may occur.
- Supervise ambulation. Adverse reactions such as drowsiness and ataxia are more likely to

occur in older adults and debilitated or those receiving larger doses. Dosage adjustment may be necessary.

- Monitor I&O ratio, including urinary and bowel elimination.
- Note: Psychic and physical dependence may occur in patients on long-term high dosage therapy, in those with histories of alcohol or drug addiction, or in those who self-medicate.
- Monitor lab tests: Periodic CBC and LFTs during prolonged therapy.

**Patient & Family Education**

- Avoid alcohol and other CNS depressants during therapy unless otherwise advised by prescriber. Concomitant use of these agents can cause severe drowsiness, respiratory depression, and apnea.
- Do not drive or engage in other potentially hazardous activities or those requiring mental precision until reaction to drug is known.
- Tell prescriber if you become or intend to become pregnant during therapy; drug may need to be discontinued.
- Take drug as prescribed; do not change dose or dose intervals.

---

**DIAZOXIDE**
(dye-az-ox'ide)
**Proglycem**

**Classifications:** GLUCOSE ELEVATING AGENT
Therapeutic; HYPOGLYCEMIC

**AVAILABILITY** Oral suspension

**ACTION & *THERAPEUTIC EFFECT***
Causes dose-related increase in blood glucose level caused by inhibition of insulin release from

Common adverse effects in *italic;* life-threatening effects <u>underlined</u>; generic names in **bold;** classifications in SMALL CAPS; ♣ Canadian drug name; ⓟ Prototype drug

485

the pancreas. *Increases blood glucose level.*

**USES** Orally in treatment of various diagnosed hypoglycemic states due to hyperinsulinism when other medical treatment or surgical management has been unsuccessful or is not feasible.

**CONTRAINDICATIONS** Hypersensitivity to diazoxide or other thiazides; cerebral bleeding, eclampsia; aortic coarctation; AV shunt, significant coronary artery disease; pheochromocytoma; functional hypoglycemia; lactation. Use in presence of increased bilirubin in newborns.

**CAUTIOUS USE** Diabetes mellitus; impaired cerebral or cardiac circulation; impaired renal function; patients taking corticosteroids or estrogen–progestogen combinations; hyperuricemia, history of gout, uremia; pregnancy (category C).

**ROUTE & DOSAGE**

**Hypoglycemia**
*Adult/Child:* **PO** 3–8 mg/kg divided every 8–12 h
*Neonate/Infant:* **PO** 8–15 mg/ kg/day divided q8–12h

**ADMINISTRATION**
**Oral**
▪ Do not give darkened solutions. Store at 2°–30° C (36°–86° F) unless otherwise directed. Protect from light, heat, and freezing.

**ADVERSE EFFECTS** (≥1%) **CNS:** Headache, weakness, malaise, *dizziness,* polyneuritis, sleepiness, insomnia, euphoria, anxiety, extrapyramidal signs. **CV:** Palpitations, atrial and ventricular arrhythmias, flushing, shock; *orthostatic hypotension,* CHF, transient hypertension. **Special Senses:** Tinnitus, momentary hearing loss; blurred vision, transient cataracts, subconjunctival hemorrhage, ring scotoma, diplopia, lacrimation, papilledema. **GI:** *Nausea, vomiting,* abdominal discomfort, diarrhea, constipation, ileus, anorexia, transient loss of taste, impaired hepatic function. **Hematologic:** Transient neutropenia, eosinophilia, decreased Hgb/Hct, decreased IgG. **Body as a Whole:** Hypersensitivity (rash, fever, leukopenia); chest and back pain, muscle cramps. **Urogenital:** Decreased urinary output, nephrotic syndrome (reversible), hematuria, increased nocturia, proteinuria, azotemia; inhibition of labor. **Skin:** Monilial dermatitis, herpes, hirsutism; loss of scalp hair, sweating, sensation of warmth, burning, or itching. **Endocrine:** Advance in bone age (children), *hyperglycemia, sodium and water retention, edema,* hyperuricemia, glycosuria, enlargement of breast lump, galactorrhea; decreased immunoglobulinemia, hirsutism.

**DIAGNOSTIC TEST INTERFERENCE** Diazoxide can cause false-negative response to ***glucagon.***

**INTERACTIONS Drug:** SULFO-NYLUREAS antagonize effects; THIAZIDE DIURETICS may intensify hyperglycemia and antihypertensive effects; **phenytoin** increases risk of hyperglycemia, and diazoxide may increase **phenytoin** metabolism, causing loss of seizure control.

**PHARMACOKINETICS Onset:** 1 h. **Duration:** 8 h. **Distribution:** Crosses blood–brain barrier and placenta. **Metabolism:** Partially metabolized in the liver. **Elimination:** In urine. **Half-Life:** 21–45 h.

Common adverse effects in *italic;* life-threatening effects underlined; generic names in **bold;** classifications in SMALL CAPS; ♣ Canadian drug name; ◍ Prototype drug

## NURSING IMPLICATIONS
### Assessment & Drug Effects
- Monitor closely for S&S of CHF (e.g., development of edema, weight gain). Sodium and fluid retention may precipitate CHF in those with preexisting cardiac disease.
- Report promptly any change in I&O ratio.
- Oral administration usually does not produce marked effects on BP. However, do make periodic measurements of BP and vital signs.
- Monitor lab tests: Baseline and periodic blood glucose, urine for glucose and ketones, serum electrolytes, CBC with differential, Hct, platelet count, AST, and serum uric acid.

### Patient & Family Education
- Note: Drug may cause hyperglycemia and glycosuria. Closely monitor blood and urine glucose; report any abnormalities to prescriber.
- Report palpitations, chest pain, dizziness, fainting, or severe headache.

## DIBUCAINE
(dye'byoo-kane)
Nupercainal
**Classification:** ANESTHETIC, LOCAL (AMIDE-TYPE)
Therapeutic: LOCAL ANESTHETIC
**Prototype:** Procaine

## AVAILABILITY Ointment

## ACTION & THERAPEUTIC EFFECT
Inhibits initiation and conduction of nerve impulses by reducing permeability of nerve cell membrane to sodium ions. *Relief of pain and itching due to inhibiting conduction of nerve impulses.*

## USES
Fast, temporary relief of pain and itching due to hemorrhoids and other anorectal disorders, nonpoisonous insect bites, sunburn, minor burns, cuts, and scratches.

## CONTRAINDICATIONS
Hypersensitivity to amide-type anesthetics.

## CAUTIOUS USE
Pregnancy (category C); lactation; children younger than 12 y.

## ROUTE & DOSAGE

| Itching Due to Insect Bites or Hemorrhoids |
| --- |
| *Adult:* **Topical** Apply skin cream or ointment to affected area as needed [max: 1 oz (28 g)/24 h]; insert rectal ointment morning and evening and after each bowel movement |
| *Child:* **Topical** Apply skin cream or ointment to affected area as needed [max: 1/4 oz (7 g)/24 h] |

## ADMINISTRATION
### Topical
- Apply cream preparation after bathing or swimming (water soluble).
- Store at 15°–30° C (59°–86° F) in tight, light-resistant containers.

## ADVERSE EFFECTS (≥1%)
**Skin:** Irritation, contact dermatitis; rectal bleeding (suppository).

## PHARMACOKINETICS
**Absorption:** Poorly absorbed from intact skin; readily absorbed from mucous membranes or abraded skin. **Onset:** 15 min. **Duration:** 2–4 h.

## NURSING IMPLICATIONS
### Patient & Family Education
- Discontinue if irritation or rectal bleeding (following use of rectal preparations) develops and consult prescriber.

---

Common adverse effects in *italic*; life-threatening effects <u>underlined</u>; generic names in **bold**; classifications in SMALL CAPS; ♣ Canadian drug name; ⊘ Prototype drug

487

**D**

- Prescriber may prescribe sitz baths 3–4 × day to reduce the swelling and pain of hemorrhoids.
- Note: Medication is intended for temporary relief of mild to moderate itching or pain. Seek medical advice for continuing discomfort, pain, bleeding, or sensation of rectal pressure.

## DICLOFENAC
(di-klo'fen-ak)
Zorvolex

## DICLOFENAC SODIUM
PENNSAID, Solaraze, Voltaren, Voltaren-XR

## DICLOFENAC POTASSIUM
Cambia, Cataflam, Zipsor

## DICLOFENAC EPOLAMINE
Flector

**Classifications:** NONSTEROIDAL ANALGESIC, ANTI-INFLAMMATORY DRUG (NSAID)
Therapeutic: ANALGESIC, NSAID; ANTIPYRETIC
**Prototype:** Ibuprofen

**AVAILABILITY** **Diclofenac:** Capsule. **Diclofenac Sodium:** Delayed release tablet; sustained release tablet; ophthalmic solution; gel; transdermal solution. **Diclofenac Potassium:** Tablet; powder for solution. **Diclofenac Epolamine:** Transdermal patch

## ACTION & *THERAPEUTIC EFFECT*
Diclofenac competitively inhibits both cyclooxygenase (COX) isoenzymes, COX-1 and COX-2, by blocking arachidonic acid conversion to other chemicals, thus leading to its analgesic, antipyretic, and anti-inflammatory effects. As a potent inhibitor of cyclooxygenase, it decreases the synthesis of prostaglandins. *Nonsteroidal anti-inflammatory drug (NSAID) with analgesic and antipyretic activity.*

**USES** Analgesic and antipyretic effects in symptomatic treatment of rheumatoid arthritis, osteoarthritis, and ankylosing spondylitis. Also acute gout; juvenile rheumatoid arthritis; various rheumatic conditions. **Ophthalmic:** Cataract surgery; photophobia associated with refractive surgery. **Topical:** Treatment of actinic keratosis. **Transdermal:** Acute pain.

**CONTRAINDICATIONS** Hypersensitivity to diclofenac, NSAIDS, or salicylate or bovine protein; patients in whom asthma, urticaria, angioedema, bronchospasm results from use of aspirin or other NSAIDS; GI bleeding or ulcer; hepatic porphyria; perioperative CABG pain; pregnancy (category D); 30 wk gestation or more with use of **PO** form; lactation; **gelatin** form use in individuals with previous history of hypersensitivity.

**CAUTIOUS USE** Patients receiving anticoagulant therapy; DM; asthma; history of GI disease or bleeding; hepatic disease; GU tract problems such as dysuria, cystitis, hematuria, impaired renal function; nephritis, nephrotic syndrome, patients who must restrict their sodium intake; dehydration; impaired hepatic function; SLE; heart failure or reduced left ventricular ejection fraction; cardiac disease; fluid retention; hypertension; older adults; pregnancy (category C), children.

## ROUTE & DOSAGE

### Mild/Moderate Pain
*Adult:* **PO Zipsor** 25 mg q.i.d. **Zorvolex** 18 or 35 mg t.i.d. **Immediate release tablet:** 50 mg t.i.d.

Common adverse effects in *italic;* life-threatening effects <u>underlined;</u> generic names in **bold;** classifications in SMALL CAPS; ♣ Canadian drug name; ⊙ Prototype drug

**D**

### Rheumatoid Arthritis

*Adult:* **PO** 150–200 mg/day in 3–4 divided doses or 75 mg delayed release daily or 100 mg sustained release daily
*Child:* **PO** 25 mg b.i.d. or t.i.d.

### Osteoarthritis

*Adult:* **PO** 100–150 mg/day in 3–4 divided doses; 75 mg delayed release daily; 100 mg sustained release daily; **Topical (gel)** 4 g for each knee, ankle or foot q.i.d. **(solution)** 40 drops to each affected knee q.i.d.

### Ankylosing Spondylitis

*Adult:* **PO** 25 mg q.i.d. and 25 mg at bedtime

### Actinic Keratosis

*Adult:* **Topical** Apply to affected area b.i.d. for 60–90 days

### Acute Pain (Flector)

*Adult:* **Transdermal** Apply one patch to most painful area b.i.d.

## ADMINISTRATION

### Oral

- Ensure that sustained release forms of drug are not chewed or crushed. **Must be** swallowed whole.
- Minimize gastric irritation by administering it with a full glass of milk or food.
- Store at 15°–30° C (59°–86° F) away from heat and direct light.

### Topical/Transdermal

- Do not apply gel or patch to areas of skin irritation.
- Massage gel into skin of entire affected area. Do not wash area within 1 hr of application.

- Avoid application of any other topical products to treated area.
- Do not apply external heat or occlusive dressing to treated area.

**ADVERSE EFFECTS** (≥1%) **CNS:** Dizziness, headache, drowsiness. **Special Senses:** Tinnitus. **Skin:** Rash, pruritus. **GI:** *Dyspepsia,* nausea, vomiting, abdominal pain, cramps, constipation, diarrhea, indigestion, abdominal distension, flatulence, peptic ulcer. **CV:** *Fluid retention,* hypertension, CHF. **Respiratory:** Asthma. **Body as a Whole:** Back, leg, or joint pain. **Endocrine:** Hyperglycemia, increased transaminase. **Hematologic:** Prolonged bleeding time; inhibits platelet aggregation.

**DIAGNOSTIC TEST INTERFERENCE**
*Liver function test* values may be increased. *Liver function test* abnormalities may return to normal despite continued use; however, if significant abnormalities occur, clinical signs and symptoms consistent with liver disease develop, or systemic manifestations such as eosinophilia or rash occur, the medication should be discontinued. *Serum uric acid* concentrations may be decreased because of increased *renal clearance.*

**INTERACTIONS Drug:** Increases **cyclosporine**-induced nephrotoxicity; increases **methotrexate** levels (increases toxicity); may decrease BP-lowering effects of DIURETICS; may increase levels and toxicity of **lithium;** may increase **digoxin** levels. **Herbal: Feverfew, garlic, ginger, ginkgo** may increase risk of bleeding.

**PHARMACOKINETICS Absorption:** Readily absorbed from GI

Common adverse effects in *italic;* life-threatening effects <u>underlined</u>; generic names in **bold;** classifications in SMALL CAPS; ♣ Canadian drug name; ☻ Prototype drug

489

tract; 50–60% reaches systemic circulation. **Peak:** 2–3 h. **Distribution:** Widely distributed including synovial fluid and into breast milk; 99% protein bound. **Metabolism:** Extensively metabolized in liver. **Elimination:** 50–70% in urine, 30–35% in feces. **Half-Life:** 1.2–2 h (PO); 12 h (transdermal).

## NURSING IMPLICATIONS

### Black Box Warning

*Diclofenac has been associated with increased risk of serious, potentially fatal, CV thrombotic events (i.e., MI and stroke). Risk may increase with duration of use and may be greater in those with risk factors for CV disease.*

### Assessment & Drug Effects

- Monitor for signs and symptoms of GI irritation and ulceration especially in the the older adult.
- Monitor for and report promptly S&S of CV thrombotic events (i.e., angina, MI, TIA, or stroke).
- Monitor BP for new onset or worsening of preexisting hypertension.
- Monitor diabetics closely for loss of diabetic glycemic control.
- Monitor for increased serum sodium and potassium in patients receiving potassium-sparing diuretics.
- Monitor for S&S of CHF, including weight gains greater than 1 kg (2 lb)/24 h.
- Monitor lab tests: Periodic LFTs, serum uric acid, Hct, PT/INR, and blood glucose.

### Patient & Family Education

- Seek immediate medical attention if you experience S&S of adverse cardiovascular effects, such as chest pain, shortness of breath, weakness, or slurring of speech.
- Report immediately to prescriber S&S of serious GI irritation, such as stomach pain, frequent indigestion, tarry stools, or vomiting blood.
- Be alert for S&S of adverse skin reactions. Report promptly development of rash, blisters, or other skin reactions.
- Do not take aspirin or other OTC analgesics without permission of the prescriber.
- Avoid alcohol or other CNS depressants.
- Do not drive or engage in other potentially hazardous activities until reaction to drug is known.
- Diabetics should monitor blood glucose carefully for loss of glycemic control.

## DICLOXACILLIN SODIUM
(dye-klox-a-sill'in)

**Classification:** PENICILLIN ANTIBIOTIC, PENICILLINASE-RESISTANT PENICILLIN
**Therapeutic:** PENICILLIN ANTIBIOTIC
**Prototype:** Oxacillin sodium

## AVAILABILITY Capsule

## ACTION & *THERAPEUTIC EFFECT*

It inhibits the final stage of bacterial cell wall synthesis by preferentially binding to specific penicillin-binding proteins (PBPs) that are located inside bacterial cell wall; this leads to cell death. *Effective against penicillinase-producing staphylococci.*

## USES Primarily in systemic infections caused by penicillinase-producing staphylococci and penicillin-resistant staphylococci.

**CONTRAINDICATIONS** Hypersensitivity to penicillins.

**CAUTIOUS USE** History of or suspected atopy or allergy (asthma, eczema, hives, hay fever); history of hypersensitivity to cephalosporins or carbapenem; GI disease, colitis; renal or hepatic impairment; pregnancy (category B); lactation.

## ROUTE & DOSAGE

**Mild to Moderate Infections**
*Adult:* **PO** 125–250 mg q6h
*Child (weight less than 40 kg).* **PO** 12.5–25 mg/kg q6h (max: 4 g/day)

## ADMINISTRATION

**Oral**

- Give on an empty stomach at least 1 h before or 2 h after meals. Food reduces drug absorption.
- Store capsules at room temperature in tight containers unless otherwise directed.

**ADVERSE EFFECTS** (≥1%) **Body as a Whole:** Hypersensitivity (pruritus, urticaria, rash, wheezing, sneezing, anaphylaxis; eosinophilia). **GI:** Nausea, vomiting, flatulence, *diarrhea*, abdominal pain. **Other:** Transient elevations of ALT, superinfections.

**INTERACTIONS Drug: Probenecid** decreases dicloxacillin elimination.

**PHARMACOKINETICS Absorption:** 35–76% absorbed from GI tract. **Peak:** 0.5–2 h. **Duration:** 4–6 h. **Distribution:** Distributed throughout body with highest concentrations in liver and kidney; low CSF penetration; crosses placenta; distributed into breast milk. **Metabolism:** In liver. **Elimination:** Primarily in urine with some elimination through bile. **Half-Life:** 30–60 min.

## NURSING IMPLICATIONS

### Assessment & Drug Effects

- Note: Take care to establish previous exposure and sensitivity to penicillins and cephalosporins as well as other allergic reactions of any kind before initiating therapy.
- Obtain C&S prior to initiation of therapy to determine susceptibility of causative organism. Therapy may begin pending test results.
- Monitor lab tests: Baseline C&S, weekly WBC with differential, and periodic LFTs.

### Patient & Family Education

- Take medication around the clock. Do not miss a dose and continue taking medication until it is all gone, unless otherwise directed by prescriber.
- Check with prescriber if GI side effects appear.
- Watch for and report the signs of hypersensitivity reactions and superinfections (see Appendix F).

## DICYCLOMINE HYDROCHLORIDE
(dye-sye'kloe-meen)

Bentyl, Bentylol ◆, Formulex ◆, Lomine ◆
**Classifications:** ANTICHOLINERGIC; ANTISPASMODIC
Therapeutic: GI ANTISPASMODIC
**Prototype:** Atropine

**AVAILABILITY** Capsule; tablet; syrup; solution for injection

## ACTION & *THERAPEUTIC EFFECT*

Relieves smooth muscle spasm by direct effect on the muscles as well as by antagonism of bradykinin and histamine-induced spasm in GI tract. *Exerts antispasmodic effect on the GI tract.*

Common adverse effects in *italic;* life-threatening effects underlined; generic names in **bold;** classifications in SMALL CAPS; ◆ Canadian drug name; ☻ Prototype drug

491

**USES** Irritable bowel syndrome.

**CONTRAINDICATIONS** Hypersensitivity to anticholinergic drugs; obstructive diseases of GU and GI tracts, paralytic ileus, intestinal atony, biliary tract disease; closed-angle glaucoma; unstable cardiovascular status; severe ulcerative colitis, toxic megacolon, esophagitis; myasthenia gravis; peripheral neuropathy; lactation; infants younger than 6 mo.

**CAUTIOUS USE** Prostatic hypertrophy; autonomic neuropathy; hyperthyroidism; coronary heart disease, CHF, arrhythmias, hypertension; hepatic or renal disease; GERD, hiatal hernia associated with esophageal reflux; older adults; pregnancy (category B); children.

## ROUTE & DOSAGE

**Irritable Bowel Disorders**
*Adult/Adolescent:* **PO** 20–40 mg q.i.d.; **IM** 20 mg q4–6h.

## ADMINISTRATION

**Oral**
- Give 30 min before meals and at bedtime.

**Intramuscular**
- Give deep IM into a large muscle. **Do not** give IV.
- Store below 30° C (86° F) unless otherwise directed.

**ADVERSE EFFECTS** (≥1%) **All:** Dose related. **Body as a Whole:** Allergic reactions; curare-like effect (cyanosis, apnea, respiratory arrest); decreased sweating; suppression of lactation; urticaria. **CNS:** Lightheadedness, drowsiness, headache, insomnia, brief euphoria, fever, restlessness, irritability, coma, seizures. **CV:** Fluctuations

in heart rate, palpitation, tachycardia. **GI:** *Dry mouth,* nausea, *constipation,* paralytic ileus, vomiting, diminished sense of taste, bloated feeling. **Urogenital:** Urinary hesitancy, *urinary retention,* impotence. **Special Senses:** Blurred vision.

**PHARMACOKINETICS Absorption:** Readily from GI tract. **Onset:** 1–2 h. **Duration:** 4 h. **Metabolism:** In liver. **Elimination:** 80% in urine, 10% in feces. **Half-Life:** 9–10 h.

## NURSING IMPLICATIONS

### Assessment & Drug Effects

- Monitor for adverse effects especially in infants. Treatment of infant colic with dicyclomine includes some risk, especially in infants younger than 2 mo of age. Infants younger than 6 wk have developed respiratory symptoms as well as seizures, fluctuations in heart rate, weakness, and coma within minutes after taking syrup formulation. Symptoms generally last 20–30 min and are believed to be due to local irritation.
- Monitor I&O to assess for urinary retention.
- If drug produces drowsiness and light-headedness, supervision of ambulation and other safety precautions are warranted.

### Patient & Family Education

- Exercise caution in hot weather. Dicyclomine may increase risk of heatstroke by decreasing sweating, especially in older adults.
- Do not drive or engage in other potentially hazardous activities until reaction to drug is known.
- Report changes in urine volume, voiding pattern.

## DIDANOSINE (DDI)
(di-dan′o-sine)
Videx, Videx EC

---

Common adverse effects in *italic;* life-threatening effects underlined; generic names in **bold;** classifications in SMALL CAPS; ♣ Canadian drug name; ◐ Prototype drug

**Classifications:** ANTIRETROVIRAL; NUCLEOSIDE REVERSE TRANSCRIPTASE INHIBITOR (NRTI)
Therapeutic: ANTIRETROVIRAL (NRTI)
**Prototype:** Lamivudine

**AVAILABILITY** Delayed release capsule; powder for oral solution

**ACTION & THERAPEUTIC EFFECT**
DDI interferes with the HIV RNA-dependent DNA polymerase (reverse transcriptase), thus preventing replication of the virus. *Synthetic purine nucleotide that inhibits replication of HIV.*

**USES** Advanced HIV infection in patients who are intolerant to zidovudine (AZT) or who demonstrate significant clinical or immunologic deterioration during zidovudine therapy.

**CONTRAINDICATIONS** Hypersensitivity to any of the components in the formulation; suspected or confirmed pancreatitis; lactic acidosis; severe hepatomegaly; portal hypertension; development of peripheral neuropathy; PKU; lactation.

**CAUTIOUS USE** Individuals with peripheral vascular disease, history of neuropathy, chronic pancreatitis, renal impairment, or any liver impairment; risk of liver disease; patients on sodium restriction; renal failure, renal impairment; alcoholism; older adults; gout; concurrent use with stavudine in pregnancy; pregnancy (category B).

**ROUTE & DOSAGE**

**HIV Infection**

*Adult/Adolescent/Child:* **PO**
*Weight 60 kg or more:* 400 mg tablets daily or 200 mg b.i.d.; *weight 25–60 kg:* 250 mg tablets daily or 125 mg b.i.d.; *weight 20–25 kg:* 200 mg daily

*Child/Infant (8 mo or older):*
**PO (solution)** 120 mg/m$^2$ b.i.d.
*Neonate/Infant (2 wk to younger than 8 mo):* **PO** 100 mg/m$^2$ b.i.d.

**Renal Impairment Dosage Adjustment**

Varies based on patient weight and dosage form used; see package insert

**ADMINISTRATION**
**Oral**
- Give drug on an empty stomach. Food should not be consumed within 15–30 min of drug administration.
- Give with water. **Do not** give with fruit juice or any other acid-containing liquid.
- Ensure that delayed release forms are swallowed whole. They must not be crushed or chewed.
- Mix powder for oral solution (buffered) with at least 120 mL (4 oz) of water, stir until dissolved (requires 2–3 min), and immediately swallow.
- Dosage reduction may be indicated in those with renal impairment.
- Store reconstituted liquid in a tightly closed container in refrigerator for up to 30 days.

**ADVERSE EFFECTS** (≥1%) **CV:** Palpitations, thrombophlebitis, arrhythmias, *vasodilation.* **CNS:** *Headache, dizziness, nervousness, insomnia, peripheral neuropathy,* lethargy, poor coordination, seizures. **Special Senses:** Retinal depigmentation, photophobia, blurred vision, optic neuritis, diplopia, blindness. **GI:** *Abdominal pain, nausea, vomiting, diarrhea,* constipation, stomatitis, dry mouth, pancreatitis, increased liver enzymes. **Hematologic:** Increased WBC, neutrophil, lymphocyte, and platelet counts;

---

Common adverse effects in *italic;* life-threatening effects underlined; generic names in **bold;** classifications in SMALL CAPS; ✦ Canadian drug name; ⓟ Prototype drug

493

increased Hgb, <u>thrombocytopenia</u>, ecchymosis, hemorrhage, petechiae. **Metabolic:** Hypocalcemia, hypokalemia, hypomagnesemia, hyperuricemia (asymptomatic), *hypertriglyceridemia,* <u>pancreatitis,</u> <u>lactic acidosis.</u> **Musculoskeletal:** Muscle atrophy, myalgia, arthritis, decreased strength. **Respiratory:** *Asthma, cough, dyspnea, epistaxis, rhinitis, rhinorrhea,* hypoventilation, pharyngitis, rhonchi or rales, sinusitis, congestion. **Skin:** Rash, impetigo, eczema, *pruritus, sweating,* erythema.

**INTERACTIONS Drug:** ALUMINUM- and MAGNESIUM-CONTAINING ANTACIDS may increase the aluminum- and magnesium-associated adverse effects of tablets. The effectiveness of **dapsone** in prophylaxis of *Pneumocystis carinii* pneumonia may be reduced by concomitant didanosine. May cause additive neuropathy with **zalcitabine** (ddC). Reduce dose when used with **tenofovir. Food:** Absorption is significantly decreased by food. Take on an empty stomach.

**PHARMACOKINETICS Absorption:** Rapidly absorbed from GI tract when administered to fasting patient with antacids; 23–40% reaches systemic circulation. **Peak:** 0.6–1 h. **Distribution:** Distributed primarily to body water; 21% reaches CSF; crosses placenta. **Elimination:** 36% in urine. **Half-Life:** 0.8–1.5 h.

## NURSING IMPLICATIONS

### Black Box Warning

*Didanosine has been associated with fatal and nonfatal pancreatitis, lactic acidosis, and hepatomegaly with steatosis.*

### Assessment & Drug Effects

- Monitor for S&S of pancreatitis (e.g., abdominal pain, nausea,

vomiting, elevated serum amylase). Report immediately to prescriber and withhold drug until ruled out.
- Monitor for S&S of peripheral neuropathy (e.g., numbness, tingling, burning, pain in hands or feet). Report to prescriber; dose reduction may be indicated.
- Monitor patients with renal impairment for drug toxicity and hypermagnesemia manifested by muscle weakness and confusion.
- Monitor lab tests: Periodic CBC with differential, serum electrolytes, uric acid, and lipid profile.

### Patient & Family Education

- Report immediately to prescriber any of the following: Abdominal pain, nausea, or vomiting.
- Do not breast-feed while taking this drug.

## DIETHYLPROPION HYDROCHLORIDE ⓟ

(dye-eth-il-proe'pee-on)

Nobesine ♦

**Classification:** ANOREXIANT
**Therapeutic:** ANOREXIANT
**Controlled Substance:** Schedule IV

**AVAILABILITY** Tablet; sustained release tablet

## ACTION & *THERAPEUTIC EFFECT*

Anorexigenic action is probably secondary to direct (CNS) stimulation of appetite control center in hypothalamus and limbic regions. *Suppresses appetite as a result of drug action on CNS appetite control center.*

**USES** As short-term (a few weeks) adjunct in a regimen of weight reduction based on caloric restriction in obesity management.

**CONTRAINDICATIONS** Known hypersensitivity or idiosyncrasy to sympathomimetic amines; severe hypertension, advanced arteriosclerosis, hyperthyroidism; glaucoma; history of drug abuse; agitated states; within 14 days of MAOI therapy; pulmonary hypertension.

**CAUTIOUS USE** Hypertension, valvular heart disease; cardiac arrhythmia; symptomatic cardiovascular disease; psychosis, mania, epilepsy; diabetes mellitus; older adults; renal failure or impairment; seizure disorder; pregnancy (category B); lactation. Safe use in children younger than 16 y is not known.

## ROUTE & DOSAGE

**Obesity**
*Adult/Adolescent:* PO 25 mg t.i.d.
30–60 min a.c. or 75 mg sustained
release daily midmorning

## ADMINISTRATION

### Oral
- Give on an empty stomach, 30 min–1 h before meals
- Store at 15°–30° C (59°–86° F) in well-closed container unless otherwise specified.

## ADVERSE EFFECTS (≥1%) **Body as a Whole:** Hypersensitivity (urticaria, rash, erythema); muscle pain, dyspnea, hair loss, blurred vision, severe dermatoses (chronic intoxication), increased sweating. **CNS:** Mild euphoria, restlessness, *nervousness,* dizziness, headache, irritability, hyperactivity, insomnia, drowsiness, mood changes, lethargy, increase in convulsive episodes in patients with epilepsy. **CV:** Palpitation, tachycardia, precordial pain, rise in BP. **GI:** Nausea, vomiting, diarrhea, constipation, dry mouth, unpleasant taste. **Urogenital:** Impotence, changes in libido, gynecomastia, menstrual irregularities; polyuria, dysuria.

## INTERACTIONS **Drug:** **Acetazolamide, sodium bicarbonate** decreases diethylpropion elimination; **ammonium chloride, ascorbic acid** increases diethylpropion elimination; a BARBITURATE and diethylpropion taken together may antagonize the effects of both drugs; **furazolidone** may increase blood pressure effects of AMPHETAMINES, and interaction may persist for several weeks after discontinuation of **furazolidone; guanethidine** antagonizes antihypertensive effects; MAO INHIBITORS, **selegiline** can cause hypertensive crisis (fatalities reported)—AMPHETAMINES should not be administered at the same time or within 14 days of these drugs; PHENOTHIAZINES may inhibit mood-elevating effects of AMPHETAMINES; TRICYCLIC ANTIDEPRESSANTS enhance AMPHETAMINES' effects by increasing **norepinephrine** release; BETA AGONISTS increase cardiovascular adverse effects.

## PHARMACOKINETICS **Absorption:** Readily from GI tract. **Duration:** 4 h, regular tablets; 10–14 h, sustained release. **Elimination:** In urine. **Half-Life:** 4–6 h.

## NURSING IMPLICATIONS

### Assessment & Drug Effects
- Observe patients with epilepsy closely for reduction in seizure control.
- Monitor diabetics for loss of glycemic control.
- Note: Varying degrees of psychologic and rarely physical dependence can occur.

### Patient & Family Education
- Swallow sustained release tablets whole; **do not** chew.

Common adverse effects in *italic;* life-threatening effects underlined; generic names in **bold;** classifications in SMALL CAPS; ♣ Canadian drug name; ⊕ Prototype drug

495

**D**

- Do not drive or engage in other potentially hazardous activities until reaction to drug is known.
- If diabetic, closely monitor blood glucose values.

## DIFLORASONE DIACETATE

(dye-flor'a-sone)

Florone, Florone E, Maxiflor, Psorcon

**See Appendix A-4.**

## DIFLUNISAL

(dye-floo'ni-sal)

**Classifications:** ANALGESIC, NONSTEROIDAL ANTI-INFLAMMATORY DRUG (NSAID)

Therapeutic: ANALGESIC, NSAID; ANTI-RHEUMATIC

**Prototype:** Ibuprofen

**AVAILABILITY** Tablet

### ACTION & *THERAPEUTIC EFFECT*

Has peripheral analgesic properties due to interfering with prostaglandin synthesis by inhibiting cyclooxygenase (COX) isoenzymes, COX-1 and COX-2. *Has analgesic and anti-inflammatory properties.*

**USES** Treatment of osteoarthritis and rheumatoid arthritis; mild to moderate pain.

**CONTRAINDICATIONS** Patients in whom aspirin or other NSAIDs precipitate an acute asthmatic attack (bronchospasm), urticaria, angioedema, severe rhinitis, or shock; active peptic ulcer, GI bleeding; severe salicylate hypersensitivity; treatment of perioperative pain in CABG care; pregnancy (category D third trimester).

**CAUTIOUS USE** History of upper GI disease; preexisting renal disease; impaired renal or hepatic function; alcoholics; compromised cardiac function, and other conditions associated with fluid retention; bone marrow suppression; geriatric patients; hypertension; patients who may be adversely affected by prolonged bleeding time; elderly; pregnancy (category C first and second trimester); lactation. Safe use in children younger than 12 y not established.

## ROUTE & DOSAGE

### Arthritis/Pain Conditions

*Adult:* **PO** 250–500 b.i.d. (max: 1500 mg/day)

## ADMINISTRATION

### Oral

- Give with water, milk, or food to reduce GI irritation. Food causes slight reduction in absorption rate, but does not affect total amount absorbed.
- Store at 15°–30° C (59°–86° F) in tightly closed containers unless otherwise directed.

**ADVERSE EFFECTS** (≥1%) **Body as a Whole:** Hypersensitivity syndrome (fever, chills, rash, eosinophilia, changes in renal and hepatic function, <u>anaphylactic reactions with bronchospasm</u>). **CNS:** Headache, drowsiness, insomnia, dizziness, vertigo, light-headedness, fatigue, weakness, nervousness, confusion, disorientation. **CV:** Palpitation, tachycardia, *peripheral edema.* **Special Senses:** Tinnitus, hearing loss; blurred vision, reduced visual acuity, changes in color vision, scotomas, corneal deposits, retinal disturbances. **GI:** *Nausea,* GI pain, flatulence, GI bleeding, peptic ulcer, anorexia,

Common adverse effects in *italic;* life-threatening effects <u>underlined</u>; generic names in **bold;** classifications in SMALL CAPS; ♣ Canadian drug name; ☯ Prototype drug

eructation, cholestatic jaundice. **Urogenital:** Hematuria, proteinuria, interstitial nephritis, <u>renal failure</u>. **Hematologic:** Prolonged PT, anemia, decreased serum uric acid, transient elevations of liver function tests. **Skin:** Rash, toxic epidermal necrolysis, exfoliative dermatitis, urticaria. **Other:** Weight gain, hyperventilation, dyspnea, photosensitivity.

## DIAGNOSTIC TEST INTERFERENCE
False elevation of **serum salicylate levels.**

## INTERACTIONS
**Drug:** ANTACIDS decrease diflunisal absorption; **aspirin** and other NSAIDS increase risk of GI bleeding; increases risk of **warfarin**-induced hypoprothrombinemia; increases **methotrexate** levels and toxicity.

## PHARMACOKINETICS
**Absorption:** Readily from GI tract. **Onset:** 1 h. **Peak:** 2–3 h. **Duration:** 12 h. **Distribution:** Probably crosses placenta; distributed into breast milk. **Metabolism:** In liver. **Elimination:** In urine. **Half-Life:** 8–12 h.

## NURSING IMPLICATIONS

### Black Box Warning

*Diflunisal has been associated with increased risk of serious, potentially fatal, CV thrombotic events (i.e., MI and stroke). Risk may increase with duration of use and may be greater in those with risk factors for CV disease.*

### Assessment & Drug Effects
- Monitor for and report promptly S&S of CV thrombotic events (i.e., angina, MI, TIA, or stroke).
- Note: Although the antipyretic effect is mild, chronic or high doses may mask fever in some patients.

- Monitor lab tests: Periodic Hgb and Hct, PT/INR, and renal function tests with prolonged use.

### Patient & Family Education
- Seek immediate medical attention if you experience S&S of adverse cardiovascular effects, such as chest pain, shortness of breath, weakness, or slurring of speech.
- Report to prescriber onset of visual or auditory problems.
- Check for and report peripheral edema and unusual weight gain.
- Report immediately to prescriber S&S of serious GI irritation, such as stomach pain, frequent indigestion, tarry stools, or vomiting blood.
- Be alert for S&S of adverse skin reactions. Report promptly development of rash, blisters, or other skin reactions.
- Do not drive or engage in other potentially hazardous activities until reaction to drug is known.
- Do not take aspirin or other OTC analgesics without permission of the prescriber.

## DIGOXIN ◔
(di-jox'in)
Lanoxin
**Classifications:** CARDIAC GLYCOSIDE; INOTROPIC
**Therapeutic:** CARDIAC GLYCOSIDE; ANTIARRYTHMIC

**AVAILABILITY** Tablet; oral solution; solution for injection

## ACTION & *THERAPEUTIC EFFECT*
Inhibits the sodium pump (NaK-ATPase), causing increased availability of intracellular calcium in the myocardium and conduction system, resulting in increased inotropy and automaticity, and reduced conduction velocity; indirectly causes parasympathetic stimulation of the autonomic nervous system resulting in a variety

Common adverse effects in *italic*; life-threatening effects <u>underlined</u>; generic names in **bold**; classifications in SMALL CAPS; ♣ Canadian drug name; ◔ Prototype drug

497

of effects on the CV system (e.g., decreased conduction through the AV node). *Increases contractility of heart muscle (positive inotropic effect). Has antiarrhythmic properties that result from its effects on the AV node.*

**USES** Rapid digitalization and for maintenance therapy in CHF, atrial fibrillation, atrial flutter, paroxysmal atrial tachycardia.

**CONTRAINDICATIONS** Digitalis hypersensitivity, sick sinus syndrome, Wolff-Parkinson-White syndrome; ventricular fibrillation, ventricular tachycardia unless due to CHF; hypocalcemia; myocarditis. Full digitalizing dose not given if patient has received digoxin during previous week or if slowly excreted cardiotonic glycoside has been given during previous 2 wk.

**CAUTIOUS USE** Renal insufficiency, hypokalemia, advanced heart disease, cardiomyopathy, acute MI, incomplete AV block, cor pulmonale; hypothyroidism; lung disease; older adults, or debilitated patients; pregnancy (category C); lactation; premature, children.

## ROUTE & DOSAGE

### Atrial Fibrillation/ Digitalizing Dose

Give ½ dose initially followed by ¼ at 8–12 h intervals
*Adult:* **PO** 0.75–1.5 mg;
**IV** 0.5–1 mg
*Child (2 to younger than 10 y):*
**IV** 20–35 mcg/kg; *10 y or older:*
8–12 mcg/kg; **PO** *2 to younger than 10 y:* 30–40 mcg/kg; *10 y or older:* 10–15 mcg/kg
*Infant:* **IV** 30–50 mcg/kg; **PO** 35–60 mcg/kg
*Neonate (Preterm):* **IV** 15–25 mcg/kg; *full-term:* 20–30 mcg/kg

### Maintenance Dose

*Adult/Adolescent/Child (10 y or older):* **IV** 2.4–3.6 mcg/kg/day; **PO** 3.4–5.1 mcg/kg/day
*Child (5 to younger than 10 y):* **IV** 4.6–9 mcg/kg/day in divided doses; **PO** 6.4–12 mcg/kg/day in divided doses
*Child (2–4 y):* **IV** 7.6–10.6 mcg/kg/day in divided doses
*Child (younger than 2 y):* 9–15 mcg/kg/day in divided doses

### Renal Impairment Dosing Adjustment

See package insert for adjustment based on CrCl and lean body weight

## ADMINISTRATION

### Oral

- Give without regard to food. Administration after food may slightly delay rate of absorption, but total amount absorbed is not affected.
- Crush and mix with fluid or food if patient cannot swallow it whole.

### Intravenous

*PREPARE:* **Direct:** Give undiluted or diluted in 4 mL of sterile water, D5W, or NS (using less diluent than 4 mL per 1 mL digoxin may cause precipitation).
*ADMINISTER:* **Direct:** Give each dose over at least 5 min. ▪ Monitor IV site frequently. Infiltration of parenteral drug into subcutaneous tissue can cause local irritation and sloughing.
*INCOMPATIBILITIES:* **Solution/additive: Dobutamine. Y-site: Amiodarone, amphotericin B cholesteryl complex, capsofungin, dantrolene, daunorubicin, diazepam, diazoxide, doxorubicin, fluconazole, foscarnet, gemtuzumab, idarubicin,**

Common adverse effects in *italic;* life-threatening effects <u>underlined</u>; generic names in **bold;** classifications in SMALL CAPS; ♣ Canadian drug name; ⊙ Prototype drug

**D**

lansoprazole, minocycline, mitoxantrone, paclitaxel, pentamidine, phenytoin, propofol, quinipristin/dalfopristin, sulfamethoxazole/trimethoprim, telavancin, propofol.

▪ Store tablets, elixir, and injection solution at 25° C (77° F) or at 15°–30° C (59°–86° F).

## ADVERSE EFFECTS (≥1%) CNS: Fatigue, muscle weakness, headache, facial neuralgia, mental depression, paresthesias, hallucinations, confusion, drowsiness, agitation, dizziness. CV: Arrhythmias, hypotension, AV block. Special Senses: Visual disturbances. GI: Anorexia, *nausea*, vomiting, diarrhea. Other: Diaphoresis, recurrent malaise, dysphagia.

## INTERACTIONS Drug: ANTACIDS, cholestyramine, colestipol decrease digoxin absorption; DIURETICS, CORTICOSTEROIDS, amphotericin B, LAXATIVES, sodium polystyrene sulfonate may cause hypokalemia, increasing the risk of digoxin toxicity; calcium IV may increase risk of arrhythmias if administered together with digoxin, quinidine, verapamil, amiodarone, atorvastatin, captoril, diltiazem, erythromycin, alprazolam, BETA BLOCKERS, cyclosporine, ranolazine, ssris, telmisartan flecainide significantly increase digoxin levels, and digoxin dose should be decreased; succinylcholine may potentiate arrhythmogenic effects; nefazodone may increase digoxin levels. Food: High fiber intake may decrease absorption. Herbal: Ginseng increase digoxin toxicity; ma huang, ephedra may induce arrhythmias; St. John's wort decreases plasma concentration. Lab Test: Panax ginseng can falsely elevate concentrations with fluorescence polarization immunoassay (FPIA) or falsely lower concentrations with microparticle enzyme immunoassay (MEIA).

## PHARMACOKINETICS Absorption: 70% Onset: 1–2 h PO; 5–30 min IV. Peak: 6–8 h PO; 1–5 h IV. Duration: 3–4 days in fully digitalized patient. Distribution: Widely distributed; tissue levels significantly higher than plasma levels; crosses placenta. Metabolism: 14% in liver. Elimination: 80–90% by kidneys; may appear in breast milk. Half-Life: 34–44 h.

## NURSING IMPLICATIONS
### Assessment & Drug Effects
▪ Take apical pulse for 1 full min, noting rate, rhythm, and quality before administering drug.
▪ Withhold medication and notify prescriber if apical pulse falls below ordered parameters (e.g., less than 50 or 60/min in adults and less than 60 or 70/min in children).
▪ Be familiar with patient's baseline data (e.g., quality of peripheral pulses, blood pressure, clinical symptoms, serum electrolytes, creatinine clearance) as a foundation for making assessments.
▪ Monitor for S&S of drug toxicity: In children, cardiac arrhythmias are usually reliable signs of early toxicity. Early indicators in adults (anorexia, nausea, vomiting, diarrhea, visual disturbances) are rarely initial signs in children.
▪ Monitor I&O ratio during digitalization, particularly in patients with impaired renal function. Also monitor for edema daily and auscultate chest for rales.
▪ Monitor serum digoxin levels closely during concurrent antibiotic–digoxin therapy, which can precipitate toxicity because of altered intestinal flora.

D

- Observe patients closely when being transferred from one preparation (tablet, parenteral) to another.
- Monitor lab tests: Baseline and periodic serum digoxin, potassium, magnesium, and calcium.

**Patient & Family Education**

- Report to prescriber if pulse falls below 60 or rises above 110 or if you detect skipped beats or other changes in rhythm, when digoxin is prescribed for atrial fibrillation.
- Suspect toxicity and report to prescriber if any of the following occur: Anorexia, nausea, vomiting, diarrhea, or visual disturbances.
- Weigh each day under standard conditions. Report weight gain greater than 1 kg (2 lb)/day.
- Take digoxin PRECISELY as prescribed. Do not skip or double a dose or change dose intervals, and take it at same time each day.
- Do not take OTC medications, especially those for coughs, colds, allergy, GI upset, or obesity, without prior approval of prescriber.
- Continue with brand originally prescribed unless otherwise directed by prescriber.

# DIGOXIN IMMUNE FAB (OVINE)

(di-jox'in)

Digibind, DigiFab

**Classification:** ANTIDOTE
**Therapeutic:** ANTIDOTE

**AVAILABILITY** Solution for injection

## ACTION & *THERAPEUTIC EFFECT*

Fab acts by selectively complexing with circulating digoxin or digitoxin, thereby preventing drug from binding at receptor sites; the complex is then eliminated in urine. *Used as an antidote for digitalis toxicity.*

**USES** Treatment of potentially life-threatening digoxin or digitoxin intoxication in carefully selected patients.

**CONTRAINDICATIONS** Hypersensitivity to sheep products; renal or cardiac failure.

**CAUTIOUS USE** Prior treatment with sheep antibodies or ovine Fab fragments; mannitol hypersensitivity; history of allergies; impaired renal function or renal failure; older adults; pregnancy (category C); lactation.

## ROUTE & DOSAGE

**Serious Digoxin Toxicity Secondary to Overdose**

*Adult/Child:* **IV** Dosages vary according to amount of digoxin to be neutralized; dosages are based on total body load or steady state serum digoxin concentrations (see package insert); some patients may require a second dose after several hours

## ADMINISTRATION

**Intravenous**

**PREPARE: Direct:** Dilute each vial with 4 mL of sterile water for injection to yield 9.5 mg/mL for Digibind and 10 mg/mL for DigiFab; mix gently. **IV Infusion:** Dilute further with any volume of NS compatible with cardiac status. ▪ For those receiving less than 3 mg, further dilute to a concentration of 1 mg/mL by adding an additional 34 mL of NS to Digibind or 36 mL of NS to DigiFab. ▪ For very small doses for infants, reconstitute to a concentration of 10 mg/mL.
**ADMINISTER: Direct:** Give undiluted bolus only if cardiac arrest is

imminent. **IV Infusion:** Give IV infusion over 30 min, preferably through a 0.22-micron membrane filter if Digibind is being infused. ▪ For administration to infants: Reconstitute as for direct IV and administer with a tuberculin syringe. ▪ For small doses (e.g., 2 mg or less), dilute the reconstituted 40 mg vial with 36 mL of NS to yield 1 mg/mL. ▪ Closely monitor for fluid overload.

▪ Use reconstituted solutions promptly or refrigerate at 2°–8° C (36°–46° F) for up to 4 h.

## ADVERSE EFFECTS (>1%)
Adverse reactions associated with use of digoxin immune Fab are related primarily to the effects of **digitalis** withdrawal on the heart (see Nursing Implications). Allergic reactions have been reported rarely. Hypokalemia.

## DIAGNOSTIC TEST INTERFERENCE
Digoxin immune Fab may interfere with **serum digoxin** determinations by immunoassay tests.

## PHARMACOKINETICS
**Onset:** Less than 1 min after IV administration. **Elimination:** In urine over 5–7 days. **Half-Life:** 14–20 h.

## NURSING IMPLICATIONS

### Assessment & Drug Effects
▪ Perform skin testing for allergy prior to administration of immune Fab, particularly in patients with history of allergy or who have had previous therapy with immune Fab.
▪ Keep emergency equipment and drugs immediately available before skin testing is done or first dose is given and until patient is out of danger.
▪ Monitor for therapeutic effectiveness: Reflected in improvement in cardiac rhythm abnormalities, mental orientation and other neurologic symptoms, and GI and visual disturbances. S&S of reversal of digitalis toxicity occurs in 15–60 min in adults and usually within minutes in children.
▪ Baseline and frequent vital signs and EGG during administration.
▪ Note: Serum potassium is particularly critical during first several hours following administration of immune Fab. Monitor closely.
▪ Monitor closely: Cardiac status may deteriorate as inotropic action of digitalis is withdrawn by action of immune Fab. CHF, arrhythmias, increase in heart rate, and hypokalemia can occur.
▪ Make sure serum digoxin levels and ECG readings are obtained for at least 2–3 wk.
▪ Monitor lab tests: Baseline serum digoxin and serum creatinine; baseline serum potassium, then hourly for 4–6 hr, and at least daily thereafter.

### Patient & Family Education
▪ Tell prescriber about all other medications you are taking, including non-prescription medications, nutritional supplements, or herbal products.
▪ Check with your prescriber before stopping or starting any of your medicines.

## DIHYDROERGOTAMINE MESYLATE
(dye-hye-droe-er-got'a-meen)
D.H.E. 45, Migranal
**Classifications:** ALPHA-ADRENERGIC ANTAGONIST; ERGOT ALKALOID
**Therapeutic:** ANTIMIGRAINE
**Prototype:** Ergotamine

Common adverse effects in *italic*; life-threatening effects underlined; generic names in **bold**; classifications in SMALL CAPS; ♣ Canadian drug name; ⊚ Prototype drug

501

# DIHYDROERGOTAMINE MESYLATE

**AVAILABILITY** Nasal spray; solution for injection

## ACTION & *THERAPEUTIC EFFECT*
Alpha-adrenergic blocking agent and ergot alkaloid with direct constricting effect on smooth muscle of peripheral and cranial blood vessels. Acts as selective serotonin agonists at the 5-HT$_1$ receptors located on intracranial blood vessels, which may also cause vasoconstriction of large intracranial conductance arteries; this correlates with relief of migraine headaches. *Reduces rate of serotonin-induced platelet aggregation. Has somewhat weaker vasoconstrictor action than ergotamine but greater adrenergic blocking activity, resulting in relief from migraine headaches.*

**USES** To prevent or abort headache or migraine.

**UNLABELED USES** To treat postural hypotension.

**CONTRAINDICATIONS** History of hypersensitivity to ergot preparations; peripheral vascular disease, coronary heart disease, MI, hypertension; peptic ulcer; severely impaired hepatic or renal function; sepsis; concurrent treatment with potent CYP3A4 inhibitors, including protease inhibitors, and macrolide antibiotics; within 48 h of surgery; pregnancy (category X); lactation.

**CAUTIOUS USE** Moderate or mild renal or hepatic impairment; obesity; diabetes mellitus; postmenopausal women; males older than 40 y; pulmonary heart disease; valvular heart disease; smokers. Safe use in children younger than 6 y is not established.

## ROUTE & DOSAGE

**Migraine Headache**
*Adult:* **IV/IM/Subcutaneous** 1 mg, may be repeated at 1 h intervals to a total of 3 mg **IM** or 2 mg **IV/Subcutaneous** (max: 6 mg/wk); **Intranasal** 1 spray (0.5 mg) in each nostril, may repeat with additional spray in 15 min if no relief (max: 4 sprays/attack); wait 6–8 h before treating another attack (max: 8 sprays/24 h, 24 sprays/wk)

## ADMINISTRATION

**Intranasal**
- Give at first warning of migraine headache.

**Intramuscular/Subcutaneous**
- Give at first warning of migraine headache.
- Withdraw IM or subcutaneous dose directly from ampule. Do not dilute.
- Note: Onset of action is about 20 min; when rapid relief is required, the IV route is prescribed.

**Intravenous**

*PREPARE:* **Direct:** Give undiluted.
*ADMINISTER:* **Direct:** Give at a rate of 1 mg/60 sec.

- Store at 15°–30° C (59°–86° F) unless otherwise directed. ▪ Protect ampules from heat and light; do not freeze. ▪ Discard ampule if solution appears discolored.

**ADVERSE EFFECTS** (≥1%) **CV** Vaso-spasm: Coldness, numbness and tingling in fingers and toes, muscle pains and weakness of legs, precordial distress and pain, transient tachycardia or bradycardia, hypertension (large doses). **GI:** *Nausea, vomiting.* **Body as a**

**Whole:** Dizziness, dysphoria, *localized edema and itching;* ergotism (excessive doses).

### INTERACTIONS Drug: BETA-BLOCKERS, **erythromycin** increase peripheral vasoconstriction with risk of ischemia; increased **ergotamine** toxicity with drugs that inhibit CYP3A4 (e.g., PROTEASE INHIBITORS, **amprenavir, ritonavir, nelfinavir, indinavir, saquinavir**), MACROLIDE ANTIBIOTICS **(erythromycin, azithromycin, clarithromycin),** AZOLE ANTIFUNGALS **(ketoconazole, itraconazole, fluconazole, clotrimazole), nefazodone, fluoxetine, fluvoxamine. Food:** Grapefruit juice may increase toxicity.

### PHARMACOKINETICS Onset:
15–30 min IM; less than 5 min IV. **Duration:** 3–4 h. **Distribution:** Probably distributed into breast milk. **Metabolism:** In liver by CYP3A4. **Elimination:** Primarily in urine; some in feces. **Half-Life:** 21–32 h.

### NURSING IMPLICATIONS

#### Black Box Warning

*Serious and life-threatening peripheral ischemia have been associated with concurrent administration of dihydroergotamine with potent CYP3A4 inhibitors such as protease inhibitors and macrolide antibiotics.*

#### Assessment & Drug Effects
- Monitor cardiac status, especially when large doses are given.
- Monitor for and report numbness and tingling of fingers and toes, extremity weakness, muscle pain, or intermittent claudication.

#### Patient & Family Education
- Take at first warning of migraine headache.

- Lie down in a quiet, darkened room for several hours after drug administration for best results.
- Report immediately if any of the following S&S develop: Chest pain, nausea, vomiting, change in heartbeat, numbness, tingling, pain or weakness of extremities, edema, or itching.
- Women should use effective means of contraception while using this drug. Notify prescriber if you become pregnant.

---

## DILTIAZEM
(dil tye'a-zem)

Cardizem, Cardizem CD, Cardizem LA, Cartia XT, Dilacor XR, Dilt-CD, Dilt-XR, Matzim LA, Taztia XT, Tiazac

**Classifications:** CALCIUM CHANNEL BLOCKING AGENT; ANTIANGINAL; ANTIHYPERTENSIVE
**Therapeutic:** ANTIANGINAL; ANTIARRHYTHMIC; ANTIHYPERSENSITIVE
**Prototype:** Verapamil

### AVAILABILITY
Tablet; sustained release tablet; extended release capsule; extended release tablet; solution for injection

### ACTION & *THERAPEUTIC EFFECT*
Inhibits calcium ion influx through slow channels into cell of myocardial and arterial smooth muscle. Improves myocardial perfusion, and reduces left ventricular workload. *Slows SA and AV node conduction (antiarrhythmic effect). Dilates coronary arteries and arterioles and inhibits coronary artery spasm; thus myocardial oxygen delivery is increased (antianginal effect). By vasodilation of peripheral arterioles, drug decreases total peripheral vascular resistance and reduces arterial BP at rest (antihypertensive effect).*

---

Common adverse effects in *italic;* life-threatening effects underlined; generic names in **bold;** classifications in SMALL CAPS; ♣ Canadian drug name; ⊙ Prototype drug

503

**USES** Vasospastic angina (Prinzmetal's variant or at rest angina), chronic stable (classic effort-associated) angina, essential hypertension. **IV form:** Atrial fibrillation, atrial flutter, supraventricular tachycardia.

**UNLABELED USES** Prevention of reinfarction in non-Q-wave MI.

**CONTRAINDICATIONS** Known hypersensitivity to drug; sick sinus syndrome (unless pacemaker is in place and functioning); acute MI; pulmonary congestion; severe hypotension (systolic less than 90 mm Hg or diastolic less than 60 mm Hg); heart failure; patients undergoing intracranial surgery; bleeding aneurysms; lactation.

**CAUTIOUS USE** Sinoatrial nodal dysfunction, sick sinus syndrome with functioning pacemaker; left ventricular dysfunction, CHF, severe bradycardia; hypertrophic obstructive cardiomyopathy; conduction abnormalities; renal or hepatic impairment; older adults; pregnancy (category C); children.

## ROUTE & DOSAGE

### Angina
*Adult:* **PO** 30 mg q.i.d., may increase q1–2 days as required (usual range: 180–360 mg/day in divided doses); **PO Extended release** 120–180 mg daily **PO (Cardizem LA)** 180 mg daily

### Hypertension
*Adult/Adolescent:* **PO Extended release (once daily formulations)** 120–240 mg daily or 20–120 mg b.i.d

### Atrial Fibrillation/Flutter
*Adult:* **IV** 0.25 mg/kg IV bolus over 2 min, if inadequate response, may repeat in 15 min with 0.35 mg/kg, followed by a continuous infusion of 5–10 mg/h (max: 15 mg/h for 24 h)

## ADMINISTRATION

### Oral
- Do not crush sustained release capsules or tablets. They **must be** swallowed whole.
- Withhold if systolic BP is less than 90 mm Hg or diastolic is less than 60 mm Hg.
- Give before meals and at bedtime.
- Store at 15°–30° C (59°–86° F).

### Intravenous

***PREPARE:*** **Direct:** Give undiluted. **Continuous:** For IV infusion, add to a volume of D5W, NS, or D5/0.45% NaCl (e.g., 100–500 mL) that can be administered in 24 h or less.

***ADMINISTER:*** **Direct:** Give as a bolus dose over 2 min. A second bolus may be given after 15 min. **Continuous:** Give at a rate 10–15 mg/h. Infusion duration longer than 24 h and infusion rate greater than 15 mg/h are not recommended.

***INCOMPATIBILITIES:*** **Y-site: Acetazolamide, acyclovir, allopurinol, aminophylline, amphotericin B, ampicillin, ampicillin/sulbactam, cefepime, cefoperazone, ceftobiprole, chloramphenicol, dantrolene, diazepam, doxorubicin, fluorouracil, furosemide, ganciclovir, gemtuzumab, heparin, hydrocortisone, insulin, ketorolac, lansoprazole, methotrexate, methylprednisolone, micafungin, mitomycin, nafcillin, pantoprazole, pentobarbital, phenobarbital, phenytoin, piperacillin/tazobactam, procainamide, rifampin, sodium bicarbonate.**

## ADVERSE EFFECTS (≥1%) CNS:
*Headache,* fatigue, dizziness, asthenia,

D

drowsiness, nervousness, insomnia, confusion, tremor, gait abnormality. **CV:** Edema, arrhythmias, angina, second- or third-degree AV block, bradycardia, CHF, flushing, hypotension, syncope, palpitations. **GI:** Nausea, constipation, anorexia, vomiting, diarrhea, impaired taste, weight increase. **Skin:** Rash.

## INTERACTIONS
**Drug:** BETA-BLOCKERS, **digoxin** may have additive effects on av node conduction prolongation; may increase **digoxin** or **quinidine** levels; **cimetidine** may increase diltiazem levels, thus increasing effects; may increase **cyclosporine** levels. May increase STATIN levels, monitor closely. Do not use more than 10 mg of **simvastatin** concurrently. Do not use with **lomidapide**. **Herbal:** Monitor carefully if used with hawthorn.

## PHARMACOKINETICS
**Absorption:** Approximately 80% from GI tract, with 40% reaching systemic circulation. **Peak:** 2–3 h; 6–11 h sustained release; 11–18 h Cardizem LA. **Distribution:** Into breast milk. **Metabolism:** In liver (CYP3A4). **Elimination:** Primarily in urine with some elimination in feces. **Half-Life:** Oral 3.5–9 h, IV 2 h.

## NURSING IMPLICATIONS
### Assessment & Drug Effects
- Check BP and ECG before initiation of therapy and monitor particularly during dosage adjustment period.
- Monitor for and report S&S of CHF.
- Monitor for headache. An analgesic may be required.
- Supervise ambulation as indicated.

### Patient & Family Education
- Make position changes slowly and in stages; light-headedness and dizziness (hypotension) are possible.
- Do not drive or engage in other potentially hazardous activities until reaction to drug is known.

## DIMENHYDRINATE
(dye-men-hye'dri-nate)
Calm-X, Dimenhydrinate Injection, Dramamine
**Classifications:** ANTIHISTAMINE (H₁-RECEPTOR ANTAGONIST); ANTIVERTIGO
**Therapeutic:** ANTIVERTIGO; ANTIEMETIC
**Prototype:** Diphenhydramine

**AVAILABILITY** Tablet; chewable tablet; solution for injection; liquid

## ACTION & THERAPEUTIC EFFECT
H₁-receptor antagonist with antiemetic action thought to involve ability to inhibit cholinergic stimulation in vestibular and associated neural pathways. *Has antiemetic and antivertigo activity.*

**USES** Chiefly in prevention and treatment of motion sickness. Also has been used in management of vertigo, nausea, and vomiting associated with radiation sickness, labyrinthitis, Ménière's syndrome, stapedectomy, anesthesia, and various medications.

**CONTRAINDICATIONS** Narrow-angle glaucoma, BPH; GI obstruction; urinary tract obstruction; CNS depression; lactation; neonates.

**CAUTIOUS USE** Convulsive disorders; asthma; COPD; severe hepatic disease; PKU; history of porphyria; closed-angle glaucoma; older adults; pregnancy (category B). Safe use in children younger than 2 y not established.

## ROUTE & DOSAGE

**Motion Sickness**
*Adult:* **PO** 50–100 mg q4–6h (max: 400 mg/24 h); **IV/IM** 50 mg as needed

*Child (2–6 y):* **PO** up to 25 mg q6–8h (max: 75 mg/24 h); *6–12 y:* 25–50 mg q6–8h (max: 150 mg/24 h); **IM** 1.25 mg/kg q.i.d. up to 300 mg/day

## ADMINISTRATION

- First dose should be given 30–60 min before starting activity.

### Oral

- Ensure that chewable tablets are chewed and not swallowed whole.

### Intramuscular

- Give undiluted and inject deep IM into a large muscle.

### Intravenous

**PREPARE: Direct:** Dilute each 50 mg in 10 mL of NS.

**ADMINISTER: Direct:** Give each 50 mg or fraction thereof over 2 min.

**INCOMPATIBILITIES: Solution/additive: Aminophylline, amobarbital, chlorpromazine, glycopyrrolate, hydrocortisone, hydroxyzine, pentobarbital, phenobarbital, phenytoin, prochlorperazine, promazine, promethazine.**

- Store preferably at 15°–30° C (59°–86° F), unless otherwise directed by manufacturer. • Examine parenteral preparation for particulate matter and discoloration. Do not use unless absolutely clear.

## ADVERSE EFFECTS (≥1%) CNS:
*Drowsiness,* headache, incoordination, dizziness, blurred vision, nervousness, restlessness, *insomnia (especially children).* **CV:** Hypotension, palpitation. **GI:** Dry mouth, nose, throat; anorexia, constipation or diarrhea. **Urogenital:** Urinary frequency, dysuria.

## DIAGNOSTIC TEST INTERFERENCE
***Skin testing*** procedures should not be performed within 72 h after use of an antihistamine.

## INTERACTIONS Drug: Alcohol
and other CNS DEPRESSANTS enhance CNS depression, drowsiness; TRICYCLIC ANTIDEPRESSANTS compound anticholinergic effects.

## PHARMACOKINETICS Absorption: Readily absorbed from GI tract. **Onset:** 15–30 min PO; immediate IV; 20–30 min IM. **Duration:** 3–6 h. **Distribution:** Distributed into breast milk. **Elimination:** In urine.

## NURSING IMPLICATIONS

### Assessment & Drug Effects

- Use fall precautions and supervise ambulation; drug produces high incidence of drowsiness.
- Note: Tolerance to CNS depressant effects usually occurs after a few days of drug therapy; some decrease in antiemetic action may result with prolonged use.
- Monitor for dizziness, nausea, and vomiting; these may indicate drug toxicity.

### Patient & Family Education

- Do not drive or engage in other potentially hazardous activities until response to drug is known.
- Take 30–60 min before departure to prevent motion sickness; repeat before meals and upon retiring.

## DIMERCAPROL
(dye-mer-kap′role)
BAL in Oil

**Classifications:** CHELATING AGENT; ANTIDOTE

Therapeutic: ANTIDOTE

**AVAILABILITY** Solution for injection

## ACTION & *THERAPEUTIC EFFECT*
Combines with ions of various heavy metals to form relatively

stable, nontoxic, soluble complexes called chelates, which can be excreted; inhibition of enzymes by toxic metals is thus prevented. *Neutralizes the effects of various heavy metals.*

**USES** Acute poisoning by arsenic, gold, and mercury; as adjunct to edetate calcium disodium (EDTA) in treatment of lead encephalopathy.

**UNLABELED USES** Chromium dermatitis; ocular and dermatologic manifestations of arsenic poisoning, as adjunct to penicillamine to increase rate of copper excretion in Wilson's disease, and for poisoning with heavy metals.

**CONTRAINDICATIONS** Hepatic insufficiency (with exception of postarsenical jaundice); history of peanut oil hypersensitivity; severe renal insufficiency; poisoning due to cadmium, iron, selenium, or uranium; lactation

**CAUTIOUS USE** Hypertension; oliguria; patients with G6PD deficiency; preexisting renal disease; rheumatoid arthritis; pregnancy (category C).

## ROUTE & DOSAGE

### Arsenic or Gold Poisoning
*Adult/Child.* **IM** 2.5–3 mg/kg q4h for first 2 days, then q.i.d. on third day, then b.i.d. for 10 days

### Mercury Poisoning
*Adult/Child:* **IM** 5 mg/kg initially, followed by 2.5 mg/kg 1–2 × day for 10 days

### Acute Lead Encephalopathy
*Adult/Child:* **IM** 4 mg/kg initially, then 3–4 mg/kg q4h with EDTA for 2–7 days depending on response

## ADMINISTRATION

**Intramuscular**
- Initiate therapy ASAP (within 1–2 h) after ingestion of the poison because irreversible tissue damage occurs quickly, particularly in mercury poisoning.
- Give by deep IM injection only. Local pain, gluteal abscess, and skin sensitization possible. Rotate injection sites and observe daily.
- Determine if a local anesthetic may be given with the injection to decrease injection site pain.
- Handle with caution; contact of drug with skin may produce erythema, edema, dermatitis.

**ADVERSE EFFECTS** (≥1%) **CNS:** Headache, anxiety, muscle pain or weakness, restlessness, paresthesias, tremors, *convulsions, shock* **CV:** *Elevated BP,* tachycardia. **Special Senses:** Rhinorrhea; burning sensation, feeling of pain and constriction in throat. **GI:** Nausea, *vomiting;* burning sensation in lips and mouth, halitosis, salivation; abdominal pain, metabolic acidosis. **Urogenital:** Burning sensation in penis, renal damage. **Other:** Pain in chest or hands, pain and sterile abscess at injection site, sweating, reduction in polymorphonuclear leukocytes, dental pain.

**DIAGNOSTIC TEST INTERFERENCE** $I^{131}$ *thyroid uptake* values may be decreased if test is done during or immediately following dimercaprol therapy.

**INTERACTIONS Drug:** Iron, **cadmium, selenium, uranium** form toxic complexes with dimercaprol.

**PHARMACOKINETICS Peak:** 30–60 min. **Distribution:** Distributed mainly in intracellular spaces, including brain; highest concentrations in liver and kidneys. **Elimination:** Completely excreted in urine and bile within 4 h. **Half-Life:** Short.

---

Common adverse effects in *italic;* life-threatening effects underlined; generic names in **bold**; classifications in SMALL CAPS; ✦ Canadian drug name; ⊕ Prototype drug

507

## NURSING IMPLICATIONS

### Assessment & Drug Effects

- Monitor vital signs. Elevations of systolic and diastolic BPs accompanied by tachycardia frequently occur within a few minutes following injection and may remain elevated up to 2 h.
- Note: Fever occurs in approximately 30% of children receiving treatment and may persist throughout therapy.
- Monitor I&O. Drug is potentially nephrotoxic. Report oliguria or change in I&O ratio to prescriber.
- Check urine daily for albumin, blood, casts, and pH. Blood and urinary levels of the metal serve as guides for dosage adjustments.
- Minor adverse reactions generally reach maximum 15–20 min after drug administration and subside in 30–90 min.

### Patient & Family Education

- Drink as much fluid as the prescriber will permit.

## DIMETHYL FUMARATE

(dye-meth'il fue'ma-rate)

Tecfidera

**Classifications:** NEUROPROTECTIVE; ANTI-INFLAMMATORY

Therapeutic: NEUROPROTECTIVE; ANTI-INFLAMMATORY

**AVAILABILITY** Delayed release capsule

## ACTION & *THERAPEUTIC EFFECT*

Mechanism of action is unknown but believed to be associated with activation of a pathway involved in the cellular response to oxidative stress. *DMF decreases inflammation in neurologic tissue thus exerting a protective effect.*

**USES** Treatment of patients who have relapsing forms of multiple sclerosis.

**CONTRAINDICATIONS** Serious infections.

**CAUTIOUS USE** Drug-related lymphopenia; QT prolongation; pregnancy (category C); lactation.

## ROUTE & DOSAGE

| Multiple Sclerosis |
|---|
| *Adult:* **PO** 120 mg b.i.d. for 7 days, then 240 mg b.i.d. |

## ADMINISTRATION

### Oral

- May be given irrespective of food.
- Capsules **must be** swallowed whole. They should not be opened or chewed.
- Store at 15°–30° C (59°–86° F). Protect from light.

**ADVERSE EFFECTS** (>2%) **Body as a Whole:** *Flushing, infection.* **GI:** *Abdominal pain, diarrhea,* dyspepsia, *nausea, vomiting.* **Hematological:** Lymphopenia. **Metabolic:** ALT/AST increased. **Skin:** Erythema, pruritus, rash.

**PHARMACOKINETICS Peak:** 2–2.5 h. **Distribution:** 27–45% plasma protein bound. **Metabolism:** In liver to active metabolite, monomethyl fumarate (MMF). **Elimination:** Exhalation of $CO_2$ (60%) and renal (16%). **Half-Life:** 1 h.

## NURSING IMPLICATIONS

### Assessment & Drug Effects

- Monitor response to therapy.
- Monitor for adverse events: Flushing and GI reactions (abdominal pain, diarrhea, and nausea) are

Common adverse effects in *italic;* life-threatening effects <u>underlined;</u> generic names in **bold;** classifications in SMALL CAPS; ♣ Canadian drug name; ◎ Prototype drug the most common reactions, especially in early therapy, and may decrease over time.

- Monitor lab tests: Baseline CBC (within first 6 mo), then annually thereafter.

### Patient & Family Education

- Store in original container.
- Discard opened container of medication after 90 days.
- Inform prescriber if you are pregnant or plan to become pregnant.

# DIMETHYL SULFOXIDE

(dye-meth′il sul-fox′ide)

**DMSO, Rimso-50**

**Classifications:** GENITOURINARY; LOCAL ANTI-INFLAMMATORY

**Therapeutic:** INTERSTITIAL CYSTITIS AGENT

## AVAILABILITY Solution

## ACTION & *THERAPEUTIC EFFECT*

Reported effects include anti-inflammatory effects, membrane penetration, collagen dissolution, vasodilation, muscle relaxation, diuresis, initiation of histamine release at administration site, cholinesterase inhibition. *Has symptomatic relief of interstitial cystitis with local anti-inflammatory properties.*

## USES Symptomatic treatment of interstitial cystitis.

## UNLABELED USES Topical treatment of a variety of musculoskeletal disorders, arthritis, scleroderma, tendinitis, breast and prostate malignancies, retinitis pigmentosa, herpesvirus infections, head and spinal cord injuries, shock, and as a carrier to enhance penetration and absorption of other drugs. Also used to protect living cells and tissues during cold storage (cryoprotection). Widely used as an industrial solvent and in veterinary medicine for treatment of musculoskeletal injuries.

## CONTRAINDICATIONS Urinary tract malignancy; lactation.

## CAUTIOUS USE Hepatic or renal dysfunction; pregnancy (category C). Safe use in children is not established.

## ROUTE & DOSAGE

### Interstitial Cystitis

*Adult:* **Instillation** 50 mL of 50% solution instilled slowly into urinary bladder and retained for 15 min; may repeat q2wk until maximum relief obtained, then increase intervals between treatments

## ADMINISTRATION

### Instillation

- Apply analgesic lubricant such as lidocaine jelly to urethra to facilitate insertion of catheter.
- Instruct patient to retain instillation for 15 min and then expel it by spontaneous voiding.
- Note: Discomfort associated with instillation usually lessens with repeated administration. Prescriber may prescribe an oral analgesic or suppository containing belladonna and an opiate prior to instillation to reduce bladder spasm.
- Store at 15°–30° C (59°–86° F) unless otherwise directed. Protect from strong light. Avoid contact with plastics.

## ADVERSE EFFECTS (≥1%) **Special Senses:** Transient disturbances in color vision, photophobia. **GI:** Nausea, diarrhea. Hypersensitivity: Local or generalized rash, erythema, pruritus, urticaria, swelling of face, dyspnea (<u>anaphylactoid reaction</u>). **Other:** Nasal congestion, headache, sedation, drowsiness. **Following instillation:** *Garlic-like odor on*

Common adverse effects in *italic;* life-threatening effects <u>underlined</u>; generic names in **bold;** classifications in SMALL CAPS; ✦ Canadian drug name; ⊘ Prototype drug

509

**D**

*breath and skin; garlic-like taste;* discomfort during administration; transient cystitis. **Following topical application:** Vesicle formation.

**INTERACTIONS Drug:** Decreases effectiveness of **sulindac,** possibly causing severe peripheral neuropathy.

**PHARMACOKINETICS Absorption:** Readily absorbed systemically. **Peak:** 4–8 h. **Distribution:** Widely distributed in tissues and body fluids; penetrates blood–brain barrier; distributed into breast milk. **Metabolism:** Metabolized to dimethyl sulfide (garlic breath) and dimethyl sulfone. **Elimination:** Dimethyl sulfide excreted through lungs and skin; dimethyl sulfone may remain in serum longer than 2 wk and is excreted in urine and feces.

**NURSING IMPLICATIONS**

**Assessment & Drug Effects**

▪ Monitor and report level of bladder discomfort. In cases of severe discomfort prescriber may elect to do instillation under anesthesia.
▪ Monitor for visual disturbances. Complete eye evaluation, including slit-lamp examination, is recommended prior to and at regular intervals during therapy.

**Patient & Family Education**

▪ Note: Garlic-like taste may be experienced within minutes after drug instillation and may last for several hours. Garlic-like odor on breath and skin may last as long as 72 h.

## DINOPROSTONE (PGE₂, PROSTAGLANDIN E₂)
(dye-noe-prost'one)
Cervidil, Prostin E₂, Prepidil

**Classification:** OXYTOCIC
Therapeutic: PROSTAGLANDIN;
OXYTOCIC
**Prototype:** Oxytocin

**AVAILABILITY** Vaginal suppository; **Prepidil:** Vaginal gel; **Cervidil:** Vaginal insert

**ACTION & THERAPEUTIC EFFECT**
Synthetic prostaglandin E₂ that appears to act directly on myometrium and vascular smooth muscle. Stimulation of gravid uterus in early weeks of gestation is more potent than that of oxytocin. *Contractions are qualitatively similar to those that occur during term labor. Has high success rate when used as abortifacient before twentieth week and for stimulation of labor in cases of intrauterine fetal death.*

**USES** To terminate pregnancy from twelfth week through second trimester; cervical ripening prior to labor induction.

**CONTRAINDICATIONS** Acute pelvic inflammatory disease; abnormal fetal position; history of pelvic surgery, cervical stenosis, active cardiac, pulmonary, renal, or hepatic disease.

**CAUTIOUS USE** History of hypertension, hypotension, asthma, epilepsy, anemia, diabetes mellitus; jaundice, history of hepatic, renal, or cardiovascular disease; glaucoma or raised intraocular pressure; cervicitis, acute vaginitis, infected endocervical lesion; previous history of caesarean section; pregnancy (category C). Safety and efficacy in children or adolescents not established.

**ROUTE & DOSAGE**

**Induction of Labor**
*Adult:* **Endocervical** Place **Prepidil** 0.5 mg endocervically, may

Common adverse effects in *italic;* life-threatening effects underlined; generic names in **bold;** classifications in SMALL CAPS; ♣ Canadian drug name; ⊙ Prototype drug

repeat q6h (max: 1.5 mg); place **Cervidil** insert 10 mg transversely in the posterior fornix of the vagina, remove on onset of active labor or 12 h after insertion

**Evacuation of Uterus/Abortion**

*Adult:* **Intravaginal** Insert 20 mg suppository high in vagina, repeat q3–5h until abortion occurs or membranes rupture (max total dose: 240 mg)

## ADMINISTRATION

### Endocervical & Intravaginal

- **Do not** exceed recommended dose.
- Antiemetic and antidiarrheal medication may be prescribed to be given before dinoprostone to minimize GI side effects.
- Place vaginal insert in the vagina immediately after removal from the foil package. **Do not** use without retrieval system.
- Keep patient in supine position for 10 min after administration of suppository to prevent expulsion and enhance absorption.
- Store suppositories in freezer at temperature not exceeding –20° C (–4° F) unless otherwise specified.

## ADVERSE EFFECTS (≥1%) **CNS:**
Headache, tremor, tension. **CV:** Transient hypotension, flushing, cardiac arrhythmias. **GI:** *Nausea, vomiting, diarrhea.* **Urogenital:** Vaginal pain, endometritis, uterine contractions, uterine rupture. **Respiratory:** Dyspnea, cough, hiccups. **Body as a Whole:** *Chills, fever,* dehydration, diaphoresis, rash, localized warm feeling, back pain.

## INTERACTIONS **Drug:** OXYTOCICS used with extreme caution.

## PHARMACOKINETICS **Absorption:** Slowly absorbed from vagina;

Cervidil insert releases approximately 0.3 mg/h. **Onset:** 10 min. **Duration:** 2–3 h. **Distribution:** Widely distributed in body. **Metabolism:** Rapidly metabolized in lungs, kidneys, spleen, and other tissues. **Elimination:** Mainly in urine; some in feces.

## NURSING IMPLICATIONS

### Black Box Warning

*Recommended doses of dinoprostone should not be exceeded.*

### Assessment & Drug Effects

- Observe patient carefully, after insertion of the drug. Rupture of the membranes is not a contraindication to drug, but be aware that profuse bleeding may result in expulsion of the suppository. Report wheezing, chest pain, dyspnea, and significant changes in BP and pulse to the prescriber.
- Monitor uterine contractions and observe for and report excessive vaginal bleeding and cramping pain.
- Monitor vital signs. Fever is a physiologic response of the hypothalamus to use of dinoprostone and occurs within 15–45 min after insertion of suppository. Temperature returns to normal within 2–6 h after discontinuation of medication.

### Patient & Family Education

- Continue taking your temperature (late afternoon) for a few days after discharge. Contact prescriber with onset of fever, bleeding, abdominal cramps, abnormal or foul-smelling vaginal discharge.
- Avoid douches, tampons, intercourse, and tub baths for at least 2 wk. Clarify with prescriber.

## DINUTUXIMAB
(di-nu-tux′-i-mab)
Unituxin

Common adverse effects in *italic*; life-threatening effects underlined; generic names in **bold**; classifications in SMALL CAPS; ◆ Canadian drug name; ⊘ Prototype drug

511

**Classifications:** ANTINEOPLASTIC; IMMUNOMODULATOR; MONOCLONAL ANTIBODY
**Therapeutic:** ANTINEOPLASTIC
**Prototype:** Basiliximab

**AVAILABILITY** Solution for injection

**ACTION & THERAPEUTIC EFFECT**
Binds to the glycolipid GD2 that is expressed on neuroblastoma cells and induces cell lysis of GD2-expressing cells through antibody-dependent cell-mediated cytotoxicity (ADCC) and complement-dependent cytotoxicity (CDC). *Kills neuroblastoma cells and slows tumor growth.*

**USES** Treatment of pediatric patients with high-risk neuroblastoma who achieve at least a partial response to prior first-line multi-agent, multimodality therapy; used in combination with granulocyte-macrophage colony-stimulating factor (GM-CSF), interleukin-2 (IL-2) and 13-cis-retinoic acid (RA).

**CONTRAINDICATIONS** History of anaphylaxis to dinutuximab; severe unresponsive pain, severe sensory neuropathy, or moderate to severe peripheral motor neuropathy; atypical hemolytic uremic syndrome; severe capillary leak syndrome; pregnancy; lactation.

**CAUTIOUS USE** Infusion reactions; pain and peripheral neuropathy; capillary leak syndrome; hypotension; infection; neurologic disorders of the eye; electrolyte imbalance.

**ROUTE & DOSAGE**

**Neuroblastoma**
*Child/Adolescent:* **IV** 17.5 mg/m²/d for 10–20 h for 4 consecutive days; repeat for a total of 5 cycles (max infusion rate: 1.75 mg/m²/h); cycles 1, 3, and 5 are 24 days with infusions on days 4–7; cycles 2–4 are 32 days with infusions on days 8–11

**Adverse Reactions/Toxicity Dosage Adjustments**
See manufacturer's information for adjustments

**ADMINISTRATION**

**Intravenous**

**PRE-TREATMENT:**
- Hydration: Administer IV NS 10 mL/kg over 1 h just prior to initiating each infusion.
- Analgesics: Morphine sulfate or similar opioid is required before/during dinutuximab infusion to control pain.
- Antihistamine: Diphenhydramine or similar antihistamine is required before/during dinutuximab infusion to reduce risk of infusion reaction.
- Antipyretics: Acetaminophen is required before/during dinutuximab infusion to control fever.

**PREPARE: IV Infusion:** Withdraw required volume from vial and inject into a 100 mL bag of NS. Mix by gentle inversion but do not shake. Discard unused contents of the vial.
**ADMINISTER: IV Infusion:** Initiate at 0.875 mg/m²/h for 30 min; then rate can be gradually increased as tolerated (max: 1.75 mg/m²/h).

- Store undiluted vials under refrigeration. Initiate infusion within 4 h of preparation.

**ADVERSE EFFECTS** (≥10%) **Body as a Whole:** Device-related infection, *arthralgia,* back pain, *angioedema,* *infusion reactions, pain, pyrexia,* sepsis. **CNS:** Peripheral neuropathy. **CV:** *Capillary leak syndrome,* hemorrhage, hypotension, hypertension, tachycardia, angioedema. **GI:** *Diarrhea,* nausea, anorexia, *vomiting, abdominal pain.* **Hematological:** *Anemia, lymphopenia, neutropenia, thrombocytopenia.* **Metabolic:** Hyperglycemia, hypertriglyceridemia, *hypoalbuminemia, hypocalcemia, hypokalemia,* hypomagnesemia, *hyponatremia, hypophosphatemia, increased ALT/AST,* increased serum creatinine, increased weight. **Respiratory:** *Hypoxia,* bronchospasm, wheezing. **Skin:** *Urticaria.* **Urogenital:** Proteinuria.

## PHARMACOKINETICS Half-Life: 10 d.

## NURSING IMPLICATIONS

### Black Box Warning

*Dinutuximab has been associated with potentially life-threatening infusion reactions, and is known to cause severe neuropathic pain.*

### Assessment & Drug Effects

- Monitor patients closely for S&S of an infusion reaction or other serious adverse effects during and for at least 4 h after infusion. Immediately interrupt infusion and notify prescriber for severe infusion reactions (see Adverse Effects).
- Monitor vital signs during and for at least 4 h after infusion. Stop infusion and notify prescriber for symptomatic hypotension, systolic BP less than lower limit of normal for age or decreased by more than 15% of baseline.
- Monitor pain level frequently.
- Monitor for signs of severe motor neuropathy or ocular

neurological disorders (e.g., blurred vision, photophobia, mydriasis, fixed or unequal pupils, eyelid ptosis).
- Monitor lab tests: Baseline and periodic CBC with differential, serum electrolytes, renal function tests, and LFTs.

### Patient & Family Education

- Report immediately symptoms such as facial or lip swelling, hives, difficulty breathing, lightheadedness or dizziness that occur during or within 24 h following the infusion.
- Report promptly severe or worsening pain, and S&S of neuropathy (e.g., numbness, tingling, burning, or weakness).
- Report promptly problems with the eyes (e.g., blurred vision, photophobia, double vision, drooping eyelid).
- Women should use effective contraception during therapy and for 2 mo after the last dose.
- Do not breast-feed while taking this drug.

# DIPHENHYDRAMINE HYDROCHLORIDE 

(dye-fen-hye'dra-meen)

Allerdryl ◆, Benadryl, Benadryl Dye-Free, Sleep-Eze 3, Sominex Formula 2, Tusstat, Twilite, Valdrene

**Classifications:** CENTRALLY ACTING CHOLINERGIC ANTAGONIST; ANTIHISTAMINE; H$_1$-RECEPTOR ANTAGONIST

Therapeutic: ANTIHISTAMINE; SEDATIVE-HYPNOTIC; ANTIPARKINSON; ANTIDYSKINETIC; NONNARCOTIC ANTITUSSIVE

## AVAILABILITY Capsules; tablet; syrup; solution for injection

Common adverse effects in *italic;* life-threatening effects underlined; generic names in **bold;** classifications in SMALL CAPS; ◆ Canadian drug name; ⊕ Prototype drug

513

**D**

## ACTION & *THERAPEUTIC EFFECT*

Competes for $H_1$-receptor sites on effector cells, thus blocking histamine release. Effects in parkinsonism and drug-induced extrapyramidal symptoms are apparently related to its ability to suppress central cholinergic activity and to prolong action of dopamine by inhibiting its reuptake and storage. *Has antihistamine, antivertigo, antiemetic, antianaphylactic, antitussive, antidyskinetic, and sedative-hypnotic effects.*

## USES
Temporary symptomatic relief of various allergic conditions and to treat or prevent motion sickness, vertigo, and reactions to blood or plasma in susceptible patients. Also used in anaphylaxis as adjunct to epinephrine and other standard measures after acute symptoms have been controlled; in treatment of parkinsonism and drug-induced extrapyramidal reactions; as a nonnarcotic cough suppressant; as a sedative-hypnotic; and for treatment of intractable insomnia.

## CONTRAINDICATIONS
Hypersensitivity to antihistamines of similar structure; lower respiratory tract symptoms (including acute asthma); narrow-angle glaucoma; prostatic hypertrophy, bladder neck obstruction; GI obstruction or stenosis; lactation, premature neonates, and neonates.

## CAUTIOUS USE
History of asthma; COPD; convulsive disorders; increased IOP; hyperthyroidism; hypertension, cardiovascular disease; hepatic disease; diabetes mellitus; older adults, infants, and young children; pregnancy (category C). Use as a nighttime sleep aid in children younger than 2 y not established.

## ROUTE & DOSAGE

**Allergy Symptoms, Antiparkinsonism, Motion Sickness, Nighttime Sedation**

*Adult:* **PO** 25–50 mg t.i.d. or q.i.d. (max: 300 mg/day); **IV/IM** 10–50 mg q4–6h (max: 400 mg/day)
*Child (2–6 y):* **PO** 6.25 mg q4–6h (max: 300 mg/24 h); *6–12 y:* 12.5–25 mg q4–6h (max: 300 mg/24 h); **IV/IM** 5 mg/kg/day divided into 4 doses (max: 300 mg/day)

**Nonproductive Cough**

*Adult:* **PO** 25 mg q4–6h (max: 100 mg/day)
*Child (2–6 y):* **PO** 6.25 mg q4–6h (max: 25 mg/24 h); *6–12 y:* 12.5 mg q4–6h (max: 50 mg/24 h)

## ADMINISTRATION

### Oral
- Give with food or milk to lessen GI adverse effects.
- For motion sickness: Give the first dose 30 min before exposure to motion; give remaining doses before meals and at bedtime.

### Intramuscular
- Give IM injection deep into large muscle mass; alternate injection sites. Avoid perivascular or subcutaneous injections because of its irritating effects.
- Note: Hypersensitivity reactions (including anaphylactic shock) are more likely to occur with parenteral than PO administration.

### Intravenous

*PREPARE:* **Direct:** Give undiluted.
*ADMINISTER:* **Direct:** Give at a rate of 25 mg or a fraction thereof over 1 min.
*INCOMPATIBILITIES:* **Solution/additive: Amphotericin B, dexame-**

thasone, iodipamide, loraze-pam, methylprednisolone, metoclopramide, pentobarbital, phenobarbital, phenytoin. Y-site: Allopurinol, amiophylline, amphotericin B cholesteryl complex, ampicillin, azathioprine, cefmandole, cefazolin, cefepime, cefmetazole, cefonicid, cefperazone, cefotaxime, cefotetan, cefoxitin, ceftazidime, ceftobiprole, ceftriaxone, cefuroxime, cephalothin, chloramphenicol, dantrolene, diazepam, diazoxide, fluorouracil, foscarnet, furosemide, ganciclovir, indomethacin, insulin, ketorolac, lansoprazole, methylprednisolone, mezlocillin, nitroprusside, pantoprazole, pentobarbital, phenobarbital, phenytoin, sulfamethoxazole/trimethoprim.

- Store in tightly covered containers at 15°–30° C (59°–86° F) unless otherwise directed by manufacturer. Keep injection and elixir formulations in light-resistant containers.

## ADVERSE EFFECTS (>1%) CNS:
*Drowsiness,* dizziness, headache, fatigue, disturbed coordination, tingling, heaviness and weakness of hands, tremors, euphoria, nervousness, restlessness, insomnia, confusion; (especially in children): Excitement, fever. **CV:** Palpitation, *tachycardia,* mild hypotension or hypertension, cardiovascular collapse. **Special Senses:** Tinnitus, vertigo, dry nose, throat, nasal stuffiness; blurred vision, diplopia, photosensitivity, dry eyes. **GI:** *Dry mouth,* nausea, epigastric distress, anorexia, vomiting, constipation, or diarrhea. **Urogenital:** Urinary frequency or retention, dysuria. **Body as a Whole:** Hypersensitivity (skin rash, urticaria, photosensitivity, anaphylactic shock). **Respiratory:** Thickened bronchial secretions, wheezing, sensation of chest tightness.

## DIAGNOSTIC TEST INTERFERENCE
Diphenhydramine should be discontinued 4 days prior to *skin testing* procedures for allergy because it may obscure otherwise positive reactions.

## INTERACTIONS Drug: Alcohol
and other CNS DEPRESSANTS, MAO INHIBITORS compound CNS depression.

## PHARMACOKINETICS Absorption:
Readily absorbed from GI tract but only 40–60% reaches systemic circulation. **Onset:** 15–30 min. **Peak:** 1–4 h. **Duration:** 4–7 h. **Distribution:** Crosses placenta; distributed into breast milk. **Metabolism:** In liver; some degradation in lung and kidney. **Elimination:** Mostly in urine within 24 h.

## NURSING IMPLICATIONS
### Assessment & Drug Effects
- Monitor cardiovascular status especially with preexisting cardiovascular disease.
- Monitor for adverse effects especially in children and the older adult.
- Supervise ambulation and institute fall precautions as necessary. Drowsiness is most prominent during the first few days of therapy and often disappears with continued therapy. Older adults are especially likely to manifest dizziness, sedation, and hypotension.

### Patient & Family Education
- Do not use alcohol and other CNS depressants because of the possible additive CNS depressant effects with concurrent use.
- Do not drive or engage in other potentially hazardous activities until the response to drug is known.
- Increase fluid intake, if not contraindicated; drug has an atropine-like drying effect (thickens bronchial secretions) that may make expectoration difficult.

**D**

# DIPHENOXYLATE HYDROCHLORIDE WITH ATROPINE SULFATE
(dye-fen-ox'i-late)

Diphenatol, Lofene, Lomanate, Lomotil, Lonox, Lo-Trol, Low-Quel, Nor-Mil

**Classification:** ANTIDIARRHEAL
**Therapeutic:** ANTIDIARRHEAL
**Controlled Substance:** Schedule V

**AVAILABILITY** Tablet; liquid

## ACTION & *THERAPEUTIC EFFECT*
A synthetic narcotic opiate agonist that inhibits mucosal receptors responsible for peristaltic reflex, thereby reducing GI motility. *Reduces peristalsis thereby stopping or diminishing diarrhea.*

## USES Adjunct in symptomatic management of diarrhea.

## CONTRAINDICATIONS Hypersensitivity to diphenoxylate or atropine; severe dehydration or electrolyte imbalance, advanced liver disease, obstructive jaundice, diarrhea caused by pseudomembranous enterocolitis; diarrhea induced by poisons; glaucoma; lactation.

## CAUTIOUS USE Advanced hepatic disease, abnormal liver function tests; renal function impairment, MAOI therapy; addiction-prone individuals, or those whose history suggests drug abuse; ulcerative colitis; children; pregnancy (category C). Safe use in children younger than 2 y not established.

## ROUTE & DOSAGE

### Diarrhea
*Adult:* **PO** 1–2 tablets or 1–2 teaspoons full (5 mL) 3–4 × day (each tablet or 5 mL contains 2.5 mg diphenoxylate HCl and 0.025 mg atropine sulfate)
*Child (2–12 y):* **PO** 0.3–0.4 mg/kg/day of liquid in divided doses

## ADMINISTRATION
### Oral
- Crush tablet if necessary and give with fluid of patient's choice.
- Reduce dosage as soon as initial control of symptoms occurs.
- Withhold drug in presence of severe dehydration or electrolyte imbalance until appropriate corrective therapy has been initiated.
- Note: Treatment is generally continued for 24–36 h before it is considered ineffective.
- Store in tightly covered, light-resistant container, preferably 15°–30° C (59°–86° F), unless otherwise directed by manufacturer.

## ADVERSE EFFECTS (≥1%) **Body as a Whole:** Hypersensitivity (pruritus, angioneurotic edema, giant urticaria, rash). **CNS:** Headache, sedation, drowsiness, dizziness, lethargy, numbness of extremities; restlessness, euphoria, mental depression, weakness, general malaise. **CV:** Flushing, palpitation, tachycardia. **Special Senses:** Nystagmus, mydriasis, blurred vision, miosis (toxicity). **GI:** Nausea, vomiting, anorexia, dry mouth, abdominal discomfort or distension, paralytic ileus, toxic megacolon. **Other:** Urinary retention, swelling of gums.

## INTERACTIONS **Drug:** MAO INHIBITORS may precipitate hypertensive crisis; **alcohol** and other CNS DEPRESSANTS may enhance CNS effects; also see **atropine.**

## PHARMACOKINETICS **Absorption:** Readily absorbed from GI

tract. **Onset:** 45–60 min. **Peak:** 2 h. **Duration:** 3–4 h. **Distribution:** Distributed into breast milk. **Metabolism:** Rapidly metabolized to active and inactive metabolites in liver. **Elimination:** Slowly through bile into feces; small amount in urine. **Half-Life:** 4.4 h.

## NURSING IMPLICATIONS

### Assessment & Drug Effects

- Assess GI function; report abdominal distention and signs of decreased peristalsis.
- Monitor for S&S of dehydration (see Appendix F). It is essential to monitor young children closely; dehydration occurs more rapidly in this age group and may influence variability of response to diphenoxylate and predispose patient to delayed toxic effects.
- Monitor frequency and consistency of stools.

### Patient & Family Education

- Take medication only as directed by prescriber.
- Notify prescriber if diarrhea persists or if fever, bloody stools, palpitation, or other adverse reactions occur.
- Do not drive or engage in other potentially hazardous activities until response to drug is known.

## DIPYRIDAMOLE

(dye-peer-id'a-mole)

Apo-Dipyridamole ♦, Persantine

**Classifications:** ANTIPLATELET; PLATELET AGGREGATE INHIBITOR

Therapeutic: PLATELET AGGREGATE INHIBITOR

**AVAILABILITY** Tablet; solution for injection

## ACTION & *THERAPEUTIC EFFECT*

Nonnitrate coronary vasodilator that increases coronary blood flow by selectively dilating coronary arteries, thereby increasing myocardial oxygen supply. Additionally, it exhibits antiplatelet aggregation activity. *Reduces the risk of thromboembolism.*

**USES** To prevent postoperative thromboembolic complications associated with prosthetic heart valves and as adjunct for thallium stress testing.

**UNLABELED USES** To reduce rate of reinfarction following MI; to prevent TIAs (transient ischemic attacks) and coronary bypass graft occlusion.

**CAUTIOUS USE** Hypotension, anticoagulant therapy; aspirin sensitivity; elderly; severe hepatic dysfunction; syncope; pregnancy (category B); lactation. Safety and efficacy in children younger than 12 y not established.

## ROUTE & DOSAGE

**Prevention of Thromboembolism In Cardiac Valve Replacement**

*Adult:* PO 75–100 mg q.i.d
*Child:* PO 1–2 mg t.i.d.

**Thromboembolic Disorders**

*Adult:* PO 150–400 mg/day in divided doses

**Thallium Stress Test**

*Adult:* IV 0.142 mg/kg/min for 4 min

## ADMINISTRATION

### Oral

- Give on an empty stomach at least 1 h before or 2 h after meals, with a full glass of water. Prescriber may prescribe with food if gastric distress persists.

Common adverse effects in *italic*; life-threatening effects <u>underlined</u>; generic names in **bold**; classifications in SMALL CAPS; ♦ Canadian drug name; ⊙ Prototype drug

517

## Intravenous

**PREPARE: Direct:** Dilute to at least a 1:2 ratio with 0.45% NaCl, NS, or D5W to yield a final volume of 20–50 mL.
**ADMINISTER: Direct:** Give a single dose over 4 min (0.142 mg/kg/min).

- Store in a tightly closed container at 15°–30° C (59°–86° F) unless otherwise directed. Protect injection from direct light.

**ADVERSE EFFECTS** (≥1%) Usually dose related, minimal, and transient. **CNS:** Headache, dizziness, faintness, syncope, weakness. **CV:** Peripheral vasodilation, flushing. **GI:** Nausea, vomiting, diarrhea, abdominal distress. **Skin:** Skin rash, pruritus.

**INTERACTIONS Drug:** Other ANTICOAGULANTS can increase bleeding risk. **Herbal: Evening primrose oil, ginseng** can increase bleeding risk.

**PHARMACOKINETICS Absorption:** Readily absorbed from GI tract. **Peak:** 45–150 min. **Distribution:** Small amount crosses placenta. **Metabolism:** In liver. **Elimination:** Mainly in feces. **Half-Life:** 10–12 h.

## NURSING IMPLICATIONS

### Assessment & Drug Effects

- Monitor therapeutic effectiveness. Clinical response may not be evident before second or third month of continuous therapy. Effects include reduced frequency or elimination of anginal episodes, improved exercise tolerance, reduced requirement for nitrates.

### Patient & Family Education

- Notify prescriber of any adverse effects.
- Make all position changes slowly and in stages, especially from recumbent to upright posture, if postural hypotension or dizziness is a problem.

# DISOPYRAMIDE PHOSPHATE

(dye-soe-peer′a-mide)

Norpace, Norpace CR, Rythmodan ♦, Rythmodan-LA ♦
**Classification:** CLASS IA ANTIARRHYTHMIC
Therapeutic: CLASS IA ANTIARRHYTHMIC
**Prototype:** Procainamide

**AVAILABILITY** Capsule; sustained release capsule

## ACTION & *THERAPEUTIC EFFECT*

Decreases myocardial conduction velocity and excitability in the atria, ventricles, and accessory pathways. It prolongs the QRS and QT intervals in normal sinus rhythm and atrial arrhythmias. *Acts as myocardial depressant by reducing rate of spontaneous diastolic depolarization in pacemaker cells, thereby suppressing ectopic focal activity.*

**USES** Treatment of ventricular tachycardia.

**UNLABELED USES** To treat or prevent serious refractory arrhythmias. To convert atrial fibrillation, atrial flutter, and paroxysmal atrial tachycardia to normal sinus rhythm.

**CONTRAINDICATIONS** Cardiogenic shock, preexisting 2nd or 3rd degree AV block (if no pacemaker is present); sick sinus syndrome (bradycardia-tachycardia); Wolff-Parkinson-White (WPW) syndrome or bundle branch block, history of torsades de pointes; cardiogenic shock; QT prolongation; uncompensated or inadequately compensated CHF, hypotension (unless secondary to cardiac arrhythmia), hypokalemia.

**D**

**CAUTIOUS USE** Myocarditis or other cardiomyopathy, underlying cardiac conduction abnormalities; hepatic or renal impairment; urinary tract disease (especially prostatic hypertrophy); diabetes mellitus; myasthenia gravis; older adults; narrow-angle glaucoma; family history of glaucoma; pregnancy (category C); lactation.

## ROUTE & DOSAGE

### Arrhythmias

*Adult (weight greater than 50 kg):* **PO** 100–200 mg q6h or 300 mg loading dose; *weight less than 50 kg:* 100 mg q6h
*Adolescent:* **PO** 6–15 mg/kg/day in divided doses q6h
*Child (younger than 1 y):* **PO** 10–30 mg/kg/day in divided doses q6h; *1 to younger than 4 y:* 10–20 mg/kg/day in divided doses q6h; *4–12 y:* 10–15 mg/kg/day in divided doses q6h

## ADMINISTRATION

### Oral

- Start drug 6–12 h after last quinidine dose and 3–6 h after last procainamide dose for patients who have been receiving either quinidine or procainamide.
- Give sustained release capsules whole.
- Do not use sustained release capsules in loading doses when rapid control is required or in patients with creatinine clearance of 40 mL/min or less.
- Start sustained release capsules 6 h after last dose of conventional capsule if change in drug form is made.
- Store at 15°–30° C (59°–86° F) unless otherwise directed.

**ADVERSE EFFECTS** (≥1%) **Body as a Whole:** Hypersensitivity (pruritus, urticaria, rash, photosensitivity, <u>laryngospasm</u>). **CNS:** Dizziness, headache, fatigue, muscle weakness, convulsions, paresthesias, nervousness, acute psychosis, peripheral neuropathy. **CV:** *Hypotension,* chest pain, edema, dyspnea, syncope, bradycardia, tachycardia; worsening of CHF or cardiac arrhythmia; <u>cardiogenic shock, heart block</u>; edema with weight gain. **Special Senses:** *Blurred vision,* dry eyes, increased IOP, precipitation of acute angle-closure glaucoma. **GI:** *Dry mouth, constipation,* epigastric or abdominal pain, cholestatic jaundice. **Urogenital:** *Hesitancy* and *retention,* urinary frequency, urgency, renal insufficiency. **Other:** Dry nose and throat, drying of bronchial secretions, initiation of uterine contractions (pregnant patient); muscle aches, precipitation of myasthenia gravis, <u>agranulocytosis</u> (rare), <u>thrombocytopenia</u>.

**INTERACTIONS Drug:** ANTICHOLINERGIC DRUGS (e.g., TRICYCLIC ANTIDEPRESSANTS, ANTIHISTAMINES) compound anticholinergic effects; other ANTIARRHYTHMICS compound toxicities; **phenytoin, rifampin** may increase disopyramide metabolism and decrease levels; may increase **warfarin**-induced hypoprothrombinemia.

**PHARMACOKINETICS Absorption:** Readily from GI tract; 60–83% reaches systemic circulation. **Onset:** 30 min–3.5 h. **Peak:** 1–2 h. **Duration:** 1.5–8.5 h. **Distribution:** Distributed in extracellular fluid; crosses placenta; distributed into breast milk. **Metabolism:** In liver. **Elimination:** 80% in urine, 10% in feces. **Half-Life:** 4–10 h.

---

Common adverse effects in *italic;* life-threatening effects underlined; generic names in **bold**; classifications in SMALL CAPS; ♣ Canadian drug name; ⊙ Prototype drug

519

**D**

## NURSING IMPLICATIONS

### Black Box Warning

*Disopyramide should only be used in patients with life-threatening ventricular arrhythmias.*

### Assessment & Drug Effects

- Check apical pulse before administering drug. Withhold drug and notify prescriber if pulse rate is slower than 60 bpm, faster than 120 bpm, or if there is any unusual change in rate, rhythm, or quality.
- Monitor ECG closely. The following signs are indications for drug withdrawal: Prolongation of QT interval and worsening of arrhythmia interval, QRS widening (greater than 25%).
- Monitor for rapid weight gain or other signs of fluid retention.
- Monitor BP closely in all patients during periods of dosage adjustment and in those receiving high dosages.
- Monitor I&O, particularly in older adults and patients with impaired renal function or prostatic hypertrophy. Persistent urinary hesitancy or retention may necessitate lower dosage or discontinuation of drug.
- Report S&S of hyperkalemia (see Appendix F); it enhances drug's toxic effects.
- Monitor for S&S of CHF.
- Monitor lab tests: Baseline and periodic blood glucose and serum potassium.

### Patient & Family Education

- Take drug precisely as prescribed to maintain regularity of heartbeat.
- Weigh daily under standard conditions and check ankles for edema. Report to prescriber a weekly weight gain of 1–2 kg (2–4 lb) or more.
- Make position changes slowly, particularly when getting up from lying down because of the possibility of hypotension; dangle legs for a few minutes before walking, and do not stand still for prolonged periods.
- Do not drive or engage in other potentially hazardous activities until response to drug is known.

## DISULFIRAM

(dye-sul'fi-ram)

Antabuse

**Classifications:** ENZYME INHIBITOR; ANTIALCOHOL AGENT
Therapeutic: ALCOHOL ABUSE DETERRANT

**AVAILABILITY** Tablet

## ACTION & *THERAPEUTIC EFFECT*

Inhibits the enzyme acetaldehyde dehydrogenase, which normally metabolizes alcohol in the body. *When a small amount of alcohol is ingested, a complex of highly unpleasant symptoms known as the disulfiram reaction occurs, which serves as a deterrent to further drinking.*

**USES** Management of chronic alcoholism.

**CONTRAINDICATIONS** Severe myocardial disease; cardiac disease; psychosis; patients who have recently ingested alcohol, metronidazole, paraldehyde; multiple drug dependence.

**CAUTIOUS USE** Diabetes mellitus; epilepsy; seizure disorders; hypothyroidism; coronary artery disease, cerebral damage; chronic and acute nephritis; renal disease; hepatic cirrhosis or insufficiency; abnormal EEG; pregnancy (category B); lactation.

## ROUTE & DOSAGE

**Alcoholism**
*Adult:* **PO** 500 mg/day for 1–2 wk, then 125–500 mg/day (max: 500 mg/day)

## ADMINISTRATION

### Oral

- Daily dose may be given at bedtime to minimize sedative effect of the drug. Decrease in dose may also reduce sedative effect.
- Make sure patient has abstained from alcohol and alcohol-containing preparations for at least 12 h and preferably 48 h before initiating therapy. **Never** give to a person who is intoxicated.
- Store at 15°–30° C (59°–86° F) unless otherwise directed. Protect tablets from light.

**ADVERSE EFFECTS** (≥1%) **Reaction with alcohol ingestion:** Flushing of face, chest, arms, pulsating headache, nausea, violent vomiting, thirst, sweating, marked uneasiness, confusion, weakness, vertigo, blurred vision, pruritic skin rash, hyperventilation, abnormal gait, slurred speech, disorientation, confusion, personality changes, bizarre behavior, psychoses, tachycardia, palpitation, chest pain, hypotension to shock level arrhythmias, acute congestive failure. **Severe reactions:** Marked respiratory depression, unconsciousness, convulsions, sudden death. **Body as a Whole:** Hypersensitivity (allergic or acneiform dermatitis; urticaria, fixed-drug eruption). **CNS:** Drowsiness, fatigue, restlessness, headache, tremor, psychoses (usually with high doses), polyneuritis, peripheral neuropathy, optic neuritis. **GI:** Mild GI disturbances, garlic-like or metallic taste, hepatotoxicity, hypersensitivity hepatitis.

## DIAGNOSTIC TEST INTERFERENCE

Disulfiram can reduce **uptake of** $I^{131}$; or decreases **PBI** test results (rare).

**INTERACTIONS Drug: Alcohol** (including in liquid OTC drugs, **IV nitroglycerin, IV cotrimoxazole), metronidazole, paraldehyde** will produce disulfiram reaction; **isoniazid** can produce neurologic symptoms; may increase blood levels and toxicity of **warfarin, paraldehyde,** BARBITURATES, **phenytoin.** Do not use with **tinidazole.**

**PHARMACOKINETICS Absorption:** Slowly absorbed from GI tract **Onset:** Up to 12 h. **Duration:** Up to 2 wk after last dose. **Distribution:** Initially deposited in fat. **Metabolism:** Metabolized slowly in liver. **Elimination:** 5–20% excreted in feces; 20% remains in body for 1–2 wk; some may be excreted in breath as carbon disulfide.

## NURSING IMPLICATIONS

### Black Box Warning

*Disulfiram should not be given to anyone in a state of alcohol intoxication or without their full knowledge.*

### Assessment & Drug Effects

- Note: Disulfiram reaction occurs within 5–10 min following ingestion of alcohol and may last 30 min to several hours. Intensity of reaction varies with each individual, but is generally proportional to the amount of alcohol ingested.
- Treat patient with severe disulfiram reaction as though in shock. Monitor potassium levels, especially if patient has diabetes mellitus.

■ Monitor lab tests: Baseline and periodic LFTs.

**Patient & Family Education**

■ Patient should understand fully the possible dangers if alcohol is ingested during disulfiram treatment. Carry identification card indicating use of disulfiram.

■ Report promptly to prescriber the onset of nausea with right upper quadrant pain or discomfort, itching, jaundiced sclerae or skin, dark urine, clay-colored stools. Withhold drug pending liver function tests.

■ Note: Ingestion of even small amounts of alcohol or use of external applications that contain alcohol may be sufficient to produce a reaction. Read all labels and avoid use of anything containing alcohol.

■ Alcohol sensitivity may last as long as 2 wk after disulfiram has been discontinued.

■ Note: Adverse effects of drug are often experienced during first 2 wk of therapy; symptoms usually disappear with continued therapy or with dose reduction.

■ Do not drive or engage in other potentially hazardous activities until response to drug is known.

# DOBUTAMINE HYDROCHLORIDE

(doe-byoo'ta-meen)

Dobutrex

**Classifications:** ADRENERGIC AGONIST; VASOPRESSOR

Therapeutic: CARDIAC STIMULANT; IONOTROPIC

**Prototype:** Isoproterenol

**AVAILABILITY** Solution for injection

**ACTION & *THERAPEUTIC EFFECT***
Stimulates beta₁-receptors in the heart, increasing contractility and cardiac output. It also has weak beta₂ activity, and alpha₁ selective activity. Sympathetic nervous system effects increase cardiac output and decrease pulmonary wedge pressure and total systemic vascular resistance. Also increases conduction through AV node, and has lower potential for precipitating arrhythmias than dopamine. *In CHF or cardiogenic shock it increases cardiac output, enhances renal perfusion, increases renal output, and renal sodium excretion.*

**USES** Inotropic support in short-term treatment of adults with cardiac decompensation due to depressed myocardial contractility (cardiogenic shock) resulting from either organic heart disease or from cardiac surgery.

**UNLABELED USES** To augment cardiovascular function in children undergoing cardiac catheterization, stress thallium testing.

**CONTRAINDICATIONS** History of hypersensitivity to other sympathomimetic amines or sulfites, ventricular tachycardia, idiopathic hypertrophic subaortic stenosis; hypovolemia.

**CAUTIOUS USE** Preexisting hypertension, hypotension; atrial fibrillation; acute MI; unstable angina, severe coronary artery disease; pregnancy (category C). Safe use in children younger than 2 y is not established.

**ROUTE & DOSAGE**

| Cardiac Decompensation |
| --- |
| *Adult:* **IV** 0.5–1 mcg/kg/min then titrate up to 2.5–15 mcg/kg/min (max: 40 mcg/kg/min) |
| *Adolescent/Child:* **IV** 2–20 mcg/kg/min |

Common adverse effects in *italic;* life-threatening effects <u>underlined;</u> generic names in **bold;** classifications in SMALL CAPS; ♣ Canadian drug name; ⊙ Prototype drug

## ADMINISTRATION

### Intravenous

*PREPARE:* **Continuous:** Dilute 250 mg/20 mL vial or 500 mg/40 mL vial of dobutamine in at least 50 mL or 100 mL, respectively, of compatible IV solution. ▪ Use IV solutions within 24 h.

*ADMINISTER:* **Continuous:** Rate of infusion is determined by body weight and controlled by an infusion pump (preferred) or a microdrip IV infusion set. ▪ IV infusion rate and duration of therapy are determined by heart rate, blood pressure, ectopic activity, urine output, and whenever possible, by measurements of cardiac output and central venous or pulmonary wedge pressures.

*INCOMPATIBILITIES:* **Solution/additive:** Acyclovir, alteplase, aminophylline, bumetanide, calcium chloride, calcium gluconate, diazepam, digoxin, furosemide, heparin, insulin, magnesium sulfate, phenytoin, potassium chloride, potassium phosphate, sodium bicarbonate. **Y-site:** Acyclovir, alteplase, aminophylline, amphotericin B cholesteryl sulfate, cefepime, foscarnet, furosemide, heparin, indomethacin, lansoprazole, pantoprazole, pemetrexed, phytonadione, piperacillin/tazobactam, warfarin.

▪ Refrigerate reconstituted solution at 2°–15° C (36°–59° F) for 48 h or store for 6 h at room temperature.

## ADVERSE EFFECTS (≥1%) **All:**
Generally dose related. **CNS:** Headache, tremors, paresthesias, mild leg cramps, nervousness, fatigue (with overdosage). **CV:** *Increased heart rate and BP,* premature ventricular beats, palpitation, *anginal pain.* **GI:** Nausea, vomiting. **Other:** Nonspecific chest pain, shortness of breath.

## INTERACTIONS **Drug:** GENERAL ANESTHETICS (especially **cyclopropane** and **halothane**) may sensitize myocardium to effects of CATECHOLAMINES such as dobutamine and lead to serious arrhythmias—use with extreme caution; BETA-ADRENERGIC BLOCKING AGENTS (e.g., **metoprolol, propranolol**) may make dobutamine ineffective in increasing cardiac output, but total peripheral resistance may increase—concomitant use generally avoided; MAO INHIBITORS, TRICYCLIC ANTIDEPRESSANTS potentiate pressor effects—use with extreme caution.

## PHARMACOKINETICS **Onset:** 2–10 min. **Peak:** 10–20 min. **Metabolism:** Metabolized in liver and other tissues by COMT. **Elimination:** In urine. **Half-Life:** 2 min

## NURSING IMPLICATIONS

### Assessment & Drug Effects

▪ Correct hypovolemia by administration of appropriate volume expanders prior to initiation of therapy.
▪ Monitor therapeutic effectiveness. At any given dosage level, drug takes 10–20 min to produce peak effects.
▪ Monitor ECG and BP continuously during administration.
▪ Note: Marked increases in blood pressure (systolic pressure is the most likely to be affected) and heart rate, or the appearance of arrhythmias or other adverse cardiac effects are usually reversed promptly by reduction in dosage.
▪ Observe patients with preexisting hypertension closely for exaggerated pressor response.

---

Common adverse effects in *italic;* life-threatening effects <u>underlined;</u> generic names in **bold;** classifications in SMALL CAPS; ♣ Canadian drug name; ⊘ Prototype drug

523

- Monitor I&O ratio and pattern. Urine output and sodium excretion generally increase because of improved cardiac output and renal perfusion.

**Patient & Family Education**
- Report anginal pain to prescriber promptly.

## DOCETAXEL
(doc-e-tax'el)

Taxotere

**Classifications:** ANTINEOPLASTIC; TAXANE

Therapeutic: ANTINEOPLASTIC
**Prototype:** Paclitaxel

**AVAILABILITY** Solution for injection

**ACTION & THERAPEUTIC EFFECT**
A semisynthetic analog of paclitaxel that binds to the microtubule network essential for interphase and mitosis of the cell cycle. *Docetaxel stabilizes the microtubules involved in cell division and prevents their normal functioning; this results in inhibiting mitosis in cancer cells.*

**USES** Breast cancer, gastric cancer, prostate cancer, head/neck cancer, non-small cell lung cancer.

**CONTRAINDICATIONS** Hypersensitivity to docetaxel or other drugs formulated with polysorbate 80, paclitaxel; neutrophil count less than 1500 cells/mm$^3$, biliary tract disease, hepatic disease, jaundice, intramuscular injections, thrombocytopenia, acute infection, pregnancy (category D); lactation.

**CAUTIOUS USE** Bone marrow suppression, bone marrow transplant patients; CHF, ascites, peripheral edema, pleural effusion; radiation therapy; pulmonary disorders, acute bronchospasm; cardiac tamponade; dental disease, dental work, herpes infection; hypotension, elderly; infection. Safety and efficacy in children younger than 18 y not established.

## ROUTE & DOSAGE

**Breast Cancer**

*Adult:* **IV** 60–100 mg/m$^2$ q3wk (premedicate patients with dexamethasone 8 mg b.i.d. × 5 days, starting 1 day prior to docetaxel)

**Prostate Cancer**

*Adult:* **IV** 75 mg/m$^2$ q21days plus prednisone (5 mg PO twice daily) for 10 cycles (premedicate patients with dexamethasone 8 mg 12h, 3h, and 1h prior to starting docetaxel infusion)

**Non–Small-Cell Lung Cancer**

*Adult:* **IV** 75 mg/m$^2$ q3wk

**Head/Neck Cancer**

*Adult:* **IV** 75 mg/m$^2$ q21 days × 4 cycles

## ADMINISTRATION

- Note: If drug contacts skin during preparation, wash immediately with soap and water.

**Intravenous**

***PREPARE:*** **IV Infusion:** Preparation instructions vary by manufacturer; refer to specific prescribing information.

***ADMINISTER:*** **IV Infusion** Give at a constant rate over 1 h. ▪ Administer ONLY after premedication with corticosteroids to prevent hypersensitivity. ▪ Reduce dose by 25% following severe neutropenia (less than 500 cells/mm$^3$) for 7 days or longer for febrile

D

neutropenia, severe cutaneous reactions, or severe peripheral neuropathy.

*INCOMPATIBILITIES:* Y-site: **Amphotericin B, doxorubicin, methylprednisolone, nalbuphine.**

• Refrigerate vials at 2°–8° C (36°–46° F). Protect from light. Do not store in PVC bags. • Store diluted solutions in refrigerator or at room temperature for 8 h.

## ADVERSE EFFECTS (≥1%) CNS:
Paresthesia, pain, burning sensation, weakness, confusion. **CV:** Hypotension, *fluid retention (peripheral edema, weight gain),* pleural effusion. **GI:** *Nausea, vomiting, diarrhea, stomatitis,* abdominal pain; increased liver function tests (AST or ALT). **Hematologic:** <u>Neutropenia</u>, leukopenia, <u>thrombocytopenia, anemia</u>, febrile neutropenia. **Skin:** Rash, localized eruptions, desquamation, *alopecia,* nail changes (hyper/hypopigmentation, onycholysis). **Body as a Whole:** *Hypersensitivity reactions,* infusion site reactions (hyperpigmentation, inflammation, redness, dryness, phlebitis, extravasation).

## INTERACTIONS Drug: Possible
interaction with other drugs metabolized by CYP3A4.

## PHARMACOKINETICS Distribution: 97% protein bound. Metabolism: In liver by CYP3A4. Elimination: 80% in feces, 20% renally. Half-Life: 11.1 h.

## NURSING IMPLICATIONS

### Black Box Warning

*Docetaxel has been associated with increased mortality in persons with abnormal liver function,* *non-small cell lung cancer, and those receiving higher doses. Docetacel can cause severe neutropenia, hypersensitivity reactions, and marked fluid retention.*

### Assessment & Drug Effects
• Monitor for S&S of hypersensitivity (see Appendix F), which may develop within a few minutes of initiation of infusion. It is usually not necessary to discontinue infusion for minor reactions (i.e., flushing or local skin reaction).
• Assess throughout the course of therapy and report cardiovascular dysfunction, respiratory distress; fluid retention; development of neurosensory symptoms, severe, cutaneous eruptions on feet, hands, arms, face, or thorax; and S&S of infection.
• Monitor lab tests: LFTs prior to each drug cycle; frequent CBCs with differential.

### Patient & Family Education
• Learn common adverse effects and measures to control or minimize them when possible. Report immediately any distressing adverse effects.
• Report promptly to prescriber any of the following: Fever, edema in lower extremities, weight gain, shortness of breath, muscle pain, or skin reactions.
• Note: It is extremely important to comply with corticosteroid therapy and monitoring of lab values.
• Avoid pregnancy during therapy.

## DOCOSANOL
(doc'os-a-nol)

Abreva

**Classification:** ANTIVIRAL
**Therapeutic:** ANTIVIRAL

Common adverse effects in *italic*; life-threatening effects <u>underlined</u>; generic names in **bold**; classifications in SMALL CAPS; ♣ Canadian drug name; ◯ Prototype drug

525

**D**

## AVAILABILITY Cream

## ACTION & *THERAPEUTIC EFFECT*
Docosanol inhibits viral replication by interfering with the early intracellular events surrounding viral entry into target cells. *Believed to exert its antiviral effect by inhibiting fusion of the HSV (herpes virus) envelope with the human cell plasma membrane, therefore making it difficult for the virus to enter the cell and replicate.*

## USES Treatment of herpes simplex infections of the face and lips (i.e., cold sores).

## CONTRAINDICATIONS Hypersensitivity to docosanol or any of the inactive ingredients in the cream; immunosuppressant patients; lactation.

## CAUTIOUS USE Pregnancy (category C). Safety and efficacy in children not established.

## ROUTE & DOSAGE

### Herpes Simplex Infections
*Adult:* **Topical** Apply to lesions 5 × day for up to 10 days, starting at onset of symptoms

## ADMINISTRATION
### Topical
- Apply cream only to the affected areas using a gloved finger. Rub in gently but completely.
- Do not apply near or in the eyes.
- Avoid application to the mucous membranes inside of the mouth.
- Store at 20°–25° C (68°–77° F).

## ADVERSE EFFECTS (≥1%) CNS:
Headache. **Skin:** Skin irritation, burning.

## INTERACTIONS Drug: No clinically significant interactions established.

## NURSING IMPLICATIONS
### Assessment & Drug Effects
- Monitor severity and extent of infection.
- Notify prescriber if improvement is not seen within 10 days of initiating treatment

### Patient & Family Education
- Wash hands before and after applying cream.
- Do not share this cream with any other individual as this may spread the herpes virus.
- Report to prescriber if your condition worsens or does not improve within 10 days of beginning treatment.

---

# DOCUSATE CALCIUM (DIOCTYL CALCIUM SULFOSUCCINATE) ℗
(dok'yoo-sate)
DCS, PMS-Docusate Calcium, Pro-Cal-Sof, Surfak

# DOCUSATE POTASSIUM
Dialose, Diocto-K, Kasof

# DOCUSATE SODIUM
Colace, Colace Enema, Dio-Sul, Disonate, DGSS, D-S-S, Duosol, Lax-gel, Laxinate 100, Modane, Pro-Sof, Regulax ◆, Regutol, Therevac-Plus, Therevac-SB

**Classification:** STOOL SOFTENER
**Therapeutic:** STOOL SOFTENER

## AVAILABILITY Docusate Calcium:
Capsule. **Docusate Potassium:** Tablet; capsule. **Docusate Sodium:** Tablet; capsule; syrup

## ACTION & *THERAPEUTIC EFFECT*
Anionic surface-active agent with emulsifying and wetting properties. *Detergent action lowers surface tension, permitting water and fats to*

Common adverse effects in *italic;* life-threatening effects <u>underlined</u>; generic names in **bold**; classifications in SMALL CAPS; ◆ Canadian drug name; ℗ Prototype drug *penetrate and soften stools for easier passage.*

**USES** Prophylactically in patients who should avoid straining during defecation and for treatment of constipation associated with hard, dry stools (e.g., following anorectal surgery, MI).

**CONTRAINDICATIONS** Atonic constipation, nausea, vomiting, abdominal pain, fecal impaction, structural anomalies of colon and rectum, intestinal obstruction or perforation; use of docusate sodium in patients on sodium restriction; use of docusate potassium in patients with renal dysfunction.

**CAUTIOUS USE** History of CHF, edema, diabetes mellitus; pregnancy (category C).

## ROUTE & DOSAGE

**Stool Softener**

*Adult:* **PO** 50–500 mg/day **PR** 50–100 mg added to enema fluid
*Child (younger than 3 y):* **PO** 10–40 mg/day; *3 to younger than 6 y:* 20–60 mg/day; *6–12 y:* 40–120 mg/day

## ADMINISTRATION

### Oral

- Give with a full glass of water if allowed.
- Store syrup formulations in tight, light-resistant containers at 15°–30° C (59°–86° F) unless directed otherwise.

### Rectal

- Microenema: Insert full length of nozzle (half length for children) into the rectum. Squeeze entire contents of tube and remove completely before releasing grip on tube.
- Store in tightly covered containers.

**ADVERSE EFFECTS** (≥1%) **GI:** Occasional mild abdominal cramps, *diarrhea,* nausea, bitter taste. **Other:** Throat irritation (liquid preparation), rash.

**INTERACTIONS Drug:** Docusate will increase systemic absorption of **mineral oil.**

## NURSING IMPLICATIONS

### Assessment & Drug Effects

- Withhold drug if diarrhea develops and notify prescriber.
- Therapeutic effectiveness: Usually apparent 1–3 days after first dose.

### Patient & Family Education

- Take sufficient liquid with each dose and increase fluid intake during the day, if allowed. Oral liquid (**not** syrup) may be administered in milk, fruit juice, or infant formula to mask bitter taste.
- Do not take concomitantly with mineral oil.
- Do not take for prolonged periods in lieu of proper dietary management or treatment of underlying causes of constipation.

# DOFETILIDE

(do-fe-ti'lyde)

Tikosyn

**Classifications:** CLASS III ANTIARRHYTHMIC, POTASSIUM CHANNEL BLOCKER
**Therapeutic:** CLASS III ANTI-ARRHYTHMIC
**Prototype:** Amiodarone HCl

**AVAILABILITY** Capsule

## ACTION & THERAPEUTIC EFFECT

Prolongs the cardiac action potential by blocking potassium channels and thus one or more potassium currents. Action results in suppression of arrhythmias dependent

Common adverse effects in *italic;* life-threatening effects underlined; generic names in **bold;** classifications in SMALL CAPS; ♣ Canadian drug name; ⊘ Prototype drug

527

upon reentry of potassium ions. *Effectiveness indicated by correction of atrial arrhythmias.*

**USES** Symptomatic atrial fibrillation and flutter.

**CONTRAINDICATIONS** Hypersensitivity to dofetilide; QT prolongation; ventricular arrhythmias; history of torsades de pointes; electrolyte imbalances (e.g., hypokalemia, hypomagnesemia, etc.); renal failure; lactation.

**CAUTIOUS USE** Atrioventricular block, bradycardia, CHF, concurrent administration of potassium depleting diuretics, hepatic or renal impairment; history of moderate $QT_c$ interval prolongation; moderate to severe hypertension; recent MI or unstable angina; vascular heart disease; older adults; pregnancy (category C). Safety and efficacy in children younger than 18 y not established.

## ROUTE & DOSAGE

Dosing of dofetilide must be done very carefully. Dofetilide can cause serious cardiac arrhythmias, particularly, ventricular tachycardia of the torsades de pointes type. Ecg and renal function must be assessed prior to beginning therapy. Clinicians who are unfamiliar with the use of this drug should read the package insert.

**Atrial Fibrillation/Flutter**

*Adult:* **PO** Based on creatinine clearance (CrCl) and $QT_c$ interval, if $QT_c$ increases by more than 15% from baseline or is greater than 500 milliseconds 2–3 h after initial dose. Decrease subsequent doses by 50%.

**Renal Impairment Dosage Adjustment**

*CrCl greater than 60 mL/min:* 500 mcg b.i.d.; *40–60 mL/min:* 250 mcg b.i.d.; *20–39 mL/min:* 125 mcg b.i.d.

## ADMINISTRATION

**Oral**

- Administer with or without food.
- Do not give dofetilide if $QT/QT_c$ interval greater than 420 milliseconds (or greater than 500 milliseconds with ventricular conduction abnormalities).
- Administer only with continuous ECG monitoring.
- Do not initiate therapy until 3 mo after withdrawal of previous antiarrhythmic therapy.
- Do not initiate therapy until 3 mo after amiodarone has been withdrawn or plasma level is less than 0.3 mcg/mL.
- Store at 15°–30° C (59°–86° F); protect from moisture and humidity.

**ADVERSE EFFECTS** (≥1%) **Body as a Whole:** Flu-like syndrome, back pain. **CNS:** *Headache,* dizziness, insomnia. **CV:** <u>*Torsades de pointes arrhythmia, ventricular arrhythmias,*</u> AV block, *chest pain* v.tach, v.fibrillation, **GI:** Nausea, diarrhea, abdominal pain. **Respiratory:** Respiratory infection, dyspnea. **Skin:** Rash.

**INTERACTIONS Drug: Dofetilide** levels increased by **verapamil, cimetidine, trimethoprim, ketoconazole, prochlorperazine, megestrol;** do not give with drugs known to increase the $QT_c$ interval such as **bepridil,** PHENOTHIAZINES, TRICYCLIC ANTIDEPRESSANTS, ORAL MACROLIDES, other ANTIARRHYTHMICS. Do not use with BETA-AGONISTS.

Common adverse effects in *italic;* life-threatening effects <u>underlined;</u> generic names in **bold;** classifications in SMALL CAPS; ♣ Canadian drug name; ⊕ Prototype drug

**PHARMACOKINETICS Absorption:** Greater than 90% bioavailable. **Peak:** 2–3 h. **Distribution:** 60–70% protein bound. **Metabolism:** In liver. **Elimination:** Primarily excreted unchanged in urine. **Half-Life:** 10 h.

## NURSING IMPLICATIONS

### Assessment & Drug Effects

- Monitor ECG continuously during first 3 days of therapy; then periodically.
- Do not discharge patient until 12 h after conversion to normal sinus rhythm.
- Notify prescriber immediately of electrolyte imbalances, especially hypokalemia and hypomagnesemia.
- Monitor lab tests: Baseline and periodic serum electrolytes and creatinine clearance; periodic CBC and routine blood chemistry.

### Patient & Family Education

- Report immediately conditions that cause potassium loss (e.g., prolonged vomiting, diarrhea, excessive sweating).
- **Do not** take concurrently cimetidine, verapamil, ketoconazole, trimethoprim.

## DOLASETRON MESYLATE

(dol a-se'tron)

**Anzemet**

**Classifications:** SELECTIVE SEROTONIN (5-HT$_3$) RECEPTOR ANTAGONIST; ANTIEMETIC
**Therapeutic:** ANTIEMETIC
**Prototype:** Ondansetron

**AVAILABILITY** Solution for injection

## ACTION & *THERAPEUTIC EFFECT*

A selective serotonin (5-HT$_3$) receptor antagonist. Serotonin receptors affected are located in the chemoreceptor trigger zone (CTZ) of the brain and peripherally on the vagal nerve terminal. Serotonin, released from the cells of the small intestine, activate 5-HT$_3$ receptors located on vagal efferent neurons, thus initiating the vomiting reflex. *Has effective antiemetic properties.*

**USES** Prevention of nausea and vomiting from emetogenic chemotherapy, prevention and treatment of postoperative nausea and vomiting.

**CONTRAINDICATIONS** Hypersensitivity to dolasetron. **IV route:** Nausea and vomiting associated with cancer chemotherapy; congenital QT prolongation syndrome; uncorrected hypokalemia or hypomagnesemia.

**CAUTIOUS USE** Patients who have or may develop prolongation of cardiac conduction intervals, particularly QT$_c$ (i.e., patients with potential hypokalemia, hypomagnesemia, diuretics; patients taking antiarrhythmic drugs and high-dose anthracycline therapy, etc.), pregnancy (category B); lactation. Safety and efficacy in children younger than 2 y not established.

## ROUTE & DOSAGE

### Prevention of Chemotherapy-Induced Nausea and Vomiting

*Adult/Child (2 y or older):* **PO** 100 mg 1 h prior to chemotherapy

### Pre-/Postoperative Nausea and Vomiting

*Adult:* **IV** 12.5 mg 15 min before cessation of anesthesia or when postoperative nausea and vomiting occurs; **PO** 100 mg within 2 h prior to surgery
*Child (2 y or older):* **IV** 0.35 mg/kg up to 12.5 mg 15 min before cessation of anesthesia or when postoperative nausea and

Common adverse effects in *italic;* life-threatening effects underlined; generic names in **bold;** classifications in SMALL CAPS; ♣ Canadian drug name; ⓟ Prototype drug

529

vomiting occurs; **PO** 1.2 mg/kg up to 100 mg starting 2 h prior to surgery (may also mix IV formulation in apple or apple-grape juice and administer orally)

## ADMINISTRATION

### Oral
- Give within 2 h before surgery, when used for postoperative nausea.

### Intravenous

*PREPARE:* **Direct:** Give undiluted. **IV Infusion:** Dilute in 50 mL of any of the following: NS, D5W, D5/0.45% NaCl, LR.

*ADMINISTER:* **Direct:** Inject undiluted drug over 30 sec. **IV Infusion:** Infuse diluted drug over 15 min.
*INCOMPATIBILITIES:* **Solution/additive: Potassium chloride.**

- Store at 20°–25° C (66°–77° F) and protect from light. ▪ Diluted IV solution may be stored refrigerated up to 48 h.

## ADVERSE EFFECTS (≥1%) **Body as a Whole:** Fever, fatigue, pain, chills or shivering. **CNS:** *Headache,* dizziness, drowsiness. **CV:** Hypertension. **GI:** *Diarrhea,* increased LFTs, abdominal pain. **Genitourinary:** Urinary retention.

## INTERACTIONS **Drugs:** Avoid use with **apomorphine** due to hypotension; **ziprasidone** may prolong QT interval.

## PHARMACOKINETICS **Absorption:** Rapidly absorbed from GI tract. **Peak:** 0.6 h IV, 1 h PO. **Distribution:** Crosses placenta, distributed into breast milk. **Metabolism:** Metabolized to hydrodolasetron by carbonyl reductase. Hydrodolasetron is metabolized in the liver by CYP2D6. **Elimination:** Primarily in urine as hydrodolasetron. **Half-Life:** 10 min dolasetron, 7.3 h hydrodolasetron.

## NURSING IMPLICATIONS

### Assessment & Drug Effects
- Monitor closely cardiac status especially with vomiting, excess diuresis, or other conditions that may result in electrolyte imbalances.
- Monitor lab results and report promptly development of hypokalemia or hypomagnesemia.
- Monitor ECG, especially in those taking concurrent antiarrhythmic or other drugs that may cause QT prolongation.
- Monitor for and report signs of bleeding (e.g., hematuria, epistaxis, purpura, hematoma).
- Monitor lab tests: Baseline serum electrolytes before initiating drug.

### Patient & Family Education
- Headache requiring analgesic for relief is a common adverse effect.

## DOLUTEGRAVIR

(doe'loo-teg'ra-vir)
Tivicay
**Classifications:** ANTIRETROVIRAL; INTEGRASE INHIBITOR
Therapeutic: ANTIRETROVIRAL
**Prototype:** Raltegravir

## AVAILABILITY Tablet

## ACTION & *THERAPEUTIC EFFECT*
Dolutegravir binds to an enzyme (integrase) necessary for HIV-1 viral DNA integration and HIV replication. *Inhibits the HIV viral replication cycle.*

## USES In combination with other retroviral agents for the treatment of HIV-1 infection in adults and children aged 12 y and older and weighing at least 40 kg.

**CONTRAINDICATIONS** Hypersensitivity to dolutegravir; coadministration with dofetilide; severe hepatic impairment; lactation.

**CAUTIOUS USE** Patients with hepatitis B or C co-infections; mild-to-moderate hepatic impairment; older adults; children younger than 12 y or weighing less than 40 mg; pregnancy (category B).

## ROUTE & DOSAGE

**HIV-1 Infection**

*Adult:* **PO** 50 mg once daily
*Child (12 y or older and weight at least 40 kg):* **PO** 50 mg once daily

**Concurrent Potent UGT1A/
CYP3A Inducer Dosage
Adjustment**
50 mg b.i.d.

**Known or Suspected INSTI
Resistance Dosage Adjustment**
50 mg b.i.d.

**Hepatic Impairment
Dosage Adjustment**

*Severe hepatic impairment
(Child-Pugh class C):* Not
recommended

## ADMINISTRATION

**Oral**
- May be given without regard to food.
- Store at 15°–30° C (59°–86° F).

**ADVERSE EFFECTS** (>1%) **Body as a Whole:** Fatigue, hepatitis, hypersensitivity reactions. **CNS:** Dizziness, headache, insomnia **GI:** Abdominal pain, abdominal discomfort, flatulence, nausea, vomiting. **Hematological:** Neutropenia. **Metabolic:** Hyperglycemia, increased ALT/AST, increased bilirubin, increased cholesterol, increased creatine kinase, increased lipase, increased triglycerides. **Musculoskeletal:** Abdominal discomfort, myositis, upper abdominal pain. **Skin:** Pruritus. **Urogenital:** Renal impairment.

**INTERACTIONS Drug:** Dolutegravir may increase the levels of coadministered drugs that require the renal organic cation transporter (OCT2). Coadministration of UGT inhibitors and inducers may increase or decrease the levels of dolutegravir, respectively. **Carbamazepine, efavirenz, ctravirine, fosamprenavir, nevirapine, oxcarbazepine, phenobarbital, phenytoin, rifampin, ritonavir, tipranavir** decrease the levels of dolutegravir. **Metformin** increases the levels of dolutegravir. BUFFERED MEDICATIONS, **calcium supplements,** CATION-CONTAINING ANTACIDS or LAXATIVES, **iron supplements, sucralfate. Herbal:** St. **John's wort** decreases the levels of dolutegravir.

**PHARMACOKINETICS Peak:** 2–3 h. **Distribution:** Greater than 98.9% plasma protein bound. **Metabolism:** In liver. **Elimination:** Fecal (53%) and renal (31%). **Half-Life:** 14 h.

## NURSING IMPLICATIONS

**Assessment & Drug Effects**
- Monitor for S&S of hypersensitivity (see Appendix F).
- Withhold drug and notify prescriber if a rash appears.
- Monitor for S&S of hepatotoxicity (see Appendix F).
- Monitor lab tests: Baseline and periodic LFTs, viral load, CD4 count, and lipid profile.

**Patient & Family Education**
- Report promptly development of a rash accompanied by any of the following: Fever, extreme tiredness,

**D**

muscle or joint aches, blisters, swelling about the face, difficulty breathing.
- Report promptly S&S of liver damage: Yellowing of skin or whites of eyes, dark urine, pale stools, nausea or vomiting, loss of appetite, right-sided abdominal pain.
- Notify prescriber immediately if you suspect a pregnancy.
- Do not breast-feed while taking this drug.

## DONEPEZIL HYDROCHLORIDE ℗

(don-e′pe-zil)

**Aricept, Aricept ODT**

**Classifications:** CENTRAL ACTING CHOLINERGIC; CHOLINESTERASE INHIBITOR
**Therapeutic:** ANTIDEMENTIA; ALZHEIMER'S AGENT

**AVAILABILITY** Tablet; orally disintegrating tablet

## ACTION & *THERAPEUTIC EFFECT*

A cholinesterase inhibitor, presumably elevates acetylcholine concentration in the cerebral cortex by slowing degrading acetylcholine released by remaining intact neurons. *Improves global function, cognition, and behavior of patients with mild to moderate Alzheimer's.*

## USES
Mild, moderate, or severe dementia of Alzheimer's type.

## UNLABELED USES
Vascular dementia, poststroke aphasia, memory improvement in multiple sclerosis patients, traumatic brain injury.

## CONTRAINDICATIONS
Hypersensitivity to donepezil, or piperidine derivatives; GI bleeding, jaundice; lactation; children.

**CAUTIOUS USE** Anesthesia, sick sinus rhythm, AV block, bradycardia, cardiac arrhythmias, cardiac disease, hypotension; hyperthyroidism, history of ulcers, abnormal liver function; history of asthma or obstructive pulmonary disease, history of seizures, urinary tract obstruction, intestinal obstruction; diarrhea, emesis, GI disease, renal failure, renal impairment, surgery; pregnancy (category C).

## ROUTE & DOSAGE

**Alzheimer's Disease-Related Dementia**
*Adult:* **PO** 5–10 mg at bedtime (may increase to 23 mg daily after 3 mo)

## ADMINISTRATION

**Oral**
- Give immediately before going to bed.
- Dosage increase from 5 to 10 mg is usually made only after 4–6 wk of therapy.
- Store at 15°–30° C (59°–86° F).

**ADVERSE EFFECTS** (≥1%) **Body as a Whole:** *Headache,* fatigue, infection. **CNS:** *Insomnia,* dizziness, depression, tremor, irritability, vertigo, ataxia. **CV:** Syncope, hypertension, atrial fibrillation, hot flashes, hypotension. **GI:** *Nausea, diarrhea, vomiting, muscle cramps, anorexia,* GI bleeding, bloating, fecal incontinence, epigastric pain. **Respiratory:** Dyspnea. **Skin:** Pruritus, sweating, urticaria. **Other:** Accidental injury, ecchymoses, muscle cramps, dehydration, blurred vision, urinary incontinence, nocturia.

**INTERACTIONS Drug: Ketoconazole, quinidine** may inhibit donepezil metabolism; **carbamazepine, dexamethasone, phenobarbital, phenytoin, rifampin**

Common adverse effects in *italic*; life-threatening effects <u>underlined</u>; generic names in **bold**; classifications in SMALL CAPS; ♣ Canadian drug name; ℗ Prototype drug may increase donepezil elimination; donepezil may interfere with the action of ANTICHOLINERGIC AGENTS. Do not use with **dofetilide, dronderarone, ziprasidone** due to increased QT prolongation.

**PHARMACOKINETICS Absorption:** Rapidly from GI tract. **Peak:** 3–4 h. **Distribution:** 96% protein bound. **Metabolism:** In liver by CYP2D6 and CYP3A4. **Elimination:** Primarily in urine. **Half-Life:** 70 h.

## NURSING IMPLICATIONS

### Assessment & Drug Effects

- Monitor closely for S&S of GI ulceration and bleeding, especially with concurrent use of NSAIDs.
- Monitor carefully patients with a history of asthma or obstructive pulmonary disease.
- Monitor cardiovascular status; drug may have vagotonic effect on the heart, causing bradycardia, especially in presence of conduction abnormalities.
- Assess bladder adequacy prior to treatment.

### Patient & Family Education

- Exercise caution. Fainting episodes related to slowing the heart rate may occur.
- Report immediately to prescriber any S&S of GI ulceration or bleeding (e.g., "coffee-ground" emesis, tarry stools, epigastric pain).

## DOPAMINE HYDROCHLORIDE

(doe'pa-meen)

**Classifications:** ALPHA- AND BETA-ADRENERGIC AGONIST; IONOTROPIC
**Therapeutic:** CARDIAC STIMULANT; VASOPRESSOR
**Prototype:** Epinephrine

**AVAILABILITY** Solution for injection

## ACTION & *THERAPEUTIC EFFECT*

Major cardiovascular effects produced by direct action on alpha- and beta-adrenergic receptors and on specific dopaminergic receptors in mesenteric and renal vascular beds. Positive inotropic effect on myocardium increases cardiac output with increase in systolic and pulse pressure. Improves circulation to renal vascular bed by decreasing renal vascular resistance with resulting increase in GFR and urinary output. *Due to its potential for inotropic, chronotropic, and vasopressor effects, dopamine has several clinical uses, including decreased cardiac output as well as correction of hypotension associated with cardiogenic and septic shock.*

**USES** To correct hemodynamic imbalance in shock syndrome due to MI (cardiogenic shock), trauma, endotoxic septicemia (septic shock), open heart surgery, and heart failure.

**UNLABELED USES** Acute renal failure; cirrhosis; hepatorenal syndrome; barbiturate intoxication.

**CONTRAINDICATIONS** Pheochromocytoma; uncorrected tachyarrhythmias or ventricular fibrillation; persistent hypotension.

**CAUTIOUS USE** Patients with history of occlusive vascular disease (e.g., Buerger's or Raynaud's disease); CAD; cold injury; acute MI; diabetic endarteritis; arterial embolism; pregnancy (category C); lactation, children younger than 2 y.

## ROUTE & DOSAGE

### Shock/Surgery

*Adult:* **IV** 2–5 mcg/kg/min increased gradually up to 20 mcg/kg/min if necessary

---

Common adverse effects in *italic;* life-threatening effects <u>underlined</u>; generic names in **bold;** classifications in SMALL CAPS; ♣ Canadian drug name; ⊕ Prototype drug

533

**D**

*Adolescent/Child:* **IV** 1–5 mcg/kg/min increased gradually up to 20 mcg/kg/min

**Heart Failure**

*Adult:* **IV** 3–10 mcg/kg/min

## ADMINISTRATION

### Intravenous

*PREPARE:* **Continuous:** Dilute just prior to administration. ▪ Dilute contents of 1 or more vials in either 250 or 500 mL of the following: D5W, D5/NS, D5/LR, D5/0.45% NaCl, NS.

*ADMINISTER:* **Continuous:** Infusion rate is based on body weight. ▪ Infusion rate and guidelines for adjusting rate relative changes in blood pressure are prescribed by prescriber. ▪ Microdrip and other reliable metering device should be used for accuracy of flow rate.

*INCOMPATIBILITIES:* **Solution/additive: Acyclovir, alteplase, amphotericin B, ampicillin, metronidazole, penicillin G, sodium bicarbonate. Y-site: Acyclovir, alteplase, amphotericin B cholesteryl complex, cefepime, doxycycline, furosemide, indomethacin, insulin, lansoprazole, sodium bicarbonate.**

▪ Correct hypovolemia, if possible, with either whole blood or plasma before initiation of dopamine therapy. ▪ Monitor infusion continuously for free flow, and take care to avoid extravasation, which can result in tissue sloughing and gangrene. Use a large vein of the antecubital fossa. ▪ Antidote for extravasation: Stop infusion promptly and remove needle. Immediately infiltrate the ischemic area with 5–10 mg

phentolamine mesylate in 10–15 mL of NS, using syringe and fine needle. Pediatric dosage of phentolamine should be 0.1–0.2 mg/kg (max: 10 mg per dose).

▪ Protect dopamine from light. Discolored solutions should not be used.

▪ Store reconstituted solution for 24 h at 2°–15° C (36°–59° F) or 6 h at room temperature 15°–30° C.

## ADVERSE EFFECTS (≥1%) CV:

*Hypotension,* ectopic beats, *tachycardia,* anginal pain, palpitation, vasoconstriction (indicated by disproportionate rise in diastolic pressure), cold extremities; <u>Aberrant conduction</u>, <u>bradycardia</u>, <u>widening of QRS complex</u>, elevated blood pressure. **GI:** Nausea, vomiting. **CNS:** Headache, anxiety. **Skin:** Necrosis, tissue sloughing with extravasation, <u>gangrene</u>, piloerection. **Other:** Azotemia, dyspnea, dilated pupils (high doses), increased serum glucose.

## DIAGNOSTIC TEST INTERFERENCE

Dopamine may modify test response when histamine is used as a control for *intradermal skin tests.*

## INTERACTIONS Drug: MAO IN-

HIBITORS, ERGOT ALKALOIDS, increase alpha-adrenergic effects (headache, hyperpyrexia, hypertension); **guanethidine, phenytoin** may decrease dopamine action; BETA-BLOCKERS antagonize cardiac effects; ALPHA BLOCKERS antagonize peripheral vasoconstriction; **halothane, cyclopropane** increase risk of hypertension and ventricular arrhythmias.

## PHARMACOKINETICS Onset: Less

than 5 min. **Duration:** Less than 10 min. **Distribution:** Widely distributed; does not cross blood–brain barrier. **Metabolism:** Inactive in the liver, kidney, and plasma by monoamine

Common adverse effects in *italic;* life-threatening effects <u>underlined;</u> generic names in **bold;** classifications in SMALL CAPS; ♣ Canadian drug name; ◉ Prototype drug oxidase and COMT. **Elimination:** In urine. **Half-Life:** 2 min.

## NURSING IMPLICATIONS

### Black Box Warning

*Dopamine extravasation may cause necrosis and sloughing of surrounding tissue.*

### Assessment & Drug Effects

- Monitor infusion continuously for free flow, and take care to avoid extravasation, which can result in tissue sloughing and gangrene.
- Monitor blood pressure, pulse, peripheral pulses, and urinary output at intervals prescribed by prescriber. Precise measurements are essential for accurate titration of dosage.
- Report the following indicators promptly to prescriber for use in decreasing or temporarily suspending dose: Reduced urine flow rate in absence of hypotension; ascending tachycardia; dysrhythmias; disproportionate rise in diastolic pressure (marked decrease in pulse pressure); signs of peripheral ischemia (pallor, cyanosis, mottling, coldness, complaints of tenderness, pain, numbness, or burning sensation).
- Monitor therapeutic effectiveness. In addition to improvement in vital signs and urine flow, other indices of adequate dosage and perfusion of vital organs include loss of pallor, increase in toe temperature, adequacy of nail bed capillary filling, and reversal of confusion or comatose state.

## DORIPENEM

(dor-i-pen'em)

Doribax

**Classifications:** BETA-LACTAM ANTIBIOTIC; CARBAPENEM ANTIBIOTIC
**Therapeutic:** ANTIBIOTIC
**Prototype:** Imipenem-cilastatin

**AVAILABILITY** Powder for injection

## ACTION & *THERAPEUTIC EFFECT*

Inhibits essential penicillin-binding proteins resulting in inhibition of bacterial cell wall synthesis, resulting in bacterial cell death. *Bactericidal against aerobic and anaerobic gram-negative and gram-positive bacteria, and effectively resolves infection.*

**USES** Single-agent treatment of complicated intra-abdominal infections and urinary tract infections, including pyelonephritis caused by susceptible organisms.

**UNLABELED USES** Hospital-acquired pneumonia.

**CONTRAINDICATIONS** Hypersensitivity to doripenem, or beta-lactam antibiotics; multiple allergies; ventilator-assisted pneumonia; inhalation route.

**CAUTIOUS USE** Hypersensitivity to cephalosporins, penicillins; moderate to severe renal impairment; GI disease, colitis, IBD; history of a seizure disorder; stroke; bacterial meningitis; older adults; pregnancy (category B); lactation. Safe use in children and adolescents is not established.

## ROUTE & DOSAGE

### Complicated Intra-Abdominal Infection
*Adult:* **IV** 500 mg q8h × 5–14 days

**D**

### Complicated UTI, Including Pyelonephritis

*Adult:* **IV** 500 mg q8h × 10 days

### Renal Impairment Dosage Adjustment

*CrCl 30–50 mL/min:* 250 mg q8h; *greater than 10 mL/min but less than 30 mL/min:* 250 mg q12h

## ADMINISTRATION

Intravenous

*PREPARE:* **Intermittent:** Add 10 mL of sterile water for injection or NS to the 500 mg or 250 mg vial, gently shake to form suspension; yields 50 mg/mL (500 mg vial) or 25 mg/mL (250 mg vial). ▪ **Preparation of 500 mg dose:** Withdraw contents of 500 mg vial with a 21-gauge needle and add to infusion bag of 100 mL of NS or D5W, gently shake until clear. Final concentration is approximately 4.5 mg/mL. ▪ **Preparation of 250 mg dose:** Withdraw contents of 250 mg vial with a 21-gauge needle and add to infusion bag of 50 or 100 mL of NS or D5W, gently shake until clear. Final concentration is approximately 4.2 mg/mL (50 mL bag) or 2.3 mg/mL (100 mL bag).
*ADMINISTER:* **Intermittent:** Infuse over 60 min.
*INCOMPATIBILITIES:* **Solution/additive:** Do not combine with any other drug. **Y-site:** **Amphotericin B, amphotericin B lipid, diazepam, potassium, propofol.** ▪ Transfer reconstituted suspension to IV bag within 1 h of preparation.

## ADVERSE EFFECTS (≥1%) Body as a Whole: Anaphylaxis, hypersensitivity reactions. **CNS:** *Headache,* seizures. **CV:** Phlebitis. **GI:**

Diarrhea, nausea, oral candidiasis. **Hematologic:** Anemia. **Metabolic:** Elevated hepatic enzymes. **Skin:** Rash. **Urogenital:** Vulvomycotic infection

## INTERACTIONS Drug: Doripenem decreases plasma levels of **valproic acid. Probenecid** increases doripenem plasma levels.

## PHARMACOKINETICS Distribution: Minimal protein binding. **Metabolism:** In liver (18%) to inactive metabolite. **Elimination:** Urine (primarily unchanged). **Half-Life:** 1 h.

## NURSING IMPLICATIONS

### Assessment & Drug Effects

▪ Determine history of hypersensitivity reactions to other beta-lactams, cephalosporins, penicillins, or other drugs.
▪ Discontinue drug and immediately report S&S of hypersensitivity (see Appendix F).
▪ Report S&S of superinfection or pseudomembranous colitis (see Appendix F).
▪ Monitor lab tests: Baseline C&S; periodic LFTs, Hct, and Hgb.

### Patient & Family Education

▪ Learn S&S of hypersensitivity, superinfection, and pseudomembranous colitis; report any of these to prescriber promptly.

## DORNASE ALFA

(dor'naze)

Pulmozyme

**Classifications:** RESPIRATORY ENZYME; MUCOLYTIC
Therapeutic: MUCOLYTIC

## AVAILABILITY Solution for inhalation

Common adverse effects in *italic*; life-threatening effects <u>underlined</u>; generic names in **bold**; classifications in SMALL CAPS; ✤ Canadian drug name; ⊘ Prototype drug

## ACTION & *THERAPEUTIC EFFECT*

In cystic fibrosis (CF) viscous, purulent secretions in the airway reduce pulmonary function and lead to exacerbations of infection. Purulent pulmonary secretions contain very high concentrations of DNA released by degenerating leukocytes that are present in response to infection. Dornase alfa hydrolyzes the DNA present in sputum/mucus of cystic fibrosis patients and reduces viscosity in the lungs. *Promotes improved clearance of secretions from the respiratory tract.*

## USES
In combination with standard therapies to reduce the frequency of respiratory infections in patients with CF and to improve pulmonary function.

## UNLABELED USES
Chronic bronchitis, management of atelectasis.

## CONTRAINDICATIONS
Hypersensitivity to dornase or hamster protein; lactation.

## CAUTIOUS USE
Decreased pulmonary function, pregnancy (category D). Safe use in children younger than 3 mo not established.

## ROUTE & DOSAGE

### Cystic Fibrosis

*Adult/Child (3 mo or older):*
**Inhalation** 2.5 mg (1 ampule) inhaled once daily using a recommended nebulizer, may increase to twice daily (do not mix with other agents in nebulizer)

## ADMINISTRATION

**Inhalation**
- Do not dilute or mix with any other drugs or solutions in the nebulizer.

- Use only with nebulizer systems recommended by the drug manufacturer.
- Do not shake ampules; do not use ampules that have been at room temperature longer than 24 h or have become cloudy or discolored.
- Store refrigerated at 2°–8° C (36°–46° F) in protective foil pouch.

## ADVERSE EFFECTS (≥1%)
**Respiratory:** Hoarseness, sore throat, voice alterations, pharyngitis, laryngitis, cough, rhinitis. **Other:** Conjunctivitis, chest pain, rash.

## PHARMACOKINETICS
**Absorption:** Minimal systemic absorption. **Onset:** 3–8 days. **Duration:** Benefit lasts up to 4 days after discontinuing treatment.

## NURSING IMPLICATIONS

### Assessment & Drug Effects
- Monitor for improvement in dyspnea and sputum clearance.
- Monitor for S&S of hypersensitivity (see Appendix F). Patients with a history of hypersensitivity to bovine pancreatic dornase are at high risk.
- Monitor for adverse effects; rarely, dosage adjustments may be required.

### Patient & Family Education
- Report rash, hives, itching, or other S&S of hypersensitivity to prescriber immediately.
- Know potential adverse effects and report those that are bothersome or do not disappear.
- Take a missed dose as soon as possible; if it is almost time for the next dose, skip the missed dose.

---

# DORZOLAMIDE HYDROCHLORIDE
(dor-zol′a-mide)
Trusopt
**Classifications:** EYE PREPARATION; CARBONIC ANHYDRASE INHIBITOR

---

**D**

Therapeutic: ANTIGLAUCOMA;
OCULAR ANTIHYPERTENSIVE
**Prototype:** Acetazolamide

**AVAILABILITY** Opth solution

**ACTION & *THERAPEUTIC EFFECT***
Dorzolamide is a sulfonamide
that inhibits carbonic anhydrase
in the eye, thus reducing the rate
of aqueous humor formation with
subsequent lowering of IOP. Elevated IOP is a major risk factor
in the pathogenesis of optic nerve
damage and visual field loss due to
glaucoma. *Lowers IOP in glaucoma
or ocular hypertension.*

**USES** Ocular hypertension, open-
angle glaucoma.

**CONTRAINDICATIONS** Previous
hypersensitivity to dorzolamide.

**CAUTIOUS USE** History of hypersensitivity to other carbonic anhydrase inhibitors, sulfonamides, or
thiazide diuretics; ocular infection
or inflammation; recent ocular surgery; moderate to severe renal or
hepatic insufficiency; angle-closure
glaucoma; corneal abrasion; older
adults, pregnancy (category C).

**ROUTE & DOSAGE**

**Glaucoma, Ocular Hypertension**

*Adult/Adolescent/Child/Infant:*
**Ophthalmic** 1 drop in affected
eye t.i.d.

**ADMINISTRATION**
**Instillation**
▪ Apply gentle pressure to lacrimal
sac during and immediately following drug instillation for about
1 min to lessen degree of systemic
absorption.

▪ Administer at least 10 min apart, if
another ophthalmic drug is being
used concurrently.
▪ Store at 15°–30° C (59°–86° F).

**ADVERSE EFFECTS** (≥1%) **CNS:**
Headache. **GI:** Bitter taste, nausea.
**Special Senses:** *Transient burning or stinging, transient blurred
vision,* superficial punctate keratitis,
tearing, dryness, photophobia, ocular
allergic reaction. **Skin:** Rash.

**PHARMACOKINETICS Absorp-
tion:** Some systemic absorption.
**Onset:** 2 h. **Duration:** 8–12 h. **Distribution:** Into red blood cells.
**Elimination:** In urine. **Half-Life:** RBC
elimination about 4 mo.

**NURSING IMPLICATIONS**
**Assessment & Drug Effects**
▪ Inquire about previous hypersensitivity to sulfonamides prior to
therapy.
▪ Withhold drug and notify prescriber if S&S of local or systemic
hypersensitivity occur (see
Appendix F).
▪ Withhold the drug and notify the
prescriber if ocular irritation occurs.

**Patient & Family Education**
▪ Learn proper technique for applying eyedrops.
▪ Do not allow tip of drug dispenser
to come in contact with the eye.
▪ Discontinue drug and report to
prescriber: Ocular irritation, infection, or S&S of systemic hypersensitivity occur (see Appendix F).

---

# DOXAPRAM HYDROCHLORIDE
(dox'a-pram)

Dopram
**Classifications:** CEREBRAL
STIMULANT; RESPIRATORY STIMULANT
Therapeutic: CEREBRAL STIMULANT;
RESPIRATORY STIMULANT
**Prototype:** Caffeine

---

Common adverse effects in *italic;* life-threatening effects <u>underlined</u>; generic names
in **bold;** classifications in SMALL CAPS; ✤ Canadian drug name; ⊘ Prototype drug

**D**

**AVAILABILITY** Solution for injection

**ACTION & *THERAPEUTIC EFFECT***
Short-acting stimulant capable of stimulating all levels of the cerebro-spinal axis. Respiratory stimulation by direct medullary action increases tidal volume and slightly increases respiratory rate. Decreases $Pco_2$ and increases $Po_2$ by increasing alveolar ventilation. *Effectively used to stimulate respiration postanesthesia, for drug-induced CNS depression, and for chronic pulmonary disease associated with acute hypercapnia.*

**USES** Short-term adjunctive therapy to alleviate postanesthesia and drug-induced respiratory depression. Also as a temporary measure (approximately 2 h) in hospitalized patients with COPD associated with acute respiratory insufficiency as an aid to prevent elevation of $Paco_2$ during administration of oxygen. (Not used with mechanical ventilation.)

**UNLABELED USES** Neonatal apnea refractory to xanthine therapy.

**CONTRAINDICATIONS** Epilepsy and other convulsive disorders; head injury, cerebral edema; ventilatory disorders, pulmonary fibrosis, flail chest, pneumothorax, air way obstruction, extreme dyspnea, or acute bronchial asthma; severe hypertension, severe coronary artery disease, uncompensated heart failure, CVA; lactation.

**CAUTIOUS USE** History of bronchial asthma, COPD; cardiac disease, severe tachycardia, arrhythmias, hypertension; renal or hepatic impairment; hyperthyroidism; pheochromocytoma; increased intracranial pressure; peptic ulcer, patients undergoing gastric surgery; acute agitation; older adults; pregnancy (category C). Safe use in children younger than 12 y not established.

**ROUTE & DOSAGE**

**Postanesthesia**

*Adult:* **IV** 0.5–1 mg/kg single injection (not more than 1.5 mg/kg), may repeat q5min up to 2 mg/kg total dose; infusion of 0.5–1 mg/kg (max total dose: 4 mg/kg)

**Drug-Induced CNS Depression**

*Adult:* **IV** 1–2 mg/kg repeat in .5 min, then q1–2h until patient awakens [if relapse occurs, resume q1–2h injections (max total dose: 3 g), if no response after priming dose, may give 1–3 mg/min for up to 2 h until patient awakens]

**Chronic Obstructive Pulmonary Disease**

*Adult:* **IV** 0.5–2 mg/kg OR 1–2 mg/min for a max of 2 h (max rate: 3 mg/min)

**ADMINISTRATION**

▪ IV administration to neonates: Verify correct IV concentration and rate of infusion with prescriber. Generally do not use in newborns because doxapram contains benzyl alcohol.
▪ Ensure adequacy of airway and oxygenation before initiation of doxapram therapy.

**Intravenous**

*PREPARE:* **Direct:** Give undiluted. **IV Infusion for CNS Depression:** Dilute 250 mg (12.5 mL) in 250 mL of D5W or NS. **IV Infusion for COPD:** Add 400 mg doxapram to 180 mL of D5W, D10W, or NS to yield 2 mg/mL.
*ADMINISTER:* **Direct for CNS Depression:** Give undiluted over 5 min. **IV Infusion for CNS Depression:** Give at a rate of 1–3 mg/min, depending on patient response. Never exceed 3 mg/min.

---

Common adverse effects in *italic*; life-threatening effects underlined; generic names in **bold;** classifications in SMALL CAPS; ◆ Canadian drug name; ⊕ Prototype drug

**D**

- Infusion should not be administered for longer than 2 h. **IV Infusion for COPD:** Infuse at 0.5–1.5 mL/min. *INCOMPATIBILITIES:* Solution/additive: **Aminophylline, ascorbic acid,** CEPHALOSPORINS, **dexamethasone, diazepam, digoxin, dobutamine, folic acid, furosemide, hydrocortisone, ketamine, methylprednisolone, minocycline, ticarcillin.** Y-site: **Clindamycin.**

- Store at 15°–30° C (59°–86° F) unless otherwise directed.

**ADVERSE EFFECTS** (≥1%) **CNS:** Dizziness, sneezing, apprehension, confusion, *involuntary movements,* hyperactivity, paresthesias; feeling of warmth and burning, especially of genitalia and perineum; flushing, sweating, hyperpyrexia, headache, pilomotor erection, pruritus, muscle tremor, rigidity, convulsions, *increased deep-tendon reflexes,* bilateral Babinski sign, *carpopedal spasm,* pupillary dilation, mild delayed narcosis. **CV:** *Mild to moderate increase in BP, sinus tachycardia,* bradycardia, extrasystoles, lowered T waves, PVCs, chest pains, tightness in chest. **GI:** Nausea, vomiting, diarrhea, salivation, sour taste. **Urogenital:** Urinary retention, frequency, incontinence. **Respiratory:** Dyspnea, tachypnea, cough, <u>laryngospasm, bronchospasm,</u> hiccups, rebound hypoventilation, hypocapnia with tetany. **Other:** Local skin irritation, thrombophlebitis with extravasation; decreased Hgb, Hct, and RBC count; elevated BUN; albuminuria.

**INTERACTIONS Drug:** MAO INHIBITORS, SYMPATHOMIMETIC AGENTS add to pressor effects.

**PHARMACOKINETICS Onset:** 20–40 s. **Peak:** 1–2 min. **Duration:** 5–12 min. **Metabolism:** Rapidly metabolized. **Elimination:** In urine as metabolites.

**NURSING IMPLICATIONS**
**Assessment & Drug Effects**
- Monitor IV site frequently. Extravasation or use of same IV site for prolonged periods can cause thrombophlebitis (see Appendix F) or tissue irritation.
- Monitor carefully and observe accurately: BP, pulse, deep tendon reflexes, airway, and arterial blood gases. All are essential guides for determining minimum effective dosage and preventing overdosage. Make baseline determinations for comparison.
- Discontinue doxapram if arterial blood gases show evidence of deterioration and when mechanical ventilation is initiated.
- Observe patient continuously during therapy and maintain vigilance until patient is fully alert (usually about 1 h) and protective pharyngeal and laryngeal reflexes are completely restored.
- Notify prescriber immediately of any adverse effects. Be alert for early signs of toxicity: Tachycardia, muscle tremor, spasticity, hyperactive reflexes.
- Note: A mild to moderate increase in BP commonly occurs.
- Discontinue if sudden hypotension or dyspnea develops.
- Monitor lab tests: Arterial $Po_2$, $Pco_2$ and $O_2$ saturation prior to both initiation of doxapram infusion and oxygen administration in patients with COPD, and then at least every 30 min during infusion.

**DOXAZOSIN MESYLATE**
(dox-a′zo-sin)
Cardura, Cardura XL
**Classification:** ALPHA₁-ADRENERGIC ANTAGONIST
Therapeutic: ANTIHYPERTENSIVE
**Prototype:** Prazosin

**AVAILABILITY** Tablet; extended release tablet

**ACTION & *THERAPEUTIC EFFECT***
By selective competitive inhibition
of alpha$_1$-adrenoreceptors, it produces vasodilation in both arterioles and veinous vessels resulting
in both peripheral vascular resistance and reduced blood pressure.
*Long-acting effect of lowering blood
pressure in supine or standing
individuals with most pronounced
effect on diastolic pressure. Also
used for benign prostatic, hyperplasia.*

**USES** Mild to moderate hypertension, benign prostatic hypertrophy.

**UNLABELED USES** CHF.

**CONTRAINDICATIONS** Hypersensitivity to doxazosin, prazosin, and terazosin; hypotension,
syncope.

**CAUTIOUS USE** Hepatic impairment or disease; renal disease, impairment, or failure; older adults
due to high incidence of orthostatic
hypotension; pregnancy (category
C); lactation. Safe use in children
not established.

**ROUTE & DOSAGE**

**Hypertension**

*Adult:* **PO** Start with 1 mg at
bedtime and titrate up to
maximum of 16 mg/day in 1–2
divided doses

**BPH**

*Adult:* **PO Immediate release** 1 mg
daily, may titrate to max of 8/day;
**Extended release** 4 mg daily may
titrate to max of 8 mg/day

**ADMINISTRATION**
**Oral**
- Give initial dose of immediate release tablet at bedtime to
minimize problems with postural
hypotension and syncope.
- Individualize maintenance dose according to the standing BP response.
- Store at 15°–30° C (59°–86° F).

**ADVERSE EFFECTS** (≥1%) **CV:** *Orthostatic hypotension,* edema. **CNS:**
*Vertigo, headache, dizziness,* somnolence, fatigue, nervousness, anxiety. **GI:** Nausea, abdominal pain.
**Hematologic:** Leukopenia. **Skin:**
Pruritus, eczema.

**INTERACTIONS Drug: Sildenafil,
vardenafil, avanafil, nifedipine,**
and **tadalafil** may enhance hypotensive effects. Do not use with
**boceprevir,** ALPHA-BLOCKERS or **tranylcypromine. Herbal: Ma huang**
or **yohimbine** may decrease effect.

**PHARMACOKINETICS Absorp-
tion:** Readily from GI tract; 62–69%
reaches systemic circulation. **Peak:**
2–6 h. **Duration:** Up to 24 h. **Distribution:** Highly protein bound (98–
99%). **Metabolism:** Approximately
35% of dose is metabolized in liver.
**Elimination:** 9% in urine, 63% in
feces. **Half-Life:** 9–12 h.

**NURSING IMPLICATIONS**
**Assessment & Drug Effects**
- Monitor BP with patient lying
down and standing; doses above
4 mg increase the risk of postural
hypotension.
- Monitor BP 2–6 h after initial dose
or any dose increase. This is when
postural hypotension is most likely
to occur.

**Patient & Family Education**
- Do not drive or engage in other
potentially hazardous activities

Common adverse effects in *italic;* life-threatening effects underlined; generic names
in **bold;** classifications in SMALL CAPS; ♣ Canadian drug name; ⦾ Prototype drug

541

**D**

for 12–24 h after the first dose or an increase in dosage or when medication is restarted after an interruption in dosage.

- Use caution when rising from a sitting or supine position in order to avoid orthostatic hypotension and syncope; make position and directional changes slowly and in stages.
- Report to the prescriber episodes of dizziness or palpitations. These will require a dosage adjustment.

## DOXEPIN HYDROCHLORIDE
(dox′e-pin)

Prudoxin, Silenor, Triadapin ◆, Zonalon

**Classifications:** TRICYCLIC ANTIDEPRESSANT; ANXIOLYTIC
**Therapeutic:** ANTIDEPRESSANT; ANTIANXIETY
**Prototype:** Imipramine

**AVAILABILITY** Capsule; oral concentrate; tablet, cream

**ACTION & *THERAPEUTIC EFFECT***
Dibenzoxepin is a tricyclic antidepressant (TCA) that inhibits serotonin reuptake from the synaptic gap; also inhibits norepinephrine reuptake to a moderate degree. *Effective for treatment of both depression and anxiety.*

**USES** Anxiety; depression; insomnia; atopic dermatitis; eczema; lichen simplex.

**UNLABELED USES** Migraine prophylaxis, neuralgia, irritable bowel syndrome.

**CONTRAINDICATIONS** Hypersensitivity to doxepin, dibenzoxepins; during acute recovery phase following MI; bundle branch block, cardiac arrhythmias, QT prolongation; ileus; urinary retention; glaucoma; increased intraocular pressure; prostatic hypertrophy; tendency for urinary retention; suicidal ideation; within 14 days of MAOI drug use; lactation.

**CAUTIOUS USE** Patients receiving electroconvulsive therapy, history of suicidal tendency, head trauma; alcoholism; bipolar disorder, schizophrenia, psychosis; depression; diabetes mellitus; GI disease; GERD; narrow angle glaucoma risk factors; history of insomnia; risk factors for bone fractures; risk factors for orthostatic hypotension; Parkinson's disease; seizure disorders; cardiovascular, or hepatic dysfunction; older adults; IADH syndrome; risk factors for hyponatremia; pregnancy (category C). Safe use in children younger than 18 y not established.

## ROUTE & DOSAGE

### Depression/Anxiety

*Adult:* **PO** 25–150 mg/day in divided doses, may increase up to 300 mg/day (use lower doses in older adult patients)
*Geriatric:* **PO** 10–50 mg/day may increase to 150 mg/day

### Insomnia (Silenor)

*Adult:* **PO** 3–6 mg at bedtime
*Geriatric:* **PO** 3 mg at bedtime

### Dermatitis

*Adult:* **Topical** Apply a thin film q.i.d. with at least 3–4 h between applications, may use up to 8 days

### *Pharmacogenetic Dosage Adjustment*

*CYP2D6 Poor metabolizers:* Give 40% of normal starting oral dose

Common adverse effects in *italic;* life-threatening effects underlined; generic names in **bold**; classifications in SMALL CAPS; ◆ Canadian drug name; ⊙ Prototype drug

## ADMINISTRATION
### Oral
- Give oral concentrate diluted with approximately 120 mL water, milk, or fruit juice.
- Empty capsule and swallow contents with fluid or mix with food as necessary if it cannot be swallowed whole.
- Inform prescriber if daytime sedation is pronounced. Entire daily dose (up to 150 mg) may be prescribed for bedtime administration.

### Topical
- Apply a thin film to affected areas; allow 3–4 h between applications.
- Store all forms at 15°–30° C (59°–86° F) in tightly closed, light-resistant container.

## ADVERSE EFFECTS (≥1%) All:
Anticholinergic. **CNS:** *Drowsiness,* dizziness, weakness, fatigue, headache, hypomania, confusion, tremors, paresthesias. **CV:** *Orthostatic hypotension,* palpitation, hypertension, tachycardia, ECG changes. **Special Senses:** Mydriasis, blurred vision, photophobia. **GI:** *Dry mouth,* sour or metallic taste, epigastric distress, constipation. **Urogenital:** Urinary retention, delayed micturition, urinary frequency. **Other:** Increased perspiration, tinnitus, weight gain, photosensitivity reaction, skin rash, agranulocytosis, *burning or stinging at application site,* edema.

## INTERACTIONS Drug:
May decrease some antihypertensive response to ANTIHYPERTENSIVES; CNS DEPRESSANTS, **alcohol,** HYPNOTICS, BARBITURATES, SEDATIVES potentiate CNS depression; may increase hypoprothrombinemic effect of ORAL ANTICOAGULANTS; **levodopa,** SYMPATHOMIMETICS (e.g., **epinephrine, norepinephrine**) introduce

possibility of sympathetic hyperactivity with hypertension and hyperpyrexia; MAO INHIBITORS introduce possibility of severe reactions, toxic psychosis, cardiovascular instability; **methylphenidate** or **cimetidine** increases plasma levels; THYROID AGENTS may increase possibility of arrhythmias; be cautious with other drugs that prolong the QT interval (e.g., ANTIARRYTHMICS). **Herbal: Ginkgo** may decrease seizure threshold; **St. John's wort** may cause **serotonin** syndrome.

## PHARMACOKINETICS Absorption:
Rapidly from GI sites and through intact skin. **Peak:** 2 h. **Distribution:** Crosses placenta; distributed into breast milk. **Metabolism:** In liver. **Elimination:** Primarily in urine. **Half-Life:** 6–8 h.

## NURSING IMPLICATIONS

### Black Box Warning

*Doxepin has been associated with increased risk of suicidal thinking and behavior in children, adolescents, and young adults.*

### Assessment & Drug Effects
- Monitor for clinical worsening, suicidality, or unusual changes in behavior, especially at initiation of therapy and with children, adolescents, and young adults.
- Monitor use of other CNS depressants, including alcohol. Danger of overdosage or suicide attempt is increased when patient uses excessive amounts of alcohol.
- Be alert to changes in voiding and evaluate patient for constipation and abdominal distention; drug has moderate to strong anticholinergic effects.

### Patient & Family Education
- Monitor closely during initial treatment and when the dose is

Common adverse effects in *italic;* life-threatening effects underlined; generic names in **bold;** classifications in SMALL CAPS; ♣Canadian drug name; Ⓟ Prototype drug

543

adjusted up or down for worsening of depression or suicidal thoughts and behavior. Report promptly to prescriber.

- Be alert for and report to prescriber emergence of anxiety, agitation, panic attacks, insomnia, irritability, hostility, aggressiveness, restlessness or other unusual changes in behavior.
- Maintain established dosage regimen and avoid change of intervals, doubling, reducing, or skipping doses.
- Consult prescriber about safe amount of alcohol, if any, that can be taken. The actions of both alcohol and doxepin are potentiated when used together and for up to 2 wk after doxepin is discontinued.
- Do not drive or engage in other potentially hazardous activities until response to drug is known.

# DOXERCALCIFEROL
(dox-er-kal'si-fe-rol)
Hectorol
**Classification:** VITAMIN D ANALOG
Therapeutic: ANTIHYPERPARATHYROID;
VITAMIN D ANALOG
**Prototype:** Calcitriol

**AVAILABILITY** Capsule; solution for injection

## ACTION & *THERAPEUTIC EFFECT*
Vitamin $D_2$ analog that is activated by the liver. Activated vitamin D is needed for absorption of dietary calcium in the intestine, and the parathyroid hormone (PTH), which mobilizes calcium from the bone tissue. *Regulates the blood calcium level.*

**USES** Hyperparathyroidism.

**CONTRAINDICATIONS** Hypersensitivity to doxercalciferol or other vitamin D analogs; recent hypercalcemia, recent hyperphosphatemia, hypervitaminosis D.

**CAUTIOUS USE** Renal or hepatic insufficiency; renal osteodystrophy with hyperphosphatemia, prolonged hypercalcemia; pregnancy (category B); lactation. Safety and efficacy in children not established.

## ROUTE & DOSAGE

**Secondary Hyperparathyroidism**
*Adult:* **PO** 10 mcg 3 × wk at dialysis, adjust dose as needed to lower iPTH into the range of 150–300 pg/mL by increasing the dose in 2.5 mcg increments every 8 wk (max: 60 mcg/wk) **IV** 4 mcg 3 × wk at end of dialysis (max: 18 mcg/wk)

## ADMINISTRATION

**Oral**
- Give at time of dialysis.
- Withhold drug and notify prescriber if any of the following occurs: iPTH less than 100 pg/mL, hypercalcemia, hyperphosphatemia, or product of serum calcium × serum phosphorus greater than 70.
- Store at 20°–25° C (66°–77° F); excursions to 15°–30° C (59°–86° F) are permitted.

**Intravenous**

*PREPARE:* **Direct:** No dilution is needed.
*ADMINISTER:* **Direct:** Give a bolus injection at the end of dialysis sessions.

- Store at 15°–20° C (59°–77° F).

**ADVERSE EFFECTS** (≥1%) **Body as a Whole:** Abscess, *headache, malaise,* arthralgia. **CNS:** *Dizziness,* sleep disorder. **CV:** Bradycardia,

Common adverse effects in *italic;* life-threatening effects <u>underlined;</u> generic names in **bold;** classifications in SMALL CAPS; ♣ Canadian drug name; ⊕ Prototype drug

*edema*. **GI:** Anorexia, constipation, dyspepsia, *nausea, vomiting*. **Respiratory:** *Dyspnea*. **Skin:** Pruritus. **Other:** Weight gain.

**INTERACTIONS Drug: Cholestyramine, mineral oil** may decrease absorption; MAGNESIUM-CONTAINING ANTACIDS may cause hypermagnesemia; other VITAMIN D ANALOGS may increase toxicity and hypercalcemia.

**PHARMACOKINETICS Absorption:** Absorbed from GI tract and is activated in the liver. **Peak:** 11–12 h. **Metabolism:** Activated by CYP27 to form 1alpha, 25-$(OH)_2D_2$ (major metabolite) and 1alpha, 24-dihydroxy vitamin $D_2$ (minor metabolite). **Half-Life:** 32–37 h.

### NURSING IMPLICATIONS

#### Assessment & Drug Effects
- Monitor for S&S of hypercalcemia (see Appendix F).
- Monitor lab tests: Baseline and weekly during dose titration iPTH, serum calcium, serum phosphorus; then periodically thereafter.

#### Patient & Family Education
- Do not take antacids without consulting the prescriber.
- Notify the prescriber if you become pregnant while taking this drug.
- Do not use mineral oil on the days doxercalciferol is taken. Mineral oil may decrease absorption of drug.
- Do not take nonprescription drugs containing magnesium while taking doxercalciferol.
- Report S&S of hypercalcemia immediately: Bone or muscle pain, dry mouth with metallic taste, rhinorrhea, itching, photophobia, conjunctivitis, frequent urination, anorexia, and weight loss.

# DOXORUBICIN HYDROCHLORIDE ℗⊕
(dox-oh-roo'bi-sin)
Adriamycin

# DOXORUBICIN LIPOSOME
Doxil

**Classifications:** ANTINEOPLASTIC; ANTHRACYCLINE; (ANTIBIOTIC)
Therapeutic: ANTINEOPLASTIC

**AVAILABILITY** Powder for injection; solution for injection; liposomal injection

**ACTION & *THERAPEUTIC EFFECT*** Cytotoxic agent with wide spectrum of antitumor activity. Intercalates with preformed DNA residues, blocking effective DNA and RNA transcription. A potent radiosensitizer capable of enhancing radiation reactions. *Highly destructive to rapidly proliferating cells and slowly developing carcinomas; selectively toxic to cardiac tissue.*

**USES** Adjuvant therapy in breast cancer, disseminated neoplastic conditions.

**CONTRAINDICATIONS** History of hypersensitive reactions to conventional or liposomal doxorubicin; severe hepatic impairment; severe myelosuppression; severe arrhythmias, recent MI; obstructive jaundice, previous treatment with complete cumulative doses of doxorubicin or daunorubicin; pregnancy (category D); lactation.

**CAUTIOUS USE** Impaired hepatic or renal function; patients who have received cyclophosphamide or pelvic irradiation or radiotherapy to areas surrounding heart; preexisting heart disease; history of atopic dermatitis; children.

Common adverse effects in *italic;* life-threatening effects <u>underlined</u>; generic names in **bold**; classifications in SMALL CAPS; ◆ Canadian drug name; ⊘ Prototype drug

545

**D**

## ROUTE & DOSAGE

### CONVENTIONAL DOXORUBICIN

**Acute Lymphatic Leukemia**

*Adult/Child:* **IV** 30 mg/m² weekly × 4 wk

**Acute Myelogenous Leukemia**

*Adult/Child:* **IV** 30 mg/m² × 3 days (with cytarabine)

**Breast Cancer**

*Adult:* **IV** 60 mg/m² on day 1 of 21 day cycle × 4 cycles.

**Transitional Bladder Cell Cancer**

*Adult:* **IV** 30 mg/m²/dose once monthly

**Hodgkin's Disease**

*Adult/Child:* **IV** 25 mg/m² days 1 and 15, repeat q28days

**Thyroid Cancer**

*Adult/Child:* **IV** 60–75 mg/m² q3wk

**Other Neoplasms**

*Adult:* **IV** 40–50 mg/m² usually in combination with other agents (max total cumulative lifetime dose: 500–550 mg/m²)
*Child:* **IV** 35–75 mg/m² as single dose, repeat at 21-day interval, or 20–30 mg/m² once weekly (max total cumulative lifetime dose: 500–550 mg/m²)

**Hepatic Impairment Dosage Adjustment**

*Bilirubin 1.2–3 mg/dL:* Reduce dose by 50%; bilirubin 3–5 mg/dL: Reduce dose by 75%
*Bilirubin greater than 5 mg/dL:* Stop therapy

### DOXORUBICIN LIPOSOME

**Kaposi's Sarcoma**

*Adult:* **IV** 20 mg/m² q3wk. Infuse over 30 min (do not use in-line filters).

**Progressive/Refractory Ovarian Cancer**

*Adult:* **IV** 50 mg/m² q4wk, minimum of 4 courses

**Relapsed/Refractory Multiple Myeloma**

*Adult:* **IV** 45 mg/m² q4wk, up to 6 cycles

**Hepatic Impairment Dosage Adjustment**

*Bilirubin 1.2–3 mg/dL:* Reduce dose 50%; bilirubin 3–5 mg/dL: Reduce dose by 75%

## ADMINISTRATION

### Intravenous

▪ IV administration to children: Verify correct IV concentration and rate of infusion with prescriber. ▪ Wear gloves and use caution when preparing drug solution. If powder or solution contacts skin or mucosa, wash copiously with soap and water.

### Conventional Doxorubicin

**PREPARE: Direct:** *Vial reconstitution:* Dilute with 1 mL of nonbacteriostatic NS for each 2 mg of doxorubicin to yield a final concentraion of 2 mg/mL. ▪ For each mL of NS added, withdraw an equal volume of air from vial to minimize pressure buildup. Shake to dissolve. ▪ *Doxorubicin solutions:* Solutions of 2 mg/mL are available that can be further diluted in 50 mL or more of NS or D5W.
**ADMINISTER: Direct:** Give bolus dose slowly into Y-site of freely running IV infusion of NS or D5W. ▪ If possible, use IV tubing attached to a needle inserted into a larger vein with a butterfly needle. ▪ Usually infused over 3–10 min or longer. ▪ Monitor for red streaking along

vein or facial flushing which indicates need to slow infusion rate.

### Lyophilized Doxorubicin

*PREPARE:* **IV Infusion:** Dilute doses up to 90 mg in 250 mL of D5W and doses greater than 90 mg in 500 mL D5W. Solution will be translucent but not clear, and will be red in color. ▪ **Do not** use filters during preparation or administration.

*ADMINISTER:* **IV Infusion: Do not** give bolus injection or undiluted solution. ▪ Infuse at 1 mg/min initially; may increase rate to complete infusion in 1 h if no adverse reactions occur. Slow infusion rate as warranted if an adverse reaction occurs. ▪ Do not use a filter.

*INCOMPATIBILITIES:* **Solution/additive:** *Conventional doxorubicin:* **Aminophylline, diazepam, fluorouracil. Y-site:** *Conventional doxorubicin.* **Allopurinol, amphotericin B cholesteryl sulfate, cefepime, gallium ganciclovir, lansoprazole, pemetrexed, prochlorperazine, propofol, TPN.** *Doxorubicin liposome:* **Amphotericin B, amphotericin B cholesteryl complex, hydroxyzine, mannitol, meperidine, metoclopramide, mitoxantrone, morphine, paclitaxel, piperacillin/tazobactam, promethazine, sodium bicarbonate.**

▪ Facial flushing and local red streaking along the vein may occur if drug is administered too rapidly. ▪ Avoid using antecubital vein or veins on dorsum of hand or wrist, if possible, where extravasation could damage underlying tendons and nerves. ▪ Also avoid veins in extremity with compromised venous or lymphatic drainage.

▪ Store reconstituted solution for 24 h at room temperature; refrigerated at 4°–10° C (39°–50° F) for 48 h. Protect from sunlight; discard unused solution.

**ADVERSE EFFECTS** (≥1%) **Body as a Whole:** Hypersensitivity (red flare around injection site, erythema, skin rash, pruritus, angioedema, urticaria, eosinophilia, fever, chills, anaphylactoid reaction). **CV:** Serious, irreversible myocardial toxicity with delayed CHF, ventricular arrhythmias, acute left ventricular failure, hypertension, hypotension, cardiomyopathy. **GI:** *Stomatitis,* esophagitis with ulcerations, nausea, vomiting, anorexia, inanition, diarrhea. **Hematologic:** *Severe myelosuppression* (60–85% of patients); leukopenia *(principally granulocytes),* thrombocytopenia, anemia. **Skin:** Hyperpigmentation of nail beds, tongue, and buccal mucosa (especially in blacks); *complete alopecia* (reversible), hyperpigmentation of dermal creases (especially in children), rash, *recall phenomenon (skin reaction due to prior radiotherapy).* **Other:** Lacrimation, drowsiness, fever, facial flush with too rapid IV infusion rate, microscopic hematuria, hyperuricemia, *hand-foot syndrome.* **With extravasation:** *severe cellulitis, vesication, tissue necrosis,* lymphangitis, phlebosclerosis.

**INTERACTIONS Drug:** BARBITURATES may decrease effects by increasing its hepatic metabolism; **streptozocin** may prolong doxorubicin half-life; agents affecting QT interval (e.g., **Bepridil, droperidol, erythromycin, haloperidol, methadone,** PHENOTHIAZINES, etc.) may increase risk of cardiac side effects. Conventional doxorubicin: Avoid use with **zidovudine,** monitor **warfarin** carefully.

Common adverse effects in *italic;* life-threatening effects underlined; generic names in **bold;** classifications in SMALL CAPS; ◆ Canadian drug name; ⊘ Prototype drug

547

**PHARMACOKINETICS** **Distribution:** Widely distributed; does not cross blood–brain barrier; 75% protein binding; does not cross placenta; passes into breast milk. **Metabolism:** In liver to active metabolite. **Elimination:** Primarily in bile. **Half-Life:** 30–50 h. *Doxorubicin Liposome:* **Distribution:** Vascular fluid. **Metabolism:** In plasma and liver. **Elimination:** In urine. **Half-Life:** 44–55 h.

## NURSING IMPLICATIONS

### Black Box Warning

*Doxorubicin can cause severe local tissue necrosis if extravasation occurs. Doxorubicin has been associated with cardiotoxicity, severe bone marrow suppression, and development of secondary malignancies (i.e., acute myelogenous leukemia or myelodysplastic syndrome).*

### Assessment & Drug Effects

- Care should be taken to avoid extravasation. Stop infusion, remove IV needle, and notify prescriber promptly if patient complains of stinging or burning sensation at the injection site.
- Monitor any area of extravasation closely for 3–4 wk. If ulceration begins (usually 1–4 wk after extravasation), a plastic surgeon should be consulted.
- Establish baseline data. Include temperature, pulse, respiration, BP, body weight, laboratory values, and I&O ratio and pattern.
- Cardiac function must be evaluated prior to initiation of therapy, at regular intervals, and at end of therapy.
- Be alert to and report early signs of cardiotoxicity (see Appendix F). Acute life-threatening arrhythmias may occur within a few hours of drug administration.

- Report promptly objective signs of hepatic dysfunction (jaundice, dark urine, pruritus) or kidney dysfunction (altered I&O ratio and pattern, local discomfort with voiding).
- Report signs of superinfection (see Appendix F) promptly; these may result from antibiotic therapy during leukopenic period.
- Avoid rectal medications and use of rectal thermometer; rectal trauma is associated with bloody diarrhea resulting from an antiblastic effect on rapidly growing intestinal mucosal cells.
- Monitor lab tests: Baseline and periodic LFTs, renal function, CBC with differential.

### Patient & Family Education

- Complete loss of hair (reversible) is an expected adverse effect. It may also involve eyelashes and eyebrows, beard and mustache, pubic and axillary hair. Regrowth of hair usually begins 2–3 mo after drug is discontinued.
- Drug turns urine red for 1–2 days after administration.
- Keep hands away from eyes to prevent conjunctivitis. Increased tearing for 5–10 days after a single dose is possible.
- Maintain fastidious oral hygiene, especially before and after meals. Stomatitis, generally maximal in second week of therapy, frequently begins with a burning sensation accompanied by erythema of oral mucosa that may progress to ulceration and dysphagia in 2 or 3 days.
- Exposure to doxorubicin during the first trimester of pregnancy can result in fetal abnormalities or fetal loss.

## DOXYCYCLINE HYCLATE
(dox-i-sye′kleen)

Apo-Doxy ✦, Doryx, Doxy,
Doxycin ✦, Monodox,
Vibramycin

**Classifications:** ANTIBIOTIC;
TETRACYCLINE
**Therapeutic:** ANTIBIOTIC
**Prototype:** Tetracycline

**AVAILABILITY** Capsule, tablet; solution for injection

## ACTION & THERAPEUTIC EFFECT

Semisynthetic broad-spectrum long-acting tetracycline antibiotic that is more lipophilic than the other tetracyclines allowing it to pass through the lipid layer of bacteria where reversible binding to the 30 S ribosomal subunits of bacteria occurs. This blocks the binding of transfer RNA (tRNA) to the messenger RNA (mRNA) of bacteria, resulting in inhibition of bacterial protein synthesis. *Primarily bacteriostatic against both gram-positive and gram-negative bacteria.*

**USES** Similar to those of tetracycline (e.g., chlamydial and mycoplasmal infections); gonorrhea, syphilis in penicillin-allergic patients; rickettsial diseases, acute exacerbations of chronic bronchitis.

**UNLABELED USES** Treatment of acute PID, leptospirosis, prophylaxis for rape victims, suppression and chemoprophylaxis of chloroquine-resistant *Plasmodium falciparum* malaria, short-term prophylaxis and treatment of travelers' diarrhea caused by enterotoxigenic strains of *Escherichia coli.* Intrapleural administration for malignant pleural effusions, post-exposure anthrax treatment and prophylaxis.

**CONTRAINDICATIONS** Sensitivity to any of the tetracyclines; use during period of tooth development including last half of pregnancy; pregnancy (category D); lactation, infants, and children younger than 8 y except for use in anthrax exposure (causes permanent yellow discoloration of teeth, enamel hypoplasia, and retardation of bone growth).

**CAUTIOUS USE** Alcoholism; hepatic disease; GI disease; sulfite hypersensitivity; sunlight (UV) exposure.

## ROUTE & DOSAGE

### Skin/Skin Structure Infections
*Adult/Adolescent/Child (8 y or older, weight 45 kg or more):*
**IV** 200 mg on day 1 then 100–200 mg daily
*Child (8 y or older, weight 45 kg or less):* **IV** 4.4 mg/kg on day 1 then 2.2–4.4 mg/kg/day in divided doses

### UTI
*Adult/Adolescent:* **PO** 100 mg q12h × 1 day then 100 mg daily; **IV** 200 mg on day 1 then 100–200 mg daily

### Gonorrhea
*Adult:* **PO** 100 mg b.i.d. × 7 days

### Primary and Secondary Syphilis
*Adult:* **PO** 100 mg b.i.d. × 14 days

### Acute Pelvic Inflammatory Disease
*Adult:* **IV** 100 mg q12h until improved, then 100 mg **PO** b.i.d. to complete 14 days

### Acne
*Adult:* **PO** 100 mg q12h on day 1, then 100 mg daily
*Child (8 y or older, weight greater than 45 kg):* **PO** 100 mg q12h on day 1, then 100 mg daily; *weight less than 45 kg:* **PO** 2.2 mg/kg q12h on day 1, then 2.2 mg/kg/daily

Common adverse effects in *italic;* life-threatening effects underlined; generic names in **bold;** classifications in SMALL CAPS; ✦ Canadian drug name; ⊕ Prototype drug

549

D

**Anthrax Post-Exposure**

*Adult/Adolescent/Child (8 y or older, weight greater than 45 kg):*
**IV** 100 mg q12h, then switch to **PO** for a total of 60
*Child (8 y or less or weight 45 kg or less)* **IV** 2.2 mg/kg q12h, then switch to **PO** for a total of 60

## ADMINISTRATION
### Oral
- Check expiration date. Degradation products of tetracycline are toxic to the kidneys.
- Give with food or a full glass of milk to minimize nausea without significantly affecting bioavailability of drug (unlike most **tetracyclines**). Patient should sit up for at least 30–120 min after administration to reduce the risk of esophageal irritation and ulceration.
- Consult prescriber about ordering the oral suspension for patients who are bedridden or have difficulty swallowing.

### Intravenous

*PREPARE:* **Intermittent:** Reconstitute by adding 10 mL sterile water for injection, or D5W, NS, LR, D5/LR, or other diluent recommended by manufacturer, to each 100 mg of drug. • Further dilute with 100–1000 mL (per 100 mg of drug) of compatible infusion solution to produce concentrations ranging from 0.1 to 1 mg/mL.
*ADMINISTER:* **Intermittent:** Duration of infusion varies with dose but is usually 1–4 h. • Recommended minimum infusion time for 100 mg of 0.5 mg/mL solution is 1 h. Infusion should be completed within 12 h of dilution. • When diluted with LR or D5/LR, infusion **must be** completed within 6 h to ensure adequate stability. • Protect all solutions from direct sunlight during infusion.

*INCOMPATIBILITIES:* Solution/additive: **Potassium phosphate.** Y-site: **Allopurinol, heparin, meropenem, premetrexed disodium, piperacillin/tazobactam, TPN.**

- Store oral and parenteral forms (prior to reconstitution) in tightly covered, light-resistant containers at 15°–30° C (59°–86° F) unless otherwise directed. • Refrigerate reconstituted solutions for up to 72 h. After this time, infusion **must be** completed within 12 h.

## ADVERSE EFFECTS (≥1%) Special
**Senses:** Interference with color vision. **Cardiac:** Hypertension. **CNS:** Pain, anxiety. **Genitourinary:** Dymenorrhea. **Neuromuscular and Skeletal:** Arthralgia **GI:** Anorexia, *nausea, vomiting, diarrhea,* enterocolitis; esophageal irritation (oral capsule and tablet). **Respiratory:** Nasopharyngitis, bronchitis, sinusitis, nasal congestion. **Skin:** Rashes, photosensitivity reaction. **Other:** Thrombophlebitis (IV use), superinfections.

## DIAGNOSTIC TEST INTERFERENCE
Like other **tetracyclines,** doxycycline may cause false increases in *urinary catecholamines* (fluorometric methods); false decreases in *urinary urobilinogen;* false-negative *urine glucose* with *glucose oxidase methods* (e.g., *Clinistix, TesTape*); parenteral doxycycline (containing ascorbic acid) may cause false-positive determinations using *Benedict's reagent* or *Clinitest.*

## INTERACTIONS Drug: ANTACIDS,
**iron** preparation, **calcium, magnesium, zinc, kaolinpectin, sodium bicarbonate** can significantly decrease absorption; effects of both doxycycline and **desmopressin** antagonized; increases **digoxin**

absorption, thus increasing risk of **digoxin** toxicity; **methoxyflurane** increases risk of renal failure. Do not use with **acitretin** or **isotretinoin**.

## PHARMACOKINETICS Absorption: Completely absorbed from GI tract. **Peak:** 1.5–4 h. **Distribution:** Penetrates eye, prostate, and CSF; crosses placenta; distributed into breast milk. **Metabolism:** In GI tract. **Elimination:** Mainly in feces. **Half-Life:** 14–24 h.

## NURSING IMPLICATIONS

### Assessment & Drug Effects

- Report sudden onset of painful or difficult swallowing promptly to prescriber. Doxycycline (capsule and tablet forms) is associated with a comparatively high incidence of esophagitis, especially in patients older than 40 y.
- Report evidence of superinfections (see Appendix F).

### Patient & Family Education

- Take capsule or tablet forms with a full glass (240 mL) of water to ensure passage into stomach and prevent esophageal ulceration. Avoid taking capsule or tablet within 1 h of lying down or retiring.
- Avoid exposure to direct sunlight and ultraviolet light during and for 4 or 5 days after therapy is terminated to reduce risk of phototoxic reaction. Phototoxic reaction appears like an exaggerated sunburn. Sunscreens provide little protection.

## DRONABINOL
(droe-nab'i-nol)
**Marinol**
**Classifications:** CANNABINOID; ANTIEMETIC
**Therapeutic:** ANTIEMETIC; APPETITE STIMULANT
**Controlled Substance:** Schedule III

## AVAILABILITY Capsule

## ACTION & *THERAPEUTIC EFFECT*
Synthetic derivative of tetrahydrocannabinol (THC), the principal psychoactive constituent of marijuana *(Cannabis sativa)*. Inhibits vomiting through the control mechanism in the medulla oblongata, producing potent antiemetic effect. Risk of drug abuse is high. *Produces potent antiemetic effect and is used to treat chemotherapy-induced nausea and vomiting. For use of appetite stimulant in the treatment of anorexia associated with weight loss.*

## USES To treat chemotherapy-induced nausea and vomiting in cancer patients. Appetite stimulant for AIDS patients.

## UNLABELED USES Glaucoma.

## CONTRAINDICATIONS Nausea and vomiting caused by other than chemotherapeutic agents; hypersensitivity to dronabinol or sesame oil; lactation.

## CAUTIOUS USE First exposure, especially in the older adult or cardiac patient; hypertension, hypotension, cardiovascular disorders; epilepsy; psychiatric illness, patient receiving other psychoactive drugs; severe hepatic dysfunction; pregnancy (category C); children due to psychoactive effects.

## ROUTE & DOSAGE

| Chemotherapy-Induced Nausea |
|---|
| *Adult/Child:* **PO** 5 mg/m$^2$ 1–3 h before administration of chemotherapy, then q2–4h after chemotherapy for a total of 4–6 doses, dose may be increased by 2.5 mg/m$^2$ (max: 15 mg/m$^2$ if necessary) |

Common adverse effects in *italic;* life-threatening effects underlined; generic names in **bold**; classifications in SMALL CAPS; ♣ Canadian drug name; ❍ Prototype drug

551

**D**

**Appetite Stimulant**
*Adult:* **PO** 2.5 mg b.i.d., before lunch and dinner

## ADMINISTRATION
### Oral
- Do not repeat dose following a CNS adverse reaction until patient's mental state has returned to normal and the circumstances have been evaluated.
- Store capsules at 8°–15° C (46°–59° F).

## ADVERSE EFFECTS (≥1%) CNS:
*Drowsiness,* psychologic high, dizziness, anxiety, confusion, euphoria, sensory or perceptual difficulties, impaired coordination, depression, irritability, headache, ataxia, memory lapse, paresthesias, paranoia, depersonalization, disorientation, tinnitus, nightmares, speech difficulty, facial flush, diaphoresis. **CV:** Tachycardia, orthostatic hypotension, hypertension, facial flushing, syncope. **GI:** Dry mouth, abdominal pain, nausea, vomiting, diarrhea, fecal incontinence. **Other:** Muscular weakness.

## INTERACTIONS Drug: **Alcohol** and
other CNS DEPRESSANTS may exaggerate psychoactive effects of dronabinol; TRICYCLIC ANTIDEPRESSANTS, **atropine** may cause tachycardia. Do not use with **nabilone** due to increased psychotoxic effects.

## PHARMACOKINETICS **Absorption:** Rapidly absorbed from GI tract, with bioavailability of 10–20%. **Peak:** 2–3 h. **Distribution:** Fat soluble; distributed to many organs; distributed into breast milk; 97% protein bound. **Metabolism:** In liver; extensive first-pass metabolism. **Elimination:** Principally in bile; 50% in feces within 72 h; 10–15% in urine. **Half-Life:** 25–36 h.

## NURSING IMPLICATIONS
### Assessment & Drug Effects
- Monitor patients with hypertension or heart disease for BP and cardiac status.
- Response to dronabinol is varied, and previous uneventful use does not guarantee that adverse reactions will not occur. Effects of drug may persist an unpredictably long time (days). Extended use at therapeutic dosage may cause accumulation of toxic amounts of dronabinol and its metabolites.
- Watch for disturbing psychiatric symptoms if dose is increased: Altered mental state, loss of coordination, evidence of a psychologic high (easy laughing, elation and heightened awareness), or depression.
- Note: Abrupt withdrawal is associated with symptoms (within 12 h) of irritability, insomnia, restlessness. Peak intensity occurs at about 24 h: Hot flashes, diaphoresis, rhinorrhea, watery diarrhea, hiccups, anorexia. Usually, syndrome is over in 96 h.

### Patient & Family Education
- Do not drive or engage in other potentially hazardous activities that require alertness and judgment because of high incidence of dizziness and drowsiness.
- Understand potential (reversible) for drug-induced mood or behavior changes that may occur during dronabinol use.
- Do not ingest alcohol during period of systemic dronabinol effect. Effect on blood ethanol levels is complex and unpredictable.

## DRONEDARONE
(dro-ne′da-rone)
Multaq
**Classification:** CLASS III ANTIARRHYTHMIC

**Therapeutic:** CLASS III
ANTIARRHYTHMIC

## AVAILABILITY Tablet

## ACTION & *THERAPEUTIC EFFECT*

Antiarrhythmic class III drug known to inhibit potassium currents, sodium channels, and slow-L type calcium channels. *Reduces risk of hospitalization in patients with recent paroxysmal or persistent atrial fibrillation (AF).*

## USES Recent episode of paroxysmal or persistent atrial fibrillation.

## CONTRAINDICATIONS NYHA

Class IV HF or NYHA Class II-III HF with a recent decompensation requiring hospitalization or referral to a specialized HF clinic; permanent atrial fibrillation; second and third degree AV block or sick sinus syndrome (except with used in conjunction with a functioning pacemaker); bradycardia less than 40 bpm; QT$_c$ interval elongation; severe hepatic impairment; pregnancy (category X); lactation.

## CAUTIOUS USE HF; prolonged QT interval; hypokalemia, hypomagnesium; potassium-depleting diuretics; moderate liver impairment; women of child-bearing age. Safety and efficacy in children younger than 18 y not established.

## ROUTE & DOSAGE

### Atrial Fibrillation
*Adult:* **PO** 400 mg b.i.d. with meals

## ADMINISTRATION
### Oral
- Give with morning and evening meal. **Do not** give with grapefruit juice.
- Store at 15°–3° C (56°–89° F).

## ADVERSE EFFECTS (≥1%) **Body as a Whole:** Asthenia. **CV:** Bradycardia, *QT$_c$ prolongation.* **GI:** Abdominal pain, diarrhea, dyspepsia, nausea, vomitting. **Metabolic:** *Increased serum creatinine,* hepatic injury. **Skin:** Dermatitis, eczema, erythematous, macula-papular rash, pruritus.

## INTERACTIONS **Drug:** Concomitant use of CYP3A4 inducers (e.g., **rifampin, phenobarbital, carbamazepine, phenytoin**) can increase the levels of dronedarone. **Ketoconazole, itraconazole, clarithromycin**, and other inhibitors of CYP3A4 can increase the levels of dronedarone. Dronedarone can increase the levels of **digoxin** and other compounds requiring P-glycoprotein (P-gp) transport. BETA-BLOCKERS may provoke excessive bradycardia. **Verapamil** and **diltiazem** can potentiate dronedarone's effects on conduction. Use cautiously with **dabigatran. Food: Grapefruit juice** can increase the levels of dronedarone. **Herbal: St. John's wort** can decrease the levels of dronedarone.

## PHARMACOKINETICS **Peak:** 3–6 h. **Distribution:** 98% plasma protein bound. **Metabolism:** Extensive hepatic metabolism to active and inactive compounds. **Elimination:** 84% in the feces; 6% in the urine. **Half-Life:** 13–19 h.

## NURSING IMPLICATIONS
### Assessment & Drug Effects
- Monitor vital signs and ECG. Report promptly prolongation of the QT$_c$ interval.
- Monitor for S&S of hepatic toxicity (see Appendix F).
- Report promptly S&S of worsening HF (e.g., rapid weight gain, dependent edema, increasing shortness of breath).
- Withhold drug and notify prescriber if hypokalemia or hypomagnesemia develops.

---

Common adverse effects in *italic;* life-threatening effects <u>underlined</u>; generic names in **bold**; classifications in SMALL CAPS; ♣Canadian drug name; ⓟ Prototype drug

- Monitor lab tests: Baseline and periodic potassium and magnesium levels; periodic serum creatinine.

**Patient & Family Education**

- Report immediately any of the following: Shortness of breath, wheezing, chest tightness, coughing up frothy sputum, rapid weight gain, requiring more pillows to sleep at night.
- Women of childbearing age should use effective contraception while on this drug.
- Avoid grapefruit and grapefruit juice while taking this drug.

## DROPERIDOL

(droe-per'i-dole)

**Classifications:** BUTYROPHENONE; MISCELLANEOUS ANTIEMETIC; ANXIOLYTIC
Therapeutic: ANTIEMETIC; ANTIANXIETY
**Prototype:** Aprepitant

**AVAILABILITY** Solution for injection

**ACTION & *THERAPEUTIC EFFECT***
Antagonizes emetic effects of morphine-like analgesics and other drugs that act on chemoreceptor trigger zone. *Sedative property reduces anxiety and motor activity without necessarily inducing sleep; patient remains responsive. Has antiemetic properties.*

**USES** To reduce nausea/vomiting association with surgery/diagnostic procedures.

**UNLABELED USES** Chemotherapy-induced nausea-vomiting.

**CONTRAINDICATIONS** Known or suspected QT elongation; history of torsades de pointes; known intolerance to droperidol; hypokalemia, hypomagnesia; lactation.

**CAUTIOUS USE** Older adult, debilitated, alcoholism, and other poor-risk patients; MAOI therapy; Parkinson's disease; cardiac disease; cardiac bradyarrhythmias, cardiac arrhythmias, CHF, hypotension; liver and kidney impairment or disease; pregnancy (category C). Safe use in children younger than 2 y is not established.

## ROUTE & DOSAGE

**Postoperative Nausea and Vomiting Prevention Using Continual ECG Monitoring**

*Adult:* **IV/IM** 2.5 mg; additional doses of 1.25 mg may be given
*Child:* **IV/IM** 0.1 mg/kg (max: 2.5 mg)

**Renal Impairment Dosage Adjustment**

Due to increased risk of QT prolongation and torsades de points continuous monitoring is required

## ADMINISTRATION

**Intramuscular**
- Give undiluted.
- Give deep IM into a large muscle.

**Intravenous**
IV administration to infants and children: Verify correct rate of IV injection with prescriber.

**PREPARE: Direct:** Give undiluted.
**ADMINISTER: Direct:** *Adult:* Give at a rate of 2.5 mg or fraction thereof over 1–2 min. *Child:* Give a single dose over at least 2 min.
**INCOMPATIBILITIES:** Solution/additive: BARBITURATES. **Y-site: Allopurinol, amphotericin B cholesteryl complex, cefepime, cefotetan, fluorouracil, foscarnet, furosemide, heparin, leucovorin, methotrexate, nafcillin, piperacillin/tazobactam.**

Common adverse effects in *italic;* life-threatening effects underlined; generic names in **bold;** classifications in SMALL CAPS; ♣ Canadian drug name; ❂ Prototype drug

- Store at 15°–30° C (59°–86° F), unless otherwise directed by manufacturer. Protect from light.

## ADVERSE EFFECTS (≥1%) CNS:

*Postoperative drowsiness, extrapyramidal symptoms:* dystonia, akathisia, oculogyric crisis; dizziness, restlessness, anxiety, hallucinations, mental depression. **CV:** *Hypotension, tachycardia,* irregular heartbeats *(prolonged QT$_c$ interval even at low doses).* **Other:** Chills, shivering, laryngospasm, bronchospasm.

## INTERACTIONS Drugs: Additive

effect with CNS depressants, **metoclopramide** may increase extrapyramidal symptoms, closely monitor other drugs affecting QT interval.

## PHARMACOKINETICS Onset: 3–10

min. **Peak:** 30 min. **Duration:** 2–4 h; may persist up to 12 h. **Distribution:** Crosses placenta. **Metabolism:** In liver. **Elimination:** In urine and feces.

## NURSING IMPLICATIONS

### Black Box Warning

*Droperidol has been associated with development of QT prolongation and/or torsade de pointes.*

### Assessment & Drug Effects

- Monitor ECG throughout therapy. Report immediately prolongation of QT$_c$ interval.
- Monitor vital signs closely. Hypotension and tachycardia are common adverse effects.
- Exercise care in moving medicated patients because of possibility of severe orthostatic hypotension. Avoid abrupt changes in position.
- Observe patients for signs of impending respiratory depression carefully when receiving a concurrent narcotic analgesic.

- Note: EEG patterns are slow to return to normal during the postoperative period.
- Observe carefully and report promptly to prescriber early signs of acute dystonia: Facial grimacing, restlessness, tremors, torticollis, oculogyric crisis. Extrapyramidal symptoms may occur within 24–48 h postoperatively.
- Note: Droperidol may aggravate symptoms of acute depression.

## DROXIDOPA

(drox-i-dop′a)

Northera

**Classifications:** DOPAMINE RECEPTOR AGONIST; HYPERTENSIVE

Therapeutic: HYPERTENSIVE

**Prototype:** Carbidopa

## AVAILABILITY Gelatin capsules

## ACTION & *THERAPEUTIC EFFECT*

Droxidopa is directly metabolized to norepinephrine. Believed to exert its pharmacological effects through norepinephrine which *increases BP by inducing peripheral arterial and venous vasoconstriction.*

## USES Treatment of neurogenic

orthostatic hypotension caused by primary autonomic failure (Parkinson's disease, multiple system atrophy, and pure autonomic failure), dopamine beta-hydroxylase deficiency, and non-diabetic autonomic neuropathy.

## CONTRAINDICATIONS Lactation.

## CAUTIOUS USE Supine hyperten-

sion; neuroleptic malignant syndrome; ischemic heart disease; CHF; arrhythmias; hypersensitivity to tartrazine (especially in those with aspirin hypersensitivity); severe renal impairment; pregnancy (category C).

## ROUTE & DOSAGE

### Neurogenic Orthostatic Hypotension

*Adult:* **PO** 100 mg t.i.d. initially; can titrate in 100 mg increments q24–48h (max: 600 mg t.i.d.)

## ADMINISTRATION

### Oral

- Give capsule whole. It should not be crushed or chewed.
- Give consistently with/without food, upon arising in a.m., at midday, and in late afternoon at least 3 h before bedtime (to reduce risk of supine hypertension during sleep).
- Store at 15° C–30° C (59° F–86° F).

## ADVERSE EFFECTS (≥ 1%) **Body as a Whole:** *Falling,* headache. **CNS:** Dizziness. **CV:** Hypertension, *syncope.* **GI:** Nausea. **Urogenital:** *Urinary tract infection.*

## INTERACTIONS **Drug: Carbidopa** may decrease the levels of droxidopa's active metabolite. Other drugs that increase blood pressure (**ephedrine, midodrine,** SEROTONIN 5-HT1D RECEPTOR AGONISTS).

## PHARMACOKINETICS **Peak:** 1–4 h. **Distribution:** Plasma protein binding is dose related. **Metabolism:** Bioactivated to norepinephrine. **Elimination:** Primarily renal. **Half-Life:** 2.5 h.

## NURSING IMPLICATIONS

### Black Box Warning

*Droxidopa has been associated with severe, potentially fatal supine hypertension.*

### Assessment & Drug Effects

- Elevate the head of the bed to lessen risk of supine hypertension.
- Monitor supine BP (with head of bed elevated) prior to and during treatment and more frequently when increasing doses.
- If supine hypertension cannot be managed by elevation of the head of the bed, report to prescriber as dose should be reduced or drug discontinued.

### Patient & Family Education

- Rest and sleep in an upper-body elevated position.
- Monitor blood pressure and report promptly to prescriber significant elevations when supine.
- Be consistent when taking drug with respect to food (see ADMINISTRATION).

## DULAGLUTIDE

(du-la-glu'tide)

*Trulicity*

**Classifications:** ANTIDIABETIC; INCRETIN MIMETIC; GLUCAGON–LIKE PEPTIDE-1

**Therapeutic:** ANTIDIABETIC

**Prototype:** Exenatide

## AVAILABILITY Single-dose pen and prefilled syringe

## ACTION & *THERAPEUTIC EFFECT*

Improves glycemic control in type 2 diabetes mellitus by mimicking the functions of incretin, a glucagon-like peptide-1 (GLP-1), which enhances glucose-dependent insulin secretion by pancreatic beta-cells, suppresses inappropriately elevated glucagon secretion, and slows gastric emptying. *Improves glycemic control by reducing fasting and postprandial glucose concentrations.*

## USES Type 2 diabetes mellitus in combination with diet and exercise.

## CONTRAINDICATIONS Serious hypersensitivity to dulaglutide or

556

Common adverse effects in *italic;* life-threatening effects <u>underlined</u>; generic names in **bold**; classifications in SMALL CAPS; ♣ Canadian drug name; ● Prototype drug component of the formulation; personal or family history of medullary thyroid carcinoma; multiple endocrine neoplasia (MEN); pancreatitis; lactation.

**CAUTIOUS USE** Hepatic impairment; renal impairment; preexisting, severe GU disease; gastroparesis; history of pancreatitis; pregnancy (category C). Safety and efficacy in children younger than 18 y not established.

## ROUTE & DOSAGE

### Type 2 Diabetes Mellitus
*Adult:* **Subcutaneous** 0.75 mg once weekly; may increase to 1.5 mg once weekly

## ADMINISTRATION

### Subcutaneous
- Administer weekly on the same day each wk, without regard to meals or time of day.
- May change injection day as long as the last dose was administered at least 3 days prior.
- Inject into the upper arm, thigh, or abdomen.
- Use a different injection site each week.
- Store at 2°–8° C (36°–46° F). Do not freeze. Protect from light. Single-dose pen or prefilled syringe can be kept at room temperature, up to 30° C (86° F), for 14 days.

**ADVERSE EFFECTS** (≥ 1%) **Body as a Whole:** Asthenia, fatigue, hypersensitivity reactions, malaise. **CV:** Tachycardia. **GI:** Abdominal distension, abdominal pain, constipation, decreased appetite, diarrhea, dyspepsia, eructation, flatulence, gastroesophageal reflux disease, gastrointestinal pain, nausea. **Hematological:** Hypoglycemia. **Metabolic:** Increased amylase and lipase levels.

**INTERACTIONS Drug:** Concomitant use with **insulin** or an INSULIN SECRETAGOGUE may result in additive effects on blood glucose. Dulaglutide slows gastric emptying and has the potential to decrease the rate of absorption of other co-administered oral drugs.

**PHARMACOKINETICS Peak:** 24–72 h. **Metabolism:** In liver. **Elimination:** Primarily in urine. **Half-Life:** 5 days.

## NURSING IMPLICATIONS

### Black Box Warning

*Dulaglutide may pose a risk of thyroid C-cell tumor development, although a direct link has not been established.*

### Assessment & Drug Effects
- Monitor for and report S&S of significant GI distress, including nausea, vomiting, and diarrhea.
- Monitor for S&S of hypoglycemia and S&S of acute pancreatitis (acute abdominal pain with/without vomiting). If pancreatitis is suspected, withhold drug and notify prescriber immediately.
- Monitor for and report immediately site injection reactions such as cellulitis, abscess, and skin necrosis.
- Monitor lab tests: Frequent fasting and postprandial plasma glucose and periodic HbA1C; baseline and periodic renal function tests.

### Patient & Family Education
- If a weekly dose is missed, administer it as soon as possible as long as next scheduled dose is due at least 3 days later.
- Dulaglutide may cause decreased appetite and some weight loss.
- Report significant GI distress to prescriber. Report promptly persistent,

---

**D**

severe abdominal pain that may be accompanied by vomiting.

▪ Report symptoms of thyroid tumors (e.g., a lump in the neck, hoarseness, dysphagia, dyspnea).

▪ Do not breast-feed while taking this drug.

## DULOXETINE HYDROCHLORIDE

(du-lox'e-teen)

Cymbalta, Irenka

**Classifications:** ANTIDEPRESSANT; SEROTONIN NOREPINEPHRINE REUPTAKE INHIBITOR (SNRI)

**Therapeutic:** ANTIDEPRESSANT; SNRI; ANTIANXIETY; NEUROPATHIC PAIN RELIEVER

**Prototype:** Venlafaxine

**AVAILABILITY** Delayed-release capsule

**ACTION & THERAPEUTIC EFFECT** Potentiates serotonergic and noradrenergic activity in the CNS. Antidepressant and antianxiety effects are presumed to be due to its dual inhibition of CNS presynaptic neuronal uptake of serotonin and norepinephrine, thus increasing the serum levels of both substances. *Effective as an antidepressant, antianxiety, and neuropathic pain reliever.*

**USES** Treatment of major depression, generalized anxiety, fibromyalgia, diabetic peripheral neuropathy, musculoskeletal pain.

**UNLABELED USES** Stress urinary incontinence, osteoarthritis.

**CONTRAINDICATIONS** Concurrent administration of MAOI therapy or within 14 days of use; initiation of MAOI within 5 days of starting duloxetine; suicidal ideation; uncontrolled narrow-angle glaucoma; alcoholism; severe skin reaction to duloxetine; bipolar depression; end-stage renal disease; hepatitis; jaundice; abrupt discontinuation; pregnancy (category D in third trimester).

**CAUTIOUS USE** Anorexia nervosa, bipolar disease; history of mania, history of suicidal tendencies; cardiac disease; renal impairment or renal failure; hepatic impairment; impaired gastric mobility; DM; hypertension; risk factors for hyponatremia or SIADH; older adults; pregnancy (category C in first and second trimester); lactation. Safe use in children younger than 18 y not established.

## ROUTE & DOSAGE

| Depression |
| --- |
| *Adult:* **PO** 40–60 mg/day in one or two divided doses |
| **Generalized Anxiety/Diabetic Neuropathy/Musculoskeletal Pain** |
| *Adult:* **PO** 60 mg once daily |
| **Fibromyalgia** |
| *Adult:* **PO** 30 mg/day × 1 wk then 60 mg/day |

## ADMINISTRATION

**Oral**

▪ Do not initiate therapy within 14 days of the last dose of an MAOI.

▪ **Must be** swallowed whole. Do not cut, chew, or crush. Do not sprinkle on food or mix with liquids.

▪ Store at 15°–30° C (59°–86° F).

**ADVERSE EFFECTS** (≥1%) **Body as a Whole:** Fatigue, hot flashes. **CNS:** Dizziness, somnolence, tremor, *insomnia.* **GI:** *Nausea, dry mouth, constipation,* diarrhea, vomiting. **Metabolic:** Decreased appetite, weight loss. **Skin:** Increased sweating. **Special Senses:** Blurred vision. **Urogenital:** Decreased libido, abnormal orgasm, erectile dysfunction, ejaculatory

Common adverse effects in *italic*; life-threatening effects <u>underlined</u>; generic names in **bold**; classifications in SMALL CAPS; ✦ Canadian drug name; ⊘ Prototype drug dysfunction. Cholestatic jaundice and hepatitis.

**INTERACTIONS Drug: Alcohol** may result in increased liver function tests; MAOIS may result in hyperthermia, rigidity, mental status changes, myoclonus, autonomic instability, features resembling neuroleptic malignant syndrome; **cimetidine, fluoxetine, fluvoxamine, paroxetine, quinidine,** QUINOLONES may increase levels and half-life of duloxetine; may increase levels and toxicity of **thioridazine,** TRICYCLIC ANTIDEPRESSANTS. **Amphetamine, dextroamphetamine, buspirone, cocaine, dexfenfluramine, fenfluramine, lithium, phentermine, sibutramine, nefazodone,** SSRIS, TRIPTANS, **tramadol, trazodone** may cause serotonin syndrome. **Herbal: St. John's wort, tryptophan** may cause serotonin syndrome.

**PHARMACOKINETICS Peak:** 6 h. **Metabolism:** In the liver by CYP2D6 and CYP1A2. **Elimination:** 70% in urine, 20% in feces. **Half-Life:** 12 h (8–17 h).

**NURSING IMPLICATIONS**
**Assessment & Drug Effects**
- Ensure that a complete list of all concurrent medications is obtained.
- Monitor for S&S of numerous drug-drug interactions (see Interaction section).
- Monitor closely for and report suicide ideation, especially when drug is initiated or dosage changed.
- Report emergence of any of the following: Anxiety, agitation, panic attacks, insomnia, irritability, hostility, psychomotor restlessness, hypomania, and mania.
- Monitor BP, especially in those being treated for hypertension.
- Monitor lab tests: Periodic serum creatinine, blood urea nitrogen, and LFTs.

**Patient & Family Education**
- The beneficial effects of this drug may not be felt for approximately 4 wk.
- Report any of the following: Suicidal ideation (especially early in treatment or when dosage is changed), palpitations, anxiety, hyperactivity, agitation, panic attacks, insomnia, irritability, hostility, restlessness.
- Do not abruptly discontinue taking this drug. Notify prescriber if side effects are bothersome.
- Avoid or minimize use of alcohol while taking this drug.
- Do not self-treat for coughs, colds, or allergies. Consult prescriber.

**DUPILUMAB**
(doo-pil´ue-mab)
Dupixent
**Classifications:** SKIN AND MUCOUS MEMBRANE AGENT; MONOCLONAL ANTIBODY; INTERLEUKIN-4 RECEPTOR ANTAGONIST
Therapeutic: ANTIECZEMA AGENT

**AVAILABILITY** Subcutaneous injection; prefilled syringe

**ACTION & *THERAPEUTIC EFFECT*** Human monoclonal IgG4 antibody that inhibits interleukin-4 and interleukin 13 signaling by binding to the subunit, thus inhibiting the cytokine-induced responses including proinflammatory cytokines. *Reduces inflammatory response in moderate to severe eczema (atopic dermatitis).*

**USES** Treatment of moderate to severe eczema (atopic dermatitis) when topical therapies have failed or contraindicated.

**CONTRAINDICATIONS** Hypersensitivity to dupilumab or components of the injection.

**CAUTIOUS USE** Hypersensitivity to dupilumab; pregnancy; lactation. Safety and efficacy in children not established.

## ROUTE & DOSAGE

**Atopic Dermatitis**
*Adult:* **Subcutaneous** 600 mg at first dose, then 300 mg every other wk

## ADMINISTRATION

**Subcutaneous**
- Allow prefilled syringe to reach room temperature for approx 45 min prior to use.
- Administer subcutaneously into the thigh, lower abdomen, or outer upper arm. Do not inject into tissue that is tender, bruised, red, hard, scaly, or affected by psoriasis.
- Rotate injection sites.

**ADVERSE EFFECTS** (≥ 2%) **GI:** Oral herpes. **Immunologic:** *Antibody development.* **Integumentary:** *Injection site reaction.* **Ophthalmic:** *Conjunctivitis,* eye pruritis.

**INTERACTIONS DRUG:** Avoid use with live vaccines; avoid use with other monoclonal antibodies.

**PHARMACOKINETICS Absorption:** 64% bioavailability. **Onset:** Peak effect in 1 wk. **Metabolism:** Catabolism to small peptides and amino acids, similar to endogenous IgG. **Elimination:** Nondetectable 10 wk post-discontinuation.

## NURSING IMPLICATIONS

### Assessment & Drug Effects
- Monitor for signs of hypersensitivity reaction and ocular adverse effects.

### Patient & Family Education
- Notify prescriber if you experience signs or symptoms of allergic reaction such as rash, hives, itching, shortness of breath, wheezing, cough, swelling of the face, lips, tongue, or throat; or any other signs.

# DUTASTERIDE
(du-tas'ter-ide)
Avodart
**Classifications:** ANTIANDROGEN; 5-ALPHA REDUCTASE INHIBITOR
**Therapeutic:** BENIGN PROSTATIC HYPERPLASIA (BPH) AGENT
**Prototype:** Finasteride

**AVAILABILITY** Capsule

**ACTION & *THERAPEUTIC EFFECT***
Specific inhibitor of the steroid 5-alpha-reductase, an enzyme necessary to convert testosterone into the potent androgen 5-alpha-dihydrotestosterone (DHT) in the prostate gland. *Decreases the production of testosterone in the prostate gland.*

**USES** Treatment of benign prostatic hypertrophy (BPH).

**UNLABELED USE** Alopecia.

**CONTRAINDICATIONS** Hypersensitivity to dutasteride or finasteride; women of child bearing potential; pregnancy (category X); lactation.

Common adverse effects in *italic;* life-threatening effects <u>underlined;</u> generic names in **bold;** classifications in SMALL CAPS; ◆ Canadian drug name; ⊘ Prototype drug

**CAUTIOUS USE** Hepatic impairment, obstructive uropathy; older adult males.

## ROUTE & DOSAGE

**BPH**
*Adult:* **PO** 0.5 mg once daily

## ADMINISTRATION

### Oral

- Do not handle capsules if you are or may become pregnant because of the potential for absorption of dutasteride and the subsequent risk to a developing male fetus.
- Do not open or crush capsules. They **must be** swallowed whole.
- Store at 15°–30° C (59°–86° F).

## ADVERSE EFFECTS (>1%) **Endocrine:** Gynecomastia. **Urogenital:** Ejaculation dysfunction, impotence, decreased libido, prostate cancer.

## DIAGNOSTIC TEST INTERFERENCE

**Lab Test:** Dutasteride affects the **serum PSA levels**, so levels should be established after 3–6 mo of therapy.

## INTERACTIONS **Drug:** **Diltiazem, verapamil** may decrease clearance of dutasteride. **Herbal:** May see exaggerated effects with **saw palmetto.**

## PHARMACOKINETICS **Absorption:** Rapidly; 60% bioavailability. **Peak:** 2–3 h. **Distribution:** 99% protein bound. **Metabolism:** In liver by CYP3A4. **Elimination:** Primarily in feces. **Half-Life:** 5 wk.

## NURSING IMPLICATIONS

### Assessment & Drug Effects

- Monitor voiding patterns, assessing for ease of starting a stream, frequency, and urgency.

- Monitor lab tests: Baseline and periodic PSA.

### Patient & Family Education

- Do not donate blood until at least 6 mo following last dose to prevent administration of dutasteride to a pregnant female transfusion recipient.
- Ejaculate volume might be decreased during treatment but this does not seem to interfere with normal sexual function.
- Note that the incidence of most drug-related sexual adverse events (impotence, decreased libido, and ejaculation disorder) typically decrease with duration of treatment.

## DYPHYLLINE
(dye'fi-lin)
**Dylix, Lufyllin, Protophylline ◆**
**Classifications:** RESPIRATORY SMOOTH MUSCLE RELAXANT, XANTHINE; BRONCHODILATOR
**Therapeutic:** BRONCHODILATOR; ANTIASTHMATIC
**Prototype:** Theophylline

## AVAILABILITY Tablet, elixir

## ACTION & *THERAPEUTIC EFFECT*
Xanthine derivative of theophylline causes bronchodilation, myocardial stimulation, and smooth muscle relaxation. *Effective bronchodilator and antiasthmatic agent.*

## USES Acute bronchial asthma and reversible bronchospasm associated with chronic bronchitis and emphysema.

## CONTRAINDICATIONS Hypersensitivity to xanthine compounds; apnea in newborns.

Common adverse effects in *italic;* life-threatening effects <u>underlined</u>; generic names in **bold;** classifications in SMALL CAPS; ◆ Canadian drug name; ❷ Prototype drug

561

**E**

**CAUTIOUS USE** Severe cardiac disease, hypertension, acute myocardial injury; renal or hepatic dysfunction; glaucoma; seizure disorders; hyperthyroidism; peptic ulcer; older adults; children; pregnancy (category C); lactation. Safe use in children under 6 y is not established.

## ROUTE & DOSAGE

**Asthma**
*Adult:* **PO** Up to 15 mg/kg q.i.d.

## ADMINISTRATION

### Oral

- Give oral preparation with a full glass of water on an empty stomach (e.g., 1 h before or 2 h after meals) to enhance absorption. However, administration after meals may help to relieve gastric discomfort.
- Exercise care in the amount of elixir given to children because it has a high alcohol content (18–20%).

**ADVERSE EFFECTS** (≥1%) **CNS:** Headache, irritability, restlessness, dizziness, insomnia, light-headedness, muscle twitching, <u>convulsions</u>. **CV:** Palpitation, *tachycardia,* extrasystoles, flushing, hypotension. **GI:** *Nausea,* vomiting, diarrhea, anorexia, epigastric distress. **Respiratory:** Tachypnea. **Other:** Albuminuria, fever, dehydration.

**INTERACTIONS** **Drug:** BETA-BLOCKERS may antagonize bronchodilating effects of dyphylline; **halothane** increases risk of cardiac arrhythmias; **probenecid** may decrease dyphylline elimination.

**PHARMACOKINETICS** **Absorption:** Readily from GI tract. **Peak:** 1 h. **Metabolism:** In liver (but not to theophylline). **Elimination:** In urine. **Half-Life:** 2 h.

## NURSING IMPLICATIONS

### Assessment & Drug Effects

- Monitor therapeutic effectiveness; usually occurs at a blood level of at least 12 mcg/mL.
- Note: Toxic dyphylline plasma levels, although rare with normal dosage, are a risk in patients with a diminished capacity for dyphylline clearance (e.g., those with CHF or hepatic impairment or who are older than 55 y or younger than 1 y).

### Patient & Family Education

- Take medication consistently with or without food at the same time each day.
- Notify prescriber of adverse effects: Nausea, vomiting, insomnia, jitteriness, headache, rash, severe GI pain, restlessness, convulsions, or irregular heartbeat.
- Avoid alcohol and also large amounts of coffee and other xanthine-containing beverages (e.g., tea, cocoa, cola) during therapy.
- Consult prescriber before taking OTC preparations. Many OTC drugs for coughs, colds, and allergies contain nervous system stimulants.

## ECHOTHIOPHATE IODIDE

(ek-oh-thye′oh-fate)
Phospholine Iodide
See Appendix A-1.

---

Common adverse effects in *italic;* life-threatening effects <u>underlined;</u> generic names in **bold;** classifications in SMALL CAPS; ♦ Canadian drug name; ◉ Prototype drug

# ECONAZOLE NITRATE
(e-kone'a-zole)

Ecostatin ◆, Spectazole

**Classifications:** ANTIBIOTIC;
AZOLE ANTIFUNGAL
Therapeutic: ANTIFUNGAL
**Prototype:** Fluconazole

## AVAILABILITY Cream

## ACTION & *THERAPEUTIC EFFECT*
Disrupts normal fungal cell membrane permeability resulting in cell death. *Active against dermatophytes, yeasts, and many other fungi.*

## USES Topically for treatment of tinea pedis (athlete's foot or ringworm of foot), tinea cruris ("jock itch" or ringworm of groin), tinea corporis (ringworm of body), tinea versicolor, and cutaneous candidiasis (moniliasis).

## UNLABELED USES Has been used for topical treatment of erythrasma and with corticosteroids for fungal or bacterial dermatoses associated with inflammation.

## CONTRAINDICATIONS Infants younger than 3 mo.

## CAUTIOUS USE Pregnancy (category C); lactation.

## ROUTE & DOSAGE

**Tinea Cruris, Tinea Corporis, Tinea Pedis, Cutaneous Candidiasis**

*Adult/Child:* **Topical** Apply sufficient amount to affected areas twice daily, morning and evening

**Tinea Versicolor**

*Adult:* **Topical** Apply sufficient amount to affected areas once daily

## ADMINISTRATION
**Topical**
- Cleanse skin with soap and water and dry thoroughly before applying medication (unless otherwise directed by prescriber). Wash hands thoroughly before and after treatments.
- Do not use occlusive dressings unless prescribed by prescriber.
- Store at less than 30° C (86° F) unless otherwise directed.

## ADVERSE EFFECTS (≥1%) **Skin:**
Burning, stinging sensation, pruritus, erythema.

## PHARMACOKINETICS **Absorption:** Minimal percutaneous absorption through intact skin; increased absorption from denuded skin. **Peak:** 0.5–5 h. **Elimination:** Less than 1% of applied dose is eliminated in urine and feces.

## NURSING IMPLICATIONS
**Patient & Family Education**
- Use medication for the prescribed time even if symptoms improve and report to prescriber skin reactions suggestive of irritation or sensitization.
- Notify prescriber if full course of therapy does not result in improvement. Diagnosis should be reevaluated.
- Do not apply the topical cream in or near the eyes or intravaginally.

# EDETATE CALCIUM DISODIUM
(ed'e-tate)

Calcium Disodium Versenate

**Classification:** CHELATING AGENT
Therapeutic: CHELATING AGENT;
ANTIPOISON

---

Common adverse effects in *italic;* life-threatening effects <u>underlined</u>; generic names in **bold;** classifications in SMALL CAPS; ◆ Canadian drug name; ☉ Prototype drug

**AVAILABILITY** Solution for injection

## ACTION & *THERAPEUTIC EFFECT*

Combines with divalent and trivalent metals to form stable, nonionizing soluble complexes that can be readily excreted by kidneys. Action is dependent on ability of heavy metal to displace the less strongly bound calcium in drug molecules. *Chelating agent that binds with heavy metals such as lead to form a soluble complex that can be excreted through the kidney, thereby ridding the body of the poisonous substance.*

**USES** As adjunct in treatment of acute and chronic lead poisoning (plumbism). Generally used in combination with dimercaprol (BAL) in treatment of lead encephalopathy or when blood lead level exceeds 100 mcg/dL. Also used to diagnose suspected lead poisoning.

**UNLABELED USES** Treatment of poisoning from other heavy metals such as chromium, manganese, nickel, zinc, and possibly vanadium; removal of radioactive and nuclear fission products such as plutonium, yttrium, uranium. Not effective in poisoning from arsenic, gold, or mercury.

**CONTRAINDICATIONS** Severe kidney disease, active renal disease, anuria, oliguria; hepatitis; IV use in patients with lead encephalopathy not generally recommended (because of possible increase in intracranial pressure).

**CAUTIOUS USE** Kidney dysfunction; active tubercular lesions; history of gout; cardiac arrhythmias; pregnancy (category B); lactation.

## ROUTE & DOSAGE

### Diagnosis of Lead Poisoning

*Adult:* **IV/IM** 500 mg/m² (max: 1 g) over 1 h, then collect urine for 24 h (if mcg lead:mg EDTA ratio in urine is greater than 1, the test is positive)
*Child:* **IM** 50 mg/kg (max: 1 g), then collect urine for 6–8 h, (if mcg lead:mg EDTA ratio in urine is greater than 0.5, the test is positive)

### Treatment of Lead Poisoning

*Adult/Child:* **IV** 1–1.5 g/m²/day infused over 8–24 h for up to 5 days; **IM** 1–1.5 g/m²/day divided q8–12h

### Asymptomatic Lead Poisoning

*Adult/Child:* **IV** 1 g/m²/day infused over 8–24 h for up to 5 days

### *Lead Nephropathy/Renal Impairment Dosage Adjustment*

*Adult (Based on serum CrCl less than 2 mg/dL):* **IV** 1 g/m²/day × 5 days; *2–3 mg/dL:* 500 mg/m²/day × 5 days; *3.1–4 × 3 doses mg/dL:* 500 mg/m² q48h; *greater than 4 mg/dL:* 500 mg/m² once/wk. Infuse over 8–24 h, may repeat monthly

## ADMINISTRATION

- **Never** give higher than recommended doses.

### Intramuscular

- IM route preferred for symptomatic children and recommended for patients with incipient or overt lead-induced encephalopathy.
- Add Procaine HCl to minimize pain at injection site (usually 1 mL of procaine 1% to each 1 mL of concentrated drug). Consult prescriber.

**E**

## Intravenous

*PREPARE:* **IV Infusion:** Dilute the total daily dose in 250–500 mL of NS or D5W.

*ADMINISTER:* **IV Infusion:** Warning: Rapid IV infusion may be LETHAL by suddenly increasing intracranial pressure in patients who already have cerebral edema. ▪ Manufacturer recommends total daily dose over 8–12 h. Consult prescriber for specific rate.

*INCOMPATIBILITIES:* Solution/additive: **Amphotericin B, D10W hydralazine, lactated Ringer's.**

## ADVERSE EFFECTS (≥1%) CV:

Hypotension, thrombophlebitis. **GI:** Anorexia, nausea, vomiting, diarrhea, abdominal cramps, cheilosis. **Hematologic:** Transient bone marrow depression, depletion of blood metals. **Urogenital:** <u>Nephrotoxicity</u> (renal tubular necrosis), proteinuria, hematuria. **Body as a Whole:** *Febrile reaction* (excessive thirst, fever, chills, severe myalgia, arthralgia, GI distress), *histamine-like reactions* (flushing, throbbing headache, sweating, sneezing, nasal congestion, lacrimation, postural hypotension, tachycardia).

## DIAGNOSTIC TEST INTERFERENCE

Edetate calcium disodium may decrease **serum cholesterol, plasma lipid** levels (if elevated), and **serum potassium** values. **Glycosuria** may occur with toxic doses.

## PHARMACOKINETICS Absorption:

Well absorbed IM. **Onset:** 1 h. **Peak:** Peak chelation 24–48 h. **Distribution:** Distributed to extracellular fluid; does not enter CSF. **Metabolism:** Not metabolized. **Elimination:** Chelated lead excreted in urine; 50% excreted in 1 h. **Half-Life:** 20–60 min IV, 90 min IM.

## NURSING IMPLICATIONS

### Black Box Warning

*Edeta calcium has been associated with potentially fatal effects, especially when higher doses are used or when it is continued after toxic effects appear.*

### Assessment & Drug Effects

▪ Determine adequacy of urinary output prior to therapy. This may be done by administering IV fluids before giving first dose.

▪ Increase fluid intake to enhance urinary excretion of chelates. Avoid excess fluid intake, however, in patients with lead encephalopathy because of the danger of further increasing intracranial pressure. Consult prescriber regarding allowable intake.

▪ Monitor I&O. Since drug is excreted almost exclusively via kidneys, toxicity may develop if output is inadequate. Stop therapy if urine flow is markedly diminished or absent. Report any change in output or I&O ratio to prescriber.

▪ Be alert for occurrence of febrile reaction that may appear 4–8 h after drug infusion (see ADVERSE EFFECTS).

▪ Monitor lab tests: Before each course of therapy, urinalysis and urine sediment, renal and hepatic function and serum electrolytes, repeat after the 2nd and 5th day of therapy, or daily in severe cases.

## EDOXABAN

(e-dox'a-ban)

Savaysa

**Classifications:** ANTICOAGULANT; ANTITHROMBOTIC; SELECTIVE FACTOR XA INHIBITOR
**Therapeutic:** ANTITHROMBOTIC
**Prototype:** Rivaroxaban

---

Common adverse effects in *italic*; life-threatening effects <u>underlined</u>; generic names in **bold;** classifications in SMALL CAPS; ✦ Canadian drug name; ⊙ Prototype drug

**E**

## AVAILABILITY Tablet

## ACTION & *THERAPEUTIC EFFECT*
Inhibits free FXa and prothrombinase activity, and inhibits thrombin-induced platelet aggregation. *Inhibition of FXa in the coagulation cascade reduces thrombin generation which reduces thrombus formation.*

## USES Treatment of deep vein thrombosis (DVT) and pulmonary embolism (PE) and reduction of the risk of stroke and systemic embolism (SE) in patients with nonvalvular atrial fibrillation (NVAF).

## CONTRAINDICATIONS Active pathological bleeding; atrial fibrillation if CrCL greater than 95 mL/min; severe renal impairment; CrCl less than 15mL/min; concomitant use of rifampin or other anticoagulants.

## CAUTIOUS USE Nonvalvular atrial fibrillation; moderately impaired renal function (dose adjustment for CrCl 15–50 mL/min); moderate or severe hepatic impairment (Child-Pugh class B and C); patients with low body weight, 60 kg or less; concomitant use of drugs affecting hemostasis; spinal/epidural anesthesia or spinal/epidural puncture; mechanical heart valves or moderate to severe mitral stenosis; pregnancy; lactation. Safety and efficacy in children not established.

## ROUTE & DOSAGE

**Nonvalvular Atrial Fibrillation**
*Adult:* **PO** 60 mg once daily

**Deep Vein Thrombosis and Pulmonary Embolism**
*Adult (60 kg or less):* **PO** 30 mg daily following 5–10 days of therapy with a parenteral anticoagulant

*Adult (over 60 kg):* **PO** 60 mg once daily following 5–10 days of therapy with a parenteral anticoagulant

**Renal Impairment Dosage Adjustment**
*CrCL 15 to 50 mL/min:* 30 mg once daily
*CrCl greater than 95 mL/min:* Avoid use

## ADMINISTRATION
**Oral**
- May be given without regard to food.
- Store at 15°–30° C (59°–86° F).

## ADVERSE EFFECTS (>1%) **Body as a Whole:** Puncture site bleeding. **GI:** Epistaxis, gastrointestinal bleeding. **Hematological:** Anemia, increased bleeding tendencies. **Metabolic:** Abnormal liver function tests. **Respiratory:** Oral/pharyngeal bleeding. **Skin:** Cutaneous soft tissue bleeding, rash. **Urogenital:** Macroscopic hematuria/urethral, vaginal bleeding.

## INTERACTIONS **Drug:** Concurrent use of other ANTICOAGULANTS, ANTIPLATELETS, and THROMBOLYTICS may increase the risk of bleeding. **Rifampin** should not be used with edoxaban.

## PHARMACOKINETICS **Absorption:** 62% bioavailable. **Peak:** 1–2 h. **Metabolism:** Minimal, primarily excreted unchanged. **Elimination:** Primarily renal. **Half-Life:** 10–14 h.

## NURSING IMPLICATIONS

### Black Box Warning

*Edoxaban has reduced efficacy in nonvalvular atrial fibrillation patients with CrCl greater than 95 mL/min; it should not be used in*

Common adverse effects in *italic;* life-threatening effects <u>underlined</u>; generic names in **bold;** classifications in SMALL CAPS; ♣ Canadian drug name; ⊙ Prototype drug

E

*these patients. Premature discontinuation of edoxaban increases the risk of ischemic events. Edoxaban has been associated with hematomas that may result in long-term or permanent paralysis when used in patients treated with spinal or epidural anesthesia or puncture.*

### Assessment & Drug Effects
- Monitor closely for S&S of frank or occult bleeding.
- Monitor for and report promptly S&S of neurologic impairment, especially following any invasive spinal or epidural procedure.
- Monitor lab tests: Baseline and periodic CrCl; baseline LFTs, periodic Hgb and Hct.

### Patient & Family Education
- Report promptly S&S of bleeding.
- Do not abruptly stop taking this drug unless advised to do so by prescriber.
- Do not take aspirin containing products or non-steroidal anti-inflammatory drugs (NSAIDs) without discussing their use with your prescriber.
- Following spinal anesthesia or spinal puncture while taking edoxaban: Report immediately back pain, tingling, numbness (especially in your legs and feet), muscle weakness, loss of control of the bowels or bladder.
- Women of childbearing age should discuss with prescriber potential risks associated with pregnancy.
- Do not breast-feed while taking this drug without consulting prescriber.

## EDROPHONIUM CHLORIDE
(ed-roe-foe'nee-um)
Enlon
**Classifications:** CHOLINERGIC MUSCLE STIMULANT; CHOLINESTERASE INHIBITOR

**Therapeutic:** ANTICHOLINESTERASE; MUSCLE STIMULANT
**Prototype:** Neostigmine

**AVAILABILITY** Solution for injection

**ACTION & *THERAPEUTIC EFFECT***
Facilitates transmission of impulses across the myoneural junction by inhibiting the destruction of acetylcholine by cholinesterase. *Acts as antidote to curariform drugs by displacing them from muscle cell receptor sites, thus permitting resumption of normal transmission of neuromuscular impulses.*

**USES** Differential diagnosis and as adjunct in evaluation of treatment requirements of myasthenia gravis; curare antagonist.

**CONTRAINDICATIONS** Hypersensitivity to anticholinesterase agents; cholinesterase inhibitor toxicity; intestinal and urinary obstruction; aplastic anemia; lactation.

**CAUTIOUS USE** Sulfite hypersensitivity; bronchial asthma; epilepsy; recent coronary occlusion; renal impairment; cardiac arrhythmias; bradycardia; peptic ulcer disease; hypotension; patients receiving digitalis; chronic hepatitis C infection; hepatic impairment; older adults; history of thromboembolism; patients with high risk of cataracts; East-Asian ethnicity; women of child bearing age; pregnancy (category C).

**ROUTE & DOSAGE**

### Myasthenia Gravis Diagnosis
*Adult:* **IV** Prepare 10 mg in a syringe; inject 2 mg over 15–30 sec, if no reaction after 45 sec, inject the remaining 8 mg, may

Common adverse effects in *italic*; life-threatening effects <u>underlined</u>; generic names in **bold**; classifications in SMALL CAPS; ◆ Canadian drug name; ⊕ Prototype drug

567

**E**

repeat test after 30 min; **IM** Inject 10 mg, if cholinergic reaction occurs, retest after 30 min with 2 mg to rule out false-negative reaction *Child (weight 34 k or less):* **IV** 1 mg, if no response after 45 sec, dose may be titrated up to 5 mg; **IM** 2 mg; *weight greater than 34 kg:* **IV** 2 mg, if no response after 45 sec, dose may be titrated up to 10 mg; **IM** 5 mg

**Evaluation of Myasthenia Treatment**

*Adult:* **IV** 1–2 mg administered 1 h after last PO dose of anticholinesterase medication

**Curare Antagonist**

*Adult:* **IV** 1 mL (10 mg) over 30–45 sec, repeat as necessary [max dose: 4 mL (40 mg)]

## ADMINISTRATION

- Note: Have antidote (atropine sulfate) immediately available and facilities for endotracheal intubation, tracheostomy, suction, assisted respiration, and cardiac monitoring for treatment of cholinergic reaction.

**Intramuscular**

- Give undiluted. IM route used if IV route not accessible.

**Intravenous**

*PREPARE:* **Direct/Infusion:** May be given undiluted or diluted in D5W or NS for infusion.
*ADMINISTER:* **Direct:** Inject 2 mg (adult and child weighing more than 34 kg) or 1 mg (child weighing 34 kg or less) over 15–30 sec; if no reaction after 45 sec, inject additional 8 mg (adult) or titrate up to a total of 8 mg additional (child weighing more than 34 kg) or titrate in 1 mg increments up to a total of 4 mg additional (child

weighing 34 kg or less), may repeat test after 30 min. ▪ If cholinergic reaction (increased muscle weakness) is obtained after initial 1 or 2 mg, discontinue test and give atropine IV (as ordered). **IV Infusion:** Infuse over 1 h.

## ADVERSE EFFECTS (≥1%) **Body as a Whole:** Severe adverse effects uncommon with usual doses. **CNS:** Weakness, muscle cramps, dysphoria, fasciculations, incoordination, dysarthria, dysphagia, convulsions, <u>respiratory paralysis</u>. **CV:** Bradycardia, irregular pulse, hypotension, pulmonary edema. **Special Senses:** Miosis, blurred vision, diplopia, lacrimation. **GI:** *Diarrhea, abdominal cramps, nausea, vomiting, excessive salivation.* **Respiratory:** Increased bronchial secretions, <u>bronchospasm, laryngospasm</u>, pulmonary edema. **Other:** Excessive sweating, urinary frequency, incontinence.

## INTERACTIONS **Drug: Procainamide, quinidine** may antagonize the effects of edrophonium; DIGITALIS GLYCOSIDES increase the sensitivity of the heart to edrophonium; **succinylcholine, decamethonium** may prolong neuromuscular blockade.

## PHARMACOKINETICS **Onset:** 30–60 sec IV; 2–10 min IM. **Duration:** 5–10 min IV; 5–30 min IM.

## NURSING IMPLICATIONS

### Assessment & Drug Effects

- Monitor vital signs. Observe for signs of respiratory distress. Patients older than 50 y are particularly likely to develop bradycardia, hypotension, and cardiac arrest.
- Edrophonium test for myasthenia gravis: All cholinesterase inhibitors (anticholinesterases) should be discontinued for at least 8 h before test. Positive response to edrophonium test consists of brief

Common adverse effects in *italic;* life-threatening effects <u>underlined</u>; generic names in **bold;** classifications in SMALL CAPS; ♣ Canadian drug name; ⊙ Prototype drug

improvement in muscle strength unaccompanied by lingual or skeletal muscle fasciculations.

- Evaluation of myasthenic treatment: *Myasthenic response* (immediate subjective improvement with increased muscle strength, absence of fasciculations; generally indicates that patient requires larger dose of anticholinesterase agent or longer-acting drug); *Cholinergic response* [muscarinic adverse effects (lacrimation, diaphoresis, salivation, abdominal cramps, diarrhea, nausea, vomiting; accompanied by decrease in muscle strength; usually indicates over-treatment with cholinesterase inhibitor)]; *Adequate response* [no change in muscle strength; fasciculations may be present or absent; minimal cholinergic adverse effects (observed in patients at or near optimal dosage level)].

## EFAVIRENZ ⊕

(e-fa'vi-renz)

*Sustiva*

**Classifications:** ANTIRETROVIRAL; NONNUCLEOSIDE REVERSE TRANSCRIPTASE INHIBITOR (NNRTI)
*Therapeutic:* ANTIRETROVIRAL; NNRTI (including first trimester)

**AVAILABILITY** Capsule; tablet

**ACTION & *THERAPEUTIC EFFECT***
Binds directly to reverse transcriptase and blocks RNA polymerase activities of the HIV-1 virus, thus preventing replication of the virus. *Prevents replication of the HIV-1 virus. Resistant strains appear rapidly. Effectiveness is indicated by reduction in viral load (plasma level HIV RNA).*

**USES** HIV-1 infection in combination with other antiretroviral agents.

**CONTRAINDICATIONS** Hypersensitivity to efavirenz; suicidal ideation; pregnancy (category D, including fetal harm in first trimester), lactation.

**CAUTIOUS USE** Liver disease, alcoholism, hepatitis B or C, hypertriglyceridemia, hypercholesterolemia, substance abuse; moderate to severe hepatic impairment; antimicrobial resistance, bipolar disorder, depression, suicidal tendencies, psychiatric disorders related to use of efavirenz; drug or alcohol abuse; exfoliative dermatitis; females of childbearing age, CNS disorders; history of seizures; older adults. Safety and efficacy in children younger than 3 mo or who weigh less than 3.5 kg (8 lb) not established.

## ROUTE & DOSAGE

**HIV Infection (with other antiretrovirals)**

*Adult/Adolescent:* **PO** 600 mg daily
*Child/Infant (3 mo or older, weight 3.5 kg to less than 5 kg):* **PO** 100 mg daily; *weight 5 kg to less than 7.5 kg:* 150 mg daily; *weight 7.5 to less than 15 kg:* 200 mg daily; *weight 15 to less than 20 kg:* 250 mg daily; *weight 20 to less than 25 kg:* 300 mg daily; *weight 25 to less than 32.5 kg:* 350 mg daily; *weight 32.5 to less than 40 kg:* 400 mg daily; *weight greater than 40 kg:* 600 mg daily

## ADMINISTRATION

**Oral**
- Use bedtime dosing to increase tolerability of CNS adverse effects.

**E**

- Give exactly as ordered. Do not skip a dose or discontinue therapy without consulting the prescriber.
- Do not give efavirenz following a high fat meal.
- Store at 15°–30° C (59°–86° F) in a tightly closed container and protect from light.

**ADVERSE EFFECTS** (≥1%) **Body as a Whole:** Fatigue, fever. **CNS:** Dizziness, headache, hypoesthesia, impaired concentration, insomnia, abnormal dreams, somnolence, depression, nervousness, adverse psychiatric experiences. **Endocrine:** *Hypercholesterolemia.* **GI:** *Nausea,* vomiting, *diarrhea,* dyspepsia, abdominal pain, flatulence, anorexia, increased *liver function tests* (ALT, AST). **Respiratory:** Cough. **Skin:** *Rash* (erythematous rash, pruritus, *maculopapular rash,* <u>erythema multiforme, Stevens–Johnson syndrome, toxic epidermal necrolysis</u>), increased sweating. **Urogenital:** Renal calculus, hematuria. **CV:** <u>Prolonged QT interval.</u>

**DIAGNOSTIC TEST INTERFERENCE** False-positive *urine tests* for **marijuana.**

**INTERACTIONS Drug:** Decreased concentrations of **clarithromycin, indinavir, nelfinavir, saquinavir, voriconazole, ponatinib, ketoconazole, amprenavir, saquinavir,** increased concentrations of **ritonavir, azithromycin.** Efavirenz levels are increased by **ritonavir, fluconazole, voriconazole** and decreased by **saquinavir, rifampin, carbamazepine, nevirapine.** Additional drugs not recommended for administration with efavirenz include **midazolam, triazolam,** ERGOT DERIVATIVES, **warfarin. Herbal:** St. John's wort may decrease antiretroviral activity.

**PHARMACOKINETICS Peak:** 5 h; steady-state 6–10 days. **Distribution:**

99% protein bound. **Metabolism:** In liver by cytochrome P450 3A4 and 2B6; can induce (increase) its own metabolism. **Elimination:** 14–34% in urine, 16–61% in feces. **Half-Life:** 52–76 h after single dose, 40–55 h after multiple doses.

**NURSING IMPLICATIONS**

**Assessment & Drug Effects**
- Monitor for suicidal ideation in patients who are depressed, or who have a history of depression.
- Monitor GI status and evaluate ability to maintain a normal diet.
- Monitor lab tests: Periodic LFTs and lipid profile.

**Patient & Family Education**
- Contact prescriber promptly if any of the following occurs: Skin rash, delusions, inappropriate behavior, suicidal ideation.
- Avoid pregnancy because of fetal harm in first trimester of pregnancy.
- Use or add barrier contraception if using hormonal contraceptive.
- Notify prescriber immediately if you become pregnant.
- Do not drive or engage in potentially hazardous activities until response to the drug is known. Dizziness, impaired concentration, and drowsiness usually improve with continued therapy.

**EFLORNITHINE HYDROCHLORIDE**
(e-flor′ni-theen)
Vaniqa
**Classification:** DERMATOLOGIC
**Therapeutic:** FACIAL HIRSUTISM AGENT

**AVAILABILITY** Cream

**ACTION & *THERAPEUTIC EFFECT***
Inhibits enzyme activity in the skin that is required for hair growth.

*Results in retarding the rate of facial hair growth.*

**USES** Reduction of unwanted facial hair in women.

**CONTRAINDICATIONS** Hypersensitivity to eflornithine or its components.

**CAUTIOUS USE** Bone marrow suppression; HIV; hearing impairment, renal impairment or failure; pregnancy (category C); lactation. Safe use in children younger than 12 y is not established.

**ROUTE & DOSAGE**

| Hair Removal |
| --- |
| *Adult:* **Topical** Apply thin layer b.i.d. (at least 8 h apart) to affected areas of the face |

**ADMINISTRATION**

**Topical**
- Apply thin layer to affected skin areas on face and under chin and rub in thoroughly.
- Do not wash treated areas for at least 8 h after application.
- Store at 15°–30° C (59°–86° F).

**ADVERSE EFFECTS** (≥1%) **Body as a Whole** Facial edema. **CNS** Dizziness, headache. **GI:** Dyspepsia, anorexia. **Skin:** *Acne, pseudofolliculitis barbae,* stinging, burning, pruritus, erythema, tingling, irritation, rash, alopecia, folliculitis, ingrown hair.

**PHARMACOKINETICS Absorption:** Less than 1% absorbed through intact skin. **Metabolism:** Not metabolized. **Elimination:** Primarily in urine. **Half-Life:** 8 h.

**NURSING IMPLICATIONS**

**Assessment & Drug Effects**
- Monitor for and report skin irritation.

- Note: Drug slows growth of facial hair, but is not a depilatory.

**Patient & Family Education**
- Note: Effect of drug is usually not apparent for 4–8 wk.
- Reduce frequency of drug application to once daily if skin irritation occurs. If irritation continues, contact prescriber.

---

## ELETRIPTAN HYDROBROMIDE
(e-le-trip′tan)
Relpax
**Classification:** SEROTONIN 5-HT$_1$ RECEPTOR AGONIST
Therapeutic: ANTIMIGRAINE
**Pregnancy Category:** C

**AVAILABILITY** Tablet

**ACTION & *THERAPEUTIC* EFFECT**
Eletriptan stimulates presynaptic 5-HT$_{1D}$ receptors inhibiting dural vasodilation and agonizes vascular 5-HT$_{1B}$ receptors causing vasoconstriction of intracranial extracerebral vessels. *Inhibits dural vasodilation and inflammation, and causes vasoconstriction of painfully dilated intracranial extra-cerebral vessels, thus relieving the migraine headache. Also relieves photophobia, phonophobia, and nausea and vomiting associated with migraine attacks.*

**USES** Treatment of acute migraine attacks with or without aura.

**CONTRAINDICATIONS** Hypersensitivity to eletriptan; history of CAD; ischemic or vasospastic CAD, arteriosclerosis, history of MI; ischemic colititis, Raynaud's disease uncontrolled hypertension; CVA or TIA; within 24 h of administering of another ergotamine; lactation within 24 h after dose; severe hepatic insufficiency; hemiplegic or basilar

Common adverse effects in *italic*; life-threatening effects underlined; generic names in **bold**; classifications in SMALL CAPS; ♣Canadian drug name; ⊙ Prototype drug

571

E

migraine; peripheral vascular disease; concurrent MAOI therapy.

**CAUTIOUS USE** Hypotension in the elderly; older adults; mild to moderate hepatic impairment; diabetes, obesity, smoking, high cholesterol; men older than 40 y; postmenopausal women; pregnancy (category C); lactation. Safe use in children younger than 18 y not established.

## ROUTE & DOSAGE

### Acute Migraine
*Adult:* **PO** 20 mg or 40 mg at onset of migraine (max: 40 mg/dose and 80 mg/day), may repeat dose in 2 h if partial response

### Hepatic Impairment Dosage Adjustment
*Severe Hepatic Impairment:* Not recommended

## ADMINISTRATION

### Oral
- Give one tablet as soon as the migraine begins.
- May give 2nd tablet if headache improves but returns after 2 h.
- If 1st tablet is ineffective, do not give a 2nd without consulting prescriber.
- Do not give within 72 h of potent CYP3A4 inhibitors (see INTERACTIONS).
- Store at 15°–30° C (59°–86° F). Protect from light and moisture.

**ADVERSE EFFECTS** (≥1%) **Body as a Whole:** *Asthenia,* paresthesia, flushing, back pain, chills. **CNS:** Dizziness, drowsiness, headache, somnolence, hypertonia, hypesthesia. **CV:** Chest tightness/pressure, palpitation, hypertension. The following are rare, usually seen in patients with cardiovascular disease risk factors: Coronary vasospasm, transient myocardial ischemia, <u>MI</u>, ventricular tachycardia, atrial fibrillation, ventricular fibrillation. **GI:** Abdominal pain, dyspepsia, dysphagia, nausea, vomiting, dry mouth. **Respiratory:** Pharyngitis. **Skin:** Sweating.

**INTERACTIONS Drug:** Drugs that inhibit CYP3A4 may increase eletriptan levels and toxicity, do not administer eletriptan within 72 h of AZOLE ANTIFUNGALS (especially **itraconazole, ketoconazole, voriconazole**), **amiodarone, cimetidine, dalfopristin, quinupristin, diltiazem, metronidazole, nicardipine, norfloxacin, quinine, verapamil, zafirlukast, zileuton,** MACROLIDE ANTIBIOTICS, NONNUCLEOTIDE REVERSE TRANSCRIPTASE INHIBITORS, PROTEASE INHIBITORS, SELECTIVE SEROTONIN REUPTAKE INHIBITORS, **sibutramine;** ERGOT ALKALOIDS may prolong vasospastic adverse reactions (do not use within 24 h of ergot-containing drugs); do not administer within 24 h of other 5-HT$_1$ AGONISTS (increases adverse effects). **Food: Grapefruit juice** may increase eletriptan levels and toxicity. **Herbal: echinacea, St. John's wort** may increase triptan toxicity.

**PHARMACOKINETICS Absorption:** Rapid with 50% reaching systemic circulation. **Onset:** 1–2 h. **Peak:** 1.5 h. **Distribution:** 85% protein bound. **Metabolism:** In liver by CYP3A4. **Elimination:** Nonrenal routes. **Half-Life:** 4–5 h.

## NURSING IMPLICATIONS

### Assessment & Drug Effects
- Monitor CV status carefully following first dose in patients at risk for coronary artery disease (e.g., history of hypertension, postmenopausal women, men older than 40 y, persons with known CAD

risk factors) or who have coronary artery vasospasms.

▪ Report immediately chest pain, tightness in chest or throat that is severe or does not quickly resolve following a dose of eletriptan.

▪ Monitor therapeutic effectiveness. Pain relief is usually achieved within 1 h.

**Patient & Family Education**

▪ Note: If first dose is ineffective, do not take a second dose as it will not work for the same attack.

▪ Inform prescriber of all prescription, nonprescription, and herbal drugs you are taking. Do not add additional drugs without informing prescriber as many drugs interact with eletriptan.

▪ Report promptly any of the following: Headache more severe than usual, migraine; dizziness, faintness, blurred vision; chest, neck, or throat pain; irregular heart beat, palpitations; shortness of breath, wheezing, difficulty breathing; tingling, pain, or numbness in the face, hands, or feet; seizures; severe stomach pain, cramping, or bloody diarrhea.

▪ Do not drive or engage in any potentially hazardous task until reaction to drug is known.

# ELUXADOLINE

(e-lux'a-do-line)

Viberzi

**Classifications:** PERIPHERAL MU-RECEPTOR AGONIST; ANTISECRETORY AGENT

Therapeutic: ANTISECRETORY AGENT

**AVAILABILITY** Tablet

**ACTION & *THERAPEUTIC EFFECT***
A mixed mu-opioid receptor agonist, delta opioid receptor antagonist, and kappa opioid receptor agonist. *Acts locally to reduce abdominal pain*

*and diarrhea in patients with IBS-D without constipating side effects.*

**USES** Indicated for the treatment of irritable bowel syndrome with diarrhea (IBS-D) in adults.

**CONTRAINDICATIONS** Severe hepatic impairment (Child-Pugh class C); history of chronic or severe constipation or sequelae from constipation, or known or suspected mechanical GI obstruction; known or suspected biliary duct obstruction or sphincter of Oddi disease or dysfunction; history of pancreatitis or structural diseases of the pancreas, including known or suspected pancreatic duct obstruction; alcoholism, alcohol abuse, or alcohol addiction, or consumption of more than 3 alcoholic beverages per day.

**CAUTIOUS USE** Older adults; severe constipation; patients with a history of substance abuse; concomitant use of strong CYP inhibitors; pregnancy; lactation. Safety and efficacy in children not established.

## ROUTE & DOSAGE

### IBS-D

*Adult:* **PO** 100 mg b.i.d.; decrease to 75 mg b.i.d. if not tolerated or if patient doesn't have a gallbladder

***Hepatic Impairment Dosage Adjustment***

*Mild (Child-Pugh class A) or moderate (Child-Pugh class B) impairment:* Decrease to 75 mg b.i.d.
*Severe (Child-Pugh class C) impairment:* Contraindicated

## ADMINISTRATION

**Oral**

▪ Give with food.
▪ Store at 15°–30° C (59°–86° F).

---

**ADVERSE EFFECTS** (≥1%) **Body as a Whole:** Euphoric mood, fatigue, sedation, somnolence. **CNS:** Dizziness. **GI:** Abdonimal distension, abdominal pain, *constipation*, flatulence, nausea, viral gastroenteritis, vomiting. **Metabolic:** Increased ALT/AST. **Respiratory:** Asthma, bronchospasm, bronchitis, nasopharyngitis, <u>respiratory failure</u>, upper respiratory tract infection, wheezing. **Skin:** Rash.

**INTERACTIONS Drug:** Co-administration with organic anion transporting polypeptide 1B1 (OATP1B1) inhibitors (e.g., **cyclosporine, eltrombopag, gemfibrozil**, HIV PROTEASE INHIBITORS, **rifampin**) may increase the levels of eluxadoline. Strong CYP inhibitors (e.g., **bupropion, ciprofloxacin, clarithromycin, fluconazole, gemfibrozil, paroxetine**) may increase the levels of eluxadoline. **Aloserton**, ANTICHOLINERGICS, and OPIOIDS may cause serious adverse effects related to constipation. Eluxadoline may increase the levels of co-administered substrates for OATP1B1 and breast cancer resistance protein (BCRP) (e.g., **rosuvastatin**). Eluxadoline may increase the levels of co-administered CYP3A substrates with a narrow therapeutic index (e.g., **alfentanil, cyclosporine, dihydroergotamine, ergotamine, fentanyl, pimozide, quinidine, sirolimus, tacrolimus**).

**PHARMACOKINETICS Peak:** 1.5 h. **Distribution:** 81% plasma protein bound. **Metabolism:** In liver. **Elimination:** Primarily fecal (82%). **Half-Life:** 3.7–6 h.

## NURSING IMPLICATIONS

### Assessment & Drug Effects
- Monitor for and report promptly S&S of symptoms of sphincter of Oddi spasm (e.g., acute worsening of epigastric or biliary-type abdominal pain, increased pancreatic enzymes, or increased hepatic transaminases), especially in patients without a gallbladder.
- Monitor patients with hepatic impairment for impaired mental or physical abilities and other adverse drug reactions.
- Monitor lab tests: Baseline and periodic LFTs; periodic pancreatic enzymes.

### Patient & Family Education
- Stop taking this drug and notify prescriber if experiencing new or worsening abdominal pain or pain in the upper right side of abdomen that radiates to the back or shoulder, with or without nausea and vomiting.
- Limit use of alcohol while taking this drug.
- Stop taking this drug and notify prescriber if experiencing constipation that lasts more than 4 days.
- In cases with liver impairment, do not drive or engage in other dangerous activities until response to drug is known.
- Women of childbearing age should discuss with prescriber potential risks associated with taking this drug.
- Do not breast-feed while taking this drug without consulting prescriber.

# ELVITEGRAVIR/COBICISTAT/ EMTRICITABINE/TENOFOVIR DISOPROXIL FUMARATE

(el-vi-te-gra′vir) (co-bi-ci′stat) (em-tri′ci-ta-been) (ten-o-fo′vir)

Stribild

**Classification:** ANTIRETROVIRAL; INTEGRASE STRAND INHIBITOR; NUCLEOSIDE REVERSE TRANSCRIPTASE INHIBITOR

**Therapeutic:** ANTIRETROVIRAL

**Prototype:** Raltegravir and zidovudine

**AVAILABILITY** Elvitegravir 150 mg/cobicistat 150 mg/emtricitabine 200 mg/tenofovir disoproxil fumarate 300 mg tablets

## ACTION & THERAPEUTIC EFFECT
**Elvitegravir:** Inhibits activity of HIV-1 integrase, an HIV-1 encoded enzyme that is required for viral replication. *Blocks formation of the HIV-1 provirus and propagation of the viral infection.* **Cobicistat:** Inhibits CYP3A-mediated metabolism of elvitegravir, thus increasing the bioavailability and prolonging the half-life of elvitegravir. *Increases the efficacy of elvetegravir.* **Emtricitabine:** See separate monograph for emtricitabine. **Tenofovir:** See separate monograph for tenofovir.

**USES** Used for the treatment of HIV 1 infection in adults who are antiretroviral treatment-naive.

**CONTRAINDICATIONS** Lactic acidosis; coinfection with chronic hepatitis B virus (HBV); severe hepatic impairment; acute renal failure; creatinine clearance below 50 mL/min; lactation.

**CAUTIOUS USE** Mild-to-moderate hepatic impairment; renal impairment; history of or risk for pancreatitis; older adults; pregnancy (category B). Safety and efficacy in children younger than 18 y not established.

## ROUTE & DOSAGE

**HIV-1 Infection**
*Adult:* One combination tablet daily

**Hepatic Impairment Dosage Adjustment**
*Child-Pugh class C (Severe impairment):* Not recommended

**Renal Impairment Dosage Adjustment**
*CrCl less than 70 mL/min:* Do not initiate treatment.
*CrCl less than 50 mL/min:* Discontinue if CrCl falls below 50 mL/min during treatment

## ADMINISTRATION
**Oral**
- Give with food.
- Store at 15°–30° C (59°–86° F).

**ADVERSE EFFECTS (≥1%) Body as a Whole:** Fever, lactic acidosis, paresthesia, peripheral neuropathy, severe acute exacerbations of hepatitis B, pain, severe hepatomegaly with stenosis. **CNS:** Abnormal dreams, anxiety, depression, dizziness, fatigue, headache, insomnia, somnolence. **GI:** *Diarrhea,* flatulence, dyspepsia, *nausea,* vomiting. **Hematological:** Immune reconstitution syndrome. **Metabolic:** Alterations in serum glucose, decrease bone mineral density, elevated amylase, elevated alkaline phosphatase, elevated ALT and AST, elevated bilirubin, elevated creatine kinase, elevated cholesterol, elevated creatinine, glycosuria, elevated triglycerides, hematuria, neutropenia. **Musculoskeletal:** Abdominal pain, arthralgia, back pain, myalgia. **Respiratory:** Increased cough, nasopharyngitis, pneumonia, rhinitis, sinusitis, upper respiratory tract infection. **Skin:** Rash. **Urogenital:** Onset or worsening of renal impairment.

**INTERACTIONS Drug:** Elvitegravir/cobicistat/emtricitabine/tenofovir disoproxil fumarate can increase the levels of other compounds that require CYP3A4 (**amiodarone, disopyramide**) or CYP2D6 (**paroxetine,** BETA BLOCKERS, **risperidone**) for metabolism or are substrates for

Common adverse effects in *italic;* life-threatening effects underlined; generic names in **bold**; classifications in SMALL CAPS; ♣Canadian drug name; ◐ Prototype drug

575

P-glycoprotein. Strong (i.e., **ataza-navir, clarithromycin, indina-vir, itraconazole, ketoconazole, nefazodone, nelf-inavir, rito-navir, saquinavir, telithromycin**) and moderate (i.e., **aprepitant, diltiazem, erythromycin, flu-conazole, fosamprenavir, vera-pamil**) inhibitors of CYP3A4 can increase the levels of elvitegravir and cobicistat. Strong (i.e., **car-bamazepine, dexamethasone, phenobarbital, phenytoin, ri-fabutin, rifampin, rifapentine**) and moderate (i.e., **bosentan, efavirenz, etravirine, modafinil, nafcillin**) CYP3A4 inducers may decrease the levels of elvitegravir and cobicistat. Elvitegravir levels are lowered if used in combina-tion with ANTACIDS. Elvitegravir/cobicistat/emtricitabine/tenofovir disoproxil fumarate can increase the levels of **warfarin, colchicine, fluti-casone**, and **norgestimate.** Elvite-gravir/cobicistat/emtricitabine/tenofovir disoproxil fumarate can increase adverse effects associated with PHOSPHODIESTERASE-5 INHIBITORS (**sildenafil, tadalafil, vardenar-il**).**Food: Grapefruit** or **grapefruit juice** may increase the levels of elvitegravir and cobicistat. **Herbal: St. John's wort** may decrease the levels of elvitegravir and cobicistat.

## PHARMACOKINETICS **Peak:**
Elvitegravir 4 h; cobicistat and emtricitabine 3 h; tenofovir 2 h. **Distribution:** Elvitegravir and co-bicistat 97–99% plasma protein bound; emtricitabine and teno-fovir minimally bound to plasma proteins. **Metabolism:** Cobicistat, elvitegravir, and emtricitabine in the liver; tenofovir is not signifi-cantly metabolized. **Elimination:** Elvitegravir and cobicistat primar-ily fecal; emtricitibine and tenofo-vir primarily renal. **Half-Life:** 12.6 h.

(elvitegravir); 3.5 h. (cobicistat); 10 h. (emtricitabine); 17 h. (tenofovir).

## NURSING IMPLICATIONS
Note: Consult individual monographs for emtricitabine and tenofovir diso-proxil fumarate for additional nurs-ing implications.

### Black Box Warning

*This combination of drugs has been associated with severe, and potentially fatal, lactic acidosis and hepatomegaly.*

### Assessment & Drug Effects
- Monitor for and report S&S of lactic acidosis and hepatic impairment. Withhold drug and report to pre-scriber if either is suspected.
- Monitor for signs of bone frac-tures as bone mineral density may be diminished.
- Monitor lab tests: Baseline and pe-riodic renal function tests, urine for glucose and protein, serum electrolytes, alkaline phosphatase, LFTs, and parathyroid hormone.

### Patient & Family Education
- Ensure that prescriber has a com-plete list of all prescription and OTC drugs you are taking.
- Exercise caution with potentially harmful physical activities as de-creased bone density may predis-pose to fractures.
- Notify prescriber if you experi-ence unexplained nausea, vomit-ing, or stomach discomfort.
- Do not breast-feed while taking this drug.

## EMEDASTINE DIFUMARATE ℗
(em-e-das'teen di-foom'a-rate)
Emadine
**Classifications:** OCULAR; ANTIHISTAMINE; H₁-RECEPTOR ANTAGONIST

Common adverse effects in *italic;* life-threatening effects <u>underlined</u>; generic names in **bold;** classifications in SMALL CAPS; ♣ Canadian drug name; ⊙ Prototype drug

**Therapeutic:** OCULAR ANTIHISTA-MINE

**AVAILABILITY** Ophthalmic solution

**ACTION & *THERAPEUTIC EFFECT***
It blocks $H_1$-receptors and inhibits histamine-stimulated vascular permeability in the conjunctiva. *Relieves ocular pruritus related to allergic response to histamine.*

**USES** Temporary relief of seasonal allergic conjunctivitis.

**CONTRAINDICATIONS** Hypersensitivity to emedastine.

**CAUTIOUS USE** Hypersensitivity to other antihistamines, soft contact lenses; pregnancy (category B); lactation. Safety and efficacy in children younger than 3 y not established.

**ROUTE & DOSAGE**

**Allergic Conjunctivitis**
*Adult /Adolescent/Child (older than 3 y):* **Ophthalmic** 1 drop in affected eye q.i.d.

**ADMINISTRATION**

**Instillation**
- Wash hands before and after use.
- Shake well before using. Apply drops in the center of the lower conjunctival sac. Do not touch eyelids with dropper.
- Gently close eyes for 1–2 min after installation of drops.
- Wait 10 min after installation of drug before inserting soft lenses into eyes.
- Store in a tightly closed bottle. Protect the solution from light.
- Do not use if discolored.

**ADVERSE EFFECTS** (≥1%) **CNS:** Headache. **Special Senses:** *Ocular*

*irritation, mild transient stinging and burning,* conjunctival congestion, eyelid edema, eye pain, photophobia, abnormal lacrimation.

**INTERACTIONS Drug:** No clinically significant interactions established.

**PHARMACOKINETICS Absorption:** Minimal. **Half-Life:** 3–4 h.

**NURSING IMPLICATIONS**

**Assessment & Drug Effects**
- Monitor for S&S of hypersensitivity to the drug (see Appendix F).
- Evaluate safety of engaging in hazardous activities since drowsiness is a potential adverse effect.

**Patient & Family Education**
- Learn potential adverse responses to emedastine.
- Eye drops contain benzalkonium chloride, which may damage soft contact lenses. After instillation of drops, wait 10 min before inserting these contact lenses into the eye.
- Contact your prescriber if symptoms do not start to improve in 2 or 3 days.

## EMLA (EUTECTIC MIXTURE OF LIDOCAINE AND PRILOCAINE)
**EMLA Cream**
**Classification:** LOCAL ANESTHETIC
**Therapeutic:** LOCAL ANESTHETIC
**Prototype:** Procaine

**AVAILABILITY** Cream

**ACTION & *THERAPEUTIC EFFECT***
EMLA cream is a mixture of lidocaine and prilocaine. *EMLA is a topical analgesic.*

**USES** Topical anesthetic on normal intact skin for local anesthesia.

**UNLABELED USES** Topical anesthetic prior to leg ulcer debridement; treatment of postherpetic neuralgia.

Common adverse effects in *italic;* life-threatening effects <u>underlined;</u> generic names in **bold;** classifications in SMALL CAPS; ◆Canadian drug name; ❷ Prototype drug

577

**E**

**CONTRAINDICATIONS** Patients with known sensitivity to local anesthetics; patients with congenital or idiopathic methemoglobinemia; tympanic membrane perforation.

**CAUTIOUS USE** Acutely ill, debilitated, or older adult patients; severe liver disease; pregnancy (category B); lactation. Safe use in children younger than 1 mo not established.

## ROUTE & DOSAGE

**Topical Anesthetic**

*Adult/Child (1 mo or older):*
**Topical** Apply 2.5 g of cream (½ of 5-g tube) over 20–25 cm² of skin, cover with occlusive dressing and wait at least 1 h, then remove dressing and wipe off cream, cleanse area with an antiseptic solution and prepare patient for the procedure.

## ADMINISTRATION

**Topical**

- Apply a thick layer to skin (approximately ½ of 5-g tube/20–25 cm² or 2 × 2 in) at site of procedure. Apply an occlusive dressing. Do not spread out cream. Seal edges of dressing well to avoid leakage.
- Apply EMLA cream 1 h before routine procedure and 2 h before painful procedure.
- Remove EMLA cream prior to skin puncture and clean area with an aseptic solution.
- Store at room temperature 15°–30° C (59°–86° F).

## ADVERSE EFFECTS (≥1%) **Hematologic:** Methemoglobinemia, especially in infants, small children, and patients with G6PD deficiency. **Skin:** *Blanching and redness,* itching, heat sensation. **Body as a Whole:** Edema, sore-

ness, aching, numbness, heaviness. **Other:** The adverse effects of lidocaine could occur with large doses or if there is significant systemic absorption.

**INTERACTIONS Drug:** May cause additive toxicity with CLASS I ANTIARRHYTHMICS; may increase risk of developing methemoglobin when used with **acetaminophen, chloroquine, dapsone, fosphenytoin,** NITRATES and NITRITES, **nitric oxide, nitrofurantoin, nitroprusside, pamaquine, phenobarbital, phenytoin, primaquine, quinine,** or SULFONAMIDES.

**PHARMACOKINETICS Absorption:** Penetrates intact skin. **Onset:** 15–60 min. **Peak:** 2–3 h. **Duration:** 1–2 h after removal of cream. **Distribution:** Crosses blood–brain barrier and placenta, distributed into breast milk. **Metabolism:** In liver. **Elimination:** 98% of absorbed dose is excreted in urine. **Half-Life:** 60–150 min.

## NURSING IMPLICATIONS

### Assessment & Drug Effects

- Monitor for local skin reactions including erythema, edema, itching, abnormal temperature sensations, and rash. These reactions are very common and usually disappear in 1–2 h.
- Note: Patients taking Class I antiarrhythmic drugs may experience toxic effects on the cardiovascular system. EMLA should be used with caution in these patients.
- Wash immediately with water or saline if contact with the eye occurs; protect the eye until sensation returns.

### Patient & Family Education

- Skin analgesia lasts for 1 h following removal of the occlusive dressing. Analgesia may be accompanied by temporary loss of all sensation in the treated skin. Advise caution until sensation returns.

# EMPAGLIFLOZIN
(em-pa-gli-flo'sin)
Jardiance

**Classifications:** ANTIDIABETIC; SODIUM-GLUCOSE CO-TRANSPORTER 2 (SGLT2) INHIBITOR
Therapeutic: ANTIDIABETIC
**Prototype** Canagliflozin

## AVAILABILITY Tablet

## ACTION & *THERAPEUTIC EFFECT*
Inhibits the sodium-glucose cotransporter 2 (SGLT2) in the proximal renal tubules that is responsible for the majority of the reabsorption of filtered glucose in the kidney. *Empagliflozin inhibits SGLT2 thus allowing more glucose to be removed from the blood stream and excreted by the kidney.*

## USES An adjunct to diet and exercise to improve glycemic control in adults with type 2 diabetes mellitus.

## CONTRAINDICATIONS Hypersensitivity to canagliflozin or any component of the formulation; severe renal impairment (GFR less than 30 mL/minute/1.73 m²), end-stage renal disease, or on dialysis; lactation.

## CAUTIOUS USE Mild or moderate renal impairment; low systolic pressure; increased LDL-C; older adults; pregnancy (category C). Safety and efficacy in children younger than 18 y not established.

## ROUTE & DOSAGE

**Type 2 Diabetes Mellitus**
*Adult:* **PO** 10 mg once daily in a.m.; can increase to 25 mg once daily

**Renal Impairment Dosage Adjustment**
*GFR less than 45 mL/min/1.73 m²:* Do not initiate
*GFR consistently falls to less than 45 mL/min/1.73 m²:* Discontinue

## ADMINISTRATION
**Oral**
- Give in the morning without regard to food.
- Store at 15°–30° C (59°–86° F).

## ADVERSE EFFECTS ($\geq$ 1%) Body as a Whole: Polydipsia, volume depletion. GI: Nausea. Hematological: Decreased hematocrit. Metabolic: Dyslipidemia, hypoglycemia, increased serum creatinine. Musculoskeletal: Arthralgia. Urogenital: Genital mycotic infections, increased urination, *urinary tract infection.*

## DIAGNOSTIC TEST INTERFERENCE
Empagliflozin increases urinary glucose excretion and will lead to positive **urine glucose tests.** *Empagliflozin will interfere with an 1,5 anhydroglucitol (1,5 AG) assay.*

## INTERACTIONS Drug: Coadministration with DIURETICS may cause volume depletion. Coadministration with **insulin** or INSULIN SECRETAGOGUES increases the risk for hypoglycemia.

## PHARMACOKINETICS Peak: 1.5 h. Distribution: 86% plasma protein bound. Metabolism: In liver. Elimination: Renal (54%) and fecal (41%). Half-Life: 12.4 h.

## NURSING IMPLICATIONS
**Assessment & Drug Effects**
- Monitor BP throughout therapy as drug causes intravascular volume depletion.

Common adverse effects in *italic;* life-threatening effects <u>underlined</u>; generic names in **bold**; classifications in SMALL CAPS; ♣ Canadian drug name; ⊘ Prototype drug

579

**E**

- Monitor for symptomatic hypotension especially at the initiation of therapy and in the older adult or those taking other drugs that lower BP.
- Monitor for S&S of genital fungal infections.
- Monitor lab tests: Baseline and periodic renal function tests; periodic HbA1C and lipid profile.

**Patient & Family Education**

- Monitor blood sugar as directed by prescriber. Note that this drug will cause sugar to appear in your urine.
- Report to prescriber if you experience S&S of hypoglycemia (see Appendix F).
- Report to prescriber any S&S of an allergic reaction (e.g., rash, hives).
- Maintain adequate fluid intake as drug can cause dehydration. Inform prescriber if you experience dizziness upon standing.
- Yeast infections of the vagina and penis (especially in uncircumcised men) may occur. Report promptly for treatment.
- Report to prescriber if a pregnancy is suspected.
- Discontinue breast-feeding while taking this drug.

---

# EMTRICITABINE
(em-tri'ci-ta-been)
*Emtriva*
**Classifications:** ANTIRETROVIRAL; NUCLEOSIDE REVERSE TRANSCRIPTASE INHIBITOR (NRTI)
**Therapeutic:** ANTIRETROVIRAL, NRTI
**Prototype:** Zidovudine

**AVAILABILITY** Capsule; oral solution

## ACTION & *THERAPEUTIC EFFECT*
It inhibits HIV-1 reverse transcriptase (RT), both by competing with the natural DNA nucleoside and by incorporation into viral DNA, which

terminates the formation of the viral DNA chain. *The viral load is decreased as measured by an increase in CD4 leukocyte count and suppression of viral RNA.*

**USES** Treatment of HIV in combination with other antiretroviral agents.

**UNLABELED USES** Treatment of chronic hepatitis B in HIV-positive patients, HIV prophylaxis.

**CONTRAINDICATIONS** Hypersensitivity to emtricitabine; suicidal ideation; chronic HBV infection; development of lactic acidosis or hepatomegaly; pregnancy (category B); lactation.

**CAUTIOUS USE** Renal impairment, and with end-stage renal disease; hepatic impairment; history of mental illness including bipolar disorder, psychosis; history of suicidal tendencies; alcoholism; substance abuse; seizure disorders; hypercholesterolemia, hypertriglyceridemia; older adults; children less than 3 mo.

## ROUTE & DOSAGE

**HIV**

*Adult/Adolescent/Child (weight greater than 33 kg):* **PO** 200 mg (capsule) or 240 mg (solution) once/day
*Child (3 mo–17 y):* **PO** 6 mg/kg days (max: 240 mg/day)
*Neonate/Infant (younger than 3 mo):* 3 mg/kg daily

**Renal Impairment Dosage Adjustment**

*CrCl 30–49 mL/min:* 200 mg q48h; *15–29 mL/min:* 200 mg q72h; *less than 15 mL/min:* 200 mg q96h

---

Common adverse effects in *italic;* life-threatening effects <u>underlined</u>; generic names in **bold**; classifications in SMALL CAPS; ♣ Canadian drug name; ⊘ Prototype drug

## ADMINISTRATION

### Oral

- Give at the same time daily.
- Store at 15°–30° C (59°–86° F) in a tightly closed container.

## ADVERSE EFFECTS (≥1%) Body as a Whole: Asthenia, neuropathy, peripheral neuritis *infection in pediatric patients.* CNS: *Headache,* depression, dizziness, insomnia. GI: *Diarrhea, nausea,* dyspepsia, abdominal pain, hepatomegaly. **Metabolic:** Lactic acidosis. Musculoskeletal: Arthralgia, myalgia, paresthesias. **Respiratory:** Cough, rhinitis. Skin: *Rash, hyperpigmentation* of palms and soles of feet.

## PHARMACOKINETICS Absorption: 93% reaches systemic circulation. Peak: 1–2 h. Distribution: 4% protein bound. Metabolism: In liver. Elimination: Urine. Half-Life: 10 h (active metabolite has intracellular half-life of 39 h).

## NURSING IMPLICATIONS

### Assessment & Drug Effects

- Monitor closely for S&S of lactic acidosis, especially in persons with known risk factors such as female gender, obesity, alcoholism, or hepatic disease.
- Withhold drug and notify prescriber if S&S suggestive of lactic acidosis or hepatotoxicity occur.
- Monitor closely for severe exacerbation of hepatitis B in coinfected patients if this drug is discontinued.
- Monitor lab tests: Baseline renal function tests; frequent LFTs and serum electrolytes during the last trimester of pregnancy; complete blood chemistry if lactic acidosis is suspected; and periodic lipid profile.

### Patient & Family Education

- May cause serious CNS effects. Avoid driving or operating machinery until individual reaction to the drug is known.
- Report any of the following to the prescriber: Difficulty breathing, shortness of breath, fast or irregular heartbeat; weight gain with fullness around waist and/or face; vomiting or diarrhea; unexplained muscle aches, pains, weakness, or fatigue; yellow eyes or skin.
- Avoid alcoholic drinks while taking this drug.
- Do not self-treat nausea, vomiting, or stomach pain. Contact prescriber for guidance.

## ENALAPRIL MALEATE ℗

(e-nal′a-pril)

Vasotec, Epaned

## ENALAPRILAT

**Classifications:** ANGIOTENSIN-CONVERTING ENZYME (ACE) INHIBITOR; ANTIHYPERTENSIVE
Therapeutic: ANTIHYPERTENSIVE

**AVAILABILITY** Tablet; oral solution; solution for injection

## ACTION & THERAPEUTIC EFFECT

Angiotensin-converting enzyme (ACE) inhibitor that catalyzes the conversion of angiotensin I to angiotensin II, therefore decreases angiotensin II levels, thus decreasing vasopressor activity and aldosterone secretion. Both actions achieve an antihypertensive effect by suppression of the renin–angiotensin–aldosterone system. ACE inhibitors also reduce peripheral arterial resistance (afterload), pulmonary capillary wedge pressure (PCWP), a measure of preload, pulmonary vascular resistance, and improve cardiac output. *Antihypertensive effect lowers blood pressure. Improvement in cardiac output results in increased exercise tolerance.*

---

Common adverse effects in *italic;* life-threatening effects underlined; generic names in **bold;** classifications in SMALL CAPS; ◆ Canadian drug name; ℗ Prototype drug

**E**

**USES** Management of hypertension, proteinuria, and heart failure.

**UNLABELED USES** Hypertension or renal crisis in scleroderma, diabetic nephropathy, persistent albuminuria.

**CONTRAINDICATIONS** Hypersensitivity to enalapril or captopril; uncorrected hypotension; heredity of idiopathic angioedema; history of angioedema related to an ACE inhibitor; acute renal failure; co-admistration of aliskiren in diabetics. There has been evidence of fetotoxicity and kidney damage in newborns exposed to ACE inhibitors during pregnancy including first trimester. (category D); lactation.

**CAUTIOUS USE** Renal impairment, renal artery stenosis; history of angioedema; patients with hypovolemia, receiving diuretics; undergoing dialysis; hepatic disease; bone marrow suppression; patients in whom excessive hypotension would present a hazard (e.g., cerebrovascular insufficiency); CHF; aortic stenosis, cardiomyopathy; hepatic impairment; DM; women of childbearing age; infants and children with CrCl less than 30 mL/min/1.73 m².

## ROUTE & DOSAGE

### Hypertension
*Adult:* **PO** 2.5–5 mg/day, may increase to 10–40 mg/day in 1–2 divided doses; **IV** 0.625–1.25 mg q6h, may give up to 5 mg q6h in hypertensive emergencies.
*Child/Infant (1 mo or older):* **PO** 0.08 mg/kg/day, may increase (max: 5 mg/kg/day).

### Heart Failure
*Adult:* **PO** 2.5 mg b.i.d., may increase up to 5–20 mg/day in 1–2 divided doses (max: 40 mg/day).

### Proteinuria
*Adolescent/Child:* **PO** 0.2–0.6 mg/kg/day in divided doses

### Renal Impairment Dosage Adjustment
*Enalapril:* *CrCl less than 30 mL/min:* Start with 2.5 mg dose then titrate
*Enalaprilat:* *CrCl less than 30 mL/min:* Start with dose of 0.625 mg q6h then titrate

### Hemodialysis Dosage Adjustment
Adjust for clinical response

## ADMINISTRATION

### Oral
- Discontinue diuretics, if possible, for 2–3 days prior to initial oral dose to reduce incidence of hypotension. If the diuretic cannot be discontinued, give an initial dose of 2.5 mg. Keep patient under medical supervision for at least 2 h and until BP has stabilized for at least an additional hour.
- Give with food or drink of patient's choice.
- Protect from heat and light. Expiration date: 30 mo following date of manufacture if stored at less than 30° C.
- Store tablets at 30° C (86° F); protect from heat and light.

### Intravenous
Note: Verify correct IV concentration and rate of infusion/injection with prescriber for neonates, infants, children.

*PREPARE:* **Direct:** May be given undiluted or diluted with up to 50 mL of a compatible diluent. For neonates, mix 1 mL (1.25 mg) in 49 mL D5W or NS to yield 0.025 mg/mL. **Intermittent:** Dilute in 50 mL of D5W, NS, D5/NS, D5/LR.

Common adverse effects in *italic;* life-threatening effects underlined; generic names in **bold;** classifications in SMALL CAPS; ♣ Canadian drug name; ⦾ Prototype drug

*ADMINISTER:* **Direct/Intermittent:** Give direct IV slowly over at least 5 min through a port of a free flowing infusion of D5W or NS or as an infusion over 5 min.
▪ Longer infusion time decreases risk of severe hypotension.

*INCOMPATIBILITIES:* **Y-site:** **Amphotericin B, amphotericin B cholesteryl, ampicillin, caspofungin, cefepime, dantrolene, diazepam, diazoxide, gemtuzumab, haloperidol, hydralazine, lansoprazole, nesiritide, pantoprazole, phenytoin, SMZ/TMP.**

**ADVERSE EFFECTS** (≥1%) **CNS:** *Headache, dizziness,* fatigue, nervousness, paresthesias, asthenia, insomnia, somnolence. **CV:** *Hypotension including postural hypotension,* syncope, palpitations, chest pain. **GI:** Diarrhea, nausea, abdominal pain, loss of taste, dyspepsia. **Hematologic:** Decreased Hgb and Hct. **Urogenital:** Acute kidney failure, deterioration in kidney function. **Skin:** Pruritus with and without *rash,* angioedema, erythema. **Metabolic:** Hyperkalemia. **Respiratory:** Cough. **Whole Body:** Angioedema.

**INTERACTIONS Drug: Indomethacin** and other NSAIDS may decrease antihypertensive activity; POTASSIUM SUPPLEMENTS, POTASSIUM-SPARING DIURETICS may cause hyperkalemia; use with other ACE INHIBITORS or ARBS does not provide additional benefit compared to monotherapy; may increase **lithium** levels and toxicity. **Pregabalin** may cause angioedema. Do not use with **azathioprine.**

**PHARMACOKINETICS Absorption:** 70% from GI tract. **Onset:** 1 h PO; 15 min IV. **Peak:** 4–8 h PO; 4 h IV. **Duration:** 12–24 h PO; 6 h IV. **Distribution:** Limited amount crosses blood–brain barrier; crosses placenta. **Metabolism:** PO dose undergoes first-pass metabolism in liver to active form, enalaprilat. **Elimination:** 60% in urine, 33% in feces within 24 h. **Half-Life:** 2 h.

## NURSING IMPLICATIONS

### Black Box Warning

*Enalapril has been associated with fetal injury and death.*

### Assessment & Drug Effects

▪ Monitor for therapeutic effectiveness. Peak effects after the first IV dose may not occur for up to 4 h; peak effects of subsequent doses may exceed those of the first.
▪ Maintain bedrest and monitor BP for the first 3 h after the initial IV dose. First-dose phenomenon (i.e., a sudden exaggerated hypotensive response) may occur within 1–3 h of first IV dose, especially in the patient with very high blood pressure or one on a diuretic and controlled salt intake regimen. An IV infusion of normal saline for volume expansion may be ordered to counteract the hypotensive response. This initial response is not an indicator to stop therapy.
▪ Monitor BP for first several days of therapy. If antihypertensive effect is diminished before 24 h, the total dose may be given as 2 divided doses.
▪ Report transient hypotension with lightheadedness. Older adults are particularly sensitive to drug-induced hypotension. Supervise ambulation until BP has stabilized.
▪ Monitor for hyperkalemia. Patients who have diabetes, impaired kidney function, or CHF are at risk of developing hyperkalemia during enalapril treatment.
▪ Monitor lab tests: Baseline and periodic serum potassium and renal function tests.

---

Common adverse effects in *italic;* life-threatening effects underlined; generic names in **bold;** classifications in SMALL CAPS; ♣Canadian drug name; ☻ Prototype drug

**E**

**Patient & Family Education**

- Notify prescriber immediately if a pregnancy is suspected. Drug should be discontinued as soon as possible.
- Full antihypertensive effect may not be experienced until several weeks after enalapril therapy starts.
- When drug is discontinued due to severe hypotension, the hypotensive effect may persist a week or longer after termination because of long duration of drug action.
- Do not follow a low-sodium diet (e.g., low-sodium foods or low-sodium milk) without approval from prescriber.
- Avoid use of salt substitute (principal ingredient: potassium salt) and potassium supplements because of the potential for hyperkalemia.
- Notify prescriber of a persistent nonproductive cough, especially at night, accompanied by nasal congestion.
- Report to prescriber promptly if swelling of face, eyelids, tongue, lips, or extremities occurs. Angioedema is a rare adverse effect and, if accompanied by laryngeal edema, may be fatal.
- Do not drive or engage in other potentially hazardous activities until response to drug is known.

## ENASIDENIB
(en-a-sid′a-nib)

Idhifa

**Classifications:** ANTINEOPLASTIC AGENT; IDH2 INHIBITOR
Therapeutic: ANTINEOPLASTIC AGENT

**AVAILABILITY** Tablet

**ACTION & *THERAPEUTIC EFFECT***
Small molecule inhibitor that reduces abnormal histone hypermethylation, restores myeloid differentiation, reduces blast counts, and increases percentages of mature myeloid cells. *Antineoplastic agent used to treat relapsed or refractory acute myeloid leukemia.*

**USES** For the treatment of relapsed or refractory acute myeloid leukemia in patients with isocitrate dehydrogenase-2 (IDH2) mutation.

**CAUTIOUS USE** Pregnancy; lactation. Safety and efficacy in children not established.

## ROUTE & DOSAGE

**Acute Myeloid Leukemia**
*Adult:* **PO** 100 mg daily

**Hepatic Impairment Dosage Adjustment**
*Total bilirubin greater than 3 × ULN for more than 2 wk:* 50 mg daily; *once billirubin decreases to less than 2 × ULN:* Resume 100 mg daily

## ADMINISTRATION

**Oral**
- Administer orally once daily with or without food at approximately the same time each day.
- Swallow whole with a glass of water.
- Do not split or crush tablets.

**ADVERSE EFFECTS (≥ 2%) Body as a Whole:** *Cytokine release syndrome.* **Endocrine and Metabolic:** *Decreased serum calcium, decreased serum potassium.* **GI:** *Nausea, diarrhea, decreased appetite, vomiting, dysgeusia.* **Hematologic:** *Abnormal phosphorus levels,* leukocytosis, tumor lysis syndrome. **Hepatic:** *Increased serum bilirubin.*

**Respiratory:** Acute respiratory distress, pulmonary edema.

## PHARMACOKINETICS **Absorption:** 57% bioavailability, 98.5% protein bound. **Onset:** Peak effect in 4 h. **Metabolism:** Hepatic via multiple CYP enzymes and UGTs. **Elimination:** 89% in feces, 11% in urine. **Half-Life:** 137 h.

## NURSING IMPLICATIONS

### Black Box Warning

*Enasidenib has been associated with symptoms of differentiation syndrome, which if left untreated is fatal. Symptoms include fever, hypotension, and dyspnea.*

### Assessment & Drug Effects

- Monitor for signs of differentiation syndrome including fever, cough, dyspnea, bone pain, rapid weight gain, edema, and lymphadenopathy as well as tumor lysis syndrome.
- Obtain CBC and electrolytes prior to therapy and every 2 wk for the first 3 mo of therapy.
- Monitor lab tests: Baseline and routine monitoring of IDH2 mutation, LFTs, renal function tests, and pregnancy tests.

### Patient & Family Education

- Notify prescriber if you have signs of differentiation syndrome including bone pain, cough, fever, shortness of breath, sudden weight gain, swelling in the arms or legs, or swollen gland(s).
- Notify prescriber right away if you have signs of kidney problems such as inability to urinate, change in appearance of urine, change in amount of urine, or blood in the urine.

- Call prescriber if you have signs of liver problems including dark urine, feeling tired, upset stomach, stomach pain, light-colored stools, vomiting, or yellow skin or eyes.
- Tell your doctor Notify prescriber if you experience signs or symptoms of allergic reaction such as rash, hives, itching, shortness of breath, wheezing, cough, swelling of the face, lips, tongue, or throat; or any other signs.
- Use effective birth control while on this medication and for 1 mo after stopping this drug.

## ENFUVIRTIDE
(en-fu-vir'tide)

Fuzeon

**Classifications:** ANTIRETROVIRAL; FUSION INHIBITOR
**Therapeutic:** ANTIRETROVIRAL

**AVAILABILITY** Solution for injection

## ACTION & *THERAPEUTIC EFFECT*
Enfuvirtide interferes with entry of HIV-1 into host cells by inhibiting fusion of the virus with the host cell membranes. In order for HIV-1 to enter and infect a human cell, the viral surface glycoprotein (gp41) must bind to the host CD4+ cells. Then, the viral glycoprotein undergoes a change in shape facilitating the fusion of viral membranes with the host cell membrane. Prevents entry of the HIV-1 virus into host cells. *Effectiveness is measured in reduction of viral load as measured by an increase in CD4 leucocyte count and suppression of viral RNA.*

**USES** Treatment of advanced HIV disease with evidence of resistance to other therapies.

Common adverse effects in *italic;* life-threatening effects <u>underlined;</u> generic names in **bold;** classifications in SMALL CAPS; ♣ Canadian drug name; ◐ Prototype drug

585

E

## CONTRAINDICATIONS

Hypersensitivity to enfuvirtide or any of its components; HIV/HBV co-infected patients; severe hepatomegaly; lactation.

## CAUTIOUS USE

Hypersensitivity to mannitol; renal and hepatic impairment; renal clearance of less than 35 mL/min; bacterial pneumonia, low initial CD4 count, past history of lung disease, high initial viral load, IV drug use; history of pulmonary disease; pregnancy (category C).

## ROUTE & DOSAGE

### Advanced HIV Disease

*Adult/Adolescent (16 y or older or weight 42.6 kg or more):*
**Subcutaneous** 90 mg b.i.d.
*Child/Adolescent (6–16 y or weight less than 42.6 kg):*
**Subcutaneous** 2 mg/kg (up to 90 mg) b.i.d.

## ADMINISTRATION

#### Subcutaneous

- Reconstitute by adding 1.1 mL sterile water for injection into vial. Mix by gently tapping vial for 10 sec, then gently rolling in palms of hands. Ensure that no drug is remaining on vial wall. Allow vial to stand until powder completely dissolves (up to 45 min). Solution should be clear, colorless, and without bubbles or particulate matter.
- Bring refrigerated reconstituted solution to room temperature before injection. Ensure that powder is fully dissolved and solution is clear, colorless, and without bubbles or particulate matter.
- Inject into upper arm, abdomen, or anterior thigh.
- Rotate injection sites and inject in an area with no current injection site reaction.

- Store unreconstituted vials at 15°–30° C (59°–86° F) or refrigerated at 2°–6° C (3°–46° F); do not freeze.

## ADVERSE EFFECTS (≥1%) 

**Body as a Whole:** Injection site reactions (pain, induration, erythema, nodules, cysts, pruritus, ecchymoses), infection at injection site, fatigue, systemic hypersensitivity reactions, Guillain-Barré syndrome, asthenia, herpes simplex infections, influenza, lymphadenopathy, myalgia, peripheral neuropathy. **CNS:** Anxiety, depression, insomnia. **GI:** Diarrhea, nausea, abdominal pain, anorexia, constipation, dysgeusia, pancreatitis, weight loss. **Hematologic:** Eosinophilia, anemia. **Metabolic:** Increased amylase, increased lipase, increased ALT and AST, hypertriglyceridemia. **Respiratory:** Bacterial pneumonia, acute respiratory distress syndrome, cough, sinusitis. **Skin:** Pruritus, skin papilloma. **Special Senses:** Conjunctivitis. **Urogenital:** Glomerulonephritis.

## INTERACTIONS

Increases levels of **tripranavir** (dose adjustment not needed).

## PHARMACOKINETICS

**Absorption:** 84.3% absorbed from subcutaneous site. **Peak:** Average 4–8 h. **Distribution:** 92% protein bound. **Metabolism:** Catabolized into constituent amino acids. **Half-Life:** 4 h.

## NURSING IMPLICATIONS

#### Assessment & Drug Effects

- Inspect subcutaneous sites for S&S of site reactions (e.g., itching, swelling, redness, pain, tenderness, or hardened skin) that usually last for less than 7 days postinjection.
- Monitor closely for S&S of pneumonia, especially with low initial

Common adverse effects in *italic;* life-threatening effects <u>underlined;</u> generic names in **bold;** classifications in SMALL CAPS; ✚ Canadian drug name; ⊘ Prototype drug

CD4 count, high initial viral load, IV drug use, smoking, or prior history of lung disease.
- Monitor lab tests: Periodic LFTs, serum lipase and amylase, lipid profile, and CBC with differential.

**Patient & Family Education**
- Report promptly S&S of infection at subcutaneous injection sites: Increased heat, redness, pain, or oozing.
- Report promptly S&S of pneumonia: Cough with fever, rapid breathing, shortness of breath.

# ENOXAPARIN ⓟ

(e-nox'a-pa-rin)

Lovenox

**Classifications:** ANTICOAGULANT; LOW MOLECULAR WEIGHT HEPARIN
Therapeutic: ANTICOAGULANT; ANTITHROMBOTIC

**AVAILABILITY** Solution for injection

## ACTION & THERAPEUTIC EFFECT
Low molecular weight heparin with antithrombotic properties. Does affect thrombin time (TT) and activated thromboplastin time (aPTT) up to 1.8 × the control value. Antithrombotic properties are due to its antifactor Xa and antithrombin (antifactor IIa) in the coagulation activities. *An effective anticoagulation agent, it is used for prophylactic treatment as an antithrombotic agent following certain types of surgery.*

## USES
Prevention of deep vein thrombosis (DVT) after hip, knee, or abdominal surgery, treatment of DVT and pulmonary embolism, management of acute ST elevation myocardial infarction (STEMI), unstable angina, non-Q wave MI.

## CONTRAINDICATIONS
Hypersensitivity to enoxaprin, porcine protein hypersensitivity, active major bleeding, GI bleeding, hemophilia, heparin hypersensitivity, heparin-induced thrombocytopenia (HIT), thrombocytopenia associated with an antiplatelet antibody in the presence of enoxaparin, bleeding disorders, idiopathic thrombocytopenic purpura (ITP).

## CAUTIOUS USE
Uncontrolled arterial hypertension, recent history of GI disease, conditions or surgery with increased risk of bleeding; history of spinal deformity or spinal surgery; percutaneous coronary revascularization procedures; hepatic disease, hypertension, coagulopathy, thrombocytopenia; dental disease; diabetic retinopathy; dialysis, diverticulitis, inflammatory bowel disease, peptic ulcer disease; endocarditis; renal impairment, stroke, surgery, older adults; pregnancy (category B); lactation. Safe use in neonates, infants, and children has not been established.

## ROUTE & DOSAGE

**Prevention of DVT after Hip or Knee Surgery**
*Adult:* **Subcutaneous** 30 mg b.i.d. for 10–14 days starting 12–24 h post-surgery

**Prevention of DVT after Abdominal Surgery**
*Adult:* **Subcutaneous** 40 mg daily starting 2 h before surgery and continuing for 7–10 days (max: 12 days)

**Treatment of DVT and Pulmonary Embolus**
*Adult:* **Subcutaneous** 1 mg/kg q12h or 1.5 mg/kg/day

---

Common adverse effects in *italic;* life-threatening effects underlined; generic names in **bold;** classifications in SMALL CAPS; ♣ Canadian drug name; ⓟ Prototype drug

E

### Non-Q Wave MI

*Adult:* **Subcutaneous** 1 mg/kg q12h for 2–8 days, give concurrently with aspirin 100–325 mg/day

### Acute STEMI/Unstable Angina

*Adult:* **IV** 30 mg bolus plus 1 mg/kg subcutaneously, then 1 mg/kg q12h subcutaneously

### Renal Impairment Dosage Adjustment

*CrCl less than 30 mL/min:* 30 mg or 1 mg/kg q24h

## ADMINISTRATION

### Subcutaneous

- Use a TB syringe or prefilled syringe to ensure accurate dosage.
- Do not expel the air bubble from the 30- or 40-mg prefilled syringe before injection.
- Place patient in a supine position for injection of the drug.
- Alternate injections between left and right anterolateral and posterolateral abdominal wall.
- Hold the skin fold between the thumb and forefinger and insert the whole length of the needle into the skin fold. Hold skin fold throughout the injection. Do not rub site post-injection.
- Store at 15°–30° C (59°–86° F).

### Intravenous

*PREPARE:* **Direct:** Give undiluted.
*ADMINISTER:* **Direct:** Give bolus dose direct IV through an IV line. Flush before and after with NS or D5W to ensure that the IV line has been cleared. Do not mix with any other drugs or solutions.

## ADVERSE EFFECTS (≥1%) **Body as a Whole:** Allergic reactions

(rash, urticaria), fever, <u>angioedema</u>, arthralgia, pain and inflammation at injection site, peripheral edema, fever. **Digestive:** Abnormal liver function tests. **Hematologic:** <u>Hemorrhage</u>, thrombocytopenia, ecchymoses, anemia. **Respiratory:** Dyspnea. **Skin:** Rash, pruritus.

## INTERACTIONS **Drug:** Aspirin, NSAIDs, **warfarin** can increase risk of hemorrhage. **Herbal: Garlic, ginger, ginkgo, feverfew** may increase risk of bleeding.

## PHARMACOKINETICS **Absorption:** 91% from subcutaneous injection site. **Peak:** 3 h. **Duration:** 4.6 h. **Distribution:** Accumulates in liver, kidneys, and spleen. Does not cross placenta. **Elimination:** Primarily in urine. **Half-Life:** 4.6 h.

## NURSING IMPLICATIONS

### Assessment & Drug Effects

- Monitor platelet count closely. Withhold drug and notify prescriber if platelet count less than 100,000/mm$^3$.
- Monitor closely patients with renal insufficiency and older adults who are at higher risk for thrombocytopenia.
- Monitor for and report immediately any sign or symptom of unexplained bleeding.
- Monitor for and report promptly S&S of neurological impairment.
- Monitor lab tests: Periodic CBC, platelet count, urine and stool for occult blood.

### Patient & Family Education

- Report to prescriber promptly signs of unexplained bleeding such as: Pink, red, or dark brown urine; red or dark brown vomitus; bleeding gums or bloody sputum; dark, tarry stools.
- Do not take any OTC drugs without first consulting prescriber.

# ENTACAPONE
(en-ta'ca-pone)

Comtan

**Classifications:** CATECHOLAMINE
O-METHYLTRANSFERASE (COMT)
INHIBITOR; ANTIPARKINSON
**Therapeutic:** ANTIPARKINSON
**Prototype:** Tolcapone

## AVAILABILITY Tablet

## ACTION & THERAPEUTIC EFFECT

Selective inhibitor of catecholamine O-methyltransferase (COMT). COMT is responsible for metabolizing levodopa to an intermediate compound 3-O-methyldopa, a chemical which interferes with the availability of levodopa to the brain. Therefore, it increases availability of levodopa in CNS. *Taken with levodopa, it decreases formation of 3-O-methyldopa, thus increasing the duration of the motor response of the brain to levodopa in Parkinson's disease, diminishing its manifestations.*

**USES** Adjunct to levodopa/carbidopa to treat Parkinson's disease.

## CONTRAINDICATIONS Hypersensitivity to entacapone; concurrent use of nonselective MAO inhibitors; major psychiatric disorders; individuals with suspicious, undiagnosed skin lesions or history of melanoma; children.

## CAUTIOUS USE Hepatic impairment; biliary obstruction; history of hypotension or syncope; sleep disorders; pregnancy (category C); lactation.

## ROUTE & DOSAGE

**Parkinson's Disease**
*Adult:* **PO** 200 mg administered with each dose of levodopa/carbidopa (max: 1600 mg/day)

## ADMINISTRATION

### Oral
- Give simultaneously with each levodopa/carbidopa dose.
- **Must be** tapered if discontinued. Never discontinue abruptly.
- Do not administer to patients receiving nonselective MAO inhibitors.
- Store at 15°–30° C (59°–86° F).

## ADVERSE EFFECTS (≥1%) **Body as a Whole:** Back pain, fatigue, asthenia. **CNS:** *Dyskinesia, hyperkinesia,* hypokinesia, dizziness, anxiety, somnolence, agitation. **GI:** Taste perversion, *nausea, diarrhea,* abdominal pain, constipation, vomiting, dry mouth, dyspepsia, flatulence, gastritis. **Respiratory:** Dyspnea. **Skin:** Increased sweating. **Other:** *Urine discoloration,* purpura.

## INTERACTIONS Drug: Extreme caution **must be** used if administered with a nonselective MAOI; **bitolterol, dobutamine, dopamine, epinephrine, isoetharine, isoproterenol, methyldopa, norepinephrine** may increase heart rates, possibly cause arrhythmias, excessive changes in BP. May increase risk of bleeding when used with **warfarin.**

## PHARMACOKINETICS Absorption: Rapidly absorbed, 35% bioavailable. **Peak:** 1 h. **Distribution:** Highly protein bound. **Metabolism:** Extensively metabolized in plasma and erythrocytes. **Elimination:** Primarily in feces. **Half-Life:** 2.4 h (terminal).

## NURSING IMPLICATIONS

### Assessment & Drug Effects
- Monitor carefully for hyperpyrexia, confusion, or emergence of Parkinson's S&S during drug withdrawal.
- Monitor for orthostatic hypotension and worsening of dyskinesia or hyperkinesia.

**E**

### Patient & Family Education
- Take with levodopa/carbidopa; not effective alone.
- Do not discontinue abruptly; gradually reduce dosage.
- Exercise caution when rising from a sitting or lying position because faintness/dizziness can occur.
- Exercise caution with hazardous activities until reaction to the drug is known.
- Harmless brownish-orange discoloration of urine is possible.
- Report unusual adverse effects (e.g., hallucinations/unexplained diarrhea).

## ENTECAVIR
(en-te'ca-vir)
Baraclude
**Classifications:** ANTIRETROVIRAL; NUCLEOSIDE REVERSE TRANSCRIPTASE INHIBITOR (NRTI)
Therapeutic: ANTIRETROVIRAL; NRTI
**Prototype:** Lamivudine

**AVAILABILITY** Tablet; oral solution

**ACTION & *THERAPEUTIC EFFECT***
Inhibits hepatitis B viral (HBV) DNA polymerase by inhibiting viral reverse transcriptase of messenger RNA that ultimately results in inhibiting the synthesis of HBV DNA. *The antiviral activity of entecavir inhibits HBV DNA synthesis.*

**USES** Hepatitis B infection.

**CONTRAINDICATIONS** Hypersensitivity to entecavir; lactic acidosis; severe hepatomegaly; HIV/HVB co-infected patients, if HIV is not being treated with highly active antiretroviral therapy; lactation.

**CAUTIOUS USE** Liver transplant patients; HIV patients; renal impairment,

ESRF, dialysis; older adults; labor and delivery; pregnancy (category C). Safety and efficacy in children younger than 16 y not established.

## ROUTE & DOSAGE

**Chronic Hepatitis B (nucleoside-treatment–naïve patients)**
*Adult/Adolescent (16 y or older):*
**PO** 0.5 mg daily

**Chronic Hepatitis B (lamivudine- or telbivudine-resistant patients/ chronic hepatitis B with decompensated liver disease)**
*Adult/Adolescent (16 y or older):*
**PO** 1 mg daily

***Renal Impairment Dosage Adjustment***
*CrCl 30–49 mL/min:* Decrease dose by 50%; *10–29 mL/min:* Decrease dose by 70%; *less than 10 mL/min:* Decrease dose by 90%

## ADMINISTRATION
### Oral
- Give on an empty stomach (at least 2 h before/after a meal).
- Administer after hemodialysis.
- Store in a tightly closed container at 15°–30° C (59°–86° F).

**ADVERSE EFFECTS** (≥1%) **CNS:** Dizziness, fatigue, headache, insomnia, somnolence. **GI:** Diarrhea, dyspepsia, nausea, vomiting. **Metabolic:** Elevated liver enzymes (ALT, AST), hyperamylasemia, elevated lipase concentration, hyperbilirubinemia, fasting hyperglycemia, glycosuria, hematuria, lactic acidosis.

**INTERACTIONS Drug:** Use of entecavir with drugs that reduce renal function or compete for active tubular secretion may increase serum concentrations of either drug. **Food: *High fat*** meal reduces oral absorption.

## PHARMACOKINETICS **Peak:** 0.5–1 h. **Distribution:** 13% protein bound. **Metabolism:** Minimal. **Elimination:** Primarily in the urine. **Half-Life:** 128–149 h.

## NURSING IMPLICATIONS

### Black Box Warning

*Entecavir has been associated with severe, and potentially fatal, lactic acidosis and hepatomegaly.*

### Assessment & Drug Effects
- Monitor closely for adverse reactions when drugs that are known to affect renal function are taken concurrently.
- Monitor for S&S of lactic acidosis, including respiratory distress, tachycardia, and irregular HR.
- Monitor lab tests: Periodic LFTs during treatment and for several months after drug is discontinued; periodic fasting plasma glucose.

### Patient & Family Education
- Follow directions for taking the drug (see ADMINISTRATION).
- Do not discontinue medication without consent of prescriber.
- Do not drive or engage in potentially hazardous activities until response to drug is known.
- Inform prescriber if you are or plan to become pregnant.
- Report any of the following to a health care provider: Unexplained tiredness or weakness, unusual muscle pain, difficulty breathing, cold extremities, dizziness or lightheadedness, irregular heartbeat, loss of appetite, stomach pain, nausea, vomiting, clay-colored stool, dark urine, or jaundice.

# ENZALUTAMIDE
(en-za-loo'ta-mide)
Xtandi

**Classification:** ANTINEOPLASTIC; ANDROGEN RECEPTOR INHIBITOR; ANTIANDROGEN
**Therapeutic:** ANTINEOPLASTIC
**Prototype:** Flutamide

## AVAILABILITY Capsule

## ACTION & *THERAPEUTIC EFFECT*
Competitively inhibits androgen binding to androgen receptors and inhibits androgen receptor-mediated nuclear translocation and interaction with DNA. *Decreases proliferation and induces cell death of prostate cancer cells.*

## USES Metastatic castration-resistant prostate cancer in patients who have previously received docetaxel.

## CONTRAINDICATIONS Pregnancy (category X); lactation.

## CAUTIOUS USE History of seizures, TIA within 12 mo, or CVA; brain metastases; severe renal or hepatic impairment. Safety and efficacy in children younger than 18 y not established.

## ROUTE & DOSAGE

### Prostate Cancer
*Adult:* **PO** 160 mg once daily
*Grade 3 or Greater Toxicity:* Withhold drug for 1 wk or until symptoms improve to Grade 2 or better; resume at the same or a reduced dose
*Concomitant Therapy with a Strong CYP2C8 Inhibitor:* Decrease dose to 80 mg once daily

**E**

## ADMINISTRATION

### Oral
- Give without regard to food.
- Ensure that capsules are swallowed whole and not chewed or opened.
- Store at 15°–30° C (59°–86° F).

## ADVERSE EFFECTS (≥2%) **Body as a Whole:** *Asthenia, fatigue, peripheral edema.* **CNS:** Anxiety, dizziness, hallucinations, *headache,* hypesthesia, insomnia, mental impairment disorders, paresthesia, spinal cord compression, and cauda equina syndrome. **CV:** *Hot flush,* hypertension. **GI:** *Diarrhea.* **Hematological:** Neutropenia. **Metabolic:** Elevated ALT, elevated bilirubin. **Musculoskeletal:** *Arthralgia, back pain,* fall, *muscular weakness, musculoskeletal pain,* musculoskeletal stiffness, nonpathologic fractures. **Respiratory:** Epistaxis, lower respiratory tract and lung infection, *upper respiratory tract infection.* **Skin:** Dry skin, pruritus. **Urogenital:** Hematuria, pollakiuria.

## INTERACTIONS **Drug:** Strong inhibitors of CYP2C8 (e.g., **gemfibrozil**) or CYP3A4 (e.g., **itraconazole**) increase the levels of enzalutamide. Strong or moderate inducers of CYP2C8 (e.g., **rifampin**) or CYP3A4 (e.g., **carbamazepine, phenobarbital, phenytoin, rifabutin, rifampin, rifapentine, bosentan, efavirenz, etravirine, modafinil, nafcillin**) may decrease the levels of enzalutamide. Enzalutamide may decrease the levels of other drugs that require CYP2C9, CYP2C19, or CYP3A4 for metabolism; therefore drugs with narrow therapeutic indexes that require these isoforms for metabolism (e.g., **alfentanil, cyclosporine, dihydroergotamine,**

**ergotamine, fentanyl, phenytoin, pimozide, quinidine, sirolimus, tacrolimus, warfarin**) should not be used in combination with enzalutamide. **Food: Grapefruit** or **grapefruit juice** may increase the levels of enzalutamide. **Herbal: St. John's wort** may decrease the levels of enzalutamide.

## PHARMACOKINETICS **Peak:** 1 h. **Distribution:** 97–98% plasma protein bound. **Metabolism:** In liver. **Elimination:** Renal (71%) and fecal (14%). **Half-Life:** 5.8 days.

## NURSING IMPLICATIONS

### Assessment & Drug Effects
- Monitor ambulation as drug may cause dizziness and predisposition to falls.
- Monitor cognitive status and report signs of mental impairment.
- Monitor lab tests: Baseline and periodic CBC with differential and LFTs.

### Patient & Family Education
- Take drug at the same time each day.
- Exercise caution with potentially dangerous activities until response to drug is known.
- Use a condom and another effective method of birth control during and for 3 mo after treatment if having sex with a woman of childbearing potential.

## EPHEDRINE SULFATE
(e-fed′rin sul-fate)

**Classifications:** ALPHA- AND BETA-ADRENERGIC AGONIST; BRONCHODILATOR
**Therapeutic:** BRONCHODILATOR
**Prototype:** Epinephrine HCl

## AVAILABILITY Capsule; solution for injection

## ACTION & *THERAPEUTIC EFFECT*

Both indirect- and direct-acting sympathomimetic amine thought to act indirectly by releasing tissue stores of norepinephrine and directly by stimulation of alpha-, beta$_1$-, and beta$_2$-adrenergic receptors. Like epinephrine, contracts dilated arterioles of nasal mucosa, thus reducing engorgement and edema and facilitating ventilation and drainage. *Ephedrine relaxes bronchial smooth muscle, relieving mild bronchospasm, improving air exchange and increasing vital capacity.*

## USES

In treatment of mild cases of acute asthma and in patients with chronic asthma requiring continuing treatment and for temporary support of ventricular rate in Adams-Stokes syndrome.

## CONTRAINDICATIONS

History of hypersensitivity to ephedrine or other sympathomimetics; narrow-angle glaucoma; angina pectoris, coronary insufficiency, chronic heart disease, uncontrolled hypertension, cardiac arrhythmias, cardiomyopathy; hypovolemia; concurrent MAOI therapy; lactation.

## CAUTIOUS USE

Hypertension, arteriosclerosis, closed-angle glaucoma; diabetes mellitus; hyperthyroidism; prostatic hypertrophy; renal impairment; unstable vasomotor symptoms; pregnancy (category C).

## ROUTE & DOSAGE

### Bronchodilator, Nasal Decongestant

*Adult:* **PO** 25–50 mg q3–4h prn (max: 150 mg/24 h); **IM/IV/Subcutaneous** 12.5–25 mg

*Child (2 y or older):* **PO** 2–3 mg/kg/day in 4–6 divided doses

### Hypotension

*Adult:* **IM/Subcutaneous/IV** 5–25 mg slow IV, may repeat in 5–10 min if necessary (max: 150 mg/24 h)
*Child:* **IM/Subcutaneous** 0.5 mg/kg or 16.7 mg/m$^2$ q4–6h

### Narcolepsy

*Adult:* **PO** 25–50 mg q3–4h

### Enuresis

*Adult:* **PO** 25 mg at bedtime

## ADMINISTRATION

### Oral

- Administer last dose a few hours before bedtime, if possible, to minimize insomnia.
- Store at 15°–30° C (59°–86° F) in tightly closed, light-resistant containers unless otherwise directed by the manufacturer.

### Subcutaneous/Intramuscular

- Give undiluted.

### Intravenous

**PREPARE: Direct:** Dilute in 5 or 10 mg/mL with D5W or NS.
**ADMINISTER: Direct:** Direct IV at a rate of 10 mg or fraction thereof over 30–60 sec.
**INCOMPATIBILITIES: Solution/additive: Hydrocortisone, pentobarbital, phenobarbital, secobarbital. Y-site: Amphotericin B liposome, azathioprine, caspofungin, dantrolene, diazepam, diazoxide, ganciclovir, garenoxacin mesylate, pantoprazole, pentamidine, phenytoin sodium, SMZ/TMP, thiopental sodium.**

---

**E**

- Store in tightly closed, light-resistant containers. Do not use liquid formulation unless it is absolutely clear.

## ADVERSE EFFECTS (≥1%) CNS:
Headache, insomnia, *nervousness,* anxiety, tremulousness, confusion, hallucination, delerium, insomnia giddiness. **CV:** Palpitation, bradycardia, cardiac arrhythmia, hypertension tachycardia. **Urogenital: GU:** Difficult or painful urination, acute urinary retention (especially older men with prostatism). **GI:** Nausea, vomiting, anorexia. **Respiratory:** Dyspnea. **Body as a Whole:** Sweating, thirst, overdosage: Euphoria, confusion, delirium, convulsions, pyrexia, hypertension, rebound hypotension, respiratory difficulty. **Skin:** Fixed-drug eruption. **Topical Use:** *Burning, stinging,* dryness of nasal mucosa, sneezing, rebound congestion.

## DIAGNOSTIC TEST INTERFERENCE
Ephedrine is generally withdrawn at least 12 h before *sensitivity tests* are made to prevent false-positive reactions.

## INTERACTIONS Drug: MAO IN-HIBITORS, TRICYCLIC ANTIDEPRESSANTS, **furazolidone, guanethidine** may increase alpha-adrenergic effects (headache, hyperpyrexia, hypertension); **sodium bicarbonate** decreases renal elimination of ephedrine, increasing its CNS effects; **epinephrine, norepinephrine** compound sympathomimetic effects; effects of ALPHA and BETA-BLOCKERS and ephedrine antagonized.

## PHARMACOKINETICS Absorption:
Readily absorbed from GI tract. **Peak:** 15 min–1 h. **Duration:** Bronchodilation 2–4 h; cardiac and pressor effects up to 4 h PO and 1 h IV. **Distribution:** Widely distributed; crosses blood–brain barrier and placenta; distributed into breast milk. **Metabolism:** Small amounts metabolized in liver. **Elimination:** In urine. **Half-Life:** 3–6 h.

## NURSING IMPLICATIONS
### Assessment & Drug Effects
- Supervise continuously patients receiving ephedrine IV. Take baseline BP and other vital signs. Check BP repeatedly during first 5 min, then q3–5min until stabilized.
- Monitor I&O ratio and pattern, especially in older male patients. Encourage patient to void before taking medication (see ADVERSE EFFECTS).

### Patient & Family Education
- Note: Ephedrine is a commonly abused drug. Learn adverse effects and dangers; take medication ONLY as prescribed.
- Do not take OTC medications for coughs, colds, allergies, or asthma unless approved by prescriber. Ephedrine is a common ingredient in these preparations.

## EPINASTINE HYDROCHLORIDE
(e-pi-nas'teen)
Elestat
**See Appendix A-1.**

## EPINEPHRINE 🅟
(ep-i-ne'frin)
Akovaz, Corphedra,
Epinephrine Pediatric,
EpiPen Auto-Injector,
Symjepi

## EPINEPHRINE BITARTRATE
AsthmaHaler, Bronkaid Mist
Suspension, Bronitin Mist
Suspension, Epitrate

Common adverse effects in *italic;* life-threatening effects <u>underlined;</u> generic names in **bold;** classifications in SMALL CAPS; ♣ Canadian drug name; 🅟 Prototype drug

E

# EPINEPHRINE HYDROCHLORIDE

Adrenalin Chloride, Bronkaid Mistometer, Dysne-Inhal, Epifrin, SusPhrine ♣

# EPINEPHRINE, RACEMIC

Vaponefrin ♣

**Classifications:** ALPHA- AND BETA-ADRENERGIC AGONIST; CARDIAC STIMULANT; VASOPRESSOR
Therapeutic: ANTI-ANAPHYLACTIC; VASOPRESSOR

**AVAILABILITY** Solution for inhalation; spray; suspension; nasal solution

**ACTION & *THERAPEUTIC EFFECT***
A catecholamine that acts directly on both alpha and beta receptors; it is the most potent activator of alpha receptors. Strengthens myocardial contraction; increases systolic but may decrease diastolic blood pressure; increases cardiac rate and cardiac output. Constricts bronchial arterioles and inhibits histamine release, thus reducing congestion and edema and increasing tidal volume and vital capacity. Relaxes uterine smooth musculature and inhibits uterine contractions. *Reverses anaphylatic reactions and provides temporary relief from acute asthmatic attack. Restores normal cardiac rhythm.*

**USES** Temporary relief of bronchospasm, acute asthmatic attack, hypotension during anesthesia, hypersensitivity and anaphylactic reactions, syncope due to heart block or carotid sinus hypersensitivity, and to restore cardiac rhythm in cardiac arrest.

**CONTRAINDICATIONS** There are no absolute contraindications to the use of injectable epinephrine in a life-threatening situation. Hypersensitivity to sympathomimetic amines; narrow-angle glaucoma; hemorrhagic, traumatic, or cardiogenic shock; cardiac dilatation, cerebral arteriosclerosis, coronary insufficiency, arrhythmias, organic heart or brain disease; during second stage of labor; for local anesthesia of fingers, toes, ears, nose, genitalia.

**CAUTIOUS USE** Older adults or debilitated patients; prostatic hypertrophy; hypertension; diabetes mellitus; hyperthyroidism; Parkinson's disease; tuberculosis; psychoneurosis; in patients with long-standing bronchial asthma and emphysema with degenerative heart disease; pregnancy (category C); lactation.

## ROUTE & DOSAGE

### Anaphylaxis

*Adult:* **Subcutaneous** 0.1–0.5 mg q10–15min prn; **IV** 0.1–0.25 mg q5–15min
*Child:* **Subcutaneous** 0.01 mL/kg of, 1:1000 q10–15min prn; **IV** 0.01 mL/kg of 1:1000 q10–15min
*Neonate:* **IV Intratracheal** 0.01–0.05 mg/kg q3–5min prn

### Cardiac Arrest

*Adult:* **IV** 1 mg q3–5min as needed; **Intracardiac** 0.1–1 mg
*Child:* **IV** 0.01 mg/kg q3–5min as needed; (max: 1 mg); **Intracardiac** 0.05–0.1 mg/kg

### Asthma

*Adult:* **Subcutaneous** 0.1–0.5 mg q20min–4h; **Inhalation** 1 inhalation q4h prn

---

Common adverse effects in *italic*; life-threatening effects <u>underlined</u>; generic names in **bold**; classifications in SMALL CAPS; ♣Canadian drug name; ⊕ Prototype drug

*Child:* **Subcutaneous** 0.01 mL/kg of 1:1000 q20min–4h; **Inhalation** 1 inhalation q4h prn

**Hypotension During Anesthesia**

*Adult:* **IV** 5-25 mg, may repeat in 5-10 min (max: 50 mg); **IM/ Subcutaneous** 10-50 mg, may repeat if needed

**Nasal Hemostasis**

*Adult/Child:* **Instillation** 1–2 drops 0.1% ophthalmic or 0.1% nasal solution

**Topical Hemostatic**

*Adult/Child:* **Topical** 1:50,000–1:1000 applied topically or 1:500,000–1:50,000 mixed with a local anesthetic

## ADMINISTRATION

### Inhalation

- Have patient in an upright position when aerosol preparation is used. The reclining position can result in overdosage by producing large droplets instead of fine spray.
- Instruct patient to rinse mouth and throat with water immediately after inhalation to avoid swallowing residual drug (may cause epigastric pain and systemic effects from the propellant in the aerosol preparation) and to prevent dryness of oropharyngeal membranes.

### Instillation (Nasal)

- Instill nose drops with head in lateral, head-low position to prevent entry of drug into throat.
- Instruct patient to rinse nose dropper or spray tip with hot water after each use to prevent contamination of solution with nasal secretions.

### Instillation (Ocular)

- Remove soft contact lenses before instilling eye drops.
- Instruct patient to apply gentle finger pressure against nasolacrimal duct immediately after drug is instilled for at least 1 or 2 min following instillation to prevent excessive systemic absorption.

### Subcutaneous

- Use tuberculin syringe to ensure greater accuracy in measurement of parenteral doses.
- Protect epinephrine injection from exposure to light at all times. Do not remove ampule or vial from carton until ready to use.
- Shake vial or ampule thoroughly to disperse particles before withdrawing epinephrine suspension into syringe; then inject promptly.
- Aspirate carefully before injecting epinephrine. Inadvertent IV injection of usual subcutaneous doses can result in sudden hypertension and possibly cerebral hemorrhage.
- Rotate injection sites and observe for signs of blanching. Vascular constriction from repeated injections may cause tissue necrosis.

### Intravenous

Note: Verify correct rate of IV injection to neonates, infants, children with prescriber.

Note: 1:1000 solution contains 1 mg/1 mL. 1:10,000 solution contains 0.1 mg/1 mL.

***PREPARE:* Direct:** Dilute each 1 mg of 1:1000 solution with 10 mL of NS to yield 1:10,000 solution. • The 1:10,000 solution may be given undiluted. **IV Infusion:** Dilute required dose in 250–500 mL of D5W.

***ADMINISTER:* Direct:** Give each 1 mg over 1 min or longer; may give more rapidly in cardiac ar-

E

rest. **IV Infusion:** 1–10 mcg/min titrated according to patient's condition.

*INCOMPATIBILITIES:* Solution/additive: **Aminophylline, cephapirin, hyaluronidase, me-phentermine, sodium bicar-bonate, warfarin.** Y-site: **Acyclovir, alemtuzumab, amphotericin B, ampicillin, azathioprine sodium, carmustine, dacarbazine, dantrolene sodium, diazepam, diazoxide, fluorouracil, fosfomycin sodium, ganciclovir sodium, gemtuzumab ozogamicin, indomethacin sodium trihydrate, micafungin sodium, pentobarbitol sodium, phenobarbitol sodium, phenytoin sodium, sodium bicaronate sulfamethoxazole-trimethoprim, thiopental sodium.** ▪ If extravasation occurs, stop infusion immediately and disconnect (leave cannula/needle in place); gently aspirate extravasated solution (**Do not** flush the line); remove needle/cannula; elevate extremity. Initiate antidote and apply dry warm compresses.

## ADVERSE EFFECTS (≥1%) Special Senses: *Nasal burning or stinging,* dryness of nasal mucosa, sneezing, rebound congestion. *Transient stinging or burning of eyes,* lacrimation, brow ache, headache, rebound conjunctival hyperemia, allergy, iritis; with prolonged use: Melanin-like deposits on lids, conjunctiva, and cornea; corneal edema; loss of lashes (reversible); maculopathy with central scotoma in aphakic patients (reversible). **Body as a Whole:** *Nervousness,* restlessness, sleeplessness, fear, anxiety, *tremors,* severe headache, cerebrovascular accident, weakness, dizziness, syncope, pallor, sweating, dyspnea. **GI:** Nausea, vomiting. **CV:** Precordial pain, *palpitations,* hypertension, <u>MI</u>, tachy-arrhythmias including <u>ventricular fibrillation</u>. **Respiratory:** Bronchial and <u>pulmonary edema</u>. **Urogenital:** Urinary retention. **Skin:** Tissue necrosis with repeated injections. **Metabolic:** Metabolic acidoses, elevated serum lactic acid, transient elevations of blood glucose, hypoglycemia, hypokalemia. **CNS:** Altered state of perception and thought, psychosis.

## INTERACTIONS Drug: May increase hypotension in circulatory collapse or hypotension caused by PHENOTHIAZINES, **oxytocin, entacapone.** Additive toxicities with other SYMPATHOMIMETICS **(albuterol, dobutamine, dopamine, isoproterenol, metaproterenol, norepinephrine, phenylephrine, phenylpropanolamine, pseudoephedrine, ritodrine, salmeterol, terbutaline),** MAO INHIBITORS, TRYCYCLIC ANTIDEPRESSANTS, ALPHA- AND BETA-ADRENERGIC BLOCKING AGENTS (e.g., **ergotamine, propranolol**) antagonize effects of epinephrine. GENERAL ANESTHETICS increase cardiac irritability.

## PHARMACOKINETICS Absorption: Inactivated in GI tract. **Onset:** 3–5 min, 1 h on conjunctiva. **Peak:** 20 min, 4–8 h on conjunctiva. **Duration:** 12–24 h topically. **Distribution:** Widely distributed; does not cross blood–brain barrier; crosses placenta. **Metabolism:** In tissue and liver by monoamine oxidase (MAO) and catecholamine-methyltransferase (COMT). **Elimination:** Small amount unchanged in urine; excreted in breast milk.

## NURSING IMPLICATIONS

### Assessment & Drug Effects

- Check BP repeatedly when epinephrine is administered IV during first 5 min, then q3–5min until stabilized.
- Monitor BP, pulse, respirations, and urinary output and observe patient closely following IV administration. Continuous cardiac monitoring is recommended during IV infusion. If disturbances in cardiac rhythm occur, withhold epinephrine and notify prescriber immediately.
- Keep prescriber informed of any changes in intake-output ratio.
- Advise patient to report bronchial irritation, nervousness, or sleeplessness. Dosage should be reduced.
- Monitor blood glucose and HbA1C for loss of glycemic control if diabetic.

### Patient & Family Education

- Report to prescriber if symptoms of asthma are not relieved in 20 min or if they become worse following inhalation.
- Be aware intranasal application may sting slightly.
- Administer ophthalmic drug at bedtime or following prescribed miotic to minimize mydriasis, with blurred vision and sensitivity to light (possible in some patients being treated for glaucoma).
- Transitory stinging may follow initial ophthalmic administration and that headache and browache occur frequently at first but usually subside with continued use. Notify prescriber if symptoms persist.
- Discontinue epinephrine eye drops and consult a prescriber if signs of hypersensitivity develop (edema of lids, itching, discharge, crusting eyelids).
- Learn how to administer epinephrine subcutaneously. Keep medication and equipment available for home emergency. Confer with prescriber.
- Advise patient to report bronchial irritation, nervousness, or sleeplessness. Dosage should be reduced.
- Report tolerance to prescriber; may occur with repeated or prolonged use. Continued use of epinephrine in the presence of tolerance can be dangerous.
- Take medication only as prescribed and immediately notify prescriber of onset of systemic effects of epinephrine.
- Discard discolored or precipitated solutions.

## EPIRUBICIN HYDROCHLORIDE
(e-pi-roo′bi-sin)
Ellence
**Classifications:** ANTINEOPLASTIC; ANTRACYCLINE; (ANTIBIOTIC)
Therapeutic: ANTINEOPLASTIC
**Prototype:** Doxorubicin HCl

**AVAILABILITY** Intravenous solution

**ACTION & THERAPEUTIC EFFECT**
Cytotoxic antibiotic with wide spectrum of antitumor activity and strong immunosuppressive properties. Complexes with DNA causing the DNA helix to change shape, thus blocking effective DNA and RNA transcription. *Highly destructive to rapidly proliferating cells. Effectiveness indicated by tumor regression.*

**USES** Adjunctive therapy for axillary node-positive breast cancer.

**CONTRAINDICATIONS** Hypersensitivity to epirubicin and other related drugs; marked myelosuppression with neutrophil count less than 1500 cells/mm$^3$;

severely impaired cardiac function, cardiomyopathy; severe cardiac arrhythmias, recent MI; severe hepatic disease, jaundice; previous treatment with maximum doses of epirubicin, doxorubicin, or daunorubicin; pregnancy (category D); lactation.

**CAUTIOUS USE** Arrhythmias, CHF; mild or moderate liver dysfunction; severe renal insufficiency or renal failure; females 70 y and older.

## ROUTE & DOSAGE

### Breast Cancer

*Adult:* **IV** 100–120 mg/m² infused on day 1 of a 3–4 wk cycle or 50–60 mg/m² on day 1 and 8 of a 3–4 wk cycle (max cumulative dose: 900 mg/m²)

### Hepatic Impairment Dosage Adjustment

*Bilirubin 1.2–3 mg/dL:* Give 50% of dose; *bilirubin over 3 mg/dL:* Give 25% of dose; *bilirubin greater than 5 mg/dL:* Skip dose

### Toxicity Dosage Adjustment

Reduce dose by 25% if platelets less than 50,000/mm³, ANC less than 250/mm³, neutropenic fever, or grade 3 or 4 hematologic toxicity

## ADMINISTRATION

### Intravenous

Note: Pregnant women **should not** prepare or administer this drug. Wear protective goggles, gowns and disposable gloves and masks when handling this drug. **Discard all** equipment used in preparation of this drug in high-risk, waste-disposal bags for incineration. Treat accidental contact with skin or eyes by rinsing with copious amounts of water followed by prompt medical attention.

*PREPARE:* **IV Infusion:** Epirubicin is manufactured as a preservative-free ready-to-use solution. The contents of a vial **must be** used within 24 h of first penetrating the rubber stopper. Discard unused solution.

*ADMINISTER:* **IV Infusion:** Measure ordered dose and inject into a port of a freely flowing IV solution of D5W or NS over 3–20 min. ▪ **Do not** give by direct IV push into a vein. ▪ Avoid IV sites that enter small veins or repeated injections into the same vein. ▪ Monitor IV site closely for S&S of extravasation and if suspected, notify prescriber immediately.

*INCOMPATIBILITIES:* Solution/additive: ALKALINE SOLUTIONS (including **sodium bicarbonate**), **fluorouracil, heparin.** Y-site: **Acyclovir, allopurinol, aminophylline, amphotericine B, ampicillin, azithromycin, cefepime, cefoperazone, cefotetan, cefoxitin, ceftazidime, ceftriaxone, cefuroxime, dexmethasone, diazepam, ertapenem, fluorouracil, foscarnet, fosphenytoin, furosemide, gallium, ganciclovir, gemtuzumab, heparin, hydrocortisone, ketorolac, leucovorin, magnesium, meropenem, methohexital, methylprenisolone, nafcillin, pantoprazole, pemetrexed, pentobarbital, phenobarbital, phenytoin, piperacillin, potassium, sodium bicarbonate, sulfamethoxazole/trimethoprim, thopental, ticarcillin, tigecycline.**

▪ Store at 2°–8° C (36°–46° F). Protect from light.

---

Common adverse effects in *italic;* life-threatening effects underlined; generic names in **bold;** classifications in SMALL CAPS; ✦ Canadian drug name; ⊙ Prototype drug

599

E

## ADVERSE EFFECTS (≥1%) Body as a Whole: *Lethargy,* fever. CV: Asymptomatic decrease in LVEF, CHF. GI: *Nausea, vomiting, mucositis, diarrhea,* anorexia. Hematologic: Leukopenia, neutropenia, anemia, thrombocytopenia, AML. Skin: *Alopecia, injection site reaction,* rash, itching, skin changes. Other: *Amenorrhea, hot flashes, infection, conjunctivitis/keratitis,* secondary acute myelogenous leukemia (related to cumulative dose).

## INTERACTIONS Drug: Cimetidine increases epirubicin levels; concomitant use with cardioactive drugs (e.g., CALCIUM CHANNEL BLOCKERS) may affect cardiac function.

## PHARMACOKINETICS Distribution: Widely distributed, 77% protein bound, concentrated in red blood cells. Metabolism: Extensively in liver, blood and other organs. Clearance is reduced in patients with hepatic impairment. Elimination: Primarily in bile, some urinary excretion; clearance decreases in older adult female patients. Half-Life: 33 h.

## NURSING IMPLICATIONS

### Black Box Warning

*Epiruibicin extravasation can cause severe local tissue necrosis. Epirubicin has been associated with cardiac toxicity (including fatal CHF during or long after termination of therapy), hepatic impairment, myelosuppression, and secondary AML.*

### Assessment & Drug Effects

- Withhold drug and notify prescriber of any of the following: Neutrophil count less than 1500 cells/mm$^3$, recent MI, suspicion of severe myocardial insufficiency.
- Obtain baseline and periodic (before each cycle of therapy) cardiac evaluation: Left ventricular ejection fraction, ECG and ECHO (tests are recommended especially in the presence of risk factors of cardiac toxicity).
- Monitor cardiac status closely throughout therapy as the risk of developing severe CHF increases rapidly when cumulative doses approach 900 mg/m$^2$. Report significant ECG changes immediately. Report immediately S&S of the following: Tachycardia, gallop rhythm, pleural effusion, pulmonary edema, dependent edema, ascites, or hepatomegaly.
- Monitor lab tests: Baseline and before each cycle of therapy CBC with differential and platelet count, serum eletrolytes, LFTs, and serum creatinine.

### Patient & Family Education

- Review all literature regarding the adverse effects of epirubicin therapy carefully.
- Report any of the following to prescriber immediately: Pain at the site of IV infusion, chest pain, palpitations, shortness of breath or difficulty breathing, sudden weight gain, swelling of hands, feet or legs, or any unexplained bleeding.
- Be aware that your urine may turn red for 1–2 days after receiving this drug. This change is expected and harmless.
- Do not take OTC cimetidine or any other OTC drug without consulting prescriber.
- Use effective means of contraception (both men and women) while on epirubicin therapy.

Common adverse effects in *italic;* life-threatening effects underlined; generic names in **bold;** classifications in SMALL CAPS; ✦ Canadian drug name; ⊘ Prototype drug

# EPLERENONE

(e-ple're-none)

Inspra

**Classifications:** ELECTROLYE & WATER BALANCE AGENT; SELECTIVE ALDOSTERONE RECEPTOR ANTAGONIST (SARA); ANTIHYPERTENSIVE
Therapeutic: ANTIHYPERTENSIVE; DIURETIC; SARA
**Prototype:** Spironolactone

## AVAILABILITY Tablet

## ACTION & *THERAPEUTIC EFFECT*

Binds to mineralocorticoid receptors and blocks the binding of aldosterone, a component of the renin angiotensin-aldosterone system (RAAS). Thus, eplerenone blocks the primary effect of aldosterone which is sodium reabsorption. *Lowers blood pressure by inhibiting sodium and water retention, thus reducing total plasma volume.*

**USES** Treatment of hypertension. Adjunctive therapy for post MI heart failure.

**CONTRAINDICATIONS** Serum potassium greater than 5.5 mEq/L; type 2 diabetes with microalbuminuria; serum creatinine greater than 2 mg/dL in males or greater than 1.8 mg/dL in females; CrCl less than 30 mL/min; type II diabetics do not use if CrCl is less than 50 mL/min; severe hepatic impairment; lactation.

**CAUTIOUS USE** Hepatic impairment; hepatic disease; diabetics with CHF post MI; CHF; renal impairment; older adults; pregnancy (category B). Safety and efficacy in children, infants, or neonates not established.

## ROUTE & DOSAGE

### Hypertension

*Adult:* **PO** 50 mg once daily, may be increased to 50 mg b.i.d., if inadequate response after 4 wk

### Heart Failure/Post MI

*Adult:* **PO** 25 mg then titrate to 50 mg daily

#### Renal Impairment Dosage Adjustment

*CrCl less than 50 mL/min (hypertension patient):* Do not administer
*CrCl less than 30 mL/min (heart failure patients):* Do not administer

## ADMINISTRATION

Oral
- Do not administer in combination with potassium supplements or potassium-sparing diuretics.
- Manufacturer recommends dosage reduction to 25 mg once daily with concurrent administration of erythromycin, saquinavir, verapamil, or fluconazole.
- Store at 15°–30° C (59°–86° F).

**ADVERSE EFFECTS** (≥1%) **Body as a Whole:** Fatigue, flu-like syndrome. **CNS:** Headache, dizziness. **CV:** Angina, MI. **GI:** Diarrhea, abdominal pain. **Endocrine:** Gynecomastia. **Metabolic:** *Hyperkalemia,* increased GGT, hypercholesterolemia, hypertriglyceridemia, decreased sodium levels. **Respiratory:** Cough. **Urogenital:** Albuminuria, abnormal vaginal bleeding.

**INTERACTIONS Drug:** ACE INHIBITORS, ANGIOTENSIN II RECEPTOR BLOCKERS, AZOLE ANTIFUNGALS (e.g., **fluconazole,**

**E**

itraconazole, ketoconazole), **erythromycin, saquinavir, verapamil, spironolactone** may increase risk of hyperkalemia. **Food: Potassium-**containing SALT SUBSTITUTES may increase risk of hyperkalemia.

## PHARMACOKINETICS
**Absorption:** Rapidly absorbed. **Peak:** 1.5 h. **Distribution:** 50% protein bound, primarily to alpha$_1$-acid glycoproteins. **Metabolism:** In liver by CYP3A4. **Elimination:** 32% in feces, 67% in urine. **Half-Life:** 4–6 h.

## NURSING IMPLICATIONS

### Assessment & Drug Effects

- Monitor cardiovascular status with frequent BP determinations. Note that BP lowering usually occurs within 2 wk with maximal antihypertensive effects achieved within 4 wk.
- Concurrent drugs: Monitor serum potassium levels more frequently when patient also receiving an ACE inhibitor or an angiotensin II receptor antagonist. Monitor frequently for lithium toxicity with concurrent use.
- Withhold drug and notify prescriber for any of the following: Serum potassium greater than 5.5 mEq/L, serum creatinine greater than 2 mg/dL in males or greater than 1.8 mg/dL in females, creatinine clearance less than 50 mL/min, microalbuminuria in type 2 diabetics.
- Monitor lab tests: Baseline serum potassium, repeat within the 1st wk, again at 1 mo or after dosage adjustment, then periodically thereafter.

### Patient & Family Education

- Do not use potassium supplements, salt substitutes containing potassium, or contraindicated drugs (e.g., ketoconazole, itraconazole) without consulting prescriber.
- Do not use OTC nonsteroidal anti-inflammatory drugs without consulting prescriber.
- Do not drive or operate machinery until reaction to drug is known. It may cause dizziness.

## EPOETIN ALFA (HUMAN RECOMBINANT ERYTHROPOIETIN) ◉

(e-po-e-tin)

**Epogen, Eprex ♦, Procrit**

**Classification:** HEMATOPOIETIC GROWTH FACTOR

**Therapeutic:** ANTIANEMIC; HUMAN ERYTHROPOIETIN

**AVAILABILITY** Solution for injection

## ACTION & *THERAPEUTIC EFFECT*

Human erythropoietin is produced in the kidney and stimulates bone marrow production of RBCs (erythropoiesis). Hypoxia and anemia generally increase the production of erythropoietin. Epoetin alpha stimulates RBC production. *Stimulates the production of RBCs in the bone marrow of severely anemic patients.*

**USES** Treatment of anemia.

## CONTRAINDICATIONS
Uncontrolled hypertension and known hypersensitivity to mammalian cell–derived products and albumin (human); hamster protein hypersensitivity; iron-deficiency anemia; pure red cell aplasia associated with erythropoietin protein drugs.

## CAUTIOUS USE
Leukemia, sickle cell disease; coagulopathy; seizure disorders; pregnancy (category C); lactation; infants; neonates.

---

Common adverse effects in *italic;* life-threatening effects <u>underlined</u>; generic names in **bold;** classifications in SMALL CAPS; ♦ Canadian drug name; ◉ Prototype drug

## ROUTE & DOSAGE

### Anemia of CKD

*Adult:* **Subcutaneous/IV** Start with 50–100 units/kg/dose until target Hct range of 30–33% (max: 36%) is reached; if Hgb increases more than 1 g/dL and approaches 12 g/dL, reduce dose by 25%. If after 4 wk there is less than 1 g/dL, increase dose by 25%.
*Child/Infant:* **IV/Subcutaneous** 50 units/kg 3 × wk (adjust as above)

### Anemia Related to Chemotherapy

*Adult:* **Subcutaneous** 150 units/kg 3 × wk or 40,000 units once/wk when Hgb below 10 g/dL
*Adolescent/Child (older than 5 y):* **IV** 600 units/kg/wk when Hgb below 10 g/dL

## ADMINISTRATION

### Subcutaneous
- Do not shake solution. Shaking may denature the glycoprotein, rendering it biologically inactive.
- Inspect solution for particulate matter prior to use. Do not use if solution is discolored or if it contains particulate matter.
- Use only one dose/vial, and do not reenter vial.
- Do not give with any other drug solution.

### Intravenous

*PREPARE:* **Direct:** Give undiluted.
*ADMINISTER:* **Direct:** Give direct IV as a bolus dose over 1 min.
*INCOMPATIBILITIES:* **Solution/additive:** D10W, normal saline.
- Discard any unused portion of the vial. It contains no preservatives.

- Store at 2°–8° C (36°–46° F). Do not freeze or shake.

## ADVERSE EFFECTS (≥1%) CNS:
Seizures, *headache.* **CV:** *Hypertension.* **GI:** Nausea, diarrhea. **Hematologic:** *Iron deficiency,* thrombocytosis, pure red cell aplasia, *clotting of AV fistula.* **Other:** Sweating, bone pain, arthralgias.

## INTERACTIONS Drug: Do not give concurrently with **darbepoetin alfa.**

## PHARMACOKINETICS Onset:
7–14 days. **Metabolism:** In serum. **Elimination:** Minimal recovery in urine. **Half-Life:** 4–13 h.

## NURSING IMPLICATIONS

### Black Box Warning

*Epoetin Alfa has been associated with increased risk of death, MI, stroke, venous thrombosis, vascular access thrombosis, and tumor progression.*

### Assessment & Drug Effects
- Control BP adequately prior to initiation of therapy and closely monitor and control during therapy. Hypertension is an adverse effect that **must be** controlled.
- Be aware that BP may rise during early therapy as Hct increases. Notify prescriber of a rapid rise in Hct (more than 4 points in 2 wk). Dosage will need to be reduced because of risk of serious hypertension.
- Monitor for hypertensive encephalopathy in patients with CRF during period of increasing Hct.
- Monitor for premonitory neurologic symptoms (i.e., aura) and report their appearance

**E**

promptly). The potential for seizures exists during periods of rapid Hct increase (more than 4 points in 2 wk).

- Monitor closely for thrombotic events (e.g., MI, CVA, TIA), especially for patients with CRF.
- Monitor lab tests: Baseline transferrin and serum ferritin; Hgb at least weekly; periodic CBC with differential and platelet count, BUN, creatinine, and serum electrolytes.

### Patient & Family Education

- Important for those with CDK to comply with antihypertensive medication and dietary restrictions.
- Do not drive or engage in other potentially hazardous activity during the first 90 days of therapy because of possible seizure activity.
- Understand that headache is a common adverse effect. Report if severe or persistent, may indicate developing hypertension.

## EPOPROSTENOL SODIUM ⓟ

(e-po-pros'te-nol)

Flolan

**Classifications:** PROSTAGLANDIN; PULMONARY ANTIHYPERTENSIVE

Therapeutic: PULMONARY ANTIHYPERTENSIVE

**AVAILABILITY** Powder for injection

## ACTION & *THERAPEUTIC EFFECT*

Naturally occurring prostaglandin that reduces right and left ventricular afterload, increases cardiac output, and increases stroke volume through its vasodilation effect. Potent pulmonary vasodilator that reduces pulmonary hypertension. *Potent vasodilator of pulmonary and systemic arterial vascular beds and an inhibitor of platelet aggregation.*

**USES** Long-term treatment of primary pulmonary hypertension in NYHA Class III and IV patients.

**CONTRAINDICATIONS** Hypersensitivity to **epoprostenol** or related compounds; chronic use with left ventricular systolic dysfunction in CHF patients; long-term use in patients who develop pulmonary edema during dose initiation; lactation.

**CAUTIOUS USE** Patients with risk factors for bleeding; older adults, pregnancy (category B). Safety and efficacy in children not established.

## ROUTE & DOSAGE

### Primary Pulmonary Hypertension

*Adult (acute dose):* **IV** Initiate with 2 ng/kg/min, increase by 2 ng/kg/min q15min until dose-limiting effects occur (e.g., nausea, vomiting, headache, hypotension, flushing); **Chronic administration** Start infusion at 4 ng/kg/min less than the maximum tolerated infusion; if maximum tolerated infusion is 5 ng/kg/min or less, start *maintenance infusion* at 50% of maximum tolerated dose

### Intravenous

***PREPARE:*** **Continuous** Note: **Must be** reconstituted using sterile diluent for epoprostenol; must not be mixed with any other medications or solution prior to or during administration. • To make 100 mL of 3000 ng/mL, add 5 mL of the supplied diluent to one 0.5 mg vial; withdraw 3 mL and add to enough diluent to make a total of 100 mL. ▪ To make 100 mL of 5000 ng/mL, add 5 mL of diluent to one 0.5 mg vial; withdraw contents of vial and add to enough diluent to make a total of 100 mL. ▪ To make 100 mL of 10,000 ng/mL, add 5 mL of diluent to each of two 0.5 mg vials; withdraw contents of each vial and add to enough diluent to make a total of 100 mL. ▪ To make 100 mL of 15,000 ng/mL, add 5 mL of diluent to a 1.5 mg vial; withdraw contents of vial and add to enough diluent to make a total of 100 mL.

*ADMINISTER:* **Continuous:** Give at ordered rate using an infusion control device. Avoid abrupt infusion interruption or large dosage reduction.

*INCOMPATIBILITIES:* **Solution/additive:** Do not mix or infuse with any other parenteral drugs or solutions prior to or during administration.

▪ Store unopened vials at 15°–25° C (59°–77° F). Protect from light. ▪ See manufacturer's directions for stability or storage of reconstituted solutions.

## ADVERSE EFFECTS (≥1%) CNS:
*Chills, fever, flu-like syndrome, dizziness,* syncope, *headache, anxiety/nervousness,* agitation, hyperesthesia, paresthesia, dizziness. **CV:** *Tachycardia, hypotension, flushing, chest pain,* bradycardia. **GI:** *Diarrhea, nausea, vomiting, anorexia,* abdominal pain. **Musculoskeletal:** *Jaw pain, myalgia, nonspecific musculoskeletal pain.* **Respiratory:** Dyspnea. **Dermatologic:** Dermal ulcer, eczema, skin rash, urticaria. **Other:** Dose-limiting effects.

## INTERACTIONS Drug: Hypotension if administered with other VASODILATORS or ANTIHYPERTENSIVES.

## PHARMACOKINETICS Peak: Approximately 15 min. Metabolism:
Rapidly hydrolyzed at neutral pH in blood; also subject to enzyme degradation. **Elimination:** 82% in urine. **Half-Life:** Approximately 6 min.

## NURSING IMPLICATIONS
### Assessment & Drug Effects
▪ Assess carefully for development of pulmonary edema during dose ranging.
▪ Monitor respiratory and cardiovascular status frequently during entire period of chronic use of epoprostenol.
▪ Monitor for and report recurrence or worsening of symptoms associated with primary pulmonary hypertension (e.g., dyspnea, dizziness, exercise intolerance) or adverse effects of drug; dosage adjustments may be needed.

### Patient & Family Education
▪ Learn correct techniques for storage, reconstitution, and administration of drug, and maintenance of catheter site (see ADMINISTRATION).
▪ Notify prescriber immediately of S&S of worsening primary pulmonary hypertension, adverse drug reactions, and S&S of infection at catheter site or sepsis.

# EPROSARTAN MESYLATE
(e-pro-sar'tan)

**Classifications:** RENIN ANGIOTENSIN SYSTEM ANTAGONIST; ANGIOTENSIN II RECEPTOR ANTAGONIST, ANTIHYPERTENSIVE
**Therapeutic:** ANTIHYPERTENSIVE
**Prototype:** Losartan potassium

## AVAILABILITY Tablet

## ACTION & *THERAPEUTIC EFFECT*
Selectively blocks the binding of angiotensin II to the $AT_1$ receptors

Common adverse effects in *italic;* life-threatening effects <u>underlined;</u> generic names in **bold;** classifications in SMALL CAPS; ◆Canadian drug name; ⊚ Prototype drug

605

E

found in many tissues. This blocks vasoconstricting and aldosterone-secreting effects of angiotensin II, thus resulting in an antihypertensive effect. *It decreases both the systolic and diastolic BP.*

**USES** Treatment of hypertension.

**CONTRAINDICATIONS** Hypersensitivity to eprosartan, losartan, or other angiotensin II receptor antagonists; pregnancy (category D second and third trimester); lactation.

**CAUTIOUS USE** Angioedema, aortic or mitral value stenosis, coronary artery disease, cardiomyopathy, hypotension, CHF; biliary obstruction; older adults; severe hepatic dysfunction, renal artery stenosis, renal disease, renal impairment; pregnancy (category C first trimester; discontinue as soon as pregnancy is detected). Safe use in children younger than 18 y not established.

## ROUTE & DOSAGE

### Hypertension
*Adult:* **PO** 600 mg daily (range 400–800 mg) (max: 900 mg/day)

## ADMINISTRATION

### Oral
- Correct volume depletion prior to therapy to prevent hypotension.
- Store at 20°–25° C (68°–77° F); protect from moisture and direct light.

**ADVERSE EFFECTS** (≥1%) **Body as a Whole:** Viral infection, fatigue, arthralgia, edema. **CNS:** Depression, dizziness, fatigue. **GI:** Abdominal pain, diarrhea, hypertriglyceridemia. **Respiratory:** Upper respiratory infection, rhinitis, pharyngitis, cough. **Hematologic:** Neutropenia.

**INTERACTIONS Drug:** Use of another ARB does not provide any additional benefits. Use caution with **lithium** due to increased lithium toxicity risk. Use of DIURETICS may increase hypotension risk.

**PHARMACOKINETICS Absorption:** Only 13% of oral dose reaches systemic circulation. **Peak:** 1–2 h. **Metabolism:** Minimal metabolism. **Elimination:** 61% in feces and 37% in urine. **Half-Life:** 5–9 h.

## NURSING IMPLICATIONS

### Black Box Warning

*Eprosartan has been associated with fetal injury and death.*

### Assessment & Drug Effects
- Monitor BP periodically; do trough readings just before scheduled dose when possible.
- Monitor for S&S of angioedema (may occur within 30 min or as long as 30 days after initial dose).
- Monitor lab tests: Periodic LFTs, BUN and creatinine, serum potassium, sodium, CBC with differential.

### Patient & Family Education
- Inform prescriber immediately of pregnancy. Drug should be discontinued as soon as possible.
- Report episodes of dizziness especially associated with position changes.
- Report swelling of lips, tongue, face, or feeling of obstruction in neck immediately.

## EPTIFIBATIDE
(ep-ti-fib′a-tide)
Integrilin
**Classifications:** ANTIPLATELET; PLATELET GLYCOPROTEIN (GP IIB/IIIA) INHIBITOR
Therapeutic: ANTIPLATELET
**Prototype:** Abciximab

**AVAILABILITY** Solution for injection

## ACTION & *THERAPEUTIC EFFECT*
Binds to the glycoprotein IIb/IIIa (GPIIb/IIIa) receptor sites of platelets. *Inhibits platelet aggregation by preventing fibrinogen, von Wille-brand's factor, and other molecules from adhering to GPIIb/IIIa receptor sites on platelets.*

**USES** Treatment of acute coronary syndromes (unstable angina, non-Q-wave MI) and patients undergoing percutaneous coronary interventions (PCIs).

**CONTRAINDICATIONS** Hypersensitivity to eptifibatide; active bleeding; GI or GU bleeding within 6 wk; thrombocytopenia; renal failure requiring dialysis; coagulopathy; recent major surgery or trauma; intracranial neoplasm, intracranial bleeding within 6 mo; severe hypertension (systolic blood pressure greater than 200 mm Hg or diastolic blood pressure greater than 110 mm Hg), aneurysm.

**CAUTIOUS USE** Hypersensitivity to related compounds (e.g., abciximab, tirofiban, lamifiban); pregnancy (category B); lactation. Safety and efficacy in children not established.

## ROUTE & DOSAGE

**Acute Coronary Syndromes (ACS)**

*Adult:* **IV** 180 mcg/kg initial bolus (max: 22.6 mg) followed by 2 mcg/kg/min until hospital discharge or up to 72 h

**Percutaneous Coronary Interventions (PCI)**

*Adult:* **IV** 180 mcg/kg initial bolus followed by 2 mcg/kg/min; after 10 min, a second 180 mcg/kg

bolus should be given; the infusion should continue up to 24 h after the end of the procedure

**Renal Impairment Dosage Adjustment**

*CrCl 10–49 mL/min:* Give 1 mcg/kg/min continuous infusion

## ADMINISTRATION
- Note: Review contraindications to administration prior to giving this drug.

**Intravenous**

*PREPARE:* **Direct:** Give undiluted.
*ADMINISTER:* **Direct:** Give bolus doses IV push over 1–2 min. **Continuous** Start continuous infusion immediately following bolus dose. ▪ Give undiluted directly from the 100-mL vial (at a rate based on patient's weight) using a vented infusion set. ▪ May be given in the same IV line with NS or D5/NS (either solution may contain up to 60 mEq KCl).

▪ Store unopened vials at 2°–8° C (36°–46° F) and protect from light. Discard any unused portion in opened vial.

**ADVERSE EFFECTS** (≥1%) **CNS:** Intracranial bleed (rare). **GI:** GI bleeding. **Hematologic:** *Bleeding* (major bleeding 4.4–11%), anemia, thrombocytopenia.

**INTERACTIONS Drug:** ORAL ANTICOAGULANTS, NSAIDS, **dipyridamole, ticlopidine, dextran** may increase risk of bleeding.

**PHARMACOKINETICS Duration:** 6–8 h after stopping infusion. **Metabolism:** Minimally metabolized. **Elimination:** 50% in urine. **Half-Life:** 2.5 h.

E

Common adverse effects in *italic*; life-threatening effects underlined; generic names in **bold**; classifications in SMALL CAPS; ♣ Canadian drug name; ⓟ Prototype drug

607

E

## NURSING IMPLICATIONS
### Assessment & Drug Effects

- Prior to infusion determine PT/aPTT and INR, activated clotting time (ACT) for those undergoing percutaneous coronary intervention (PCI); Hct or Hgb; platelet count; and serum creatinine.
- Minimize all vascular and other trauma during treatment. When obtaining IV access, avoid using a noncompressible site such as the subclavian vein.
- Monitor carefully for and immediately report S&S of bleeding (e.g., femoral artery access site bleeding, intracerebral hemorrhage, GI bleeding).
- Immediately stop infusion of eptifibatide and heparin if bleeding at the arterial access site cannot be controlled by pressure.
- Achieve hemostasis at the arterial access site by standard compression for a minimum of 4 h prior to hospital discharge following discontinuation of eptifibatide and heparin.
- Monitor lab tests: Baseline and periodic aPTT and INR (target aPPT, 50–70 sec); during PCI (target ACT, 300–350 sec).

## ERGOCALCIFEROL
(er-goe-kal-si′fe-role)
Activated Ergosterol,
Calcidol, Drisdol, D-ViSol,
Ostoforte ♦, Radiostol ♦,
Radiostol Forte ♦, Vitamin D₂
**Classification:** VITAMIN D ANALOG
Therapeutic: VITAMIN D ANALOG
**Prototype:** Calcitriol

**AVAILABILITY** Oral liquid; capsule, tablet; solution for injection

## ACTION & *THERAPEUTIC EFFECT*
The name vitamin D encompasses two related fat-soluble substances. Vitamin D acts like a hormone in that it is distributed through the circulation and plays a major regulatory role. Responsible for regulation of serum calcium level. *Maintains normal blood calcium and phosphate ion levels by enhancing their intestinal absorption and by promoting mobilization of calcium from bone and renal tubular resorption of phosphate.*

**USES** Familial hypophosphatemia (vitamin D–resistant rickets), osteomalacia (adult rickets), anticonvulsant-induced rickets and osteomalacia, osteoporosis, renal osteodystrophy, hypocalcemia associated with hypoparathyroidism; prophylaxis and treatment of nutritional rickets. Also hypophosphatemia in Fanconi's syndrome.

**UNLABELED USES** With varying clinical results in lupus vulgaris, psoriasis, and rheumatoid arthritis.

**CONTRAINDICATIONS** Hypersensitivity to vitamin D, hypervitaminosis D, hypercalcemia, hyperphosphatemia, renal osteodystrophy with hyperphosphatemia, malabsorption syndrome, decreased kidney function.

**CAUTIOUS USE** Coronary disease; arteriosclerosis (especially in older adults); history of kidney stones; biliary tract disease; lactation. Safe use of amounts in excess of 400 international units (10 mcg) daily during pregnancy (category C) is not established.

## ROUTE & DOSAGE

| Nutritional Rickets, Osteomalacia |
| --- |
| *Adult:* **PO** 25–125 mcg/day for 6–12 wk, may need up to 7.5 mg/day in patients with malabsorption |
| *Child:* **PO** 50–125 mcg/day, may need up to 250–625 mcg/day in patients with malabsorption |

### Vitamin D–Dependent Rickets

*Adult:* **PO** 250 mcg–1.5 mg/day, may need up to 12.5 mg/day (prolonged therapy with greater than 2.5 mg/day increases risk of toxicity)
*Child:* **PO** 75–125 mcg/day, may need up to 1.5 mg/day

### Hypoparathyroidism, Pseudohypoparathyroidism

*Adult:* **PO** 625 mcg–5 mg/day, may need up to 10 mg/day (prolonged therapy with greater than 2.5 mg/day increases risk of toxicity)
*Child:* **PO** 1.25–5 mg/day, (prolonged therapy with greater than 2.5 mg/day increases risk of toxicity)

## ADMINISTRATION

### Oral

- Preserve in tightly covered, light-resistant containers. Drug decomposes when exposed to light and air.

## ADVERSE EFFECTS (≥1%) **Body as a Whole:** Fatigue, weakness, vertigo, tinnitus, ataxia, muscle and joint pain, hypotonia (infants), exanthema, rhinorrhea; pruritus; mild acidosis. **CNS:** Headache, drowsiness, convulsions. **GI:** Metallic taste, dry mouth, anorexia, nausea, vomiting, diarrhea, constipation, abdominal cramps. **Hematologic:** Anemia. **Musculoskeletal:** Calcification of soft tissues (kidneys, blood vessels, myocardium, lungs, skin). **Urogenital:** Nephrotoxicity (polyuria, hyposthenuria, polydipsia, nocturia, casts, albuminuria, hematuria), kidney failure. **CV:** Hypertension, cardiac arrhythmias. **Special Senses:** Conjunctivitis (calcific); photophobia. **Metabolic:** Osteoporosis (adults); weight loss,

chronic hypervitaminosis D in children (mental and physical retardation, suppression of linear growth).

## DIAGNOSTIC TEST INTERFERENCE

Vitamin D may cause false increase in *serum cholesterol* measurements *(Zlatkis-Zak reaction)*.

## INTERACTIONS **Drug: Cholestyramine, colestipol, mineral oil** may decrease absorption of vitamin D.

## PHARMACOKINETICS **Absorption:** Readily from GI tract. **Peak:** After 4 wk. **Duration:** 2 mo or more. **Distribution:** Most of drug first appears in lymph, stored chiefly in liver and in skin, brain, spleen, and bones. **Metabolism:** In liver and kidney to active metabolites. **Elimination:** About 50% of PO dose in bile; may be stored in tissues for months. **Half-Life:** 12–24 h.

## NURSING IMPLICATIONS

### Assessment & Drug Effects

- Monitor closely patients receiving therapeutic doses of vitamin D; must remain under close medical supervision.
- Monitor for hypercalcemia; in patients with osteomalacia a decrease in serum alkaline phosphatase may signal the onset of hypercalcemia.
- Monitor lab tests: Baseline and periodic serum calcium and phosphorus.

### Patient & Family Education

- Avoid magnesium-containing antacids and laxatives with chronic kidney failure when receiving vitamin D preparations since vitamin D increases the risk of magnesium intoxication than other patients.
- Do not use OTC medications unless approved by prescriber.

Common adverse effects in *italic;* life-threatening effects underlined; generic names in **bold;** classifications in SMALL CAPS; ♣ Canadian drug name; ⊙ Prototype drug

609

**E**

## ERGOTAMINE TARTRATE 🄿🄳
(er-got′a-meen)

~~Ergomar~~

**Classifications:** ALPHA-ADRENERGIC ANTAGONIST; ERGOT ALKALOID

~~Therapeutic:~~ ANTIMIGRAINE

**AVAILABILITY** Sublingual tablet

## ACTION & *THERAPEUTIC EFFECT*

Natural amino acid alkaloid of ergot. Alpha-adrenergic blocking agent with direct-stimulating action on cranial and peripheral vascular smooth muscles and depressant effect on central vasomotor centers. *In vascular headache, exerts vasoconstrictive action on previously dilated cerebral vessels, reduces amplitude of arterial pulsations, and antagonizes effects of serotonin.*

**USES** As single agent or in combination with caffeine to prevent or abort migraine, cluster headache (histamine cephalalgia), and other vascular headaches.

**CONTRAINDICATIONS** Hypersensitivity to ergotamine; sepsis, obliterative vascular disease, thromboembolic disease, prolonged use of excessive dosage, liver and kidney disease, severe pruritus, diabetes mellitus; marked arteriosclerosis, history of MI, peripheral vascular disease; coronary artery disease, angina; basilar/hemiplegic migraine; hepatic disease; biliary tract disease; cholestasis; hypertension; infectious states, anemia, malnutrition; concurrent administration of potent CYP3A4 inhibitors (e.g., protease inhibitors and macrolide antibiotics); pregnancy (category X).

**CAUTIOUS USE** Older adult patients; lactation. Safe use in children not established.

## ROUTE & DOSAGE

**Vascular Headaches**

*Adult:* **SL** 1–2 mg followed by 1–2 mg q30min until headache abates or until max of 6 mg/24 h or 10 mg/wk

## ADMINISTRATION

**Sublingual**

- Instruct patient to allow sublingual (SL) tablet to dissolve under tongue and not to drink, eat, or smoke while tablet is in place. Do not crush SL tablets.

**ADVERSE EFFECTS** (≥1%) **Body as a Whole:** Paresthesias; pain (spasms) of facial muscles, tongue, limbs, and lumbar region with difficulty in walking; muscle pains, *weakness,* numbness, coldness and cyanosis of digits (Raynaud's phenomenon). **CNS:** Delirium; convulsive seizures; confusion; depression; drowsiness. **GI:** *Nausea; vomiting;* diarrhea; abdominal pain; unquenchable thirst; partial necrosis of tongue, disagreeable aftertaste. **CV:** Rapid, weak, or irregular pulse; intermittent claudication, complete absence of medium- and large-vessel pulsations in extremities; precordial distress and pain; angina pectoris, transient bradycardia or tachycardia; elevated or lowered BP. **Skin:** Itching and cold skin; gangrene of nose, digits, ears. **Urogenital:** Kidney failure. **Other:** Symptoms of ergotism.

**INTERACTIONS Drug:** With high doses of BETA-ADRENERGIC BLOCKERS, SYMPATHOMIMETICS, possibility of additive vasoconstrictor effects; **erythromycin, troleandomycin** may cause severe peripheral vasospasm. **Eletriptan, naratriptan, rizatriptan, sumatriptan, or zolmitriptan** may

Common adverse effects in *italic;* life-threatening effects <u>underlined;</u> generic names in **bold;** classifications in SMALL CAPS; ♣ Canadian drug name; 🄿 Prototype drug increase risk of coronary ischemia, separate drugs by 24 h; AZOLE ANTI-FUNGALS **(ketoconazole, itraconazole, fluconazole, clotrimazole), nefazodone, fluoxetine, fluvoxamine, amprenavir, delavirdine, efavirenz, indinavir, nelfinavir, ritonavir, and saquinavir,** may inhibit ergot metabolism and increase toxicity; **sibutramine, dexfenfluramine, nefazodone, fluvoxamine** may increase risk of serotonin syndrome. **Food: Grapefruit juice** may increase toxicity.

## PHARMACOKINETICS Absorption:
Variable. **Peak:** 0.5–3 h. **Distribution:** Crosses blood–brain barrier. **Metabolism:** Extensive first-pass metabolism in liver. **Elimination:** 96% in feces; excreted in breast milk. **Half-Life:** 2.7 h initial phase, 21 h terminal phase.

## NURSING IMPLICATIONS
### Assessment & Drug Effects
- Monitor adverse GI effects. Nausea and vomiting are adverse reactions that occur in about 10% of patients after they take ergotamine. Patient may need an antiemetic. Consult with prescriber.
- Monitor patients with PVD carefully for development of peripheral ischemia.
- Monitor long-term effectiveness. Patients receiving high ergotamine doses for prolonged periods may experience increased frequency of headaches, fatigue, and depression. Discontinuation of the drug in these patients results in severe withdrawal headache that may last a few days.
- Overdose symptoms: Nausea, vomiting, weakness, and pain in legs, numbness and tingling in fingers and toes, tachycardia or bradycardia, hypertension or hypotension, and localized edema.

### Patient & Family Education
- Begin drug therapy as soon after onset of migraine attack as possible, preferably during migraine prodrome (scintillating scotomas, visual field defects, nausea, paresthesias usually on side opposite to that of the migraine).
- Notify prescriber if migraine attacks occur more frequently or are not relieved.
- Lie down in a quiet, dark room for 2–3 h after drug administration.
- Report muscle pain or weakness of extremities, cold or numb digits, irregular heartbeat, nausea, or vomiting. Carefully protect extremities from exposure to cold temperatures; provide warmth, but not heat, to ischemic areas.
- **Do not** increase dosage without consulting prescriber; overdosage is the chief cause of adverse effects from the drug.

# ERIBULIN MESYLATE
(er-e-bu'lin)
Halaven
**Classifications:** ANTINEOPLASTIC; MITOTIC INHIBITOR
**Therapeutic:** ANTINEOPLASTIC

## AVAILABILITY Solution for injection

## ACTION & *THERAPEUTIC EFFECT*
A microtubule inhibitor that blocks completion of the cell cycle and prevents cell replication resulting in apoptotic cell death. *Interferes with mitosis and cell replication thus reducing growth and metastatic spread of cancer cells.*

## USES Treatment of metastatic breast cancer in patients who have previously received at least two previous chemotherapeutic regimens that included an anthracycline and a taxane in either the adjuvant or metastatic setting.

---

Common adverse effects in *italic;* life-threatening effects <u>underlined;</u> generic names in **bold;** classifications in SMALL CAPS; ♣ Canadian drug name; ❷ Prototype drug

E

**CONTRAINDICATIONS** Congenital long QT syndrome; ANC less than 1000 mm³; platelets less than 75,000 mm³; Grade 3 or 4 nonhematologic toxicities; pregnancy (category D).

**CAUTIOUS USE** Neutropenia; peripheral neuropathy; QT prolongation; hepatic impairment; renal impariment; lactation. Safety and efficacy in children not established.

## ROUTE & DOSAGE

**Metastatic Breast Cancer**

*Adult:* **IV** 1.4 mg/m² days 1 and 8 of a 21-day cycle. Repeat cycle as needed or until unacceptable toxicities arise

**Delay Doses for Any of the Following**

*If ANC less than 1000/mm³, platelets less than 75,000/mm³, or Grade 3 or 4 nonhematological toxicities:* Do not administer eribulin; the day 8 dose may be delayed a max of 1 wk

*If toxicities do not resolve to Grade 2 or better by day 15:* Omit the dose

*If toxicities resolve or improve to Grade 2 or better by day 15:* Administer eribulin at a reduced dose and initiate the next cycle no sooner than 2 wk later

**Hematologic Toxicity Dosage Adjustment**

*If ANC less than 500/mm³ for more than 7 days, ANC less than 1000/mm³ with fever or infection, platelets less than 25,000/mm³ or less than 50,000/mm³ requiring transfusion or day 8 of previous cycle omitted or delayed:* Permanently reduce dose to 1.1 mg/m²

*If while receiving 1.1 mg/m², recurrence of hematologic event occurs, or if day 8 of previous cycle omitted or delayed:* Permanently reduce dose to 0.7 mg/m²

*If while receiving 0.7 mg/m², recurrence of hematologic event occurs, or if day 8 of previous cycle omitted or delayed:* Discontinue eribulin

**Nonhematologic Toxicity Dosage Adjustment**

*If Grade 3 or 4 nonhematologic toxicity or if day 8 of previous cycle omitted or delayed:* Permanently reduce dose to 1.1 mg/m²

*While receiving 1.1 mg/m², if recurrence of Grade 3 or 4 nonhematologic toxicity occurs, or if day 8 of previous cycle omitted or delayed:* Permanently reduce dose to 0.7 mg/m²

*While receiving 0.7 mg/m², if recurrence of Grade 3 or 4 nonhematologic toxicity occurs, or if day 8 of previous cycle omitted or delayed:* Discontinue eribulin

**Hepatic Impairment Dosage Adjustment**

*Mild hepatic impairment (Child-Pugh class A):* Reduce dose to 1.1 mg/m²

*Moderate hepatic impairment (Child-Pugh class B):* Reduce dose to 0.7 mg/m²

**Renal Impairment Dosage Adjustment**

*CrCl 30–50 mL/min:* Reduce dose to 1.1 mg/m²

Common adverse effects in *italic;* life-threatening effects underlined; generic names in **bold;** classifications in SMALL CAPS; ♣ Canadian drug name; ◉ Prototype drug

## ADMINISTRATION

### Intravenous

- Correct hypokalemia or hypomagnesemia prior to initiating eribulin.

*PREPARE:* **IV Infusion:** May be given undiluted or diluted in 100 mL of NS. Do not dilute with dextrose.

*ADMINISTER:* **IV Infusion:** Give over 2–5 min. Do not administer in same IV line as dextrose or any other required medication.

*INCOMPATIBILITIES:* **Solution/additive:** Incompatible with D5W for dilution.

- Store unopened at 15°–30° C (59°–86° F). Store undiluted in a syringe or diluted in NL for up to 4 h at room temperature or for up to 24 h under refrigeration.

## ADVERSE EFFECTS (≥1%) Body as a Whole: Mucosal inflammation, pyrexia. **CNS:** *Asthenia/fatigue*, depression, dizziness, *headache*, insomnia, *peripheral neuropathy*. **GI:** Abdominal pain, *constipation*, *diarrhea*, dry mouth, dyspepsia, *nausea*, stomatitis, vomiting. **Hematological:** *Anemia*, febrile neutropenia, *neutropenia*, thrombocytopenia. **Metabolic:** *Anorexia*, *decreased weight*, hypokalemia, *increased ALT*, peripheral edema. **Musculoskeletal:** *Arthralgia*, *back pain*, bone pain, muscle spasms, muscle weakness, *myalgia*, pain in extremitiy. **Respiratory:** Cough, *dyspnea*, upper respiratory tract infection. **Skin:** *Alopecia*, rash. **Special Senses:** Dysgeusia, increased lacrimation. **Urogenital:** Urinary tract infection.

## INTERACTIONS Drug: Eribulin has been associated with QT prolongation. Coadministration of another drug that prolongs the QT interval (e.g., **disopyramide, procainamide, amiodarone, bretylium, clarithromycin, levofloxacin**) may cause additive effects.

## PHARMACOKINETICS Distribution: 49–65% plasma protein bound. **Metabolism:** Minimal. **Elimination:** Fecal (82%) and renal (9%). **Half-Life:** 40 h.

## NURSING IMPLICATIONS

### Assessment & Drug Effects

- Monitor ECG in those with CHF, bradyarrhythmias, concurrent use of Class Ia and III antiarrhythmics, and electrolyte imbalances.
- Monitor closely for S&S of peripheral motor and sensory neuropathy.
- Monitor temperature. Report fever and/or S&S of infection.
- Withhold drug and notify prescriber of the following: Grade 3 or 4 peripheral neuropathy, hypokalemia or hypomagnesemia; prolonged QT interval.
- Monitor lab tests: Baseline and periodic serum electrolytes; CBC with differential prior to each dose and more often with Grade 3 or 4 cytopenia; periodic LFTs.

### Patient & Family Education

- Report promptly fever (100.5° F or greater) or other S&S of infection.
- Report S&S of peripheral neuropathy, including: Tingling, numbness, deep pain in the feet, legs, or arms; weakness or problems with balance; or difficulty with fine motor skills.
- Effective methods of birth control are recommended during therapy. Notify prescriber immediately if a pregnancy develops.

E

- Do not breast-feed while taking this drug without consulting prescriber.

# ERLOTINIB 🅟⏷
(er-lo'ti-nib)

Tarceva

**Classifications:** ANTINEOPLASTIC; KINASE INHIBITOR; EPIDERMAL GROWTH FACTOR RECEPTOR INHIBITOR

Therapeutic: ANTINEOPLASTIC

## AVAILABILITY Tablet

## ACTION & *THERAPEUTIC EFFECT*

Erlotinib is a human epidermal growth factor receptor type 1 (HER1/EGFR) inhibitor. Antitumor action is believed to be due to inhibition of phosphorylation of tyrosine kinase associated with the EGFR present on the cell surface of both normal and cancer cells. *Inhibition of EGFR in cancer cells diminishes their capacity for cell proliferation, cell survival, and decreases metastases.*

## USES Treatment of patients with locally advanced or metastatic non-small-cell lung cancer (NSCLC), pancreatic cancer.

## CONTRAINDICATIONS Hypersensitivity to erlotinib; severe hepatic impairment; acute/worsening of ocular disorders such as eye pain; GI perforation; interstitial lung disease; severe renal impairment; exfoliative skin reaction; pregnancy (category D); lactation.

## CAUTIOUS USE Mild or moderate hepatic or renal impairment; history of peptic ulcers or diverticular disease; myelosuppression; ocular toxicities (corneal ulcer). Safety and efficacy in children not established.

## ROUTE & DOSAGE

**Metastatic Non–Small-Cell Lung Cancer**
*Adult:* **PO** 150 mg once daily

**Pancreatic Cancer (with Gemcitabine)**
*Adult:* **PO** 100 mg daily × 7 wk with one wk rest (each cycle)

*Hepatic Impairment Dosage Adjustment*
Discontinue use in patient with severe change in liver function

## ADMINISTRATION

### Oral
- Give at least 1 h before or 2 h after eating.
- Store at 15°–30° C (59°–86° F). Keep container tightly closed. Protect from light.

## ADVERSE EFFECTS (≥1%) **Body as a Whole:** Infection, muscle pain, *weight loss.* **GI:** *Diarrhea, anorexia, fatigue,* nausea, vomiting, stomatitis, abdominal pain. **Metabolic:** Increased LFTs. **Respiratory:** *Dyspnea,* cough, interstitial lung disease. **Skin:** *Acneiform rash,* alopecia, pruritus, dry skin. **Special Senses:** Conjunctivitis, dry eyes. **CV:** *Edema.* **CNS:** Anxiety, depression.

## INTERACTIONS **Drug:** Dose will need to be adjusted with concurrent strong **CYP3A4 inducers (e.g., carbamazepine, nevirapine, phenobarbital, phenytoin). Atazanavir, clarithromycin, indinavir, itraconazole, ketoconazole, nefazodone, nelfinavir, ritonavir, saquinavir, telithromycin, troleandomycin, voriconazole** may increase erlotinib

Common adverse effects in *italic;* life-threatening effects <u>underlined;</u> generic names in **bold;** classifications in SMALL CAPS; ♣ Canadian drug name; 🄌 Prototype drug levels and toxicity; increased bleeding with **warfarin. Herbal: St. John's wort** may decrease erlotinib levels.

## PHARMACOKINETICS **Absorption:** 60% absorbed; food can increase to 100%. **Peak:** 4 h. **Metabolism:** In liver by CYP3A4. **Elimination:** In feces (83%). **Half-Life:** 36.2 h.

## NURSING IMPLICATIONS

### Assessment & Drug Effects
- Monitor closely changes in pulmonary function.
- Withhold drug and notify prescriber for acute onset of new or progressive pulmonary symptoms (e.g., dyspnea, cough, or fever) or significant changes in liver functions as indicated by elevated transaminases, bilirubin, and alkaline phosphatase.
- Monitor lab tests: Periodic LFTs

### Patient & Family Education
- Report promptly any of the following. Severe or persistent diarrhea, nausea, anorexia, or vomiting; onset or worsening of unexplained shortness of breath or cough; eye irritation.
- Monitor closely PT/INR values with concurrent warfarin therapy.
- Women should use effective means to avoid pregnancy while taking this drug.

## ERTAPENEM SODIUM
(er-ta-pen′em)

Invanz

**Classification:** BETA-LACTAM ANTIBIOTIC
**Therapeutic:** ANTIBIOTIC
**Prototype:** Imipenem-cilastatin

**AVAILABILITY** Solution for injection

## ACTION & *THERAPEUTIC EFFECT*
Broad-spectrum carbapenem antibiotic that inhibits the cell wall synthesis of gram-positive and gram-negative bacteria by its strong affinity for penicillin-binding proteins (PBPs) of the bacterial cell wall. *Effective against both gram-positive and gram-negative bacteria. Highly resistant to most bacterial beta-lactamases.*

## USES Complicated intra-abdominal infections, complicated skin and skin structure infections, community-acquired pneumonia, complicated UTI (including pyelonephritis), and acute pelvic infections due to susceptible bacteria.

## CONTRAINDICATIONS Hypersensitivity to ertapenem, penicillins, or carbapenem antibiotics; hypersensitivity to amide-type local anesthetics such as lidocaine; hypersensitivity to meropenem or imipenem.

## CAUTIOUS USE Hypersensitivity to other beta-lactam antibiotics (penicillins, cephalosporins); hypersensitivity to other allergens; renal impairment; history of CNS disorders; history of seizures; meningitis; older adults; pregnancy (category B); lactation (bottle feed during and for 5 days after therapy ends). Safe use in infants younger than 3 mo not established.

## ROUTE & DOSAGE

| **Community-Acquired Pneumonia; Complicated UTI** |
| --- |
| *Adult/Adolescent:* **IV/IM** 1 g daily × 10–14 days; may switch to appropriate **PO** antibiotic after 3 days if responding |
| *Child/Infant (3 mo or older):* **IV/IM** 15 mg/kg q12h × 10–14 days (max: 1 g/day) |

Common adverse effects in *italic;* life-threatening effects <u>underlined</u>; generic names in **bold;** classifications in SMALL CAPS; ♣Canadian drug name; ⊕ Prototype drug

615

E

### Intra-Abdominal Infection

*Adult/Adolescent:* **IV/IM** 1 g daily × 5–14 days
*Child/Infant (3 mo or older):* **IV/IM** 15 mg/kg b.i.d. × 5–14 days (max: 1 g/day)

### Skin and Skin Structure Infections

*Adult/Adolescent:* **IV/IM** 1 g daily × 7–14 days
*Child/Infant (3 mo or older):* **IV/IM** 15 mg/kg b.i.d. × 7–14 days (max: 1 g/day)

### Acute Pelvic Infections

*Adult:* **IV/IM** 1 g daily × 3–10 days

### Renal Impairment Dosage Adjustment

*CrCl less than 30 mL/min:* Reduce dose to 500 mg daily

## ADMINISTRATION

### Intramuscular

- Reconstitute 1 g vial with 3.2 mL of 1% lidocaine HCl injection (without epinephrine). Shake vial thoroughly to form solution. Use immediately.
- Inject deep IM into a large muscle mass (such as the gluteal muscles or lateral part of the thigh).
- The reconstituted IM solution should be used within 1 h after preparation. Note: **Do not** use this solution for IV administration.

### Intravenous

**PREPARE: Intermittent for Adult/Child:** Reconstitute 1 g vial with 10 mL of sterile water for injection, NS, or bacteriostatic water for injection. Shake well to dissolve. **Intermittent for Adult/Child (13 y or older):** Immediately after reconstitution, transfer contents to 50 mL of NS injection solution. **Intermit-**

tent for Child (3 mo–12 y): Immediately after reconstitution, transfer required dose to enough NS injection solution to yield a final concentration of 20 mg/mL or less. *ADMINISTER:* **Intermittent:** Infuse over 30 min. Note: Infusion should be completed within 6 h of reconstitution.
*INCOMPATIBILITIES:* Solution/additive: **Mannitol, sodium bicarbonate. Y-site: Alemtuzumab, allopurinol, amiodarone, amphotericin B, anidulafungin, caspofungin, chlorpromazine, dantrolene, daunorubicin, diazepam, dobutamine, doxorubicin, droperidol, epirubicin, hydralazine, hydroxyzine, idarubicin, midazolam, minocycline, mitoxantrone, nicardipine, ondansetron, pentamidine, phenytoin, prochlorperazine, promethazine, quinidine, quinupristin/dalfopristin, thiopental, topotecan, verapamil.**

- Store lyophilized powder above 25° C (77° F). ▪ Must use reconstituted solution stored at room temperature (not above 25° C/77° F) within 6 h. ▪ May store for 24 h under refrigeration. Use within 4 h of removal from refrigeration. ▪ Do not freeze.

## ADVERSE EFFECTS (≥1%) **Body as a Whole:** Phlebitis or thrombosis at injection site, asthenia, fatigue, <u>death</u>, fever, leg pain. **CNS:** Anxiety, altered mental status, dizziness, headache, insomnia. **CV:** Chest pain, hypertension, hypotension, tachycardia, edema. **GI:** Abdominal pain, *diarrhea*, acid regurgitation, constipation, dyspepsia, nausea, vomiting, increased AST and ALT. **Respiratory:** Cough, dyspnea, pharyngitis, rales/rhonchi, and respiratory distress. **Skin:** Erythema, pruritus, rash. **Urogenital:** Vaginitis.

Common adverse effects in *italic;* life-threatening effects <u>underlined;</u> generic names in **bold;** classifications in SMALL CAPS; ♣ Canadian drug name; ◎ Prototype drug

**INTERACTIONS Drug: Probenecid** decreases renal excretion. **Valproic acid** levels may be decreased.

**PHARMACOKINETICS Absorption:** 90% from IM site. **Peak:** 2.3 h. **Distribution:** 95% protein bound, distributes into breast milk. **Metabolism:** Hydrolysis of beta-lactam ring. **Elimination:** 80% in urine, 10% in feces. **Half-Life:** 4.5 h.

**NURSING IMPLICATIONS**

**Assessment & Drug Effects**

- Determine history of hypersensitivity reactions to other beta-lactams, cephalosporins, penicillins, or other drugs.
- Discontinue drug and immediately report S&S of hypersensitivity (see Appendix F).
- Report S&S of superinfection or pseudomembranous colitis (see Appendix F).
- Monitor for seizures especially in older adults and those with renal insufficiency.
- Monitor lab tests: Periodic LFTs, CBC, platelet count, and routine blood chemistry during prolonged therapy.

**Patient & Family Education**

- Learn S&S of hypersensitivity, superinfection, and pseudomembranous colitis (see Appendix F); report any of these to prescriber promptly.

## ERYTHROMYCIN ⦿

(er-ith-roe-mye'sin)

Eryc, EryPed, EryTab, Erythrocin, Erythromid ♦, Erythromycin Base, Novo-Rythro ♦, PCE

## ERYTHROMYCIN STEARATE

**Classification:** MACROLIDE ANTIBIOTIC
**Therapeutic:** ANTIBIOTIC

**AVAILABILITY Erythromycin:** Tablet; delayed release tablet; capsule; topical solution; gel; ointment pledgets; ophthalmic ointment. **Erythromycin Stearate:** Tablet

**ACTION & THERAPEUTIC EFFECT** Macrolide antibiotic that binds to the 50S ribosomal subunit, thus inhibiting bacterial protein synthesis. *More active against gram-positive organisms than against gram-negative organisms due to its superior penetration into gram-positive organisms.*

**USES** Pneumococcal pneumonia, *Mycoplasma pneumoniae* (primary atypical pneumonia), acute pelvic inflammatory disease caused by *Neisseria gonorrhoeae* in females sensitive to penicillin, infections caused by susceptible strains of staphylococci, streptococci, and certain strains of *Haemophilus influenzae*. Also used in intestinal amebiasis, Legionnaires' disease, uncomplicated urethral, endocervical, and rectal infections caused by *Chlamydia trachomatis,* for prophylaxis of ophthalmia neonatorum caused by *N. gonorrhoeae, C. trachomatis,* and for chlamydial conjunctivitis in neonates. Alternative to penicillin for treatment of streptococcal pharyngitis, for prophylaxis of rheumatic fever and bacterial endocarditis, for treatment of diphtheria as adjunct to antitoxin and for carrier state, and as alternate choice in treatment of primary syphilis in patients allergic to penicillins. **Topical applications:** Pyodermas, acne vulgaris, and external ocular infections, including neonatal chlamydial conjunctivitis and gonococcal ophthalmia.

**CONTRAINDICATIONS** Hypersensitivity to erythromycins or other macrolide antibiotics; congenital QT

Common adverse effects in *italic;* life-threatening effects underlined; generic names in **bold;** classifications in SMALL CAPS; ♦Canadian drug name; ⦿ Prototype drug

617

prolongation; electrolyte imbalances. **Estolate:** History of hepatotoxicity in patients with hepatic disease.

**CAUTIOUS USE** Impaired liver function; seizure disorders; history of GI disorders; pregnancy (category B).

## ROUTE & DOSAGE

### Moderate to Severe Infections

*Adult:* **PO** 250–500 mg q6h; 333 mg q8h (ethylsuccinate form) *Child:* **PO** 30–50 mg/kg/day divided q6h; **Topical** Apply ointment to infected eye 1 or more × day
*Neonate:* **PO** *7 days or younger:* 10 mg/kg q12h; *7 days or older:* 10 mg/kg q8–12h; **Topical** 0.5–1 cm in conjunctival sac once

### *Chlamydia* Conjuctivitis

*Neonate:* **PO** 50 mg/kg/day divided into 4 daily doses × 14d

## ADMINISTRATION

### Oral

- Erythromycin base or stearate should be given on an empty stomach 2 h before or after a meal. Do not give with, or immediately before or after, fruit juices.
- Enteric-coated tablets may be given without regard to meals.
- Ensure that capsules and tablets are not chewed or crushed. They **must be** swallowed whole.

### Topical

- Prophylaxis for neonatal eye infection: Ribbon of ointment approximately 1 cm long is placed into lower conjunctival sac of neonate shortly after birth. Use a new tube of erythromycin for each neonate.
- Store all forms at 20°–25° C (68°–77° F) in tightly capped containers unless otherwise directed by manufacturer.

**ADVERSE EFFECTS** (≥1%) **GI:** *Nausea, vomiting, abdominal cramping,* diarrhea, heartburn, anorexia. **CV:** Torsade de pointes, <u>ventricular arrhythmia</u>, ventricular tachycardia. **Body as a Whole:** Fever, eosinophilia, urticaria, skin eruptions, fixed drug eruption, anaphylaxis. Superinfections by nonsusceptible bacteria, yeasts, or fungi. **Special Senses:** Ototoxicity: Reversible bilateral hearing loss, tinnitus, vertigo. **Digestive:** (Estolate) Cholestatic hepatitis syndrome. **Skin:** (Topical use) Erythema, desquamation, burning, tenderness, dryness or oiliness, pruritus.

**DIAGNOSTIC TEST INTERFERENCE** False elevations of ***urinary catecholamines, urinary steroids,*** and ***AST, ALT*** (by ***colorimetric methods***).

**INTERACTIONS Drug:** Serum levels and toxicities of **alfentanil, bexarotene, carbamazepine, cevimeline, cilostazol, clozapine, cyclosporine, disopyramide, estazolam, fentanyl, midazolam, methadone, modafinil, quinidine, sirolimus, digoxin, theophylline, triazolam, warfarin** are increased. Use is contraindicated with **eliglustat, ezetimibe, filbanserin, itaconazole, ketoconazole, lomitapide, lovastatin, pimozide, simvastatin, ergotamine, dihydroergotamine** may increase peripheral vasospasm. Do not use with drugs that prolong QT interval (e.g., **abarelix, asenapine, bepridil, chloroquine, clozapine, disopyramide, dofetilide, dronedarone, droperidol, fluconazole, levomethadyl, nilotinib, posaconazole, saquinavir, thioridazine, ziprasidone**). **Food: Grapefruit juice** may increase side effects.

## PHARMACOKINETICS **Absorption:** Most erythromycins are absorbed in small intestine. **Peak:** 1–4 h PO. **Distribution:** Widely distributed to most body tissues; low concentrations in CSF; concentrates in liver and bile; crosses placenta. **Metabolism:** Partially in liver. **Elimination:** Primarily in bile; excreted in breast milk. **Half-Life:** 1.5–2 h.

## NURSING IMPLICATIONS

### Assessment & Drug Effects

- Report onset of GI symptoms after PO administration. These are dose related; if symptoms persist after dosage reduction, prescriber may prescribe drug to be given with meals in spite of impaired absorption.
- Monitor for adverse GI effects. Pseudomembranous enterocolitis (see Appendix F), a potentially life-threatening condition, may occur during or after antibiotic therapy.
- Observe for S&S of superinfection by overgrowth of nonsusceptible bacteria or fungi. Emergence of resistant staphylococcal strains is highly predictable during prolonged therapy.
- Monitor for S&S of hepatotoxicity. Premonitory S&S include: Abdominal pain, nausea, vomiting, fever, leukocytosis, and eosinophilia; jaundice may or may not be present. Symptoms may appear a few days after initiation of drug but usually occur after 1–2 wk of continuous therapy. Symptoms are reversible with prompt discontinuation of erythromycin.
- Monitor for ototoxicity that appears to develop most frequently in patients receiving 4 g/day or more, older adults, female patients, and patients with kidney or liver dysfunction. It is reversible with prompt discontinuation of drug.

- Monitor lab tests: Periodic LFTs during prolonged therapy.

### Patient & Family Education

- Notify prescriber for S&S of superinfection (see Appendix F).
- Notify prescriber immediately for S&S of pseudomembranous enterocolitis (see Appendix F), which may occur even after the drug is discontinued.
- Report any ototoxic effects including dizziness, vertigo, nausea, tinnitus, roaring noises, hearing impairment (see Appendix F).

# ERYTHROMYCIN ETHYLSUCCINATE

(er-ith-roe-mye'sin)

Apo-Erythro-ES ♦, E.E.S., E.E.S.-200, E.E.S.-400, EryPed

**Classification:** MACROLIDE ANTIBIOTIC
**Therapeutic:** ANTIBIOTIC
**Prototype:** Erythromycin

## AVAILABILITY Tablet, suspension

## ACTION & *THERAPEUTIC EFFECT*
Macrolide antibiotic that binds to the 50S ribosomal subunit of bacteria, thus inhibiting bacterial protein synthesis. *More active against gram-positive than gram-negative bacteria.*

## USES See ERYTHROMYCIN.

## CONTRAINDICATIONS Hypersensitivity to erythromycins or any macrolide antibiotic; history of erythromycin-associated hepatitis; preexisting liver disease; congenital QT prolongation; electrolyte imbalances.

## CAUTIOUS USE Myasthenia gravis; history of GI disease; seizure disorders; pregnancy (category B).

Common adverse effects in *italic*; life-threatening effects underlined; generic names in **bold**; classifications in SMALL CAPS; ♦ Canadian drug name; ⊚ Prototype drug

619

E

## ROUTE & DOSAGE

### Infection

*Adult:* **PO** 400 mg q6h up to 4 g/day according to severity of infection

*Child:* **PO** 30–50 mg/kg/day in 4 divided doses (max: 100 mg/kg/day) for severe infections

## ADMINISTRATION

- Note: 400 mg erythromycin ethylsuccinate is approximately equal to 250 mg erythromycin base.

### Oral

- Suspensions are stable for 14 days at room temperature unless otherwise stated by manufacturer. Note expiration date.
- Store tablets in tight containers unless otherwise directed.

## ADVERSE EFFECTS (≥1%) GI:
Diarrhea, *nausea,* vomiting, stomatitis, *abdominal cramps,* anorexia, hepatotoxicity. **Skin:** Skin eruptions. **Special Senses:** Ototoxicity. **Body as a Whole:** Potential for superinfections.

## INTERACTIONS Drug: Serum levels and toxicities of **alfentanil, bexarotene, carbamazepine, cevimeline, cilostazol, clozapine, cyclosporine, disopyramide, estazolam, fentanyl, midazolam, methadone, modafinil, quinidine, sirolimus, digoxin, theophylline, triazolam, warfarin** are increased. **Ergotamine** may increase peripheral vasospasm and may increase risk of arrhythmias.

## PHARMACOKINETICS Absorption: Readily absorbed from GI tract. **Peak:** 2 h. **Distribution:** Concentrates in liver; crosses placenta; distributed into breast milk. **Metabolism:** In liver.

**Elimination:** Primarily in bile and feces. **Half-Life:** 2–5 h.

## NURSING IMPLICATIONS

### Assessment & Drug Effects

- Cholestatic hepatitis syndrome is most likely to occur in adults who have received erythromycin estolate for more than 10 days or who have had repeated courses of therapy. The condition generally clears within 3–5 days after cessation of therapy.
- Monitor lab tests: Baseline C&S.

### Patient & Family Education

- Advise patient to report immediately the onset of adverse reactions and to be on the alert for signs and symptoms associated with jaundice (see Appendix F).
- Ototoxicity is most likely to occur in patients receiving high dosage or who have impaired kidney function. Report immediately the onset of tinnitus, vertigo, or hearing impairment.

## ERYTHROMYCIN LACTOBIONATE

(er-ith-roe-mye'sin lak'toe-bye'oh-nate)

Erythrocin Lactobionate-I.V.

**Classification:** MACROLIDE ANTIBIOTIC

Therapeutic: ANTIBIOTIC

**Prototype:** Erythromycin

## AVAILABILITY Solution for injection

## ACTION & *THERAPEUTIC EFFECT*
Soluble salt of erythromycin that binds to the 50S ribosome subunits of susceptible bacteria, resulting in the suppression of protein synthesis of bacteria. *More active against gram-positive than gram-negative bacteria.*

Common adverse effects in *italic;* life-threatening effects <u>underlined;</u> generic names in **bold;** classifications in SMALL CAPS; ♣ Canadian drug name; ◑ Prototype drug

**USES** When oral administration is not possible or the severity of infection requires immediate high serum levels. See erythromycin.

**CONTRAINDICATIONS** Hypersensitivity to erythromycin or macrolide antibiotics; congenital QT prolongation; electrolyte imbalances.

**CAUTIOUS USE** Impaired liver function; seizure disorders; pregnancy (category B); children.

## ROUTE & DOSAGE

**Infections**
*Adult/Child:* **IV** 15–20 mg/kg/day in 4 divided doses
**Legionnaires' Disease**
*Adult:* **IV** 0.5–1 g q6h × 21 days
**Pelvic Inflammatory Disease**
*Adult:* **IV** 500 mg q6h × 3d, then convert to PO

## ADMINISTRATION

Intravenous

*PREPARE:* **Intermittent/Continuous:** Initial solution is prepared by adding 10 mL sterile water for injection without preservatives to each 500 mg or fraction thereof. ▪ Shake vial until drug is completely dissolved. **Intermittent:** Further dilute each 1 g dose in 100–250 mL of LR or NS. **Continuous (preferred):** Further dilute each 1 g in 1000 mL LR or NS. ▪ Give within 4 h.
*ADMINISTER:* **Intermittent:** Give 1 g or fraction thereof over 20–60 min. ▪ Slow rate if pain develops along course of vein. **Continuous (preferred):** Continuous infusion is administered slowly, usually over 6–24 h.

*INCOMPATIBILITIES:* **Solution/additive: Dextrose**-containing solutions, **ascorbic acid, colistimethate, clindamycin, furosemide, heparin, linezolid, metaraminol, metoclopramide, tetracycline, vitamin B complex with C. Y-site: Cefepime, ceftazidime, fluconazole.**

▪ Store: **Glucceptate,** reconstituted solution is stable up to 7 days if refrigerated at 2°–8° C (36°–46° F); use solution diluted for infusion within 4 h. **Lactobionate,** reconstituted solution is stable up to 14 days if refrigerated at 2°–8° C (36°–46° F); use solution diluted for infusion within 8 h.

**ADVERSE EFFECTS** (≥1%) **Body as a Whole:** *Pain and venous irritation after IV injection;* allergic reactions, <u>anaphylaxis</u> (rare); superinfections. **GI:** *Nausea,* vomiting, diarrhea, *abdominal cramps,* variations in liver function tests following prolonged or repeated therapy. (See also ERYTHROMYCIN.)

**INTERACTIONS** **Drug:** Serum levels and toxicities of **alfentanil, bex-arotene, carbamazepine, cev-imeline, cilostazol, clozapine, cyclosporine, disopyramide, estazolam, fentanyl, midazolam, methadone, modafinil, quinidine, sirolimus, digoxin, theophylline, triazolam, warfarin** are increased. **Ergotamine** may increase peripheral vasospasm, and may increase risk of arrhythmias.

**PHARMACOKINETICS** **Peak:** 1 h. **Distribution:** Concentrates in liver; crosses placenta; distributed into breast milk. **Metabolism:** In liver. **Elimination:** Primarily in bile and feces; 12–15% in urine. **Half-Life:** 3–5 h.

Common adverse effects in *italic;* life-threatening effects <u>underlined</u>; generic names in **bold;** classifications in SMALL CAPS; ♣ Canadian drug name; ☻ Prototype drug

621

**E**

## NURSING IMPLICATIONS

### Assessment & Drug Effects

- Monitor for hearing impairment which may occur with large doses of this drug. It may occur as early as the second day and as late as the third week of therapy.
- Monitor for S&S of thrombophlebitis (see Appendix F). IV infusion of large doses is reported to increase risk.
- Monitor lab tests: Baseline C&S.

### Patient & Family Education

- Notify prescriber immediately of tinnitus, dizziness, or hearing impairment.

## ESCITALOPRAM OXALATE

(es-ci-tal'o-pram)

**Lexapro**

**Classifications:** ANTIDEPRESSANT; SELECTIVE SEROTONIN REUPTAKE INHIBITOR (SSRI)

**Therapeutic:** ANTIDEPRESSANT; SSRI

**Prototype:** Fluoxetine

### AVAILABILITY Liquid

### ACTION & THERAPEUTIC EFFECT

Selective serotonin reuptake inhibitor (SSRI) in the CNS. Antidepressant effect is presumed to be linked to its inhibition of CNS presynaptic neuronal uptake of serotonin. *Selective serotonin reuptake inhibition mechanism results in the antidepressant activity with or without anxiety symptoms.*

### USES Depression, generalized anxiety disorder.

### UNLABELED USES Treatment of panic disorders, social anxiety disorders.

### CONTRAINDICATIONS Hypersensitivity to citalopram; concurrent use of MAOIS or use within 14

days of discontinuing MAOIS; abrupt discontinuation; suicidal ideations; mania; bipolar depression; volume depleted.

### CAUTIOUS USE Hypersensitivity to other SSRIs; suicidal tendencies; bipolar disorder; obsessive-compulsive disorder, major depressive disorder, all major psychiatric disorders especially pediatric patients; depression, history of mania, hypomania; hyponatremia, ethanol intoxication, ECT, dehydration, severe renal impairment, hepatic disease; older adults; history of seizure disorders; older adults; pregnancy (category C); lactation (not within 4 h of drug ingestion). Safety and efficacy in children younger than 12 y not established.

## ROUTE & DOSAGE

### Depression, Generalized Anxiety

*Adult/Adolescent:* **PO** 10 daily, may increase to 20 mg daily if needed after 1 wk
*Geriatric:* **PO** 10 mg daily

### Panic Disorder

*Adult:* **PO** 5 daily, may increase to 20 mg daily if needed after 1 wk

### Hepatic Impairment Dosage Adjustment

*Adult:* **PO** 10 daily

## ADMINISTRATION

### Oral

- Do not begin this drug within 14 days of stopping an MAOI.
- Dose increments should be separated by at least 1 wk.
- Store at 15°–30° C (59°–86° F) in tightly closed container and protect from light.

Common adverse effects in *italic;* life-threatening effects <u>underlined;</u> generic names in **bold;** classifications in SMALL CAPS; ♣ Canadian drug name; ☉ Prototype drug

## ADVERSE EFFECTS (≥1%) **Body as a Whole:** Fatigue, fever, arthralgia, myalgia. **CV:** Palpitation, hypertension. **GI:** *Nausea,* diarrhea, dyspepsia, abdominal pain, dry mouth, vomiting, flatulence, reflux. **CNS:** Dizziness, *insomnia, somnolence,* paresthesia, migraine, tremor, vertigo. **Metabolic:** Increased or decreased weight, hyponatremia. **Respiratory:** URI, rhinitis, sinusitis. **Skin:** Increased sweating. **Urogenital:** Dysmenorrhea, decreased libido, ejaculation disorder, impotence, menstrual cramps.

## INTERACTIONS **Drug:** Combination with MAOI could result in hypertensive crisis, hyperthermia, rigidity, myoclonus, autonomic instability; **cimetidine** may increase escitalopram levels; **linezolid** may cause serotonin syndrome. Use with drugs affecting hemostasis (**aspirin, warfarin**) increases bleeding risk. **Herbal:** **St. John's wort** may cause serotonin syndrome.

## PHARMACOKINETICS **Absorption:** Rapidly absorbed from GI tract. **Onset:** Approximately 1 wk. **Peak:** 3 h. **Distribution:** 80% protein bound; crosses placenta; distributed into breast milk. **Metabolism:** In liver by CYP3A4, 2C19, and 2D6 enzymes. **Elimination:** 20% in urine, 80% in bile. **Half-Life:** 25 h.

## NURSING IMPLICATIONS

### Black Box Warning

*Escitalopram has been associated with suicidal thinking and behavior in children, adolescents, and young adults.*

### Assessment & Drug Effects
- Closely observe for worsening of depression or emergence of suici-dality, especially in adolescents or children.
- Monitor periodically HR and BP, and carefully monitor complete cardiac status in person with known or suspected cardiac disease.
- Monitor closely older adult patients for adverse effects, especially with doses greater than 20 mg/day.
- Monitor lab tests: Periodic lithium levels when given concurrently.

### Patient & Family Education
- Report promptly changes in behavior such as anxiety, agitation, depression, panic attacks, aggressiveness, and suicidal ideation.
- Do not engage in hazardous activities until reaction to this drug is known.
- Avoid using alcohol while taking escitalopram.
- Inform prescriber of commonly used OTC drugs as there is potential for drug interactions. The use of aspirin and NSAIDs can affect coagulation and cause increased risk of bleeding.
- Report distressing adverse effects including any changes in sexual functioning or response.
- Periodic ophthalmology exams are advised with long-term treatment.

## ESLICARBAZEPINE ACETATE
(es-li-car′ba-ze-peen)

Aptiom

**Classifications:** ANTICONVULSANT; TRICYCLIC
**Therapeutic:** ANTICONVULSANT
**Prototype:** Carbamazepine

## AVAILABILITY Tablet

## ACTION & *THERAPEUTIC EFFECT*
Mechanism of action thought to involve inhibition of voltage-gated sodium channels. *Decreases frequency of partial-onset seizures.*

Common adverse effects in *italic;* life-threatening effects underlined; generic names in **bold;** classifications in SMALL CAPS; ◆ Canadian drug name; ◉ Prototype drug

623

**E**

**USES** Adjunctive treatment of partial-onset seizures.

**CONTRAINDICATIONS** Hypersensitivity to eslicarbazepine or oxycarbazepine including anaphylactic reactions and angioedema; drug reaction with eosinophilia and systemic symptoms (DRESS)/multiorgan reaction; hypersensitivity or previous such reaction with oxycarbazepine; severe hematologic reactions; suicidal ideation or worsening of depression; jaundice and drug-induced hepatic injury; severe hepatic impairment; severe hyponatremia; lactation.

**CAUTIOUS USE** Depression or other psychiatric conditions; history of suicidal thoughts; renal impairment; hyponatremia or patients at risk for hyponatremia symptoms; mild to moderate hepatic impairment; thyroid disorders; pregnancy (category C).

## ROUTE & DOSAGE

**Partial-Onset Seizures**

*Adult:* **PO** 400 mg daily, may increase to 800 mg and then to 1200 mg daily in one wk intervals

**Hepatic Impairment Dosage Adjustment**

*Severe Impairment:* Not recommended

**Renal Impairment Dosage Adjustment**

*Moderate to Severe Impairment (CrCl less than 50 mL/min):* 200 mg once daily, may increase to 400–600 mg once daily after 2 wk

## ADMINISTRATION

**Oral**

- May give without regard to food.
- Tablets must be swallowed whole. They should not be crushed or chewed.
- When drug is discontinued, dose should be reduced gradually.
- Store at 15°–30° C (59°–86° F).

**ADVERSE EFFECTS** (≥1%) **Body as a Whole:** Asthenia, fall, *fatigue*, gait disturbance, peripheral edema. **CNS:** *Ataxia*, balance disorder, depression, *dizziness*, dysarthria, *headache*, insomnia, memory impairment, *somnolence, tremor, vertigo.* **CV:** Hypertension. **GI:** Abdominal pain, constipation, diarrhea, gastritis, *nausea, vomiting.* **Metabolic:** Decreased hemoglobin and hematocrit, hyponatremia, increased creatine phosphokinase, increased LDL, increased total cholesterol, increased tricylcerides. **Respiratory:** Cough. **Skin:** Rash. **Special Senses:** *Blurred vision, diplopia,* nystagmus, visual impairment. **Urogenital:** Urinary tract infection. **Other:** Multiorgan hypersensitivity/DRESS (Drug Reaction with Eosinophilia and Systemic Symptoms); anaphylaxis hypersensitivity reaction; suicidal ideation.

**DIAGNOSTIC TEST INTERFERENCE** Dose-dependent decreases in *serum T3* and *serum T4 (free* and *total).*

**INTERACTIONS Drug:** Other ANTIEPILEPTIC DRUGS (e.g., **carbamazepine, phenobarbital, phenytoin, primidone**) may decrease the levels of eslicarbazepine. Eslicarbazepine can increase the levels of other drugs that are metabolized by CYP2C19 (e.g., **clobazam, omeprazole, phenytoin**). Eslicarbazepine can decrease the levels of other drugs that are metabolized by CYP3A4 (e.g., **rosuvastatin, simvastatin**). Eslicarbazepine decreases the levels of **ethinylestradiol** and **levonorgestrel.**

Common adverse effects in *italic;* life-threatening effects <u>underlined</u>; generic names in **bold;** classifications in SMALL CAPS; ✦ Canadian drug name; ⊘ Prototype drug

## PHARMACOKINETICS Absorption: Greater than 90% bioavailable. **Peak:** 1–4 h. **Distribution:** Less than 40% plasma protein bound. **Metabolism:** Rapidly hydrolyzed to active metabolite; inactivated via conjugation. **Elimination:** Primarily renal. **Half-Life:** 13–20 h.

## NURSING IMPLICATIONS
### Assessment & Drug Effects
- Monitor for and report promptly suicidal thoughts or behavior.
- Withhold drug and notify prescriber immediately for any of the following: Manifestations of hypersensitivity (e.g., swelling of the face, eyes, lips, tongue, or difficulty in swallowing or breathing, fever, lymphadenopathy), rash or any other dermatologic reaction.
- Monitor for dizziness, ataxia, vertigo, balance disorder, gait disturbance, and abnormal coordination. Institute safety precautions as needed.
- Monitor for and report promptly signs of hyponatremia (see Appendix F).
- Monitor lab tests: Periodic serum sodium and LFTs.

### Patient & Family Education
- Do not abruptly stop taking this drug. Doing so may trigger increased seizure frequency and status epilepticus.
- Report immediately emergence or worsening of depression, unusual changes in mood or behavior, or the emergence of suicidal thoughts or behavior.
- Report promptly to prescriber: Development of a rash or other skin reaction; signs of low serum sodium (e.g., tiredness, irritability, confusion, muscle weakness spasms, more frequent or more severe seizures).
- Do not drive or engage in other potentially dangerous activities until response to drug is known.

- Notify prescriber immediately if you become or suspect you are pregnant. Women who do not wish to become pregnant should use additional or alternative non-hormonal birth control.
- Do not breast-feed while taking this drug.

E

# ESMOLOL HYDROCHLORIDE
(ess'moe-lol)
Brevibloc
**Classification:** BETA-ADRENERGIC ANTAGONIST; ANTIARRHYTHMIC
**Therapeutic:** ANTIARRHYTHMIC
**Prototype:** Propranolol

**AVAILABILITY** Solution for injection

## ACTION & *THERAPEUTIC EFFECT*
Ultrashort-acting beta$_1$-adrenergic blocking agent with cardioselective properties. Inhibits the agonist effect of catecholamines by competitive binding at beta-adrenergic receptors. Antiarrhythmic properties occur at the AV node. *Effective as an antiarrhythmic agent on the AV-nodal conduction system. Blocks sympathetically mediated increases in cardiac rate and BP since it binds predominantly to beta$_1$-receptors in cardiac tissue.*

## USES Supraventricular tachyarrhythmias (SVT) in perioperative and postoperative periods or in other critical situations. Also short-term treatment of noncompensating sinus tachycardia and in the control of heart rate for patients with MI.

## UNLABELED USES Moderate postoperative hypertension; treatment of intense transient adrenergic response to surgical stress in cardiac as well as noncardiac surgery.

## CONTRAINDICATIONS Hypersensitivity to esmolol; heart block

Common adverse effects in *italic;* life-threatening effects underlined; generic names in **bold;** classifications in SMALL CAPS; ✦Canadian drug name; ➊ Prototype drug

625

greater than first degree, severe sinus bradycardia, cardiogenic shock; decompensated HF or cardiac shock; acute bronchospasm.

**CAUTIOUS USE** History of allergy; CHF; pulmonary disease such as bronchial asthma, COPD, or pulmonary edema; diabetes mellitus; pheochromocytoma; renal impairment; hyperthyroidism; older adults; pregnancy (category C); lactation. Safe use in children younger than 18 y not established.

## ROUTE & DOSAGE

### Supraventricular Tachyarrhythmias

*Adult:* **IV** 500 mcg/kg loading dose followed by 50 mcg/kg/min, may increase dose q5–10min prn if response inadequate, may repeat loading dose followed by 100 mcg/kg/min × 4 min; may continue repeating loading dose and increasing 4-min dose by 50 mcg/kg/min prn (max: 200 mcg/kg/min)

### Intraoperative/Postoperative Tachycardia

*Adult:* **IV** 80 mg bolus followed by 150 mcg/kg/min; increase if needed (max: 300 mcg/kg/min)

## ADMINISTRATION

Intravenous

*PREPARE:* **Direct:** Use the 10 mg/mL vial undiluted for the loading dose. **IV Infusion:** Prepare maintenance infusion by adding 2.5 g to 250 mL or 5 g to 500 mL or 10 mg to 1000 mL of IV solution to yield 10 mg/mL. Compatible diluents include D5W, D5/LR, D5/NS, D5/.45NS, LR.

*ADMINISTER:* **Direct:** Give loading dose over 1 min. **IV Infusion:** • Give maintenance infusion over 4 min. • If adequate response is noted, continue maintenance infusion with periodic adjustments as needed.

*INCOMPATIBILITIES:* **Solution/additive: Diazepam, procainamide. Y-site: Acyclovir, amphotericin B cholesteryl, azathioprine, cefmandole, cefotetan, dantrolene, dexamethasone, diazepam, diazoxide, furosemide, ganciclovir, gemtuzumab, inamrinone, idomethacin, ketorolac, lansoprazole, milrinone, minocycline, oxacillin, pantoprazole, phenobarbital, warfarin.**

• Diluted infusion solution is stable for at least 24 h at room temperature.

**ADVERSE EFFECTS** (≥1%) **CNS:** Headache, *dizziness,* somnolence, confusion, agitation. **CV:** *Hypotension* (dose related), cold hands and feet, bradyarrhythmias, flushing, myocardial depression. **GI:** Nausea, vomiting. **Respiratory:** Dyspnea, chest pain, rhonchi, <u>bronchospasm</u>. **Skin:** *Infusion site inflammation* (redness, swelling, induration).

**INTERACTIONS** **Drug:** May increase **digoxin** IV levels 10–20%; **morphine** IV may increase esmolol levels by 45%; **succinylcholine** may prolong neuromuscular blockade.

**PHARMACOKINETICS** **Onset:** Less than 5 min. **Peak:** 10–20 min. **Duration:** 10–30 min. **Metabolism:** Hydrolyzed by RBC esterases. **Elimination:** In urine. **Half-Life:** 9 min.

## NURSING IMPLICATIONS

### Assessment & Drug Effects

- Monitor BP, pulse, ECG, during esmolol infusion. Hypotension may have its onset during the initial titration phase; thereafter the risk increases with increasing doses. Usually the hypotension experienced during esmolol infusion is resolved within 30 min after infusion is reduced or discontinued.

- Change injection site if local reaction occurs. IV site reactions (burning, erythema) or diaphoresis may develop during infusion. Both reactions are temporary. Blood chemistry abnormalities have not been reported.

- Overdose symptoms: Discontinue administration if the following symptoms occur: Bradycardia, severe dizziness or drowsiness, dyspnea, bluish-colored fingernails or palms of hands, seizures.

## ESOMEPRAZOLE MAGNESIUM

(e-so-me′pra-zole)

Nexium

**Classification:** PROTON PUMP INHIBITOR
**Therapeutic** ANTIULCER
**Prototype:** Omeprazole

**AVAILABILITY** Capsule; powder for injection; oral suspension

## ACTION & *THERAPEUTIC EFFECT*

Isomer of omeprazole, a weak base that is converted to the active form in the highly acidic environment of the gastric parietal cells. Inhibits the enzyme $H^+ K^+$-ATPase (the acid pump), thus suppressing gastric acid secretion. *Due to inhibition of the $H^+K^+$-ATPase, esomeprazole substantially decreases both basal and stimulated acid secretion through inhibition of the acid pump in parietal cells.*

**USES** Erosive esophagitis, gastrointestinal reflux disease (GERD), hypersecretory diseases, duodenal ulcer associated with *H. pylori* in combination with antibiotics.

**CONTRAINDICATIONS** Hypersensitivity to esomeprazole, magnesium, omeprazole, or other proton pump inhibitors; gastric malignancy; lactation.

**CAUTIOUS USE** Severe renal insufficiency; severe hepatic impairment; treatment for more than a year; gastric ulcers; elderly; IBD, GI disease; pregnancy (category B). Safe use in infants younger than 1 mo has not been established.

## ROUTE & DOSAGE

### Healing of Erosive Esophagitis

*Adult/Adolescent:* **PO/IV** 20–40 mg daily at least 1 h before meals × 4–8 wk
*Child/Infant:* **PO** 2.5–10 mg daily × 6 wk (see package insert for weight based dose)

### GERD, Erosive Esophagitis Maintenance

*Adult/Adolescent:* **PO/IV** 20–40 mg daily at least 1 h before meals × 4–8 wk
*Child (1 y or older):* **PO** 20 kg or greater: 10–20 mg daily at least 1 h before meals up to 8 wk; *weight less than 20 kg:* 10 mg daily at least 1 h before meals up to 8 wk

### Duodenal Ulcer

*Adult:* **PO** 40 mg daily × 10 days

### Hypersecretory Disease (Zollinger-Ellison)

*Adult:* **PO** 40 mg b.i.d.

### NSAID Ulcer Prophylaxis

*Adult:* **PO** 20–40 mg daily

---

Common adverse effects in *italic*; life-threatening effects <u>underlined</u>; generic names in **bold**; classifications in SMALL CAPS; ◆Canadian drug name; ◐ Prototype drug

E

## GERD Associated with History or Erosive Esophagitis

*Adult:* **IV** 20–40 daily × 10 days
*Adolescent/Child (greater than 55 kg):* **IV** 20 mg daily
*Adolescent/Child (less than 55 kg):* 10 mg daily
*Infant (older than 1 mo):* 0.5 mg/kg daily

### Hepatic Impairment Dosage Adjustment

*Child-Pugh class C:* Do not exceed 20 mg/day

## ADMINISTRATION

### Oral

- Give at least 1 h before eating.
- Do not crush or chew capsule. **Must be** swallowed whole.
- Open capsule and mix pellets with applesauce (cold or room temperature) if patient cannot swallow capsules. **Do not** crush pellets. Applesauce should be swallowed immediately after mixing without chewing.
- May take with antacids.
- Store in the original blister package 15°–30° C (59°–86° F).

### Intravenous

**PREPARE: Direct:** Reconstitute powder with 5 mL of NS. **IV Infusion:** Further dilute reconstituted solution in 50 mL of NS, LR, or D5W.

**ADMINISTER: Direct:** Withdraw required dose from reconstituted solution and give over no less than 3 min. **Do not** give direct IV to children. **IV Infusion:** Give IV solution over 10–30 min.

**INCOMPATIBILITIES:** Do not give simultaneously with any other medication through the same IV site or line.

- Flush IV line with NS, LR, or D5W before/after infusion.
- Store reconstituted solution at room temperature up to 30° C (86° F); give within 12 h of reconstitution with NS or LR and within 6 h of reconstitution with D5W.

## ADVERSE EFFECTS (≥1%) CNS:
Headache. **GI:** Nausea, vomiting, diarrhea, constipation, abdominal pain, flatulence, dry mouth.

## INTERACTIONS Drug: May increase **diazepam, phenytoin, warfarin** levels. May decrease levels of **atazanavir** and **nelfinavir. Food:** Food decreases absorption by up to 35%.

## PHARMACOKINETICS Absorption: Destroyed in acidic environment, therefore capsules are designed for delayed absorption in the small intestine. 70% reaches systemic circulation. **Metabolism:** In liver by CYP2C19. **Elimination:** Inactive metabolites excreted in both urine and feces. **Half-Life:** 1.5 h.

## NURSING IMPLICATIONS

### Assessment & Drug Effects

- Monitor for S&S of adverse CNS effects (vertigo, agitation, depression) especially in severely ill patients.
- Monitor phenytoin levels with concurrent use.
- Monitor INR/PT with concurrent warfarin use.
- Monitor lab tests: Periodic serum magnesium with drugs, such as diuretics, that might lower magnesium levels.

### Patient & Family Education

- Report any changes in urinary elimination such as pain or discomfort associated with urination to prescriber.

---

Common adverse effects in *italic;* life-threatening effects <u>underlined</u>; generic names in **bold;** classifications in SMALL CAPS; ♣ Canadian drug name; ⊙ Prototype drug

- Report severe diarrhea. Drug may need to be discontinued.

# ESTAZOLAM
(es-ta-zo'lam)

**Classifications:** SEDATIVE-HYPNOTIC, NONBARBITUATE; BENZODIAZEPINE
Therapeutic: SEDATIVE
**Prototype:** Triazolam
**Controlled Substance:** Schedule IV

## AVAILABILITY Tablet

## ACTION & *THERAPEUTIC EFFECT*

Benzodiazepine whose effects (anxiolytic, sedative, hypnotic, skeletal muscle relaxant) are mediated by the inhibitory neurotransmitter gamma-aminobutyric acid (GABA). GABA acts at the thalamic, hypothalamic, and limbic levels of CNS. *Benzodiazepines generally decrease the number of awakenings from sleep. Stage 2 sleep is increased with all benzodiazepines. Estazolam shortens stages 3 and 4 (slow-wave sleep), and REM sleep is shortened. The total sleep time, however, is increased.*

## USES Short-term management of insomnia.

## CONTRAINDICATIONS Known sensitivity to benzodiazepines; acute closed-angle glaucoma, primary depressive disorders or psychosis; abrupt discontinuation; coma, shock, acute alcohol intoxication; pregnancy (category X); lactation.

## CAUTIOUS USE Renal and hepatic impairment, renal failure; organic brain syndrome, alcoholism, benzodiazepine dependence, suicidal ideations, CNS depression, seizure disorder, status epilepticus; substance abuse; shock, coma; dementia, mania, psychosis; myasthenia gravis, Parkinson's disease; sleep apnea; open-angle glaucoma, GI disorders, older adult and debilitated patients; limited pulmonary reserve, pulmonary disease, COPD. Safe use in children younger than 18 y not established.

## ROUTE & DOSAGE

### Insomnia
*Adult:* **PO** 1 mg at bedtime, may increase up to 2 mg if necessary (older adult patients may start with 0.5 mg at bedtime)

## ADMINISTRATION

### Oral
- For older adult patients in good health, a 1 mg dose is indicated; reduce initial dose to 0.5 mg for debilitated or small older adult patients.
- Dosage reduction also may be needed in the presence of hepatic impairment.

## ADVERSE EFFECTS (≥1%) CNS:
Headache, dizziness, impaired coordination, hypokinesia, *somnolence*, hangover, weakness. **CV:** Palpitations, arrhythmias, syncope (all rare). **Hematologic:** <u>Leukopenia</u>, <u>agranulocytosis</u>. **GI:** Constipation, xerostomia, anorexia, flatulence, vomiting. **Musculoskeletal:** Arthritis, arthralgia, myalgia, muscle spasm.

## INTERACTIONS Drug: Cimetidine
may decrease metabolism of estazolam and increase its effects; **alcohol** and other CNS DEPRESSANTS may increase drowsiness; CYP3A4 inhibitors (**ketoconazole, itraconazole, nefazodone, diltiazem, fluvoxamine, cimetidine, isoniazid, erythromycin**) can increase concentrations

Common adverse effects in *italic;* life-threatening effects <u>underlined;</u> generic names in **bold;** classifications in SMALL CAPS; ♣Canadian drug name; ⏻ Prototype drug

629

and toxicity of estazolam; **carbamaz-epine, phenytoin, rifampin,** BARBITURATES may decrease estazolam concentrations. **Food: Grapefruit juice** greater than 1 quart may increase toxicity. **Herbal: Kava, valerian** may potentiate sedation.

## PHARMACOKINETICS **Absorption:** Rapidly absorbed from GI tract. **Onset:** 20–30 min. **Peak:** 2 h. **Distribution:** Crosses rapidly into brain; crosses placenta; distributed into breast milk. **Metabolism:** Extensively in liver. **Elimination:** In urine. **Half-Life:** 10–24 h.

## NURSING IMPLICATIONS

### Assessment & Drug Effects

- Monitor for improvement in S&S of insomnia.
- Assess for excess CNS depression or daytime sedation.
- Assess for safety, especially with older adult or debilitated patients, as dizziness and impaired coordination are known adverse effects.

### Patient & Family Education

- Learn adverse effects and report those experienced to the prescriber.
- Avoid using this drug in combination with other CNS depressant drugs or alcohol.
- Do not drive or engage in other potentially hazardous activities until response to drug is known.

# ESTRADIOL 🅟

(ess-tra-dye′ole)

Alora, Climara, Divigel, Elestrin, Estrace, Estring, EstroGel, Evamist, Menostar, Minivelle, Vivelle, Vivelle DOT, Vagifem

# ESTRADIOL ACETATE

Femring

# ESTRADIOL CYPIONATE

Depo-Estradiol

# ESTRADIOL VALERATE

Delestrogen

**Classification:** ESTROGEN
**Therapeutic:** ESTROGEN REPLACEMENT

**AVAILABILITY Estradiol:** Oral tablet; topical gel; topical spray; transdermal patch; vaginal cream; vaginal tablet. **Cypionate:** Solution for injection. **Valerate:** Solution for injection

## ACTION & *THERAPEUTIC EFFECT*

Estrogens exert their effects by binding to and activating intracellular estrogen receptors which modulate expression of many genes. Estradiol is the predominant estrogen during reproductive years. It acts as a growth hormone which stimulates and maintains tissue in reproductive organs and it reduces bone resorption and increases bone formation. *Estradiol is effective in controlling symptoms of menopause due to natural decline of circulating endogenous estrogens.*

## USES Natural or surgical menopausal symptoms, kraurosis vulvae, atrophic vaginitis, primary ovarian failure, female hypogonadism, castration. Used adjunctively with diet, calcium, and physical therapy to prevent and treat postmenopausal osteoporosis; also for palliation in advanced prostatic carcinoma and inoperable metastatic breast cancer in women at least 5 y after menopause. Combined with progestins in many oral contraceptive formulations.

## CONTRAINDICATIONS Estrogenic-dependent neoplasms, breast cancer (except in selected patients being treated for metastatic disease). History of thromboembolic disorders; history of stroke; active

Common adverse effects in *italic;* life-threatening effects <u>underlined</u>; generic names in **bold**; classifications in SMALL CAPS; ♣ Canadian drug name; 🅟 Prototype drug arterial thrombosis, antithrombin deficiency, or thrombophilic disorders; undiagnosed abnormal genital bleeding; uterine fibroids; endometriosis; history of cholestatic disease; hepatic dysfunction or disease; thyroid dysfunction; blood dyscrasias; known protein C, protein S, or antithrombin deficiency; hypercalcemia; lupus (SLE); known or suspected pregnancy (category X).

**CAUTIOUS USE** Adolescents with incomplete bone growth; endometriosis; hypertension, cardiac insufficiency; diseases of calcium and phosphate metabolism (metabolic bone disease); cerebrovascular disease; mental depression; benign breast disease, family history of breast or genital tract neoplasm; DM; CAD; SLE; gallbladder disease; preexisting leiomyoma, abnormal mammogram, history of idiopathic jaundice of pregnancy; varicosities; asthma; epilepsy; migraine headaches; liver or kidney dysfunction; jaundice, acute intermittent porphyria, pyridoxine deficiency.

## ROUTE & DOSAGE

**Menopause, Atrophic Vaginitis, Kraurosis Vulvae**

*Adult:* **PO** 0.5–2 mg/day; **Topical** 2–4 g vaginal cream intravaginally once/day for 1–2 wk, then 1–2 g/day for 1–2 wk, then 1 g 1–3 × wk; **Transdermal patch** Weekly or twice a week depending on product directions; **EstroGel** Apply 1.25 g (one-half applicatorful) to one arm every day (usually in the morning). **IM Cypionate** 1–5 mg once q3–4wk; **Valerate** 10–25 mg once q4wk; **Divigel** Apply one packet to upper thigh daily (alternate legs); **Evamist** Apply one spray to inner forearm daily, dose may be increased to 2–3 sprays daily

**Metastatic Breast Cancer**

*Adult:* **PO** 10 mg t.i.d. × 3 mo

**Prostatic Cancer**

*Adult:* **PO** 1–2 mg t.i.d. **IM Valerate** 30 mg once q1–2wk

## ADMINISTRATION

### Oral

- Give with or immediately after solid food to reduce nausea.
- Protect tablets from light and moisture in well-closed container. Protect from freezing, unless otherwise directed by manufacturer.

### Intravaginal

- Insert calibrated dosage applicator approximately 5 cm (2 in.) into vagina, directing it slightly back toward sacrum. Instill medication by pushing plunger. Patient should remain in recumbent position about 30 min to prevent losing the medication. Observe perineal area before each administration: If mucosa is red, swollen, or excoriated or if there is a change in vaginal discharge, report to prescriber.

### Topical

- Cleanse and dry selected skin area. Apply as directed under Route & Dosage.

### Transdermal

- Cleanse and dry selected skin area on trunk of body, preferably the abdomen. Avoid application to the breasts, to an irritated, abraded, oily area, or to the waistline. If system falls off, it may be reapplied, or if necessary, a new one can be applied. Return to original treatment schedule. Rotate application site with an interval of at least 1 wk between applications to a particular site.

Common adverse effects in *italic*; life-threatening effects underlined; generic names in **bold**; classifications in SMALL CAPS; ✤ Canadian drug name; ⊕ Prototype drug

631

**E**

## Intramuscular

- Give deep with at least a 21-gauge needle in the gluteal muscle.
- Store at 15°–30° C (59°–86° F); protect from light and freezing.

## ADVERSE EFFECTS (≥1%) CNS:
Headache, migraine, dizziness, mental depression, chorea, convulsions, increased risk of dementia. **CV:** <u>Thromboembolic disorders</u>, stroke, CAD, hypertension. **Special Senses:** Intolerance to contact lenses, worsening of myopia or astigmatism, scotomas. **GI:** *Nausea,* vomiting, anorexia, increased appetite, diarrhea, abdominal cramps or pain, constipation, bloating, colitis, acute pancreatitis, cholestatic jaundice, benign hepatoadenoma. **Urogenital:** Mastodynia, breast secretion, spotting, changes in menstrual flow, dysmenorrhea, amenorrhea, cervical erosion, altered cervical secretions, premenstrual-like syndrome, vaginal candidiasis, endometrial cystic hyperplasia, reactivation of endometriosis, increased size of preexisting fibromyomas, cystitis-like syndrome, hemolytic uremic syndrome, change in libido; in men: Gynecomastia, testicular atrophy, feminization, impotence (reversible). **Metabolic:** Reduced carbohydrate tolerance, hyperglycemia, hypercalcemia, folic acid deficiency, fluid retention. **Skin:** Dermatitis, pruritus, seborrhea, oily skin, acne; photosensitivity, chloasma, loss of scalp hair, hirsutism. **Body as a Whole:** Pain and postinjection flare at injection site; sterile abscess; leg cramps, weight changes. **Hematologic:** Acute intermittent porphyria.

## DIAGNOSTIC TEST INTERFERENCE
Estradiol reduces response of *metyrapone* test and excretion of *pregnanediol*. *Increases: BSP* retention, norepinephrine-induced *platelet aggregability, hydrocortisone, PBI, T₄, sodium, thyroxine-binding globulin (TBG), prothrombin and factors VII, VIII, IX,* and *X; serum triglyceride,* and *phospholipid* concentrations, *renin* substrate. *Decreases: Antithrombin III, pyridoxine,* and *serum folate* concentrations, serum *cholesterol,* values for the $T_3$ *resin uptake* test, *glucose tolerance.* May cause false-positive test for *LE cells* or *antinuclear antibodies (ANA).*

## INTERACTIONS Drug: BARBITURATES, **bosentan, phenytoin, rifampin** decrease estrogen effect by increasing its metabolism; ORAL ANTICOAGULANTS may decrease hypoprothrombinemic effects; interfere with effects of **bromocriptine;** may increase levels and toxicity of **cyclosporine,** TRICYCLIC ANTIDEPRESSANTS, **theophylline;** decrease effectiveness of **amprenavir, clofibrate.**

## PHARMACOKINETICS Absorption:
Rapid from GI tract; readily through skin and mucous membranes; slow from IM injections. **Distribution:** Throughout body tissues, especially in adipose tissue; crosses placenta. **Metabolism:** Primarily in liver. **Elimination:** In urine; in breast milk.

## NURSING IMPLICATIONS

### Assessment & Drug Effects
- Monitor for and promptly report any of the following: Abnormal vaginal

bleeding; S&S of CV problems (e.g., shortness of breath, chest pain, calf tenderness, dizziness, visual changes); abdominal pain or other signs of gall bladder disease.

- Monitor adverse GI effects. Nausea, frequently at breakfast time, usually disappears after 1 or 2 wk of drug use.
- Check BP on a regular basis in patients with cardiac or kidney dysfunction or hypertension; monitored carefully.
- Note: Severe hypercalcemia (greater than 15 mg/dL) may be caused by estradiol therapy in patients with breast cancer and bone metastasis.

**Patient & Family Education**

- Notify prescriber of intermittent breakthrough bleeding, spotting, bleeding, or unexplained and sudden pain.
- Determine weight under standard conditions 1 or 2 × wk; report sudden weight gain or other signs of fluid retention.
- Notify prescriber of calf pain upon flexing foot and the following symptoms of thromboembolic disorders: Tenderness, swelling, and redness in extremity; sudden, severe headache or chest pain; slurring of speech; change in vision; tenderness, pain, sudden shortness of breath.
- Learn breast self-examination and perform every month.
- Report persistent or recurrent upper abdominal pain as it may indicate gall bladder problems.
- Monitor blood glucose for loss of glycemic control if diabetic.
- Decrease caffeine intake, since estrogen depresses caffeine metabolism.
- Learn self-examination of breasts and follow a monthly schedule.
- Estrogen-induced feminization and impotence in male patients are reversible with termination of therapy.

# ESTRAMUSTINE PHOSPHATE SODIUM

(ess-tra-muss'teen)

Emcyt

**Classifications:** ANTINEOPLASTIC; ALKYLATING AGENT; NITROGEN MUSTARD

**Therapeutic:** ANTINEOPLASTIC

**Prototype:** Cyclophosphamide

**AVAILABILITY** Capsule

**ACTION & *THERAPEUTIC EFFECT***
Conjugate of estradiol and the carbamate of nitrogen mustard. Incorporation of estramustine in tumor tissues is probably due to the presence of estramustine-binding protein (EMBP), which is found in prostate carcinoma, glioma, melanoma, and breast carcinoma. Binds to proteins and microtubulin resulting in microtubule changes in the cell division cycle, thus arresting cell division in the G2/M phase of the cell cycle. *Major effectiveness reported to be in patients who have been refractory to estrogen therapy alone.*

**USES** Prostate cancer.

**CONTRAINDICATIONS** Hypersensitivity to either estradiol or nitrogen mustard; active thrombophlebitis or thromboembolic disorders; pregnancy (category D); lactation.

**CAUTIOUS USE** History of thrombophlebitis, thromboses, or thromboembolic disorders; cerebrovascular or coronary artery disease; gallstones or peptic ulcer; impaired liver function; metabolic bone diseases associated with hypercalcemia; diabetes mellitus; hypertension; conditions that might be aggravated by fluid retention (e.g., epilepsy, migraine, kidney dysfunction); older adults.

---

Common adverse effects in *italic;* life-threatening effects underlined; generic names in **bold;** classifications in SMALL CAPS; ◆Canadian drug name; ☯ Prototype drug

**E**

## ROUTE & DOSAGE

**Prostate Cancer**

*Adult:* **PO** 14 mg/kg/day or 600 mg/m²/day in 3–4 divided doses

## ADMINISTRATION

**Oral**

- Give with meals to reduce incidence of GI adverse effects. Some patients require drug withdrawal because of intolerable GI effects.
- Store at 2°–8° C (38°–46° F) in tight, light-resistant containers, unless otherwise directed by manufacturer.

## ADVERSE EFFECTS (≥1%) **CNS:**
Lethargy, emotional lability, insomnia, headache, anxiety. **CV:** CVA, <u>MI</u>, *thrombophlebitis,* CHF, *peripheral edema.* **GI:** *Nausea,* diarrhea, anorexia, flatulence, vomiting, thirst, GI bleeding. **Hematologic:** <u>Leukopenia</u>, <u>thrombocytopenia</u>, *abnormalities in liver function tests,* hypercalcemia, <u>bone marrow depression</u> (rare). **Respiratory:** Hoarseness, burning sensation in throat, dyspnea, upper respiratory discharge, <u>pulmonary emboli</u>. **Skin:** Rash, pruritus, urticaria, dry skin, easy bruising, flushing, peeling skin and fingertips, thinning hair. **Special Senses:** Tearing of eyes. **Urogenital:** Gynecomastia, breast tenderness, impotence. **Endocrine:** Decrease in glucose tolerance. **Musculoskeletal:** Leg cramps.

## INTERACTIONS **Food:** Milk, dairy products, calcium supplements may decrease estramustine absorption.

## PHARMACOKINETICS **Absorption:** Readily absorbed from GI tract. **Peak:** 2–3 h. **Metabolism:** Dephosphorylated in intestines to estramustine, estradiol, and nitrogen mustard; further metabolized in liver. **Elimination:** In feces via bile. **Half-Life:** 20 h.

## NURSING IMPLICATIONS

### Assessment & Drug Effects

- Monitor weight and examine for peripheral edema. Be mindful that drug can cause CHF.
- Monitor I&O ratio and pattern to prevent dehydration and electrolyte imbalance, especially with vomiting or diarrhea.
- Observe diabetics closely because of possibility of estramustine-induced reduction in glucose tolerance.
- Monitor lab tests: Baseline and periodic LFTs and bilirubin; repeat after drug has been discontinued for 2 mo.

### Patient & Family Education

- Eat small meals at frequent intervals to reduce drug-induced nausea, eat slowly, and try cold food if food odors are offensive.
- Drink liquids 1 h before or 1 h after rather than with meals; clear liquids may be more palatable.

## ESTROGEN-PROGESTIN COMBINATIONS (CONTRACEPTIVES)
**Oral**

**Monophasic:** Apri, Alesse, Aviane, Balziva, Brevicon, Cryselle, Demulen, Desogen, Gencept, Junel, Lessina, Levlite, Levora, Loestrin, Lo/Ovral, Low-Ogestrel, Microgestin, Modicon, Nordette, Norethin, Norinyl, Nortrel, Ogestrel, Ortho-Cept, Ortho-Cyclen, Ortho-Novum, Ovcon, Portia, Previfem, Seasonale, Sprintec, Yasmin, Yaz, Zovia
**Biphasic:** LoSeasonique, Kariva, Mircette, Ortho-Novum 10/11
**Triphasic:** Aranelle, Cydessa, Enpresse, Estrostep, Estrostep Fe, Lybrel, Ortho-Novum 7/7/7, Ortho Tri-Cyclen, Ortho Tri-Cyclen

---

Common adverse effects in *italic;* life-threatening effects <u>underlined</u>; generic names in **bold;** classifications in SMALL CAPS; ✤ Canadian drug name; ⦿ Prototype drug

Lo, Tri-Norinyl, Tri-Previfem, Tri-Sprintec, Triphasil, Trivora, Velivet
**Four-Phasic:** Natazia, Quartette
**Postcoital Contraceptives (levonogesterol):** Plan B, My-Way, Next Choice One Dose

**Transdermal**
Ortho Evra
**Intravaginal**
NuvaRing
**Classification:** ESTROGEN-PROGESTIN COMBINATIONS
Therapeutic: CONTRACEPTIVE
**Prototype:** Estradiol, Norethindrone

**AVAILABILITY** Oral tablet; transdermal; intravaginal

## ACTION & *THERAPEUTIC EFFECT*

Three types of estrogen-progestin combinations are available: (1) monophasic, fixed dosage of estrogen-progestin throughout the cycle; (2) biphasic, amount of estrogen remains the same throughout cycle, less progestin in first half of cycle and increased progestin in second half; (3) triphasic, estrogen amount is the same or varies throughout cycle, progestin amount varies. *Fixed combination of estrogen and progestin produces contraception by preventing ovulation and rendering reproductive tract structures hostile to sperm penetration and zygote implantation.*

**USES** To prevent conception and to treat hypermenorrhea and endometriosis; postcoital contraceptive or "morning after pill"; moderate acne in females 15 y or older (Tri-Cyclen).

## CONTRAINDICATIONS

Familial or personal history of or existence of breast or other estrogen-dependent neoplasm, recurrent chronic cystic mastitis, patients at high risk of arterial or venous thrombotic diseases; DM with vascular disease; history of or existence of thrombophlebitis or thromboembolic disorders, cerebral vascular or coronary artery disease, MI, hepatic tumor or disease; family history of hepatic porphyria, undiagnosed abnormal vaginal bleeding, women age 35 and over who smoke, adolescents with incomplete epiphyseal closure; pregnancy (category X); lactation.

**CAUTIOUS USE** History of depression, preexisting hypertension, or cardiac or renal disease; impaired liver function, history of migraine, convulsive disorders, or asthma; multiparous women with grossly irregular menses, DM, or familial history of diabetes; gallbladder disease, lupus erythematosus, hereditity angioedema; rheumatic disease, varicosities, smokers.

## ROUTE & DOSAGE

### Contraception

*Adult:* **PO** 1 active tablet daily for 21 days, then placebo tablet or no tablets for 7 days, repeat cycle; **Continuous regimen** (Seasonale) 1 tablet daily × 84 consecutive days. Wait 7 days for withdrawal bleeding before starting next cycle; **Topical** Apply one patch once weekly for 3 wk, then have 1 wk patch-free before repeating the cycle; **Intravaginal** Insert 1 ring on or before day 5 of the cycle. Remove ring after 3 wk, followed by a 1 wk rest. Then insert new ring.

### Postcoital Contraception (levonorgesterol)

*Adult:* **PO** 1 tablet within 72 h of intercourse, some products also require a second dose 12 h later

---

Common adverse effects in *italic*; life-threatening effects <u>underlined</u>; generic names in **bold**; classifications in SMALL CAPS; ✦Canadian drug name; ☻ Prototype drug

635

E

## ADMINISTRATION

### Oral
- Give without regard to meals.
- Do not exceed 24-h intervals between the daily doses; taking with a meal or at bedtime is a helpful reminder.

### Topical
- Apply transdermal patch immediately after removing from pouch.
- Apply the adhesive side to a clean, dry area of the lower abdomen or upper quadrant of buttock.

## ADVERSE EFFECTS (≥1%) **Body as a Whole:** Paresthesias. **CV:** Malignant hypertension, thrombotic and thromboembolic disorders, *mild to moderate increase in BP*, increase in size of varicosities, edema. **Endocrine:** Estrogen excess (*nausea*, bloating, menstrual tension, cervical mucorrhea, polyposis, *chloasma, hypertension,* migraine headache, breast fullness or tenderness, edema); estrogen deficiency (hypomenorrhea, *early or mid-cycle breakthrough bleeding,* increased spotting); progestin excess (hypomenorrhea, breast regression, *vaginal candidiasis,* depression, fatigue, weight gain, increased appetite, acne, oily scalp, hair loss); progestin deficiency (late-cycle breakthrough bleeding, amenorrhea). **GI:** *Nausea,* cholelithiasis, gallbladder disease, cholestatic jaundice, benign hepatic adenomas; diarrhea, constipation, abdominal cramps. **Metabolic:** *Decreased glucose tolerance,* pyridoxine deficiency (see also diagnostic test interferences), acute intermittent porphyria. **Skin:** Rash (allergic), photosensitivity (photoallergy or phototoxicity), irritation from patch. **Special Senses:** Unexplained loss of vision, optic neuritis, proptosis, diplopia, change in corneal curvature (steepening), intolerance to contact lenses, retinal thrombosis, papilledema. **Urogenital:** Ureteral dilation, increased incidence of urinary tract infection, hemolytic uremia syndrome, renal failure, increased risk of congenital anomalies, decreased quality and quantity of breast milk, dysmenorrhea, increased size of preexisting uterine fibroids, *menstrual disorders.* Foreign body sensation, coital problems, device expulsion, vaginal discomfort, vaginitis, leukorrhea from ring.

## DIAGNOSTIC TEST INTERFERENCE

ORAL CONTRACEPTIVES (OCS) increase **BSP** retention, **prothrombin** and **coagulation factors II, VII, VIII, IX, X; platelet agregability, thyroid-binding globulin, PBI, $T_4$; transcortin; corticosteroid, triglyceride** and **phospholipid** levels; **ceruloplasmin, aldosterone, amylase, transferrin; renin** activity, **vitamin A.** OCS decrease **antithrombin III, $T_3$** resin uptake, **serum folate, glucose tolerance, albumin, vitamin $B_{12}$** and reduce the **metyrapone** test response.

## INTERACTIONS **Drug: Aminocaproic acid** may increase clotting factors, leading to hypercoagulable state; BARBITURATES, ANTICONVULSANTS, ANTIBIOTICS, **rifampin,** ANTIFUNGALS reduce efficacy of OCS and increase incidence of breakthrough bleeding and risk of pregnancy. May decrease efficacy of **lamotrigine. Herbal: St. John's wort** may decrease efficacy of OCS.

## PHARMACOKINETICS **Absorption:** Oral: Readily from GI tract; or from transdermal patch placed on abdomen, buttock, upper outer arm and upper torso (excluding breast). Vaginal insert: Norgestrel 100% absorbed. **Peak:** Patch: 48 h. **Duration:**

Patch: 1 wk. **Distribution:** Widely distributed; crosses placenta; small amount distributed into breast milk. **Metabolism:** In liver. **Elimination:** In urine and feces. **Half-Life:** 6–45 h oral. Following removal of the patch: Norelgestromin 28 h, vaginal ring: Norgestrel 29 h.

## NURSING IMPLICATIONS

### Black Box Warning

*Estrogen use in postmenopausal women has been associated with increased risk of endometrial cancer, MI, stroke, breast cancer, PE, DVT, and dementia.*

### Assessment & Drug Effects

- Monitor for and promptly report any of the following: Abnormal vaginal bleeding; S&S of CV problems (e.g., shortness of breath, chest pain, calf tenderness, dizziness, visual changes); abdominal pain or other signs of gall bladder disease.
- Check BP periodically. In some women, changes in BP occur within each cycle; in others, slow increase of pressure, particularly diastolic, over several months is significant. Drug-induced BP elevation is usually reversible with cessation of OCs.
- *Nausea* with or without vomiting occurs in approximately 10% of patients during the first cycle and is reportedly one of the major reasons for voluntary discontinuation of therapy. Most adverse effects tend to disappear in third or fourth cycle of use. Instruct patient to report symptoms that persist after fourth cycle. Dose adjustment or a different product may be indicated.
- *Hirsutism and loss of hair* are reversible with discontinuation of OCs or by change of selected combination.

- Acne may improve, worsen, or develop for first time. In women on OCs for at least 1 y, postcontraceptive acne sometimes occurs 3–4 mo after stopping drug and may continue for 6–12 mo.
- Anovulation or amenorrhea following termination of OC regimen may persist more than 6 mo. The user with pretreatment oligomenorrhea or secondary amenorrhea is most apt to have oversuppression syndrome.

### Patient & Family Education

- Use an additional method of birth control during the first week of the initial cycle.
- Consult patient information supplied with drug for management of missed doses.
- Ovulation is unlikely with omission of 1 daily dose; however, the possibility of escaped ovulation, spotting, or breakthrough bleeding increases with each missed dose.
- Discontinue medication if intra-cycle bleeding resembling menstruation occurs. Begin taking tablets from a new compact on day 5. If bleeding persists, see prescriber.
- Transdermal patches: Apply only one patch at a time and never cut or otherwise alter a patch prior to application.
- See prescriber to rule out pregnancy if 2 consecutive periods are missed, before continuing on OCs.
- Learn breast self-examination and do every month.
- Record frequent weight checks to permit early recognition of fluid retention.
- Understand the increased risk of thromboembolic and cardiovascular problems and increased incidence of gallbladder disease with OC use. Be alert to manifestations of thrombotic or thromboembolic disorders: Severe headache (especially if persistent and

E

recurrent), dizziness, blurred vision, leg or chest pain, respiratory distress, unexplained cough. Discontinue drug if any of these symptoms appear and report them promptly to prescriber.

- Report sudden abdominal pain immediately to prescriber in order to rule out ectopic pregnancy.
- Stop drug and contact prescriber if unexplained partial or complete, sudden or gradual loss of vision, protrusion of eyeballs, or blurred vision occurs.
- If OC use is accompanied by vaginal itching and irritation, report to prescriber promptly to rule out candidiasis.
- Monitor blood glucose closely if diabetic. Adjustment of antidiabetic medication may be necessary.
- Use alternate method of birth control when breast-feeding until infant is weaned.

## ESTROGENS, CONJUGATED

(ess'tro-jenz)

C.E.S. ◆, Enjuvia, Premarin

**Classification:** ESTROGENS
**Therapeutic:** FEMALE HORMONE REPLACEMENT THERAPY (HRT)
**Prototype:** Estradiol

**AVAILABILITY** Tablet; solution for injection; solution for injection; vaginal cream

## ACTION & *THERAPEUTIC EFFECT*

Circulating estrogens modulate the pituitary secretion of the gonadotropins luteinizing hormone (LH) and follicle stimulating hormone (FSH) through a negative feedback mechanism. Estrogens act to reduce the elevated levels of these gonadotropins seen in postmenopausal women. *Binds to intracellular receptors that stimulate DNA and RNA to synthesize proteins responsible for effects of estrogen.*

**USES** Atrophic vaginitis, kraurosis vulvae, and abnormal bleeding (hormonal imbalance); also female hypogonadism, primary ovarian failure, vasomotor symptoms associated with menopause; to retard progression of osteoporosis and as palliative therapy of breast and prostatic carcinomas.

**UNLABELED USES** Infertility, hyperparathyroidism.

**CONTRAINDICATIONS** History of breast cancer, except for palliative therapy; known anaphylactic reaction or angioedema to conjugated estrogens; vaginal and cervical cancers; endometrial cancer; endometrial hyperplasia; abnormal vaginal bleeding; hepatic disease or cancer; CAD; hepatic impairment; history of cholestatic jaundice associated with use of estrogen or pregnancy; hypercalcemia; ovarian cancer; history of thromboembolic disease; known protein C, protein S, or antithrombin deficiency; known or suspected pregnancy (category X).

**CAUTIOUS USE** Hypertension; gallbladder disease; DM; heart failure; kidney dysfunction.

## ROUTE & DOSAGE

| Menopause, Osteoporosis, Atrophic Vaginitis, Kraurosis Vulvae |
| --- |
| *Adult:* **PO** 0.3–1.25 mg/day for 21 days each month, adjust to lowest level that gives symptom control (0.625 mg/day or less); **IV/IM** 25 mg, repeated in 6–12 h if needed; **Topical** 2–4 g of cream/day |
| **Female Hypogonadism** |
| *Adult:* **PO** 2.5–7.5 mg/day in 1–3 divided doses for 20 days, followed by a 10-day rest period |

Common adverse effects in *italic;* life-threatening effects <u>underlined;</u> generic names in **bold;** classifications in SMALL CAPS; ◆ Canadian drug name; ❽ Prototype drug

**Breast Cancer**
*Adult:* **PO** 10 mg t.i.d. for at least 3 mo
**Prostatic Cancer Palliation**
*Adult:* **PO** 1.25–2.5 mg t.i.d.

## ADMINISTRATION

### Oral
- Give at the same time each day.

### Topical
- Use calibrated dosage applicator dispensed with the cream.

### Intramuscular
- Reconstitute by first removing approximately 5 mL of air from the dry-powder vial, then slowly inject the supplied diluent to the vial by aiming it at the side of the vial. Gently agitate to dissolve but **do not shake.**
- Use within a few hours of reconstitution.

### Intravenous

**PREPARE: Direct:** Reconstitute as for IM injection.
**ADMINISTER: Direct:** Give slowly at a rate of 5 mg/min. • Estrogen solution is compatible with D5W and NS and may be added to IV tubing just distal to the needle if necessary.
**INCOMPATIBILITIES:** Solution/additive: **Ascorbic acid.** Y-site: **Pantoprazole.**

- Store ampule and reconstituted solution at 2°–8° C (38°–46° F) and protected from light; stable for 60 days. • Discard precipitated or discolored solution.

## ADVERSE EFFECTS (≥1%) CNS:
Headache, dizziness, depression, *libido changes.* **CV:** <u>Thromboembolic disorders</u>, hypertension. **GI:** *Nausea,* vomiting, diarrhea, bloating, cholestatic jaundice. **Urogeni-** **tal:** Mastodynia, spotting, changes in menstrual flow, dysmenorrhea, amenorrhea. **Metabolic:** Reduced carbohydrate tolerance, fluid retention. **Other:** Leg cramps, intolerance to contact lenses.

## INTERACTIONS Drug: BARBITURATES, **carbamazepine, phenytoin, rifampin** decrease estrogen effect by increasing its metabolism; ORAL ANTICOAGULANTS may decrease hypoprothrombinemic effects; interfere with effects of **bromocriptine;** may increase levels and toxicity of **cyclosporine,** TRICYCLIC ANTIDEPRESSANTS, **theophylline;** decrease effectiveness of **clofibrate.**

## PHARMACOKINETICS Absorption: Rapid absorption from GI tract; readily absorbed through skin and mucous membranes (including vaginal mucosa); slow absorption from IM injections. **Distribution:** Distributed throughout body tissues, especially in adipose tissue; crosses placenta, excreted in breast milk. Conjugated estrogens are bound primarily to albumin. **Metabolism:** Metabolized primarily in liver to glucuronide and sulfate conjugates of estradiol, and estriol. **Elimination:** In urine. **Half-Life:** 4–18 h.

## NURSING IMPLICATIONS

### Black Box Warning

*Estrogen use in postmenopausal women has been associated with increased risk of endometrial cancer, MI, stroke, breast cancer, PE, DVT, and dementia.*

### Assessment & Drug Effects
- See additional implications under estradiol.
- Monitor for and report breakthrough vaginal bleeding.

Common adverse effects in *italic;* life-threatening effects <u>underlined</u>; generic names in **bold;** classifications in SMALL CAPS; ✦ Canadian drug name; ⓟ Prototype drug

639

**E**

- Assess for relief of menopausal symptoms.
- Monitor bone density annually when used for osteoporosis prophylaxis.
- Monitor lab tests: Periodic serum phosphatase levels with prostate cancer.

**Patient & Family Education**

- Be aware of importance of taking drug exactly as prescribed: Specifically, do not omit, increase, or decrease doses without advice of prescriber.
- Intravaginal administration: For self-administration, wash hands well before and after application, and avoid contact of denuded areas with the cream. Do not use tampons while on vaginal cream therapy.
- Notify prescriber promptly of adverse symptoms.
- Know signs of thrombophlebitis (see Appendix F) and report promptly if suspected.
- Review package insert to ensure understanding of estrogen therapy.

# ESTROGENS, ESTERIFIED

(ess'tro-jenz)

Estratab, Menest, Menrium, Neo-Estrone ✦

**Classification:** ESTROGEN
**Therapeutic:** ESTROGEN; FEMALE HORMONE REPLACEMENT THERAPY (HRT)
**Prototype:** Estradiol

**AVAILABILITY** Tablet

## ACTION & THERAPEUTIC EFFECT

At the cellular level, estrogens increase cervical secretions, result in proliferation of the endometrium, and increase uterine tone. Estrogens also can affect bone calcium deposition and accelerate epiphyseal closure. Estrogens appear to prevent osteoporosis associated with the onset of menopause; they generally do not reverse bone density loss that has already developed. *Binds to intracellular receptors that stimulate DNA and RNA to synthesize proteins responsible for effects of estrogen.*

**USES** Atrophic vaginitis, kraurosis vulvae and abnormal bleeding (hormonal imbalance), female hypogonadism, castration, primary ovarian failure, vasomotor symptoms associated with menopause, palliative therapy of breast and prostatic carcinomas; prevention of osteoporosis.

**CONTRAINDICATIONS** Breast cancer except as treatment; cervical cancer; endometrial cancer; endometrial hyperplasia; prostate cancer; hepatic disease or cancer; hypercalcemia; lupus (SLE); abnormal genital bleeding; thromboembolic disorders; known or suspected pregnancy (category X); lactation.

**CAUTIOUS USE** Hypertension; history of depression; gallbladder disease; DM; heart failure; risk of thromboembolic or thrombotic disease; impaired liver function; kidney dysfunction; migraine headaches; seizure disorders; women over 65 y.

## ROUTE & DOSAGE

**Menopause**

*Adult:* **PO** 0.3–1.25 mg/day for 21 days each month, adjust to lowest level that gives symptom control (0.625 mg/day or less)

**Female Hypogonadism, Primary Ovarian Failure, Female Castration**

*Adult:* **PO** 2.5–7.5 mg/day in 1–3 divided doses for 20 days followed by a 10-day rest period, during last 5 days of estrogen, give a PO progestin

**Breast Cancer**

*Adult:* **PO** 10 mg t.i.d. for 2–3 mo

**Prostatic Cancer (palliation)**

*Adult:* **PO** 1.25–2.5 mg t.i.d. for several weeks

**Prevention of Osteoporosis**

*Adult:* **PO** 0.3 mg daily

## ADMINISTRATION

### Oral

- Give with food or fluid of patient's choice.
- Store tablets at 15°–30° C (59°–86° F) in a tightly closed container.

## ADVERSE EFFECTS (≥1%) CNS:

Headache, dizziness, depression, *libido changes*. **CV:** Thromboembolic disorders, hypertension. **GI:** *Nausea,* vomiting, diarrhea, bloating, cholestatic jaundice. **Urogenital:** Mastodynia, spotting, changes in menstrual flow, dysmenorrhea, amenorrhea. **Metabolic:** Reduced carbohydrate tolerance, fluid retention. **Other:** Leg cramps, intolerance to contact lenses.

## INTERACTIONS Drug:

BARBITURATES, **phenytoin, rifampin** decrease estrogen effect by increasing its metabolism; ORAL ANTICOAGULANTS may decrease hypoprothrombinemic effects; interfere with effects of **bromocriptine;** may increase levels and toxicity of **cyclosporine,** TCAS, **theophylline;** decrease effectiveness of **clofibrate.**

## PHARMACOKINETICS Absorption:

Well absorbed with first pass metabolism. **Metabolism:** Metabolized in GI mucosa and liver to estrone, further metabolized to inactive metabolites. **Elimination:** In urine and bile. **Half-Life:** 4–18.5 h.

## NURSING IMPLICATIONS

### Black Box Warning

*Estrogen use in postmenopausal women has been associated with increased risk of endometrial cancer, MI, stroke, breast cancer, PE, DVT, and dementia.*

### Assessment & Drug Effects

- See nursing implications under estradiol.
- Monitor for and report breakthrough vaginal bleeding.
- Assess for relief of menopausal symptoms.
- Monitor bone density annually when used for osteoporosis prophylaxis.
- Monitor lab tests: Periodic serum phosphatase levels with prostate cancer.

### Patient & Family Education

- Be aware of importance of taking drug exactly as prescribed: Specifically, do not omit, increase, or decrease doses without advice of prescriber. Know what to do when a dose is missed.
- Review package insert to ensure understanding of estrogen therapy.

## ESTROPIPATE

(es-troe-pi'pate)

**Ogen, Ortho-Est**

**Classification:** ESTROGEN

**Therapeutic:** ESTROGEN; FEMALE HORMONE REPLACEMENT THERAPY (HRT)

**Prototype:** Estradiol

## AVAILABILITY Tablet; cream

## ACTION & *THERAPEUTIC EFFECT*

Estrogens exert their effects by binding to and activating intracellular

Common adverse effects in *italic;* life-threatening effects underlined; generic names in **bold;** classifications in SMALL CAPS; ♣ Canadian drug name; ✪ Prototype drug

641

estrogen receptors which modulate expression of many genes. Estrogens act as growth hormones which stimulate and maintain tissue in reproductive organs and reduce bone resorption and increase bone formation. Estrone is the predominant estrogen during post menopausal years. *Estrone is effective in controlling symptoms of menopause due to natural decline of circulating endogenous estrogens. Replaces estrogen in postmenopausal women relieving symptoms of menopause.*

**USES** Atrophic vaginitis, kraurosis vulvae, and abnormal bleeding (hormonal imbalance); also female hypogonadism, primary ovarian failure, vasomotor symptoms associated with menopause, and as palliative therapy of prostatic carcinoma.

**CONTRAINDICATIONS** Estrogen hypersensitivity; breast cancer; vaginal cancer; endometrial hyperplasia; thromboembolic disease; known or suspected pregnancy (category X); lactation.

**CAUTIOUS USE** Hypertension; gallbladder disease; DM; heart failure; kidney dysfunction; liver impairment; seizure disorders; women over 65 y.

## ROUTE & DOSAGE

### Menopause, Atrophic Vaginitis, Kraurosis Vulvae
*Adult:* **PO** 0.75–6 mg/day for 21 days each month; adjust to lowest level that gives symptom control; **Intravaginal** 2–4 g of cream once/day in a cyclic regimen

### Female Hypogonadism, Primary Ovarian Failure, Female Castration
*Adult:* **PO** 1.5–9 mg/day in 1–3 divided doses for 21 days,

followed by an 8–10-day drug-free period

## ADMINISTRATION
### Oral
- Give with food or fluid of patient's choice.

### Intravaginal
- Apply vaginal cream using calibrated dosage applicator dispensed with drug. Squeeze tube of cream to force sufficient amount into applicator so that number on plunger indicating prescribed dose is level with top of barrel.
- Store at 15°–30° C (59°–86° F) in tightly closed containers unless otherwise directed.

**ADVERSE EFFECTS** (≥1%) **CNS:** Headache, dizziness, depression, *libido changes.* **CV:** <u>Thromboembolic disorders</u>, edema, hypertension. **GI:** *Nausea,* vomiting, diarrhea, bloating, cholestatic jaundice. **Urogenital:** Mastodynia, spotting, changes in menstrual flow, dysmenorrhea, amenorrhea. **Metabolic:** Reduced carbohydrate tolerance, fluid retention. **Other:** Leg cramps, intolerance to contact lenses.

**INTERACTIONS Drug:** Carbamazepine, phenytoin, rifampin decrease estrogen levels because they increase its metabolism; may enhance steroid effects of CORTICOSTEROIDS; may decrease anticoagulant effects of ORAL ANTICOAGULANTS. **Herbal:** St. John's wort may decrease blood levels. **Dong quai, red clover, black cohosh,** and **saw palmetto** may have additive hormonal effects.

**PHARMACOKINETICS Absorption:** Absorbed with some metabolism occuring in GI tract. Some systemic absorption from vaginal administration. **Metabolism:** In GI tract and liver. **Half-Life:** 4–18.5 h.

## NURSING IMPLICATIONS

### Black Box Warning

*Estrogen use in postmenopausal women has been associated with increased risk of endometrial cancer, MI, stroke, breast cancer, PE, DVT, and dementia.*

### Assessment & Drug Effects
- See nursing implications under estradiol.
- Monitor for and report breakthrough vaginal bleeding.
- Assess for relief of menopausal symptoms.
- Monitor lab tests: Periodic serum phosphatase levels with prostate cancer.

### Patient & Family Education
- Do not use tampons while on vaginal cream therapy.
- Intravaginal administration: For self-administration, wash hands well before and after application.
- Pull plunger out of barrel and wash applicator in warm soapy water after use.
- Note: Sudden discontinuation of vaginal cream after high dosage or prolonged use may evoke withdrawal bleeding.

## ESZOPICLONE
(es-zo'pi clone)
Lunesta

**Classifications:** SEDATIVE-HYPNOTIC
**Therapeutic:** SEDATIVE-HYPNOTIC
**Controlled Substance:** Schedule IV

## AVAILABILITY Tablet

## ACTION & *THERAPEUTIC EFFECT*
Mechanism of action believed to result from its interaction with GABA-receptor complexes at binding sites close to or coupled to benzodiazepine receptors in the brain. *Improves sleep maintenance in transient insomnia.*

**USES** Treatment of insomnia.

**CONTRAINDICATIONS** Hypersensitivity to eszopiclone; alcohol intoxication; alcoholism; eszopiclone induced angioedema; suicidal tendencies or ideation; lactation.

**CAUTIOUS USE** Hepatic impairment; debilitated patients; signs and symptoms of depression; compromised respiratory function; COPD; older adults; pregnancy (category C). Safe use in children younger than 18 y is not established.

## ROUTE & DOSAGE

### Insomnia
*Adult:* **PO** 1 mg at bedtime; may increase if needed
*Geriatric:* **PO** 1 mg at bedtime (max: 2 mg)

### Severe Hepatic Impairment Dosage Adjustment
Max dose: 2 mg

## ADMINISTRATION
### Oral
- Give immediately prior to bedtime.
- Store at 15°–30° C (59°–86° F).

**ADVERSE EFFECTS** (≥1%) **CNS:** Anxiety, confusion, depression, dizziness, hallucinations, *headache,* irritability, decreased libido, nervousness, *somnolence.* **CV:** *Tachycardia,* pericardial infusion, left ventricular systolic dysfunction (LVSD). **GI:** Dry mouth, dyspepsia, nausea, vomiting. **Urogenital:** Dysmenorrhea, gynecomastia. **Respiratory:** Infection. **Skin:** Rash, pruritus. **Special Senses:** *Unpleasant taste.*

E

Common adverse effects in *italic;* life-threatening effects <u>underlined;</u> generic names in **bold;** classifications in SMALL CAPS; ♦ Canadian drug name; ❷ Prototype drug

643

**INTERACTIONS Drug:** Do not use with **amiodarone,** ANTIRETROVIRAL PROTEASE INHIBITORS, **aprepitant, clarithromycin, dalfopristin/ quinupristin, delavirdine, diltiazem, efavirenz, erythromycin, fluconazole, fluoxetine, fluvoxamine, itraconazole, ketoconazole, mifepristone, nefazodone, norfloxacin,** other systemic AZOLE ANTIFUNGALS (**miconazole** and **voriconazole**), **troleandomycin, zafirlukast** due to increased eszopiclone levels. **Ethanol** and other CNS DEPRESSANT agents can produce additive effects in combination with eszopiclone. **Herbal: St. John's wort** can increase eszopiclone levels.

**PHARMACOKINETICS Absorption:** Rapidly absorbed from GI tract. **Distribution:** 52–59% protein bound. **Peak:** 1 h. **Metabolism:** Extensive hepatic metabolism. **Elimination:** Primarily in the urine. **Half-Life:** 5–6 h.

**NURSING IMPLICATIONS**

**Assessment & Drug Effects**

- Monitor for and report worsening insomnia and cognitive or behavioral changes.
- Monitor for suicidal ideation in depressive patients.
- Monitor for S&S of CNS depression when other CNS depressants are used concurrently.
- Supervise ambulation if patient is out of bed after taking eszopiclone.

**Patient & Family Education**

- Follow directions for taking the drug (see Administration).
- Do not take this drug unless you can get at least 8 h of sleep.
- Do not consume alcohol while taking this drug.

- Do not drive or engage in potentially hazardous activities until response to drug is known.
- Report any of the following to a health care provider: Worsening insomnia, cognitive or behavioral changes, problem with reproductive function.

## ETANERCEPT ℗

(e-tan'er-cept)

Enbrel

**Classifications:** BIOLOGIC RESPONSE MODIFIER; IMMUNOMODULATOR; TUMOR NECROSIS FACTOR (TNF) MODIFIER
**Therapeutic:** DISEASE-MODIFYING ANTIRHEUMATIC (DMARD); ANTIPSORIATIC

**AVAILABILITY** Solution for injection; prefilled syringe

**ACTION & THERAPEUTIC EFFECT**
Fusion protein produced by recombinant DNA technology that binds specifically to tumor necrosis factor (TNF) and blocks it from attaching to cell surface TNF receptors. This naturally occurring cytokine (e.g., TNF) is part of the normal immune and inflammatory response. TNF mediates inflammation and modulates cellular immune responses. Elevated levels of TNF are found in the synovial fluids of rheumatoid arthritis (RA) patients. *Effectiveness is indicated by improved RA symptomatology and/ or decreased inflammation in other inflammatory disorders.*

**USES** Reduction of the signs and symptoms of RA and psoriatic RA in adults, and polyarticular juvenile RA (JRA) in children with inadequate response to other disease-modifying antirheumatic drugs. Treatment of ankylosing spondylitis, moderate-severe chronic plaque psoriasis.

Common adverse effects in *italic;* life-threatening effects <u>underlined;</u> generic names in **bold;** classifications in SMALL CAPS; ♣ Canadian drug name; ⦿ Prototype drug

## CONTRAINDICATIONS

Hypersensitivity to etanercept; malignancy; benzyl alcohol; benzyl alcohol hypersensitivity; patients with sepsis or other active infection; agranulocytosis; malignancy; bleeding, hematologic disease, intramuscular administration, intravenous administration; latex hypersensitivity; sepsis; varicella; lactation.

## CAUTIOUS USE

Immunosuppression; autoimmune disease, bone marrow suppression; diabetes mellitus; hamster protein hypersensitivity; heart failure; multiple sclerosis, neoplastic disease, neurologic disease, seizure disorder, seizures; vaccination, varicella, vasculitis; pregnancy (category B). Safety and efficacy in children younger than 2 y not established.

## ROUTE & DOSAGE

**Rheumatoid Arthritis, Psoriatic Arthritis, Ankylosing Spondylitis**

Adult: **Subcutaneous** 50 mg once weekly

**Juvenile RA**

Adolescent/Child (2–17 y): **Subcutaneous** 0.8 mg/kg weekly (max: 50 mg/week)

**Plaque Psoriasis**

Adult: **Subcutaneous** 50 twice weekly (3–4 days apart) for 3 mo, then 50 mg weekly

## ADMINISTRATION

**Subcutaneous**

- Reconstitute by slowly injecting the supplied diluent into the vial. Swirl gently to dissolve and do not shake. Reconstituted solution should be clear and colorless. Use within 6 h.
- Inject into thigh, abdomen, upper arm; rotate injection sites and never inject into an old injection site or where skin is tender, bruised, red, or hard.
- Store reconstituted solution up to 6 h refrigerated at 2°–8° C (36°–46° F). Store unopened dose tray refrigerated at 2°–8° C (36°–46° F).

## ADVERSE EFFECTS (≥1%)

**Body as a Whole:** Asthenia, *influenza*, serious *infections*, sepsis fever, monitor for reactivation of tuberculosis, increased malignancy risk. **CNS:** Headache, dizziness, cerebral ischemia, depression, demyelinating disorders (multiple sclerosis, myelitis, optic neuritis). **CV:** Heart failure, MI, myocardial ischemia, hypertension, hypotension. **GI:** Abdominal pain, diarrhea, dyspepsia, cholecystitis, pancreatitis diarrhea, GI hemorrhage. **Respiratory:** Rhinitis, URI, *pharyngitis*, cough, respiratory disorder, *sinusitis*, dyspnea may reactivate latent tuberculosis (TB). **Skin:** Rash; injection site reactions (*erythema, itching, pain, swelling*). **Musculoskeletal:** Bursitis. **Hematologic:** Pancytopenia.

## INTERACTIONS

**Drug:** Concurrent or recent use with **azathioprine, cyclophosphamide, leflunomide, methotrexate** has been associated with pancytopenia. Do not use with DMARDS due to increased risk of infection.

## PHARMACOKINETICS

**Onset:** 1–2 wk. **Peak:** 72 h. **Half-Life:** 115 h.

## NURSING IMPLICATIONS

### Black Box Warning

*Etanercept has been associated with serious, potentially fatal infections especially in those taking immunosuppressants, and with development of lymphomas and other malignancies in children and adolescents.*

Common adverse effects in *italic;* life-threatening effects underlined; generic names in **bold;** classifications in SMALL CAPS; ✦ Canadian drug name; ⊙ Prototype drug

645

### Assessment & Drug Effects
- Monitor carefully for and immediately report S&S of infection.

### Patient & Family Education
- A PPD test is recommended before starting therapy to check for TB.
- Discard all needles and syringes after use; do not reuse.
- Withhold etanercept and notify prescriber before resuming drug if you develop an infection or are exposed to varicella virus.
- Avoid vaccinations, in general, and live vaccines, in particular, while on etanercept.
- Note: Injection site reactions (e.g., redness, pain, swelling) are common in the first month of therapy but generally decrease over time.

# ETELCALCETIDE
(e-tel-kals′se-tide)
Parsabiv
**Classifications:** CALCIMIMETIC; ENDOCRINE AGENT
Therapeutic: ANTIPARATHYROID AGENT

**AVAILABILITY** Solution for injection

## ACTION & *THERAPEUTIC EFFECT*
A synthetic peptide calcimimetic that activates the calcium-sensing receptor of the parathyroid gland. *Results in decreased PTH secretion, serum calcium, and serum phosphorus levels in patients with secondary hyperparathyroidism on hemodialysis.*

**USES** Treatment of secondary hyperparathyroidism in patients with chronic kidney disease on hemodialysis.

## CONTRAINDICATIONS Hypersensitivity to etelcalcetide or components of the injection.

## CAUTIOUS USE Hypersensitivity to etelcalcetide; heart failure; seizure disorder; pregnancy; lactation. Safety and efficacy in children not established.

## ROUTE & DOSAGE

**Hyperparathyroidism**

*Adult:* **IV** 5 mg bolus 3 × wk at the end of hemodialysis; titration scenarios available in package insert (max: 15 mg 3 × wk)

## ADMINISTRATION
### Intravenous

***PREPARE:*** Do not mix or dilute prior to administration. Do not use vial if particulate matter or discoloration is observed.
***ADMINISTER:*** Administer intravenously as an undiluted IV bolus into venous line of the dialysis circuit at the end of hemodialysis during or after rinse back.
***INCOMPATIBILITIES:*** Do not mix with other IV medications.

- Store in original carton in refrigerator at 2°–8° C (36°–46° F) to protect from light. Do not expose to temparatures greater than 25° C (77° F). Use within 7 days if stored in the original carton. Use within 4 h and do not expose to direct sunlight if removed from the original carton.

## ADVERSE EFFECTS (≥ 2%) CNS:
Headache, paresthesia. **Endocrine and Metabolic:** *Decreased serum calcium, hypophosphatemia,* hypocalcemia, hyperkalemia. **GI:** *Nausea, diarrhea,* vomiting. **Muscular:** *Muscle spasm,* myalgia. **Cardiac:** Prolonged QT interval, cardiac failure. **Immunologic:** Antibody development.

## PHARMACOKINETICS Onset:
Effect seen within 30 min.

Common adverse effects in *italic*; life-threatening effects <u>underlined</u>; generic names in **bold**; classifications in SMALL CAPS; ♣ Canadian drug name; ⊙ Prototype drug

**Metabolism:** Biotransformed in blood; forms conjugates with serum albumin. **Elimination:** 60% in dialysate, 3% in urine, 4.5% in feces. **Half-Life:** 3–4 days (hemodialysis patients).

## NURSING IMPLICATIONS

### Assessment and Drug Effects

- Monitor for signs of hypocalcemia, worsening of heart failure, GI bleeding or ulceration, QT interval prolongation, and ventricular arrhythmia.
- Monitor lab tests: Baseline and routine monitoring of serum calcium and PTH levels.

### Patient & Family Education

- Notify prescriber if you have symptoms of low calcium levels such as muscle cramps or spasms, numbness or tingling, or seizures.
- Notify prescriber if you experience signs or symptoms of allergic reaction such as rash, hives, itching, shortness of breath, wheezing, cough, swelling of the face, lips, tongue, or throat; or any other signs.

## ETHACRYNIC ACID

(eth-a-krin'ik)

Edecrin

## ETHACRYNATE SODIUM

**Classifications:** ELECTROLYTIC AND WATER BALANCE AGENT; LOOP DIURETIC
**Therapeutic:** LOOP DIURETIC
**Prototype:** Furosemide

**AVAILABILITY** Tablet; solution for injection

**ACTION & THERAPEUTIC EFFECT** Inhibits sodium and chloride reabsorption in proximal tubule and most segments of loop of Henle. Promotes significant fluid excretion by inhibiting reabsorption of a large proportion of filtered sodium. *Rapid and potent diuretic effect resulting in hypotensive effect. Fluid and electrolyte loss may exceed that caused by thiazides.*

**USES** Severe edema associated with CHF, hepatic cirrhosis, ascites of malignancy, kidney disease, nephrotic syndrome, lymphedema.

**UNLABELED USES** Treatment of nephrogenic diabetes insipidus, hypercalcemia, mild to moderate hypertension, and as adjunct in therapy of hypertensive crisis complicated by pulmonary edema.

**CONTRAINDICATIONS** History of hypersensitivity to ethacrynic acid; increasing azotemia, anuria; hepatic coma, severe diarrhea, dehydration, electrolyte imbalance, hypotension, lactation.

**CAUTIOUS USE** Hepatic cirrhosis, history of hepatic encephalopathy; severe myocardial disease; older adults, cardiac patients; diabetes mellitus; history of gout; pulmonary edema associated with acute MI; diabetic mellitus; hyperaldosteronism; nephrotic syndrome; history of pancreatitis; pregnancy (category B). **IV:** Safe use in children, infants and neonates not established.

## ROUTE & DOSAGE

### Edema

*Adult:* **PO** 50–100 mg 1–2 × day, may increase by 25–50 mg prn up to 400 mg/day; **IV** 0.5–1 mg/kg or 50 mg up to 100 mg, may repeat if necessary
*Child:* **PO** 1 mg/kg daily, may increase to 3 mg/kg/day

Common adverse effects in *italic;* life-threatening effects <u>underlined</u>; generic names in **bold;** classifications in SMALL CAPS; ♣ Canadian drug name; ⊕ Prototype drug

647

## ADMINISTRATION

### Oral

- Give after a meal or food to prevent gastric irritation.
- Schedule doses to avoid nocturia and thus sleep interference. Avoid administration within at least 4 h of bedtime, if possible. This recommendation may not apply to the patient who accumulates fluid and develops respiratory symptoms during sleep.

### Intravenous

*PREPARE:* **Direct:** Reconstitute by adding 50 mL of D5W or NS to vial. ▪ Use solution within 24 h. ▪ Vials reconstituted with D5W may turn cloudy; if so, discard the vial.

*ADMINISTER:* **Direct:** Give at a rate of 10 mg/min. May give through tubing of a freely flowing, compatible infusion. ▪ If a second IV dose is required, a new site should be selected to prevent thrombophlebitis.

*INCOMPATIBILITIES:* **Solution/additive: Hydralazine, procainamide, ranitidine, tolazoline, triflupromazine.**

- Store oral and parenteral form at 15°–30° C (59°–86° F) unless otherwise directed.

## ADVERSE EFFECTS (≥1%) **CNS:**
Headache, fatigue, apprehension, confusion. **CV:** *Postural hypotension* (dizziness, light-headedness). **Metabolic:** Hyponatremia, *hypokalemia,* hypochloremic alkalosis, hypomagnesemia, hypocalcemia, hypercalciuria, hyperuricemia, hypovolemia, hematuria, glycosuria, hyperglycemia, gynecomastia, elevated BUN, creatinine, and urate levels. **Special Senses:** Vertigo, tinnitus, sense of fullness in ears, temporary or permanent deafness. **GI:** Anorexia, diarrhea, nausea, vomiting, dysphagia, abdominal discomfort or pain, GI bleeding (IV use), abnormal liver function tests. **Hematologic:** Thrombocytopenia, agranulocytosis (rare), severe neutropenia (rare). **Skin:** Skin rash, pruritus. **Body as a Whole:** Fever, chills, acute gout; local irritation and thrombophlebitis with IV injection.

## INTERACTIONS **Drug:** THIAZIDE DIURETICS increase potassium loss; increased risk of **digoxin** toxicity from hypokalemia; CORTICOSTEROIDS, **amphotericin B** increases risk of hypokalemia; decreased **lithium** clearance, so increased risk of lithium toxicity; SULFONYLUREA effect may be blunted, causing hyperglycemia; ANTIHYPERTENSIVE AGENTS increase risk of orthostatic hypotension; AMINOGLYCOSIDES may increase risk of ototoxicity; **warfarin** potentiates hypoprothrombinemia.

## PHARMACOKINETICS **Absorption:** Rapidly absorbed from GI tract. **Onset:** 30 min PO; 5 min IV. **Peak:** 2 h PO; 15–30 min IV. **Duration:** 6–8 h PO; 2 h IV. **Distribution:** Does not cross CSF. **Metabolism:** Metabolized to cysteine conjugate. **Elimination:** 30–65% in urine; 35–40% in bile. **Half-Life:** 30–70 min.

## NURSING IMPLICATIONS

### Assessment & Drug Effects

- Observe closely following IV infusion. Rapid, copious diuresis following IV administration can produce hypotension.
- Monitor IV site closely. Extravasation of IV drug causes local pain and tissue irritation from dehydration and blood volume depletion.
- Monitor BP during initial therapy. Because orthostatic hypotension can occur, supervise ambulation.
- Monitor BP and pulse throughout therapy in patients with impaired cardiac function. Diuretic-induced hypovolemia may reduce cardiac

Common adverse effects in *italic;* life-threatening effects underlined; generic names in **bold;** classifications in SMALL CAPS; ♣ Canadian drug name; ⊙ Prototype drug

output, and electrolyte loss promotes cardiotoxicity in those receiving digitalis (cardiac) glycosides.

- Establish baseline weight prior to start of therapy; weigh patient under standard conditions. Keep prescriber informed of weight loss or gain in excess of 1 kg (2 lb)/day.
- Monitor I&O ratio. Report promptly excessive diuresis, oliguria, hematuria, or sudden profuse diarrhea. Report signs to prescriber.
- Observe for and report S&S of electrolyte imbalance. Anorexia, nausea, vomiting, thirst, dry mouth, polyuria, oliguria, weakness, fatigue, dizziness, faintness, headache, muscle cramps, paresthesias, drowsiness, mental confusion.
- Report immediately possible signs of thromboembolic complications (see Appendix F).
- Impaired glucose tolerance with hyperglycemia and glycosuria has occurred in patients receiving doses in excess of 200 mg/day.
- Monitor lab tests: Baseline and periodic serum electrolytes, $CO_2$, BUN, and creatinine.

**Patient & Family Education**

- Learn S&S of hypokalemia and hyponatremia (see Appendix F), and report any of these promptly to prescriber.
- Make position changes slowly, particularly from lying to upright posture.
- Notify prescriber immediately of any evidence of impaired hearing. Hearing loss may be preceded by vertigo, tinnitus, or fullness in ears; it may be transient, lasting 1–24 h, or it may be permanent.

# ETHAMBUTOL HYDROCHLORIDE

(e-tham'byoo-tole)

Etibi ♦, Myambutol

**Classification:** ANTITUBERCULOSIS
**Therapeutic:** ANTITUBERCULAR
**Prototype:** Isoniazid

**AVAILABILITY** Tablet

**ACTION & THERAPEUTIC EFFECT**
Appears to inhibit RNA synthesis and thus arrests multiplication of tubercle bacilli. The emergence of resistant strains is delayed by administering ethambutol in combination with other antituberculosis drugs. *Synthetic antituberculosis agent that is also effective against atypical mycobacterial infections.*

**USES** In conjunction with other antituberculosis agents in treatment of pulmonary tuberculosis.

**UNLABELED USES** Atypical mycobacterial infections.

**CONTRAINDICATIONS** Hypersensitivity to ethambutol; optic neuritis, patients unable to report changes in vision (young children, or unconscious patients).

**CAUTIOUS USE** Renal impairment, hepatic disease, gout; ocular defects (e.g., cataract, recurrent ocular inflammatory conditions, diabetic retinopathy); pregnancy (category B). Safe use in children younger than 6 y not established.

**ROUTE & DOSAGE**

**Tuberculosis**

*Adult:* **PO** 15 mg/kg q24h; for retreatment start with 25 mg/kg/day for 60 days, then decrease to 15 mg/kg/day
*Child (6–12 y):* **PO** 10–15 mg/kg/day

Common adverse effects in *italic;* life-threatening effects <u>underlined;</u> generic names in **bold;** classifications in SMALL CAPS; ♦ Canadian drug name; ⦾ Prototype drug

649

**E**

## ADMINISTRATION

### Oral

▪ Give with food if GI irritation occurs.
▪ Protect ethambutol from light, moisture, and excessive heat. Store at 15°–30° C (59°–86° F) in tightly closed container unless otherwise directed.

## ADVERSE EFFECTS (≥1%) CNS:

Headache, dizziness, confusion, hallucinations, paresthesias, joint pains. **Special Senses:** Ocular toxicity: *Retrobulbar optic neuritis;* possibility of anterior optic neuritis with decrease in visual acuity, temporary loss of vision, constriction of visual fields, red–green color blindness, central and peripheral scotomas, eye pain, photophobia; retinal hemorrhage and edema. **GI:** Anorexia, nausea, vomiting, abdominal pain. **Body as a Whole:** Hypersensitivity (pruritus, dermatitis, anaphylaxis).

## INTERACTIONS Drug: Aluminum-containing antacids can decrease absorption.

## PHARMACOKINETICS Absorption:

70–80% from GI tract. **Peak:** 2–4 h. **Distribution:** Distributes to most body tissues; highest concentrations in erythrocytes, kidney, lungs, saliva; crosses placenta; distributed into breast milk. **Metabolism:** In liver. **Elimination:** 50% in urine within 24 h; 20–22% in feces. **Half-Life:** 3–4 h.

## NURSING IMPLICATIONS

### Assessment & Drug Effects

▪ Perform C&S prior to and periodically throughout therapy.
▪ Ophthalmoscopic examination is recommended prior to and at monthly intervals during therapy.
▪ Monitor I&O ratio in patients with renal impairment. Report oliguria or any significant changes in ratio or in laboratory reports of kidney

function. Systemic accumulation with toxicity can result from delayed drug excretion.
▪ Monitor lab tests: Periodic LFTs, renal function tests, and CBC.

### Patient & Family Education

▪ Adhere to drug regimen exactly and keep follow-up appointments.
▪ Notify prescriber promptly of the onset of blurred vision, changes in color perception, constriction of visual fields, or any other visual symptoms. Have eyes checked periodically. Ethambutol can cause irreversible blindness due to optic neuritis.

## ETHIONAMIDE

(e-thye-on-am′ide)
Trecator
**Classifications:** ANTITUBERCULOSIS; ANTILEPROSY (SULFONE)
Therapeutic: ANTITUBERCULAR; ANTI-LEPROSY
**Prototype:** Isoniazid

## AVAILABILITY Tablet

## ACTION & *THERAPEUTIC EFFECT*

Ethionamide appears to inhibit mycolic acid synthesis, which disrupts the formation of the mycobacterial cell wall. *Effective against human and bovine strains of* Mycobacterium tuberculosis *and M. kansasii and some strains of* Mycobacterium avium-intracellulare *complex. Also active against M. leprae.*

## USES Active tuberculosis infection (with other agents).

## UNLABELED USES Atypical mycobacterial infections and tuberculous meningitis.

## CONTRAINDICATIONS Hypersensitivity to ethionamide and chemically related drugs [e.g.,

isoniazid, niacin (nicotinamide)]; severe liver damage; hepatic encephalopathy.

**CAUTIOUS USE** Diabetes mellitus, liver dysfunction, history of psychiatric illnesses including depression; history of thyroid disease; pregnancy (category C); lactation, children younger than 12 y.

## ROUTE & DOSAGE

### Tuberculosis
Adult: **PO** 15–20 mg/kg/day
Child: **PO** 15–20 mg/kg/day in 2–3 equally divided doses (max: 1 g/day)

## ADMINISTRATION
### Oral
- Give with or after meals to minimize GI adverse effects. Some patients tolerate ethionamide best when it is taken as a single dose after the evening meal or as a single dose at bedtime.
- About 50% of patients cannot tolerate a single dose larger than 500 mg because of GI adverse effects.
- Store in a cool, dry place at 8°–15° C (46°–59° F) in a tightly closed container unless otherwise directed.

## ADVERSE EFFECTS (≥1%) **CNS:** Headache, restlessness, mental depression, drowsiness, dizziness, ataxia, hallucinations, paresthesias, convulsions. **GI:** Dose related and frequent; symptoms may be due to CNS stimulation rather than to GI irritation: Anorexia, *epigastric distress, nausea, vomiting,* metallic taste, *diarrhea,* stomatitis, sialorrhea. **Metabolic:** Elevated ALT, AST; hepatitis (with jaundice), hypothyroidism. **Urogenital:** Menorrhagia, impotence. **Body as a Whole:** Postural hypotension.

## INTERACTIONS **Drug: Cycloserine, isoniazid** may increase neurotoxic effects.

## PHARMACOKINETICS **Absorption:** 80% absorbed from GI tract. **Peak:** 3 h. **Duration:** 9 h. **Distribution:** Widely distributed including CSF; crosses placenta; distribution into breast milk unknown. **Metabolism:** In liver. **Elimination:** In urine. **Half-Life:** 3 h.

## NURSING IMPLICATIONS
### Assessment & Drug Effects
- Report onset of skin rash. Progression to exfoliative dermatitis can occur if drug is not promptly discontinued.
- Monitor blood glucose closely in the diabetic until response to drug is established. Diabetics appear to be especially prone to hepatotoxicity (see Appendix F).
- Monitor lab tests: Baseline C&S. Baseline and periodic LFTs, CBC, renal function tests, and serum glucose.

### Patient & Family Education
- Avoid alcohol or use in moderation because ethionamide may increase potential for liver dysfunction.
- Notify prescriber of S&S of hepatotoxicity (see Appendix F); generally reversible if drug is promptly withdrawn.
- Make position changes slowly and in stages, particularly from lying to upright posture if experiencing hypotension.

## ETHOSUXIMIDE ⊙
(eth-oh-sux'i-mide)
Zarontin
**Classification:** SUCCINIMIDE ANTICONVULSANT
Therapeutic: ANTICONVULSANT

---

Common adverse effects in *italic;* life-threatening effects <u>underlined;</u> generic names in **bold;** classifications in SMALL CAPS; ♣ Canadian drug name; ⊙ Prototype drug

**AVAILABILITY** Capsule; syrup

## ACTION & *THERAPEUTIC EFFECT*

Succinimide anticonvulsant that reduces the current in T-type calcium channel found on primary afferent neurons. Activation of the T channel causes low-threshold calcium spikes in neurons, believed to play a role in the spike-and-wave pattern observed during absence (petit mal) seizures. *Reduces frequency of epileptiform attacks, apparently by depressing motor cortex and elevating CNS threshold to stimuli.*

## USES
Management of absence (petit mal) seizures, myoclonic seizures, and akinetic epilepsy. May be administered with other anticonvulsants when other forms of epilepsy coexist with petit mal.

## CONTRAINDICATIONS
Hypersensitivity to succinimides; severe liver or kidney disease; bone marrow suppression; use alone in mixed types of epilepsy (may increase frequency of grand mal seizures).

## CAUTIOUS USE
Hematologic disease; preexisting hepatic disease; intermittent porphyria; renal disease; pregnancy (undetermined). Safe use in children younger than 3 y not established.

## ROUTE & DOSAGE

### Absence Seizures

*Adult/Child (6–12 y):* **PO** 250 mg b.i.d., may increase q4–7days prn (max: 1.5 g/day)
*Child (3–6 y):* **PO** 250 mg/day, may increase q4–7days prn (max: 1.5 g/day)

## ADMINISTRATION

### Oral
▪ Give with food if GI distress occurs.

▪ Store all forms at 15°–30° C (59°–86° F); capsules in tight containers, and syrup in light-resistant containers; avoid freezing.

## ADVERSE EFFECTS (≥1%)
**CNS:** Drowsiness, hiccups, ataxia, dizziness, headache, euphoria, restlessness, irritability, anxiety, hyperactivity, aggressiveness, inability to concentrate, lethargy, confusion, sleep disturbances, night terrors, hypochondriacal behavior, muscle weakness, fatigue. **Special Senses:** Myopia. **GI:** Nausea, vomiting, *anorexia, epigastric distress,* abdominal pain, *weight loss,* diarrhea, constipation, gingival hyperplasia. **Urogenital:** Vaginal bleeding. **Hematologic:** Eosinophilia, leukopenia, thrombocytopenia, agranulocytosis, pancytopenia, aplastic anemia, positive direct Coombs' test. **Skin:** Hirsutism, pruritic erythematous skin eruptions, urticaria, alopecia, erythema multiforme, exfoliative dermatitis.

## INTERACTIONS
**Drug: Carbamazepine** decreases ethosuximide levels; **isoniazid** significantly increases ethosuximide levels; levels of both **phenobarbital** and ethosuximide may be altered with increased seizure frequency. **Herbal: Ginkgo** may decrease anticonvulsant effectiveness.

## PHARMACOKINETICS
**Absorption:** Readily from GI tract. **Peak:** 4 h; steady state: 4–7 days. **Metabolism:** In liver. **Elimination:** In urine; small amounts in bile and feces. **Half-Life:** 30 h (child), 60 h (adult).

## NURSING IMPLICATIONS

### Assessment & Drug Effects
▪ Monitor adverse drug effects. GI symptoms, drowsiness, ataxia, dizziness, and other neurologic adverse effects occur frequently

Common adverse effects in *italic;* life-threatening effects underlined; generic names in **bold;** classifications in SMALL CAPS; ♣ Canadian drug name; ⚫ Prototype drug and indicate the need for dosage adjustment.

- Observe closely during period of dosage adjustment and whenever other medications are added or eliminated from the drug regimen. Therapeutic serum levels: 40–80 mcg/mL.
- Observe patients with prior history of psychiatric disturbances for behavioral changes. Close supervision is indicated. Drug should be withdrawn slowly if these symptoms appear.
- Monitor lab tests: Baseline and periodic hematologic studies, LFTs and renal function tests.

**Patient & Family Education**
- Discontinue drug only under prescriber supervision; abrupt withdrawal of ethosuximide (whether used alone or in combination therapy) may precipitate seizures or petit mal status.
- Do not drive or engage in other potentially hazardous activities until response to drug is known.
- Monitor weight on a weekly basis. Report anorexia and weight loss to prescriber; may indicate need to reduce dosage.

## ETIDRONATE DISODIUM ℗

(e-ti-droe'nate)

**Classifications:** BISPHOSPHONATE; BONE METABOLISM REGULATOR
Therapeutic: BONE METABOLISM REGULATOR

**AVAILABILITY** Tablet

## ACTION & *THERAPEUTIC EFFECT*

Inhibits bone resorption, primarily through effect on osteoclasts. Contributes to increases in bone mass and maintenance of trabecular integrity by significantly decreasing

frequency of new bone-remodeling cycles, and significantly decreasing resorption bone cavity depth without reducing the ability of osteoblasts to fill resorption cavities with normal bone. *Inhibits bone resorption and increases bone mass.*

**USES** Symptomatic Paget's disease, hypercalcemia due to malignant neoplasm, and heterotopic ossification.

**UNLABELED USES** Prevention and treatment of corticosteroid-induced osteoporosis.

**CONTRAINDICATIONS** Hypersensitivity to etidronate; clinically overt osteomalacia, abnormalities of the esophagus; pathologic fractures; renal failure; osteonecrosis of the jaw.

**CAUTIOUS USE** Renal impairment; asthma; colitis; dysphagia; esophagitis; gastritis; patients on restricted calcium and vitamin D intake; older adults; pregnancy (category C); lactation. Safe use in children younger than 18 y not established.

## ROUTE & DOSAGE

### Paget's Disease

*Adult:* **PO** 5–10 mg/kg/day for up to 6 mo or 11–20 mg/kg/day for up to 3 mo, may repeat after 3–6 mo off the drug if necessary

### Heterotopic Ossification Due to Spinal Cord Injury

*Adult:* **PO** 20 mg/kg/day for 2 wk, then 10 mg/kg/day for an additional 10 wk

### Heterotopic Ossification Due to Total Hip Arthroplasty

*Adult:* **PO** 20 mg/kg/day starting 1 mo before the procedure and continuing for 3 mo after

Common adverse effects in *italic;* life-threatening effects underlined; generic names in **bold;** classifications in SMALL CAPS; ♣ Canadian drug name; ◉ Prototype drug

653

E

## ADMINISTRATION

### Oral

- Give as single dose on empty stomach 2 h before meals with full glass of water or juice to reduce gastric irritation. Instruct patient to stay upright after taking the medication.
- Relieve GI adverse effects by dividing total oral daily dose.

## ADVERSE EFFECTS (≥1%) GI:
*Nausea,* diarrhea, *loose bowel movements,* metallic or altered taste. **Musculoskeletal:** Bone pain, increased risk of fractures in patient with Paget's disease. **Metabolic:** Hypocalcemia, hyperphosphatemia, elevated serum phosphatase, suppressed mineralization of uninvolved skeleton (focal osteomalacia). **CV:** Agranulocytosis. **Urogenital:** Renal insufficiency (high doses).

## INTERACTIONS Drug: CALCIUM SUPPLEMENTS, ANTACIDS, IRON, AND OTHER MINERAL SUPPLEMENTS may decrease absorption of etidronate (give etidronate 2 h before other drugs). **Food:** Food will decrease bioavailability of etidronate (give 2 h before meals).

## PHARMACOKINETICS Absorption: Variably from GI tract. **Distribution:** 50% distributed to bone. **Metabolism:** Not metabolized. **Elimination:** 50% in urine. **Half-Life:** 6 h.

## NURSING IMPLICATIONS

### Assessment & Drug Effects

- Report persistent nausea or diarrhea; GI adverse effects may interfere with adequate nutritional status and need to be treated promptly.
- Monitor I&O ratio, serum creatinine, or BUN of patient with impaired renal function.
- Monitor for signs of hypocalcemia. Latent tetany (hypocalcemia) may be detected by Chvostek's and Trousseau's signs and a serum calcium value of 7–8 mg/dL.
- Note: Serum phosphate levels generally return to normal 2–4 wk after medication is discontinued.
- Monitor lab tests: Periodic serum calcium and phosphate.

### Patient & Family Education

- Avoid eating 2 h before or after taking etidronate. Drug absorption is decreased by food, especially milk, milk products, and other foods high in calcium, mineral supplements, and antacids.
- Notify prescriber promptly of sudden onset of unexplained pain. Risk of pathological fractures increases when daily dose of 20 mg/kg is taken longer than 3 mo.
- Report promptly if bone pain, restricted mobility, heat over involved bone site occur.

## ETODOLAC
(e-to′do-lac)

**Classifications:** ANALGESIC, NONSTEROIDAL ANTI-INFLAMMATORY AGENT (NSAID); DISEASE-MODIFYING ANTIRHEUMATIC DRUG (DMARD)
Therapeutic: ANALGESIC, NSAID; DMARD; ANTIPYRETIC
**Prototype:** Ibuprofen

## AVAILABILITY Tablet; capsule; sustained release tablet

## ACTION & *THERAPEUTIC EFFECT*
Inhibits cyclooxygenase (COX-1 and COX-2) enzyme activity and prostaglandin synthesis. NSAIDs may also suppress production of rheumatoid factor. *Produces analgesic, antipyretic, and anti-inflammatory effects of an NSAID.*

**USES** Osteoarthritis and acute pain, rheumatoid arthritis, arthralgia, juvenile rheumatoid arthritis.

**CONTRAINDICATIONS** Hypersensitivity to NSAIDS, salicylates; ulceration or inflammation; perioperative CABG pain; asthma, urticaria, or other allergic reactions to aspirin or other NSAIDs; S&S of developing liver disease; use in labor and delivery; pregnancy (category D third trimester).

**CAUTIOUS USE** Renal impairment, liver function impairment, GI disorders, history of GI ulceration, GI bleeding; cardiac disorders including fluid retention, hypertension, heart failure; dehydration; asthma; preexisting hematologic diseases (e.g., coagulopathy and hemophilia) or thrombocytopenia; IM injections, dental work; DM; surgery when hemostasis is required; immunosuppression, neutropenia; patients over 65 y, pregnancy (category C first and second trimester); lactation. Safe use in children younger than 6 y not established.

## ROUTE & DOSAGE

**Acute Pain**
*Adult:* **PO** 200–400 mg q6–8h prn

**Osteoarthritis/Rheumatoid Arthritis**
*Adult:* **PO** 600–1200 mg/day in divided doses, (max: 1200 mg/day; **Extended release** 400–1000 mg daily

**Juvenile Rheumatoid Arthritis**
*Adolescent/Child (older than 6 y), weight 20–30 kg)* **PO**
*20–30 kg:* 400 mg daily; *31–45 kg:* 600 mg daily; *46–60 kg:* 800 mg daily; *over 60 kg:* 1000 mg daily

## ADMINISTRATION
### Oral
- Give with food or milk to reduce risk of GI ulceration.
- Ensure that sustained release form of drug is not chewed or crushed. It **must be** swallowed whole.
- Store at 15°–25° C (59°–77° F); tablets and capsules in bottles; sustained release capsules in unit-dose packages. Protect all forms from moisture.

**ADVERSE EFFECTS** (≥1%) **CV:** Fluid retention, edema. **CNS:** Dizziness, asthenia, depression, headache, drowsiness, insomnia, nervousness. **GI:** *Dyspepsia, nausea, vomiting, diarrhea,* indigestion, heartburn, abdominal pain, constipation, flatulence, gastritis, melena, peptic ulcer, GI bleeding. **Hematologic:** Thrombocytopenia, increased bleeding time. **Skin:** Rash, pruritus. **Urogenital:** Dysuria, polyuria. **Metabolic:** Hepatotoxicity, chills. **Special Senses:** Blurred vision; tinnitus. **Respiratory:** Asthma. **Muscular:** Weakness.

**DIAGNOSTIC TEST INTERFERENCE** May cause a false-positive *urinary bilirubin* test and a false-positive *ketone* test done with the dipstick method. May cause a small decrease (1 to 2 mg/dL) in *serum uric acid* levels.

**INTERACTIONS Drug:** May reduce effects of **diuretics** and antihypertensive effects of **beta-blockers** and other ANTIHYPERTENSIVE MEDICATIONS. May increase **digoxin** and **lithium** levels and nephrotoxicity due to **cyclosporine.** Do not use with **cidofovir** or with other NSAIDS. **Herbal: Feverfew, garlic, ginger, ginkgo** may increase bleeding.

**PHARMACOKINETICS Absorption:** Readily from GI tract. **Onset:** 30 min. **Peak:** 1–2 h. **Duration:** 4–12 h.

Common adverse effects in *italic;* life-threatening effects <u>underlined</u>; generic names in **bold;** classifications in SMALL CAPS; ✦ Canadian drug name; ✪ Prototype drug

655

**Distribution:** Widely distributed; 99% protein bound; not known if crosses placenta or if distributed into breast milk. **Metabolism:** Extensively in liver. **Elimination:** 72% in urine, 16% in feces. **Half-Life:** 6–7 h.

## NURSING IMPLICATIONS

### Black Box Warning

*Etodolac has been associated with increased risk of serious, potentially fatal GI bleeding and cardiovascular events (e.g., MI & CVA); risk may increase with duration of use and may be greater in the older adult and those with risk factors for CV disease.*

### Assessment & Drug Effects

- Assess for signs of GI ulceration and bleeding. Risk factors include high doses of etodolac, history of peptic ulcer disease, alcohol use, smoking, and concomitant use of aspirin.
- Monitor for and report promptly S&S of CV thrombotic events (i.e., angina, MI, TIA, or stroke).
- Assess carefully for fluid retention by monitoring weight and observing for edema in patients with a history of CHF.
- Monitor for decreased BP control in hypertensive patients.
- Monitor for drug toxicity when used concurrently with either digoxin or lithium.
- Monitor for rhinitis, urticaria, or other signs of allergic reactions.
- Monitor carefully increases in etodolac dosage with older adult patients; adverse effects are more pronounced.
- Monitor lab tests: Periodic CBC, renal function tests, and LFTs.

### Patient & Family Education

- Learn S&S of GI ulceration. Stop medication in presence of bleeding and contact the prescriber immediately.

- Stop taking drug and report promptly to prescriber if you experience chest pain, shortness of breath, weakness, slurring of speech, or other signs of a cardiac or neurologic problem.
- Do not take aspirin, which may potentiate ulcerogenic effects.

## ETOPOSIDE
(e-toe-po'side)

Etopophos, Toposar

**Classifications:** ANTINEOPLASTIC; MITOTIC INHIBITOR
**Therapeutic:** ANTINEOPLASTIC, CELL-CYCLE SPECIFIC
**Prototype:** Vincristine

**AVAILABILITY** Capsule; solution for injection; lyophilized powder for injection

### ACTION & THERAPEUTIC EFFECT

Produces cytotoxic action by arresting $G_2$ (resting or premitotic) phase of cell cycle; also acts on S phase of DNA synthesis. High doses cause lysis of cells entering mitotic phase, and lower doses inhibit cells from entering prophase. *Antineoplastic effect is due to its ability to arrest mitosis (cell division).*

**USES** Lung cancer, testicular cancer, small cell lung cancer.

**UNLABELED USES** Hodgkin's and non-Hodgkin's lymphomas, acute myelogenous (nonlymphocytic) leukemia, ovarian cancer, thyoma, trophoblastic disease.

**CONTRAINDICATIONS** Severe bone marrow depression; severe hepatic or renal impairment; existing or recent viral infection, bacterial infection; intraperitoneal, intrapleural, or intrathecal administration; pregnancy (category D); lactation.

Common adverse effects in *italic;* life-threatening effects underlined; generic names in **bold;** classifications in SMALL CAPS; ♣ Canadian drug name; ☻ Prototype drug

**CAUTIOUS USE** Impaired kidney or liver function; gout; radiation therapy. Safe use in children not established.

## ROUTE & DOSAGE

### Testicular Carcinoma

*Adult:* **IV** 100 mg/m²/day for 5 consecutive days or 100 mg/m² on days 1, 3, and 5 q3–4wk for 3–4 courses; **PO** Twice the IV dose rounded to the nearest 50 mg

### Small Cell Lung Carcinoma

*Adult:* **IV** 35 mg/m²/day for 4 consecutive days to 50 mg/m²/day for 5 consecutive days q3–4wk; **PO** Twice the IV dose rounded to the nearest 50 mg

### Hepatic Impairment Dosage Adjustment

*Total bilirubin 1.5–3 mg/dL:* Decrease by 50%; *3.1–5 mg/dL:* Decrease by 75%; *over 5 mg/dL:* Hold dose

### Renal Impairment Dosage Adjustment

*CrCl 45–60 mL/min:* Reduce dose 15%; *30–44 mL/min:* Reduce dose 20%; *less than 30 mL/min:* Reduce dose 25%

## ADMINISTRATION

### Oral

- Oral dose is usually in the range of 70–100 mg/m² daily, rounded to nearest 50 mg.
- Refrigerate capsules at 2°–8° C (36°–46° F) unless otherwise directed. Do not freeze.

### Intravenous

This drug is a cytotoxic agent and caution should be used to prevent any contact with the drug. Follow institutional or standard guidelines for preparation, handling, and disposal of cytotoxic agents.

**PREPARE: IV Infusion:** *Etoposide concentration for injection:* Each 100 mg **must be** diluted with 250–500 mL of D5W or NS to produce final concentrations of 0.2–0.4 mg/mL. *Etoposide phosphate:* Add 5 or 10 mL of sterile water for injection, D5W, NS, bacteriostatic water for injection, or bacteriostatic NS for injection to yield 20 or 10 mg/mL etoposide, respectively. ■ May be given as prepared or further diluted to as low as 0.1 mg/mL in either D5W or NS.

**ADMINISTER: IV Infusion:** Give by slow IV infusion over 30–60 min to reduce risk of hypotension and bronchospasm. ■ Before administration, inspect solution for particulate matter and discoloration. Solution should be clear and yellow. If crystals are present, discard.

**INCOMPATIBILITIES: Y-site: Cefepime, dantrolene, diazepam, filgrastim, gallium, gemtuzumab, idarubicin, indomethacin, lansoprazole, pantoprazole, phenytoin.**

■ Diluted solutions with concentration of 0.2 mg/mL are stable for 96 h, and the 0.4 mg/mL solutions are stable for 24 h under normal room fluorescent light in glass or plastic (PVC) containers. ■ Phosphate solution is stable for 24 h at room temperature or refrigerated.

**ADVERSE EFFECTS** (≥1%) **Body as a Whole:** Hypersensitivity (sweating, chills, fever, coryza, tachycardia; throat, back and general body pain; abdominal cramps, flushing, substernal chest pain, dyspnea,

Common adverse effects in *italic*; life-threatening effects underlined; generic names in **bold**; classifications in SMALL CAPS; ✦ Canadian drug name; ⊙ Prototype drug

657

bronchospasm, pulmonary edema, anaphylactoid reaction). **CNS:** Peripheral neuropathy, paresthesias, weakness, somnolence, unusual tiredness, transient confusion. **CV:** Transient hypotension; thrombophlebitis with extravasation. **GI:** *Nausea, vomiting,* dyspepsia, anorexia, diarrhea, constipation, stomatitis. **Hematologic:** <u>Leukopenia *(principally granulocytopenia), thrombocytopenia,* severe myelosuppression,</u> *anemia, pancytopenia, neutropenia.* **Respiratory:** Pleural effusion, bronchospasm. **Skin:** *Reversible alopecia* (can progress to total baldness); radiation recall dermatitis; necrosis, *pain at IV site*.

**INTERACTIONS Drug:** ANTICOAGULANTS, ANTIPLATELET AGENTS, NSAIDS, **aspirin** may increase risk of bleeding. Avoid concurrent use of LIVE VACCINES. **Food: Grapefruit juice** may decrease effect.

**PHARMACOKINETICS Absorption:** Approximately 50% from GI tract. **Peak:** 1–1.5 h. **Distribution:** Variable penetration into CSF. **Metabolism:** In liver. **Elimination:** 44–60% in urine, 2–16% in feces over 3 days. **Half-Life:** 5–10 h.

## NURSING IMPLICATIONS

### Black Box Warning

*Etoposide has been associated with severe myelosuppression with resulting infection and/or bleeding.*

### Assessment & Drug Effects

- Check IV site during and after infusion. Extravasation can cause thrombophlebitis and necrosis.
- Be prepared to treat an anaphylactoid reaction (see Appendix F). Stop infusion immediately if the reaction occurs.

- Monitor vital signs during and after infusion. Stop infusion immediately if hypotension or tachycardia develop.
- Withhold therapy when an absolute neutrophil count is below $500/mm^3$ or a platelet count below $50,000/mm^3$.
- Be alert to evidence of patient complaints that might suggest development of leukopenia (see Appendix F), infection (immunosuppression), and bleeding.
- Protect patient from any trauma that might precipitate bleeding during period of platelet nadir particularly. Withhold invasive procedures if possible.
- Monitor lab tests: Prior to each cycle and at frequent intervals CBC with platelet count; periodic renal function and LFTs.

### Patient & Family Education

- Learn possible adverse effects of etoposide, such as blood dyscrasias, alopecia, carcinogenesis, before treatment begins.
- Make position changes slowly, particularly from lying to upright position because transient hypotension after therapy is possible.
- Inspect mouth daily for ulcerations and bleeding. Avoid obvious irritants such as hot or spicy foods, smoking, and alcohol.

## ETRAVIRINE

(e-tra'vi-reen)
Intelence
**Classifications:** ANTIRETROVIRAL; NONNUCLEOSIDE REVERSE TRANSCRIPTASE INHIBITOR (NNRTI)
Therapeutic: ANTIRETROVIRAL; NNRTI
**Prototype:** Efavirenz

**AVAILABILITY** Tablet

## ACTION & *THERAPEUTIC EFFECT*

Prevents replication of HIV-1 viruses by binding directly to reverse transcriptase, thus blocking RNA- and DNA-dependent polymerase activities. *Effectiveness is indicated by reduction in viral load (plasma level HIV RNA).*

## USES
HIV-1 infection in combination with other antiretroviral agents.

## CONTRAINDICATIONS
Severe skin reactions; lactation.

## CAUTIOUS USE
Severe hepatic impairment (Child-Pugh class C); concurrent hepatitis B or C, dyslipidemia; older adults; pregnancy (category B). Safety and efficacy in children not established.

## ROUTE & DOSAGE

### HIV Infection

*Adults/Adolescent/Child (6 y or older, weight 30 kg or more*
**PO** 200 mg b.i.d.
*Adolescent/Child (6 y or older, weight 25–29 kg):*
**PO** 150 mg b.i.d.; *weight 20–24 kg:* 125 mg b.i.d.; *weight 16–19 kg:* 100 mg b.i.d.

## ADMINISTRATION

### Oral
- Give after a meal. Ensure that tablets are not chewed.
- May dissolve in water if patient cannot swallow tablets. Once dissolved, should be swallowed immediately. Rinse glass several times and instruct to swallow each time to ensure entire dose has been administered.

- Store at 15°–30° C (59°–86° F). Keep bottles closed tightly to protect from moisture. Do not remove desiccant pouches from bottle.

## ADVERSE EFFECTS (≥1%) **Body as a Whole:** Peripheral neuropathy, rhabdomyolysis, **CNS:** Fatigue, headache. **CV:** Hypertension, hemorrhagic stroke. **GI:** Abdominal pain, *diarrhea, nausea,* vomiting. **Metabolic:** Elevated creatinine, elevated LDL, elevated total cholesterol, elevated triglycerides, elevated glucose, elevated ALT, hepatic failure. **Skin:** *Rash.*

## INTERACTIONS
**Drug:** Compounds that inhibit CYP3A4, CYP2C9, and/or CYP2C19 (e.g., **itraconazole, ketoconazole**) may increase plasma levels of etravirine. Compounds that induce CYP3A4, CYP2C9, and/or CYP2C19 (e.g., **carbamazepine, phenobarbital, phenytoin**) may decrease plasma levels of etravirine. Etravirine may decrease the plasma levels of other compounds that require CYP3A4 for metabolism (e.g., HIV PROTEASE INHIBITORS) and may increase the plasma levels of other compounds that require CYP2C9 and/or CYP2C19 for metabolism (e.g., **diazepam, warfarin**). **Herbal: St. John's wort, echinacea** may decrease etravirine efficacy.

## PHARMACOKINETICS
**Peak:** 2.5 to 4 h. **Distribution:** 99.9% protein bound. **Metabolism:** In liver by CYP2C9, CYP2C19, and CYP3A4. **Elimination:** 93.7% in feces, 1.2% in urine. **Half-Life:** 41 h.

## NURSING IMPLICATIONS

### Assessment & Drug Effects
- Monitor for and report promptly potentially serious adverse reactions, including skin hypersensitivity

Common adverse effects in *italic;* life-threatening effects underlined; generic names in **bold;** classifications in SMALL CAPS; ♣ Canadian drug name; ● Prototype drug

659

reactions, muscle pain indicative of rhabdomyolysis, and S&S of hepatic dysfunction.
- Monitor for and report S&S of opportunistic infections.
- Monitor lab tests: Periodic CD4+ T cell count, plasma HIV RNA, CBC with platelet count, serum amylase, LFTs, renal function tests, and lipid profile.

**Patient & Family Education**
- Do not take on an empty stomach.
- Do not remove drying-agent pouches from medication bottle.
- Report promptly any of the following: Rash, S&S of infection, or unexplained muscle pain.
- Report use of all prescription and nonprescription medications, as well as herbs, to prescriber.

# EVEROLIMUS
(e-ver-o-li′mus)
Afinitor, Zortress
**Classifications:** BIOLOGIC RESPONSE MODIFIER; IMMUNOMODULATOR; ANTINEOPLASTIC; KINASE INHIBITOR
Therapeutic: ANTINEOPLASTIC; IMMUNOSUPPRESSANT
**Prototype:** Erlotinib

**AVAILABILITY** Tablet; oral suspension

**ACTION & THERAPEUTIC EFFECT**
Binds to an intracellular protein of several types of cancer cells and inhibits a major dysfunctional kinase pathway in cancer development. It also reduces the expression of vascular endothelial growth factor (VEGF) in these cells. *Reduces cell proliferation, angiogenesis, and glucose uptake in renal and several other types of carcinoma cells.*

**USES** Zortress only: Prophylaxis of kidney/liver transplant rejection Afinitor only: HER2 negative breast

cancer, astrocytomia, pancreatic tumors, advanced renal carcinoma, renal angiomyolipoma with tuberous sclerosis.

**CONTRAINDICATIONS** Hypersensitivity to everolimus, or other rapamycin derivatives; use in heart transplants, hypersensitivity to sirolimus (**Zortess**) only. Severe hepatic impairment (Child-Pugh class C); acute renal failure; within 30 days of liver transplant; severe noninfection pneumonitis; fungal infection; live vaccine; severe hereditary problems of galactose intolerance; pregnancy (category D); lactation.

**CAUTIOUS USE** Child-Pugh class B hepatic impairment; renal impairment; severe refractory hyperlipidemia; DM; older adults.

**ROUTE & DOSAGE**

| **Renal Cell Cancer (Afinitor)** |
|---|
| *Adult:* **PO** 10 mg once daily. 15–20 mg daily for patients taking a strong CYP3A4 inducer. |
| **PNET/HERS 2 Negative Breast Cancer** |
| *Adult:* **PO** 10 mg daily |
| **Astrocytomia (Affinitor only)** |
| *Adult/Adolescent/Child (over 3):* PO 4.5 mg/m2 qd |
| *Hepatic Impairment Dosage Adjustment* |
| *Moderate impairment (Child-Pugh class B):* Reduce to 5 mg once daily. |
| **Kidney Transplant Rejection Prophylaxis (Zortress only)** |
| *Adult:* **PO** 0.75 mg q12h |
| **Liver Transplant (Zortress only)** |
| *Adult:* **PO** 1 mg b.i.d. |

## ADMINISTRATION

**Oral**

- Give at the same time each day with/without food.
- Ensure that the tablet is swallowed whole. It should not be crushed or chewed.
- Store at 15°–30° C (59°–86° F). Protect from light and moisture.

## ADVERSE EFFECTS (≥3%) Body
as a Whole: *Asthenia,* chest pain, chills, epistaxis, *fatigue, infection,* peripheral edema, pyrexia. CNS: Dizziness, dysgeusia, headache, insomnia, pareshesia. CV: Hypertension, tachycardia. GI: Abdominal pain, *diarrhea,* dry mouth, dysphagia, hemorrhoids, *mucosal inflammation,* nausea, *stomatitis,* vomiting. Hematologic: *Anemia, decreased hemoglobin,* decreased neutrophils, decreased platelets, *lymphopenia,* hemorrhage. Metabolic: Decreased weight, elevated AST and ALT, elevated bilirubin, elevated creatinine, *hypercholesterolemia, hypertriglyceridemia, hyperglycemia, hypophosphatemia.* Musculoskeletal: Jaw pain, pain in extremity. Respiratory: Alveolitis, bronchitis, *cough, dyspnea,* interstitial lung disease, lung infiltration, nasopharyngitis, pneumonia, *pneumonitis,* pulmonary alveolar hemorrhage, pulmonary effusion, pharyngolaryngeal pain, rhinorrhea, sinusitis. Skin: Acneiform dermatitis, dry skin, erythema, hand-foot syndrome, nail disorder, onychoclasis, pruritus, *rash,* skin lesion. Special Senses: Eyelid edema. Urogenital: <u>Renal failure</u>.

## INTERACTIONS Drug: Strong inhibitors of CYP3A4 and P-glycoprotein (e.g., **ketoconazole, erythromymin, veramapil**) increase everolimus levels. Strong inducers (e.g., **rifampin**) decrease everolimus levels.

## PHARMACOKINETICS Peak:
1–2 h. **Distribution:** 74% plasma protein bound. **Metabolism:** In liver to inactive metabolites. **Elimination:** Fecal (80%) and renal (5%). **Half-Life:** 30 h.

## NURSING IMPLICATIONS

### Black Box Warning

*Everolimus has been associated with increased risk of malignancies, graft thrombosis, nephrotoxicity, and serious infection following heart transplant.*

### Assessment & Drug Effects

- Monitor for and promptly report S&S of a hypersensitivity reaction (e.g., anaphylaxis, dyspnea, flushing, chest pain, angioedema).
- Monitor renal function and promptly report S&S of nephrotoxicity.
- Monitor pulmonary status and report promptly unexplained cough, shortness of breath, pain on inspiration, or diminished breath sounds.
- Monitor for and promptly report S&S of infection.
- Monitor lab tests: Baseline and periodic CBC with differential, renal function tests, blood glucose, and lipid profile.

### Patient & Family Education

- Report promptly any signs of infections, including sore throat, fever, and flu-like symptoms.
- Avoid live vaccinations and close contact with those who have received live vaccines.
- Practice meticulous oral hygiene. Do not use mouthwashes that contain alcohol or peroxide.
- Women should use adequate means of contraception to avoid pregnancy while on this drug and for 8 wk after ending treatment.

---

Common adverse effects in *italic;* life-threatening effects <u>underlined</u>; generic names in **bold**; classifications in SMALL CAPS; ♣ Canadian drug name; ◯ Prototype drug

# EVOLOCUMAB
(e-vo-loc′u-mab)
Repatha
**Classifications:** MONOCLONAL ANTIBODY; PROPROTEIN CONVERTASE SUBTILISIN KEXIN TYPE 9 (PCSK9) INHIBITOR; ANTILIPIDEMIC; LIPID LOWERING
Therapeutic: ANTILIPIDEMIC

**AVAILABILITY** Prefilled syringe for injection

## ACTION & *THERAPEUTIC EFFECT*
Binds to the enzyme, human proprotein convertase subtilisin kexin 9 (PCSK9), and inhibits circulating PCSK9 from binding to the LDL receptor (LDLR), preventing PCSK9-mediated LDLR degradation. *Increases the number of LDLRs available to clear LDL from the blood, thereby lowering LDL-C levels.*

**USES** Adjunct treatment of adults with heterozygous familial hypercholesterolemia (HeFH), homozygous familial hypercholesterolemia (HoFH), or clinical atherosclerotic cardiovascular disease (CVD), primary hyperlipidemia.

**CONTRAINDICATIONS** History of a serious hypersensitivity reaction to evolocumab; concomitant use of belimumab; pregnancy (second and third trimester).

**CAUTIOUS USE** Allergic reactions (e.g., rash, urticaria), pregnancy (first trimester); lactation. Safety and efficacy not established in children with HoFH who are younger than 13 y or who have primary hyperlipidemia or HeFH.

## ROUTE & DOSAGE

**Heterozygous Familial Hypercholesterolemia or Atherosclerotic Disease**

*Adult:* **Subcutaneous** 140 mg q2wk or 420 mg once monthly
**Homozygous Familial Hypercholesterolemia**
*Adult:* **Subcutaneous** 420 mg once monthly

## ADMINISTRATION
**Subcutaneous**
- Allow evolocumab to warm to room temperature for at least 30 min if refrigerated.
- Administer into abdomen, thigh, or upper arm; avoid areas that are tender, bruised, red, or indurated. Rotate injection sites.
- To administer the 420 mg dose, give three 140 mg injections consecutively within 30 min.
- Store refrigerated or at room temperature [up to 25° C (77° F)] in the original carton. If kept at room temperature, must be used within 30 days.

**ADVERSE EFFECTS** (≥1%) **Body as a Whole:** Dizziness, fatigue, hypersensitivity reactions, influenza, injection site reactions. **CNS:** Headache. **CV:** Hypertension. **GI:** Diarrhea, gastroenteritis, nausea. **Musculoskeletal:** Arthralgia, back pain, musculoskeletal pain, muscle spasms, myalgia. **Respiratory:** Cough, *nasopharyngitis*, sinusitis, upper respiratory tract infection. **Urogenital:** Urinary tract infection.

**PHARMACOKINETICS Peak:** 3–4 days. **Metabolism:** Peptide degradation. **Half-Life:** 11–17 days.

## NURSING IMPLICATIONS
**Assessment & Drug Effects**
- Monitor for and report S&S of an allergic reaction. Withhold drug and notify prescriber for S&S of a serious allergic reaction.
- Monitor lab tests: Baseline and periodic lipid profile.

### Patient & Family Education

- If a dose is missed, administer as soon as possible if there are more than 7 days until the next scheduled dose, or omit the missed dose and administer the next dose according to the original schedule.
- Women of childbearing age should discuss potential risks of pregnancy with prescriber.
- Do not breast-feed without consulting prescriber.

---

# EXEMESTANE
(ex-e-mes'tain)
Aromasin
**Classifications:** ANTINEOPLASTIC; AROMATASE INHIBITOR
**Therapeutic:** ANTINEOPLASTIC
**Prototype:** Anastrozole

---

## AVAILABILITY Tablet

## ACTION & THERAPEUTIC EFFECT

Steroidal aromatase inhibitor that suppresses the plasma estrogens, estradiol and estrone. The enzyme, aromatase, converts estrone to estradiol. *Tumor regression is possible in postmenopausal women with estrogen dependent breast cancer. Effectiveness is indicated by evidence of reduction in tumor size.*

## USES Estrogen-receptor positive early breast cancer following treatment with tamoxifen, treatment of advanced breast cancer in postmenopausal women whose disease has progressed following tamoxifen therapy.

## UNLABELED USES Risk reduction for invasive breast cancer in postmenopausal women.

## CONTRAINDICATIONS Hypersensitivity to exemestane; coadministration of estrogen-containing drugs; women who are or may become

pregnant; premenopausal women; lactation; pregnancy (category X).

## CAUTIOUS USE Hepatic or renal insufficiency; GI disorders; cardiovascular disease; hyperlipidemia. Safe use in children not established.

## ROUTE & DOSAGE

### Early and Advanced Breast Cancer
*Adult:* **PO** 25 mg daily

## ADMINISTRATION

### Oral
- Give following a meal.
- Store at 15°–30° C (59°–86° F).

## ADVERSE EFFECTS (≥1%) **Body as a Whole:** *Fatigue, hot flashes, pain,* flu-like symptoms; edema; fever; paresthesia. **CNS:** *Depression, insomnia, anxiety; dizziness;* headache. **CV:** Hypertension. **GI:** *Nausea,* vomiting, abdominal pain, anorexia, constipation, diarrhea, increased appetite. **Respiratory:** Dyspnea, cough, bronchitis, sinusitis. **Skin:** Increased sweating, rash, itching. **Other:** UTI; lymphedema.

## PHARMACOKINETICS **Absorption:** Rapidly, approximately 42% reaches systemic circulation. **Distribution:** Extensive tissue distribution, 90% protein bound. **Metabolism:** Extensively in liver (CYP3A4). **Elimination:** Equally in urine and feces. **Half-Life:** 24 h.

## NURSING IMPLICATIONS

### Assessment & Drug Effects
- Monitor lab tests: Baseline LFTs, BUN and creatinine; periodic WBC with differential, lipid profile, and routine blood chemistry.

### Patient & Family Education
- Review manufacturer's patient literature thoroughly to reinforce understanding of likely adverse effects.

---

Common adverse effects in *italic;* life-threatening effects <u>underlined</u>; generic names in **bold;** classifications in SMALL CAPS; ✦ Canadian drug name; ⊘ Prototype drug

- Report bothersome adverse effects to prescriber.

## EXENATIDE ℗

(e-xe'na-tide)

**Byetta, Bydureon**

**Classification:** ANTIDIABETIC, INCRETIN MIMETIC

**Therapeutic:** ANTIDIABETIC

**AVAILABILITY** Solution for injection, extended release suspension for injection

**ACTION & *THERAPEUTIC EFFECT***
Improves glycemic control in type 2 diabetes mellitus by mimicking the functions of incretin, a glucagon-like peptide-1 (GLP-1). Exenatide enhances glucose-dependent insulin secretion by pancreatic beta-cells, suppresses inappropriately elevated glucagon secretion, and slows gastric emptying. These actions decrease glucagon stimulation of hepatic glucose output and decrease insulin demand. *Improves glycemic control by reducing fasting and postprandial glucose concentrations in patients with type 2 diabetes.*

**USES** Type 2 diabetes mellitus in combination with diet/exercise.

**CONTRAINDICATIONS** Hypersensitivity to exenatide; type I diabetes; severe GI disease, diabetic ketoacidosis; gastroparesis; history of pancreatitis; severe GI disease or gastroparesis; end-stage renal disease, severe renal impairment (CrCl less than 30 mL/min). Extend release exenatide is contraindicated in family/personal history of medullary thyroid carcinoma and multiple endocrine neoplasia syndrome type 2.

**CAUTIOUS USE** Renal impairment; renal disease; thyroid disease; older adults; pregnancy (category C); lactation. Safety and efficacy in children not established.

## ROUTE & DOSAGE

### Type 2 Diabetes Mellitus

*Adult:* **Subcutaneous** Initial dose of 5 mcg b.i.d., within 60 min prior to the morning and evening meal. After 1 mo, may increase to 10 mcg b.i.d., within 60 min prior to the morning and evening meal; **Extended release** 2 mcg each week.

## ADMINISTRATION

**Subcutaneous**

- Give daily dose subcutaneously into thigh, abdomen, or upper arm within 60 min before the morning and evening meals. Do not administer after a meal.
- Extended release (ER) form: May be given any time of day without regard to meals. The day of weekly dosing may be changed as needed if last dose given at least 3 days prior.
- Do not give within 1 h of oral antibiotics or an oral contraceptive.
- Store at 2°–8° C (36°–46° F) and protect from light. Discard pen 30 days after first use. Do not use if pen has been frozen. After first use, pen may be kept at or below 25° C (77° F).

**ADVERSE EFFECTS** (≥1%) **CNS:** Asthenia, dizziness, restlessness, jittery feeling. **GI:** Nausea, vomiting, diarrhea, constipation, dyspepsia, anorexia, gastroesophageal reflux. **Metabolic:** Hypoglycemia, excessive sweating (hyperhidrosis or diaphoresis). **Body as a Whole:** Injection site reaction.

**INTERACTIONS Drug:** Owing to its ability to slow gastric emptying, exenatide can decrease the rate and/or serum levels of oral medications that require GI absorption, increased risk of hypoglycemia with other INSULIN products.

## PHARMACOKINETICS **Peak:** 2 h (immediate release); 2 wk (extended release). **Elimination:** Primarily in urine. **Half-Life:** 2.4 h.

## NURSING IMPLICATIONS

### Black Box Warning

*Exenatide may pose a risk of thyroid C-cell tumor development, although a direct link has not been established.*

### Assessment & Drug Effects

- Monitor for and report S&S of significant GI distress, including NV&D.
- Monitor for S&S of hypoglycemia and S&S of acute pancreatitis (acute abdominal pain with/without vomiting). If pancreatitis is suspected, withhold drug and notify prescriber immediately.
- Monitor for and report immediately site injection reactions such as cellulitis, abscess, and skin necrosis.
- Monitor lab tests: Frequent fasting and postprandial plasma glucose, and periodic HbA1C; baseline and periodic renal function tests.

### Patient & Family Education

- If a scheduled daily dose is missed, wait for the next scheduled dose.
- If a weekly dose is missed, administer it as soon as possible as long as next scheduled dose is due at least 3 days later.
- Discard any pen that has been in use for greater than 30 days.
- Exenatide may cause decreased appetite and some weight loss.
- Report significant GI distress to prescriber. Report promptly persistent, severe abdominal pain

that may be accompanied by vomiting.
- Report promptly discomfort and/or irritation at injection sites.
- Report symptoms of thyroid tumors (e.g., a lump in the neck, hoarseness, dysphagia, dyspnea).

## EZETIMIBE
(e-ze-ti'mibe)

Zetia, Ezetrol ♦

**Classifications:** ANTILIPEMIC; CHOLESTEROL ABSORPTION INHIBITOR

Therapeutic: CHOLESTEROL LOWERING

## AVAILABILITY Tablet

## ACTION & *THERAPEUTIC EFFECT*

Inhibits absorption of cholesterol at the brush border of the small intestine leading to a decreased delivery of cholesterol to the liver, reduction of hepatic cholesterol stores and an increased clearance of cholesterol from the blood. *Decreases total cholesterol, LDL cholesterol, apo B, and triglycerides while increasing HDL cholesterol.*

## USES Treatment of primary hypercholesterolemia alone or with an HMG-CoA reductase inhibitor (statin); treatment of homozygous sitosterolemia as an adjunct to diet.

## CONTRAINDICATIONS Hypersensitivity to ezetimibe; concurrent use with HMG-CoA reductase inhibitor (statin) in patients with active liver disease or elevated serum transaminases; moderate to severe hepatic disease; myopathy; lactation.

## CAUTIOUS USE Mild hepatic insufficiency; severe renal impairment; older adults pregnancy (category C). Safe use in children younger than 10 y not established.

Common adverse effects in *italic;* life-threatening effects underlined; generic names in **bold**; classifications in SMALL CAPS; ♦ Canadian drug name; ⊙ Prototype drug

665

## ROUTE & DOSAGE

**Hypercholesterolemia**
*Adult:* **PO** 10 mg daily

## ADMINISTRATION

### Oral
- Give no sooner than 2 h before or 4 h after administration of a bile acid sequestrant such as cholestyramine.
- Store at 15°–30° C (59°–86° F). Protect from moisture.

### ADVERSE EFFECTS (≥1%) **Body as a Whole:** Fatigue, arthralgia, back pain, myalgia, angioedema, myopathy. **CNS:** Dizziness, headache. **GI:** Abdominal pain, diarrhea. **Respiratory:** Pharyngitis, sinusitis, cough. **Hematologic:** Thrombocytopenia. **Skin:** Rash. **Other:** Hepatitis, pancreatitis, rhabdomyolysis.

### INTERACTIONS Drug: BILE ACID SEQUESTRANTS (e.g., **cholestyramine**) may decrease absorption (give ezetimibe 2 h before or 4 h after these drugs); **cyclosporine** or FIBRIC ACID DERIVATIVES can significantly increase ezetimibe levels.

### PHARMACOKINETICS Absorption: Well absorbed from the small intestine. **Peak:** 4–12 h. **Distribution:** Ezetimibe-glucuronide is 99% protein bound. **Metabolism:** Extensively conjugated to an active glucuronide compound (ezetimibe-glucuronide). Metabolized in small intestine and liver. **Elimination:** Primarily in feces. **Half-Life:** 22 h.

## NURSING IMPLICATIONS

### Assessment & Drug Effects
- Assess for and report unexplained muscle pain, especially when used in combination with a statin drug.
- Monitor closely patients who take both ezetimibe and cyclosporine.
- Monitor lab tests: Baseline and periodic lipid profile; baseline LFTs and, when used with a statin, periodic LFTs in accordance with the monitoring schedule for that statin.

### Patient & Family Education
- Report unexplained muscle pain, tenderness, or weakness.
- Females should use effective methods of contraception to prevent pregnancy while taking this drug in combination with a statin.

# EZOGABINE
(e-zog' a-been)
**Potiga**
**Classifications:** ANTICONVULSANT; POTASSIUM CHANNEL OPENER
**Therapeutic:** ANTICONVULSANT

## AVAILABILITY Tablet

## ACTION & *THERAPEUTIC EFFECT*
Mechanism of action thought to be related to enhancement of transmembrane potassium currents resulting in stabilization of the resting membrane and reduced brain excitability. May also augment GABA-mediated currents. *Reduces frequency of partial onset seizures.*

## USES Adjunctive therapy in the treatment of partial onset seizures.

## CONTRAINDICATIONS Suicidal ideations.

## CAUTIOUS USE Urinary hesitation or retention; history of hepatic or renal impairment; confusional states, psychotic symptoms (including suicidal tendencies or behavior), depression; hallucinations; dizziness and somnolence; BPH; prolonged QT interval or history of; CHF; ventricular hypertrophy; hypokalemia or hypomagnesemia; older adults; pregnancy (category C) and lactation.

Safety and efficacy in children under 18 y not established.

## ROUTE & DOSAGE

### Partial Seizures

*Adult 65 y or younger:* **PO** 100 mg t.i.d. initially, may increase by 50 mg/wk to 200–400 mg t.i.d. *Adult older than 65 y:* **PO** 50 mg t.i.d. initially, may increase by 50 mg/wk to 250 mg t.i.d.

### Hepatic Impairment Dosage Adjustment

*Moderate impairment (Child-Pugh score 7 or higher up to 9):* Same as adult over 65 y
*Severe impairment (Child-Pugh score greater than 9):* 50 mg t.i.d. initially, may increase by 50 mg/wk to 200 mg t.i.d.

### Renal Impairment Dosage Adjustment

*CrCl less than 50 mL/min:* 50 mg t.i.d. initially, may increase by 50 mg/wk to 200 mg t.i.d.

## ADMINISTRATION

### Oral

- May be given with or without food.
- Tablets should be swallowed whole and not crushed or chewed.
- Ezogabine is ordinarily discontinued over a period of three weeks.
- Store at −15°–30° C (59°– 86° F).

## ADVERSE EFFECTS (≥2%) **Body as a Whole:** Increased weight, influenza. **CNS:** Abnormal coordination, amnesia, anxiety, aphasia, asthenia, attention disturbance, balance disorder, *confusion*, *dizziness*, dysrthria, dysphasia, *fatigue*, gait disturbances, *memory impairment*, paresthesia, *somnolence*, tremor, vertigo. **GI:** Constipation, dyspepsia, nausea. **Special Senses:** Blurred vision, diplopia. **Urogenital:** Chromaturia, dysuria, hematuria, urinary hesitation.

## DIAGNOSTIC TEST INTERFERENCE
False elevations of ***serum*** and ***urine bilirubin.***

## INTERACTIONS **Drug: Carbamazepine** and **phenytoin** decrease the plasma levels of ezogabine. Ezogabine may increase the plasma levels of **digoxin** and decrease the plasma levels of **lamotrigine.** Ezogabine may cause an additive effect with other drugs that prolong the QT interval (e.g., **amiodarone, procainamide, droperidol, mesoridazine, moxifloxacin, pimozide, thioridazine**). **Food: Alcohol** may increase the levels of ezogabine.

## PHARMACOKINETICS **Peak:** 0.5–2 h. **Distribution:** 80% plasma protein bound. **Metabolism:** In the liver to inactive metabolites. **Elimination:** Renal (86%) and fecal (14%). **Half-Life:** 7–11 h.

## NURSING IMPLICATIONS

### Black Box Warning

*Ezogabine has been associated with retinal abnormalities resulting in loss of vision.*

### Assessment & Drug Effects

- Monitor for and report immediately: Suicidal ideation or any other psychiatric symptom, confusional states, dizziness, or somnolence.
- Monitor urinary output especially in those with BPH, cognitive impairment, or concurrent anticholinergic drugs. Report promptly signs of urinary retention.
- Monitor for S&S of digoxin toxicity with concurrent therapy.

Common adverse effects in *italic;* life-threatening effects underlined; generic names in **bold;** classifications in SMALL CAPS; ♣ Canadian drug name; ⊘ Prototype drug

667

- Vision should be assessed at baseline and every 6 mo.
- Monitor lab tests: Baseline and periodic LFTs and renal function tests; periodic serum digoxin with concurrent therapy.

### Patient & Family Education

- Report immediately: Suicidal thoughts, altered mental status, confusion, excessive drowsiness or dizziness, or decreased ability to urinate.
- Do not abruptly stop taking ezogabine unless told to do so by prescriber.
- Report promptly any changes in vision.
- Avoid alcohol while taking this drug.
- Do not drive or engage in potentially hazardous activities until response to drug is known.
- Notify prescriber if you become pregnant or intend to become pregnant during therapy.
- Do not breast-feed while taking this drug without consulting prescriber.

## FAMCICLOVIR
(fam-ci′clo-vir)
Famvir
**Classification:** ANTIVIRAL
Therapeutic: ANTIVIRAL
**Prototype:** Acyclovir

### AVAILABILITY Tablet

### ACTION & *THERAPEUTIC EFFECT*

Prodrug of the antiviral agent penciclovir that prevents viral replication by inhibition of DNA synthesis in herpes virus–infected cells. *Effectiveness is indicated by decreasing pain and crusting of lesions followed by loss of vesicles, ulcers, and crusts. Interferes with DNA synthesis of herpes simplex virus type 1 and 2 (HSV-1 and HSV-2) infections, varicella-zoster virus, and cytomegalovirus.*

**USES** Management of acute herpes zoster, genital herpes, recurrent episodes of genital herpes in immunocompromised adults.

**UNLABELED USES** Bell's palsy, post herpetic neuralgia prophylaxis.

**CONTRAINDICATIONS** Hypersensitivity to famciclovir; lactation.

**CAUTIOUS USE** Renal or hepatic impairment, carcinoma, older adults, pregnancy (category B). Safety in children younger than 18 y not established.

### ROUTE & DOSAGE

**Herpes Zoster, Treatment**

*Adult:* **PO** 500 mg q8h for 7 days, start within 48–72 h of onset of rash

**Renal Impairment Dosage Adjustment**

*CrCl 40–59 mL/min:* 500 mg q12h; *20–39 mL/min:* 500 mg q24h

**Treatment of Recurrent Genital Herpes**

*Adult:* **PO** 125 mg b.i.d. × 5 days OR 1000 mg b.i.d.

**Suppression of Recurrent Genital Herpes**

*Adult:* **PO** 250 mg b.i.d. for up to 1 y

### ADMINISTRATION

#### Oral

- Most effective when given within 72 h of appearance of a rash or within 6 h of onset of a genital lesion.
- Store at room temperature, 15°–30° C (59°–86° F).

**ADVERSE EFFECTS** (≥1%) **CNS:** *Headache,* somnolence, dizziness, paresthesias, fatigue, fever, rigors. **Hematologic:** Purpura. **GI:** Nausea, diarrhea, vomiting, constipation, anorexia, abdominal pain. **Body as a Whole:** Pharyngitis, sinusitis, pruritus.

**INTERACTIONS Drug: Probenecid** may decrease elimination; famciclovir may increase **digoxin** levels.

**PHARMACOKINETICS Absorption:** Readily absorbed from GI tract and rapidly converted to penciclovir in intestinal and liver tissue. **Onset:** Median times to full crusting of lesions, loss of vesicles, loss of ulcers, and loss of crusts were 6, 5, 7, and 19 days, respectively; median time to loss of acute pain was 21 days. **Peak:** 1 h. **Distribution:** Distributes into breast milk of animals. **Metabolism:** Metabolized in liver and intestinal tissue to penciclovir, which is the active antiviral agent. **Elimination:** Approximately 60% recovered in urine as penciclovir. **Half-Life:** Penciclovir 2–3 h.

## NURSING IMPLICATIONS

### Assessment & Drug Effects
- Monitor lab tests: Baseline and periodic CBC and routine blood chemistry.

### Patient & Family Education
- Learn potential adverse effects and report those that are bothersome to prescriber.
- Be aware that a full therapeutic response may take several weeks.

---

## FAMOTIDINE
(fa-moe'ti-deen)
Pepcid, Pepcid AC
**Classification:** ANTISECRETORY (H₂-RECEPTOR ANTAGONIST)
Therapeutic: ANTIULCER
**Prototype:** Cimetidine

**AVAILABILITY** Tablet; oral suspension; solution for injection

## ACTION & *THERAPEUTIC EFFECT*
Competitive inhibitor of histamine at $H_2$ receptor sites in gastric parietal cells. Inhibits gastric acid secretion as well as pepsin secretion. *Reduces parietal cell output of hydrochloric acid; thus, detrimental effects of acid on gastric mucosa are diminished.*

**USES** Short-term treatment of active duodenal ulcer, gastric ulcer, dyspepsia or heartburn. Maintenance therapy for duodenal ulcer patients on reduced dosage after healing of an active ulcer. Treatment of pathologic hypersecretory conditions (e.g., Zollinger-Ellison syndrome). Treatment of gastroesophageal reflux disease (GERD), gastritis.

**UNLABELED USES** Stress ulcer prophylaxis, aspiration prophylaxis, NSAID-induced ulcer prophylaxis.

**CONTRAINDICATIONS** Hypersensitivity to famotidine or other H₂-receptor antagonists; sudden GI bleeding; lactation.

**CAUTIOUS USE** Renal insufficiency; renal failure; PKU; hepatic disease vitamin B12 deficiency; older adults; pregnancy (category B).

## ROUTE & DOSAGE

### Duodenal Ulcer
*Adult:* **PO** 40 mg at bedtime or 20 mg b.i.d.; **PO Maintenance Therapy** 20 mg at bedtime; **IV** 20 mg q12h
*Child:* **PO/IV** 0.25–0.5 mg/kg q12h (max: 40 mg/day)

### Pathological Hypersecretory Conditions
*Adult:* **PO** 20–160 mg q6h; **IV** 20 mg q6h

### GERD, Gastritis
*Adult:* **PO** 20 mg b.i.d.

---

Common adverse effects in *italic*; life-threatening effects underlined; generic names in **bold**; classifications in SMALL CAPS; ♣ Canadian drug name; ⊘ Prototype drug

669

F

*Child:* **PO** 0.5 mg/b.i.d. (max: 40 mg b.i.d.)

*Infant (3 mo–1 yr):* **PO** 0.5 mg/kg b.i.d. for up to 8 wk

**Heartburn/Dyspepsia Prevention (self treatment)**

*Adult:* **PO** 10 mg 15 min prior to meal (max dose: 20 mg/day)

*Renal Impairment Dosage Adjustment*

*CrCl less than 50 mL/min:* 50% of usual dose or usual dose q36–48h

## ADMINISTRATION

### Oral

- Give with liquid or food of patient's choice; an antacid may also be given if patient is also on antacid therapy.
- Shake suspension vigorously before use.
- Do not chew tablet; dose may be taken 10-60 min before eating food or drinking beverages known to cause heartburn.
- Store at 15°–30° C (59°–86° F). Protect from moisture and strong light; do not freeze.

### Intravenous

Note: Verify correct IV concentration and rate of infusion/injection with prescriber before administration to infants or children.

*PREPARE:* **Direct:** Dilute each 20 mg (2 mL) famotidine IV solution (containing 10 mg/mL) with D5W, NS, or other compatible IV diluent (see manufacturer's directions) to a total volume of 5 or 10 mL. **Intermittent:** Dilute required dose with 100 mL compatible IV solution.

*ADMINISTER:* **Direct:** Give over not less than 2 min. **Intermittent:** Infuse over 15–30 min.

*INCOMPATIBILITIES:* **Y-site:** Amphotericin B cholesteryl complex, azithromycin, cefepime, piperacillin/tazobactam.

- Store IV solution at 2°–8° C (36°–46° F); reconstituted IV solution is stable for 48 h at room temperature 15°–30° C (59°–86° F).

**ADVERSE EFFECTS** (≥1%) **CNS:** Dizziness, headache, confusion, agitation, depression. **GI:** Constipation, diarrhea, vomiting. **Skin:** Rash, acne, pruritus, dry skin, flushing. **Hematologic:** Thrombocytopenia. **Urogenital:** Increases in BUN and serum creatinine.

**INTERACTIONS Drug:** May inhibit absorption of **itraconazole** or **ketoconazole.** Do not use with **dasatinib.** Can affect serum concentrations of other medications requiring acid environment for absorption (i.e., **atazanavir, budesonide, erlotinib**).

**PHARMACOKINETICS Absorption:** Incompletely from GI tract (40–50% reaches systemic circulation). **Onset:** 1 h. **Peak:** 1–3 h PO; 0.5–3 h IV. **Duration:** 10–12 h. **Metabolism:** In liver. **Elimination:** In urine. **Half-Life:** 2.5–4 h.

## NURSING IMPLICATIONS

### Assessment & Drug Effects

- Monitor for improvement in GI distress.
- Monitor for signs of GI bleeding.
- Monitor CBC, gastric pH, occult blood with GI bleeding.

### Patient & Family Education

- Be aware that pain relief may not be experienced for several days after starting therapy.

## FAT EMULSION, INTRAVENOUS

(fat e-mul'sion)

Intralipid, Liposyn II, Nutrilipid, Smoflipid

**Classifications:** CALORIC AGENT; LIPID EMULSION

Therapeutic: NUTRITIONAL SUPPLEMENT; LIPID

**AVAILABILITY** Emulsion

## ACTION & *THERAPEUTIC EFFECT*
Provides the essential fatty acids (e.g., linoleic acid and alpha linolenic acid) necessary for normal structure and function of cell membranes. *Used as a nutritional supplement.*

**USES** Fatty acid deficiency treatment or prophyalxis. Also to supply fatty acids and calories in high-density form to patients receiving prolonged TPN therapy who cannot tolerate high dextrose concentrations or when fluid intake **must be** restricted.

**CONTRAINDICATIONS** Hyperlipemia; bone marrow dyscrasias; impaired fat metabolism as in pathological hyperlipemia, lipoid nephrosis, acute pancreatitis accompanied by hyperlipemia.

**CAUTIOUS USE** Severe hepatic or pulmonary disease; coagulation disorders; anemia; when danger of fat embolism exists; history of gastric ulcers; diabetes mellitus; thrombocytopenia; newborns, premature neonates, infants with hyperbilirubinemia, pregnancy (category C); preterm neonates

## ROUTE & DOSAGE

**Prevention of Essential Fatty Acid Deficiency**

*Adult:* **IV** 500 mL of 10% or 250 mL of 20% solution twice/wk (max: rate of 100 mL/h)
*Child:* **IV** 5–10 mL/kg/day twice/wk (max: 3–4 g/kg/day; max: rate of 100 mL/h)

**Essential Fatty Acid Deficiency Treatment**

*Adult/Child/Infant/Neonate:* **IV** 8–10% of caloric intake

**Calorie Source in Fluid-Restricted Patients**

*Adult:* **IV** 1–2 g/kg/day up to 2.5 g/kg or no more than 60% of nonprotein calories daily (max: rate of 100 mL/h)
*Child (11–17 y):* **IV** 1 g/kg/day up to 2.5 g/kg/day or no more than 60% of nonprotein calories daily (max: rate of 100 mL/h)
*Child/Infant (1–10 yrs):* **IV** 1–2 g/kg/day, up to 3 g/kg/day (no more than 60% of nonprotein calories daily)
*Neonate:* **IV** 0.5–1 g/kg/day, increase by 0.5 g/kg/day (max: 3 g/kg/day; max: infusion 0.15 g/kg/h)

## ADMINISTRATION
**Intravenous**

Do not use if oil appears to be separating out of the emulsion.

*PREPARE:* **IV Infusion** Allow preparations that have been refrigerated to stand at room temperature for about 30 min before using whenever possible. ▪ Check with a pharmacist before mixing fat emulsions with electrolytes, vitamins, drugs, or other nutrient solutions.
*ADMINISTER:* Check specific manufacturer's guidelines regarding use of in-line filter for infusion. **IV Infusion for Adult:** *10% emulsion:* Infuse at 1 mL/min for first 15–30 min; increase to 2 mL/min if no adverse reactions. ▪ *20% emulsion:* Infuse at 0.5 mL/min for first 15–30 min; increase to 2 mL/min if no adverse reactions occur. **IV Infusion for Child:** *10% emulsion:* Infuse at 0.1 mL/min for first 10–15 min; give as slow as possible and NEVER exceed 1 g/kg in 4 h. ▪ Do not exceed 100 mL/h. ▪ *20% emulsion:* Infuse at 0.05 mL/min for first 10–15 min; increase to 1 g/kg in 4 h if no

Common adverse effects in *italic;* life-threatening effects <u>underlined</u>; generic names in **bold**; classifications in SMALL CAPS; ♣ Canadian drug name; ⊙ Prototype drug

671

adverse reactions occur. ▪Do not exceed 50 mL/h. **IV Infusion for Premature Neonate:** Infuse at rate not to exceed 0.15 g/kg/h. **IV Infusion for All Patients:** Give fat emulsions via a separate peripheral site or by piggyback into same vein receiving amino acid injection and dextrose mixtures or give by piggyback through a Y-connector near infusion site so that the two solutions mix only in a short piece of tubing proximal to needle. ▪ Must hang fat emulsions higher than hyperalimentation solution bottle to prevent backup of fat emulsion into primary line. ▪ Do not use an in-line filter because size of fat particles is larger than pore size. ▪ Control flow rate of each solution by separate infusion pumps. ▪ Use a constant rate over 20–24 h to reduce risk of hyperlipemia in neonates and prematures because they tend to metabolize fat slowly.
*INCOMPATIBILITIES:* **Solution/additive: Aminophylline, amphotericin B, ampicillin, calcium chloride, calcium gluconate, dextrose 10%, gentamicin, hetastarch, magnesium chloride, penicillin G, phenytoin, ranitidine, vitamin B complex. Y-site: Acyclovir, albumin, amphotericin B, cyclosporine, doxorubicin, doxycycline, droperidol, ganciclovir, haloperidol, heparin, hetastarch, hydromorphone, levorphanol, lorazepam, midazolam, minocycline, nalbuphine, ondansetron, pentobarbital, phenobarbital, potassium phosphate, sodium phosphate.**

▪ Discard contents of partly used containers. ▪ Store, unless otherwise directed by manufacturer, Intralipid 10% and Liposyn 10% at room temperature [25° C (77° F) or below]; refrigerate Intralipid 20%. Do not freeze.

## ADVERSE EFFECTS (≥1%) Body as a Whole: Hypersensitivity reactions (to egg protein), irritation at infusion site. **Hematologic:** Hypercoagulability, <u>thrombocytopenia</u> in neonates. **GI:** *Nauesea, transient increases in liver function tests, hypertriglyceridemia.* **Long-Term Administration:** Sepsis, jaundice (cholestasis), hepatomegaly, kernicterus (infants with hyperbilirubinemia), <u>shock</u> (rare), alumnimum toxicity.

## DIAGNOSTIC TEST INTERFERENCE
Blood samples drawn during or shortly after fat emulsion infusion may produce abnormally high ***hemoglobin MCH and MCHC*** values. Fat emulsions may cause transient abnormalities in ***liver function tests*** and may interfere with estimations of ***serum bilirubin*** (especially in infants).

## INTERACTIONS Drug: No clinically significant interactions established.

## NURSING IMPLICATIONS

### Black Box Warning

*Fat emulsion infusion has been associated with deaths in preterm infants.*

### Assessment & Drug Effects
▪ Monitor closely infusion rate and total daily dose. Strict adherence to the recommended total daily dose is mandatory; hourly infusion rate should be as slow as possible and should not exceed 1 g/kg in 4 h.
▪ Observe patient closely. Acute reactions tend to occur within the first 2½ h of therapy.
▪ Note: Lipemia must clear after each daily infusion. Degree of lipemia is measured by serum.

triglycerides and cholesterol levels 4–6 h after infusion has ceased.

- Neonate lab tests: Obtain daily platelet counts in neonates during first week of therapy, then every other day during second week, and 3 × a week thereafter because newborns are prone to develop thrombocytopenia.
- Monitor lab tests: Baseline hematologic studies; baseline and periodic LFTs, renal function tests, and lipid profile.

### Patient & Family Education
- Report difficulty breathing, nausea, vomiting, or headache to prescriber.

# FEBUXOSTAT
(fee-bux'o-stat)
Uloric

**Classifications:** ANTIGOUT; XANTHINE OXIDASE INHIBITOR
**Therapeutic:** ANTIGOUT
**Prototype:** Allopurinol

## AVAILABILITY Tablet

## ACTION & *THERAPEUTIC EFFECT*
Febuxostat decreases serum uric acid by inhibiting the enzyme needed to convert xanthine to uric acid (end product of protein catabolism). *Effectiveness is measured by decreasing serum uric acid level to less than 6 mg/dL.*

## USES Management of hyperuricemia in patients with chronic gout.

## CONTRAINDICATIONS Asymptomatic hyperuricemia; concurrent use with **azathioprine** or **mercaptopurine**.

## CAUTIOUS USE History of MI or stroke; severe renal impairment (CrCl less than 30 mL/min); severe hepatic dysfunction (Child-Pugh class C); pregnancy (category C); lactation. Safety and efficacy in children younger than 18 y not established.

## ROUTE & DOSAGE

### Gout
*Adult:* **PO** 40 mg once daily; can be increased to 80 mg once daily

### Renal Impairment Dosage Adjustment
*CrCl 15 to 29 mL/minute:* Do not exceed 40 mg daily; *CrCl less than 15 mL/minute:* Use with caution

## ADMINISTRATION
### Oral
- Administer with or without food or antacids.
- Concurrent therapy with an NSAID or colchicine is recommended to prevent gout flares during the first 6 mo of therapy.
- Store at 15°–30° C (59°–86° F) away from light.

## ADVERSE EFFECTS (≥1%) **CV:** <u>Atrial fibrillation, AV block, thromboembolic events.</u> **GI:** Nausea. **Metabolic:** Elevated AST and ALT levels. **Musculoskeletal:** Arthralgia. **Skin:** Rash. **Whole Body:** <u>Rhabdomyolysis.</u>

## INTERACTIONS **Drug:** Febuxostat will increase the levels of drugs requiring xanthine oxidase for normal metabolism (e.g., **6-mercaptopurine, azathioprine**). Use with cytotoxic ANTINEOPLASTIC agents may cause nephropathy.

## PHARMACOKINETICS **Absorption:** 49%. **Peak:** 1–1.5 h. **Distribution:** Greater than 99% plasma protein bound. **Metabolism:** Extensive hepatic metabolism via oxidation and glucuronide conjugation. **Elimination:** Renal (49%) and fecal (45%). **Half-Life:** 5–8 h.

## NURSING IMPLICATIONS
### Assessment & Drug Effects
- Monitor for and report gout flares.

Common adverse effects in *italic;* life-threatening effects <u>underlined;</u> generic names in **bold;** classifications in SMALL CAPS; ♣ Canadian drug name; ⊘ Prototype drug

673

F

- Monitor CV status throughout therapy.
- Monitor for signs/symptoms of hypersensitivity or severe skin reactions.
- Monitor lab tests: Baseline serum uric acid and at 2 wk, and periodically thereafter. Baseline and periodic LFTs.

### Patient & Family Education
- Notify prescriber if you experience a gout flare, but do not stop taking this drug.
- NSAIDs are typically used to control gout flares. Consult prescriber.

## FELBAMATE
(fel'ba-mate)
Felbatol
**Classification:** ANTICONVULSANT; HYDANTOIN
**Therapeutic:** ANTICONVULSANT
**Prototype:** Phenytoin

**AVAILABILITY** Tablet; suspension

**ACTION & *THERAPEUTIC EFFECT***
Anticonvulsant that blocks repetitive firing of neurons and increases seizure threshold; prevents seizure spread. *Increases seizure threshold and prevents seizure spread.*

**USES** Treatment of Lennox–Gastaut syndrome and partial seizures.

**UNLABELED USES** Treatment of generalized tonic/clonic seizures.

**CONTRAINDICATIONS** Hypersensitivity to felbamate, history of blood dyscrasia or hepatic dysfunction; bone marrow depression; active liver disease; elevated serum AST or ALT; severe anemia.

**CAUTIOUS USE** Hypersensitivity to other carbamates; renal impairment, renal failure; thrombocytopenia;

iron-deficiency anemia; older adults; pregnancy (category C); lactation. Safety and efficacy in children other than those with Lennox–Gastaut syndrome not established.

## ROUTE & DOSAGE

### Partial Seizures
*Adult:* **PO** Initiate with 1200 mg/day in 3–4 divided doses, may increase by 600 mg/day q2wk (max: 3600 mg/day); when converting to monotherapy, reduce dose of concomitant anticonvulsants by 1/3 when initiating felbamate, then continue to decrease other anticonvulsants by 1/3 with each increase in felbamate q2wk; when using as adjunctive therapy, decrease other anticonvulsants by 20% when initiating felbamate and note that further reductions in other anticonvulsants may be required to minimize side effects and drug interactions

### Lennox–Gastaut Syndrome
*Child:* **PO** Start at 15 mg/kg/day in 3 or 4 divided doses, reduce concurrent antiepileptic drugs by 20%, further reductions may be required to minimize side effects due to drug interactions, may increase felbamate by 15 mg/kg/day at weekly intervals (max: 45 mg/kg/day)

## ADMINISTRATION
### Oral
- Titrate dose under close clinical supervision.
- Shake suspension well before giving a dose.
- Store in airtight container at room temperature, 15°–30° C (59°–86° F).

Common adverse effects in *italic;* life-threatening effects <u>underlined;</u> generic names in **bold;** classifications in SMALL CAPS; ♣ Canadian drug name; ⓞ Prototype drug

## ADVERSE EFFECTS (≥1%) CNS:
Mild tremors, headache, dizziness, ataxia, diplopia, blurred vision; agitation, aggression, hallucinations, fatigue, psychological disturbances. **Endocrine:** Slight elevation of serum cholesterol, hyponatremia, hypokalemia, weight gain and loss. **GI:** *Nausea and vomiting,* anorexia, constipation, hiccup, taste disturbance, indigestion, esophagitis, increased appetite, acute liver failure. **Hematologic:** <u>Aplastic anemia.</u>

## INTERACTIONS Drug:
Felbamate reduces serum **carbamazepine** levels by a mean of 25%, but increases levels of its active metabolite, increases serum **phenytoin** levels approximately 20%, and increases **valproic acid** levels. **Herbal: Gingko** may decrease anticonvulsant effectiveness.

## PHARMACOKINETICS Absorption:
90% from GI tract. Absorption of tablet not affected by food. **Onset:** Therapeutic effect approximately 14 days. **Peak:** Peak plasma levels at 1–6 h. **Distribution:** 20–25% protein bound, readily crosses the blood–brain barrier. **Metabolism:** In the liver via the cytochrome P450 system. **Elimination:** 40–50% excreted unchanged in urine, rest excreted in urine as metabolites. **Half-Life:** 20–23 h.

## NURSING IMPLICATIONS

### Black Box Warning

*Felbamate has been associated with a development of acute liver failure and a marked increase in risk of aplastic anemia.*

### Assessment & Drug Effects
- Report immediately any hematologic abnormalities.
- Note: When used concomitantly with either phenytoin or carbamazepine, carefully monitor serum levels of these drugs when felbamate is added, when adjustments in felbamate dosing are made, or when felbamate is discontinued.
- Monitor weight, because both weight gain and loss have been reported.
- Monitor for S&S of drug toxicity including GI distress, liver dysfunction, and CNS toxicity. Withhold drug and notify prescriber if any liver function test parameters exceed the ULN.
- Monitor lab tests: Baseline and periodic LFTs and complete hematologic studies; periodic serum sodium and potassium.

### Patient & Family Education
- Report promptly signs of liver dysfunction including jaundice, anorexia, GI discomfort, and fatigue.
- Report promptly signs of bone marrow suppression including infection, bleeding, easy bruising or signs of anemia.

## FELODIPINE
(fel-o'di peen)

**Classifications:** CALCIUM CHANNEL BLOCKER; ANTIHYPERTENSIVE
**Therapeutic:** ANTIHYPERTENSIVE
**Prototype:** Nifedipine

## AVAILABILITY
Sustained release tablet

## ACTION & *THERAPEUTIC EFFECT*
Calcium channel antagonist with high vascular selectivity that reduces systolic, diastolic, and mean arterial pressure at rest and during exercise. Felodipine inhibits influx of extracellular calcium across myocardial and vascular smooth muscle cell membranes. Resultant decrease in intracellular calcium inhibits contractility of smooth muscle, resulting in dilation of coronary and systemic arteries. *BP reduction*

Common adverse effects in *italic;* life-threatening effects <u>underlined</u>; generic names in **bold;** classifications in SMALL CAPS; ◆ Canadian drug name; ⊕ Prototype drug

675

*is due to reduction in peripheral vascular resistance (afterload) against which the heart works. This reduces oxygen demand by the heart and may account for its effectiveness in chronic stable angina.*

**USES** Treatment of hypertension.

**UNLABELED USES** Angina.

**CONTRAINDICATIONS** Hypersensitivity to felodipine; sick sinus rhythm or second- or third-degree heart block except with the use of a pacemaker; abnormal aortic stenosis; hypotension; bradycardia; cardiogenic shock; acute MI; left ventricular dysfunction.

**CAUTIOUS USE** Hypotension, CHF, angina; aortic stenosis, cardiomyopathy; older adults; GERD; hiatal hernia; hepatic impairment; older adults; pregnancy (category C); lactation. Safety and efficacy in children not established.

## ROUTE & DOSAGE

### Hypertension

*Adult:* **PO** 5 mg once/day can increase if needed (max: 10 mg/day)
*Geriatric:* **PO** 2.5 mg once daily; may increase if needed

## ADMINISTRATION

### Oral

- Give tablet whole. Do not crush or chew tablets.
- Store at or below 30° C (86° F) in a tightly closed, light-resistant container.

**ADVERSE EFFECTS** (≥1%) **Body as a Whole:** Most adverse effects appear to be dose dependent. **CV:** Tachycardia, *palpitations, flushing, peripheral edema.* **CNS:** *Dizziness, fatigue,* headache. **GI:** Nausea, flatulence, diarrhea, dyspepsia. **Hematologic:** Small but significant decreases in Hct, Hgb, and RBC count.

**DIAGNOSTIC TEST INTERFERENCE** Serum *alkaline phosphatase* may be slightly but significantly increased. Plasma total and ionized *calcium* levels rise significantly. Serum *gamma-glutamyl transferase* may increase.

**INTERACTIONS Drug:** Do not use with **itraconazole, ketaconazole, clarithromycin** due to increased levels of felodipine. **Adenosine** may cause prolonged bradycardia if it is used to treat patients with toxic concentrations of CALCIUM CHANNEL BLOCKERS. **Carbamazepine, phenobarbital, phenytoin** may decrease felodipine effect. **Cimetidine** may increase felodipine bioavailability and adverse effect risk. Concomitant felodipine and **digoxin** administration produces only transient increases in plasma **digoxin** concentrations (35–40% increase), which are not sustained with continued administration. **Food: Grapefruit juice** may increase adverse effects.

**PHARMACOKINETICS Absorption:** Completely from GI tract; it undergoes extensive first-pass metabolism with only about 15% of dose reaching systemic circulation. **Onset:** Less than 1 h. **Peak:** 2–4 h. **Duration:** 20–24 h (sustained release formulation). **Distribution:** Greater than 99% bound to plasma proteins. **Metabolism:** Metabolized via hepatic cytochrome P-450 mixed function oxidase system. **Elimination:** 60–70% of metabolites are excreted in urine within 72 h. **Half-Life:** 10 h.

## NURSING IMPLICATIONS

### Assessment & Drug Effects

- Monitor BP carefully, especially at initiation of drug therapy, in patients older than 64 y, and in those with impaired liver function.

- Anticipate BP reduction with possible reflex heart rate increase (5–10 bpm) 2–5 h after dosing.
- Report sustained hypotension promptly; more common with concurrent beta-blocker therapy.
- Assess for and report reflex tachycardia; may precipitate angina.
- Monitor patients for possible digoxin toxicity when taking concurrent digoxin.

**Patient Education**

- Report peripheral edema, headache, or flushing to prescriber. These may necessitate discontinuation of drug.
- Get up from lying down slowly and in stages; there is potential for dizziness and hypotension.

## FENOFIBRATE ℗

(fen-o-fi'brate)

Antara, Lofibra, Tricor, Triglide, TriLipix

**Classifications:** ANTILIPEMIC; FIBRATE
**Therapeutic:** CHOLESTEROL-LOWERING

**AVAILABILITY** Tablet; capsule; delayed release capsule

## ACTION & *THERAPEUTIC EFFECT*

Fibric acid derivative with lipid-regulating properties. Lowers plasma triglycerides by inhibiting triglyceride synthesis and, as a result, lowers VLDL production as well as stimulates the catabolism of triglyceride-rich lipoprotein (e.g., VLDL). Produces a moderate increase in HDL cholesterol levels in most patients. *Effectiveness indicated by reduction in the level of serum triglycerides and VLDL production*.

**USES** Adjunctive therapy to diet for patients with high triglycerides.

**CONTRAINDICATIONS** Hypersensitivity to fenofibrate or other fibric acid derivatives (e.g., clofibrate, benzofibrate); liver or severe kidney dysfunction; unexplained liver function abnormality; preexisting hepatic disease; primary biliary cirrhosis; preexisting gallbladder disease; thrombocytopenia; lactation.

**CAUTIOUS USE** Renal impairment, older adults; history of bleeding disorders; myelosuppression; pregnancy (category C). Safety and efficacy in children not established.

## ROUTE & DOSAGE

**Hypertriglyceridemia**
*Adult:* **PO** 43–200 mg/day depending on product

## ADMINISTRATION

**Oral**

- Drug is usually discontinued after 2 mo if adequate lipid reduction is not achieved with the maximum recommended dose.
- Give at least 1 h before or 4–6 h after cholestyramine.
- Store at 15°–30° C (59°–86° F) in a tightly closed container and protect from light.

**ADVERSE EFFECTS** (≥1%) **Body as a Whole:** Asthenia, fatigue, infections, flu-like syndrome, localized pain, arthralgia. **CNS:** Headache, paresthesia, dizziness, insomnia. **CV:** Arrhythmia. **GI:** Dyspepsia, eructation, flatulence, nausea, vomiting, abdominal pain, constipation, diarrhea, increased appetite. **Respiratory:** Cough, rhinitis, sinusitis. **Skin:** Pruritus, rash. **Special Senses:** Earache, eye floaters, blurred vision, conjunctivitis,

Common adverse effects in *italic*; life-threatening effects underlined; generic names in **bold**; classifications in SMALL CAPS; ♣ Canadian drug name; ℗ Prototype drug

677

eye irritation, **Urogenital:** Decreased libido, polyuria, vaginitis.

**INTERACTIONS**   **Drug:** May potentiate anticoagulant effects of **warfarin;** combination with an HMG-COA REDUCTASE INHIBITOR (STATIN) may result in rhabdomyolysis; **cholestyramine, colestipol** may decrease absorption (give fenofibrate 1 h before or 4–6 h after BILE ACID SEQUESTRANTS); may increase risk of nephrotoxicity of **cyclosporine.**

**PHARMACOKINETICS   Absorption:** Well absorbed from the GI tract; increased with food. **Peak:** 6–8 h. **Distribution:** 99% protein bound; excreted in breast milk. **Metabolism:** Rapidly hydrolyzed by esterases to active metabolite, fenofibric acid. **Elimination:** 60% in urine, 25% in feces. **Half-Life:** 20 h.

## NURSING IMPLICATIONS

### Assessment & Drug Effects

- Assess for muscle pain, tenderness, or weakness and, if present, monitor CPK level. Withdraw drug with marked elevations of CPK or if myopathy is suspected.
- Monitor patients on coumarin-type drugs closely for prolongation of PT/INR.
- Monitor lab tests: Periodic lipid levels, LFTs, and CBC with differential.

### Patient & Family Education

- Contact prescriber immediately if any of the following develops: Unexplained muscle pain, tenderness, or weakness, especially with fever or malaise; yellowing of skin or eyes; nausea or loss of appetite; skin rash or hives.
- Inform prescriber regarding concurrent use of cholestyramine, oral anticoagulants, or cyclosporine.

# FENOLDOPAM MESYLATE

(fen-ol'do-pam mes'y-late)

**Corlopam**

**Classifications:** NON-NITRATE VASODILATOR; DOPAMINE AGONIST; ANTIHYPERTENSIVE

**Therapeutic:** ANTIHYPERTENSIVE

**AVAILABILITY** Solution for injection

**ACTION & *THERAPEUTIC EFFECT***
Rapid-acting vasodilator that is a dopamine $D_1$-like receptor agonist. Exerts hypotensive effects by decreasing peripheral vascular resistance while increasing renal blood flow, diuresis, and natriuresis. Effectiveness *indicated by rapid reduction in BP. Decreases both systolic and diastolic pressures.*

**USES** Short-term (up to 48 h) management of severe hypertension.

**CONTRAINDICATIONS** Hypersensitivity to fenoldopam.

**CAUTIOUS USE** Asthmatic patients; hepatic cirrhosis, portal hypertension, or variceal bleeding; arrhythmias, tachycardia, or angina, particularly unstable angina; elevated IOP; angular-closure glaucoma; hypotension; hypokalemia; acute cerebral infarct or hemorrhage; pregnancy (category B); lactation.

## ROUTE & DOSAGE

| Severe Hypertension |
| --- |
| *Adult:* **IV** 0.1–0.3 mcg/kg/min by continuous infusion for up to 48 h, may increase by 0.05–0.1 mcg/kg/min q15min (dosage range: 0.01–1.6 mcg/kg/min)<br>*Child:* **IV** 0.2 mcg/kg/min, may increase to 0.3–0.5 mcg/kg/min |

Common adverse effects in *italic;* life-threatening effects underlined; generic names in **bold;** classifications in SMALL CAPS; ♣ Canadian drug name; ⊙ Prototype drug

## ADMINISTRATION

### Intravenous

*PREPARE:* **Continuous for Adult:** Dilute to a final concentration of 40 mcg/mL by adding 1 mL (10 mg), 2 mL (20 mg), or 3 mL (30 mg) of fenoldopam to 250, 500, or 1000 mL, respectively, of NS or D5W. **Continuous for Child:** Dilute to a final concentration of 60 mcg/mL by adding 0.6 mL (6 mg), 1.5 mL (15 mg) or 3 mL (3 mg) of fenoldopam to 100, 250, or 500 mL, respectively, of NS or D5W.

*ADMINISTER:* **Continuous for Adult/Child:** Give only by continuous infusion; never give a direct or bolus dose. ▪ Titrate initial dose up or down no more frequently than q15min.

*INCOMPATIBILITIES:* **Y-site: Acyclovir, aminophylline, amphotericin B, ampicillin, bumetanide, cefoxitin, dantrolene, dexamethasone, diazepam, fosphenytoin, furosemide, ganciclovir, gemtuzumab, hetastarch, ketorolac, meropenem, mesna, methohexital, methylprednisolone, mitomycin, pantoprazole, pentobarbital, phenytoin, prochlorperazine, sodium bicarbonate.**

▪ Note: Diluted solution is stable under normal room temperature and light for 24 h. Discard any unused solution after 24 h. ▪ Store at 15°–30° C (59°–86° F) in a tightly closed container and protect from light.

## ADVERSE EFFECTS (≥1%) Body as a Whole: Injection site reaction, pyrexia, nonspecific chest pain. CNS: Headache, nervousness, anxiety, insomnia, dizziness. CV: *Hypotension, tachycardia,* T-wave inversion, flushing, postural hypotension, extrasystoles, palpitations, bradycardia, heart failure, ischemic heart disease, MI, angina. GI: Nausea, vomiting, abdominal pain or fullness, constipation, diarrhea. Metabolic: Increased creatinine, BUN, glucose, transaminases, LDH; hypokalemia. Respiratory: Nasal congestion, dyspnea, upper respiratory disorder. Skin: Sweating. Other: UTI, leukocytosis, bleeding.

## INTERACTIONS Use with BETA-BLOCKERS increases risk of hypotension.

## PHARMACOKINETICS Onset: 5 min. Peak: 15 min. Duration: 15–30 min. Distribution: Crosses placenta. Metabolism: Conjugated in liver. Elimination: 90% in urine, 10% in feces. Half-Life: 5 min.

## NURSING IMPLICATIONS

### Assessment & Drug Effects

▪ Monitor BP and HR carefully at least q15min or more often as warranted; expect dose-related tachycardia.

▪ Monitor lab tests: Frequent serum electrolytes.

# FENOPROFEN CALCIUM

(fen-oh-proe'fen)

Nalfon

**Classifications:** ANALGESIC, NONSTEROIDAL ANTI-INFLAMMATORY DRUG (NSAID)

Therapeutic: ANALGESIC; NSAID; ANTIARTHRITIC; ANTIPYRETIC

**Prototype:** Ibuprofen

## AVAILABILITY Tablet; capsule

## ACTION & *THERAPEUTIC EFFECT*

Fenoprofen competitively inhibits both cyclooxygenase COX-1 and COX-2 enzymes by blocking arachidonate binding to prostaglandin $G_2$ resulting in its pharmacologic effects. *Has nonsteroidal, anti-inflammatory, antipyretic, antiarthritic properties that provide relief from mild to severe pain.*

Common adverse effects in *italic*; life-threatening effects underlined; generic names in **bold**; classifications in SMALL CAPS; ♣ Canadian drug name; ⓟ Prototype drug

679

**USES** Rheumatoid arthritis; osteoarthritis; relief of mild to moderate pain.

**UNLABELED USES** Juvenile rheumatoid arthritis, acute gouty arthritis, ankylosing spondylitis.

**CONTRAINDICATION** Hypersensitivity to fenoprofen or other NSAIDs; salicylate; history of nephrotic syndrome associated with aspirin or other NSAIDS; patient in whom urticaria, severe rhinitis, bronchospasm, angioedema, nasal polyps are precipitated by aspirin or other NSAIDS; preexisting asthma; severe renal or hepatic dysfunction; GI bleeding, ulceration, or perforation; perioperative pain associated in CABG; pregnancy (category D starting 30 wk gestation).

**CAUTIOUS USE** History of GI tract disorders; lupus; renal failure; renal impairment; hemophilia or other bleeding tendencies; compromised cardiac function; risk factors for CAD; CHF; hypertension; fluid retention; impaired hearing; older adults; pregnancy (category C before 30 wk gestation); lactation. Safety in children less than 18 y not established.

## ROUTE & DOSAGE

### RA/OA
*Adult:* **PO** 400–600 mg t.i.d. or q.i.d. (max: 3200 mg/day)

### Mild to Moderate Pain
*Adult:* **PO** 200 mg q4–6h prn

## ADMINISTRATION

### Oral
- Give on an empty stomach 30–60 min before or 2 h after meals. Give with meals, milk, or antacid (prescribed) if patient experiences GI disturbances.
- May crush tablets or empty capsule and mix with fluid or mix with food.

- Store capsules and tablets in tightly closed containers at 15°–30° C (59°–86° F); avoid freezing.

**ADVERSE EFFECTS** (≥1%) **CNS:** *Headache, drowsiness,* dizziness, asthenia, fatigue, lassitude, tremor, confusion, insomnia, nervousness, depression. **Special Senses:** Tinnitus, decreased hearing, deafness; blurred vision. **GI:** *Indigestion, nausea, vomiting,* anorexia, *constipation,* diarrhea, flatulence, abdominal pain, dry mouth; infrequent: Gastritis, peptic ulcer, GI bleeding. **Urogenital:** Dysuria, cystitis, hematuria, oliguria, azotemia, anuria, allergic nephritis, papillary necrosis, nephrotoxicity (rare). **Hematologic:** (Infrequent) Thrombocytopenia, hemolytic anemia, agranulocytosis, pancytopenia. **CV:** Palpitations, atrial fibrillation. **Skin:** (May or may not be hypersensitivity reaction) Pruritus, rash, purpura, increased sweating, urticaria. **Body as a Whole:** Dyspnea, malaise, anaphylaxis, edema.

**INTERACTIONS Drug:** Fenoprofen may prolong bleeding time; should not be given with ORAL ANTICOAGULANTS, **heparin;** action and side effects of **phenytoin,** SULFONYLUREAS, SULFONAMIDES, and fenoprofen may be potentiated. **Herbal: Feverfew, garlic, ginger, gingko** may increase bleeding potential.

**DIAGNOSTIC TEST INTERFERENCE** May elevate Amerlex-M assay values for *thyroid tests.*

**PHARMACOKINETICS Absorption:** 80% from GI tract, 99% protein bound. **Onset:** 2 h. **Peak:** 2 h. **Duration:** 4–6 h. **Distribution:** Small amounts into breast milk. **Metabolism:** In liver. **Elimination:** Primarily in urine; some biliary excretion. **Half-Life:** 3 h.

## NURSING IMPLICATIONS

### Black Box Warning

*Etodolac has been associated with increased risk of serious, potentially fatal GI bleeding and cardiovascular events (e.g., MI & CVA); risk may increase with duration of use and may be greater in the older adult and those with risk factors for CV disease.*

### Assessment & Drug Effects

- Baseline and periodic auditory and ophthalmic examinations are recommended in patients receiving prolonged or high-dose therapy.
- Monitor for S&S of GI bleeding. Significant GI bleeding may occur without prior warning.
- Monitor for and report promptly S&S of CV thrombotic events (i.e., angina, MI, TIA, or stroke).
- Monitor lab tests: Baseline Hct and Hgb, renal function tests and LFTs.

### Patient & Family Education

- Do not drive or engage in potentially hazardous activities until response to drug is known, fenoprofen may cause dizziness and drowsiness.
- Report immediately the onset of unexplained fever, rash, arthralgia, oliguria, edema, weight gain to prescriber. Possible symptoms of nephrotic syndrome are rapidly reversible if drug is promptly withdrawn.
- Understand that alcohol and aspirin may increase risk of GI ulceration and bleeding tendencies; avoid both unless otherwise advised by prescriber.

## FENTANYL CITRATE

(fen′ta-nil)

Abstral, Actiq, Duragesic, Fentora, Ionsys, Lazanda, Onsolis, Sublimaze, Subsys

**Classifications:** ANALGESIC; NARCOTIC (OPIATE AGONIST)
Therapeutic: NARCOTIC ANALGESIC
**Prototype:** Morphine
**Controlled Substance:** Schedule II

**AVAILABILITY** Solution for injection; lozenge; lozenge on a stick; transdermal patch; buccal tablet; buccal film; sublingual tablet; nasal spray

## ACTION & *THERAPEUTIC EFFECT*

Synthetic, potent narcotic agonist that causes analgesia and sedation. Its alterations in respiratory rate and alveolar ventilation may persist beyond the analgesic effect. *Provides analgesia for moderate to severe pain as well as sedation.*

**USES** Short-acting analgesic during operative and perioperative periods, moderate or severe pain.

**UNLABELED USES** Dyspnea, sedation maintenance.

**CONTRAINDICATIONS** Hypersensitivity to **fentanyl;** patients who have received MAO inhibitors within 14 days; substance abuse; patients who are not opioid tolerant; acute pain; out-patient surgery; significant respiratory compromise including acute or severe bronchial asthma; myasthenia gravis; labor and delivery; have or are suspected of having paralytic ileus; lactation. **Transdermal patch:** Patients not opioid tolerant; acute pain or short-term use; postoperative pain; mild pain; intermittent pain. **Sublingual:** Acute or postoperative pain, including headache/migraine and in patients not opioid tolerant.

**CAUTIOUS USE** Head injuries, increased intracranial pressure; older adults, debilitated, poor-risk patients; cardiac diseases, angina, hypotension, or cardiac arrhythmias;

Common adverse effects in *italic;* life-threatening effects underlined; generic names in **bold;** classifications in SMALL CAPS; ♣ Canadian drug name; ● Prototype drug

681

F

COPD, other respiratory problems; liver and kidney dysfunction; history of drug addition; family history of substance abuse; bradyarrhythmias; children; pregnancy (category C) .

## ROUTE & DOSAGE

### General Anesthesia Induction

*Adult:* **IV** 50–100 mcg 30–60 min before surgery

### Post-Operative Pain Management

*Adult/Adolescent/Child (older than 1 y):* **IV/IM** 1–2 mcg/kg

### Breakthrough Cancer Pain

*Adult:* **PO Actiq** only: 200 mcg over 15 min
**Fentora** only: 100 mcg over 30 min
**Onsolis** only: 200 mcg initial dose, may titrate up by 200 mcg in each subsequent episode (max: 4 simultaneous doses)
**Abstral** only: 100 mcg until dissolved, may repeat after 30 min, do not repeat for at least 2 h
**Intranasal Lazanda** only: 100 mcg spray, do not repeat for at least 2 h

### Postoperative Pain in Recovery Room

*Adult:* **IM/IV** 50–100 mcg q1–2h prn

### Chronic Pain

*Adult:* **Transdermal** Individualize and regularly reassess doses of transdermal fentanyl; for patient not already receiving an opioid, the initial dose is 25 mcg/h patch q3days; for patients already on opioids, see package insert for conversions; **Stick lozenge (Actiq)** 200 mcg (**Actiq** only) as breakthrough agent; **IV/IM** 50–110 mcg
*Child (over 2):* **Transdermal** Individualize and reassess regularly

## ADMINISTRATION

### Buccal

- *Buccal tablet:* Do not push tablet through blister, as this may cause damage to tablet.
- *Buccal film:* Place film on inside of cheek with the pink side against the mucous membrane. Hold film against cheek for 5 sec. Film should be left in place until it dissolves (15–30 min). Liquids may be consumed after 5 min but solids should not be eaten until film dissolves.

### Oral

- *Lozenge:* Place unit between cheek and lower gum, moving it from one side to the other using the handle. Instruct the patient to suck, not chew, the lozenge. Should be consumed over a 15-min period.

### Sublingual

- *Sublingual tablet:* Note that Abstral tablets are not equivalent on a mcg/mcg basis with other fentanyl products. Place tablet under tongue immediately after removal from blister pack. Instruct patient not to chew, suck, or swallow tablet, and allow to completely dissolve in the sublingual cavity before eating or drinking.
- *Sublingual tablet and spray:* Note that the sublingual spray and tablet are not interchangable on a dosage basis.

### Intranasal

- *Nasal spray:* Lazanda is not equivalent to other fentanyl products on a mcg/mcg basis.

### Intramuscular

- Inject undiluted into a large muscle.

### Transdermal

- Place on nonirritated flat surface (e.g., chest, back, upper arm). The upper back is preferred to minimize unintended patch removal. Clip (not shave) hair at application site prior to system application. If needed, clean site prior to application only with clear water. Press patch in place for 30 sec. If gel from patch leaks out and contacts skin of patient or caregiver, wash thoroughly with water.

- Do not expose the fentanyl application site and surrounding area to any direct external heat source (e.g., heating pad or electric blanket, heat or tanning lamp, sauna, hot bath).

### Intravascular

*PREPARE:* **Direct:** Give parenteral doses undiluted or diluted in 5 mL sterile water or NS.
*ADMINISTER:* **Direct:** Inject slowly over 1–3 min.
*INCOMPATIBILITIES:* **Solution/additive: Fluorouracil, levobupivacaine, lornoxicam, ropivacaine. Y-site: Amiodarone, amphotericin B conventional, ampicillin, azithromycin, dantrolene, diazepam, diazoxide, gemtuzumab, haloperidol, hydralazine, hydroxycobalamine, pantoprazole, phenytoin, SMZ/TMP.**

- Store at 15°–30° C (59°–86° F) unless otherwise directed. Protect drug from light.

### ADVERSE EFFECTS (≥1%) CNS:
*Sedation,* euphoria, dizziness, diaphoresis, delirium, convulsions with high doses. **CV:** Hypotension, bradycardia, <u>circulatory depression, cardiac arrest</u>. **Special Senses:** Miosis, blurred vision. **GI:** *Nausea,* vomiting, constipation, ileus. **Respiratory:** Laryngospasm, bronchoconstriction, <u>respiratory depression or arrest</u>. **Body as a Whole:** Muscle rigidity, especially muscles of respiration after rapid IV infusion, urinary retention. **Skin:** Rash, contact dermatitis from patch.

### INTERACTIONS Drug: Alcohol
and other CNS DEPRESSANTS potentiate effects; MAO INHIBITORS may precipitate hypertensive crisis.

### PHARMACOKINETICS Absorption:
Absorbed through the skin, leveling off between 12–24 h. **Onset:** Immediate IV; 7–15 min IM; 12–24 h transdermal. **Peak:** 3–5 min IV; 24–72 h transdermal. **Duration:** 30–60 min IV; 1–2 h IM; 72 h transdermal. **Metabolism:** In liver by CYP3A4. **Elimination:** In urine. **Half-Life:** 17 h transdermal.

## NURSING IMPLICATIONS

### Black Box Warning

*Fentanyl has been associated with severe, potentially fatal, respiratory depression.*

#### Assessment & Drug Effects

- Monitor vital signs and observe patient for signs of skeletal and thoracic muscle (depressed respirations) rigidity and weakness.
- Watch closely for respiratory depression and for movements of various groups of skeletal muscle in extremities, external eye, and neck during postoperative period. These movements may present patient management problems; report promptly.
- Note: Duration of respiratory depressant effect may be considerably longer than narcotic analgesic effect. Have immediately available oxygen, resuscitative and intubation equipment, and an opioid antagonist such as naloxone.

#### Patient & Family Education

- Follow exactly instructions for taking fentanyl and for disposal of unit provided in patient information.
- Exercise caution when engaging in hazardous activities until reaction to drug is known.

Common adverse effects in *italic*; life-threatening effects <u>underlined</u>; generic names in **bold**; classifications in SMALL CAPS; ♣ Canadian drug name; ⦾ Prototype drug

683

- Do not apply any source of direct, external heat to skin area to which patch is attached.
- Children exposed to buccal tablets are at high risk for respiratory depression. Keep out of reach of children.

## FERROUS SULFATE ⓟ
(fer′rous sul′fate)

Feosol, Fer-In-Sol, Fer-Iron, Ferospace, Ferralyn, Fesofor, Mol-Iron, Novoferrosulfa ♦, Slow-Fe, Slow Iron

## FERROUS FUMARATE
(fer′rous foo′ma-rate)

Femiron, Hemocyte, Neo-Fer-50 ♦, Novofumar ♦, Palafer ♦

## FERROUS GLUCONATE
(fer′rous gloo′koe-nate)

Ferate, Fergon, Fertinic ♦, Novoferrogluc ♦

**Classification:** IRON PREPARATION
Therapeutic: ANTIANEMIC; IRON SUPPLEMENT

## AVAILABILITY Ferrous Sulfate:
Tablet; sustained release tablet; syrup; elixir; **Ferrous Fumarate:** Tablet; extended release tablet; **Ferrous Gluconate:** Tablet

## ACTION & THERAPEUTIC EFFECT
**Ferrous sulfate:** Standard iron preparation that corrects erythropoietic abnormalities induced by iron deficiency but does not stimulate erythropoiesis. **Ferrous gluconate:** Claimed to cause less gastric irritation and be better tolerated than ferrous sulfate. *Effectiveness is experienced within 48 h as a sense of well-being, increased vigor, improved appetite, and decreased irritability (in children). Reticulocyte response begins in about 4 days;* *it usually peaks in 7–10 days and returns to normal after 2 or 3 wk.*

**USES** To correct simple iron deficiency and to treat iron deficiency anemias. May be used prophylactically during periods of increased iron needs, as in infancy, childhood, and pregnancy.

**CONTRAINDICATIONS** Peptic ulcer, regional enteritis, ulcerative colitis; hemolytic anemias (in absence of iron deficiency), hemochromatosis, hemosiderosis, patients receiving repeated transfusions, pyridoxine-responsive anemia; cirrhosis of liver.

**CAUTIOUS USE** Hepatic disease; GI diseases; sulfite hypersensitivity; pregnancy (category A).

## ROUTE & DOSAGE

**Ferrous Sulfate (20% elemental iron)**
**Ferrous Fumarate (33% elemental iron)**
**Ferrous Gluconate (12% elemental iron)**
**Treatment of Iron Deficiency Anemia**

*Adult:* **PO** 60 mg elemental iron 1–3 × daily for 4 wk
*Infant/Child:* **PO** 3–6 mg elemental iron/kg/day (divide doses) for 4 wk

## ADMINISTRATION
### Oral
- Give on an empty stomach if possible because oral iron preparations are best absorbed then (i.e., between meals). Minimize gastric distress if needed by giving with or immediately after meals with adequate liquid.
- Do not crush tablet or empty contents of capsule when administering.

Common adverse effects in *italic;* life-threatening effects underlined; generic names in **bold;** classifications in SMALL CAPS; ♦ Canadian drug name; ⓟ Prototype drug

- Do not give tablets or capsules within 1 h of bedtime.
- Consult prescriber about prescribing a liquid formulation or a less corrosive form, such as ferrous gluconate, if the patient experiences difficulty in swallowing tablet or capsule.
- Dilute liquid preparations well and give through a straw or placed on the back of tongue with a dropper to prevent staining of teeth and to mask taste. Instruct the patient to rinse mouth with clear water immediately after ingestion.
- Mix ferosol elixir with water; not compatible with milk or fruit juice. Fer-In-Sol (drops) may be given in water or in fruit or vegetable juice, according to manufacturer.
- Do not use discolored tablets.
- Store in tightly closed containers and protect from moisture. Store at 15° 30° C (59°–86° F).

**ADVERSE EFFECTS** (≥1%) **GI:** *Nausea, heartburn,* anorexia, *constipation,* diarrhea, epigastric pain, abdominal distress, *black stools.* **Special Senses:** Yellow-brown discoloration of eyes and teeth (liquid forms). **Large Chronic Doses in Infants:** Rickets (due to interference with phosphorus absorption). **Massive Overdosage:** Lethargy, drowsiness, nausea, vomiting, abdominal pain, diarrhea, local corrosion of stomach and small intestines, pallor or cyanosis, metabolic acidosis, <u>shock, cardiovascular collapse</u>, convulsions, <u>liver necrosis</u>, coma, renal failure, <u>death</u>.

**DIAGNOSTIC TEST INTERFERENCE**
By coloring feces black, large iron doses may cause false-positive tests for *occult blood with orthotoluidine (Hematest, Occultist, Labstix); guaiac reagent benzidine test* is reportedly not affected.

**INTERACTIONS Drug:** ANTACIDS decrease iron absorption; iron

decreases absorption of TETRACYCLINES, **ciprofloxacin, ofloxacin; chloramphenicol** may delay iron's effects; iron may decrease absorption of **penicillamine. Food:** Food decreases absorption of iron; **ascorbic acid (vitamin C)** may increase iron absorption.

**PHARMACOKINETICS Absorption:** 5–10% absorbed in healthy individuals; 10–30% absorbed in iron-deficiency; food decreases amount absorbed. **Distribution:** Transported by transferrin to bone marrow, where it is incorporated into hemoglobin; crosses placenta. **Elimination:** Most of iron released from hemoglobin is reused in body; small amounts are lost in desquamation of skin, GI mucosa, nails, and hair; 12–30 mg/mo lost through menstruation.

**NURSING IMPLICATIONS**
**Assessment & Drug Effects**
- Continue iron therapy for 2–3 mo after the hemoglobin level has returned to normal (roughly twice the period required to normalize hemoglobin concentration).
- Monitor bowel movements as constipation is a common adverse effect.
- Monitor lab tests: Periodic Hgb and reticulocyte counts.

**Patient & Family Education**
- Note: Ascorbic acid increases absorption of iron. Consuming citrus fruit or tomato juice with iron preparation (except the elixir) may increase its absorption.
- Be aware that milk, eggs, or caffeine beverages when taken with the iron preparation may inhibit absorption.
- Be aware that iron preparations cause dark green or black stools.
- Report constipation or diarrhea to prescriber; symptoms may be

Common adverse effects in *italic*; life-threatening effects <u>underlined</u>; generic names in **bold**; classifications in SMALL CAPS; ♣ Canadian drug name; ⊘ Prototype drug

685

relieved by adjustments in dosage or diet or by change to another iron preparation.

# FESOTERODINE

(fes'oh-ter'oh-deen)

Toviaz

**Classifications:** ANTICHOLINERGIC; MUSCARINIC RECEPTOR ANTAGONIST; BLADDER ANTISPASMODIC

**Therapeutic:** BLADDER ANTISPAS-MODIC

**Prototype:** Oxybutynin

**AVAILABILITY** Extended release tablet

## ACTION & *THERAPEUTIC EFFECT*

A muscarinic receptor antagonist that reduces urinary incontinence, urgency, and frequency. It helps regulate the involuntary contractions of the bladder associated with sudden urges to urinate. *It controls urinary incontinence or overactive bladder (OAB).*

**USES** Treatment of overactive bladder in patients with urinary incontinence, urgency.

**CONTRAINDICATIONS** Severe hepatic impairment (Child-Pugh class C); gastric obstruction, paralytic ileus, uncontrolled narrow-angle glaucoma; urinary retention; severe BPH; lactation.

**CAUTIOUS USE** Cross-sensitivity to tolterodine; mild to moderate hepatic impairment (Child-Pugh class A and B); renal insufficiency; history of constipation; bladder outlet obstruction; history of decreased GI motility; severe constipation; palpitations; narrow-angle glaucoma; myasthenia gravis; pregnancy (category C). Safe use in children not established.

## ROUTE & DOSAGE

### Overactive Bladder

*Adult:* **PO** 4–8 mg daily. Do not exceed 4 mg daily with concurrent potent CYP3A4 inhibitors.

### Hepatic Impairment Dosage Adjustment

*Severe hepatic impairment (Child-Pugh class C):* Not recommended

### Renal Impairment Dosage Adjustment

*CrCl less than 30 mL/min:* Do not exceed 4 mg

## ADMINISTRATION

### Oral

- Give with water without regard to food.
- Do not break or crush extended release tablet. Ensure that it is swallowed whole.
- Store at 15°–30° C (59°–86° F).

**ADVERSE EFFECTS** (≥1%) **Body as a Whole:** Peripheral edema, upper respiratory tract infection, urinary tract infection, angioedema. **CNS:** Insomnia. **GI:** Constipation, *dry mouth*, dyspepsia, nausea. **Metabolic:** Elevated ALT levels, elevated GGT levels. **Musculoskeletal:** Back pain. **Respiratory:** Cough, dry throat. **Skin:** Rash. **Special Senses:** Dry eyes. **Urogenital:** Dysuria, urinary retention, urinary tract infection.

**INTERACTIONS Drug:** Potent CYP-3A4 INHIBITORS (e.g., **clarithromycin, itraconazole, ketoconazole, nefazodone, nelfinavir,** and **ritonavir**) increase fesoterodine levels. INDUCERS OF CYP3A4 (e.g., **rifampin**) can decrease fesoterodine levels.

**PHARMACOKINETICS Absorption:** 52% bioavailable. **Peak:** 5 h. **Distribution:** 50% plasma protein bound. **Metabolism:** Hepatic metabolism to active and inactive metabolites. **Elimination:** Renal (70%) and fecal (7%). **Half-Life:** 7 h.

## NURSING IMPLICATIONS

### Assessment & Drug Effects

- Monitor bowel and bladder function as urinary retention and constipation are potential adverse effects. Older adults are at greater risk for adverse effects, especially with the 8 mg dose.
- Monitor for and report bothersome anticholinergic effects (see Appendix F).

### Patient & Family Education

- Use caution in hot environments to avoid heat prostration as fesoterodine causes decreased sweating and reduces body cooling in excessive heat.
- Exercise caution with hazardous activities until response to drug is known.
- Moderate alcohol consumption as it may enhance drowsiness caused by fesoterodine.

## FEXOFENADINE

(fex-o-fen'a-deen)
Allegra

**Classifications:** NONSEDATING; ANTIHISTAMINE; $H_1$-RECEPTOR ANTAGONIST
**Therapeutic:** NONSEDATING ANTIHISTAMINE
**Prototype:** Loratadine

## AVAILABILITY
Tablet; capsule; orally disintegrating tablet; oral suspension

## ACTION & *THERAPEUTIC EFFECT*
Competes with histamine for binding at the $H_1$-receptor. This blocks effects of histamine on $H_1$-receptors resulting in decreased formation of edema, flare, and pruritus. *Inhibits antigen-induced bronchospasm*

*and histamine release from mast cells. Efficacy is indicated by reduction of the following: Nasal congestion and sneezing; watery or red eyes; itching nose, palate, or eyes.*

**USES** Relief of symptoms associated with seasonal allergic rhinitis, and chronic urticaria.

**CONTRAINDICATIONS** Hypersensitivity to fexofenadine or terfenadine; neonates.

**CAUTIOUS USE** Mild to severe renal and hepatic insufficiency, hypertension, diabetes mellitus, ischemic heart disease, increased ocular pressure, hyperthyroidism, renal impairment, prostatic hypertrophy; elderly, pregnancy (category C); lactation; young children.

## ROUTE & DOSAGE

### Allergic Rhinitis

*Adult/Adolescent:* **PO** 60 mg b.i.d. OR 180 mg daily
*Child (2–11 y):* **PO** 30 mg b.i.d.
*Child (6–11 y):* **PO** (oral disintegrating tablet) 30 mg b.i.d.

### Chronic Urticaria

*Adult:* **PO** 60 mg b.i.d. OR 180 mg daily
*Child (2–11 y):* **PO** 30 mg b.i.d.
*Child (6–11 y):* **PO** (oral disintegrating tablet) 30 mg b.i.d.
*Child (younger than 2 y)/Infant (6 mo or older):* **PO** 15 mg b.i.d.

### *Renal Impairment Dosage Adjustment*

*CrCl less than 80 mL/min.* Give normal dose only once/day

## ADMINISTRATION

### Oral

- Reduce starting dose for those with decreased kidney function.

---

Common adverse effects in *italic;* life-threatening effects <u>underlined</u>; generic names in **bold;** classifications in SMALL CAPS; ♣ Canadian drug name; ⓟ Prototype drug

687

- Do not give within 15 min of an aluminum- or magnesium-containing antacid.
- Store at 20°–25° C (68°–77° F). Protect from excess moisture.

## ADVERSE EFFECTS (≥1%) CNS:
*Headache,* drowsiness, fatigue. **GI:** Nausea, dyspepsia, throat irritation.

## INTERACTIONS Drug: ANTACIDS
will decrease serum level of fexofenadine. **Herbal: St. John's wort** will decrease serum level of fexofenadine. **Food: Grapefruit juice** or **apple juice** may decrease efficacy.

## PHARMACOKINETICS Absorption:
Rapidly from GI tract, 33% reaches systemic circulation. **Onset:** 1 h. **Peak:** 2–3 h. **Duration:** At least 12 h. **Distribution:** 60–70% bound to plasma proteins. **Metabolism:** Only 5% of dose metabolized in liver. **Elimination:** 80% in urine, 11% in feces. **Half-Life:** 14.4 h.

## NURSING IMPLICATIONS

### Assessment & Drug Effects
- Monitor therapeutic effectiveness, which is indicated by decreased nasal congestion, sneezing, watery or red eyes, and itching nose, palate, or eyes.

### Patient & Family Education
- Note: Drug is well tolerated and causes minimal adverse effects.

## FIDAXOMICIN
(fye-dax'oh-mye'sin)
Dificid
**Classifications:** MACROLIDE ANTIBIOTIC
Therapeutic: ANTIBIOTIC
**Prototype:** Erythromycin

## AVAILABILITY Tablet

## ACTION & *THERAPEUTIC EFFECT*
Macrolide antibiotic that inhibits RNA-synthesis by RNA polymerases. *Bactericidal action on* Clostridium difficile *in the GI tract.*

## USES
Treatment of pseudomembranous colitis or *Clostridium difficile*-associated diarrhea (CDAD).

## CAUTIOUS USE
Not for use in systemic infections; hyperglycemia; metabolic acidosis; pregnancy; lactation. Safety and efficacy in children younger than 18 y not established.

## ROUTE & DOSAGE

### Clostridium Difficile–Associated Diarrhea
*Adult:* **PO** 200 mg b.i.d. for 10 d

## ADMINISTRATION

### Oral
- May give without regard to food.
- Store at 15°–30° C (59°–86° F).

## ADVERSE EFFECTS (≥2%) GI:
Abdominal pain, GI hemorrhage, *nausea, vomiting.* **Hematological:** Anemia, neutropenia.

## PHARMACOKINETICS Absorption:
Minimal systemic absorption. **Peak:** 2 h. **Distribution:** Primarily confined to GI tract. **Metabolism:** Hydrolysis in GI tract to active metabolite. **Elimination:** Primarily fecal (92%). **Half-Life:** 11.7 h.

## NURSING IMPLICATIONS

### Assessment & Drug Effects
- Note that fidaxomicin is not effective for treatment of systemic infections.
- Monitor GI symptoms of CDAD (*C. difficile*-associated disease) and report increasing GI distress.

- Effectiveness is indicated by decreasing diarrhea and improvement in other S&S of GI distress.
- Monitor lab tests: CBC with differential as needed.

**Patient & Family Education**
- It is common to feel better soon after beginning treatment, however, do not stop taking the drug until the full course of treatment is completed.

## FILGRASTIM ⓟ

(fil-gras′tim)

Neupogen, Zarxio

**Classification:** HEMATOPOIETIC GROWTH FACTOR
Therapeutic: ANTINEUTROPENIC, GRANULOCYTE COLONY-STIMU-LATING FACTOR (G-CSF)

**AVAILABILITY** Solution for injection

## ACTION & THERAPEUTIC EFFECT

Human granulocyte colony-stimulating factor (G-CSF) produced by recombinant DNA technology. Endogenous G-CSF regulates production of neutrophils within the bone marrow; primarily affects neutrophil proliferation, differentiation, and selected end-cell functional activity (including enhanced phagocytic activity and antibody-dependent killing). *Increases neutrophil proliferation and differentiation within the bone marrow.*

**USES** Treatment of chemotheraphy induced neutropenia, neutropenia, peripheral blood stem cell mobilization, radiation exposure.

## CONTRAINDICATIONS Hypersensitivity to *Escherichia coli*–derived proteins, concurrent administration with chemotherapy, radiation; ARDS.

**CAUTIOUS USE** Sickle cell disease; renal impairment; respiratory insufficiency; pregnancy (category C); lactation.

## ROUTE & DOSAGE

### Neutropenia Prophylaxis
*Adult/Adolescent/Child:* **IV** 5 mcg/kg/day by 30 min infusion, may increase by 5 mcg/kg/day (max: 30 mcg/kg/day); **Subcutaneous** 5 mcg/kg/day as single dose, may increase based on pt response

### Bone Marrow Transplant
*Adult:* **IV** 10 mcg/kg/day given 24 h after cytotoxic therapy and 24 h after bone marrow transfusion

### Radiation Exposure
*Adult/Adolescent/Child/Infant (older than 7 mo):* **Subcutaenous** 10 mcg/kg/day

## ADMINISTRATION

**Subcutaneous & Intravenous**
- Do not administer filgrastim 24 h before or after cytotoxic chemotherapy or while undergoing radiation therapy. - Use only one dose/vial; do not reenter the vial.
- Prior to injection, filgrastim may be allowed to reach room temperature for a maximum of 6 h.
- Discard any vial left at room temperature for longer than 6 h.

**Subcutaneous**
- Inject into the outer upper arm, abdomen (except within 2 inches of navel), front middle thigh, or the upper outer buttocks area.

**Intravenous**
**PREPARE: Intermittent/Continuous:** May dilute with 10–50 mL D5W to yield 15 mcg/mL or greater. ■ If more diluent is used

Common adverse effects in *italic;* life-threatening effects underlined; generic names in **bold;** classifications in SMALL CAPS; ◆ Canadian drug name; ⓟ Prototype drug

689

F

to yield concentrations of 5–15 mcg/mL, 2 mL of 5% human albumin **must be** added for each 50 mL D5W (prior to adding filgrastim) to prevent adsorption to plastic IV infusion materials.

*ADMINISTER:* **Intermittent:** Give a single dose over 15–30 min. ▪ Flush line before/after with D5W. **Continuous:** Give a single dose over 4–24 h. ▪ Flush line before/after with D5W.

*INCOMPATIBILITIES:* **Y-site: Aminocaproic acid, amphotericin B, cefepime, cefoperazone, cefotaxime, cefoxitin, ceftaroline, ceftizoxime, ceftobiprole, ceftriaxone, cefuroxime, clindamycin, dactinomycin, etoposide, fluorouracil, furosemide, gentamicin, heparin, imipenem, mannitol, methylprednisolone, metronidazole, mitomycin, piperacillin, prochlorperazine, thiotepa.**

▪ Store refrigerated at 2°–8° C (36°–46° F). Do not freeze. Avoid shaking.

## ADVERSE EFFECTS (≥1%) **CV:**
Abnormal ST segment depression, chest pain. **CNS:** *Dizziness, fatigue, headache.* **Hematologic:** Anemia. **Metabolic:** *Increased uric acid, increased lactate dehydrogenase, increased serum alkaline phosphatase.* **GI:** *Nausea,* anorexia. **Respiratory:** Cough, dyspnea. **Body as a Whole:** *Bone pain,* hyperuricemia, *thrombocytopenia, splenomegaly fever.* **Integumentary:** Rash.

## DIAGNOSTIC TEST INTERFERENCE
Elevations in **leukocyte alkaline phosphatase, serum alkaline phosphatase, lactate dehydrogenase,** and **uric acid** have been reported. These elevations appear to be related to increased bone marrow activity.

## INTERACTIONS **Drug:** Can interfere with activity of CYTOTOXIC AGENTS, do not use 24 h before or after CYTOTOXIC AGENTS.

## PHARMACOKINETICS **Absorption:** Readily from subcutaneous site. **Onset:** 4 h. **Peak:** 1 h. **Elimination:** Probably in urine. **Half-Life:** 1.4–7.2 h.

## NURSING IMPLICATIONS

### Assessment & Drug Effects
▪ Discontinue filgrastim if absolute neutrophil count exceeds 10,000/mm³ after the chemotherapy-induced nadir. Neutrophil counts should then return to normal.
▪ Assess degree of bone pain if present. Consult prescriber if nonnarcotic analgesics do not provide relief.
▪ Monitor lab tests: Baseline and twice weekly CBC with differential and platelet count.

### Patient & Family Education
▪ Report bone pain and, if necessary, to request analgesics to control pain.
▪ Some patients (or caregivers) are candidates for self-administration using the prefilled syringe form with proper training.
▪ Note: Proper drug administration and disposal are important. A puncture-resistant container for the disposal of used syringes and needles should be available to the patient.

## FINAFLOXACIN
(fin-a-flox′a-sin)

Xtoro

**Classifications:** QUINOLONE ANTIBIOTIC
Therapeutic: ANTIBIOTIC
**Prototype:** Ciprofloxacin

## AVAILABILITY Otic suspension

## ACTION & *THERAPEUTIC EFFECT*
An antimicrobial effective against

Common adverse effects in *italic;* life-threatening effects <u>underlined</u>; generic names in **bold;** classifications in SMALL CAPS; ♦ Canadian drug name; ◔ Prototype drug most strains of *Pseudomonas aeruginosa* and *Staphylococcus aureus*. *Effective in controlling external ear infections.*

**USES** Treatment of acute otitis externa caused by susceptible strains of *Pseudomonas aeruginosa* and *Staphylococcus aureus* in patients 1 y and older.

**CAUTIOUS USE** Allergic reactions to finafloxacin or other quinolones; prolonged use (may lead to overgrowth of nonsusceptible organisms).

## ROUTE & DOSAGE

**Otitis externa**

*Adult/Child (1 y or older):* **Otic 4 drops b.i.d. into affected ear(s) for 7 days; if using otowick, initial dose can be doubled**

## ADMINISTRATION

**Otic**

- Warm suspension by holding bottle in the hand for 1–2 min prior to dosing. Shake bottle well before use.
- Place patient with the affected ear upward, instill the drops, and maintain the position for 60 sec.
- Store at 2°–25° C (36°–77° F).

**ADVERSE EFFECTS** (>1%) **GI:** Nausea. **Special Senses:** Ear pruritus.

## NURSING IMPLICATIONS

**Assessment & Drug Effects**

- Monitor for and report promptly rash or other allergic reaction.

**Patient & Family Education**

- Warm by holding bottle in hand for 1–2 min before instillation. Instilling a cold solution may cause dizziness.
- Have patient lie with the affected ear upward, instill the drops, and maintain the position for 60 sec.

- Report promptly to prescriber if an allergic reaction occurs.

# FINASTERIDE ℗

(fin-as'te-ride)

Propecia, Proscar

**Classifications:** ANTIANDROGEN; 5-ALPHA REDUCTASE INHIBITOR
**Therapeutic:** ANTIANDROGEN

**AVAILABILITY** Tablet

## ACTION & *THERAPEUTIC EFFECT*

Specific inhibitor of the steroid 5-alpha-reductase, an enzyme necessary to convert testosterone into potent androgen 5-alpha-dihydrotestosterone (DHT) in the prostate gland. *Decreases the production of testosterone in the prostate gland.*

**USES** Benign prostatic hypertrophy, male pattern hair loss (androgenetic alopecia).

**CONTRAINDICATIONS** Hypersensitivity to finasteride; females, pregnancy (category X), lactation, children.

**CAUTIOUS USE** Hepatic impairment, obstructive uropathy.

## ROUTE & DOSAGE

**Benign Prostatic Hypertrophy**

*Adult:* **PO** 5 mg/day

**Male Pattern Hair Loss**

*Adult:* **PO** 1 mg daily

## ADMINISTRATION

**Oral**

- Crush tablets if necessary. Pregnant women should not handle the crushed drug; if absorbed through the skin it may be harmful to a male fetus.
- Store at 15°–30° C (59°–86° F) unless otherwise directed.

---

Common adverse effects in *italic*; life-threatening effects <u>underlined</u>; generic names in **bold**; classifications in SMALL CAPS; ◆ Canadian drug name; ℗ Prototype drug

**ADVERSE EFFECTS** (≥1%) **Uro-genital:** Impotence, decreased libido, decreased volume of ejaculate. **CV:** Postural hypotension. **Body as a Whole:** Asthenia.

**DIAGNOSTIC TEST INTERFERENCE** Depresses levels of **DHT** and **prostate-specific antigen (PSA).** **Testosterone** levels usually are increased.

**INTERACTIONS Drug:** No clinically significant interactions established. **Herbal: Saw palmetto** may potentiate effects of finasteride.

**PHARMACOKINETICS Absorption:** Readily from GI tract. **Onset:** 3–6 mo. **Duration:** 5–7 days. **Elimination:** 39% in urine, 57% in feces. **Half-Life:** 5–7 h.

## NURSING IMPLICATIONS

### Assessment & Drug Effects

- Evaluate carefully any sustained increase in serum PSA levels while patient is taking finasteride. It may indicate the presence of prostate cancer or noncompliance with the therapy.
- Monitor patients with a large residual urinary volume or decreased urinary flow. These patients may not be candidates for this therapy.

### Patient & Family Education

- Use a barrier contraceptive to prevent pregnancy in a sexual partner.
- Be aware that impotence and decreased libido may occur with treatment.
- Report promptly any of the following: breast tenderness or enlargement; testicular pain; rash, itching, or swelling about the face and lips.

## FINGOLIMOD

(fin-go'-li-mod)
Gilenya

**Classification:** BIOLOGIC RESPONSE MODIFIER; IMMUNOMODULATOR; SPHINGOSINE 1-PHOSPHATE RECEPTOR MODULATOR
**Therapeutic:** IMMUNOMODULATOR

**AVAILABILITY** Capsule

**ACTION & THERAPEUTIC EFFECT** Reduces the number of lymphocytes leaving lymph nodes and entering the peripheral blood stream. Mechanism of action in MS is unknown but may involve reduction in the migration of lymphocytes into the CNS. *Reduces the frequency of exacerbations in relapsing MS and slows development of physical disability.*

**USES** Treatment of relapsing forms of multiple sclerosis.

**CONTRAINDICATIONS** Sensitivity to fingolimod, MI, unstable angina, stroke, transient ischemic attack, decompensated heart failure requiring hospitalization, or class III/IV heart failure in the past 6 mo; Mobitz type II second-degree heart block and Mobitz type II third-degree heart block or sick sinus syndrome, unless patient has a functioning pacemaker; baseline QTc interval 500 msec or more; PML.

**CAUTIOUS USE** Bradyarrhythmia, sick sinus syndrome, prolonged QT interval, ischemic cardiac disease, congestive heart failure, or hypertension; risk factors for hypotension; concurrent immunosuppressive or immune modulating therapies; infection; varicella zoster antibody testing/vaccination; macula edema; decreased respiratory function; hepatic dysfunction; renal impairment; age 65 y or older; pregnancy

---

692  Common adverse effects in *italic;* life-threatening effects underlined; generic names in **bold;** classifications in SMALL CAPS; ♣ Canadian drug name; ℗ Prototype drug

(category C); lactation. Safety and efficacy in children younger than 18 y not established.

## ROUTE & DOSAGE

### Multiple Sclerosis
Adult: PO 0.5 mg once daily

### Hepatic Impairment Dosage Adjustment

Mild or moderate hepatic impairment: No dosage adustment needed
Severe hepatic impairment (Child-Pugh class C, total score greater than 10): Monitor closely due to increased risk of adverse effects.

## ADMINISTRATION

### Oral

- May be given with or without food.
- Monitor closely for 6 h after first dose for S&S of bradycardia. If fingolimod is discontinued for more than 2 wk then reinitiated, observe for bradycardia for 6 h following reinitiated dose.
- Store at 15°–30°C (59°–86°F).

## ADVERSE EFFECTS (≥1%) Body as a Whole: Asthenia, *infection*, influenza, herpes infections. CNS: *Headache*, depression, dizziness, migraine, paresthesia. CV: Bradycardia, hypertension, AV block. GI: Diarrhea nausea, abdominal pain, gastroenteritis, abdominal pain, nausea. Hematologic: <u>Leukopenia</u>, lymphopenia. Metabolic: *Increased ALT and AST,* increased GGT, increased triglycerides, weight loss. Musculoskeletal: Back pain, leg pain, weakness. Respiratory: Bronchitis, cough, dyspnea, sinusitis. Skin: Alopecia, eczema, pruritus, tinea infections. Special Senses: Blurred vision, eye pain.

## INTERACTIONS Drug: Ketoconazole increases levels of fingolimod; ANTINEOPLASTIC, IMMUNOSUPPRESSIVE or IMMUNOMODULATING agents may increase the risk of immunosuppresion; fingolimod causes an additional reduction of heart rate when used with **atenolol;** CLASS IA and CLASS III ANTIARRHYTMICS may increase risk of serious rhythm disturbances and BETA BLOCKERS may cause increased bradycardia during fingolimod initiation.

## PHARMACOKINETICS Absorption: 93% bioavailable. Peak: 12–16 h. Distribution: 99.7% plasma protein bound. Metabolism: Phosphorylated to active metabolite; oxidized by multiple CYP450 enzymes. Elimination: Renal (81%) and fecal (2.5%). Half-Life: 6–9 d.

## NURSING IMPLICATIONS

### Assessment & Drug Effects

- Baseline ECG is recommended to identify risk factors for bradycardia and AV block especially in those with known cardiac risk factors or concurrent antiarrhythmic drugs including beta blockers and calcium channel blockers.
- Monitor HR and BP at baseline and for 6 h after the first dose. HR declines within 1 h and is maximal at approximately 6 h. Monitor HR during first month of therapy during which time a return to baseline should be seen.
- Monitor for and report promptly S&S of the following: Infection, hepatic dysfunction (e.g., unexplained nausea, vomiting, abdominal pain, fatigue, anorexia, or jaundice and/or dark urine), or dyspnea.
- Baseline ophthalmologic exam is recommended and should be performed if patient reports visual disturbances at any time while taking this drug.

---

- Monitor lab tests: Baseline and periodic CBC, bilirubin.

**Patient & Family Education**
- Those who have not had chickenpox or received the vaccination should consider receiving the VZV vaccine prior to starting treatment with fingolimod.
- Promptly report any of the following: S&S of infection; visual disturbances; new onset or worsening dyspnea; unexplained nausea, vomiting, abdominal pain, fatigue, loss of appetite, jaundice, and/or dark urine.
- Women of childbearing age should use effective contraception during and for 2 mo following discontinuation of fingolimod.
- Notify prescriber immediately if a pregnancy occurs.

# FLAVOXATE HYDROCHLORIDE
(fla-vox'ate)
**Classifications:** ANTICHOLINERGIC; SMOOTH MUSCLE RELAXANT
Therapeutic: URINARY TRACT ANTISPASMODIC
**Prototype:** Oxybutynin

**AVAILABILITY** Tablet

## ACTION & *THERAPEUTIC EFFECT*
Exerts spasmolytic action on smooth muscle. Increases urinary bladder capacity in patients with spastic bladder, possibly by direct action on detrusor muscle. Also demonstrates local anesthetic and analgesic action. *Has antispasmodic action on the urinary bladder.*

**USES** Symptomatic relief of dysuria, overactive bladder, urinary urgency/ incontinence.

**CONTRAINDICATIONS** Pyloric or duodenal obstruction, obstructive intestinal lesions, ileus, acha-lasia, GI hemorrhage; obstructive uropathies of lower urinary tract.

**CAUTIOUS USE** Suspected or closed-angle glaucoma; myasthenia gravis; autonomic neuropathy; dehydration; older adults; pregnancy (category B). Safety in children younger than 12 y not established.

## ROUTE & DOSAGE

**Dysuria, Nocturia, Incontinence/ OAB**
*Adult/Adolescent:* PO 100–200 mg t.i.d. or q.i.d.

## ADMINISTRATION
**Oral**
- Give without regard to meals.
- Store at 15°–30° C (59°–86° F) unless otherwise directed.

**ADVERSE EFFECTS** (≥1%) **CNS:** Headache, vertigo, drowsiness, mental confusion (especially in older adults). **CV:** Palpitation, tachycardia. **Special Senses:** Blurred vision, increased intraocular tension, disturbances of eye accommodation. **GI:** Nausea, vomiting, dry mouth (and throat), constipation (with high doses). **Skin:** Dermatosis, urticaria. **Other:** Dysuria, hyperpyrexia, eosinophilia, leukopenia (rare).

**INTERACTIONS Drug:** May antagonize the GI motility effects of **met-oclopramide,** may add to GI slowing caused by ANTIDIARRHEALS.

**PHARMACOKINETICS Elimination:** 10–30% in urine within 6 h.

## NURSING IMPLICATIONS
**Assessment & Drug Effects**
- Monitor heart rate. Report tachycardia.
- Those with suspected glaucoma should be closely monitored for increased intraocular tension.

Common adverse effects in *italic;* life-threatening effects underlined; generic names in **bold;** classifications in SMALL CAPS; ♣ Canadian drug name; ⦿ Prototype drug

**Patient & Family Education**

- Do not drive or engage in potentially hazardous activities until response to drug is known.
- Report adverse reactions to prescriber as well as clinical improvement or the lack of a favorable response.

## FLECAINIDE ℗
(fle-kay'nide)
Tambocor
**Classification:** CLASS IC
ANTIARRHYTHMIC
**Therapeutic:** CLASS IC ANTI-
ARRHYTHMIC

**AVAILABILITY** Tablet

## ACTION & *THERAPEUTIC EFFECT*
Local (membrane) anesthetic and antiarrhythmic with electrophysiologic properties similar to other class IC antiarrhythmic drugs. Slows conduction velocity throughout myocardial conduction system, increases ventricular refractoriness. *Is an effective suppressant of PVCs and a variety of atrial and ventricular arrhythmias.*

**USES** Life-threatening ventricular arrhythmias.

**UNLABELED USES** Atrial tachycardia and other arrhythmias unresponsive to standard agents (e.g., quinidine), Wolff-Parkinson-White syndrome, and recurrent ventricular tachycardias.

**CONTRAINDICATIONS** Hypersensitivity to flecainide; preexisting second- or third-degree AV block, right bundle branch block when associated with a left hemiblock unless a pacemaker is present; cardiogenic shock, left ventricular dysfunction; recent acute MI; QT prolongation syndromes; electrolyte imbalances.

**CAUTIOUS USE** Hypersensitivity to amide local anesthetics; atrial fibrillation; cardiac arrhythmias; cardiac disease; sick sinus syndrome; severe or moderate hepatic or renal impairment; older adults; pregnancy (category C); children and infants.

## ROUTE & DOSAGE

**Life-Threatening Ventricular Arrhythmias**
*Adult:* **PO** 100 mg q12h, may increase by 50 mg b.i.d. q4days (max: 400 mg/day)
*Child:* **PO** 1–3 mg/kg/day in 3 divided doses (max: 8 mg/kg/day)

## ADMINISTRATION
**Oral**
- Do not increase dosage more frequently than every 4 days.
- Store in tightly covered, light-resistant containers at 15°–30° C (59°–86° F) unless otherwise directed.

**ADVERSE EFFECTS** (≥1%) **CNS:** *Dizziness,* headache, light-headedness, unsteadiness, paresthesias, fatigue. **CV:** Arrhythmias, chest pain, worsening of CHF. **Special Senses:** *Blurred vision, difficulty in focusing,* spots before eyes. **GI:** *Nausea,* constipation, change in taste perception. **Body as a Whole:** Dyspnea, fever, edema.

**INTERACTIONS Drug: Cimetidine** may increase flecainide levels; may increase **digoxin** levels 15–25%; BETA-BLOCKERS may have additive negative inotropic effects.

**PHARMACOKINETICS Absorption:** Readily from GI tract. **Peak:** 2–3 h. **Distribution:** Crosses placenta; distributed into breast milk. **Metabolism:** In liver. **Elimination:** Mainly in urine. **Half-Life:** 7–22 h.

---

Common adverse effects in *italic;* life-threatening effects <u>underlined</u>; generic names in **bold;** classifications in SMALL CAPS; ♣ Canadian drug name; ℗ Prototype drug

695

## NURSING IMPLICATIONS

### Black Box Warning

*Flecainide has ventricular proar-rhythmic effects in patients with atrial fibrillation/flutter.*

### Assessment & Drug Effects

- Correct preexisting hypokalemia or hyperkalemia before treatment is initiated.
- ECG monitoring, including Holter monitor for ambulating patients, is recommended because of the possibility of drug-induced arrhythmias.
- Note: Effective trough plasma levels are between 0.7–1 mcg/mL. The probability of adverse reactions increases when trough levels exceed 1 mcg/mL.
- Monitor carefully during period of dose adjustment.
- Monitor lab tests: Periodic flecainide plasma level, especially in patients with severe CHF or renal failure.

### Patient & Family Education

- Note: It is VERY important to take this drug at the prescribed times.
- Report visual disturbances to prescriber.

## FLOXURIDINE

(flox-yoor′i-deen)

**Classifications:** ANTINEOPLASTIC; ANTIMETABOLITE, PYRIMIDINE
Therapeutic: ANTINEOPLASTIC
**Prototype:** Fluorouracil

**AVAILABILITY** Powder for injection

## ACTION & *THERAPEUTIC EFFECT*

Pyrimidine antagonist and cell-cycle specific that is catabolized to fluorouracil in the body; highly toxic because it blocks an enzyme essential to normal DNA and RNA synthesis.

*Proliferative cells of neoplasms are affected more than healthy tissue cells.*

**USES** Palliative agent in management of selected patients with GI metastasis to liver.

**UNLABELED USES** Carcinoma of breast, ovary, cervix, urinary bladder, and prostate not responsive to other antimetabolites.

**CONTRAINDICATIONS** Existing or recent viral infections; pregnancy (category D); lactation.

**CAUTIOUS USE** Poor nutritional status, bone marrow depression, serious infections; high-risk patients: prior high-dose pelvic irradiation, impaired kidney or liver function.

## ROUTE & DOSAGE

### Carcinoma

*Adult:* **Intra-Arterial** 0.1–0.6 mg/kg/day by continuous intra-arterial infusion

## ADMINISTRATION

Intra-arterial Infusion

*PREPARE:* **Direct:** Reconstitute with 5 mL sterile distilled water for injection; further dilute with D5W or NS injection to a volume appropriate for the infusion apparatus to be used.

*ADMINISTER:* **Direct:** It is administered by pump to overcome pressure in large arteries and to ensure a uniform rate. ▪ Examine infusion site frequently for signs of extravasation. If this occurs, stop infusion and restart in another vessel.

*INCOMPATIBILITIES:* Y-site: **Allopurinol, cefepime.**

- Keep reconstituted solutions, which are stable at 2°–8° C (36°–46° F), for no more than 2 wk.

Common adverse effects in *italic;* life-threatening effects underlined; generic names in **bold;** classifications in SMALL CAPS; ♣ Canadian drug name; ⊘ Prototype drug

- Store at 15°–30° C (59°–86° F) unless otherwise directed.

**ADVERSE EFFECTS** (≥1%) **CNS:** Vertigo, convulsions, depression, hemiplegia. **CV:** Myocardial ischemia, angina. **GI:** *Nausea, vomiting, stomatitis,* diarrhea, cramps, anorexia, enteritis, gastritis, esophagopharyngitis. **Hematologic:** <u>Leukopenia</u>, <u>thrombocytopenia</u>. **Skin:** Dermatitis, alopecia (usually reversible), *erythema* or increased skin pigmentation (photosensitivity), dry skin, pruritic ulcerations, rash. **Body as a Whole:** Hiccups, fever, epistaxis, decreased resistance to disease. **Urogenital:** Renal insufficiency.

**INTERACTIONS Drug:** Metronidazole may increase general floxuridine toxicity; may increase or decrease serum levels of **phenytoin, fosphenytoin; hydroxyurea** can decrease conversion to active metabolite.

**PHARMACOKINETICS Distribution:** Distributed to tumor, intestinal mucosa, bone marrow, liver, and CSF; probably crosses placenta. **Metabolism:** Rapidly metabolized in liver to fluorouracil. **Elimination:** 15% in urine, 60–80% through lungs as carbon dioxide. **Half-Life:** 16 min.

**NURSING IMPLICATIONS**

### Black Box Warning

*Because floxuridine has been associated with severe toxic reactions, patient should be hospitalized for the first course of therapy.*

**Assessment & Drug Effects**
- Discontinue therapy promptly with onset of any of the following: Stomatitis, esophagopharyngitis, intractable vomiting, diarrhea,

leukopenia (WBC less than 3500/mm³), or rapidly falling WBC count, thrombocytopenia (platelets 100,000/mm³), GI bleeding, hemorrhage from any site.
- Monitor lab tests: Baseline and periodic total and differential WBC counts, and platelet count.

**Patient & Family Education**
- Be aware that floxuridine sometimes causes temporary thinning of hair.

## FLUCONAZOLE ⓟ
(flu-con'a-zole)

Diflucan

**Classification:** AZOLE ANTIFUNGAL
Therapeutic: ANTIFUNGAL

**AVAILABILITY** Tablet; oral suspension; solution for injection

**ACTION & *THERAPEUTIC EFFECT***
Interferes with formation of ergosterol, the principal sterol in the fungal cell membrane leading to cell death. *Antifungal properties are related to the drug effect on the functioning of fungal cell membrane.*

**USES** Cryptococcal meningitis and oropharyngeal and systemic candidiasis, both commonly found in AIDS and other immunocompromised patients; vaginal candidiasis.

**CONTRAINDICATIONS** Hypersensitivity to fluconazole; S&S of drug-inducted liver disease; lacatation.

**CAUTIOUS USE** Hypersensitivity to other azole antifungals; AIDS or malignancy; hepatic impairment; structural cardiac disease; history of torsades de pointes or QT prolongation; renal impairment or failure; pregnancy (category C).

Common adverse effects in *italic*; life-threatening effects <u>underlined</u>; generic names in **bold**; classifications in SMALL CAPS; ♥ Canadian drug name; ⓟ Prototype drug

697

F

## ROUTE & DOSAGE

### Oropharyngeal Candidiasis

*Adult:* **PO/IV** 200 mg day 1, then 100 mg/day × 14 days
*Child:* **PO/IV** 3–6 mg/kg/day × 14 days

### Esophageal Candidiasis

*Adult:* **PO/IV** 200 mg day 1, then 100 mg daily × 3 wk
*Child/Infant:* **PO/IV** 3–6 mg/kg/day × 21 days

### Systemic Candidemia

*Adult:* **PO/IV** 400 mg day 1, then 200 mg daily × 4 wk
*Child/Infant/Nenonate (14 days or older):* **PO/IV** 6 mg/kg q12h × 28 days
*Neonate (0–14 days):* **IV** 6 mg/kg q72h

### Vaginal Candidiasis

*Adult:* **PO** 150 mg × 1 dose

### Cryptococcal Meningitis

*Adult:* **PO/IV** 400 mg day 1, then 200 mg daily × 10–12 wk
*Child/Infant/Neonate:* **PO/IV** 12 mg/kg day 1, then 6–12 mg/kg/day × 10–12 wk

### Renal Impairment Dosage Adjustment

*CrCl 50 mL/min or less (without concurrent dialysis):* Give 50% of maintenance dose

### Hemodialysis Dosage Adjustment

Administer full dose post-dialysis

## ADMINISTRATION

### Oral

- Take this medication for the full course of therapy, which may take weeks or months.
- Take next dose as soon as possible if you miss a dose; however, do not take a dose if it is almost time for next dose. Do not double dose.

### Intravenous

*PREPARE:* **Continuous:** Packaged ready for use as a 2 mg/mL solution. Remove wrapper just prior to use.

*ADMINISTER:* **Continuous:** Give at a maximum rate of approximately 200 mg/h. Give after hemodialysis is completed. ▪ Do not use IV admixtures of fluconazole and other medications.

*INCOMPATIBILITIES:* **Solution/additive:** Trimethoprim-sulfamethoxazole. **Y-site:** Amphotericin B, amphotericin B cholesteryl, ampicillin, calcium gluconate, cefotaxime, ceftazidime, ceftriaxone, cefuroxime, chloramphenicol, clindamycin, dantrolene, diazepam, diazoxide, digoxin, furosemide, gemtuzumab, haloperidol, hydralazine, hydroxyzine, imipenem-cilastatin, pantoprazole, pentamidine, phenytoin, piperacillin, SMZ/TMP ticarcillin.

**ADVERSE EFFECTS** (≥1%) **CNS:** Headache. **GI:** Nausea, vomiting, abdominal pain, diarrhea, increase in AST in patients with cryptococcal meningitis and AIDS. **Skin:** Rash.

**INTERACTIONS Drug:** Increased PT in patients on **warfarin;** may increase **alosetron, bexarotene, phenytoin, cevimeline, cilostazol, cyclosporine, dihydroergotamine, ergotamine, dofetilide, haloperidol, levobupivacaine, modafinil, zonisamide** levels and toxicity; hypoglycemic reactions with ORAL SULFONYLUREAS; decreased fluconazole levels with **rifampin, cimetidine;** may prolong the effects of **fentanyl, alfentanil, methadone.**

## PHARMACOKINETICS **Absorption:** 90% from GI tract. **Peak:** 1–2 h. **Distribution:** Widely distributed, including CSF. **Metabolism:** 11% of dose metabolized in liver. **Elimination:** In urine. **Half-Life:** 20–50 h.

## NURSING IMPLICATIONS

### Assessment & Drug Effects
- Monitor for allergic response. Patients allergic to other azole antifungals may be allergic to fluconazole.
- Note: Drug may cause elevations of the following laboratory serum values: ALT, AST, alkaline phosphatase, bilirubin.
- Monitor for S&S of hepatotoxicity.
- Monitor lab tests: Periodic LFTs, renal function tests, and serum potassium.

### Patient & Family Education
- Monitor carefully for loss of glycemic control if diabetic.
- Inform prescriber of all medications being taken.

## FLUCYTOSINE
(floo-sye'toe-seen)
Ancobon
**Classification:** ANTIFUNGAL
**Therapeutic:** ANTIFUNGAL
**Prototype:** Fluconazole

## AVAILABILITY Capsule

## ACTION & *THERAPEUTIC EFFECT*
Selectively penetrates fungal cell and is converted to fluorouracil, an antimetabolite believed to be responsible for antifungal activity. *Has antifungal activity against* Cryptococcus *and* Candida *as well as chromomycosis.*

## USES Alone or in combination with amphotericin B for serious systemic infections caused by susceptible strains of *Cryptococcus* and *Candida* species.

## UNLABELED USES *Chromomycosis.*

## CONTRAINDICATIONS Hypersensitivity to flucytosine; lactation.

## CAUTIOUS USE Hepatic disease; electrolyte imbalance; bone marrow depression, hematologic disorders, patients being treated with or having received radiation or bone marrow depressant drugs; dental disease; extreme caution in impaired kidney function; pregnancy (category C); children.

## ROUTE & DOSAGE

### Fungal Infection
*Adult:* **PO** 50–150 mg/kg/day divided q6h

## ADMINISTRATION
### Oral
- Lower dosages with longer dosage intervals are recommended in patients with serum creatinine of 1.7 mg/dL or higher. Check with prescriber.
- Give capsules a few at a time over 15 min to decrease incidence and severity of nausea and vomiting.
- Store in light-resistant containers at 15°–30° C (59°–86° F).

## ADVERSE EFFECTS (≥1%) **CNS:** Confusion, hallucinations, headache, sedation, vertigo. **GI:** Nausea, vomiting, diarrhea, abdominal bloating, enterocolitis. **Hematologic:** Hypoplasia of bone marrow: Anemia, leukopenia, thrombocytopenia, agranulocytosis, eosinophilia. **Skin:** Rash. **Metabolic:** Elevated levels of serum alkaline phosphatase, AST, ALT, BUN, serum creatinine. **GI:** Hepatomegaly, hepatitis.

## DIAGNOSTIC TEST INTERFERENCE
False elevations of **serum creatinine.**

Common adverse effects in *italic;* life-threatening effects underlined; generic names in **bold;** classifications in SMALL CAPS; ♣ Canadian drug name; ☺ Prototype drug

699

**INTERACTIONS Drug: Amphotericin B** can increase flucytosine toxicity. **Cytosine** may decrease activity of flucytosine.

**PHARMACOKINETICS Absorption:** Readily from GI tract. **Peak:** 2 h. **Distribution:** Widely distributed in body tissues including aqueous humor and CSF; crosses placenta. **Metabolism:** Minimal. **Elimination:** 75–90% in urine unchanged. **Half-Life:** 3–5 h.

## NURSING IMPLICATIONS

### Black Box Warning

*Flucytosine is associated with severe hematologic, renal, and hepatic adverse reactions.*

### Assessment & Drug Effects

- Monitor renal status closely because renal impairment can cause increased serum concentration of drug with greater adverse effects.
- Frequent assays of blood drug level are recommended, especially in patients with impaired kidney function to determine adequacy of drug excretion (therapeutic range: 25–120 mg/mL).
- Monitor I&O. Report change in I&O ratio or pattern. Because most of drug is eliminated unchanged by kidneys, compromised function can lead to drug accumulation.
- C&S tests should be performed before initiation of therapy and at weekly intervals during therapy. Organism resistance has been reported.
- Monitor lab tests: Baseline and periodic WBC and platelet count, renal function tests and LFTs.

### Patient & Family Education

- Report fever, sore mouth or throat, and unusual bleeding or bruising tendency to prescriber.
- Be aware that the general duration of therapy is 4–6 wk, but it may continue for several months.

# FLUDROCORTISONE ACETATE ●

(floo-droe-kor'ti-sone)

Florinef Acetate

**Classifications:** ADRENOCORTICAL STEROID; MINERALOCORTICOID
Therapeutic: MINERALOCORTICOID; ANTI-INFLAMMATORY

**AVAILABILITY** Tablet

## ACTION & *THERAPEUTIC EFFECT*

Long-acting synthetic steroid with potent mineralocorticoid activity. Small doses produce marked sodium retention, increased urinary potassium excretion, and elevated BP. *Synthetic corticosteroid replacement product for adrenocortical insufficiency.*

**USES** Partial replacement therapy for adrenocortical insufficiency and for treatment of salt-losing forms of congenital adrenogenital syndrome.

**UNLABELED USES** To increase systolic and diastolic blood pressure in patients with severe hypotension secondary to diabetes mellitus or to levodopa therapy.

**CONTRAINDICATIONS** Hypersensitivity to glucocorticoids, idiopathic thrombocytopenic purpura, psychoses, acute glomerulonephritis, viral or bacterial diseases of skin, systemic fungal infections; infections not controlled by antibiotics, active or latent amebiasis, hypercorticism, smallpox vaccination or other immunologic procedures.

**CAUTIOUS USE** Diabetes mellitus; chronic, active hepatitis positive for hepatitis B surface antigen; hyperlipidemia; cirrhosis; stromal herpes simplex; glaucoma, tuberculosis of eye; osteoporosis; convulsive disorders; hypothyroidism; diverticulitis; nonspecific ulcerative colitis; fresh intestinal anastomoses; active or latent peptic ulcer; gastritis; esophagitis; thromboembolic disorders; CHF; metastatic carcinoma; hypertension; renal insufficiency; history of allergies; active or arrested tuberculosis; myasthenia gravis; history of psychosis; pregnancy (category C); lactation; children.

## ROUTE & DOSAGE

**Adrenocortical Insufficiency**

*Adult:* **PO** 0.1 mg/day, may range from 0.1 mg 3 × wk to 0.2 mg/day
*Child:* **PO** 0.05–0.1 mg/day

**Salt-Losing Adrenogenital Syndrome**

*Adult:* **PO** 0.1–0.2 mg/day
*Child:* **PO** 0.05–0.1 mg/day

## ADMINISTRATION

**Oral**

- Note: Concomitant oral cortisone or hydrocortisone therapy may be advisable to provide substitute therapy approximating normal adrenal activity.
- Store in airtight containers at 15°–30° C (59°–86° F). Protect from light.

## ADVERSE EFFECTS (≥1%) CNS:
Vertigo, headache, nystagmus, increased intracranial pressure with papilledema (usually after discontinuation of medication), mental disturbances, aggravation of preexisting psychiatric conditions, insomnia, ataxia (rare). **CV:** CHF, hypertension, thromboembolism (rare), tachycardia. **Endocrine:** Suppressed linear growth in children, decreased glucose tolerance; hyperglycemia, manifestations of latent diabetes mellitus; hypocorticism; amenorrhea

and other menstrual difficulties. **Special Senses:** Posterior subcapsular cataracts (especially in children), glaucoma, exophthalmos, increased intraocular pressure with optic nerve damage, perforation of the globe. **Metabolic:** Hypocalcemia; *sodium and fluid retention;* hypokalemia and hypokalemic alkalosis, negative nitrogen balance, decreased serum concentration of vitamins A and C. **GI:** *Nausea,* increased appetite, ulcerative esophagitis, pancreatitis, abdominal distension, peptic ulcer with perforation and hemorrhage, melena. **Hematologic:** Thrombocytopenia. **Musculoskeletal:** (Long-term use) Osteoporosis, compression fractures, muscle wasting and weakness, tendon rupture, aseptic necrosis of femoral and humeral heads. **Skin:** Skin thinning and atrophy, *acne, impaired wound healing;* petechiae, ecchymosis, easy bruising; suppression of skin test reaction; hypopigmentation or hyperpigmentation, hirsutism, acneiform eruptions, subcutaneous fat atrophy; allergic dermatitis, urticaria, angioneurotic edema, increased sweating. **Body as a Whole:** Anaphylactoid reactions (rare), aggravation or masking of infections; malaise, weight gain, obesity. **Urogenital:** Increased or decreased motility and number of sperm.

## INTERACTIONS Drug: The antidiabetic effects of **insulin** and SULFONYLUREAS may be diminished; **amphotericin B,** DIURETICS may increase **potassium** loss; **warfarin** may decrease prothrombin time; **indomethacin, ibuprofen** can potentiate the pressor effect of fludrocortisone; ANABOLIC STEROIDS increase risk of edema and acne; **rifampin** may increase the hepatic metabolism of fludrocortisone.

## PHARMACOKINETICS Absorption: Readily from GI tract. **Peak:**

Common adverse effects in *italic;* life-threatening effects underlined; generic names in **bold;** classifications in SMALL CAPS; ♣ Canadian drug name; ☺ Prototype drug

701

1.7 h. **Metabolism:** In liver. **Half-Life:** 3.5 h.

## NURSING IMPLICATIONS

### Assessment & Drug Effects

- Monitor weight and I&O ratio to observe onset of fluid accumulation, especially if patient is on unrestricted salt intake and without potassium supplement. Report weight gain of 2 kg (5 lb)/wk.
- Monitor and record BP daily. If hypertension develops as a consequence of therapy, report to prescriber. Usually, the dose will be reduced to 0.05 mg/day.
- Check BP q4–6h and weight at least every other day during periods of dosage adjustment.
- Monitor for S&S of hypokalemia and hyperkalemic metabolic alkalosis (see Appendix F).
- Monitor lab tests: Periodic serum electrolytes.

### Patient & Family Education

- Report signs of hypokalemia (see Appendix F).
- Be aware of signs of potassium depletion associated with high sodium intake: Muscle weakness, paresthesias, circumoral numbness; fatigue, anorexia, nausea, mental depression, polyuria, delirium, diminished reflexes, arrhythmias, cardiac failure, ileus, ECG changes.
- Eat foods with high potassium content.
- Signs of edema should be reported immediately. Sodium intake may or may not require regulation, depending on individual needs and clinical situation.
- Weigh daily under standard conditions and report steady weight gain.
- Report intercurrent infection, trauma, or unexpected stress of any kind promptly when taking maintenance therapy.
- Carry medical identification at all times.

# FLUMAZENIL ⓟ

(flu-ma′ze-nil)

Mazicon ◆, Romazicon

**Classification:** BENZODIAZEPINE ANTAGONIST

**Therapeutic:** BENZODIAZEPINE ANTIDOTE

**AVAILABILITY** Solution for injection

**ACTION & *THERAPEUTIC EFFECT*** Antagonizes the effects of benzodiazepine on the CNS, including sedation, impairment of recall, and psychomotor impairment. *Reverses the action of a benzodiazepine.*

**USES** Reversal of sedation induced by benzodiazepine for anesthesia or diagnostic or therapeutic procedures as well as through overdose.

**UNLABELED USES** Seizure disorders, alcohol intoxication, hepatic encephalopathy, facilitation of weaning from mechanical ventilation.

**CONTRAINDICATIONS** Hypersensitivity to flumazenil or to benzodiazepines; patients given a benzodiazepine for control of a life-threatening condition; patients showing signs of cyclic antidepressant overdose; seizure-prone individuals; during labor and delivery.

**CAUTIOUS USE** Hepatic function impairment, older adults, intensive care patients, head injury, anxiety or pain disorder; drug- and alcohol-dependent patients, and physical dependence upon benzodiazepines; pregnancy (category C); lactation; children.

Common adverse effects in *italic;* life-threatening effects <u>underlined</u>; generic names in **bold;** classifications in SMALL CAPS; ◆ Canadian drug name; ⓟ Prototype drug

## ROUTE & DOSAGE

### Reversal of Sedation

*Adult:* **IV** 0.2 mg over 15 sec, may repeat 0.2 mg each min for 4 additional doses or a cumulative dose of 1 mg
*Child:* **IV** 0.01 mg/kg may repeat each min (max: 1 mg)

### Benzodiazepine Overdose

*Adult:* **IV** 0.2 mg over 30 sec, if no response after 30 sec, then 0.3 mg over 30 sec, may repeat with 0.5 mg each min (max cumulative dose: 3 mg)

## ADMINISTRATION

### Intravenous

**PREPARE: Direct:** May give undiluted or diluted. If diluted use D5W, lactated Ringer's, NS
**ADMINISTER: Direct:** Ensure patency of IV before administration of flumazenil, since extravasation will cause local irritation. • Do not give as bolus dose. Give through an IV that is freely flowing into a large vein. **Direct for Reversal of Anesthesia or Sedation:** Give each dose slowly over 15 sec. • In high-risk patients, slow the rate to provide the smallest effective dose. **Direct for Benzodiazepine Overdose:** Give each dose slowly over 30 sec.

• Use all diluted solutions within 24 h of dilution.

## ADVERSE EFFECTS (≥1%) CNS:
Emotional lability, headache, *dizziness,* agitation, *resedation,* seizures, blurred vision. **GI:** *Nausea, vomiting,* hiccups. **Other:** Shivering, pain at injection site, hypoventilation.

## INTERACTIONS Drug: May antagonize effects of **zaleplon, zolpidem;**

may cause convulsions or arrhythmias with TRICYCLIC ANTIDEPRESSANTS.

## PHARMACOKINETICS Onset:
1–5 min. **Peak:** 6–10 min. **Duration:** 2–4 h. **Metabolism:** In the liver to inactive metabolites. **Elimination:** 90–95% in urine, 5–10% in feces within 72 h. **Half-Life:** 54 min.

## NURSING IMPLICATIONS

### Black Box Warnings

*Flumazenil has been associated with the occurrence of seizures.*

### Assessment & Drug Effects
• Monitor respiratory status carefully until risk of resedation is unlikely (up to 120 min). Drug may not fully reverse benzodiazepine-induced ventilatory insufficiency.
• Monitor carefully for seizures and take appropriate precautions.

### Patient & Family Education
• Do not drive or engage in potentially hazardous activities until at least 18–24 h after discharge following a procedure.
• Do not ingest alcohol or nonprescription drugs for 18–24 h after flumazenil is administered or if the effects of the benzodiazepine persist.

## FLUNISOLIDE
(floo-niss'oh-lide)
AeroBid, Nasalide, Nasarel
**See Appendix A-3.**

## FLUOCINOLONE ACETONIDE
(floo-oh-sin'oh-lone)
Fluoderm ◆, Synalar
**Prototype:** Hydrocortisone
**See Appendix A-4.**

## FLUOCINONIDE
(floo-oh-sin'oh-nide)

Common adverse effects in *italic;* life-threatening effects underlined; generic names in **bold;** classifications in SMALL CAPS; ◆ Canadian drug name; ⊙ Prototype drug

703

Lidemol, Lidex, Lidex-E,
Lyderm, Topsyn, Vanos
**See Appendix A-4.**

## FLUOROMETHOLONE
(flure-oh-meth'oh-lone)
Flarex, FML Forte, FML
Liquifilm
**See Appendix A-1.**

## FLUOROURACIL
## [5-FLUOROURACIL (5-FU)] ⓟ
(flure-oh-yoor'a-sil)
Carac, Efudex, Fluoroplex
**Classifications:** ANTINEOPLASTIC;
ANTIMETABOLITE, PYRIMIDINE
Therapeutic: ANTINEOPLASTIC

**AVAILABILITY** Solution for injection; topical solution; topical cream

**ACTION & *THERAPEUTIC EFFECT***
Pyrimidine antagonist and cell-cycle specific agent that blocks action of enzymes essential to normal DNA and RNA synthesis; unbalanced growth and death of cell follow. Exhibits higher affinity for tumor tissue than healthy tissue. *Highly toxic, especially to proliferative cells in neoplasms, bone marrow, and intestinal mucosa.*

**USES** Systemically as single agent or in combination with other antineoplastics for treatment of patients with inoperable neoplasms of breast, colon or rectum, stomach, pancreas, urinary bladder, ovary, cervix, liver. Also topically for solar or actinic keratoses and superficial basal cell carcinoma.

**UNLABELED USES** To induce repigmentation in vitiligo; actinic cheilitis; malignant effusions; mucosal leukoplakia.

**CONTRAINDICATIONS** Hypersensitivity to any fluorouracil components; poor nutritional status; myelosuppression; patients with dihydropyrimidine dehydrogenase (DPD) enzyme deficiency; women who are or may become pregnant; pregnancy (category D); lactation.

**CAUTIOUS USE** Major surgery during previous month; history of high-dose pelvic irradiation, metastatic cell infiltration of bone marrow, previous use of alkylating agents; cardiac disease, CAD, angina; men and women in childbearing ages; hepatic or renal impairment. Safety and efficacy in children younger than 18 y not established.

## ROUTE & DOSAGE

**Cancer Therapy**

Dose depends on concurrent medication and stage/location of cancer. See package insert for specific dosing.

**Actinic and Solar Keratosis**

*Adult:* **Topical** Apply cream or solution b.i.d. for 2–6 wk; apply **Carac** once daily

**Superficial Basal Cell Carcinoma**

*Adult:* **Topical** Apply 5% cream b.i.d. for 3–6 wk

*Obesity Dosage Adjustment*

Dose patient based on lean body mass

## ADMINISTRATION

**Topical**

▪ Use gloved fingers to apply topical drug.
▪ Do not use occlusive dressings with topical drug. Use a porous gauze dressing for cosmetic purposes.
▪ Store at 15°–30° C (59°–86° F) unless otherwise directed. Protect from light and freezing.

Common adverse effects in *italic;* life-threatening effects <u>underlined</u>; generic names in **bold;** classifications in SMALL CAPS; ♣ Canadian drug name; ⓟ Prototype drug

**Intravenous**

This drug is a cytotoxic agent and caution should be used to prevent any contact with the drug. Follow institutional or standard guidelines for preparation, handling, and disposal of cytotoxic agents.

**PREPARE: Direct/Infusion:** This drug may be given undiluted or further diluted in D5W or NS for infusion. ▪ If a precipitate forms, redissolve drug by heating to 60° C (140° F) and shake vigorously. Allow to cool to body temperature before administration.

**ADMINISTER: Direct/Infusion:** Give by direct IV injection over 1–2 min. ▪ Infuse over 2–24 h as ordered. **IV Extravasation:** Inspect injection site frequently; avoid extravasation. If it occurs, stop infusion and restart in another vein. ▪ Ice compresses may reduce danger of local tissue damage from infiltrated solution.

**INCOMPATIBILITIES: Solution/additive: Carboplatin, ciprofloxacin, cisplatin, cytarabine, diazepam, doxorubicin, epirubicin, fentanyl, leucovorin, metoclopramide, morphine. Y-site: Aldesleukin, amiodarone, amphotericin B cholesteryl, buprenorphine, calcium chloride, caspofungin, chlorpromazine, ciprofloxacin, diazepam, diltiazem, diphenhydramine, dobutamine, dolasetron, doxycycline, droperidol, epinephrine, epirubicin, filgrastim, gallium, haloperidol, hydroxyzine, idarubicin, irinotecan, lansoprazole, levofloxacin, lorazepam, methadone, midazolam, minocycline, nicardipine, ondansetron, pentamidine, phenytoin, prochlorperazine, promethazine, quinupristin/dalfopristin, topotecan, TPN, vancomycin, verapamil, vinorelbine.**

▪ Fluorouracil solution is normally colorless to faint yellow. Slight discoloration during storage does not appear to affect potency or safety. ▪ Discard dark yellow solution.

## ADVERSE EFFECTS (≥1%)

**CNS:** Euphoria, acute cerebellar syndrome (dysmetria, nystagmus, ataxia, severe mental deterioration); pustular contact hypersensitivity **CV:** Cardiotoxicity (rare), angina. **GI:** Anorexia, *nausea, vomiting, stomatitis,* esophagopharyngitis, medicinal taste, *diarrhea,* proctitis. **Hematologic:** Anemia, leukopenia, thrombocytopenia, eosinophilia. **Body as a Whole:** Hypersensitivity· Pustular contact eruption, edema of face, eyes, tongue, legs. **Skin:** SLE-like dermatitis, *alopecia,* photosensitivity, erythema, increased pigmentation, skin dryness and fissuring, pruritic maculopapular rash. **Topical:** Local pain, pruritus, hyperpigmentation, burning at site of application, dermatitis, suppuration, swelling, scarring, toxic granulation.

## DIAGNOSTIC TEST INTERFERENCE

Fluorouracil may decrease *plasma albumin* (because of drug-induced protein malabsorption).

## INTERACTIONS

**Drug: Metronidazole** may increase general floxuridine toxicity; may increase or decrease serum levels of **phenytoin, fosphenytoin; hydroxyurea** can decrease conversion to active metabolite.

## PHARMACOKINETICS

**Distribution:** Distributed to tumor, intestinal mucosa, bone marrow, liver, and CSF; probably crosses placenta. **Metabolism:** In liver. **Elimination:** 15% in urine, 60–80% through lungs as carbon dioxide. **Half-Life:** 16 min.

---

Common adverse effects in *italic;* life-threatening effects underlined; generic names in **bold;** classifications in SMALL CAPS; ♣ Canadian drug name; ⊘ Prototype drug

705

## NURSING IMPLICATIONS
### Assessment & Drug Effects
- Use protective isolation of patient during leukopenic period (WBC less than 3500/mm³).
- Watch for and report signs of abnormal bleeding from any source during thrombocytopenic period (day 7–17); inspect skin for ecchymotic and petechial areas. Protect patient from trauma.
- Report disorientation or confusion; drug should be withdrawn immediately.
- Indications to discontinue drug: Severe stomatitis, leukopenia (WBC less than 3500/mm³ or rapidly decreasing count), intractable vomiting, diarrhea, thrombocytopenia (platelets less than 100,000/mm³), and hemorrhage from any site.
- Inspect patient's mouth daily. Promptly report cracked lips, xerostomia, white patches, and erythema of buccal membranes.
- Report development of maculopapular rash; it usually responds to symptomatic treatment and is reversible.
- Be aware of expected response of lesion to topical 5-FU: Erythema followed in sequence by vesiculation, erosion, ulceration, necrosis, epithelialization. Applications of drug are continued until ulcerative stage is reached (2–6 wk after initial applications) and then discontinued.
- Monitor lab tests: Total and differential WBC counts before each dose. Baseline and periodic Hct, LFTs, renal function tests.

### Patient & Family Education
- Understand that it is very important to report the first signs of toxicity: Anorexia, vomiting, nausea, stomatitis, diarrhea, GI bleeding.
- Avoid exposure to sunlight or ultraviolet lamp treatments. Protect exposed skin. Photosensitivity usually subsides 2–3 mo after last dose.
- Report promptly to prescriber any difficulty in maintaining balance while ambulating.
- Use contraception during 5-FU treatment. If you suspect you are pregnant, tell your prescriber.

# FLUOXETINE HYDROCHLORIDE ℗
(flu'ox-e-tine)
Prozac, Prozac Weekly, Sarafem

**Classifications:** SELECTIVE SEROTONIN REUPTAKE INHIBITOR (SSRI); ANTIDEPRESSANT
Therapeutic: ANTIDEPRESSANT; SSRI

## AVAILABILITY
Tablet; capsule; solution; sustained release capsule

## ACTION & THERAPEUTIC EFFECT
A selective serotonin reuptake inhibitor (SSRI). Antidepressant effect is presumed to be linked to its inhibition of CNS neuronal uptake of serotonin, a neurotransmitter. *Effectiveness may take from several days to 5 wk to develop fully. Drug has antidepressant, antiobsessive-compulsive, and antibulimic actions.*

## USES
Depression, obsessive-compulsive disorder (OCD), bipolar depression, bulimia nervosa, premenstrual dysphoric disorder, panic disorder.

## UNLABELED USES
Obesity, fibromyalgia, hot flashes, PTSD, social anxiety disorder.

## CONTRAINDICATIONS
Hypersensitivity to fluoxetine or other SSRI drugs; bipolar disorder; hyponatremia; concurrent administration with MAOIs, pimozide or thioridazine; children younger than 7 y for OCD, children younger than 8 y for depression.

Common adverse effects in *italic*; life-threatening effects underlined; generic names in **bold**; classifications in SMALL CAPS; ♣ Canadian drug name; ℗ Prototype drug

**CAUTIOUS USE** Hepatic and renal impairment, renal failure, abrupt discontinuation, anorexia nervosa, mania, bleeding; hyponatremia, cardiac disease, dehydration, DM, patients with history of suicidal ideations or current suicidal tendencies; history of QT prolongation, or congenital long QT syndrome; seizure disorders, ECT, hepatic disease. Older adults may require dose adjustments; pregnancy (category C); lactation.

## ROUTE & DOSAGE

### Depression

*Adult:* **PO Immediate release** 20 mg/day may increase by 20 mg/day at weekly intervals (max: 80 mg/day); when stable may switch to 90 mg sustained release capsule qwk
*Child (8 y or older):* **PO** 10–20 mg/day in a.m.
*Geriatric:* **PO** Start with 10 mg/day

### Obsessive Compulsive Disorder

*Adult.* **PO** 20 mg daily may increase if needed (max: 80 mg/day)
*Adolescent/Child (7 y or older):* **PO** 10 mg/day may increase to 20 mg/day

### Premenstrual Dysphoric Disorder

*Adult:* **PO** 20 mg daily (max: 60 mg/day)

### Bulimia Nervosa

*Adult:* **PO** 60 mg daily

### Panic Disorder

*Adult:* **PO** 10 mg daily may increase to 20 mg daily

### *Pharmacogenetic Dosage Adjustment*

*CYP2D6 poor metabolizers:* Start at 80% of normal dose

## ADMINISTRATION

### Oral

- Give as a single dose in morning. Give in two divided doses; one in a.m. and one at noon to prevent insomnia, when more than 20 mg/day prescribed.
- Provide suicidal or potentially suicidal patient with small quantities of prescription medication.
- Monitor for worsening of depression or expression of suicidal ideations.
- Store at 15°–25° C (59°–77° F).

**ADVERSE EFFECTS** (≥1%) **CNS:** *Headache, nervousness, anxiety, insomnia,* drowsiness, fatigue, tremor, dizziness, yawning. **CV:** Palpitations, hot flushes, chest pain. **GI:** *Nausea, diarrhea,* anorexia, dyspepsia, increased appetite, dry mouth. **Skin:** Rash, pruritus, sweating, hypersensitivity reactions. **Special Senses:** Blurred vision. **Body as a Whole:** Myalgias, arthralgias, flu-like syndrome, hyponatremia. **Urogenital:** Sexual dysfunction, menstrual irregularities. **Respiratory:** Pharyngitis.

**INTERACTIONS Drug:** Concurrent use of **tryptophan** may cause agitation, restlessness, and GI distress; MAO INHIBITORS, **selegiline** may increase risk of severe hypertensive reaction and death; increases half-life of **diazepam;** may increase toxicity of TRICYCLIC ANTIDEPRESSANTS; AMPHETAMINES, **cilostazol, nefazodone, pentazocine, propafenone, sibutramine, tramadol, venlafaxine** may increase risk of serotonin syndrome; may inhibit metabolism of **carbamazepine, phenytoin, ritonavir;**

Common adverse effects in *italic;* life-threatening effects <u>underlined</u>; generic names in **bold;** classifications in SMALL CAPS; ♣ Canadian drug name; ● Prototype drug

707

increased ergotamine toxicity with **dihydroergotamine, ergotamine.** Do not use with agents that cause QT prolongation (**pimozide, ziprasidone**). **Herbal: St. John's wort** may cause serotonin syndrome.

**PHARMACOKINETICS Absorption:** 60–80% from GI tract. **Onset:** 1–3 wk. **Peak:** 4–8 h. **Distribution:** Widely distributed, including CNS. **Metabolism:** In liver to active metabolite, norfluoxetine. **Elimination:** Greater than 80% in urine; 12% in feces. **Half-Life:** Fluoxetine 2–3 days, norfluoxetine 7–9 days.

## NURSING IMPLICATIONS

### Assessment & Drug Effects

- Monitor children and adolescents for changes in behavior and suicidal ideation.
- Use with caution in the older adult patient or patient with impaired renal or hepatic function (may need lower dose).
- Supervise patients closely who are high suicide risks; especially during initial therapy.
- Monitor for S&S of anaphylactoid reaction (see Appendix F).
- Monitor serum sodium level for development of hyponatremia, especially in patients who are taking diuretics or are otherwise hypovolemic.
- Monitor diabetics for loss of glycemic control; hypoglycemia has occurred during initiation of therapy, and hyperglycemia during drug withdrawal.
- Weigh weekly to monitor weight loss, particularly in the older adult or nutritionally compromised patient. Report significant weight loss to prescriber.
- Observe for and promptly report rash or urticaria and S&S of fever, leukocytosis, arthralgias, carpal

tunnel syndrome, edema, respiratory distress, and proteinuria.

- Observe for dizziness and drowsiness and employ safety measures as indicated.
- Monitor for and report increased anxiety, nervousness, or insomnia; may need modification of drug dose.
- Monitor for seizures in patients with a history of seizures. Use appropriate safety precautions.
- Taper dosage slowly when discontinuing.
- Monitor lab tests: Periodic serum electrolytes; frequent plasma glucose in diabetics.

### Patient & Family Education

- Notify prescriber of any rash; possible sign of a serious group of adverse effects.
- Do not drive or engage in potentially hazardous activities until response to drug is known; especially if dizziness noted.
- Monitor blood glucose for loss of glycemic control if diabetic.
- Note: Drug may increase seizure activity in those with history of seizure.

# FLUPHENAZINE DECANOATE
(floo-fen'a-zeen)
Modecate Decanoate ♦

# FLUPHENAZINE HYDROCHLORIDE
Moditen HCl ♦

**Classifications:** ANTIPSYCHOTIC; PHENOTHIAZINE
**Therapeutic:** ANTIPSYCHOTIC
**Prototype:** Chlorpromazine

**AVAILABILITY** Tablet; elixir; oral concentrate; solution for injection; **Decanoate:** Solution for injection

## ACTION & *THERAPEUTIC EFFECT*
Potent phenothiazine, antipsychotic agent that blocks postsynaptic

dopamine receptors in the brain. Similar to other phenothiazines with the following exceptions: More potent/weight, higher incidence of extrapyramidal complications, and lower frequency of sedative, hypotensive, and antiemetic effects. *Effective for treatment of antipsychotic symptoms including schizophrenia.*

**USES** Management of manifestations of psychotic disorders.

**CONTRAINDICATIONS** Known hypersensitivity to fluphenazine, older adults with dementia-related psychosis; suspected or subcortical brain damage, comatose or severely depressed states, blood dyscrasias, liver damage; renal or hepatic disease; NMS; lactation; children younger than 12 y.

**CAUTIOUS USE** Older adults, previously diagnosed breast cancer; closed-angle glaucoma; GI disorders; significant pulmonary disease; renal failure; seizure disorders; history of suicidal ideation or high risk for suicide attempt; cardiovascular diseases; pheochromocytoma; history of convulsive disorders; patients exposed to extreme heat or phosphorous insecticides; peptic ulcer; respiratory impairment; older adults; pregnancy (category undetermined).

## ROUTE & DOSAGE

**Psychosis**
*Adult:* **PO** 2.5–10 mg/day in 2–3 divided doses (max: of 20 mg/day); **IM** 2.5–10 mg/day divided q6–8h (max: 10 mg/day);
**Decanoate IM/Subcutaneous** 12.5–25 mg q1–4wk

## ADMINISTRATION

### Oral
- Dilute oral concentrate in fruit juice, water, carbonated beverage, milk, soup. Avoid caffeine-containing beverages (cola, coffee) as a diluent, also tannic acid (tea) or pectinates (apple juice).
- Protect all preparations from light and freezing. Solutions may safely vary in color from almost colorless to light amber. Discard dark or otherwise discolored solutions.
- Store in tightly closed container at 15°–30° C (59°–86° F) unless otherwise specified by manufacturer. Protect all forms from light.

### Intramuscular/Subcutaneous
- Fluphenazine hydrochloride (HCl) is given IM and fluphenazine decanoate may be given IM or subcutaneously.

**ADVERSE EFFECTS** (≥1%) **CNS:** *Extrapyramidal symptoms* (resembling Parkinson's disease), <u>tardive dyskinesia</u>, sedation, drowsiness, dizziness, headache, mental depression, catatonic-like state, <u>impaired thermoregulation</u>, grand mal seizures. **CV:** Tachycardia, hypertension, hypotension. **GI:** Dry mouth, nausea, epigastric pain, constipation, fecal impaction, cholecystic jaundice. **Urogenital:** Urinary retention, polyuria, inhibition of ejaculation. **Hematologic:** Transient <u>leukopenia</u>, <u>agranulocytosis</u>. **Skin:** Contact dermatitis **Body as a Whole:** Peripheral edema. **Special Senses:** Nasal congestion, blurred vision, increased intraocular pressure, *photosensitivity.* **Endocrine:** Hyperprolactinemia.

**INTERACTIONS Drug: Alcohol** and other CNS DEPRESSANTS may potentiate depressive effects; decreases seizure threshold, may need to adjust

Common adverse effects in *italic;* life-threatening effects <u>underlined</u>; generic names in **bold;** classifications in SMALL CAPS; ♣ Canadian drug name; ⊘ Prototype drug

709

dosage of ANTICONVULSANTS. Do not use with drugs that prolong QT interval. **Herbal: Kava** may increase risk and severity of dystonic reactions.

## PHARMACOKINETICS **Absorption:** HCl is readily absorbed PO and IM; decanoate has delayed IM absorption. **Onset:** 1 h HCl; 24–72 h decanoate. **Peak:** 0.5 h PO; 1.5–2 h IM HCl. **Duration:** 6–8 h HCl; 1–6 wk decanoate. **Distribution:** Crosses blood–brain barrier and placenta. **Metabolism:** In liver. **Half-Life:** 15 h HCl; 7–10 days decanoate.

## NURSING IMPLICATIONS

### Black Box Warning

*Fluphenazine has been associated with increased mortality in older adults with dementia-related phychosis.*

### Assessment & Drug Effects

- Monitor very closely older adults with dementia. Report immediately onset of mental depression and extrapyramidal symptoms.
- Be alert for appearance of acute dystonia (see Appendix F). Symptoms can be controlled by reducing dosage or by adding an antiparkinsonism drug such as benztropine.
- Monitor BP during early therapy. If systolic drop is more than 20 mm Hg, inform prescriber.
- Monitor I&O ratio and bowel elimination pattern. Check for abdominal distension and pain. Monitor for xerostomia and constipation.
- Monitor lab tests: Periodic renal function tests with long-term treatment; periodic WBC with differential, and LFTs.

### Patient & Family Education

- Do not drive or engage in potentially hazardous activities until response to drug is known.
- Do not stop taking drug abruptly.
- Inform prescriber promptly if following symptoms appear: Light-colored stools, changes in vision, sore throat, fever, cellulitis, rash, any interference with movement.
- Avoid exposure to sun; wear protective clothing and cover exposed skin surfaces with sun screen.
- Avoid alcohol while on fluphenazine therapy.
- Note: Fluphenazine may discolor urine pink to red or reddish brown.
- Periodic ophthalmologic exams are recommended.

## FLURANDRENOLIDE
(flure-an-dren'oh-lide)
Cordran, Cordran SP, Drenison ♦
See Appendix A-4.

## FLURAZEPAM HYDROCHLORIDE
(flure-az'e-pam)
Apo-Flurazepam ♦, Novoflupam ♦
**Classifications:** SEDATIVE-HYPNOTIC, NONBARBITUATE; BENZODIAZEPINE
Therapeutic: SEDATIVE
**Prototype:** Triazolam
**Controlled Substance:** Schedule IV

## AVAILABILITY Capsule

## ACTION & *THERAPEUTIC EFFECT*
Benzodiazepine derivative that enhances the GABA-benzodiazepine receptor complex. GABA is an inhibitory neurotransmitter involved in anxiolytic and sedative effects.

Flurazepam appears to act at the limbic and subcortical levels of CNS to produce sedation. *Reduces sleep induction time; produces marked reduction of stage 4 sleep (deepest sleep stage) while at the same time increasing duration of total sleep time.*

**USES** Hypnotic in management of all kinds of insomnia (e.g., difficulty in falling asleep, frequent nocturnal awakening or early morning awakening or both). Also for treatment of poor sleeping habits.

## CONTRAINDICATIONS

Prolonged administration; benzodiazepine hypersensitivity; ethanol intoxication; COPD, sleep apnea; respiratory depression; shock; coma; major depression or psychosis; intermittent porphyria; pregnancy (category X), lactation.

## CAUTIOUS USE

Impaired renal or hepatic function; glaucoma; mental depression, psychoses, history of suicidal tendencies, bipolar disorder; intermittent porphyria; addiction-prone individuals; older adult or debilitated patients; COPD; children younger than 15 y.

## ROUTE & DOSAGE

**Sedative, Hypnotic**

*Adult (15 y or older):* **PO** 15–30 mg at bedtime
*Geriatric:* **PO** 15 mg at bedtime

## ADMINISTRATION

### Oral

- Give once patient is in bed and ready to fall asleep.
- Store in light-resistant container with childproof cap at 15°–30° C (59°–86° F) unless otherwise specified.

## ADVERSE EFFECTS (≥1%) CNS:

*Residual sedation, drowsiness,* light-headedness, dizziness, ataxia, headache, nervousness, apprehension, talkativeness, irritability, depression, hallucinations, nightmares, confusion, paradoxic reactions: Excitement, euphoria, hyperactivity, disorientation, coma (overdosage). **Special Senses:** Blurred vision, burning eyes. **GI:** Heartburn, nausea, vomiting, diarrhea, abdominal pain. **Body as a Whole:** Immediate allergic reaction, hypotension, granulocytopenia (rare), jaundice (rare).

## DIAGNOSTIC TEST INTERFERENCE

Flurazepam may increase serum levels of *total and direct bilirubin, alkaline phosphatase, AST,* and *ALT.* False-negative *urine glucose* reactions may occur with *Clinistix* and *Diastix;* no effect with *TesTape.*

## INTERACTIONS

**Drug: Alcohol,** CNS DEPRESSANTS, ANTICONVULSANTS potentiate CNS depression; **cimetidine, disulfiram** may increase flurazepam levels, thus increasing its toxicity. **Herbal: Kava, valerian** may potentiate sedation.

## PHARMACOKINETICS

**Absorption:** Readily from GI tract. **Onset:** 15–45 min. **Duration:** 7–8 h. **Distribution:** Crosses blood–brain barrier and placenta; distributed into breast milk. **Metabolism:** In liver to active metabolites. **Elimination:** Primarily in urine. **Half-Life:** 47–100 h.

## NURSING IMPLICATIONS

### Assessment & Drug Effects

- Monitor effectiveness. Hypnotic effect is apparent on second or third night of consecutive use and continues 1–2 nights after drug is stopped (drug has a long half-life).

---

Common adverse effects in *italic;* life-threatening effects underlined; generic names in **bold;** classifications in SMALL CAPS; ♣ Canadian drug name; ⊘ Prototype drug.

711

- Supervise ambulation. Residual sedation and drowsiness are relatively common. Excessive drowsiness, ataxia, vertigo, and falling occur more frequently in older adults or debilitated patients.
- Be aware that withdrawal symptoms have occurred 3 days after abrupt discontinuation after prolonged use and include worsening of insomnia, dizziness, blurred vision, anorexia, GI upset, nasal congestion, paresthesias.

**Patient & Family Education**

- Avoid potentially hazardous activities until response to drug is known.
- Avoid alcohol. Concurrent ingestion with flurazepam intensifies CNS depressant effects; symptoms may occur even when alcohol is ingested as long as 10 h after last flurazepam dose.
- Be aware of the possible additive depressant effects when drug is combined with barbiturates, tranquilizers, or other CNS depressants.

# FLURBIPROFEN SODIUM

(flure-bi'proe-fen)

Ocufen

**Classifications:** ANALGESIC, NONSTEROIDAL ANTI-INFLAMMATORY DRUG (NSAID); COX-1 AND COX-2 INHIBITOR; ANTIPYRETIC
**Therapeutic:** ANALGESIC, NSAID
**Prototype:** Ibuprofen

**AVAILABILITY** Tablet; ophthalmic solution

**ACTION & *THERAPEUTIC EFFECT***
Inhibits prostaglandin synthesis including in the conjunctiva and uvea by inhibiting the COX-1 or COX-2 enzymes. Ocular flurbiprofen reduces miosis, permitting maintenance of drug-induced mydriasis during surgical procedures.

*An anti-inflammatory, nonsteroidal analgesic. Additionally, it inhibits migration of leukocytes into inflamed tissues, depresses monocyte function, and may inhibit platelet aggregation. Reduces miosis intraoperatively.*

**USES** Inhibition of intraoperative miosis; arthritis and other inflammatory diseases; mild to moderate pain.

**UNLABELED USES** Management of postoperative ocular inflammation, prevention of postcystoid macular edema.

**CONTRAINDICATIONS** Hypersensitivity to NSAIDs, or salicylates; perioperative pain from CABG; pregnancy (category D third trimester); lactation.

**CAUTIOUS USE** Patient who may be adversely affected by prolonged bleeding time; patient in whom asthma, rhinitis, or urticaria is precipitated by aspirin or other NSAIDs; pregnancy (category B first and second trimester). Safe use in children not established.

## ROUTE & DOSAGE

| **Inflammatory Disease** |
| --- |
| *Adult:* **PO** 200–300 mg/day in 2–4 divided doses (max: 300 mg/day) |
| **Mild to Moderate Pain** |
| *Adult:* **PO** 50–100 mg q6–8h |
| **Inhibition of Intraoperative Miosis** |
| *Adult:* **Topical** 1 drop in eye approximately q30min beginning 2 h before surgery for a total of 4 drops/affected eye |

Common adverse effects in *italic;* life-threatening effects underlined; generic names in **bold;** classifications in SMALL CAPS; ♣ Canadian drug name; ⊘ Prototype drug

## ADMINISTRATION

### Topical

- Instill ophthalmic preparation with great care to avoid contamination of solution. Do not touch eye surface with dropper.

### Oral

- Use the 300 mg dose for initiation of therapy or for acute exacerbations of disease.
- May be given with food, milk, or antacids.
- Store at 15°–30° C (59°–86° F) in tight, light-resistant container.

## ADVERSE EFFECTS (≥1%) Special

**Senses:** *Mild ocular stinging,* burning, itching, or foreign body sensation (transient). **Other:** Slowed corneal healing; increased bleeding time. **For adverse effects to oral preparations, see ibuprofen.**

## INTERACTIONS Drug: ORAL ANTI-

COAGULANTS, **heparin** may prolong bleeding time; actions and side effects of **phenytoin**, SULFONYLUREAS, or SULFONAMIDES may be potentiated. Do not use with **cidofovir** or **ketorlac. Herbal: Feverfew, garlic, ginger, gingko** may increase bleeding potential.

## PHARMACOKINETICS Absorp-

**tion:** 80% absorbed from GI tract. **Onset:** 2 h. **Peak:** 2 h. **Duration:** 6–8 h. **Distribution:** Small amounts distributed into breast milk. **Metabolism:** In liver. **Elimination:** Primarily in urine; some biliary excretion. **Half-Life:** 5 h.

## NURSING IMPLICATIONS

### Black Box Warning

*Flurbiprofen has been associated with increased risk of serious,* *potentially fatal GI bleeding and cardiovascular events (e.g., MI & CVA); risk may increase with duration of use and may be greater in the older adult and those with risk factors for CV disease.*

### Assessment & Drug Effects

- Observe patients with history of cardiac decompensation closely for evidence of fluid retention and edema.
- Monitor for and report promptly S&S of CV thrombotic events (i.e., angina, MI, TIA, or stroke).
- Lab tests: Baseline and periodic evaluations of Hgb, renal function tests, LFTs.
- Auditory and ophthalmologic examinations are recommended with prolonged or high-dose therapy.
- Monitor for GI distress and S&S of GI bleeding.

### Patient & Family Education

- Report ocular irritation that persists after flurbiprofen use during surgery (tearing, dry eye sensation, dull eye pain, photophobia) to prescriber.
- Be alert for bleeding tendency and report unexplained bleeding, prolongation of bleeding time, or bruises.
- Notify prescriber immediately of passage of dark tarry stools, "coffee ground" emesis, frankly bloody emesis, or other GI distress, as well as blood or protein in urine, and onset of skin rash, pruritus, jaundice.
- Monitor for and report promptly S&S of CV thrombotic events (i.e., angina, MI, TIA, or stroke).
- Do not drive or engage in potentially hazardous activities until response to the drug is known.
- Avoid alcohol. Concurrent use may increase risk of GI ulceration and bleeding tendencies.

Common adverse effects in *italic*; life-threatening effects underlined; generic names in **bold**; classifications in SMALL CAPS; ♣ Canadian drug name; ❶ Prototype drug

713

## FLUTAMIDE ⊘

(flu'ta-mide)

Eulexin

**Classifications:** ANTINEOPLASTIC;
ANTIANDROGEN
Therapeutic: ANTINEOPLASTIC;
ANTIANDROGEN

**AVAILABILITY** Capsule

### ACTION & THERAPEUTIC EFFECT

Nonsteroidal, nonhormonal, antiandrogenic drug that inhibits androgen uptake or binding of androgen to target tissues (i.e., prostatic cancer cells). *Interferes with the binding of both testosterone and dihydrotestosterone to target tissue (i.e., prostate cancer cells).*

**USES** In combination with luteinizing hormone-releasing hormone agonists (i.e., leuprolide) or castration for early stage and metastatic prostate cancer.

**CONTRAINDICATIONS** Hypersensitivity to flutamide; severe liver impairment if ALT is equal to twice the normal value; females; pregnancy (category D); lactation.

**CAUTIOUS USE** Lactase deficiency.

### ROUTE & DOSAGE

**Prostate Cancer**
*Adult:* **PO** 250 mg (2 caps) q8h

### ADMINISTRATION

**Oral**
- Use with caution in patients with severe hepatic impairment.
- Store at 2°–30° C (36°–86° F) in a tightly closed, light-resistant container.

**ADVERSE EFFECTS** (≥1%) **CNS:** Drowsiness, confusion, depression, anxiety, nervousness. **GI:** Diarrhea, nausea, vomiting, anorexia, hepatitis, cholestatic jaundice, encephalopathy, hepatic necrosis, acute hepatic failure, may increase ALT, AST, bilirubin. **Urogenital:** *Hot flashes, loss of libido, impotence.* **Hematologic:** Anemia, leukopenia, thrombocytopenia. **Skin:** Rash. **Body as a Whole:** Edema. **Endocrine:** Gynecomastia, galactorrhea.

**INTERACTIONS Drug:** May increase INR in patients on **warfarin.**

**PHARMACOKINETICS Absorption:** Readily absorbed from GI tract. **Onset:** Antiandrogenic activity 2.2 h; symptomatic relief 2–4 wk. **Duration:** 3 mo–2.5 y, with an average of 10.5 mo. **Metabolism:** Metabolized in liver to at least 10 different metabolites; the major metabolite, 2-hydroxyflutamide (SCH-16423), is an alpha-hydroxylated derivative that is biologically active. **Elimination:** 98% in urine. **Half-Life:** 5–6 h.

## NURSING IMPLICATIONS

### Black Box Warning

*Flutamide has been associated with severe, potentially fatal, liver injury.*

### Assessment & Drug Effects
- Monitor for symptomatic relief of bone pain.
- Assess for development of gynecomastia and galactorrhea; if these become bothersome, dosage reduction may be warranted.
- Lab tests: Monitor LFTs and serum bilirubin periodically.
- Monitor for and report promptly S&S of liver dysfunction or development of a lupus-like syndrome.

Common adverse effects in *italic;* life-threatening effects underlined; generic names in **bold;** classifications in SMALL CAPS; ♣ Canadian drug name; ⊘ Prototype drug

### Patient & Family Education

- Be aware of potential adverse effects of therapy.
- Notify prescriber immediately of the following: Pain in upper abdomen, yellowing of skin and eyes, dark urine, respiratory problems, rashes on face, difficulty urinating, sore throat, fever, chills.

## FLUTICASONE

(flu-ti-ca'sone)

Advair, Flonase, Flovent, Flovent HFA, Cutivate, Veramyst

**See Appendixes A-3, A-4.**

## FLUVASTATIN

(flu-vah-stat'in)

Lescol, Lescol XL

**Classifications:** HMG-COA REDUCTASE INHIBITOR (STATIN); ANTIHYPERLIPEMIC

Therapeutic: CHOLESTEROL-LOWERING (STATIN)

**Prototype:** Lovastatin

**AVAILABILITY** Capsule; extended release tablet

### ACTION & *THERAPEUTIC EFFECT*

Inhibits reductase 3-hydroxy-3-methylglutaryl coenzyme A (HMG-CoA) that is essential to hepatic production of cholesterol. Cholesterol-lowering effect triggers induction of LDL receptors, which promotes removal of LDL and VLDL remnants (precursors of LDL) from plasma. *Results in an increase in plasma HDL concentration. HDLs collect excess cholesterol from body cells and transport it to the liver for excretion.*

**USES** Adjunct to diet for the reduction of elevated total LDL cholesterol in patients with primary hypercholesterolemia (types IIa and IIb).

**UNLABELED USES** Other types of hyperlipidemias.

**CONTRAINDICATIONS** Hypersensitivity to fluvastatin, lovastatin, pravastatin, or simvastatin; active liver disease or unexplained persistent elevated liver function tests; pregnancy (category X); lactation.

**CAUTIOUS USE** Patients who consume substantial quantities of alcohol; history of severe liver impairment; renal impairment. Safe use in children younger than 10 y not established.

### ROUTE & DOSAGE

**Hypercholesterolemia**

*Adult/Adolescent/Child (10 y and older):* **PO** 20–40 mg at bedtime, may increase up to 80 mg/day in 1–2 doses

### ADMINISTRATION

**Oral**

- Ensure the extended release tablet is not chewed or crushed. It **must be** swallowed whole.
- Separate doses of this drug and bile-acid resin (e.g., cholestyramine) by at least 2 h when given concomitantly.
- Note: Dosage adjustments may be required in patients with significant renal or hepatic impairment.
- Store at room temperature, 15°–30° C (59°–86° F).

**ADVERSE EFFECTS** (≥1%) **CNS:** Headache, fatigue, insomnia. **Body as a Whole:** Myalgia. **GI:** Dyspepsia, abdominal pain, diarrhea. **Skin:** Rash.

**INTERACTIONS Drug:** May increase risk of bleeding with **warfarin;**

Common adverse effects in *italic;* life-threatening effects <u>underlined</u>; generic names in **bold;** classifications in SMALL CAPS; ♣ Canadian drug name; ☻ Prototype drug

715

**cholestyramine** decreases fluvastatin absorption; **rifampin** increases metabolism of fluvastatin; may increase risk of myopathy and rhabdomyolysis with **gemfibrozil, fenofibrate, clofibrate.**

## PHARMACOKINETICS Absorption:
Readily from GI tract; about 24% reaches systemic circulation after first-pass metabolism. **Onset:** 3–6 wk. **Peak:** Serum level 0.5–1 h. **Distribution:** 98% protein bound; distributed into breast milk. **Metabolism:** In liver. **Elimination:** 95% in bile; 5% in urine. **Half-Life:** 0.5–1 h.

## NURSING IMPLICATIONS

### Assessment & Drug Effects
- Lab tests: Monitor lipoprotein levels; maximal lipid-lowering effect occurs in 4–6 wk. Monitor serum transaminase and CPK levels every 3–4 mo for the first year and periodically thereafter.
- Monitor PT and INR in patients on concurrent warfarin therapy; PT & INR may be prolonged.

### Patient & Family Education
- Take fluvastatin at bedtime.
- Be alert and report signs of bleeding immediately when also taking warfarin.
- Notify prescriber immediately of the following: Fever; rash; muscle pain, weakness, tenderness, or cramping.
- Reduce or eliminate alcohol consumption while taking fluvastatin.

## FLUVOXAMINE
(flu-vox′a-meen)
Luvox
**Classifications:** SELECTIVE SEROTONIN REUPTAKE INHIBITOR (SSRI); ANTIDEPRESSANT
Therapeutic: ANTIDEPRESSANT; SSRI
**Prototype:** Fluoxetine

**AVAILABILITY** Tablet; extended release capsule

## ACTION & *THERAPEUTIC EFFECT*
Antidepressant with potent, selective, inhibitory activity on neuronal (5-HT) serotonin reuptake (SSRI). *Effective as an antidepressant and for control of obsessive-compulsive disorder and social anxiety.*

**USES** Treatment of obsessive-compulsive disorders.

**UNLABELED USES** Post-traumatic stress disorder, depression, panic attacks, eating disorder, social anxiety disorder, major depressive disorder.

**CONTRAINDICATIONS** Hypersensitivity to fluvoxamine or fluoxetine; suicidal ideation; concurrent MAOI therapy or within 14 days of use; bipolar depression; lactation.

**CAUTIOUS USE** Liver disease, renal impairment, abrupt discontinuation; cardiac disease, dehydration, hyponatremia, older adults, ECT, seizure disorders, history of suicidal tendencies, tobacco smoking; pregnancy (category C). Safety and efficacy in children younger than 8 y for obsessive compulsive disorder not established.

## ROUTE & DOSAGE

**Obsessive-Compulsive Disorder**

*Adult:* **PO** Start with 50 mg daily, may increase slowly up to 300 mg/day given every night or divided b.i.d. OR **Extended release** 100 mg every night, may increase up (max: 300 mg/day)
*Adolescent:* **PO** Start with 25 mg daily, may increase by 25 mg

q4–7days up to 300 mg/day in divided doses

*Child (8–11 y):* **PO** Start with 25 mg every night, may increase by 25 mg q4–7days (max: 200 mg/day in divided doses)

***Pharmacogenetic Dosage Adjustment***

*Poor CYP2D6 metabolizers:* Start with 70% of dose

## ADMINISTRATION

### Oral

- Do not open extended release capsules. They **must be** swallowed whole.
- Give starting doses at bedtime to improve tolerance to nausea and vomiting; both are common early in therapy.
- Store at room temperature, 15°–30° C (59°–86° F), away from moisture and light.

## ADVERSE EFFECTS (≥1%) **CNS:**
*Somnolence, headache, agitation, insomnia, dizziness,* seizures. **CV:** Orthostatic hypotension, slight bradycardia. **GI:** *Nausea, vomiting, dry mouth, constipation, anorexia,* diarrhea. **Urogenital:** Sexual dysfunction. **Skin:** Stevens–Johnson syndrome, toxic epidermal necrolysis (rare).

## DIAGNOSTIC TEST INTERFERENCE
***Gamma-glutamyl transferase*** increased by more than 3-fold following 3 wk of therapy.

## INTERACTIONS **Drug:** Increases plasma levels of **amitriptyline, clomipramine,** and other TRI-CYCLIC ANTIDEPRESSANTS. May antagonize the blood pressure-lowering effects of **atenolol** and other BETA-BLOCKERS. May increase levels and toxicity of **carbamazepine, mexiletine.** May increase **lithium** levels causing neurotoxicity, serotonin syndrome, somnolence, and mania. Increases prothrombin time in patients on **warfarin;** increased ergotamine toxicity with **dihydroergotamine, ergotamine.** Use with CYP1A2 IN-HIBITORS **(thioridazine, pimozide, alosetron, tizanidine, ramelteon)** increases **fluvoxamine** levels and toxicity. **Food: Grapefruit juice** may increase risk of side effects. **Herbal: Melatonin** may increase and prolong drowsiness; **St. John's wort** may cause serotonin syndrome.

## PHARMACOKINETICS **Absorption:** Almost completely absorbed from GI tract. **Onset:** 4–7 days. **Distribution:** Approximately 77% bound to plasma proteins; excreted in human breast milk but in an amount that poses little risk to the nursing infant. **Metabolism:** In liver. **Elimination:** Completely in urine. **Half-Life:** 16–24 h.

## NURSING IMPLICATIONS

### Black Box Warning

*Fluvoxamine has been associated with increased risk of suicidal thinking and behavior in children, adolescents, and young adults.*

### Assessment & Drug Effects
- Monitor for worsening of depression or emergence of suicidal ideations especially in adolescents and children.
- Monitor for significant nausea and vomiting, especially during initial therapy.
- Assess safety; drowsiness and dizziness are common adverse effects.

Common adverse effects in *italic;* life-threatening effects <u>underlined</u>; generic names in **bold;** classifications in SMALL CAPS; ♣ Canadian drug name; ⦿ Prototype drug

717

- Monitor PT and INR carefully with concurrent warfarin therapy; adjust warfarin as needed.

### Patient & Family Education
- Note: Nausea and vomiting are common in early therapy. Notify prescriber if these adverse effects last more than a few days.
- Exercise caution with hazardous activity until response to the drug is known.

## FOLIC ACID (VITAMIN B₉, PTEROYLGLUTAMIC ACID)
(fol'ic)

Apo-Folic ◆, Folacin, Novofolacid ◆

## FOLATE SODIUM
Folvite Sodium

**Classification:** VITAMIN B₉
**Therapeutic:** VITAMIN SUPPLEMENT

**AVAILABILITY** Tablet; solution for injection

## ACTION & *THERAPEUTIC EFFECT*
Vitamin B₉ essential for nucleoprotein synthesis and maintenance of normal erythropoiesis. Acts to correct folic acid deficiency that results in production of defective DNA that leads to megaloblast formation and arrest of bone marrow maturation. *Stimulates production of RBCs, WBCs, and platelets in patients with megaloblastic anemias.*

## USES
Folate deficiency, macrocytic anemia, and megaloblastic anemias associated with malabsorption syndromes, alcoholism, primary liver disease, inadequate dietary intake, pregnancy, infancy, and childhood.

## CONTRAINDICATIONS
Folic acid alone for pernicious anemia or other vitamin B₁₂ deficiency states; normocytic, refractory, aplastic, or undiagnosed anemia; neonates.

**CAUTIOUS USE** Pregnancy (category A).

## ROUTE & DOSAGE

**Therapeutic**

*Adult:* **PO/IM/Subcutaneous/IV** 1 mg/day or less
*Child:* **PO/IM/Subcutaneous/IV** 1 mg/day or less

**Maintenance**

*Adult:* **PO/IM/Subcutaneous/IV** 0.4 mg/day or less
*Child (4 y or younger):* **PO/IM/Subcutaneous/IV** Up to 0.3 mg/day; *4 y or older:* up to 0.1 mg/day
*Infant:* **PO/IM/Subcutaneous/IV** 0.1 mg/day

## ADMINISTRATION
### Oral
- Oral route is preferred to other routes.

### Intramuscular/Subcutaneous
- Give undiluted. Use caution not to inject intradermally.

### Intravenous

***PREPARE:*** **Direct/Continuous:** Given undiluted.
***ADMINISTER:*** **Direct/Continuous:** Give over 30–60 sec. ▪ May also add to a continuous infusion.
***INCOMPATIBILITIES:*** **Solution/additive: Calcium gluconate, chlorpromazine, dextrose 40% in water, doxapram.**

- Store at 15°–30° C (59°–86° F) in tightly closed containers protected from light, unless otherwise directed.

## ADVERSE EFFECTS (≥1%)
Reportedly nontoxic. Slight flushing and feeling of warmth following IV administration.

## DIAGNOSTIC TEST INTERFERENCE

Falsely low serum *folate levels* may occur with *Lactobacillus casei assay* in patients receiving antibiotics such as TETRACYCLINES.

## INTERACTIONS Drug: Chloramphenicol may antagonize effects of **folate** therapy; **phenytoin** metabolism may be increased, thus decreasing its levels.

## PHARMACOKINETICS Absorption: Readily from proximal small intestine. Peak: 30–60 min PO. Distribution: Distributed to all body tissues; high concentrations in CSF; crosses placenta; distributed into breast milk. Metabolism: In liver to active metabolites. Elimination: Small amounts in urine in folate-deficient patients; large amounts excreted in urine with high doses.

## NURSING IMPLICATIONS

### Assessment & Drug Effects

- Obtain a careful history of dietary intake and drug and alcohol usage prior to start of therapy.
- Keep prescriber informed of patient's response to therapy.
- Monitor patients on phenytoin for subtherapeutic plasma levels.

### Patient & Family Education

- Remain under close medical supervision while taking folic acid therapy. Adjustment of maintenance dose should be made if there is threat of relapse.

## FONDAPARINUX SODIUM

(fon-da-par'i-nux)

Arixtra

**Classification:** ANTICOAGULANT, SELECTIVE FACTOR XA INHIBITOR
**Therapeutic:** ANTICOAGULANT; ANTITHROMBOTIC
**Prototype:** RIVAROXABAN

## AVAILABILITY Syringe

## ACTION & THERAPEUTIC EFFECT

Fondaparinux sodium causes antithrombin III (ATIII)-mediated selective inhibition of Factor Xa. It potentiates the innate neutralization of Factor Xa by ATIII. This interrupts the blood coagulation cascade, inhibiting thrombin formation and, thus, thrombus development. *Effective in the prevention and treatment of deep-vein thrombosis measured by the laboratory value of the amount of anti-Xa assay expressed in mg.*

## USES Prophylaxis for DVT or pulmonary embolism (PE) in patients undergoing hip or knee replacement surgery or abdominal surgery; treatment of acute DVT without PE with warfarin, treatment of PE with warfarin.

## UNLABELED USES Acute coronary syndrome, unstable angina/non-ST-elevation MI.

## CONTRAINDICATIONS Hypersensitivity to fondaparinux; active bleeding; GI bleeding; severe renal impairment with a creatinine clearance of less than 30 mL/min; weight less than 50 kg; active major bleeding; bacterial endocarditis; intramuscular administration; thrombocytopenia associated with fondaparinux.

## CAUTIOUS USE Renal impairment or disease; indwelling epidural catheter; dental disease, dental work; diabetic retinopathy; diverticulitis; endocarditis, epidural anesthesia; hemophilia, heparin-induced thrombocytopenia (HIT), hepatic impairment; hypertension, idiopathic thrombocytopenia purpura (ITP); inflammatory bowel disease, lumbar puncture, spinal anesthesia; stroke, surgery; thrombocytopenia, thrombolytic therapy; vaginal bleeding, menstruation; peptic ulcer disease; bleeding disorders including a history of GI ulceration, etc.,

Common adverse effects in *italic;* life-threatening effects underlined; generic names in **bold;** classifications in SMALL CAPS; ♣ Canadian drug name; ⊘ Prototype drug

719

history of heparin-induced thrombo-cytopenia; older adults; pregnancy (category B); lactation. Safety and efficacy in children not established.

## ROUTE & DOSAGE

### DVT, Pulmonary Embolism Prophylaxis

*Adult (weight greater than 50 kg):*
**Subcutaneous** 2.5 mg daily starting at least 6 h postsurgery × 5–9 days; *for hip fracture patients:* up to 24 days additional use

### Treatment of DVT, Pulmonary Embolism

*Adult (weight less than 50 kg):*
**Subcutaneous** 5 mg; *weight 50–100 kg:* 7.5 mg; *weight greater than 100 kg:* 10 mg once daily × 5–9 days

### Renal Impairment Dosage Adjustment

*CrCl 30–50 mL/min:* Use with caution; *less than 30 mL/min:* Use is contraindicated

## ADMINISTRATION

### Subcutaneous

- Give no sooner than 6 h after surgery.
- Inspect visually for particulate matter and discoloration prior to administration.
- Do not expel the air bubble from the syringe before the injection.
- Use prefilled syringe to inject into fatty tissue, alternating injection sites (e.g., between L and R abdominal wall).
- Store at 25° C (77° F); excursions permitted to 15°–30° C (59°–86° F).

## ADVERSE EFFECTS (≥1%) **Body as a Whole:** Fever, edema. **CNS:** Insomnia, dizziness, confusion, headache. **CV:** Hypotension. **GI:** Nausea, constipation, vomiting, diarrhea, dyspepsia, elevated LFTs. **Endocrine:** Hypokalemia. **Hematologic:** Hemorrhage, *anemia*, hematoma. **Skin:** Irritation at injection site, rash, purpura, bullous eruption. **Urogenital:** UTI, urinary retention.

## INTERACTIONS **Drug:** ANTICOAGULANTS, ANTIPLATELETS, NSAIDS, **aspirin** may increase risk of bleeding. **Herbal: Feverfew, ginkgo, ginger, evening primrose oil** may potentiate bleeding.

## PHARMACOKINETICS **Absorption:** Rapidly and completely absorbed from subcutaneous injection site. **Peak:** 2–3 h. **Distribution:** Primarily in blood. **Metabolism:** Negligible metabolism. **Elimination:** In urine. **Half-Life:** 18 h.

## NURSING IMPLICATIONS

### Black Box Warning

*Fondaparinux has been associated with development of epidural and spinal hematomas.*

### Assessment & Drug Effects

- Monitor frequently for S&S of neurologic impairment; if noted, urgent treatment is necessary.
- Monitor for S&S of bleeding or hemorrhage. If noted, withhold fondaparinux and notify prescriber immediately.
- Withhold fondaparinux and notify prescriber if platelet count falls below 100,000/mm³.
- Monitor lab tests: Baseline and periodic renal function tests; periodic CBC with platelet count, and serum creatinine.

### Patient & Family Education

- Report any of the following to a health care provider: Signs of unexplained bleeding such as: Pink, red, or dark brown urine; red or dark brown vomitus; bleeding

gums or bloody sputum; dark, tar-ry stools.
- Learn proper injection technique if you are to self-administer this drug.
- Do not take any OTC drugs without first consulting prescriber.

## FORMOTEROL FUMARATE

(for-mo-ter'ol)

Foradil Aerolizer, Perforomist

**Classifications:** BETA-ADRENERGIC AGONIST; BRONCHODILATOR

Therapeutic: BRONCHODILATOR

**Prototype:** Albuterol

**AVAILABILITY** Inhalation capsule; solution for inhalation

## ACTION & THERAPEUTIC EFFECT

Long-acting selective beta$_2$-adrenergic receptor agonist that stimulates production of intracellular cyclic AMP, which causes relaxation of bronchial smooth muscle. It also inhibits release of mediators of immediate hypersensitivity (e.g., histamine and leukotrienes) from mast cells in the lung. *Acts locally in lung as a bronchodilator; prevents bronchoconstriction that occurs during an asthma attack.*

**USES** Treatment of asthma, bronchitis, prevention of exercise-induced asthma, prevention of bronchospasm in COPD.

## CONTRAINDICATIONS Hyper-
sensitivity to formoterol; significantly worsening or acutely deteriorating asthma; status asthmaticus or other severe asthmatic attacks; acute episode of COPD where extensive measures are required; paradoxical bronchospasm.

## CAUTIOUS USE Cardiovascu-
lar disorders (especially coronary insufficiency, cardiac arrhythmias, and hypertension), QT prolongation; convulsive disorders; thyrotoxicosis; heightened responsiveness to sympathomimetic amines; diabetes mellitus; pregnancy (category C); lactation. Safe use in children younger than 5 y has not been established.

## ROUTE & DOSAGE

**Treatment of Asthma, COPD, Bronchitis/Emphysema**

*Adult/Child (5 y or older):*
**Inhaled** Inhale contents of 1 capsule q12h

**Prevention of Exercise-Induced Asthma**

*Adult/Child (12 y or older):* **Inhaled** Inhale contents of 1 capsule at least 15 min before exercise, do not repeat for at least 12 h

## ADMINISTRATION

**Oral Inhalation**
- Remove capsule from blister IMMEDIATELY before use.
- Avoid exposing capsules to moisture.
- Give capsules only by the oral inhalation route and only by using the Aerolizer Inhaler™. Review use of the Aerolizer Inhaler in *Patient Instructions for Use* provided by manufacturer. Do not use a spacer with the Aerolizer.
- Instruct patient not to swallow capsule and not to exhale into the Aerolizer.
- Store capsules in the blister at 20°–25° C (86°–77° F).

**ADVERSE EFFECTS** (≥1%) **Body as a Whole:** *Viral infections,* chest infection, chest pain, fatigue. **CNS:** Headache, tremor, dizziness, insomnia. **GI:** Abdominal pain,

Common adverse effects in *italic;* life-threatening effects <u>underlined;</u> generic names in **bold;** classifications in SMALL CAPS; ♣ Canadian drug name; ⓟ Prototype drug

721

dyspepsia, nausea. **Respiratory:** Pharyngitis, bronchitis, dyspnea, tonsillitis, dysphonia, <u>fatal exacerbation of asthma</u>. **Skin:** Rash.

**INTERACTIONS Drug:** Effects may be antagonized by NONSELECTIVE BETA-BLOCKERS; XANTHINES, STEROIDS; DIURETICS may potentiate hypokalemia. Avoid use with MAOIs. Use with **dronderone** is contraindicated.

**PHARMACOKINETICS Absorption:** Rapidly absorbed. **Onset:** 1–3 min. **Peak:** 1–3 h. **Metabolism:** Metabolized by glucuronidation in the liver. **Elimination:** 60% in urine, 33% in feces. **Half-Life:** 10 h.

## NURSING IMPLICATIONS

### Black Box Warning

*Formoterol has been associated with increased risk of asthma-related hospitalizations and deaths.*

### Assessment & Drug Effects

- Monitor cardiovascular status with periodic ECG, BP, and HR determinations.
- Withhold drug and notify prescriber immediately of S&S of bronchospasm.
- Monitor diabetics closely for loss of glycemic control.
- Monitor lab tests: Periodic serum potassium and blood glucose.

### Patient & Family Education

- Do not take this drug more frequently than every 12 h.
- Use a short-acting inhaler if symptoms develop between doses of formoterol.
- Seek medical care immediately if a previously effective dosage regimen fails to provide the usual response, or if swelling about the face and neck and difficulty breathing develop.

- Report any of the following immediately to the prescriber: Rash, hives, palpitations, chest pain, rapid heart rate, tremor or nervousness.
- Diabetics should monitor blood glucose levels carefully for hyperglycemia.

---

# FOSAMPRENAVIR CALCIUM

(fos-am-pre′na-vir)

Lexiva

**Classifications:** ANTIRETROVIRAL; PROTEASE INHIBITOR
**Therapeutic:** PROTEASE INHIBITOR
**Prototype:** Saquinavir

**AVAILABILITY** Tablet; oral suspension

## ACTION & *THERAPEUTIC EFFECT*

Fosamprenavir is a prodrug rapidly converted to amprenavir. Amprenavir is an HIV-1 protease inhibitor that binds to the active site of HIV-1 protease. Binding prevents processing of viral Gag and Gag-Pol polyprotein precursors, resulting in formation of immature noninfectious viral particles. *Inhibits normal replication of the HIV virus rendering the virus noninfectious.*

**USES** Treatment of HIV infection in combination with other antiretroviral agents.

**UNLABELED USES** HIV prophylaxis (occupational exposure).

**CONTRAINDICATIONS** Hypersensitivity to amprenavir or sulfonamide severe or life-threatening skin reactions; severe hepatic impairment; lactation.

**CAUTIOUS USE** Sulfonamide allergy; mild to moderate hepatic impairment; hypercholesterolemia, hypertriglycerolemia; DM; diabetic ketoacidosis; older adults; autoimmune diseases; hemophilia; pregnancy (category C), children/infant.

## ROUTE & DOSAGE

### HIV Infection

*Adult/Adolescent:* **PO** 700 mg b.i.d. in combination with 100 mg **ritonavir** b.i.d. (preferred if previously on a protease inhibitor); or 1400 mg b.i.d.; or 1400 mg daily in combination with 200 mg ritonavir daily *Child/Infant (weight greater than 20 kg):* (All with concurrent **ritonavir** use) **PO** 18 mg/kg b.i.d.; *weight 15–20 kg:* 23 mg/kg b.i.d; *weight 11–14 kg:* 20 mg/kg b.i.d; *weight less than 11 kg:* 45 mg/kg b.i.d (max: 700 mg/dose)

### Hepatic Impairment Dosage Adjustment

*Mild to moderate impairment (Child-Pugh score 5–6):* Reduce dose to 700 mg b.i.d. without *ritonavir; Severe hepatic impairment (Child-Pugh score 10–15):* 350 mg b.i.d. (without ritonavir) or 300 mg b.i.d. (with ritonavir).

## ADMINISTRATION

### Oral

- Ensure that patient is not receiving drugs contraindicated with fosamprenavir.
- Oral suspension should be administered to adults without food and to pediatric patients with food.
- Store at 15°–30° C (59°–86° F) in a tightly closed container.

## ADVERSE EFFECTS (≥1%) **Body as a Whole:** Fatigue. **CNS:** *Oral/* *perioral paresthesia,* peripheral paresthesia, depression, mood disorders. **GI:** *Nausea, vomiting, diarrhea,* abdominal pain, taste disorders, increased triglycerides, and hyperglycemia. **Skin:** *Rash,* pruritus, <u>Stevens–Johnson syndrome</u>.

## INTERACTIONS Note: Interaction profile can be significantly affected by coadministration with ritonavir. Metabolite is a strong inhibitor of CYP3A4. **Drug:** Administration with **amiodarone, bepridil, dihydroergotamine, ergotamine, flecainide, itraconazole, ketoconazole, lidocaine, midazolam, pimozide, propafenone, quinidine, triazolam,** and TRICYCLIC ANTIDEPRESSANTS may cause life-threatening reactions; **rifampin, rifabutin,** ORAL CONTRACEPTIVES, **phenobarbital, phenytoin, carbamazepine** decrease **amprenavir** concentrations; **amprenavir** may increase **dihydroergotamine, ergotamine, sildenafil** concentrations and toxicity; **amprenavir** may decrease **methadone** levels, monitor INR with **warfarin;** increased risk of myopathy and rhabdomyolysis with **lovastatin, simvastatin;** may decrease antiviral effectiveness of **delavirdine** or **lopinavir/ritonavir.** Avoid with **boceprevir. Herbal: St. John's wort** may decrease antiretroviral activity.

## PHARMACOKINETICS **Absorption:** Rapidly hydrolyzed to amprenavir (active component) by gut enzymes. **Peak:** 2.5 h. **Metabolism:** In liver by CYP3A4. **Elimination:** 14% in urine, 75% in feces. **Half-Life:** 7.7 h.

## NURSING IMPLICATIONS

### Assessment & Drug Effects

- Ensure that patient has provided a complete list of all prescription, nonprescription, or herbal drugs being used.

---

Common adverse effects in *italic;* life-threatening effects <u>underlined</u>; generic names in **bold;** classifications in SMALL CAPS; ◆ Canadian drug name; ⊘ Prototype drug

723

- Monitor closely diabetics for loss of glycemic control.
- Monitor males taking PDE5 inhibitors for erectile dysfunction for adverse events including hypotension, visual changes, and priapism. Report promptly.
- Monitor lab tests: Baseline and periodic LFTs and CD4 count; periodic lipid profile and blood glucose.

**Patient & Family Education**

- If you miss a dose by more than 4 h, wait and take the next dose at the regular time.
- Do not take other prescription, nonprescription, or herbal drugs without consulting prescriber.
- Monitor blood glucose more often than usual if diabetic.
- To prevent pregnancy, use a barrier contraceptive in addition to hormonal contraception.

## FOSCARNET
(fos'car-net)

**Classification:** ANTIVIRAL
**Therapeutic:** ANTIVIRAL

**AVAILABILITY** Solution for injection

**ACTION & *THERAPEUTIC EFFECT***
Selectively inhibits the viral-specific DNA polymerases and reverse transcriptases of susceptible viruses, thus preventing elongation of the viral DNA chain. *Effective against cytomegalovirus (CMV), herpes simplex virus types 1 and 2 (HSV-1, HSV-2), human herpesvirus 6 (HHV-6), Epstein-Barr virus (EBV), and varicella-zoster virus (VZV).*

**USES** CMV retinitis, mucocutaneous HSV, acyclovir-resistant HSV in immunocompromised patients.

**UNLABELED USES** Other CMV infections, herpes zoster infections in AIDS patients.

**CONTRAINDICATIONS** Hypersensitivity to foscarnet; lactation.

**CAUTIOUS USE** Renal impairment, cardiac disease; mineral and electrolyte imbalances, seizures, older adults; pregnancy (category C); children.

## ROUTE & DOSAGE

**CMV Retinitis**
*Adult:* **IV Induction** 60 mg/kg q8h for 2–3 wk **or** 90 mg/kg q12h for 2–3 wk; induction may be repeated if relapse occurs

**Recurrent CMV Retinitis**
*Adult:* **IV** 90–120 mg/kg/day

**Acyclovir-Resistant HSV in Immunocompromised Patients**
*Adult:* **IV** 40 mg/kg q8–12h for up to 3 wk or until lesions heal

***Renal Impairment Dosage Adjustment***
See package insert.

## ADMINISTRATION

- Note: Dose **must be** adjusted for renal insufficiency. See package insert for specific dosing adjustment.

**Intravenous**

***PREPARE:* Direct:** Given undiluted (24 mg/mL) through a central line. ■ For peripheral infusion, dilute to 12 mg/mL with D5W or NS. ■ Do not give other IV solution or drug through the same catheter with foscarnet.
***ADMINISTER:* Direct:** Give at a constant rate not to exceed 1 mg/kg/min over the specified period of infusion with an infusion pump. ■ Do not increase the rate of infusion or shorten the specified

interval between doses. ▪ Use prepared IV solutions within 24 h.
*INCOMPATIBILITIES:* Solution/additive: **Lactated Ringer's** Y-site: **Acyclovir, allopurinol, amiodarone, amphotericin B, calcium chloride, caspofungin, chlorpromazine, ciprofloxacin, dantrolene, daunorubicin, diazepam, digoxin, diphenhydramine, dobutamine, dolasetron, doxorubicin, droperidol, epirubicin, ganciclovir, haloperidol, hydralazine, idarubicin, labetalol, leucovorin, lorazepam, methylprednisolone, midazolam, mitoxantrone, mycophenolate, nicardipine, norepinephrine, ondansetron, pentamidine, phenytoin, prochlorperazine, promethazine, quinupristine/dalfopristin, SMZ/TMP, thiopental, topotecan, trimetrexate, vancomycin, verapamil, vinorelbine.**

▪ Prehydrate and continue daily hydration with 2.5 L of NS to reduce nephrotoxicity. ▪ Store according to manufacturer's directions.

## ADVERSE EFFECTS (>1%) **CV:**
Thrombophlebitis if infused through a peripheral vein. **CNS:** Tremor, muscle twitching, *headache*, weakness, fatigue, confusion, anxiety. **Endocrine:** *Hypophosphatemia, hypokalemia, hypomagnesemia, hypocalcemia.* **GI:** Nausea, vomiting, *diarrhea.* **Urogenital:** Penile ulceration. **Hematologic:** *Anemia*, leukopenia, thrombocytopenia. **Renal:** *Nephrotoxicity* (acute renal failure, tubular necrosis). **Skin:** Fixed drug eruption, rash.

## DIAGNOSTIC TEST INTERFERENCE
May cause increase or decrease in serum ***calcium, phosphorus,*** and

***magnesium.*** Decreases ***Hct*** and ***Hgb.*** Increased serum ***creatinine.***

## INTERACTIONS **Drug:** AMINO-GLYCOSIDES, **amphotericin B, vancomycin** may increase risk of nephrotoxicity. **Etidronate, pamidronate, pentamidine (IV)** may exacerbate hypocalcemia.

## PHARMACOKINETICS **Onset:**
3–7 days. **Duration:** Relapse usually occurs 3–4 wk after end of therapy. **Distribution:** 3–28% of dose may be deposited in bone; variable penetration into CSF; crosses placenta; distributed into breast milk. **Metabolism:** Not metabolized. **Elimination:** 73–94% in urine. **Half-Life:** 3–4 h.

## NURSING IMPLICATIONS

### Black Box Warning

*Foscarnet has been associated with severe renal impairment and seizures associated with mineral and electrolyte imbalances.*

### Assessment & Drug Effects
▪ Monitor for electrolyte imbalances.
▪ Monitor for seizures and take appropriate precautions.
▪ Question patients regarding local irritation of the penile or vulvovaginal epithelium. If either occurs, increase hydration and better personal hygiene.
▪ Monitor lab tests: Periodic CBC, serum electrolytes, serum creatinine, and creatinine clearance.

### Patient & Family Education
▪ Report perioral tingling, numbness, and paresthesia to prescriber immediately.
▪ Understand that drug is not a cure for CMV retinitis; regular ophthalmologic exams are necessary.
▪ Note: Good hydration is important to maintain adequate output of urine.

F

# FOSFOMYCIN TROMETHAMINE

(fos-fo-my'sin)

Monurol

**Classification:** ANTIBIOTIC
**Therapeutic:** URINARY TRACT
ANTI-INFECTIVE
**Prototype:** Nitrofurantoin

## AVAILABILITY Packets

## ACTION & *THERAPEUTIC EFFECT*

Synthetic, broad-spectrum, bacte-ricidal agent that blocks the first steps in bacterial cell wall synthe-sis. *Acts as a bactericidal agent against* Enterococcus faecalis, E. faecium, *and* Escherichia coli. *In addition, it is effective against* Klebsiella, Proteus, *and* Serratia. *Effectiveness is indicated by im-provement in cystitis symptoms within 2–3 days.*

**USES** Treatment of uncomplicated UTIs in women.

**CONTRAINDICATIONS** Hyper-sensitivity to fosfomycin.

**CAUTIOUS USE** Pregnancy (cat-egory B); lactation. Safety and efficacy in children younger than 12 y not established.

## ROUTE & DOSAGE

### UTI

*Adult:* **PO** 3 g sachet dissolved in 3–4 oz of water as a single dose given once

## ADMINISTRATION

### Oral

- Pour entire contents of a single dose into 3–4 oz water (not hot), stir to dissolve completely, and give immediately. Drug must not be taken in the dry form.
- Store at 15°–30° C (59°–86° F).

**ADVERSE EFFECTS** (≥1%) **Body as a Whole:** Pain. **CNS:** *Head-ache,* dizziness. **GI:** *Diarrhea,* nau-sea, abdominal pain, dyspepsia. **Respiratory:** Rhinitis, pharyngitis. **Urogenital:** Vaginitis, dysmenor-rhea.

**INTERACTIONS Drug: Metoclo-pramide** may decrease urinary ex-cretion of fosfomycin.

**PHARMACOKINETICS Absorp-tion:** Rapidly from GI tract, 37% of dose reaches systemic circulation as free acid. **Peak Urine Concentra-tion:** 2–4 h. **Distribution:** Not protein bound, distributed to kidneys, blad-der wall, prostate, and seminal vesi-cles. **Elimination:** Primarily in urine. **Half-Life:** 5.7 h.

## NURSING IMPLICATIONS

### Assessment & Drug Effects

- Monitor lab tests: Urine C&S be-fore and after therapy.

### Patient & Family Education

- Notify prescriber if symptoms do not improve in 2–3 days.

# FOSINOPRIL

(fos-in'o-pril)

Monopril

**Classifications:** ANGIOTENSIN-CONVERTING ENZYME (ACE) INHIBITOR; ANTIHYPERTENSIVE
**Therapeutic:** ANTIHYPERTENSIVE; ACE INHIBITOR
**Prototype:** Enalapril

## AVAILABILITY Tablet

## ACTION & *THERAPEUTIC EFFECT*

Lowers BP by interrupting con-version sequences initiated by renin that leads to formation of

Common adverse effects in *italic;* life-threatening effects underlined; generic names in **bold;** classifications in SMALL CAPS; ♣ Canadian drug name; ● Prototype drug

726

angiotensin II, a potent vasocon-strictor. Inhibition of ACE also leads to decreased circulating aldosterone, a secretory response to angiotensin II stimulation. *Lowers blood pressure and reduces peripheral arterial resistance (afterload) and improves cardiac output as well as activity tolerance.*

**USES** Mild to moderate hypertension, CHF.

**CONTRAINDICATIONS** Hypersensitivity to fosinopril or any other ACE inhibitor(s); angioedema; renal artery stenosis; pregnancy (category D); lactation.

**CAUTIOUS USE** Impaired kidney function, autoimmune disease; collagen-vascular disease; hepatic disease; hyperkalemia, or surgery and anesthesia; history of angioedema; black patients; aortic stenosis or cardiomyopathy; dialysis; older adult; pregnancy (category C in first trimester; however, discontinue as soon as pregnancy is suspected). Safety in children not established.

## ROUTE & DOSAGE

### Hypertension
*Adult:* **PO** 10 mg once/day may increase to 20–40 mg (max: 80 mg/day)

### Heart Failure
*Adult:* **PO** 5–10 mg daily; may increase to 20–40 mg

## ADMINISTRATION
### Oral
▪ An initial 5 mg dose is preferred in HF patients with moderate to severe renal failure or in those who have been recently diuresed.
▪ Store at 15°–30° C (59°–86° F) and protect from moisture.

**ADVERSE EFFECTS** (≥1%) **CV:** Hypotension. **CNS:** Headache, fatigue, dizziness. **Endocrine:** Hyperkalemia. **GI:** Nausea, vomiting, diarrhea. **Urogenital:** Proteinuria. **Respiratory:** Cough. **Skin:** Rash.

**INTERACTIONS Drug:** NSAIDS may decrease antihypertensive effects of fosinopril. POTASSIUM SUPPLEMENTS, POTASSIUM-SPARING DIURETICS increase risk of hyperkalemia. ACE inhibitors may increase **lithium** levels and toxicity.

**PHARMACOKINETICS Absorption:** Readily absorbed from GI tract; converted to its active form, fosinoprilat, in the liver. **Peak:** 3 h. **Duration:** 24 h. **Distribution:** Approximately 90% protein bound; crosses placenta. **Metabolism:** Hydrolyzed by intestinal and hepatic esterases to its active form, fosinoprilat. **Elimination:** 44% in urine, 46% in feces. **Half-Life:** 3–4 h (fosinoprilat).

## NURSING IMPLICATIONS

### Black Box Warning

*Fosinopril can cause fetal injury and death when used during the second and third trimesters.*

### Assessment & Drug Effects
▪ Monitor for at least 2 h after initial dose for first-dose hypotension, especially in salt- or volume-depleted patients.
▪ Monitor BP at the time of peak effectiveness, 2–6 h after dosing and at the end of the dosing interval just before next dose.

---

Common adverse effects in *italic;* life-threatening effects underlined; generic names in **bold;** classifications in SMALL CAPS; ♣ Canadian drug name; ⊘ Prototype drug

727

- Report diminished antihypertensive effect toward the end of the dosing interval. An inadequate trough response may be an indication for dividing the daily dose.
- Observe for S&S of hyperkalemia (see Appendix F).
- Monitor lab tests: Periodic BUN, serum creatinine, and serum potassium.

**Patient & Family Education**
- Discontinue fosinopril and report to prescriber any of the following: S&S of angioedema (e.g., swelling of face or extremities, difficulty breathing or swallowing); syncope; chronic, nonproductive cough.
- Maintain adequate fluid intake and avoid potassium supplements or salt substitutes unless specifically prescribed by the prescriber.
- Report promptly if pregnancy is suspected.
- Report vomiting or diarrhea to prescriber immediately.

## FOSPHENYTOIN SODIUM
(fos-phen'i-toin)

Cerebyx

**Classification:** ANTICONVULSANT; HYDANTOIN
**Therapeutic:** ANTICONVULSANT
**Prototype:** Phenytoin

**AVAILABILITY** Solution for injection

**ACTION & THERAPEUTIC EFFECT**
Prodrug of phenytoin that converts to the anticonvulsant phenytoin that modulates the sodium channels of neurons, calcium flux across neuronal membranes, and enhances the sodium–potassium ATPase activity of neurons and glial cells. *Effective as an anticonvulsant agent by preventing seizure activity.*

**USES** Control of generalized convulsive status epilepticus and the prevention and treatment of seizures during neurosurgery, or as a parenteral short-term substitute for oral phenytoin.

**UNLABELED USES** Antiarrhythmic agent especially in treatment of digitalis-induced arrhythmia; treatment of trigeminal neuralgia (tic douloureux).

**CONTRAINDICATIONS** Hypersensitivity to hydantoin products, rash, seizures due to hypoglycemia, sinus bradycardia, complete or incomplete heart block; Adams-Stokes syndrome; pregnancy (category D).

**CAUTIOUS USE** Impaired liver or kidney function, alcoholism, hypotension, heart block, bradycardia, severe CAD, diabetes mellitus, hyperglycemia, respiratory depression, acute intermittent porphyria; children; lactation.

**ROUTE & DOSAGE**

**Status Epilepticus**

*Adult:* **IV Loading Dose** 15–20 mg PE/kg (PE = phenytoin sodium equivalents) administered at 100–150 mg PE/min;
**IV Maintenance Dose** 4–6 mg PE/kg/day

**Substitution for Oral Phenytoin Therapy**

*Adult:* **IV/IM** Substitute fosphenytoin at the same total daily dose in mg PE as the oral dose at a rate of infusion not greater than 150 mg PE/min

Common adverse effects in *italic*; life-threatening effects underlined; generic names in **bold;** classifications in SMALL CAPS; ♦ Canadian drug name; ❷ Prototype drug

### Seizure Prevention during Surgery

*Adult:* **IV/IM** 10–20 mg PE/kg then 4–6 mg PE/kg/day

## ADMINISTRATION

▪ Note: All dosing is expressed in phenytoin sodium equivalents (PE) to avoid the need to calculate molecular weight adjustments between fosphenytoin and phenytoin sodium doses. **Always** prescribe and fill fosphenytoin in PE units.

### Intramuscular

▪ Follow institutional policy regarding maximum volume to inject into one IM site.

### Intravenous

*PREPARE:* **Direct:** Dilute in D5W or NS to a concentration of 1.5–25 mg PE/mL.
*ADMINISTER:* **Direct:** Give 100–150 mg PE/min. Do **NOT** administer at a rate greater than 150 mg PE/min.
*INCOMPATIBILITIES:* **Y-site: Fenol-dopam, midazolam.**

▪ Store at 2°–8° C (36°–46° F); may store at room temperature not to exceed 48 h.

## ADVERSE EFFECTS (≥1%) CNS:

Usually dose related. Paresthesia, tinnitus, *nystagmus, dizziness, somnolence, drowsiness,* ataxia, mental confusion, tremors, insomnia, headache, seizures, increased reflexes, dysarthria, intracranial hypertension. **CV:** Bradycardia, tachycardia, asystole, hypotension, hypertension, cardiovascular collapse, cardiac arrest, heart block, ventricular fibrillation, phlebitis. **Special Senses:** Photophobia, conjunctivitis, diplopia, blurred vision. **GI:** *Gingival hyperplasia,* nausea, vomiting, constipation, epigastric pain, dysphagia, loss of taste, weight loss, hepatitis, liver necrosis. **Hematologic:** Thrombocytopenia, leukopenia, leukocytosis, agranulocytosis, pancytopenia, eosinophilia; megaloblastic, hemolytic, or aplastic anemias. **Metabolic:** Fever, hyperglycemia, glycosuria, weight gain, edema, transient increase in serum thyrotropic (TSH) level, hyperkalemia, osteomalacia, or rickets associated with hypocalcemia and elevated alkaline phosphatase activity. **Skin:** Alopecia, hirsutism (especially in young female); rash: Scarlatiniform, maculopapular, urticarial, morbilliform (may be fatal); bullous, exfoliative, or purpuric dermatitis; Stevens–Johnson syndrome, toxic epidermal necrolysis, keratosis, neonatal hemorrhage, *pruritus.* **Urogenital:** Acute renal failure, Peyronie's disease. **Respiratory:** Acute pneumonitis, pulmonary fibrosis. **Musculoskeletal:** Periarteritis nodosum, acute systemic lupus erythematosus, craniofacial abnormalities (with enlargement of lips). **Other:** Lymphadenopathy, injection site pain, chills.

## DIAGNOSTIC TEST INTERFERENCE

Fosphenytoin may produce lower than normal values for ***dexamethasone*** or ***metyrapone*** tests; may increase serum levels of ***glucose, BSP,*** and ***alkaline phosphatase*** and may decrease ***PBI*** and ***urinary steroid*** levels.

## INTERACTIONS Drug: Alcohol

decreases effects; OTHER ANTICONVULSANTS may increase or decrease fosphenytoin levels; fosphenytoin increases metabolism of CORTICOSTEROIDS, ORAL ANTICOAGULANTS, and ORAL CONTRACEPTIVES, decreasing their effectiveness; **amiodarone, chloramphenicol, omeprazole** increase fosphenytoin levels; antituberculosis

Common adverse effects in *italic;* life-threatening effects underlined; generic names in **bold;** classifications in SMALL CAPS; ♣ Canadian drug name; ⓟ Prototype drug

729

F

agents, **voriconazole** decrease fosphenytoin levels. Do not use with **delviradine. Food: Folic acid, calcium, vitamin D** absorption may be decreased by fosphenytoin; fosphenytoin absorption may be decreased by enteral nutrition supplements. **Herbal: Ginkgo** may decrease anticonvulsant effectiveness.

## PHARMACOKINETICS **Absorption:** Completely absorbed after IM administration. **Peak:** 30 min IM. **Distribution:** 95–99% bound to plasma proteins, displaces phenytoin from protein binding sites; crosses placenta, small amount in breast milk. **Metabolism:** Converted to phenytoin by phosphatases; phenytoin is oxidized in liver to inactive metabolites. **Elimination:** Half-life 15 min to convert fosphenytoin to phenytoin, 22 h phenytoin; phenytoin metabolites excreted in urine.

## NURSING IMPLICATIONS

### Black Box Warning

*Fosphenytoin infusion has been associated with risk of severe hypotension and cardiac arrhythmias, especially if infusion rate exceeds 150 mg (PE)/min.*

Note: See **phenytoin** for additional Nursing Implications.

### Assessment & Drug Effects

- Monitor ECG, BP, and respiratory function continuously during and for 10–20 min after infusion.
- Discontinue infusion and notify prescriber if rash appears. Be prepared to substitute alternative therapy rapidly to prevent withdrawal-precipitated seizures.
- Allow at least 2 h after IV infusion and 4 h after IM injection before monitoring total plasma phenytoin concentration.

- Monitor diabetics for loss of glycemic control.
- Monitor carefully for adverse effects, especially in patients with renal or hepatic disease or hypoalbuminemia.
- Monitor lab tests: Periodic CBC with differential, platelet count, serum electrolytes, and blood glucose.

### Patient & Family Education

- Be aware of potential adverse effects. Itching, burning, tingling, or paresthesia are common during and for some time following IV infusion.

## FROVATRIPTAN
(fro-va-trip'tan)
Frova
**Classification:** SEROTONIN 5-HT$_1$ RECEPTOR AGONIST
Therapeutic: ANTIMIGRAINE
**Prototype:** Sumatriptan

## AVAILABILITY Tablet

## ACTION & *THERAPEUTIC EFFECT*
Selective agonist that binds with high affinity to 5-HT$_{1D}$, 5-HT$_{1B}$, 5-HT$_{1F}$ serotonin receptors, which are found on extracerebral and intracranial blood vessels, and on other structures in the CNS. This results in vasoconstriction and agonist effects on nerve terminals in the trigeminal system. *Activation of 5-HT$_1$ receptors results in constriction of cranial vessels that become dilated during a migraine attack, and reduced signal transmission in the pain pathways.*

## USES Treatment of migraine headache with or without aura.

## CONTRAINDICATIONS Hypersensitivity to frovatriptan; significant cardiovascular disease such as ischemic

heart disease, coronary artery vaso-spasms, peripheral vascular disease, history of cerebrovascular events, or uncontrolled hypertension; within 24 h of receiving another 5-HT₁ agonist or an ergotamine-containing or ergot-type drug; basilar or hemiplegic migraine.

**CAUTIOUS USE** Significant risk factors for coronary artery disease unless a cardiac evaluation has been done; hypertension; risk factors for cerebrovascular accident; impaired liver or kidney function; pregnancy (category C); lactation. Safe use in children younger than 18 y has not been established.

## ROUTE & DOSAGE

### Migraine Headache

*Adult:* **PO** 2.5 mg. If headache returns, may repeat after at least 2 h (max: 7.5 mg/24 h).

## ADMINISTRATION

### Oral

- Do not give within 24 h of an ergot-containing drug.
- Administer any time after symptoms of migraine appear.
- Do not administer a second dose without consulting the prescriber for any attack during which the FIRST dose did **not** work.
- Give a second dose if headache was relieved by first dose but symptoms return; however, wait at least 2 h after the first dose before giving a second dose.
- Do not give more than two doses in 24 h.
- Store at 15°–30° C (59°–86° F).

**ADVERSE EFFECTS** (≥1%) **Body as a Whole:** Fatigue, hot or cold sensation, flushing. **CNS:** Dizziness, headache, paresthesia, somnolence, insomnia, anxiety. **CV:**

Chest pain, palpitation. **GI:** Dyspepsia, nausea, vomiting, diarrhea, dry mouth. **Musculoskeletal:** Skeletal pain. **Special Senses:** Abnormal vision. **Skin:** Sweating.

**INTERACTIONS Drug: Dihydro-ergotamine, methysergide,** other 5-HT₁ AGONISTS may cause prolonged vasospastic reactions; SSRIS, **sibutramine** have rarely caused weakness, hyperreflexia, and incoordination; MAOIS should not be used with 5-HT₁ AGONISTS. **Herbal: Gingko, ginseng, echinacea, St. John's wort** may increase triptan toxicity.

**PHARMACOKINETICS Absorption:** 20–30% bioavailability. **Peak:** 2–4 h. **Distribution:** 15% protein bound. **Metabolism:** In liver by CYP1A2. **Elimination:** 30% renally, 60% in feces. **Half-Life:** 26 h.

## NURSING IMPLICATIONS

### Assessment & Drug Effects

- Monitor cardiovascular status carefully following first dose in patients at relatively high risk for coronary artery disease (e.g., post-menopausal women, men older than 40 y, persons with known CAD risk factors), or who have coronary artery vasospasms.
- Report to prescriber immediately chest pain or tightness in chest or throat that is severe, or does not quickly resolve following a dose of frovatriptan.
- Pain relief usually begins within 10 min of ingestion, with complete relief in approximately 65% of all patients within 2 h.
- Monitor BP, especially in those being treated for hypertension.

### Patient & Family Education

- Review patient information leaflet provided by the manufacturer carefully.

---

Common adverse effects in *italic;* life-threatening effects <u>underlined</u>; generic names in **bold;** classifications in SMALL CAPS; ♣ Canadian drug name; ⊙ Prototype drug

731

- Notify prescriber immediately if symptoms of severe angina (e.g., severe or persistent pain or tightness in chest, back, neck, or throat) or hypersensitivity (e.g., wheezing, facial swelling, skin rash, itching, or hives) occur.
- Do not take any other serotonin receptor agonist (e.g., Imitrex, Maxalt, Zomig, Amerge) within 24 h of taking frovatriptan.
- Report any other adverse effects (e.g., tingling, flushing, dizziness) at next prescriber visit.

# FULVESTRANT
(ful-ves′trant)
Faslodex

**Classifications:** ANTINEOPLASTIC; ANTIESTROGEN
**Therapeutic:** ANTINEOPLASTIC; ANTIESTROGEN
**Prototype:** Tamoxifen citrate

**AVAILABILITY** Solution for injection

**ACTION & THERAPEUTIC EFFECT**
Fulvestrant is an estrogen receptor antagonist that selectively binds to the estrogen receptors (ER) of breast cancer cells. Estrogen stimulates the tumor growth of estrogen-sensitive breast tissue cancer cells in postmenopausal women. *In postmenopausal women, many breast cancers have positive estrogen receptors (ERs), and the growth of these tumors is stimulated by estrogen. Therefore, fulvestrant decreases estrogen-sensitive breast tissue tumor growth.*

**USES** Treatment of hormone receptor-positive metastatic breast cancer in postmenopausal women.

**CONTRAINDICATIONS** Hypersensitivity to fulvestrant; pregnancy (category D); lactation.

**CAUTIOUS USE** Moderate liver impairment; biliary disease; coagulopathy; anticoagulant therapy; older adults. Safety and efficacy in children not established.

## ROUTE & DOSAGE

**Metastatic Breast Cancer**
*Adult:* **IM** 500 mg on days 1, 15, and 29; then 500 mg monthly

**Hepatic Impairment Dosage Adjustment**
*Moderate hepatic impairment (Child-Pugh class B):* **IM** administer 250 mg on days 1, 15, 29, and once monthly thereafter

## ADMINISTRATION

**Intramuscular**
- Break the seal of the white plastic cover on the syringe luer connector to remove the cover with the attached rubber tip cap. Twist to lock the needle to the luer connector. Remove excess gas from the syringe (a small gas bubble may remain).
- Administer slowly in the buttock.
- Immediately activate needle protection device upon withdrawal from patient by pushing lever arm completely forward until needle tip is fully covered.
- Store in a refrigerator, 2°–8° C (36°–46° F) in original container.

**ADVERSE EFFECTS (≥1%) Body as a Whole:** *Asthenia, pain, injection site pain,* flu-like syndrome, fever, peripheral edema, infection. **CNS:** Dizziness, headache, insomnia, paresthesia, depression, anxiety, fatigue. **CV:** *Vasodilation.* **GI:** *Nausea, vomiting, constipation, diarrhea,* anorexia, stomatitis. **Hematologic:** Anemia. **Musculoskeletal:** *Bone pain,* arthritis. **Respiratory:**

*Pharyngitis, dyspnea, cough.* **Skin:** Rash, sweating. **Hepatic:** Increased liver enzymes.

## PHARMACOKINETICS **Peak:** 7 days. **Duration:** 1 mo. **Distribution:** 99% protein bound. **Metabolism:** In liver via CYP3A4. **Elimination:** 90% in feces. **Half-Life:** 40 days.

## NURSING IMPLICATIONS
### Assessment & Drug Effects
- Monitor for S&S of tumor progression.
- Monitor lab tests: Periodic CBC with differential, LFTs, and pregnancy testing.

### Patient & Family Education
- Use two methods of contraception while taking this drug. Immediately notify prescriber if you think you are pregnant.
- Report vaginal bleeding to prescriber. Understand the possibility of drug-induced menstrual irregularities before starting treatment.

## FUROSEMIDE ⊕
(fur oh'se-mide)

**Fumide ♦, Furomide ♦, Lasix, Luramide ♦**

**Classifications:** ELECTROLYTIC AND WATER BALANCE AGENT; LOOP DIURETIC; ANTIHYPERTENSIVE
**Therapeutic:** LOOP DIURETIC; ANTIHYPERTENSIVE

## AVAILABILITY Tablet; oral solution; solution for injection

## ACTION & *THERAPEUTIC EFFECT*
Rapid-acting potent sulfonamide "loop" diuretic and antihypertensive. Inhibits reabsorption of sodium and chloride primarily in loop of Henle and also in proximal and distal renal tubules. *An antihypertensive that decreases edema and intravascular volume, which lowers blood pressure.*

## USES Treatment of edema associated with CHF, cirrhosis of liver, and kidney disease, including nephrotic syndrome. May be used for management of hypertension, alone or in combination with other antihypertensive agents, and for treatment of hypercalcemia.

## CONTRAINDICATIONS History of hypersensitivity to furosemide or sulfonamides; increasing oliguria, anuria, fluid and electrolyte depletion states; hepatic coma; preeclampsia, eclampsia.

## CAUTIOUS USE Hepatic disease; hepatic cirrhosis; renal disease, nephrotic syndrome; cardiogenic shock associated with acute MI; ventricular arrhythmias, CHF, diarrhea; history of SLE, history of gout; DM; older adults; pregnancy (category C); lactation, infants.

## ROUTE & DOSAGE

### Edema
*Adult:* **PO** 20–80 mg in 1 or more divided doses up to 600 mg/day if needed; **IV/IM** 20–40 mg in 1 or more divided doses up to 600 mg/day
*Child:* **PO** 2 mg/kg, may be increased by 1–2 mg/kg q6–8h (max: 6 mg/kg/dose); **IV/IM** 1–2 mg/kg, may be increased by 1 mg/kg q2h if needed (max: 6 mg/kg/dose)
*Neonate:* **PO** 1–4 mg/kg q12–24h; **IV/IM** 1 mg/kg q12–24h

### Hypertension
*Adult:* **PO** 10–40 mg b.i.d. (max: 480 mg/day)

---

Common adverse effects in *italic;* life-threatening effects underlined; generic names in **bold**; classifications in SMALL CAPS; ♣ Canadian drug name; ⊕ Prototype drug

## ADMINISTRATION

### Oral

- Give with food or milk to reduce possibility of gastric irritation.
- Schedule doses to avoid sleep disturbance (e.g., a single dose is generally given in the morning; twice-a-day doses at 8 a.m. and 2 p.m.).
- Store tablets at controlled room temperature, preferably at 15°–30° C (59°–86° F) unless otherwise directed. Protect from light.
- Store oral solution in refrigerator, preferably at 2°–8° C (36°–46° F). Protect from light and freezing.

### Intramuscular

- Protect syringes from light once they are removed from package.
- Discard yellow or otherwise discolored injection solutions.

### Intravenous

Note: Verify correct IV concentration and rate of infusion/injection with prescriber before administration to infants or children.

**PREPARE: Direct:** Give undiluted. For high-dose therapy, dilute in NS or other compatible solution.

**ADMINISTER: Direct:** Give undiluted at a rate of 20 mg or a fraction thereof over 1 min. ▪ With high doses a rate of 4 mg/min is recommended to decrease risk of ototoxicity.

**INCOMPATIBILITIES: Solution/additive: Amiodarone, buprenorphine, chlorpromazine, diazepam, dobutamine, erythromycin, fructose, gentamicin, isoproterenol, meperidine, metoclopramide, milrinone, netilmicin, pancuronium, papaveretum, prochlorperazine, promethazine, quinidine, thiamine. Y-site: Alemtuzumab, amphotericin B, amrinone, amsacrine, atracurium, azithromycin, benztropine, bupernophine, butorphanol, caspofungin, chlorpromazine, ciprofloxacin, cisatracurium, clarithromycin, codeine, dantrolene, daunorubicin, dexrazoxane, diazepam, diazoxide, diltiazem, dimenhdrinate, diphenhydramine, dobutamine, dopamine, doxorubicin, doxycycline, drotrecogin, droperidol, epirubicin, esmolol, famotidine, fenoldopam, filgrastim, fluconazole, gatifloxacin, gemcitabine, gemtuzumab, gentamicin, haloperidol, heparin, hydralazine, hydroxyzine, idarubicin, insulin, isoproterenol, labetalol, lansoprazole, levofloxacin, magnesium, meperidine, metoclopramide, midazolam, milrinone, minocycline, mivacurium, morphine, mycophenolate, nalbuphine, nestiritide, netilmicin, nicardipine, nitroglycerine, norepinephrine, ondansetron, pancuronium, pantoprazole, papaverine, phenytoin, prochlorperazine, promethazine, protamine, pyridoxine, quinidine, quinupristin/dalfopristin, rituximab, SMZ/TMP, telavancin, thiamine, tetracycline, vancomycin, vecuronium, verapamil, vinblastine, vincristine, vinorelbine, TPN.**

- Use infusion solutions within 24 h.
- Store parenteral solution at controlled room temperature, preferably at 15°–30° C (59°–86° F) unless otherwise directed. Protect from light.

## ADVERSE EFFECTS (≥1%) CV:

Postural hypotension, dizziness with excessive diuresis, acute hypotensive episodes, circulatory collapse. **Metabolic:** Hypovolemia,

Common adverse effects in *italic;* life-threatening effects underlined; generic names in **bold;** classifications in SMALL CAPS; ✦ Canadian drug name; ● Prototype drug dehydration, hyponatremia, *hypokalemia,* hypochloremia, metabolic alkalosis, hypomagnesemia, hypocalcemia (tetany), hyperglycemia, glycosuria, elevated BUN, hyperuricemia. **GI:** Nausea, vomiting, oral and gastric burning, anorexia, diarrhea, constipation, abdominal cramping, acute pancreatitis, jaundice. **Urogenital:** Allergic interstitial nephritis, irreversible renal failure, urinary frequency. **Hematologic:** Anemia, leukopenia, thrombocytopenic purpura, aplastic anemia, agranulocytosis (rare). **Special Senses:** Tinnitus, vertigo, feeling of fullness in ears, hearing loss (rarely permanent), blurred vision. **Skin:** Pruritus, urticaria, exfoliative dermatitis, purpura, photosensitivity, porphyria cutanea tarda, necrotizing angiitis (vasculitis). **Body as a Whole:** Increased perspiration; paresthesias; activation of SLE, muscle spasms, weakness; thrombophlebitis, pain at IM injection site.

### DIAGNOSTIC TEST INTERFERENCE

Furosemide may cause elevations in *BUN, serum amylase, cholesterol, triglycerides, uric acid,* and *blood glucose* levels, and may decrease *serum calcium, magnesium, potassium,* and *sodium* levels.

### INTERACTIONS Drug: OTHER DIURETICS enhance diuretic effects; with **digoxin** increased risk of toxicity because of hypokalemia; NON-DEPOLARIZING NEUROMUSCULAR BLOCKING AGENTS (e.g., **tubocurarine**) prolong neuromuscular blockage; CORTICOSTEROIDS, **amphotericin B** potentiate hypokalemia; decreased **lithium** elimination and increased toxicity; SULFONYLUREAS, **insulin** blunt hypoglycemic effects; NSAIDS may attenuate diuretic effects.

### PHARMACOKINETICS Absorption: 60% PO dose from GI tract. **Peak:** 60–70 min PO; 20–60 min IV. **Onset:** 30–60 min PO; 5 min IV. **Duration:** 2 h. **Distribution:** Crosses placenta. **Metabolism:** Small amount in liver. **Elimination:** Rapidly in urine; 50% of oral dose and 80% of IV dose excreted within 24 h; excreted in breast milk. **Half-Life:** 30 min.

## NURSING IMPLICATIONS

### Black Box Warning

*Furosemide has been associated with profound diuresis and water and electrolyte depletion.*

### Assessment & Drug Effects

- Observe patients receiving parenteral drug carefully; closely monitor BP and vital signs. Sudden death from cardiac arrest has been reported.
- Monitor for S&S of hypokalemia (see Appendix F).
- Monitor BP during periods of diuresis and through period of dosage adjustment.
- Observe older adults closely during period of brisk diuresis. Sudden alteration in fluid and electrolyte balance may precipitate significant adverse reactions. Report symptoms to prescriber.
- Monitor urine and blood glucose and HbA1C closely in diabetics and patients with decompensated hepatic cirrhosis. Drug may cause hyperglycemia.
- Monitor I&O ratio and pattern. Report decrease or unusual increase in output. Excessive diuresis can result in dehydration and hypovolemia, circulatory collapse, and hypotension. Weigh patient daily under standard conditions.
- Monitor lab tests: Frequent blood count, serum and urine

---

Common adverse effects in *italic;* life-threatening effects underlined; generic names in **bold**; classifications in SMALL CAPS; ♣ Canadian drug name; ● Prototype drug

735

electrolytes, $CO_2$, BUN, blood sugar, and uric acid during first few months of therapy and periodically thereafter.

**Patient & Family Education**
- Consult prescriber regarding allowable salt and fluid intake.
- Ingest potassium-rich foods daily (e.g., bananas, oranges, peaches, dried dates) to reduce or prevent potassium depletion.
- Learn S&S of hypokalemia (see Appendix F). Report muscle cramps or weakness to prescriber.
- Make position changes slowly because high doses of antihypertensive drugs taken concurrently may produce episodes of dizziness or imbalance.
- Avoid replacing fluid losses with large amounts of water.
- Avoid prolonged exposure to direct sun.

## GABAPENTIN ℗

(gab-a-pen'tin)
Gralise, Horizant, Neurontin
**Classifications:** ANTICONVULSANT; GABA ANALOG
Therapeutic: ANTICONVULSANT; PAINFUL NEUROPATHY

**AVAILABILITY** Capsule; tablet; extended release tablet

**ACTION & *THERAPEUTIC EFFECT***
Gabapentin is a GABA neurotransmitter analog; however, it does not inhibit GABA uptake or degradation. It appears to interact with GABA cortical neurons, but its relationship to functional activity as an anticonvulsant is unknown. *Used in conjunction with other anticonvulsants to control certain types of seizures in patients with epilepsy. Effective in controlling painful neuropathies.*

**USES** Adjunctive therapy for partial seizures with or without secondary generalization in adults, post-herpetic neuralgia, restless leg syndrome.

**UNLABELED USES** Add-on therapy for generalized seizures, peripheral neuropathy, migraine prophylaxis.

**CONTRAINDICATIONS** Hypersensitivity to gabapentin; suicidal ideations; lactation.

**CAUTIOUS USE** Status epilepticus, renal impairment, history of suicidal tendencies; psychiatric disorders; older adults; pregnancy (category C). Safety and efficacy in infants and children younger than 3 y not established.

## ROUTE & DOSAGE

### Adjunctive Therapy for Seizure Disorder

*Adult/Child (12 y or older):*
**PO** Start 300 mg on day 1, 300 mg b.i.d. on day 2, 300 mg t.i.d. on day 3, and continue to increase over a week to an initial total dose of 400 mg t.i.d. (1200 mg/day); may increase to 1800–2400 mg/day depending on response (most patients receive 900–1800 mg/day in 3 divided doses) 400 mg t.i.d. (1200 mg/day)
*Child (3–12 y):* **PO** Start 10–15 mg/kg/day in 3 divided doses, titrate q3days to target dose of 40 mg/kg/day in pts 3–4 y or 25–35 mg/kg/day in pts 5 y or older in 3 divided doses

### Post-Herpetic Neuralgia

*Adult:* **PO** Start 300 mg day 1, 300 mg b.i.d. day 2, and 300 mg t.i.d. day 3; may increase up to 600 mg t.i.d. if needed

Common adverse effects in *italic*; life-threatening effects underlined; generic names in **bold**; classifications in SMALL CAPS; ♣ Canadian drug name; ℗ Prototype drug

**Gralise only:** Titrate to 1800 mg which will be taken daily

**Restless Leg Syndrome (Horizant only)**

*Adult:* **PO** 600 mg qd at 5 p.m.

**Renal Impairment Dosage Adjustment**

*CrCl greater than 60 mL/min:* 400 mg t.i.d.; *30–60 mL/min:* 300 mg b.i.d.; *15–30 mL/min:* 300 mg daily; *less than 15 mL/min:* 300 mg every other day

**Hemodialysis Dosage Adjustment** 200–300 mg following dialysis

## ADMINISTRATION

### Oral

- Ensure that extended release tablet is swallowed whole, and not crushed or chewed.
- Separate doses of gabapentin and antacids by 2 h.
- Withdraw drug gradually over 1 wk; abrupt discontinuation may cause status epilepticus.
- Store at 15°–30° C (59°–86° F); protect from heat, moisture, and direct light.

## ADVERSE EFFECTS (≥1%) CNS:
*Drowsiness, fatigue,* dizziness, tremor, slurred speech, impaired concentration, headache, increased frequency of partial seizures. **Endocrine:** Weight gain. **GI:** Nausea, gastric upset, vomiting. **Special Senses:** Blurred vision, nystagmus. **Skin:** Rash, eczema.

## INTERACTIONS Drug: Increase in
**phenytoin** levels at higher doses (300–600 mg/day gabapentin). Does not affect serum levels of other ANTICONVULSANTS. ANTACIDS reduce absorption of gabapentin. **Herbal: Ginkgo** may decrease effectiveness.

## PHARMACOKINETICS Absorption:
50–60% from GI tract. **Peak:** Peak level 1–3 h; peak effect 2–4 wk. **Distribution:** Crosses the blood–brain barrier; readily passes into cerebrospinal fluid; not bound to plasma proteins; highest concentrations found in pancreas and kidneys. **Metabolism:** Does not appear to be metabolized. **Elimination:** 76–81% unchanged in 96 h; 10–23% recovered in feces. **Half-Life:** 5–6 h.

## NURSING IMPLICATIONS

### Assessment & Drug Effects

- Monitor for therapeutic effectiveness; may not occur until several weeks following initiation of therapy.
- In those treated for seizure disorders, assess frequency of seizures: In rare cases, the drug has increased the frequency of partial seizures.
- Monitor for and report dizziness, somnolence, or other signs of CNS depression. Assess safety: Vision, concentration, and coordination impairment increase the risk for injury.
- Monitor for changes in behavior that may be indicative of suicidal ideation.

### Patient & Family Education

- Learn potential adverse effects of drug.
- Notify prescriber immediately if any of the following occur: Increased seizure frequency, visual changes, unusual bruising or bleeding.
- Do not drive or engage in other potentially hazardous activities until response to drug is known.
- Do not abruptly discontinue use of drug; do not take drug within 2 h of an antacid.

---

Common adverse effects in *italic;* life-threatening effects underlined; generic names in **bold;** classifications in SMALL CAPS; ♣ Canadian drug name; ⊙ Prototype drug

## GALANTAMINE HYDROBROMIDE

(ga-lan'ta-meen)

**Razadyne, Razadyne ER**

**Classifications:** CENTRALLY ACTING CHOLINERGIC; CHOLINESTERASE INHIBITOR; ANTIDEMENTIA

**Therapeutic:** ANTIALZHEIMER'S; ANTIDEMENTIA

**Prototype:** Donezepril HCl

**AVAILABILITY** Tablet; extended release capsule; oral solution

**ACTION & THERAPEUTIC EFFECT**
Competitive and reversible inhibitor of acetylcholinesterase, which is the enzyme responsible for the hydrolysis (breakdown) of the neurotransmitter, acetylcholine. The cholinergic system is used in processing needed for attention, memory as well as modulation of excitatory neurotransmission. *In Alzheimer's disease cholinesterase inhibitors are designed to offset loss of presynaptic cholinergic function, slowing decline of memory and maintaining ability to perform functions of daily living.*

**USES** Treatment of mild to moderate dementia of Alzheimer's type.

**UNLABELED USES** Vascular dementia.

**CONTRAINDICATIONS** Hypersensitivity to galantamine; CrCl less than 9 mL/min; severe hepatic impairment or in children.

**CAUTIOUS USE** Bradycardia, heart block, or other cardiac conduction disorders; asthma, COPD; potential bladder outflow obstruction; a history of seizures or GI bleeding; Alzheimer disease; renal impairment; mild or moderate hepatic impairment; pregnancy (category B); lactation.

## ROUTE & DOSAGE

### Alzheimer's Disease

*Adult:* **PO** Initiate with 4 mg b.i.d. × at least 4 wks, if tolerated may increase by 4 mg b.i.d. q4wk to target dose of 12 mg b.i.d. (8–16 mg b.i.d.)

**Hepatic Impairment Dosage Adjustment**

Not recommended with severe hepatic impairment

**Renal Impairment Dosage Adjustment**

*CrCl less than 9 mL/min:* Not recommended

## ADMINISTRATION

### Oral

- Give with meals (breakfast and dinner) to reduce the risk of nausea.
- Extended release capsules should be swallowed whole and not crushed or chewed.
- Make increases in dosage increments at 4-wk intervals.
- If drug is interrupted for several days or more, restart at the lowest dose and gradually increase to the current dose.
- Store at 15°–30° C (59°–86° F).

**ADVERSE EFFECTS** (≥1%) **Body as a Whole:** Weight loss, fatigue, rhinitis, syncope, malaise, asthenia, fever. **CNS:** Dizziness, headache, depression, insomnia, somnolence, tremor. **CV:** Bradycardia, chest pain. **GI:** *Nausea, vomiting,* diarrhea, anorexia, abdominal pain, dyspepsia, flatulence.

**Hematologic:** Anemia. **Urogenital:** UTI, hematuria, incontinence. **Nervous System:** Tinnitus, leg cramps. **Other:** <u>Increased mortality in patients with mild cognitive impairment</u>.

**INTERACTIONS Drug:** Additive effects with other CHOLINESTERASE INHIBITORS (e.g., **succinylcholine, bethanecol**); **cimetidine, erythromycin, ketoconazole, paroxetine** may increase levels and toxicity.

**PHARMACOKINETICS Absorption:** Rapidly and completely. **Peak:** 1 h. **Distribution:** Mainly distributes to red blood cells. **Metabolism:** In liver by CYP2D6 and CYP3A4. **Elimination:** 95% in urine. **Half-Life:** 7 h (4.4–10 h).

## NURSING IMPLICATIONS

### Assessment & Drug Effects
- Monitor cardiovascular status including baseline and periodic EKG and BP readings. Assess for postural hypotension.
- Monitor I&O rates and pattern for urinary incontinence or urinary retention.
- Monitor appetite and food intake. Weigh weekly and report significant weight loss.

### Patient & Family Education
- Report any of the following to a health care provider immediately: Loss of weight, urinary retention, chest pain, palpitations, difficulty breathing, fainting, dark stools, blood in the urine.

## GANCICLOVIR
(gan-ci'clo-vir)
Cytovene, Vitrasert, Zirgan
**Classification:** ANTIVIRAL; PURINE NUCLEOSIDE

Therapeutic: ANTIVIRAL
**Prototype:** Acyclovir

**AVAILABILITY** Powder for injection; opthalmic gel; solution for injection

**ACTION & THERAPEUTIC EFFECT**
A synthetic purine nucleoside analog that inhibits the replication of CMV DNA. *Sensitive human viruses include CMV, herpes simplex virus-1 and -2 (HSV-1, HSV-2), Epstein-Barr virus, and varicella-zoster virus.*

**USES** CMV retinitis, prophylaxis and treatment of systemic CMV infections; dendritic keratitis.

**UNLABELED USES** CMV pneumonitis, encephalitis, herpes simplex virus, varicella infection.

**CONTRAINDICATIONS** Hypersensitivity to ganciclovir or acyclovir. **IV form:** Lactation.

**CAUTIOUS USE** Valacyclovir or penciclovir hypersensitivity; renal impairment, bone marrow suppression; chemotherapy; radiation therapy; dehydration; preexisting cytopenias; secondary malignancy; older adults; pregnancy (category C).

## ROUTE & DOSAGE

**Induction Therapy for CMV**

*Adult:* **IV** 5 mg/kg q12h for 14–21 days (doses may range from 2.5–5 mg/kg q8–12h for 10–35 days)

**Maintenance Therapy for CMV**

*Adult:* **IV** 5 mg/kg daily 7 days/wk or 6 mg/kg daily 5 days/wk

Common adverse effects in *italic*; life-threatening effects <u>underlined</u>; generic names in **bold**; classifications in SMALL CAPS; ♣ Canadian drug name; ⊙ Prototype drug

739

**Prevention of CMV Disease in Patients at Risk**

*Adult:* **IV** 5 mg/kg q12h 7–14 days, then 5 mg/kg daily or 6 mg/kg/day 5 days/wk

**Dendritic Keratitis**

*Adult/Adolescent/Child (older than 2 y):* **Opthalmic** 1 drop in affected eye 5 × daily until healed then 1 drop in affected eye t.i.d. × 7 days

**Renal Impairment Dosage Adjustment**

*CrCl 50–70 mL/min:* Use 50% of dose; *25–50 mL/min:* Use 50% of dose and q24h interval (induction) and 25% of dose and q24h interval (maintenance); *10–25 mL/min:* Use 25% of dose and q24h interval (induction) and 12.5% of dose and q24h interval (maintenance)

**Hemodialysis Dosage Adjustment**

Give dose post-dialysis

## ADMINISTRATION

▪ Avoid direct contact with skin and mucous membranes. Wash thoroughly with soap and water if contact occurs.

### Opthalmic

▪ Place one drop in the conjunctival sac.

### Intravenous

▪ Note: Do not administer if neutrophil count falls below 500/mm³ or platelet count falls below 25,000/mm³.

*PREPARE:* **Intermittent** Reconstitute the 500-mg vial using only 10 mL of sterile water (supplied) for injection immediately before use to yield 50 mg/mL. ▪ Shake well to dissolve. ▪ Withdraw the ordered amount and add to 100 mL of NS, D5W, or LR (volume less than 100 mL may be used, but the final concentration should be less than 10 mg/mL).

*ADMINISTER:* **Intermittent:** Give at a constant rate over 1 h. ▪ Avoid rapid infusion or bolus injection.

*INCOMPATIBILITIES:* Solution/additive: Amino acid solutions (TPN), bacteriostatic water for injection, **foscarnet.** Y-site: Aldes-leukin, amifostine, amikacin, aminocaproic acid, aminophylline, amphotericin B colloidal, ampicillin, ampicillin/sulbactam, amsacrine, ascorbic acid, atracurium, azathioprine, aztreonam, benztropine, bumetanide, butorpha-nol, cefamandole, cefazolin, cefepime, cefmetazole, cefonicid, cefoperazone, cefotaxime, cefotetan, cefoxitin, ceftazidime, ceftizoxime, ceftriaxone, cefuroxime, cefphalothin, cephapirin, chloramphenicol, chlorpromazine, cimetidine, clindamycin, codeine, cytarabine, dantrolen, diaze-pam, diltiazem, diphenhydramine, dobutamine, dopa-mine, doxorubicin, doxycy-cline, ephedrine, epinephrine, epirubicin, erythromycin, esmolol, famotidine, fenoldo-pam, foscarnet, gemcitabine, gemtuzumab, gentamicin, haloperidol, hydralazine, hydrocortisone, hydroxyzine, idarubicin, imipenem/cilastin, irinotecan, isoproterenol, ketorolac, lidocaine, meperidine, metaraminol, methoxamine, methyldopate, methyl-prednisolone, metoclopramide, metronidazole, mezlocillin, midazolam, minocycline, morphine, mycophenolate, nalbuphine, netilmicin, norepine-phrine, ondansetron, palonosetron, papaverine, penicillin G, pentazocine, phentolamine, phenylephrine, phenytoin, piperacillin/tazobactam, procainamide, prochlorperazine, promethazine, pyridoxine, quinidine, quinupristin/dalfopristin, sargramostim, sodium bicarbonate, streptokinase, succinylcholine, SMZ/TMP, tacrolimus, thiamine, ticarcillin, TPN, tobramycin, vancomycin, vercuronium, verapamil, vino-relbine.

- Store reconstituted solutions refrigerated at 4° C; use within 12 h.
- Store infusion solution refrigerated up to 24 h of preparation.

## ADVERSE EFFECTS (≥1%) CNS: *Fever,* headache, disorientation, mental status changes, ataxia, coma, confusion, dizziness, paresthesia, nervousness, somnolence, tremor. CV: Edema, phlebitis. GI: *Nausea, diarrhea,* anorexia, elevated liver enzymes. Hematologic: Bone marrow suppression, thrombocytopenia, granulocytopenia, eosinophilia, leukopenia, hyperbilirubinemia. Metabolic: Hyperthermia, hypoglycemia. Urogenital: Infertility. Skin: Rash. Opthalmic: Blurred vision, eye irritation, keratitis, conjunctival hyperemia.

## INTERACTIONS Drug: ANTINEOPLASTIC AGENTS, **amphotericin B, didanosine, trimethoprim-sulfamethoxazole (TMP-SMZ), dapsone, pentamidine, probenecid, zidovudine** may increase bone marrow suppression and other toxic effects of ganciclovir; may increase risk of nephrotoxicity from **cyclosporine;** may increase risk of seizures due to **imipenem-cilastatin.** Oral product increases **didanosine** levels.

## PHARMACOKINETICS Onset: 3–8 days. Duration: Clinical relapse can occur 14 days to 3.5 mo after stopping therapy; positive blood and urine cultures recur 12–60 days after therapy. Distribution: Distributes throughout body including CSF, eye, lungs, liver, and kidneys; crosses placenta in animals; not known if distributed into breast milk. Metabolism: Not metabolized. Elimination: Unchanged in urine. Half-Life: 2.5–4.2 h.

## NURSING IMPLICATIONS

### Black Box Warning

*Ganciclovir has been associated with severe bone marrow suppression.*

### Assessment & Drug Effects

- Inspect IV insertion site throughout infusion for signs and symptoms of phlebitis.
- Monitor lab tests: Neutrophil and platelet counts at least every other day during twice-daily dosing and weekly thereafter; serum creatinine or creatinine clearance at least q2wk; periodic renal function tests in the older adult.

### Patient & Family Education

- Note: Drug is not a cure for CMV retinitis; follow regular ophthalmologic examination schedule.
- Drink lots of fluids during therapy.
- Use barrier contraception throughout therapy and for at least 90 days afterward.
- Maintain frequent hematologic monitoring.

## GANIRELIX ACETATE 🄿

(gan-i-rel′ix)

Antagon

Common adverse effects in *italic;* life-threatening effects underlined; generic names in **bold;** classifications in SMALL CAPS; ♣ Canadian drug name; 🄿 Prototype drug

741

**Classification:** GONADOTROPIN-RELEASING HORMONE (GnRH) ANTAGONIST
Therapeutic: GnRH ANTAGONIST; INFERTILITY AGENT
**Prototype:** Ganirelix

## AVAILABILITY Syringe

## ACTION & *THERAPEUTIC EFFECT*
It acts by competitively blocking the GnRH receptors on the pituitary inducing a rapid, reversible suppression of gonadotropin secretion, and subsequent suppression of pituitary LH and FSH secretion. *Upon discontinuation of the drug, LH and FSH levels are fully recovered within 48 h increasing fertility.*

## USES Infertility treatment.

## CONTRAINDICATIONS Prior hypersensitivity to ganirelix, LHRH, or other LHRH analogs, mannitol hypersensitivity; ovarian cyst; primary ovarian failure; pregnancy (category X); lactation.

## CAUTIOUS USE History of current allergic disorders (e.g., asthma, hay fever, urticaria, eczema) or a history of allergic reactions to medications; renal/hepatic dysfunction; endocrine disorders; alcohol consumption.

## ROUTE & DOSAGE

### Infertility
*Adult:* **Subcutaneous** After initiating follicle-stimulating hormone (FSH) therapy on day 2 or 3 of the cycle, give 250 mcg once daily during the early-to-mid-follicular phase

## ADMINISTRATION
- Note: The packaging of the product, Antagon, contains natural rubber latex which may cause allergic reactions.

### Subcutaneous
- Inject into subcutaneous tissue in the abdomen around the umbilicus or into the upper thigh.
- Rotate injection sites.
- Store at 5°–30° C (59°–86° F) and protect from light.

## ADVERSE EFFECTS (≥1%) CNS: Headache. GI: Abdominal pain, nausea. Endocrine: Ovarian hyperstimulation syndrome. Skin: Injection site reaction. Urogenital: Vaginal bleeding.

## PHARMACOKINETICS Absorption: 91% from subcutaneous site. Peak: 1 h. Distribution: 81% protein bound. Elimination: 75% in feces; 22% in urine. Half-Life: 13–16 h.

## NURSING IMPLICATIONS
### Assessment & Drug Effects
- Exercise caution with patients with hypersensitivity to GnRH or with known allergic disorders (e.g., asthma, hay fever). These patients should be carefully monitored after the first injection for S&S of an anaphylactic reaction.
- Monitor lab tests: Baseline and periodic CBC with differential, and periodic total bilirubin.

### Patient & Family Education
- Report menstrual disorders (e.g., spotting, frank vaginal bleeding) to prescriber.
- Notify prescriber immediately if you think you are pregnant.

# GEMCITABINE HYDROCHLORIDE
(gem-ci′ta-been)
Gemzar

Common adverse effects in *italic;* life-threatening effects <u>underlined</u>; generic names in **bold**; classifications in SMALL CAPS; ♣ Canadian drug name; ⊘ Prototype drug

**Classifications:** ANTINEOPLASTIC; ANTIMETABOLITE, PYRIMIDINE
Therapeutic: ANTINEOPLASTIC
**Prototype:** Fluorouracil

**AVAILABILITY** Solution for injection; powder for injection

**ACTION & *THERAPEUTIC EFFECT***
A pyrimidine analog that inhibits DNA polymerase and ribonucleotide reductase, enzymes necessary for DNA synthesis in tumor cells. It is also incorporated into tumor cell DNA causing the DNA to malfunction, resulting in the initiation of apoptotic cell death. *Gemcitabine induces DNA fragmentation in dividing cells, resulting in cell death of tumor cells.*

**USES** Locally advanced or metastatic adenocarcinoma of the pancreas, non–small-cell lung cancer, breast cancer, ovarian cancer.

**CONTRAINDICATIONS** Hypersensitivity to gemcitabine; drug-induced pulmonary toxicity; pregnancy (category D); lactation.

**CAUTIOUS USE** Myelosuppression, neutropenia; renal or hepatic dysfunction; history of bleeding disorders, infection, previous cytotoxic or radiation treatment; older adults. Safety and efficacy in children 18 y or younger not established.

**ROUTE & DOSAGE**

**Pancreatic Cancer**
*Adult:* **IV** 1000 mg/m$^2$ dose, frequency differs based on concurrent antineoplastic agents
**Non–Small-Cell Lung Cancer**
*Adult:* **IV** 1000 mg/m$^2$ on days 1, 8, 15 of 28-day cycle OR 1250 mg/m$^2$ on days 1 and 8 of 21-day cycle. Given with cisplatin.

**Breast Cancer**
*Adult:* **IV** 1250 mg/m$^2$ on days 1 and 8 of 21-day cycle. Given with paclitaxel.
**Ovarian Cancer**
*Adult:* **IV** 1000 mg/m$^2$ on days 1 and 8 of 21 day cycle

**ADMINISTRATION**

**Intravenous**

This drug is a cytotoxic agent and caution should be used to prevent any contact with the drug. Follow institutional or standard guidelines for preparation, handling, and disposal of cytotoxic agents. Gloves (single) **must be** worn during receiving, unpacking, and placing in storage. Double glove and gown when administering.

*PREPARE:* **IV Infusion:** Dilute with NS without preservatives by adding 5 mL or 25 mL to the 200 mg or 1 g vial, respectively, to yield 38 mg/mL. ▪ Shake to dissolve ▪ Dilute further if necessary with NS to concentrations as low as 0.1 mg/mL.
*ADMINISTER:* **IV Infusion:** Infuse over 30 min. Infusion time greater than 60 min is associated with increased toxicity.
*INCOMPATIBILITIES:* **Y-site: Acyclovir, amphotericin B, cefepime hydrochloride, cefoperazone, cefotaxime, chloramphenicol, dantrolene, daptomycin, diazepam, doxorubicin hydrochloride liposomal, furosemide, ganciclovir, imipenem/cilastatin, irinotecan, ketorolac, lansoprazole, methotrexate, methylprednisolone, mitomycin, nafcillin, pantoprazole, pemetrexed, phenytoin, piperacillin/tazobactam, prochlorperazine, thiopental sodium.**

Common adverse effects in *italic;* life-threatening effects underlined; generic names in **bold**; classifications in SMALL CAPS; ♣ Canadian drug name; ⦿ Prototype drug

743

▪ Store reconstituted solutions unrefrigerated at 20°–25° C (68°–77° F). Use within 24 h of reconstitution.

**ADVERSE EFFECTS** (≥1%) **CNS:** *Fever, flu-like syndrome (anorexia, headache, cough, chills, myalgia)*, paresthesias, drowsiness. **GI:** *Nausea, vomiting, diarrhea,* stomatitis, *transient elevations of liver transaminases.* **Hematologic:** <u>*Myelosuppression (anemia, leukopenia, neutropenia,* thrombocytopenia)</u>. **Skin:** Bullous skin eruption, desquamation, *alopecia*. **Urogenital:** Mild proteinuria and hematuria. **Other:** *Dyspnea, edema, peripheral edema, infection*, elevated liver function tests.

**INTERACTIONS Drug:** May increase effect of **warfarin** or ORAL ANTICOAGULANTS or NSAIDS. Do not use with **sargramostin** or **filgrastim.**

**PHARMACOKINETICS Peak:** Peak concentrations reached 30 min after infusion; lower clearance in women and older adult results in higher concentrations at any given dose. **Distribution:** Crosses placenta, distributed into breast milk. **Metabolism:** Intracellularly by nucleoside kinases to active diphosphate and triphosphate nucleosides. **Elimination:** 92–98% recovered in urine within 1 wk. **Half-Life:** 32–94 min.

**NURSING IMPLICATIONS**

**Assessment & Drug Effects**

▪ Monitor lab tests: CBC with differential and platelet count prior to each dose. Baseline and periodic renal function tests and LFTs.

**Patient & Family Education**

▪ Learn about common adverse effects and measures to control or minimize when possible. Notify prescriber immediately of any distressing adverse effects.

▪ Note: Fever with flu-like symptoms, rash, and GI distress are very common.

▪ Females should use reliable contraception while taking this drug.

**GEMFIBROZIL**
(gem-fi'broe-zil)
Lopid
**Classifications:** ANTILIPEMIC; FIBRATE
Therapeutic: CHOLESTEROL-LOWERING
**Prototype:** Fenofibrate

**AVAILABILITY** Tablet

**ACTION & *THERAPEUTIC EFFECT*** Fibric acid derivative with lipid regulating properties. Blocks lipolysis of stored triglycerides in adipose tissue and inhibits hepatic uptake of fatty acids. *Decreases VLDL and therefore triglyceride synthesis. Produces a moderate increase in HDL cholesterol levels and reduces levels of total and LDL cholesterol and triglycerides.*

**USES** Patients with very high serum triglyceride levels (above 750 mg/dL) (type IV and V hyperlipidemia) who have not responded to intensive diet restriction and are at risk of pancreatitis and abdominal pain. Also severe familial hypercholesterolemia (type IIa or IIb) that developed in childhood and has failed to respond to dietary control or to other cholesterol-lowering drugs.

**CONTRAINDICATIONS** Gallbladder disease, biliary cirrhosis, hepatic, or severe renal dysfunction.

**CAUTIOUS USE** Diabetes mellitus, hypothyroidism; renal impairment, cholelithiasis; pregnancy (category C); lactation. Safety and

Common adverse effects in *italic;* life-threatening effects <u>underlined;</u> generic names in **bold;** classifications in SMALL CAPS; ♣ Canadian drug name; ⦿ Prototype drug

efficacy in children younger than 18 y not established.

## ROUTE & DOSAGE

### Hypertriglyceridemia
*Adult:* **PO** 600 mg b.i.d. 30 min before morning and evening meal, may increase up to 1500 mg/day

## ADMINISTRATION
### Oral
- Give 30 min before breakfast and evening meal.
- Store at 15°–30° C (59°–86° F) unless otherwise directed.

## ADVERSE EFFECTS (≥1%) CNS:
Headache, dizziness, blurred vision. **GI:** *Abdominal* or *epigastric pain*, diarrhea, nausea, vomiting, flatulence. **Hematologic:** Eosinophilia, mild decreases in Hct, Hgb. **Musculoskeletal:** Painful extremities, back pain, muscle cramps, myalgia, arthralgia, swollen joints. **Skin:** Rash, dermatitis, pruritus, urticaria. **Endocrine:** Hypokalemia, moderate hyperglycemia.

## INTERACTIONS Drug:
May potentiate hypoprothrombinemic effects of ORAL ANTICOAGULANTS; **lovastatin** increases risk of myopathy and rhabdomyolysis; may increase hypoglycemic effects of ANTIDIABETIC MEDICATIONS.

## PHARMACOKINETICS Absorption:
Readily from GI tract. **Peak:** 1–2 h. **Metabolism:** Undergoes enterohepatic circulation. **Elimination:** In urine; 6% in feces. **Half-Life:** 1.3–1.5 h.

## NURSING IMPLICATIONS
### Assessment & Drug Effects
- Note: Mild decreases in WBC, Hgb, Hct may occur during early

stage of treatment but generally stabilize with continued therapy.
- Note: Drug is usually withdrawn if lipid response is inadequate after 3 mo of therapy.
- Notify prescriber if patient presents S&S suggestive of cholelithiasis or cholecystitis; gallbladder studies may be indicated. Symptoms often occur during the night or early morning; jaundice may or may not be present.
- Monitor lab tests: Baseline and periodic lipid profile, CBC, blood glucose, and LFTs.

### Patient & Family Education
- Do not drive or engage in other potentially hazardous activities until response to drug is known.
- Report promptly if you develop jaundice, pruritus, or unexplained upper abdominal discomfort.

## GEMIFLOXACIN
(gem-i-flox'a-cin)
**Factive**
**Classifications:** QUINOLONE ANTIBIOTIC
**Therapeutic:** ANTIBIOTIC
**Prototype:** Ciprofloxacin HCl

## AVAILABILITY Tablet

## ACTION & THERAPEUTIC EFFECT
Gemifloxacin inhibits bacterial DNA gyrases (topoisomerase II), enzymes essential in replication, transcription, and repair of bacterial DNA. *Gemifloxacin is active against a wide range of gram-positive and gram-negative bacteria.*

## USES Treatment of acute exacerbations of chronic bronchitis, mild to moderate community-acquired pneumonia.

## UNLABELED USES Acute sinusitis, UTI, acute pyelonephritis, gonorrhea.

---

Common adverse effects in *italic;* life-threatening effects <u>underlined</u>; generic names in **bold;** classifications in SMALL CAPS; ♣ Canadian drug name; ⊙ Prototype drug

745

**CONTRAINDICATIONS** Hypersensitivity to gemifloxacin or other fluoroquinolone antibiotics; known QT prolongation; tendon pain; viral disease; history of myasthenia gravis; history of peripheral neuropathy; lactation.

**CAUTIOUS USE** Hypokalemia, hypomagnesemia, or concurrent use of Class IA or III antiarrhythmic agents; history of OT prolongation; bradycardia, acute myocardial ischemia; renal disease or impairment; hepatic disease; central nervous system disorders such as epilepsy; glucose 6-phosphate dehydrogenase deficiency; tendinitis; older adults; pregnancy (category C). Safe use in children 18 y or younger not established.

## ROUTE & DOSAGE

### Acute Exacerbation of Chronic Bronchitis

*Adult:* **PO** 320 mg daily × 5 days

### Community-Acquired Pneumonia

*Adult:* **PO** 320 mg daily × 5–7 days

### Renal Impairment Dosage Adjustment

*CrCl 40 mL/min or less:* 160 mg daily

## ADMINISTRATION

### Oral

- Give 2 h before or 3 h after drugs containing aluminum, magnesium, iron, zinc, or buffered tablets of any type.
- Give at least 2 h before sucralfate.
- Store at 15°–30° C (59°–86° F) and protect from light.

**ADVERSE EFFECTS** (≥1%) **CNS:** Headache. **GI:** Nausea, vomiting, diarrhea, elevated liver enzymes. **Skin:** Rash.

**INTERACTIONS Drug:** ANTACIDS, **didanosine (tablets and powder), iron, sevelamer, sulcralfate** decrease absorption; may prolong the QT interval with **amiodarone, bepridil, bretylium, chlorprocaine, disopyramide, dofetilide, dronedarone, ibutilide, quinidine, pimozide, procainamide, sotalol, ziprasidone** leading to arrhythmias; may augment phototoxicity of RETINOIDS.

**PHARMACOKINETICS Absorption:** 71% absorbed. **Distribution:** 50–75% protein bound. **Peak:** 0.5–2 h. **Metabolism:** Minimally in liver. **Elimination:** Primarily renal. **Half-Life:** 7 h.

## NURSING IMPLICATIONS

### Black Box Warning

*Gemifloxacin has been associated with increased risk of tendinitis and tendon rupture, and with exacerbation of muscle weakness in those with MG.*

### Assessment & Drug Effects

- Monitor cardiac status with concurrent use of drugs that may prolong the QT interval. Report immediately bradycardia or S&S of heart failure.
- Withhold drug and report to prescriber any of the following: Tremors, restlessness, lightheadedness, confusion, hallucinations, paranoia, depression, nightmares, and insomnia.
- Lab tests: C&S prior to initiation of therapy; baseline and periodic serum electrolytes; serum creatinine, BUN; LFTs. frequent blood glucose levels in diabetics; CBC with differential and platelet count with prolonged treatment.

### Patient & Family Education

- Warn patient to report hallucinations, depression, suicidal thoughts, or convulsions.

Common adverse effects in *italic;* life-threatening effects <u>underlined;</u> generic names in **bold;** classifications in SMALL CAPS; ♣ Canadian drug name; ☉ Prototype drug

- Use sunscreen and protective clothing outdoors. Avoid sun lamps.
- Stop gemifloxacin and notify prescriber for pain or swelling of a tendon or around a joint.
- Drink fluid liberally (unless contraindicated) while taking this drug.
- Do not drive or engage in other hazardous activities until reaction to drug is known.

## GENTAMICIN SULFATE ℞

(jen-ta-mye'sin)

Garamycin Ophthalmic, Genoptic

**Classification:** AMINOGLYCOSIDE ANTIBIOTIC
Therapeutic: ANTIBIOTIC

**AVAILABILITY** Ointment; cream; ophthalmic solution; ophthalmic ointment; solution for injection

## ACTION & THERAPEUTIC EFFECT

Broad-spectrum aminoglycoside antibiotic that binds irreversibly to 30S subunit of bacterial ribosomes, blocking a vital step in protein synthesis, and attachment of RNA molecules to bacterial ribosomes resulting in cell death. *Active against a wide variety of aerobic gram-negative but not anaerobic gram-negative bacteria. Also effective against certain gram-positive organisms, particularly penicillin-sensitive bacteria.*

**USES** Parenteral use restricted to treatment of serious infections of GI, respiratory, and urinary tracts, CNS, bone, skin, and soft tissue (including burns) when other less toxic antimicrobial agents are ineffective or are contraindicated. Has been used in combination with other antibiotics. Also used topically for primary and secondary skin infections and for superficial infections of external eye and its adnexa.

**UNLABELED USES** Prophylaxis of bacterial endocarditis in patients undergoing operative procedures or instrumentation.

**CONTRAINDICATIONS** History of hypersensitivity to, or toxic reaction with any aminoglycoside antibiotic; pregnancy (category D); lactation.

**CAUTIOUS USE** Impaired renal function; history of eighth cranial (acoustic) nerve impairment; preexisting vertigo or dizziness or tinnitus; dehydration, fever; renal impairment, dehydration; hypocalcemia; HF; Fabry disease; older adults, obesity, neuromuscular disorders: MG; parkinsonian syndrome; premature infants, neonates, infants; children. **Topical:** Applied to widespread areas.

## ROUTE & DOSAGE

### Moderate to Severe Infection

*Adult:* **IV/IM** 1–2 mg/kg loading dose followed by 3–5 mg/kg/day in 3 divided doses; **Intrathecal** 4–8 mg preservative free daily; **Ophthalmic** 1–2 drops of solution in eye q4h up to 2 drops q1h; **Topical** small amount of ointment b.i.d. or t.i.d.
*Child:* **IV/IM** 6–7.5 mg/kg/day in 3 divided doses;
*3 mo or older:* **Intrathecal** 1–2 mg preservative free daily
*Neonate:* **IV/IM** 2.5 mg/kg/day

### Prophylaxis of Bacterial Endocarditis

*Adult:* **IV/IM** 1.5 mg/kg 30 min before procedure, may repeat in 8 h
*Child (weight less than 27 kg):* **IV/IM** 2 mg/kg 30 min before procedure, may repeat in 8 h

---

Common adverse effects in *italic;* life-threatening effects underlined; generic names in **bold;** classifications in SMALL CAPS; ♣ Canadian drug name; ● Prototype drug

747

**G**

***Obesity Dosage Adjustment***
Dose based on IBW, in morbid obesity use IBW + 0.4 (TBW–IBW)

***Renal Impairment Dosage Adjustment***
Reduce dose or extend dosing interval

## ADMINISTRATION

### Ophthalmic
- Apply pressure to inner canthus for 1 min immediately after instillation of drops.
- Have patient keep eyes closed for 1–2 min after administration of ophthalmic ointment to assure medication contact. Caution patient that vision will be blurred for a few minutes.

### Topical
- Wash affected area with mild soap and water, rinse, and dry thoroughly. Gently apply small amount of medication to lesions; cover with sterile gauze.
- Do not apply topical preparations, particularly cream, to large denuded body surfaces because systemic absorption and toxicity are possible.

### Intramuscular
- Give deep into a large muscle.
- Do not use solutions that are discolored or that contain particulate matter; drug for IV or IM is clear and colorless or slightly yellow.

### Intrathecal
- Note: Intrathecal formulation is a clear and colorless solution.
- Use promptly after opening; contains no preservatives and any unused portion should be discarded.

### Intravenous

***PREPARE: Intermittent:*** Dilute a single dose with 50–200 mL of D5W or NS. ▪ For pediatric patients, amount of infusion fluid may be proportionately smaller depending on patient's needs but should be sufficient to be infused over the same time period as for adults. ▪ Note: Premixed, single-dose containers are ready to use and require no dilution.

***ADMINISTER: Intermittent:*** Give over 30 min–1 h. May extend infusion time to 2 h for a child.

***INCOMPATIBILITIES:*** **Solution/additive:** Fat emulsion, **TPN, amphotericin B, ampicillin,** CEPHALOSPORINS, **cytarabine, heparin, ticarcillin. Y-site: Allopurinol, amphotericin B cholesteryl, azithromycin, furosemide, heparin, hetastarch, idarubicin, indomethacin, iodipamide, propofol, warfarin.**

- Store all gentamicin solutions at 2°–30° C (36°–86° F) unless otherwise directed by manufacturer.

## ADVERSE EFFECTS (≥1%) **Special Senses:** Ototoxicity (vestibular disturbances, impaired hearing), optic neuritis. **CNS:** Neuromuscular blockade: Skeletal muscle weakness, apnea, respiratory paralysis (high doses); arachnoiditis (intrathecal use). **CV:** Hypotension or hypertension. **GI:** Nausea, vomiting, transient increase in AST, ALT, and serum LDH and bilirubin; hepatomegaly, splenomegaly. **Hematologic:** Increased or decreased reticulocyte counts; granulocytopenia, thrombocytopenia (fever, bleeding tendency), thrombocytopenic purpura, anemia. **Body as a Whole:** Hypersensitivity (rash, pruritus, urticaria, exfoliative dermatitis, eosinophilia, burning sensation of skin, drug fever, joint pains, laryngeal edema, anaphylaxis). **Urogenital:** Nephrotoxicity: Proteinuria, tubular necrosis, cells or casts in urine, hematuria, rising BUN, nonpro-

tein nitrogen, serum creatinine; *decreased creatinine clearance.* **Other:** Local irritation and pain following IM use; thrombophlebitis, abscess, superinfections, syndrome of hypocalcemia (tetany, weakness, hypokalemia, hypomagnesemia). **Topical and Ophthalmic:** Photosensitivity, sensitization, erythema, pruritus; burning, stinging, and lacrimation (ophthalmic formulation).

**INTERACTIONS Drug: Amphotericin B, capreomycin, cisplatin, methoxyflurane, polymyxin B, vancomycin, ethacrynic acid,** and **furosemide** increase risk of nephrotoxicity. GENERAL ANESTHETICS and NEUROMUSCULAR BLOCKING AGENTS (e.g., **succinylcholine**) po tentiate neuromuscular blockade. **Indomethacin** may increase gentamicin levels in neonates.

**PHARMACOKINETICS Absorption:** Well absorbed from IM site. **Peak:** 30–90 min IM. **Distribution:** Widely distributed in body fluids, including ascitic, peritoneal, pleural, synovial, and abscess fluids; poor CNS penetration; concentrates in kidney and inner ear; crosses placenta. **Metabolism:** Not metabolized. **Elimination:** Excreted unchanged in urine; small amounts accumulate in kidney and are eliminated over 10–20 days; small amount excreted in breast milk. **Half-Life:** 2–4 h.

**NURSING IMPLICATIONS**

### Black Box Warning

*Gentamicin has been associated with nephrotoxicity and ototoxicity.*

### Assessment & Drug Effects

- Lab tests: Perform C&S and renal function tests prior to first dose and periodically during therapy. Determine creatinine clearance

and serum drug concentrations at frequent intervals.

- Note: Dosages are generally adjusted to maintain peak serum gentamicin concentrations of 4–10 mcg/mL, and trough concentrations of 1–2 mcg/mL. Prolonged peak concentrations above 12 mcg/mL and trough concentrations above 2 mcg/mL are associated with toxicity.
- Draw blood specimens for peak serum gentamicin concentration 30 min–1 h after IM administration, and 30 min after completion of a 30–60 min IV infusion. Draw blood specimens for trough levels just before the next IM or IV dose.
- Monitor vital signs and I&O. Keep patient well hydrated to prevent chemical irritation of renal tubules. Report oliguria, unusual appearance of urine, change in I&O ratio or pattern, and presence of edema (prolongs elimination time).
- Watch for S&S of bacterial overgrowth (opportunistic infections) with resistant or nonsusceptible organisms (diarrhea, anogenital itching, vaginal discharge, stomatitis, glossitis).

### Patient & Family Education

- Report promptly S&S of ototoxic effect (e.g., headache, dizziness or vertigo, nausea and vomiting with motion, ataxia, nystagmus, tinnitus, roaring noises, sensation of fullness in ears, hearing impairment).
- Note: When using topical applications: Avoid excessive exposure to sunlight because of danger of photosensitivity; withhold medication and notify prescriber if condition fails to improve within 1 wk, worsens, or signs of irritation or sensitivity occur; and apply medication as directed and only for length of time prescribed (overuse can result in superinfections).

Common adverse effects in *italic;* life-threatening effects underlined; generic names in **bold;** classifications in SMALL CAPS; ✦ Canadian drug name; ◎ Prototype drug

749

# GLATIRAMER ACETATE

(gla-tir′a-mer)

**Copaxone, Glatopa**

**Classifications:** BIOLOGIC
RESPONSE MODIFIER; IMMUNOLOGIC
**Therapeutic:** IMMUNOSUPPRESSANT

**AVAILABILITY** Solution for injection

## ACTION & *THERAPEUTIC EFFECT*

Mechanism of action is not fully understood. Thought to modify immune processes that are responsible for the pathogenesis of multiple sclerosis. *Its function is to reduce the relapse rate of multiple sclerosis (MS), a demyelinating disease of the CNS.*

**USES** Reduce frequency of relapses in patients with relapsing–remitting multiple sclerosis.

**CONTRAINDICATIONS** Hypersensitivity to glatiramer acetate or mannitol.

**CAUTIOUS USE** Immunosuppression, history of asthma or other respiratory disorders; angina; pregnancy (category B); lactation. Safe use in children younger than 18 y has not been established.

## ROUTE & DOSAGE

### Multiple Sclerosis

*Adult:* **Subcutaneous** 20 mg daily or 40 mg 3 × wk at least 48 h apart

## ADMINISTRATION

### Subcutaneous

- Use recommended subcutaneous injection sites: Arms, abdomen, hips, and thighs.
- Give 40 mg dose on same 3 days each wk.
- Allow prefilled syringe to stand at room temperature for 20 min prior to injection.

- Note that glatiramer 20 mg/mL and 40 mg/mL formulations are not interchangeable.
- Store vials at −20° to −10° C (−4° to −14° F).

**ADVERSE EFFECTS** (≥1%) **Body as a Whole:** *Asthenia, back pain,* chills, facial edema, fever, *flu-like syndrome, infection, pain, arthralgia.* **CNS:** Migraine, agitation, *anxiety, hypotonia.* **CV:** *Chest pain, palpitations,* syncope, tachycardia, *vasodilation.* **GI:** *Diarrhea, nausea,* anorexia, gastroenteritis, vomiting. **Respiratory:** *Dyspnea, rhinitis,* bronchitis. **Skin:** *Rash, pruritus, sweating.* **Other:** *Postinjection reaction (flushing, chest pain, palpitations, anxiety, dyspnea, constriction of throat, urticaria), injection site reactions (erythema, hemorrhage, pain, pruritus, urticaria, swelling),* ecchymoses, *lymphadenopathy,* ear pain, dysmenorrhea, urinary urgency.

## NURSING IMPLICATIONS

### Assessment & Drug Effects

- Monitor for therapeutic effectiveness: Indicated by longer remission periods and reduced frequency of attacks.
- Assess for systemic postinjection reactions (see PATIENT & FAMILY EDUCATION). Assure patient that reaction is self-limiting. Assess for local reactions at injection sites including erythema, itching, induration, and soreness.
- Monitor for S&S of compromised immune response (e.g., increasing frequency of infections).

### Patient & Family Education

- Note: Systemic postinjection reaction with chest pain, palpitations, flushing, urticaria, anxiety, dyspnea, and laryngeal constriction may occur immediately after

Common adverse effects in *italic*; life-threatening effects <u>underlined</u>; generic names in **bold**; classifications in SMALL CAPS; ♣ Canadian drug name; ◯ Prototype drug injection. These symptoms are transient (lasting from 30 sec to 30 min), require no treatment, and resolve spontaneously.

- Report any distressing adverse drug effects.

# GLIMEPIRIDE
(gli-me'pi-ride)

**Amaryl**

**Classifications:** ANTIDIABETIC; SULFONYLUREA
**Therapeutic:** ANTIDIABETIC
**Prototype:** Glyburide

## AVAILABILITY Tablet

## ACTION & THERAPEUTIC EFFECT
Second-generation sulfonylurea hypoglycemic agent that directly stimulates functioning pancreatic beta cells to secrete insulin, leading to a direct drop in blood glucose. Indirect action leads to increased sensitivity of peripheral insulin receptors, resulting in increased insulin binding in peripheral tissues. *Lowers blood sugar by increasing secretion of insulin from pancreatic beta cells. Glimepiride improves postprandial glycemic control.*

## USES Adjunct to diet and exercise in patients with type 2 diabetes.

## CONTRAINDICATIONS Hypersensitivity to glimepiride, diabetic ketoacidosis; nondiabetic patients with renal glycosuria; lactation.

## CAUTIOUS USE Previous hypersensitivity to other sulfonylureas, sulfonamides, or thiazide diuretics; hypoglycemia or conditions predisposing to hypoglycemia (e.g., prolonged nausea and vomiting, alcohol ingestion, surgery; renal or hepatic function impairment, severe infections); pregnancy (category C). Safe use in children is not established.

## ROUTE & DOSAGE

### Type 2 Diabetes Mellitus

*Adult:* **PO** Start with 1–2 mg once daily with breakfast or first main meal, may increase to usual maintenance dose of 1–4 mg once daily (max: 8 mg/day)

## ADMINISTRATION

### Oral
- Give with breakfast or first main meal.
- Note: Maximum starting dose is 2 mg or less. With renal or hepatic insufficiency, initial recommended dose is 1 mg.
- Store in tightly closed container at 15°–30° C (59°–86° F)

## ADVERSE EFFECTS (≥1%) CNS:
Dizziness, asthenia, headache, blurred vision, changes in accommodation. **GI:** Nausea, vomiting, diarrhea, abdominal pain. **Hematologic:** Leukopenia, agranulocytosis (rare), thrombocytopenia. **Metabolic:** Hypoglycemia. **Skin:** Rash, pruritus, erythema, urticaria, maculopapular eruptions.

## INTERACTIONS Drug: Hypoglycemic effects may be potentiated by other protein-bound drugs (e.g., ADRENERGIC ANTAGONISTS, **chloramphenicol,** MAO INHIBITORS, NSAIDS, **probenecid,** SALICYLATES, SULFONAMIDES, **warfarin**). CORTICOSTEROIDS, **phenytoin, isoniazid, nicotinic acid,** SYMPATHOMIMETIC AMINES, THIAZIDE DIURETICS may attenuate effects of glimepiride. **Herbal:** Ginseng, garlic may increase hypoglycemic effects.

## PHARMACOKINETICS Absorption: Completely absorbed from GI tract. **Onset:** 1 h. **Peak:** 2–3 h. **Distribution:** Greater than 99.5% protein bound; probably secreted into

Common adverse effects in *italic;* life-threatening effects underlined; generic names in **bold;** classifications in SMALL CAPS; ♣ Canadian drug name; ⊘ Prototype drug

751

breast milk. **Metabolism:** In liver by CYP2C9. **Elimination:** 60% in urine, 40% in feces. **Half-Life:** 5–9 h.

## NURSING IMPLICATIONS

### Assessment & Drug Effects

- Monitor for hypoglycemia especially with concurrent drugs which enhance hypoglycemic effects.
- Monitor lab tests: Frequent fasting and postprandial blood glucose, HgbA1C every 3–6 mo.

### Patient & Family Education

- Take a missed dose as soon as possible unless it is almost time for next dose; NEVER take two doses at the same time.
- Avoid drinking alcohol or using OTC drugs without informing prescriber.
- Learn about adverse reactions and drug interactions.

## GLIPIZIDE

(glip'i-zide)

Glucotrol, Glucotrol XL

**Classifications:** ANTIDIABETIC; SULFONYLUREA

Therapeutic: ANTIDIABETIC

**Prototype:** Glyburide

**AVAILABILITY** Tablet; sustained release tablet

## ACTION & *THERAPEUTIC EFFECT*

Second-generation sulfonylurea hypoglycemic agent that directly stimulates functioning pancreatic beta cells to secrete insulin, leading to an acute drop in blood glucose. Indirect action leads to altered numbers and sensitivity of peripheral insulin receptors, resulting in increased insulin binding. It also causes inhibition of hepatic glucose production and reduction in serum glucagon levels. *It lowers blood glucose level by stimulating pancreatic beta cells.*

*Glipizide improves postprandial glycemic control.*

**USES** Adjunct to diet for control of hyperglycemia in patient with type 2 diabetes mellitus.

**CONTRAINDICATIONS** Hypersensitivity to sulfonylureas; diabetic ketoacidosis; lactation.

**CAUTIOUS USE** Impaired renal and hepatic function; thyroid disease; debilitated, malnourished patients; G6PD deficiency; trauma; surgery; patients with adrenal or pituitary insufficiency; older adults. **Extended release form:** Severe GI narrowing; pregnancy (category C). Safe use in children has not been established.

## ROUTE & DOSAGE

### Control of Hyperglycemia

*Adult:* **PO** 2.5–5 mg/day 30 min before breakfast, may increase by 2.5–5 mg q1–2wk; greater than 15 mg/day in divided doses 30 min before morning and evening meal (max: 40 mg/day); 5–10 mg sustained release tablets once/day

## ADMINISTRATION

### Oral

- Give once daily dosing 30 min before the first meal of the day.
- Ensure that sustained release form of drug is not chewed or crushed. It **must be** swallowed whole.
- Store in tightly closed, light-resistant container at 15°–30° C (59°–86° F).

**ADVERSE EFFECTS** (≥1%) **GI:** Nausea, diarrhea, constipation, gastralgia, cholestatic jaundice (rare). **Metabolic:** Hepatic porphyria, hypoglycemia. **Skin:** Erythema, morbilliform or maculopapular rash, pruritus, urticaria, eczema (transient). **Body as a Whole:** Hypersensitivity (fatigue, drowsiness, hunger, GI distress with heartburn, abdominal pain, anorexia). **CNS:** Transient drowsiness, headache, anxiety, ataxia, confusion; seizures, coma. **CV:** Tachycardia. **Special Senses:** Visual disturbances.

**INTERACTIONS Drug: Alcohol** produces **disulfiram**-like reaction in some patients; ORAL ANTI-COAGULANTS, **chloramphenicol, clofibrate, phenylbutazone,** MAO INHIBITORS, SALICYLATES, **probenecid,** SULFONAMIDES may potentiate hypoglycemic actions; THIAZIDES may antagonize hypoglycemic effects; **cimetidine** may increase glipizide levels, causing hypoglycemia. **Herbal: Ginseng, garlic** may increase hypoglycemic effects.

**PHARMACOKINETICS Absorption:** Readily from GI tract. **Onset:** 15–30 min. **Peak:** 1–2 h. **Duration:** Up to 24 h. **Metabolism:** Metabolized extensively in liver. **Elimination:** Mainly in urine with some excretion via bile in feces. **Half-Life:** 3–5 h.

**NURSING IMPLICATIONS**
**Assessment & Drug Effects**
- Observe response to the initial dose, especially in older adult or debilitated patients; early signs of hypoglycemia are easily overlooked.
- Patients transferred from a sulfonylurea with a long half-life (e.g., chlorpropamide, half-life: 30–40 h) **must be** made aware of the potential for hypoglycemic responses (see Appendix F) for 1–2 wk because of potential overlapping of drug effect.
- Note: The first signs of hypoglycemia may be hard to detect in patients receiving concurrent beta-blockers or older adults.

- Monitor lab tests: Periodic fasting and postprandial blood glucose, and HgbA1C.

**Patient & Family Education**
- Treat mild hypoglycemia (reaction without loss of consciousness or neurologic symptoms) with PO glucose and adjustment of dosage and meal pattern; monitor closely for at least 5–7 days to assure reestablishment of safe control. Severe hypoglycemia requires emergency hospitalization to permit treatment to maintain a blood glucose level above 100 mg/dL.
- Test fasting and postprandial blood glucose frequently.
- Keep all follow-up medical appointments and adhere to dietary instructions, regular exercise program, and scheduled and blood testing.
- When a drug that affects the hypoglycemic action of sulfonylureas (see DRUG INTERACTIONS) is withdrawn or added to the glipizide regimen, be alert to the added danger of loss of control. Urine and blood glucose tests and test for ketone bodies should be carefully monitored.
- Report promptly severe skin rash and pruritus as these may indicate a need for discontinuation of drug. Symptoms usually subside rapidly when drug is withdrawn.

## GLUCAGON
(gloo'ka-gon)
GlucaGen
**Classification:** ANTIHYPOGLYCEMIC
**Therapeutic:** ANTIHYPOGLYCEMIC; DIAGNOSTIC TEST AID

**AVAILABILITY** Powder for injection

**ACTION & THERAPEUTIC EFFECT**
Recombinant glucagon identical to glucagon produced by alpha cells of

Common adverse effects in *italic*; life-threatening effects <u>underlined</u>; generic names in **bold**; classifications in SMALL CAPS; ♣ Canadian drug name; ⊙ Prototype drug

753

islets of Langerhans. Stimulates uptake of amino acids and their conversion to glucose precursors. Promotes lipolysis in liver and adipose tissue with release of free fatty acid and glycerol, which further stimulates ketogenesis and hepatic gluconeogenesis. Action in hypoglycemia relies on presence of adequate liver glycogen stores. *Increases blood glucose secondary to gluconeogenesis, which is the breakdown of glycogen to glucose in the liver.*

**USES** Hypoglycemia, radiologic studies of GI tract.

**UNLABELED USES** GI disturbances associated with spasm, cardiovascular emergencies, and to overcome cardiotoxic effects of beta-blockers, quinidine, tricyclic antidepressants; as an aid in abdominal imaging; choking due to esophageal foreign body impaction.

**CONTRAINDICATIONS** Hypersensitivity to glucagon or protein compounds; depleted glycogen stores in liver; insulinemia; pheochromocytoma.

**CAUTIOUS USE** Cardiac disease, CAD; adrenal insufficiency; malnutrition; children; pregnancy (category B); lactation.

## ROUTE & DOSAGE

### Hypoglycemia

*Adult/Adolescent/Child (greater than 25 kg):* **IM/IV/Subcutaneous** 1 mg, may repeat q5–20min if no response for 1–2 more doses
*Child (younger than 8y, weight less than 25 kg):* **IM/IV/Subcutaneous** 0.5 mg (max: 1 mg)

### Diagnostic Aid to Relax Stomach or Upper GI Tract

*Adult:* **IV** 0.2–0.5 mg **IM** 1 mg

### Diagnostic Aid for Colon Exam

*Adult:* **IV** 0.5–0.75 mg; **IM** 1–2 mg

## ADMINISTRATION

Note: 1 mg = 1 unit

### Subcutaneous/Intramuscular
- Dilute 1 unit (1 mg) of glucagon with 1 mL of diluent supplied by manufacturer.
- Use immediately after reconstitution of dry powder. Discard any unused portion.
- Note: Glucagon is incompatible in syringe with any other drug.

### Intravenous
***PREPARE:* Direct:** Prepare as noted for intramuscular injection. Do not use a concentration greater than 1 unit/mL.
***ADMINISTER:* Direct:** Give 1 unit or fraction thereof over 1 min.
- May be given through a Y-site D5W (not NS) infusing. Note: Rapid injection may be associated with increased nausea and vomiting; place patient in lateral recumbent position to protect airway.
***INCOMPATIBILITIES:* Solution/additive: Sodium chloride.**

- Store unreconstituted vials and diluent at 20°–25° C (68°–77° F).

**ADVERSE EFFECTS** (≥1%) **GI:** Nausea and vomiting. **Body as a Whole:** Hypersensitivity reactions. **Skin:** Stevens–Johnson syndrome (erythema multiforme). **Metabolic:** Hyperglycemia, hypokalemia.

**INTERACTIONS Drug:** May enhance effect of ORAL ANTICOAGULANTS.

**PHARMACOKINETICS Onset:** 5–20 min. **Peak:** 30 min. **Duration:** 1–1.5 h. **Metabolism:** In liver, plasma, and kidneys. **Half-Life:** 3–10 min.

## NURSING IMPLICATIONS
### Assessment & Drug Effects
- Be prepared to give IV glucose if patient fails to respond to glucagon. Notify prescriber immediately.
- Note: Patient usually awakens from (diabetic) hypoglycemic coma 5–20 min after glucagon injection. Give PO carbohydrate as soon as possible after patient regains consciousness.
- Note: After recovery from hypoglycemic reaction, symptoms such as headache, nausea, and weakness may persist.

### Patient & Family Education
- Note: Prescriber may request that a responsible family member be taught how to administer glucagon subcutaneously or IM for patients with frequent or severe hypoglycemic reactions. Notify prescriber promptly whenever a hypoglycemic reaction occurs so the reason for the reaction can be determined.
- Review package insert and directions (see ADMINISTRATION).

## GLYBURIDE ⊙
(glye'byoor-ide)
Euglucon ♣, Glynase
**Classifications:** ANTIDIABETIC; SULFONYLUREA
Therapeutic: ANTIDIABETIC

## AVAILABILITY Tablet; micronized tablet

## ACTION & *THERAPEUTIC EFFECT*
One of the most potent of the second-generation sulfonylurea hypoglycemic agents. Appears to lower blood sugar concentration by sensitizing pancreatic beta cells to release insulin in the presence of elevated serum glucose levels and by reducing glucose output from the liver as well as increasing insulin sensitivity in peripheral target sites. *Blood glucose-lowering effect persists during long-term glyburide treatment, but there is a gradual decline in meal-stimulated secretion of endogenous insulin toward pretreatment levels.*

## USES
Adjunct to diet and exercise to lower blood glucose in patients with type 2 diabetes mellitus.

## CONTRAINDICATIONS
Hypersensitivity to glyburide or sulfonylureas; diabetic ketoacidosis; type I diabetes mellitus; major surgery; severe trauma; severe infection; withhold 14 days before labor and delivery; lactation, elderly.

## CAUTIOUS USE
History of sulfonamide hypersensitivity; renal and hepatic impairment; cardiovascular disease; thyroid disease; mild renal impairment or hepatic disease; adrenal or pituitary insufficiency; older adults, debilitated, or malnourished patients; pregnancy (category C); children.

## ROUTE & DOSAGE

### Control of Hyperglycemia
*Adult:* **PO** 2.5–5 mg/day with breakfast, may increase by 2.5 mg q1–2wk; greater than 10 mg/day should be given in divided doses (max: 20 mg/day); **Micronized** 1.5–3 mg/day (max: 12 mg/day)

## ADMINISTRATION
### Oral
- Give once daily in the morning with breakfast or with first main meal.

- Store in tightly closed, light-resistant container at 15°–30° C (59°–86° F).

## ADVERSE EFFECTS (≥1%) Metabolic: Hypoglycemia. GI: Epigastric fullness, heartburn, nausea, vomiting. Skin: Pruritus, erythema, urticarial or cholestatic jaundice (rare), morbilliform eruptions. Special Senses: Blurred vision. Body as a Whole: Weight gain.

## INTERACTIONS Drug: Alcohol causes disulfiram-like reaction in some patients; ORAL ANTICOAGULANTS, chloramphenicol, clofibrate, phenylbutazone, MAO INHIBITORS, SALICYLATES, probenecid, SULFONAMIDES, clarithromycin may potentiate hypoglycemic actions; THIAZIDES may antagonize hypoglycemic effects; cimetidine may increase glyburide levels, causing hypoglycemia. Contraindicated with bosentan. Herbal: Ginseng, garlic may increase hypoglycemic effects.

## PHARMACOKINETICS Absorption: Readily absorbed from GI tract. Onset: 15–60 min. Peak: 1–2 h. Duration: Up to 24 h. Distribution: Distributed in highest concentrations in liver, kidneys, and intestines; crosses placenta. Metabolism: Extensively in liver. Elimination: Equally in urine and feces. Half-Life: 10 h.

## NURSING IMPLICATIONS

### Assessment & Drug Effects

- Monitor blood glucose levels carefully during the dangerous early treatment period when dosage is being individualized. Older adults are especially vulnerable to glyburide-induced hypoglycemia (see Appendix F) because the antidiabetic agent is long-acting.
- Note: The first signs of hypoglycemia may be hard to detect when the patient is also receiving a beta-blocker or is an older adult.

- Monitor lab tests: Frequent fasting and postprandial blood glucose, periodic HbA1C.

### Patient & Family Education

- Eat or drink some form of sugar (e.g., corn syrup, orange juice with 2 or 3 tsp of table sugar) when symptoms of hypoglycemia occur. Report reaction to prescriber promptly.
- Remember that loss of control of diabetes may result from stress such as fever, surgery, trauma, or infection. Check blood glucose more frequently during stress periods.
- Keep all follow-up medical appointments and adhere to dietary instructions, regular exercise program, and scheduled blood testing.
- Report blurred vision to prescriber.

## GLYCERIN
(gli′ser-in)

Fleet Babylax, Glycerol, Osmoglyn

## GLYCERIN ANHYDROUS
Ophthalgan

**Classifications:** HYPEROSMOTIC LAXATIVE; ANTIGLAUCOMA

Therapeutic: HYPEROSMOTIC LAXATIVE; ANTIGLAUCOMA; OCULAR OSMOTIC DIURETIC

## AVAILABILITY Oral solution; suppositories; ophthalmic solution

## ACTION & THERAPEUTIC EFFECT

**Oral:** Glycerin raises plasma osmotic pressure by withdrawing fluid from extravascular spaces; lowers ocular tension by decreasing volume of intraocular fluid. May also reduce CSF pressure. **Ocular topic application:** Reduces edema by hydroscopic effect. **Glycerin suppositories:** Apparently work by causing dehydration of exposed tissue, which produces an irritant effect, and by absorbing water from tissues, thus creating more bowel mass. Both actions stimulate peristalsis in the large bowel. *Reduces intraocular pressure by lowering intraocular fluid. Relieves constipation by absorption of water and stimulation of peristalsis.*

**USES** Orally to reduce elevated intraocular pressure (IOP) before or after surgery in patients with acute narrow-angle glaucoma, retinal detachment, or cataract and to reduce elevated CSF pressure. Sterile glycerin (anhydrous) is used topically to reduce superficial corneal edema resulting from trauma, surgery, or disease and to facilitate ophthalmoscopic examination. Used rectally (suppository or enema) to relieve constipation.

**UNLABELED USES** To reduce mortality due to strokes in older adults.

**CONTRAINDICATIONS** Diabetic ketoacidosis; moderate or severe renal impairment (CrCl less than 50 mL/min), renal failure.

**CAUTIOUS USE** Cardiac disease; mild renal impairment; hepatic disease; diabetes mellitus; thyroid disease; dehydrated or older adults; pregnancy (category C); lactation.

## ROUTE & DOSAGE

### Decrease IOP

*Adult/Child:* **PO** 1–1.8 g/kg 1–1.5 h before ocular surgery, may repeat q5h

### Constipation

*Adult/Child (6 y or older):* **PR** Insert 1 suppository or 5–15 mL of enema high into rectum and retain for 15 min

*Child (younger than 6 y):* **PR** Insert 1 infant suppository or 2–5 mL of enema high into rectum and retain for 15 min

*Neonate:* **PR** 0.5 mL of rectal solution (enema)

### Reduction of Corneal Edema

*Adult:* **Topical** 1–2 drops instilled into eye q3–4h

## ADMINISTRATION

### Oral

- Pour oral solution over crushed ice and have patient sip through a straw.
- Prevent or relieve headache (from cerebral dehydration) by having patient lie down during and after administration of drug.

### Rectal

- Ensure that suppository is inserted beyond rectal sphincter.

## ADVERSE EFFECTS (≥1%) **CNS:** Headache, dizziness, disorientation. **CV:** Irregular heartbeat. **GI:** Nausea, vomiting, thirst, diarrhea, abdominal cramps, rectal discomfort, hyperemia of rectal mucosa. **Metabolic:** Hyperglycemia, glycosuria, dehydration, hyperosmolar nonketotic coma.

## PHARMACOKINETICS **Absorption:** Readily absorbed from GI tract after oral administration; rectal preparations are poorly absorbed. **Onset:** 10 min PO. **Peak:** 30 min–2 h. **Duration:** 4–8 h. **Metabolism:** 80% metabolized in liver; 10–20% metabolized in kidneys to $CO_2$ and water or utilized in glucose or glycogen synthesis. **Elimination:** 7–14% excreted unchanged in urine. **Half-Life:** 30–40 min.

## NURSING IMPLICATIONS
### Assessment & Drug Effects

- Consult prescriber regarding fluid intake in patients receiving drug for elevated IOP. Although

---

hypotonic fluids will relieve thirst and headache caused by the dehydrating action of glycerin, these fluids may nullify its osmotic effect.

- Monitor glycemic control in diabetics. Drug may cause hyperglycemia (see Appendix F).

**Patient & Family Education**

- Evacuation usually comes 15–30 min after administration of glycerin rectal suppository or enema.
- Note: Slight hyperglycemia and glycosuria may occur with PO use; adjustment in antidiabetic medication dosage may be required.

# GLYCOPYRROLATE

(glye-koe-pye′roe-late)

Cuvposa, Robinul, Robinul Forte

**Classifications:** ANTICHOLINERGIC; ANTIMUSCARINIC; ANTISPASMODIC
**Therapeutic:** GI ANTISPASMODIC
**Prototype:** Atropine

**AVAILABILITY** Oral solution; tablet; solution for injection

**ACTION & THERAPEUTIC EFFECT**
An anticholinergic (antimuscarinic) agent that inhibits the action of acetylcholine on smooth muscle, cardiac muscle, the SA and AV nodes, and exocrine glands (including salivary). Its effect on gastric glands diminishes the volume and acidity of gastric secretions and, in the respiratory tract, controls excessive pharyngeal, tracheal, and bronchial secretions. *Inhibits motility of GI and genitourinary tract; it also decreases volume of gastric and pancreatic secretions, saliva, and perspiration.*

**USES** Adjunctive management of peptic ulcer and other GI disorders associated with hyperacidity, hypermotility, spasm and for sialorrhea. Also used parenterally as preanesthetic and intraoperative medication and to reverse neuromuscular blockade.

**CONTRAINDICATIONS** Glaucoma; asthma; prostatic hypertrophy, obstructive uropathy; obstructive lesions or atony of GI tract; achalasia; severe ulcerative colitis; myasthenia gravis; BPH; urinary tract obstruction; during cyclopropane anesthesia.

**CAUTIOUS USE** Autonomic neuropathy, hepatic or renal disease; cardiac arrhythmias; pregnancy (category B); lactation; children.

## ROUTE & DOSAGE

**Peptic/Duodenal Ulcer**
*Adult:* **PO** 1 mg t.i.d or 2 mg b.i.d. or t.i.d. in equally divided intervals (max: 8 mg/day), then decrease to 1 mg b.i.d.; **IM/IV** 0.1–0.2 mg 3–4 × day

**Sialorrhea**
*Child/Adolescent (3 y or older):* **PO** 0.02 mg/kg t.i.d.; titrate to response (max: 0.1 mg/kg)

**Reversal of Neuromuscular Blockade**
*Adult/Child:* **IV** 0.2 mg administered with 1 mg of neostigmine or 5 mg pyridostigmine

## ADMINISTRATION

**Oral**
- Give without regard to meals.

**Intramuscular**
- Give undiluted, deep into a large muscle.

**Intravenous**
*PREPARE:* **Direct:** Give undiluted.
- Inspect for cloudiness and discoloration. Discard if present.

Common adverse effects in *italic;* life-threatening effects underlined; generic names in **bold;** classifications in SMALL CAPS; ♣ Canadian drug name; ⊘ Prototype drug

*ADMINISTER:* **Direct:** Give 0.2 mg or fraction thereof over 1–2 min.
*INCOMPATIBILITIES:* **Solution/additive:** **Methylprednisolone. Y-site: Amphotericin B, ampicillin, dantrolene, diazepam, diazoxide, fluorescein, furosemide, haloperidol, hydroxyzine, indomethacin, insulin, irinotecan, mitomycin, pantoprazole, phenytoin, pipercillin, sulfamethoxazole/ trimethoprim.**

- Store at 20°–25° C (68°–77° F).

## ADVERSE EFFECTS (≥1%) **Body as a Whole:** *Decreased sweating,* weakness. **CNS:** Dizziness, drowsiness, overdosage (<u>neuromuscular blockade</u> with curare-like action leading to muscle weakness and <u>paralysis</u> is possible). **CV:** Palpitation, tachycardia. **GI:** *Xerostomia,* constipation. **Urogenital:** *Urinary hesitancy or retention.* **Special Senses:** Blurred vision, mydriasis.

## INTERACTIONS **Drug: Amantadine,** ANTIHISTAMINES, TRICYCLIC ANTIDEPRESSANTS, **quinidine, disopyramide, procainamide** compound anticholinergic effects; decreases **levodopa** effects; **methotrimeprazine** may precipitate extrapyramidal effects; decreases antipsychotic effects (decreased absorption) of PHENOTHIAZINES.

## PHARMACOKINETICS **Absorption:** Poorly and incompletely absorbed. **Onset:** 1 min IV; 15–30 min IM/Subcutaneous; 1 h PO. **Peak:** 30–45 min IM/Subcutaneous; 1 h PO. **Duration:** 2–7 h IM/Subcutaneous; 8–12 h PO. **Distribution:** Crosses placenta. **Metabolism:** Minimally in liver. **Elimination:** 85% in urine. **Half-Life:** 30–70 min (adult), 20–99 min (child), 20–120 min (infant).

## NURSING IMPLICATIONS
### Assessment & Drug Effects
- Incidence and severity of adverse effects are generally dose related.
- Monitor I&O ratio and pattern particularly in older adults. Watch for urinary hesitancy and retention.
- Monitor vital signs, especially when drug is given parenterally. Report any changes in heart rate or rhythm.

### Patient & Family Education
- Avoid high environmental temperatures (heat prostration can occur because of decreased sweating).
- Do not drive or engage in other potentially hazardous activities requiring mental alertness until response to drug is known.
- Use good oral hygiene, rinse mouth with water frequently and use a saliva substitute to lessen effects of dry mouth.

## GOLD SODIUM THIOMALATE
(thye-oh-mah′late)
Myochrysine ♦
**Classifications:** BIOLOGICAL RESPONSE MODIFIER; IMMUNOMODULATOR; DISEASE-MODIFYING ANTIRHEUMATIC DRUG (DMARD)
**Therapeutic:** ANTIRHEUMATIC; GOLD COMPOUND
**Prototype:** Auranofin

## AVAILABILITY Solution for injection

## ACTION & *THERAPEUTIC EFFECT*
Mechanism of action is unknown. Appears to act by suppression of phagocytosis, altered immune responses, and possibly by inhibition of prostaglandin synthesis. *Has immunomodulatory and anti-inflammatory effects.*

## USES Selected patients (adults and juveniles) with acute rheumatoid arthritis.

---

Common adverse effects in *italic;* life-threatening effects <u>underlined;</u> generic names in **bold;** classifications in SMALL CAPS; ♦ Canadian drug name; ⊙ Prototype drug

759

**UNLABELED USES** Psoriatic arthritis, Felty's syndrome.

**CONTRAINDICATIONS** History of severe toxicity from previous exposure to gold or other heavy metals; severe debilitation; SLE, Sjögren's syndrome in rheumatoid arthritis; renal disease; hepatic dysfunction, history of infectious hepatitis; uncontrolled diabetes or CHF.

**CAUTIOUS USE** History of drug allergies or hypersensitivity; marked hypertension; history of blood dyscrasias such as granulocytopenia or anemia caused by drug sensitivity; CHF; diabetes mellitus; previous kidney or liver disease; colitis, IBD; compromised cerebral or cardiovascular circulation; pregnancy (category C); children.

## ROUTE & DOSAGE

### Rheumatoid Arthritis

*Adult:* **IM** 10 mg wk 1, 25 mg wk 2, then 25–50 mg/wk to a cumulative dose of 1 g (if improvement occurs, continue at 25–50 mg q2wk for 2–20 wk, then q3–4wk indefinitely or until adverse effects occur)
*Child:* **IM** 10 mg test dose, then 1 mg/kg/wk or 2.5–5 mg for wk 1 and 2, followed by 1 mg/kg q1–4wk (max single dose: 50 mg)

## ADMINISTRATION

**Intramuscular**

- Agitate vial before withdrawing dose to ensure uniform suspension.
- Give deep into upper outer quadrant of gluteus maximus with patient lying down. Patient should remain recumbent for at least 15 min after injection because of the danger of "nitritoid reaction" (transient giddiness, vertigo, facial flushing, fainting).

- Observe for allergic reactions.
- Store in tight, light-resistant containers at 15°–30° C (59°–86° F). Do not use if any darker than pale yellow.

**ADVERSE EFFECTS** (≥1%) **CNS:** Dizziness, syncope, sweating, flushing. **CV:** Bradycardia. **GI:** Hepatitis, metallic taste, *stomatitis,* nausea, vomiting. **Hematologic:** Agranulocytosis, aplastic anemia, eosinophilia (all rare). **Urogenital:** Nephrotic syndrome, glomerulitis with hematuria, *proteinuria.* **Skin:** Transient pruritus, *erythema, dermatitis,* fixed drug eruption, alopecia, shedding of nails, gray to blue pigmentation of skin (chrysiasis). **Special Senses:** Gold deposits in ocular tissues, *photosensitivity.* **Body as a Whole:** Peripheral neuritis, angioneurotic edema, interstitial pneumonitis, anaphylaxis (rare). **Respiratory:** Pulmonary fibrosis.

**INTERACTIONS Drug:** ANTIMALARIALS, IMMUNOSUPPRESSANTS, **penicillamine, phenylbutazone** increased risk of blood dyscrasias.

**PHARMACOKINETICS Absorption:** Slowly and irregularly absorbed from IM site. **Peak:** 3–6 h. **Distribution:** Widely distributed, especially to synovial fluid, kidney, liver, and spleen; does not cross blood–brain barrier; crosses placenta. **Metabolism:** Not studied. **Elimination:** 60–90% of dose ultimately excreted in urine; also eliminated in feces; traces may be found in urine for 6 mo. **Half-Life:** 3–168 days.

**NURSING IMPLICATIONS**

### Black Box Warning

*Gold sodium thiomalate has been associated with severe and potentially fatal adverse reactions.*

Common adverse effects in *italic*; life-threatening effects <u>underlined</u>; generic names in **bold**; classifications in SMALL CAPS; ♣ Canadian drug name; ❻ Prototype drug

## Assessment & Drug Effects

- Note: Rapid reduction in hemoglobin level, WBC count below 4000/mm$^3$, eosinophil count above 5%, and platelet count below 100,000/mm$^3$ signify possible toxicity.
- Interview and examine patient before each injection to detect occurrence of transient pruritus or dermatitis (both are common early indications of toxicity), stomatitis (sore tongue, palate, or throat), metallic taste, indigestion, or other signs and symptoms of possible toxicity. Interrupt treatment immediately and notify prescriber if any of these reactions occurs.
- Observe for allergic reaction, which may occur almost immediately after injection, 10 min after injection, or at any time during therapy. Withhold drug and notify prescriber if observed. Keep antidote dimercaprol (BAL) on hand during time of injection.
- Monitor lab tests: Prior to each injection, urinalysis for protein, blood, and sediment. Baseline Hgb and RBC, WBC count with differential, and platelet count before initiation of therapy and at regular intervals.

## Patient & Family Education

- Therapeutic effects may not appear until after 2 mo of therapy.
- Notify prescriber of rapid improvement in joint swelling; this is indicative that you are closely approaching drug tolerance level.
- Use protective measures in sunlight. Exposure to sunlight may aggravate gold dermatitis.
- Notify prescriber at the appearance of unexplained skin bruising; this is always an indication for doing a platelet count.
- Know possible adverse reactions and report any symptom suggestive of toxicity immediately to prescriber.

# GOLIMUMAB
(go-li-mu'mab)

**Simponi, Simponi Aria**

**Classifications:** MONOCLONAL ANTIBODY; IMMUNOLOGIC; IMMUNODULATOR; TUMOR NECROSIS FACTOR (TNF) MODIFIER; DISEASE-MODIFYING ANTIRHEUMATIC DRUG (DMARD)

**Therapeutic:** IMMUNOMODULATOR; ANTIRHEUMATIC (DMARD); ANTIPSORIATIC

**Prototype:** Etanercept

**AVAILABILITY** Solution for injection

## ACTION & *THERAPEUTIC EFFECT*

A monoclonal antibody that binds to TNF-alpha, thus preventing it from binding to its receptors. TNF is a cytokine that plays an important role in the immune and inflammatory responses. Elevated levels of TNF are found in the synovial fluids, joints, and blood of rheumatoid arthritis (RA) patients. *Effectiveness is indicated by improved RA symtomatology and/or decreased inflammation in other inflammatory disorders.*

**USES** Treatment of moderately to severely active rheumatoid arthritis, active ankylosing spondylitis, active psoriatic arthritis and ulcerative colitis.

**CONTRAINDICATIONS** Hypersensitivity to golimumab; <u>serious infection or sepsis</u>; live vaccines; agranulocytosis; lactation.

**CAUTIOUS USE** History of hepatitis B; history of TB or opportunistic infection; chronic or recurrent infections; history of HBV infection or carriers of HBV; malignancy; CHF; central or peripheral demyelization disorders, MS; cytopenias; older adults; pregnancy (category B). Safe use in children not established.

Common adverse effects in *italic;* life-threatening effects <u>underlined;</u> generic names in **bold;** classifications in SMALL CAPS; ♣ Canadian drug name; ☻ Prototype drug

761

## ROUTE & DOSAGE

### Rheumatoid Arthritis/Anklyosing Spondylitis/Psoriatic Arthritis

*Adult:* **Subcutaneous** 50 mg qmo;
**IV (Simponi Aria)** 2 mg/kg then
repeat at 4 wk and then q8 wk

### Ulcerative Colitis

*Adult:* **Subcutaneous** 200 mg then
100 mg 2 wk later for induction,
then 100 mg q4wk (starting
week 6)

### Rheumatoid Arthritis (Simponi Aria)

*Adult:* **IV** 2 mg/kg, repeat at 4 wk
then q8wk

## ADMINISTRATION

### Subcutaneous

- Allow prefilled syringe/autoinjector to come to room temperature for 30 min prior to injection. Do not warm any other way.
- Do not shake the autoinjector at any time. After injection, do not pull autoinjector away from skin until a second click sound (3–15 sec after the first sound) is heard.
- Rotate injection sites. Do not inject into areas that are tender, bruised, red, or hard.
- Do not initiate treatment in anyone with an active infection.

### Intravenous

*PREPARE:* **IV Infusion:** Dilute required volume of golimumab in NS to a final volume of 100 mL. Mix gently, do not shake. Diluted solution may be stored at room temperature for 4 h.
*ADMINISTER:* **IV Infusion:** Give over 30 min through a nonpyrogenic, low-protein-binding filter, pore size 0.22 micrometer or less.
*INCOMPATIBILITIES:* Do not infuse in same IV line with other agents.

- Store refrigerated at 2°–8° C (36°–46° F) and protect from light by keeping in carton until use.

**ADVERSE EFFECTS** (≥1%) **Body as a Whole:** Influenza, infection, injection site erythema. **CNS:** Dizziness, pyrexia. **CV:** Hypertension. **GI:** Oral herpes, constipation. **Metabolic:** Elevated ALT and AST levels. **Respiratory:** Bronchitis, *nasopharyngitis,* sinusitis, *upper respiratory tract infection.* **Skin:** Paraesthesia.

**INTERACTIONS Drug: Abatacept, anakinra** and other TNF-ALPHA BLOCKERS may increase the risk of serious infection.

**PHARMACOKINETICS Peak:** 2–6 days. **Half-Life:** 2 wk.

## NURSING IMPLICATIONS

### Black Box Warning

*Golimumab has been associated with severe, potentially fatal, infections, and development of malignancies in children and adolescents.*

### Assessment & Drug Effects

- Monitor closely for S&S of infection.
- Withhold drug and notify prescriber if symptoms of an infection develop.
- Monitor for and report new-onset and exacerbations of psoriasis.
- Monitor lab tests: Baseline and periodic TB tests, periodic LFTs.

### Patient & Family Education

- Contact prescriber immediately for any of the following: Symptoms of infection; jaundice; extreme fatigue; poor appetite or vomiting; or pain in the upper, right abdomen.
- If a case of pre-existing psoriasis worsens or if a new rash develops, contact prescriber.

## GOSERELIN ACETATE

(gos-er'e-lin)

Common adverse effects in *italic;* life-threatening effects <u>underlined;</u> generic names in **bold;** classifications in SMALL CAPS; ♣ Canadian drug name; ⊙ Prototype drug

GOSERELIN ACETATE

Zoladex
**Classification:** ANTINEOPLASTIC; GONADOTROPIN-RELEASING HORMONE (GnRH) ANALOG
**Therapeutic:** ANTINEOPLASTIC; GnRH ANALOG
**Prototype:** Leuprolide

**AVAILABILITY** Subcutaneous implant

**ACTION & THERAPEUTIC EFFECT**
A synthetic form of luteinizing hormone-releasing hormone (LHRH or GnRH) that inhibits pituitary gonadotropin secretion. *With chronic administration, serum testosterone levels in males fall into the range normally seen with surgically castrated men.*

**USES** Prostate cancer, breast cancer. Endometrial thinning agent prior to endometrial ablation for dysfunctional uterine bleeding, endometriosis, prevention of early menopause during chemotherapy.

**UNLABELED USES** Benign prostatic hyperplasia, uterine leiomyomas, prevention of early menopause during chemotherapy.

**CONTRAINDICATIONS** Known hypersensitivity to an LHRH, hypercalcemia; pregnancy (category X for endometriosis, endometrial thinning, category D for breast cancer); lactation.

**CAUTIOUS USE** Renal impairment; family history of osteoporosis; osteoporosis; prostate cancer; patients at risk for spinal cord compression; DM; CVD; obesity; low BMI. Safety and efficacy in children not established.

**ROUTE & DOSAGE**

**Prostate Cancer, Breast Cancer, Endometriosis**
*Adult:* **Subcutaneous** 3.6 mg q28days, 10.8 mg depot q12wk

**Endometrial Thinning Prior to Endometrial Ablation**
*Adult:* **Subcutaneous** 3.6 mg (procedure performed 4 wk after administration) if second injection required then surgery performed 2–4 wk after that dose

**ADMINISTRATION**
**Subcutaneous**
- Follow manufacturer's directions exactly for implanting the drug subcutaneously in the upper abdominal wall.
- Store at room temperature not to exceed 25° C (77° F).

**ADVERSE EFFECTS** (≥1%) **CNS:** Headache, tumor flare, depression, insomnia. **Endocrine:** Gynecomastia, breast swelling and tenderness, *postmenopausal symptoms* (*hot flashes*, vaginal dryness). **GI:** Nausea. **Skin:** *Acne, diaphoresis, seborrhea.* **Urogenital:** Vaginal spotting, breakthrough bleeding, decreased libido, *impotence.* **Musculoskeletal:** Bone pain, bone loss **CV:** Increased risk of MI (men only), *peripheral edema, vasodilation.*

**DIAGNOSTIC TEST INTERFERENCE** Interferes with pituitary gonadotropic and gonadal function tests during and for 12 wk after treatment.

**PHARMACOKINETICS Absorption:** Rapidly absorbed following subcutaneous administration. **Duration:** 29 days. **Elimination:** Excreted by kidneys. **Half-Life:** 4.9 h.

**NURSING IMPLICATIONS**
**Assessment & Drug Effects**
- Monitor carefully during the first month of therapy for S&S of spinal cord compression or ureteral obstruction in patients with prostate cancer. Report immediately to prescriber.

- Anticipate a transient worsening of symptoms (e.g., bone pain) during the first weeks of therapy in patients with prostate cancer.
- Monitor lab tests: Periodic fasting blood glucose.

**Patient & Family Education**
- Note: Sexual dysfunction in men and hot flashes may accompany drug use.
- Notify prescriber immediately of symptoms of spinal cord compression or urinary obstruction.

# GRANISETRON
(gran'i-se-tron)
Sancuso, Sustol
**Classifications:** ANTIEMETIC; 5-HT$_3$ ANTAGONIST
Therapeutic: ANTIEMETIC
**Prototype:** Ondansetron

**AVAILABILITY** Tablet; solution for injection; oral solution; transdermal patch; extended release injection

**ACTION & THERAPEUTIC EFFECT** Granisetron is a selective serotonin (5-HT$_3$) receptor antagonist. Serotonin receptors of the 5-HT$_3$ type are located centrally in the chemoreceptor trigger zone, and peripherally on the vagal nerve terminals. Serotonin released from the wall of the small intestine stimulates these vagal afferent neurons through the serotonin receptors, and initiates vomiting reflex. *Effective in preventing nausea and vomiting associated with cancer chemotherapy.*

**USES** Chemotherapy-induced nausea/vomiting treatment and prophylaxis; radiation-induced nausea/vomiting prophylaxis.

**CONTRAINDICATIONS** Hypersensitivity to granisetron, or benzyl alcohol; GI obstruction; neonates.

**CAUTIOUS USE** Hypersensitivity to ondansetron or similar drugs;

liver disease; patients with long QT interval; pregnancy (category B); lactation; children 2 y or younger.

## ROUTE & DOSAGE

**Chemotherapy-Related Nausea and Vomiting**

*Adult/Child (2 y or older):* **IV** 10 mcg/kg, beginning at least 30 min before initiation of chemotherapy (up to 40 mcg/kg/dose has been used); **PO** 1 mg b.i.d., start 1 mg up to 1 h prior to chemotherapy, then second tab 12 h later OR 2 mg daily

*Adult:* **Transdermal** Apply 1 patch q5days

**Radiation-Induced Nasuea/Vomiting**

*Adult:* **PO** 2 mg dose within 1 h of radiation

**Renal Impairment Dosage Adjustment**

*Crl Cl 30–59 mL/min:* **Extended release injection** Do not administer more frequently than every 14 days

## ADMINISTRATION
**Oral**
- Give only on the day of chemotherapy. one hour prior to chemotherapy.

**Transdermal**
- Apply patch to upper outer arm 24–48 h before start of chemotherapy.
- Remove patch no sooner than 24 h after completion of chemotherapy.
- Patch may be left in place for up to 7 days.

**Intravenous**

**PREPARE: Direct:** Give undiluted. **IV Infusion:** Dilute in NS or D5W to a total volume of 20–50 mL.
- Prepare infusion at time of

administration; do not mix in solution with other drugs.

***ADMINISTER:* Direct:** Give a single dose over 30 sec. **IV Infusion:** Infuse diluted drug over 5 min or longer; complete infusion 20–30 min prior to initiation of chemotherapy.

***INCOMPATIBILITIES:* Y-site:** **Amphotericin B, dantrolene sodium, diazepam, gemtuzumab ozogamcin, lansprazone, phenytoin sodium.**

• Store at 15°–30° C (59°–86° F) for 24 h after dilution under normal lighting conditions.

## ADVERSE EFFECTS (≥1%) CNS:
*Headache,* dizziness, *somnolence,* insomnia, labile mood, anxiety, fatigue. **GI:** *Constipation,* nausea, diarrhea, elevated liver function tests. **Body as a Whole:** Injection site reaction.

## INTERACTIONS Drug: Ketoconazole
may inhibit metabolism. Contraindicated with medications that prolong the QT interval (e.g., **bepridil, dofetilide, fluconazole**).

## PHARMACOKINETICS  Onset:
Several minutes. **Duration:** Approximately 24 h. **Distribution:** Widely distributed in body tissues. **Metabolism:** Appears to be metabolized in liver. **Elimination:** Excreted in urine as metabolites. **Half-Life:** 10–11 h in cancer patients, 4–5 h in healthy volunteers.

## NURSING IMPLICATIONS
### Assessment & Drug Effects
• Monitor the frequency and severity of nausea and vomiting.
• Monitor for constipation and for decreased bowel activity.
• Assess for headache, which usually responds to nonnarcotic analgesics.
• Monitor lab tests: Periodic LFTs.

### Patient & Family Education
• Note: Headache requiring an analgesic for relief is a common adverse effect.
• Learn ways to manage constipation.

## GRISEOFULVIN MICROSIZE
(gri-see-oh-ful′vin)
Fulvicin-U/F, Grifulvin V, Grisactin, Grisovin-FP ♣

## GRISEOFULVIN ULTRAMICROSIZE
Fulvicin P/G, Grisactin Ultra, Gris-PEG
**Classification:** ANTIFUNGAL ANTIBIOTIC
Therapeutic: ANTIFUNGAL

## AVAILABILITY  Griseofulvin Microsize:
Tablet; capsule; suspension. **Griseofulvin Ultramicrosize:** Tablet

## ACTION & *THERAPEUTIC EFFECT*
Arrests metaphase of cell division by disrupting mitotic spindle structure in fungal cells. Deposits in keratin precursor cells and has special affinity for diseased tissue. It is tightly bound to new keratin of skin, hair, and nails that becomes highly resistant to fungal invasion. *Effective against various species of* Epidermophyton, Microsporum, *and* Trichophyton *(has no effect on other fungi, including* Candida, *bacteria, and yeasts).*

## USES Mycotic disease of skin, hair,
and nails not amenable to conventional topical measures. Concomitant use of appropriate topical agent may be required, particularly for tinea pedis.

## UNLABELED USES Raynaud's disease,
angina pectoris, and gout.

---

**CONTRAINDICATIONS** Hypersensitivity to griseofulvin; porphyria; hepatocellular failure; SLE; serious skin reaction to drug; pregnancy (X); lactation, prophylaxis against fungal infections.

**CAUTIOUS USE** Penicillin-sensitive patients (possibility if cross-sensitivity with penicillin exists; however, reportedly penicillin-sensitive patients have been treated without difficulty); hepatic impairment; children 2 y or younger.

## ROUTE & DOSAGE

**Tinea Corporis, Tinea Cruris, Tinea Capitis**

*Adult:* **PO** 500 mg microsize or 330–375 mg ultramicrosize daily in single or divided doses
*Child:* **PO** 10–20 mg/kg/day microsize or 5–10 mg/kg/day ultramicrosize in single or divided doses

**Tinea Pedis, Tinea Unguium**

*Adult:* **PO** 0.75–1 g microsize or 660–750 mg ultramicrosize daily in single or divided doses (decrease microsize dose to 500 mg/day after response is noted)
*Child:* **PO** 10–20 mg/kg/day microsize or 5–10 mg/kg/day ultramicrosize in single or divided doses

## ADMINISTRATION

### Oral

- Give with or after meals to allay GI disturbances.
- Give the microsize formulations with a high fat content meal (increases drug absorption rate) to enhance serum levels. Consult prescriber.
- Store at 15°–30° C (59°–86° F) in tightly covered containers unless otherwise directed.

**ADVERSE EFFECTS** (≥1%) **Body as a Whole:** Hypersensitivity (urticaria, photosensitivity, skin rashes, Stevens–Johnson syndrome, pruritus, fixed drug eruption, serum sickness syndromes, severe angioedema). **CNS:** *Severe headache,* insomnia, fatigue, mental confusion, impaired performance of routine functions, psychotic symptoms, vertigo. **GI:** Heartburn, nausea, vomiting, diarrhea, flatulence, dry mouth, thirst, decreased taste acuity, anorexia, unpleasant taste, furred tongue, oral thrush. **Hematologic:** <u>Leukopenia</u>, neutropenia, granulocytopenia, punctate basophilia, monocytosis. **Urogenital:** Nephrotoxicity (proteinuria); hepatotoxicity; estrogen-like effects (in children); aggravation of SLE. **Other:** Overgrowth of nonsusceptible organisms; candidal intertrigo.

**INTERACTIONS Drug: Alcohol** may cause flushing and tachycardia; BARBITURATES may decrease activity of griseofulvin; may decrease hypoprothrombinemic effects of ORAL ANTICOAGULANTS; may increase **estrogen** metabolism, resulting in breakthrough bleeding, and decrease contraceptive efficacy of ORAL CONTRACEPTIVES.

**PHARMACOKINETICS Absorption:** Absorbed primarily from duodenum; microsize is variably and unpredictably absorbed; ultramicrosize is almost completely absorbed. **Peak:** 4–8 h. **Distribution:** Concentrates in skin, hair, nails, fat, and skeletal muscle; crosses placenta. **Metabolism:** In liver. **Elimination:** Mainly in urine; some excretion in perspiration. **Half-Life:** 9–24 h.

## NURSING IMPLICATIONS

### Assessment & Drug Effects

- Inquire about history of sensitivity to griseofulvin, penicillins, or other allergies prior to initiating treatment.

Common adverse effects in *italic;* life-threatening effects <u>underlined;</u> generic names in **bold;** classifications in SMALL CAPS; ♣ Canadian drug name; ⊙ Prototype drug

- Monitor food intake. Drug may alter taste sensations, and this may cause appetite suppression and inadequate nutrient intake.
- Monitor lab tests: WBC with differential at least once weekly during first month of therapy; periodic renal function tests and LFTs.

### Patient & Family Education
- Continuing treatment as prescribed to prevent relapse, even if you experience symptomatic relief after 48–96 h of therapy.
- Note: Duration of treatment depends on time required to replace infected skin, hair, or nails, and thus varies with infection site. Average duration of treatment for tinea capitis (scalp ringworm), 4–6 wk; tinea corporis (body ringworm), 2–4 wk, tinea pedis (athlete's foot), 4–8 wk; tinea unguium (nail fungus), at least 4 mo for fingernails, depending on rate of growth, and 6 mo or more for toenails.
- Avoid exposure to intense natural or artificial sunlight, because photosensitivity-type reactions may occur.
- Note: Headaches often occur during early therapy but frequently disappear with continued drug administration.
- Avoid alcohol while taking this drug. Disulfiram-type reaction (see Appendix F) are possible with ingestion of alcohol during therapy.
- Pharmacologic effects of oral contraceptives may be reduced. Breakthrough bleeding and pregnancy may occur. Alternative forms of birth control should be used during therapy.

# GUAIFENESIN ℗
(gwye-fen'e-sin)
Anti-Tuss, GG-Cen, Glyceryl Guaiacolate, Glycotuss, Glytuss, Guiatuss, Humibid, Hytuss, Malotuss, Mytussin, Mucinex, Resyl ✦, Robitussin

**Classification:** EXPECTORANT
Therapeutic: EXPECTORANT

**AVAILABILITY** Syrup; oral liquid; tablet; sustained release tablet

## ACTION & *THERAPEUTIC EFFECT*
Reduces viscosity of respiratory secretions and increases sputum volume, thus increasing the efficiency of the cough reflex and of ciliary action in removing accumulated secretions from the trachea and bronchi. *Increases respiratory tract fluid secretions and helps to loosen phlegm and bronchial secretions.*

**USES** To combat dry, nonproductive cough associated with colds and bronchitis. A common ingredient in cough mixtures.

**CONTRAINDICATIONS** Hypersensitivity to guaifenesin; cough due to CHF, ACE inhibitor therapy, or tobacco smoking.

**CAUTIOUS USE** Chronic cough; asthma; pregnancy (category C); lactation; children younger than 6 y.

## ROUTE & DOSAGE

| Cough |
|---|
| *Adult/Adolescent:* **PO Immediate release** 200–400 mg q4h up to 2.4 g/day; **Extended release** 600–1200 mg q12h up to 2.4 g/day |
| *Child (6–11 y):* **PO** 100–200 mg q4h up to 1.2 g/day or **Extended release** 600 mg q12h |
| *Child (2–5 y):* **PO Immediate release** 50–100 mg q4h; **PO Extended release** 300 mg q12h |

---

## ADMINISTRATION

### Oral

- Ensure that sustained release form of drug is not chewed or crushed. It **must be** swallowed whole.
- Follow dose with a full glass of water if not contraindicated.
- Carefully observe maximum daily doses for adults and children.

## ADVERSE EFFECTS (≥1%) GI: Low incidence of nausea. CNS: Drowsiness.

## DIAGNOSTIC TEST INTERFERENCE

May produce color interference with determinations of *urinary 5-hydroxyindoleacetic acid (5-HIAA)* and *vanillylmandelic acid (VMA).*

## PHARMACOKINETICS Absorption: Well absorbed. Elimination: In urine

## NURSING IMPLICATIONS

### Assessment & Drug Effects

- Monitor for therapeutic effectiveness. Persistent cough may indicate a serious condition requiring further diagnostic work.
- Notify prescriber if high fever, rash, or headaches develop.

### Patient & Family Education

- Increase fluid intake to help loosen mucus; drink at least 8 glasses of fluid daily.
- Contact prescriber if cough persists beyond 1 wk.
- Contact prescriber if high fever, rash, or headache develops.

## GUANFACINE HYDROCHLORIDE

(gwahn'fa-seen)

**Intuniv, Tenex**

**Classifications:** ALPHA-ADRENERGIC AGONIST; CENTRAL-ACTING ANTIHYPERTENSIVE

**Therapeutic:** ANTIHYPERTENSIVE

**Prototype:** Methyldopa

## AVAILABILITY Tablet; extended release tablet

## ACTION & *THERAPEUTIC EFFECT*

In cerebral cortex, stimulation of alpha$_2$-adrenoreceptors triggers inhibitory neurons to reduce central sympathetic outflow (i.e., impulses from vasomotor center to heart and blood vessels). **Extended release form:** Targets ADHD symptoms through central alpha$_2$-receptor activity in the prefrontal cortex. *Results in decreased peripheral vascular resistance, thus lowering blood pressure, and a slightly reduced (5 bpm) heart rate. Minimizes the signs and symptoms of ADHD in children.*

## USES Management of mild-to-moderate hypertension; attention deficit hyperactivity disorder (ADHD) (**extended release form** only).

## UNLABELED USES Adjunct in heroin withdrawal; Tourette's syndrome.

## CONTRAINDICATIONS Hypersensitivity to guanfacine; treatment of acute hypertension associated with toxemia of pregnancy; psychiatric disorders that mimic ADHD.

## CAUTIOUS USE Severe coronary insufficiency, recent MI, cerebrovascular disease; chronic renal or hepatic failure; older adult; pregnancy (category B); lactation; children younger than 6 y (**extended release form**).

## ROUTE & DOSAGE

### Hypertension

*Adult:* **PO** 1 mg/day at bedtime, may be gradually increased to 3 mg/day if needed

### Attention Deficit Hyperactivity Disorder

*Adolescent/Child (6 y or older):* **PO** Extended release 1 mg daily,

Common adverse effects in *italic;* life-threatening effects <u>underlined;</u> generic names in **bold;** classifications in SMALL CAPS; ♣ Canadian drug name; ⊙ Prototype drug

titrate up based on response
(normal range: 1–4 mg daily)

## ADMINISTRATION
### Oral
- Ensure that extended release tablets are swallowed whole and not crushed or chewed.
- Usually given as a single dose at bedtime to reduce effect of somnolence.
- Discontinue treatment gradually with planned tapering of schedule.
- Store tablets at 15°–30° C (59°–86° F) in tightly closed container; protect from light.

## ADVERSE EFFECTS (≥1%) CNS:
Confusion, amnesia, mental depression, drowsiness, *dizziness*, *sedation*, headache, asthenia, *fatigue*, insomnia, nightmares. **CV:** Bradycardia, palpitation, substernal pain, arrhythmia exacerbation. **Special Senses:** Rhinitis, tinnitus, taste change; vision disturbances, conjunctivitis, iritis. **GI:** *Dry mouth*, *constipation*, abdominal pain, diarrhea, dysphagia, nausea. **Respiratory:** Bronchospasm. **Urogenital:** *Impotence*, testicular disorder, urinary incontinence. **Musculoskeletal:** Leg cramps, hypokinesia. **Skin:** Dermatitis, pruritus, purpura, sweating. **Other:** Dyspnea.

## INTERACTIONS Drug: Alcohol
and other CNS DEPRESSANTS compound sedation and CNS depression. May increase **valproic acid** levels. Use cautiously with MAO INHIBITORS or CYP3A4 INHIBITORS or INDUCERS. **Conivaptan** can cause increased hypotension.

## PHARMACOKINETICS Absorption:
Readily absorbed from GI tract; 70% protein bound. **Onset:** 2 h; 6 h (extended release). **Peak:** 6 h. **Duration:** Up to 24 h. **Distribution:** Crosses placenta. **Metabolism:** In liver. **Elimination:** 80% ActHIB, Hiberix, Liquid PedvaxHIB in the urine in 24 h. **Half-Life:** 17 h.

## NURSING IMPLICATIONS
### Assessment & Drug Effects
- Do not discontinue abruptly; may cause plasma and urinary catecholamine increases leading to symptoms of tachycardia, insomnia, anxiety, nervousness. Rebound hypertension (i.e., increases in BP to levels significantly greater than those before therapy) may occur 2–7 days after abrupt drug withdrawal, but serious effects rarely develop.
- Monitor BP until it is stabilized. Report a rise in pressure that occurs toward end of dose interval; a divided dose schedule may be ordered.
- Assess mental status and alertness. Adverse effects tend to be dose dependent, increasing significantly with doses above 3 mg/day.

### Patient & Family Education
- Continue drug even after you feel well. This is a maintenance dosage regimen (dose and dose intervals). If 2 or more doses are missed, consult prescriber about how to reestablish dosage regimen.
- Employ measures to keep mouth moist; saliva substitutes (e.g., Moi-Stir, Xero-Lube) are available OTC. If dry mouth persists longer than 2 wk, patient should check with dentist.
- Do not drive or engage in other potentially hazardous tasks requiring alertness until response to drug is known.
- Avoid alcohol and do not self-medicate with OTC drugs such as sleeping medications, or cough medications without consulting prescriber.

Common adverse effects in *italic*; life-threatening effects underlined; generic names in **bold**; classifications in SMALL CAPS; ♣ Canadian drug name; ● Prototype drug

769

# GUSELKUMAB
(gue-sel-koo'mab)
Tremfya

**Classifications:** ANTIPSORIATIC AGENT; MONOCLONAL ANTIBODY; INTERLEU-KIN-23 INHIBITOR
Therapeutic: ANTIPSORIATIC

**AVAILABILITY** Subcutaneous injection, prefilled syringe

**ACTION & *THERAPEUTIC EFFECT***
Human monoclonal IgG1 antibody that selectively binds with interleukin-23 receptor to inhibit the release of proinflammatory cytokines and chemokines. *Reduces inflammatory response in adults with moderate to severe plaque psoriasis.*

**USES** Treatment of moderate to severe plaque psoriasis in patients who are candidates for systemic therapy or phototherapy.

**CAUTIOUS USE** Pregnancy; lactation. Safety and efficacy in children not established.

**ROUTE & DOSAGE**

**Psoriasis**

*Adult:* **Subcutaneous** 100 mg at wk 0, 4, and then every 8 wk thereafter

**ADMINISTRATION**

**Subcutaneous**
- Allow prefilled syringe to reach room temperature for approximately 30 min prior to use.
- Administer subcutaneously into the thigh, abdomen more than 2 in from umbilicus, or outer upper arm.
- Do not inject into tissue that is tender, bruised, red, hard, scaly, or affected by psoriasis.

**ADVERSE EFFECTS** (≥ 2%)
**Body as a Whole:** *Infection.* **CNS:**
Headache. **GI:** Diarrhea, gastroenteritis. **Hepatic:** Increased liver enzymes. **Integumentary:** Tinea, injection site reaction. **Muscular:** Arthralgia. **Respiratory:** *URI.* **Immunologic:** Antibody development, herpes simplex infection.

**INTERACTIONS: Drug:** Avoid use of live vaccines in patients treated with guselkumab. Potential interaction for drugs metabolized by CYP450 enzymes, however no specific medications identified in clinical studies.

**PHARMACOKINETICS Absorption:** 49% bioavailability. **Onset:** Peak in 5.5 days. **Metabolism:** Similar to endogenous IgG. **Half-Life:** 15–18 days.

**NURSING IMPLICATIONS**

**Assessment & Drug Effects**
- Evaluate for tuberculosis infection prior to treatment.
- Monitor for signs of infection including active tuberculosis.

**Patient & Family Education**
- Notify prescriber if you experience signs or symptoms of allergic reaction such as rash, hives, itching, shortness of breath, wheezing, cough, swelling of the face, lips, tongue, or throat; or any other signs.
- Prior to initiating treatment, notify prescriber if you have active TB.

# HAEMOPHILUS b CONJUGATE VACCINE (Hib)
(hee-mof'il-us)
ActHIB, Hiberix, PedvaxHIB
**See Appendix J.**

# HALCINONIDE
(hal-sin'oh-nide)
Halog

**Classifications:** ANTI-INFLAM-
MATORY; FLUORINATED STEROID
Therapeutic: ANTI-INFLAMMATORY
**Prototype:** Hydrocortisone

**AVAILABILITY** Ointment; cream;
solution

**ACTION & *THERAPEUTIC EFFECT***
Fluorinated steroid with substituted
17-hydroxyl group. Crosses cell
membranes, complexes with nuclear
DNA and stimulates synthesis of enzymes thought to be responsible for
anti-inflammatory effects. *Exhibits
anti-inflammatory, antipyretic, and
vasocontrictive properties*.

**USES** Relief of pruritic and inflammatory manifestations of corticosteroid-responsive dermatoses.

**CONTRAINDICATIONS** Use on
large body surface area; long-term
use; infection; acne vulgaris, acne
rosacea, perioral dermatitis.

**CAUTIOUS USE** Hypersensitivity
to corticosteroids; diabetes mellitus; older adults; skin abrasion,
pregnancy (category C); lactation.

## ROUTE & DOSAGE

**Inflammation**

*Adult:* **Topical** Apply thin layer
b.i.d. or t.i.d.
*Child:* **Topical** Apply thin layer
once/day

## ADMINISTRATION

### Topical
- Wash skin gently and dry thor
oughly before each application.
- Note: Ointment is preferred for
dry scaly lesions. Moist lesions are
best treated with solution.
- Do not apply in or around the eyes.
- Do not apply occlusive dressings
over areas covered with halci-

nonide unless specifically prescribed.
- Store at 15°–30° C (59°–86° F).

**ADVERSE EFFECTS** (≥1%) **Endocrine:** Reversible HPA axis suppression, hyperglycemia, glycosuria.
**Skin:** Burning, itching, irritation,
erythema, dryness, folliculitis, hypertrichosis, pruritus, acneiform
eruptions, hypopigmentation, perioral dermatitis, allergic contact dermatitis, stinging cracking/tightness
of skin, secondary infection, skin atrophy, striae, miliaria, telangiectasia.

**PHARMACOKINETICS** **Absorption:** Minimum through intact skin;
increased from axilla, eyelid, face,
scalp, scrotum, or with occlusive
dressing.

## NURSING IMPLICATIONS

### Assessment & Drug Effects
- Discontinue if signs of infection
or irritation occur.
- Monitor for systemic corticosteroid effects that may occur with
occlusive dressings or topical applications over large areas of skin.

### Patient & Family Education
- Do not use an occlusive dressing
with this drug unless specifically
directed to do so by prescriber.
- Wash your hands before and after
applying this topical medicine.
- Do not get any of the medication
in your eyes. If you do, rinse it out
with plenty of cool tap water.

## HALOPERIDOL ⏵
(ha-loe-per′i-dole)
Haldol, Peridol ♦

## HALOPERIDOL DECANOATE
Haldol LA

**Classification:** ANTIPSYCHOTIC;
BUTYROPHENONE
Therapeutic: ANTIPSYCHOTIC

Common adverse effects in *italic*; life-threatening effects underlined; generic names
in **bold**; classifications in SMALL CAPS; ♦ Canadian drug name; ⏵ Prototype drug
771

# HALOPERIDOL

**AVAILABILITY** Tablet; oral solution; solution for injection

## ACTION & *THERAPEUTIC EFFECT*
Blocks postsynaptic dopamine (D$_2$) receptors in the limbic system of the brain. Decrease in dopamine neurotransmission has been correlated with its antipsychotic effects, and its higher instance of extrapyramidal effects. *Decreases psychotic manifestations and exerts strong antiemetic effect.*

**USES** Management of manifestations of psychotic disorders and Tourette's syndrome; for treatment of agitated states in acute and chronic psychoses; ADHD, oppositional defiant disorder.

**UNLABELED USES** Cancer chemotherapy as an antiemetic in doses smaller than those required for antipsychotic effects; treatment of autism; alcohol dependence; agitation; mania.

**CONTRAINDICATIONS** Parkinson's disease, seizure disorders, coma; older adults with dementia-related psychosis; severe toxic CNS depression; Parkinson disease; severe neutropenia (ANC less than 1000/mm³); alcoholism; severe mental depression, CNS depression; signs and symptoms of neuroleptic malignant syndrome (NMS); bronchopneumonia; lactation.

**CAUTIOUS USE** Cyclic mood disorders; older adult or debilitated patients, urinary retention, pulmonary disease; history of hypocalcemia; glaucoma, severe cardiovascular disorders, long QT syndrome, AV block, bundle-branch block, cardiac arrhythmias, uncompensated heart failure, recent acute MI; hematologic disease; thyrotoxicosis, or hypothyroidism; older adults;

debilitated patients; pregnancy (category C). Safe use in children younger than 3 y is not established.

## ROUTE & DOSAGE

### Schizophrenia
*Adult:/Adolescent* PO 0.5–2 mg 2–3 × day IM 2–10 mg repeated q4h prn; **Decanoate:** 10–20 × previous dose in oral **haloperidol** equivalents (see package insert for conversion tables)
*Child (3–12 y and 15–40 kg):* PO 0.5 mg/day in 2–3 divided doses, may be increased by 0.5 mg q5–7days to 0.05–0.15 mg/kg/day

### ADHD/Oppositional Defiant Disorder
*Child (3–12 y; weight 15–40 kg):* PO 0.5 mg/day in 2–3 divided doses

### Severe Psychosis
*Adult:* IM 2–5 mg, may repeat qh prn

### Tourette's Disorder
*Adult:* PO 0.25–2 mg b.i.d. or t.i.d.
*Child:* PO 0.25–0.5 mg per day titrate slowly to effect (usual dose 1–4 mg/day)

### *Pharmacogenetic Dosage Adjustment*
*CYP3D6 poor metabolizers:* Start with 75% of initial dose

## ADMINISTRATION
### Oral
- Give with a full glass (240 mL) of water or with food or milk.
- Taper dosing regimen when discontinuing therapy. Abrupt termination can initiate extrapyramidal symptoms.

H

Common adverse effects in *italic;* life-threatening effects underlined; generic names in **bold;** classifications in SMALL CAPS; ✦ Canadian drug name; ⊕ Prototype drug

**Intramuscular**

- Give by deep injection into a large muscle. Do not exceed 3 mL/ injection site. A 21-guage needle is recommended.
- Have patient recumbent at time of parenteral administration and for about 1 h after injection. Assess for orthostatic hypotension.
- Store in light-resistant container at 15°–30° C (59°–86° F), unless otherwise specified by manufacturer. Discard darkened solutions.

## ADVERSE EFFECTS (≥1%) CNS:
*Extrapyramidal reactions:* Parkinsonian symptoms, dystonia, akathisia, tardive dyskinesia (after long-term use); insomnia, restlessness, anxiety, euphoria, agitation, drowsiness, mental depression, lethargy, fatigue, weakness, tremor, ataxia, headache, confusion, vertigo; neuroleptic malignant syndrome, hyperthermia, grand mal seizures, exacerbation of psychotic symptoms, tremor. **CV:** Tachycardia, ECG changes, hypotension, hypertension (with overdosage). **Endocrine:** Menstrual irregularities, galactorrhea, lactation, gynecomastia, impotence, increased libido, hyponatremia, hyperglycemia, hypoglycemia. **Special Senses:** Blurred vision. **Hematologic:** Mild transient leukopenia, agranulocytosis (rare). **GI:** Dry mouth, anorexia, nausea, vomiting, constipation, diarrhea, hypersalivation. **Urogenital:** Urinary retention, priapism. **Respiratory:** Laryngospasm, bronchospasm, increased depth of respiration, bronchopneumonia, respiratory depression. **Skin:** Diaphoresis, maculopapular and acneiform rash, photosensitivity. **Other:** Cholestatic jaundice, variations in liver function tests, decreased serum cholesterol, weight gain.

## INTERACTIONS Drug: CNS DEPRESSANTS, OPIATES, **alcohol** increase CNS

depression; may antagonize activity of ORAL ANTICOAGULANTS; ANTICHOLINERGICS may increase intraocular pressure; **methyldopa** may precipitate dementia.

## PHARMACOKINETICS Absorption:
Well absorbed from GI tract; 60% reaches systemic circulation; 92% protein bound. **Onset:** 30–45 min IM. **Peak:** 4–6 h PO; 10–20 min IM; 6–7 days decanoate. **Distribution:** Distributes mainly to liver with lower concentration in brain, lung, kidney, spleen, heart. **Metabolism:** In liver. **Elimination:** 40% excreted in urine within 5 days; 15% eliminated in feces; excreted in breast milk. **Half-Life:** 12–38 h.

## NURSING IMPLICATIONS

### Black Box Warning

*Haloperidol has been associated with increased mortality in older adults with dementia-related psychosis.*

### Assessment & Drug Effects

- Monitor for therapeutic effectiveness. Because of long half-life, therapeutic effects are slow to develop in early therapy or when established dosing regimen is changed. "Therapeutic window" effect (point at which increased dose or concentration actually decreases therapeutic response) may occur after long period of high doses. Close observation is imperative when doses are changed.
- Monitor patient's mental status daily. Target symptoms expected to decrease with successful haloperidol treatment include hallucinations, insomnia, hostility, agitation, and delusions.
- Monitor for neuroleptic malignant syndrome (NMS) (see Appendix F), especially in those with hypertension or taking lithium. Symptoms

Common adverse effects in *italic;* life-threatening effects underlined; generic names in **bold;** classifications in SMALL CAPS; ✦ Canadian drug name; ⊘ Prototype drug

773

of NMS can appear suddenly after initiation of therapy or after months or years of taking neuroleptic (antipsychotic) medication. Immediately discontinue drug if NMS suspected.

- Monitor for parkinsonism and tardive dyskinesia (see Appendix F). Risk of tardive dyskinesia appears to be greater in women receiving high doses and in older adults. It can occur after long-term therapy and even after therapy is discontinued.
- Monitor for extrapyramidal (neuromuscular) reactions that occur frequently during first few days of treatment. Symptoms are usually dose related and are controlled by dosage reduction or concomitant administration of antiparkinson drugs.
- Be alert for behavioral changes in patients who are concurrently receiving antiparkinson drugs.
- Monitor for exacerbation of seizure activity.
- Observe patients closely for rapid mood shift to depression when haloperidol is used to control mania or cyclic disorders. Depression may represent a drug adverse effect or reversion from a manic state.
- Monitor lab tests: Periodic WBC with differential urinalysis and LFTs with prolonged therapy.

### Patient & Family Education

- Avoid use of alcohol during therapy.
- Do not drive or engage in other potentially hazardous activities until response to drug is known.
- Discuss oral hygiene with health care provider; dry mouth may promote dental problems. Drink adequate fluids.
- Avoid overexposure to sun or sunlamp and use a sunscreen;

drug can cause a photosensitivity reaction.

## HEPARIN SODIUM ⊙⁺
(hep′a-rin)
Hepalean ♦, Heparin Sodium Lock Flush Solution, Hep-Lock
**Classification:** ANTICOAGULANT
Therapeutic: ANTICOAGULANT

**AVAILABILITY** Solution for injection

**ACTION & THERAPEUTIC EFFECT**
Exerts direct effect on the cascade of blood coagulation by enhancing the inhibitory actions of antithrombin III (heparin cofactor) on several factors essential to normal blood clotting. This blocks the conversion of prothrombin to thrombin and fibrinogen to fibrin. *Inhibits formation of new clots. Has rapid anticoagulant effect. Does not lyse already existing thrombi but may prevent their extension and propagation.*

**USES** Prophylaxis and treatment of venous thrombosis and pulmonary embolism and to prevent thromboembolic complications arising from cardiac and vascular surgery, frostbite, and during acute stage of MI. Also used in treatment of disseminated intravascular coagulation (DIC), atrial fibrillation with embolization, and as anticoagulant in blood transfusions, extracorporeal circulation, and dialysis procedures.

**UNLABELED USES** Prophylaxis in hip and knee surgery. Heparin Sodium Lock Flush Solution is used to maintain potency of indwelling IV catheters in intermittent IV therapy or blood sampling. It is not intended for anticoagulant therapy.

**CONTRAINDICATIONS** History of hypersensitivity to heparin (white clot syndrome); uncontrollable bleeding state, except when due to DIC; active bleeding, severe thrombocytopenia; patients in whom suitable blood coagulation tests cannot be performed; ascorbic acid deficiency; active or angiodysplasitic GI disorders including ulcerative lesions; suspected intracranial hemorrhage, severe uncontrolled hypertension, shock; pregnancy when using formulation with bentyl alcohol; lactation for premature infants or neonates if using formulation with bentyl alcohol.

**CAUTIOUS USE** Alcoholism; history of allergy; immediate postpartum period; high risk factors for bleeding including subacute bacterial endocarditis, congenital or acquired bleeding disorders; history of hemorrhagic stroke; advanced kidney, liver, or biliary disease; active tuberculosis; bacterial endocarditis; recent GI bleeding; recent evasive surgery; recent surgery of eye, brain, spinal cord or spinal tap; patients older than 60 y especially women; reduced bone density; patients in hazardous occupations; cerebral embolism; pregnancy (category C); lactation; children.

## ROUTE & DOSAGE

### Treatment of Arterial Thromboembolism

*Adult:* **IV** 80 units/kg bolus then 18 units/kg/h infusion dose adjusted to maintain desired aPTT; **Subcutaneous** 10,000–20,000 units followed by 8000–20,000 units q8–12h

*Child:* **IV** 50 units/kg bolus, then 20,000 units/m²/24 h or 50–100 units/kg q4h

### Open Heart Surgery

*Adult:* **IV** 150–400 units/kg

### Prophylaxis of Embolism

*Adult:* **Subcutaneous** 5000 units q8–12h until patient is ambulatory

## ADMINISTRATION

- Note: Before administration, check coagulation test values; if results are not within therapeutic range, notify prescriber for dosage adjustment.
- Do not use solutions of heparin or heparin lock-flush that contain benzyl alcohol preservative in neonates.

**Subcutaneous**
- Use more concentrated heparin solutions for subcutaneous injection.
- Make injections into the fatty layer of the abdomen or just above the iliac crest. Avoid injecting within 5 cm (2 in.) of umbilicus or in a bruised area. Insert needle into tissue roll perpendicular to skin surface. Do not withdraw plunger to check entry into blood vessel.
- Systematically rotate injection sites and keep record.
- Exercise caution to avoid IM injection.

**Intravenous**

*PREPARE:* **Direct:** Give undiluted. **Intermittent/Continuous:** May add to any amount of NS, D5W, or LR for injection. ▪ Invert IV solution container at least 6 × to ensure adequate mixing.

*ADMINISTER:* **Direct:** Give a single dose over 60 sec. **Intermittent/Continuous (preferred):** Use infusion pump to give at ordered rate.

*INCOMPATIBILITIES:* **Solution/additive: Alteplase, amikacin, atracurium, ciprofloxacin, codeine, cytarabine, daunorubicin,**

Common adverse effects in *italic;* life-threatening effects <u>underlined;</u> generic names in **bold;** classifications in SMALL CAPS; ◆ Canadian drug name; ◐ Prototype drug

775

**H**

dobutamine, epirubicin, erythromycin, gentamicin, hyaluronidase, hydrocortisone, kanamycin, levorphanol, meperidine, morphine, netilmicin, polymyxin B, promethazine, streptomycin, tobramycin, vancomycin. **Y-site:** Alteplase, amiodarone, amphotericin B cholesteryl, amsacrine, capreomycin, caspofungin, ciprofloxacin, clarithromycin, dacarbazine, dantrolene, daunorubicin, diazepam, diazoxide, dimenhydrinate, dobutamine, dolasetron, doxorubicin, doxycycline, droperidol, epirubicin, ergotamine, filgrastim, garenoxacin, gatifloxacin, gentamicin, haloperidol, hydroxyzine, idarubicin, isosorbide, ketamine, levofloxacin, methotrimeprazine, mexiletine, mitoxantrone, mycophenolate, netilmicin, oritavancin, palifermin, papaverine, pentamidine, phenytoin, polymyxin B, posaconazole, propafenone, protamine, quinupristin/dalfoprisin, retaplase, streptomycin, tobramycin, tramadol, triflupromazine, vancomycin, vinorelbine.

▪ Store at 15°–30° C (59°–86° F). Protect from freezing.

## ADVERSE EFFECTS (≥1%) **Hematologic:** Spontaneous bleeding, _transient_ thrombocytopenia, hypofibrinogenemia, "white clot syndrome." **Body as a Whole:** Fever, chills, urticaria, pruritus, skin rashes, itching and burning sensations of feet, numbness and tingling of hands and feet, elevated BP, headache, nasal congestion, lacrimation, conjunctivitis, chest pains, arthralgia, bronchospasm, anaphylactoid reactions. **Endocrine:** Osteoporosis, hypoaldosteronism, suppressed renal function, hyperkalemia;

rebound hyperlipidemia (following termination of heparin therapy). **GI:** Increased AST, ALT. **Urogenital:** Priapism (rare). **Skin:** Injection site reactions: Pain, itching, ecchymoses, tissue irritation and sloughing; cyanosis and pains in arms or legs (vasospasm), reversible transient alopecia (usually around temporal area).

## DIAGNOSTIC TEST INTERFERENCE

Notify laboratory that patient is receiving heparin, when a test is to be performed. Possibility of false-positive rise in **BSP** test and in **serum thyroxine;** and increases in **resin $T_3$ uptake;** false-negative $^{125}I$ **fibrinogen uptake.** Heparin prolongs **PT.** Valid readings may be obtained by drawing blood samples at least 4–6 h after an IV dose (but at any time during heparin infusion) and 12–24 h after a subcutaneous heparin dose.

## INTERACTIONS **Drug:** May prolong PT, which is used to monitor therapy with ORAL ANTICOAGULANTS; **aspirin,** NSAIDS increase risk of bleeding; **nitroglycerin** IV may decrease anticoagulant activity; **protamine** antagonizes effects of heparin. **Herbal: Evening primrose oil, feverfew, ginkgo, ginger** may potentiate bleeding.

## PHARMACOKINETICS **Onset:** 20–60 min subcutaneous. **Peak:** Within minutes. **Duration:** 2–6 h IV; 8–12 h subcutaneous. **Distribution:** Does not cross placenta; not distributed into breast milk. **Metabolism:** In liver and by reticuloendothelial system. **Elimination:** In urine. **Half-Life:** 90 min.

## NURSING IMPLICATIONS

### Assessment & Drug Effects

▪ Monitor aPTT levels closely.
▪ Note: In general, dosage is adjusted to keep aPTT between 1.5–2.5 × normal control level.

- Draw blood for coagulation test 30 min before each scheduled subcutaneous or intermittent IV dose and approximately q4h for patients receiving continuous IV heparin during dosage adjustment period. After dosage is established, tests may be done once daily.
- Patients vary widely in their reaction to heparin; risk of hemorrhage appears greatest in women, all patients older than 60 y, and patients with liver disease or renal insufficiency.
- Monitor vital signs. Report fever, drop in BP, rapid pulse, and other S&S of hemorrhage.
- Observe all needle sites daily for hematoma and signs of inflammation (swelling, heat, redness, pain).
- Antidote: Have on hand protamine sulfate (1% solution), specific heparin antagonist.
- Monitor lab tests: Baseline coagulation tests, Hct, Hgb, RBC, and platelet counts prior to initiation of therapy and at regular intervals throughout therapy.

### Patient & Family Education

- Protect from injury and notify prescriber of pink, red, dark brown, or cloudy urine; red or dark brown vomitus; red or black stools; bleeding gums or oral mucosa; ecchymoses, hematoma, epistaxis, bloody sputum; chest pain; abdominal or lumbar pain or swelling; unusual increase in menstrual flow; pelvic pain; severe or continuous headache, faintness, or dizziness.
- Note: Menstruation may be somewhat increased and prolonged; usually, this is not a contraindication to continued therapy if bleeding is not excessive.
- Learn correct technique for subcutaneous administration if discharged from hospital on heparin.

- Engage in normal activities such as shaving with a safety razor in the absence of a low platelet (thrombocyte) count. Usually, heparin does not affect bleeding time.
- Caution: Smoking and alcohol consumption may alter response to heparin and are not advised.
- Do not take aspirin or any other OTC medication without prescriber's approval.

## HEPATITIS A VACCINE

(hep′a-ti-tis)

Havrix, Vaqta

See Appendix J.

## HEPATITIS B IMMUNE GLOBULIN

(hep′a-ti-tis)

HepaGam B, HyperHep, Nabi-HB

See Appendix J.

## HEPATITIS B VACCINE (RECOMBINANT) ⓟ

(hep′a-ti-tis)

Engerix-B, Recombivax HB

See Appendix J.

## HETASTARCH

(het′a-starch)

Hespan

**Classification:** PLASMA EXPANDER
**Therapeutic:** PLASMA EXPANDER
**Prototype:** Albumin

**AVAILABILITY** Solution for injection

**ACTION & *THERAPEUTIC EFFECT***
Synthetic starch closely resembling human glycogen. Acts much like albumin and dextran but is claimed to

Common adverse effects in *italic;* life-threatening effects <u>underlined;</u> generic names in **bold;** classifications in SMALL CAPS; ♣ Canadian drug name; ⓟ Prototype drug

777

be less likely to produce anaphylaxis or to interfere with cross matching or blood typing procedures. *May prolong the aPTT and PT. In hypovolemic patients, it increases arterial and venous pressures, heart rate, cardiac output, urine output, as well as colloidal osmotic pressure.*

**USES** Treatment of hypovolemia, leukapheresis.

**UNLABELED USES** As a priming fluid in pump oxygenators for perfusion during extracorporeal circulation and as a cryoprotective agent for long-term storage of whole blood.

**CONTRAINDICATIONS** Hypersensitivity to hetastarch; severe bleeding disorders, CHF, severe liver disease; treatment of shock not accompanied by hypovolemia; critically ill adult patients; renal disease with oliguria or anuria not related to hypovolemia; intracranial bleeding; critically ill including those with sepsis.

**CAUTIOUS USE** Hepatic or renal insufficiency, pulmonary edema in the very young or older adults, fluid overload; CABG surgery; patients on sodium restriction; pregnancy (category C); lactation. Safe use in children is not established.

## ROUTE & DOSAGE

### Hypovolemia
*Adult:* **IV** 500–1000 mL or 20 mL/ kg/day (max: 1500 mL/day)

### Leukapheresis
*Adult:* **IV** 250–750 mL infused at a constant fixed ratio of 1:8 to venous whole blood

### *Renal Impairment Dosage Adjustment*
*CrCl less than 10 mL/min:* Use original initial dose, then reduce doses by 25–50%

## ADMINISTRATION
**Intravenous**

*PREPARE:* **IV Infusion:** Use undiluted as prepared by manufacturer.
*ADMINISTER:* **IV Infusion:** Specific flow rate is prescribed by prescriber. Rate may be as high as 20 mL/ kg/h in acute hemorrhagic shock.
▪ Rate is usually reduced in patients with burns or septic shock.
*INCOMPATIBILITIES:* **Y-site:** Varies based on manufacturer consult package insert.

▪ Store at room temperature; avoid extremes of heat or cold. ▪ Discard partially used bags.

**ADVERSE EFFECTS** (≥1%) **CV:** Peripheral edema, <u>circulatory overload, heart failure</u>. **Hematologic:** With large volumes, prolongation of PT, PTT, clotting time, and bleeding time; decreased Hct, Hgb, platelets, calcium, and fibrinogen; dilution of plasma proteins, hyperbilirubinemia, increased sedimentation rate. **Body as a Whole:** Pruritus, <u>anaphylactoid reactions</u> (periorbital edema, urticaria, wheezing), vomiting, mild fever, chills, influenza-like symptoms, headache, muscle pains, submaxillary and parotid glandular swelling.

**PHARMACOKINETICS Duration:** 24–36 h. **Distribution:** Remains in intravascular space. **Metabolism:** In reticuloendothelial system. **Elimination:** In urine with some biliary excretion.

## NURSING IMPLICATIONS
**Assessment & Drug Effects**

### Black Box Warning

*Hetastarch has been associated with increased mortality in critically ill patients, including those with sepsis.*

Common adverse effects in *italic*; life-threatening effects <u>underlined</u>; generic names in **bold**; classifications in SMALL CAPS; ♣ Canadian drug name; ⊘ Prototype drug

- Monitor for S&S of hypersensitivity reaction (see Appendix F).
- Measure and record I&O. Report oliguria or significant changes in I&O ratio.
- Monitor BP and vital signs and observe patient for unusual bruising or bleeding.
- Observe for signs of circulatory overload (see Appendix F).
- Check laboratory reports of Hct values. Notify prescriber if there is an appreciable drop in Hct or if value approaches 30% by volume. Hct should not be allowed to drop below 30%.
- Monitor lab tests: Periodic WBC count with differential, platelet count; and PT & PTT during leukapheresis.

**Patient & Family Education**
- Notify prescriber for any of the following: Difficulty breathing, nausea, chills, headache, itching.

## HOMATROPINE HYDROBROMIDE ⓟ
(hoe-ma'troe-peen)

Isopto Homatropine

**See Appendix A-1.**

## HUMAN PAPILLOMAVIRUS BIVALENT VACCINE ⓟ
(hu'man pap-ih-lo'ma-vye'rus)

Cervarix

**See Appendix J.**

## HUMAN PAPILLOMAVIRUS QUADRIVALENT VACCINE ⓟ
(hu'man pap-ih-lo'ma-vye'rus)

Gardasil

**See Appendix J.**

## HYALURONIDASE, OVINE
(hi-a-lu-ron'i-dase)

Amphadase, Hylenex, Vitrase

**Classifications:** HYALURONIC ACID DERIVATIVE; ABSORPTION AND DISPERSING ENHANCER
**Therapeutic:** ABSORPTION AND DISPERSING ENHANCER

**AVAILABILITY** Solution for injection

**ACTION & *THERAPEUTIC EFFECT***
Hyaluronidase is a diffusing substance that modifies the permeability of connective tissue through the hydrolysis of hyaluronic acid found in the intercellular substance of connective tissue. *It increases the absorption and dispersion of solutions in the intercellular spaces.*

**USES** Adjunct to increase the absorption and dispersion of other injected drugs; hypodermoclysis; adjunct in subcutaneous urography for improving resorption of radiopaque agents.

**UNLABELED USES** Adjunct for ophthalmic anesthesia, treatment of vitreous hemorrhage and diabetic retinopathy.

**CONTRAINDICATIONS** Hypersensitivity to hyaluronidase or any other ingredient in formulation; injection into infected or acutely inflamed area, area of swelling due to bites or stings; corneal injection; injection by IV.

**CAUTIOUS USE** Pregnancy (category C), lactation.

**ROUTE & DOSAGE**

**Adjuvant to Increase the Absorption and Dispersion of Other Drugs**
*Adult/Adolescent/Child:* 150

units (range: 50–300) added to solution

**Hypodermoclysis**
*Adult/Adolescent/Child:* 150 units

**Subcutaneous Urography**
*Adult/Adolescent/Child:*
**Subcutaneous** 75 units prior to contrast medium

## ADMINISTRATION

### Subcutaneous

- Give subcutaneously prior to contrast media. Do not inject near an infected or acutely inflamed area.
- Store unopened vial at 2°–8° C (35°–46° F). After reconstitution, store at 20°–25° C (59°–77° F), and use within 6 h. Protect from light.

## ADVERSE EFFECTS (≥1%) CV:
Edema. **Other:** Injection site reaction (e.g., erythema, irritation); enhanced adverse events associated with coadministered drugs.

## INTERACTIONS Drug: SALICYLATES,
CORTICOSTEROIDS, ESTROGENS, or H₁-BLOCKERS may confer partial resistance to the action of hyaluronidase in some tissues.

## NURSING IMPLICATIONS

### Assessment & Drug Effects

- Monitor for S&S of hypersensitivity: Urticaria, erythema, chills, nausea, vomiting, dizziness, tachycardia, and hypotension. Withhold and notify prescriber if hypersensitivity occurs.
- Note: Those receiving large doses of salicylates, cortisone, ACTH, estrogens, or antihistamines may require larger amounts of hyaluronidase for equivalent dispersing effect.

### Patient & Family Education

- Report immediately any of the following: Rash, itching, chills, nausea, vomiting, dizziness, or palpitations.

# HYDRALAZINE HYDROCHLORIDE ℗

(hye-dral'a-zeen)

**Classifications:** NONNITRATE VASODILATOR; ANTIHYPERTENSIVE
**Therapeutic:** ANTIHYPERTENSIVE

**AVAILABILITY** Tablet; solution for injection

## ACTION & *THERAPEUTIC EFFECT*
Reduces BP mainly by direct effect on vascular smooth muscles of arterial-resistance vessels, resulting in vasodilatation. *Reduces BP with diastolic response often being greater than systolic response. Vasodilation reduces peripheral resistance and substantially improves cardiac output, and renal and cerebral blood flow.*

## USES In management of hypertension.

## UNLABELED USES Treatment of acute CHF.

## CONTRAINDICATIONS Monotherapy for CHF, mitral valvular rheumatic heart disease, MI, tachycardia.

## CAUTIOUS USE Coronary heart disease; cerebrovascular accident, advanced renal impairment, coronary heart disease, renal disease; renal failure; SLE; use with MAO inhibitors; pregnancy (category C); children; lactation.

## ROUTE & DOSAGE

### Hypertension

*Adult:* **PO** 10–50 mg q.i.d.; **IM** 10–50 mg q4–6h; **IV** 10–20 mg q4–6h, switch to oral ASAP

*Renal Impairment Dosage Adjustment*
CrCl 10–50 mL/min: Dose q8h

## ADMINISTRATION

### Oral

- Give with food; bioavailability is increased by taking it with food.
- Discontinue gradually to avoid sudden rise in BP and acute heart failure.
- Inform patients of the dangers of abrupt withdrawal.

### Intramuscular

- Give deep into a large muscle.

### Intravenous

*PREPARE:* **Direct:** Give undiluted. Use immediately after being drawn into syringe. ▪ Do not add to IV solutions.
*ADMINISTER:* **Direct:** Give each 10 mg or fraction thereof over 1 min.
*INCOMPATIBILITIES:* **Solution/additive:** Aminophylline, ampicillin, chlorothiazide, edetate calcium disodium, ethacrynate, hydrocortisone, mephentermine, methohexital, nitroglycerin, phenobarbital, verapamil, D5W. **Y-site:** Acyclovr, alfetnanil, amikacin, aminophylline, amphotericin B, ampicillin, ascorbic acid, atracurium, atropine, azathioprine, aztreonam, benztropine, bretylium, bumetanide, CEPHALOSPORINS, chlorthiazide, dantrolene, diazepam, diazoxide, doxorubicin, ertapenem, folic acid, foscarnet, furosemide, ganciclovir, gemtuzumab, haloperidol, indomethacin, lorazepam, methohexital, methylprednisolone, nafcillin, nitroprusside, oxacillin, pantoprazole, pemetrexed, pentobarbital, phenytoin, piperacillin/tazobactam, SMZ/TMP, ticarcillin, tigecycline.

- Store at 15°–30° C (59°–86° F) in tight, light-resistant containers unless otherwise directed. Avoid freezing.

## ADVERSE EFFECTS (≥1%) **Body as a Whole:** Hypersensitivity (rash, urticaria, pruritus, fever, chills, arthralgia, eosinophilia, cholangitis, hepatitis, obstructive jaundice). **CNS:** *Headache,* dizziness, tremors. **CV:** *Palpitation,* angina, *tachycardia,* flushing, paradoxical pressor response. Overdose: Arrhythmia, shock. **Special Senses:** Lacrimation, conjunctivitis. **GI:** Anorexia, nausea, vomiting, diarrhea, constipation, abdominal pain, paralytic ileus. **Urogenital:** Difficulty in urination, glomerulonephritis. **Hematologic:** Decreased hematocrit and hemoglobin, anemia, agranulocytosis (rare). **Other:** Nasal congestion, muscle cramps, SLE-like syndrome, fixed drug eruption, edema.

## DIAGNOSTIC TEST INTERFERENCE

Positive *direct Coombs' tests* in patients with hydralazine-induced SLE. Hydralazine interferes with urinary *17-OHCS* determinations *(modified Glenn-Nelson technique).*

## INTERACTIONS **Drug:** BETA-BLOCKERS and other ANTIHYPERTENSIVE AGENTS compound hypotensive effects.

## PHARMACOKINETICS **Absorption:** Readily absorbed from GI tract. **Onset:** 20–30 min. **Peak:** 2 h. **Duration:** 2–6 h. **Distribution:** Crosses placenta; distributed into breast milk. **Metabolism:** In liver. **Elimination:** 90% in urine; 10% in feces. **Half-Life:** 2–8 h.

Common adverse effects in *italic;* life-threatening effects underlined; generic names in **bold;** classifications in SMALL CAPS; ♣ Canadian drug name; ⓟ Prototype drug

781

## NURSING IMPLICATIONS

### Assessment & Drug Effects

- Monitor BP and HR closely. Check every 5 min until it is stabilized at desired level, then every 15 min thereafter throughout hypertensive crisis.
- Monitor for S&S of SLE, especially with prolonged therapy.
- Monitor I&O when drug is given parenterally and in those with renal dysfunction.
- Monitor lab tests: Baseline and periodic BUN, creatinine clearance, uric acid, serum potassium, and blood glucose. Baseline and periodic antinuclear antibody titer with prolonged therapy.

### Patient & Family Education

- Monitor weight, check for edema, and report weight gain to prescriber.
- Note: Some patients experience headache and palpitations within 2–4 h after first PO dose; symptoms usually subside spontaneously.
- Make position changes slowly and avoid standing still, hot baths/showers, strenuous exercise, and excessive alcohol intake.
- Do not drive or engage in other potentially hazardous activities until response to drug is known.

## HYDROCHLOROTHIAZIDE (HCTZ) ℗

(hye-droe-klor-oh-thye′a-zide)

Apo-Hydro ♣, Microzide

**Classifications:** ELECTROLYTIC AND WATER BALANCE; THIAZIDE DIURETIC

Therapeutic: DIURETIC

**AVAILABILITY** Capsule; tablet; oral solution

## ACTION & *THERAPEUTIC EFFECT*

Diuretic action is associated with drug interference with reabsorption of sodium ions across the distal renal tubular segment of the nephron. This enhances excretion of sodium, chloride, potassium, bicarbonates, and water. It also decreases cardiac output and reduces plasma and extracellular fluid volume. *Therapeutic effectiveness is measured by decrease in edema and lowering of blood pressure.*

**USES** Adjunct in treatment of edema associated with CHF, hepatic cirrhosis, renal failure, and in the management of hypertension.

**UNLABELED USES** Nephrogenic diabetes insipidus, hypercalciuria, and treatment of electrolyte disturbances associated with renal tubular acidosis.

**CONTRAINDICATIONS** Hypersensitivity to thiazides or other sulfonamides; anuria; electrolyte imbalance.

**CAUTIOUS USE** Bronchial asthma, allergy; hepatic cirrhosis; hepatic impairment; renal impairment; acid/base imbalance; CHF; stroke, CVA; history of gout, SLE; DM; latent DM; post sympathectomy; older adults; excessive sunlight UV exposure; neonates with jaundice; pregnancy (category B); lactation.

## ROUTE & DOSAGE

### Edema

*Adult:* **PO** 25–100 mg/day in 1–3 divided doses (max: 200 mg/day)

Common adverse effects in *italic;* life-threatening effects <u>underlined</u>; generic names in **bold;** classifications in SMALL CAPS; ♣ Canadian drug name; ℗ Prototype drug

### Hypertension

*Adult/Adolescent:* **PO** 12.5–25 mg/day in 1–2 divided doses; may titrate up
*Child/Infant (6 mo and older):* **PO** 1–2 mg/kg/day in 2 divided doses
*Neonate (younger than 6 mo):* **PO** 2–3.3 mg/kg/day in 2 divided doses

### ADMINISTRATION

**Oral**

- Give with food or milk to reduce GI upset.
- Schedule doses to avoid nocturia and interrupted sleep. If given in 2 doses, schedule second dose no later than 3 p.m.
- Store tablets in tightly closed container at 15°–30° C (59°–86° F) unless otherwise directed.

### ADVERSE EFFECTS (≥1%) CNS:

Mood changes, unusual tiredness or weakness, dizziness, lightheadedness, paresthesias. **CV:** Irregular heartbeat, weak pulse, orthostatic hypotension. **GI:** Dry mouth, increased thirst, nausea, vomiting, anorexia, diarrhea, pancreatitis, jaundice. **Hematologic:** Agranulocytosis, thrombocytopenia, aplastic anemia, leukopenia. **Metabolic:** *Hyperglycemia,* glycosuria, *hyperuricemia, hypokalemia.* **Other:** Hypersensitivity reactions, photosensitivity, blurred vision, yellow vision (xanthopsia), muscle spasm.

### DIAGNOSTIC TEST INTERFERENCE

May interfere with *parathyroid function tests, tyramine/phentolamine tests, histamine tests for pheochromocytoma.*

### INTERACTIONS Drug: Amphotericin B, CORTICOSTEROIDS

increase hypokalemic effects; SULFONYLUREAS, **insulin** may antagonize hypoglycemic effects; BILE ACID SEQUESTRANTS decrease THIAZIDE absorption; **diazoxide** intensifies hypoglycemic and hypotensive effects; increased **potassium** and **magnesium** loss may cause **digoxin** toxicity; decreases **lithium** excretion and increases toxicity; increases risk of NSAID-induced renal failure and may attenuate diuresis; **amiodarone** may increase risk of arrythmia. Do not use with **dofetilide.** Withhold dose for 24 h prior to **amifostine** usage. Monitor with **topiramate.**

### PHARMACOKINETICS Absorption:

Incompletely absorbed. **Onset:** 2 h. **Peak:** 4 h. **Duration:** 6–12 h. **Distribution:** Distributed throughout extracellular tissue; concentrates in kidney; crosses placenta; distributed in breast milk. **Metabolism:** Does not appear to be metabolized. **Elimination:** In urine. **Half-Life:** 45–120 min.

### NURSING IMPLICATIONS

**Assessment & Drug Effects**

- Monitor for therapeutic effectiveness. Antihypertensive effects may be noted in 3–4 days; maximal effects may require 3–4 wk.
- Check BP at regular intervals.
- Monitor closely for hypokalemia; it increases the risk of digoxin toxicity.
- Monitor I&O and check for edema.
- Note: Drug may cause hyperglycemia and loss of glycemic control in diabetics.
- Note: Drug may cause orthostatic hypotension, dizziness.

H

---

Common adverse effects in *italic;* life-threatening effects underlined; generic names in **bold;** classifications in SMALL CAPS; ♥ Canadian drug name; ☯ Prototype drug

783

- Monitor lab tests: Baseline and periodic serum electrolytes, blood counts, BUN, blood glucose, uric acid, $CO_2$.

**Patient & Family Education**
- Monitor weight daily.
- Note: Diabetic patients need to monitor blood glucose closely. This drug causes impaired glucose tolerance.
- Report signs of hypokalemia (see Appendix F) to prescriber.
- Change positions slowly; avoid hot baths or showers, extended exposure to sunlight, and sitting or standing still for long periods.
- Note: Photosensitivity reaction may occur 10–14 days after initial sun exposure.

# HYDROCODONE BITARTRATE

(hye-droe-koe'done)
Hysingla ER, Zohydro ER
**Classifications:** NARCOTIC (OPIATE AGONIST) ANALGESIC; ANTITUSSIVE
**Therapeutic:** NARCOTIC ANALGESIC; ANTITUSSIVE
**Prototype:** Morphine
**Controlled Substance:** Schedule II

**AVAILABILITY** Usually formulated with acetaminophen, ibuprofen, or homatropine. Extended release tablet; extended release capsule

**ACTION & THERAPEUTIC EFFECT** CNS depressant with moderate to severe relief of pain. Suppresses cough reflex by direct action on cough center in medulla. *CNS depressant with moderate to severe relief of pain. Effective in cough suppression.*

**USES** Symptomatic relief of hyperactive or nonproductive cough and for relief of moderate to moderately severe pain. A common ingredient in a variety of proprietary mixtures.

**CONTRAINDICATIONS** Hypersensitivity to hydrocodone; acute or severe asthmatic bronchitis; COPD; upper airway obstruction; paralytic ileus (known or suspected), GI obstruction; lactation.

**CAUTIOUS USE** Respiratory depression, asthma, emphysema; history of drug abuse or dependence; postoperative patients; congenital long QT syndrome; drug-inducted QT prolongation; history of seizure disorder; BPH; adrenal insufficiency; hepatic impairment; renal impairment; G6PD deficiency; GI disease; patients with preexisting increased ICP, head trauma; CNS depression; older adults, debilitated patients; pregnancy (category C). Safety and efficacy in children not established.

## ROUTE & DOSAGE

**Chronic/Severe Pain**
*Adult:* **PO** 10 mg q12h in opioid-tolerant patients

## ADMINISTRATION

**Oral**
- Give with food or milk to prevent GI irritation.
- Preserve in tight, light-resistant containers.
- Do not crush, chew, or dissolve, as these actions may lead to an uncontrolled delivery of a fatal dose.

**ADVERSE EFFECTS** (≥1%) **GI:** Dry mouth, *constipation, nausea,* vomiting, abdominal pain. **CV:** Peripheral edema. **CNS:** Light-headedness,

H

sedation, anxiety, dizziness, *drowsiness,* euphoria, anxiety dysphoria. **Respiratory:** *Respiratory depression.* **Skin:** Urticaria, rash, pruritus.

**INTERACTIONS Drug: Alcohol** and other CNS DEPRESSANTS compound sedation and CNS depression. **Herbal: St. John's wort** increases sedation.

**PHARMACOKINETICS Onset:** 10 20 min. **Duration:** 3–6 h. **Distribution:** Crosses placenta; distributed into breast milk. **Metabolism:** In liver. **Elimination:** In urine. **Half-Life:** 3.8 h.

## NURSING IMPLICATIONS

### Black Box Warning

*Hydrocodone has been associated with high potential for abuse and addiction, life-threatening respiratory depression, and neonatal opioid withdrawal syndrome. The risk of potentially fatal overdose increases with coingestion of alcohol.*

### Assessment & Drug Effects
- Monitor for effectiveness of drug for pain relief.
- Monitor for nausea and vomiting, especially in ambulatory patients.
- Monitor respiratory status and bowel elimination.

### Patient & Family Education
- Avoid hazardous activities until response to drug is determined.
- Do not use alcohol or other CNS depressants; may cause additive CNS depression.
- Drink plenty of liquids for adequate hydration.
- Do not take larger doses than prescribed since abuse potential is high.

# HYDROCORTISONE ●
(hye-droe-kor'ti-sone)
Cetacort, Cortaid, Cortenema, Dermolate, Hytone, Rectocort ✦, Synacort

# HYDROCORTISONE ACETATE
Anusol HC, Carmol HC, Cortaid, Cort-Dome, Corticaine, Cortifoam, Cortiment ✦, Epifoam

# HYDROCORTISONE CYPIONATE
Cortef

# HYDROCORTISONE SODIUM SUCCINATE
A-Hydrocort, Solu-Cortef

# HYDROCORTISONE VALERATE
Westcort

# HYDROCORTISONE BUTYRATE
Locoid

**Classification:** ADRENOCORTICAL STEROID
**Therapeutic:** ANTI-INFLAMMATORY; IMMUNOSUPPRESSANT; ANTIPSORIATIC

**AVAILABILITY Hydrocortisone:** Tablet; cream, lotion, ointment, spray. **Hydrocortisone Acetate:** Oral suspension; cream; ointment. **Hydrocortisone Cypionate:** Tablet. **Hydrocortisone Sodium Succinate:** Solution for injection. **Hydrocortisone Valerate:** Cream; ointment. **Hydrocortisone Butyrate:** Cream; ointment; topical solution

## ACTION & THERAPEUTIC EFFECT
Short-acting synthetic steroid with both glucocorticoid and mineralo-corticoid properties that affect

Common adverse effects in *italic;* life-threatening effects <u>underlined;</u> generic names in **bold;** classifications in SMALL CAPS; ✦ Canadian drug name; ● Prototype drug

785

nearly all systems of the body. **Anti-inflammatory (glucocorticoid) action:** Stabilizes leukocyte lysosomal membranes; inhibits phagocytosis and release of allergic substances; suppresses fibroblast formation and collagen deposition; reduces capillary dilation and permeability; and increases responsiveness of cardiovascular system to circulating catecholamines. **Immunosuppressive action:** Modifies immune response to various stimuli; reduces antibody titers; and suppresses cell-mediated hypersensitivity reactions. **Mineralocorticoid action:** Promotes sodium retention, but under certain circumstances (e.g., sodium loading), enhances sodium excretion; promotes potassium excretion; and increases glomerular filtration rate (GFR). **Metabolic action:** Promotes hepatic gluconeogenesis, protein catabolism, redistribution of body fat, and lipolysis. *Has anti-inflammatory, immunosuppressive, and metabolic functions in the body.*

**USES** Replacement therapy in adrenocortical insufficiency; to reduce serum calcium in hypercalcemia, to suppress undesirable inflammatory or immune responses, to produce temporary remission in nonadrenal disease, and to block ACTH production in diagnostic tests. Use as anti-inflammatory or immunosuppressive agent largely replaced by synthetic glucocorticoids that have minimal mineralocorticoid activity. Topically for atopic dermatitis or inflammatory conditions.

**CONTRAINDICATIONS** Hypersensitivity to glucocorticoids, idiopathic thrombocytopenic purpura, psychoses, acute glomerulonephritis, viral or bacterial diseases of skin, infections not controlled by antibiotics, active or latent amebiasis, hypercorticism (Cushing's syndrome), smallpox vaccination or other immunologic procedures; acne: lactation (except for topical use). **Topical steroids:** Presence of varicella, vaccinia, on surfaces with compromised circulation.

**CAUTIOUS USE** Diabetes mellitus; chronic, active hepatitis positive for hepatitis B surface antigen; hyperlipidemia; cirrhosis; stromal herpes simplex; glaucoma, tuberculosis of eye; osteoporosis; convulsive disorders; hypothyroidism; diverticulitis; nonspecific ulcerative colitis; fresh intestinal anastomoses; active or latent peptic ulcer; gastritis; esophagitis; thromboembolic disorders; CHF; metastatic carcinoma; hypertension; renal insufficiency; history of allergies; active or arrested tuberculosis; systemic fungal infection; myasthenia gravis; older adults; pregnancy (category C); children and infants.

## ROUTE & DOSAGE

### Adrenal Insufficiency, Anti-Inflammatory

*Adult:* **PO** 10–320 mg/day in 3–4 divided doses; **IV/IM** 15–800 mg/day in 3–4 divided doses (max: 2 g/day); **Subcutaneous** Sodium phosphate only, 15–240 mg/day
*Child:* **PO** 2.5–10 mg/kg/day in 3–4 divided doses; **IV/IM** 1–5 mg/kg/day divided q12–24h

### Intra-Articular, Intralesional (Acetate Salt)

*Adult:* **IM** 5–50 mg q3–5days for bursae; 5–50 mg once q1–4wk for joints

**Anti-Inflammatory Agent**

*Adult:* **Topical** Apply a small amount to the affected area 1–4 × day; **PR** Insert 1% cream, 10% foam, 10–25 mg suppository, or 100 mg enema nightly

**Atopic Dermatitis**

*Adult/Adolescent/Child/Infant (3 mo or older):* **Topical** Apply sparingly b.i.d.

## ADMINISTRATION

Note: Hydrocortisone phosphate may be given subcutaneously, IM, or IV. Hydrocortisone succinate may be given IM or IV.

### Oral
- Give oral drug with food.

### Rectal
- Administer retention enema preferably after a bowel movement; retain at least 1 h or all night if possible.

### Topical
- Apply medication sparingly, rub until it disappears, and then reapply, leaving a thin coat over lesion. Cover area with transparent plastic or other occlusive device or vehicle only when so ordered.
- Avoid covering a weeping or exudative lesion.
- Note: Occlusive dressings usually are not applied to face, scalp, scrotum, axilla, and groin.
- Inspect skin carefully between applications for ecchymotic, petechial, and purpuric signs, maceration, secondary infection, skin atrophy, striae or miliaria; if present, stop medication and notify prescriber.
- Store medication at 15°–30° C (59°–86° F) unless otherwise directed by manufacturer; protect from light and freezing.

### Intramuscular
- Inject deep into gluteal muscle.

### Intravenous
IV administration to infants, children: Verify correct IV concentration and rate of infusion/injection with prescriber.

*PREPARE:* **Direct (preferred):** Give undiluted. **Intermittent:** Dilute in 50–1000 mL of D5W, NS, or D5/NS.

*ADMINISTER:* **Direct:** Give over 30 sec (e.g., 100 mg) to 10 min (e.g., 500 mg or more). **Intermittent:** Give over 10 min.

*INCOMPATIBILITIES:* Solution/additive: **Amobarbital, ampicillin, bleomycin, colistimethate, dimenhydrinate, doxapram, doxorubicin, ephedrine, heparin, hydralazine, metaraminol, methicillin, nafcillin, pentobarbital, phenobarbital, prochlorperazine, promethazine, secobarbital, tetracycline.** Y-site: **Ergotamine, phenytoin.**
- Administer solutions that have been diluted for IV infusion within 24 h.

## ADVERSE EFFECTS (≥1%) **Body as a Whole:** Hypersensitivity or anaphylactoid reactions; aggravation or masking of infections; malaise, weight gain, obesity; urogenital urinary frequency and urgency, enuresis increased or decreased motility and number of sperm. **CNS:** Vertigo, headache, nystagmus, ataxia (rare), increased intracranial pressure with papilledema (usually after discontinuation of medication), mental disturbances, aggravation of preexisting psychiatric conditions, insomnia, anxiety, mental confusion, depression. **CV:** Syncopal episodes, thrombophlebitis, thromboembolism or fat embolism, palpitation, tachycardia,

Common adverse effects in *italic;* life-threatening effects underlined; generic names in **bold;** classifications in SMALL CAPS; ♣ Canadian drug name; ☉ Prototype drug

787

necrotizing angiitis, CHF, hypertension edema. **Endocrine:** Suppressed linear growth in children, decreased glucose tolerance; hyperglycemia, manifestations of latent diabetes mellitus; hypocorticism; amenorrhea and other menstrual difficulties; moon facies. **Special Senses:** Posterior subcapsular cataracts (especially in children), glaucoma, exophthalmos, increased intraocular pressure with optic nerve damage, perforation of the globe, fungal infection of the cornea, decreased or blurred vision. **Metabolic:** Hypocalcemia; *sodium* and *fluid retention;* hypokalemia and hypokalemic alkalosis decreased serum concentration of vitamins A and C; hyperglycemia, hypernatremia. **GI:** Cramping, bleeding, *nausea,* increased appetite, ulcerative esophagitis, pancreatitis, abdominal distention, peptic ulcer with perforation and hemorrhage, melena. **Hematologic:** Thrombocytopenia, polycythemia, ecchymoses. **Musculoskeletal:** Osteoporosis, compression fractures, muscle wasting and weakness, tendon rupture, aseptic necrosis of femoral and humeral heads. **Skin:** Skin thinning and atrophy, *acne, impaired wound healing;* petechiae, ecchymosis, easy bruising; suppression of skin test reaction; hypopigmentation or hyperpigmentation, hirsutism, acneiform eruptions, subcutaneous fat atrophy; allergic dermatitis, urticaria, angioneurotic edema, increased sweating. With parenteral therapy at IV site–pain, irritation, necrosis, atrophy, sterile abscess; Charcot-like arthropathy following intra-articular use; burning and tingling in perineal area (after IV injection).

## DIAGNOSTIC TEST INTERFERENCE

Hydrocortisone (corticosteroids) may increase serum *cholesterol,* *blood glucose,* serum *sodium, uric acid* (in acute leukemia) and *calcium* (in bone metastasis). It may decrease serum *calcium, potassium, PBI, thyroxin (T₄), triiodothyronine (T₃) and reduce thyroid I 131* uptake. It increases *urine glucose* level and *calcium* excretion; decreases *urine 17-OHCS* and *17-KS* levels. May produce false-negative results with *nitroblue tetrazolium test* for systemic bacterial infection and may suppress reactions to skin tests.

## INTERACTIONS **Drug:** BARBITURATES, **phenytoin, rifampin** may increase hepatic metabolism, thus decreasing cortisone levels; ESTROGENS potentiate the effects of hydrocortisone; NSAIDS compound ulcerogenic effects; **cholestyramine, colestipol** decrease hydrocortisone absorption; DIURETICS, **amphotericin B** exacerbate hypokalemia; ANTICHOLINESTERASE AGENTS (e.g., **neostigmine**) may produce severe weakness; immune response to VACCINES and TOXOIDS may be decreased.

## PHARMACOKINETICS **Absorption:** Readily from GI tract and IM injection site. **Onset:** 1–2 h PO; immediately IV; 3–5 days PR. **Peak:** 1 h PO; 4–8 h IM. **Duration:** 1–1.5 days PO/IM; 0.5–4 wk intra-articular. **Distribution:** Distributed primarily to muscles, liver, skin, intestines, kidneys; crosses placenta. **Metabolism:** In liver. **Elimination:** HPA suppression 8–12 h; metabolites excreted in urine; excreted in breast milk. **Half-Life:** 1.5–2 h.

## NURSING IMPLICATIONS

### Assessment & Drug Effects

- Establish baseline and continuing data on BP, weight, fluid and electrolyte balance, and blood glucose.

Common adverse effects in *italic;* life-threatening effects underlined; generic names in **bold;** classifications in SMALL CAPS; ♣ Canadian drug name; ⊙ Prototype drug

- Monitor for adverse effects. Older adults and patients with low serum albumin are especially susceptible to adverse effects.
- Be alert to signs of hypocalcemia (see Appendix F).
- Ophthalmoscopic examinations are recommended every 2–3 mo, especially if patient is receiving ophthalmic steroid therapy.
- Monitor for persistent backache or chest pain; compression and spontaneous fractures of long bones and vertebrae present hazards.
- Monitor for and report changes in mood and behavior, emotional instability, or psychomotor activity, especially with long-term therapy.
- Be alert to possibility of masked infection and delayed healing (anti-inflammatory and immunosuppressive actions).
- Note: Dose adjustment may be required if patient is subjected to severe stress (serious infection, surgery, or injury).
- Note: Single doses of corticosteroids or use for a short period (less than 1 wk) do not produce withdrawal symptoms when discontinued, even with moderately large doses.
- Monitor lab tests: Periodic serum electrolytes, blood glucose, Hct and Hgb, platelet count, and WBC with differential.

### Patient & Family Education

- Expect a slight weight gain with improved appetite. After dosage is stabilized, notify prescriber of a sudden slow but steady weight increase [2 kg (5 lb)/wk].
- Avoid alcohol and caffeine; may contribute to steroid-ulcer development in long-term therapy.
- Do not ignore dyspepsia with hyperacidity. Report symptoms to prescriber and **do not** self-medicate to find relief.
- **Do not** use aspirin or other OTC drugs unless prescribed specifically by the prescriber.
- Note: A high protein, calcium, and vitamin D diet is advisable to reduce risk of corticosteroid-induced osteoporosis.
- Notify prescriber of slow healing, any vague feeling of being sick, or return to pretreatment symptoms.
- Do not abruptly discontinue drug; doses are gradually reduced to prevent withdrawal symptoms.
- Report exacerbation of disease during drug withdrawal.
- Apply topical preparations sparingly in small children. The hazard of systemic toxicity is higher because of the greater ratio of skin surface area to body weight.

## HYDROMORPHONE HYDROCHLORIDE

(hye-droe-mor'fone)

Dilaudid, Dilaudid HP, Exalgo

**Classifications:** NARCOTIC (OPIATE AGONIST); ANALGESIC
**Therapeutic:** NARCOTIC ANALGESIC; ANTITUSSIVE
**Prototype:** Morphine
**Controlled Substance:** Schedule II

**AVAILABILITY** Tablet; oral liquid; solution for injection; extended release tablet; rectal suppository

### ACTION & *THERAPEUTIC EFFECT*

Potent opiate receptor agonist that does not alter pain threshold but changes the perception of pain in the CNS. *An effective narcotic analgesic that controls mild to moderate pain. Also has antitussive properties.*

**USES** Relief of moderate to severe pain.

**CONTRAINDICATIONS** Intolerance to opiate agonists; opiate-naïve

Common adverse effects in *italic;* life-threatening effects <u>underlined;</u> generic names in **bold;** classifications in SMALL CAPS; ◆ Canadian drug name; ⊕ Prototype drug

789

patients; severe respiratory depression; acute or severe asthma, bronchial asthma, status asthmaticus in an unmonitored setting or in absence of resuscitative equipment; upper airway obstruction, GI obstruction; ileus; obstetrical analgesia; pregnancy (category D in high doses at term); lactation. **Extended release form:** Preexisting severe narrowing of any portion of GI tract.

**CAUTIOUS USE** Abrupt discontinuation, alcoholism or history of drug abuse; angina; biliary tract disease; epidural administration; GI disease; head trauma, other intracranial lesions, preexisting increase intracranial lesions; or increased ICP; heart failure; hepatic disease; hypotension, hypovolemia, oliguria, BPH; pulmonary disease; significant COPD; respiratory depression; disease, renal impairment; increased inflammatory bowel disease, ulcerative colitis; adrenal insufficiency; bladder obstruction; cardiac arrhythmias, cardiac disease; history of seizures; history of substance abuse; surgery of biliary tract, GI surgery; urethral stricture, urinary retention; debilitated patients; older adults; pregnancy (category C); children.

## ROUTE & DOSAGE

### Moderate to Severe Pain

*Adult:* **PO** 2–4 mg q4–6h prn in opioid naïve patients or 2.5–10 mg q3–6h (liquid form); **Subcutaneous/IM** 1–2 mg q2–3h depending on patient response and previous opioid exposure; **IV** 0.2–1 mg q2–3h; **Rectal** 3mg q6–8h titrate to relief

## ADMINISTRATION

### Oral
▪ Ensure that extended release tablet is swallowed whole and not crushed or chewed.

▪ For chronic pain, around-the-clock dosing is recommended.

### Rectal
▪ Insert beyond the rectal sphincter to ensure retention.

### Subcutaneous/Intramuscular
▪ **Do not** confuse Dilaudid-HP Injection (a concentrated formulation) with Dilaudid Injection. Overdose and death could result.
▪ Store at room 15°–30° C (59°–86° F) and protect from light.

### Intravenous

IV administration to children: Verify correct IV concentration and rate of infusion with prescriber.

*PREPARE:* **Direct:** May be given undiluted or diluted in 5 mL of sterile water or NS. **IV Infusion:** Solution typically diluted to 1 mg/mL (specific concentration is ordered by prescriber) in D5W, NS, or other compatible solution. ▪ **For Dilaudid-HP:** Reconstitute 250 mg dry powder vial immediately prior to use with 25 mL sterile water for injection to yield 10 mg/mL. ▪ Final dilution of Dilaudid-HP 250 and HP 500 (supplied 500 mg/50 mL) **must be** ordered by prescriber.

*ADMINISTER:* **Direct:** Give 2 mg or fraction thereof over 3–5 min. **IV Infusion:** Both final volume and rate of infusion **must be** ordered by prescriber.

*INCOMPATIBILITIES:* Solution/additive: **Prochlorperazine, sodium bicarbonate, thiopental.** Y-site: **Amphotericin B cholesteryl, cefazolin, ceftobiprole, dantrolene, dimenhydrinate, diazepam, gallium, lansoprazole, minocycline, pantoprazole, phenobarbital, phenytoin, sargramostim, thiopental.**

▪ A slight discoloration in ampules or multidose vials causes no loss of

Common adverse effects in *italic;* life-threatening effects <u>underlined;</u> generic names in **bold;** classifications in SMALL CAPS; ✦ Canadian drug name; ⊙ Prototype drug

potency. ▪ Store in tight, light-resistant containers at 15°–30° C (59°–86° F).

## ADVERSE EFFECTS (≥1%) GI:
Nausea, vomiting, constipation. **CNS:** Euphoria, dizziness, sedation, *drowsiness.* **CV:** Hypotension, bradycardia or tachycardia. **Respiratory:** <u>Respiratory depression</u>. **Special Senses:** Blurred vision.

## INTERACTIONS Drug: Alcohol
and other CNS DEPRESSANTS compound sedation and CNS depression. **Herbal: St. John's wort, kava** may increase sedation.

## PHARMACOKINETICS Absorption:
60% absorbed from GI tract. **Onset:** 15 min IV, 30 min PO. **Peak:** 30–90 min. **Duration:** 3–4 h; higher AUC in geriatric patients. **Distribution:** Crosses placenta; distributed into breast milk. **Metabolism:** In liver. **Elimination:** In urine. **Half-Life:** 2–3 h.

## NURSING IMPLICATIONS

### Black Box Warning

*Hydromorphone has been associated with respiratory depression and substance abuse.*

### Assessment & Drug Effects
▪ Note baseline respiratory rate, rhythm, and depth and size of pupils before administration. Respirations of 12/min or less and mitosis are signs of toxicity. Withhold drug and promptly notify prescriber.
▪ Monitor vital signs at regular intervals. Drug-induced respiratory depression may occur even with small doses and increases progressively with higher doses.
▪ Assess effectiveness of pain relief 30 min after medication administration.

▪ Monitor drug effects carefully in older adult or debilitated patients and those with impaired renal and hepatic function.
▪ Assess effectiveness of cough. Drug depresses cough and sigh reflexes and may induce atelectasis, especially in postoperative patients and those with pulmonary disease.
▪ Note: Nausea and orthostatic hypotension most often occur in ambulatory patients or when a supine patient assumes the head-up position.
▪ Monitor I&O ratio and pattern. Assess lower abdomen for bladder distension. Report oliguria or urinary retention.
▪ Monitor bowel pattern; drug-induced constipation may require treatment.

### Patient & Family Education
▪ Request medication at the onset of pain and do not wait until pain is severe.
▪ Use caution with activities requiring alertness; drug may cause drowsiness, dizziness, and blurred vision.
▪ Hydromorphone may be habit forming and has the potential for abuse.
▪ Avoid alcohol and other CNS depressants while taking this drug.

## HYDROQUINONE
(hyc'droc-kwin-one)

Aclaro, Eldopaque, Eldoquin, Esoterica Regular, Lustra, Melanex, Porcelana, Solaquin

**Classifications:** PIGMENT AGENT; DEPIGMENTOR
Therapeutic: DEPIGMENTOR

## AVAILABILITY Cream; gel; solution

Common adverse effects in *italic*; life-threatening effects <u>underlined</u>; generic names in **bold**; classifications in SMALL CAPS; ♣ Canadian drug name; ⓟ Prototype drug

791

## ACTION & *THERAPEUTIC EFFECT*

Causes reversible bleaching of hyperpigmented skin due to increased melanin. Interferes with formation of new melanin but does not destroy existing pigment. Depresses melanin synthesis and melanocytic growth, possibly by increasing excretion of melanin from melanocytes. *Interferes with formation of new melanin but does not destroy existing pigment.*

**USES** Gradual bleaching of hyperpigmented skin conditions.

**CONTRAINDICATIONS** Hyersensitivity to hydroquinone, PABA, paraben, or sulfite; prickly heat, sunburn, irritated skin, depilatory usage.

**CAUTIOUS USE** Pregnancy (category C), lactation. Safe use in children younger than 12 y not established.

## ROUTE & DOSAGE

**Bleaching of Hyperpigmented Skin**

*Adult:* **Topical** Apply thin layer and rub into hyperpigmented skin b.i.d., a.m. and p.m.

## ADMINISTRATION

**Topical**

- Test skin for sensitivity before treatment is initiated. Apply small amount of drug (about 25 mm in diameter) to an unbroken patch of skin and check in 24 h. Do not use drug if vesicle formation, itching, or excessive inflammation occur. Minor redness is not a contraindication.
- Limit applications to an area no larger than that of face and neck.

**ADVERSE EFFECTS** (≥1%) **Skin:** Dryness and fissuring of paranasal and infraorbital areas, inflammatory reaction, erythema; stinging, tingling, burning sensations; irritation, sensitization, and contact dermatitis.

## NURSING IMPLICATIONS

### Assessment & Drug Effects

- Monitor for therapeutic effectiveness: In general, complete depigmentation occurs in 1–4 mo and lasts 2–6 mo after hydroquinone is discontinued. Once desired results are obtained, reduce amount and frequency of applications to the least that will maintain depigmentation.
- Discontinue if bleaching or skin lightening does not occur after 2 or 3 mo of therapy.

### Patient & Family Education

- Use a sunscreen agent or a hydroquinone formulation containing a sunscreen for daytime applications.
- Wash drug off if rash or irritation develops and consult prescriber.
- Avoid contact with the eyes and not to use on open lesions, sunburned, irritated, or otherwise damaged skin.
- Continue use of protective clothing and sunscreening agent after treatment is terminated to reduce possibility of repigmentation.

## HYDROXOCOBALAMIN (VITAMIN B₁₂ ALPHA)

(hye-drox-oh-koe-bal′a-min)

Hydrobexan, Hydroxo-12, LA-12

**Classification:** VITAMIN SUPPLEMENT
Therapeutic: VITAMIN B₁₂ REPLACEMENT
**Prototype:** Cyanocobalamin

**AVAILABILITY** Solution for injection

## ACTION & *THERAPEUTIC EFFECT*

Cobalamin derivative similar to cyanocobalamin (vitamin B₁₂).

Essential for normal cell growth, cell reproduction maturation of RBCs, myelin synthesis, and believed to be involved in protein synthesis. *Effective in vitamin $B_{12}$ deficiency that results in megaloblastic anemia.*

**USES** Treatment of vitamin $B_{12}$ deficiency.

**UNLABELED USES** Cyanide poisoning and tobacco amblyopia.

**CONTRAINDICATIONS** History of sensitivity to vitamin $B_{12}$, other cobalamins, or cobalt; indiscriminate use in folic acid deficiency.

**CAUTIOUS USE** Pregnancy (category A; category C in greater than RDA); lactation; children.

## ROUTE & DOSAGE

**Vitamin B₁₂ Deficiency**
*Adult:* **IM** 30 mcg/day for 5–10 days and then 100–200 mcg/mo or 1000 mcg every other day until remission and then 1000 mcg/mo
*Child:* **IM** 100 mcg doses to a total of 1–5 mg over 2 wk and then 30–50 mcg/mo

## ADMINISTRATION

**Intramuscular**
▪ Give deep into a large muscle.

**INTERACTIONS Drug: Chloramphenicol** may interfere with therapeutic response to hydroxocobalamin.

**PHARMACOKINETICS Distribution:** Widely distributed; principally stored in liver, kidneys, and adrenals; crosses placenta.

**Metabolism:** Converted in tissues to active coenzymes; enterohepatically cycled. **Elimination:** 50–95% of doses 100 mcg or greater are excreted in urine in 48 h; excreted in breast milk.

## NURSING IMPLICATIONS

### Assessment & Drug Effects

▪ Monitor for therapeutic effectiveness: Response to drug therapy is usually dramatic, occurring within 48 h. Effectiveness is measured by laboratory values and improvement in manifestations of vitamin $B_{12}$ deficiency.
▪ Obtain a careful history of sensitivities. Sensitization can take as long as 8 y to develop.
▪ Monitor potassium levels during the first 48 h, particularly in patients with Addisonian pernicious anemia or megaloblastic anemia. Conversion to normal erythropoiesis can result in severe hypokalemia and sudden death.
▪ Monitor vital signs in patients with cardiac disease and be alert to symptoms of pulmonary edema; generally occur early in therapy.
▪ Monitor bowel function. Bowel regularity is essential for consistent absorption of oral preparations.
▪ Monitor lab tests: Prior to therapy reticulocyte and erythrocyte counts, Hgb, Hct, vitamin $B_{12}$, and serum folate levels; repeated 5–7 days after start of therapy and at regular intervals during therapy.

### Patient & Family Education

▪ Notify prescriber of any intercurrent disease or infection. Increased dosage may be required.
▪ Note: It is imperative to understand that drug therapy **must be** continued throughout life for

Common adverse effects in *italic;* life-threatening effects <u>underlined</u>; generic names in **bold;** classifications in SMALL CAPS; ✦ Canadian drug name; ⊙ Prototype drug

793

pernicious anemia to prevent irreversible neurologic damage.

- Neurologic damage is considered irreversible if there is no improvement after 1–1.5 y of adequate therapy.
- Dietary deficiency of vitamin B$_{12}$ has been observed in strict vegetarians (vegans) and their breast-fed infants as well as in the elderly.

## HYDROXYCHLOROQUINE

(hye-drox-ee-klor′oh-kwin)

Plaquenil

**Classifications:** BIOLOGIC RESPONSE MODIFIER; ANTIMALARIAL; DISEASE MODIFYING RHEUMATIC DRUG (DMARD)

Therapeutic: ANTIMALARIAL; ANTI-RHEUMATIC

**Prototype:** Chloroquine

### AVAILABILITY Tablets

### ACTION & *THERAPEUTIC EFFECT*

Antimalarial activity results from forming complexes with DNA of parasite, thereby inhibiting replication and transcription to RNA and DNA synthesis of the parasite. *Effective against* Plasmodium vivax *and* Plasmodium malariae. *Also is effective as second line of defense for treatment of rheumatoid arthritis and SLE.*

### USES Suppressive prophylaxis and treatment of acute malarial attacks due to all forms of susceptible malaria, treatment of systemic lupus erythematous, rheumatoid arthritis.

### UNLABELED USES Porphyria cutanea tarda.

### CONTRAINDICATIONS Known hypersensitivity to retinal or visual field changes associated with quinoline compounds; psoriasis, porphyria, G6PD deficiency; long-term therapy in children.

### CAUTIOUS USE Hepatic disease; alcoholism, use with hepatotoxic drugs; impaired renal function, porphoria; metabolic acidosis; patients with tendency to dermatitis; pregnancy (category C).

## ROUTE & DOSAGE

Note: Doses are expressed in terms of hydroxychloroquine base: 400 mg tablet = 310 mg base; 800 mg tablet = 620 mg base

### Acute Malaria

*Adult:* **PO** 620 mg base followed by 310 mg base at 6, 18, and 24 h
*Child (weight greater than 30 kg):* **PO** 10 mg base/kg, then 5 mg base/kg at 6, 18, and 24 h

### Malaria Prophylaxis

*Adult:* **PO** 310 mg base the same day each week starting 2 wk before exposure and continuing for 4–6 wk after leaving the area of exposure
*Child: (weight greater than 30 kg):* **PO** 5 mg base/kg the same day each week starting 2 wk before exposure and continuing for 4–8 wk after leaving the area of exposure

### Lupus Erythematosus

*Adult:* **PO** 155 mg–310 mg base 1–2 × day

### Rheumatoid Arthritis

*Adult:* **PO** 400–600 mg/day until response, then decrease to lowest maintenance levels possible

## ADMINISTRATION

### Oral

- Give drug with meals or milk to reduce incidence of GI distress.
- Give antacids and laxatives at least 4 h before or after hydroxychloroquine.
- Do not crush or divide film-coated tablets.
- Store at 15°–30° C (59°–86° F) unless otherwise directed.

## ADVERSE EFFECTS (≥1%) CNS:

Fatigue, vertigo, headache, mood or mental changes, anxiety, *retinopathy*, blurred vision, difficulty focusing, suicidal ideation. **GI:** Anorexia, nausea, vomiting, diarrhea, abdominal cramps, weight loss. **Hematologic:** Hemolysis in patients with G6PD deficiency, agranulocytosis (rare), aplastic anemia (rare), thrombocytopenia, cadiomyopathy. **Skin:** Bleaching or loss of hair, unusual pigmentation (blue-black) of skin or inside mouth, skin rash, itching. **Other:** Hepatic failure.

## INTERACTIONS Drug: Alu-

**minum-** and **magnesium**-containing ANTACIDS and LAXATIVES decrease hydroxychloroquine absorption; separate administrations by at least 4 h; hydroxychloroquine may interfere with response to **rabies vaccine.** Do not use with other agents that prolong the QT interval.

## PHARMACOKINETICS Absorption:

Rapidly and almost completely absorbed. **Peak:** 1–2 h. **Distribution:** Widely distributed; concentrates in lungs, liver, erythrocytes, eyes, skin, and kidneys; crosses placenta. **Metabolism:** Partially in liver to active metabolite. **Elimination:** In urine; excreted in breast milk. **Half-Life:** 70–120 h.

## NURSING IMPLICATIONS

### Assessment & Drug Effects

- Monitor for therapeutic effectiveness; may not appear for several weeks, and maximal benefit may not occur for 6 mo.
- Withhold drug and notify prescriber if weakness, visual symptoms, hearing loss, unusual bleeding, bruising, or skin eruptions occur.
- Monitor lab tests: Periodic blood cell counts with long-term therapy.

### Patient & Family Education

- Learn about adverse effects and their symptoms when taking prolonged therapy.
- Follow drug regimen exactly as prescribed by the prescriber.

# HYDROXYPROGESTERONE CAPROATE

(hye-drox'ee-proe-jes'ter-one kap'roe-ate)

Makena

**Classifications:** HORMONE; PROGESTIN
**Therapeutic:** PROGESTIN
**Prototype:** Progesterone

**AVAILABILITY** Solution for injection

## ACTION & *THERAPEUTIC EFFECT*

The mechanism by which hydroxyprogesterone reduces the risk of preterm birth is unknown. *Decreases risk of recurrent preterm births.*

**USES** Decrease risk of premature birth in women with a singleton pregnancy who have a history of singleton spontaneous preterm birth.

**UNLABELED USES** Amenorrhea, dysfunctional uterine bleeding, endometrial cancer, test for endogenous estrogen production.

---

Common adverse effects in *italic;* life-threatening effects underlined; generic names in **bold;** classifications in SMALL CAPS; ♣ Canadian drug name; ⊘ Prototype drug

795

## CONTRAINDICATIONS
Current/history of thrombosis or thromboembolic disorders; current/history of breast cancer or other hormone-sensitive cancer; undiagnosed abnormal vaginal bleeding not related to pregnancy; cholestatic jaundice of pregnancy; benign or malignant liver tumors or other active liver disease; uncontrolled hypertension; postmenopausal status.

## CAUTIOUS USE
Hypersensitivity; diabetes or prediabetes; conditions exacerbated by fluid retention (e.g., preeclampsia, seizure disorder, migraine, asthma, cardiac or renal dysfunction); hypertension; jaundice; depression. Safety and efficacy in children under 16 y not established.

## ROUTE & DOSAGE

**Prevention of Premature Birth**

*Adult:* **IM** 250 mg weekly. Begin between 16 wk 0 d to 20 wk 6 d of pregnancy. Continue until wk 37 or delivery whichever occurs first.

## ADMINISTRATION

### Intramuscular
- Draw up 1 mL using an 18-guage needle. Change to a 21-gauge 1½ inch needle.
- Slowly inject (over at least 1 min) into the upper outer quadrant of the gluteus maximus.
- Store at 15°–30° C (59°–86° F) upright and protect from light. Discard vial 5 wk after first use.

## ADVERSE EFFECTS (≥1%)
**Body as a Whole:** Hypersensitivity reactions, injection-site nodule, *injection-site pain*, injection-site pruritus, *injection-site swelling*, miscarriage, stillbirth. **CV:** Gestational hypertension or preeclampsia, thromboembolic disorders. **GI:** Diarrhea, nausea. **Metabolic:** Decreased glucose tolerance, fluid retention, gestational diabetes. **Skin:** Pruritus, *urticaria*.

## INTERACTIONS
**Drug:** Hydroxyprogesterone can decrease the plasma levels of drugs that are substrates for CYP1A2 (e.g., **clozapine, theophylline, tizanidine**), CYP2A6 (e.g., **acetaminophen, nicotine**), or CYP2B6 (i.e., **bupropion, efavirenz, methadone**). Do not use with **bosentan.**

## PHARMACOKINETICS
**Peak:** 3–7 d. **Distribution:** Extensively bound to plasma proteins. **Metabolism:** In liver. **Elimination:** Fecal (50%) and renal (30%). **Half-Life:** 7.8 d.

## NURSING IMPLICATIONS

### Assessment & Drug Effects
- Monitor periodically: BP, weight, and mental status.
- Monitor diabetics closely for loss of glycemic control.
- Promptly report development of any of the following: New onset hypertension; S&S of thromboembolic disorder; unexplained vaginal bleeding; sudden weight gain; jaundice; depression; S&S of hypersensitivity (see Appendix F).

### Patient & Family Education
- Report to prescriber if injection site becomes inflamed or increasingly painful over time.
- Diabetics should frequently monitor blood sugar and report significant changes to the prescriber.

Common adverse effects in *italic;* life-threatening effects underlined; generic names in **bold;** classifications in SMALL CAPS; ♣ Canadian drug name; ⊘ Prototype drug

# HYDROXYUREA
(hye-drox′ee-yoo-ree-ah)
**Hydrea, Droxia**
**Classifications:** ANTINEOPLASTIC;
ANTIMETABOLITE
**Therapeutic:** ANTINEOPLASTIC

## AVAILABILITY Capsule

## ACTION & *THERAPEUTIC EFFECT*
A cell-cycle-phase antineoplastic that
causes an immediate inhibition of
DNA synthesis by acting as an RNA
reductase inhibitor necessary for
DNA synthesis but without interfering with the synthesis of RNA or protein. *Cytotoxic effect limited to tissues
with high rates of cell proliferation.*

## USES Palliative treatment of meta-
static melanoma, chronic myelocytic
leukemia; recurrent metastatic, or inoperable ovarian cancer. Also used
as adjunct to x-ray therapy for treatment of advanced primary squamous cell (epidermoid) carcinoma
of head (excluding lip), neck, lungs.

## UNLABELED USES Psoriasis; com-
bination therapy with radiation of
lung carcinoma; sickle cell anemia.

## CONTRAINDICATIONS Severe
myelosuppression; severe anemia, thrombocytopenia; pregnancy (category D); lactation.

## CAUTIOUS USE Recent use of
other cytotoxic drugs or irradiation; bone marrow depression; renal dysfunction; HIV patients; older
adults; history of gout. Safe use in
children not established.

## ROUTE & DOSAGE

### Palliative Therapy
*Adult:* **PO** 80 mg/kg q3days or
20–30 mg/kg/day

### Sickle Cell Disease
*Adult:* **PO** 15 mg/kg/day, may
increase by 5 mg/kg/day (max:
35 mg/kg/day or until toxicity
develops)

### Renal Impairment Dosage Adjustment
*CrCl 10–50 mL/min:* Administer
50% of dose; *less than 10 mL/
min:* Administer 20% of dose

### Hemodialysis Dosage Adjustment
Administer dose after
hemodialysis; no supplemental
dose needed

## ADMINISTRATION
### Oral
- Open, mix with water, and give
  immediately when patient has difficulty swallowing capsule
- Store in tightly covered container
  at 15°–30° C (59°–86° F) unless
  otherwise directed.

## ADVERSE EFFECTS (≥1%) CNS:
Rare: Headache, dizziness, hallucinations, convulsions. **GI:** Stomatitis, anorexia, nausea, vomiting,
diarrhea, constipation. **Hematologic:** Bone marrow suppression
(leukopenia, anemia, thrombocytopenia), megaloblastic erythropoiesis. **Skin:** Maculopapular rash,
facial erythema, postirradiation erythema. **Urogenital:** Renal tubular
dysfunction, elevated BUN, serum,
creatinine levels, hyperuricemia.
**Body as a Whole:** Fever, chills, malaise.

## INTERACTIONS Drug: No clini-
cally significant interactions established.

## PHARMACOKINETICS Absorp-
tion: Readily absorbed from GI tract.
**Peak:** 2 h. **Distribution:** Crosses

Common adverse effects in *italic*; life-threatening effects underlined; generic names
in **bold**; classifications in SMALL CAPS; ♣ Canadian drug name; ● Prototype drug

797

blood–brain barrier. **Metabolism:** In liver. **Elimination:** As respiratory $CO_2$ and as urea in urine.

## NURSING IMPLICATIONS

### Assessment & Drug Effects

- Interrupt therapy if WBC drops to 2500/mm$^3$ or platelets to 100,000/mm$^3$.
- Monitor I&O. Advise patients with high serum uric acid levels to drink at least 10–12 240 mL (8 oz) glasses of fluid daily to prevent uric acid nephropathy.
- Note: Patients with marked renal dysfunction may rapidly develop visual and auditory hallucinations and hematologic toxicity.
- Monitor lab tests: Baseline and periodic renal function tests, LFTs, and bone marrow function tests; hemoglobin, CBC with differential, platelet counts at least once weekly.

### Patient & Family Education

- Notify prescriber of fever, chills, sore throat, nausea, vomiting, diarrhea, loss of appetite, and unusual bruising or bleeding.
- Use barrier contraceptive during therapy. Drug is teratogenic.

## HYDROXYZINE HYDROCHLORIDE 🅿ʳ

(hye-drox'i-zeen)

Atarax Syrup, Hyzine-50, Vistaril Intramuscular, Vistacon, Vistaject-25 & -50

## HYDROXYZINE PAMOATE

Vistaril Oral

**Classifications:** ANTIHISTAMINE; H$_1$-RECEPTOR ANTAGONIST

Therapeutic: ANTIPRURITIC; ANTIANXIETY; ANTIEMETIC

**AVAILABILITY** **Hydroxyzine HCl:** Tablets; syrup; oral suspension; solution for injection. **Hydroxyzine Pamoate:** Capsule; liquid suspension

## ACTION & *THERAPEUTIC EFFECT*

H$_1$-receptor antagonist effective in treatment of histamine-mediated pruritus or other allergic reactions. Its tranquilizing effect is produced primarily by depression of hypothalamus and brainstem reticular formation, rather than cortical areas. *Effective as an antianxiety agent and sedative. Additionally, it is an effective agent for pruritus and as an antiemetic agent.*

**USES** Emotional or psychoneurotic states characterized by anxiety, tension, or psychomotor agitation; to relieve anxiety, control nausea and emesis, and reduce narcotic requirements before or after surgery or delivery. Also used in management of pruritus due to allergic conditions (e.g., chronic urticaria), atopic and contact dermatoses, and in treatment of acute and chronic alcoholism with withdrawal symptoms or delirium tremens.

**CONTRAINDICATIONS** Known hypersensitivity to hydroxyzine; use as sole treatment in psychoses or depression; lactation.

**CAUTIOUS USE** History of allergies; GI disorders; cardiac disease; COPD; older adults; pregnancy (category C); children.

## ROUTE & DOSAGE

| Anxiety |
| --- |
| *Adult:* **PO** 50–100 mg t.i.d. or q.i.d.; **IM** 50–100 mg q4–6h *Child (younger than 6 y):* **PO** 50 mg/day in divided doses; *6 y* |

*or older:* 50 mg/day in divided doses; **IM** 1.1 mg/kg q4–6h

**Pruritus**

*Adult:* **PO** 25 mg t.i.d. or q.i.d.; **IM** 25 mg q4–6h
*Geriatric:* **PO** 10 mg 3–4 × daily
*Child (6 y or older):* **PO** 50–100 mg/day in divided doses;
*younger than 6 y:* 50 mg/day in divided doses; **IM** 1.1 mg/kg q4–6h

**Nausea**

*Adult:* **IM** 25–100 mg q4–6h
*Child:* **IM** 1.1 mg/kg q4–6h

## ADMINISTRATION

### Oral

- Note: Tablets may be crushed and taken with fluid of patient's choice. Capsule may be emptied and contents swallowed with water or mixed with food. Liquid formulations are available.

### Intramuscular

- Give deep into body of a relatively large muscle. The Z-track technique of injection is recommended to prevent subcutaneous infiltration.
- Recommended site: In adult, the gluteus maximus or vastus lateralis; in children, the vastus lateralis.
- Protect all forms from light. Store at 15°–30° C (59°–86° F) unless otherwise specified.

*INCOMPATIBILITIES:* Solution/additive: **Aminophylline, amobarbital, chloramphenicol, dimenhydrinate, penicillin G, pentobarbital, phenobarbital.**

## ADVERSE EFFECTS (≥1%) **CNS:**
*Drowsiness* (usually transitory), sedation, dizziness, headache. **CV:** Hypotension. **GI:** *Dry mouth.* **Body as a Whole:** Urticaria, dyspnea, chest tightness, wheezing, involuntary motor activity (rare). **Hematologic:** Phlebitis, hemolysis, thrombosis. **Skin:** Erythematous macular eruptions, erythema multiforme, digital gangrene from inadvertent IV or intra-arterial injection, injection site reactions.

## DIAGNOSTIC TEST INTERFERENCE
Possible false positive *serum TCA screen.*

## INTERACTIONS **Drug:** Alcohol and CNS DEPRESSANTS add to CNS depression; TRICYCLIC ANTIDEPRESSANTS and other ANTICHOLINERGICS have additive anticholinergic effects; may inhibit pressor effects of **epinephrine.**

## PHARMACOKINETICS **Absorption:** Readily from GI tract. **Onset:** 15–30 min PO. **Duration:** 4–6 h. **Distribution:** Not known if it crosses placenta or is distributed into breast milk. **Metabolism:** In liver. **Elimination:** In bile.

## NURSING IMPLICATIONS

### Assessment & Drug Effects

- Evaluate alertness. Drowsiness may occur and usually disappears with continued therapy or following reduction of dosage.
- Monitor condition of oral membranes daily when patient is on high dosage of hydroxyzine.
- Reduce dosage of the depressant up to 50% when CNS depressants are prescribed concomitantly.

### Patient & Family Education

- Do not drive or engage in other potentially hazardous activities until response to drug is known.
- **Do not** take alcohol and hydroxyzine at the same time.
- Relieve dry mouth by frequent warm water rinses, increasing fluid intake, and use of a salivary substitute (e.g., Moi-Stir, Xero-Lube).

Common adverse effects in *italic;* life-threatening effects underlined; generic names in **bold;** classifications in SMALL CAPS; ♣ Canadian drug name; ⊙ Prototype drug

799

- Give teeth scrupulous care. Avoid irritation or abrasion of gums and other oral tissues.

# HYOSCYAMINE SULFATE

(hye-oh-sye′a-meen)

Anaspaz, Cystospaz, Levsin, Levsinex, NuLev

**Classifications:** ANTICHOLINERGIC; ANTIMUSCARINIC; ANTISPASMODIC
Therapeutic: GI ANTISPASMODIC
**Prototype:** Atropine

**AVAILABILITY** Tablet; sublingual tablet; sustained release capsule; orally disintegrating tablet; oral solution; elixir; solution for injection

## ACTION & *THERAPEUTIC EFFECT*
Competitive inhibitor of acethycholine at autonomic postganglionic cholinergic receptors. It decreases motility (smooth muscle tone) in GI, biliary, and urinary tracts. *Effective as a GI antispasmodic.*

## USES GI tract disorders caused by
spasm and hypermotility, as conjunct therapy with diet and antacids for peptic ulcer management, and as an aid in the control of gastric hypersecretion and intestinal hypermotility. Also symptomatic relief of biliary and renal colic, as a "drying agent" to relieve symptoms of acute rhinitis, to control preanesthesia salivation and respiratory tract secretions, to treat symptoms of parkinsonism, and to reduce pain and hypersecretion in pancreatis.

## CONTRAINDICATIONS Hypersensitivity to belladonna alkaloids, prostatic hypertrophy, obstructive diseases of GI or GU tract, ulcerative colitis, paralytic ileus or intestinal atony; MG.

**CAUTIOUS USE** Diabetes mellitus, cardiac disease, cardiac arrhythmias; autonomic neuropathy; closed-angle glaucoma; GERD, hiatal hernia; pulmonary disease; renal or hepatic disease; pregnancy (category C); lactation; children younger than 2 y.

## ROUTE & DOSAGE

**GI Spasms**

*Adult:* **IV/IM/Subcutaneous**
0.25–0.5 mg q4h; **PO/Sublingual**
0.125–0.25 mg t.i.d. or q.i.d. prn
*Child (2–12 y):* **PO** 0.0625–0.125
mg q4h prn (max: 0.75 mg/day)

## ADMINISTRATION
- Note: Dose for older adults may need to be less than the standard adult dose. Observe patient carefully for signs of paradoxic reactions.

### Oral
- Give immediate release and sublingual tablets 30 min to 1 h ac.
- Orally disintegrating tablets may be chewed or placed on tongue for disintegration.
- Ensure that sustained release form of drug is not chewed or crushed. It **must be** swallowed whole.

### Intramuscular/Subcutaneous
- May be given undiluted.

### Intravenous

*PREPARE:* **Direct:** Give undiluted.
*ADMINISTER:* **Direct:** Give a single dose over 60 sec.
- Store at 15°–30° C (59°–86° F).

## ADVERSE EFFECTS (≥1%) CNS:
Headache, unusual tiredness or weakness, confusion, *drowsiness,* excitement in older adult patients.
**CV:** Palpitations, tachycardia. **Special Senses:** *Blurred vision,* increased

intraocular tension, cycloplegia, mydriasis. **GI:** *Dry mouth, constipation,* paralytic ileus. **Other:** *Urinary retention,* anhidrosis, suppression of lactation.

### INTERACTIONS **Drug: Amantadine,** ANTIHISTAMINES, TRICYCLIC ANTI-DEPRESSANTS, **quinidine, disopyramide, procainamide** add anticholinergic effects; decreases **levodopa** effects; **methotrimeprazine** may precipitate extrapyramidal effects; decreases antipsychotic effects of PHENOTHIAZINES (decreased absorption).

### PHARMACOKINETICS **Absorption:** Well absorbed from all administration sites. **Onset:** 2–3 min IV; 20–30 min PO. **Peak:** 15–30 min IV; 30–60 min PO. **Duration:** 4–6 h (up to 12 h with sustained release form). **Distribution:** Distributed in most body tissues; crosses blood–brain barrier and placenta; distributed in breast milk. **Metabolism:** In liver. **Elimination:** In urine. **Half-Life:** 3.5–13 h.

### NURSING IMPLICATIONS

#### Assessment & Drug Effects
- Monitor bowel elimination; may cause constipation.
- Monitor urinary output.
- Lessen risk of urinary retention by having patient void prior to each dose.
- Assess for dry mouth and recommend good practices of oral hygiene.

#### Patient & Family Education
- Avoid excessive exposure to high temperatures; drug-induced heatstroke can develop.
- Do not drive or engage in other potentially hazardous activities until response to drug is known.
- Use dark glasses if experiencing blurred vision, but if this adverse effect persists, notify prescriber for dose adjustment or possible drug change.

# IBANDRONATE SODIUM
**Boniva**

**Classifications:** BISPHOSPHONATE; BONE METABOLISM REGULATOR
**Therapeutic:** BONE METABOLISM REGULATOR
**Prototype:** Etidronate

### AVAILABILITY Tablet

### ACTION & *THERAPEUTIC EFFECT*
It inhibits activity of osteoclasts and reduces bone resorption and turnover in the matrix of the bone. *In postmenopausal women, it reduces the rate of bone turnover, resulting in a net gain in bone mass.*

### USES Prevention and treatment of osteoporosis in postmenopausal women.

### UNLABELED USES Treatment of metastatic bone disease in breast cancer.

### CONTRAINDICATIONS Hypersensitivity to ibandronate; severe renal impairment; hypocalcemia, vitamin D deficiency; inability to stand or sit up straight for 60 min; achalasia, esophageal stricture, dysphagia; signs and symptoms of bone fracture due to ibandronate use; severe renal impairment (CrCl less than 30 mL/min).

### CAUTIOUS USE Hypersensitivity to other bisphosphanates; mild or moderate renal impairment; history of GI bleeding or disease, esophagitis, esophageal or gastric ulcers; older adults; pregnancy (category C); lactation. Safe use in children younger than 18 y not established.

### ROUTE & DOSAGE

| Postmenopausal Osteoporosis |
| --- |
| *Adult:* **PO** 2.5 mg daily or 150 mg once monthly on the same day each month; **IV** 3 mg every 3 mo |

Common adverse effects in *italic;* life-threatening effects underlined; generic names in **bold;** classifications in SMALL CAPS; ◆ Canadian drug name; ⊙ Prototype drug

801

*Renal Impairment
Dosage Adjustment*

*CrCl less than 30 mL/min:* Use not recommended

## ADMINISTRATION

### Oral

- Correct hypocalcemia before administering ibandronate.
- Give at least 60 min before food, beverage, or other medications (including vitamins).
- Instruct to swallow whole with a full glass of plain water (180–240 mL; 6–8 oz) while standing or sitting in an upright position.
- Keep patient sitting up or ambulating for 60 min after taking drug.

### Intravenous

*PREPARE: Direct:* Give undiluted. *ADMINISTER:* **Direct:** Give over 15–30 sec.

- Store at 15°–30° C (59°–86° F).

## ADVERSE EFFECTS (≥1%) CNS:
Dizziness, headache, nerve root lesion, vertigo. **GI:** Dyspepsia, constipation, diarrhea, esophagitis, gastritis, pharyngitis, nausea, vomiting. **Respiratory:** Upper respiratory infection, pharyngitis. **Skin:** Rash. **Body as a Whole:** Back pain. **Other:** Tooth disorder.

## DIAGNOSTIC TEST INTERFERENCE
Interferes with the use of bone-imaging agents.

## INTERACTIONS Drug: Concurrent administration of **calcium, magnesium,** or **iron** reduces ibandronate adsorption. **Food:** Food reduces ibandronate absorption (ibandronate should be taken in a fasting state).

## PHARMACOKINETICS Absorption: Bioavailability poor (0.6%). **Peak:** 0.5–2 h. **Distribution:** 86–99%

protein bound. **Metabolism:** None. **Elimination:** Renal. **Half-Life:** 10–60 h.

## NURSING IMPLICATIONS

### Assessment & Drug Effects

- Withhold drug and notify prescriber if the CrCl less than 30 mL/min.
- Diagnostic test: Bone density scan every 12–18 mo.
- Monitor for S&S of upper GI distress, especially with concurrent use of NSAIDs or aspirin.
- Monitor lab tests: Periodic albumin-adjusted serum calcium, serum phosphate, serum alkaline phosphatase, fasting and 24 h urinary calcium, and serum electrolytes; baseline and periodic renal function.

### Patient & Family Education

- Take the monthly dose on the same day each month. Carefully follow directions for taking the drug (see ADMINISTRATION).
- If a monthly dose is missed, and the next scheduled dose is more than 7 days away, take one 150 mg tablet the next morning, then resume the original monthly schedule. Do not take two 150 mg tablets in the same week.
- Report to prescriber any of the following: Severe bone, joint, or muscle pain; heartburn, pain behind the sternum, difficulty or pain with swallowing.

## IBRUTINIB
(i-brut'i-nib)

Imbruvica

**Classifications:** ANTINEOPLASTIC AGENT; KINASE INHIBITOR
**Therapeutic:** ANTINEOPLASTIC AGENT
**Prototype:** Erlotinib

## AVAILABILITY Capsule

## ACTION & *THERAPEUTIC EFFECT*

A potent and irreversible inhibitor of Bruton tyrosine kinase (BTK), an enzyme that is an integral component of the B-cell receptor (BCR) and cytokine receptor pathways; activation of B-cell receptor signaling is important for survival of malignant B cells; *BTK inhibition results in decreased malignant B-cell proliferation and survival.*

**USES** Treatment of patients with mantle cell lymphoma (MCL) or patients with chronic lymphocytic leukemia (CLL) who have received at least one prior therapy; Waldenström macroglobulinemia; graft-versus-host disease.

**CONTRAINDICATIONS** Strong CYP3A4 inhibitors; severe renal impairment (CrCl less than 25 mL/min); pregnancy (category D); lactation.

**CAUTIOUS USE** Neutropenia, thrombocytopenia, anemia; mild to moderate renal impairment; hyperuricemia; mild hepatic impairment; arrhythmias; older adults. Safety and efficacy in children younger than 18 y not established.

## ROUTE & DOSAGE

**Mantle Cell Lymphoma (MCL)**

*Adult:* **PO** 560 mg once daily at approximately the same time daily

**Chronic Lymphocytic Leukemia (CLL)/Waldenström Macroglobulinemia**

*Adult:* **PO** 420 mg once daily at approximately the same time each day until disease progression

**Graft-Versus-Host disease (GVHD)**

*Adult:* **PO** 420 mg daily until GVHD progression.

*Adverse Reactions Dosage Adjustment*

Interrupt therapy for any Grade 3 or greater non-hematological, Grade 3 or greater neutropenia with infection or fever, or Grade 4 hematological toxicities. *After recovery to baseline or Grade 1 toxicity, restart—First occurrence:* 560 mg daily MCL or 420 mg daily CLL; *Second occurrence:* 420 mg daily MCL or 280 mg daily CLL; *Third occurrence:* 280 mg daily MCL or 140 mg daily CLL; *Fourth occurrence:* Discontinue.

### Use with CYP3A4 Inhibitors

*Strong CYP3A4 inhibitors:* Avoid use.
*Moderate CYP3A4 inhibitors:* Decrease dose to 140 mg daily

### *Hepatic Impairment Dosage Adjustment*

*Child-Pugh class A:* Reduce dose to 140 mg daily
*Child-Pugh class B/C:* Do not use

## ADMINISTRATION

### Oral

- Give with water at approximately the same time every day.
- Capsules **must be** swallowed whole; they should not be opened or chewed.
- Store in original container at 15°–30° C (59°–86° F).

**ADVERSE EFFECTS** (≥ 1%) **Body as a Whole:** Fever, infection. **CNS:** Anxiety, chills, dizziness, *fatigue*, headache, insomnia, laceration, malignant neoplasm, *peripheral neuropathy*. **CV:** Atrial fibrillation, hypertension, *peripheral edema*. **GI:** *Abdominal pain, constipation, decreased appetite, diarrhea*, dyspepsia, *nausea*, stomatitis, vomiting. **Hematological:** *Anemia, bruise*, carcinoma, decreased hemoglobin, *decreased platelet count*, hemorrhage, *neu-*

Common adverse effects in *italic;* life-threatening effects underlined; generic names in **bold;** classifications in SMALL CAPS; ♣ Canadian drug name; ⊕ Prototype drug

803

*tropenia,* thrombocytopenia, petechia. **Metabolic:** Dehydration, hyperuricemia hypoalbuminuria, hypokalemia, increased serum creatinine. **Musculoskeletal:** *Arthralgia,* muscle spasm, *musculoskeletal pain,* weakness. **Respiratory:** Cough, *dyspnea,* epistaxis, oropharyngeal pain, pneumonia, sinusitis, *upper respiratory tract infection.* **Skin:** *Skin rash,* skin infection, pruritis. **Urogenital:** Urinary tract infection. **Special senses:** Dry eye syndrome, blurred vision.

**INTERACTIONS Drug:** Ibrutinib may enhance the adverse effects of drugs with antiplatelet activity (e.g., p2y12 INHIBITORS, SSRIS, **aspirin**). Inhibitors of CYP3A4 (e.g., **ketoconazole, itraconazole, voriconazole, posaconazole, clarithromycin, telithromycin**) may increase the levels of ibrutinib. Inducers of CYP3A4 (e.g., **carbamazepine, rifampin, phenytoin**) may decrease the levels of ibrutinib. **Food: Grapefruit** and **grapefruit juice** may increase the levels of ibrutinib. **Herbal: St. John's wort** may decrease the levels of ibrutinib.

**PHARMACOKINETICS Peak:** 1–2 h. **Distribution:** 97% plasma protein bound. **Metabolism:** Extensive hepatic metabolism. **Elimination:** Fecal (80%) and renal (10%). **Half-life:** 4-6 h.

## NURSING IMPLICATIONS

### Assessment & Drug Effects
- Monitor BP, heart rate, and temperature.
- Monitor ECG, especially with new-onset dyspnea.
- Report irregular heart rate and suspected arrhythmias (e.g., atrial fibrillation or flutter).
- Monitor fluid status and maintain adequate hydration.
- Monitor for and report promptly S&S of bleeding or infection (e.g., UTI, upper respiratory tract infection).

- Monitor lab tests: Baseline and monthly (or as necessary) CBC with differential, platelet count, renal function tests, and LFTs; uric acid clinically indicated.

### Patient & Family Education
- Do not consume grapefruit, grapefruit juice or Seville oranges during therapy.
- Report immediately to prescriber any of the following: Temperature 100.5° F or higher, chest pain or palpitations, unexplained bleeding, or shortness of breath.
- Report GI adverse effects including mouth ulcers, severe reflux or dyspepsia, or severe diarrhea.
- Report excessive weight gain, edema, or numbness or tingling of extremities.
- Women of childbearing potential should use effective means of contraception while taking this drug.
- Do not breast-feed while taking this drug.

## IBUPROFEN ⓟ
(eye-byoo′proe-fen)

Advil, Amersol ✣ Caldolor, Children's Motrin, Motrin, Nuprin

**Classifications:** ANALGESIC, NONSTEROIDAL ANTI-INFLAMMATORY DRUG (NSAID) (COX-1 AND COX-2 INHIBITOR); ANTIPYRETIC
Therapeutic: ANALGESIC, NSAID; ANTI-INFLAMMATORY; ANTIPYRETIC

**AVAILABILITY** Tablet; chewable tablet; suspension; drops; solution for injection

**ACTION & *THERAPEUTIC EFFECT***
(COX-1 and COX-2) NSAID inhibitor with nonsteroidal anti-inflammatory activity that blocks prostaglandin synthesis. Its activity also includes modulation of T-cell function, inhibition of inflammatory

cell chemotaxis, decreased release of superoxide radicals, or increased scavenging of these compounds at inflammatory sites. *Has nonsteroidal anti-inflammatory, analgesic, and antipyretic effects. Inhibits platelet aggregation and prolongs bleeding time.*

**USES** Chronic, symptomatic rheumatoid arthritis and osteoarthritis; relief of mild to moderate pain; primary dysmenorrhea; reduction of fever.

**UNLABELED USES** Gout, juvenile rheumatoid arthritis, psoriatic arthritis, ankylosing spondylitis, vascular headache.

**CONTRAINDICATIONS** Hypersensitivity to ibuprofen; patient in whom urticaria, severe rhinitis, bronchospasm, angioedema, nasal polyps are precipitated by aspirin or other NSAIDs; active peptic ulcer, bleeding abnormalities; perioperative pain related to CABG surgery; signs and symptoms of renal toxicity to ibuprofen; severe hepatic reactions to ibuprofen; development of signs and symptoms of meningitis while taking ibuprofen, salicylate hypersensitivity.

**CAUTIOUS USE** History of GI ulceration or GI bleeding; intrinsic coagulation defects; DM; impaired hepatic or renal function, chronic renal failure; hypertension, history of CAD; angina, MI, cardiac decompensation; patients with SLE, and related connective tissue disorders; adults older than 60 y; pregnancy (category C). Safe use in children younger than 6 mo not established.

## ROUTE & DOSAGE

### Inflammatory Disease
*Adult:* **PO** 400–800 mg t.i.d. or q.i.d. (max: 3200 mg/day)

*Child (weight less than 20 kg):* **PO** Up to 400 mg/day in divided doses; *weight 20 kg to less than 30 kg:* Up to 600 mg/day in divided doses; *weight 30–40 kg:* Up to 800 mg/day in divided doses

### Dysmenorrhea
*Adult:* **PO** 400 mg q4–6h up to 1200 mg/day

### Mild to Moderate Pain
*Adult:* **PO** 400 mg q4–6h up to 1200 mg/day **IV** 400 mg q4–6h prn or 100–200 mg q4h prn

### Fever
*Adult:* **PO** 200–400 mg t.i.d. or q.i.d. (max: 1200 mg/day) *Child (6 mo–12 y):* **PO** 5–10 mg/kg q4–6h up to 40 mg/kg/day

## ADMINISTRATION

### Oral
- Give on an empty stomach, 1 h before or 2 h after meals. May be taken with meals or milk if GI intolerance occurs.
- Ensure that chewable tablets are chewed or crushed before being swallowed.
- Note: Tablet may be crushed if patient is unable to swallow it whole and mixed with food or liquid before swallowing.
- Store in tightly closed, light-resistant container unless otherwise directed by manufacturer.

### Intravenous
Patients should be well hydrated before IV infusion to prevent renal damage.

***PREPARE: Infusion:*** Dilute required dose with NS, D5W or LR to a final concentration of 4 mg/mL or less.

***ADMINISTER: Infusion:*** Infuse over at least 30 min.

---

**ADVERSE EFFECTS** (≥1%) **CNS:** Headache, dizziness, light-headedness, anxiety, emotional lability, fatigue, malaise, drowsiness, confusion, depression, aseptic meningitis. **CV:** Hypertension, palpitation, congestive heart failure (patient with marginal cardiac function); <u>thrombotic events (MI, stroke)</u>; peripheral edema. **Special Senses:** Amblyopia (blurred vision, decreased visual acuity, scotomas, changes in color vision); nystagmus, visual-field defects; tinnitus, impaired hearing. **GI:** Dry mouth, gingival ulcerations, dyspepsia, *heartburn, nausea,* vomiting, anorexia, diarrhea, constipation, bloating, flatulence, epigastric or abdominal discomfort or pain, GI ulceration, *occult blood loss.* **Hematologic:** <u>Thrombocytopenia,</u> neutropenia, hemolytic or <u>aplastic anemia, leukopenia</u>; decreased Hgb, Hct; transitory rise in AST, ALT, serum alkaline phosphatase; rise in (Ivy) bleeding time. **Urogenital:** Acute renal failure, polyuria, azotemia, cystitis, hematuria, nephrotoxicity, decreased creatinine clearance. **Skin:** Maculopapular and vesicobullous skin eruptions, erythema multiforme, pruritus, rectal itching, acne. **Body as a Whole:** Fluid retention with edema, Stevens–Johnson syndrome, <u>toxic hepatitis,</u> hypersensitivity reactions, <u>anaphylaxis,</u> bronchospasm, serum sickness, SLE, angioedema.

**INTERACTIONS Drug:** ORAL ANTICOAGULANTS, **heparin** may prolong bleeding time; avoid other NSAIDs; may increase **lithium** and **methotrexate** toxicity. Do not use **cidofovir** due to toxicity risk. **Herbal: Feverfew, garlic, ginger, ginkgo** may increase bleeding potential.

**PHARMACOKINETICS Absorption:** 80% from GI tract (oral product). **Onset:** 1 h (antipyretic). **Peak:** 1–2 h. **Duration:** 6–8 h. **Metabolism:** In liver. **Elimination:** Primarily in urine; some biliary excretion. **Half-Life:** 2–4 h.

## NURSING IMPLICATIONS

### Black Box Warning

*Ibuprofen has been associated with increased risk of serious, potentially fatal GI bleeding and cardiovascular events (e.g., MI & CVA); risk may increase with duration of use and may be greater in the older adult and those with risk factors for CV disease.*

### Assessment & Drug Effects

- Monitor for and report promptly S&S of CV thrombotic events (i.e., angina, MI, TIA, or stroke).
- Observe patients with history of cardiac decompensation closely for evidence of fluid retention and edema.
- Monitor for and report promptly S&S of GI ulceration or bleeding. Significant GI bleeding may occur without prior warning.
- Auditory and ophthalmologic examinations are recommended in patients receiving prolonged or high-dose therapy.
- Note: Symptoms of acute toxicity in children include apnea, cyanosis, response only to painful stimuli, dizziness, and nystagmus.
- Monitor lab tests: Baseline and periodic Hgb, renal function tests, and LFTs.

### Patient & Family Education

- Stop taking drug and report promptly to prescriber if you experience chest pain, shortness of breath, weakness, slurring of speech, or other signs of a cardiac or neurologic problem.
- Notify prescriber immediately of passage of dark tarry stools, "coffee ground" emesis, frankly

bloody emesis, or other GI distress, as well as blood or protein in urine, and onset of skin rash, pruritus, jaundice.

- Do not drive or engage in other potentially hazardous activities until response to the drug is known.
- Do not self-medicate with ibuprofen if taking prescribed drugs or being treated for a serious condition without consulting prescriber.
- Do not give to children younger than 3 mo or for longer than 2 days without consulting prescriber.
- Do not take aspirin concurrently with ibuprofen.
- Avoid alcohol and NSAIDs unless otherwise advised by prescriber. Concurrent use may increase risk of GI ulceration and bleeding tendencies.

# IBUTILIDE FUMARATE

(i-bu'ti-lide)

Corvert

**Classification:** CLASS III ANTIARRHYTHMIC
**Therapeutic:** CLASS III ANTIARRHYTHMIC
**Prototype:** Amiodarone HCl

**AVAILABILITY** Solution for injection

## ACTION & THERAPEUTIC EFFECT

Ibutilide is a Class III antiarrhythmic that prolongs cardiac action potential and increases both atrial and ventricular refractoriness without affecting conduction. *Effective in treating recently occurring atrial arrhythmias. It may produce proarrhythmic effects that can be life threatening.*

**USES** Rapid conversion of atrial fibrillation or atrial flutter of recent onset.

## CONTRAINDICATIONS Hypersensitivity to ibutilide, hypokalemia, hypomagnesemia.

**CAUTIOUS USE** History of CHF, cardiac ejection fraction of 35% or less, recent MI, prolonged QT intervals, ventricular arrhythmias; renal or liver disease, cardiovascular disorder other than atrial arrhythmias; pregnancy (category C); lactation. Safe use in children younger than 18 y not established.

## ROUTE & DOSAGE

**Atrial Fibrillation or Flutter**

*Adult (weight less than 60 kg):* **IV** 0.01 mg/kg, may repeat in 10 min if inadequate response; *weight 60 kg or greater:* 1 mg, may repeat in 10 min if inadequate response

## ADMINISTRATION

- Hypokalemia and hypomagnesemia should be corrected prior to treatment with ibutilide.

Intravenous

*PREPARE:* **Direct:** Give undiluted **IV Infusion:** Contents of 1 mg vial may be diluted in 50 mL of D5W or NS to yield 0.017 mg/mL.
*ADMINISTER:* **Direct/IV Infusion:** Give a single dose by direct injection or infusion over 10 min.
- Stop injection/infusion as soon as presenting arrhythmia is terminated or with appearance of ventricular tachycardia or marked prolongation of QT or QT$_c$.

- Store diluted solution up to 24 h at 15°–30° C (59°–86° F) or 48 h refrigerated at 2°–8° C (36°–46° F).

**ADVERSE EFFECTS** (≥1%) **CNS:** Headache. **CV:** Proarrhythmic effects (sustained and nonsustained polymorphic ventricular tachycardia), AV block, bundle branch block, ventricular extrasystoles, hypotension,

Common adverse effects in *italic;* life-threatening effects <u>underlined</u>; generic names in **bold;** classifications in SMALL CAPS; ♣ Canadian drug name; ⊘ Prototype drug

807

postural hypotension, bradycardia, tachycardia, palpitations, prolonged QT segment. **GI:** Nausea.

**INTERACTIONS Drug:** Increased potential for proarrhythmic effects when administered with PHENO-THIAZINES, TRICYCLIC ANTIDEPRESSANTS, **amiodarone, disopyramide, quinidine, procainamide, sotalol** may cause prolonged refractoriness if given within 4 h of ibutilide.

**PHARMACOKINETICS Onset:** 30 min. **Metabolism:** In liver. **Elimination:** 82% in urine, 19% in feces. **Half-Life:** 6 h (range 2–21 h).

## NURSING IMPLICATIONS

### Black Box Warning

*Ibutilide has been associated with potentially fatal arrhythmias usually, but not always, in association of QT prolongation.*

### Assessment & Drug Effects

- Observe with continuous ECG, BP, and HR monitoring during and for at least 4 h after infusion or until QT$_c$ has returned to baseline. Monitor for longer periods with liver dysfunction or if proarrhythmic activity is observed.
- Hypokalemia and hypomagnesemia should be corrected prior to beginning treatment with ibutilide.
- Monitor for therapeutic effectiveness. Conversion to normal sinus rhythm normally occurs within 30 min of initiation of infusion.
- Monitor lab tests: Baseline serum potassium and magnesium.

### Patient & Family Education

- Consult prescriber and understand the potential risks of ibutilide therapy.

# IDARUBICIN

(i-da-roo'bi-cin)

**Idamycin PFS**

**Classifications:** ANTINEOPLASTIC; ANTHRACYCLINE (ANTIBIOTIC)

**Therapeutic:** ANTINEOPLASTIC

**Prototype:** Doxorubicin

**AVAILABILITY** Solution for injection

## ACTION & THERAPEUTIC EFFECT

Cytotoxic anthracycline that exhibits inhibitory effects on DNA topoisomerase II, an enzyme responsible for repairing faulty sections of DNA. It results in breaks in the helix of the DNA, and thus it affects RNA and protein synthesis in rapidly dividing cells. *Has antineoplastic and cytotoxic action on cancer cells that results in cell death.*

**USES** In combination with other antineoplastic drugs for treatment of AML.

**UNLABELED USES** Breast cancer, other solid tumors.

**CONTRAINDICATIONS** Myelo-suppression, hypersensitivity to idarubicin or doxorubicin, pregnancy (category D), lactation.

**CAUTIOUS USE** Impaired renal or hepatic function; patients who have received irradiation or radiotherapy to areas surrounding heart; cardiac disease. Safe use in children younger than 2 y not established.

## ROUTE & DOSAGE

### Acute Myelogenous Leukemia (AML)

*Adult:* **IV** 12 mg/m$^2$ daily for 3 days injected slowly over 10–15 min

**Acute Nonlymphocytic Leukemia, Acute Lymphocytic Leukemia**

*Child:* **IV** 10–12 mg/m²/day for 3 days

**Renal Impairment Dosage Adjustment**

*Creatinine greater than 2 mg/dL:* Give 75% of dose

**Hepatic Impairment Dosage Adjustment**

*Bilirubin 1.5–5 mg/dL:* Give 50% of dose; *if greater than 5 mg/dL:* Do not use drug

## ADMINISTRATION

**Intravenous**

IV administration to infants, children: Verify correct IV concentration and rate of infusion with prescriber.

This drug is a cytotoxic agent and caution should be used to prevent any contact with the drug. Follow institutional or standard guidelines for preparation, handling, and disposal of cytotoxic agents.

*PREPARE:* **IV Infusion:** Further dilution is not required.

*ADMINISTER:* **IV Infusion:** Give slowly over 10–15 min into tubing of free flowing IV of NS or D5W. ▪ If extravasation is suspected, immediately stop infusion, elevate the arm, and apply ice pack for 30 min then q.i.d. for 30 min × 3 days.

*INCOMPATIBILITIES:* Solution/additive: ALKALINE SOLUTIONS (i.e., **sodium bicarbonate**), **heparin.**
Y-site: **Acyclovir, allopurinol, ampicillin/sulbactam, cefazolin, cefepime, ceftazidime, clindamycin, dexamethasone, etoposide, furosemide, gentamicin, heparin, hydrocortisone, imipenem/cilastatin, lorazepam, meperidine, methotrexate, mezlocillin, piperacillin/tazobactam, sargramostim, sodium bicarbonate, teniposide, vancomycin, vincristine.**

▪ Store reconstituted solutions up to 7 days refrigerated at 2°–8° C (36°–46° F) and 72 h at room temperature 15°–30° C (59°–86° F).

## ADVERSE EFFECTS (≥1%) **CV:** CHF, atrial fibrillation, chest pain, MI. **GI:** *Nausea, vomiting, diarrhea, abdominal pain,* mucositis. **Hematologic:** *Anemia, leukopenia,* thrombocytopenia. **Other:** Nephrotoxicity, hepatotoxicity, *alopecia,* rash.

## INTERACTIONS **Drug:** IMMUNOSUPPRESSANTS cause additive bone marrow suppression; ANTICOAGULANTS, NSAIDS, SALICYLATES, **aspirin,** THROMBOLYTIC AGENTS increase risk of bleeding; idarubicin may blunt the effects of **filgrastim, sargramostim.**

## PHARMACOKINETICS **Onset:** Median time to remission 28 days. **Peak:** Serum level 4 h. **Duration:** Serum levels 120 h. **Distribution:** Concentrates in nucleated blood and bone marrow cells. **Metabolism:** In liver to idarubicinol, which may be as active as idarubicin. **Elimination:** 16% in urine; 17% in bile. **Half-Life:** Idarubicin 15–45 h, idarubicinol 45 h.

## NURSING IMPLICATIONS

### Black Box Warning

*Idarubicin can cause severe local tissue necrosis if extravasation occurs and it has been associated with severe myelosuppression.*

Common adverse effects in *italic*; life-threatening effects underlined; generic names in **bold**; classifications in SMALL CAPS; ✦ Canadian drug name; ◐ Prototype drug

809

## Assessment & Drug Effects

- Monitor infusion site closely, as extravasation can cause severe local tissue necrosis. Notify prescriber if pain, erythema, or edema develops at insertion site.
- Monitor cardiac status closely, especially in older adult patients or those with preexisting cardiac disease.
- Monitor hematologic status carefully; during the period of myelosuppression, patients are at high risk for bleeding and infection.
- Monitor for development of hyperuricemia secondary to lysis of leukemic cells.
- Monitor lab tests: Periodic LFTs and renal function tests, CBC with differential, and coagulation studies.

## Patient & Family Education

- Learn all potential adverse reactions to idarubicin.
- Anticipate possible hair loss.
- Discuss interventions to minimize nausea, vomiting, diarrhea, and stomatitis with health care providers.

# IDARUCIZUMAB

(i-dare'you-scis-ooh-mab)

Praxbind

**Classifications:** MONOCLONAL ANTIBODY; COAGULATION REVERSAL AGENT

Therapeutic: COAGULATION REVERSAL AGENT

**AVAILABILITY** Solution for injection

## ACTION & *THERAPEUTIC EFFECT*

A humanized monoclonal antibody fragment (Fab) that binds to dabigatran and its acylglucuronide metabolites with higher affinity than dabigatran binds to thrombin. *This action neutralizes dabigatran as well as its active metabolites, thus reversing their anticoagulant effect.*

**USES** Indicated for the reversal of the anticoagulant effects of dabigatran in patients requiring emergency surgery or other urgent procedures, and in patients with life-threatening or uncontrolled bleeding.

**CAUTIOUS USE** Hereditary fructose intolerance, thromboembolic disease, pregnancy, lactation.

## ROUTE & DOSAGE

**Reversal of Dabigatran Effects**
*Adult:* **IV** 5 gram

## ADMINISTRATION

Intravenous

*PREPARE:* **IV Infusion:** Flush the line with 0.9% sodium chloride prior to infusion. Recommended dose provided is 2 vials each containing 2.5 g/50 mL.
*ADMINISTER:* **IV Infusion:** Administer 5 g dose as either 2 consecutive infusions or inject both vials consecutively via syringe. A pre-existing intravenous line may be used for administration.
*INCOMPATIBILITIES* Solution/additive: None listed; however, the solution should not be mixed with other medicinal products or solutions.

- Store refrigerated at 2–8° C (36-46° F).
- Do not freeze; do not shake.
- Prior to use, the unopened vial may be kept at room temperature 25° C (77°F) for up to 48 h if stored in the original package in order to protect from light or up to 6 h when exposed to light.
- Administer within 1 h after solution has been removed from the vial.

**ADVERSE EFFECTS** (≥4%) **Body as a Whole:** Hypersensitivity reactions, pneumonia. **CNS:** Delirium, headache. **CV:** Thromboembolic events. **GI:** Constipation. **Metabolic:** Hypokalemia.

Common adverse effects in *italic;* life-threatening effects underlined; generic names in **bold;** classifications in SMALL CAPS; ♣ Canadian drug name; ⊙ Prototype drug

**PHARMACOKINETICS Metabolism:** Biodegradation of monoclonal antibody. **Elimination:** Primarily renal. **Half-Life:** 10.3 h.

## NURSING IMPLICATIONS

### Assessment & Drug Effects

- Obtain baseline aPTT, repeat at 2 h and then every 12 h until aPTT returns to normal.
- Assess for S&S of bleeding and thromboembolism in patients with hereditary fructose intolerance.

### Patient & Family Education

- This drug is used to undo the effects of a blood thinner. The chance of blood clots may be raised after using this drug. Follow instructions from your health care provider about prevention of blood clots.
- Report signs or symptoms of a blood clot immediately such as chest pain or pressure; coughing up blood; swelling, warmth, numbness, change of color, or pain in a leg or arm; or trouble breathing or talking.

## IDELALISIB

(i-del-a-li'sib)
Zydelig

**Classifications:** ANTINEOPLASTIC; KINASE INHIBITOR
**Therapeutic:** ANTINEOPLASTIC
**Prototype:** Erlotinib

## AVAILABILITY Tablets

## ACTION & *THERAPEUTIC EFFECT*

Potent inhibitor of the enzyme, phosphatidylinositol 3-kinase (PI3Kδ), which is highly expressed in malignant lymphoid B-cells. *PI3Kδ inhibition results in apoptosis of malignant tumor cells, thus reducing the number of malignant lymphocytes.*

**USES** Treatment of patients with relapsed chronic lymphocytic leukemia (CLL), relapsed follicular B-cell non-Hodgkin lymphoma (FL), and relapsed small lymphocytic lymphoma (SLL).

**CONTRAINDICATIONS** History of serious allergic reactions including anaphylaxis and toxic epidermal necrolysis; intestinal perforation; concurrent CYP3A inducers or substrates; recurrent hepatotoxicity, life-threatening diarrhea, or pneumonitis due to idelalisib; pregnancy (category D), lactation.

**CAUTIOUS USE** Neutropenia, thrombocytopenia, anemia; preexisting liver impairment; pulmonary toxicity; colitis; older adults. Safety and efficacy in children less than 18 y not established.

## ROUTE & DOSAGE

**Chronic Lymphocytic Leukemia, B-Cell Non-Hodgkin Lymphoma, Small Lymphocytic Lymphoma**

*Adult:* **PO** 150 mg b.i.d.

*Hepatic Impairment Dosage Adjustment*

*ALT/AST greater than 5 to 20 × ULN or bilirubin greater than 3 to 10 × ULN:* Interrupt therapy; monitor LFTs at least weekly until ALT/AST and/or bilirubin is ULN or less, then restart therapy at 100 mg b.i.d. *ALT/AST greater than 20 × ULN, bilirubin greater than 10 × ULN, or recurrent hepatotoxicity:* Permanently discontinue.

*Toxicity Dosage Adjustment*

*Severe diarrhea or diarrhea requiring hospitalization:* Interrupt therapy, monitor at least weekly, restart at 100 mg b.i.d., when

Common adverse effects in *italic*; life-threatening effects <u>underlined</u>; generic names in **bold**; classifications in SMALL CAPS; ♣ Canadian drug name; ⊙ Prototype drug

811

diarrhea has resolved. *Life-threatening diarrhea:* Permanently discontinue

*Neutropenia ANC less than 500 cells/mm³:* Interrupt therapy, monitor ANC at least weekly, then restart at 100 mg b.i.d. when ANC 500 cells/mm³ or greater

*Thrombocytopenia platelet count less than 25,000 cells/mm³:* Interrupt therapy, monitor platelet count at least weekly, then restart at 100 mg b.i.d. when platelet count 25,000 cells/mm³ or greater

*Symptomatic pneumonitis (any severity):* Discontinue

*Other severe or life-threatening toxicities:* Interrupt therapy until toxicity is resolved; resume treatment at 100 mg b.i.d. Permanently discontinue for any recurrence after re-challenge.

## ADMINISTRATION

### Oral

- Give without regard to food.
- Tablets **must be** swallowed whole. They must not be crushed or chewed.
- May give a missed dose if within 6 h of usual dosing time. If more than 6 h, skip the missed dose and resume with the next scheduled dose.
- Store at 15°–30° C (59°–86° F).

## ADVERSE EFFECTS (≥ 2%) **Body as a Whole:** Asthenia, *chills, fatigue,* night sweats, pain, peripheral edema, *pyrexia,* sepsis *fever.* **CNS:** Headache, insomnia. **GI:** *Abdominal pain, diarrhea,* gastroesophageal reflux disease, *nausea,* stomatitis, vomiting. **Metabolic:** Altered glucose level (increase and decrease), altered lymphocyte count (increase and decrease), decreased appetite, decreased hemoglobin, <u>decreased neutrophils, decreased platelets,</u> hypertriglyceridemia, hyponatremia, *increased ALT and AST,* increase gamma glutamyl transpeptidase. **Musculoskeletal:** Arthralgia. **Respiratory:** Bronchitis, cough, *dyspnea,* nasal congestion, *pneumonia,* sinusitis, upper respiratory infection. **Skin:** Rash. **Urogenital:** Urinary tract infection.

## INTERACTIONS **Drug:** Coadministration with other drugs that inhibit CYP3A4 (e.g., **erythromycin, itraconazole, ketoconazole**) may increase the levels of idelalisib. Coadministration with other drugs that induce CYP3A4 (e.g., **carbamazepine, phenytoin, rifampin**) may decrease the levels of idelalisib. Idelalisib may increase the levels of other drugs that require CYP3A4 for metabolism. **Food: Grapefruit** and **grapefruit juice** may increase the levels of idelalisib. **Herbal: St. John's wort** may decrease the levels of idelalisib.

## PHARMACOKINETICS **Peak:** 1.5 h. **Distribution:** 84% plasma protein bound. **Metabolism:** In liver. **Elimination:** Renal (14%) and fecal (78%). **Half-Life:** 8.2 h.

## NURSING IMPLICATIONS

### Black Box Warning

*Idelalisib has been associated with severe and sometimes fatal cases of hepatotoxicity, diarrhea, colitis, pneumonitis, and intestinal perforation.*

### Assessment & Drug Effects

- Monitor for and report promptly any of the following: S&S of severe diarrhea/colitis, intestinal

Common adverse effects in *italic*; life-threatening effects <u>underlined</u>; generic names in **bold**; classifications in SMALL CAPS; ♣ Canadian drug name; ⊕ Prototype drug

perforation, pneumonitis (e.g., cough, dyspnea, hypoxia), dermatologic toxicity (i.e., dermatitis or rash), and hypersensitivity reactions. Withhold drug for any of the foregoing until prescriber is consulted.

- Monitor lab tests: LFTs q2wk first 3 mo, q4wk next 3 mo, then q1–3 mo thereafter, or as necessary; CBC with differential and platelet count q2wk first 3 mo, and at least weekly with neutropenia, or as necessary.

### Patient & Family Education

- Report immediately if you develop a fever or any signs of infection.
- Report immediately to prescribed if you experience signs of intestinal toxicity or perforation such as abdominal pain, chills, fever, nausea, vomiting, or severe diarrhea (i.e., six or more bowel movements per day).
- Report signs of skin toxicity including rash with or without itching.
- Report signs of liver damage including jaundice, bruising, abdominal pain, or bleeding.
- Report new or worsening respiratory symptoms including cough or dyspnea.
- Women of childbearing age should use effective means of contraception while taking this drug and for at least 1 mo after ending treatment.
- Do not breast-feed while taking this drug.

## IFOSFAMIDE
(i-fos′fa-mide)

**Classifications:** ANTINEOPLASTIC; ALKYLATING AGENT
Therapeutic: ANTINEOPLASTIC
**Prototype:** Cyclophosphamide

**AVAILABILITY** Solution for injection

## ACTION & *THERAPEUTIC EFFECT*
Interacts with DNA as a cell cycle nonspecific agent. Antineoplastic action is primarily due to crosslinking of strands of DNA and RNA as well as inhibition of protein synthesis. *It has antineoplastic and cytotoxic action on cancer cells that results in cell death*.

**USES** In combination with other agents in various regimens for germ cell testicular cancer.

**CONTRAINDICATIONS** Previous hypersensitivity to ifosfamide; severe bone marrow depression; dehydration; pregnancy (category D); lactation.

**CAUTIOUS USE** Impaired renal function, renal failure; hepatic disease; prior radiation or prior therapy with other cytotoxic agents.

## ROUTE & DOSAGE

### Antineoplastic

*Adult:* **IV** 1.2 g/m²/day for 5 consecutive days; repeat q3wk or after recovery from hematologic toxicity (platelets 100,000/mm³ or greater; WBC 4000/mm³ or greater)

## ADMINISTRATION

### Intravenous

This drug is a cytotoxic agent and caution should be used to prevent any contact with the drug. Follow institutional or standard guidelines for preparation, handling, and disposal of cytotoxic agents.

*PREPARE:* **IV Infusion:** Reconstitute each 1 g or 3 g vial with 20 mL or 60 mL, respectively, of sterile water or bacteriostatic water to yield 50 mg/mL. ▪ Shake

Common adverse effects in *italic;* life-threatening effects underlined; generic names in **bold**; classifications in SMALL CAPS; ♣ Canadian drug name; ⦿ Prototype drug

813

well to dissolve. ■May be further diluted with D5W, NS, or LR to achieve concentrations of 0.6–20 mg/mL. ■ Use solution prepared with sterile water within 6 h.
***ADMINISTER:* IV Infusion:** Give slowly over 30 min. ■ Note: Mesna is always given concurrently with ifosfamide; never give ifosfamide alone.
***INCOMPATIBILITIES:* Y-site: Cefepime, methotrexate.**

■Store reconstituted solution prepared with bacteriostatic solution up to a week at 30° C (86° F) or 6 wk at 5° C (41° F).

**ADVERSE EFFECTS** (≥1%) **CNS:** *Somnolence, confusion, hallucinations,* coma, dizziness, seizures, cranial nerve dysfunction. **GI:** *Nausea, vomiting,* anorexia, diarrhea, metabolic acidosis, hepatic dysfunction. **Hematologic:** <u>Neutropenia, thrombocytopenia.</u> **Urogenital:** <u>Hemorrhagic cystitis, nephrotoxicity.</u> **Skin:** *Alopecia,* skin necrosis with extravasation.

**INTERACTIONS Drug:** HEPATIC ENZYME INDUCERS (BARBITURATES, **phenytoin**) may increase hepatic conversion of ifosfamide to active metabolite; CORTICOSTEROIDS may inhibit conversion to active metabolites.

**PHARMACOKINETICS Distribution:** Distributed into breast milk. **Metabolism:** In liver via CYP3A4. **Elimination:** 70–86% in urine. **Half-Life:** 7–15 h.

**NURSING IMPLICATIONS**

**Black Box Warning**

*Ifosfamide has been associated with hemorrhagic cystitis and CNS toxicities.*

**Assessment & Drug Effects**
■ Hold drug and notify prescriber if WBC count is below 2000/mm³ or platelet count is below 50,000/mm³.
■ Reduce risk of hemorrhagic cystitis by hydrating with 3000 mL of fluid daily prior to therapy and for at least 72 h following treatment to ensure ample urine output.
■ Monitor for and repost promptly any of the following CNS symptoms: Somnolence, confusion, depressive psychosis, and hallucinations.
■ Monitor lab tests: CBC with differential prior to each dose and at regular intervals; urinalysis prior to each dose for microscopic hematuria.

**Patient & Family Education**
■ Void frequently to lessen contact of irritating chemical with bladder mucosa by keeping well hydrated.
■ Note: Susceptibility to infection may increase. Avoid people with infection. Notify prescriber of any infection, fever or chills, cough or hoarseness, lower back or side pain, painful or difficult urination.
■ Check with prescriber immediately if there is any unusual bleeding or bruising, black tarry stools, or blood in urine or if pinpoint red spots develop on skin.
■ Discuss possible adverse effects (e.g., alopecia, nausea, and vomiting) and measures that can minimize them with health care provider.

**ILOPERIDONE**
(i-lo-per'i-done)
Fanapt
**Classification:** ATYPICAL ANTIPSYCHOTIC
Therapeutic: ANTIPSYCHOTIC
**Prototype:** Clozapine

## AVAILABILITY Tablet

## ACTION & *THERAPEUTIC EFFECT*

Mechanism of action is unknown, however, thought to be both a dopamine ($D_2$) and serotonin (5-$HT_2$) antagonist. *Effective in treating acute schizophrenia uncontrolled by other agents.*

## USES Acute treatment of schizophrenia.

## CONTRAINDICATIONS Hypersensitivity to iloperidone; older adults with dementia-related psychosis; suicidal ideation; neuroleptic malignant syndrome (NMS); severe hepatic impairment; recent acute MI; ANC less than 100 mm³; lactation.

## CAUTIOUS USE Congenital long QT syndrome; history of cardiac arrhythmias; history of suicidal tendencies; cardiovascular disease; CVA; CHF; cerebrovascular disease; risk for aspiration pneumonia; tardive dykinesia; DM; history of seizures; history of leukopenia/neutropenia; moderate hepatic impairment; patients at risk for aspiration pneumonia; older adults; pregnancy (category C). Safety and efficacy in children not established.

## ROUTE & DOSAGE

### Schizophrenia

*Adult:* **PO** Initial 1 mg b.i.d., then titrate.

*Titration schedule:* Increase each b.i.d. dose by 2 mg a day from day 2 through 7 or until desired dose reached (max: 12 mg b.i.d.). **Note:** Reduce dose by 50% with concurrent use of a strong CYP2D6 inhibitor (e.g., fluoxetine or paroxetine) or strong CYP3A4 inhibitor (e.g., ketoconazole or clarithromycin).

### *Pharmacogenetic Dosage Adjustment*

Reduce dose 50% for poor CYP2D6 metabolizers

## ADMINISTRATION

### Oral

- Note that gradual dose titration is recommended initially and whenever patient has been off drug for more than 3 days.
- Store at 15°–30° C (59°–86° F) and protect from light.

## ADVERSE EFFECTS (≥1%) Body as a Whole: Fatigue. CNS: *Dizziness,* extrapyramidal disorder, lethargy, *somnolence,* tremor. CV: Hypotension, orthostatic hypotension, *tachycardia.* GI: Abdominal discomfort, diarrhea, *dry mouth, nausea.* Metabolic: Increased weight. Musculoskeletal: Arthralgia, musculoskeletal stiffness. Respiratory: Dyspnea, nasal congestion, nasopharyngitis, upper respiratory infection. Skin: Rash. Special Senses: Blurred vision. Urogenital: Ejaculation failure.

## INTERACTIONS Drug: Potential additive QT prolongation if used in combination with drugs with similar effects (e.g., **disopyramide, procainamide, amiodarone**). Inhibitors of CYP3A4 (e.g., **ketoconazole, itraconazole, clarithromycin**) or CYP2D6 (e.g., **fluoxetine, paroxetine**) can increase iloperidone levels. Do not use with **saquinavir** due to risk of torsades de pointes. Food: Grapefruit juice may increase iloperidone levels.

## PHARMACOKINETICS Peak: 2–4 h. Distribution: 95% plasma protein bound. Metabolism: Extensive hepatic metabolism to active and inac-

Common adverse effects in *italic*; life-threatening effects underlined; generic names in **bold**; classifications in SMALL CAPS; ✚ Canadian drug name; ⑦ Prototype drug

815

tive metabolites. **Elimination:** Renal (major) and fecal. **Half-Life:** 18–33 h.

## NURSING IMPLICATIONS

### Black Box Warning

*Iloperidone has been associated with increased mortality in older adults with dementia-related psychosis.*

### Assessment & Drug Effects

- Monitor for suicidal ideation and report promptly if suspected.
- Monitor BP, HR, and weight. Monitor orthostatic vital signs with concurrent antihypertensive therapy or any condition that predisposes to hypotension (e.g., advanced age, dehydration).
- Monitor for orthostatic hypotension and syncope, especially early in therapy.
- Monitor ECG for prolongation of the $QT_c$ interval.
- Monitor diabetics and those at risk for diabetes for loss of glycemic control.
- Monitor lab tests: Baseline and periodic CBC with differential.

### Patient & Family Education

- Be alert for and report worsening of condition, including ideas of suicide.
- Make position changes slowly, especially from a lying or sitting position to a standing position.
- If diabetic, monitor blood sugar closely for loss of control.
- Stop taking the drug and report immediately any of the following: Feeling faint or fainting, high fever, muscle rigidity, altered mental status, or palpitations.
- Do not drink alcohol while taking this drug.
- Avoid engaging in hazardous activities until response to drug is known.

# IMATINIB MESYLATE
(i-ma′ti-nib)

Gleevec

**Classifications:** ANTINEOPLASTIC; MONOCLONAL ANTIBODY; EPIDERMAL GROWTH FACTOR RECEPTOR; KINASE INHIBITOR
Therapeutic: ANTINEOPLASTIC
**Prototype:** Erlotinib

## AVAILABILITY Tablet

## ACTION & *THERAPEUTIC EFFECT*
Epidermal growth factor receptor-tyrosine kinase inhibitor (EGFR-TKI) that interferes with intracellular signaling pathways that are involved in the development of malignancies. Imatinib inhibits abnormal Bcr-Abl tyrosine kinase created by the Philadelphia chromosome abnormality in chronic myeloid leukemia (CLM). *Inhibits WBC cell proliferation and induces cell death in Bcr-Abl tyrosine kinase positive cells as well as in newly formed leukemic cells. Thus, it interferes with progression of chronic myeloid leukemia (CML). Additionally, imatinib inhibits proliferation and induces cell death in gastrointestinal stomal tumor (GIST) that express a mutation of an activated cKit tyrosine kinase.*

## USES Treatment of CML in blast crisis, or in chronic phase after failure of interferon-alpha therapy; unresectable and/or metastatic malignant gastrointestinal stromal tumors (GISTs), acute lymphoblastic leukemia; hypereosinophillic syndrome.

## UNLABELED USES Acute lymphocytic leukemia (ALL), soft tissue sarcoma, recurrence of stomach and intestinal tumors.

## CONTRAINDICATIONS Pregnancy (category D), lactation.

---

Common adverse effects in *italic;* life-threatening effects <u>underlined</u>; generic names in **bold;** classifications in SMALL CAPS; ♣ Canadian drug name; ⊕ Prototype drug

**CAUTIOUS USE** History of hypersensitivity to other monoclonal antibodies; hepatic or renal impairment; bleeding, bone marrow suppression; cardiac disease; fungal infections; GI bleeding; history of gastric surgery; heart failure; hepatic disease; infection; jaundice; peripheral edema; renal disease; history of viral infection older adults; females of childbearing age. Safe use in children younger than 3 y not established.

## ROUTE & DOSAGE

### CML Chronic Phase

*Adult:* **PO** 400 mg daily with a meal and large glass of water

*Child (3 y or older):* **PO** 260 or 340 mg/m²/day in 1 or 2 divided dose(s)

### CML Accelerated Phase or Blast Crisis

*Adult:* **PO** 600 mg daily with a meal and large glass of water

### Philadelphia Chromosome–Positive Acute Lymphoblastic Leukemia

*Child (1 y or older):* **PO** 340 mg/m²/day

### Acute Lymphoblastic Leukemia

*Adult:* **PO** 600 mg/day until disease progression

### GISTs/Hyereosinophilic Syndrome

*Adult:* **PO** 400 mg daily

### *Hepatic Impairment Dosage Adjustment*

Reduce dose to 300–400 mg daily

### *Toxicity Dosage Adjustment*

*Bilirubin greater than 3 × ULN:* Withhold therapy until levels have returned to less than 1.5 × ULN
*Liver transaminase greater than 5 × ULN:* Withhold therapy until levels have returned to less than 2.5 × ULN
*Hematologic toxicity:* Adjust based on disease state being treated and ANC: See package insert for adjustments

## ADMINISTRATION

### Oral

- Give with meal and large glass of water (at least 8 oz).
- Store at 15°–30° C (59°–86° F).

**ADVERSE EFFECTS** (≥1%) **Body as a Whole:** *Fluid retention, edema, fatigue,* ascites, weight gain, *fever,* night sweats, weakness. **CNS:** CNS hemorrhage, *headache,* anxiety, dizziness, insomnia, depression, taste disorder, paresthesia. **GI:** *Nausea, vomiting, diarrhea,* GI hemorrhage, dyspepsia, *abdominal pain, constipation, anorexia,* increased AST, ALT, and bilirubin. **Hematologic:** Hemorrhage, *neutropenia,* petechiae, epistaxis, pancytopenia (rare), thrombocytopenia (rare). **Metabolic:** Hypokalemia. **Musculoskeletal:** *Muscle cramps, pain, arthralgia,* myalgia. **Respiratory:** *Cough, dyspnea,* pharyngitis, pneumonia. **Skin:** *Rash,* pruritus. **Cardiac:** Hypotension, chest pain.

**INTERACTIONS Drug: Clarithromycin, erythromycin, ketoconazole, itraconazole** may increase imatinib levels and toxicity; **carbamazepine, dexamethasone, phenobarbital, phenytoin, rifampin** may decrease imatinib levels; may increase levels of BENZODIAZEPINES, DIHYDROPYRIDINE, CALCIUM CHANNEL BLOCKERS (e.g., **nifedipine**), **warfarin. Herbal: St. John's wort** may decrease imatinib levels.

**PHARMACOKINETICS Absorption:** Well absorbed, 98% reaches systemic circulation. **Peak:** 2–4 h.

Common adverse effects in *italic;* life-threatening effects underlined; generic names in **bold**; classifications in SMALL CAPS; ✦ Canadian drug name; ❶ Prototype drug

817

**Metabolism:** Primarily by CYP3A4 in liver. **Elimination:** Primarily in feces. **Half-Life:** 18 h imatinib, 40 h active metabolite.

## NURSING IMPLICATIONS

### Assessment & Drug Effects

- Monitor for S&S of fluid retention. Weigh daily and report rapid weight gain immediately.
- Withhold drug and notify prescriber for any of the following: Bilirubin greater than 3 × ULN, AST/ALT greater than 5 × ULN; treatment may be reinstituted when bilirubin less than 1.5 × ULN and AST/ALT less than 2.5 × ULN.
- Monitor lab tests: CBC with platelet count and differential weekly × 1 mo, biweekly for the 2nd mo, periodically thereafter as clinically indicated; baseline and monthly LFTs; periodic serum creatinine, TSH, and electrolytes.

### Patient & Family Education

- Do not take any OTC drugs (e.g., acetaminophen, St. John's wort) without consulting prescriber.
- Report any S&S of bleeding immediately to prescriber (e.g., black tarry stool, bright red or cola-colored urine, bleeding from gums).
- Report immediately to prescriber any unexplained change in mental status.
- Use effective means of contraception while taking this drug. Women of childbearing age should avoid becoming pregnant.

---

# IMIPENEM-CILASTATIN SODIUM ℗

(i-mi-pen'em sye-la-stat'in)

Primaxin

**Classification:** BETA-LACTAM ANTIBIOTIC
**Therapeutic:** ANTIBIOTIC

**AVAILABILITY** Solution for injection

## ACTION & *THERAPEUTIC EFFECT*

Fixed combination of imipenem, a beta-lactam antibiotic, and cilastatin. Action of imipenem: Inhibition of mucopeptide synthesis in bacterial cell walls leading to cell death. Cilastatin increases the serum half-life of imipenem. *Effectively used for severe or resistant infections. Acts synergistically with aminoglycoside antibiotics against some isolates of* Pseudomonas aeruginosa.

## USES Treatment of serious infections caused by susceptible organisms in the urinary tract, lower respiratory tract, bones and joints, skin and skin structures; also intraabdominal, gynecologic, and mixed infections; bacterial septicemia and endocarditis.

## UNLABELED USES Infective endocarditis.

## CONTRAINDICATIONS Hypersensitivity to any component of product, multiple allergens; renal impairment with CrCl of less than or equal to 5 mL/min/1.73m².

## CAUTIOUS USE Hypersensitivity to another carbapenen or penicillin, or cephalosporin; patients with CNS disorders (e.g., seizures, brain lesions, history of recent head injury); renal impairment; older adults; pregnancy (category C); lactation.

## ROUTE & DOSAGE

### Serious Infections

*Adult:* **IV** 250–500 mg q6–8h (max: 4 g/day); **IM:** 500 or 750 mg q12h (max: 4 g/day)
*Child (3 mo or older):* **IV** 15–25 mg/kg q6h; *1–3 mo:* 25 mg/kg q6–12h
*Neonate (weight greater than 1500 g):* **IV** 25 mg/kg q8–12h

---

Common adverse effects in *italic;* life-threatening effects <u>underlined;</u> generic names in **bold;** classifications in SMALL CAPS; ♣ Canadian drug name; ℗ Prototype drug

*Renal Impairment Dosage Adjustment*

Make adjustments/package insert (based on *CrCl*)

## ADMINISTRATION

Caution: IM and IV solutions are **not** interchangeable; **do not** give IM solution by IV, and **do not** give IV solution as IM.

### Intramuscular

- Reconstitute powder for IM injection as follows: Add 2 mL or 3 mL of 1% lidocaine HCl solution without epinephrine, respectively, to the 500 mg vial or the 750 mg vial. Agitate to form a suspension then withdraw and inject entire contents of the vial IM.
- Give IM suspension by deep injection into the gluteal muscle or lateral thigh.
- Use reconstituted IM injection within 1 h after preparation.

### Intravenous

*PREPARE:* **Intermittent:** Reconstitute each dose with 10 mL of D5W, NS, or other compatible infusion solution. ▪ Agitate the solution until clear. Color should range from colorless to yellow. ▪ Further dilute with 100 mL of same solution used for initial dilution.

*ADMINISTER:* **Intermittent:** Give each 500 mg or fraction thereof over 20–30 min. Infuse larger doses over 40–60 min. ▪ **Do not** give as a bolus dose. ▪ Nausea appears to be related to infusion rate, and if it presents during infusion, slow the rate (occurs most frequently with 1-g doses).

*INCOMPATIBILITIES:* Solution/additive: **Amoxicillin, lactated Ringer's, mannitol,** some **dextrose**-containing solutions, **potassium chloride, sodium bicarbonate, TPN.** Y-site: **Alemtuzumab, allopurinol, amiodarone, amphotericin B cholesteryl, azathioprine, azithromycin, ceftriaxone, chlorpromazine, dacarbazine, dantrolene, daptomycin, daunorubicin, diazepam, diazoxide, drotrecogin, etoposide, fluconazole, gallium, ganciclovir, garenoxacin, gemcitabine, haloperidol, inamrinone, lansoprazole, lorazepam, mannitol, mechlorethamine, metaraminol, meperidine, methyldopa midzolam, milrinone, minocycline, mycophenolate, nalbuphine, nicardipine, palonosetron, peritoneal dialysis solution, phenytoin, prochlorperazine, pyridoxine, quinpristin/dalfopristin, sargramostim, sodium bicarbonate, SMZ/TMP, temocillin, thiamine, topotecan, vecuronium.**

- Store according to manufacturer's recommendations; stability of IV solutions depends on diluent used for reconstitution. ▪ Most IV solutions retain potency for 4 h at 15°–30° C (59°–86° F) or for 24 h if refrigerated at 4° C (39° F). Avoid freezing.

## ADVERSE EFFECTS (≥1%) Body as a Whole:
Hypersensitivity (rash, fever, chills, dyspnea, pruritus), weakness, oliguria/anuria, polyuria, polyarthralgia; *phlebitis and pain at injection site,* superinfections. **CNS:** Seizures, dizziness, confusion, somnolence, encephalopathy, myoclonus, tremors, paresthesia, headache. **GI:** *Nausea, vomiting,* diarrhea, <u>pseudomembranous colitis</u>, hemorrhagic colitis, gastroenteritis, abdominal pain, glossitis, heartburn. **Respiratory:** Chest discomfort, hyperventilation, dyspnea. **Skin:** Rash, pruritus, urticaria, candidiasis, flushing,

---

Common adverse effects in *italic;* life-threatening effects <u>underlined</u>; generic names in **bold;** classifications in SMALL CAPS; ✦ Canadian drug name; ⊙ Prototype drug

819

increased sweating, skin texture change, facial edema. **Metabolic:** Hyponatremia, hyperkalemia alkaline phosphatase, AST, ALT BUN, LDH, creatinine. **Hematologic:** increased WBC, *decreased Hgb, Hct,* eosinophilia, thrombocytopenia. **Special Senses:** Transient hearing loss.

**INTERACTIONS Drug: Aztreonam, cephalosporins, penicillins** may antagonize the antibacterial effects. May affect **cyclosporine** levels.

**PHARMACOKINETICS Distribution:** Widely distributed; limited concentrations in CSF; crosses placenta; in breast milk. **Elimination:** 70% in urine within 10 h. **Half-Life:** 1 h.

## NURSING IMPLICATIONS

### Assessment & Drug Effects

- Determine previous hypersensitivity reaction to beta-lactam antibiotics (penicillins and cephalosporins) or to other allergens.
- Monitor for S&S of hypersensitivity (see Appendix F). Discontinue drug and notify prescriber if S&S occur.
- Monitor closely patients vulnerable to CNS adverse effects.
- Notify prescriber if focal tremors, myoclonus, or seizures occur; dosage adjustment may be needed.
- Monitor for S&S of superinfection (see Appendix F).
- Notify prescriber promptly to rule out pseudomembranous enterocolitis if severe diarrhea accompanied by abdominal pain and fever occurs (see Appendix F).
- Note: Sodium content derived from drug is high; consider in patient on restricted sodium intake.
- Monitor renal, hematologic, and liver function periodically.

### Patient & Family Education

- Notify prescriber immediately to report pruritus or symptoms of respiratory distress.
- Report pain or discomfort at IV infusion site.
- Report loose stools or diarrhea promptly.

## IMIPRAMINE HYDROCHLORIDE ℗

(im-ip′ra-meen)

Tofranil

## IMIPRAMINE PAMOATE

**Classification:** TRICYCLIC ANTIDEPRESSANT (TCA)
**Therapeutic:** ANTIDEPRESSANT

**AVAILABILITY** Tablet **Imipramine pamoate:** Capsule

## ACTION & *THERAPEUTIC EFFECT*

TCAs potentiate both norepinephrine and serotonin in the CNS by blocking their reuptake by presynaptic neurons. Imipramine decreases number of awakenings from sleep, markedly reduces time in REM sleep, and increases stage 4 sleep. Relief of nocturnal enuresis is due to anticholinergic activity and to nervous system stimulation, resulting in earlier arousal to sensation of full bladder. *Effective as an antidepressant. Relieves nocturnal enuresis in children.*

**USES** Depression, enuresis.

**UNLABELED USES** ADHD, bulimia nervosa, neuropathic pain, panic disorders, postherpetic neuralgia, overactive bladder, urinary incontinence.

**CONTRAINDICATIONS** Hypersensitivity to tricyclic drugs; concomitant use of MAOIs within 14 days; suicidal ideation; acute recovery period after MI; pregnancy (category D); lactation.

**CAUTIOUS USE** History of suicidal thoughts; respiratory difficulties; cardiovascular, hepatic, or GI diseases; blood disorders; increased intraocular pressure, narrow-angle glaucoma; schizophrenia, MDD, bipolar disorder; electroshock therapy; hypomania or manic episodes, patient with suicidal tendencies, seizure disorders; CHF; conductions defects, arrhythmias; strokes, tachycardia; BPH; urinary retention; older adults; adolescents, children younger than 6 y.

## ROUTE & DOSAGE

**Depression**

*Adult:* **PO** 75 mg/day titrate to response (150 mg/day in divided dose)
*Adolescent:* **PO** 30–40 mg/day; may titrate based on response

**Enuresis in Childhood**

*Adolescent:* **PO** 25 mg at bedtime, may titrate up (max: 75 mg)
*Child (6–12):* **PO** 10–25 mg at bedtime, may titrate up (max: 50 mg)

**Pharmacogenetic Dosage Adjustment**

*Poor CYP2D6 metabolizers:* Start at 30% of normal dose

## ADMINISTRATION

**Oral**

- Give with or immediately after food.
- Note: Single doses can be given at bedtime or q.a.m., respectively, if drowsiness or insomnia results.

**ADVERSE EFFECTS** (≥1%) **Body as a Whole:** Hypersensitivity (skin rash, erythema, petechiae, urticaria, pruritus, photosensitivity, angioedema of face, tongue, or generalized; drug fever). **CNS:** *Sedation, drowsiness,* dizziness, headache, fatigue, numbness, tingling (paresthesias) of extremities; incoordination, ataxia, tremors, peripheral neuropathy, extrapyramidal symptoms (including parkinsonism effects and tardive dyskinesia); lowered seizure threshold, altered EEG patterns, delirium, disturbed concentration, confusion, hallucinations, anxiety, nervousness, insomnia, vivid dreams, restlessness, agitation, shift to hypomania, mania; exacerbation of psychoses; hyperpyrexia. **CV:** *Orthostatic hypotension,* mild sinus tachycardia; *arrhythmias,* hypertension or hypotension, palpitation, MI, CHF, *heart block,* ECG changes, stroke, flushing, cold cyanotic hands and feet (peripheral vasospasm). **Endocrine:** Testicular swelling, gynecomastia (men), galactorrhea and breast enlargement (women), increased or decreased libido, ejaculatory and erectile disturbances, delayed or absent orgasm (male and female); elevation or depression of blood glucose levels. **Special Senses:** Nasal congestion, tinnitus; *blurred vision,* disturbances of accommodation, *slight mydriasis,* nystagmus. **GI:** *Dry mouth,* constipation, heartburn, excessive appetite, weight gain, nausea, vomiting, diarrhea, slowed gastric emptying time, flatulence, abdominal cramps, esophageal reflux, anorexia, stomatitis, increased salivation, black tongue, peculiar taste, paralytic ileus. **Urogenital:** *Urinary retention,* delayed micturition, nocturia, paradoxic urinary frequency. **Hematologic:** Bone marrow depression; agranulocytosis, eosinophilia, thrombocytopenia. **Other:** Excessive perspiration, cholestatic jaundice, precipitation of acute intermittent porphyria; dyspnea, changes in heat and cold tolerance, hair loss, syndrome of inappropriate anti-diuretic hormone secretion (SIADH).

---

**INTERACTIONS Drug:** MAO INHIBITORS may precipitate hyperpyrexic crisis, tachycardia, or seizures; ANTIHYPERTENSIVE AGENTS potentiate orthostatic hypotension; CNS DEPRESSANTS, **alcohol** add to CNS depression; **norepinephrine** and other SYMPATHOMIMETICS may increase cardiac toxicity; **cimetidine** decreases hepatic metabolism, thus increasing imipramine levels; **methylphenidate** inhibits metabolism of imipramine and thus may increase its toxicity. Do not use with other drugs that might prolong the QT interval. **Herbal: Ginkgo** may decrease seizure threshold; **St. John's wort** may cause serotonin syndrome.

**PHARMACOKINETICS Absorption:** Completely absorbed from GI tract. **Peak:** 1–2 h. **Metabolism:** Metabolized to the active metabolite desipramine in liver. **Elimination:** Primarily in urine, small amount in feces; crosses placenta; may be secreted in breast milk. **Half-Life:** 8–16 h.

## NURSING IMPLICATIONS

### Black Box Warning

*Imipramine has been associated with increased risk of suicidal thinking and behavior in children, adolescents, and young adults.*

### Assessment & Drug Effects

- Monitor children, adolescents, and young adults for increase in suicidality.
- Be alert for and report new or worsening symptoms such as anxiety, agitation, panic attacks, insomnia, irritability, hostility, aggressiveness, impulsivity, hypomania, and mania.
- Monitor HR and BP frequently. Orthostatic hypotension may be marked in pretreatment hypertensive or cardiac patients.
- Monitor CV status especially in the older adult and those with preexisting CV disease.
- Monitor older adults for excessive sedation.
- Monitor urinary and bowel elimination, at least until maintenance dosage is stabilized, to detect urinary retention or frequency, constipation, or paralytic ileus.
- Notify prescriber of extrapyramidal symptoms (tremors, twitching, ataxia, incoordination, hyperreflexia, drooling) in patients receiving large doses and especially in older adults.
- Monitor diabetic patients for loss of glycemic control. Hyperglycemia or hypoglycemia (see Appendix F) occur in some patients.
- Monitor lab tests: CBC with differential if fever and sore throat develop.

### Patient & Family Education

- Report promptly signs of a worsening condition, suicidal ideation, or unusual changes in behavior, especially in children and adolescents.
- Older adults should change position slowly and in stages, especially from lying down to upright posture and dangle legs over bed for a few minutes before walking.
- **Do not** use OTC drugs while on a TCA without prescriber approval.
- Do not drive or engage in other potentially hazardous activities until response to drug is known.
- Avoid exposure to strong sunlight because of potential photosensitivity.

# IMIQUIMOD
(i-mi′qui-mod)
Zyclara
**Classifications:** KERATOLYTIC; IMMUNOMODULATOR
**Therapeutic:** IMMUNE RESPONSE MODIFIER; KERATOLYTIC

**AVAILABILITY** Cream

**ACTION & *THERAPEUTIC EFFECT***
An immune response modifier thought to induce cytokine production, including interferon-alfa, which may interfere with viral replication. *Despite destruction of HPV warts, latent or subclinical HPV infection can persist, and recurrence of visible warts is common.*

**USES** Treatment of external genital and perianal warts *(Condylomata acuminata)*, actinic keratosis on the face and scalp of immunocompetent adults, and superficial basal cell carcinoma.

**UNLABELED USES** Treatment of common warts, herpes simplex virus.

**CONTRAINDICATIONS** Occlusive dressing; ocular exposure; excessive sun exposure or sunburn; UV exposure; surgery or drug treatment on affected area.

**CAUTIOUS USE** Hypersensitivity to benzyl alcohol or paraben; HIV infection; pregnancy (category C); lactation. Safe use in children younger than 12 y not established.

**ROUTE & DOSAGE**

**Genital and Perianal Warts**

*Adult/Adolescent (12 y or older):*
**Topical** Apply a thin layer to the affected areas once daily 3 × wk just before bedtime. Wash off cream after 6–10 h (max: 16 wk therapy).

**Actinic Keratosis**

*Adult:* **Topical** Apply a thin layer to the affected areas once daily 2 × wk just before sleep for 16 wk. Wash off cream after 8 h.

**Superficial Basal Cell Carcinoma**

*Adult:* **Topical** Apply a thin layer to the affected areas once daily 5 × wk just before sleep for 6 wk. Wash off cream after 8 h.

**ADMINISTRATION**

**Topical**
- Handwashing before and after application is recommended.
- Wash treatment area with soap and water and allow to dry thoroughly (at least 10 min).
- Single-use packets contain sufficient cream to cover an area of up to 20 cm$^2$ (approx. 8 in. by 8 in.).
- Instruct patient to apply a thin layer of cream (avoid using excessive cream), and work into area until no longer visible. Do not occlude the application site.
- After each treatment period, remove the cream by washing the treated area with soap and water.
- Avoid ocular exposure.
- Store below 25° C (77° F).

**ADVERSE EFFECTS** (≥1%) **Body as a Whole:** Fungal infections, flu-like symptoms, myalgia. **CNS:** Headache. **Skin:** *Application site reactions, pruritus,* burning, bleeding, stinging, redness, tenderness, irritation, *erythema,* edema, weeping/exudates, dry skin, scabbing/crusting, hyperkeratosis, inflammatory reaction of female external genitalia, dermal ulceration or excoriation. **Respiratory:** Upper respiratory tract infection.

**PHARMACOKINETICS Absorption:** Minimal through intact skin.

Common adverse effects in *italic;* life-threatening effects underlined; generic names in **bold;** classifications in SMALL CAPS; ✦ Canadian drug name; ⊘ Prototype drug

823

## NURSING IMPLICATIONS

### Assessment & Drug Effects

- Monitor for and report promptly severe local inflammatory reactions on female external genitalia.

### Patient & Family Education

- Uncircumcised males with warts under the foreskin: Pull back the foreskin and clean the area daily to help avoid penile skin reactions.
- Females should not apply cream directly into the vagina. Application to the labia may cause pain or swelling and may cause difficulty in passing urine.
- When being treated for actinic keratosis, avoid or minimize UV light exposure (artificial and sunlight). Wear protective clothing. If sunburn develops, avoid using imiquimod cream until fully recovered.

---

# IMMUNE GLOBULIN INTRAMUSCULAR [IGIM, GAMMA GLOBULIN, IMMUNE SERUM GLOBULIN (ISG)] ℗

(im'mune glob'u-lin)

BayGam

# IMMUNE GLOBULIN INTRAVENOUS (IGIV)

Flebogamma, Gammagard, Gammar-P IV, IGIV, Iveegam, Octagam

# IMMUNE GLOBULIN SUBCUTANEOUS (IGSC, SCIG)

Hizentra, Vivaglobin

**Classifications:** BIOLOGIC RESPONSE MODIFIER; IMMUNOGLOBULIN
Therapeutic: IMMUNOGLOBULIN

**AVAILABILITY IGIM:** Solution for injection. **IGIV:** Solution for injection; powder for injection. **Subcutaneous:** Solution

## ACTION & *THERAPEUTIC EFFECT*

Concentrated solution containing globulin (primarily IgG) from human plasma of either venous or placental origin and processed by a special fractionating technique. *Like hepatitis B immune globulin (H-BIG), contains antibodies specific to hepatitis B surface antigen but in lower concentrations. Therefore, not considered treatment of first choice for postexposure prophylaxis against hepatitis B but usually an acceptable alternative when H-BIG is not available.*

## USES **IGIM:** Provides passive immunity or to modify severity of certain infectious diseases [e.g., rubeola (measles), rubella (German measles), varicella-zoster (chickenpox), type A (infectious) hepatitis], and as replacement therapy in congenital agammaglobulinemia or IgG deficiency diseases. May be used as an alternative to H-BIG to provide passive immunity in hepatitis B infection. Also for postexposure prophylaxis of hepatitis non-A, non-B, and nonspecific hepatitis. **IGIV:** Principally as maintenance therapy in patients unable to manufacture sufficient quantities of IgG antibodies, in patients requiring an immediate increase in immunoglobulin levels, and when IM injections are contraindicated as in patients with bleeding disorders or who have small muscle mass. Also in chronic autoimmune thrombocytopenia and idiopathic thrombocytopenic purpura (ITP). Treatment of primary immunodeficiency disorders associated with defects in humoral immunity. **IGSC:** Primary immune deficiency.

## UNLABELED USES Kawasaki syndrome, chronic lymphocytic leukemia, AIDS, premature and low-birth-weight

neonates, autoimmune neutropenia, HIV-associated thrombocytopenia, or hemolytic anemia.

**CONTRAINDICATIONS** History of anaphylaxis or severe reaction to human immune serum globulin (IG) or to any ingredient in the formulations; persons with clinical hepatitis A; IGIV for patients with class-specific anti IgA deficiencies; IGIM in severe thrombocytopenia or other bleeding disorders.

**CAUTIOUS USE** Dehydration, diabetes mellitus, children, older adults, hypovolemia, IgA deficiency, infection; renal disease, renal impairment; sepsis; sucrose hypersensitivity; vaccination, viral infection; pregnancy (category C); lactation.

## ROUTE & DOSAGE

**Hepatitis A Exposure**

*Adult/Child:* **IM** 0.02 mL/kg as soon as possible after exposure; if period of exposure will be 3 mo or longer, give 0.05–0.06 mL/kg once q4–6mo

**Hepatitis B Exposure**

*Adult/Child:* **IM** 0.02–0.06 mL/kg as soon as possible after exposure if H-BIG is unavailable

**Rubella Exposure**

*Adult:* **IM** 20 mL as single dose in susceptible pregnant women

**Rubeola Exposure**

*Adult/Child:* **IM** 0.25 mL/kg within 6 days of exposure

**Varicella-Zoster Exposure**

*Adult/Child:* **IM** 0.6–1.2 mL/kg promptly

**Immunoglobulin Deficiency**

*\*Dosages may vary between brands and formulations (see package insert)*
*Adult/Child:* **IV** 200–400 mg/kg monthly; **IM** 1.2 mL/kg followed by 0.6 mL/kg q2–4wk

**Idiopathic Thrombocytopenia Purpura**

*Adult/Child:* **IV** 400 mg/kg/day for 5 consecutive days or 1 g/kg × 1–2 days

**Obesity Dosage Adjustment**

Dose based on IBW or adjusted IBW

## ADMINISTRATION

- Note: In hepatitis A (infectious hepatitis), immune globulin is most effective when given before or as soon as possible after exposure but not more than 2 wk after (incubation period for hepatitis A is 15–50 days). - Do not give immune globulin to those presenting clinical manifestations of hepatitis A. - For hepatitis B (serum hepatitis), give immune globulin within 24 h and not more than 7 days after exposure. - Note: IGIM and IGIV formulations are **not** interchangeable.

### Intramuscular

- Give adults and older children injections into deltoid or anterolateral aspect of thigh; neonates and small children, into anterolateral aspect of thigh.
- Avoid gluteal injections; however, when large volumes of immune globulin are prescribed or when large doses **must be** divided into several injections, the upper outer quadrant of the gluteus has been used in adults.

### Intravenous

***PREPARE: IV Infusion:*** Refer to manufacturer's directions for information on the specific

Common adverse effects in *italic;* life-threatening effects <u>underlined;</u> generic names in **bold;** classifications in SMALL CAPS; ✤ Canadian drug name; ⊙ Prototype drug

825

product. Allow refrigerated product to come to room temperature.
**ADMINISTER: IV Infusion:** Flow rates vary with product being infused. Refer to manufacturer's directions for the specific product.
▪ Most products may be infused at a rate of 0.5 mg/kg/min for the first 10 min, then increased q20min, if tolerated, by 0.8 mg/kg/min (max rate: 6 mg/kg/min).
**INCOMPATIBILITIES:** Do not mix other drugs with immunoglobulin.

▪ Store as directed by manufacturer for specific product. Avoid freezing.
▪ Do not use if turbidity has occurred or if product has been frozen.

**ADVERSE EFFECTS** (≥1%) **Body as a Whole:** *Pain, tenderness, muscle stiffness at IM site;* local inflammatory reaction, erythema, urticaria, angioedema, headache, malaise, fever, arthralgia, nephrotic syndrome, hypersensitivity (fever, chills, anaphylactic shock), infusion reactions (*nausea, flushing, chills,* headache, chest tightness, wheezing, skeletal pain, back pain, abdominal cramps, anaphylaxis), renal dysfunction, renal failure.

**INTERACTIONS Drug:** May interfere with antibody response to LIVE VIRUS VACCINES (measles/mumps/rubella); give VACCINES 14 days before or 3 mo after IMMUNOGLOBULINS.

**PHARMACOKINETICS Peak:** 2 days. **Distribution:** Rapidly and evenly distributed to intravascular and extravascular fluid compartments. **Half-Life:** 21–23 days.

## NURSING IMPLICATIONS

### Black Box Warning

*IV immune globulin has been associated with renal dysfunction, acute renal failure, osmotic nephropathy, and death.*

### Assessment & Drug Effects
▪ Make sure emergency drugs and appropriate emergency facilities are immediately available for treatment of anaphylaxis or sensitization.
▪ Monitor for S&S adverse reaction to infusion (e.g., nausea, chills, headache, chest tightness); these are indications to slow rate of infusion.
▪ Note: Hypersensitivity reactions (see Appendix F) are most likely in patients receiving large IM doses, repeated injections, or rapid IV infusion.
▪ Monitor vital signs and infusion rate closely when patient is receiving IGIV.
▪ Monitor for and report S&S of renal dysfunction (e.g., decreased urine output, sudden weight gain, fluid retention/edema).

### Patient & Family Education
▪ Report immediately S&S of hypersensitivity (see Appendix F).
▪ Report promptly to prescriber signs of kidney damage such as decreased urine output, sudden weight gain, edema, shortness of breath.

## INDACATEROL MALEATE
(in'da-ka'ter-ol mal'ee-ate)

*Arcapta*

**Classifications:** BRONCHODILATOR; RESPIRATORY SMOOTH MUSCLE RELAXANT; BETA-ADRENERGIC AGONIST
**Therapeutic:** BRONCHODILATOR; RESPIRATORY SMOOTH MUSCLE RELAXANT
**Prototype:** Albuterol

**AVAILABILITY** Capsule containing powder for inhalation

## ACTION & *THERAPEUTIC EFFECT*
Acts primarily on beta$_2$-adrenergic

Common adverse effects in *italic;* life-threatening effects <u>underlined</u>; generic names in **bold;** classifications in SMALL CAPS; ✦ Canadian drug name; ❶ Prototype drug receptors in bronchial smooth muscle and, possibly on the small percentage of $beta_2$-adrenergic receptors found in cardiac muscle. *Causes relaxation of bronchial smooth muscle and bronchodilation.*

**USES** Prophylactic, maintenance treatment of chronic obstructive pulmonary disorder (COPD), including chronic bronchitis and emphysema

**CONTRAINDICATIONS** Asthma (without concurrent use of a long-term asthma control drug); acutely deteriorating COPD; acute episodes of bronchospasm.

**CAUTIOUS USE** Paradoxical bronchospasms; cardiovascular disease including hypertension; seizure disorder; thyrotoxicosis; sensitivity to sympathomimetic drugs; concurrent use of other drugs containing long-acting $beta_2$-agonist; pregnancy (category C); lactation. Safety and efficacy in children not established.

## ROUTE & DOSAGE

### Chronic Obstructive Pulmonary Disorder

*Adult:* **PO Inhalation** 75 mcg once daily

## ADMINISTRATION

### Oral Inhalation

- Capsules should be removed from blister immediately before use.
- Capsules should be used only with the neohaler device. Capsules must not be swallowed.
- The Arcapta neohaler should be administered at the same time each day.
- Store at 15°–30° C (59°–86° F) in foil package until ready to use.

**ADVERSE EFFECTS** (≥2%) **Body as a Whole:** Peripheral edema. **CNS:** Headache. **GI:** Nausea. **Metabolic:** Hyperglycemia. **Musculoskeletal:** Muscle spasms, musculoskeletal pain. **Respiratory:** Cough, nasopharyngitis, oropharyngeal pain, sinusitis, upper respiratory tract infection, COPD exacerbation.

**INTERACTIONS Drug:** ADRENERGIC AGONISTS and MONOAMINE OXIDASE INHIBITORS may potentiate indacaterol. BETA-BLOCKERS may interfere with the actions of indacaterol. CORTICOSTEROIDS (e.g., **prednisone, dexamethasone**), **theophylline,** THIAZIDE DIURETICS OR LOOP DIURETICS may increase risk of hypokalemia. CYP3A4 inhibitors and/or P-gp efflux transporters (e.g., **ketoconazole,** HIV PROTEASE INHIBITORS, **erythromycin**) may increase the levels of indacaterol. Indacaterol has been associated with QT prolongation. Drugs that prolong the QT interval (e.g., **disopyramide, procainamide, amiodarone, bretylium, clarithromycin, levofloxacin**) may cause additive effects. TRICYCLIC ANTIDEPRESSANTS (e.g., **amitriptyline**) may potentiate cardiovascular effects of indacaterol.

**PHARMACOKINETICS Absorption:** 43–45% bioavailable. **Peak:** 15 min. **Distribution:** 94–96% plasma protein bound. **Metabolism:** In the liver. **Elimination:** Primarily fecal. **Half-Life:** 45.5–126 h.

## NURSING IMPLICATIONS

### Black Box Warning

*Indacaterol has been associated with increased risk of asthma-related death.*

---

## Assessment & Drug Effects

- Monitor HR, BP, and respiratory status. Report immediately deterioration in respiratory condition or development of paradoxical bronchospasms following inhalation.
- Periodic ECG monitoring with concurrent use of other drugs associated with QT prolongation.
- Monitor lab tests: Periodic serum potassium; blood glucose in diabetics or prediabetics.

## Patient & Family Education

- Do not use for relief of acute symptoms.
- Discontinue drug use and immediately notify prescriber of any of the following: Symptoms of COPD are worsening; indacaterol no longer controls the symptoms of COPD; breathing is worsened following inhalation of indacaterol; the concurrently prescribed short-acting beta$_2$-agonist drug becomes less effective, or more inhalations of the short-acting drug are required.
- Diabetics should monitor blood glucose level more frequently for loss of glycemic control.

# INDAPAMIDE
(in-dap'a-mide)
Lozide ◆
**Classifications:** ELECTROLYTIC AND WATER BALANCE; DIURETIC
**Therapeutic:** THIAZIDE-LIKE DIURETIC; ANTIHYPERTENSIVE
**Prototype:** Hydrochlorothiazide

## AVAILABILITY Tablet

## ACTION & *THERAPEUTIC EFFECT*

Sulfonamide derivative that has both diuretic and direct vascular effects. Acts on the proximal portion of the distal renal tubules. Enhances excretion of sodium, potassium, and water by interfering with sodium transfer across renal epithelium of tubules. *Hypotensive activity appears to result from a decrease in plasma and extracellular fluid volume, decreased peripheral vascular resistance, direct arteriolar dilation, and calcium channel blockade.*

**USES** Hypertension or edema related to heart failure.

**CONTRAINDICATIONS** Hypersensitivity to indapamide or other sulfonamide derivatives, anuria, lactation.

**CAUTIOUS USE** Electrolyte imbalance, hypokalemia, severe renal impairment; impaired hepatic function or progressive liver disease; prediabetic and type II diabetic patient, history of gout; pregnancy (category B). Safe use in children is not established.

## ROUTE & DOSAGE

### Edema
*Adult:* **PO** 2.5 mg once/day, may increase to 5 mg/day if needed

### Hypertension
*Adult:* **PO** 1.25 mg once daily, may increase to 2.5 mg daily after 1 mo (max: 5 mg/day)

## ADMINISTRATION

### Oral

- Give with food or milk to reduce GI irritation.
- Administer in a.m. to prevent nocturia.
- Store in a tight, light-resistant container unless otherwise directed.

**ADVERSE EFFECTS** (≥1%) **CNS:** Headache, dizziness, fatigue, weakness, muscle cramps or spasm, paresthesia, tension, anxiety, nervousness, agitation, vertigo, insomnia, mental depression, blurred vision, drowsiness. **CV:** Orthostatic hypotension, PVCs, dysrhythmias, flushing, palpitation. **GI:** Dry mouth, anorexia, nausea, vomiting, diarrhea, constipation, abdominal cramps or pain. **Urogenital:** Urinary frequency, nocturia, polyuria, glycosuria, impotence or reduced libido. **Skin:** Rash, hives, pruritus, vasculitis, photosensitivity. **Metabolic:** Dilutional hyponatremia, *hyperuricemia,* exacerbation of gout; *hypokalemia,* hyperglycemia, *hypochloremia,* hypercalcemia, increased BUN or creatinine, weight loss, exacerbation of SLE, increased cholesterol.

**DIAGNOSTIC TEST INTERFERENCE** Since indapamide may cause hypercalcemia (and hypophosphatemia), it is generally withheld before tests for *parathyroid function* are performed.

**INTERACTIONS Drug:** Effects of **diazoxide** and indapamide intensified; increased risk of **digoxin** toxicity with hypokalemia; decreased renal **lithium** clearance may increase risk of **lithium** toxicity. May increase hypotensive effect with ACE INHIBITORS. Hyponatremic effect may be enhanced by SSRIs.

**PHARMACOKINETICS Absorption:** Readily from GI tract; 70–79% plasma bound. **Peak:** 2–2.5 h. **Duration:** Up to 36 h. **Metabolism:** In liver. **Elimination:** 60% in urine; 16–23% in feces. **Half-Life:** 14–18 h.

**NURSING IMPLICATIONS**
**Assessment & Drug Effects**
- Monitor BP periodically throughout therapy.
- Monitor for digitalis toxicity with concurrent therapy.
- Note: Electrolyte imbalances may be clinically serious with protracted vomiting and diarrhea, excessive sweating, GI drainage, and paracentesis.
- Report promptly signs of hyponatremia or hypokalemia (see Appendix F).
- Monitor diabetics for loss of glycemic control.
- Monitor lab tests: Baseline and periodic BUN, serum creatinine, uric acid, blood glucose, and serum electrolytes.

**Patient & Family Education**
- Notify prescriber of decreased urine output, dizziness, weakness or muscle cramps, nausea, jaundice, or blurred vision.
- Take precautions from sun exposure because of risk of photosensitivity.
- Record weight at least every other day; inspect ankles and legs for edema. Report unexplained, progressive weight gain [e.g., 1–1.5 kg (2–3 lb) in 2–3 days].

**INDINAVIR SULFATE**
(in din'a-vir)
Crixivan
**Classifications:** ANTIRETROVIRAL; PROTEASE INHIBITOR
**Therapeutic:** PROTEASE INHIBITOR
**Prototype:** Saquinavir

**AVAILABILITY** Capsule

**ACTION & *THERAPEUTIC EFFECT*** Indinavir is an HIV protease inhibitor. HIV protease is

Common adverse effects in *italic;* life-threatening effects underlined; generic names in **bold;** classifications in SMALL CAPS; ♣ Canadian drug name; ☺ Prototype drug

829

an enzyme required to produce the polyprotein precursors of the functional proteins in infectious HIV. Indinavir binds to the protease active site and thus inhibits its activity. *Protease inhibitors prevent cleavage of HIV viral polyproteins, resulting in formation of immature noninfectious virus particles.*

**USES** Treatment of HIV infection, in combination with other agents.

**CONTRAINDICATIONS** Hypersensitivity to indinavir; severe leukocyturia of greater than 100 cells/high power field; hemolytic anemia; lactation.

**CAUTIOUS USE** Hepatic dysfunction, hepatitis; renal impairment, history of nephrolithiasis, diabetes mellitus; hyperglycemia; concurrent HBV infection; history of adverse responses to other protease inhibitors; autoimmune disease; older adults; pregnancy (category C). Optimal dosing regimen for use in children has not been established.

## ROUTE & DOSAGE

| HIV (dose varies based on concurrent HAART) |
|---|
| *Adult:* **PO** 800 mg q8h |

## ADMINISTRATION

### Oral

- Give with water on an empty stomach 1 h before or 2 h after meal; if needed, may be given with a very light meal or beverage.
- Note: When didanosine and indinavir are ordered concurrently, give each on empty stomach at least 1 h apart.
- Do not administer concurrently with midazolam or triazolam.

- Store tightly closed with desiccant in original bottle.

**ADVERSE EFFECTS** (≥1%) **CNS:** Fatigue, headache, insomnia, dizziness, somnolence, nervousness, agitation, anxiety, paresthesia, peripheral neuropathy, tremor, vertigo. **CV:** Palpitations. **Hematologic:** Anemia, splenomegaly, lymphadenopathy. **GI:** *Nausea,* diarrhea, abdominal discomfort, dyspepsia, stomatitis, anorexia, dry mouth, cholecystitis, cholestasis, constipation, flatulence. **Skin:** Body odor, rash, pruritus, seborrhea, skin ulceration, dry skin, sweating, urticaria. **Other:** Myalgia, allergic reaction, bronchitis, cough, rhinitis, taste alterations, visual disturbances, hyperglycemia, diabetes, kidney stones.

**INTERACTIONS Drug: Rifabutin, rifampin** significantly decrease indinavir levels. **Ketoconazole** significantly increases indinavir levels. Indinavir could inhibit the metabolism and increase the toxicity of **amiodarone, midazolam, sildenafil, tadalafil, trazodone, triazolam, vardenafil.** Indinavir and **didanosine** should be administered at least 1 h apart on empty stomach to permit full absorption of each; increased **ergotamine** toxicity with indinavir. **Rosuvastatin, simvastatin** should not be used concurrently. **Herbal: St. John's wort,** garlic decreases ANTIRETROVIRAL activity of indinavir. **Food:** Avoid taking with high fat food.

**PHARMACOKINETICS Absorption:** Rapidly from GI tract; a meal high in calories, fat, and protein significantly reduces absorption. **Distribution:** 60% protein bound. **Metabolism:** In liver by CYP3A4. **Elimination:** Primarily in feces (greater than 80%), 20% in urine.

## NURSING IMPLICATIONS

### Assessment & Drug Effects

- Assess for S&S of renal dysfunction, respiratory dysfunction, GI distress, and other common adverse effects.
- Monitor lab tests: Periodic blood glucose and urinalysis.

### Patient & Family Education

- Learn drug interactions and potential adverse reactions. Drink plenty of liquids to minimize risk of renal stones.
- Notify prescriber of flank pain, hematuria, S&S of jaundice, or other distressing adverse effects.

## INDOMETHACIN

(in-doe-meth'a-sin)

Indocid ♦, Indocin, Indocin SR

**Classification:** ANALGESIC, NONSTEROIDAL ANTI-INFLAMMATORY (NSAID)

**Therapeutic:** ANALGESIC, NSAID; ANTIRHEUMATIC

**Prototype:** Ibuprofen

**AVAILABILITY** Capsule; sustained release capsule; oral suspension; suppositories; solution for injection

## ACTION & *THERAPEUTIC EFFECT*

Potent nonsteroidal compound that competes with COX-1 and COX-2 enzymes, thus interfering with formation of prostaglandin. Appears to reduce motility of polymorphonuclear leukocytes, development of cellular exudates, and vascular permeability in injured tissue resulting in its anti-inflammatory effects. Inhibition of prostaglandins is thought to promote closure of the patency of the ductus arterious. Antipyretic and anti-inflammatory actions may be related to its ability to inhibit prostaglandin biosynthesis. *It is a potent analgesic, anti-inflammatory, and antipyretic agent. Promotes closure of persistent patent ductus arteriosus.*

**USES** Palliative treatment in active stages of moderate to severe rheumatoid arthritis, ankylosing rheumatoid spondylitis, acute gouty arthritis, and osteoarthritis of hip in patients intolerant to or unresponsive to adequate trials with salicylates and other therapy. Also used IV to close patent ductus arteriosus in the premature infant.

**UNLABELED USES** To relieve biliary pain and dysmenorrhea, Paget's disease, athletic injuries, juvenile arthritis, idiopathic pericarditis.

**CONTRAINDICATIONS** Allergy to indomethacin, aspirin, or other NSAID; nasal polyps associated with angioedema; history of asthma; history of recurrent GI lesions; perioperative pain with CABG; serious skin reactions to indomethacin; severe hepatic impairment due to indomethacin; pregnancy (D third trimester); lactation; neonates with significant renal failure.

**CAUTIOUS USE** History of psychiatric illness, epilepsy, parkinsonism; impaired renal or hepatic function; history of ulcer disease or GI bleeding; infection; coagulation disorders; infection, CV disease; CHF, hypertension; fluid retention; preexisting asthma; older adults, persons in hazardous occupations; pregnancy (category C first and second trimester); lactation; children, infants.

Common adverse effects in *italic;* life-threatening effects <u>underlined</u>; generic names in **bold;** classifications in SMALL CAPS; ♦ Canadian drug name; ❷ Prototype drug

831

## ROUTE & DOSAGE

### Rheumatoid Arthritis

*Adult:* **PO** 25–50 mg b.i.d or t.i.d. (max: 200 mg/day) or 75 mg sustained release 1–2 × day

### Pediatric Arthritis

*Child:* **PO** 1–2 mg/kg/day in 2–4 divided doses (max: 4 mg/kg/day) or 150–200 mg/day

### Acute Gouty Arthritis

*Adult:* **PO/PR** 50 mg t.i.d. until pain is tolerable, then rapidly taper

### Bursitis

*Adult:* **PO** 25–50 mg t.i.d. or q.i.d. (max: 200 mg/day) or 75 mg sustained release 1–2 × day

### Close Patent Ductus Arteriosus

*Premature neonate (younger than 48 h):* IV 0.2 mg/kg followed by 2 doses of 0.1 mg/kg q12–24h; *2–7 days:* 0.2 mg/kg followed by 2 doses of 0.2 mg/kg q12–24h; *younger than 7 days:* 0.2 mg/kg followed by 2 doses of 0.25 mg/kg q12–24h

## ADMINISTRATION

### Oral

- Give immediately after meals, or with food, milk, or antacid (if prescribed) to minimize GI side effects.

### Rectal

- Indomethacin rectal suppository use is contraindicated with history of proctitis or recent bleeding.

### Intravenous

*PREPARE:* **Direct:** Dilute 1 mg with 1 mL of NS or sterile water for injection without preservatives. Resulting concentration (1 mg/mL) may be further diluted with an additional 1 mL for each 1 mg to yield 0.5 mg/mL.

*ADMINISTER:* **Direct:** Give by direct IV with a single dose given over 20–30 min.

*INCOMPATIBILITIES:* **Y-site: Amikacin, amino acid, atracurium, aztreonam, benztropine, buprenorphine, butorphanol, calcium chloride, calcium gluconate, cefoperazone, cefotetan, chlorpromazine, cimetidine, dactinomycin, dantrolene, daunorubicin, dexamethasone, diazepam, diazoxide, diphenhydramine, dobutamine, dopamine, doxycycline, epinephrine, erythromycin, esmolol, etoposide, famotidine, gentamicin, glycopyrrolate, haloperidol, hydralazine, isoproterenol, labetalol, levofloxacin, magnesium sulfate, meperidine, metaraminol, methyldopate, midazolam, minocycline, morphine, nalbuphine, netilmicin, norepinephrine, ondansetron, oxytocin, paclitaxel, pantoprazole, papaverine, pentamidine, pentazocine, phenylephrine, phenytoin, polymyxin B sulfate, prochlorperazine, promethazine, propranolol, protamine, pyridoxine, quinidine, succinylcholine chloride, sufentanil, citrate, SMZ/TMP, thiamine tobramycin, tolazoline, vancomycin, vasopressin, verapamil.**

- Avoid extravasation or leakage; drug can be irritating to tissue. - Discard any unused drug, since it contains no preservative.

- Store oral and rectal forms in tight, light-resistant containers unless otherwise directed. Do not freeze.

## ADVERSE EFFECTS (≥1%) Body as a Whole: Hypersensitivity (rash, purpura, pruritus, urticaria,

angioedema, angiitis, rapid fall in blood pressure, dyspnea, asthma syndrome in aspirin-sensitive patients), edema, weight gain, flushing, sweating. **CNS:** Headache, *dizziness,* vertigo, light-headedness, syncope, fatigue, muscle weakness, ataxia, insomnia, nightmares, drowsiness, confusion, coma, convulsions, peripheral neuropathy, psychic disturbances (hallucinations, depersonalization, depression), aggravation of epilepsy, parkinsonism. **CV:** Elevated BP, palpitation, chest pains, tachycardia, bradycardia, CHF, increased risk of MI. **Special Senses:** Blurred vision, lacrimation, eye pain, visual field changes, corneal deposits, retinal disturbances including macula, *tinnitus,* hearing disturbances, epistaxis. **GI:** *Nausea, vomiting,* diarrhea, anorexia, bloating, abdominal distention, ulcerative stomatitis, proctitis, rectal bleeding, GI ulceration, hemorrhage, perforation, toxic hepatitis. **Hematologic:** Hemolytic anemia, aplastic anemia (sometimes fatal), agranulocytosis, leukopenia, thrombocytopenic purpura, inhibited platelet aggregation. **Urogenital:** Renal function impairment, hematuria, urinary frequency; vaginal bleeding, breast changes. **Skin:** Hair loss, exfoliative dermatitis, erythema nodosum, tissue irritation with extravasation. **Metabolic:** Hyponatremia, hypokalemia, hyperkalemia, hypoglycemia or hyperglycemia, glycosuria (rare).

## DIAGNOSTIC TEST INTERFERENCE
Increased *AST, ALT, bilirubin, BUN;* positive direct *Coombs' test.*

## INTERACTIONS **Drug:** ORAL ANTICOAGULANTS, **heparin, alcohol** may prolong bleeding time; may increase **lithium** toxicity; effects of ORAL ANTICOAGULANTS, **phenytoin,** SALICYLATES, SULFONAMIDES, SULFONYLUREAS increased because of protein-binding displacement; increased toxicity including GI bleeding with SALICYLATES, NSAIDS; may blunt effects of ANTIHYPERTENSIVES and DIURETICS. **Herbal: Feverfew, garlic, ginger, ginkgo** may increase bleeding potential.

## PHARMACOKINETICS **Absorption:** Completely absorbed from GI tract. **Onset:** 1–2 h. **Peak:** 3 h. **Duration:** 4–6 h. **Metabolism:** In liver. **Elimination:** Primarily in urine. **Half-Life:** 2.5–124 h.

## NURSING IMPLICATIONS

### Black Box Warning

*Indomethacin has been associated with increased risk of serious, potentially fatal GI bleeding and cardiovascular events (e.g., MI & CVA); risk may increase with duration of use and may be greater in the older adult and those with risk factors for CV disease.*

### Assessment & Drug Effects
- Monitor for therapeutic effectiveness: In acute gouty attack, relief of joint tenderness and pain is usually apparent in 24–36 h; swelling generally disappears in 3–5 days. In rheumatoid arthritis: Reduced fever, increased strength, reduced stiffness, and relief of pain, swelling, and tenderness.
- Monitor BP closely throughout therapy.
- Monitor for and report promptly S&S of CV thrombotic events (i.e., angina, MI, TIA, or stroke).
- Monitor for and report promptly S&S of GI ulceration or bleeding. Significant GI bleeding may occur without prior warning.

Common adverse effects in *italic;* life-threatening effects underlined; generic names in **bold**; classifications in SMALL CAPS; ✦ Canadian drug name; ☉ Prototype drug

833

- Observe patients carefully; instruct to report adverse reactions promptly to prevent serious and sometimes irreversible or fatal effects.
- Monitor weight and observe dependent areas for signs of edema in patients with underlying cardiovascular disease.
- Monitor I&O closely and keep prescriber informed during IV administration for patent ductus arteriosus. Significant impairment of renal function is possible; urine output may decrease by 50% or more. Also monitor BUN, serum creatinine, glomerular filtration rate, creatinine clearance, and serum electrolytes.
- Monitor lab tests: Periodic renal function tests, LFTs, and CBC with differential.

### Patient & Family Education
- Stop taking drug and report promptly to prescriber if you experience S&S of GI ulceration: Stomach pain, frequent indigestion and nausea, bloody or tarry stools, vomit with blood or coffee-ground appearance.
- Stop taking drug and report promptly to prescriber if you experience chest pain, shortness of breath, weakness, slurring of speech, or other signs of a cardiac or neurologic problem.
- Do not take aspirin or other NSAIDs; they increase possibility of ulcers.
- Note: Frontal headache is the most frequent CNS adverse effect; if it persists, dosage reduction or drug withdrawal may be indicated. Take drug at bedtime with milk to reduce the incidence of morning headache.
- Do not drive or engage in other potentially hazardous activities until response to drug is known.

# INFLIXIMAB
(in-flix′i-mab)

Inflectra, Remicade

**Classifications:** BIOLOGIC RESPONSE MODIFIER; MONOCLONAL ANTIBODY (IgG); TUMOR NECROSIS FACTOR (TNF) MODIFIER

Therapeutic: IMMUNOMODULATOR; ANTI-INFLAMMATORY; DISEASE-MODIFYING ANTIRHEUMATIC DRUG (DMARD)

**Prototype:** Enteracept

## AVAILABILITY Powder for injection

## ACTION & THERAPEUTIC EFFECT
Inhibits binding of TNF-alpha with its receptors thus preventing the following: Induction of proinflammatory cytokines (such as interleukins 1 & 6); enhancement of leukocyte migration out of the vascular system; activation of neutrophil and eosinophil inflammatory activity; and induction of acute inflammatory phase reactants. *Decreases GI inflammation in Crohn's and related diseases. It is also effectively used as a disease-modifying antirheumatic drug (DMARD).*

## USES Moderately to severely active Crohn's disease, including fistulizing Crohn's disease, rheumatoid arthritis, psoriatic arthritis, ankylosing spondylitis, ulcerative colitis, plaque psoriasis.

## CONTRAINDICATIONS Severe hypersensitivity to infliximab; serious infection, sepsis; heart failure; murine protein hypersensitivity; lactation.

## CAUTIOUS USE History of allergic phenomena or untoward responses to monoclonal antibody preparation; chronic infections; previous history of TB infection; history of HBV infection; renal or hepatic impairment; multiple sclerosis (potential exacerbation); fungal

infection; human antichimeric antibody (HACA); leukopenia, thrombocytopenia; immunosuppressed patients; autoimmune disorders; neoplastic disease; vasculitis; neurologic disease; neutropenia; seizure disorder; preexisting CNS demyelinating disorders; moderate to severe COPD; history of malignancy; older adults; pregnancy (category B); children.

## ROUTE & DOSAGE

### Crohn's Disease

*Adult:* **IV** 5 mg/kg infused over at least 2 h, repeat at 2 and 6 wk for fistulizing disease, then q8wk
*Child:* **IV** 5 mg/kg at weeks 0, 2, and 6, then 5 mg/kg q8wk

### Rheumatoid Arthritis

*Adult:* **IV** 3 mg/kg at weeks 0, 2, and 6, then q8wk

### Ulcerative Colitis

*Adult/Adolescent/Child (6 y or older):* **IV** 5 mg/kg at weeks 0, 2, and 6, then 5 mg/kg q8wk

### Ankylosing Spondylitis

*Adult:* **IV** 5 mg/kg at weeks 0, 2, and 6, then 5 mg/kg q6wk

### Plaque Psoriasis

*Adult:* **IV** 5 mg/kg at wk 0,2, and 6 and then 5 mg/kg q8wk

## ADMINISTRATION

▪ Note: Do not administer to a patient who has known or suspected sepsis.

### Intravenous

***PREPARE:*** **IV Infusion:** Reconstitute each 100 mg vial with 10 mL of sterile water for injection using a 21-gauge or smaller syringe. Inject sterile water against wall of vial, then gently swirl to dissolve but do not shake. ▪ Let stand for 5 min. ▪ Solution should be colorless to

light yellow with a few translucent particles. Discard if particles are opaque. ▪ Further dilute by first removing from a 250-mL IV bag of NS a volume of NS equal to the volume of reconstituted infliximab to be added to the IV bag. Slowly add the total volume of reconstituted infliximab solution to the 250-mL infusion bag and gently mix. ▪ Infusion concentration should be 0.4 to 4 mg/mL. ▪ Begin infusion within 3 h of preparation.

***ADMINISTER:*** **IV Infusion:** Give over at least 2 h using a polyethylene-lined infusion set with an in-line, low-protein-binding filter (pore size 1.2 micron or less). ▪ Flush infusion set before and after with NS to ensure delivery of total drug dose. ▪ Discard unused infusion solution.

***INCOMPATIBILITIES:*** **Y-site:** Do not infuse with any other drugs.

▪ Store unopened vials at 2°–8° C (36°–46° F).

## ADVERSE EFFECTS (≥1%) **Body as a Whole:** Fatigue, fever, pain, myalgia, back pain, chills, hot flashes, arthralgia; infusion-related reactions (fever, chills, pruritus, urticaria, chest pain, hypotension, hypertension, dyspnea). Increased risk of lymphoma and opportunistic infections, including tuberculosis. **CNS:** *Headache,* dizziness, involuntary muscle contractions, paresthesias, vertigo, anxiety, depression, insomnia. **CV:** Chest pain, peripheral edema, hypotension, hypertension, tachycardia, anemia, CHF, pericardial effusion, systemic and cutaneous vasculitis. **GI:** *Nausea,* diarrhea, *abdominal pain,* vomiting, constipation, dyspepsia, flatulence, intestinal obstruction, ulcerative stomatitis, increased hepatic enzymes. **Hematologic:** Leukopenia, neutrope-

Common adverse effects in *italic;* life-threatening effects underlined; generic names in **bold;** classifications in SMALL CAPS; ♣ Canadian drug name; ⊙ Prototype drug

835

nia, <u>thrombocytopenia</u>, pancytopenia. **Respiratory:** URI, pharyngitis, bronchitis, rhinitis, coughing, *sinusitis,* dyspnea. **Skin:** Rash, pruritus, acne, alopecia, fungal dermatitis, eczema, dry skin, increased sweating, urticaria. **Other:** Infections, development of autoantibodies, lupus-like syndrome, conjunctivitis, dysuria, urinary frequency, abscess.

**INTERACTIONS Drug:** May blunt effectiveness of VACCINES given concurrently. Do not give with TUMOR NECROSIS FACTOR MODIFIERS (e.g., **adalimumab, etanercept, infliximab,** or **certolizumab pegol**) or with drugs that block interleukin 1 (**canakinumab, rilonacept**).

**PHARMACOKINETICS Distribution:** Distributed primarily to the vascular compartment. **Half-Life:** 9.5 days.

## NURSING IMPLICATIONS

### Black Box Warning

*Infliximab has been associated with increased risk of serious, potentially fatal, infections and malignancies.*

### Assessment & Drug Effects

- Discontinue IV infusion and notify prescriber for fever, chills, pruritus, urticaria, chest pain, dyspnea, hypo/hypertension.
- Monitor for up to 2 h post-infusion for an acute infusion reaction (e.g., chest pain, hypotension, hypertension, dyspnea).
- Monitor for and immediately report S&S of generalized infection.
- Monitor lab tests: Obtain CBC with differential, LFTs, and HBV screen prior to treatment.

### Patient & Family Education

- Seek medical evaluation immediately if you suspect an infection.

# INGENOL MEBUTATE
(in'ge-nol)
Picato

**Classification:** DERMATOLOGIC; CELL DEATH INDUCER; ANTIKERATOSIS AGENT
**Therapeutic:** ANTIKERATOSIS AGENT

## AVAILABILITY Gel

## ACTION & *THERAPEUTIC EFFECT*
The mechanism of action is unknown. *Induces cell death in actinic keratosis lesions.*

## USES Topical treatment of actinic keratosis.

## CONTRAINDICATIONS Healing surgical wound; severe skin reaction beyond the treated area.

## CAUTIOUS USE Eye disorders; pregnancy (category C). Safety and efficacy in children younger than 18 y not established.

## ROUTE & DOSAGE

### Acne Keratosis of Face and Scalp
*Adult:* **Topical** 0.015% gel once daily to affected area for 3 d

### Acne Keratosis of Trunk and Extremities
*Adult:* **Topical** 0.05% gel once daily to affected area for 2 d

## ADMINISTRATION

### Topical
- Spread evenly over treatment area and allow to dry for 15 min.
- Patients who self-apply should wash hands immediately after application.
- Store refrigerated.

## ADVERSE EFFECTS (≥1%) **Body as a Whole:** Application-site reactions (infection, irritation, pain, pruritus),

headache, periorbital edema. **Respiratory:** Nasopharyngitis. **Skin:** *Crusting, erosion/ulceration, erythema, flaking/scaling, swelling, vesiculation/postulation.*

## NURSING IMPLICATIONS

### Assessment & Drug Effects

- Monitor for and report severe local skin reactions (e.g., erythema, crusting, swelling, vesiculation, pustulation, erosions, and ulceration).

### Patient & Family Education

- Treated area should not be washed or touched for 6 h after application.
- Avoid activities that cause excessive sweating for 6 h after application.
- Avoid sun exposure or use sun protection.

---

## INSULIN ASPART

(in'su-lyn)

NovoLog, NovoLog 70/30

**Classifications:** ANTIDIABETIC; RAPID-ACTING INSULIN
**Therapeutic:** RAPID-ACTING INSULIN
**Prototype:** Insulin injection

**AVAILABILITY** Solution for injection

## ACTION & *THERAPEUTIC EFFECT*

A recombinant insulin analog that is more rapidly absorbed than human insulin, with a more rapid onset and shorter duration than regular human insulin. Insulin acts via specific membrane-bound receptors on target tissues to regulate metabolism of carbohydrate, protein, and fats. Target organs for insulin include the liver, skeletal muscle, and adipose tissue. *Provides better blood glucose control than regular human insulin when given before a meal.*

**USES** Treatment of diabetes mellitus.

**CONTRAINDICATIONS** Systemic allergic reactions; history of allergic reactions to insulin; hypoglycemia.

**CAUTIOUS USE** Fever, hyperthyroidism, surgery or trauma; decreased insulin requirements due to diarrhea, nausea, or vomiting, malabsorption; renal or hepatic impairment, hypokalemia; pregnancy [category B **(NovoLog)** and category C **(NovoLog 70/30)**]; lactation. Safe use in children younger than 2 y is not established.

## ROUTE & DOSAGE

### Diabetes

*Adult/Adolescent/Child (older than 2 y):* **Subcutaneous** 0.5–1 unit/kg/day; **IV** Dose should be individualized

## ADMINISTRATION

- Use only if solution is absolutely clear.

### Subcutaneous

- **Must be given no sooner** than 5–10 min before a meal.
- Draw up insulin aspart first when mixing with NPH insulin. Give injection immediately after it is mixed.
- Store refrigerated at 2°–8° C (36°–46° F); may be stored at room temperature, 15°–30° C (59°–86° F) for up to 28 days. Do not expose to excessive heat or sunlight, and do not freeze.

### Intravenous

Use only under close medical supervision in a clinical setting.

**PREPARE: Infusion:** Dilute with NS or D5W in a polypropylene infusion bag to a final concentration of 0.05–1 unit/mL.
**ADMINISTER: Infusion:** Give at rate ordered by prescriber.

**ADVERSE EFFECTS** (≥1%) **Body as a Whole:** Allergic reactions.

---

Common adverse effects in *italic;* life-threatening effects underlined; generic names in **bold**; classifications in SMALL CAPS; ♣ Canadian drug name; ⊕ Prototype drug

837

**Endocrine:** Hypoglycemia, hypokalemia. **Skin:** Injection site reaction, lipodystrophy, pruritus, rash.

**INTERACTIONS Drug:** ORAL ANTIDIABETIC AGENTS, ACE INHIBITORS, **disopyramide, fluoxetine,** MAO INHIBITORS, **propoxyphene,** SALICYLATES, SULFONAMIDE ANTIBIOTICS, **octreotide** may enhance hypoglycemia; CORTICOSTEROIDS, **niacin, danazol,** DIURETICS, SYMPATHOMIMETIC AGENTS, PHENOTHIAZINES, THYROID HORMONES, ESTROGENS, PROGESTOGENS, **isoniazid, somatropin** may decrease hypoglycemic effects; BETA-BLOCKERS, **clonidine, lithium, alcohol** may either potentiate or weaken effects of insulin; **pentamidine** may cause hypoglycemia followed by hyperglycemia. **Herbal: Garlic, ginseng** may potentiate hypoglycemic effects. See INSULIN INJECTION.

**PHARMACOKINETICS Absorption:** Rapidly absorbed from subcutaneous injection site. **Onset:** 15 min. **Peak:** 1–3 h. **Duration:** 3–5 h. **Distribution:** Low protein binding. **Metabolism:** In liver with some metabolism in the kidneys. **Half-Life:** 81 min.

## NURSING IMPLICATIONS

### Assessment & Drug Effects

- Monitor for S&S of hypoglycemia (see Appendix F). Initial hypoglycemic response begins within 15 min and peaks 45–90 min after injection.
- Withhold drug and notify prescriber if patient is hypokalemic.
- Monitor lab tests: Periodic postprandial blood glucose and HbA1C.

### Patient & Family Education

- Eat immediately after injecting insulin aspart because it has a fast onset and short duration of action.
- Do not inject into areas with redness, swelling, itching, or dimpling.

- Ingest some form of sugar (e.g., orange juice, dissolved table sugar, honey) if symptoms of hypoglycemia develop, and seek medical assistance.
- Check blood sugar as prescribed, especially postprandial values; make note of and notify prescriber of fasting blood glucose less than 80 and greater than 120 mg/dL.
- Notify the prescriber of any of the following: Fever, infection, trauma, diarrhea, nausea or vomiting. Dosage adjustment may be needed.
- Do not take any other medication unless approved by the prescriber.

# INSULIN DEGLUDEC
(in'su-lin de-glu'dec)

Tresiba

**Classifications:** ANTIDIABETIC; LONG-ACTING INSULIN
**Therapeutic:** ANTIDIABETIC
**Prototype:** Insulin injection

**AVAILABILITY** Prefilled disposable pens with solution for injection

**ACTIONS & THERAPEUTIC EFFECT** Slowly absorbed after injection; stimulates peripheral glucose uptake especially in muscle and fat tissue; inhibits hepatic glucose production and stimulates hepatic glycogen synthesis. *Lowers blood glucose levels over an extended period of time and prevents the conversion of glycogen to glucose in the liver.*

**USES** Treatment of type 1 and type 2 diabetes.

**CONTRAINDICATIONS** Episodes of severe hypoglycemia; hypersensitivity to insulin degludec or one of its components.

**CAUTIOUS USE** Changes in meal pattern, level of physical activity, or

Common adverse effects in *italic;* life-threatening effects <u>underlined;</u> generic names in **bold;** classifications in SMALL CAPS; ◆ Canadian drug name; ⊘ Prototype drug

co-administered drugs; concomitant use of thiazolidinediones (i.e., may cause fluid retention and CHF); regimens designed to achieve tight glycemic control; episodes of mild-to-moderate hypoglycemia; hypokalemia; renal impairment; hepatic impairment; pregnancy; lactation. Safety and efficacy in children and adolescents under 18 y not established.

## ROUTE & DOSAGE

### Type 1 Diabetes

*Adult:* **Subcutaneous** *Insulin-naïve patients:* Initial dose of 1/3 to 1/2 of total daily insulin dose; use short-acting insulin for remainder of dose
*Insulin-experienced patients:* Use same unit dose as current long or intermediate-acting insulin unit; adjust according to patient's needs

### Type 2 Diabetes

*Adult:* **Subcutaneous** Initial dose of 10 units once daily; adjust according to patient's needs

## ADMINISTRATION

### Subcutaneous

- Inject into the thigh, upper arm, or abdomen.
- Rotate injection sites, and do not inject into areas with redness, swelling, itching, or dimpling.
- Do not mix with any other insulin products or solution.
- **Do not** transfer TRESIBA® from the TRESIBA® pen into a syringe for administration.
- Store not-in-use (unopened) disposable prefilled pen in refrigerator. Store in-use pen at room temperature (below 86° F [30° C]) away from direct heat and light (may be used for up to 56 days (8 wk) after being opened, if it is kept at room temperature.

## ADVERSE EFFECTS (≥1%) **Body as a Whole:** Injection site reaction, peripheral edema. **CNS:** *Headache.* **GI:** Diarrhea, gastroenteritis. **Metabolic:** *Hypoglycemia,* weight gain. **Respiratory:** *Nasopharyngitis,* sinusitis, *upper respiratory tract infection.*

## INTERACTIONS **Drug:** ANTIDIABETIC AGENTS, ACE INHIBITORS, ANGIOTENSIN II RECEPTOR BLOCKERS, DDP-4 INHIBITORS, **disopyramide,** FIBRATES, **fluoxetine,** GLP-1 RECEPTOR AGONISTS, MONOAMINE OXIDASE INHIBITORS, **pentoxifylline, pramlintide, propoxyphene,** SALICYLATES, SGLT-2 INHIBITORS, SOMATOSTATIN ANALOGS, and SULFONAMIDE ANTIBIOTICS may increase the risk of hypotension. ATYPICAL ANTIPSYCHOTICS (e.g., **clozapine, olanzapine**), CORTICOSTEROIDS, **danazol,** DIURETICS, ESTROGENS, **glucagon, isoniazid, niacin,** ORAL CONTRACEPTIVES, PHENOTHIAZINES, PROGESTINS, PROTEASE INHIBITORS, **somatropin,** SYMPATHOMIMETIC AGENTS (e.g., **albuterol, epinephrine, terbutaline**), and THYROID HORMONES can interfere with the glucose lowering effects of insulin degludec. **Alcohol,** BETA-BLOCKERS, **clonidine, lithium,** and **pentamidine** may either increase or decrease the glucose lowering effects of insulin degludec. BETA-BLOCKERS, **clonidine, guanethidine,** and **reserpine** may blunt the signs and symptoms of hypoglycemia.

## PHARMACOKINETICS **Onset:** 1 h. **Peak:** 3–4 days. **Distribution:** Greater than 99% plasma protein bound. **Metabolism:** Protein degradation to inactive metabolites. **Half-Life:** 25 h.

## NURSING IMPLICATIONS

### Assessment & Drug Effects

- Monitor for S&S of hypoglycemia (see Appendix F), especially after changes in insulin dose.

---

Common adverse effects in *italic;* life-threatening effects <u>underlined;</u> generic names in **bold;** classifications in SMALL CAPS; ♣ Canadian drug name; ⊙ Prototype drug

839

- Monitor for S&S of hypokalemia (see Appendix F).
- Withhold drug and notify prescriber if patient is hypoglycemic or hypokalemic (see Appendix F).
- Monitor lab tests: Periodic fasting blood glucose and HbA1C; periodic serum potassium.

### Patient & Family Education

- Do not take drug and notify prescriber if experiencing episodes of low blood sugar (hypoglycemia). S&S of hypoglycemia include: Dizziness or light-headedness, sweating, confusion, fast heartbeat, blurred vision, slurred speech, shakiness, anxiety, irritability, or mood changes, and headache.
- Check blood sugar as prescribed; notify prescriber if fasting blood glucose is frequently less than 80 and greater than 120 mg/dL.
- Notify the prescriber of any of the following: Fever, infection, trauma, diarrhea, nausea, or vomiting. Dosage adjustment may be needed.
- Do not take any other medication unless approved by prescriber.
- Women of childbearing age should discuss with prescriber potential risks associated with pregnancy.
- Do not breast-feed while taking this drug without consulting prescriber.

## INSULIN DETEMIR
(in'su-lyn det'e-mir)
Levemir
**Classifications:** ANTI-DIABETIC; LONG-ACTING INSULIN
Therapeutic LONG-ACTING INSULIN
**Prototype:** Insulin injection

**AVAILABILITY** Solution for injection

## ACTION & THERAPEUTIC EFFECT
Insulin detemir, a long-acting human insulin, exerts its action by binding to insulin receptors. Receptor-bound insulin lowers blood glucose by facilitating cellular uptake of glucose into skeletal muscle and fat, and inhibiting the output of glucose from the liver. *Insulin detemir is effective as a glucose-lowering agent, with glycemic control equivalent to that of NPH insulin.*

**USES** Treatment of diabetes mellitus.

**CONTRAINDICATIONS** Hypersensitivity to insulin detemir, or cresol; use in insulin infusion pumps; diabetic ketoacidosis, coma, hyperosmolar hyperglycemic state, hypoglycemia.

**CAUTIOUS USE** Renal and hepatic impairment; older adults; cardiac disease, CHF, illness, stress; pregnancy (category B); lactation. Safe and effective use in children younger than 2 y has not been established.

## ROUTE & DOSAGE

### Diabetes

*Adult/Child:* **Subcutaneous**
Insulin-naïve patients: 0.1–0.2 units/kg daily in evening or 10 units daily or b.i.d. in evenly spaced doses. For those taking a basal insulin product (i.e., NPH insulin, insulin glargine), a unit-to-unit dose conversion can be used.

## ADMINISTRATION

### Subcutaneous

- Once-daily injections should be given with the evening meal or at bedtime. With twice-daily dosing, the evening dose may be given with the evening meal, at bedtime, or 12 h after the morning dose.

Common adverse effects in *italic*; life-threatening effects <u>underlined</u>; generic names in **bold**; classifications in SMALL CAPS; ◆ Canadian drug name; ⊙ Prototype drug

- Do not administer IV or IM. With thin patients, inject at a 45-degree angle into a pinched fold of skin to avoid IM injection.
- Do not mix with any other type of insulin. Do not use with an insulin infusion pump.
- Store unopened vials under refrigeration at 2°–8° C (36°–46° F). Once removed from refrigeration, pens, cartridges, and other delivery devices **must be** kept at room temperature (not to exceed 30° C or 85° F) and either used within 42 days or discarded.

***INCOMPATIBILITIES:* Solution/additive:** Insulin detemir should not be mixed with any other insulin preparations.

### ADVERSE EFFECTS (≥1%) See
INSULIN (REGULAR). **Body as a Whole:** Allergic reactions. **Metabolic:** Hypoglycemia, weight gain. **Skin:** Lipodystrophy, pruritus, rash.

### DIAGNOSTIC TEST INTERFERENCE
See INSULIN INJECTION (REGULAR).

### INTERACTIONS Drug: See INSULIN
INJECTION (REGULAR). **Herbal:** See INSULIN INJECTION.

### PHARMACOKINETICS Absorption:
Slow, prolonged absorption over 24 h. **Peak:** 6–8 h. **Distribution:** 98–99% protein bound. **Half-Life:** 5–7 h.

### NURSING IMPLICATIONS

#### Assessment & Drug Effects
- Monitor for S&S of hypoglycemia (see Appendix F), especially after changes in insulin dose or type.
- Monitor weight periodically.
- Monitor lab tests: Periodic fasting blood glucose and HbA1C; periodic serum potassium with concurrent potassium-lowering drugs.

#### Patient & Family Education
- Follow directions for taking the drug (see Administration). Rotate injection sites and never inject into an area with redness, swelling, itching, or dimpling.
- Know parameters for withholding drug. Check blood sugar as prescribed; notify prescriber of fasting blood glucose below 80 or above 120 mg/dL.
- Ingest some form of sugar (e.g., orange juice, dissolved table sugar, honey) if symptoms of hypoglycemia develop; and seek medical assistance.
- Notify the prescriber of any of the following: Fever, infection, trauma, diarrhea, nausea, or vomiting.
- Do not take any other medication unless approved by prescriber.

## INSULIN GLARGINE
(in'su-lyn glar'geen)

**Lantus, Lantus SoloStar, Toujeo SoloStar**
**Classifications:** ANTIDIABETIC; LONG-ACTING INSULIN
**Therapeutic:** LONG-ACTING INSULIN
**Prototype:** Insulin injection

**AVAILABILITY** Solution for injection

### ACTION & *THERAPEUTIC EFFECT*
A recombinant human insulin analog with a long duration of action. Lowers blood glucose levels over an extended period of time by stimulating peripheral glucose uptake especially in muscle and fat tissue. In addition, insulin inhibits hepatic glucose production. *Lowers blood glucose levels over an extended period of time. It also prevents the conversion of glucagon to glucose in the liver.*

**USES** Bedtime dosing of adults and children with type 1 diabetes, or adults with type 2 diabetes.

Common adverse effects in *italic*; life-threatening effects underlined; generic names in **bold**; classifications in SMALL CAPS; ♣ Canadian drug name; ⓟ Prototype drug

841

**CONTRAINDICATIONS** Prior hypersensitivity to insulin glargine; during episodes of hypoglycemia.

**CAUTIOUS USE** Renal and hepatic impairment; risks for hypokalemia; older adults; illness; emotional disturbances; stress; pregnancy (category C); lactation. Safety and efficacy in children younger than 6 y of age not established.

## ROUTE & DOSAGE

### Type 1 Diabetes

*Adult* **Subcutaneous** Approximately 1/3–1/2 of the total daily insulin requirements adjust based on patient need and concurrent medications
*Child (6 y or older):* **Lantus** formulation only **Subcutaneous** Approximately ⅓ of the total daily insulin requirements; adjust based on patient needs

### Type 2 Diabetes

*Adult/Child (6 y or older):*
**Subcutaneous** 0.2 units/kg (max: 10 units) once daily and adjust according to patient needs

## ADMINISTRATION

**Subcutaneous**
- Give subcutaneous only. Do not use if solution is cloudy or viscous.
- Give at same time each day (usually at bedtime) and do not mix with any other insulin product.
- Do not share insulin pens among patients.
- Rotate administration sites.
- Administer at room temperature.
- Store in refrigerator at 2°–8° C (36°–46° F), may store at room temperature, 15°–30° C (59°–86° F). Discard opened refrigerated vials after 28 days and unrefrigerated vials after 14 days. Do not expose to excessive heat or sunlight, and do not freeze.

**ADVERSE EFFECTS** (≥1%) **Body as a Whole:** Allergic reactions, hypertension, peripheral edema, infection UTI. **Endocrine:** Hypoglycemia, hypokalemia. **Skin:** Injection site reaction, lipodystrophy, pruritus, rash. **CNS:** Depression. **GI:** Diarrhea. **Musculoskeletal:** Arthralgia, back pain, limb pain. **Special Senses:** Cataract, retinopathy. **Respiratory:** URI, sinusitis, cough.

**INTERACTIONS Drug:** ORAL ANTIDIABETIC AGENTS, ACE INHIBITORS, **disopyramide, fluoxetine,** MAO INHIBITORS, **propoxyphene,** SALICYLATES, SULFONAMIDE ANTIBIOTICS, **octreotide** may enhance hypoglycemia; CORTICOSTEROIDS, **niacin, danazol,** DIURETICS, SYMPATHOMIMETIC AGENTS, PHENOTHIAZINES, THYROID HORMONES, ESTROGENS, PROGESTOGENS, **isoniazid, somatropin** may decrease hypoglycemic effects; BETA-BLOCKERS, **clonidine, lithium, alcohol** may either potentiate or weaken effects of insulin; **pentamidine** may cause hypoglycemia followed by hyperglycemia. **Herbal: Garlic, green tea** may potentiate hypoglycemic effects.

**PHARMACOKINETICS Absorption:** Slowly absorbed from subcutaneous injection site. **Onset:** 1.5 h. **Duration:** 10.4–24 h. **Metabolism:** In liver to active metabolites.

## NURSING IMPLICATIONS

### Assessment & Drug Effects
- Monitor for S&S of hypoglycemia (see Appendix F), especially after changes in insulin dose or type.
- Withhold drug and notify prescriber if patient is hypokalemic.
- Monitor lab tests: Periodic fasting blood glucose and HbA1C.

Common adverse effects in *italic;* life-threatening effects <u>underlined</u>; generic names in **bold;** classifications in SMALL CAPS; ✚ Canadian drug name; ⊘ Prototype drug

## Patient & Family Education

- Do not inject into areas with redness, swelling, itching, or dimpling.
- Ingest some form of sugar (e.g., orange juice, dissolved table sugar, honey) if symptoms of hypoglycemia develop and seek medical assistance.
- Instruct patient and caregivers on proper insulin preparation and administration.
- Check blood sugar as prescribed; notify prescriber of fasting blood glucose less than 80 and greater than 120 mg/dL.
- Notify the prescriber of any of the following: Fever, infection, trauma, diarrhea, nausea, or vomiting. Dosage adjustment may be needed.
- Do not take any other medication unless approved by prescriber.

# INSULIN GLULISINE

(in'su-lyn glu-li'seen)

**Apidra, Apidra SoloSTAR**

**Classifications:** ANTIDIABETIC; RAPID-ACTING INSULIN

**Therapeutic:** RAPID-ACTING INSULIN

**Prototype:** Insulin injection (Regular)

**AVAILABILITY** Multidose vials; cartridge system

## ACTION & *THERAPEUTIC EFFECT*

Insulin glulisine, formed by recombinant DNA, is a rapid-acting insulin. Insulin lowers blood glucose by stimulating peripheral glucose uptake by skeletal muscle and fat and by inhibiting hepatic glucose production. Insulin causes lipolysis in the adipocytes, inhibits proteolysis, and enhances protein synthesis. *Insulin glulisine has a more rapid onset of action and a shorter duration of action than regular human insulin; thus, it provides good postprandial blood glucose control.*

**USES** Treatment of diabetes mellitus; type I diabetes mellitus in children.

**CONTRAINDICATIONS** Hypoglycemia; systemic allergy to insulin.

**CAUTIOUS USE** Renal impairment, hepatic dysfunction; thyroid disease; fever; older adults; pregnancy (category C); lactation, children. Safe use in children younger than 4 y not established.

## ROUTE & DOSAGE

### Diabetes

*Adult/Adolescent/Child (4 y or older):* **Subcutaneous** 5–10 units within 15 min before starting a meal or within 20 min after starting a meal. Dose should be individualized.

*Adult/Adolescent/Child:* **IV** 0.05–1 unit/mL via infusion

## ADMINISTRATION

### Subcutaneous

- Give within 15 min before or up to 20 min after a meal.
- Store refrigerated at 36°–46° F (2°–8° C). Discard vial if frozen. Protect from light.

### Intravenous

Use only under close medical supervision in a clinical setting.

***PREPARE:* Infusion:** Dilute with NS in a PVC bag to a final concentration of 0.05–1 unit/mL.

***ADMINISTER:* Infusion:** Give at rate ordered by prescriber.

**ADVERSE EFFECTS** (≥1%) See INSULIN (REGULAR). **Body as a Whole:** Allergic reactions. **Metabolic:** Hypoglycemia. **Skin:** Injection site reactions, lipodystrophy, pruritus, rash.

**DIAGNOSTIC TEST INTERFERENCE** See INSULIN INJECTION (REGULAR).

Common adverse effects in *italic;* life-threatening effects underlined; generic names in **bold;** classifications in SMALL CAPS; ♣ Canadian drug name; ⊘ Prototype drug

843

**PHARMACOKINETICS** **Absorption:** 70% bioavailable from injection sites. **Onset:** 15–30 min. **Peak:** 55 min. **Duration:** 3–4 h. **Metabolism:** In liver with some metabolism in the kidney. **Half-Life:** 42 min subcutaneous.

## NURSING IMPLICATIONS

### Assessment & Drug Effects

- Monitor for S&S of hypoglycemia (see Appendix F). Initial hypoglycemic response begins within 15 min and peaks, on average, 40–60 min after injection.
- Monitor lab tests: Periodic fasting and postprandial blood glucose, and HbA1C.

### Patient & Family Education

- Follow exactly directions for timing injection in relation to each meal.
- Do not inject into areas with redness, swelling, itching, or dimpling.
- If mixing with NPH human insulin, draw up insulin glulisine first. Inject immediately after mixing.
- Ingest some form of sugar (e.g., orange juice, dissolved table sugar, honey) if symptoms of hypoglycemia develop, and seek medical assistance.
- Check blood sugar as prescribed, especially postprandial values; notify prescriber of fasting blood glucose less than 80 and greater than 140 mg/dL.
- Notify the prescriber of any of the following: Fever, infection, trauma, diarrhea, nausea, or vomiting. Dosage adjustment may be needed.
- Do not take any other medication unless approved by the prescriber.

## INSULIN (REGULAR) ℗

(in'su-lyn)

Humulin R, Novolin R

**Classifications:** ANTIDIABETIC; SHORT-ACTING INSULIN

**Therapeutic:** SHORT-ACTING INSULIN

**AVAILABILITY** Solution for injection

**ACTION & *THERAPEUTIC EFFECT*** Insulin lowers blood glucose by stimulating peripheral glucose uptake by skeletal muscle and fat and inhibiting hepatic glucose production. Insulin inhibits lipolysis, proteolysis, and gluconeogenesis, and enhance protein synthesis and conversion of excess glucose into fat. *It lowers blood glucose levels by increasing peripheral glucose uptake and by inhibiting the liver from changing glycogen to glucose.*

**USES** Emergency treatment of diabetic ketoacidosis or coma, to initiate therapy in patient with insulin-dependent diabetes mellitus, and in combination with intermediate-acting or long-acting insulin to provide better control of blood glucose concentrations in the diabetic patient. Used IV to stimulate growth hormone secretion (glucose counter-regulatory hormone) to evaluate pituitary growth hormone reserve in patient with known or suspected growth hormone deficiency. Other uses include promotion of intracellular shift of potassium in treatment of hyperkalemia (IV) and induction of hypoglycemic shock as therapy in psychiatry.

**CONTRAINDICATIONS** Hypersensitivity to insulin.

**CAUTIOUS USE** Renal impairment, renal failure; hepatic impairment, fever, thyroid disease; older adults; pregnancy (category B); children.

## ROUTE & DOSAGE

**Diabetes Mellitus**

*Adult:* **Subcutaneous** 5–10 units 30–60 min a.c. and at bedtime (dose adjustments based on blood glucose determinations)

Common adverse effects in *italic;* life-threatening effects <u>underlined</u>; generic names in **bold;** classifications in SMALL CAPS; ♣ Canadian drug name; ℗ Prototype drug

*Child:* **Subcutaneous** 2–4 units 30–60 min a.c. and at bedtime (dose adjustments based on blood glucose determinations)

**Ketoacidosis**

*Adult:* **IV** 0.15 unit/kg bolus, followed by 0.1 unit/kg/hr continuous infusion

*Child:* **IV** 0.1 units/kg loading dose, followed by 0.1 units/h continuous infusion

## ADMINISTRATION

▪Note: Insulins should not be mixed unless prescribed by prescriber. In general, regular insulin is drawn up into syringe first. ▪Any change in the strength (e.g., U-40, U-100), brand (manufacturer), purity, type (regular, etc.), species (pork, human), or sequence of mixing two kinds of insulin is made by the prescriber only, since a simultaneous change in dosage may be necessary.

**Subcutaneous**

▪ Use an insulin syringe.

▪ Give regular insulin 30–60 min before a meal.

▪ Avoid injection of cold insulin; it can lead to lipodystrophy, reduced rate of absorption, and local reactions.

▪ Common injection sites: Upper arms, thighs, abdomen [avoid area over urinary bladder and 2 in. (5 cm) around navel], buttocks, and upper back (if fat is loose enough to pick up). Rotate sites.

**Intravenous**

*PREPARE:* **Direct:** Give undiluted. **Infusion:** *Humulin R U-100* should be used at a concentration of 0.1 to 1 unit/mL in IV systems with NS in polyvinyl chloride IV bags. *Novolin R* should be used at concentrations of 0.05 to 1 unit/mL

in IV systems using propylene IV bags with NS, D5W, or D10W+KCl 40 mmol/L.

*ADMINISTER:* **Direct:** Give 50 units or a fraction thereof over 1 min. **Infusion:** Rate **must be** ordered by prescriber.

*INCOMPATIBILITIES:* Solution/additive: **Aminophylline, amobarbital, chlorothiazide, cytarabine, dobutamine, octreotide, pentobarbital, phenobarbital, phenytoin, sodium bicarbonate.** Y-site: **Amiodarone, butorphanol, cefoperazone, cefoxitin, ccfobiprole, chlorpromazine, cisplatin, dantrolene, diazepam, diazoxide, diphenhydramine, drotrecogin, dobutamine, gemtuzumab, glycopyrrolate, hydroxyzine, inamrinone, isoproterenol, ketamine, micafungin, minocycline, mitomycin, nestiritide, pentamidine, phentolamine, phenylephrine, phenytoin, piperacillin/tazobactam, polymyxin B, prochlorperazine, propranolol, protamine, quinidine, quinprustin/dalfopristin, rocuronium, SMZ/TMP.**

▪ Regular insulin may be adsorbed into the container or tubing when added to an IV infusion solution. ▪ Amount lost is variable and depends on concentration of insulin, infusion system, contact duration, and flow rate. ▪ Monitor patient response closely.

▪ Insulin is stable at room temperature up to 1 mo. Avoid exposure to direct sunlight or to temperature extremes [safe range is wide: 5°–38° C (40°–100° F)]. Refrigerate but do not freeze stock supply. Insulin tolerates temperatures above 38° C with less harm than freezing.

Common adverse effects in *italic;* life-threatening effects underlined; generic names in **bold;** classifications in SMALL CAPS; ✚ Canadian drug name; ⊙ Prototype drug

845

## ADVERSE EFFECTS (≥1%) **Body as a Whole:** Most adverse effects are related to hypoglycemia; <u>anaphylaxis</u> (rare), hyperinsulinemia (*profuse sweating,* hunger, headache, *nausea, tremulousness,* tremors, *palpitation,* tachycardia, weakness, fatigue, nystagmus, circumoral pallor); numb mouth, tongue, and other paresthesias; visual disturbances (diplopia, blurred vision, mydriasis), staring expression, confusion, personality changes, ataxia, incoherent speech, apprehension, irritability, inability to concentrate, personality changes, uncontrolled yawning, loss of consciousness, delirium, hypothermia, convulsions, Babinski reflex, <u>coma</u>. (Urine glucose tests will be negatives.) **CNS:** With overdose, psychic disturbances (i.e., aphasia, personality changes, maniacal behavior). **Metabolic:** Posthypoglycemia or rebound hyperglycemia (Somogyi effect), lipoatrophy and lipohypertrophy of injection sites; insulin resistance. **Skin:** Localized allergic reactions at injection site; generalized urticaria or bullae, lymphadenopathy.

## DIAGNOSTIC TEST INTERFERENCE
Large doses of insulin may increase urinary excretion of *VMA.* Insulin can cause alterations in ***thyroid function tests*** and ***liver function test*** and may decrease ***serum potassium*** and ***serum calcium.***

## INTERACTIONS **Drug: Alcohol,** ANABOLIC STEROIDS, MAO INHIBITORS, **guanethidine,** SALICYLATES, ORAL ANTIDIABETIC agents may potentiate hypoglycemic effects; **dextrothyroxine,** CORTICOSTEROIDS may antagonize hypoglycemic effects; **furosemide,** THIAZIDE DIURETICS increase **serum glucose** levels; **propranolol** and other BETA-BLOCKERS may mask symptoms of hypoglycemic reaction. **Herbal: Garlic, ginseng** may potentiate hypoglycemic effects.

## PHARMACOKINETICS **Absorption:** Rapidly absorbed from IM and subcutaneous injections. **Onset:** 0.5–1 h. **Peak:** 2–4 h. **Duration:** 5–7 h. **Distribution:** Throughout extracellular fluids. **Metabolism:** In liver with some metabolism in kidneys. **Elimination:** Less than 2% excreted in urine. **Half-Life:** Biological, up to 13 h.

## NURSING IMPLICATIONS
### Assessment & Drug Effects
- Note: Frequency of blood glucose monitoring is determined by the insulin regimen and health status of the patient.
- Notify prescriber promptly for markedly elevated blood sugar or presence of acetone with sugar in the urine; may indicate onset of ketoacidosis.
- Monitor for hypoglycemia (see Appendix F) at time of peak action of insulin. Onset of hypoglycemia (blood sugar: 50–40 mg/dL) may be rapid and sudden.
- Check BP, I&O ratio, and blood glucose and ketones every hour during treatment for ketoacidosis with IV insulin.
- Patients with severe hypoglycemia are usually treated with glucagon, epinephrine, or IV glucose 10–50%. As soon as patient is fully conscious, oral carbohydrate (e.g., orange juice with sugar, Gatorade, or Pedialyte) to prevent secondary hypoglycemia may be used.
- Monitor lab tests: Periodic fasting and postprandial blood glucose and HbA1C; urine for ketones in new, unstable, and type 1 diabetes or if patient has lost weight, exercises vigorously, or has an

Common adverse effects in *italic;* life-threatening effects <u>underlined</u>; generic names in **bold;** classifications in SMALL CAPS; ♣ Canadian drug name; ⊙ Prototype drug

illness and whenever blood glucose is substantially elevated.

**Patient & Family Education**

- Learn correct injection technique.
- Inject insulin into the abdomen rather than a near muscle that will be heavily taxed, if engaged in active sports.
- Notify prescriber of local reactions at injection site; may develop 1–3 wk after therapy starts and last several hours to days, usually disappear with continued use.
- Do not change prescription lenses during early period of dosage regulation; vision stabilizes, usually 3–6 wk.
- Check your blood glucose often as directed by the prescriber. Hypoglycemia can result from excess insulin, insufficient food intake, vomiting, diarrhea, unaccustomed exercise, infection, illness, nervous or emotional tension, or overindulgence in alcohol.
- Respond promptly to beginning symptoms of hypoglycemia. Severe hypoglycemia is an emergency situation. Take 4 oz (120 mL) of any fruit juice or regular carbonated beverage [1.5–3 oz (45–90 mL) for child] followed by a meal of longer-acting carbohydrate or protein food. Failure to show signs of recovery within 30 min indicates need for emergency treatment.
- Carry some form of fast-acting carbohydrate (e.g., lump sugar, Life-Savers, or other candy) at all times to treat hypoglycemia.
- Check blood glucose regularly during menstrual period; loss of diabetes control (hyperglycemia or hypoglycemia) is common; adjust insulin dosage accordingly, as prescribed by prescriber.

- Notify prescriber immediately of S&S of diabetic ketoacidosis.
- Continue taking insulin during an illness, go to bed, and drink non-caloric liquids liberally (every hour if possible). Consult prescriber for insulin regulation if unable to eat prescribed diet.
- Avoid OTC medications unless approved by prescriber.

# INSULIN, ISOPHANE (NPH)

(in'su-lyn)

**Humulin N, Novolin N, ReliOn N**

**Classifications:** ANTIDIABETIC; INTERMEDIATE-ACTING INSULIN
**Therapeutic:** INTERMEDIATE ACTING INSULIN
**Prototype:** Insulin

**AVAILABILITY** Solution for injection

**ACTION & *THERAPEUTIC EFFECT***
Insulin lowers blood glucose levels by stimulating peripheral glucose uptake, especially by skeletal muscle and fat, and by inhibiting hepatic glucose production. Insulin inhibits lipolysis in the adipocyte, inhibits proteolysis, and enhances protein synthesis. NPH human insulin contains protamine and zinc, providing an intermediate-acting insulin with a slower onset and a longer duration of activity. *Usually without supplemental doses of insulin injection.*

**USES** Used to control hyperglycemia in the diabetic patient. Mixtard and Novolin 70/30 are fixed combinations of purified regular insulin 30% and NPH 70%.

**CONTRAINDICATIONS** During episodes of hypoglycemia or in patients sensitive to any ingredient in the formulation; intravenous route;

Common adverse effects in *italic;* life-threatening effects underlined; generic names in **bold;** classifications in SMALL CAPS; ◆ Canadian drug name; ⊙ Prototype drug

847

diabetic ketoacidosis; hyperosmolar hyperglycemic state.

**CAUTIOUS USE** In insulin-resistant patients, hyperthyroidism or hypothyroidism; fever; older adults, renal or hepatic impairment; pregnancy (category B); children.

## ROUTE & DOSAGE

### Diabetes Mellitus
*Adult:* **Subcutaneous** Individualized doses (see INSULIN, REGULAR)

## ADMINISTRATION
**Subcutaneous**
- Give isophane insulin 30 min before first meal of the day. If necessary, a second smaller dose may be prescribed 30 min before supper or at bedtime.
- Ensure complete dispersion by mixing thoroughly by gently rotating vial between palms and inverting it end to end several times. Do not shake.
- **Do not** mix insulins unless prescribed by prescriber. In general, when insulin injection (regular insulin) is to be combined, it is drawn first.
- Store unopened vial at 2°–8° C (36°–46° F). Avoid freezing and exposure to extremes in temperature or to direct sunlight.

**ADVERSE EFFECTS** (≥1%) See INSULIN (REGULAR).

**INTERACTIONS** See INSULIN (REGULAR).

**PHARMACOKINETICS Onset:** 1–2 h. **Peak:** 4–12 h NPH. **Duration:** 18–24 h NPH. **Metabolism:** In liver and kidney. **Elimination:** Less than 2% excreted unchanged in urine. **Half-Life:** Up to 13 h.

## NURSING IMPLICATIONS

See INSULIN (REGULAR).

**Assessment & Drug Effects**
- Suspect hypoglycemia if fatigue, weakness, sweating, tremor, or nervousness occur.

**Patient & Family Education**
- If insulin was given before breakfast, a hypoglycemic episode is most likely to occur between mid-afternoon and dinnertime, when insulin effect is peaking. Advise to eat a snack in mid-afternoon and to carry sugar or candy to treat a reaction. A snack at bedtime will prevent insulin reaction during the night.
- Learn the S&S of hypoglycemia and hyperglycemia (see Appendix F).

## INSULIN LISPRO
(in'su-lyn lis'pro)
Humalog
**Classifications:** ANTIDIABETIC; RAPID-ACTING INSULIN
Therapeutic: RAPID-ACTING INSULIN

**AVAILABILITY** Solution for injection

**ACTION & *THERAPEUTIC EFFECT***
Insulin lispro of recombinant DNA origin is a human insulin that is a rapid-acting, glucose-lowering agent of shorter duration than human regular insulin. It lowers blood glucose levels by increasing peripheral glucose uptake, especially by skeletal muscle and fat tissue, and by inhibiting the liver from changing glycogen to glucose. *It lowers blood glucose levels and inhibits liver from changing glycogen to glucose.*

**USES** Treatment of diabetes mellitus.

**CONTRAINDICATIONS** During episodes of hypoglycemia or in

patients sensitive to any ingredient in the formulation.

**CAUTIOUS USE** In insulin-resistant patients, hyperthyroidism or hypothyroidism; use of alcohol; risk for hypokalemia; renal or hepatic impairment; older adults; pregnancy (category B); lactation; children.

## ROUTE & DOSAGE

### Diabetes Mellitus (type 1)

*Adult/Adolescent/Child (older than 3 y):* **Subcutaneous** 05.–1 unit/kg/day (dose adjustments based on blood glucose determinations)
*Humalog Mix Formulation:* Individualize dosage

**Renal Impairment Dosage Adjustment**

*CrCl 10–50 mL/min:* Administer at 75% of normal dose
*CrCl less than 10 mL/min:* Administer at 50% of dose and monitor closely

## ADMINISTRATION

**Subcutaneous**
- Give within 15 min before or immediately after a meal. Give only if solution is clear and colorless.
- Note: May be given in same syringe with longer-acting insulins but absorption may be delayed.

**ADVERSE EFFECTS** (≥1%) See INSULIN INJECTION (REGULAR).

**INTERACTIONS** See INSULIN INJECTION (REGULAR).

**PHARMACOKINETICS Absorption:** Rapidly absorbed from IM and subcutaneous injection sites. **Onset:** Less than 15 min. **Peak:** 0.5–1 h. **Duration:** 3–4 h. **Distribution:** Throughout extracellular

fluids. **Metabolism:** Metabolized in liver with some metabolism in kidneys. **Elimination:** Less than 2% excreted in urine. **Half-Life:** 1 h.

## NURSING IMPLICATIONS

See INSULIN INJECTION (REGULAR).

### Assessment & Drug Effects
- Assess for hypoglycemia from 1 to 3 h after injection.
- Assess highly insulin-dependent patients for need for increases in intermediate/long-acting insulins.

### Patient & Family Education
- Note: Risk of hypoglycemia is greatest 1–3 h after injection.

# INTERFERON ALFA-2b

(in-ter-feer'on)

Intron A

**Classifications:** BIOLOGICAL RESPONSE MODIFIER; IMMUNOMODULATOR; INTERFERON; ANTINEOPLASTIC
Therapeutic ANTINEOPLASTIC; IMMUNOMODULATOR; INTERFERON; ANTIVIRAL
**Prototype:** Peginterferon alfa-2a

**AVAILABILITY** Solution for injection

## ACTION & *THERAPEUTIC EFFECT*

Interferon (IFN) alfa-2b, one of 4 types of alpha interferons, is a highly purified protein and natural product of human leukocytes within 4–6 h after viral stimulation. Produced by recombinant DNA technology. **Antiviral action:** Reprograms virus-infected cells to inhibit various stages of virus replication. **Antitumor action:** Suppresses cell proliferation. **Immunomodulating action:** Enhances phagocytic activity of macrophages and augments specific cytotoxicity of lymphocytes for target cells. The immune system and the

Common adverse effects in *italic;* life-threatening effects underlined; generic names in **bold**; classifications in SMALL CAPS; ♣ Canadian drug name; ☻ Prototype drug

849

interferon system of defense are complementary. *Has a broad spectrum of antiviral, cytotoxic, and immunomodulating activity (i.e., favorably adjusts immune system to better combat foreign invasion of antigens, cancers, and viruses).*

**USES** Hairy cell leukemia, chronic hepatitis B or C, malignant melanoma, condylomata acuminata, follicular lymphoma, AIDS-related Kaposi's sarcoma.

**UNLABELED USES** Multiple sclerosis, condylomata acuminata.

**CONTRAINDICATIONS** Hypersensitivity to interferon alfa-2b or to any components of the product; patients with or development of decompensated liver disease, chronic hepatis B or C; autoimmune hepatitis; development of hemorrhagic or ischemic cerebrovascular event; patients with visceral AIDS-related Kaposi sarcoma. Coadministration with ribavirin in pregnant women, in men with pregnant partners, thalassemia major, sickle-cell anemia, CrCl less than 50 mL/min or hypersensitivity to ribavirin; pancreatitis; suicidal ideation; lactation; neonates.

**CAUTIOUS USE** Severe, preexisting cardiac, renal, or hepatic disease; pulmonary disease (e.g., COPD); DM; preexisting thyroid disorders; patients prone to ketoacidosis; coagulation disorders; preexisting myelosuppression; previous dysrhythmias; history of pulmonary disease; autoimmune disorders; hypertriglyceridemia; history of depression or suicidal tendencies; or other neuropsychiatric disorders; substance abuse disorders; debilitating conditions; ocular disorders;

pregnancy (category C); lactation. Safety and efficacy in children younger than 18 y not established for indications other than chronic hepatitis B. Safety for chronic hepatis B in children younger than 1 y not established.

## ROUTE & DOSAGE

### Hairy Cell Leukemia

*Adult:* **IM/Subcutaneous** 2 million units/m² 3 × wk

### Kaposi's Sarcoma

*Adult:* **IM/Subcutaneous** 30 million units/m² 3 × wk
*Child (1–17 y):* **Subcutaneous** 3 million units/m² 3 × wk, then increase to 6 million units/m²

### Condylomata Acuminata

*Adult:* **IM/Subcutaneous** 1 million units/lesion 3 × wk

### Chronic Hepatitis B or C

*Adult:* **Subcutaneous** 3 million units 3 × wk × 16–24 mo

### Malignant Melanoma

*Adult:* **IV** 20 million international units/m² daily for 5 days/wk × 4 wk; maintenance dose is 10 million international units/m² given subcutaneously weekly × 48 wk

### Follicular Lymphoma

*Adult:* **SQ** 5 million units 3 × wk

### Renal Impairment Dosage Adjustment

Not removed by dialysis

## ADMINISTRATION

**Subcutaneous/Intramuscular**
- Reconstitution: The final concentration with the amount of required diluent is determined by the condition being treated (see

manufacturer's directions). Inject diluent (bacteriostatic water for injection) into interferon alfa-2b vial; gently agitate solution before withdrawing dose with a sterile syringe.

- Make sure reconstituted solution is clear and colorless to light yellow and free of particulate material; discard if there are particles or solution is discolored.
- Store vials and reconstituted solutions at 2°–8° C (36°–46° F); remains stable for 1 mo. Discard any remaining drug in reconstituted vials.

**Intravenous**

*PREPARE:* **IV Infusion:** Prepare **immediately** before use. Select the appropriate number of vials (i.e., 10, 18, or 50 million international units) of recombinant powder for injection and add to each the 1 mL of supplied diluent. Swirl gently to dissolve but do not shake. • Further dilute by adding the required dose to 100 mL of NS. • The final concentration should not be less than 10 million international units/100 mL.
*ADMINISTER:* **IV Infusion:** Infuse over 20 min.
*INCOMPATIBILITIES:* **Solution/additive: Dextrose**-containing solutions.

**ADVERSE EFFECTS** (≥1%) **Body as a Whole:** *Flu-like syndrome (fever, chills) associated with myalgia and arthralgia,* leg cramps. **CNS:** Depression, nervousness, anxiety, confusion, *dizziness, fatigue,* somnolence, insomnia, altered mental states, ataxia, tremor, paresthesias, *headache.* **CV:** Hypertension, dyspnea, *hot flushes.* **Special Senses:** Epistaxis, pharyngitis, sneezing; abnormal vision. **GI:** Taste alteration, *anorexia,* weight loss, *nausea,* vomiting, stomatitis, *diarrhea,* flatulence. **Hematologic:** Mild thrombo-

cytopenia, transient granulocytopenia, anemia, *neutropenia,* leukemia. **Skin:** Mild pruritus, mild alopecia, rash, dry skin, herpetic eruptions, nonherpetic cold sores, urticaria.

**INTERACTIONS Drug:** May increase **theophylline** levels; additive myelosuppression with ANTINEO-PLASTICS, **zidovudine** may increase hematologic toxicity, increase **doxorubicin** toxicity, increase neurotoxicity with **vinblastine**. Use with **ribavirin** increases risk of hemolytic anemia; do not use in combination with **ribavirin** if CrCl less than 50 mL/min.

**PHARMACOKINETICS Peak:** 6–8 h. **Metabolism:** In kidneys. **Half-Life:** 6–7 h.

## NURSING IMPLICATIONS

**Black Box Warnings**

*Interferon alfa-2b has been associated with fatal or life-threatening neuropsychiatric, autoimmune, ischemic, and infectious disorders.*

**Assessment & Drug Effects**
- Monitor for and report any of the following S&S immediately: Depression, suicidal ideation, suicide attempt, or other indications of psychiatric disturbance.
- Assess hydration status; patient should be well hydrated, especially during initial stage of treatment and if vomiting or diarrhea occurs.
- Monitor for and promptly report any of the following: Chest pain, dyspnea, ecchymoses, petechiae, fever, severe abdominal pain, or psychic disturbances.
- Assess for flu-like symptoms, which may be relieved by acetaminophen (if prescribed).

Common adverse effects in *italic;* life-threatening effects underlined; generic names in **bold;** classifications in SMALL CAPS; ◆ Canadian drug name; ● Prototype drug

851

- Monitor level of GI distress and ability to consume fluids and food.
- Monitor mental status and alertness; implement safety precautions if needed.
- Monitor lab tests: Baseline and periodic CBC with differential, platelet count, serum electrolytes, LFTs, and TSH.

**Patient & Family Education**
- Seek medical attention promptly for any of the following: Chest pain, shortness of breath, easy bruising, persistent fever, decrease or loss of vision, severe abdominal pain, depression or suicidal ideation.
- Note: If flu-like symptoms develop, take acetaminophen as advised by prescriber and take interferon at bedtime.
- Use caution with hazardous activities until response to drug is known.
- Learn about adverse effects and notify prescriber about those that cause significant discomfort.

# INTERFERON ALFACON-1
(in-ter-fer′on al′fa-con)
Infergen
**Classifications:** BIOLOGICAL RESPONSE MODIFIER; IMMUNOMODULATOR; INTERFERON; ANTIVIRAL
**Therapeutic:** ANTIVIRAL; INTERFERON
**Prototype:** Peginterferon alfa-2a

**AVAILABILITY** Solution for injection

**ACTION & *THERAPEUTIC EFFECT***
Its antiviral, antiproliferative, and natural killer (NK) cell activity is five × greater than interferon alpha-2b. *Effectiveness is measured by normalization of ALT level and serum HCV RNA less than 100* copies/mL. Type 1 interferons bind to the cell surface receptors inducing biological responses including antiviral, antiproliferative, and immunomodulatory activities.

**USES** Treatment of chronic hepatitis C.

**CONTRAINDICATIONS** Hypersensitivity to alpha interferons or *E. coli* products; decompensated liver disease such as jaundice, ascites, etc.; suicidal ideations or severe psychiatric disorder; lactation.

**CAUTIOUS USE** History of severe psychiatric disorder, depression, or suicidal tendencies; preexisting cardiac disease, elderly, myelosuppression, previous hypersensitivity to interferon therapy; history of endocrine disorders; ophthalmic disorders or autoimmune disorders; pregnancy (category C). Safe use in children younger than 18 y not established.

## ROUTE & DOSAGE

| Chronic Hepatitis C |
|---|
| *Adult:* **Subcutaneous** 9 mcg 3 × wk × 24 wk |

## ADMINISTRATION
**Subcutaneous**
- Allow at least 24 h to elapse between doses of interferon alfacon-1.
- Give only one dose/vial or dose/prefilled syringe. Enter each vial only once. Discard unused portion of a vial or prefilled syringe immediately.
- Store vials and syringes at 2°–8° C (36°–46° F). Avoid direct sunlight and vigorous shaking.

**ADVERSE EFFECTS** (≥1%) **Body as a Whole:** *Asthenia, headache,*

---

Common adverse effects in *italic;* life-threatening effects underlined; generic names in **bold;** classifications in SMALL CAPS; ♣ Canadian drug name; ⊕ Prototype drug

*fatigue, fever, chills, injection site reaction (pain, edema, hemorrhage, inflammation), pain, myalgia, arthralgia,* increased sweating. **CNS:** *Insomnia, depression, dizziness, paresthesia, nervousness, depression, anxiety,* agitation. **CV:** Hypertension, palpitation. **GI:** *Nausea, diarrhea, abdominal pain, anorexia, vomiting, dyspepsia,* constipation, flatulence, toothache, hemorrhoids, weight loss, hepatotoxicity. **Hematologic:** *Granulocytopenia, thrombocytopenia, leukopenia,* ecchymosis, lymphadenopathy, lymphocytosis. **Respiratory:** *Cough, bronchitis, dyspnea, pneumonia, rhinitis,* pharyngitis. **Skin:** *Alopecia, rash,* dry skin, *pruritus,* erythema. **Urogenital:** Dysmenorrhea, vaginitis, menstrual disorder.

**INTERACTIONS** No clinically significant interactions established.

**PHARMACOKINETICS Peak:** 24–36 h.

## NURSING IMPLICATIONS

### Black Box Warning

*Interferon alfacon-1 has been associated with fatal or life-threatening neuropsychiatric, autoimmune, ischemic, and infectious disorders.*

### Assessment & Drug Effects

- Monitor for and report any of the following S&S immediately: Depression, suicidal ideation, suicide attempt, or other indications of psychiatric disturbance.
- Withhold drug and notify prescriber if symptoms of hepatic-decompensation such as jaundice or ascites develop. Withhold drug and notify prescriber if any other severe adverse reaction occurs.
- Monitor lab tests: Baseline, 2 wk after initiation of therapy, and

periodically thereafter: Platelet count, Hgb and Hct, WBC and ANC, serum creatinine, serum albumin, bilirubin, thyroid function, and triglyceride; periodic LFTs.

### Patient & Family Education

- Report immediately any signs of psychiatric disturbance including depression, thoughts of suicide, nervousness, anxiety, agitation, apathy, or significant mood swings to prescriber.

## INTERFERON BETA-1a

(in-ter-fer'on)

**Avonex, Rebif**

**Classifications:** BIOLOGIC RESPONSE MODIFIER; IMMUNOMODULATOR; INTERFERON

**Therapeutic:** IMMUNOMODULATOR; INTERFERON

**Prototype:** Peginterferon alfa-2a

**AVAILABILITY Avonex:** Solution for injection; prefilled syringe. **Rebif:** Solution for injection

## ACTION & *THERAPEUTIC EFFECT*

Interferon beta-1a is produced by recombinant DNA technology. Interferon beta-1a inhibits expression of pro-inflammatory cytokines including INF-G, thought to be a major factor in triggering the autoimmune reaction that leads to multiple sclerosis. It is believed that INF-G stimulates cytotoxic T-cells and causes degradation by macrophages' enzymes on the myelin sheath of neurons in the spinal cord. *Effective in improving time of onset of progression in disability; it was significantly longer in patients treated with interferon beta-1a.*

**USES** Relapsing-remitting multiple sclerosis.

Common adverse effects in *italic*; life-threatening effects underlined; generic names in **bold**; classifications in SMALL CAPS; ♦ Canadian drug name; ⓟ Prototype drug

853

**CONTRAINDICATIONS** Previous hypersensitivity to interferon-beta or human albumin, albumin hypersensitivity, hamster protein hypersensitivity; lactation (using **Rebif**).

**CAUTIOUS USE** Suicidal tendencies, depression, preexisting psychiatric disorders; bone marrow depression; cardiac disease; seizure disorders; thyroid disease; hepatic impairment; pregnancy (category C); lactation (using **Avonex**). Safety and efficacy in children younger than 18 y not established.

## ROUTE & DOSAGE

**Multiple Sclerosis**
*Adult:* **IM Avonex** 30 mcg qwk; **Subcutaneous Rebif** 22 or 44 mcg 3 × wk

## ADMINISTRATION

### Intramuscular
- **Avonex:** Reconstitute single use Avonex vial (33 mcg of lyophilized powder) with 1.1 mL of supplied diluent and swirl gently to dissolve.
- Withdraw 1 mL for administration.
- Discard any residual drug as the product contains no preservatives.
- Use within 6 h of reconstitution.

### Subcutaneous
- **Rebif:** Give at the same time each day (preferably in the late afternoon or evening) on the same three days of the week at least 48 h apart each week.
- Inject subcutaneously using either a 22 or 44 mcg prefilled syringe. Discard any residual drug as the product contains no preservatives.
- Store unreconstituted vials or prefilled syringes at 2°–8° C (36°–46° F).

- May store for up to 30 days at room temperature up to 25° C (77° F). Do not use beyond expiration date.

**ADVERSE EFFECTS** (≥1%) **Body as a Whole:** Alopecia, myalgias, *flu-like syndrome*, anaphylaxis. **CNS:** Headache, *fever*, fatigue, lethargy, depression, somnolence, weakness, agitation, malaise, confusion or reduced ability to concentrate, anxiety, dementia, emotional lability, depersonalization, suicide attempts, worsening of psychiatric disorders. **CV:** Tachycardia, CHF (rare). **GI:** Nausea, vomiting, *diarrhea, hepatic injury.* **Hematologic:** <u>Leukopenia</u>, anemia, pancytopenia (rare), <u>thrombocytopenia</u> (rare). **Metabolic:** Hypocalcemia, elevated serum creatinine, elevated liver transaminases. **Skin:** Local skin necrosis at injection site, *pain at injection site.*

**PHARMACOKINETICS** **Peak: Avonex** 7.8–9.8 h; **Rebif** 16 h. **Metabolism:** Rapidly inactivated in body fluids and tissue. **Half-Life: Avonex** 8.6–10 h; **Rebif** 69 h.

## NURSING IMPLICATIONS

### Assessment & Drug Effects
- Withhold drug and notify prescriber if depression or suicidal ideation develops or if there is a worsening of psychiatric symptoms.
- Monitor patients with cardiac disease carefully for worsening cardiac function.
- Monitor lab tests: Periodic LFTs, renal function tests, routine blood chemistry, and CBC with differential, and platelet count; thyroid function tests q6mo with preexisting thyroid dysfunction or when clinically indicated.

## Patient & Family Education

- Take a missed dose as soon as possible but not within 48 h of next scheduled dose.
- Learn about common adverse effects, especially flu-like syndrome (headache, fatigue, fever, rigors, chest pain, back pain, myalgia).
- Withhold drug and notify prescriber of depression or suicidal ideation or exacerbation of a pre-existing seizure disorder.
- Women who become pregnant should notify prescriber promptly.

# INTERFERON BETA-1b

(in-ter-fer'on)

Betaseron, Extavia

**Classifications:** BIOLOGIC RESPONSE MODIFIER; IMMUNOMODU-LATOR; INTERFERON
**Therapeutic:** IMMUNOMODULATOR; INTERFERON
**Prototype:** Peginterferon alfa-2a

**AVAILABILITY** Solution for injection

## ACTION & THERAPEUTIC EFFECT

Interferon beta-1b is a glycoprotein produced by recombinant DNA technique. It is thought to inhibit expression of pro-inflammatory cytokines including INF-G, thought to be a major factor in triggering the autoimmune reaction. It is believed that INF-G stimulates cytotoxic T-cells and causes degradation by macrophages' enzymes on the myelin sheath of neurons in the spinal cord. *Possess antiviral, antiproliferative, antitumor, and immunomodulatory activity. The effectiveness of interferon beta-1b for multiple sclerosis (MS) is based on the assumption that MS is an immunologically mediated illness.*

**USES** Relapsing and relapsing-remitting multiple sclerosis.

**CONTRAINDICATIONS** Previous hypersensitivity to interferon beta-1b or human albumin, mannitol hypersensitivity; suicidal ideation; jaundice due to hepatic injury; worsening of CHF.

**CAUTIOUS USE** History of suicidal tendencies or mental disorders especially chronic depression; seizures; cardiac disease; hepatic impairment; pregnancy (category C) but may cause a spontaneous abortion; lactation. Safety and efficacy in children younger than 18 y not established.

## ROUTE & DOSAGE

### Multiple Sclerosis

*Adult:* **Subcutaneous** 62.5 mcg every other day during wk 1 and 2; 125 mcg every other day during wk 3 and 4; 187.5 mcg every other day during wk 5 and 6; then 250 mcg every other day

## ADMINISTRATION

### Subcutaneous

- Reconstitute by adding 1.2 mL of the supplied diluent (0.54% NaCl) to vial and gently swirl. **Do not** shake. The resultant solution contains 0.25 mg (8 million units)/mL.
- Discard reconstituted solution if it contains particulate matter or is discolored. Also discard unused solution.
- Rotate injection sites; use 27-gauge needle to administer drug.
- Store vials under refrigeration, 2°–8° C (36°–46° F) or at room temperature.

## ADVERSE EFFECTS (≥1%) CNS:
Headache, *fever,* fatigue, dizziness, lethargy, depression, somnolence, weakness, agitation, malaise, confusion or reduced ability to

Common adverse effects in *italic*; life-threatening effects underlined; generic names in **bold**; classifications in SMALL CAPS; ♣ Canadian drug name; ✪ Prototype drug

855

concentrate, anxiety, dementia, emotional lability, depersonalization, suicide attempts, hypertonia, chills. **CV:** Tachycardia, peripheral edema, CHF (rare). **GI:** Nausea, vomiting, *diarrhea,* abdominal pain. **Hematologic:** Leukopenia, thrombocytopenia, anemia. **Metabolic:** Hypocalcemia, elevated serum creatinine, elevated liver transaminases, autoimmune hepatitis, hepatic failure. **Skin:** Local skin necrosis at injection site, rash, *pain at injection site.* **Body as a Whole:** Alopecia, myalgias, *flu-like syndrome.*

**INTERACTIONS Drug:** Use with NRTIs or PROTEASE INHIBITORS should be done with caution.

**PHARMACOKINETICS Absorption:** About 50% absorbed from subcutaneous sites. **Distribution:** Penetrates intact blood–brain barrier poorly; crosses placenta; distributed into breast milk. **Metabolism:** Rapidly inactivated in body fluids and tissue.

**NURSING IMPLICATIONS**

**Assessment & Drug Effects**

▪ Monitor vital signs, neurologic status, and neuropsychiatric status frequently during therapy.
▪ Assess for and promptly treat flu-like symptom complex (fever, chills, myalgia, etc.).
▪ Assess injection sites; pain and redness are common reactions. Report tissue ulceration promptly.
▪ Monitor lab tests: LFTs at 1, 3, and 6 mo after initiation of therapy and as clinically warranted thereafter; periodic renal function tests, CBC, thyroid function, and serum electrolytes.

**Patient & Family Education**

▪ Learn and understand potential adverse drug reactions.

▪ Learn proper technique for solution preparation and injection.
▪ Self-medicate with acetaminophen (if not contraindicated) if flu-like symptom complex develops.
▪ Avoid prolonged exposure to sunlight.
▪ Use caution when performing hazardous activities until response to drug is known.

## IODOQUINOL

(eye-oh-do-kwin'ole)
Yodoxin
**Classification:** AMEBICIDE
Therapeutic: AMEBICIDE
**Prototype:** Emetine

**AVAILABILITY** Tablet

**ACTION & *THERAPEUTIC EFFECT***
Direct-acting (contact) amebicide. *Effective against both trophozoites and cyst forms of* Entamoeba histolytica *in intestinal lumen.*

**USES** Intestinal amebiasis and for asymptomatic passers of cysts. Commonly used either concurrently or in alternating courses with another intestinal amebicide.

**CONTRAINDICATIONS** Hypersensitivity to any 8-hydroxyquinoline or to iodine-containing preparations or foods; hepatic or renal damage; lactation.

**CAUTIOUS USE** Severe thyroid disease; minor self-limiting problems; prolonged high-dosage therapy; preexisting optic neuropathy; pregnancy (category C).

Common adverse effects in *italic;* life-threatening effects underlined; generic names in **bold;** classifications in SMALL CAPS; ♣ Canadian drug name; ⦿ Prototype drug

## ROUTE & DOSAGE

### Intestinal Amebiasis

*Adult:* **PO** 650 mg t.i.d. for 20 days (max: 2 g/day); may repeat after a 2–3 wk drug-free interval
*Child:* **PO** 30–40 mg/kg/day in 2–3 divided doses for 20 days (max: 1.95 g/day); may repeat after a 2–3 wk drug-free interval

## ADMINISTRATION

### Oral

- Give drug after meals. If patient has difficulty swallowing tablet, crush and mix with applesauce.

## ADVERSE EFFECTS (≥1%) **Body as a Whole:** Hypersensitivity (urticaria, pruritus). **CNS:** Headache, agitation, retrograde amnesia, vertigo, ataxia, peripheral neuropathy (especially in children); muscle pain, weakness usually below T12 vertebrae, dysesthesias especially of lower limbs, paresthesias, increased sense of warmth. **Special Senses:** Blurred vision, optic atrophy, optic neuritis, permanent loss of vision. **GI:** Nausea, vomiting, anorexia, abdominal cramps, diarrhea, constipation, rectal irritation and itching. **Skin:** Discoloration of hair and nails, acne, hair loss, urticaria, various forms of skin eruptions. **Hematologic:** Agranulocytosis (rare). **Endocrine:** Thyroid hypertrophy, iodism [generalized furunculosis (iodine toxiderma), skin eruptions, fever, chills, weakness].

## DIAGNOSTIC TEST INTERFERENCE

Iodoquinol can cause elevations of **PBI** and decrease of **I-131 uptake** (effects may last for several weeks to 6 mo even after discontinuation of therapy). **Ferric chloride test for PKU** (phenylketonuria) may yield false-positive results if iodoquinol is present in urine.

## PHARMACOKINETICS **Absorption:** Small amount from GI tract. **Elimination:** In feces.

## NURSING IMPLICATIONS

### Assessment & Drug Effects

- Monitor I&O ratio. Record characteristics of stools: Color, consistency, frequency, presence of blood, mucus, or other material.
- Note: Ophthalmologic examinations are recommended at regular intervals during prolonged therapy
- Monitor and report immediately the onset of blurred or decreased vision or eye pain. Also report symptoms of peripheral neuropathy: Pain, numbness, tingling, or weakness of extremities.

### Patient & Family Education

- Report any of the following: Skin rash, blurred vision, fever or other signs of infection.
- Complete full course of treatment. Stool needs to be examined again 1, 3, and 6 mo after termination of treatment.
- Note: Intestinal amebiasis is spread mainly by contaminated water, raw fruits or vegetables, flies, roaches, and hand-to-mouth transfer of infected feces. It is very important to wash hands after defecation and before eating.

## IPILIMUMAB

(ip'i-lim'ue-mab)

Yervoy

**Classifications:** MONOCLONAL ANTIBODY; ANTINEOPLASTIC
**Therapeutic:** ANTINEOPLASTIC

**AVAILABILITY** Solution for injection

Common adverse effects in *italic;* life-threatening effects underlined; generic names in **bold;** classifications in SMALL CAPS; ♦ Canadian drug name; ☻ Prototype drug

857

## ACTION & *THERAPEUTIC EFFECT*

A recombinant, human monoclonal antibody thought to augment T-cell activation and proliferation thus enhancing T-cell mediated antitumor immune responses. *Enhances the immune system's ability to seek out and destroy metastatic melanoma cells.*

## USES
Treatment of unresectable or metastatic malignant melanoma.

## CAUTIOUS USE
Immune-mediated hepatitis, dermatitis, neuropathies, endocrinopathies, nephritis, pneumonitis, meningitis, pericarditis, uveitis, iritis, and hemolytic anemia; pregnancy (category C); lactation. Safety and efficacy in children not established.

## ROUTE & DOSAGE

### Malignant Melanoma

*Adult:* IV 3 mg/kg q3wks for a total of 4 doses

### *Adverse Reaction Dosage Adjustment*

*Moderate immune-mediated adverse reaction or for symptomatic endocrinopathy:* Withhold dose
*If the adverse reaction completely or partial resolves (Grade 0–1) and if patient is receiving less than 7.5 mg prednisone or equivalent/ day:* Resume at 3 mg/kg q3wks until all 4 doses are given or 16 wks from first dose, whichever comes first.

*If treatment course not completed within 16 wk; or if moderate adverse reactions are persistent; or if corticosteroid dose cannot be reduced to 7.5 mg prednisone; or if severe or life-threatening adverse reactions occur:* Permanently discontinue ipilimumab

## ADMINISTRATION

### Intravenous

*PREPARE:* **IV Infusion:** Place vials at room temperature for 5 min. Do not shake. Withdraw required volume and add to an IV bag with enough NS or D5W to yield a final concentration of 1–2 mg/mL. Gently invert IV bag to mix.
*ADMINISTER:* **IV Infusion:** Give over 90 min through an IV line containing a low-protein-binding in-line filter. Flush line with NS or D5W after each dose.
*INCOMPATIBILITIES:* **Solution/additive:** Do not mix ipilimumab, or administer as an infusion with other drugs or compounds.

- Store at 2°–8°C (36°–46° F). Protect from light. May store diluted solution for up to 24 h under refrigeration or at 20°–25°C (68°–77°F). Discard partially used vials.

## ADVERSE EFFECTS (≥1%)
**Body as a Whole:** *Fatigue.* **Hepatic:** AST or ALT greater 5 × the ULN or total bilirubin greater than 3 × the ULN. **GI:** *Diarrhea;* enterocolitis; GI hemorrhage; GI perforation. **Skin:** *Pruritus, rash;* Stevens–Johnson syndrome, toxic epidermal necrolysis.

## PHARMACOKINETICS
**Half-Life:** 14.7 d.

## NURSING IMPLICATIONS

### Black Box Warning

*Ipilimumab has been associated with severe immune-mediated adverse reactions including enterocolitis, hepatitis, dermatitis, neuropathy, and endocrinopathy.*

### Assessment & Drug Effects

- Use the *Nursing Immune-Mediated Adverse Reaction Symptom Check-*

Common adverse effects in *italic*; life-threatening effects <u>underlined</u>; generic names in **bold**; classifications in SMALL CAPS; ✦ Canadian drug name; ❷ Prototype drug *list* (found on the product web site) to assess the patient.

- Monitor closely for and report immediately severe adverse reactions that may occur during or after (weeks to months) infusing. These include but are not limited to: Severe motor or sensory neuropathy; severe skin reactions; colitis with abdominal pain, fever, ileus, peritoneal signs, increased stool frequency (7 or more over baseline) or stool incontinence, need for intravenous hydration for more than 24 h, and GI hemorrhage.
- Report immediately ALT elevations of more than 5 × the ULN or total bilirubin elevations more than 3 × the ULN.
- Monitor lab tests: Baseline and before each dose: LFTs and thyroid function tests, periodic renal function tests.

### Patient & Family Education

- Read the *Medication Guide* for ipilimumab prior to each infusion.
- Report immediately to prescriber any adverse reaction experienced during or after (weeks to months) infusion.
- Women should inform prescriber if they become pregnant.

## IPRATROPIUM BROMIDE

(i-pra-troe′pee-um)

**Atrovent, Atrovent HFA**

**Classifications:** ANTICHOLINERGIC; ANTIMUSCARINIC; BRONCHODILATOR
**Therapeutic:** BRONCHODILATOR
**Prototype:** Atropine

**AVAILABILITY** Solution for inhalation; inhaler; nasal spray

**ACTION & *THERAPEUTIC EFFECT***
Results in bronchodilation by inhibiting acetylcholine at its receptor sites, thereby blocking cholinergic bronchomotor tone (bronchoconstriction); also abolishes vagally mediated reflex bronchospasm triggered by such nonspecific agents as cigarette smoke, inert dusts, cold air, and a range of inflammatory mediators (e.g., histamine). *Produces local, site-specific effects on the larger central airways including bronchodilation and prevention of bronchospasms.*

**USES** Maintenance therapy in COPD including chronic bronchitis and emphysema; nasal spray for perennial rhinitis and symptomatic relief of rhinorrhea associated with the common cold.

**UNLABELED USES** Perennial nonallergic rhinitis.

**CONTRAINDICATIONS** Hypersensitivity to atropine, bromides, peanut oils, soy lecithin; paradoxical bronchospasm.

**CAUTIOUS USE** Narrow-angle glaucoma; BPH; bladder neck obstruction; pregnancy (category B), lactation; children.

## ROUTE & DOSAGE

### COPD

*Adult:* **Inhalation** 2 inhalations of MDI t.i.d. to q.i.d. not more often than q4h (max: 12 inhalations in 24 h) **Nebulizer** 500 mcg (1 unit dose vial) q6–8h

### Rhinitis

*Adult/Adolescent/Child (6 y or older):* **Intranasal**
2 sprays of 0.03% each nostril b.i.d. or t.i.d.

Common adverse effects in *italic;* life-threatening effects underlined; generic names in **bold;** classifications in SMALL CAPS; ◆ Canadian drug name; ⊘ Prototype drug

859

## ADMINISTRATION

### Intranasal/Inhalation/Nebulizer

- Demonstrate aerosol use and check return demonstration.
- Wait 3 min between inhalations if more than one inhalation/dose is ordered.
- Avoid contact with eyes.
- Instruct patient to rinse mouth with water to minimize dry mouth.

## ADVERSE EFFECTS (≥1%) **Special Senses:** Blurred vision (especially if sprayed into eye), difficulty in accommodation, acute eye pain, worsening of narrow-angle glaucoma. **GI:** Bitter taste, dry oropharyngeal membranes. With higher doses: Nausea, constipation. **Respiratory:** *Cough,* bronchitis, dyspnea, hoarseness, exacerbation of symptoms, drying of bronchial secretions, mucosal ulcers, epistaxis, nasal dryness, sinusitis. **Skin:** Rash, hives. **Urogenital:** Urinary retention. **CNS:** Headache, dizziness.

## PHARMACOKINETICS **Absorption:** 10% of inhaled dose reaches lower airway; approximately 0.5% of dose is systemically absorbed. **Peak:** 1.5–2 h. **Duration:** 4–6 h. **Elimination:** 48% of dose excreted in feces; less than 5% excreted in urine. **Half-Life:** 1.5–2 h.

## NURSING IMPLICATIONS

### Assessment & Drug Effects

- Monitor respiratory status; auscultate lungs before and after inhalation.
- Report treatment failure (exacerbation of respiratory symptoms) to prescriber.

### Patient & Family Education

- Note: This medication is not an emergency agent because of its delayed onset and the time required to reach peak bronchodilation.

- Review patient information sheet on proper use of nasal spray.
- Allow 30–60 sec between puffs for optimum results. Do not let medication contact your eyes.
- Wait 5 min between this and other inhaled medications. Check with prescriber about sequence of administration.
- Take medication only as directed, noting some leniency in number of puffs within 24 h. Supervise child's administration until certain all of dose is being administered.
- Rinse mouth after medication puffs to reduce bitter taste.
- Discuss changes in normal urinary pattern with the prescriber (more common in older adults).
- Call prescriber if you note changes in sputum color or amount, ankle edema, or significant weight gain.

# IRBESARTAN

(ir-be-sar′tan)

Avapro

**Classifications:** ANGIOTENSIN II RECEPTOR ANTAGONIST; ANTIHYPERTENSIVE

Therapeutic: ANTIHYPERTENSIVE
**Prototype:** Losartan

## AVAILABILITY Tablet

## ACTION & *THERAPEUTIC EFFECT*

Irbesartan is an angiotensin II receptor (type $AT_1$) antagonist. Irbesartan selectively blocks the binding of angiotensin II to the $AT_1$ receptors found in many tissues (e.g., vascular smooth muscle, adrenal glands), resulting in vasodilation of vascular smooth muscle. *This blocks vasoconstricting and aldosterone-secreting effects of angiotensin II, thus resulting in an antihypertensive effect.*

## USES Hypertension, treatment of diabetic nephropathy in patients with hypertension and type 2 diabetes.

**UNLABELED USES** CHF.

**CONTRAINDICATIONS** Hypersensitivity to irbesartan, losartan, or valsartan; hypovolemia; pregnancy (category D second and third trimester); lactation.

**CAUTIOUS USE** Arterial stenosis of the renal artery, hepatic disease; severe CHF, African American patients; pregnancy (category C first trimester). Safe use in children not established.

## ROUTE & DOSAGE

**Hypertension**
*Adult:* **PO** Start with 150 mg once daily, may increase to 300 mg/day

## ADMINISTRATION

**Oral**
- Correct volume depletion prior to initiation of therapy to prevent hypotension. Titrate daily dose up to 300 mg; larger doses, however, are not likely to provide additional benefit.
- Give without regard to food.
- Store at 15°–30° C (59°–86° F).

**ADVERSE EFFECTS** (≥1%) **Body as a Whole:** Edema, fatigue, pain. **CNS:** Dizziness, headache, anxiety, nervousness. **CV:** Tachycardia, chest pain. **GI:** Diarrhea, dyspepsia, nausea, vomiting, abdominal pain. **Respiratory:** Upper respiratory infection, cough, sinus disorder, pharyngitis, rhinitis. **Skin:** Rash. **Other:** UTI, hepatitis.

**PHARMACOKINETICS Absorption:** Rapidly absorbed from GI tract, 60–80% bioavailability. **Distribution:** 90% protein bound. **Metabolism:** In the liver primarily by CYP2C9. **Elimination:** Primarily in feces. **Half-Life:** 11–15 h.

## NURSING IMPLICATIONS

### Black Box Warning

*Irbesartan has been associated with fetal injury and death.*

**Assessment & Drug Effects**
- Monitor for therapeutic effectiveness: Maximum pressure-lowering effect may not be evident for 6–12 wk; indicated by decreases in systolic and diastolic BP.
- Monitor BP periodically; trough readings, just prior to the next scheduled dose, should be made when possible.
- Monitor lab tests: Periodic BUN and creatinine, serum potassium, and CBC with differential.

**Patient & Family Education**
- Inform prescriber immediately if you become pregnant.
- Notify prescriber of episodes of dizziness, especially when making position changes.

## IRINOTECAN HYDROCHLORIDE

(eye ri-no'te can)

Camptosar

**Classifications:** ANTINEOPLASTIC; CAMPTOTHECIN ANALOG
**Therapeutic:** ANTINEOPLASTIC
**Prototype:** Topotecan

**AVAILABILITY** Solution for injection

## ACTION & *THERAPEUTIC EFFECT*

Antitumor activity due to inhibition of the intranuclear enzyme topoisomerase I (DNA-gyrase). By inhibiting topoisomerase I, irinotecan and its active metabolite, SN-38, cause double-stranded DNA damage during the synthesis (S) phase of DNA synthesis. *Irinotecan inhibits both DNA and RNA synthesis.*

Common adverse effects in *italic*; life-threatening effects underlined; generic names in **bold**; classifications in SMALL CAPS; ♣ Canadian drug name; ● Prototype drug

861

**USES** Metastatic carcinoma of colon or rectum.

**UNLABELED USES** Gastric cancer, malignant glioma, non-small cell lung cancer, pancreatic cancer.

**CONTRAINDICATIONS** Previous hypersensitivity to irinotecan, topotecan, or other camptothecin analogs; hereditary fructose intolerance; interstitial pulmonary disease; previous pelvic/abdominal radiation recipients; acute infection, severe diarrhea, bowel obstruction; pregnancy (category D); lactation.

**CAUTIOUS USE** Gastrointestinal disorders, myelosuppression, renal or hepatic impairment, history of bleeding disorders, previous cytotoxic or radiation therapy; older adults. Safe use in children not established.

## ROUTE & DOSAGE

### Metastatic Carcinoma

*Adult:* IV 125 mg/m² once weekly for 4 wk, then a 2-wk rest period (future courses may be adjusted to range from 50 to 150 mg/m² depending on tolerance; see complete prescribing information for specific dosage adjustment recommendations based on toxic effects)

### Pharmacogenetic Dosage Adjustment

Patients with UGT1A1*28 allele have increased risk of side effects, start with decreased dose

## ADMINISTRATION

### Intravenous

Administer only after premedication (at least 30 min prior) with an antiemetic.

• Wash immediately with soap and water if skin contacts drug during preparation.

*PREPARE:* **IV Infusion:** Dilute the ordered dose in enough D5W (preferred) or NS to yield a concentration of 0.12–2.8 mg/mL. • Typical amount of diluent used is 250–500 mL.

*ADMINISTER:* **IV Infusion:** Infuse over 90 min. • Closely monitor IV site; if extravasation occurs, immediately flush with sterile water and apply ice.

*INCOMPATIBILITIES:* **Y-site:** Acyclover, allopurinol, amphotericin B, cefepime, cefotaxime, ceftriaxone, chloramphenicol, chlorpromazine, dantrolene, dexmedetomidine, diazepam, droperidol, fluorouracil, fosphenytoin, furosemide, ganciclovir, gemcitabine, glycopyrrolate, methothexital, methylprenisolone, mitomycin, nafcillin, nitroprusside, premetrexed, phenytoin, piperacillin/tazobactam, trastuzumab.

• Store undiluted at 15°–30° C (59°–86° F) and protect from light. Use reconstituted solutions within 24 h.

**ADVERSE EFFECTS** (≥1%) **Body as a Whole:** *Asthenia, fever, pain,* chills, edema, abdominal enlargement, back pain. **CNS:** Headache, *insomnia, dizziness.* **CV:** Vasodilation/flushing. **GI:** *Diarrhea (early and late onset), dehydration, nausea, vomiting, anorexia, weight loss, constipation, abdominal cramping and pain,* flatulence, stomatitis, dyspepsia, increased alkaline phosphatase and AST. **Hematologic:** Leukopenia, neutropenia, *anemia.* **Respiratory:** *Dyspnea,* cough, rhinitis. **Skin:** *Alopecia,* sweating, rash.

Common adverse effects in *italic;* life-threatening effects underlined; generic names in **bold;** classifications in SMALL CAPS; ♣ Canadian drug name; ⊙ Prototype drug

**INTERACTIONS Drug:** ANTICOAGU-
LANTS, ANTIPLATELET AGENTS, NSAIDS
may increase risk of bleeding; **carbamazepine, phenytoin, phenobarbital** may decrease irinotecan levels. **Herbal: St. John's wort**
may decrease irinotecan levels.

**PHARMACOKINETICS Peak:** 1 h.
**Distribution:** Irinotecan is 30%
protein bound; active metabolite
SN-38 is 95% protein bound.
**Metabolism:** In liver by carboxy-
lesterase enzyme to active metabolite SN-38. **Elimination:** 10 h for SN-
38; 20% excreted in urine. **Half-Life:**
10–20 h.

**NURSING IMPLICATIONS**

**Black Box Warning**

*Irinotecan has been associated
with severe, potentially life-threatening diarrhea that may occur
during or shortly after infusion, or
more than 24 h after infusion.*

**Assessment & Drug Effects**
▪ Monitor closely for fluid and electrolyte imbalance. If severe diarrhea occurs during infusion, stop
infusion and notify prescriber.
▪ Monitor for acute GI distress, especially early diarrhea (within
24 h of infusion), which may be
preceded by diaphoresis and
cramping, and late diarrhea (more
than 24 h after infusion).
▪ Monitor lab tests. Prior to each
dose, WBC with differential, Hgb,
platelet count, and serum electrolytes especially during periods of
diarrhea.

**Patient & Family Education**
▪ Learn about common adverse effects and measures to control or
minimize when possible.

▪ Notify prescriber immediately
when you experience diarrhea,
vomiting, and S&S of infection.
Diarrhea requires prompt treatment to prevent serious fluid and
electrolyte imbalances.

# IRON DEXTRAN
(i'ern dek'stran)

DexFerrum, INFeD,
Proferdex

**Classifications:** BLOOD FORMER,
IRON SUPPLEMENT; ANTIANEMIC
**Therapeutic:** ANTIANEMIC; IRON
SUPPLEMENT
**Prototype:** Ferrous sulfate

**AVAILABILITY** Solution for injection

**ACTION & *THERAPEUTIC EFFECT***
A complex of ferric hydroxide
with dextran in solution for injection. Reticuloendothelial cells
of liver, spleen, and bone marrow dissociate iron (ferric ion)
from iron dextran complex. The
released ferric ion combines with
transferrin and is transported to
bone marrow where it is incorporated into hemoglobin. *Effective in replacement of iron needed
in iron deficiency anemia, thus
replenishing hemoglobin and depleted iron stores.*

**USES** Only in patients with clearly
established iron deficiency anemia
when oral administration of iron is
unsatisfactory or impossible.

**CONTRAINDICATIONS** Hypersensitivity to the product; all anemias
except iron-deficiency anemia; acute
phase of infectious renal disease.

**CAUTIOUS USE** Rheumatoid
arthritis, ankylosing spondylitis; renal
disease; SLE; impaired hepatic function; cardiac disease; history of aller-

gies or asthma; pregnancy (category C); lactation. Use not recommended in infants younger than 4 mo old.

## ROUTE & DOSAGE

### Iron Deficiency

*Adult:* **IM/IV** Dose is individualized and determined based on patient's weight and hemoglobin (see package insert); do not administer more than 100 mg (2 mL) of iron dextran within 24 h

*Child (weight less than 5 kg):* **IM/IV** No more than 0.5 mL (25 mg)/day; *weight 5–10 kg:* No more than 1 mL (50 mg)/day; *weight greater than 10 kg:* No more than 2 mL (100 mg)/day

## ADMINISTRATION

*Dexferrum* should be administered IV only; *INFeD* may be administered IV or IM.

### Test Dose

- Prior to the first *INFeD* IM dose, administer an IM test dose of 0.5 mL.
- Prior to the first IV dose, administer a 0.5 mL test dose at a gradual rate over at least 30 seconds (**INFeD**) or over at least 5 min (**Dexferrum**).
- Note: Although anaphylactic reactions (see Appendix F) usually occur within a few minutes after injection, it is recommended that 1 h or more elapse before remainder of initial dose is given following test dose.

### Intramuscular

- Give injection only into the muscle mass in upper outer quadrant of buttock (never in the upper arm). In small child, use the lateral thigh. Use a 2- or 3-inch, 19- or 20-gauge needle. The Z-track

technique is recommended. Use one needle to withdraw drug from container and another needle for injection.

- Note: If patient is receiving IM in standing position, patient should be bearing weight on the leg opposite the injection site; if in bed, patient should be in the lateral position with injection site uppermost.

### Intravenous

*PREPARE:* **Direct:** Give undiluted. **IV Infusion:** Dilute in 250–1000 mL of NS.

*ADMINISTER:* **Direct** *Test Dose:* A test dose is given before the first IV therapeutic dose. *DexFerrum:* Give test dose of 25 mg (0.5 mL) slowly over 5 min. *INFeD:* Give test dose over 30 sec. Wait 1–2 h and if no adverse reaction occurs, give the remainder of the first dose by IV infusion. **IV Infusion:** Infuse at a rate not to exceed 50 mg (1 mL) or fraction thereof over 60 sec. Avoid rapid infusion.

*INCOMPATIBILITIES:* **Solution/additive: TPN.**

- After infusion is completed, flush vein with 10 mL of NS.
- Have patient remain in bed for at least 30 min after IV administration to prevent orthostatic hypotension. Monitor BP and pulse.

- Store below 30° C (86° F) unless otherwise directed.

## ADVERSE EFFECTS (≥1%) **Body as a Whole:** Hypersensitivity (urticaria, skin rash, allergic purpura, pruritus, fever, chills, dyspnea, arthralgia, myalgia; anaphylaxis). **CNS:** Headache, shivering, transient paresthesias, syncope, dizziness, coma, seizures. **CV:** *Peripheral vascular flushing (rapid IV), hypotension,* precordial pain or pressure sensation,

tachycardia, <u>fatal cardiac arrhythmias,</u> <u>circulatory collapse.</u> **GI:** Nausea, vomiting, transient loss of taste perception, metallic taste, diarrhea, melena, abdominal pain, hemorrhagic gastritis, intestinal necrosis, hepatic damage. **Skin:** Sterile abscess and brown skin discoloration (IM site), local phlebitis (IV site), lymphadenopathy, *pain at IM injection site.* **Metabolic:** Hemosiderosis, metabolic acidosis, hyperglycemia, reactivation of quiescent rheumatoid arthritis, exogenous hemosiderosis. **Hematologic:** Bleeding disorder with severe toxicity.

## DIAGNOSTIC TEST INTERFERENCE

Falsely elevated *serum bilirubin* and falsely decreased *serum calcium* values may occur. Large doses of iron dextran may impart a brown color to serum drawn 4 h after iron administration. *Bone scans* involving Tc-99m diphosphonate have shown dense areas of activity along contour of iliac crest 1–6 days after IM injections of iron dextran.

## INTERACTIONS

May decrease absorption of oral **iron, chloramphenicol** may decrease effectiveness of iron, a toxic complex may form with **dimercaprol.**

## PHARMACOKINETICS

**Absorption:** 60% from IM site by 3 days; 90% absorbed by 1–3 wk. **Distribution:** Crosses placenta; distributed into breast milk. **Metabolism:** In reticuloendothelial system. **Half-Life:** 6 h.

## NURSING IMPLICATIONS

### Black Box Warning

*Iron dextran has been associated with anaphylactic-type reactions.*

### Assessment & Drug Effects

- Monitor closely for hypersensitivity-type reaction. Report immediately

urticaria, rash, pruitus, chills, dyspnea or other S&S of hypersensitivity.
- Systemic reactions may occur over 24 h after parenteral iron has been administered. Large IV doses are associated with increased frequency of adverse effects.
- Monitor lab tests: Periodic Hgb, Hct, and reticulocyte count.

### Patient & Family Education

- Do not take oral iron preparations when receiving iron injections.
- Eat foods high in iron and vitamin C.
- Notify prescriber of any of the following: Backache or muscle ache, chills, dizziness, fever, headache, nausea or vomiting, paresthesias, pain or redness at injection site, skin rash or hives, or difficulty breathing.

# IRON SUCROSE

(i'ron su'crose)

**Venofer, Velphoro**

**Classifications:** BLOOD FORMER; IRON REPLACEMENT; ANTIANEMIC

**Therapeutic:** ANTIANEMIC; IRON DEFICIENCY REPLACEMENT

**Prototype:** Ferrous sulfate

## AVAILABILITY

Solution for injection; chewable tablet

## ACTION & THERAPEUTIC EFFECT

A complex of iron (ferric) (III) hydroxide in sucrose. It is dissociated by the reticuloendothelial system (RES) into iron and sucrose. Normal erythropoiesis depends on the concentration of iron and erythropoietin available in the plasma; both are decreased in renal failure. *Increases serum iron level in chronic renal failure patients, and results in increased hemoglobin level.*

## USES

Treatment of iron deficiency anemia, hyperphosphatemia

Common adverse effects in *italic;* life-threatening effects <u>underlined</u>; generic names in **bold;** classifications in SMALL CAPS; ♣ Canadian drug name; ● Prototype drug

865

**CONTRAINDICATIONS** Patients with iron overload, hypersensitivity to Venofer, or for anemia not caused by iron deficiency; hemochromatosis.

**CAUTIOUS USE** Patients with a history of hypotension; older adults, decreased renal, hepatic, or cardiac function; pregnancy (category B); lactation. Safety and efficacy in children or infants not established.

## ROUTE & DOSAGE

**Iron Deficiency Anemia**

*Adult:* **IV Hemodialysis dependent (HDD-CKD):** 100 mg elemental iron given at least 15 min/hemodialysis session (cumulative dose: 1000 mg); **Non-hemodialysis dependent (NDD-CKD):** 200 mg elemental iron on 5 different occasions within the 14-day period; **Peritoneal dialysis dependent (PDD-CKD):** 300 mg on days 1 and 15, then 400 mg 14 days later

**Hyperphosphatemia**

*Adult:* **PO** 500 mg t.i.d.

## ADMINISTRATION

**Intravenous**

*PREPARE:* **Direct/Infusion: HDD-CKD:** Give direct IV undiluted or diluted immediately prior to infusion in a maxiumum of 100 mL NS. **■NDD-CKD:** Give direct IV undiluted. **■ PDD-CKD:** Dilute 300–400 mg in a maximum of 250 mL of NS for infusion.

*ADMINISTER:* **Direct:** Give the undiluted solution slowly by direct IV over 2–5 min. **IV Infusion ■**Infusion diluted solution for **HDD-CKD patient** over at least 15 min and for **PDD-CKD patient** over 90 min. ■Avoid rapid infusion.

*INCOMPATIBILITIES:* **Solution/additive:** Do not mix with other medications or parenteral nutrition solutions.

■ Store unopened vials preferably at 25° C (77° F), but room temperature permitted. Discard unused portion in opened vial.

**ADVERSE EFFECTS** (≥1%) **Body as a Whole:** Fever, pain, asthenia, malaise, <u>anaphylactoid reactions</u>. **Cardiovascular:** *Hypotension,* chest pain, hypertension, hypervolemia. **GI:** Nausea, vomiting, diarrhea, stool discoloration, abdominal pain, elevated liver function tests. **Musculoskeletal:** *Leg cramps,* muscle pain. **CNS:** Headache, dizziness. **Respiratory:** Dyspnea, pneumonia, cough, URI. **Skin:** Pruritus, injection site reaction.

**INTERACTIONS Drug:** May reduce absorption of ORAL IRON PREPARATIONS. May decrease absorption of **levothyroxine**.

**PHARMACOKINETICS Peak:** 4 wk. **Distribution:** Primarily to blood with some distribution to liver, spleen, bone marrow. **Metabolism:** Dissociated to iron and sucrose in reticuloendothelial system. **Elimination:** Sucrose is eliminated in urine, 5% of iron excreted in urine. **Half-Life:** 6 h.

## NURSING IMPLICATIONS

**Assessment & Drug Effects**

■ Withhold drug and notify prescriber when serum ferritin level equals or exceeds established guidelines.

■ Stop infusion and notify prescriber for S&S overdosage or infusing too rapidly: Hypotension, edema; headache, dizziness, nausea, vomiting, abdominal pain, joint or muscle pain, and paresthesia.

■ Monitor patient carefully during the first 30 min after initiation of IV

therapy for signs of hypersensitivity and anaphylactoid reaction (see Appendix F).
- Monitor lab tests: Periodic serum ferritin, transferrin saturation, Hct, and Hgb.

**Patient & Family Education**
- Report any of the following promptly: Itching, rash, chest pain, headache, dizziness, nausea, vomiting, abdominal pain, joint or muscle pain, and numbness and tingling.

## ISAVUCONAZONIUM SULFATE
(i-sa-vu-con'a-zo-ni-um)
Cresemba
**Classifications:** AZOLE ANTIFUNGAL
Therapeutic: ANTIFUNGAL
**Prototype:** Fluconazole

**AVAILABILITY** Capsules; solution for injection

**ACTION & THERAPEUTIC EFFECT**
Inhibits the synthesis of ergosterol, a key component of the fungal cell membrane, through the inhibition of a cytochrome P-450 dependent enzyme (lanosterol 14-alpha-demethylase). *Depletion of ergosterol within the fungal cell membrane weakens the membrane structure and impairs its function, inhibiting fungal growth.*

**USES** Treatment of invasive aspergillosis and invasive mucormycosis in patients 18 y or older.

**UNLABELED USES** Treatment of esophageal candidiasis.

**CONTRAINDICATIONS** Known hypersensitivity to isavuconazole; coadministration of strong CYP3A4 inhibitors; coadministration with strong CYP3A4 inhibitors (e.g., ketoconazole or high-dose ritonavir);

coadministration with strong CYP3A4 inducers (e.g., rifampin, carbamazepine, St. John's wort, or long acting barbiturates); patients with familial short QT syndrome; lactation.

**CAUTIOUS USE** Severe hepatic impairment; infusion-related reactions; concurrent immunosuppressants; concurrent drugs with narrow therapeutic window that are P-gp substrates (e.g., digoxin); pregnancy. Safety and efficacy in patients younger than 18 y not established.

## ROUTE & DOSAGE

**Invasive Aspergillosis or Mumormycosis**
*Adult:* **PO/IV** Loading dose of 372 mg q8h for 6 doses; then 372 mg; **PO** once daily

## ADMINISTRATION
**Oral**
- May be given without regard to food.
- Capsules must be swallowed whole; do not crush, dissolve, or open.
- Store at 15°–30° C (59°–86°F).

**Intravenous**

*PREPARE:* **IV Infusion:** Reconstitute by adding 5 mL of SW to vial to yield 1.5 mg/mL; shake gently to dissolve. Remove solution from vial and add to 250 mL of NS or D5W. Mix gently and do not shake bag.
*ADMINISTER:* **IV Infusion:** Infuse over at least 1 h using an infusion set with an in-line filter (pore size 0.2 to 1.2 micron).
*INCOMPATIBILITIES:* **Solution/additive:** Do not mix with any other medication. Should only be administered with NS or D5W.

Common adverse effects in *italic;* life-threatening effects underlined; generic names in **bold;** classifications in SMALL CAPS; ♣ Canadian drug name; ⊙ Prototype drug

867

- Storage: Reconstituted solution may be stored below 25° C (77° F) for maximum 1 h prior to preparation of infusion solution. Infusion should be completed within 6 h of dilution at room temperature. If this is not possible, immediately refrigerate at 2°–8° C (36°–46°F) the infusion solution after dilution and complete the infusion within 24 h.

## ADVERSE EFFECTS (≥1%) Body as a Whole:
Chest pain, chills, decreased appetite, fatigue, hypersensitivity, injection site reactions, malaise, *peripheral edema*. **CNS:** Anxiety, confusion, convulsion, depression, dysgeusia, encephalopathy, hallucination, *headache*, hypoesthesia, insomnia, migraine, peripheral neuropathy, paraesthesia, somnolence, stupor, syncope, tremor delirium. **CV:** Atrial fibrillation, atrial flutter, bradycardia, cardiac arrest, hypotension, palpitations, reduced QT interval, supraventricular extrasystoles, supraventricular tachycardia, thrombophlebitis, ventricular extrasystoles. **GI:** Abdominal distension, abdominal pain, *constipation*, *diarrhea*, dyspepsia, gastritis, gingivitis, *nausea*, stomatitis, *vomiting*. **Hematological:** Agranulocytosis, leukopenia, pancytopenia. **Metabolic:** Hypoalbuminemia, hypoglycemia, *hypokalemia*, hypomagnesemia, hyponatremia, increased ALT/AST, increased blood alkaline phosphatase, increased blood bilirubin, increased gamma-glutamyltransferase. **Musculoskeletal:** *Back pain*, bone pain, neck pain. **Respiratory:** Acute respiratory failure, bronchospasm, *cough*, *dyspnea*, tachypnea. **Skin:** Alopecia, dermatitis, exfoliative dermatitis, erythema, petechiae, pruritus, rash, urticaria. **Special Senses:** Optic neuropathy, tinnitus, vertigo. **Urogenital:** Hematuria, proteinuria, renal failure.

## INTERACTIONS Drug:
Co-administration with CYP3A4 inhibitors (e.g., **ketoconazole, lopinavir, ritonavir**) increases the levels of isavuconazole. Co-administration with CYP3A4 inducers (e.g., **rifampin**) decreases the levels of isavuconazole. Isavuconazole decreases the levels of **bupropion,** and **lopinavir/ritonavir,** and increases the levels of **atorvastatin, cyclosporine, digoxin, midazolam, mycophenolate mofetil, sirolimus,** and **tacrolimus.**

## PHARMACOKINETICS Absorption:
98% bioavailable. **Peak:** 2–3 h. **Distribution:** Greater than 99% plasma protein bound. **Metabolism:** In liver after conversion to isavuconazole (active drug). **Elimination:** Renal (45.5%) and fecal (46.1%) **Half-Life:** 130 h.

## NURSING IMPLICATIONS

### Assessment & Drug Effects
- Monitor baseline ECG and frequently monitor BP during IV infusion.
- Monitor closely for infusion-related reactions (e.g., hypotension, dyspnea, chills, dizziness, paresthesia) or hypersensitivity reactions (e.g., severe skin reactions, Stevens–Johnson syndrome). Discontinue the infusion and notify prescriber if these reactions occur.
- Monitor lab tests: Baseline and periodic LFTs; serum electrolytes as indicated.

### Patient & Family Education
- Report immediately if experiencing any of the following during IV infusion: Difficulty breathing, chills, dizziness, numbness and tingling, changes in sense of touch, skin rash.
- Report to prescriber if signs of liver injury develop (e.g., itchy skin,

Common adverse effects in *italic;* life-threatening effects underlined; generic names in **bold;** classifications in SMALL CAPS; ♣ Canadian drug name; ⊘ Prototype drug

nausea or vomiting, yellowing of eyes, extreme fatigue, flu-like symptoms).
- Women who are or plan to become pregnant should consult prescriber regarding potential risks to fetus.
- Use effective means of contraception while taking this drug.
- Do not breast-feed while taking this drug.

## ISOCARBOXAZID

(eye-soe-kar-box'a-zid)

Marplan

**Classifications:** ANTIDEPRESSANT; MONOAMINE OXIDASE INHIBITOR (MAOI)

Therapeutic: ANTIDEPRESSANT

**Prototype:** Phenelzine

## AVAILABILITY Tablet

## ACTION & *THERAPEUTIC EFFECT*

Inhibits monoamine oxidase, the enzyme involved in the catabolism of catecholamine neurotransmitters and serotonin. *Effectiveness as an antidepressant is due to its inhibition of MAO.*

## USES Symptomatic treatment of depressed patients refractory to or intolerant of TCAs or electroconvulsive therapy.

## CONTRAINDICATIONS Hypersensitivity to MAO inhibitors; pheochromocytoma; children (younger than 16 y); older adults (over 60 y) or debilitated patients; cardiac arrhythmias, hypertension, CVA; severe renal or hepatic impairment; history of headache; increased intracranial pressure, surgery; stroke, head trauma; suicidal ideation; lactation.

## CAUTIOUS USE Hyperthyroidism, parkinsonism, epilepsy, schizophrenia; bipolar disorder; psychosis;

suicidal risks; dental work; pregnancy (category C). Safety and efficacy in children not established.

## ROUTE & DOSAGE

**Refractory Depression**
*Adult:* **PO** 10–30 mg/day in 1–3 divided doses (max: 30 mg/day)

## ADMINISTRATION

### Oral
- Note: Dosage is individualized on the basis of patient response. Lowest effective dosage should be used.
- Store in a tight, light-resistant container.

## ADVERSE EFFECTS (≥1%) CNS:
Dizziness, light-headedness, tiredness, weakness, *drowsiness,* vertigo, headache, *overactivity,* hyperreflexia, muscle twitching, tremors, mania hypomania, *insomnia,* confusion, memory impairment. **CV:** *Orthostatic hypotension,* paradoxical hypertension, palpitation, tachycardia, other arrhythmias. **Special Senses:** *Blurred vision,* nystagmus, glaucoma. **GI:** Increased appetite, weight gain, *nausea,* diarrhea, *constipation, anorexia,* black tongue, *dry mouth,* abdominal pain. **Urogenital:** Dysuria, *urinary retention,* incontinence, sexual disturbances. **Body as a Whole:** Peripheral edema, excessive sweating, chills, skin rash, hepatitis, jaundice.

## INTERACTIONS Drug: TRICYCLIC ANTIDEPRESSANTS, **fluoxetine,** AMPHETAMINES, **ephedrine, reserpine, guanethidine, buspirone, methyldopa, dopamine, levodopa, tryptophan** may precipitate hypertensive crisis, headache, or hyperexcitability; **alcohol** and other CNS DEPRESSANTS compound CNS depressant

Common adverse effects in *italic;* life-threatening effects <u>underlined</u>; generic names in **bold;** classifications in SMALL CAPS; ♣ Canadian drug name; ⊘ Prototype drug

869

effects; **meperidine** can cause fatal cardiovascular collapse; ANESTHETICS exaggerate hypotensive and CNS depressant effects; **metrizamide** increases risk of seizures; compounds hypotensive effects of DIURETICS and other ANTIHYPERTENSIVE AGENTS. **Food:** All **tyramine**-containing foods (aged cheeses, processed cheeses, sour cream, wine, champagne, beer, pickled herring, anchovies, caviar, shrimp, liver, dry sausage, figs, raisins, overripe bananas or avocados, chocolate, soy sauce, bean curd, yeast extracts, yogurt, papaya products, meat tenderizers, broad beans) may precipitate hypertensive crisis. **Herbal: Ginseng, ephedra, ma huang, St. John's wort** may precipitate hypertensive crisis.

## PHARMACOKINETICS Duration:
Up to 2 wk. **Metabolism:** In liver.

## NURSING IMPLICATIONS

### Black Box Warning

*Isocarboxazid has been associated with suicidal thinking and behavior in children, adolescents, and young adults.*

### Assessment & Drug Effects

- Monitor for and report promptly signs of clinical deterioration or suicidal ideation. Children, adolescents and young adults are at particular risk.
- Monitor for therapeutic effectiveness: May be apparent within 1 wk or less, but in some patients there may be a time lag of 3–4 wk before improvement occurs.
- Monitor BP. Monitor for orthostatic hypotension by evaluating BP with patient recumbent and standing.

- Check for peripheral edema daily and monitor weight several times weekly.
- Note: Toxic symptoms from overdosage or from ingestion of contraindicated substances (e.g., foods high in tyramine) may occur within hours.
- Monitor I&O and bowel elimination patterns.

### Patient & Family Education

- Monitor closely behavior of children, adolescents and young adults; report immediately unusual changes in behavior or suicidal ideation.
- Make position changes slowly and in stages; lie down or sit down if faintness occurs.
- Use caution when performing potentially hazardous activities.
- Consult prescriber before self-medicating with OTC agents (e.g., cough, cold, hay fever, or diet medications).
- Avoid alcohol and excessive caffeine-containing beverages and tryptophan and tyramine-containing foods including cheeses, yeast, meat extracts, smoked or pickled meat, poultry, or fish, fermented sausages, and overripe fruit.

## ISOMETHEPTENE/
## DICHLORALPHENAZONE/
## ACETAMINOPHEN

(i-so-meth'ep-tene/di-chlor-al-phen'a-zone/a-cet'a-min-o-phen)

Duradrin, Nodolor, Migragesic IDA

**Classifications:** SYMPATHOMIMETIC; NONNARCOTIC ANALGESIC
**Therapeutic:** ANTIMIGRAINE; NONNARCOTIC ANALGESIC
**Controlled Substance:** Schedule C-IV

Common adverse effects in *italic;* life-threatening effects <u>underlined</u>; generic names in **bold;** classifications in SMALL CAPS; ♣ Canadian drug name; ⊕ Prototype drug

**AVAILABILITY** Capsule

**ACTION & *THERAPEUTIC EFFECT***
Isometheptene is a sympathomimetic amine that acts by constricting cranial and cerebral arterioles. Isometheptene relieves vascular headaches. Dichloralphenazone is a mild sedative that helps reduce headache pain. Acetaminophen is a mild analgesic. *Effective as a mild sedative, reduces headache pain as well as being a mild analgesic.*

**USES** Relief for tension, vascular, and migraine headaches.

**CONTRAINDICATIONS** Patients with glaucoma; severe renal disease; organic heart disease; hepatic disease; concurrent MAO inhibitors.

**CAUTIOUS USE** Hypertension; peripheral vascular disease, and recent cardiovascular attacks; older adults; pulmonary disease; pregnancy (category C); lactation; children.

**ROUTE & DOSAGE**

**Tension Headache**
*Adult:* **PO** 1–2 capsules q4h up to 8 capsules/24 h
**Migraine Headache**
*Adult:* **PO** 2 capsules at onset, then 1 capsule qh until relief (max: 5 capsules/12 h)

**ADMINISTRATION**
**Oral**
- Do not give this drug to anyone who is concurrently using an MAOI. Allow 14 days to elapse between discontinuation of the MAOI and administration of this drug.
- Do not give more than 8 capsules in a 24 h period.

- Store at 15°–30° C (59°–86° F) in a dry place.

**ADVERSE EFFECTS** (≥1%) **CNS:** Transient dizziness. **GI:** Acetaminophen hepatotoxicity. **Skin:** Rash.

**INTERACTIONS Drug:** MAOIS may cause hypertensive crisis; other **acetaminophen**-containing drugs (including OTC) may increase risk of hepatotoxicity.

**PHARMACOKINETICS Absorption:** Rapidly absorbed. **Metabolism:** Dichloralphenazone is metabolized to an antipyrine. See ACETAMINOPHEN and for more detail. **Elimination:** Renal and hepatic. **Half-Life:** 12 h.

**NURSING IMPLICATIONS**
**Assessment & Drug Effects**
- Monitor BP closely with preexisting hypertension.
- Monitor lower extremity perfusion with a history of PVD.

**Patient & Family Education**
- Avoid, or moderate, alcohol use while taking this drug.
- Do not drive or engage in other potentially hazardous activities until response to drug is known.
- Report any decrease in tolerance to walking if you have a history of PVD.

**ISONIAZID (ISONICOTINIC ACID HYDRAZIDE)** ⊘
(eye-soe-nye'a-zid)
INH, Isotamine ◆, Laniazid, Nydrazid, PMS Isoniazid ◆
**Classifications:** ANTI-INFECTIVE; ANTITUBERCULOSIS
**Therapeutic:** ANTITUBERCULOSIS

**AVAILABILITY** Tablet; syrup; solution for injection

Common adverse effects in *italic;* life-threatening effects <u>underlined</u>; generic names in **bold;** classifications in SMALL CAPS; ◆ Canadian drug name; ⊘ Prototype drug

871

## ACTION & *THERAPEUTIC EFFECT*

Hydrazide of isonicotinic acid with highly specific action against *Mycobacterium tuberculosis*. Postulated to act by interfering with biosynthesis of bacterial proteins, nucleic acid, and lipids. *Exerts bacteriostatic action against actively growing tubercle bacilli; may be bactericidal in higher concentrations.*

**USES** Treatment of all forms of active tuberculosis caused by susceptible organisms and as preventive in high-risk persons (e.g., household members, persons with positive tuberculin skin test reactions). May be used alone or with other tuberculostatic agents.

**UNLABELED USES** Treatment of atypical mycobacterial infections; tuberculous meningitis; action tremor in multiple sclerosis.

**CONTRAINDICATIONS** History of isoniazid-associated hypersensitivity reactions, including hepatic injury; acute liver damage of any etiology; lactation.

**CAUTIOUS USE** Chronic liver disease; HIV infection; hepatitis; severe renal dysfunction; history of convulsive disorders; chronic alcoholism; persons older than 50 y; pregnancy (category C).

## ROUTE & DOSAGE

### Treatment of Active Tuberculosis

*Adult:* **PO/IM** 5 mg/kg (max: 300 mg/day)
*Child:* **PO/IM** 10–20 mg/kg (max: 300–500 mg/day)

### Preventive Therapy

*Adult:* **PO** 300 mg/day
*Child:* **PO** 10 mg/kg up to 300 mg/day or 15 mg/kg 3 × wk

## ADMINISTRATION

### Oral

- Give on an empty stomach at least 1 h before or 2 h after meals. If GI irritation occurs, drug may be taken with meals.

### Intramuscular

- Note: Isoniazid solution for IM injection tends to crystallize at low temperatures; if this occurs, solution should be allowed to warm to room temperature to redissolve crystals before use.
- Give deep into a large muscle and rotate injection sites; local transient pain may follow IM injections.
- Store in tightly closed, light-resistant containers.

**ADVERSE EFFECTS** (≥1%) **Body as a Whole:** Drug-related fever, rheumatic and lupus erythematosus-like syndromes, irritation at injection site; hypersensitivity (fever, chills, skin eruption, vasculitis). **CNS:** *Paresthesias, peripheral neuropathy,* headache, unusual tiredness or weakness, tinnitus, dizziness, hallucinations. **Special Senses:** Blurred vision, visual disturbances, optic neuritis, atrophy. **GI:** Nausea, vomiting, epigastric distress, dry mouth, constipation; hepatotoxicity (*elevated AST, ALT;* bilirubinemia, jaundice, <u>hepatitis</u>). **Hematologic:** <u>Agranulocytosis</u>, hemolytic or <u>aplastic anemia</u>, <u>thrombocytopenia</u>, eosinophilia, methemoglobinemia. **Metabolic:** Decreased vitamin $B_{12}$ absorption, pyridoxine (vitamin $B_6$) deficiency, pellagra, gynecomastia, hyperglycemia, glycosuria, hyperkalemia, hypophosphatemia, hypocalcemia, acetonuria, metabolic acidosis, proteinuria. **Other:** Dyspnea, urinary retention (males).

## DIAGNOSTIC TEST INTERFERENCE

Isoniazid may produce false-positive results using *copper sulfate tests* (e.g., *Benedict's solution, Clinitest*) but not with *glucose oxidase methods* (e.g., *Clinistix, Dextrostix, TesTape*).

## INTERACTIONS Drug: Cycloserine, ethionamide enhance CNS toxicity; may increase phenytoin levels, resulting in toxicity; ALUMINUM-CONTAINING ANTACIDS decrease GI absorption; disulfiram may cause coordination difficulties or psychotic reactions; alcohol increases risk of hepatotoxicity. Food: Food decreases rate and extent of isoniazid absorption, should be taken 1 h before meals.

## PHARMACOKINETICS Absorption: Readily from GI tract; food may reduce rate and extent of absorption. Peak: 1–2 h. Distribution: Distributed to all body tissues and fluids including the CNS; crosses placenta. Metabolism: Inactivated by acetylation in liver. Elimination: 75–96% in urine in 24 h; excreted in breast milk. Half-Life: 1–4 h.

## NURSING IMPLICATIONS

### Black Box Warning

*Isoniazid has been associated with severe, potentially fatal hepatitis.*

### Assessment & Drug Effects

- Withhold drug and notify prescriber immediately of a hypersensitivity reaction; generally occurs within 3–7 wk after initiation of therapy.

- Monitor for and report promptly signs of hepatic toxicity (see Appendix F).
- Monitor for and report promptly signs of peripheral neuritis (e.g., paresthesias of feet and hands with numbness, tingling, burning).
- Monitor BP during period of dosage adjustment. Some experience orthostatic hypotension; therefore, caution against rapid positional changes.
- Monitor diabetics for loss of glycemic control.
- Check weight at least twice weekly under standard conditions.
- Monitor lab tests: Periodic LFTs especially in patients 35 y or older, and in those who ingest alcohol daily.

### Patient & Family Education

- Report promptly any of the following signs of liver toxicity: Unexplained weakness, nausea/vomiting, loss of appetite, dark urine, jaundice, clay-colored stools.
- Avoid or at least reduce alcohol intake while on isoniazid therapy because of increased risk of hepatotoxicity.

# ISOPROTERENOL HYDROCHLORIDE ⓟ

(eye-soe-proe-ter'e-nole)

**Isuprel**

**Classifications:** BETA-ADRENERGIC AGONIST; BRONCHODILATOR; CARDIAC STIMULATOR

**Therapeutic:** BRONCHODILATOR; ANTIARRHYTHMIC; CARDIAC STIMULATOR

## AVAILABILITY Solution for injection

Common adverse effects in *italic*; life-threatening effects underlined; generic names in **bold**; classifications in SMALL CAPS; ♣ Canadian drug name; ⓟ Prototype drug

873

## ACTION & *THERAPEUTIC EFFECT*

Synthetic sympathomimetic amine that acts directly on $beta_1$- and $beta_2$-adrenergic receptors that relaxes bronchospasm, and, by increasing ciliary motion, facilitates expectoration of pulmonary secretions. Induces stimulation of $beta_1$-adrenergic receptors and results in increased cardiac output and cardiac workload by increasing strength of contraction through positive inotropic and chronotropic effects on the heart. It also shortens AV conduction time and its refractory period in patients with heart block. *Reverses bronchospasm and facilitates removal of bronchial secretion. Increases cardiac output and cardiac workload. Also has antiarrhythmic properties by affecting AV node conduction.*

## USES

Reversible bronchospasm induced by anesthesia. As cardiac stimulant in cardiac arrest, carotid sinus hypersensitivity, cardiogenic and bacteremic shock, Adams-Stokes syndrome, or ventricular arrhythmias. Used in treatment of shock that persists after replacement of blood volume.

## UNLABELED USES

Treatment of status asthmaticus in children.

## CONTRAINDICATIONS

Preexisting cardiac arrhythmias associated with tachycardia; tachycardia caused by digitalis intoxication, central hyperexcitability, cardiogenic shock secondary to coronary artery occlusion and MI; ventricular fibrillation.

## CAUTIOUS USE

Sensitivity to sympathomimetic amines; older adult and debilitated patients, hypertension, coronary insufficiency and other cardiovascular disorders, angina; renal dysfunction, hyperthyroidism, diabetes, prostatic hypertrophy, glaucoma, tuberculosis; pregnancy (category C); lactation.

## ROUTE & DOSAGE

**Bronchospasm**
*Adult:* **IV** 0.01–0.02 mg prn

**Cardiac Arrhythmias/Cardiac Resuscitation**
*Adult:* **IV** 0.02–0.06 mg bolus, followed by 5 mcg/min infusion
*Child:* **IV** 0.1 mcg/kg/min by continuous infusion

**Shock/Hypoperfusion**
*Adult:* **IV** 0.5–5 mcg/min

## ADMINISTRATION

**Intravenous**

Note: Maximum concentration on IV solution for both adults and children: 20 mcg/mL (0.02 mg/mL)

*PREPARE:* **Direct IV Injection for Adult with AV Block/Arrhythmia/Bradycardia/Cardiac Arrest:** Dilute 1 mL (0.2) of 1:5000 solution with 9 mL NS or D5W to produce a 1:50,000 (0.02 mg/mL) solution or use 1:50,000 solution undiluted. **Continuous Infusion for Adult with AV Block/Arrhythmia/Bradycardia/Cardiac Arrest:** Dilute 10 mL (2 mg) of 1:5000 solution in 500 mL D5W to produce a 1:250,000 (4 mcg/mL) solution. **IV Infusion for Adult with Shock Hypoperfusion:** Dilute 5 mL (1 mg) of 1:5000 solution in 500 mL D5W to produce a 1:500,000 (2 mcg/mL) solution. **Direct IV Injection**

**for Adult with Bronchospasm:**
Dilute 1 mL (0.2 mg) of 1:5000 solution with 9 mL NS or D5W to produce a 1:50,000 solution undiluted. **Continuous Infusion for Child with AV Block/Bradycardia:** Dilute to a range of 4–12 mcg/mL in 100 mL of D5W or NS.

*ADMINISTER:* **Direct IV for Adult/Child:** Give at a rate of 0.2 mg or fraction thereof over 1 min. ▪ Flush with 15–20 mL NS. **Continuous IV Infusion for Adult/Child:** Rate is adjusted according to patient response. Infusion rate is generally decreased or infusion may be temporarily discontinued if heart rate exceeds 110 bpm, because of the danger of precipitating arrhythmias. ▪ Microdrip or constant-infusion pump is recommended to prevent sudden influx of large amounts of drug. ▪ IV administration is regulated by continuous ECG monitoring. ▪ Patient **must be** observed and response to therapy **must be** monitored continuously.

*INCOMPATIBILITIES:* Solution/additive: **Aminophylline, diazepam, furosemide, sodium bicarbonate.**

▪ Isoproterenol solutions lose potency with standing. ▪ Discard if precipitate or discoloration is present.

## ADVERSE EFFECTS (≥1%)

**CNS:** Headache, mild tremors, nervousness, anxiety, insomnia, excitement, fatigue. **CV:** Flushing, palpitations, tachycardia, unstable BP, anginal pain, <u>ventricular arrhythmias</u>. **GI:** Swelling of parotids (prolonged use), bad taste, buccal ulcerations (sublingual administration), nausea. **Other:** Severe prolonged asthma attack, sweating, bronchial irritation and edema. **Acute Poisoning:** Overdosage, especially after excessive use of aerosols (*tachycardia*, palpitations, nervousness, nausea, vomiting).

## INTERACTIONS

**Drug:** **Epinephrine** and other SYMPATHOMIMETIC AMINES, TRICYCLIC ANTIDEPRESSANTS increase effects and cause cardiac toxicity. HALOGENATED GENERAL ANESTHETICS exacerbate arrhythmias; while BETA-BLOCKERS antagonize effects.

## PHARMACOKINETICS

**Absorption:** Rapidly from parenteral administration. **Onset:** Immediate. **Metabolism:** Metabolized by COMT in liver, lungs, and other tissues. **Elimination:** 40–50% unchanged in urine.

## NURSING IMPLICATIONS

### Assessment & Drug Effects

▪ Check pulse before and during IV administration. Rate greater than 110 usually indicates need to slow infusion rate or discontinue infusion. Consult prescriber for guidelines.

▪ Incidence of arrhythmias is high, particularly when drug is administered IV to patients with cardiogenic shock or ischemic heart disease, digitalized patients, or to those with electrolyte imbalance.

▪ Note: Tolerance to bronchodilating effect and cardiac stimulant effect may develop with prolonged use.

▪ Note: Once tolerance has developed, continued use can result in serious adverse effects including rebound bronchospasm.

Common adverse effects in *italic;* life-threatening effects <u>underlined;</u> generic names in **bold;** classifications in SMALL CAPS; ✚ Canadian drug name; ⊕ Prototype drug

875

# ISOSORBIDE DINITRATE

(eye-soe-sor'bide)

Coronex ✦, Dilatrate-SR, Iso-Bid, Isordil, Novosorbide ✦

**Classification:** NITRATE VASODILATOR

Therapeutic: VASODILATOR; ANTIANGINAL

**Prototype:** Nitroglycerin

**AVAILABILITY** Sublingual tablet; chewable tablet; tablet; sustained release tablet; capsule

## ACTION & *THERAPEUTIC EFFECT*

Relaxes vascular smooth muscle with resulting vasodilation. Dilation of peripheral blood vessels tends to cause peripheral pooling of blood, decreased venous return to heart, and decreased left ventricular end-diastolic pressure, with consequent reduction in myocardial oxygen consumption. *Has an antianginal effect as a result of vasodilation of the coronary arteries.*

**USES** Relief of acute anginal attacks and for management of long-term angina pectoris.

**UNLABELED USES** Alone or in combination with a cardiac glycoside or with other vasodilators (e.g., hydralazine, prazosin, for refractory CHF; diffuse esophageal spasm without gastroesophageal reflux and heart failure).

**CONTRAINDICATIONS** Hypersensitivity to nitrates or nitrites.

**CAUTIOUS USE** Glaucoma, hypotension, hypovolemia; hypertrophic cardiomyopathy; older adults; preg-

nancy (category C), lacation. Safety and efficacy in children not established.

## ROUTE & DOSAGE

### Angina Prophylaxis

*Adult:* **PO** 2.5–30 mg q.i.d. a.c. and at bedtime; **Sublingual tablet** 2.5–10 mg q4–6h; **Chewable tablet** 5–30 mg chewed q2–3h; **Sustained release tablets** 40 mg q6–12h

### Acute Anginal Attack

*Adult:* **PO Sublingual tablet** 2.5–10 mg q2–3h prn; **Chewable tablet** 5–30 mg chewed prn for relief

## ADMINISTRATION

### Oral

- Do not confuse with isosorbide, an oral osmotic diuretic.
- Give regular oral forms on an empty stomach (1 h a.c. or 2 h p.c.). If patient complains of vascular headache, however, it may be taken with meals.
- Advise patient not to eat, drink, talk, or smoke while sublingual tablet is under tongue.
- Instruct patient to place sublingual tablet under tongue at first sign of an anginal attack. If pain is not relieved, repeat dose at 5–10 min intervals to a maximum of 3 doses. If pain continues, notify prescriber or go to nearest hospital emergency room.
- Chewable tablet **must be** thoroughly chewed before swallowing.
- Do not crush sustained release form. It **must be** swallowed whole.
- Have patient sit when taking rapid-acting forms of isosorbide dinitrate (sublingual and chewable tablets) because of the possibility of faintness.

- Store in a tightly closed container in a cool, dry place. Do not expose to extremes of temperature.

## ADVERSE EFFECTS (≥1%) Body as a Whole:
Hypersensitivity reaction, paradoxical increase in anginal pain, methemoglobinemia (overdose). **CNS:** Headache, dizziness, weakness, *light-headedness*, restlessness. **CV:** Palpitation, postural hypotension, tachycardia. **GI:** Nausea, vomiting. **Skin:** *Flushing*, pallor, perspiration, rash, exfoliative dermatitis.

## INTERACTIONS Drug:
**Alcohol** may enhance hypotensive effects and lead to cardiovascular collapse, ANTIHYPERTENSIVE AGENTS, PHENOTHIAZINES add to hypotensive effects.

## PHARMACOKINETICS Absorption:
Significant first-pass metabolism with PO absorption, with 10–90% reaching systemic circulation. **Onset:** 2–5 min SL; within 1 h regular tabs; within 3 min chewable tabs; 30 min sustained release tabs. **Duration:** 1–2 h SL; 4–6 h regular tabs, 0.5–2 h chewable tabs; 6–8 h sustained release tabs. **Metabolism:** In liver. **Elimination:** 80–100% in urine within 24 h.

## NURSING IMPLICATIONS

### Assessment & Drug Effects
- Monitor effectiveness of drug in relieving angina.
- Note: Headaches tend to decrease in intensity and frequency with continued therapy but may require administration of analgesic and reduction in dosage.
- Note: Chronic administration of large doses may produce tolerance and thus decrease effectiveness of nitrate preparations.

### Patient & Family Education
- Make position changes slowly, particularly from recumbent to upright posture, and dangle feet and ankles before walking.
- Lie down at the first indication of light-headedness or faintness.
- Keep a record of anginal attacks and the number of sublingual tablets required to provide relief.
- Do not drink alcohol because it may increase possibility of light-headedness and faintness.

## ISOSORBIDE MONONITRATE
(eye-soe-sor'bide)
Ismo, Imdur, Monoket
**Classification:** NITRATE VASODILATOR
**Therapeutic:** ANTIANGINAL
**Prototype:** Nitroglycerin

## AVAILABILITY
Tablet; sustained release tablet

## ACTION & *THERAPEUTIC EFFECT*
Isosorbide mononitrate is a long-acting metabolite of the coronary vasodilator isosorbide dinitrate. It decreases preload as measured by pulmonary capillary wedge pressure (PCWP), and left ventricular end volume and diastolic pressure (LVEDV), with a consequent reduction in myocardial oxygen consumption. *It is equally or more effective than isosorbide dinitrate in the treatment of chronic, stable angina. It is a potent vasodilator with antianginal and antiischemic effects.*

## USES
Prevention of angina. Not indicated for acute attacks.

## CONTRAINDICATIONS
Hypersensitivity to nitrates.

Common adverse effects in *italic;* life-threatening effects underlined; generic names in **bold;** classifications in SMALL CAPS; ◆ Canadian drug name; ⊘ Prototype drug

877

**CAUTIOUS USE** Hypotension; hypertrophic cardiomyopathy; older adults; pregnancy (category B, C) depends on manufacturer; lactation. **Extended release form:** Should not be used in patients with GI disease (e.g., GI motility, malabsorption).

## ROUTE & DOSAGE

### Prevention of Angina

*Adult:* **PO Regular release (ISMO, Monoket)** 20 mg b.i.d. 7 h apart; **Sustained release (Imdur)** 30–60 mg every morning, may increase up to 120 mg once daily after several days if needed (max: 240 mg)

## ADMINISTRATION

### Oral

- Give first dose in morning on arising and second dose 7 h later with twice daily dosing regimen. Give in morning on arising with once daily dosing.
- Store sustained release tablets in a tight container.

## ADVERSE EFFECTS (≥1%) CNS:
Headache, agitation, anxiety, confusion, loss of coordination, hypoesthesia, hypokinesia, insomnia or somnolence, nervousness, migraine headache, paresthesia, vertigo, ptosis, tremor. **CV:** Aggravation of angina, abnormal heart sounds, murmurs, <u>MI</u>, transient hypotension, palpitations. **Hematologic:** Hypochromic anemia, purpura, <u>thrombocytopenia</u>, methemoglobinemia (high doses). **GI:** Nausea, vomiting, dry mouth, abdominal pain, constipation, diarrhea, dyspepsia, flatulence, tenesmus, gastric ulcer, hemorrhoids, gastritis, glossitis.

**Metabolic:** Hyperuricemia, hypokalemia. **Urogenital:** Renal calculus, UTI, atrophic vaginitis, dysuria, polyuria, urinary frequency, decreased libido, impotence. **Respiratory:** Bronchitis, pneumonia, upper respiratory tract infection, nasal congestion, bronchospasm, coughing, dyspnea, rales, rhinitis. **Skin:** Rash, pruritus, hot flashes, acne, abnormal texture. **Special Senses:** Diplopia, blurred vision, photophobia, conjunctivitis.

## INTERACTIONS Drug: Alcohol
may cause severe hypotension and cardiovascular collapse. **Aspirin** may increase nitrate serum levels. CALCIUM CHANNEL BLOCKERS may cause orthostatic hypotension.

## PHARMACOKINETICS Absorption:
Completely and rapidly absorbed from GI tract; 93% reaches systemic circulation. **Onset:** 1 h. **Peak:** Regular release 30–60 min; sustained release 3–4 h. **Duration:** Regular release 5–12 h; sustained release 12 h. **Metabolism:** In liver by denitration and conjugation to inactive metabolites. **Elimination:** Primarily by kidneys. **Half-Life:** 4–5 h.

## NURSING IMPLICATIONS

### Assessment & Drug Effects

- Monitor cardiac status, frequency and severity of angina, and BP.
- Assess for and report possible S&S of toxicity, including orthostatic hypotension, syncope, dizziness, palpitations, light-headedness, severe headache, blurred vision, and difficulty breathing.
- Monitor lab tests: Periodic serum electrolytes.

### Patient & Family Education

- Do not crush or chew sustained release tablets. May break tablets

in two and take with adequate fluid (4–8 oz).
- Do not withdraw drug abruptly; doing so may precipitate acute angina.
- Maintain correct dosing interval with twice daily dosing.
- Note: Geriatric patients are more susceptible to the possibility of developing postural hypotension.
- Avoid alcohol ingestion and aspirin unless specifically permitted by prescriber.

# ISOTRETINOIN (13-*cis*-RETINOIC ACID) ⓟ

(eye-soe-tret'i-noyn)

Amnesteem, Claravis, Sotret

**Classification:** ANTIACNE (RETINOID)
**Therapeutic:** ANTIACNE; ANTI-NEOPLASTIC

## AVAILABILITY Capsule

## ACTION & *THERAPEUTIC EFFECT*

Decreases sebum secretion by reducing sebaceous gland size; inhibits gland cell differentiation; blocks follicular keratinization. *Has antiacne properties and may be used as a chemotherapeutic agent for epithelial carcinomas.*

## USES Treatment of severe recalcitrant cystic or conglobate acne in patient unresponsive to conventional treatment, including systemic antibiotics.

## UNLABELED USES Lamellar ichthyosis, oral leukoplakia, hyperkeratosis, acne rosacea, scarring gram-negative folliculitis; adjuvant therapy of basal cell carcinoma of lung and cutaneous T-cell lymphoma (mycosis fungoides); psoriasis; chemoprevention for prostate cancer.

## CONTRAINDICATIONS Tinnitus; hypersensitivity to parabens (preservatives in the formulation), retinoid hypersensitivity, leukopenia, neutropenia; UV exposure; pregnancy (category X), females of childbearing age; lactation.

## CAUTIOUS USE Coronary artery disease; major depression, psychosis, history of suicides, alcoholism; hepatitis, hepatic disease; visual disturbance; rheumatologic disorders, osteoporosis; history of pancreatitis, inflammatory bowel disease; diabetes mellitus; obesity; retinal disease; elevated triglycerides, hyperlipidemia.

## ROUTE & DOSAGE

**Cystic Acne**
*Adult:* **PO** 0.5–1 mg/kg/day in 2 divided doses (max recommended dose: 2 mg/kg/day) for 15–20 wk
**Disorders of Keratinization**
*Adult:* **PO** Up to 4 mg/kg/day in divided doses

## ADMINISTRATION
**Oral**
- Give with or shortly after meals.
- Note: A single course of therapy provides adequate control in many patients. If a second course is necessary, it is delayed at least 8 wk because improvement may continue without the drug.
- Store in a tight, light-resistant container. Capsules remain stable for 2 y.

## ADVERSE EFFECTS (≥1%) **Body as a Whole:** Most are dose-related (i.e., occurring at doses greater than 1 mg/kg/day), reversible with termination of therapy. **CNS:** Lethargy, headache, fatigue, visual

Common adverse effects in *italic;* life-threatening effects underlined; generic names in **bold;** classifications in SMALL CAPS; ♣ Canadian drug name; ⓟ Prototype drug

879

disturbances, pseudotumor cerebri, paresthesias, dizziness, depression, psychosis, suicide (rare). **Special Senses:** Reduced night vision, dry eyes, papilledema, eye irritation, *conjunctivitis,* corneal opacities. **GI:** *Dry mouth,* anorexia, nausea, vomiting, abdominal pain, nonspecific GI symptoms, <u>acute hepatotoxic reactions</u> (rare), inflammation and bleeding of gums, increased AST, ALT, acute pancreatitis. **Hematologic:** Decreased Hct, Hgb, elevated sedimentation rate. **Musculoskeletal:** Arthralgia; bone, joint, and muscle pain and stiffness; chest pain, skeletal hyperostosis (especially in athletic people and with prolonged therapy), mild bruising, decreased bone mineral density. **Skin:** *Cheilitis,* skin fragility, dry skin, pruritus, peeling of face, palms, and soles; photosensitivity (photoallergic and phototoxic), erythema, skin infections, petechiae, rash, urticaria, exaggerated healing response (painful exuberant granulation tissue with crusting), brittle nails, alopecia **Respiratory:** Epistaxis, *dry nose.* **Metabolic:** Hyperuricemia, *increased serum concentrations of triglycerides by 50–70%,* serum cholesterol by 15–20%, VLDL cholesterol by 50–60%, LDL cholesterol by 15–20%.

**INTERACTIONS Drug:** vitamin a supplements increase toxicity; decreases effectiveness of estrogen hormonal contraceptives in oral form as well as topical/injectable/implantable/insertable estrogen hormonal birth control. Use with systemic corticosteroids or **phenytoin** may increase bone loss.

**PHARMACOKINETICS Absorption:** Rapid absorption after slow dissolution in GI tract; 25% of ad-

ministered drug reaches systemic circulation. **Peak:** 3.2 h. **Distribution:** Not fully understood; appears in liver, ureters, adrenals, ovaries, and lacrimal glands. **Metabolism:** In liver; enterohepatically cycled. **Elimination:** In urine and feces in equal amounts. **Half-Life:** 10–20 h.

## NURSING IMPLICATIONS

### Black Box Warning

*Isotretinoin has been associated with an extremely high risk of severe birth defects if pregnancy occurs while taking isotretinoin; it must not be used by women who are pregnant or who could become pregnant.*

### Assessment & Drug Effects

- Report signs of liver dysfunction (jaundice, pruritus, dark urine) promptly.
- Monitor closely for loss of glycemic control in diabetic and diabetic-prone patients.
- Monitor for development of depression and suicidal ideation.
- Note: Persistence of hypertriglyceridemia (levels above 500–800 mg/dL) despite a reduced dose indicates necessity to stop drug to prevent onset of acute pancreatitis.
- Monitor lab tests: Baseline lipid profile and repeat at 2 wk, 1 mo, and every month thereafter throughout course of therapy; LFTs at 2- or 3-wk intervals for 6 mo and once a month thereafter during treatment.

### Patient & Family Education

- Rule out pregnancy within 2 wk of starting treatment. Use a reliable contraceptive 1 mo before, throughout, and 1 mo after therapy is discontinued.

- Maintain drug regimen even if during the first few weeks transient exacerbations of acne occur. Recurring symptoms may signify response of deep unseen lesions.
- Discontinue medication at once and notify prescriber if visual disturbances occur along with nausea, vomiting, and headache.
- Do not self-medicate with multivitamins, which usually contain vitamin A. Toxicity of isotretinoin is enhanced by vitamin A supplements.
- Avoid or minimize exposure of the treated skin to sun or sunlamps. Photosensitivity (photoallergic and phototoxic) potential is high.
- Notify prescriber immediately of abdominal pain, rectal bleeding, or severe diarrhea, which are possible symptoms of drug-induced inflammatory bowel disease.
- Keep lips moist and softened (use thin layer of lubricant such as petroleum jelly); dry mouth and cheilitis (inflamed, chapped lips), frequent adverse effects of isotretinoin.
- Notify prescriber of joint pain, such as pain in the great toe (symptom of gout and hyperuricemia).

# ISOXSUPRINE HYDROCHLORIDE

(eye-sox′syoo-preen)

**Classifications:** BETA-ADRENERGIC AGONIST; ALPHA-ADRENERGIC RECEPTOR INHIBITOR; VASODILATOR
Therapeutic: VASODILATOR
**Prototype:** Isoproterenol

## AVAILABILITY Tablet

## ACTION & *THERAPEUTIC EFFECT*

Sympathomimetic with beta-adrenergic stimulant activity and with an inhibitory effect on alpha receptors. Vasodilating action on arteries within skeletal muscles is greater than on cutaneous vessels.

*Has both cerebral and peripheral vasodilatory properties.*

**USES** Adjunctive therapy in treatment of cerebral vascular insufficiency and peripheral vascular disease, such as Raynaud's disease.

**CONTRAINDICATIONS** Immediately postpartum; presence of arterial bleeding; parenteral use in presence of hypotension, fetal distress; intrauterine fetal death; vaginal bleeding; tachycardia; presence of rash.

**CAUTIOUS USE** Bleeding disorders; severe cerebrovascular disease, severe obliterative coronary artery disease, recent MI; pregnancy (category C); lactation.

## ROUTE & DOSAGE

**Cerebral Vascular Insufficiency, Peripheral Vascular Disease**

*Adult:* **PO** 10–20 mg t.i.d. or q.i.d.

## ADMINISTRATION

Oral
- May give without regard to meals.

**ADVERSE EFFECTS** (≥1%) **CV:** Flushing, orthostatic hypotension with light-headedness, faintness; palpitation, tachycardia. **CNS:** Dizziness, nervousness, trembling, weakness. **GI:** Nausea, vomiting, abdominal distress, abdominal distention. **Dermatologic:** Skin rash.

**INTERACTIONS** Do not use with **tranylcypromine.**

**PHARMACOKINETICS Absorption:** Readily from GI tract. **Peak:** 1 h. **Duration:** 3 h. **Distribution:** Crosses placenta. **Metabolism:** In blood. **Elimination:** In urine. **Half-Life:** 1.25 h.

Common adverse effects in *italic*; life-threatening effects underlined; generic names in **bold**; classifications in SMALL CAPS; ◆ Canadian drug name; ⊙ Prototype drug

881

## NURSING IMPLICATIONS

### Assessment & Drug Effects

- Monitor for therapeutic effectiveness: Response to treatment of peripheral vascular disorders may take several weeks. Evaluate clinical manifestations of arterial insufficiency.
- Monitor BP and pulse; may cause hypotension and tachycardia. Supervise ambulation.
- Observe both mother and baby for hypotension and irregular and rapid heartbeat if isoxsuprine is used to delay premature labor. Hypocalcemia, hypoglycemia, and ileus have been observed in babies born of mothers taking isoxsuprine.

### Patient & Family Education

- Notify prescriber of adverse reactions (skin rash, palpitation, flushing) promptly; symptoms are usually effectively controlled by dosage reduction or discontinuation of drug.
- Prevent orthostatic hypotension by making position changes slowly and in stages, particularly from lying down to sitting upright and avoid standing still.
- Note: For treatment of menstrual cramps, isoxsuprine is usually started 1–3 days before onset of menstruation and continued until pain is relieved or menstrual flow stops.

## ISRADIPINE
(is-ra′di-peen)

**Classifications:** CALCIUM CHANNEL ANTAGONIST; ANTIHYPERTENSIVE
**Therapeutic:** ANTIHYPERTENSIVE; ANTIANGINAL
**Prototype:** Nifedipine

## AVAILABILITY Capsule

## ACTION & *THERAPEUTIC EFFECT*

Inhibits calcium ion influx into cardiac muscle and smooth muscle without changing calcium concentrations, thus affecting contractility. Isradipine relaxes coronary vascular smooth muscle. It significantly decreases systemic vascular resistance. *Reduces BP at rest and during isometric and dynamic exercise. Reduces BP and has an antianginal effect.*

## USES Mild to moderate hypertension.

## UNLABELED USES Angina.

## CONTRAINDICATIONS Hypersensitivity to isradipine.

## CAUTIOUS USE CHF, heart failure; hypertrophic cardiomyopathy with outflow tract obstruction; aortic stenosis; acute MI, severe bradycardia, cardiogenic shock, ventricular dysfunction; mild renal impairment, hepatic impairment; GERD, hiatal hernia with esophageal reflux; older adult; pregnancy (category C); lactation. Safety and efficacy in children not established.

## ROUTE & DOSAGE

**Hypertension**
*Adult:* **PO** 2.5 mg b.i.d. (max: 20 mg/day)

## ADMINISTRATION

### Oral

- Note: After the first 2–4 wk of therapy, dose may be increased for improved BP control in increments of 5 mg/day at 2–4 wk intervals up to a maximum dose of 20 mg/day.
- Store in a tight, light-resistant container.

## ADVERSE EFFECTS (≥1%) CNS: Headache, dizziness, fainting, fatigue,

sleep disturbances, vertigo. **CV:** Flushing, ankle edema, palpitations, tachycardia, hypotension, chest pain, CHF. **GI:** Nausea, vomiting, abdominal discomfort, constipation, increased liver enzymes. **Respiratory:** Dyspnea. **Skin:** Rash, decreased skin sensation.

**INTERACTIONS Drug: Adenosine** may prolong bradycardia. May increase **cyclosporine** levels and toxicity. **Rifampin, phenytoin, carbamazepine** and other CYP3A4 inducers may decrease effect. **Food: Grapefruit juice** may increase side effects.

**PHARMACOKINETICS Absorption:** Rapidly and completely absorbed from GI tract, 95% protein bound, but only 15–24% reaches systemic circulation because of first-pass metabolism. **Onset:** 1 h. **Peak:** 2–3 h. **Duration:** 12 h. **Metabolism:** Extensive first-pass metabolism in liver. **Elimination:** 70% in urine as inactive metabolites; 30% in feces. **Half-Life:** 8 h.

**NURSING IMPLICATIONS**

**Assessment & Drug Effects**

- Monitor BP throughout course of therapy.
- Monitor patients with a history of CHF carefully, especially with concurrent beta-blocker use. Promptly report S&S of worsening heart failure.
- Monitor ambulation, especially with older adult patients, until response to drug is known.

**Patient & Family Education**

- Notify prescriber promptly of shortness of breath, palpitations, or other signs of adverse cardiovascular effects.
- Do not drive or engage in other potentially hazardous activities until response to drug is known.

# ITRACONAZOLE

(i-tra-con'a-zole)

Onmel, Sporanox

**Classifications:** ANTIBIOTIC; AZOLE ANTIFUNGAL

Therapeutic: AZOLE ANTIFUNGAL

**Prototype:** Fluconazole

**AVAILABILITY** Capsule; tablet; oral solution; solution for injection

**ACTION & THERAPEUTIC EFFECT** Interferes with formation of ergosterol, the principal sterol in the fungal cell membrane that, when depleted, interrupts fungal membrane functioning. *Antifungal properties affect the fungal cell membrane functioning.*

**USES** Treatment of systemic fungal infections caused by blastomycosis, histoplasmosis, aspergillosis, onychomycosis due to dermatophytes of the toenail with or without fingernail involvement; oropharyngeal and esophageal candidiasis; orally to treat superficial mycoses (*Candida, pityriasis versicolor*).

**UNLABELED USES** Systemic and vaginal candidiasis; meningitis.

**CONTRAINDICATIONS** Hypersensitivity to itraconazole; hypotension; CrCl less than 30 mL/min; ventricular dysfunction as in CHF; or history of CHF when treating onychomycosis; neuropathy; systemic candidiasis; lactation.

**CAUTIOUS USE** Hypersensitivity to other azole antifungals; achlorhydria; GERD; COPD, cystic fibrosis; dialysis; older adults, females of childbearing age; hepatic disease, hepatitis, HIV infection; hypochlorhydria; pulmonary disease;

Common adverse effects in *italic;* life-threatening effects <u>underlined;</u> generic names in **bold;** classifications in SMALL CAPS; ♣ Canadian drug name; ⊘ Prototype drug

883

renal disease, renal impairment; valvular heart disease, ventricular dysfunction; angina, cardiac disease; pregnancy (category C). Safe use in children has not been established.

## ROUTE & DOSAGE

### Blastomycosis, Aspergillosis
Adult: **PO** 200–400 mg daily mg once daily and continue for at least 3 mo

### Oropharyngeal Candidiasis (solution)
Adult: **PO** 200 mg daily for 1–2 wk

### Esophageal Candidiasis
Adult: **PO** 100 mg daily for at least 3 wk (max: 200 mg/day)

### Onychomycosis
Adult: **PO** 200 mg daily × 3 mo

### Histoplasmosis
Adult: **PO** 200 mg daily then increase to max dose of 400 mg daily × 3 mo

## ADMINISTRATION

Oral
- Give capsules with a full meal.
- Give oral solution without food. Liquid should be vigorously swished for several seconds and swallowed.
- Do not interchange oral solution and capsules.
- Do not give with proton pump inhibitors, H2-blockers, or antacids.
- Divide dosages greater than 200 mg/day into two doses.
- Store capsules at room temperature of 15°–25° C (59°–77° F). Protect from light and moisture.
- Store liquid at or below 25° C (77° F).

**ADVERSE EFFECTS** (≥1%) **CV:** Hypertension with higher doses, chest pain. **CNS:** Headache, dizziness, fatigue, somnolence, abnormal dreams, hearing loss (euphoria, drowsiness less than 1%). **Endocrine:** Gynecomastia, hypokalemia (especially with higher doses), hypertriglyceridemia. **GI:** *Nausea, vomiting, dyspepsia, abdominal pain, diarrhea, anorexia, flatulence, gastritis;* elevations of serum transaminases, alkaline phosphatase, and bilirubin. **Urogenital:** Decreased libido, impotence. **Skin:** Rash, pruritus. **Acute Poisoning:** Severe toxicity (doses exceeding 400 mg daily have been associated with higher risk of hypokalemia, hypertension, adrenal insufficiency).

**INTERACTIONS Drug:** Use with **alfuzosin, alprazolam, burprenorphine,** ERGOT ALKALOIDS, **dofetilide, donepezil, doxorubicin, dronedarone, efavirenz, flibanserin, haloperidol, isavuconazonium, ivabradine, lomitapide, loperamide, lovastatin, lurasidone, methadone,** oral **midazolam, naloxegol, nisoldipine, pimavanserin, pimozide, quinidine, ranolazine, silodosin, simvastatin, thioridazine, ticagrelor triazolam, venetoclax, ziprasidone** is contraindicated. Itraconazole may increase levels and toxicity of **alprazolam, ergotamine, dihydroergotamine,** ORAL HYPOGLYCEMIC AGENTS, **warfarin, ritonavir, indinavir, vinca alkaloids, busulfan, methylergonovine, midazolam, triazolam, diazepam, nifedipine, nicardipine, amlodipine, felodipine, lovastatin, simvastatin, cyclosporine, tacrolimus, methylprednisolone, digoxin.** Combination with **dofetilide, levomethadyl, oral midazolam, pimozide, quinidine, triazolam** may cause severe cardiac events including cardiac arrest or sudden death. Itraconazole levels are decreased by **carbamazepine, phenytoin, phenobarbital, isoniazid, rifabutin, rifampin. Herbal: St. John's wort** and **garlic** may decrease itraconazole levels.

**PHARMACOKINETICS Absorption:** Best when taken with food. **Onset:** 2 wk–3 mo. **Peak:** Peak levels at 1.5–5 h. Steady-state concentrations reached in 10–14 days. **Distribution:** Highly protein bound (greater than 99%), minimal concentrations in CSF. Higher concentrations in tissues than in plasma. **Metabolism:** Extensively in liver by CYP3A4, may undergo enterohepatic recirculation. **Elimination:** 35% in urine, 55% in feces. **Half-Life:** 34–42 h.

## NURSING IMPLICATIONS

### Black Box Warning

*Itraconazole has been associated with worsening CHF in those with ventricular dysfunction and with serious adverse cardiac effects when coadministered with other drugs metabolized by the CYP450-3A4 pathway.*

### Assessment & Drug Effects

- Monitor cardiac status and liver function throughout therapy. Withhold drug and notify prescriber immediately if S&S of CHF, other cardiac dysfunction, or signs of liver dysfunction appear.
- Monitor for digoxin toxicity when given concurrently with digoxin.
- Monitor PT and INR carefully when given concurrently with warfarin.

- Monitor for S&S of hypersensitivity (see Appendix F); discontinue drug and notify prescriber if noted.
- Monitor lab tests: Baseline C&S and periodic LFTs especially in those with preexisting hepatic abnormalities.

### Patient & Family Education

- Discontinue drug and report promptly to prescriber S&S of CHF (see Appendix F).
- Notify prescriber promptly for S&S of liver dysfunction, including anorexia, nausea, and vomiting; weakness and fatigue; dark urine and clay-colored stool.
- Note: Risk of hypoglycemia may increase in diabetics on oral hypoglycemic agents.
- Women should use effective means of contraception during and for 2 mo following termination of treatment.

# IVABRADINE
(i-va-bra'deen)
Corlanor

**Classifications:** ANTIARRHYTHMIC; HYPERPOLARIZATION-ACTIVATED CYCLIC NUCLEOTIDE-GATED (HCN) CHANNEL BLOCKER
**Therapeutic:** ANTIARRHYTHMIC

## AVAILABILITY Tablets

## ACTION & THERAPEUTIC EFFECT
Blocks the hyperpolarization-activated cyclic nucleotide-gated (HCN) channel responsible for the cardiac pacemaker current which regulates heart rate. *Reduces the resting heart rate.*

**USES** Reduction of the risk of hospitalization for worsening heart failure in patients with stable, symptomatic chronic heart failure with left ventricular ejection fraction 35% or less, who are in sinus

Common adverse effects in *italic;* life-threatening effects <u>underlined;</u> generic names in **bold;** classifications in SMALL CAPS; ♣ Canadian drug name; ⊙ Prototype drug

885

rhythm with resting heart rate of 70 or more beats per minute and either are on maximally tolerated doses of beta-blockers or have a contraindication to beta-blocker use.

## CONTRAINDICATIONS
Acute decompensated heart failure; BP less than 90/50 mm Hg; sick sinus syndrome, sinoatrial block or 3rd degree AV block, unless a functioning demand pacemaker is present; resting HR less than 60 bpm prior to treatment; severe hepatic impairment (Child-Pugh class C); pacemaker dependence; concurrent strong CYP3A4 inhibitors; pregnancy; lactation.

## CAUTIOUS USE
Atrial fibrillation; decreases in HR; bradycardia symptoms; 2nd degree AV block; concurrent moderate CYP3A4 inhibitors or CYP3A4 inducers. Safety and efficacy in children younger than 18 y not established.

## ROUTE & DOSAGE

### Heart Failure
Adult: PO 5 mg b.i.d.; adjust depending on heart rate and tolerability; with conduction defects, start with 2.5 mg b.i.d.

### Heart Rate Dosage Adjustments
Greater than 60 bpm: Increase dose by 2.5 mg up to max of 7.5 mg b.i.d.
Less than 50 bpm or S&S of bradycardia: Decrease dose by 2.5 mg; discontinue if patient is taking 2.5 mg b.i.d.

## ADMINISTRATION
### Oral
- Give with meals.
- Dose may be adjusted based on HR after 2 wk of treatment.
- Store at 15°–30° C (59°–86° F).

## ADVERSE EFFECTS (≥1%) CV:
*Atrial fibrillation, bradycardia, hypertension.* **Special Senses:** Phosphenes, visual brightness.

## INTERACTIONS
**Drug:** Concomitant use of strong CYP3A4 inhibitors (e.g., AZOLE ANTIFUNGALS, MACROLIDE ANTIBIOTICS, HIV PROTEASE INHIBITORS, **nefazodone**) and moderate CYP3A4 inhibitors (e.g., **diltiazem, verapamil**) increases the levels of ivabradine. Concomitant use of CYP3A4 inducers (e.g., BARBITURATES, **phenytoin, rifampicin**) decreases the levels of ivabradine. **Food: Grapefruit** and grapefruit juice increase the levels of ivabradine. **Herbal: St. John's wort** decreases the levels of ivabradine.

## PHARMACOKINETICS
**Absorption:** 40% bioavailable. **Peak:** 1 h. **Distribution:** 70% plasma protein bound. **Metabolism:** Extensive first-pass metabolism in liver. **Elimination:** Renal and fecal. **Half-Life:** 6 h.

## NURSING IMPLICATIONS
### Assessment & Drug Effects
- Monitor ECG regularly for atrial fibrillation.
- Report promptly symptoms of atrial fibrillation, such as heart palpitations or racing, chest pressure, or worsening shortness of breath.
- Monitor HR and BP regularly. Report promptly HR outside of the range of 50–60 bpm and BP less than 90/50 mm Hg.
- Monitor HR more frequently if dosage increased or decreased, or if receiving other negative chronotropes (e.g., amiodarone, beta-blockers, digoxin).
- Monitor for and promptly report S&S of worsening heart failure.

## Patient & Family Education

- Notify prescriber promptly of any of the following: Symptoms of heart failure worsening; BP less than 90/50 mm Hg; resting HR less than 60; heart palpitations or racing; excessive fatigue or dizziness.
- Avoid drinking grapefruit juice and taking St. John's wort during treatment.
- Luminous phenomena may occur while taking this drug; experienced as temporary brightness in field of vision, or halos, or colored bright lights, usually triggered by sudden variations in light intensity, primarily during the first 2 mo of therapy.
- Use caution when driving or using machinery in situations where sudden changes in light intensity may occur (e.g., driving at night).
- Women should use effective means of contraception and notify prescriber of a known or suspected pregnancy.
- Do not breast-feed while taking this drug without consulting prescriber.

# IVERMECTIN

(i-ver-mec'tin)

Stromectol

**Classifications:** ANTHELMINTIC

**Therapeutic:** ANTHELMINTIC; ANTIPARASITIC

**Prototype:** Praziquantel

**AVAILABILITY** Tablet; skin lotion

## ACTION & *THERAPEUTIC EFFECT*

A semisynthetic anthelmintic agent which is a broad-spectrum antiparasitic agent that causes an increase in permeability to chloride ions of the parasitic cell membrane, resulting in hyperpolarization of nerve or muscle cells of parasites. This results in their paralysis and cell death. *Causes cell death of parasites.*

**USES** Treatment of strongyloidiasis of the intestinal tract, onchocerciasis.

**CONTRAINDICATIONS** Hypersensitivity to ivermectin.

**CAUTIOUS USE** Asthma; moderate or severe hepatic disease; hyperreactive onchodermatitis; older adults; pregnancy (category C); lactation; children less than 15 kg of weight.

## ROUTE & DOSAGE

**Strongyloides**

*Adult/Child (weight 15 kg or greater):* **PO** 200 mcg/kg × 1 dose

**Onchocerciasis**

*Adult/Child (weight 15 kg or greater):* **PO** 150 mcg/kg × 1 dose, may repeat q3–12mo prn

## ADMINISTRATION

Oral

- Give tablets with water rather than any other type of liquid.
- Store below 30° C (86° F).

**ADVERSE EFFECTS** (≥1%) **Body as a Whole:** *Fever,* peripheral edema. **CNS:** Dizziness. **CV:** Tachycardia. **GI:** Diarrhea, nausea. **Skin:** *Pruritus, rash.* **Other:** Arthralgia/synovitis, lymphadenopathy.

**INTERACTIONS Drug:** May increase effect of **warfarin.**

**PHARMACOKINETICS Peak:** 4 h. **Distribution:** Distributed into breast milk. **Metabolism:** In the liver. **Elimination:** In feces over 12 days. **Half-Life:** 16 h.

Common adverse effects in *italic;* life-threatening effects underlined; generic names in **bold;** classifications in SMALL CAPS; ♣ Canadian drug name; ⓟ Prototype drug

887

## NURSING IMPLICATIONS

### Assessment & Drug Effects

- Monitor for therapeutic effectiveness: Indicated by negative stool samples.
- Monitor for cardiovascular effects such as orthostatic hypotension and tachycardia.
- Monitor for and report inflammatory conditions of the eyes.

### Patient & Family Education

- Get a follow-up stool examination to determine effectiveness of treatment. Treatment for worms does not kill adult parasites; repeated follow-up and retreatment are usually needed.
- Notify prescriber if eye discomfort develops.

## IXABEPILONE

(ix-a-be-pi'lone)

Ixempra

**Classifications:** ANTINEOPLASTIC; EPOTHILONE

Therapeutic: ANTINEOPLASTIC; ANTIMITOTIC

**AVAILABILITY** Lyophilized powder for injection

**ACTION & *THERAPEUTIC EFFECT***
Binds directly to microtubules needed to form the spindles required in mitosis of dividing cells. *Blocks new cell formation during the mitotic phase of their cell division cycle, thus leading to cancer cell death.*

**USES** Metastatic or locally advanced breast cancer alone or in combination with capecitabine in patients who have failed therapy with an anthracycline and a taxane.

**CONTRAINDICATIONS** Polyoxyethylated castor oil hypersensitivity; hepatic impairment in patients with AST or ALT greater than $10 \times$ ULN, and/or bilirubin greater than $3 \times$ ULN; neutrophil count less than $1,500/mm^3$ or platelet count less than $100,000/mm^3$; concomitant use of capecitabine and bilirubin greater than $1 \times$ ULN, or AST or ALT greater than $2.5 \times$ ULN; grade 4 neuropathy or any other grade 4 toxicity; pregnancy (category D); lactation.

**CAUTIOUS USE** Hypersensitivity to ixabepilone; monotherapy of patients with hepatic impairment baseline values of AST or ALT greater than $5 \times$ ULN.

## ROUTE & DOSAGE

### Breast Cancer

*Adult:* **IV** 40 mg/m² over 3 h q3wk

### Obesity Dosage Adjustment

*BSA greater than 2.2 m²:* Dosage should be calculated based on 2.2 m² instead of actual m²

### Dosage Adjustments

- *Grade 2 neuropathy 7 days or more, or grade 3 neuropathy less than 7 days, or grade 3 toxicity other than neuropathy:* 32 mg/m²
- *Neutrophil less than 500 cells/mm³ 7 days or more, or febrile neutropenia, or platelets less than 25,000/mm³ or platelets less than 50,000/mm³ with bleeding:* Decrease dose by 20%
- *Grade 3 neuropathy 7 days or more or disabling neuropathy, or any grade 4 toxicity:* Do not administer
- *Regimen with a strong CYP3A4 inhibitor:* 20 mg/m²

Common adverse effects in *italic*; life-threatening effects underlined; generic names in **bold**; classifications in SMALL CAPS; ✦ Canadian drug name; ❂ Prototype drug

### Hepatic Impairment Dosage Adjustment in Monotherapy

- *AST and ALT 10 × ULN or less and bilirubin 1.5 × ULN or less:* 32 mg/m²
- *AST and ALT 10 × ULN or less and bilirubin greater than 1.5 × ULN but 3 × ULN or less:* 20–30 mg/m²
- *AST and ALT greater than 10 × ULN or bilirubin greater than 3 × ULN:* Do not administer

## ADMINISTRATION

### Intravenous

This drug is a cytotoxic agent and caution should be used to prevent any contact with the drug. Follow institutional or standard guidelines for preparation, handling, and disposal of cytotoxic agents. Wear double gloves and protective gown.

*PREPARE:* **IV Infusion:** Supplied in a kit containing a powder vial and diluent vial. Allow kit to come to room temperature for 30 min before reconstitution. • Slowly inject diluent into the powder vial to yield 2 mg/mL. Swirl gently and invert vial to dissolve. • Further dilute in LR solution in DEHP-free bags. Select a volume of LR to produce a final concentration of 0.2–0.6 mg/mL. Mix thoroughly.

*ADMINISTER:* **IV Infusion:** Use DEHP-free infusion line with a 0.2–1.2 micron in-line filter. • Infuse at a rate appropriate to the total volume of solution. Complete infusion within 6 h of preparation.

*INCOMPATIBILITIES:* **Solution/additive:** Diluents other than **lactated Ringer's injection** should not be combined with ixabepilone. **Y-site:** Do not use a Y-site connection with this drug.

• Store drug kit refrigerated at 2°–8° C (36°–46° F) in original packaging. • Reconstituted solution may be stored in the vial for a maximum of only 1 h at room temperature/light. • Once further diluted with lactated Ringer's injection, solution is stable at room temperature/light for 6 h.

## ADVERSE EFFECTS (≥1%) **Body as a Whole:** Chest pain, dehydration, edema, *fatigue,* hypersensitivity reactions, pain, peripheral neuropathy, pyrexia. **CNS:** Dizziness, *headache,* insomnia, fever. **CV:** Cardiovascular edema, chest pain, flushing. **GI:** *Abdominal pain, anorexia, constipation, diarrhea,* gastroesophageal reflux disease (GERD), *mucositis, nausea, stomatitis, vomiting,* taste disorder. **Hematologic:** Anemia, leukopenia, *neutropenia,* thrombocytopenia. **Metabolic:** Weight loss. **Musculoskeletal:** *Arthralgia, myalgia, musculoskeletal pain.* **Respiratory:** Cough, dyspnea, upper respiratory tract infection. **Skin:** *Alopecia,* exfoliation, hyperpigmentation, nail disorder, palmar-plantar erythrodysesthesia syndrome, pruritus, rash. **Special Senses:** Lacrimation.

## INTERACTIONS **Drug:** Inhibitors of CYP3A4 (e.g., HIV PROTEASE INHIBITORS, MACROLIDE ANTIBIOTICS, AZOLE ANTIFUNGAL AGENTS) increase the plasma level of ixabepilone. Strong CYP3A4 inducers (e.g., **dexamethasone, phenytoin, carbamazepine, rifampin, rifabutin, phenobarbital**) decrease the plasma level of ixabepilone. Do not administer with LIVE VACCINES. Avoid **metronidazole** or **disulfiram. Food:** Grapefruit and **grapefruit juice** increase the plasma level of ixabepilone. Avoid alcohol. **Herbal:** **St. John's wort** decreases the plasma level of ixabepilone.

## PHARMACOKINETICS **Distribution:** 67–77% protein bound. **Metabolism:**

Common adverse effects in *italic;* life-threatening effects underlined; generic names in **bold**; classifications in SMALL CAPS; ♣ Canadian drug name; ⊙ Prototype drug

889

In liver (CYP3A4). **Elimination:** Stool (major) and urine (minor). **Half-Life:** 52 h.

## NURSING IMPLICATIONS

### Black Box Warning

*Ixabepilone in combination with capecitabine is contraindicated in patients with AST or ALT greater than 2.5 × ULN or bilirubin greater than 1 × ULN because of an increased risk of toxicity and neutropenia-related death.*

### Actions & Drug Effects

- Monitor for signs of an infusion-related hypersensitivity reaction.
- Monitor for and promptly report signs of neuropathy.
- Monitor lab tests: Baseline and periodic CBC with differential, platelet count, LFTs; periodic serum electrolytes.

### Patient & Family Education

- Report promptly any of the following: Numbness and tingling of the hands or feet, S&S of infection (e.g., fever of 100.5° F or greater, chills, cough, burning or pain on urination), hives, itching, rash, flushing, swelling, shortness of breath, difficulty breathing, chest tightness or pain, palpitations or unusual weight gain.
- Use effective contraceptive measures to prevent pregnancy.

## IXEKIZUMAB

(ix′e′kiz-ue-mab)

Taltz

**Classifications:** INTERLEUKIN-17A ANTAGONIST; IMMUNOSUPPRESSANT; MONOCLONAL ANTIBODY
**Therapeutic:** IMMUNOSUPPRESSANT
**Prototype:** Basiliximab

**AVAILABILITY** Solution for injection

## ACTION & *THERAPEUTIC EFFECT*

A humanized IgG4 monoclonal antibody that selectively binds with the interleukin 17A (IL-17A) cytokine and inhibits its interaction with the IL-17 receptor. *This action inhibits the release of proinflammatory cytokines and chemokines that are involved in the normal inflammatory and immune responses.*

**USES** Treatment of adults with moderate-to-severe plaque psoriasis who are candidates for systemic therapy or phototherapy.

**CONTRAINDICATIONS** Hypersensitivity to ixekizumab.

**CAUTIOUS USE** Immunosuppression, Crohn's disease, infection, inflammatory bowel disease, tuberculosis, vaccination, pregnancy, lactation, children.

## ROUTE & DOSAGE

### Psoriasis

*Adult:* **Subcutaneous** 160 mg at wk 0; then 80 mg q2wk for 6 doses; then 80 mg q4wk

## ADMINISTRATION

### Subcutaneous

- Available as a pre-filled syringe containing 80 mg ixekizumab. Each 160 mg dose is administered as 2 subcutaneous injections.
- Remove from refrigerator and allow to warm to room temperature for 30 min.
- Do not administer where skin is tender, bruised, erythematous, indurated, or affected by psoriasis.
- Rotate sites of injection.
- Discard syringe after each use.
- Store unopened pre-filled syringes in refrigerator at 2°–8° C (36°–46° F).

Common adverse effects in *italic;* life-threatening effects underlined; generic names in **bold**; classifications in SMALL CAPS; ♦ Canadian drug name; ⑩ Prototype drug

**ADVERSE EFFECTS** (≥1%) **Body as a Whole:** Hypersensitivity, injection site reactions, tinea infections. **GI:** Nausea. **Metabolic:** Neutropenia, thrombocytopenia. **Respiratory:** Upper respiratory tract infections.

**INTERACTIONS Drug:** Ixekizumab can alter the formation of CYP450 enzymes and could possibly cause interactions with other drugs requiring these enzymes for metabolism.

**PHARMACOKINETICS Absorption:** Bioavailability is 60–81%. **Peak:** 4 days. **Metabolism:** Peptide degradation. **Half-Life:** 13 days.

## NURSING IMPLICATIONS

### Assessment & Drug Effects

- Assess for signs or symptoms of hypersensitivity, infection, active tuberculosis, and inflammatory bowel disease.

### Patient & Family Education

- Notify health care provider if you have active tuberculosis or inflammatory bowel disease such as Crohn's disease or ulcerative colitis.
- You may have a greater chance of getting an infection. Wash hands often. Avoid people with colds or infections. Stay current on all of your vaccinations.
- Tell your health care provider if you are breast-feeding or if you are pregnant or planning to get pregnant.

---

## KETOCONAZOLE

(ke-to-con'a-zol)

Extina, Nizoral, Xolegel

**Classification:** AZOLE ANTIFUNGAL
**Therapeutic:** AZOLE ANTIFUNGAL
**Prototype:** Fluconazole

**AVAILABILITY** Tablet; cream; shampoo; foam; gel

## ACTION & *THERAPEUTIC EFFECT*

Interferes with formation of ergosterol, the principal sterol in the fungal cell membrane that, when depleted, interrupts membrane function by increasing its permeability. *Antifungal properties are related to the drug effect on the fungal cell membrane functioning.*

**USES Oral:** Severe systemic fungal infections. **Topical:** Tinea corporis and tinea cruris and in treatment of tinea versicolor (pityriasis), seborrheic dermatitis.

**UNLABELED USES Oral:** Onychomycosis, vaginal candidiasis, Cushing's syndrome associated with adrenal or pituitary adenoma; precocious puberty, and candidiasis prophylaxis.

**CONTRAINDICATIONS** Hypersensitivity to ketoconazole or any component in the formulation; chronic alcoholism, fungal meningitis, onychomycosis; ocular exposure, ophthalmic administration, acute or chronic liver disease; coadministration of dofetilide, quinidine, pimozide, methadone, disopyramide, dronedarone, and ranolazine.

**CAUTIOUS USE** Azole antifungal hypersensitivity; achlorhydria, hypochlorhydria; hypovolemia, asthma; alcoholism; older adult; HIV infection; hyperactive onchodermatitis; pregnancy (category C); lactation. Safe use in children younger than 2 y is not established.

## ROUTE & DOSAGE

**Fungal Infections**

*Adult:* **PO** 200–400 mg once/day; **Topical** Apply 1–2 × day to affected area and surrounding skin
*Child (2 y or older):* **PO** 3.3–6.6 mg/kg/day as single dose (do not exceed adult doses)

---

Common adverse effects in *italic;* life-threatening effects <u>underlined</u>; generic names in **bold;** classifications in SMALL CAPS; ♣ Canadian drug name; ⊕ Prototype drug

891

**Dandruff**

*Adult/Child:* **Topical** Shampoo twice a week for 4 wk with at least 3 days between shampoos; **Topical (Extina)** Apply b.i.d. × 4 wk; **(Xolegel)** Apply daily × 2 wk

## ADMINISTRATION

### Oral

- Give with water, fruit juice, coffee, or tea; drug requires an acid medium for dissolution and absorption.
- Relieve nausea and vomiting during early therapy by taking drug with food and dividing into 2 daily doses.
- Do not give with antacids.
- Store in tightly covered container at 15°–30° C (59°–86° F) unless otherwise directed.

### Topical

- Apply sufficient shampoo to produce lather to wash scalp and hair and gently massage over entire scalp area for 5 min, rinse hair thoroughly and repeat, leaving shampoo on scalp for 3 min. Rinse thoroughly.

## ADVERSE EFFECTS (≥1%) **Oral:**
**Body as a Whole:** Skin rash, erythema, urticaria, pruritus, angioedema, anaphylaxis. **CV:** Cardiac dysrhythmia, prolonged QT interval, Torsades de pointes, ventricular arrhythmia. **GI:** *Nausea, vomiting,* anorexia, dry mouth, epigastric or abdominal pain, constipation, diarrhea, transient elevation in serum liver enzymes, fatal hepatic necrosis (rare). **Hematologic:** With high doses, lowers serum testosterone and ACTH-induced corticosteroid serum levels, transient decreases in serum cholesterol and triglycerides; hyponatremia (rare). **Urogenital:** Gynecomastia (males), breast pain; uterine bleeding, loss of libido, impotence, oligospermia, hair loss. **Other:** Acute hypoadrenalism (reduction of adrenal stress syndrome), renal hypofunction. **Topical: Skin:** Mild transient erythema, severe irritation, pruritus, stinging.

## INTERACTIONS **Drug: Alcohol** may cause sunburn-like reaction; ANTACIDS, ANTICHOLINERGICS, H$_2$-RECEPTOR ANTAGONISTS decrease ketoconazole absorption; **isoniazid, rifampin** increase ketoconazole metabolism, thus decreasing its activity; levels of **phenytoin** and ketoconazole decreased; do not use with BENZODIAZEPINEs; may increase levels of **cyclosporine** or **carbamazepine,** increasing the risk of toxicity; **warfarin** may potentiate hypoprothrombinemia; may increase ergotamine toxicity of **dihydroergotamine, ergotamine;** may increase concentration and toxicity of **trazodone.** Contraindicated with medications that prolong the QT interval (i.e., **dofetilide, dolansetron, donepezil,** etc). Do not use with agents extensively metabolized by CYP 3A4 (e.g., **lovastatin, quinidine,** etc.). **Herbal: Echinacea** may increase risk of hepatotoxicity.

## PHARMACOKINETICS **Absorption:** Erratically from GI tract (needs an acid pH); minimal absorption topically. **Peak:** 1–2 h. **Distribution:** Distributed to saliva, urine, sebum, and cerumen; CSF levels unpredictable; distributed into breast milk. **Metabolism:** In liver (CYP3A4). **Elimination:** Primarily in feces, 13% in urine. **Half-Life:** 8 h.

## NURSING IMPLICATIONS

### Black Box Warning

*Ketoconazole has been associated with serious, potentially fatal, hepatotoxocity and QT prolongation when coadministered with dofetilide, quinidine, pimozide, methadone, disopyramide, dronedarone, and ranolazine.*

## Assessment & Drug Effects

- Monitor for S&S of hepatotoxicity (see Appendix F). Discontinue drug immediately to prevent irreversible liver damage and report to prescriber.
- Monitor lab tests: Baseline LFTs and repeat at least monthly throughout therapy. INR, adrenal function.

## Patient & Family Education

- Report S&S of hepatotoxicity promptly to prescriber (see Appendix F).
- Do not drive or engage in potentially hazardous activities until response to drug is known.
- Avoid OTC drugs for gastric distress, such as Rolaids, Tums, Alka-Seltzer and check with prescriber before taking any other nonprescription medicines.
- Notify prescriber if skin condition fails to respond to topical therapy or worsens or if signs of irritation or sensitivity occur.

# KETOPROFEN
(kee-toe-proe′fen)

**Classifications:** ANALGESIC, NONSTEROIDAL ANTI-INFLAMMATORY DRUG (NSAID); ANTIPYRETIC
**Therapeutic:** ANALGESIC, NSAID
**Prototype:** Ibuprofen

**AVAILABILITY** Capsule; sustained release capsule

## ACTION & *THERAPEUTIC EFFECT*
Nonsteroidal anti-inflammatory drug (NSAID) that inhibits both COX-1 and COX-2 enzymes; thus it also inhibits prostaglandin synthesis, and therefore interferes with the inflammatory process. It inhibits platelet aggregation and prolongs bleeding time. *Has analgesic, anti-inflammatory, antiarthritic, and antiplatelet properties.*

**USES** Acute or long-term treatment of rheumatoid arthritis and osteoarthritis; primary dysmenorrhea; headache; symptomatic relief of postoperative, dental, and postpartum pain; visceral pain associated with cancer.

**UNLABELED USES** Reiter's syndrome, juvenile arthritis, acute gouty arthritis, biliary pain, renal colic.

**CONTRAINDICATIONS** Patient in whom aspirin, salicylate, or another NSAID induces asthma, urticaria, bronchospasm, severe rhinitis, shock; perioperatively for CABG surgery; renal nephritis, nephrotic syndrome; pregnancy (category D third trimester); lactation.

**CAUTIOUS USE** History of GI disease, GI bleeding, active ulcer; renal or hepatic impairment, patient who may be adversely affected by prolongation of bleeding time; heart failure, fluid retention; hypertension; patient receiving diuretics; geriatric patient; anemia; dental work; myasthenia gravis; pregnancy (category C first and second trimesters). Safe use in children younger than 16 y not established.

## ROUTE & DOSAGE

### Arthritis
*Adult:* **PO** 75 mg t.i.d. or 50 mg q.i.d. (max: 300 mg/day) or 200 mg sustained release daily
*Geriatric:* **PO** Start with 75 mg b.i.d., or 50 mg t.i.d.; **Sustained release** 100–150 mg once daily

### Mild to Moderate Pain, Dysmenorrhea
*Adult:* **PO** 25–50 mg q6–8h

### Headache
*Adult:* **PO** 75 mg t.i.d.–q.i.d.

Common adverse effects in *italic;* life-threatening effects <u>underlined;</u> generic names in **bold;** classifications in SMALL CAPS; ◆ Canadian drug name; ❷ Prototype drug

893

## ADMINISTRATION

### Oral

- Ensure that extended-release capsule is swallowed whole. It should not be crushed or chewed.
- Give with food, milk, or prescribed antacid to reduce GI irritation.
- Store tablets at 15°–30° C (59°–86° F) in a tightly closed, light-resistant container unless otherwise directed.
- Store capsules and suppositories at 20°–25° C (68°–77° F). Protect from light and excessive heat and humidity.

## ADVERSE EFFECTS (≥1%) CNS:
Insomnia, nervousness, *headache,* dizziness; depression, drowsiness, confusion, migraine, vertigo. **CV:** Peripheral edema, palpitations, hypertension, tachycardia, <u>MI and CVA</u>. **Special Senses:** Visual disturbances, conjunctivitis, eye pain, retinal hemorrhage, pigmentation changes; dry nose or throat, tinnitus, hearing impairment. **GI:** *Dyspepsia,* <u>drug-induced peptic ulcer, GI bleeding,</u> nausea, vomiting, diarrhea, constipation, flatulence, stomach pain, anorexia, dry mouth, gingivitis, rectal burning and hemorrhage, melena, jaundice, elevated ALT, AST. **Hematologic:** Prolonged bleeding time, anemia, purpura, <u>agranulocytosis,</u> thrombocytosis. **Urogenital:** Urinary tract irritation (dysuria, frequency/urgency), renal impairment. **Respiratory:** <u>Laryngo-spasm, bronchospasm, laryngeal edema,</u> pharyngitis. **Skin:** Rash, pruritus, urticaria, erythema, photosensitivity. **Endocrine:** Aggravation of diabetes mellitus.

## INTERACTIONS Drug: ORAL ANTI-
COAGULANTS, **heparin** may prolong bleeding time; may increase **lithium** toxicity; may increase **methotrexate** toxicity. Avoid use of other NSAIDS. Do not use with **cidofovir** or **ketorolac**. Herbal: Feverfew, garlic, ginger, ginkgo increases bleeding potential.

## PHARMACOKINETICS Absorption:
Readily from GI tract. **Onset:** 1–2 h. **Peak:** 1–2 h. **Duration:** 4–6 h. **Metabolism:** In liver. **Elimination:** Primarily in urine, some biliary excretion. **Half-Life:** 1.1–4 h.

## NURSING IMPLICATIONS

### Black Box Warning

*Ketoprofen has been associated with increased risk of serious, potentially fatal, GI bleeding and cardiovascular thrombolytic events (e.g., MI and CVA); risk may increase with duration of use and may be greater in the older adult and those with risk factors for CV disease.*

### Assessment & Drug Effects

- Monitor for hypertension and report promptly S&S of CV thrombotic events (i.e., angina, MI, TIA, or stroke).
- Monitor for and report tinnitus, hearing impairment, and visual disturbance, especially during prolonged or high-dose therapy.
- Monitor for S&S of GI ulceration (e.g., stool for occult blood, persistent indigestion).
- Monitor lab tests: Baseline and periodic hemoglobin, renal function tests, CBC and LFTs.

### Patient & Family Education

- Report promptly signs of jaundice (see Appendix F) as well as the following: Blurred vision, tinnitus, urinary urgency or frequency, unexplained bleeding, weight gain with edema.
- Stop taking drug and report promptly to prescriber if you experience chest pain, shortness of breath, weakness, slurring of speech, or other signs of a cardiac or neurologic problem.

- Note: Alcohol, aspirin, or other NSAIDs may increase risk of GI ulceration and bleeding tendencies and therefore should be avoided.
- Do not drive or engage in potentially hazardous activities until response to drug is known.

## KETOROLAC TROMETHAMINE

(ke-tor'o-lac)

Acular, Acular LS, Acuvail, SPRIX

**Classifications:** ANALGESIC, NONSTEROIDAL ANTI-INFLAMMATORY DRUG (NSAID); ANTIPYRETIC
**Therapeutic:** NONNARCOTIC ANALGESIC; NSAID
**Prototype:** Ibuprofen

**AVAILABILITY** Tablet; solution for injection; ophthalmic solution; nasal spray

## ACTION & *THERAPEUTIC EFFECT*

It inhibits synthesis of prostaglandins by inhibiting both COX-1 and COX-2 enzymes. Is a peripherally acting analgesic. It inhibits platelet aggregation and prolongs bleeding time. *Exhibits analgesic, anti-inflammatory, and antipyretic activity. Effective in controlling acute postoperative pain.*

**USES** *Short-term* management of pain; ocular itching due to seasonal allergic conjunctivitis, reduction of postoperative pain and photophobia after refractive surgery.

**CONTRAINDICATIONS** Hypersensitivity to ketorolac; hypersensitivity reaction to aspirin, salicylates, or other NSAIDs; major surgery; severe renal impairment or at risk for renal failure due to volume depletion; perioperative use in CABG surgery for 10–14 days after; suspected or confirmed CV bleeding, hemorrhagic diathesis, incomplete hemostasis; patients with risk of bleeding; active or recent GI bleeding; history of GI bleeding or peptic ulcer; pre-op or intraoperatively; exfoliative dermatitis; in combination with other NSAIDs; during labor and delivery; lactation.

**CAUTIOUS USE** Impaired renal or hepatic function; liver disease; Crohn's disease or IBD; bleeding disorders; myelosuppressive chemotherapy, debilitated patients; DM; preexisting asthma; lactase deficiency; coagulation disorders; SLE; CHF; history of hypertension; older adults; pregnancy (category C); lactation. Safe use in children younger than 17 y for all other forms not established.

## ROUTE & DOSAGE

**Pain**

*Adult:* **IV Loading Dose** 30 mg (15 mg if less than 50 kg); **IM** 30–60 mg loading dose, then 15–30 mg q6h [max: 150 mg/day on first day, then 120 mg subsequent days (30 mg load, then 15 mg q6h if less than 50 kg)]; **PO** (continuation of IV/IM therapy) 20 mg initial dose then 10 mg q6h prn (max: 40 mg/day) max duration all routes 5 days
**Nasal Spray** 1 spray q6–8h (max: 8/day)
*Geriatric:* **IV Loading Dose** 15 mg; **IM** 30 mg loading dose, then 15 mg q6h; **PO** 5–10 mg q6h prn (max: 40 mg/day) max duration all routes 5 days
*Child:* **IM** 1 mg/kg (max: 30 mg); **IV** 0.5 mg/kg (max: 15 mg)

K

## ADMINISTRATION

WARNING: Do not administer IV, IM, or PO ketorolac longer than 5 days.

### Oral

- Give with food to reduce GI effects.

### Instillation Ophthalmic

- Do not touch container to the eye when applying ophthalmic drops.

### Intramuscular

- Inject IM drug slowly and deeply into a large muscle.
- Rotate injection sites to avoid injection site pain in patients receiving multiple doses.

### Intravenous

*PREPARE:* **Direct:** Give undiluted. *ADMINISTER:* **Direct:** Give IV bolus dose over at least 15 sec. Preferred method is to give through a Y-tube in a free-flowing IV.

*INCOMPATIBILITIES:* Solution/additive: **Haloperidol, hydroxyzine, meperidine, morphine, prochlorperazine, promethazine.** Y-site: **Acyclovir, amphotericin B, azathioprine, azithromycin, calcium chloride, capsofungin, chlorpromazine, dantrolene, diazepam, diazoxide, diltiazem, diphenhydramine, dobutamine, doxycycline, epirubicin, erythromycin, esmolol, fenoldopam, gemcitabine, gemtuzumab, haloperidol, hydroxyzine, idarubicin, labetalol, levofloxacin, metaraminol, midazolam, milrinone acetate, minocycline, nalbuphine, pantoprazole, papaverine, pentamidine, pentazocine, phentolamine, phenytoin, prochlorperazine, promethazine, protamine, pyridoxine, quinidine, quinupristin/dalfopristin, rocuronium, sulfamethoxazole/trimethoprim, tolazoline, vancomycin, vecuronium, vinorelbine.**

- Store injection at 15°–30° C (59°–86° F).
- Store tablet at 20°–25° C (68°–77° F). Protect from light and humidity.

## ADVERSE EFFECTS (≥1%) CNS:
*Drowsiness,* dizziness, headache. **GI:** *Nausea,* dyspepsia, GI pain, <u>hemorrhage</u>. **Otic:** Tinnitus. **Other:** Edema, sweating, pain at injection site.

## INTERACTIONS Drug: Do not use with other NSAIDs. Do not use with **cidofovir.** May increase **methotrexate** levels and toxicity; do not use with **pentoxifylline.** Herbal: **Feverfew, garlic, ginger, ginkgo** increased bleeding potential.

## PHARMACOKINETICS Peak:
45–60 min. **Distribution:** Into breast milk. **Metabolism:** In liver. **Elimination:** In urine. **Half-Life:** 4–6 h.

## NURSING IMPLICATIONS

### Black Box Warning

*Ketorolac has been associated with increased risk of serious, potentially fatal GI bleeding and cardiovascular events (e.g., MI & CVA); risk may be greater in the older adult and those with risk factors for CV disease. Ketorolac has also been associated with increased risk of bleeding.*

### Assessment & Drug Effects

- Correct hypovolemia prior to administration of ketorolac.
- Monitor urine output in older adults and patients with a history

of cardiac decompensation, renal impairment, heart failure, or liver dysfunction as well as those taking diuretics. Discontinuation of drug will return urine output to pretreatment level.

- Monitor for S&S of GI distress or bleeding including nausea, GI pain, diarrhea, melena, or hematemesis. GI ulceration with perforation can occur anytime during treatment. Drug decreases platelet aggregation and thus may prolong bleeding time.

- Monitor for and report promptly S&S of CV thrombotic events (i.e., angina, MI, TIA, or stroke).

- Monitor for fluid retention and edema in patients with a history of CHF.

- Monitor lab tests: CBC, periodic serum electrolytes and LFTs; urinalysis (for hematuria and proteinuria) with long-term use.

### Patient & Family Education

- Watch for S&S of GI ulceration and bleeding (e.g., bloody emesis, black tarry stools) during long-term therapy.

- Stop taking drug and report promptly to prescriber if you experience chest pain, shortness of breath, weakness, slurring of speech, or other signs of a cardiac or neurologic problem.

- Note: Possible CNS adverse effects (e.g., light-headedness, dizziness, drowsiness).

- Do not drive or engage in potentially hazardous activities until response to drug is known.

- Do not use other NSAIDs while taking this drug.

## KETOTIFEN FUMARATE

(kee-toe-tye'fen)

Zaditor

**See Appendix A-1.**

## LABETALOL HYDROCHLORIDE

(la-bet'a-lole)

Trandate

**Classifications:** ALPHA- & BETA-ADRENERGIC ANTAGONIST; ANTIHYPERTENSIVE

Therapeutic: ANTIHYPERTENSIVE

**Prototype:** Propranolol

**AVAILABILITY** Tablet; solution for injection

### ACTION & *THERAPEUTIC EFFECT*

Acts as an adrenergic receptor blocking agent that combines selective alpha activity and non-selective beta-adrenergic blocking actions. The alpha blockade results in vasodilation, decreased peripheral resistance, and orthostatic hypotension. It has beta-blocking effects on the sinus node, AV node, and ventricular muscle, which lead to bradycardia, delay in AV conduction, and depression of cardiac contractility. *Effective in reducing blood pressure by vasodilation as well as depression of cardiac contractility.*

**USES** Hypertension, hypertensive emergency, preeclampsia.

**CONTRAINDICATIONS** NSAID or salicylate hypersensitivity; bronchial asthma or obstructive airway disease; uncontrolled cardiac failure, heart block (greater than first degree), cardiogenic shock, severe bradycardia; systolic blood pressure less than 100 mm Hg; perioperative CABG pain; abrupt withdrawal; pregnancy (category D third trimester).

**CAUTIOUS USE** Renal disease, renal failure, hepatic disease; well-compensated patients with history of heart failure; CHF; acute MI;

L

Common adverse effects in *italic;* life-threatening effects underlined; generic names in **bold;** classifications in SMALL CAPS; ♣ Canadian drug name; ⊛ Prototype drug

897

coronary artery disease; pheochromocytoma; DM; major surgery; liver dysfunction, jaundice; diabetes mellitus; SLE; myasthenia gravis; PVD; older adults; pregnancy (category C); lactation. Safety and efficacy in children not established.

## ROUTE & DOSAGE

### Hypertension

*Adult:* **PO** 100 mg b.i.d., may gradually increase to 200–400 mg b.i.d. (max: 1200–2400 mg/day); **IV** 20 mg slowly over 2 min, with 40–80 mg q10min if needed up to 300 mg total or 2 mg/min continuous infusion (max: 300 mg total dose)

### Preeclampsia

*Adult/Adolescent:* **IV** Dose based on patient blood pressure, see package insert

## ADMINISTRATION

### Oral

- Give with or immediately after food consistently. Food increases drug bioavailability.

### Intravenous

Note: Amount of IV solution may be changed depending on patient status.

*PREPARE:* **Direct:** Give undiluted. **Continuous:** Dilute 200 mg in 160 mL of D5W, NS, D5/NS, LR, or other compatible IV solution to yield 1 mg/mL; or dilute 200 mg in 250 mL compatible IV fluid to yield approximately 2 mg/3mL.

*ADMINISTER:* **Direct:** Give a 20-mg dose slowly over 2 min. ▪Maximum hypotensive effect occurs 5–15 min after each administration. **Continuous:** Normal rate is 2 mg/min. ▪Controlled infusion pump device is recommended for maintaining accurate flow rate during IV infusion. ▪Keep patient supine when receiving labetalol IV. ▪Take BP immediately before administration. Rate is adjusted according to BP response. ▪Discontinue drug once the desired BP is attained.

*INCOMPATIBILITIES:* **Solution/additive:** Ceftriaxone, sodium bicarbonate, tenecteplase. **Y-site:** Acyclovir, amphotericin B cholesteryl, azathioprine, cangrelor, cefazolin, cefmandole, cefoperazone, cefotetan, cefotexime, cefoxitin, ceftaroline, ceftobiprole, ceftriaxone, cefuroxime, dantrolene, diazepam, diazoxide, furosemide, gemtuzumab, heparin, hydrocortisone, indomethacin, ketorolac, lansoprazole, micafungin, mitomycin, nafcillin, nesiritide, paclitaxel, pantoprazole, penicillin, phenytoin, piperacillin/tazobactam, SMZ/TMP, warfarin.

▪Store at 2°–30° C (36°–86° F) unless otherwise advised. Do not freeze. ▪Protect tablets from moisture.

## ADVERSE EFFECTS (≥1%) CNS:
Dizziness, fatigue/malaise, headache, tremors, transient paresthesias (especially scalp tingling), hypoesthesia (numbness) following IV, mental depression, drowsiness, sleep disturbances, nightmares. **CV:** *Postural hypotension,* angina pectoris, palpitation, bradycardia, syncope, pedal or peripheral edema, pulmonary edema, CHF, flushing, cold extremities, arrhythmias (following IV), paradoxical hypertension (patients with pheochromocytoma). **Special Senses:** Dry

Common adverse effects in *italic;* life-threatening effects underlined; generic names in **bold;** classifications in SMALL CAPS; ✦ Canadian drug name; ◑ Prototype drug eyes, vision disturbances, nasal stuffiness, rhinorrhea. **GI:** Nausea, vomiting, dyspepsia, constipation, diarrhea, taste disturbances, cholestasis with or without jaundice, increases in serum transaminases, dry mouth. **Urogenital:** Acute urinary retention, difficult micturition, impotence, ejaculation failure, loss of libido, Peyronie's disease. **Respiratory:** Dyspnea, <u>bronchospasm</u>. **Skin:** Rashes of various types, increased sweating, pruritus. **Body as a Whole:** Myalgia, muscle cramps, toxic myopathy, antimitochondrial antibodies, positive antinuclear antibodies (ANA), SLE syndrome, pain at IV injection site.

### DIAGNOSTIC TEST INTERFERENCE

False increases in *urinary catecholamines* when measured by *nonspecific trihydroxyindole (THI) reaction* (due to labetalol metabolites) but not with specific *radioenzymatic* or *high-performance liquid chromatography assay techniques*.

### INTERACTIONS Drug: Cimetidine may increase effects of labetalol; **glutethimide** decreases effects of labetalol; **halothane** adds to hypotensive effects; may mask symptoms of hypoglycemia caused by ORAL SULFONYLUREAS, **insulin;** BETA AGONISTS antagonize effects of labetalol.

### PHARMACOKINETICS Absorption: Readily from GI tract, only 25% reaches systemic circulation due to first pass metabolism. **Onset:** 20 min–2 h PO; 2–5 min IV. **Peak:** 1–4 h PO; 5–15 min IV. **Duration:** 8–24 h PO; 2–4 h IV. **Distribution:** Crosses placenta; distributed into breast milk. **Metabolism:** In liver (CYP2D6).

**Elimination:** 60% in urine, 40% in bile. **Half-Life:** 3–8 h.

## NURSING IMPLICATIONS

### Assessment & Drug Effects

- Monitor BP and pulse during dosage adjustment period. Use standing BP as indicator for making dosage adjustments for oral drugs and assessing patient's tolerance of dosage increases. Take after patient stands for 10 min Clarify with prescriber.
- Monitor BP at 5 min intervals for 30 min after IV administration; then at 30 min intervals for 2 h; then hourly for about 6 h; and as indicated thereafter.
- Monitor diabetic patients closely; drug may mask usual cardiovascular response to acute hypoglycemia (e.g., tachycardia).
- Maintain patient in supine position for at least 3 h after IV administration. Then determine patient's ability to tolerate elevated and upright positions before allowing ambulation. Manage this slowly.
- Monitor lab tests: Periodic LFTs.

### Patient & Family Education

- Note: Postural hypotension is most likely to occur during peak plasma levels (i.e., 2–4 h after drug administration).
- Make all position changes slowly and in stages, particularly from lying to upright position. Older adult patients are especially sensitive to hypotensive effects.
- Do not drive or engage in other potentially hazardous activities until response to drug is known.
- Diabetics should closely monitor blood sugar for loss of glycemic control.
- Do not abruptly stop taking this drug. It is usually discontinued gradually.

---

Common adverse effects in *italic;* life-threatening effects <u>underlined</u>; generic names in **bold;** classifications in SMALL CAPS; ♣ Canadian drug name; ⊘ Prototype drug

## LACOSAMIDE
(lac-os'a-mide)

Vimpat

**Classification:** ANTICONVULSANT
Therapeutic ANTICONVULSANT
**Controlled Substance:** Schedule V

**AVAILABILITY** Tablet; oral solution; solution for injection

**ACTION & *THERAPEUTIC EFFECT***
Lacosamide selectively enhances slow inactivation of voltage-gated sodium channels, thus stabilizing hyperexcitable membranes and inhibiting repetitive neuronal firing. *Decreases frequency of partial-onset seizures in those treated with multiple antiepileptic drugs.*

**USES** Adjunctive therapy in the treatment of partial-onset seizures.

**UNLABELED USES** Neuropathic pain.

**CONTRAINDICATIONS** Severe hepatic impairment; suicidal ideation; lactation.

**CAUTIOUS USE** History of multiorgan hypersensitivity reactions; CrCl 30 mL/min or less; renal disease; mild to moderate hepatic impairment; history of suicidal tendencies, history of chronic depression; cardiovascular disease; cardiac conduction problems (e.g., second-degree AV block); myocardial ischemia; heart failure; seizure disorders; diabetic neuropathy; older adults; pregnancy (category C). Safety and efficacy in children younger than 18 y not established.

## ROUTE & DOSAGE

**Partial-Onset Seizures**

*Adult:* **PO or IV** 50 mg b.i.d.; may increase by 100 mg/day qwk to 100–200 mg b.i.d. Note: Patients may be switched from PO to IV (or vice versa) using equivalent doses and administration frequency.

**Hepatic Impairment Dosage Adjustment**

*Mild to moderate impairment:* Max daily dose: 300 mg
*Severe impairment:* Not recommended

**Renal Impairment Dosage Adjustment**

*CrCl less than 30 mL/min:* Max daily dose: 300 mg

## ADMINISTRATION

**Oral**

- Do not abruptly stop medication; it should be withdrawn gradually, over a minimum of 1 wk.
- Store tablets at 15°–30° C (59°–86° F).

**Intravenous**

*PREPARE:* **IV Infusion:** May give undiluted or diluted in NS, D5W, LR.
*ADMINISTER:* **IV Infusion:** Give over 30–60 min.
*INCOMPATIBILITIES:* **Solution/additive:** Do not mix with other drugs.

- May be stored diluted for up to 26 h at 15°–30° C (59°–86° F).

**ADVERSE EFFECTS** (≥1%) **Body as a Whole:** Asthenia, contusion, *fatigue*, gait disturbance, injection site pain and irritation, skin laceration. **CNS:** *Ataxia*, balance

Common adverse effects in *italic;* life-threatening effects <u>underlined</u>; generic names in **bold;** classifications in SMALL CAPS; ✦ Canadian drug name; ⦿ Prototype drug disorder, depression, *dizziness, headache*, memory impairment, nystagmus, somnolence, tremor, vertigo. **GI:** Diarrhea, *nausea*, vomiting. **Skin:** Pruritus. **Special Senses:** *Blurred vision, diplopia*.

## INTERACTIONS **Drug:** May prolong QT interval when given with other drugs known to affect QT interval (e.g., ANTIARRHYTHMICS, **astemizole, bepridil, droperidol**).

## PHARMACOKINETICS **Absorption:** Approximately 100% oral absorption. **Peak:** 1–4 h. **Distribution:** Less than 15% protein bound. **Metabolism:** Hepatic oxidation to less active metabolite. **Elimination:** Primarily fecal (95%). **Half-Life:** 13 h.

## NURSING IMPLICATIONS

### Assessment & Drug Effects

- Monitor for and record all seizure activity.
- Monitor for and report promptly suicidal behavior and ideation.
- Monitor closely patients with known cardiac conduction abnormalities. Baseline and periodic ECGs are recommended
- Monitor older adults for adverse reactions after each upward dose titration. Institute safety precautions as needed to avoid injury from falls.
- Monitor lab tests: Periodic CBC with differential, especially with long-term therapy.

### Patient & Family Education

- Exercise caution with hazardous activities until reaction to drug is known.
- Report promptly feelings of depression, unusual changes in mood or behavior, or thoughts of inflicting harm to self.

- Report bothersome neurologic symptoms such as dizziness, loss of balance, and blurred vision.
- Do not abruptly stop taking this drug. It **must be** tapered off.

# LACTULOSE
(lak′tyoo-lose)
**Cephulac, Chronulac**
**Classifications:** HYPEROSMOTIC LAXATIVE; NEUROLOGIC
Therapeutic: LAXATIVE; AMMONIUM DETOXICANT

**AVAILABILITY** Oral and rectal solution; syrup

## ACTION & *THERAPEUTIC EFFECT*
Reduces blood ammonia by acidifying colon contents, thus retarding diffusion of nonionic ammonia ($NH_3$) from colon to blood while promoting its migration from blood to colon. In the acidic colon, $NH_3$ is converted to nonabsorbable ammonium ions ($NH_4^+$) and is then expelled in feces. *Osmotic effect of lactulose moves water from plasma to intestines, softening stools, and stimulates peristalsis by pressure from water content of stool* Decreases blood ammonia in a patient with hepatic encephalopathy. Effectiveness is marked by improved EEG patterns and mental state (clearing of confusion, apathy, and irritation).

## USES Prevention and treatment of portal-systemic encephalopathy (PSE), including stages of hepatic precoma and coma, and by prescription for relief of chronic constipation.

## UNLABELED USES To restore regular bowel habit posthemorrhoidectomy; to evacuate bowel in older adult patients with severe constipation after barium studies; and for treatment of chronic constipation in children.

Common adverse effects in *italic;* life-threatening effects underlined; generic names in **bold;** classifications in SMALL CAPS; ♦ Canadian drug name; ● Prototype drug

901

**CONTRAINDICATIONS** Low galactose diet.

**CAUTIOUS USE** Diabetes mellitus; concomitant use with electrocautery procedures (proctoscopy, colonoscopy); older adult and debilitated patients; pregnancy (category B); lactation; children.

## ROUTE & DOSAGE

### Prevention and Treatment of Portal-Systemic Encephalopathy

*Adult:* **PO** 30–45 mL t.i.d. or q.i.d. adjusted to produce 2–3 soft stools/day
*Adolescent/Child:* **PO** 40–90 mL/day in divided doses adjusted to produce 2–3 soft stools/day
*Infant:* **PO** 2.5–10 mL/day in 3–4 divided doses adjusted to produce 2–3 soft stools/day

### Management of Acute Portal-Systemic Encephalopathy

*Adult:* **PO** 30–45 mL q1–2h until laxation is achieved, then adjusted to produce 2–3 soft stools/day; **Rectal** 300 mL diluted with 700 mL water given via rectal balloon catheter, and retained for 30–60 min, may repeat in 4–6 h if necessary or until patient can take PO

### Chronic Constipation

*Adult:* **PO** 30–60 mL/day prn
*Child:* **PO** 7.5 mL/day after breakfast

## ADMINISTRATION

### Oral

- Give with fruit juice, water, or milk (if not contraindicated) to increase palatability. Laxative effect is enhanced by taking with ample liquids. Avoid meal times.

### Rectal

- Administer as a retention enema via a rectal balloon catheter. If solution is evacuated too soon, instillation may be promptly repeated.
- Do not freeze. Avoid prolonged exposure to temperatures above 30° C (86° F) or to direct light. Normal darkening does not affect action, but discard solution that is very dark or cloudy.

**ADVERSE EFFECTS** (≥1%) **GI:** Flatulence, borborygmi, belching, abdominal cramps, pain, and distention (initial dose); *diarrhea* (excessive dose); nausea, vomiting, colon accumulation of hydrogen gas; hypernatremia.

**INTERACTIONS Drug:** LAXATIVES may incorrectly suggest therapeutic action of lactulose.

**PHARMACOKINETICS Absorption:** Poorly absorbed from GI tract. **Metabolism:** In gut by intestinal bacteria.

## NURSING IMPLICATIONS

### Assessment & Drug Effects

- In children if the initial dose causes diarrhea, dosage is reduced immediately. Discontinue if diarrhea persists.
- Promote fluid intake (1500–2000 mL/day or greater) during drug therapy for constipation; older adults often self-limit liquids. Lactulose-induced osmotic changes in the bowel support intestinal water loss and potential hypernatremia. Discuss strategy with prescriber.

### Patient & Family Education

- Laxative action is not instituted until drug reaches the colon; therefore, about 24–48 h is needed.
- Do not self-medicate with another laxative due to slow onset of drug action.

Common adverse effects in *italic;* life-threatening effects <u>underlined</u>; generic names in **bold;** classifications in SMALL CAPS; ♣ Canadian drug name; ℗ Prototype drug

- Notify prescriber if diarrhea (i.e., more than 2 or 3 soft stools/day) persists more than 24–48 h. Diarrhea is a sign of overdosage. Dose adjustment may be indicated.

# LAMIVUDINE ⓟ
(lam-i-vu'deen)
Epivir, Epivir-HBV, Heptovir ♦
**Classifications:** ANTIRETROVIRAL; NUCLEOSIDE REVERSE TRANSCRIPTASE INHIBITOR (NRTI)
Therapeutic: ANTIRETROVIRAL; NRTI

**AVAILABILITY** Tablet; oral solution

**ACTION & *THERAPEUTIC EFFECT***
Lamivudine is a synthetic nucleoside analog reverse transcriptase inhibitor. It inhibits the transcription of the HIV viral RNA chain as well as the hepatitis B viral RNA chain. *Antiviral action is effective against HIV viruses and hepatitis B (HBV) viral infections.*

**USES** HIV infection in combination with other retroviral agents; treatment of chronic hepatitis B.

**CONTRAINDICATIONS** Hypersensitivity to lamivudine; lactic acidosis; severe hepatomegaly; exacerbation of hepatitis B; immune reconstitution syndrome; lactation.

**CAUTIOUS USE** Renal impairment, renal failure; diabetes mellitus; obesity; pregnancy (category C).

## ROUTE & DOSAGE

**HIV Infection**
*Adult/Adolescent/Child (25 kg or more):* **Epivir PO** 150 mg b.i.d. or 300 mg daily
*Child (20–24 kg):* **PO** 75 mg in morning and 150 mg in evening

*Infant/Child (3 mo or older):*
**Epivir PO** 4 mg/kg b.i.d. (max: 150 mg b.i.d.)

**Renal Impairment Dosage Adjustment**
*CrCl 30–49 mL/min:* 150 mg daily; *15–29 mL/min:* 150 mg first dose, then 100 mg daily; *5–14 mL/min:* 150 mg first dose, then 50 mg daily; *less than 5 mL/min:* 50 mg first dose, then 25 mg daily

**Chronic Hepatitis B**
*Adult:* **Epivir-HBV PO** 100 mg daily
*Adolescent/Child (2–16 y):* **PO** 4 mg/kg b.i.d. (max: 150 mg)

**Renal Impairment Dosage Adjustment**
*CrCl 30–49 mL/min:* 100 mg first dose, then 50 mg daily; *15–29 mL/min:* 100 mg first dose, then 25 mg daily; *5–14 mL/min:* 35 mg first dose, then 15 mg daily; *less than 5 mL/min:* 35 mg first dose, then 10 mg daily

## ADMINISTRATION

**Oral**
- May be administered without regard to meals.
- Give Epivir b.i.d. in combination with AZT. The recommended dose for adults who weigh less than 50 kg (110 lb) is 2 mg/kg. Give Epivir-HBV daily; **do not** give in combination with AZT.
- Store solution at 20 °–25° C (68°–77° F) tightly closed.

**ADVERSE EFFECTS** (≥1%) **CNS:** *Neuropathy, insomnia,* sleep disorders, *dizziness,* depression, *headache,* fatigue, *fever, chills.* **GI:** *Nausea, diarrhea,* vomiting, sore

L

throat, anorexia, abdominal pain, cramps, dyspepsia, pancreatitis, increased LFTs (ALT, amylase), hepatomegaly with steatosis. **Hematologic:** Neutropenia, anemia, thrombocytopenia. **Musculoskeletal:** Myalgia, arthralgia, malaise, pain. **Skin:** Rash. **Respiratory:** Nasal symptoms, cough. **Metabolic:** Lactic acidosis.

**INTERACTIONS Drug:** Do not use with other drugs containing **emtricitabine.** Avoid **zalcitabine.** Increases the $C_{max}$ of **zidovudine.** **Trimethoprim-sulfamethoxazole** increases serum levels of lamivudine. Increased risk of lactic acidosis in combination with other REVERSE TRANSCRIPTASE INHIBITORS and ANTIRETROVIRAL AGENTS. **Herbal:** Do not use with **echinacea.**

**PHARMACOKINETICS Absorption:** Rapidly absorbed from GI tract (86% reaches systemic circulation). **Distribution:** Low binding to plasma proteins. **Metabolism:** Minimal. **Elimination:** Excreted primarily unchanged in urine. **Half-Life:** 2–4 h.

**NURSING IMPLICATIONS**

**Black Box Warning**

*Lamivudine has been associated with severe, potentially fatal, lactic acidosis, hepatomegaly with steatosis, and exacerbations of hepatitis B.*

**Assessment & Drug Effects**

- Monitor children closely for S&S of hepatic dysfunction, lactic acidosis (see metabolic acidosis Appendix F), and pancreatitis; if they occur, immediately stop drug and notify prescriber.
- Monitor for and report all significant adverse reactions.
- Monitor lab tests: Periodic CBC with differential, renal function

tests, LFTs, and serum amylase throughout therapy.

**Patient & Family Education**

- Report any of the following immediately: Nausea, vomiting, anorexia, abdominal pain, jaundice.
- Note: The drug may cause redistribution or accumulation of body fat and the long-term effect of these conditions are unknown.

# LAMOTRIGINE

(la-mo′tri-geen)
Lamictal, Lamictal CD, Lamictal XR
**Classification:** ANTICONVULSANT
**Therapeutic:** ANTICONVULSANT

**AVAILABILITY** Tablet; chewable tablet; orally disintegrating tablet; extended release tablet

**ACTION & *THERAPEUTIC EFFECT*** May act by inhibiting the release of glutamate and aspartate, excitatory neurotransmitters at voltage-sensitive sodium channels, resulting in decreased seizure activity in the brain. This stabilizes neuronal membranes. *Effectiveness is measured by decreasing seizure activity.*

**USES** Adjunctive therapy for partial seizures. Generalized tonic–clonic, grand mal, or myoclonic seizures in adults, treatment of bipolar disorder (immediate release only).

**UNLABELED USES** Absence seizures, prevention of migraines.

**CONTRAINDICATIONS** Hypersensitivity to lamotrigine, development of any skin rash unless it is clearly not related to the drug; multiorganic hypersensitivity reactions;

acute mania; suicidal ideation especially if severe or abrupt in onset; aseptic meningitis; lactation. **Extended release:** not approved for children younger than 13 y.

**CAUTIOUS USE** Renal insufficiency, bipolar disorder, history of suicidal tendencies, CHF, cardiac or liver function impairment; severe renal impairment; moderate to severe hepatic impairment; older adults; pregnancy (category C); lactation. Safety and efficacy in acute treatment of a mood episode not established. Safety and efficacy in children with a mood disorder who are younger than 16 y not established. Safety and efficacy for treatment of seizures in children younger than 2 y not established.

## ROUTE & DOSAGE

### Partial Seizures, Patients Receiving Anticonvulsants Other Than Valproic Acid

*Adult/Adolescent:* **PO** Start with 50 mg daily for 2 wk, then 50 mg b.i.d. for 2 wk, may titrate up to 300–500 mg/day in 2 divided doses (max: 700 mg/day)
*Child (2–12 y):* **PO** 0.3 mg/kg/day in divided doses × 2 wk, then 0.6 mg/kg/day in divided doses × 2 wk (max: 15 mg/kg/day or 400 mg/day)

### Partial Seizures, Patients Receiving Valproic Acid

*Adult:* **PO** Start with 25 mg every other day for 2 wk, then 25 mg daily for 2 wk, may titrate up to 150 mg/day in 2 divided doses (max: 200 mg/day)
*Child (2–16 y):* **PO** 0.15 mg/kg/day in divided doses × 2 wk, then

increase to 0.3 mg/kg/day in divided doses × 2 wk (max: 5 mg/kg/day or 250 mg/day)

### Bipolar Disorder, Patients Not Receiving Valproate or Carbamazepine

*Adult:* **PO** Start with 25 mg daily for 2 wk, then 50 mg daily for 2 wk, then 100 mg/day for 1 wk, then 200 mg daily

### Bipolar Disorder, Patients Receiving Valproic Acid

*Adult/Adolescent (16 y or older):* **PO** Start with 25 mg every other day for 2 wk, then 25 mg daily for 2 wk, then 50 mg daily for 1 wk, then 100 mg daily

### Bipolar Disorder, Patients Receiving Carbamazepine

*Adult/Adolescent (16 y or older):* **PO** Start with 50 mg daily for 2 wk, then 50 mg b.i.d. for 2 wk, then 100 b.i.d. for 1 wk, then 150 mg b.i.d. for 1 wk, then 200 mg b.i.d.

### Hepatic Impairment Dosage Adjustment

Reduce dose by 25%

### Severe Hepatic Impairment and Ascites Dosage Adjustment

Reduce dose by 50%

## ADMINISTRATION

### Oral

- *Orally disintegrating tablet (ODT)* should be placed on the tongue and moved around the mouth. It will rapidly disintegrate. It may be swallowed with/without water or food.
- Ensure that *chewable tablets* are chewed or crushed before being swallowed with a liquid.
- *Chewable dispersible tablets* may be swallowed whole, chewed, or mixed in water or diluted juice.

Common adverse effects in *italic;* life-threatening effects underlined; generic names in **bold;** classifications in SMALL CAPS; ♣ Canadian drug name; ⊘ Prototype drug

905

- When discontinued, drug should be tapered off gradually over a 2-wk period, unless patient safety is at risk.

## ADVERSE EFFECTS (≥1%) CNS:
*Dizziness, ataxia, somnolence, headache,* aphasia, vertigo, confusion, slurred speech, irritability, depression, incoordination, hostility. **GI:** *Nausea,* vomiting, anorexia, abdominal pain, diarrhea, dyspepsia, constipation. **CV:** Chest pain, edema. **Urogenital:** Hematuria, dysmenorrhea, vaginitis. **Special Senses:** *Diplopia, blurred vision.* **Musculoskeletal:** Peripheral neuropathy, chills, tremor, arthralgia. **Skin:** Rash (including <u>Stevens–Johnson syndrome, toxic epidermal necrolysis</u>), urticaria, pruritus, alopecia, acne. **Respiratory:** *Rhinitis,* pharyngitis, cough.

## INTERACTIONS **Drug: Carbamazepine, phenobarbital, primidone, phenytoin, fosphenytoin, rifampin,** ORAL CONTRACEPTIVES may decrease lamotrigine levels. **Valproic acid** may increase risk of serious rash. Lamotrigine may decrease serum levels of **valproic acid.** May affect efficacy of ORAL CONTRACEPTIVES. Chronic **acetaminophen** use may affect serum concentrations of lamotrigine. **Herbal: Ginkgo** may decrease anticonvulsant effectiveness. **Evening primrose** oil may affect seizure threshold.

## PHARMACOKINETICS **Absorption:** Readily from GI tract; 98% reaches systemic circulation. **Onset:** 12 wk. **Peak:** 1–4 h. **Distribution:** 55% protein bound; crosses placenta; distributed into breast milk. **Metabolism:** In liver to inactive metabolite. **Elimination:** Can induce own metabolism; excreted in urine. **Half-Life:** 25–30 h.

## NURSING IMPLICATIONS

### Black Box Warning

*Lamotrigine has been associated with severe, potentially fatal, rashes especially during wk 2–8 of therapy.*

### Assessment & Drug Effects
- Withhold drug if rash develops and immediately report to prescriber.
- Monitor the plasma levels of lamotrigine and other anticonvulsants when given concomitantly.
- Monitor patients with bipolar disorder for worsening of their symptoms and suicidal ideation. Withhold the drug and immediately report to prescriber.
- Monitor for adverse reactions when lamotrigine is used with other anticonvulsants, especially valproic acid.
- Be aware of drug interactions and closely monitor when interacting drugs are added or discontinued.

### Patient & Family Education
- Do not take drug if a skin rash develops. Contact your prescriber immediately.
- Notify prescriber for any of the following: Worsening seizure control, skin rash, ataxia, blurred vision or diplopia, fever or flu-like symptoms.
- Do not drive or engage in other potentially hazardous activities until response to the drug is known.
- Use protection from sunlight or ultraviolet light until tolerance is known; drug increases photosensitivity.
- Women using oral contraceptives to avoid pregnancy should add a barrier contraceptive.

Common adverse effects in *italic;* life-threatening effects <u>underlined</u>; generic names in **bold;** classifications in SMALL CAPS; ✦ Canadian drug name; ⊘ Prototype drug

- Schedule periodic ophthalmologic exams with long-term use.
- Do not discontinue abruptly.

# LANSOPRAZOLE

(lan'so-pra-zole)
Prevacid, Prevacid 24 HR

# DEXLANSOPRAZOLE

DexiLant

**Classifications:** ANTISECRETORY; PROTON PUMP INHIBITOR
**Therapeutic:** ANTIULCER; ANTISECRETORY
**Prototype:** Omeprazole

**AVAILABILITY** Sustained release capsule; orally disintegrating tablet; **Dexlansoprazole (delayed release):** Capsule

**ACTION & THERAPEUTIC EFFECT** Suppresses gastric acid secretion by inhibiting the $H^+$, $K^+$-ATPase enzyme [the acid (proton $H^+$) pump] in the parietal cells. *Suppresses gastric acid formation in the stomach.*

**USES** Short-term treatment of duodenal ulcer (up to 4 wk) and erosive esophagitis (up to 8 wk), pathologic hypersecretory disorders, gastric ulcers; in combination with antibiotics for *Helicobacter pylori*. Gastroesophageal reflux disease (GERD).

**UNLABELED USES** Stress gastritis prophylaxis.

**CONTRAINDICATIONS** Hypersensitivity to lansoprazole or dexlansoprazole; proton pump inhibitors (PPIs) hypersensitivity; lactation.

**CAUTIOUS USE** Hepatic impairment; gastric malignancy; older adults; pregnancy (category B), infants.

## ROUTE & DOSAGE

### Duodenal Ulcer
*Adult:* **PO** 15 mg once daily × 4 wk (treatment) or longer (maintenance)

### Erosive Esophagitis
*Adult:* **PO** 30 mg once daily × 8 wk, then decrease to 15 mg once daily; **(dexlansoprazole)** 60 mg daily

### GERD
*Adult/Adolescent:* **PO** 15 mg once daily for up to 8 wk
*Child (1–11 y, weight 30 kg or greater):* **PO** 30 mg daily; *weight less than 30 kg:* 15 mg daily (max: 30 mg/day)

### Hypersecretory Disorder
*Adult:* **PO** 60 mg once daily (max: 120 mg/day in divided doses), may need to be adjusted for hepatic impairment; **(dexlansoprazole)** 30 mg daily

### NSAID-Associated Gastric Ulcer
*Adult:* **PO** 30 mg daily for up to 8 wk

### H. pylori
*Adult:* **PO** 30 mg b.i.d. × 2 wk, in combination with antibiotics

### Hepatic Impairment Dosage Adjustment
*Severe hepatic disease (Child-Pugh class C):* Reduce dose (max: 30 mg/day **dexlansoprazole**)

### Healing Erosive Esophagitis (Dexlansoprazole)
*Adult:* **PO** 60 mg daily for up to 8 wk

### Maintenance of Healed Erosive Esophagitis (Dexlansoprazole)
*Adult:* **PO** 30 mg daily

### Non-Erosive GERD (Dexlansoprazole)
*Adult:* **PO** 30 mg daily for 4 wk

L

---

Common adverse effects in *italic;* life-threatening effects <u>underlined</u>; generic names in **bold;** classifications in SMALL CAPS; ♣ Canadian drug name; ⊙ Prototype drug

## ADMINISTRATION

### Oral

- *All forms:* Administer dosage 30 min a.c. Give once daily dose before breakfast.
- Give at least 30 min prior to any concurrent sucralfate therapy.
- Do not crush or chew capsules. Capsules can be opened and granules sprinkled on food or mixed with 40 mL of apple juice and administered through an NG tube. Do not crush or chew granules.
- Note: Disintegrating tablets contain phenylalanine and should not be used for patients with PKU. Capsule and syrup formulations do not contain phenylalanine.

## ADVERSE EFFECTS (≥1%) CNS:
Fatigue, dizziness, headache. **GI:** Nausea, *diarrhea,* constipation, anorexia, increased appetite, thirst, elevated serum transaminases (AST, ALT). **Skin:** Rash.

## INTERACTIONS Drug: May decrease **theophylline** levels. **Sucralfate** decreases lansoprazole bioavailability. May interfere with absorption of **ketoconazole, digoxin, ampicillin,** or IRON SALTS. Use with **warfarin** may increase INR. May alter **tacrolimus** concentration. **Food:** Food reduces peak lansoprazole levels by 50%.

## PHARMACOKINETICS Absorption: Rapidly from GI tract after leaving stomach. **Onset:** Acid reduction within 2 h; ulcer relief within 1 wk. **Peak:** 1.5–3 h. Dexlansoprazole has 2 peaks, at 1–2 h then at 4–5 h. **Duration:** 24 h. **Distribution:** 97% bound to plasma proteins. **Metabolism:** In liver via CYP2C19 and 3A4. **Elimination:** 14–25% in urine; part of dose eliminated in bile and feces. **Half-Life:** 1.5 h.

## NURSING IMPLICATIONS

### Assessment & Drug Effects

- Monitor for therapeutic effectiveness of concurrently used drugs that require an acid medium for absorption (e.g., digoxin, ampicillin, ketoconazole).
- Monitor lab tests: Periodic CBC, renal function tests, LFTs, and serum gastric levels.

### Patient & Family Education

- Inform prescriber of significant diarrhea.

## LANTHANUM CARBONATE
(lan-tha′num)

Fosrenol

**Classifications:** ELECTROLYTE AND WATER BALANCE AGENT; PHOSPHATE BINDER
**Therapeutic:** PHOSPHATE BINDER
**Prototype:** Sevelamer hydrochloride

## AVAILABILITY Chewable tablet

## ACTION & *THERAPEUTIC EFFECT*
Lanthanum is used for the management of hyperphosphatemia in end-stage renal disease; it is a calcium/aluminum-free phosphate binding agent. It has a higher affinity for binding to phosphate than calcium or aluminum. Low systemic absorption minimizes the risk of aluminum intoxication and hypercalcemia. Lanthanum decreases phosphate absorption from the diet. *Lowers serum phosphate.*

## USES Reduce serum phosphate levels in patients with end-stage renal disease.

## CONTRAINDICATIONS Prior hypersensitivity to lanthanum carbonate, lactation.

**CAUTIOUS USE** Bowel obstruction, Crohn's disease, acute peptic ulcer, ulcerative colitis; pregnancy (category B); children younger than 18 y.

## ROUTE & DOSAGE

**Hyporphosphatemia**

*Adult:* **PO** 1500 mg daily in divided doses then titrate to serum phosphate less than 6 mg/dL

## ADMINISTRATION

**Oral**
- Give with or immediately after a meal.
- Tablets **must be** chewed completely before swallowing. Whole tablets should not be swallowed
- Store at 15°–30° C (59°–86° F).

## ADVERSE EFFECTS (≥1%) CNS:
Headache. **CV:** Hypotension **GI:** *Nausea, vomiting, diarrhea,* abdominal pain, constipation. **Respiratory:** Bronchitis, rhinitis. **Other:** Dialysis graft occlusion.

## PHARMACOKINETICS **Absorption:** Minimal from GI tract. **Metabolism:** Not metabolized. **Elimination:** In feces. **Half-Life:** 53 h.

## NURSING IMPLICATIONS

**Assessment & Drug Effects**
- Monitor for dialysis graft occlusion, as lanthanum therapy may increase occlusion risk.
- Monitor lab tests: Serum phosphate levels during dosage titration and regularly throughout treatment; periodic serum calcium, bicarbonate, and chloride.

**Patient & Family Education**
- Chew chewable tablets completely, then swallow.

- Report promptly any of the following: Headache, drowsiness, dizziness, fainting, confusion, irritability, nausea, vomiting, or loss of appetite.

## LAPATINIB DITOSYLATE
(la-pa'ti-nib di-toe'si-late)
Tykerb
**Classifications:** BIOLOGICAL RESPONSE MODIFIER; ANTINEOPLASTIC; EPIDERMAL GROWTH FACTOR RECEPTOR; KINASE INHIBITOR
Therapeutic: ANTINEOPLASTIC
**Prototype:** Erlotinib

## AVAILABILITY Tablet

## ACTION & THERAPEUTIC EFFECT
An inhibitor of intracellular tyrosine kinase domains of both epidermal growth factor receptors [EGFR (ErbB1) and HER2 (ErbB2)] required for cell proliferation of certain breast cancers. *Inhibits ErbB-driven tumor cell growth in those who are positive for the HER2 receptor.*

## USES Treatment of advanced or metastatic breast cancer in patients whose tumor overexpresses the human epidermal receptor type 2 (HER2) protein and who have received prior therapy.

## CONTRAINDICATIONS Hypersensitivity to lapatinib, capecitabine, doxifluridine, 5-FU; decreased left ventricular ejection fraction (LVEF) of grade 1, that is below lower limits of normal (LLN); jaundice; severe hepatotoxicity to drug; development of interstitial lung disease or pneumonitis of at least Grade 3; hypokalemia, hypomagnesemia; females of childbearing age; pregnancy (category D); lactation.

L

---

Common adverse effects in *italic*; life-threatening effects <u>underlined</u>; generic names in **bold**; classifications in SMALL CAPS; ♣ Canadian drug name; ⊘ Prototype drug

909

# LAPATINIB DITOSYLATE

**CAUTIOUS USE** Moderate to severe hepatic impairment; coronary artery disease; angina, cardiac arrhythmias, congenital $QT_c$ prolongation syndrome. Safe use in children younger than 18 y not established.

## ROUTE & DOSAGE

### Breast Cancer (HER2-Positive Metastatic)

*Adult:* **PO** 1250 mg daily on days 1– 21 with capecitabine 2000 mg/m²/day q12h on days 1–14; repeat in 21-day cycle.
*Postmenopausal women:* **PO** 1500 mg/day with letrozole 2.5 mg/day

### Breast Cancer (Hormone Receptor–Positive, HER2-Positive Metastatic)

*Adult:* **PO** 1500 mg daily in combination with letrozole

### Hepatic Impairment Dosage Adjustment

*Severe hepatic impairment (Child-Pugh class C):* Reduce dose

### Toxicity Dosage Adjustment

*Grade 2 or more (excluding cardiac):* Discontinue and restart at standard dose when toxicity improves to Grade 1
*Decreased left ventricular ejection fraction:* Discontinue treatment for at least 2 wk
*Diarrhea:* Interrupt therapy; reintroduce at lower rate.

## ADMINISTRATION
### Oral

- Give lapatinib at least 1 h before/after a meal.
- Give capecitabine with food or within 30 min after food.

- Note that concurrent use with strong CYP3A4 inhibitors/inducers should be avoided (see Drug Interactions). If concurrent use is necessary, dosage adjustments are required.
- Store at 15°–30° C (59°–86° F) in a tightly closed container.

**ADVERSE EFFECTS** (≥1%) **CNS:** Insomnia, *fatigue.* **CV:** QT prolongation. **GI:** *Diarrhea,* dyspepsia, mucosal inflammation, *nausea,* stomatitis, *vomiting.* **Hematologic:** Neutropenia, <u>thrombocytopenia</u>. **Metabolic:** Elevated ALT and AST levels, hyperbilirubinemia. **Musculoskeletal:** Back pain, pain in extremities. **Respiratory:** Dyspnea, pneumonitis. **Skin:** Dry skin, *palmar-plantar erythrodysesthesia, rash.*

**INTERACTIONS Drug:** INHIBITORS OF CYP3A4 (**ketoconazole, clarithromycin, atazanavir, indinavir, nefazodone, nelfinavir, ritonavir, saquinavir, telithromycin, voriconazole**) will increase lapatinib plasma level. INDUCERS OF CYP3A4 (**dexamethasone, phenytoin, carbamazepine, rifampin, rifabutin, rifapentine, phenobarbital**) will decrease lapatinib plasma level. Lapatinib can increase plasma levels of **theophylline** and **warfarin**. **Food: Grapefruit juice** may increase the plasma level of lapatinib; co-administration with food increases lapatinib plasma levels. **Herbal: St. John's wort** will decrease plasma levels of lapatinib.

**PHARMACOKINETICS Peak:** 4 h. **Distribution:** 9% plasma protein bound. **Metabolism:** Extensive hepatic metabolism. **Elimination:** Fecal (major) and renal (minor). **Half-Life:** 24 h.

Common adverse effects in *italic;* life-threatening effects <u>underlined;</u> generic names in **bold;** classifications in SMALL CAPS; ♣ Canadian drug name; ⊙ Prototype drug

# NURSING IMPLICATIONS

## Black Box Warning

*Lapatinib has been associated with severe, potentially fatal, hepatotoxocity.*

### Assessment & Drug Effects

- Prior to initiating therapy, hypokalemia and hypomagnesemia should be corrected.
- Monitor cardiac status (i.e., LV ejection fraction, ECG with QT measurement) throughout therapy.
- Monitor for and report severe diarrhea as it may cause dehydration and serious electrolyte imbalances.
- Withhold drug and notify prescriber if changes in LFTs parameters are significant and/or S&S of hepatotoxicity appear (see Appendix F).
- Monitor for theophylline and warfarin toxicity with concurrent use.
- Monitor lab tests: Baseline and periodic serum electrolytes; baseline and q4–6 wk LFTs; periodic CBC with differential and platelet count, Hgb, Hct.

### Patient & Family Education

- Adhere to directions regarding medication and food.
- Report promptly any of the following: Palpitations, shortness of breath, severe diarrhea.
- Do not eat grapefruit or drink grapefruit juice while taking lapatinib.
- Do not take St. John's wort or OTC medications for stomach ulcers while taking lapatinib unless approved by the prescriber.
- Women are advised to use effective means of contraception while taking lapatinib.

# LATANOPROST ⊙

(la-tan'o-prost)

Xalatan

**Classifications:** EYE PREPARATION; PROSTAGLANDIN
**Therapeutic:** PROSTAGLANDIN

## AVAILABILITY Ophthalmic solution

## ACTION & *THERAPEUTIC EFFECT*

Prostaglandin analog that is thought to reduce intraocular pressure (IOP) by increasing the outflow of aqueous humor. *Reduces elevated intraocular pressure in patients with open-angle glaucoma.*

## USES Treatment of open-angle glaucoma, ocular hypertension, and elevated intraocular pressure (IOP).

## CONTRAINDICATIONS Hypersensitivity to latanoprost, benzalkonium chloride, or another component in the solution.

## CAUTIOUS USE Active intraocular inflammation such as iritis or uveitis; ocular disease; patients at risk for macular edema; history of or active herpes simplex keratitis; hepatic or renal impairment; contact lens wearers; pregnancy (category C); lactation. Safety and efficacy in children not established.

## ROUTE & DOSAGE

### Glaucoma

*Adult:* **Ophthalmic** 1 drop in affected eye(s) daily in evening

## ADMINISTRATION

### Installation

- Ensure that contact lenses are removed prior to installation and not reinserted for 15 min after installation.
- Apply only to affected eye(s). Ensure that only one drop is instilled.

---

Common adverse effects in *italic;* life-threatening effects underlined; generic names in **bold;** classifications in SMALL CAPS; ♣ Canadian drug name; ⊙ Prototype drug

- Do not allow tip of dropper to touch eye.
- Wait at least 5 min before/after instillation of other eyedrops.
- Refrigerate at 2°–8° C (36°–46° F). Protect from light. Once opened, the container may be stored at room temperature up to 25° C (77° F) for 6 wk.

**ADVERSE EFFECTS** (≥1%) **Body as a Whole:** Headache, asthenia, flu-like symptoms. **GI:** Abnormal liver function tests. **Skin:** Rash. **Special Senses:** *Conjunctival hyperemia, growth of eyelashes, ocular pruritus,* ocular dryness, visual disturbance, ocular burning, *foreign body sensation,* eye pain, pigmentation of the periocular skin, blepharitis, cataract, superficial punctate keratitis, eyelid erythema, ocular irritation, eyelash darkening, eye discharge, tearing, photophobia, allergic conjunctivitis, increases in iris pigmentation (brown pigment), conjunctival edema.

**INTERACTIONS Drug:** Precipitation may occur if mixed with eyedrops containing **thimerosal;** space other EYE PREPARATIONS at least 5 min apart.

**PHARMACOKINETICS Absorption:** Absorbed through the cornea. **On-set:** 3–4 h. **Peak IOP Reduction:** 8–12 h. **Distribution:** Minimal systemic distribution. **Metabolism:** Hydrolyzed in aqueous humor to active form. **Elimination:** Renally excreted. **Half-Life:** 17 min.

## NURSING IMPLICATIONS

### Assessment & Drug Effects

- Withhold eyedrops and notify prescriber if acute intraocular inflammation (iritis or uveitis) or external eye inflammation are noted.
- Note that increased pigmentation of the iris and eyelid, and additional growth of eyelashes on the treated

eye are adverse effects that may develop gradually over months to years.

### Patient & Family Education

- Contact prescriber immediately if any ocular reaction occurs, especially conjunctivitis and lid reactions.
- Note: Increased pigmentation of the iris and eyelid, and additional growth of eyelashes on the treated eye, are possible adverse effects of this drug. Persons with light colored eyes receiving treatment to one eye may develop a darker eye.

# LEDIPASVIR AND SOFOSBUVIR
(le-di-pas′vir and so-fos′bu-vir)

Harvoni

**Classifications:** ANTIVIRAL; DIRECT-ACTING ANTIVIRAL; VIRAL PROTEIN INHIBITOR; ANTIHEPATITIS
Therapeutic: ANTIHEPATITIS

**AVAILABILITY** Tablet

## ACTION & *THERAPEUTIC EFFECT*
Ledipasvir inhibits a protein (HCV NS5A) necessary for viral replication. Sofosbuvir is a prodrug converted to its active form (GS-461203) which inhibits an enzyme (S5B RNA-dependent RNA polymerase), essential for viral replication. *Inhibits replication of the HCV virus.*

**USES** Treatment of chronic hepatitis C (CHC) genotype 1 infection in adults.

**CAUTIOUS USE** Concurrent use of potent P-gp inducers (e.g., rifampin, St. John's wort) or amiodarone in combination with an additional direct-acting antihepaciviral agent.

## ROUTE & DOSAGE

### Chronic Hepatitis C Infection
*Adult:* 1 tablet (90 mg ledipasvir/ 400 mg sofosbuvir) once daily for 12–24 wk

Common adverse effects in *italic;* life-threatening effects <u>underlined</u>; generic names in **bold;** classifications in SMALL CAPS; ♣ Canadian drug name; ⊘ Prototype drug

## ADMINISTRATION

### Oral

- May be given without regard to food.
- Store below 30° C (86° F).

## ADVERSE EFFECTS (≥3%) CNS:
*Fatigue, headache,* insomnia. **GI:**
Diarrhea, nausea. **Metabolic:** Elevated lipase, increased bilirubin.

## INTERACTIONS Drug: Ledipasvir may increase the levels of other drugs that require P-gp or breast cancer resistance protein (BCRP). P-gp inducers (e.g., rifampin) may decrease the levels of ledipasvir and sofosbuvir. ANTACIDS, H₂-RECEPTOR ANTAGONISTS, and PROTON PUMP INHIBITORS may decrease the levels of ledipasvir. **Carbamazepine, oxcarbazepine, phenobarbital, phenytoin,** RIFAMYCINS, **ritonavir,** and **tipranavir** may decrease the levels of ledipasvir and sofosbuvir. **Simeprevir** may increase the levels of ledipasvir and sofosbuvir. Ledipasvir and sofosbuvir may increase the levels of **digoxin, rosuvastatin,** and **tenofovir. Herbal: St John's wort** may decrease the levels of ledipasvir and sofosbuvir.

## PHARMACOKINETICS
**Peak:** Ledipasvir: 4–4.5 h.; sofosbuvir: 0.8–1 h. **Distribution:** Ledipasvir greater than 99.8% plasma protein bound; sofosbuvir is 61–65% plasma protein bound. **Metabolism:** Minimal for ledipasvir; extensive for sofosbuvir (required for formation of active metabolite). **Elimination:** Primarily fecal (86%) for ledipasvir; primarily renal (80%) for sofosbuvir. **Half-Life:** Ledipasvir, 47 h.; sofosbuvir, 27 h. (active metabolite).

## NURSING IMPLICATIONS

### Assessment & Drug Effects
- Monitor ECG during first 48 h of treatment when used in combination with amiodarone and another hepatitis C direct-acting antiviral or in patients who discontinued amiodarone just prior to initiating sofosbuvir in combination with a direct-acting anti-hepaciviral.
- Monitor lab tests: Baseline and periodic LFTs and serum creatinine; baseline and periodic serum HCV-RNA, and repeat at end of treatment and during followup.

### Patient & Family Education
- Do not take OTC drugs without consulting prescriber.
- Check heart rate daily during the first 2 wk of treatment. Report promptly if outside of the parameters set by prescriber.
- Do not breast-feed without consulting prescriber.

# LEFLUNOMIDE
(le-flu'no-mide)

Arava

**Classifications:** BIOLOGIC RESPONSE MODIFIER; IMMUNOMODULATOR; ANTI-INFLAMMATORY
**Therapeutic:** DISEASE-MODIFYING ANTIRHEUMATIC DRUG (DMARD)

## AVAILABILITY Tablet

## ACTION & *THERAPEUTIC EFFECT*
An immunomodulator that demonstrates anti-inflammatory effects. Suppression of pyrimidine synthesis in T and B lymphocytes interferes with RNA and protein synthesis in cells that are involved in the inflammatory process within affected joints. This reduces cytokine and antibody-mediated destruction of the synovial joints by decreasing the inflammatory process. *Reduces the S&S of rheumatoid arthritis (RA), retards structural joint damage, and improves physical function.*

**USES** Active RA.

**UNLABELED USES** Juvenile idiopathic arthritis, psoriasis.

**CONTRAINDICATIONS** Hepatic disease; jaundice; lactase deficiency; hypersensitivity to leflunomide; patients with positive hepatitis B or C serology; malignancy, particularly lymphoproliferative disorders; severe immunosuppression; vaccination, infants; uncontrolled infection; pregnancy (category X); lactation.

**CAUTIOUS USE** Renal insufficiency; renal failure; hepatic impairment; alcoholism; immunosuppression; lactase deficiency; infection. Use in children younger than 18 y has not been fully studied.

## ROUTE & DOSAGE

### Rheumatoid Arthritis

*Adult:* **PO** Initiate with a loading dose of 100 mg/day × 3 days, then maintenance dose of 20 mg daily, may decrease to 10 mg/day if higher dose is not tolerated

## ADMINISTRATION

### Oral
- Initiate with a 3-day loading dose followed by a lower maintenance dose.

**ADVERSE EFFECTS** (≥1%) **Body as a Whole:** Allergic reaction, asthenia, flu-like syndrome, infection, pain, back pain, arthralgia, leg cramps, synovitis, tenosynovitis. **CNS:** Dizziness, headache, paresthesias, peripheral neuropathy. **CV:** Hypertension, chest pain. **GI:** *Diarrhea,* increased LFTs (ALT and AST), abdominal pain, anorexia, dyspepsia, gastroenteritis, nausea, mouth ulcer, vomiting, weight loss, hepatotoxicity. **Metabolic:** Hypokalemia. **Respiratory:** Bronchitis, cough, *respiratory infection,* pharyngitis, pneumonia, rhinitis, sinusitis. **Skin:** Rash, alopecia, eczema, pruritus, dry skin, <u>Stevens–Johnson syndrome</u>, toxic epidermal necrolysis (rare). **Urogenital:** UTI.

**INTERACTIONS** Drug: **Rifampin** may significantly increase leflunomide levels; **cholestyramine, charcoal** decrease absorption; caution should be used with other hepatotoxic drugs. Do not use with LIVE VACCINES. Do not use with **teriflunomide**.

**PHARMACOKINETICS Absorption:** Approximately 80% reaches systemic circulation. **Peak:** 6–12 h for active metabolite. **Distribution:** Greater than 99% protein bound. **Metabolism:** Metabolized primarily to M1 (active metabolite). **Elimination:** 43% in urine, 48% in feces. **Half-Life:** 19 days for active metabolite.

## NURSING IMPLICATIONS

### Black Box Warning

*Leflunomide has been associated with severe, potentially fatal, hepatotoxicity.*

### Assessment & Drug Effects
- Monitor carefully for and report immediately S&S of infection; withhold leflunomide if infection is suspected.
- Withhold drug and notify prescriber if S&S of hepatotoxicty appear (see Appendix F).
- Monitor BP and weight periodically. Doses greater than 25 mg/day are associated with a greater incidence of side effects such as alopecia, weight loss, and elevated liver enzymes.

- Monitor lab tests: Baseline screening to rule out hepatitis B or C; baseline then monthly × 6 WBC, platelet count, H&H, then q6–8 wk thereafter; baseline and monthly LFTs × 6 mo, then every 6–8 wks thereafter.

### Patient & Family Education

- Use reliable contraception while taking leflunomide.
- Note: Both women and men need to discontinue leflunomide and undergo a drug elimination procedure prescribed by the prescriber BEFORE conception.
- Withhold drug if you develop an infection and notify the prescriber before resuming the drug.
- Notify prescriber about any of the following: Hair loss, weight loss, GI distress, rash, or itching.

## LENVATINIB
(len-va'ti-nib)
Lenvima

**Classifications:** ANTINEOPLASTIC; KINASE INHIBITOR; VASCULAR EPIDERMAL GROWTH FACTOR (VEGF) RECEPTOR INHIBITOR
**Therapeutic:** ANTINEOPLASTIC
**Prototype:** Erlotinib

### AVAILABILITY Capsules

### ACTION & THERAPEUTIC EFFECT

A tyrosine kinase inhibitor of multiple receptors including vascular endothelial growth factor receptors, fibroblast growth factor receptors, and platelet derived growth factor receptors which are implicated in tumor angiogenesis, tumor growth, and cancer progression. *Interferes with development of blood vessels and essential cell components needed for thyroid tumor growth.*

**USES** Treatment of patients with locally recurrent or metastatic, progressive, radioactive iodine-refractory differentiated thyroid cancer (DTC).

**CONTRAINDICATIONS** Life-threatening hypertension; arterial thrombotic event; hepatic failure; nephrotic syndrome; GI perforation or life-threatening fistula; pregnancy; lactation.

**CAUTIOUS USE** QT prolongation; hypertension; mild-to-moderate liver or renal impairment. Safety and efficacy in children younger than 18 y not established.

### ROUTE & DOSAGE

| Thyroid Cancer |
| --- |
| *Adult:* **PO** 24 mg once daily |
| ***Hepatic Impairment Dosage Adjustment*** |
| *Severe impairment (Child-Pugh class C):* Decrease to 14 mg once daily |
| ***Renal Impairment Dosage Adjustment*** |
| *Severe impairment (CrCL less than 30 mL/min):* Decrease to 14 mg once daily |
| ***Dose Modifications for Persistent and Intolerable Grade 2 or Grade 3 Adverse Reactions or Grade 4 Laboratory Abnormalities*** |
| Interrupt until resolved to Grade 0–1 or baseline<br>*1st occurrence:* Resume at 20 mg once daily<br>*2nd occurrence:* Resume at 14 mg once daily<br>*3rd occurrence:* Resume at 10 mg once daily |

---

Common adverse effects in *italic;* life-threatening effects underlined; generic names in **bold**; classifications in SMALL CAPS; ♣ Canadian drug name; ⊘ Prototype drug

## ADMINISTRATION

### Oral
- May give without regard to food.
- Store at room temperature 20°–25° C (68°–77° F).

## ADVERSE EFFECTS (≥2%) Body as a Whole: Dental or oral infections, *fatigue*, peripheral edema. **CNS:** Dizziness, dysgeusia, headache, insomnia. **CV:** <u>Arterial thrombotic events</u>, <u>cardiac dysfunction</u>, *hypertension*, hypotension, prolonged QT interval. **GI:** *Abdominal pain*, constipation, *diarrhea*, dry mouth, dyspepsia, fistula formation, gastrointestinal perforation, nausea, oral pain, stomatitis, vomiting. **Hematological:** <u>Hemorrhagic events</u>. **Metabolic:** Decreased appetite, dehydration, hypocalcemia, hypokalemia, increased ALT/AST, increased creatinine, increased lipase, weight loss. **Musculoskeletal:** *Arthralgia, myalgia*. **Respiratory:** Cough, *dysphonia*, epistaxis. **Skin:** Alopecia, hyperkeratosis, *palmar-plantar erythrodysesthesia*. **Urogenital:** *Proteinuria*, <u>renal failure</u>, renal impairment, urinary tract infection.

## PHARMACOKINETICS Peak: 1–4 h. **Distribution:** 98–99% plasma protein bound. **Metabolism:** In liver. **Elimination:** Fecal (64%) and renal (25%). **Half-Life:** 28 h.

## NURSING IMPLICATIONS

### Assessment & Drug Effects
- Monitor ECG at baseline and periodically thereafter; withhold drug and notify prescriber for QT prolongation or other arrhythmias.
- Monitor HR and BP and report promptly irregular heart rate and significant BP elevation.
- Withhold drug and notify prescriber for S&S of any of the following:

Hepatic impairment, proteinuria, bleeding, arterial thrombotic events, cardiac dysfunction, or GI perforation or fistula formation.
- Monitor lab tests: Baseline and periodic thyroid function tests, renal function tests, LFTs, Hct & Hgb, serum electrolytes, and serum lipase.

### Patient & Family Education
- If a dose is missed and cannot be taken within 12 h, skip that dose and take the next dose at the usual time.
- Monitor HR and BP regularly.
- Contact prescriber immediately for any of the following: S&S of cardiac impairment (e.g., shortness of breath, swelling of ankles, chest pain, or irregular heart beat); S&S of a stroke (e.g., numbness or weakness on one side of body, trouble speaking, sudden severe headache, sudden vision change); S&S of liver damage (e.g., jaundice, dark "tea colored" urine, light-colored stool); S&S of bleeding.
- Women should use an effective method of birth control during treatment and for at least 2 wk after the last dose of this drug.
- Do not breast-feed while taking this drug.

## LESINURAD
(le-sin′-ure-ad)

Zurampic

**Classifications:** ANTIGOUT; URIC ACID TRANSPORTER 1 (URAT 1) INHIBITOR

Therapeutic: ANTIGOUT

## AVAILABILITY Tablets

## ACTION & *THERAPEUTIC EFFECT*
Decreases uric acid levels by inhibiting the function of uric acid transporter 1 (URAT1) and organic anion transporter 4 (OAT4). *These*

two transporter proteins are involved in the renal reabsorption of uric acid. URAT1 is responsible for the majority of the reabsorption of filtered uric acid from the renal tubular lumen, while OAT4 is a uric acid transporter associated with diuretic-induced hyperuricemia.

**USES** Treatment of hyperuricemia associated with gout in patients who have not achieved target serum uric acid levels with a xanthine oxidase inhibitor alone. Lesinurad should be used in combination with a xanthine oxidase inhibitor.

**CONTRAINDICATIONS** Severe renal impairment (CrCL less than 30 mL/min), end stage renal disease, kidney transplant recipients, or patients on dialysis; tumor lysis syndrome or Lesch-Nyhan syndrome.

**CAUTIOUS USE** Hepatic disease, organ transplant, cardiac disease, renal impairment, secondary hyperuricemia, pregnancy, lactation.

**ROUTE & DOSAGE**

**Hyperuricemia**
Adult: PO 200 mg once daily

*Hepatic Impairment Dosage Adjustment*

Severe hepatic impairment (Child-Pugh class C): Not recommended

*Renal Impairment Dosage Adjustment*

CrCL less than 45 mL/min: Not recommended

**ADMINISTRATION**
Oral
- **Must be** co-administered with a xanthine oxidase inhibitor such as allopurinol or febuxostat.

- Administer in the morning with food and water at the same time as the morning dose of xanthine oxidase inhibitor
- If treatment with xanthine oxidase inhibitor is interrupted, lesinurad should also be interrupted. Failure to follow these instructions may increase risk of adverse renal events.
- Instruct patient to stay well-hydrated.

**ADVERSE EFFECTS** (≥1%) **Body as a Whole:** Influenza. **CNS:** Headache. **CV:** Cardiovascular death, nonfatal myocardial infarction, nonfatal stroke. **GI:** Gastroesophageal reflux disease. **Hematological:** Increased serum creatinine. **Urogenital:** Nephrolithiasis, renal failure.

**INTERACTIONS Drug:** Inhibitors of CYP2C9 (e.g., **fluconazole, amiodarone**) may increase the levels of lesinurad. Lesinurad can reduce the levels of **sildenafil** and **amlodipine** and may interfere with the actions of HORMONAL CONTRACEPTIVES **Aspirin** at doses higher than 325 mg per day may decrease the efficacy of lesinurad in combination with allopurinol.

**PHARMACOKINETICS Absorption:** Bioavailability is 100%. **Peak:** 1–4 h. **Distribution:** 98% plasma protein bound. **Metabolism:** Hepatic oxidation by CYP enzymes. **Elimination:** Renal (63%) and fecal (32%). **Half-Life:** 5 h.

**NURSING IMPLICATIONS**

**Black Box Warning**

*Lesinurad has lead to acute renal failure when given alone. It should only be used in combination with a xanthine oxidase inhibitor.*

### Assessment & Drug Effects

- Monitor serum creatinine and creatinine clearance levels. Report any signs or symptoms of nephrotoxicity.
- Monitor baseline and periodic uric acid levels.

### Patient & Family Education

- Notify health care provider if you have kidney disease or a history of kidney transplant.
- Report any signs or symptoms of kidney problems such as difficulty urinating, a change in the amount of urine, blood in the urine, or a significant weight gain.
- Report any signs or symptoms of an allergic reaction such as rash; hives; wheezing; tightness in the chest or throat; trouble breathing or talking; unusual hoarseness; or swelling of the face, lips, mouth, tongue, or throat.
- All forms of hormonal contraceptives may be less effective during therapy with lesinurad. Additional methods of contraception are recommended during therapy.
- Take this medication with a full glass of water; drink lots of non-caffeinated liquids each day unless told otherwise by your health care provider.

# LETERMOVIR
(le-term'-oh-vir)
Prevymis
**Classifications:** ANTIVIRAL
Therapeutic: ANTIVIRAL

**AVAILABILITY** Tablet; solution for injection

## ACTION & *THERAPEUTIC EFFECT*
Interferes with DNA synthesis of CMV thereby inhibiting replication. *It reduces formation of new lesions and speeds healing time.*

**USES** Prophylaxis of CMV infection.

**CONTRAINDICATIONS** Co-administration with pimozide, ergot alkaloids, or cyclosprine and pitavastatin/simvastatin.

**CAUTIOUS USE** Not recommended in severe hepatic impairment, renal impairment (CrCl less than 50 mL/min), pregnancy, lactation.

## ROUTE & DOSAGE

**CMV Prophylaxis**

*Adult:* **PO** 480 mg daily started between day 0–28 post transplant, continue through day 100 post transplant; **IV** Same as PO dose

## ADMINISTRATION

### Oral

- Swallow tablet whole. May give without regard to food.

### Intravenous

*PREPARE:* **IV Infusion:** Vials are for single use only; do not shake the vials. Dilute contents of a single-use vial with 250 mL of NS or D5W only. Diluted solution may be colorless to yellow. ▪ Diluted solution is stable for up to 24 h at room temperature or up to 48 h if refrigerated at 2°–8° C (36°–46°F); time includes storage of the diluted solution through the duration of the infusion. ▪ Do not give as an IV bolus; give only as an IV infusion. ▪ Only use infusion sets made from PVC, polyehtlylene (PE), polybutadiene (PBD), silicone rubber (SR), styrene-butadiene copolymer (SBC) styrene-butadiene-styrene (SBS) or polystyrene (PS). ▪ Only use catheters made from radiopaque polyurethane.

*ADMINISTER:* **IV** Use only in patients unable to tolerate oral thearpy. Administer infusion over 1 h via peripheral or central venous catheter. Do not administer with poly-urethane containing IV administration sets.

**INCOMPATIBILITIES: New medication.** Drug incompatibilities have not been tested. Do not use with polyurethane containing tubing.

**ADVERSE EFFECTS** (> 12%) **CV:** Peripheral edema, tachycardia, <u>atrial fibrillation</u>. **CNS:** Headache, fatigue. **GI:** *nausea*, vomiting diarrhea, abdominal pain. **Hematology:** Decreased platelet count. **Respiratory:** Cough.

**INTERACTIONS Drug:** Letermovir is a substrate and inhibitor of OATP1B1/3 transporters. Avoid use with other inhibitors/substrates of the OATP1B1/3 transporters. Letermovir acts as a CYP3A4 inhibitor; monitor use with CYP3A substrates (e.g., **fentanyl, midazolam**). Letermovir may increase plasma concentrations of **amiodarone,** ANTIDIABETIC AGENTS, **ergotamine,** HMG-CoA REDUCTASE INHIBITORS, IMMUNOSUPPRESSANTS. Letermovir may decrease plasma concentrations of PROTON PUMP INHIBITORS, **phenytoin,** and **warfarin.**

**PHARMACOKINETICS Absorption:** Oral dose has 94% bioavailability. **Distribution:** 99% protein bound. **Metabolism:** Primarily eliminated unchanged. **Elimination:** 93% in feces, 2% in urine. **Half-Life:** 12 h.

**NURSING IMPLICATIONS**

**Assessment & Drug Effects**
- Monitor for CMV reactivation.
- Closely monitor in patients with CrCl less than 50mL/min receiving IV formulation.
- Monitor lab tests: Serum creatinine/BUN.

**Patient & Family Education**
- This drug interacts with many other drugs. Report any new medications to your pharmacist/prescriber.

- If patient misses a dose, take as soon as they remember. If patient does not remember until the next dose is due, skip the missed dose and go back to the regular schedule; do not double the next dose or take more than prescribed.
- Notify prescriber if pregnant or planning a pregnancy.
- Notify prescriber if breastfeeding.
- Report promptly any of the following to prescriber: Swelling in arms/legs, signs of allergic reaction.

# LETROZOLE
(le'tro-zole)
Femara

**Classifications:** ANTINEOPLASTIC; AROMATASE INHIBITOR
**Therapeutic:** ANTINEOPLASTIC
**Prototype:** Anastrozole

**AVAILABILITY** Tablet

**ACTION & THERAPEUTIC EFFECT** Nonsteroid competitive inhibitor of aromatase, the enzyme that converts androgens to estrogens. It does not inhibit adrenal steroid synthesis. *Results in the regression of estrogen-dependent tumors.*

**USES** Treatment of breast cancer in postmenopausal women.

**CONTRAINDICATIONS** Hypersensitivity to letrozole; pregnant women, women of childbearing age, premenopausal females, hormone replacement therapy (HRT); pregnancy (category X).

**CAUTIOUS USE** Moderate to severe hepatic impairment; older adults; lactation. Safety and efficacy in children not established.

## ROUTE & DOSAGE

**Breast Cancer**
*Adult:* **PO** 2.5 mg daily

**Hepatic Impairment**
**Dosage Adjustment**
*Severe hepatic impairment (Child-Pugh class C):* Reduce the dose by 50%

## ADMINISTRATION

**Oral**
▪ Give without regard to food.

## ADVERSE EFFECTS (≥1%) Body as a Whole:
Fatigue, peripheral edema, asthenia, weight increase, *musculoskeletal pain,* arthralgia, angioedema. **CNS:** Headache, somnolence, dizziness. **CV:** Chest pain, hypertension, hypercholesterolemia. **GI:** Nausea, vomiting, constipation, diarrhea, abdominal pain, anorexia, dyspepsia. **Respiratory:** Dyspnea, cough. **Skin:** Hot flushes, rash, pruritus.

## INTERACTIONS Drug:
ESTROGENS, ORAL CONTRACEPTIVES could interfere with the pharmacologic action of letrozole.

## PHARMACOKINETICS Absorption:
Rapidly from GI tract. **Metabolism:** In liver (CYP3A4 and 2A6). **Elimination:** 90% in urine. **Half-Life:** 2 days.

## NURSING IMPLICATIONS

**Assessment & Drug Effects**
▪ Monitor carefully for S&S of thrombophlebitis or thromboembolism; report immediately.
▪ Monitor lab tests: Periodic serum calcium and CBC with differential.

**Patient & Family Education**
▪ Notify prescriber immediately if S&S of thrombophlebitis develop (see Appendix F).

## LEUCOVORIN CALCIUM
(loo-koe-vor'in)

## LEVOLEUCOVORIN
(levo-loo-koe-vor'in)

**Fusilev**

**Classifications:** BLOOD FORMER; ANTIANEMIC
**Therapeutic:** ANTIANEMIC; CHEMO-THERAPEUTIC PROTECTANT

## AVAILABILITY
Tablet; solution for injection

## ACTION & *THERAPEUTIC EFFECT*
Both leucovorin and levoleucovorin are reduced forms of folic acid. Unlike folic acid, they do not require enzymatic reduction by dihydrofolate reductase. Thus, they are readily available as an essential cell growth factor. During antineoplastic therapy, both forms of the drug prevent serious toxicity by protecting cells from the action of folic acid antagonists. *Antidote against folic acid antagonists such as methotrexate.*

## USES
Methotrexate toxicity, megalobalstic anemia, colorectal cancer.

## UNLABELED USES
Treatment of non-Hodgkin's lymphoma.

## CONTRAINDICATIONS
Pernicious anemia, or other megaloblastic anemias secondary to vitamin $B_{12}$ deficiency. **Oral form:** Stomatitis.

## CAUTIOUS USE
Inadequate hydration; history of seizures; debilitated patients; older adults; pregnancy (category C); lactation; children.

## ROUTE & DOSAGE

Note: Levoleucovorin is dosed at half the normal dose of leucovorin*

**Megaloblastic Anemia**

*Adult/Child:* IV/IM Up to 1 mg/day

**Leucovorin Rescue for Methotrexate Toxicity**

*Adult/Child:* PO/IM/IV 10 mg/m² q6h until serum methotrexate levels are reduced

**Levoleucovorin Rescue**

*Adult/Adolescent/Child (6 y or older):* IV 7.5 mg q6h × 10 doses

**Inadvertent Overdose of Methotrexate (Levoleucovorin)**

*Adult/Adolescent/Child (6 y or older):* IV 7.5 mg q6h until serum methotrexate levels are below 0.01 micromolar

**Leucovorin Rescue for Other Folate Antagonist Toxicity**

*Adult/Child:* PO/IM/IV 5–15 mg/day

**Advanced Colorectal Cancer**

*Adult:* IV 200 mg/m² followed by fluorouracil 370 mg/m²

## ADMINISTRATION

### Oral

- Note: Oral route is **not** recommended for doses higher than 25 mg or if patient is likely to vomit.

### Intramuscular

- Give deep into a large muscle.

### Intravenous

*PREPARE:* **Leucovorin Direct/IV Infusion:** For doses less than 10 mg/m², reconstitute each 50 mg in 5 mL of bacteriostatic water for injection with benzyl alcohol as a preservative to yield 10 mg/mL. • For doses greater than 10 mg/m² reconstitute, as above, but with sterile water for injection without a preservative. Final concentration is 10 mg/mL. • Further dilute in 100–500 mL of IV solutions (e.g., D5W, NS, LR) to yield a concentration of 10–20 mg/mL of IV solution. **Levoleucovorin Direct:** Reconstitute the 50-mg vial with 5.3 mL NS injection to yield 10 mg/mL. • May further dilute, immediately, in NS or D5W to 0.5–5 mg/mL. • Do not mix with other solutions or additives

*ADMINISTER:* **Leucovorin/Levoleucovorin Direct:** Give 160 mg or fraction thereof over 1 min. **Leucovorin/Levoleucovorin IV Infusion:** Do not exceed direct IV rate. • Give more slowly if the volume of IV solution to be infused is large.

*INCOMPATIBILITIES:* **Leucovorin only: Solution/additive:** Fluorouracil. **Y-site:** Amphotericin B cholesteryl complex, carboplatin, droperidol, epirubicin, foscarnet, gemtuzumab, lansoprazole, pamidronate, pantoprazole, quinpristin/dalfopristin, sodium bicarbonate.

- **Leucovorin:** Use solution reconstituted with bacteriostatic water within 7 days. • Use solution reconstituted with sterile water for injection immediately. **Levoleucovorin:** Solutions with NS may be held at 15°–30° C (59°–86° F) for up to 12 h. Solutions with D5W may be held at 15°–30° C (59°–86° F) for up to 4 h. • Protect from light.

## ADVERSE EFFECTS (≥1%) Body as a Whole: Allergic sensitization

Common adverse effects in *italic;* life-threatening effects <u>underlined</u>; generic names in **bold**; classifications in SMALL CAPS; ✦ Canadian drug name; ⓟ Prototype drug

921

(urticaria, pruritus, rash, wheezing). **Hematologic:** Thrombocytosis.

**INTERACTIONS Drug:** May enhance adverse effects of **fluorouracil;** may reverse therapeutic effects of **trimethoprim-sulfamethoxazole.**

**PHARMACOKINETICS Onset:** Within 30 min. **Peak:** 0.9 h (levoleucovorin). **Duration:** 3–6 h. **Distribution:** Crosses placenta; distributed into breast milk. **Metabolism:** In liver and intestinal mucosa to tetrahydrofolic acid derivatives. **Elimination:** 80–90% in urine, 5–8% in feces. **Half-Life:** 6 h; 0.77 h (levoleucovorin).

## NURSING IMPLICATIONS

### Assessment & Drug Effects
- Monitor neurologic status. Use of leucovorin alone in treatment of pernicious anemia or other megaloblastic anemias associated with vitamin $B_{12}$ deficiency can result in an apparent hematological remission while allowing already present neurologic damage to progress.
- Monitor lab tests: Baseline and daily serum creatinine and methotrexate level when treated for methotrexate toxicity.

### Patient & Family Education
- Notify prescriber of S&S of a hypersensitivity reaction immediately (see Appendix F).

## LEUPROLIDE ACETATE ⓟ
(loo-proe'lide)
Eligard, Lupron, Lupron Depot, Lupron Depot-Ped
**Classification:** GONADOTROPIN-RELEASING HORMONE (GnRH) ANALOG
Therapeutic: GnRH ANALOG; ANTINEOPLASTIC

**AVAILABILITY** Solution for injection; microspheres for injection (depot formulations)

## ACTION & THERAPEUTIC EFFECT
A luteinizing hormone-releasing hormone (LH-RH) and GnRH agonist; acts as a potent inhibitor of gonadotropin secretion when given continuously in therapeutic doses. **Antitumor effect:** *May inhibit growth of hormone-dependent tumors as indicated by reduction in concentrations of PSA and serum testosterone to levels equal to or less than pretreatment levels.* **Contraceptive effect:** *By inhibiting gonadotropin release, ovulation or spermatogenesis is suppressed.*

**USES** Palliative treatment of advanced prostatic carcinoma; endometriosis; anemia caused by leiomyomata; percocious puberty.

**UNLABELED USES** Breast cancer; BPH, PMS; infertility.

**CONTRAINDICATIONS** Known hypersensitivity to benzyl alcohol, GnRH analog hypersensitivity; following orchiectomy or estrogen therapy; metastatic cerebral lesions; menstruation, abnormal vaginal bleeding, pregnancy (category X); lactation.

**CAUTIOUS USE** Life-threatening carcinoma in which rapid symptomatic relief is necessary; osteoporosis; older adults.

## ROUTE & DOSAGE

### Palliative Treatment for Prostate Cancer
*Adult:* **Subcutaneous** 1 mg/day; **IM** 7.5 mg/mo or 22.5 mg q3mo or 30 mg q4mo or 45 mg q6mo (depends on specific depot preparation)

Common adverse effects in *italic;* life-threatening effects underlined; generic names in **bold;** classifications in SMALL CAPS; ◆ Canadian drug name; ⓟ Prototype drug

### Endometriosis
*Adult:* **IM** 3.75 mg qmo or 11.25 mg q3mo (max: 6 mo)

### Precocious Puberty
*Child (weight greater than 37.5 kg):* **IM** 15 mg q4wk; *weight 25–37.5 kg:* 11.25 mg q4wk; *weight less than 25 kg:* 7.5 mg q4wk

### Percocious Puberty (Depot Form)
*Child (2–11 y):* **IM** 11.25 or 30 mg q3mo

## ADMINISTRATION

### Subcutaneous
- Use double gloves and protective gown for all preparation and administration of subcutaneous and intramuscular injection. Use eye protection if there is any chance of splash or if the patient may resist.
- Do not use Depot form for subcutaneous injection.
- Assemble two-syringe mixing system. Mix as directed and allow to reach room temperature and administer within 30 min of mixing. Also available as a subcutaneous implant.
- Rotate injection sites.

### Intramuscular
- Prepare solution for Depot-Ped injection. Screw plunger into the end stopper until stopper begins to turn; hold syringe upright; slowly push (6–8 sec) until first stopper is at the blue line in the middle of the barrel to combine the diluent with microspheres; keep syringe upright while mixing suspension gently until all of the powder is completely dissolved into suspension; expel air from the syringe; use within 2 h; do not use if the powder has not dissolved into a suspension. Inject at 90° angle and inject intramuscularly immediately because suspension settles quickly.
- Do not administer parenteral drug formulation if particulate matter or discoloration is present.
- Storage directions are different for different brands. Follow package insert for each brand.

**ADVERSE EFFECTS** (≥1%) **Body as a Whole:** *Disease flare (worsening of S&S of carcinoma), injection site irritation,* asthenia, fatigue, depression, fever, facial swelling. **CNS:** Dizziness, pain, headache, fatigue, insomnia, paresthesia. **CV:** *Peripheral edema,* cardiac arrhythmias, <u>MI</u>. **Endocrine:** *Hot flushes, impotence, decreased libido,* gynecomastia, breast tenderness, amenorrhea, vaginal bleeding, thyroid enlargement, hypoglycemia. **GI:** Nausea, vomiting, constipation, anorexia, sour taste, GI bleeding, diarrhea. **Musculoskeletal:** Increased bone pain, *myalgia, fractures of vertebral column.* **Renal:** Increased hematuria, dysuria, flank pain. **Respiratory:** Pleural rub, pulmonary fibrosis flare, cough, <u>pulmonary embolism</u>. **Hematologic:** Decreased Hct, Hgb. **Skin:** Pruritus, rash, hair loss, acne.

**INTERACTIONS Drug:** ANDROGENS, ESTROGENS counteract therapeutic effects. Avoid using QT prolonging agents (e.g., **bretylium, dofetilide,** etc.).

**PHARMACOKINETICS Absorption:** Readily absorbed from subcutaneous or IM sites. **Metabolism:** By enzymes in hypothalamus and anterior pituitary. **Half-Life:** 3 h.

L

Common adverse effects in *italic;* life-threatening effects <u>underlined</u>; generic names in **bold;** classifications in SMALL CAPS; ♣ Canadian drug name; ⓟ Prototype drug

923

## NURSING IMPLICATIONS

### Assessment & Drug Effects

- Monitor PSA and testosterone levels in males with prostate cancer. A gradual rise in values after their decrease may signify treatment failure.
- Inspect injection site. If local hypersensitivity reactions occur (erythema, induration), suspect sensitivity to benzyl alcohol. Report to prescriber.
- Monitor I&O ratio and pattern. Report hematuria and decreased output. Carefully monitor voiding problems, monitor Hgb and Hct, and hemoglobin A1C within 3–6 mo of beginning therapy.

### Patient & Family Education

- When used for prostate cancer, bone pain and voiding problems (i.e., symptoms of tumor obstruction) usually increase during first several weeks of continuous treatment but are transient. Hot flushes also may be experienced.
- Notify prescriber of neurologic S&S (paresthesia and weakness in lower limbs). Exercise caution when walking without assistance.
- When used for endometriosis, continuous treatment may cause amenorrhea and other menstrual irregularities.

## LEVALBUTEROL HYDROCHLORIDE

(lev-al-bu'ter-ole)

Xopenex, Xopenex HFA

**Classifications:** SHORT-ACTING BETA-ADRENERGIC AGONIST; BRONCHODILATOR

Therapeutic: BRONCHODILATOR

**Prototype:** Albuterol

**AVAILABILITY** Inhalation solution

## ACTION & *THERAPEUTIC EFFECT*

An isomer of albuterol with beta$_2$-adrenergic agonist properties; acts on the beta$_2$ receptors of the smooth muscles of the bronchial tree, thus resulting in bronchodilation. *Effective bronchodilator that decreases airway resistance, facilitates mucous drainage, and increases vital capacity.*

**USES** Treatment or prevention of bronchospasm in patients with reversible obstructive airway disease.

**CONTRAINDICATIONS** Hypersensitivity to levalbuterol or albuterol; angioedema; lactation.

**CAUTIOUS USE** Cardiovascular disorders especially coronary insufficiency, cardiac arrhythmias, hypertension, QT elongation, convulsive disorders; diabetes mellitus, diabetic ketoacidosis; older adults; seizures, status asthmaticus, tachycardia; hypersensitivity to sympathetic amines; hyperthyroidism, thyrotoxicosis; pregnancy (category C); children. **Extended Release Form:** Children older than 12 y.

## ROUTE & DOSAGE

### Bronchospasm

*Adult:* **Inhalation** 0.63 mg by nebulization t.i.d. q6–8h, may increase to 1.25 mg t.i.d. if needed
*Child (6–11 y):* **Inhalation** 0.31 mg by nebulization t.i.d. q6–8h (max: 0.63 mg t.i.d.)

## ADMINISTRATION

### Inhalation

- Use vials within 2 wk of opening pouch. Protect vial from light and use within 1 wk after removal

Common adverse effects in *italic;* life-threatening effects <u>underlined</u>; generic names in **bold;** classifications in SMALL CAPS; ♣ Canadian drug name; ◎ Prototype drug

924

from pouch. Use only if solution in vial is colorless.

***INCOMPATIBILITIES:*** **Solution/additive:** Compatibility when mixed with other drugs in a nebulizer has not been established.

- Store at 15°–25° C (59°–77° F) in protective foil pouch.

## ADVERSE EFFECTS (>1%) **Body as a Whole:** Allergic reactions, flu syndrome, pain. **CNS:** Migraine, dizziness, nervousness, tremor, anxiety. **CV:** Tachycardia. **GI:** Dyspepsia. **Respiratory:** Increased cough, viral infection, rhinitis, sinusitis, turbinate edema, paradoxical bronchospasm. **Endocrine:** Increase in serum glucose.

## INTERACTIONS **Drug:** BETA-ADREN-ERGIC BLOCKERS may antagonize levalbuterol effects; MAOI, TRICYCLIC ANTIDEPRESSANTS may potentiate levalbuterol effects on vascular system; ECG changes or hypokalemia may be exacerbated by LOOP or THIAZIDE DIURETICS.

## PHARMACOKINETICS **Onset:** 5–15 min. **Duration:** 3–6 h. **Half-Life:** 3.3 h.

## NURSING IMPLICATIONS

### Assessment & Drug Effects
- Monitor for S&S of CNS or cardiovascular stimulation (e.g., BP, HR, respiratory status).
- Monitor diabetics for loss of glycemic control.
- Monitor lab tests: Periodic serum potassium especially with co-administered loop or thiazide diuretics.

### Patient & Family Education
- Seek medical advice immediately if a previously effective dose becomes ineffective.

- Report immediately to prescriber: Chest pain or palpitations, swelling of the eyelids, tongue, lips, or face; increased wheezing or difficulty breathing.
- Do not use drug more frequently than prescribed.
- Exercise caution with hazardous activities; dizziness and vertigo are possible side effects.
- Check with prescriber before taking OTC cold medication.

## LEVETIRACETAM
(lev-e-tir'a-ce-tam)
Keppra, Keppra XR, Spirtam

**Classification:** ANTICONVULSANT
Therapeutic: ANTICONVULSANT

## AVAILABILITY Tablet; extended release tablets; oral solution; solution for injection; oral disintegrating tablet

## ACTION & *THERAPEUTIC EFFECT*
The precise mechanism of antiepileptic effects is unknown. It is a broad spectrum antiepileptic agent that does not involve GABA inhibition. It prevents epileptiform burst firing and propagation of seizure activity. *Inhibits complex partial seizures and prevents epileptic and seizure activity.*

## USES Adjunctive therapy for partial onset, myoclonic, tonic clonic seizures.

## UNLABELED USES Status epilepticus.

## CONTRAINDICATIONS Hypersensitivity to levetiracetam; suicidal ideation; labor; lactation. Avoid use in older adults with a history of falls or fractures (unless used for seizure or mood

Common adverse effects in *italic*; life-threatening effects underlined; generic names in **bold**; classifications in SMALL CAPS; ♣ Canadian drug name; ⊘ Prototype drug

925

disorders). **Extended release tablets:** Children younger than 12.

**CAUTIOUS USE** Renal impairment; renal disease; renal failure; older adults; history of psychosis or depression, suicidal tendencies; pregnancy (category C);. **Immediate release tablet** for children younger than 4 y.

## ROUTE & DOSAGE

### Partial Onset Seizures

*Adult/Adolescent (16 y or older):*
**PO/IV** 500 mg b.i.d., may increase by 500 mg b.i.d. q2wk (max: 3000 mg/day) OR **Extended release** 1000 mg tablet daily

*Child (4–15 y):* **PO Solution form/IV** 10 mg/kg b.i.d.; may increase by 20 mg/kg q2wk up to 30 mg/kg b.i.d.

*Child/Infant (older than 6 mo):*
**PO** 10 mg/kg b.i.d. may increase to 25 mg/kg b.i.d.; **IV** 7 mg/kg b.i.d. may increase to dose of 21 mg/kg b.i.d.

### Tonic Clonic Seizures

*Adult/Adolescent (16 y or older):*
**PO/IV** 500 mg b.i.d., increase by 1000 mg q2wk to dose of 3000 mg/day

*Child (6 y or older):* **PO Immediate release** or **Solution form** 10 mg/kg b.i.d., increase by 20 mg/kg q2wk to dose of 60 mg/kg/day in 2 doses

*Adolescent/Child (6 y or older 20–40 kg):* **PO Fast melt tablet** 250 mg b.i.d. then increase dose q2wk to 750 mg b.i.d.

### Myoclonic Seizures

*Adult/Adolescent/Child (12 y and older):* **PO/IV** 500 mg b.i.d.,

increase by 1000 mg/day q2wk to recommended dose of 3000 mg/day in divided doses

### *Renal Impairment Dosage Adjustment*

*CrCl 50–80 mL/min:* **Immediate release or IV** 500–1000 mg q12h; **Extended release** 1000–2000 mg q24;

*less than 30–49 mL/min:*
**Immediate release or IV** 250–750 mg q12h, (IR or IV form); **Extended release** 500–1500 mg q24h

### *Hepatic Impairment Dosage Adjustment*

*Child-Pugh class C:* Reduce to 1/2 dose

## ADMINISTRATION

### Oral

- Ensure that extended release tablets are swallowed whole. They should not be cut or chewed.
- Dose increment changes should be made no more often than at 2-wk intervals.
- Taper dose if discontinued.
- Give supplemental doses to dialysis patients after dialysis.
- Store at 15°–30° C (59°–86° F).

### Intravenous

*PREPARE:* **Intermittent:** Levetiracetam supplied in NS needs no further dilution. If using the concentrated solution, dilute required dose in 100 mL of D5W, NS or LR.
*ADMINISTER:* **Intermittent:** Give over 15 min.
*INCOMPATIBILITIES:* **Solution/additives:** Only compatible with lorazepam, diazepam and valproate sodium.

Common adverse effects in *italic;* life-threatening effects underlined; generic names in **bold;** classifications in SMALL CAPS; ♣ Canadian drug name; ⓟ Prototype drug

- Diluted solution may be stored up to 4 h at 15°–30° C (59°–86° F).

**ADVERSE EFFECTS** (≥1%) **Body as a Whole:** *Asthenia, headache, infection,* pain. **CV:** Increased blood pressure. **CNS:** *Somnolence,* amnesia, anxiety, ataxia, depression, dizziness, emotional lability, headache, hostility, nervousness, irritability, vertigo, paradoxical increase in seizures (as add-on therapy). **GI:** Anorexia, *vomiting.* **Respiratory:** Cough, pharyngitis, rhinitis, sinusitis. **Special Senses:** Diplopia. **Other:** Increased symptoms of depression; suicidal ideation.

**INTERACTIONS Drug:** AMPHETAMINES may decrease seizure threshold. Levetiracetam does not affect **estrogen, warfarin,** or **digoxin** levels or affect levels of other antiepileptic drugs. **Sevelamer, colesevelam** may decrease effectiveness. **Herbal:** Avoid use of **kava.**

**PHARMACOKINETICS Absorption:** Rapidly and almost completely absorbed. **Peak:** 1 h; steady-state 2 days. **Distribution:** Less than 10% protein bound. **Metabolism:** Minimal hepatic metabolism. **Elimination:** Renally eliminated. **Half-Life:** 7.1 h (9.6 h in older adults).

## NURSING IMPLICATIONS

### Assessment & Drug Effects

- Monitor individuals with a history of psychosis or depression for signs and symptoms of suicidal tendencies, suicidal ideation, and suicidality. Report any of these symptoms to the prescriber.
- Monitor blood pressure.
- Monitor and notify prescriber of difficulty with gait or coordination.
- Monitor lab tests: Periodic CBC with differential, serum creatinine/BUN, Hct and Hgb, and LFTs.

### Patient & Family Education

- Monitor for signs and symptoms of suicidality, especially in children with a history of depression or psychosis.
- Do not drive or engage in potentially hazardous activities until response to drug is known.
- Do not abruptly discontinue drug. MUST use gradual dose reduction/taper.

## LEVOBUNOLOL

(lee-voe-byoo'noe-lole)

**Betagan**

**See Appendix A-1.**

## LEVOCETIRIZINE

(lev-o-ce-tir'i-zeen)

**Xyzal**

**See Cetirizine.**

## LEVODOPA (L-DOPA) ⓟ

(lee-voe-doe'pa)

**Classifications:** DOPAMINE RECEPTOR AGONIST; ANTIPARKINSON
**Therapeutic:** ANTIPARKINSON

**AVAILABILITY** No longer available as a single agent drug (only in combination with others)

## ACTION & *THERAPEUTIC EFFECT*

Levodopa readily crosses the blood–brain barrier; it is believed that the dopamine level is severely reduced in parkinsonism. Levodopa restores dopamine levels in extrapyramidal centers of the brain. *Effective in controlling the involuntary muscle movement such as tremors and rigidity associated with Parkinson's disease.*

**USES** Idiopathic Parkinson's disease, postencephalitic and arteriosclerotic

Common adverse effects in *italic;* life-threatening effects underlined; generic names in **bold;** classifications in SMALL CAPS; ♣ Canadian drug name; ⓟ Prototype drug

927

parkinsonism, and parkinsonism symptoms associated with manganese and carbon monoxide poisoning.

**UNLABELED USES** To relieve pain of herpes zoster (shingles), liver coma (caused by cirrhosis or fulminating hepatitis), bone pain in metastatic breast carcinoma, adjunctive therapy in CHF.

**CONTRAINDICATIONS** Known hypersensitivity to levodopa; narrow-angle glaucoma patients with suspicious pigmented lesion or history of melanoma; acute psychoses, within 2 wk of use of MAOIs, suicidal ideation; lactation.

**CAUTIOUS USE** Cardiovascular, kidney, liver, or endocrine disease, history of MI with residual arrhythmias; peptic ulcer; convulsions; history of suicidal tendencies; depression; bipolar disorder; psychiatric disorders; chronic wide-angle glaucoma; diabetes; pulmonary diseases; bronchial asthma; pregnancy (category C). Safe use in children not established.

## ROUTE & DOSAGE

### Parkinson's Disease

*Adult:* **PO** 500 mg to 1 g daily in 2 or more equally divided doses, may be increased by 100–750 mg q3–7days (max: 8 g/day); used in combination with carbidopa

## ADMINISTRATION

### Oral

- Administer with 6–8 oz of water at least 30 min before eating or 1 h after meals to maximize absorption. May be taken with a small nonprotein snack, such as a cracker or fruit to avoid nausea. Absorption is decreased with high-protein meals.
- Crush tablets or empty capsule content into fruit juice as needed.
- Store in tight, light-resistant containers between 15°–30° C (59°–86° F).

**ADVERSE EFFECTS** (≥1%) **CNS:** *Choreiform and involuntary movements,* increased hand tremor, bradykinetic episodes (on–off phenomena), trismus, grinding of teeth (bruxism), ataxia, muscle twitching, numbness, weakness, fatigue, headache, opisthotonos, confusion, agitation, anxiety, euphoria, insomnia, nightmares; psychotic episodes with paranoid delusions or hallucinations, severe depression, including suicidal tendencies, hypomania. **CV:** *Arrhythmias, orthostatic hypotension;* palpitations, tachycardia, hypertension. **Special Senses:** *Blepharospasm,* diplopia, blurred vision, dilated pupils. **GI:** *Anorexia, nausea, vomiting,* abdominal distress, flatulence, dry mouth, dysphagia, sialorrhea; burning sensation of tongue, bitter taste, diarrhea or constipation; GI bleeding, hepatotoxicity. **Body as a Whole:** Flushing, increased sweating, weight gain or loss, edema, dark sweat or urine. **Urogenital:** Urinary retention or incontinence, increased sexual drive, priapism, postmenopausal bleeding. **Skin:** Skin rashes, loss of hair. **Respiratory:** Rhinorrhea, bizarre breathing patterns.

**DIAGNOSTIC TEST INTERFERENCE** Elevated **BUN, AST, ALT, alkaline phosphatase, LDH, bilirubin, protein-bound iodine,** serum level of **growth hormone;** decreased **glucose tolerance; hypokalemia,** decreased **WBC, Hgb,**

Common adverse effects in *italic;* life-threatening effects <u>underlined</u>; generic names in **bold;** classifications in SMALL CAPS; ♣ Canadian drug name; Ⓟ Prototype drug

**Hct. Urine glucose:** False-negative tests may result with use of **glucose oxidase methods** (e.g., **Clinistix, TesTape**) and false-positive results with the **copper reduction method** (e.g., **Clinitest**), especially in patients receiving large doses. It is reported that **Clinistix** and **TesTape** may be used if reading is taken at margin of wet and dry tape. **Urinary ketones:** There is possibility of false-positive tests by dipsticks [e.g., **Acetest** (equivocal), **Ketostix, Labstix**]; **Serum and urinary uric acid:** False elevations by **colorimetric methods,** but not with **uricase; Urinary protein:** False increases by **Lowry method; Urinary VMA:** False decreases by **Pisano method; Urinary catecholamine:** False increases by **Hingerty method. PKU urine test:** Interference.

**INTERACTIONS Drug:** MAO INHIBITORS may precipitate hypertensive crisis; TRICYCLIC ANTIDEPRESSANTS augment postural hypotension; PHENOTHIAZINES, **haloperidol** may antagonize the therapeutic effects of levodopa; **pyridoxine** can reverse effects of levodopa; ANTICHOLINERGICS may exacerbate abnormal involuntary movements; **methyldopa** may increase toxic CNS effects; HALOGENATED GENERAL ANESTHETICS increase risk of arrhythmias; do not use with **reserpine. Food:** Food decreases the rate and extent of levodopa absorption. Vitamin B supplements can decrease therapeutic effect. **Herbal: Kava** may worsen parkinsonian symptoms.

**PHARMACOKINETICS Absorption:** Rapidly and well absorbed from GI tract; lower absorption if taken with food. **Peak:** 1–3 h. **Distribution:** Widely distributed in body. **Metabolism:** Most of drug is decarboxylated to dopamine in lumen of GI tract, liver, and serum. **Elimination:** 80–85% of dose excreted in urine in 24 h. **Half-Life:** 1 h.

## NURSING IMPLICATIONS

### Assessment & Drug Effects

- Monitor vital signs, particularly during period of dosage adjustment. Report alterations in BP, pulse, and respiratory rate and rhythm.
- Supervise ambulation as indicated. Orthostatic hypotension is usually asymptomatic, but some patients experience dizziness and syncope. Tolerance to this effect usually develops within a few months of therapy.
- Make accurate observations and report adverse reactions and therapeutic effects promptly. Rate of dosage increase is determined primarily by patient's tolerance and response to drug.
- Monitor all patients closely for behavior changes.
- Report promptly muscle twitching and spasmodic winking (blepharospasm); these are early signs of overdosage. Patients on full therapeutic doses for longer than 1 y may develop such abnormal involuntary movements as well as jerky arm and leg movements. Symptoms tend to increase if dosage is not reduced.
- Report to prescriber any S&S of the on–off phenomenon sometimes associated with chronic management: Rapid unpredictable swings in intensity of motor symptoms of parkinsonism evidenced by increase in bradykinesia (attacks of "leg freezing" or slow body movement).
- Monitor mental status for S&S of drug-induced neuropsychiatric adverse reactions.
- Monitor lab tests: Periodic CBC, Hgb and Hct, renal function tests, and LFTs.

L

Common adverse effects in *italic;* life-threatening effects <u>underlined</u>; generic names in **bold;** classifications in SMALL CAPS; ♣ Canadian drug name; ⓟ Prototype drug

## Patient & Family Education

- Do not take with high-protein foods. Also avoid high consumption of food sources of pyridoxine, including wheat germ, green vegetables, bananas, whole-grain cereals, muscular and glandular meats (especially liver), legumes.
- Do not take OTC preparations or fortified cereals unless approved by prescriber. Multivitamins, antinauseants, and fortified cereals usually contain vitamin $B_6$.
- Make positional changes slowly, particularly from lying to upright position, and dangle legs a few minutes before standing.
- Resume activities gradually, observing safety precautions to avoid injury. Elevation of mood and sense of well-being may precede objective improvement. Significant improvement usually occurs during second or third wk of therapy, but may not occur for 6 mo or more in some patients.
- Follow prescribed drug regimen. Sudden withdrawal of medication can lead to parkinsonism crisis (with return of marked rigidity, akinesia, tremor, hyperpyrexia) or neuroleptic malignant syndrome (NMS).
- A metabolite of levodopa may cause urine to darken and sweat to be dark-colored.

# LEVOFLOXACIN

(lev-o-flox'a-sin)

Levaquin

**Classifications:** QUINOLONE ANTIBIOTIC

Therapeutic: ANTIBIOTIC

**Prototype:** Ciprofloxacin

**AVAILABILITY** Tablet; oral solution; solution for injection; ophthalmic solution

## ACTION & *THERAPEUTIC EFFECT*

A broad-spectrum fluoroquinolone antibiotic that inhibits DNA-gyrase, an enzyme necessary for bacterial replication, transcription, repair, and recombination. *Effective against many aerobic gram-positive and aerobic gram-negative organisms.*

**USES** Treatment of maxillary sinusitis, acute exacerbations of bacterial bronchitis, community-acquired pneumonia, uncomplicated skin/skin structure infections, UTI, acute pyelonephritis caused by susceptible bacteria; acute bacterial sinusitis; chronic bacterial prostatitis; bacterial conjunctivitis; treatment of pneumonic and septicemic plague.

**UNLABELED USES** Epididymitis, infective carditis, tuberculosis.

**CONTRAINDICATIONS** Hypersensitivity to levofloxacin and quinolone antibiotics; tendon pain, inflammation or rupture; syphilis; viral infections; photosensitivity/phototoxicity from drug; suicidal ideation; psychotic manifestations; manifestations of peripheral neuropathy; S&S of hepatitis; hypoglycemic reaction or peripheral neuropathy to drug; MG; QT prolongation.

**CAUTIOUS USE** History of suicidal ideation; psychosis; anxiety, confusion, depression; known or suspected CNS disorders; predisposed to seizure activity; risk factors associated with potential seizures (e.g., some drug therapy, renal insufficiency), dehydration, renal impairment (CrCl less than 50 mL/min); colitis; cardiac arrhythmias; DM; older adults; pregnancy (category C); lactation. Safe use in children younger than 6 mo not established.

Common adverse effects in *italic;* life-threatening effects <u>underlined</u>; generic names in **bold;** classifications in SMALL CAPS; ♦ Canadian drug name; ◯ Prototype drug

## ROUTE & DOSAGE

### Infections

*Adult:* **PO** 500 mg q24h × 10 days; **IV** 500 mg infused over 60 min q24h × 7–14 days

### Community-Acquired Pneumonia

*Adult:* **PO/IV** 750 mg q24h × 5 days

### Uncomplicated UTI

*Adult:* **PO/IV** 250 mg q24h × 14 days

### Complicated UTI, Pyelonephritis

*Adult:* **PO/IV** 250 mg q24h × 10 days

### Acute Bacterial Sinusitis

*Adult:* **PO/IV** 750 mg daily × 5 days

### Chronic Bacterial Prostatitis

*Adult:* **PO/IV** 500 mg q24h × 28 days

### Skin & Skin Structure Infections

*Adult:* **PO** 750 mg q24h × 14 days

### Inhaled Anthrax

*Adult/Adolescent/Child (weight at least 50 kg):* **IV** 500 mg daily × 60 days
*Infant/Child (6 mo or older and weight less than 50 kg):* **IV** 8 mg/kg q12h (no more than 250 mg/dose)

### Plague

*Adult:* **PO** 500 mg daily for 10–14 days

### *Renal Impairment Dosage Adjustment*

For initial dose of 500 mg, adjust as follows: *CrCl 20–50 mL/min:* 250 mg q24h; *less than 20 mL/min:* 250 mg q48h
For initial dose of 750 mg, adjust as follows: *CrCl 20–50 mL/min:* 750 mg q48h; *10–19 mL/min:* 500 mg q48h; *less than 20 mL/min:* 250 mg q48h

## ADMINISTRATION

### Oral

- Do not give oral drug within 2 h of drugs containing aluminum or magnesium (antacids), iron, zinc, or sucralfate.

### Intravenous

*PREPARE:* **Intermittent:** Withdraw the desired dose from 500 or 750 mg (25 mg/mL) single use vial. ▪ Add to enough D5W, NS, D5/NS, D5/LR, or other compatible solutions to produce a concentration of 5 mg/mL [e.g., 500 mg (or 20 mL) added to 80 mL]. ▪ Discard any unused drug remaining in the vial.
*ADMINISTER:* **Intermittent:** Infuse 500 mg or less over 60 min. ▪ Infuse 750 mg over at least 90 min. ▪**Do not** give a bolus dose or infuse too rapidly.
*INCOMPATIBILITIES:* Y-site: Do not add any drugs to levofloxacin solution or infuse simultaneously through the same line (manufacturer recommendation).

- Store tablets in a tightly closed container. IV solution is stable for 72 h at 25° C (77° F).

## ADVERSE EFFECTS (≥1%) **CNS:** Headache, insomnia, dizziness. **GI:** Nausea, diarrhea, constipation, vomiting, abdominal pain, dyspepsia. **Skin:** Rash, pruritus. **Special Senses:** Decreased vision, foreign body sensation, transient ocular burning, ocular pain, photophobia. **Urogenital:** Vaginitis. **Body as a Whole:** Injection site pain or inflammation, chest or back pain, fever, pharyngitis. **Other:** Cartilage erosion.

Common adverse effects in *italic;* life-threatening effects underlined; generic names in **bold;** classifications in SMALL CAPS; ♣ Canadian drug name; ● Prototype drug

931

**DIAGNOSTIC TEST INTERFERENCE** May cause false positive on *opiate screening tests.*

**INTERACTIONS Drug:** **Magnesium** or **aluminum**-containing antacids, **sucralfate, iron, zinc** may decrease levofloxacin absorption; NSAIDS may increase risk of CNS reactions, including seizures; may cause hyper- or hypoglycemia in patients on ORAL HYPOGLYCEMIC AGENTS. Do not use with agents known to prolong QT interval (**bepridil, doeftilide, dronedarone, halofantrine, levomethadyl, pimozide, thioridazine, ziprasidone**).

**PHARMACOKINETICS Absorption:** Rapidly from GI tract. **Peak:** PO 1–2 h. **Distribution:** Penetrates lung tissue, 24–38% protein bound. **Metabolism:** Minimally in the liver. **Elimination:** Primarily unchanged in urine. **Half-Life:** 6–8 h.

## NURSING IMPLICATIONS

### Black Box Warning

*Levofloxacin has been associated with tendinitis and tendon rupture; drug may exacerbate muscle weakness in those with MG.*

### Assessment & Drug Effects

- Withhold therapy and report to prescriber immediately any of the following: Skin rash or other signs of a hypersensitivity reaction (see Appendix F); CNS symptoms such as seizures, restlessness, confusion, hallucinations, depression; skin eruption following sun exposure; symptoms of colitis such as persistent diarrhea; joint pain, inflammation, or rupture of a tendon.
- Monitor diabetics on oral hypolgycemic agents for loss of glycemic control.

- Monitor lab tests: C&S test prior to beginning therapy, serum creatinine/BUN, and LFTs.

### Patient & Family Education

- Discontinue drug and notify prescriber if S&S of hypersensitivity occur (e.g., skin rash, hives, rapid heartbeat, difficulty swallowing or breathing).
- If tendon pain occurs, discontinue the drug and notify the prescriber.
- Consume fluids liberally while taking levofloxacin. Failure to do so can lead to crystallization of urine.
- Allow a minimum of 2 h between drug dosage and taking any of the following: Aluminum or magnesium antacids, iron supplements, multivitamins with zinc, or sucralfate.
- Avoid exposure to excess sunlight or artificial UV light.
- Closely monitor blood glucose if taking oral hypoglycemic agents for diabetic control.

## LEVOLEUCOVORIN

(levo-loo-koe-vor'in)

Fusilev

**See Leucovorin.**

## LEVONORGESTREL-RELEASING INTRAUTERINE SYSTEM

(lee'vo-nor-jes-trel)

Kyleena, Liletta, Mirena, Skyla

**Classification:** PROGESTIN HORMONE
Therapeutic: PROGESTIN
**Prototype:** Norgestrel

**AVAILABILITY** IUD, tablet

**ACTION & *THERAPEUTIC EFFECT***
A progestogen that induces morphological changes in the endometrium

Common adverse effects in *italic;* life-threatening effects <u>underlined;</u> generic names in **bold;** classifications in SMALL CAPS; ♣ Canadian drug name; ● Prototype drug

including glandular atrophy, leukocytic infiltration, and decrease in glandular and stromal mitoses. Contraceptive effect may result by preventing follicular maturation and ovulation, thickening of the cervical mucus of the uterus, thus preventing passage of sperm into the uterus, or decreasing ability of sperm to survive in an environment of altered endometrium. *Effective contraceptive.*

**USES** Hormonal contraception, menorrhagia, postcoital contraception.

**CONTRAINDICATIONS** Hypersensitivity to any component of the product; previously inserted IUD which has not been removed; suspicion of pregnancy; history of ectopic pregnancy; history of uterine anomalies which distort the uterine cavity; acute PID; vaginal bleeding of unknown etiology; septic abortion in past 3 mo; abnormal Pap or suspected/known cervical neoplasm; known or suspected carcinoma of the breast; thrombophlebitis or thromboembolic disorders, pregnancy (category X).

**CAUTIOUS USE** Women at risk for or have a venereal disease; anemia, history of migraines, presence or history of salpingitis; genital bleeding of unknown etiology; severe arterial disease; coagulopathy; previous pelvic surgery.

## ROUTE & DOSAGE

### Contraception

*Adult:* **Intrauterine** Insert device at any point in menstrual cycle; may leave in place up to 3 y (**Skyla**), 4y (**Liletta**) or 5 y (**Mirena** or **Kyleena**)

### Post Coital Contraception

*Adult/Adolescent:* **Oral** 1 tablet as soon as possible after intercourse

## ADMINISTRATION

**Intrauterine**
- Inserted only by prescriber or other person qualified by special training in the intrauterine system.

**ADVERSE EFFECTS** (≥1%) **CV:** Hypertension. **GI:** *Abdominal pain,* nausea. **Endocrine:** Breast tenderness/pain. **Hematologic:** Anemia. **Metabolic:** Weight gain. **CNS:** Depression, emotional lability, headache (including migraine), nervousness, *fatigue.* **Skin:** *Acne,* alopecia, eczema. **Urogenital:** *Amenorrhea, intermenstrual bleeding,* dysmenorrhea, leukorrhea, decreased libido, vaginal moniliasis, vulvovaginal disorders, cervicitis, dyspareunia.

**INTERACTIONS Drug:** Do not use with **bosentan**.

**PHARMACOKINETICS Peak:** Few weeks. **Duration:** 5 y. **Distribution:** 86% protein bound. **Metabolism:** In liver. **Elimination:** In both urine and feces. **Half-Life:** 37 h.

## NURSING IMPLICATIONS

### Assessment & Drug Effects

- Monitor for decreased pulse, perspiration, or pallor during insertion. Keep patient supine until these signs have disappeared.
- Monitor BP especially with preexisting hypertension.

### Patient & Family Education

- Report S&S of PID immediately: (e.g., prolonged or heavy bleeding, unusual vaginal discharge, abdominal or pelvic pain or tenderness, painful sexual intercourse, chills, fever, and flu-like symptoms).
- Report S & S of depression.
- Report any of the following to prescriber immediately: Migraine (if not experienced before) or

Common adverse effects in *italic;* life-threatening effects underlined; generic names in **bold;** classifications in SMALL CAPS; ♣ Canadian drug name; ⊘ Prototype drug

933

exceptionally severe headache, or jaundice.

# LEVORPHANOL TARTRATE
(lee-vor'fa-nole)

**Classifications:** ANALGESIC; NARCOTIC (OPIATE AGONIST)
Therapeutic: NARCOTIC ANALGESIC
**Prototype:** Morphine sulfate
**Controlled Substance:** Schedule II

## AVAILABILITY Tablet

## ACTION & *THERAPEUTIC EFFECT*
A potent synthetic morphine derivative with agonist activity only. Reported to cause less nausea, vomiting, and constipation than equivalent doses of morphine but may produce more sedation, smooth-muscle relaxation, and respiratory depression. *More potent as an analgesic and has somewhat longer duration of action than morphine.*

## USES To relieve moderate to severe pain.

## CONTRAINDICATIONS Hypersensitivity to levorphanol; labor and delivery, pregnancy (category D with long time use or high doses); lactation.

## CAUTIOUS USE Patients with impaired respiratory reserve, or depressed respirations from another cause (e.g., severe infection, obstructive respiratory conditions, chronic bronchial asthma); head injury or increased intracranial pressure; acute MI, cardiac dysfunction; liver disease, biliary surgery, alcohol or delirium tremens; liver or kidney dysfunction, hypothyroidism, Addison's disease, toxic psychosis, prostatic hypertrophy, or urethral stricture; older adults, other vulnerable populations; pregnancy (category B, short-term use of low doses); children.

## ROUTE & DOSAGE

**Moderate to Severe Pain**
*Adult:* **PO** 2 mg q6–8h prn

## ADMINISTRATION
### Oral
▪ Give in the smallest effective dose to minimize the possibility of tolerance and physical dependence.

## ADVERSE EFFECTS (≥1%) **CNS:**
Euphoria, *sedation, drowsiness,* nervousness, confusion. **CV:** Hypotension, arrhythmias. **GI:** *Nausea,* vomiting, dry mouth, cramps, *constipation.* **Urogenital:** Urinary frequency, urinary retention, sedation. **Special Senses:** Blurred vision. **Respiratory:** Respiratory depression. **Body as a Whole:** Physical dependence.

## INTERACTIONS **Drug: Alcohol** and other CNS DEPRESSANTS compound sedation and CNS depression. **Herbal: St. John's wort** may increase sedation.

## PHARMACOKINETICS **Peak:** 60–90 min. **Duration:** 6–8 h. **Distribution:** Crosses placenta; distributed into breast milk. **Metabolism:** In liver. **Elimination:** In urine. **Half-Life:** 11–16 h.

## NURSING IMPLICATIONS
### Assessment & Drug Effects
▪ Assess degree of pain relief. Drug is most effective when peaks and valleys of pain relief are avoided.
▪ Monitor bowel function.

- Monitor ambulation, especially in older adult patients.

**Patient & Family Education**

- Do not drive or engage in other potentially hazardous activities.
- Avoid alcohol and other CNS depressants unless approved by prescriber.
- Note: Ambulation may increase frequency of nausea and vomiting.
- Increase fluid and fiber intake to offset constipating effects of the drug.

## LEVOTHYROXINE SODIUM (T₄) ⊕
(lee-voe-thye-rox′een)

Eltroxin ◆, Levoxyl, Synthroid, Unithroid

**Classification:** THYROID HORMONE REPLACEMENT
**Therapeutic:** THYROID HORMONE REPLACEMENT

**AVAILABILITY** Tablet; solution for injection

**ACTION & THERAPEUTIC EFFECT**
Synthetically prepared levo-isomer of thyroxine (T₄, principal component of thyroid gland secretions, determines normal thyroid function). Principal effects include diuresis, loss of weight and puffiness, increased sense of well-being and activity tolerance, plus rise of T₃ and T₄ serum levels toward normal. *By replacing decreased or absent thyroid hormone, it restores metabolic rate of a hypothyroid individual.*

**USES** Specific replacement therapy for diminished or absent thyroid function. Administered orally for hypothyroid state; administered IV for myxedematous coma or other thyroid dysfunctions demanding rapid replacement, as well as in failure to respond to oral therapy.

**CONTRAINDICATIONS** Hypersensitivity to levothyroxine; thyrotoxicosis; severe cardiovascular conditions, acute MI; obesity treatment; adrenal insufficiency.

**CAUTIOUS USE** Cardiac disease, angina pectoris, cardiac arrhythmias, hypertension; diabetes mellitus, older adult; impaired kidney function; pregnancy (category A).

## ROUTE & DOSAGE

**Thyroid Replacement**

*Adult:* **PO** 1.7 mcg/kg/day; about 25–50 mcg/day, gradually increased by 50–100 mcg q1–4wk to usual dose of 100–400 mcg/day; **IV** ½ established oral dose (usually 50–100 mcg daily)
*Child (3–6 mo):* **PO** 8–10 mcg/kg/day or 25–50 mcg/day; *6–12 mo:* 6–8 mcg/kg/day *1–5 y:* 5–6 mcg/kg/day *6–12 y:* 4–5 mcg/kg/day *12 y or older:* 2–3 mcg/kg/day or greater than 150 mcg/day

**Myxedematous Coma**

*Adult:* **IV** 300–500 mcg day 1, additional 100–300 mcg on day 2 if needed

## ADMINISTRATION

**Oral**

- Give as a single dose, preferably 30 min–1 h before breakfast. Give consistently with respect to meals. Administer 4 h apart from antacids, iron, and calcium supplements.
- Maintenance dosage for older adults may be 25% lower than for heavier and younger adults.

---

Common adverse effects in *italic;* life-threatening effects <u>underlined</u>; generic names in **bold;** classifications in SMALL CAPS; ◆ Canadian drug name; ⊕ Prototype drug

- Store in a tight, light-resistant container.

**Intravenous**

*PREPARE:* **Direct:** Reconstitute vial by adding 5 mL of NS for injection to each 100 mcg. Shake well to dissolve. Use immediately.
*ADMINISTER:* **Direct:** Give bolus dose over 1 min not to exceed 100 mcg per min.
*INCOMPATIBILITIES:* Do not mix with other medications.

- Store dry powder at 20°–25° C (68°–77° F).

## ADVERSE EFFECTS (≥1%) CNS:

Irritability, nervousness, *insomnia,* headache (pseudotumor cerebri in children), tremors, craniosynostosis (excessive doses in children). **CV:** Palpitations, tachycardia, arrhythmias, angina pectoris, hypertension, congestive heart failure. **GI:** Nausea, diarrhea, change in appetite. **Urogenital:** Menstrual irregularities. **Body as a Whole:** Weight loss, heat intolerance, sweating, fever, leg cramps, temporary hair loss (children).

## INTERACTIONS Drug: Choles-

**tyramine, colestipol** decrease absorption of levothyroxine; **epinephrine, norepinephrine** increase risk of cardiac insufficiency; ORAL ANTICOAGULANTS may potentiate hypoprothrombinemia. **Food:** Food can inhibit absorption so should be taken on an empty stomach.

## PHARMACOKINETICS Absorp-

**tion:** Variable and incompletely absorbed from GI tract (50–80%). **Peak:** 3–4 wk. **Duration:** 1–3 wk. **Distribution:** Gradually released into tissue cells; 99% protein bound. **Half-Life:** 6–7 days.

## NURSING IMPLICATIONS

### Black Box Warning

*In euthyroid patients, levothyroxine doses within the range of daily hormonal requirements are ineffective for weight reduction. Larger doses may produce serious or even life-threatening manifestations of toxicity, particularly when given in association with sympathomimetic amines such as those used for their anorectic effects.*

### Assessment & Drug Effects

- Monitor HR and BP. Report promptly tachycardia or suspected arrhythmias.
- Monitor for adverse effects during early adjustment. If metabolism increases too rapidly, especially in older adults and heart disease patients, symptoms of angina or cardiac failure may appear.
- Monitor bone age, growth, and psychomotor function in children.
- Some children have partial hair loss after a few months; it returns even with continued therapy.
- Synthroid 100 and 300 mcg tablets contain tartrazine, which may cause an allergic-type reaction in certain patients; particularly those who are hypersensitive to aspirin.
- Monitor lab tests: Baseline and periodic tests of thyroid function. Frequent PT/INR with concurrent anticoagulant therapy.

### Patient & Family Education

- Thyroid replacement therapy is usually lifelong.
- Notify prescriber immediately of signs of toxicity (e.g., chest pain, palpitations, nervousness).
- Avoid OTC medications unless approved by prescriber.

Common adverse effects in *italic;* life-threatening effects <u>underlined</u>; generic names in **bold;** classifications in SMALL CAPS; ♣ Canadian drug name; ⊘ Prototype drug

# LIDOCAINE HYDROCHLORIDE 🅟🅟

(lye'doe-kane)

Anestacon, Dilocaine, L-Caine, Lidoderm, Lida-Mantle, Lidoject-1, LidoPen Auto Injector, Nervocaine, Octocaine, Xylocaine, Xylocard ♣

**Classifications:** CLASS IB ANTIARRHYTHMIC; LOCAL ANESTHETIC (AMIDE TYPE)
Therapeutic: CLASS IB ANTIARRHYTHMIC; LOCAL ANESTHETIC; ANTICONVULSANT

**AVAILABILITY Antidysrhythmic:** Autoinjector; injection. **Local Anesthetic:** Injection. **Topical:** Solution; ointment; cream; gel; spray; jelly; patch; intradermal patch

## ACTION & *THERAPEUTIC EFFECT*

Exerts antiarrhythmic action (Class IB) by suppressing automaticity in His-Purkinje system. Combines with fast sodium channels in myocardial cell membranes, thus inhibiting sodium influx into myocardial cells. Thus it decreases ventricular depolarization, automaticity, and excitability during diastole. As a local anesthetic, it decreases pain through a reversible nerve conduction blockade. *Suppresses automaticity in His-Purkinje system of the heart and elevates electrical stimulation threshold of ventricle during diastole. Prompt, intense, and longer-lasting local anesthetic than procaine.*

**USES** Rapid control of ventricular arrhythmias occurring during acute MI, cardiac surgery, and cardiac catheterization and those caused by digitalis intoxication. Also as surface and infiltration anesthesia and for nerve block, including caudal and spinal block anesthesia and to relieve local discomfort of skin and mucous membranes. **Patch** for relief of pain associated with post-herpetic neuralgia.

**UNLABELED USES** Refractory status epilepticus.

**CONTRAINDICATIONS** History of hypersensitivity to amide-type local anesthetics; application or injection of lidocaine anesthetic in presence of severe trauma or sepsis, blood dyscrasias, post-MI; supraventricular arrhythmias, Stokes-Adams syndrome, untreated sinus bradycardia, severe degrees of sinoatrial, atrioventricular, and intraventricular heart block.

**CAUTIOUS USE** Liver or kidney disease, CHF, marked hypoxia, respiratory depression, hypovolemia, shock; myasthenia gravis; debilitated patients, older adults; family history of malignant hyperthermia (fulminant hypermetabolism); pregnancy (category B); lactation. **Topical use:** In eyes, over large body areas, over prolonged periods, in severe or extensive trauma or skin disorders.

## ROUTE & DOSAGE

### Ventricular Arrhythmias

*Adult:* **IV** 50–100 mg bolus at a rate of 20–50 mg/min, may repeat in 5 min, then start infusion of 1–4 mg/min immediately after first bolus, not more than 300 mg/h; **IM** 200–300 mg, may repeat once after 60–90 min
*Child:* **IV** 1 mg/kg bolus dose, then 20–50 mcg/kg/min infusion

### Anesthetic Uses

*Adult:* **Infiltration** 0.5–1% solution; **Nerve block** 1–2% solution; **Epidural** 1–2% solution **Caudal**

---

1–1.5% solution; **Spinal** 5% with glucose; **Saddle Block** 1.5% with dextrose; **Topical** 2.5–5% jelly, ointment, cream, or solution

**Post-Herpetic Neuralgia**

*Adult:* **Topical** Apply up to 3 patches over intact skin in most painful areas once for up to 12 h per 24 h period

## ADMINISTRATION

### Intramuscular
- Give in deltoid muscle as preferred site.

### Topical
- Do not apply topical lidocaine to large areas of skin or to broken or abraded surfaces. Consult prescriber about covering area with a dressing.
- Avoid topical preparation contact with eyes.

### Intravenous
- Note: Do not use lidocaine solutions containing preservatives for spinal or epidural (including caudal) block. Use ONLY lidocaine HCl injection without preservatives or epinephrine that is specifically labeled for IV injection or infusion.

*PREPARE:* **Direct:** Give undiluted. **IV Infusion:** Use D5W for infusion. For adults, add 1 g to 250 or 500 mL to yield 2 or 4 mg/mL, respectively; for children, add 120 mg to 100 m to yield 1.2 mg/mL. ▪Do not use solutions with particulate matter or discoloration.

*ADMINISTER:* **Direct:** Give at a rate of 50 mg or fraction thereof over 1 min. **IV Infusion:** Use micro-drip and infusion pump. *Adult:* Rate of flow is usually 1–4 mg/min or less. *Child:* Infuse at 20–50 mcg/kg/min.

*INCOMPATIBILITIES:* Solution/additive: Ampicillin, cefazolin, methohexital, phenytoin. Y-site: Amphotericin B cholesteryl complex, phenytoin.

▪Discard partially used solutions of lidocaine without preservatives.

## ADVERSE EFFECTS (≥1%) CNS:
Drowsiness, dizziness, light-headedness, restlessness, confusion, disorientation, irritability, apprehension, euphoria, wild excitement, numbness of lips or tongue and other paresthesias including sensations of heat and cold, chest heaviness, difficulty in speaking, <u>difficulty in breathing or swallowing</u>, muscular twitching, tremors, psychosis. With high doses: <u>Convulsions, respiratory depression and arrest.</u> **CV:** With high doses: hypotension, bradycardia, conduction disorders including heart block, <u>cardiovascular collapse, cardiac arrest</u>. **Special Senses:** Tinnitus, decreased hearing; blurred or double vision, impaired color perception. **Skin:** Site of topical application may develop erythema, edema. **GI:** Anorexia, nausea, vomiting. **Body as a Whole:** Excessive perspiration, soreness at IM site, local thrombophlebitis (with prolonged IV infusion), hypersensitivity reactions (urticaria, rash, edema, <u>anaphylactoid reactions</u>).

## DIAGNOSTIC TEST INTERFERENCE
Increases in *creatine phosphokinase (CPK)* level may occur for 48 h after IM dose and may interfere with test for presence of MI.

## INTERACTIONS Drug:
Lidocaine patch may increase toxic effects of **tocainide, mexiletine;** BARBITURATES decrease lidocaine activity; **cimetidine,** BETA-BLOCKERS, **quinidine** increase pharmacologic

effects of lidocaine; **phenytoin** increases cardiac depressant effects; **procainamide** compounds neurologic and cardiac effects.

## PHARMACOKINETICS

**Absorption:** Topical application is 3% absorbed through intact skin. **Onset:** 45–90 sec IV; 5–15 min IM; 2–5 min topical. **Duration:** 10–20 min IV; 60–90 min IM; 30–60 min topical; greater than 100 min injected for anesthesia. **Distribution:** Crosses blood–brain barrier and placenta; distributed into breast milk. **Metabolism:** In liver via CYP3A4 and 2D6. **Elimination:** In urine. **Half-Life:** 1.5–2 h.

## NURSING IMPLICATIONS

### Assessment & Drug Effects

- Stop infusion immediately if ECG indicates excessive cardiac depression (e.g., prolongation of PR interval or QRS complex and the appearance or aggravation of arrhythmias).
- Monitor BP and ECG constantly; assess respiratory and neurologic status frequently to avoid potential overdosage and toxicity.
- Auscultate lungs for basilar rales, especially in patients who tend to metabolize the drug slowly (e.g., CHF, cardiogenic shock, hepatic dysfunction).
- Watch for neurotoxic effects (e.g., drowsiness, dizziness, confusion, paresthesias, visual disturbances, excitement, behavioral changes) in patients receiving IV infusions or with high lidocaine blood levels.

### Patient & Family Education

- Swish and spit out when using lidocaine solution for relief of mouth discomfort; gargle for use in pharynx, may be swallowed (as prescribed).

- Oral topical anesthetics (e.g., Xylocaine Viscous) may interfere with swallowing reflex. **Do not** ingest food within 60 min after drug application; especially pediatric, geriatric, or debilitated patients.

# LIFITEGRAST
(lif-i-teg'-rast)

Xiidra

**Classifications:** IMMUNOMODULATOR; LYMPHOCYTE FUNCTION-ASSOCIATED ANTIGEN-1 (LFA-1) ANTAGONIST

**Therapeutic:** IMMUNOMODULATOR

## AVAILABILITY
Ophthalmic solution

## ACTION & *THERAPEUTIC EFFECT*

The exact mechanism of action is unknown; however, lifitegrast binds to the integrin lymphocyte function-associated antigen-1 (LFA-1) and blocks the interaction of LFA-1 with intercellular adhesion molecule-1 (ICAM-1). *ICAM-1 may be overexpressed in corneal and conjunctival tissues in dry eye disease.*

## USES
Treatment of the signs and symptoms of dry eye disease (DED).

## CAUTIOUS USE
Use of contact lenses, lactation, pregnancy.

## ROUTE & DOSAGE

### Dry Eye Disease
*Adult:* **Ophthalmic** 1 drop b.i.d.

## ADMINISTRATION

### Ophthalmic

- Remove contact lenses before instilling drops. Wait 15 min before re-inserting lenses.
- Avoid touching tip of dropper to the eye or any surface.

Common adverse effects in *italic;* life-threatening effects <u>underlined</u>; generic names in **bold;** classifications in SMALL CAPS; ♣ Canadian drug name; ⊘ Prototype drug

939

- Gently instill one drop onto lower eyelid. Repeat for second eye.
- Discard single-use container after instilling in each eye.

**ADVERSE EFFECTS** (≥1%) **Body as a Whole:** Dysgeusia. **CNS:** Headache. **Respiratory:** Sinusitis. **Special Senses:** Blurred vision, conjunctival hyperemia, eye discharge, eye discomfort, eye irritation, eye pruritus, increased lacrimation, instillation site irritation, reduced visual acuity.

**PHARMACOKINETICS** Due to ophthalmic administration, pharmacokinetic data is limited.

## NURSING IMPLICATIONS

### Assessment & Drug Effects
- Monitor patient for signs or symptoms of an allergic reaction such as rash; hives; itching; shortness of breath; wheezing; cough; or swelling of the face, lips, tongue, or throat.

### Patient & Family Education
- Use caution when driving or performing other tasks that require clear eyesight.
- Tell your doctor if you are breastfeeding or pregnant.
- Wash hands before instilling eye drops.
- Avoid touching tip of eyedropper to eye or any other surface.

## LINACLOTIDE
(lin'a-clo-tide)

Linzess

**Classification:** ACCELERANT OF GI TRANSIT; GUANYLATE CYCLASE-C AGONIST

**Therapeutic:** ACCELERANT OF GI TRANSIT

**AVAILABILITY** Capsule

## ACTION & *THERAPEUTIC EFFECT*
Acts on the inner surface of the intestinal epithelium to increase concentrations of cGMP. Increased intracellular cGMP results in increased intestinal fluid and accelerated transit. Increased extracellualar cGMP decreases the activity of pain-sensing nerves. *Improves bowel function by decreasing constipation and associated pain due to bowel irritation.*

**USES** Treatment of irritable bowel syndrome with constipation and chronic idiopathic constipation.

**CONTRAINDICATIONS** Severe diarrhea; known or suspected mechanical GI obstruction; children younger than 6 y.

**CAUTIOUS USE** Pregnancy (category C); lactation. Safety and efficacy in children younger than 18 y not established.

## ROUTE & DOSAGE

**Irritable Bowel Syndrome with Constipation**

*Adult:* **PO** 290 mcg once daily

**Chronic Idiopathic Constipation**

*Adult:* **PO** 145 mcg once daily

## ADMINISTRATION

### Oral
- Give on an empty stomach at least 30 min prior to first meal of day.
- Ensure that capsules are swallowed whole. They should not be opened or chewed.
- Store at 20°–25° C (68°–77° F).

**ADVERSE EFFECTS** (≥1%) **Body as a Whole:** Headache, fatigue. **GI:** Abdominal distension, abdominal

Common adverse effects in *italic;* life-threatening effects <u>underlined;</u> generic names in **bold;** classifications in SMALL CAPS; ♣ Canadian drug name; ⊙ Prototype drug

pain, *diarrhea*, dyspepsia, fecal incontinence, flatulence, gastro-esophageal reflux disease, viral gastroenteritis, vomiting. **Respiratory:** Sinusitis, upper respiratory tract infection.

## PHARMACOKINETICS **Absorption:** Minimally absorbed. **Metabolism:** In the GI tract to active metabolite. **Elimination:** Fecal.

## NURSING IMPLICATIONS

### Assessment & Drug Effects
▪ Monitor bowel pattern. Report severe abdominal pain, severe diarrhea, or passage of bloody stools.

### Patient & Family Education
▪ Stop taking drug and seek immediate medical attention if you develop unusual or severe abdominal pain, and/or severe diarrhea, especially if in combination with red blood in the stool or passage of black, tarry stool.

## LINAGLIPTIN
(lin'a glip'tin)

Tradjenta

**Classifications:** HORMONE MODIFIER; ANTIDIABETIC; INCRETIN MODIFIER; DIPEPTIDYL PEPTIDASE-4 (DPP-4) INHIBITOR
**Therapeutic:** ANTIDIABETIC; DDP-4 INHIBITOR
**Prototype:** Sitagliptin

## AVAILABILITY Tablet

## ACTION & *THERAPEUTIC EFFECT*
Slows inactivation of incretin hormones released by the intestine. When the blood glucose begins to rise, incretin hormones stimulate insulin secretion and reduce glucagon secretion, resulting in decreased hepatic glucose production. *Sitagliptin lowers both fasting and postprandial plasma glucose levels.*

## USES Treatment of type 2 diabetes mellitus in combination with diet and exercise.

## CONTRAINDICATIONS History of hypersensitivity to linagliptin (e.g., urticaria, angioedema, or bronchial hyperreactivity); acute pancreatitis.

## CAUTIOUS USE Previous history of angioedema with another DPP-4 inhibitor; concurrent use with an insulin secretagogue (e.g., sulfonylurea); history of pancreatitis; pregnancy (category B); lactation. Safety and efficacy in children not established.

## ROUTE & DOSAGE

**Type 2 Diabetes Mellitus**
*Adult:* PO 5 mg once daily

## ADMINISTRATION

### Oral
▪ May be given with or without food.
▪ Store at 15°–30° C (59°–86° F).

## ADVERSE EFFECTS (≥2%) **Body as a Whole:** Hypersensitivity reactions. **CNS:** Headache. **Metabolic:** *Hypoglycemia,* hyperlipidemia, hypertriglyceridemia, increased uric acid levels, weight gain, pancreatitis. **Musculoskeletal:** Arthralgia, back pain, myalgia. **Respiratory:** Cough, nasopharyngitis. **GI:** Constipation. **GU:** Urinary tract infection.

## INTERACTIONS **Drug:** Strong inducers of CYP3A4 (e.g., **rifampin, dexamethasone, phenytoin, phenobarbital**) or P-glycoprotein (e.g., **rifampin**) may decrease the therapeutic effect of linagliptin. Combination use with a SULFONYLUREA (e.g., **glyburide**) may increase the risk of hypoglycemia.

L

---

Common adverse effects in *italic;* life-threatening effects underlined; generic names in **bold;** classifications in SMALL CAPS; ♣ Canadian drug name; ◘ Prototype drug

941

**PHARMACOKINETICS** **Absorption:** 30% bioavailable. **Peak:** 1.5 h. **Metabolism:** Primarily excreted unchanged. **Elimination:** Enterohepatic system (80%) and renal elimination (5%). **Half-Life:** 12 h.

## NURSING IMPLICATIONS

### Assessment & Drug Effects

- Monitor for S&S of hypoglycemia when used in combination with a sulfonylurea drug or insulin.
- Monitor for serious hypersensitivity reactions (e.g., angioedema, exfoliative skin conditions). Onset may occur any time during the first 3 mo of treatment.
- Monitor lab tests: Baseline and periodic HbA1C, blood glucose, serum creatinine/BUN.

### Patient & Family Education

- Seek medical attention during periods of stress or illness as dosage adjustments may be required.
- Monitor both fasting and postprandial blood glucose levels as directed.
- Report promptly for medical evaluation if you experience any of the following: Wheezing; chest tightness; fever; itching; bad cough; blue skin color; seizures; or swelling of face, lips, tongue, or throat.
- Note that when taken alone to control diabetes, linagliptin is unlikely to cause hypoglycemia because it only works when the blood sugar is rising.

## LINCOMYCIN HYDROCHLORIDE

(lin-koe-mye′sin)

Lincocin

**Classification:** LINCOSAMIDE ANTIBIOTIC

**Therapeutic:** ANTIBIOTIC
**Prototype:** Clindamycin

**AVAILABILITY** Solution for injection

## ACTION & *THERAPEUTIC EFFECT*

Derived from *Streptomyces lincolnensis* and binds to the 50S ribosomal subunits of the bacteria inhibiting protein synthesis, eventually resulting in inhibition of bacterial cell growth or bacterial cell death. *Effective against most common gram-positive pathogens. Also effective against many anaerobic bacteria.*

**USES** Reserved for treatment of serious infections caused by susceptible bacteria in penicillin-allergic patients or patients for whom penicillin is inappropriate.

**CONTRAINDICATIONS** Previous hypersensitivity to lincomycin and clindamycin; impaired liver function, known monilial infections (unless treated concurrently); lactation.

**CAUTIOUS USE** Impaired kidney function; history of GI disease, particularly colitis; history of liver, endocrine, or metabolic diseases; history of asthma, hay fever, eczema, drug or other allergies; older adult patients, pregnancy (category B); infants younger than 1 mo.

## ROUTE & DOSAGE

### Infections

*Adult:* **IM** 600 mg q12–24 h **IV** 600 mg–1 g q8–12h (max: 8 g/day)
*Adolescent/Child/Infant (older than 1 mo):* **IM** 10 mg/kg q12–24h; **IV** 10–20 mg/kg/day divided q8–12h

Common adverse effects in *italic;* life-threatening effects <u>underlined</u>; generic names in **bold;** classifications in SMALL CAPS; ♣ Canadian drug name; ● Prototype drug

## ADMINISTRATION

### Intramuscular

- Give injection deep into large muscle mass; inject slowly to minimize pain. Rotate injection sites.

### Intravenous

*PREPARE:* **Intermittent:** Dilute each 1 g of lincomycin in at least 100 mL of D5W, NS, or other compatible solution.

*ADMINISTER:* **Intermittent:** Give at a rate of 1 g/h.

*INCOMPATIBILITIES:* Solution/additive: **Colistimethate, kanamycin, methicillin, penicillin G, phenytoin.**

- Follow manufacturer's directions for further information on reconstitution, storage time, compatible IV fluids, and IV administration rates.

**ADVERSE EFFECTS** (≥1%) **Body as a Whole:** Hypersensitivity [pruritus, urticaria, skin rashes, exfoliative and vesiculobullous dermatitis, erythema multiforme (rare), angioedema, photosensitivity, <u>anaphylactoid reaction</u>, serum sickness]; superinfections (proctitis, pruritus ani, vaginitis); vertigo, dizziness, headache, generalized myalgia, thrombophlebitis following IV use; pain at IM injection site. **CV:** Hypotension, syncope, <u>cardiopulmonary arrest</u> (particularly after rapid IV). **GI:** Glossitis, stomatitis, *nausea, vomiting,* anorexia, decreased taste acuity, unpleasant or altered taste, abdominal cramps, *diarrhea,* acute enterocolitis, <u>pseudomembranous colitis (potentially fatal)</u>. **Hematologic:** Neutropenia, <u>leukopenia</u>, <u>agranulocytosis</u>, thrombocytopenic purpura, <u>aplastic anemia</u>. **Special Senses:** Tinnitus.

**INTERACTIONS Drug: Kaolin and pectin** decrease lincomycin absorption; **tubocurarine,** **pancuronium** may enhance neuromuscular blockade.

**PHARMACOKINETICS** **Peak:** 30 min IM. **Duration:** 12–14 h IM; 14 h IV. **Distribution:** High concentrations in bone, aqueous humor, bile, and peritoneal, pleural, and synovial fluids; crosses placenta; distributed into breast milk. **Metabolism:** Partially in liver. **Elimination:** In urine and feces. **Half-Life:** 5 h.

## NURSING IMPLICATIONS

### Black Box Warning

*Lincomycin has been associated with severe, potentially fatal, C. difficile pseudomenbranous colitis.*

### Assessment & Drug Effects

- Monitor BP and pulse. Have patient remain recumbent following drug administration until BP stabilizes.
- Monitor closely and report changes in bowel frequency. Discontinue drug if significant diarrhea occurs.
- Diarrhea, acute colitis, or pseudomembranous colitis (see Appendix F) may occur up to several weeks after cessation of therapy.
- Examine IM/IV injection sites daily for signs of inflammation.
- Monitor serum drug levels closely in patients with severe impairment of kidney function.
- Monitor for S&S of superinfections that are most likely to occur when therapy exceeds 10 days (see Appendix F).
- Monitor lab tests: C&S prior to initiating therapy; periodic LFTs, renal function tests, and CBC during prolonged drug therapy.

### Patient & Family Education

- Notify prescriber immediately of symptoms of hypersensitivity (see Appendix F). Drug should be discontinued.

Common adverse effects in *italic;* life-threatening effects <u>underlined</u>; generic names in **bold**; classifications in SMALL CAPS; ✦ Canadian drug name; ◐ Prototype drug

943

- Notify prescriber promptly of the onset of perianal irritation, diarrhea, or blood and mucus in stools.

# LINDANE ℗
(lin′dane)
**Classifications:** SCABICIDE; PEDICULICIDE
Therapeutic: ANTIPARASITIC; PEDICULICIDE

## AVAILABILITY Shampoo

## ACTION & THERAPEUTIC EFFECT
Action related to its direct absorption by parasites and ova (nits). Drug absorption through the parasite exoskeleton results in death of parasites and their ova. *Has ectoparasitic and ovicidal activity against the two variants of* Pediculus humanus, Pediculus capitis *(head louse) and* Pediculus pubis *(crab louse), and the arthropod* Sarcoptes scabiei *(scabies).*

## USES To treat head and crab lice and scabies infestations and to eradicate their ova.

## CONTRAINDICATIONS Premature
neonates, patient with known seizure disorders; application to eyes, face, mucous membranes, urethral meatus, open cuts or raw, weeping surfaces; prolonged or excessive applications or simultaneous application of creams, ointments, oils; extensive dermatitis; uncontrolled seizures; lactation.

## CAUTIOUS USE History of seizures; HIV infection; history of head trauma; elderly, individuals weighing less than 50 kg (110 lbs); alcoholism; pregnancy (category C); infants, children younger than 10 y, or individuals weighing less than 110 lb.

## ROUTE & DOSAGE

### Lice and Scabies Infestation
*Adult/Child:* **Topical** Apply to all body areas except the face, leave lotion on 8–12 h, then rinse off; leave shampoo on 4 min, then rinse thoroughly; **do not** repeat in less than 1 wk

## ADMINISTRATION
Note: Caregiver needs to wear plastic disposable or rubber gloves when applying lindane (nitrile, latex with neoprene or sheer vinyl). Thoroughly clean hands after application, especially if pregnant or applying medication to more than one patient, to avoid prolonged skin contact.

### Topical
- Remove all skin lotions, creams, and oil-based hair dressings completely and allow skin to dry and cool before applying lindane; this will reduce percutaneous absorption.
- Shake cream or lotion container well. Apply thin film over the affected areas. Leave in place 8–12 h and follow with bath or shower.
- Shampoo: Hair should be dry before application. Apply to dry hair without adding water. Work drug thoroughly onto hair shafts and scalp and allow to remain in place 4 min. Immediately rinse all lather away and avoid unnecessary contact with other body surfaces. Towel dry briskly and then remove nits with nit comb or tweezers.
- Store in a tight container away from direct light and heat. Protect from freezing. Store at 20°–25° C (68°–77° F).

## ADVERSE EFFECTS (≥1%) CNS:
CNS stimulation (usually after accidental ingestion or misuse of product): Restlessness, anxiety,

dizziness, tremors, convulsions; seizures; <u>death</u>. **Body as a Whole:** Inhalation (headache, nausea, vomiting, myelosuppression, irritation of ENT). **Skin:** Eczematous eruptions.

**INTERACTIONS Drug:** No clinically significant interactions established.

**PHARMACOKINETICS Absorption:** Slowly and incompletely absorbed through intact skin; maximum absorption from face, scalp, axillae. **Distribution:** Stored in body fat. **Metabolism:** In liver. **Elimination:** In urine and feces.

## NURSING IMPLICATIONS

### Black Box Warning

*Lindane has been associated with seizures and death with repeated or prolonged application.*

### Assessment & Drug Effects

- Monitor for seizure activity in individuals with a history of seizures. Withhold drug and report to prescriber immediately.
- Exercise caution when using lindane on infants, children, the elderly, and individuals with other skin conditions (e.g., atopic dermatitis, psoriasis) and in those who weigh less than 110 lbs (50 kg) as they may be at risk of serious neurotoxicity.

### Patient & Family Education

- Lindane is highly toxic drug if topical applications are excessive or if swallowed or inhaled. Keep out of reach of children. **Do not** use more often than prescribed.
- Discontinue medication and notify prescriber if skin eruptions appear.
- Do not apply medication to face, mouth, open skin lesions, or to eyelashes; avoid contact with eyes. If accidental eye contact occurs, flush with water.

## LINEZOLID ℗

(lin-e-zo'lid)

**Zyvox, Zyvoxam ♣**

**Classification:** OXAZOLIDINONE ANTIBIOTIC

**Therapeutic:** ANTIBIOTIC

**AVAILABILITY** Tablet suspension; solution for injection

## ACTION & *THERAPEUTIC EFFECT*

Synthetic antibiotic that binds to a site on the 23S ribosomal RNA of bacteria, which prevents the bacterial RNA translation process, thus preventing further growth. *Is bactericidal against gram-positive, gram-negative, and anaerobic bacteria. Bacteriostatic against enterococci and staphylococci, and bactericidal against streptococci.*

**USES** Treatment of vancomycin-resistant *Enterococcus faecium* (VREF), nosocomial pneumonia, bacteremia, complicated and uncomplicated skin and skin structure infections, community-acquired pneumonia.

**CONTRAINDICATIONS** Hypersensitivity to linezolid; concurrent MAOI therapy.

**CAUTIOUS USE** History of thrombocytopenia, thrombocytopenia; patients on serotonin reuptake inhibitors, or adrenergic agents, active alcoholism, anemia, bleeding, bone marrow suppression, cardiac arrhythmias, cardiac disease, cerebrovascular disease, chemotherapy, coagulopathy, colitis, diarrhea, hypertension, hyperthyroidism, leukopenia, MI, radiographic contrast administration, spinal anesthesia, surgery, hypertension; phenylketonuria; carcinoid syndrome; pregnancy (category C); lactation.

L

---

Common adverse effects in *italic;* life-threatening effects <u>underlined;</u> generic names in **bold;** classifications in SMALL CAPS; ♣ Canadian drug name; ℗ Prototype drug

## ROUTE & DOSAGE

**Vancomycin-Resistant**
***Enterococcus faecium***

*Adult/Adolescent (12 y or older):*
**PO/IV** 600 mg q12h × 14–28
days
*Neonate/Infant/Child:* **PO/IV**
10 mg/kg q8h × 14–28 days

**Nosocomial or Community-
Acquired Pneumonia,
Complicated Skin Infections**

*Adult/Adolescent (12 y or older):*
**PO/IV** 600 mg q12h × 10–14
days
*Infant/Child:* **PO/IV** 10 mg/kg
q8h × 10–14 days

**Uncomplicated Skin Infections**

*Adult:* **PO** 400 mg q12h × 10–14
days
*Adolescent:* **PO** 600 mg q12h ×
10–14 days
*Infant/Child:* **PO** 10 mg/kg
q12h × 10–14 days

## ADMINISTRATION

Note: No dosage adjustment is necessary when switching from IV to
oral administration.

### Oral

- Reconstitute suspension by adding 123 mL distilled water in two
portions; after adding first half,
shake to wet all of the powder,
then add second half of water and
shake vigorously to produce a
uniform suspension with a concentration of 100 mg/5 mL.
- Before each use, mix suspension
by inverting bottle 3–5 × but **do
not shake.** Discard unused suspension after 21 days.

### Intravenous

*PREPARE:* **Intermittent:** IV solution
is supplied in a single-use,
ready-to-use infusion bag. Remove from protective wrap immediately prior to use. ▪Check for
minute leaks by firmly squeezing
bag. Discard if leaks are detected.
*ADMINISTER:* **Intermittent:** Do not
use infusion bag in a series connection. ▪Give over 30–120 min.
If IV line is used to infuse other
drugs, flush before and after with
D5W, NS, or LR.
*INCOMPATIBILITIES:* Solution/
additive: **Ceftriaxone, erythromycin, trimethoprim-
sulfamethoxazole.** Y-site:
**Amphotericin B, chlorproma-
zine, dantrolene, diazepam,
pantoprazole, pentamidine,
phenytoin.**

▪ Store at 25° C (77° F) preferred;
15°–30° C (59°–86° F) permitted.
Protect from light and keep bottles
tightly closed.

## ADVERSE EFFECTS (≥1%) **Body as
a Whole:** Fever. **GI:** Diarrhea,
nausea, vomiting, constipation,
taste alteration, abnormal LFTs,
tongue discoloration. **Hematologic:**
Thrombocytopenia, leukopenia.
**CNS:** Headache, insomnia, dizziness. **Skin:** Rash. **Urogenital:** Vaginal moniliasis.

## INTERACTIONS **Drug:** MAO IN-
HIBITORS may cause hypertensive
crisis; **pseudoephedrine** may
cause elevated BP; may cause
**serotonin** syndrome with SELEC-
TIVE SEROTONIN REUPTAKE INHIBITORS.
**Food:** Tyramine-containing food
may cause elevated BP. **Herbal:**
**Ginseng, ephedra, ma huang**
may lead to elevated BP, headache,
nervousness.

## PHARMACOKINETICS **Absorp-
tion:** Rapidly absorbed, 100%
bioavailable. **Peak:** 1–2 h PO.
**Distribution:** 31% protein bound.

Common adverse effects in *italic;* life-threatening effects underlined; generic names
in **bold;** classifications in SMALL CAPS; ✦ Canadian drug name; ◑ Prototype drug

946

**Metabolism:** By oxidation. **Elimination:** Primarily in urine. **Half-Life:** 6–7 h.

## NURSING IMPLICATIONS

### Assessment & Drug Effects

- Monitor for S&S of: Bleeding; hypertension; or pseudomembranous colitis that begins with diarrhea.
- Monitor lab tests: C&S before initiating therapy; periodic CBC, platelet count, Hgb and Hct, in those at risk for bleeding or with longer than 2 wk of linezolid therapy.

### Patient & Family Education

- Report any of the following to prescriber promptly: Onset of diarrhea; easy bruising or bleeding of any type; or S&S of superinfection (see Appendix F); S&S of seizure activity.
- Avoid foods and beverages high in tyramine (e.g., aged, fermented, pickled, or smoked foods, and beverages). Limit tyramine intake to less than 100 mg per meal (see *Information for Patients* provided by the manufacturer).
- Do not take OTC cold remedies or decongestants without consulting prescriber.
- Note for phenylketonurics: Each 5 mL oral suspension contains 20 mg phenylalanine.

## LIOTHYRONINE SODIUM (T₃)

(lye-oh-thye'roe-neen)

Cytomel, Triostat

**Classification:** THYROID HORMONE
**Therapeutic:** THYROID HORMONE REPLACEMENT
**Prototype:** Levothyroxine sodium

**AVAILABILITY** Tablet; solution for injection

## ACTION & *THERAPEUTIC EFFECT*

Synthetic form of natural thyroid hormone (T₃). Shares actions and uses of thyroid but has more rapid action and more rapid disappearance of effect, permitting quick dosage adjustment, if necessary. *Replacement therapy for absent or decreased thyroid hormone. Principal effect is an increase in the metabolic rate of all body tissues.*

**USES** Replacement or supplemental therapy for cretinism, myxedema, goiter, secondary (pituitary) or tertiary (hypothalamic) hypothyroidism, and T₃ suppression test.

**CONTRAINDICATIONS** Hypersensitivity to liothyronine; thyrotoxicosis; obesity treatment; severe cardiovascular conditions, acute MI, uncontrolled hypertension; adrenal insufficiency.

**CAUTIOUS USE** Angina pectoris, hypertension; diabetes mellitus; impaired kidney function, renal failure; older adult; pregnancy (category A); lactation; children.

## ROUTE & DOSAGE

### Thyroid Replacement

*Adult:* **PO** 25–75 mcg/day
*Geriatric:* **PO** 5 mcg/day, increase by 5 mcg/day every 1–2 wk
*Child:* **PO** 5 mcg/day gradually increased by 5 mcg/day q3–4days until desired response

### Myxedema

*Adult:* **PO** 5–100 mcg/day **IV** 25–50 mcg, may repeat between 4 and 12 h after previous dose. Target dose greater than 65 mcg/day (max: 100 mcg/day).

Common adverse effects in *italic;* life-threatening effects underlined; generic names in **bold;** classifications in SMALL CAPS; ✦ Canadian drug name; ◉ Prototype drug

947

*Geriatric:* **PO** Start at 5 mcg/day

**Goiter**

*Adult:* **PO** 5–75 mcg/day
*Geriatric:* **PO** Start at 5 mcg/day
*Child:* **PO** 5 mcg/day, increase by 5 mcg q1–2 wk (usual maintenance dose 15–20 mcg/day)

**T₃ Suppression Test**

*Adult:* **PO** 75–100 mcg/day × 7 days

## ADMINISTRATION

**Oral**

- Give daily before breakfast.

**Intravenous**

***PREPARE:*** **Direct:** Give undiluted.
***ADMINISTER:*** **Direct:** Give each 10 mcg or fraction thereof over 1 min.

- Store tablets in a heat-, light-, and moisture-proof container.

**ADVERSE EFFECTS** (≥1%) **Endocrine:** Result from overdosage evidenced as S&S of hyperthyroidism (see Appendix F). **Musculoskeletal:** Accelerated rate of bone maturation in children.

**INTERACTIONS Drug: Cholestyramine, colestipol** decrease absorption; **epinephrine, norepinephrine** increase risk of cardiac insufficiency; ORAL ANTICOAGULANTS may potentiate hypoprothrombinemia.

**PHARMACOKINETICS Absorption:** Completely absorbed from GI tract. **Peak:** 24–72 h. **Duration:** Up to 72 h. **Distribution:** Gradually released into tissue cells. **Half-Life:** 6–7 days.

## NURSING IMPLICATIONS

### Black Box Warning

*In euthyroid patients, levothyroxine doses within the range of daily hormonal requirements are ineffective for weight reduction. Larger doses may produce serious or even life-threatening manifestations of toxicity, particularly when given in association with sympathomimetic amines such as those used for their anorectic effects.*

### Assessment & Drug Effects

- Watch for possible additive effects during the early period of liothyronine substitution for another preparation, particularly in older adults, children, and patients with cardiovascular disease. Residual actions of other thyroid preparations may persist for weeks.
- Metabolic effects of liothyronine persist a few days after drug withdrawal.
- Withhold drug and notify prescriber at onset of overdosage symptoms (hyperthyroidism, see Appendix F); usually therapy can be resumed with lower dosage.

### Patient & Family Education

- Take medication exactly as ordered.
- Learn S&S of hyperthyroidism (see Appendix F); notify prescriber promptly if they appear.

## LIOTRIX (T₃-T₄)

(lye'oh-trix)

Thyrolar

**Classification:** THYROID HORMONE
**Therapeutic:** THYROID HORMONE REPLACEMENT
**Prototype:** Levothyroxine sodium

Common adverse effects in *italic*; life-threatening effects underlined; generic names in **bold**; classifications in SMALL CAPS; ♦ Canadian drug name; ⊘ Prototype drug

**AVAILABILITY** Tablet

## ACTION & *THERAPEUTIC EFFECT*

Synthetic levothyroxine (T$_4$) and liothyronine (T$_3$) that influence growth and maturation of tissues, increase energy expenditure, and affect turnover of essentially all substrates. These hormones play an integral role in metabolic processes, and are important to development of the CNS in newborns. *Increases metabolic rate of all body tissues.*

**USES** Replacement or supplemental therapy for cretinism, myxedema, goiter, and secondary (pituitary) or tertiary (hypothalamic) hypothyroidism. Also with antithyroid agents in thyrotoxicosis and to prevent goitrogenesis and hypothyroidism.

**CONTRAINDICATIONS** Untreated thyrotoxicosis, acute MI, morphologic hypogonadism, nephrosis, adrenal deficiency due to hypopituitarism; tartrazine dye hypersensitivity, obesity treatment.

**CAUTIOUS USE** Myxedema; hypertension, angina, cardiac arrhythmias, cardiac disease, coronary artery disease; older adults; hypertension; arteriosclerosis; kidney dysfunction; pregnancy (category A); lactation; neonates, infants, children.

## ROUTE & DOSAGE

### Thyroid Replacement
*Adult/Child:* **PO** 12.5–30 mcg/day, gradually increase to desired response

## ADMINISTRATION

### Oral
- Give as a single daily dose, preferably before breakfast.
- Make dose increases at 1- to 2-wk intervals.

- Store in a heat-, light-, and moisture-proof container. Shelf-life: 2 y.

**ADVERSE EFFECTS** (≥1%) **CNS:** Nervousness, headache, tremors, insomnia. **CV:** Palpitation, tachycardia, angina pectoris, cardiac arrhythmias, hypertension, CHF. **GI:** Nausea, abdominal cramps, diarrhea. **Body as a Whole:** Weight loss, heat intolerance, fever, sweating, menstrual irregularities. **Musculoskeletal:** Accelerated rate of bone maturation in infants and children.

**INTERACTIONS Drug: Cholestyramine, colestipol** decrease absorption; **epinephrine, norepinephrine** increase risk of cardiac insufficiency; ORAL ANTICOAGULANTS may potentiate hypoprothrombinemia.

## NURSING IMPLICATIONS

### Black Box Warning

*In euthyroid patients, levothyroxine doses within the range of daily hormonal requirements are ineffective for weight reduction. Larger doses may produce serious or even life-threatening manifestations of toxicity, particularly when given in association with sympathomimetic amines such as those used for their anorectic effects.*

### Assessment & Drug Effects
- Watch for possible additive effects during the early period of liothyronine substitution for another preparation, particularly in older adults, children, and patients with cardiovascular disease. Residual actions of other thyroid preparations may persist for weeks.
- Note: Metabolic effects of liotrix persist a few days after drug withdrawal.

---

- Withhold drug and notify prescriber at onset of overdosage symptoms (hyperthyroidism, see Appendix F); usually therapy can be resumed with lower dosage.
- Monitor diabetics for glycemic control; an increase in insulin or oral hypoglycemic may be required.

**Patient & Family Education**

- Notify prescriber of headache (euthyroid patients); may indicate need for dosage adjustment or change to another thyroid preparation.
- Take medication exactly as ordered.
- Learn S&S of hyperthyroidism (see Appendix F); notify prescriber if they appear.

# LIRAGLUTIDE
(lir-a-glu′tide)
Saxenda, Victoza
**Classification:** ANTIDIABETIC; GLUCAGON-LIKE PEPTIDE-1 RECEPTOR AGONIST; INCRETIN MIMETICS
Therapeutic: ANTIDIABETIC
**Prototype:** Exenatide

**AVAILABILITY** Solution for injection

**ACTION & *THERAPEUTIC EFFECT***
Liraglutide is a glucagon-like peptide-1 (GLP-1) receptor agonist that causes increased insulin release and decreased glucagon release in the presence of elevated blood glucose, and delays the rate of gastric emptying. *Liraglutide lowers postprandial blood glucose levels and helps normalize HbA1C.*

**USES** Treatment of type 2 diabetes mellitus in combination with diet and exercise; reduction of cardiovascular mortality **(Victoza)**; chronic weight management **(Saxenda)**.

**CONTRAINDICATIONS** Family or personal history of medullary thyroid carcinoma (MTC); history of multiple endocrine neoplasia syndrome type 2 (MEN 2); serious hypersensitive reaction to liraglutide; Type 1 DM except for **Saxenda;** diabetic ketoacidosis; pancreatitis; pregnacy (category X for **Saxenda**); lactation.

**CAUTIOUS USE** History of pancreatitis; alcohol abuse; history of cholelithiasis; history of severe hypoglycemia; gastroparesis; history of angioedema; renal or hepatic impairment; concurrent use with insulin secretagogues (e.g., sulfonylurea); older adults; pregnancy (category C **Victoza**). Safe use in children younger than 18 y not established.

**ROUTE & DOSAGE**

| Type 2 Diabetes Mellitus / Reduction of Cardiovascular Mortality (Victoza) |
|---|
| *Adult:* **Subcutaneous** Initial dose of 0.6 mg once daily for 1 wk. After 1 wk, increase dose to 1.2–1.8 mg once daily to achieve glycemic control. |
| **Chronic Weight Management (Saxenda only)** |
| *Adult:* **Subcutaneous** 0.6 mg daily for 1 wk then increase by 0.6 mg/day at weekly intervals to target dose of 3 mg daily |

**ADMINISTRATION**

**Subcutaneous**

- Inject into abdomen, thigh, or upper arm without regard to meals.
- Injection timing can be changed without dose adjustment (i.e., injection may be given any time of day).
- Store refrigerated until first use, then may be stored refrigerated at 15°–30°C (59°–86°F) for up to 30 days. Do not freeze.

Common adverse effects in *italic;* life-threatening effects underlined; generic names in **bold;** classifications in SMALL CAPS; ◆ Canadian drug name; ☻ Prototype drug

**ADVERSE EFFECTS** (≥1%) **Body as a Whole:** Influenza. **CNS:** Dizziness, fatigue, *headache.* **CV:** Increased blood pressure, *increased heart rate,* palpitations. **GI:** *Constipation, diarrhea, nausea, vomiting,* decreased appetite, dyspepsia. **Musculoskeletal:** Back pain. **Respiratory:** Nasopharyngitis, sinusitis, *upper respiratory tract infection.* **Urogenital:** Urinary tract infection. **Metabolic:** Hypoglycemia.

**INTERACTIONS Drug:** Due to its ability to slow gastric emptying, liraglutide can decrease absorption rate and plasma levels of oral medications.

**PHARMACOKINETICS Peak:** 8–12 h. **Distribution:** 98% plasma protein bound. **Metabolism:** Peptide hydrolysis/degradation. **Elimination:** Renal and fecal as inactive metabolites. **Half-Life:** 12–13 h.

## NURSING IMPLICATIONS

### Black Box Warning

*Liraglutide has been associated with thyroid tumors in animal studies; relevance to humans has not been established.*

### Assessment & Drug Effects

- Monitor for S&S of hypoglycemia. Note that the initial week of dosing (0.6 mg/d) is not effective for glycemic control but is designed to reduce GI distress.
- Monitor for and report S&S of significant GI distress, including nausea, vomiting, and diarrhea.
- Monitor for and promptly report S&S of acute pancreatitis (acute abdominal pain with/without vomiting). If pancreatitis is suspected, withhold drug and notify prescriber immediately.

- Monitor lab tests: Frequent fasting and postprandial plasma glucose and periodic HbA1C; periodic renal function tests and LFTs.

### Patient & Family Education

- Monitor blood glucose daily as directed. Report to prescriber significant hypoglycemia.
- Report promptly any of the following: A lump in the neck; hoarseness; difficulty swallowing or difficulty breathing; significant GI distress such as persistent, severe abdominal pain that may be accompanied by vomiting.
- Discard any pen that has been in use for greater than 30 days.
- Liraglutide may cause decreased appetite and some weight loss.

# LISDEXAMFETAMINE DIMESYLATE

(lis-dex-am-fet'a-meen)

Vyvanse

**Classifications:** CEREBRAL STIMULANT; AMPHETAMINE; ANOREXIGENIC
**Therapeutic:** STIMULANT; ANOREXIGENIC; ATTENTION DEFICIT AGENT
**Prototype:** Amphetamine
**Controlled Substance:** Schedule II

**AVAILABILITY** Capsule; chewable tablet

**ACTION & *THERAPEUTIC EFFECT***
An isomer of amphetamine that has anorexigenic action; this is thought to result from CNS stimulation and possibly from loss of acuity of smell and taste. *In hyperkinetic children, amphetamines reduce motor restlessness by an unknown mechanism.*

**USES** Treatment of attention-deficit hyperactivity disorder (ADHD); binge eating disorder.

## CONTRAINDICATIONS Hypersensitivity to sympathomimetic amines, dextroamphetamine, or amphetamine; advanced arteriosclerosis; serious structural cardiac abnormalities, cardiomyopathy, cardiac arrhythmias, or symptomatic cardiovascular disease; uncontrollable hypertension; glaucoma; agitated states; during or within 14 days of administering MAOIs; emergence of new psychotic or manic symptoms caused by amphetamine use; suicidal ideation; lactation.

## CAUTIOUS USE Controlled hypertension, heart failure, recent MI, or recent ventricular arrhythmia; preexisting psychotic disorder; suicidal tendencies; bipolar disorder, depression; history of aggressive or hostile behavior; renal impairment; Tourette syndrome/tics; history of drug abuse or alcoholism; older adults; pregnancy (category C); children younger than 6 y.

## ROUTE & DOSAGE

### Attention-Deficit Hyperactivity Disorder

*Adult/Child (6–12 y):* **PO** 30 mg daily in a.m.; may increase to 50–70 mg daily at weekly intervals (max: 70 mg daily)

### Binge Eating Disorder

*Adult:* 30 mg daily in a.m. then titrate up by 20 mg at weekly interval to target dose of 50–70 mg/day

## ADMINISTRATION

### Oral

- Give daily dose in the morning.
- Capsule may be taken whole or opened and dissolved in a glass of water, yogurt, or orange juice.

- Store at 15°–30° C (59°–86° F) and protect from light.

## ADVERSE EFFECTS (≥1%) Body as a Whole: Pyrexia. CNS: Affect lability, dizziness, *headache, insomnia, irritability,* somnolence, tic. GI: *Abdominal pain, dry mouth,* nausea, xerostomia, vomiting, *decreased appetite.* Metabolic: Decreased appetite, weight loss. Respiratory: Dyspnea Skin: Rash. CV: Increased blood pressure, increased heart rate. Urogenital: Erectile dysfunction.

## DIAGNOSTIC TEST INTERFERENCE

Can cause a significant elevation in plasma CORTICOSTEROID levels and may interfere with **urinary steroid determinations.**

## INTERACTIONS Drug: **Chlorpromazine** and **haloperidol** inhibit the CNS stimulant effects of amphetamines. **Furazolidone** and MAO INHIBITORS can increase adverse effects. **Lithium** may inhibit the effects of lisdexamfetamine. Compounds that acidify the urine lower the plasma levels of lisdexamfetamine. Lisdexamfetamine inhibits the actions of **adrenergic blockers.** Co-administration of ANTIHISTAMINES with lisdexamfetamine can counteract desired sedative effects. Lisdexamfetamine may antagonize the hypotensive effects of ANTIHYPERTENSIVE AGENTS. Lisdexamfetamine may delay the absorption of **ethosuximide** and **phenytoin.** Lisdexamfetamine may potentiate the actions of TRICYCLIC ANTIDEPRESSANTS, **meperidine** and **norepinephrine. Albuterol** can cause increased cardiovascular effects.

## PHARMACOKINETICS Absorption: Rapidly from GI tract. Peak: 1 h. Distribution: Extensive throughout body. Metabolism: Prodrug

converted in liver to dextroamphetamine. **Elimination:** Urine (96%). **Half-Life:** 1 h (lisdexamfetamine) 6–8 h (dextroamphetamine).

## NURSING IMPLICATIONS

### Black Box Warning

*Lisdexamfetamine has been associated with high potential for abuse and dependence.*

### Assessment & Drug Effects

- Monitor children, adolescents, and adults for signs and symptoms of adverse cardiac reactions (e.g., hypertension, arrhythmias). Report promptly exertional chest pain or syncope.
- Monitor closely growth rate in children.
- Typically therapy is interrupted or dosage reduced periodically to assess effectiveness in behavior disorders.
- Monitor children and adolescents for development of aggressive or abnormal behaviors.

### Patient & Family Education

- Do not drive or engage in other potentially hazardous activities until response to drug is known.
- Report promptly any of the following: Chest pain with activity, new or worse behavior or thought problems, psychotic symptoms (e.g., hearing voices, believing things that are not true).
- Taper drug gradually following long-term use to avoid extreme fatigue, mental depression, and prolonged abnormal sleep pattern.

## LISINOPRIL

(ly-sin'o-pril)

*Prinivil, Qbrelis, Zestril*

**Classifications:** ANTIHYPERTENSIVE; ANGIOTENSIN-CONVERTING ENZYME (ACE) INHIBITOR
Therapeutic: ANTIHYPERTENSIVE
**Prototype:** Enalapril

**AVAILABILITY** Tablet; oral solution

## ACTION & *THERAPEUTIC EFFECT*

Lowers BP by specific inhibition of the angiotensin-converting enzyme (ACE). This interrupts conversion sequences initiated by renin that form angiotensin II, a potent vasoconstrictor. ACE inhibition alters hemodynamics without compensatory reflex tachycardia or changes in cardiac output (except in patients with CHF). *Improves cardiac output and exercise tolerance. Aldosterone is also reduced, thus permitting a potassium-sparing effect. Migraine prophylaxis.*

**USES** Hypertension, alone or concomitantly with other classes of antihypertensive agents; CHF; to improve MI survival.

**CONTRAINDICATIONS** History of angioedema related to treatment with an ACE inhibitor, ACE inhibitor hypersensitivity; history of idiopathic or hereditary angioedema; hypotension; pregnancy (category D); lactation.

**CAUTIOUS USE** Impaired kidney function, renal artery stenosis, renal disease, renal failure, hyperkalemia, aortic stenosis, cardiomyopathy; cerebrovascular disease; collagen vascular disease; CAD; dialysis; heart failure, hyperkalemia, hypotension, hypovolemia; major surgery; African Americans; autoimmune diseases, especially systemic lupus erythematosus (SLE);

L

women of reproductive age; older adults; children younger than 6 y.

## ROUTE & DOSAGE

### Hypertension

*Adult/Adolescent:* **PO** 10 mg once/day, may increase up to 20–40 mg 1–2 × day (max: 80 mg/day)
*Child (6–16 y):* **PO** Start at 0.07 mg/kg (max: 5 mg) once/day (max: 40 mg/day)
*Geriatric:* **PO** Initial 2.5–5 mg/day, may increase by 2.5–5 mg/day every 1–2 wk (max: 40 mg/day)

### Heart Failure

*Adult:* **PO** 2.5–5 mg daily may increase to highest tolerated dose (usually 5–40 mg daily)

### Acute MI

*Adult:* **PO** 2.5 mg, then 5 mg after 24 h, 10 mg after 48 h, then 10 mg once daily

## ADMINISTRATION

### Oral

- Monitor drug effect for several hours or until the BP is stabilized for at least 1 additional hour. Concurrent administration with a diuretic may compound hypotensive effect.
- Store away from both moisture and heat.

## ADVERSE EFFECTS (≥1%) **CNS:** Headache, dizziness, fatigue. **CV:** Hypotension, chest pain. **GI:** Nausea, vomiting, diarrhea, anorexia, constipation, intestinal angioedema. **Hematologic:** Neutropenia. **Respiratory:** Dyspnea, cough. **Skin:** Rash, alopecia. **Metabolic:** Azotemia, hyperkalemia, increased BUN, and creatinine levels. **Opthalmic:** Blurred

vision, diplopia, photophobia, vision loss. **Otic:** Tinnitus.

## INTERACTIONS **Drug: Indomethacin** and other NSAIDs may decrease antihypertensive activity; POTASSIUM SUPPLEMENTS, POTASSIUM-SPARING DIURETICS may cause hyperkalemia; may increase **lithium** levels and toxicity. Do not use with **sacubitril** due to risk of angioedema. Do not use with **tranylcypromine.**

## PHARMACOKINETICS **Absorption:** 25% absorbed from GI tract. **Onset:** 1 h. **Peak:** 6–8 h. **Duration:** 24 h. **Distribution:** Limited amount crosses blood–brain barrier; crosses placenta; small amount distributed in breast milk. **Metabolism:** Is not metabolized. **Elimination:** Primarily in urine. **Half-Life:** 12 h.

## NURSING IMPLICATIONS

### Black Box Warning

*Lisinopril has been associated with fetal injury and death.*

### Assessment & Drug Effects

- Place patient in supine position and notify prescriber if sudden and severe hypotension occurs within the first 1–5 h after initial drug dose; greatest risk for hypotension is in patients who are sodium- or volume-depleted because of diuretic therapy.
- Measure BP just prior to dosing to determine whether satisfactory control is being maintained for 24 h. If the antihypertensive effect is diminished in less than 24 h, an increase in dosage may be necessary.
- Monitor closely for angioedema of extremities, face, lips, tongue, glottis, and larynx. Discontinue drug

Common adverse effects in *italic*; life-threatening effects underlined; generic names in **bold**; classifications in SMALL CAPS; ♣ Canadian drug name; ◐ Prototype drug promptly and notify prescriber if such symptoms appear; carefully monitor for airway obstruction until swelling is relieved.

- Monitor serum sodium and serum potassium levels for hyponatremia and hyperkalemia.

- Withhold therapy and notify prescriber if neutropenia (neutrophil count less than 1000/mm³) develops; kidney function tests at periodic intervals, especially in patients with severe volume or sodium replacement or those with severe CHF.

- Monitor lab tests: Baseline WBC count, then every month for the first 3–6 mo of therapy, and at periodic intervals for 1 y; serum creatinine/BUN, serum postassium, serum sodium, LFTs.

### Patient & Family Education

- Discontinue drug and contact prescriber immediately for severe hypersensitivity reaction (e.g., hoarseness, swelling of the face, mouth, hands, or feet, or sudden trouble breathing).

- Women should use reliable means of contraception throughout therapy.

- Report immediately to prescriber if a pregnancy occurs.

- Be aware of importance of proper diet, including sodium and potassium restrictions. **Do not** use salt substitute containing potassium.

- Continued compliance with high BP medication is very important. If a dose is missed, take it as soon as possible but not too close to next dose.

- Do not drive or engage in other potentially hazardous activities until response to the drug is known.

- With concomitant therapy, lisinopril increases the risk of lithium toxicity.

- Notify prescriber promptly of any indication of infection (e.g., sore throat, fever).

- Do not store drug in a moist area. Heat and moisture may cause the medicine to break down.

## LITHIUM CARBONATE ℗
(li'thee-um)
Lithobid

## LITHIUM CITRATE
**Classification:** ANTIPSYCHOTIC; MOOD STABILIZER
Therapeutic: ANTIPSYCHOTIC; ANTIMANIC; ANTIDEPRESSANT

**AVAILABILITY** **Lithium Carbonate:** Capsule; sustained release tablet. **Lithium Citrate:** Syrup

## ACTION & *THERAPEUTIC EFFECT*

Lithium competes with various physiologically important cations: Na⁺, K⁺, Ca²⁺, Mg²⁺; therefore, it affects cell membranes, body water, and neurotransmitters. At the synapse, it accelerates catecholamine destruction, inhibits the release of neurotransmitters and decreases sensitivity of postsynaptic receptors. Decreases overactivity of receptors involved in stimulating manic states. *Effective response evidenced by changed facial affect, improved posture, assumption of self-care, improved ability to concentrate, improved sleep pattern. Treatment for bipolar disorder and mania.*

**USES** Control and prophylaxis of acute mania and the acute manic phase of mixed bipolar disorder.

**UNLABELED USES** Acute and recurrent depression (unipolar affective disorder), antineoplastic

Common adverse effects in *italic;* life-threatening effects underlined; generic names in **bold;** classifications in SMALL CAPS; ♣ Canadian drug name; ℗ Prototype drug

955

drug-induced neutropenia, aplastic anemia, SIADH, cyclic neutropenia.

**CONTRAINDICATIONS** Hypersensitivity to lithium or any component of formulation; history of ACE inhibitor induced angioedema; severe cardiovascular or kidney disease, severe debilitation, sodium depletion; manifestatiions of hypercalcemia; pregnancy (category D); lactation.

**CAUTIOUS USE** Thyroid disease; hypothyroidism; epilepsy; mild to moderate cardiac disease, cardiac arrhythmias, dehydration, diarrhea; mental status changes, risk of suicidal thoughts or behavior; renal disease, renal impairment; sodium restriction, urinary retention; DM: debilitative patients; older adults; children younger than 12 y.

## ROUTE & DOSAGE

**Mania**

*Adult/Adolescent:* **PO Loading Dose** 600 mg t.i.d. or 900 mg sustained release b.i.d. or 10 mL (16 mEq) of solution t.i.d.; **PO Maintenance Dose** 300 mg t.i.d. or q.i.d. or 15–20 mL (24–32 mEq) solution in 2–4 divided doses (max: 2.4 g/day) or 900–1800 mg daily in 2–3 divided doses

## ADMINISTRATION

**Oral**

- Give with meals.
- Ensure that sustained release tablets are not chewed or crushed; **must be** swallowed whole.
- Protect from light and moisture.

**ADVERSE EFFECTS** (≥1%) **CNS:** Dizziness, *headache, lethargy,* drowsiness, *fatigue,* slurred speech, psychomotor retardation, giddiness, incontinence, restlessness, seizures, confusion, blackout spells, disorientation, *recent memory loss,* stupor, coma, EEG changes. **CV:** Arrhythmias, hypotension, vasculitis, peripheral circulatory collapse, ECG changes. **Special Senses:** Impaired vision, transient scotomas, tinnitus. **Endocrine:** Diffuse thyroid enlargement, hypothyroidism, *nephrogenic diabetes insipidus,* transient hyperglycemia, glycosuria, hyponatremia. **GI:** *Nausea, vomiting, anorexia, abdominal pain, diarrhea, dry mouth,* metallic taste. **Musculoskeletal:** *Fine hand tremors,* coarse tremors, choreoathetotic movements; fasciculations, clonic movements, incoordination including ataxia, *muscle weakness,* hyperreflexia, encephalopathic syndrome (weakness, lethargy, fever, tremors, confusion, extrapyramidal symptoms). **Skin:** Thought to be toxicity rather than allergy: Pruritus, maculopapular rash, hyperkeratosis, chronic folliculitis, transient acneiform papules (face, neck, intertriginous areas), anesthesia of skin, cutaneous ulcers, drying and thinning of hair, allergic vasculitis. **Hematologic:** *Reversible leukocytosis* (14,000 to 18,000/mm³). **Urogenital:** Albuminuria, oliguria, urinary incontinence, polyuria, polydipsia, increased uric acid excretion. **Body as a Whole:** Edema, weight gain (common) or loss, exacerbation of psoriasis; flu-like symptoms.

**INTERACTIONS Drug: Carbamazepine, haloperidol,** PHENO-THIAZINES increase risk of neurotoxicity, extrapyramidal effects, and tardive dyskinesias; DIURETICS, NSAIDS, **methyldopa, probenecid,** TETRACYCLINES decrease renal clearance of lithium, increasing pharmacologic and toxic effects;

Common adverse effects in *italic;* life-threatening effects underlined; generic names in **bold;** classifications in SMALL CAPS; ♣ Canadian drug name; ⓟ Prototype drug

THEOPHYLLINES, **urea, sodium bicarbonate, sodium** or **potassium citrate** increase renal clearance of lithium, decreasing its pharmacologic effects. BETA-BLOCKERS may mask signs of toxicity. Do not use with agents known to prolong QT interval (**bepridil, doeftilide, dronedarone, halofantrine, levomethadyl, pimozide, thioridazine, ziprasidone**).

## PHARMACOKINETICS **Absorption:** Readily absorbed from GI tract. **Peak:** 0.5–3 h carbonate; 15–60 min citrate. **Distribution:** Crosses blood–brain barrier and placenta; distributed into breast milk. **Metabolism:** Not metabolized. **Elimination:** 95% in urine, 1% in feces, 4 5% in sweat. **Half-Life:** 20–27 h.

## NURSING IMPLICATIONS

### Black Box Warning

*Lithium toxicity can occur at doses close to therapeutic levels.*

### Assessment & Drug Effects

- Monitor for S&S of lithium toxicity (e.g., vomiting, diarrhea, lack of coordination, drowsiness, muscular weakness, slurred speech when level is 1.5–2 mEq/L; ataxia, blurred vision, giddiness, tinnitus, muscle twitching, coarse tremors, polyuria when greater than 2 mEq/L). Withhold one dose and call prescriber. Drug should not be stopped abruptly.
- Monitor older adults carefully to prevent toxicity, which may occur at serum levels ordinarily tolerated by other patients.
- Be alert to and report symptoms of hypothyroidism (see Appendix F).
- Weigh patient daily; check for edema. Report changes in I&O

ratio, sudden weight gain, or edema.
- Report early signs of extrapyramidal reactions promptly to prescriber.
- Monitor lab tests: Periodic lithium levels (draw blood sample prior to next dose or 8–12 h after last dose) at least every 6 mo; periodic thyroid function tests, CBC with differential, serum electrolytes, thyroid function tests.

### Patient & Family Education

- Be alert to increased output of dilute urine and persistent thirst. Dose reduction may be indicated.
- Contact prescriber if diarrhea or fever develops. Avoid practices that may encourage dehydration: Hot environment, excessive caffeine beverages (diuresis).
- Drink plenty of liquids (2–3 L/day) during stabilization period and at least 1–1 5 L/day during ongoing therapy.
- Do not drive or engage in other potentially hazardous activities until response to drug is known. Lithium may impair both physical and mental ability.
- Use effective contraceptive measures during lithium therapy.

## LIXISENATIDE
(lix-i-sen′-a-tide)

Adlyxin

**Classifications:** ANTIDIABETIC; GLUCAGON-LIKE PEPTIDE-1 RECEPTOR AGONIST; INCRETIN MIMETIC
Therapeutic: ANTIDIABETIC
**Prototype:** Exenatide

**AVAILABILITY** Solution for injection

## ACTION & *THERAPEUTIC EFFECT*
An agonist of glucagon-like peptide-1 (GLP-1) that increases

Common adverse effects in *italic*; life-threatening effects <u>underlined</u>; generic names in **bold**; classifications in SMALL CAPS; ♣ Canadian drug name; ⊘ Prototype drug

957

glucose-dependent insulin release, decreases glucagon secretion, and slows gastric emptying. *It improves glycemic control by reducing fasting and postprandial glucose concentrations in patients with type 2 diabetes.*

**USES** Type 2 diabetes mellitus in combination with diet and exercise.

**CONTRAINDICATIONS** Hypersensitivity to lixisenatide; angioedema.

**CAUTIOUS USE** Alcoholism, type 1 diabetes mellitus, lactation, children.

## ROUTE & DOSAGE

**Type 2 Diabetes Mellitus**

*Adult:* **Subcutaneous** Initial dose of 10 mcg once daily for 14 days; increase to 20 mcg on day 15

**Renal Impairment Dosage Adjustment**

Close monitoring required with renal impairment

## ADMINISTRATION

**Subcutaneous Injection**
- Administer subcutaneously in thigh, abdomen, or upper arm; do not give IM or IV.
- Rotate injection sites.
- Available as a pre-filled pen. Activate before using the first time. Do not share injection pens between patients.
- Administer once daily 1 h before first meal of the day.

**ADVERSE EFFECTS** (≥1%) **Body as a Whole:** Immunogenicity, injection site reactions, nausea. **GI:** Abdominal distension, abdominal pain, constipation, diarrhea, dyspepsia, *nausea, vomitting.* **Metabolic:** Hypoglycemia.

**INTERACTIONS Drug:** Lixisenatide delays gastric emptying and may reduce the rate of absorption of orally administered medications. Lixisenatide increases the potential risk of hypoglycemia when used in combination with a SULFONYLUREA or **basal insulin.**

**PHARMACOKINETICS Peak:** 1–3.5 h. **Metabolism:** Peptide degradation. **Elimination:** Primarily renal. **Half-Life:** 3 h.

## NURSING IMPLICATIONS

**Assessment & Drug Effects**
- Monitor HbA1c levels at least twice annually.
- Monitor renal function.
- Monitor patient for S&S of GI effects.
- Monitor patient for S&S of hypersensitivity.

**Patient & Family Education**
- Check blood sugar levels as ordered by your health care provider.
- Watch for S&S of hypoglycemia such as feeling cold, sweaty, irritable, or confused.
- Avoid driving if blood sugar is low.
- Follow diet and exercise plan as ordered by your health care provider.
- Report S&S of injection site reaction, stomach pain, difficulty urinating, blood in the urine, or significant weight gain.
- Birth control taken by mouth should be taken at least 1 h before or 11 h after taking this drug.

## LODOXAMIDE
(lo-dox′a-mide)
Alomide
**See Appendix A-1.**

# LOMUSTINE

(loe-mus'teen)

CeeNU, CCNU

**Classifications:** ANTINEOPLASTIC; ALKYLATING AGENT; NITROSOUREA

Therapeutic: ANTINEOPLASTIC

**Prototype:** Cyclophosphamide

**AVAILABILITY** Capsule

## ACTION & THERAPEUTIC EFFECT

Has cell-cycle-nonspecific activity against rapidly proliferating cell populations. Inhibits synthesis of both DNA and RNA. *Has antineoplastic and myelosuppressive effect.*

**USES** Palliative therapy in addition to other modalities or with other chemotherapeutic agents in malignant glioma and as secondary therapy in Hodgkin's disease.

**UNLABELED USES** GI, lung, and renal carcinomas, non-Hodgkin's lymphomas, malignant melanoma, and multiple myeloma.

**CONTRAINDICATIONS** Immunization with live virus vaccines, viral infections; severe bone marrow suppression; active infection; pregnancy (category D); lactation.

**CAUTIOUS USE** Patients with decreased circulating platelets, leukocytes, or erythrocytes; kidney or liver function impairment; previous cytotoxic or radiation therapy; pulmonary disease.

## ROUTE & DOSAGE

**Palliative Therapy**

*Adult/Adolescent:* **PO** 130 mg/m² as single dose, repeated in 6 wk; subsequent doses based on hematologic response (WBC greater than 4000/mm³, platelets greater than 100,000/mm³)

*Child:* **PO** 75–150 mg/m² q6wk

## ADMINISTRATION

**Oral**

- Give on an empty stomach to reduce possibility of nausea, may also give an antiemetic before drug to prevent nausea.
- Store capsules away from excessive heat (over 40° C).

**ADVERSE EFFECTS** (≥1%) **CNS:** Lethargy, ataxia, disorientation. **GI:** Anorexia, *nausea, vomiting,* stomatitis, transient elevations of LFTs. **Hematologic:** Delayed (cumulative) myelosuppression: (Thrombocytopenia, leukopenia); anemia. **Skin:** Alopecia, skin rash, itching. **Urogenital:** Nephrotoxicity. **Respiratory:** Pulmonary toxicity (rare).

**INTERACTIONS Drug:** Cimetidine can increase bone marrow toxicity; ANTICOAGULANTS, NSAIDS, SALICYLATES increase risk of bleeding.

**PHARMACOKINETICS Absorption:** Readily absorbed from GI tract. **Peak:** 1–6 h. **Distribution:** Readily crosses blood–brain barrier; crosses placenta; distributed into breast milk. **Metabolism:** In liver to several active metabolites. **Elimination:** In urine. **Half-Life:** 16–48 h.

## NURSING IMPLICATIONS

### Black Box Warning

*Lomustine has been associated with bone marrow suppression resulting in bleeding and severe infection.*

Common adverse effects in *italic*; life-threatening effects underlined; generic names in **bold**; classifications in SMALL CAPS; ♣ Canadian drug name; ⊕ Prototype drug

959

### Assessment & Drug Effects

- A repeat course is not given until platelets have returned to above 100,000/mm³ and leukocytes to above 4000/mm³.
- Avoid invasive procedures during nadir of platelets.
- Thrombocytopenia occurs about 4 wk and leukopenia about 6 wk after a dose, persisting 1–2 wk.
- Inspect oral cavity daily for S&S of superinfections (see Appendix F) and stomatitis or xerostomia.
- Monitor lab tests: Blood counts weekly and for at least 6 wk after last dose. Periodic LFTs and renal function tests.

### Patient & Family Education

- Nausea and vomiting may occur 3–5 h after drug administration, usually lasting less than 24 h.
- Anorexia may persist for 2 or 3 days after a dose.
- Notify prescriber of signs of sore throat, cough, fever. Also report unexplained bleeding or easy bruising.
- Use reliable contraceptive measures during therapy.
- Be aware of the possibility of hair loss while taking this drug.
- A given dose may include capsules of different colors; the pharmacist prepares prescribed dose by combining various capsule strengths.

## LOPERAMIDE ⓟ
(loe-per'a-mide)
Imodium, Imodium AD, Kaopectate III, Maalox Anti-diarrheal, Pepto Diarrhea Control

**Classification:** ANTIDIARRHEAL
Therapeutic: ANTIDIARRHEAL

**AVAILABILITY** Tablet; capsule liquid

## ACTION & *THERAPEUTIC EFFECT*
Inhibits GI peristaltic activity by direct action on circular and longitudinal intestinal muscles. Prolongs transit time of intestinal contents, increases consistency of stools, and reduces fluid and electrolyte loss. *Effectiveness as an antidiarrheal agent is due to prolonging transit time in the colon.*

**USES** Acute nonspecific diarrhea, chronic diarrhea associated with inflammatory bowel disease, and to reduce fecal volume from ileostomies.

**CONTRAINDICATIONS** Conditions in which constipation should be avoided, ileus, severe colitis, bacterial gastroenteritis; acute diarrhea caused by broad-spectrum antibiotics (pseudomembranous colitis) or associated with microorganisms that penetrate intestinal mucosa (e.g., toxigenic *Escherichia coli, Salmonella,* or *Shigella*); GI bleeding; lactation.

**CAUTIOUS USE** Dehydration; diarrhea caused by invasive bacteria; ulcerative colitis; impaired liver function; prostatic hypertrophy; history of narcotic dependence; pregnancy (category C); children younger than 2 y.

## ROUTE & DOSAGE

### Acute Diarrhea

*Adult:* **PO** 4 mg followed by 2 mg after each unformed stool (max: 16 mg/day)
*Child (2 to younger than 6 y):* **PO** 1 mg t.i.d.; *6 to younger than 8y:* 2 mg b.i.d.; *8–12 y:* 2 mg t.i.d.

### Chronic Diarrhea

*Adult:* **PO** 4 mg followed by 2 mg after each unformed stool until diarrhea is controlled (max: 16 mg/day)
*Child:* **PO** 0.1 mg/kg after each unformed stool (usually 1 mg)

Common adverse effects in *italic;* life-threatening effects <u>underlined</u>; generic names in **bold**; classifications in SMALL CAPS; ♣ Canadian drug name; ⓟ Prototype drug

## ADMINISTRATION

### Oral

▪ Do not give prn doses to a child with acute diarrhea.

### ADVERSE EFFECTS (≥1%) Body as a Whole: Hypersensitivity (skin rash); fever. CNS: Drowsiness, fatigue, dizziness, CNS depression (overdosage). GI: Abdominal discomfort or pain, abdominal distention, bloating, constipation, nausea, vomiting, anorexia, dry mouth; <u>toxic megacolon</u> (patients with ulcerative colitis).

### INTERACTIONS Drug: No clinically significant interactions established.

### PHARMACOKINETICS Absorption: Poorly absorbed from GI tract. Onset: 30–60 min. Peak: 2.5 h solution; 4–5 h capsules. Duration: 4–5 h. Metabolism: In liver. Elimination: Primarily in feces, less than 2% in urine. Half-Life: 11 h.

## NURSING IMPLICATIONS

### Assessment & Drug Effects

▪ Monitor therapeutic effectiveness. Chronic diarrhea usually responds within 10 days. If improvement does not occur within this time, it is unlikely that symptoms will be controlled by further administration.
▪ Discontinue if there is no improvement after 48 h of therapy for acute diarrhea.
▪ Monitor fluid and electrolyte balance.
▪ Notify prescriber promptly if the patient with ulcerative colitis develops abdominal distention or other GI symptoms (possible signs of potentially fatal toxic megacolon).

### Patient & Family Education

▪ Notify prescriber if diarrhea does not stop in a few days or if abdominal pain, distention, or fever develops.

▪ Record number and consistency of stools.
▪ Do not drive or engage in other potentially hazardous activities until response to drug is known.
▪ Do not take alcohol and other CNS depressants concomitantly unless otherwise advised by prescriber; may enhance drowsiness.
▪ Learn measures to relieve dry mouth; rinse mouth frequently with water, suck hard candy.

## LOPINAVIR/RITONAVIR

(lop-i-na′ver/rit-o-na′ver)

Kaletra

**Classifications:** ANTIRETROVIRAL; PROTEASE INHIBITOR

**Therapeutic:** PROTEASE INHIBITOR

**Prototype:** Saquinavir mesylate

**AVAILABILITY** Tablet; oral suspension

### ACTION & *THERAPEUTIC EFFECT*

Inhibits the activity of HIV protease and prevents the cleavage of viral polyproteins essential for the maturation of HIV. Ritonavir inhibits the CYP3A metabolism of lopinavir, thereby, increasing the blood level of lopinavir. *Decreases plasma HIV RNA level; reduces viral load as a result of the combined therapy of the two drugs in HIV infected patients.*

**USES** Treatment of HIV infection in combination with other antiretroviral agents.

**CONTRAINDICATIONS** Hypersensitivity to lopinavir or ritonavir; lactation.

**CAUTIOUS USE** Hepatic impairment, patients with hepatitis B or C, cirrhosis; history of elevated

Common adverse effects in *italic;* life-threatening effects <u>underlined</u>; generic names in **bold;** classifications in SMALL CAPS; ♦ Canadian drug name; ❂ Prototype drug

961

transaminase; older adults; DM; history of pancreatitis; cardiac disease; potential for PR prolongation and QT prolongation; congenital prolongation, hypokalemia; conduction abnormalities, ischemic heart disease, and cardiomyopathy; history of triglyceride elevation; autoimmune disorders (e.g., Graves' disease, polymyositis, Guillain-Barre syndrome); elevated total cholesterol and triglycerides; hemophilia; older adults; pregnancy (category C); infants less than 14 days old.

## ROUTE & DOSAGE

### HIV Infection—Treatment Naïve

Adult: **PO** 800/200 mg or 400/100 mg b.i.d. daily

### HIV Infection—Treatment Experienced

Adult: **PO** 400/100 mg (3 tablets or 5 mL suspension) b.i.d., increase dose to 533/133 mg (4 tablets or 6.5 mL) b.i.d., with concurrent efavirenz or nevirapine

Child (6 mo–12 y, weight 7 to less than 15 kg): **PO** with concurrent efavirenz or nevirapine 12/3 mg/kg b.i.d.; weight 15–40 kg: 10/2.5 mg/kg; weight greater than 40 kg: 400/100 mg b.i.d., increase dose: weight 7 to less than 15 kg: 13/3.25 mg/kg; weight 15–40 kg: 11/2.75 mg/kg; weight greater than 40 kg: 533/133 mg b.i.d.

Adolescent/Child/Infant (6 mo to 18 y): **PO** Without concurrent efavirenz, nevirapine, fosamprenavir, or nelfinavir 230/57.5 mg/m² b.i.d.

Infant (14 days to 6 mo): **PO** 16/4 mg/kg or 300/75 mg/m² b.i.d.

## ADMINISTRATION
### Oral

- Give with a meal or light snack.
- Note: If didanosine is concurrently ordered, give didanosine 1 h before or 2 h after lopinavir/ritonavir.
- Store refrigerated at 2°–8° C (36°–46° F). If stored at room temperature 25° C (77° F) or below, discard after 2 mo.

## ADVERSE EFFECTS (≥1%) **Body as a Whole:** Asthenia, pain. **GI:** Abdominal pain, abnormal stools, *diarrhea, nausea,* vomiting. **CNS:** Headache, insomnia, abnormal taste. **Skin:** Rash. **Metabolic:** Hypercholesterolemia, increased triglycerides, ALT increased, weakness. **Hematologic:** Platelets decreased, amenorrhea.

## INTERACTIONS **Drug: Flecainide, propafenone, pimozide** may lead to life-threatening arrhythmias; **rifampin** may decrease antiretroviral response; **dihydroergotamine, ergotamine, methylergonovine** may lead to acute ergot toxicity; HMG-COA REDUCTASE INHIBITORS may increase risk of myopathy and rhabdomyolysis; BENZODIAZEPINES may have prolonged sedation or respiratory depression; **efavirenz, nevirapine,** ANTICONVULSANTS, STEROIDS may decrease lopinavir levels; **delavirdine, ritonavir** may increase lopinavir levels; may increase levels of **amprenavir, indinavir, saquinavir, ketoconazole, itraconazole, midazolam, triazolam, rifabutin, sildenafil, atorvastatin, cerivastatin,** IMMUNOSUPPRESSANTS; may decrease levels of **atovaquone, methadone,** may increase trazodone toxicity; decrease efficacy of

hormonal contraceptives, increases midazolam concentration and toxicity. Also see INTERACTIONS in **ritonavir** monograph. **Herbal: St. John's wort, garlic** may decrease effect.

## PHARMACOKINETICS Absorption: Increased absorption when taken with food. **Peak:** 4 h. **Distribution:** 98–99% protein bound. **Metabolism:** Extensively metabolized by CYP3A. **Elimination:** Primarily in feces. **Half-Life:** 5–6 h lopinavir.

## NURSING IMPLICATIONS

### Assessment & Drug Effects
- Monitor for S&S of: Pancreatitis, especially with marked triglyceride elevations; new onset diabetes or loss of glycemic control; hypothyroidism or Cushing's syndrome.
- Monitor lab tests: Periodic fasting blood glucose, LFTs, lipid profile, serum amylase, inorganic phosphorus, CBC with differential, and thyroid function tests.

### Patient & Family Education
- Report all prescription and non-prescription drugs being taken. Do not use herbal products, especially St. John's wort, without first consulting the prescriber.
- Become familiar with the potential adverse effects of this drug; report those that are bothersome to prescriber.
- Concurrent use of sildenafil (Viagra) increases risk for adverse effects such as hypotension, changes in vision, and sustained erection; promptly report any of these to the prescriber.
- Use additional or alternative contraceptive measures if estrogen-based hormonal contraceptives are being used.

# LORATADINE ⊕
(lor'a-ta-deen)

Alavert, Claritin, Claritin Reditabs

**Classifications:** NONSEDATING ANTIHISTAMINE; $H_1$-RECEPTOR ANTAGONIST
Therapeutic: NONSEDATING ANTIHISTAMINE

## AVAILABILITY Tablet; syrup

## ACTION & *THERAPEUTIC EFFECT*
Long-acting nonsedating antihistamine with selective peripheral $H_1$-receptor antagonism, thus blocking histamine release. Loratadine diminishes capillary permeability, edema formation, and constriction of respiratory, GI, and vascular smooth muscle. *Effective in relieving allergic reactions related to histamine release.*

## USES Relief of symptoms of seasonal allergic rhinitis; idiopathic chronic urticaria.

## CONTRAINDICATIONS Hypersensitivity to loratadine, or structurally related antihistamines.

## CAUTIOUS USE Hepatic and renal impairment, renal disease, renal failure; emphysema, chronic bronchitis; asthma; pregnancy (category B); lactation. **Syrup and chewable tablets:** Children 2 y and older. **Orally disintegrating tablets:** Children 6 y and older.

## ROUTE & DOSAGE

### Allergic Rhinitis
*Adult/Adolescent/Child (6 y or older):* **PO** 10 mg once/day or 5 mg q12h
*Child (2 to less than 6 y):* **PO** 5 mg daily

## ADMINISTRATION
**Oral**
- Give on an empty stomach, 1 h before or 2 h after a meal.
- Store in a tightly closed container.

## ADVERSE EFFECTS (≥1%) CNS:
Dizziness, dry mouth, fatigue, headache, somnolence, altered salivation and lacrimation, thirst, flushing, anxiety, depression, impaired concentration. **CV:** Hypotension, hypertension, palpitations, syncope, tachycardia. **GI:** Nausea, vomiting, flatulence, abdominal distress, constipation, diarrhea, weight gain, dyspepsia. **Body as a Whole:** Arthralgia, myalgia. **Special Senses:** Blurred vision, earache, eye pain, tinnitus. **Skin:** Rash, pruritus, photosensitivity.

## PHARMACOKINETICS Absorption:
Readily from GI tract. **Onset:** 1–3 h. **Peak:** 8–12 h; reaches steady state levels in 3–5 days. **Duration:** 24 h. **Distribution:** Distributed into breast milk. **Metabolism:** In liver to active metabolite, descarboethoxyloratidine. **Elimination:** In urine and feces. **Half-Life:** 12–15 h.

## NURSING IMPLICATIONS
**Assessment & Drug Effects**
- Assess carefully for and report distressing or dangerous S&S that occur after initiation of the drug. A variety of adverse effects, although not common, are possible. Some are an indication to discontinue the drug.
- Monitor cardiovascular status and report significant changes in BP and palpitations or tachycardia.

**Patient & Family Education**
- Drug may cause significant drowsiness in older adult patients and those with liver or kidney impairment.
- Note: Concurrent use of alcohol and other CNS depressants may have an additive effect.

## LORAZEPAM ℗
(lor-a'ze-pam)
Ativan
**Classifications:** ANXIOLYTIC; SEDATIVE-HYPNOTIC; BENZODIAZEPINE
**Therapeutic:** ANTIANXIETY; SEDATIVE-HYPNOTIC
**Controlled Substance:** Schedule IV

**AVAILABILITY** Tablet; oral solution; solution for injection

## ACTION & THERAPEUTIC EFFECT
Effects (antianxiety, sedative, hypnotic, and skeletal muscle relaxant) are mediated by the inhibitory neurotransmitter GABA. Action sites are thalamic, hypothalamic, and limbic levels of CNS. *Antianxiety agent that also causes mild suppression of REM sleep, while increasing total sleep time.*

**USES** Management of anxiety disorders and for short-term relief of symptoms of anxiety. Also used for preanesthetic medication to produce sedation and to reduce anxiety and recall of events related to day of surgery; for management of status epilepticus and insomnia.

**UNLABELED USES** Chemotherapy-induced nausea and vomiting.

**CONTRAINDICATIONS** Known sensitivity to benzodiazepines; acute narrow-angle glaucoma; primary depressive disorders or psychosis; COPD; coma, shock, sleep apnea; acute alcohol intoxication; dementia; intraarterial administration; respiratory depression; pregnancy (category D), and lactation.

Common adverse effects in *italic*; life-threatening effects underlined; generic names in **bold**; classifications in SMALL CAPS; ♣ Canadian drug name; ℗ Prototype drug

**CAUTIOUS USE** Renal or hepatic impairment; renal failure; organic brain syndrome; myasthenia gravis; narrow-angle glaucoma; pulmonary disease; mania; psychosis; suicidal tendency; history of seizure disorders; GI disorders; older adults and debilitated patients; children younger than 12 y.

## ROUTE & DOSAGE

### Anxiety
*Adult:* **PO** 2–3 mg/day in divided doses (max: 10 mg/day)
*Geriatric:* **PO** 1–2 mg/day (max: 2 mg/day)

### Insomnia
*Adult:* **PO** 2–4 mg at bedtime

### Preoperative Sedation Induction
*Adult:* **IM** (0.05 mg/kg) (max: 4 mg) at least 2 h before surgery; **IV** 0.044 mg/kg (max: 2 mg) 15–20 min before surgery

### Status Epilepticus
*Adult:* **IV** 4 mg injected slowly at 2 mg/min, may repeat dose once if inadequate response after 10 min

## ADMINISTRATION

### Oral
▪ Increase the evening dose when higher oral dosage is required, before increasing daytime doses.

### Intramuscular
▪ Injected undiluted, deep into a large muscle mass.

### Intravenous
▪ IV administration to neonates, infants, children: Verify correct IV concentration and rate of infusion with prescriber. ▪ Patients older than 50 y may have more profound and prolonged sedation with IV lorazepam (usual max initial dose: 2 mg).

*PREPARE:* **Direct:** Prepare lorazepam immediately before use. Dilute with an equal volume of sterile water, D5W, or NS.
*ADMINISTER:* **Direct:** Inject directly into vein or into IV infusion tubing at rate not to exceed 2 mg/min and with repeated aspiration to confirm IV entry. ▪ Take extreme precautions to PREVENT intra-arterial injection and perivascular extravasation.
*INCOMPATIBILITIES:* Solution/additive: **Dexamethasone.** Y-site: **Aldesleukin, aztreonam, fluconazole, foscarnet, gallium, idarubicin, imipenem/cilastatin, omeprazole, ondansetron, sargramostim, sufentanil, TPN with albumin.**

▪ Keep parenteral preparation in refrigerator; do not freeze. ▪ Do not use a discolored solution or one with a precipitate.

**ADVERSE EFFECTS** (≥1%) **Body as a Whole:** Usually disappear with continued medication or with reduced dosage, injection site irritation. **CNS:** Anterograde amnesia, *drowsiness, sedation,* dizziness, weakness, unsteadiness, disorientation, depression, sleep disturbance, restlessness, confusion, hallucinations. **CV:** Hypertension or hypotension. **Special Senses:** Blurred vision, diplopia; depressed hearing. **GI:** Nausea, vomiting, abdominal discomfort, anorexia.

**INTERACTIONS Drug: Alcohol,** CNS DEPRESSANTS, ANTICONVULSANTS potentiate CNS depression; **cimetidine** increases lorazepam plasma levels, increases toxicity;

---

Common adverse effects in *italic;* life-threatening effects <u>underlined</u>; generic names in **bold;** classifications in SMALL CAPS; ♣ Canadian drug name; ⊕ Prototype drug

lorazepam may decrease antiparkinsonism effects of **levodopa;** may increase **phenytoin** levels; smoking decreases sedative and antianxiety effects. **Herbal: Kava, valerian** may potentiate sedation.

## PHARMACOKINETICS **Absorption:** Readily absorbed from GI tract. **Onset:** 1–5 min IV; 15–30 min IM. **Peak:** 60–90 min IM; 2 h PO. **Duration:** 12–24 h. **Distribution:** Crosses placenta; distributed into breast milk. **Metabolism:** Not metabolized in liver. **Elimination:** In urine. **Half-Life:** 10–20 h.

## NURSING IMPLICATIONS

### Assessment & Drug Effects

- IM or IV lorazepam injection of 2–4 mg is usually followed by a depth of drowsiness or sleepiness that permits patient to respond to simple instructions whether patient appears to be asleep or awake.
- Monitor vital signs, CNS status, and ability to void following administration.
- Supervise ambulation of older adult patients for at least 8 h after lorazepam injection to prevent falling and injury.
- Supervise patient who exhibits depression with anxiety closely; the possibility of suicide exists, particularly when there is apparent improvement in mood.
- Monitor lab tests: Periodic CBC and LFTs with long-term therapy.

### Patient & Family Education

- Do not drive or engage in other hazardous activities for at least 24–48 h after receiving an injection of lorazepam.
- Do not consume alcoholic beverages for at least 24–48 h after an injection and avoid when taking an oral regimen.

- Notify prescriber if daytime psychomotor function is impaired; a change in regimen or drug may be needed.
- Terminate regimen gradually over a period of several days. Do not stop long-term therapy abruptly; withdrawal may be induced with feelings of panic, tonic–clonic seizures, tremors, abdominal and muscle cramps, sweating, and vomiting.
- Discuss discontinuation of drug with prescriber if you wish to become pregnant.

# LORCASERIN
(lor-ca′ser-in)

Belviq, Belviq XR

**Classification:** ANORECTANT; SEROTONIN 5-HT$_{2C}$ RECEPTOR AGONIST

Therapeutic: APPETITE SUPPRESSANT

## AVAILABILITY Tablet; extended release tablet

## ACTION & *THERAPEUTIC EFFECT*
A selective serotonin 5-HT$_{2C}$ receptor agonist that activates anorexigenic (appetite suppressing) neurons in the hypothalamus. *It is a mediator of satiety thus reducing appetite and calorie intake.*

## USES As an adjunct for chronic weight management.

## CONTRAINDICATIONS Pregnancy X; lactation; severe renal impairment, ESRD; dialysis; suicidal ideation.

## CAUTIOUS USE Older adults; renal impairment; severe hepatic impairment; history of depression; history of drug dependence. Safety and efficacy in children younger than 18 y not established.

Common adverse effects in *italic;* life-threatening effects underlined; generic names in **bold;** classifications in SMALL CAPS; ♣ Canadian drug name; ⊕ Prototype drug

## ROUTE & DOSAGE

**Weight Management**
*Adult:* **PO Immediate release**
10 mg b.i.d.; **Extended release**
20 mg daily

## ADMINISTRATION

### Oral
- May be given without regard to food.
- Swallow extended release tablets whole; do not chew, crush, or divide.
- Store at 15°–30° C (59°–86° F).

## ADVERSE EFFECTS (≥2%) **Body as a Whole:** Chills, seasonal allergy, toothache, worsening of diabetes mellitus. **CNS:** Anxiety, depression, cognitive impairment, *dizziness, fatigue, headache,* insomnia, psychiatric disorders, stress. **CV:** Hypertension. **GI:** *Constipation,* decreased appetite, *diarrhea, dry mouth,* gastroenteritis, *nausea,* vomiting. **Hematological:** Decreased hemoglobin, decreased lymphocyte count, decreased neutrophil count. **Metabolic:** Elevation of prolactin levels, hypoglycemia, peripheral edema. **Musculoskeletal:** Back pain, muscle spasms, musculoskeletal pain. **Respiratory:** Cough, nasopharyngitis, oropharyngeal pain, sinus congestion, upper respiratory tract infection. **Skin:** Rash. **Special Senses:** Blurred vision, dry eye, visual impairment. **Urogenital:** Urinary tract infection.

## INTERACTIONS **Drug:** Lorcaserin may increase the levels of other drugs that require CYP2D6 for metabolism (e.g., **dextromethorphan, doxepin, thioridazine**). Increased risk of serotonin syndrome if used in combination with TRIPTANS, MONOAMINE OXIDASE INHIBITORS, **linezolid,** SELECTIVE SEROTONIN REUPTAKE INHIBITORS (SSRIs), ERGOT DERIVATIVES, SELECTIVE SEROTONIN-NOREPINEPHRINE REUPTAKE INHIBITORS (SNRIs), **dextromethorphan, tricyclic antidepressants** (TCAs), **bupropion, lithium,** or **tramadol**. Do not use with **dapoxetine**. **Food:** Increased risk of serotonin syndrome if used in combination with foods that contain high amounts of **tryptophan. Herbal:** Increased risk of serotonin syndrome if used in combination with **St. John's wort.**

## PHARMACOKINETICS **Peak:** 1.5–2 h (immediate release); 10 h (extended release). **Distribution:** 70% plasma protein bound. **Metabolism:** In the liver. **Elimination:** Primarily renal (92%). **Half-Life:** 11 h (immediate release); 12 h (extended release).

## NURSING IMPLICATIONS

### Assessment & Drug Effects
- Monitor cardiac status throughout therapy. Report promptly S&S of CHF or valvular heart disease (e.g., dyspnea, dependent edema, bradycardia, or a new cardiac murmur).
- Monitor for serotonin syndrome symptoms (e.g., changes in mental status, cognitive impairment, tachycardia, labile blood pressure, hyperreflexia, GI distress).
- Monitor weight weekly.
- Assess response to therapy at 12 wk. If a weight loss of 5% or greater has not been achieved, continued use is unlikely to result in relevant weight loss.
- Monitor diabetics for loss of glycemic control (i.e., hypoglycemia).
- Monitor lab tests: Periodic CBC with differential; prolactin level if elevation suspected.

L

Common adverse effects in *italic;* life-threatening effects underlined; generic names in **bold;** classifications in SMALL CAPS; ✦ Canadian drug name; ● Prototype drug

967

**Patient & Family Education**

- Therapeutic results are possible only with concurrent adherence to calorie-restricted diet and increased physical activity. Discontinue use if 5% weight loss has not been achieved by 12 wk.
- Monitor closely fasting and postprandial blood glucose values if diabetic.
- Report promptly any of the following: Dependent edema, palpitations, shortness of breath, changes in mood or behavior, agitation, suicidal thoughts or behavior.
- Men who have an erection lasting longer than 4 h should immediately discontinue drug and seek emergency medical attention.
- Women should avoid pregnancy or breastfeeding while taking this drug.

# LOSARTAN POTASSIUM ℗

(lo-sar'tan)

Cozaar

**Classifications:** ANGIOTENSIN II RECEPTOR ANTAGONIST; ANTIHYPERTENSIVE

Therapeutic: ANTIHYPERTENSIVE

## AVAILABILITY Tablet

## ACTION & *THERAPEUTIC EFFECT*

Angiotensin II receptor (type $AT_1$) antagonist acts as a potent vasoconstrictor and primary vasoactive hormone of the renin–angiotensin–aldosterone system. Selectively blocks the binding of angiotensin II to the $AT_1$ receptors found in many tissues (e.g., vascular smooth muscle, adrenal glands). *Antihypertensive effect is due to vasodilation and inhibition of aldosterone effects on sodium and water retention.*

## USES Hypertension.

## CONTRAINDICATIONS Hypersensitivity to losartan, pregnancy (category D second and third trimester), lactation.

**CAUTIOUS USE** Patients on diuretics, heart failure; hyperkalemia; hypovolemia; renal or hepatic impairment, pregnancy (category C discontinue use as soon as detected); children younger than 6 y.

## ROUTE & DOSAGE

**Hypertension**

*Adult/Adolescent/Child (older than 6 y and over 20 kg):* **PO** 25–50 mg in 1–2 divided doses (max: 100 mg/day); start with 25 mg/day if volume depleted (i.e., on diuretics)

## ADMINISTRATION

**Oral**

- Note: Starting dose is reduced 50% in patients with possible volume depletion or a history of liver disease.

## ADVERSE EFFECTS (≥1%) CNS:

Dizziness, insomnia, headache. **GI:** Diarrhea, dyspepsia. **Musculoskeletal:** Muscle cramps, myalgia, back or leg pain. **Respiratory:** Nasal congestion, cough, upper respiratory infection, sinusitis.

## INTERACTIONS Drug: Phenobarbital decreases serum levels of losartan and its metabolite.

## PHARMACOKINETICS Absorption: Rapidly absorbed from GI tract; approximately 25–33% reaches systemic circulation. **Peak:** 6 h. **Duration:** 24 h. **Distribution:** Highly bound to plasma proteins; does not appear to cross blood–brain barrier. **Metabolism:** Extensively metabolized in liver by cytochrome P450 enzymes to an active metabolite. **Elimination:** 35%

in urine, 60% in feces. **Half-Life:** Losartan 1.5–2 h; metabolite 6–9 h.

## NURSING IMPLICATIONS

### Black Box Warning

*Losartan has been associated with fetal injury and death when used during the second and third trimesters.*

### Assessment & Drug Effects

- Monitor BP at drug trough (prior to a scheduled dose).
- Inadequate response may be improved by splitting the daily dose into twice-daily dose.
- Monitor lab tests: Periodic CBC, electrolytes, LFTs and renal function tests with long-term therapy.

### Patient & Family Education

- Do not use potassium supplements or salt substitutes without consulting prescriber.
- Notify prescriber of symptoms of hypotension (e.g., dizziness, fainting).
- Notify prescriber immediately of pregnancy.

## LOTEPREDNOL ETABONATE

(lo-te'pred-nol e ta bo'nate)

Alrex, Lotemax

**See Appendix A-1.**

## LOVASTATIN ⓟ

(loe-vah-stat'in)

Altoprev, Mevacor

**Classifications:** ANTILIPEMIC; LIPID-LOWERING; HMG-COA REDUCTASE INHIBITOR (STATIN)

**Therapeutic:** LIPID-LOWERING; STATIN

**AVAILABILITY** Tablet; extended release tablet

## ACTION & *THERAPEUTIC EFFECT*

Reduces plasma cholesterol levels by interfering with body's ability to produce its own cholesterol. This cholesterol-lowering effect triggers induction of LDL receptors, which promote removal of LDL and VLDL remnants (precursors of LDL) from plasma. Also results in an increase in plasma HDL concentrations (HDL collects excess cholesterol from body cells and transports it to liver for excretion). *Reduces plasma cholesterol levels by interfering with body's ability to produce its own cholesterol, and it also lowers LDL and VLDL cholesterol.*

**USES** Hypercholesterolemia, coronary heart disease, heterozygous familial hypercholesterolemia in adolescents, primary/secondary prevention of atherosclerotic cardiovascular disease.

**CONTRAINDICATIONS** Hypersensitivity to lovastatin; active liver disease, unexplained persistent elevations of serum transaminases; cholestasis, hepatic encephalopathy, hepatitis, jaundice; rhabdomyolysis, or myopathy; surgery, trauma; hypotension, renal failure; homozygous familial hypercholesterolemia; pregnancy (category X); lactation.

**CAUTIOUS USE** Patient who consumes substantial quantities of alcohol; history of liver disease; electrolyte imbalance, endocrine disease; infection, severe renal impairment, seizure disorder; DM; patient with risk factors predisposing to development of kidney failure secondary to rhabdomyolysis; older adults; females of child-bearing age; children younger than 10 y. **Extended release tablets:** Safety and efficacy in children not established.

L

Common adverse effects in *italic;* life-threatening effects <u>underlined</u>; generic names in **bold;** classifications in SMALL CAPS; ♣ Canadian drug name; ⓟ Prototype drug

969

## ROUTE & DOSAGE

**Hypercholesterolemia/Coronary Heart Disease**

*Adult:* **PO Extended release** 20–60 mg daily; **Immediate release** 10–80 mg daily

*Adolescent:* **PO Immediate release** 10–40 mg once/day

**Prevention of Cardiovascular Disease (Moderate-Intensity Therapy)**

*Adult:* **PO Immediate release** 40 mg daily

## ADMINISTRATION

### Oral

- Give with the evening meal if daily. Give the first of 2 daily doses with breakfast.
- Ensure that extended release tablets are not crushed or chewed. They **must be** swallowed whole.
- Store tablets at 5°–30° C (41°–86° F) in light-resistant, tightly closed container.

## ADVERSE EFFECTS (≥1%) **Body as a Whole:** Generally well tolerated. **CNS:** Dizziness, mild transient headache, insomnia, fatigue. **Special Senses:** Blurred vision. **GI:** *Dyspepsia, dysgeusia, heartburn, nausea, constipation, diarrhea, flatus, abdominal pain, and cramps.* **Metabolic:** Increases in serum transaminases, elevated creatine phosphokinase (CPK). **Skin:** Rash, pruritus.

## INTERACTIONS **Drug:** **Clarithromycin, clofibrate, cyclosporine, danazol, erythromycin, fenofibrate, fluconazole, gemfibrozil, itraconazole, ketoconazole, miconazole, niacin,** and PRO-TEASE INHIBITORS increase risk of myopathy and rhabdomyolysis; potentiate hypoprothrombinemia with **warfarin.** Do not use with **boceprevir, conivaptan, idelalisib, mifepristone, telaprevir, telithromycin. Food: Grapefruit juice** (greater than 1 qt/day) may increase risk of myopathy and rhabdomyolysis.

## DIAGNOSTIC TEST INTERFERENCE

May elevate *HgbA1C* or *fasting blood glucose.*

## PHARMACOKINETICS **Absorption:** 30% from GI tract; extensive first-pass metabolism. **Onset:** 2 wk. **Peak:** 4–6 wk. **Distribution:** Crosses blood–brain barrier and placenta; distributed into breast milk. **Metabolism:** In liver to active metabolites. **Elimination:** 83% in feces; 10% in urine. **Half-Life:** 1.1–1.7 h.

## NURSING IMPLICATIONS

### Assessment & Drug Effects

- Drug-induced increases in serum transaminases, usually not associated with jaundice or other clinical S&S, return to normal when drug is discontinued. If these values rise and remain at 3 × upper level of normal, drug will be discontinued and liver biopsy considered.
- Monitor diabetics for loss of glycemic control.
- Monitor lab tests: LFTs at 6 and 12 wk after initiation of therapy and periodically thereafter; periodic HbA1C, and lipid profile.

### Patient & Family Education

- Notify prescriber promptly of muscle tenderness or pain, especially if accompanied by fever or malaise. If CPK is elevated or if myositis is diagnosed, drug will be discontinued.
- Avoid or at least reduce alcohol consumption.

- Understand that lovastatin is not a substitute for, but an addition to, diet therapy.
- Diabetics should monitor blood glucose frequently for loss of glycemic control.

# LOXAPINE HYDROCHLORIDE
(lox'a-peen)
Adasuve
# LOXAPINE SUCCINATE
**Classification:** ANTIPSYCHOTIC
**Therapeutic:** ANTIPSYCHOTIC
**Prototype:** Clozapine

**AVAILABILITY** Capsule; powder for inhalation

## ACTION & *THERAPEUTIC EFFECT*
Blocks postsynaptic dopamine receptors in the brain; Also possesses serotonin-blocking activity. *Stabilizes emotional component of schizophrenia.*

**USES** Schizophrenia, bipolar disorder.

**UNLABELED USES** Agitation.

**CONTRAINDICATIONS** Hypersensitivity to loxapine or amoxapine including bronchospasm reaction to drug; CNS depression or coma; dementia-related psychosis in older adults; NMS; severe neutropenia; history of/current diagnosis of asthma, COPD, or other lung disease associated with bronchospasm, acute respiratory signs or symptoms; lactation.

**CAUTIOUS USE** Tardive dyskinesia; glaucoma, prostatic hypertrophy, urinary retention, history of convulsive disorders, cardiovascular disease; transient hypotensive episodes; alcoholism; brain tumor; hematologic disease; hepatic disease; renal impairment; decreased GI motility; thyroid disease;

older adults; pregnancy (category C); children younger than 16 y.

## ROUTE & DOSAGE

**Schizophrenia**

*Adult:* **PO** Start with 10 mg b.i.d. and rapidly increase to maintenance dose of 60–100 mg/day in divided doses (max: 250 mg/day)

**Agitation with Schizophrenia/ Bipolar Disorder**

*Adult:* **Inhalation** 10 mg daily

## ADMINISTRATION

### Oral
- Give with food, milk, or water to reduce possibility of stomach irritation.
- Cadasuve Inhaler: Refer to manufacturer's information for specific instructions for administration of the oral inhalation powder using the Cadasuve inhaler.

## ADVERSE EFFECTS (≥1%)
**CNS:** *Drowsiness, sedation, dizziness, syncope, EEG changes,* paresthesias, staggering gait, muscle weakness, *extrapyramidal effects,* akathisia, <u>tardive dyskinesia, neuroleptic malignant syndrome</u>. **CV:** *Orthostatic hypotension,* hypertension, tachycardia. **Special Senses:** Nasal congestion, tinnitus; blurred vision, ptosis. **GI:** Constipation, dry mouth, *dysgeusia.* **Skin:** Dermatitis, facial edema, pruritus, photosensitivity. **Urogenital:** Urinary retention, menstrual irregularities. **Body as a Whole:** Polydipsia, weight gain or loss, hyperpyrexia, transient <u>leukopenia</u>.

## INTERACTIONS **Drug: Alcohol** and other CNS DEPRESSANTS potentiate

Common adverse effects in *italic;* life-threatening effects <u>underlined</u>; generic names in **bold;** classifications in SMALL CAPS; ♣ Canadian drug name; ◐ Prototype drug

971

CNS depression; will inhibit vasopressor effects of **epinephrine**. Use caution with other ANTIPSYCHOTICS. Do not use with **metoclopramide** due to increased risk of extrapyramidal effects. Do not use with **abarelix**.

**PHARMACOKINETICS Absorption:** Readily absorbed from GI tract. **Onset:** 20–30 min. **Peak:** 1.5–3 h. **Duration:** 12 h. **Distribution:** Widely distributed; crosses placenta; distributed into breast milk; 97% protein bound. **Metabolism:** In liver. **Elimination:** 50% in urine, 50% in feces. **Half-Life:** 19 h.

## NURSING IMPLICATIONS

### Black Box Warning

*Loxapine has been associated with increased mortality in the older adult with dementia-related psychosis.*

### Assessment & Drug Effects

- Monitor baseline BP pattern prior and during therapy; both hypotension and hypertension have been reported as adverse reactions.
- Observe carefully for extrapyramidal effects such as acute dystonia (see Appendix F) during early therapy. Most symptoms disappear with dose adjustment or with antiparkinsonism drug therapy.
- Discontinue therapy and report promptly to prescriber the first signs of impending tardive dyskinesia (fine vermicular movements of the tongue) when patient is on long-term treatment.
- Monitor I&O and bowel elimination patterns and check for bladder distention. Depressed patients often fail to report urinary retention or constipation.

- Risk of seizures is increased in those with history of convulsive disorders.

### Patient & Family Education

- **Do not** change dosage regimen in any way without prescriber approval.
- Avoid self-dosing with OTC drugs unless approved by the prescriber.
- Drowsiness usually decreases with continued therapy. If it persists and interferes with daily activities, consult prescriber. A change in time of administration or dose may help.
- Avoid potentially hazardous activity until response to drug is known.
- Learn measures to relieve dry mouth; rinse mouth frequently with water, suck hard candy. Avoid commercial products that may contain alcohol and enhance drying and irritation.
- Notify prescriber of blurred or colored vision.
- Do not take drug dose and notify prescriber of following: Light-colored stools, bruising, unexplained bleeding, prolonged constipation, tremor, restlessness and excitement, sore throat and fever, rash.
- Stay out of bright sun; cover exposed skin with sunscreen.

## LUBIPROSTONE
(lu-bi-pros'tone)
*Amitiza*

**Classifications:** LAXATIVE AND STOOL SOFTENER; CHLORIDE CHANNEL ACTIVATOR
**Therapeutic:** LAXATIVE AND STOOL SOFTENER

**AVAILABILITY** Capsule

**ACTION & *THERAPEUTIC EFFECT***
Lubiprostone activates chloride channels in the intestine that

L

enhance chloride-rich intestinal fluid secretion without changing serum sodium and potassium concentrations. *The increase in intestinal fluid secretion enhances intestinal motility, thereby increasing the passage of stool and alleviating symptoms associated with chronic idiopathic constipation.*

**USES** Treatment of chronic idiopathic constipation; constipation-predominant irritable bowel syndrome (IBS-C); opioid-induced constipation.

**CONTRAINDICATIONS** Hypersensitivity to lubiprostone; history of mechanical GI obstruction; Crohn's disease, volvulus, diverticulitis, etc.; severe diarrhea; lactation.

**CAUTIOUS USE** GI disease, hepatic impairment; pregnancy (Category C); children.

## ROUTE & DOSAGE

### Chronic Idiopathic/Opioid-Induced Constipation

*Adult:* **PO** 24 mcg b.i.d.

### IBS-C

*Adult:* **PO** 8 mcg b.i.d.

### *Hepatic Dose Adjustment (for Chronic Constipation)*

*Child-Pugh class B:* Start with 16 mcg b.i.d.

*Child-Pugh class C:* Start with 8 mcg b.i.d.

### *(for IBS)*

*Child-Pugh class C:* Start with 8 mcg daily

## ADMINISTRATION

### Oral

- Administer with food to minimize nausea.

- Capsule should be swallowed whole.
- Do not administer to a patient with severe diarrhea or suspected bowel obstruction.
- Store at 15°–30° C (59°–86° F).

**ADVERSE EFFECTS** (≥1%) **Body as a Whole:** Chest pain, peripheral edema, pyrexia. **CNS:** Anxiety, depression, dizziness, fatigue, *headache,* insomnia. **CV:** Hypertension. **GI:** *Abdominal pain and discomfort,* constipation, *diarrhea,* dry mouth, dyspepsia, *flatulence,* viral gastroenteritis, gastroesophageal reflux disease, loose stools, *nausea,* vomiting. **Musculoskeletal:** Arthralgia, back pain, pain in extremities. **Respiratory:** Bronchitis, cough, dyspnea, nasopharyngitis, sinusitis, upper respiratory infection. **Urogenital:** Urinary tract infection.

**PHARMACOKINETICS Absorption:** Very low. **Peak:** 1.1 h (M3). **Distribution:** 94% protein bound. **Metabolism:** Extensive nonhepatic metabolism. **Elimination:** Urine (major) and feces. **Half-Life:** 0.9–1.4 h.

## NURSING IMPLICATIONS

### Assessment & Drug Effects

- Monitor for and report S&S of bowel obstruction.
- Monitor lab tests: Baseline and periodic LFTs.

### Patient & Family Education

- Report to prescriber if you experience severe or prolonged diarrhea, or new or worsening abdominal pain or dyspnea following dosing.
- Do not drive or engage in potentially hazardous activities until response to drug is known.

Common adverse effects in *italic;* life-threatening effects underlined; generic names in **bold;** classifications in SMALL CAPS; ♣ Canadian drug name; ⊕ Prototype drug

973

## LULICONAZOLE
(lu-li-con′a-zole)

Luzu

**Classifications:** AZOLE ANTIFUNGAL
**Therapeutic:** AZOLE ANTIFUNGAL
**Prototype:** Fluconazole

### AVAILABILITY Cream

### ACTION & *THERAPEUTIC EFFECT*

An azole antifungal that appears to inhibit an enzyme required for formation of fungal cell membranes. *Inhibits fungal cell formation and fungal growth.*

### USES Topical treatment of interdigital *tinea pedis, tinea cruris,* and *tinea corporis* caused by the organisms *Trichophyton rubrum* and *Epidermophyton floccosum,* in patients 18 y and older.

### CAUTIOUS USE Pregnancy (category C); lactation. Safety and efficacy in children younger than 18 y not established.

### ROUTE & DOSAGE

**Fungal Infection**

*Adult:* **Topical** Apply once daily to affected and immediately surrounding areas for 1 or 2 wk

### ADMINISTRATION

**Topical**
- Apply to affected area out to about 1 inch of surrounding healthy skin.
- Store at 15°–30° C (59°–86° F).

### ADVERSE EFFECTS (≥1%) **Skin:** Application site reactions, cellulitis, dermatitis.

### INTERACTIONS **Drug:** Luliconazole may increase the levels of other drugs that require CYP2C19 and CYP3A4 for oxidative metabolism.

**PHARMACOKINETICS** **Peak:** 5.8–16.9 h. **Distribution:** Greater than 99% plasma protein bound.

### NURSING IMPLICATIONS

**Assessment & Drug Effects**
- Monitor affected area for clearance of fungal infection.

**Patient & Family Education**
- Wash your hands after application to affected areas.
- Avoid contacting mucous membranes (e.g., mouth, vagina, eyes) with this cream.
- Report to prescriber if you are pregnant or plan to become pregnant.

## LURASIDONE
(lu-ra′si-done)

Latuda

**Classification:** ATYPICAL ANTIPSYCHOTIC
**Therapeutic:** ANTIPSYCHOTIC
**Prototype:** Clozapine

### AVAILABILITY Tablet

### ACTION & *THERAPEUTIC EFFECT*

The mechanism of action is unknown but the efficacy of lurasidone in schizophrenia is thought to be mediated through central dopamine Type 2 ($D_2$) and serotonin Type 2 ($5HT_{2A}$) receptor antagonism. *Controls schizophrenic ideation and behavior.*

### USES Bipolar disorder and schizophrenia.

### CONTRAINDICATIONS Hypersensitivity to lurasidone; older adults with dementia-related psychosis; suicidal ideation; severe neutropenia or leukopenia; agranulocytosis; severe suicidality; neuroleptic malignant syndrome (NMS); patients at risk for aspiration pneumonia; lactation.

Common adverse effects in *italic;* life-threatening effects underlined; generic names in **bold;** classifications in SMALL CAPS; ◆ Canadian drug name; ⊙ Prototype drug

**CAUTIOUS USE** Moderate and severe renal impairment; Child-Pugh class B and C hepatic impairment; cardiovascular disease; dyslipidemia; orthostatic hypotension; history of suicide; disorders that lower seizure threshold (e.g., Alzheimer dementia; Parkinson disease; dementia with Lewy bodies; history of drug abuse or dependence); history of seizures or NMS; tardive dyskinesia; hyperglycemia; mellitis DM or with family history of DM; history of breast cancer; infection; older adults; pregnancy (category B). Safety and efficacy in children not established.

## ROUTE & DOSAGE

### Schizophrenia

*Adult:* **PO** 40 mg daily then increase as needed (max: 160 mg)

### Bipolar Disorder

*Adult:* **PO** 20 mg daily then increase (normal range 20–120 mg/day)

### Hepatic Impairment Dosage Adjustment

*Child-Pugh class B and C:* Reduce dose (max: 40 mg once daily)

### Renal Impairment Dosage Adjustment

*CrCl less than 50 mL/min:* Reduce dose (max: 80 mg once daily)

## ADMINISTRATION

### Oral

- Give with food (at least 350 calories).
- Store at 15°–30°C (59°–86°F).

**ADVERSE EFFECTS** (≥1%) **Body as a Whole:** Agitation, anxiety, fatigue, insomnia, restlessness. **CNS:** *Akathisia,* dizziness, dystonia, *Parkinsonism, somnolence.* **CV:** Tachycardia. **GI:** Abdominal pain, diarrhea, dyspepsia, *nausea,* salivary hypersecretion, vomiting. **Metabolic:** Elevated ALT and AST levels, elevated serum creatinine, elevated serum triglycerides, increased serum cholesterol, increased serum glucose. **Musculoskeletal:** Back pain, decreased appetite. **Skin:** Pruritus, rash. **Special Senses:** Blurred vision.

**INTERACTIONS Drug:** Do not use with strong inhibitors of CYP3A4 (e.g., **ketoconazole, ritonavir, voriconazole**); with moderate CYP3A4 inhibitors (e.g., **carbamazepine, diltiazem, erythromycin, fluconazole**) start with half dose. Inducers of CYP3A4 (e.g., **rifampin**) decrease the levels of lurasidone. **Food:** Avoid **Grapefruit juice.** **Herbal: St. John's wort** can decrease the levels of lurasidone.

**PHARMACOKINETICS Absorption:** Approximately 9–19% is orally absorbed. **Peak:** 1–3 h. **Distribution:** 99% plasma protein bound. **Metabolism:** Hepatic via CYP3A4. **Elimination:** Fecal (80%) and renal (9%). **Half-Life:** 18 h.

## NURSING IMPLICATIONS

### Black Box Warning

*Lurasidone has been associated with increased mortality in older adults with dementia-related psychosis and with increased risk of suicidal thoughts and behavior in children, adolescents, and young adults.*

### Assessment & Drug Effects

- Monitor for and report promptly suicidal ideation.

---

Common adverse effects in *italic;* life-threatening effects <u>underlined</u>; generic names in **bold;** classifications in SMALL CAPS; ♣ Canadian drug name; ⊕ Prototype drug

- Monitor orthostatic vital signs, especially in those at risk for hypotension. Risk is highest at time of dose initiation or escalation.
- Monitor closely patients with neutropenia. Report promptly development of fever or other signs of infection.
- Monitor weight and report significant weight gain.
- Monitor diabetics closely for loss of glycemic control.
- Monitor for and report promptly seizure activity, S&S of NMS or tardive dyskinesia (see Appendix F).
- Taper dosage slowly when discontinuing.
- Monitor lab tests: Periodic blood glucose, lipid profile, LFTs, and CBC with differential.

**Patient & Family Education**

- Do not engage in hazardous activities until response to drug is known.
- Rise slowly from a lying or sitting position to avoid dizziness and fainting.
- Report immediately any of the following: Suicidal thoughts, fever, muscle rigidity, palpitations, signs of infection, dizziness or fainting upon standing.
- Avoid situations that may cause overheating or dehydration.
- Avoid alcohol while taking lurasidone.
- Monitor blood glucose levels frequently if diabetic.

# MAFENIDE ACETATE
(ma′fe-nide)
Sulfamylon
**Classification:** SULFONAMIDE ANTIBIOTIC
Therapeutic: ANTIBIOTIC
**Prototype:** Sulfisoxazole

**AVAILABILITY** Powder, cream

**ACTION & *THERAPEUTIC EFFECT*** Produces marked reduction of bacterial growth in vascular tissue. Active in presence of purulent matter and serum. *Bacteriostatic against many gram-positive and gram-negative organisms, including Pseudomonas aeruginosa, and certain strains of anaerobes.*

**USES** Treatment of second- and third-degree burns.

**CONTRAINDICATIONS** History of hypersensitivity to mafenide or sulfonamides; respiratory (inhalation) injury, pulmonary infection; lactation.

**CAUTIOUS USE** Impaired kidney or pulmonary function, G6PD deficiency and hemolytic anemia with DIC; burn patients with acute kidney failure; pregnancy (category C); children younger than 3 mo.

**ROUTE & DOSAGE**

**Burns**

*Adult/Adolescent/Child:* **Topical** Apply aseptically to burn areas to a thickness of approximately 15 mm ($^1/_{16}$ in) once or twice daily

**ADMINISTRATION**
**Topical**

- Apply cream or solution aseptically to cleansed, debrided burn areas with sterile gloved hand.
- Cover burn areas with cream at all times. Make reapplications to areas from which cream has been removed as necessary.
- Store in tight, light-resistant containers. Avoid extremes of temperature.

**ADVERSE EFFECTS** (≥1%) **Hypersensitivity:** Pruritus, rash, urticaria, blisters, eosinophilia.

M

**Skin:** *Intense pain, burning, or stinging at application sites,* bleeding of skin, excessive body water loss, excoriation of new skin, superinfections. **Other:** Metabolic acidosis.

## PHARMACOKINETICS **Absorption:** Rapidly from burn surface. **Peak:** 2–4 h. **Metabolism:** Rapidly inactivated in blood to a weak carbonic anhydrase inhibitor. **Elimination:** Via kidneys.

## NURSING IMPLICATIONS
### Assessment & Drug Effects
- Monitor vital signs. Report immediately changes in BP, pulse, and respiratory rate and volume.
- Monitor I&O. Report oliguria or changes in I&O ratio and pattern.
- Be alert to S&S of metabolic acidosis (see Appendix F).
- Be alert to evidence of superinfections (see Appendix F), particularly in and below burn eschar.
- Observe carefully; accuracy is critical. It is frequently difficult to distinguish between adverse reactions to mafenide and the effects of severe burns.
- Note: Allergic reactions have reportedly occurred 10–14 days after initiation of mafenide therapy. Temporary discontinuation of drug may be necessary.
- Report intense local pain to prescriber; pain caused by drug may require administration of analgesic.
- Monitor lab tests: Periodic serum electrolytes and tests for acid-base balance.

### Patient & Family Education
- Apply only a thin dressing over burns unless otherwise directed.
- Therapy is usually continued until healing is progressing well (usually 60 days) or site is ready for grafting (after about 35–40 days). It is not withdrawn while there is a possibility of infection unless adverse reactions intervene.
- Report any of the following to the prescriber immediately: Foul-smelling drainage from wounds, bleeding at wound site, unexplained fever.

# MAGNESIUM CITRATE
(mag-nes′i-um)
Citrate of Magnesia,
Citroma
**Classification:** SALINE CATHARTIC
**Therapeutic:** LAXATIVE
**Prototype:** Magnesium hydroxide

**AVAILABILITY** Solution

## ACTION & *THERAPEUTIC EFFECT*
Hyperosmotic laxative that promotes bowel evacuation by causing osmotic retention of fluid; this distends colon and stimulates peristaltic activity. *Evacuates bowels.*

**USES** To evacuate bowel prior to certain surgical and diagnostic procedures; intermittently as laxative to treat acute constipation.

## CONTRAINDICATIONS Severe renal impairment, renal failure; gastrointestinal bleeding; nausea, vomiting, diarrhea, abdominal pain, acute surgical abdomen; intestinal impaction, obstruction or perforation; rectal bleeding; use of solutions containing sodium bicarbonate in patients on sodium-restricted diets.

## CAUTIOUS USE Mild or moderate renal impairment; cardiac disease; older adults; pregnancy (category A); lactation; children younger than 2 y.

Common adverse effects in *italic;* life-threatening effects <u>underlined</u>; generic names in **bold**; classifications in SMALL CAPS; ♣ Canadian drug name; ◐ Prototype drug

977

## ROUTE & DOSAGE

**Acute Constipation**

*Adult/Adolescent:* **PO** 150–300 mL
*Child (6–12 y):* **PO** 100–150 mL;
*2–5 y:* 60–120 mL

**Bowel Prep**

*Adult /Adolescent:* **PO** 150–300
mL once
*Child (2 to younger than 6 y):* **PO**
0.5 mL/kg (max: 200 mL) under
supervision of physician; *6–12 y:*
75–150 mL one time

## ADMINISTRATION

### Oral

- Give on an empty stomach with a
full (240 mL) glass of water. Time
dosing so that it does not interfere
with sleep. Drug produces a watery
or semifluid evacuation in 2–6 h.
- Chill solution by pouring it over
ice or refrigerate it until ready to
use to increase palatability.
- Be aware that once container is
opened, effervescence will decrease. This does not effect the
quality of preparation.
- Store at 2°–30° C (36°–86° F) in
tightly covered containers.

## ADVERSE EFFECTS (≥1%) **GI:**
Abdominal cramps, nausea, flatulence, fluid and electrolyte imbalance, hypermag-nesemia (prolonged use).

## INTERACTIONS **Drug:** May de-
crease effectiveness of **digoxin,** ORAL
ANTICOAGULANTS, PHENOTHIAZINES; will
decrease absorption of **ciprofloxacin,** TETRACYCLINES; **sodium polystyrene sulfonate** will bind magnesium, decreasing its effectiveness.

## PHARMACOKINETICS **Onset:**
3–6 h.

## NURSING IMPLICATIONS

### Assessment & Drug Effects
- Monitor for dehydration, hypokalemia, and hyponatremia (see
Appendix F) since drug may
cause intense bowel evacuation.

### Patient & Family Education
- Do not use for routine treatment
of constipation (especially in older adult).
- Expect some degree of abdominal cramping.

## MAGNESIUM HYDROXIDE
(mag-nes'i-um)

Magnesia, Magnesia
Magma, Milk of Magnesia,
M.O.M.

**Classifications:** SALINE CATHARTIC;
ANTACID

Therapeutic: LAXATIVE; ANTACID

**AVAILABILITY** Tablet; suspension

## ACTION & *THERAPEUTIC EFFECT*
Aqueous suspension of magnesium
hydroxide with rapid and long-
acting neutralizing action. Causes
osmotic retention of fluid, which
distends colon, resulting in mechanical stimulation of peristaltic activity. *Acts as antacid in low
doses and as mild saline laxative at
higher doses.*

**USES** Short-term treatment of occasional constipation, for relief
of GI symptoms associated with
hyperacidity, and as adjunct in
treatment of peptic ulcer. Also has
been used in treatment of poisoning by mineral acids and arsenic,
and as mouthwash to neutralize
acidity.

**CONTRAINDICATIONS** Abdominal pain, nausea, vomiting, chronic

M

diarrhea, severe kidney dysfunction, fecal impaction, intestinal obstruction or perforation, rectal bleeding, colostomy, ileostomy.

**CAUTIOUS USE** Renal impairment, renal disease; older adults; pregnancy (category A); lactation; children younger than 2 y.

## ROUTE & DOSAGE

**Laxative**

*Adult:* **PO** 2.4–4.8 g (30–60 mL)/ day in 1 or more divided doses
*Child (2 to less than 6 y):* **PO** 0.4–1.2 g (5–15 mL)/day in 1 or more divided doses; *6–11 y:* 1.2–2.4 g (15–30 mL)/day in 1 or more divided doses

## ADMINISTRATION

**Oral**

- Shake bottle well before pouring to assure mixing of suspension.
- Follow drug with at least a full glass of water to enhance drug action for laxative effect. Administer in the morning or at bedtime. Most effective when taken on an empty stomach.
- Store at 15°–30° C (59°–86° F) in tightly covered container. Slowly absorbs carbon dioxide on exposure to air. Avoid freezing.

**ADVERSE EFFECTS** (≥1%) **GI:** Nausea, vomiting, abdominal cramps, *diarrhea.* **Urogenital:** Alkalinization of urine. **Body as a Whole:** Weakness, lethargy, mental depression, hyporeflexia, dehydration, coma. **Metabolic:** Electrolyte imbalance with prolonged use. **CV:** Hypotension, bradycardia, complete heart block and other ECG abnormalities. **Respiratory:** Respiratory depression.

**INTERACTIONS Drug:** Milk of Magnesia decreases absorption of **chlordiazepoxide, dicumarol, digoxin, isoniazid,** QUINOLONES, TETRACYCLINES.

**PHARMACOKINETICS Absorption:** 15–30% of magnesium is absorbed. **Onset:** 3–6 h. **Distribution:** Small amounts distributed in saliva and breast milk. **Elimination:** In feces; some renal excretion.

## NURSING IMPLICATIONS

**Assessment & Drug Effects**

- Evaluate the patient's continued need for drug. Prolonged and frequent use of laxative doses may lead to dependence. Additionally, even therapeutic doses can raise urinary pH and thereby predispose susceptible patients to urinary infection and urolithiasis.

**Patient & Family Education**

- Investigate the cause of persistent or recurrent constipation or gastric distress with prescriber.

M

## MAGNESIUM OXIDE

(mag-nes'i-um)

Mag-Ox, Maox, Par-Mag, Uro-Mag

**Classifications:** ANTACID; SALINE CATHARTIC
**Therapeutic:** ANTACID; MAGNESIUM SUPPLEMENT; LAXATIVE
**Prototype:** Magnesium hydroxide

**AVAILABILITY** Tablet; capsule

## ACTION & *THERAPEUTIC EFFECT*

Nonsystemic antacid with high neutralizing capacity and relatively long duration of action. *Acts as an antacid in low doses and a mild saline laxative at higher doses. Also effective as a magnesium supplement.*

**USES** Essentially the same as magnesium hydroxide. May also be used as magnesium supplement.

**CONTRAINDICATIONS** Abdominal pain, nausea, vomiting, diarrhea, severe kidney dysfunction, fecal impaction, intestinal obstruction or perforation, ileus; rectal bleeding, colostomy, ileostomy; AV block; hypermagnesia.

**CAUTIOUS USE** Cardiac disease, renal disease, renal impairment; electrolyte imbalance; pregnancy (category A); lactation.

## ROUTE & DOSAGE

**Antacid**
*Adult:* **PO** 280–1500 mg with water or milk q.i.d., p.c. and at bedtime

**Laxative**
*Adult:* **PO** 2–4 g with water or milk at bedtime

**Magnesium Supplement**
*Adult:* **PO** 400–1200 mg/day in divided doses

## ADMINISTRATION

### Oral
- Separate administration of this drug from other oral drugs by 1–2 h.
- Store at 15°–30° C (59°–86° F) in airtight containers. On exposure to air, magnesium oxide rapidly absorbs moisture and carbon dioxide.

**ADVERSE EFFECTS** (≥1%) **GI:** *Diarrhea,* abdominal cramps, nausea; hypermagnesemia, kidney stones (chronic use).

**INTERACTIONS Drug:** See magnesium hydroxide.

**PHARMACOKINETICS Absorption:** 30–50% from GI tract. **Elimination:** In urine.

## NURSING IMPLICATIONS

### Assessment & Drug Effects
- Monitor for dehydration, hypokalemia, and hyponatremia (see Appendix F) since drug may cause intense bowel evacuation.
- Monitor lab tests: Periodic serum magnesium.

### Patient & Family Education
- Liquid preparation is reportedly more effective than the tablet form, as with other antacids.

# MAGNESIUM SALICYLATE
(mag-nes'i-um)
Doan's Pills
**Classification:** ANALGESIC; NONSTEROIDAL ANTI-INFLAMMATORY DRUG (NSAID)
**Therapeutic:** NONNARCOTIC ANALGESIC, NSAID; ANTIPYRETIC
**Prototype:** Aspirin

**AVAILABILITY** Caplet

## ACTION & *THERAPEUTIC EFFECT*
Sodium-free salicylate derivative that is a nonsteroidal anti-inflammatory drug (NSAID). It inhibits prostaglandin synthesis. *In equal doses, less potent than aspirin as an analgesic and antipyretic. Has anti-inflammatory effects.*

**USES** Relief of pain and inflammation in rheumatoid arthritis, osteoarthritis, bursitis, and other musculoskeletal disorders.

**CONTRAINDICATIONS** Hypersensitivity to salicylates; erosive gastritis, peptic ulcer; advanced renal insufficiency, liver damage; thrombolytic therapy; bleeding disorders; before surgery; pregnancy (category D third trimester).

**CAUTIOUS USE** Serious acid-base imbalances; renal disease, history of GI bleeding, or peptic ulcers; SLE; history of acute bronchospasm; pregnancy (category C first and second trimester); lactation; children younger than 12 y.

## ROUTE & DOSAGE

### Analgesic/Antipyretic

*Adult:* **PO** 650 mg t.i.d. or q.i.d.
*Child (older than 2 y):* **PO** 50–75 mg/kg/day divided into 4–6 doses (max: 3.6 g/day)

### Arthritic Conditions

*Adult:* **PO** Up to 9.6 g/day in divided doses

## ADMINISTRATION
### Oral

- Give with a full glass of water, food, or milk to minimize gastric irritation.

**ADVERSE EFFECTS (≥1%) Body as a Whole:** Salicylism [dizziness, drowsiness, tinnitus, hearing loss, nausea, vomiting, hypermagnesemia (with high doses in patients with renal insufficiency)].

**INTERACTIONS Drug: Aminosalicylic acid** increases risk of SALICYLATE toxicity; **ammonium chloride** and other ACIDIFYING AGENTS decrease renal elimination and increase risk of SALICYLATE toxicity; anticoagulants— added risk of bleeding with ANTICOAGULANTS; CARBONIC ANHYDRASE INHIBITORS enhance SALICYLATE toxicity; CORTICOSTEROIDS compound ulcerogenic effects; increases **methotrexate** toxicity; low doses of SALICYLATES

may antagonize uricosuric effects of **probenecid, sulfinpyrazone.**

**PHARMACOKINETICS Absorption:** Well absorbed from the GI tract. **Peak:** 20 min. **Distribution:** Widely distributed with high levels of salicylic acid in liver and kidney, crosses placenta, excreted in breast milk. **Metabolism:** Salicylic acid is metabolized in liver. **Elimination:** In kidneys. **Half-Life:** 2–3 h with single dose, 15–30 h with chronic dosing.

## NURSING IMPLICATIONS
### Assessment & Drug Effects

- Monitor lab tests. Periodic serum magnesium if used in high dosages or with renal impairment.

### Patient & Family Education

- Report to prescriber promptly tinnitus, hearing loss, or dizziness.
- Do not take aspirin-containing drugs without consent of prescriber.
- Check ingredients. Doan's pills may contain acetaminophen plus salicylamide.

# MAGNESIUM SULFATE
(mag-nes'i-um)

**Classifications:** SALINE CATHARTIC; ELECTROLYTE REPLACEMENT; ANTICONVULSANT
**Therapeutic:** ELECTROLYTE REPLACEMENT; ANTICONVULSANT
**Prototype:** Magnesium hydroxide

**AVAILABILITY** Solution for injection

**ACTION & THERAPEUTIC EFFECT**
**Oral:** Acts as a laxative by osmotic retention of fluid, which distends colon, increases water content of feces, and causes mechanical stimulation of bowel activity. **Parenteral:** Acts as a CNS depressant and also as a depressant of smooth, skeletal, and cardiac

Common adverse effects in *italic;* life-threatening effects underlined; generic names in **bold;** classifications in SMALL CAPS; ✦ Canadian drug name; ⊙ Prototype drug

981

muscle function. Anticonvulsant properties thought to be produced by CNS depression by decreasing acetylcholine liberated from motor nerve terminals, producing peripheral neuromuscular blockade. *Effective parenterally as a CNS depressant, smooth muscle relaxant and anticonvulsant in labor and delivery, and cardiac disorders. When taken orally, it is a laxative.*

**USES** Parenterally to control seizures in toxemia of pregnancy, epilepsy, and acute nephritis and for prophylaxis and treatment of hypomagnesemia.

**UNLABELED USES** To inhibit premature labor (tocolytic action) and as adjunct in hyperalimentation, to alleviate bronchospasm of acute asthma.

**CONTRAINDICATIONS** Myocardial damage; AV heart block; cardiac arrest except for certain arrhythmias; hypermagnesemia; GI obstruction; pregnancy (category D). **IV:** For toxemia during the 2 h preceding delivery. **Oral:** In patients with abdominal pain, nausea, vomiting or other signs of appendicitis; fecal impaction, or intestinal irritation, obstruction, or perforation; magnesium-restricted diet.

**CAUTIOUS USE** Renal disease; renal failure; renal impairment; acute MI; digitalized patients; older adults. **IV:** Children.

## ROUTE & DOSAGE

**Seizures**

*Adult:* **IV** 1 g, may need to repeat dose

**Preeclampsia, Eclampsia**

*Adult:* **IM/IV** 4–5 g slowly; simultaneously, 5 g **IM** in alternate buttocks q4h

**Hypomagnesemia**

*Adult:* **IM/IV** *Mild:* 1 g q6h for 4 doses; *Severe:* 5 g infused over 3 h
*Child:* **IV** 25–50 mg/kg q4–6h prn (max single dose: 2000 mg)

**Total Parenteral Nutrition**

*Adult:* **IV** 8–24 mEq/day

## ADMINISTRATION

- Magnesium 1%, 2%, 4%, and 8% solutions are for IV route only. Both IV and IM routes are appropriate for magnesium 20% and 50%; 50% solution must be diluted prior to IV administration.

### Intramuscular

- IM injection is painful and should be reserved for patients with limited IV access and severe hypomagnesemia.
- Give deep using the 50% concentration for adults and the 20% concentration for children.

### Intravenous

Note: Verify correct IV concentration and rate of infusion for administration to infants, children with prescriber.

*PREPARE:* **Direct/IV Infusion:** Give solutions with concentrations of 20% or less undiluted. ▪ Dilute more concentrated solutions to 20% (200 mg/mL) or less with D5W or NS.

*ADMINISTER:* **Direct:** Give at a rate of 150 mg over at least 1 min. Note: 20% solution contains 200 mg/mL, 10% solution contains 100 mg/mL. **IV Infusion:** Give required dose over 4 h. Do not exceed the direct rate.

*INCOMPATIBILITIES:* **Solution/additive: 10% fat emulsion, amphotericin B, calcium, chlorpromazine, clindamycin,**

M

cyclosporine, dobutamine, hydralazine, polymyxin B, procaine, prochlorperazine, sodium bicarbonate. **Y-site:** Amiodarone, amphotericin B, cholesteryl, cefepime, ciprofloxacin, haloperidol, lansoprazole.

**ADVERSE EFFECTS** (≥1%) **Body as a Whole:** Flushing, sweating, extreme thirst, sedation, confusion, depressed reflexes or no reflexes, muscle weakness, <u>flaccid paralysis</u>, hypothermia. **CV:** Hypotension, depressed cardiac function, <u>complete heart block, circulatory collapse</u>. **Respiratory:** <u>Respiratory paralysis</u>. **Metabolic:** Hypermagnesemia, hypocalcemia, dehydration, electrolyte imbalance including hypocalcemia with repeated laxative use.

**INTERACTIONS Drug:** NEUROMUSCULAR BLOCKING AGENTS add to respiratory depression and apnea.

**PHARMACOKINETICS Onset:** 1–2 h PO; 1 h IM. **Duration:** 30 min IV; 3–4 h PO. **Distribution:** Crosses placenta; distributed into breast milk. **Elimination:** In kidneys.

**NURSING IMPLICATIONS**

**Assessment & Drug Effects**
- Observe constantly when given IV. Check BP and pulse q10–15 min or more often if indicated.
- Early indicators of magnesium toxicity (hypermagnesemia) include cathartic effect, profound thirst, feeling of warmth, sedation, confusion, depressed deep tendon reflexes, and muscle weakness.
- Monitor respiratory rate closely. Report immediately if rate falls below 12.
- Check urinary output, especially in patients with impaired kidney function. Therapy is generally not continued if urinary output is less

than 100 mL during the 4 h preceding each dose.
- Observe newborns of mothers who received parenteral magnesium sulfate within a few hours of delivery for signs of toxicity, including respiratory and neuromuscular depression.
- Observe patients receiving drug for hypomagnesemia for improvement in the following signs of deficiency: Irritability, choreiform movements, tremors, tetany, twitching, muscle cramps, tachycardia, hypertension, psychotic behavior.
- Have calcium gluconate readily available in case of magnesium sulfate toxicity.
- Monitor lab tests: Periodic serum magnesium, calcium, and phosphorus.

**Patient & Family Education**
- Drink sufficient water during the day when drug is administered orally to prevent net loss of body water.

**M**

**MANNITOL** 🄿
(man'ni-tole)
Osmitrol
**Classifications:** ELECTROLYTIC AND WATER BALANCE AGENT; OSMOTIC DIURETIC
**Therapeutic:** OSMOTIC DIURETIC

**AVAILABILITY** Solution for injection

**ACTION & *THERAPEUTIC EFFECT***
Increases rate of electrolyte excretion by the kidney, particularly sodium, chloride, and potassium. Induces diuresis by raising osmotic pressure of glomerular filtrate, thereby inhibiting tubular reabsorption of water and solutes. Reduces elevated intraocular and cerebrospinal pressures by increasing plasma osmolality, thus inducing diffusion of water from these fluids

Common adverse effects in *italic;* life-threatening effects <u>underlined;</u> generic names in **bold;** classifications in SMALL CAPS; ♣ Canadian drug name; 🄿 Prototype drug

983

back into plasma and extravascular space. *Osmotic diuretic that reduces intracranial pressure, cerebral edema, intraocular pressure, and promotes diuresis, thus preventing or treating oliguria.*

**USES** To promote diuresis in prevention and treatment of oliguric phase of acute kidney failure following cardiovascular surgery, severe traumatic injury, surgery in presence of severe jaundice, hemolytic transfusion reaction. Also used to reduce elevated intraocular (IOP) and intracranial pressure (ICP), to measure glomerular filtration rate (GFR), to promote excretion of toxic substances, to relieve symptoms of pulmonary edema, and as irrigating solution in transurethral prostatic reaction to minimize hemolytic effects of water. Commercially available in combination with sorbitol for urogenital irrigation.

**CONTRAINDICATIONS** Anuria; severe renal failure with azotemia or increasing oliguria; marked pulmonary congestion or edema; severe CHF; metabolic edema; hypovolemia; organic CNS disease, intracranial bleeding; shock, severe dehydration; concomitantly with blood.

**CAUTIOUS USE** Electrolyte imbalance; older adult; pregnancy (category B); lactation; children.

## ROUTE & DOSAGE

### Acute Kidney Failure
*Adult:* **IV Test Dose** 0.2 g/kg over 3–5 min if partial response may repeat test dose 1 time. If still negative, do not use. **Treatment** 50–100 g as 15–20% solution over 90 min to several hours
*Child:* **IV Test Dose** 0.2 g/kg (max: 12.5 g) over 3–5 min;

**Positive Response** Urine flow of 1 mL/kg/h for 1–2 h; **Maintenance** 0.25–0.5 g/kg q4–6h

### Edema, Ascites
*Adult:* **IV** 100 g as a 10–20% solution over 2–6 h

### Elevated IOP or ICP
*Adult:* **IV** 1.5–2 g/kg as a 15–25% solution over 30–60 min

### Acute Chemical Toxicity
*Adult:* **IV** 100–200 g depending on urine output

### Measurement of GFR
*Adult:* **IV** 100 mL of 20% solution diluted with 180 mL NaCl injection infused at a rate of 20 mL/min

## ADMINISTRATION

**Intravenous**
Note: Verify correct IV concentration and rate of infusion for administration to infants, children with prescriber.

*PREPARE:* **IV Infusion:** Give undiluted.
*ADMINISTER:* **IV Infusion:** Give a single dose over 30–90 min. *Oliguria:* A test dose is given to patients with marked oliguria to check adequacy of kidney function. Response is considered satisfactory if urine flow of at least 30–50 mL/h is produced over 2–3 h after drug administration; then rate is adjusted to maintain urine flow at 30–50 mL/h with a single dose usually being infused over 90 min or longer. ▪ Concentrations higher than 15% have a greater tendency to crystallize. ▪ Use an administration set with a 5 micron in-line IV filter when infusing concentrations of 15% or above.

Common adverse effects in *italic;* life-threatening effects <u>underlined;</u> generic names in **bold;** classifications in SMALL CAPS; ♣ Canadian drug name; ✪ Prototype drug

*INCOMPATIBILITIES:* Solution/additive: **Furosemide, imipenem-cilastatin, meropenem, potassium chloride, sodium chloride, whole blood.** Y-site: **Cefepime, doxorubicin liposome, filgrastim, pantoprazole.**

- Store at 15°–30° C (59°–86° F) unless otherwise directed. Avoid freezing.

## ADVERSE EFFECTS (≥1%) CNS:
Headache, tremor, convulsions, dizziness, transient muscle rigidity. **CV:** Edema, CHF, angina-like pain, hypotension, hypertension, thrombophlebitis. **Eye:** Blurred vision. **GI:** Dry mouth, nausea, vomiting. **Urogenital:** Marked diuresis, urinary retention, nephrosis, uricosuria **Metabolic:** *Fluid and electrolyte imbalance,* especially hyponatremia; dehydration, acidosis. **Other:** With extravasation (local edema, skin necrosis; chills, fever, allergic reactions).

## INTERACTIONS Drug:
Increases urinary excretion of **lithium,** SALICYLATES, BARBITURATES, **imipramine, potassium.**

## PHARMACOKINETICS Onset:
1–3 h diuresis; 30–60 min IOP; 15 min ICP. **Duration:** 4–6 h IOP; 3–8 h ICP. **Distribution:** Confined to extracellular space; does not cross blood–brain barrier except with very high plasma levels in the presence of acidosis. **Metabolism:** Small quantity metabolized to glycogen in liver. **Elimination:** Rapidly excreted by kidneys. **Half-Life:** 100 min.

## NURSING IMPLICATIONS
### Assessment & Drug Effects
- Take care to avoid extravasation. Observe injection site for signs of inflammation or edema.

- Measure I&O accurately and record to achieve proper fluid balance.
- Monitor vital signs closely. Report significant changes in BP and signs of CHF.
- Monitor for possible indications of fluid and electrolyte imbalance (e.g., thirst, muscle cramps or weakness, paresthesias, and signs of CHF).
- Be alert to the possibility that a rebound increase in ICP sometimes occurs about 12 h after drug administration. Patient may complain of headache or confusion.
- Take accurate daily weight.
- Monitor lab tests: Periodic serum electrolytes and renal function tests.

### Patient & Family Education
- Report any of the following: Thirst, muscle cramps or weakness, paresthesia, dyspnea, or headache.
- Family members should immediately report any evidence of confusion.

# MAPROTILINE HYDROCHLORIDE
(ma-proe′ti-leen)

**Classification:** TETRACYCLIC ANTIDEPRESSANT
**Therapeutic:** ANTIDEPRESSANT
**Prototype:** Mirtazapine

## AVAILABILITY Tablet

## ACTION & *THERAPEUTIC EFFECT*
It selectively inhibits reuptake of norepinephrine at CNS adrenergic synapses; this appears to produce antidepressant as well as antianxiety effects of maprotiline. *Useful in depression associated with anxiety and sleep disturbances.*

## USES Treatment
of depressive neurosis (dysthymic disorder) and

manic-depressive illness, depressed type (major depressive disorder).

**UNLABELED USES** Bulimia, pain, panic attack, enuresis.

**CONTRAINDICATIONS** Acute MI, AV block, cardiac arrhythmias, QT prolongation; MAOI therapy within 14 days; tricyclic antidepressant therapy; history of alcoholism; suicidal ideation.

**CAUTIOUS USE** History of seizure activity; psychotic disorders; history of suicidal tendencies; DM; hepatic disease; GI disease; GERD; BPH; respiratory depression; labor and delivery; pregnancy (category B); lactation; children younger than 18 y.

## ROUTE & DOSAGE

### Mild to Moderate Depression

*Adult:* **PO** Start at 75 mg/day and may increase q2wk up to 150 mg/day in single or divided doses
*Geriatric:* **PO** Start with 25 mg at bedtime may increase to 50–75 mg/day

### Severe Depression

*Adult:* **PO** Start at 100–150 mg/day may increase up to 300 mg/day in single or divided doses if needed

### *Pharmacogenetic Dosage Adjustment*

*Poor CYP2D6 metabolizers:* Start with 40% of dose

## ADMINISTRATION

### Oral

- Give as single dose or in divided doses. Initiate therapy with low dosages to reduce risk of seizures.
- Store at 15°–30° C (59°–86° F) unless otherwise specified.

**ADVERSE EFFECTS** (≥1%) **CNS:** Seizures, exacerbation of psychosis, hallucinations, tremors, excitement, confusion, dizziness, *drowsiness.* **CV:** *Orthostatic hypotension,* hypertension, tachycardia. **Special Senses:** Accommodation disturbances, blurred vision, mydriasis. **GI:** Nausea, vomiting, epigastric distress, *constipation, dry mouth.* **Urogenital:** *Urinary retention,* frequency. **Skin:** Hypersensitivity reactions (skin rash, urticaria, photosensitivity).

**INTERACTIONS Drug:** May decrease some response to ANTIHYPERTENSIVES; CNS DEPRESSANTS, **alcohol,** HYPNOTICS, BARBITURATES, SEDATIVES potentiate CNS depression; may increase hypoprothrombinemic effect of ORAL ANTICOAGULANTS; with **levodopa,** SYMPATHOMIMETICS (e.g., **epinephrine, norepinephrine**) there is possibility of sympathetic hyperactivity with hypertension and **hyperpyrexia;** with MAO INHIBITORS or **linezolid** there is possibility of severe reactions, toxic psychosis, cardiovascular instability; **methylphenidate** increases plasma TCA levels; THYROID DRUGS increase possibility of arrhythmias; **cimetidine** may increase plasma TCA levels.

**PHARMACOKINETICS Absorption:** Slowly absorbed from GI tract. **Peak:** 12 h. **Distribution:** Distributed chiefly to brain, lungs, liver, and kidneys. **Metabolism:** In liver. **Elimination:** 70% in urine, 30% in feces. **Half-Life:** 51 h.

## NURSING IMPLICATIONS

### Black Box Warning

*Maprotiline has been associated with suicidal thinking and behavior in children, adolescents, and young adults.*

M

### Assessment & Drug Effects

- Monitor for increased suicidality, unusual changes in behavior, or suicide attempt. Inform the prescriber immediately.
- Assess level of sedative effect. If recovering patient becomes too lethargic to care for personal hygiene or to maintain food intake and interactions with others, report to prescriber.
- Monitor bowel elimination pattern and I&O ratio. Severe constipation and urinary retention are potential problems, especially in the older adult. Advise increased fluid intake (at least 1500 mL/day).
- Observe seizure precautions; risk of seizures appears to be high in heavy drinkers.
- Bear in mind that if patient uses excessive amounts of alcohol, potentiated effects of maprotiline may increase the danger of overdosage or suicide attempt.

### Patient & Family Education

- Report immediately to prescriber signs of worsening mental status such as suicidal ideation, aggressiveness, agitation, anxiety, hostility, impulsivity, insomnia, irritability, panic attacks, and worsening of depression.
- Use caution with tasks that require alertness and skill; ability may be impaired during early therapy.
- Do not change dose or dose schedule without consulting prescriber.
- Do not use OTC drugs unless approved by prescriber.
- Avoid alcohol; the effects of maprotiline are potentiated when both are used together and for 2 wk after maprotiline is discontinued.

# MARAVIROC
(mar-a-vir'ok)
Selzentry

**Classifications:** ANTIRETROVIRAL; FUSION INHIBITOR; CELLULAR CHEMOKINE RECEPTOR (CCR5) ANTAGONIST
Therapeutic: ANTIRETROVIRAL

**AVAILABILITY** Tablet

**ACTION & THERAPEUTIC EFFECT**
Selectively binds to human chemokine coreceptor-5 (CCR-5) on cell membranes of helper T cell lymphocytes preventing interaction with the HIV-1 envelope protein necessary for the HIV virus to enter helper T cells. *Prevents infection of helper T cells by HIV-1 viruses with CCR-5 tropism.*

**USES** Treatment of human immunodeficiency virus (HIV-1) infection in combination with other antiretroviral agents.

**CONTRAINDICATIONS** Patients with dual/mixed, or chemokine-related receptor (CCR-4)-tropic HIV-1 virus; treatment naïve adults or children with HIV-1; S&S of hepatitis, allergic reaction to drug, or hepatoxicity; severe renal impairment in patients who are taking potent CYP3A inhibitors or inducers; immune reconstitution syndrome; lactation.

**CAUTIOUS USE** Hepatic impairment, hepatitis B or C; renal impairment; CrCl less than 50 mL/min; cardiac disease or increased risk for cardiovascular events; older adults; postural hypotension; mild to moderate renal impairment; pregnancy (category B); children younger than 16 y.

Common adverse effects in *italic;* life-threatening effects underlined; generic names in **bold;** classifications in SMALL CAPS; ♦ Canadian drug name; ❍ Prototype drug

987

## ROUTE & DOSAGE

### Regimen without CYP3A Inducers or Inhibitors

*Adult /Adolescent:* **PO** 300 mg b.i.d.

### Regimen with CYP3A Inhibitor with/without CYP3A Inducer

*Adult /Adolescent:* **PO** 150 mg b.i.d.

### Regimen with CYP3A Inducers without a Strong CYP3A Inhibitor

*Adult /Adolescent:* **PO** 600 mg b.i.d.

### Renal/Hepatic Dosage Adjustment

See package insert.

## ADMINISTRATION

### Oral

- **Must be** given in combination with other antiretroviral drugs.
- Store at 15°–30° C (59°–86° F).

## ADVERSE EFFECTS (≥1%) **Body as a Whole:** Appetite disorders, herpes infection, pain and discomfort, *pyrexia.* **CNS:** Depression, disturbances in consciousness, *sleep disorders, dizziness,* paresthesias and dysesthesias, peripheral neuropathies, sensory abnormalities. **CV:** Vascular hypertension disorders. **GI:** *Abdominal pain,* constipation, dyspepsia, stomatitis, ulceration. **Hematologic:** Neutropenia. **Metabolic:** Elevated AST levels. **Musculoskeletal:** Joint-related signs and symptoms, muscle pains, *musculoskeletal symptoms.* **Respiratory:** Breathing abnormalities, bronchitis, bronchospasm, *cough,* influenza, paranasal sinus disorder, pneumonia, respiratory tract disorders, sinusitis, *upper respiratory tract infection.* **Skin:** Apocrine and eccrine gland disorders, benign neoplasms, dermatitis, eczema, folliculitis, lipodystrophies, pruritus, *rash.* **Urogenital:** Bladder and urethral symptoms, condyloma acuminatum, urinary tract signs and symptoms.

## INTERACTIONS **Drug:** STRONG CYP3A4 INHIBITORS (HIV PROTEASE INHIBITORS with the exception of **tipranavir/ritonavir, delavirdine, ketoconazole, itrazonazole, clarithromycin**) increase maraviroc plasma level. CYP3A4 INDUCERS (**efavirenz, rifampin, carbamazepine, phenobarbital, phenytoin**) decrease maraviroc plasma level. **Food:** Coadministration with a high-fat meal decreases the plasma levels of maraviroc. **Herbal:** **St. John's wort** may decrease the plasma levels of maraviroc.

## PHARMACOKINETICS **Absorption:** Bioavailability is 23–33%. **Peak:** 0.5–4 h (dose-dependent). **Distribution:** 75% protein bound. **Metabolism:** In liver via CYP3A4. **Elimination:** Primarily in stool. **Half-Life:** 14–18 h.

## NURSING IMPLICATIONS

### Black Box Warning

*Maraviroc has been associated with severe hepatotoxicity. Severe rash or evidence of a systemic allergic reaction may occur prior to the development of hepatotoxicity.*

### Assessment & Drug Effects

- Monitor for and report promptly S&S of hepatotoxicity, hepatitis or infection.
- Report promptly rash, fever, or other signs of an allergic reaction.
- Monitor BP especially in those on antihypertensive drugs and with a history of postural hypotension.

Common adverse effects in *italic;* life-threatening effects underlined; generic names in **bold;** classifications in SMALL CAPS; ♣ Canadian drug name; ◑ Prototype drug

- Monitor CV status especially in those with preexisting conditions that cause myocardial ischemia.
- Monitor lab tests: Baseline and periodic CD4+ cell count and HIV RNA viral load; periodic LFTs and WBC with differential.

**Patient & Family Education**
- Report promptly any of the following: Itchy rash, yellow skin or eyes, nausea or vomiting, upper abdominal pain, flu-like symptoms, unexplained fatigue.
- Exercise caution when arising from a lying or sitting position. Dizziness is a common adverse effect.
- Do not engage in dangerous activities until response to drug is known.

# MECHLORETHAMINE HYDROCHLORIDE
(me-klor-eth'a-meen)

Mustargen

**Classifications:** ANTINEOPLASTIC; ALKYLATING AGENT; NITROGEN MUSTARD
Therapeutic: ANTINEOPLASTIC
**Prototype:** Cyclophosphamide

**AVAILABILITY** Powder for injection

**ACTION & THERAPEUTIC EFFECT**
Analog of mustard gas that forms highly reactive carbonium ion that causes cross-linking and abnormal base-pairing in DNA, thereby interfering with DNA replication and RNA and protein synthesis. Cell-cycle nonspecific inhibitor of DNA and RNA synthesis. *Antineoplastic agent that simulates actions of x-ray therapy, but nitrogen mustards produce more acute tissue damage and more rapid recovery.*

**USES** Generally confined to nonterminal stages of neoplastic disease, as single agent or in combination with other agents in palliative treatment of Hodgkin's disease (stages III and IV), lymphosarcoma, mycosis fungoides, polycythemia vera, bronchogenic carcinoma, chronic myelocytic or chronic lymphocytic leukemia. Also for intrapleural, intrapericardial, and intraperitoneal palliative treatment of metastatic carcinoma resulting in effusion.

**CONTRAINDICATIONS** Myelosuppression; infectious granuloma; known infectious diseases, acute herpes zoster; intracavitary use with other systemic bone marrow suppressants; pregnancy (category D); lactation.

**CAUTIOUS USE** Bone marrow infiltration with malignant cells, chronic lymphocytic leukemia; men or women in childbearing age.

## ROUTE & DOSAGE

**Advanced Hodgkin's Disease**
Adult: **IV** 6 mg/m² on day 1 and 8 of a 28 day cycle
**Other Neoplasms**
Adult: **IV** 0.4 mg/kg given as a single dose or in divided doses of 0.1–0.2 mg/kg/day, may repeat course in 3–6 wk

**Obesity Dosage Adjustment**
Dose based on IBW

## ADMINISTRATION

**Intravenous**
Wear surgical gloves during preparation and administration of solution. ▪ Avoid inhalation of vapors and dust and contact of drug with eyes and skin. ▪ Flush contaminated area immediately if drug contacts the skin. Use copious

amounts of water for at least 15 min, followed by 2% sodium thiosulfate solution. Irritation may appear after a latent period.
▪ Irrigate immediately if eye contact occurs. Use copious amounts of NS followed by ophthalmologic examination as soon as possible.

*PREPARE:* **Direct:** Reconstitute immediately before use by adding 10 mL sterile water for injection or NS injection to vial to yield 1 mg/mL. With needle still in stopper, shake vial several times to dissolve.
▪ Discard colored solution or contents of any vial with drops of moisture.

*ADMINISTER:* **Direct:** To reduce risk of severe local reactions from extravasation or high concentration of the drug, inject slowly over 3–5 min into tubing or sidearm of freely flowing IV infusion. ▪Flush vein with running IV solution for 2–5 min to clear tubing of any remaining drug. ▪Be alert for extravasation. Treat promptly with subcutaneous or intradermal injection with isotonic sodium thiosulfate solution (1/6 molar) and application of ice compresses intermittently for a 6–12 h period to reduce local tissue damage and discomfort. ▪ Tissue induration and tenderness may persist 4–6 wk, and tissue may slough.

*INCOMPATIBILITIES:* **Solution/additive:** D5W, **methohexital, normal saline. Y-site:** Allopurinol, cefepime.

## ADVERSE EFFECTS (≥1%) **CNS:**
Neurotoxicity: Vertigo, tinnitus, headache, drowsiness, peripheral neuropathy, light-headedness, paresthesias, cerebral deterioration, coma. **GI:** Stomatitis, xerostomia, anorexia, *nausea, vomiting,* diarrhea.

**Hematologic:** Leukopenia, *thrombocytopenia,* lymphocytopenia, agranulocytosis, *anemia,* hyperheparinemia. **Skin:** Pruritus, hyperpigmentation, herpes zoster, alopecia. **Urogenital:** Amenorrhea, azoospermia, chromosomal abnormalities, hyperuricemia. **Body as a Whole:** Weakness, hypersensitivity reactions. *With extravasation: Painful inflammatory reaction, tissue sloughing, thrombosis, thrombophlebitis.*

**INTERACTIONS Drug:** May reduce effectiveness of ANTIGOUT AGENTS by raising serum **uric acid** levels; dosage adjustments may be necessary; may prolong neuromuscular blocking effects of **succinylcholine;** may potentiate bleeding effects of ANTICOAGULANTS, SALICYLATES, NSAIDS, PLATELET INHIBITORS.

**PHARMACOKINETICS Metabolism:** Rapid hydrolysis and demethylation. **Elimination:** In urine. **Half-Life:** Less than 1 min.

## NURSING IMPLICATIONS

### Black Box Warning

*This drug is highly toxic and must be handled and administered with care. Inhalation of dust or vapors and contact with skin or mucous membranes, especially those of the eyes, must be avoided. Avoid exposure during pregnancy. Mechlorethamine extravasation has been associated with painful tissue inflammation and sloughing.*

### Assessment & Drug Effects
▪ Monitor infusion site closely. If infiltration is suspected, immediately DC infusion (see ADMINISTRATION).

Common adverse effects in *italic;* life-threatening effects underlined; generic names in **bold;** classifications in SMALL CAPS; ♣ Canadian drug name; ❺ Prototype drug

- Monitor and record patient's fluid losses. Prolonged vomiting and diarrhea can produce volume depletion.
- Report immediately petechiae, ecchymoses, or abnormal bleeding from intestinal and buccal membranes. Keep injections and other invasive procedures to a minimum during period of thrombocytopenia.
- Report symptoms of agranulocytosis (e.g., unexplained fever, chills, sore throat, tachycardia, and mucosal ulceration).
- Monitor lab tests: Periodic CBC with differential and platelet count. Periodic serum uric acid levels.

**Patient & Family Education**

- Report any signs of bleeding immediately.
- Avoid exposure to people with infection, especially upper respiratory tract infections.
- Use caution to prevent falls or other traumatic injuries, especially during periods of low platelet counts.
- Increase fluid intake up to 3000 mL/day if allowed to minimize risk of kidney stones. Report promptly all symptoms, including flank or joint pain, swelling of lower legs and feet, changes in voiding pattern.

---

## MECLIZINE HYDROCHLORIDE ⓟ

(mek'li-zeen)

Antivert, Antrizine, Bonamine ◆, Bonine, Dizmiss, RuVert-M

**Classification:** ANTIHISTAMINE; $H_1$-RECEPTOR ANTAGONIST; ANTIVERTIGO

Therapeutic: ANTIHISTAMINE, ANTIVERTIGO

**AVAILABILITY** Tablet; capsule

**ACTION & *THERAPEUTIC EFFECT***

An $H_1$ receptor antagonist with anticholinergic, CNS depressant, and local anesthetic effects. Its antiemetic and antivertigo effects are not fully understood. It depresses inner ear labyrinth excitability and vestibular stimulation, and it may affect chemoreceptor trigger zone in the CNS. *Exhibits antivertigo, and antiemetic effects.*

**USES** Management of nausea, vomiting, and dizziness associated with motion sickness and in vertigo associated with diseases affecting vestibular system.

**CONTRAINDICATIONS** Hypersensitivity to meclizine; GI obstruction, ileus.

**CAUTIOUS USE** Angle-closure glaucoma, older adults, asthma, prostatic hypertrophy, pregnancy (category B), lactation. Use in children younger than 12 y not recommended.

**ROUTE & DOSAGE**

**Motion Sickness**

*Adult/Adolescent:* PO 25–50 mg 1 h before travel, may repeat q24h if necessary for duration of journey

**Vertigo**

*Adult/Adolescent:* PO 25–100 mg/day in divided doses

**ADMINISTRATION**

**Oral**

- Give without regard to meals.
- Ensure that chewable tablets are chewed or crushed before being swallowed with a liquid.

**ADVERSE EFFECTS** (≥1%) **CNS:** *Drowsiness.* **GI:** Dry mouth. **Special Senses:** Blurred vision. **Body as a Whole:** Fatigue.

M

---

Common adverse effects in *italic*; life-threatening effects <u>underlined</u>; generic names in **bold**; classifications in SMALL CAPS; ◆ Canadian drug name; ⓟ Prototype drug

991

**INTERACTIONS Drug: Alcohol,** CNS DEPRESSANTS may potentiate sedative effects of meclizine.

**PHARMACOKINETICS Absorption:** Readily absorbed from GI tract. **Onset:** 1 h. **Duration:** 8–24 h. **Distribution:** Crosses placenta. **Elimination:** Primarily in feces. **Half-Life:** 6 h.

**NURSING IMPLICATIONS**

**Assessment & Drug Effects**

- Supervision of ambulation, particularly with the older adult, since drug may cause drowsiness.
- Assess effectiveness of drug and inform prescriber when prescribed for vertigo; dosage adjustment may be required.

**Patient & Family Education**

- Do not drive or engage in potentially hazardous activities until response to drug is known.
- Be aware that sedative action may add to that of alcohol, barbiturates, narcotic analgesics, or other CNS depressants.
- Take 1 h before departure when prescribed for motion sickness.

## MECLOFENAMATE SODIUM
(me-kloe-fen-am′ate)

**Classification:** ANALGESIC, NON-STEROIDAL ANTI-INFLAMMATORY DRUG (NSAID)
**Therapeutic:** ANALGESIC, NSAID; ANTIPYRETIC; ANTIRHEUMATIC
**Prototype:** Ibuprofen

**AVAILABILITY** Capsule

**ACTION & THERAPEUTIC EFFECT**
Inhibits prostaglandin synthesis by inhibiting both the COX-1 and COX-2 enzymes necessary for its synthesis and competes for binding at prostaglandin receptor sites. Does not appear to alter course of arthritis. *Palliative anti-inflammatory and analgesic activity.*

**USES** Symptomatic treatment of acute or chronic rheumatoid arthritis and osteoarthritis; treatment of dysmenorrhea.

**UNLABELED USES** Management of psoriatic arthritis, mild to moderate postoperative pain.

**CONTRAINDICATIONS** Hypersensitivity to aspirin or other NSAIDS; active peptic ulcer, ulcerative colitis; perioperative pain related to CABG surgery; renal disease; pregnancy (category D third trimester), patient designated as functional class IV rheumatoid arthritis (incapacitated, bedridden, etc).

**CAUTIOUS USE** History of upper GI tract disease; coronary artery disease; acute MI, cardiac arrhythmias; CVA; diabetes mellitus; SLE; compromised cardiac and kidney function, or other conditions predisposing to fluid retention; pregnancy (category C first and second trimester); lactation; children younger than 14 y.

**ROUTE & DOSAGE**

| Inflammatory Disease |
|---|
| *Adult:* **PO** 200–400 mg/day in 3–4 divided doses (max: 400 mg/day) |
| **Dysmennorhea** |
| *Adult:* **PO** 100 mg t.i.d. starting at onset of menstrual flow |

**ADMINISTRATION**

**Oral**

- Give with food or milk if patient complains of GI distress. An aluminum and magnesium hydroxide antacid (Maalox) also may be prescribed. Consult prescriber if symptoms persist.
- Withhold dose and report to prescriber if significant diarrhea occurs.
- Store at 15°–30° C (59°–86° F) in airtight, light-resistant container.

Common adverse effects in *italic;* life-threatening effects underlined; generic names in **bold;** classifications in SMALL CAPS; ✤ Canadian drug name; ⊙ Prototype drug

**ADVERSE EFFECTS** (≥1%) **CNS:** *Dizziness,* vertigo, lack of concentration, confusion, *headache,* tinnitus. **CV:** Edema. **GI:** *Severe diarrhea (dose-related),* peptic ulceration, <u>GI bleeding</u>, dyspepsia, abdominal pain, *nausea,* vomiting (may be severe), flatulence, eructation, pyrosis, anorexia, constipation. **GI:** *Abnormal liver function tests,* cholestatic jaundice. **Special Senses:** Blurred vision. **Urogenital:** Elevated BUN and creatinine, kidney failure. **Skin:** Rash, pruritus, urticaria.

**INTERACTIONS Drug:** ORAL ANTI-COAGULANTS, **heparin** may prolong bleeding time; may increase **lithium** toxicity; increases pharmacologic and toxic activity of **phenytoin**, SULFONYLUREAS, SULFONAMIDES, **warfarin** through protein-binding displacement. **Herbal: Feverfew, garlic, ginger, ginkgo** increase bleeding potential.

**PHARMACOKINETICS Absorption:** Rapidly and completely from GI tract. **Peak:** 1–2 h. **Duration:** 2–4 h. **Distribution:** Crosses placenta. **Metabolism:** In liver. **Elimination:** 60% in urine, 30% in feces. **Half-Life:** 2–3.3 h.

## NURSING IMPLICATIONS

### Black Box Warning

*Meclofenamate has been associated with increased risk of serious, potentially fatal, GI bleeding and cardiovascular events (e.g., MI & CVA); risk may increase with duration of use and may be greater in the older adult and those with risk factors for CV disease.*

### Assessment & Drug Effects

- Report diarrhea promptly. It is the most frequent adverse effect and usually dose related.

- Monitor I&O ratio. Encourage fluid intake of at least 8 glasses of liquid a day.
- Monitor for and report promptly S&S of CV thrombotic events (i.e., angina, MI, TIA, or stroke).
- Monitor for and report promptly S&S of GI ulceration or bleeding. Significant GI bleeding may occur without prior warning.
- Monitor lab tests: Hct and Hgb if anemia is suspected.

### Patient & Family Education

- Report immediately to prescriber any sign of bleeding (e.g., melena, epistaxis, ecchymosis) when taking concomitant oral anticoagulant.
- Stop taking drug and promptly notify the prescriber if nausea, vomiting, severe diarrhea, and abdominal pain occur.
- Report to prescriber without delay: Blurred vision, tinnitus, or taste disturbances.
- Report weight gain of more than 2.5 to 3.5 kg (3–4 lb)/wk as well as signs of edema: Swollen ankles, tibiae, hands, feet.
- Dizziness, a troublesome early side effect, frequently disappears in time. Avoid driving or potentially hazardous activities until response to drug is known.

# MEDROXYPROGESTERONE ACETATE

(me-drox'ec-proe-jess'te-rone)

Depo-Provera, Depo-subQ Provera 104, Provera

**Classification:** PROGESTIN
**Therapeutic:** PROGESTIN
**Prototype:** Progesterone

**AVAILABILITY** Tablet; suspension for injection

## ACTION & THERAPEUTIC EFFECT

Induces and maintains endometrium, preventing uterine bleeding;

M

Common adverse effects in *italic;* life-threatening effects <u>underlined;</u> generic names in **bold;** classifications in SMALL CAPS; ♣ Canadian drug name; ⊘ Prototype drug

993

inhibits production of pituitary gonadotropin, thus preventing ovulation and producing thick cervical mucus resistant to passage of sperm. *Slows release of luteinizing hormone (LH) preventing follicular maturation and ovulation.*

**USES** Dysfunctional uterine bleeding; secondary amenorrhea; endometrial hyperplasia, parenteral form **(Depo-Provera)** used in adjunctive, palliative treatment of inoperable, recurrent, and metastatic endometrial or renal carcinoma; contraception; endometriosis-associated pain.

**UNLABELED USES** Obstructive sleep apnea, treatment of hot flashes.

**CONTRAINDICATIONS** Hypersensitivity to medroxyprogesterone or any component of drug; history of arterial thromboembolic disorders; active DVT; breast cancer, vaginal cancer, uterine cancer, undiagnosed abnormal genital bleeding; hepatic impairment or disease; incomplete abortion; pregnancy (category X); lactation.

**CAUTIOUS USE** Asthma, seizure disorders, CVA; history of DVT; DM, hypercholesterolemia, hypertension, SLE, obesity, tobacco use; migraine, cardiac or kidney dysfunction. **IM:** Owing to potential for irreversible bone loss, long-term birth control use should be avoided or used in adolescents and early adulthood.

## ROUTE & DOSAGE

### Secondary Amenorrhea

*Adult:* **PO** 5–10 mg/day for 5–10 days beginning any time if endometrium is adequately estrogen primed (withdrawal bleeding occurs in 3–7 days after discontinuing therapy)

### Abnormal Bleeding Due to Hormonal Imbalance

*Adult:* **PO** 5–10 mg/day for 5–10 days beginning on the assumed or calculated 16th or 21st day of menstrual cycle; if bleeding is controlled, administer 2 subsequent cycles

### Endometrial Hyperplasia

*Adult:* **PO** 5–10 mg daily for 12–14 days/mo beginning on day 1 or 16 of cycle

### Carcinoma

*Adult:* **IM** 400–1000 mg/wk; continue at 400 mg/mo if improvement occurs and disease stabilizes

### Contraceptive

*Adult:* **IM** 150 mg q3mo
**Subcutaneous** 104 mg q3mo

## ADMINISTRATION

### Oral
- Oral drug may be given with food to minimize GI distress.

### Intramuscular
- Shake vial vigorously for at least 1 min prior to drawing up dose.
- Administer IM deep into a large muscle.
- Shake vial vigorously for at least 1 min prior to drawing up dose.
- Inject into anterior thigh or abdomen.
- Store all formulations at 15°–30° C (59°–86° F); protect from freezing.

## ADVERSE EFFECTS (≥1%) **CNS:** <u>Cerebral thrombosis or hemorrhage</u>, depression. **CV:** Hypertension, pulmonary embolism, edema. **GI:** Vomiting, nausea, cholestatic jaundice, abdominal cramps. **Urogenital:** *Breakthrough bleeding,* changes in menstrual flow, dysmenorrhea, vaginal candidiasis. **Skin:** Angioneurotic edema. **Body as a Whole:** Weight changes; *breast tenderness,* enlargement or secretion. **Musculoskeletal:** Loss of bone mineral density.

**M**

Common adverse effects in *italic;* life-threatening effects <u>underlined;</u> generic names in **bold;** classifications in SMALL CAPS; ♣ Canadian drug name; ❶ Prototype drug

INTERACTIONS Drug: **Aminoglutethimide** decreases serum concentrations of medroxyprogesterone; BARBITURATES, **carbamazepine, oxcarbazepine, phenytoin, primidone, rifampin, modafinil, rifabutin, topiramate** can increase metabolism and decrease serum levels of medroxyprogesterone. **Herbal:** Intermenstrual bleeding and loss of contraceptive efficacy may occur with **St. John's wort.**

PHARMACOKINETICS **Peak:** 2–4 h PO, 3 wk IM. **Distribution:** Greater than 90% protein bound. **Metabolism:** In liver. **Elimination:** Primarily in feces. **Half-Life:** 30 days PO, 50 days IM.

## NURSING IMPLICATIONS

### Black Box Warning

*Compounds with estrogen plus progestin have been associated with increased risk of DVT, PE, CVA, MI, dementia, and invasive breast cancer in postmenopausal women.*

### Assessment & Drug Effects

- See progesterone for numerous additional nursing implications.
- Be aware that IM injection may be painful. Monitor sites for evidence of sterile abscess. A residual lump and discoloration of tissue may develop.
- Monitor for S&S of thrombophlebitis (see Appendix F).

### Patient & Family Education

- Initially menstrual cycle may be irregular with unpredictable bleeding or spotting. Over time amenorrhea develops. Be aware that after repeated IM injections, infertility and amenorrhea may persist as long as 18 mo.

# MEFENAMIC ACID
(me-fe-nam'ik)
*Ponstel*

**Classification:** ANALGESIC, NONSTEROIDAL ANTI-INFLAMMATORY DRUG (NSAID)
**Therapeutic:** ANALGESIC, NSAID; ANTIPYRETIC
**Prototype:** Ibuprofen

AVAILABILITY Tablet

## ACTION & *THERAPEUTIC EFFECT*
NSAID that inhibits COX-1 and COX-2 enzymes necessary for prostaglandin synthesis. It affects platelet function. *Analgesic and anti-inflammatory actions.*

USES Short-term relief of mild to moderate pain including primary dysmenorrhea.

CONTRAINDICATIONS Angioedema, anaphylactic reaction or hypersensitivity to mefenamic; undiagnosed abnormal genital bleeding; breast cancer (known or suspected); DVT or PE (current or history of); active or history of arterial thromboembolic disease (e.g., stroke, MI); hepatic impairment or disease; pancreatitis; pregnancy; lactation.

CAUTIOUS USE Hypersensitivity to aspirin, history of UGI bleeding; blood dyscrasias; asthma; seizure disorders; hepatic hemangioma; migraines; porphyria; hypoparathyroidism; prior history of cholestatic jaundice; cardiac arrhythmias; hypertriglyceridemia; CHF; edema; history of DVT; DM; SLE; older adults. Longterm use increases risk of serious adverse events (see DRUG ADVERSE EFFECTS). Safety and efficacy in children younger than 14 y not established.

## ROUTE & DOSAGE

### Dysmenorrhea

*Adult/Adolescent:* **PO** 500 mg at the onset of menses then 250 mg q6h (no longer than 2–3 days)

M

---

Common adverse effects in *italic;* life-threatening effects underlined; generic names in **bold;** classifications in SMALL CAPS; ♣ Canadian drug name; ⊙ Prototype drug

995

## ADMINISTRATION

### Oral

- Give with meals, food, or milk to minimize GI adverse effects.
- Duration of therapy should not exceed 1 wk (manufacturer's warning).

## ADVERSE EFFECTS (≥1%) CNS:

Drowsiness, insomnia, dizziness, nervousness, confusion, headache. **GI:** *Severe diarrhea,* ulceration, and bleeding; *nausea, vomiting,* abdominal cramps, flatus, constipation, hepatic toxicity. **Hematologic:** Prolonged prothrombin time, severe autoimmune hemolytic anemia (long-term use), leukopenia, eosinophilia, agranulocytosis, thrombocytopenic purpura, megaloblastic anemia, pancytopenia, bone marrow hypoplasia. **Urogenital:** Nephrotoxicity, dysuria, albuminuria, hematuria, elevation of BUN. **Skin:** Urticaria, rash, facial edema. **Special Senses:** Eye irritation, loss of color vision (reversible), blurred vision, ear pain. **Body as a Whole:** Perspiration. **CV:** Palpitation. **Respiratory:** Dyspnea; acute exacerbation of asthma; bronchoconstriction (in patients sensitive to aspirin).

## DIAGNOSTIC TEST INTERFERENCE

False-positive reactions for *urinary bilirubin* (using *diazo tablet test*).

## INTERACTIONS Drug:

Mefenamic acid may prolong bleeding time with ORAL ANTICOAGULANTS, **heparin;** may increase **lithium** toxicity; increases pharmacologic and toxic activity of **phenytoin,** SULFONYLUREAS, SULFONAMIDES, **warfarin** because of protein-binding displacement. **Herbal: Feverfew, garlic, ginger, ginkgo** increase bleeding potential.

## PHARMACOKINETICS Absorption:

Rapidly and completely from GI tract. **Peak:** 2–4 h. **Duration:** 6 h. **Distribution:** Distributed in breast milk. **Metabolism:** Partially in liver. **Elimination:** 50% in urine, 50% in feces. **Half-Life:** 2 h.

## NURSING IMPLICATIONS

### Black Box Warning

*Mefenamic acid has been associated with increased risk of serious, potentially fatal, GI bleeding and cardiovascular events (e.g., MI & CVA); risk may increase with duration of use and may be greater in the older adult and those with risk factors for CV disease.*

### Assessment & Drug Effects

- Monitor for and report promptly S&S of GI ulceration or bleeding. Significant GI bleeding may occur without prior warning.
- Monitor for and report promptly S&S of CV thrombotic events (i.e., angina, MI, TIA, or stroke).
- Assess patients who develop severe diarrhea and vomiting for dehydration and electrolyte imbalance.
- Monitor lab tests: Periodic CBC, Hct and Hgb, and renal function tests.

### Patient & Family Education

- Discontinue drug promptly if diarrhea, dark stools, hematemesis, ecchymoses, epistaxis, or rash occur and do not use again. Contact prescriber.
- Notify prescriber if persistent GI discomfort, sore throat, fever, or malaise occur.
- Stop taking drug and report promptly to prescriber if you experience chest pain, shortness of breath, weakness, slurring of speech, or other signs of a cardiac or neurologic problem.
- Do not drive or engage in potentially hazardous activities until response to drug is known. It may cause dizziness and drowsiness.
- Monitor blood glucose for loss of glycemic control if diabetic.

# MEFLOQUINE HYDROCHLORIDE

(me-flo'quine)

**Classifications:** ANTIPROTOZOAL; ANTIMALARIAL
Therapeutic: ANTIMALARIAL
**Prototype:** Chloroquine

## AVAILABILITY Tablet

## ACTION & *THERAPEUTIC EFFECT*

Antimalarial agent that inhibits replication of parasites. *Effective against all types of malaria, including chloroquine-resistant malaria.*

## USES Treatment of mild to moderate acute malarial infections, prevention of chloroquine-resistant malaria caused by *Plasmodium falciparum* and *P. vivax.*

## CONTRAINDICATIONS Hypersensitivity to mefloquine or a related compound; with a calcium channel blocking agent; severe heart arrhythmias, history of QT_c prolongation, aggressive behavior; active depression, or history of depression, suicidal ideation; generalized anxiety disorder, psychosis, schizophrenia, or other major psychiatric disorders; seizure disorders; lactation.

## CAUTIOUS USE Persons piloting aircraft or operating heavy machinery.

## ROUTE & DOSAGE

Note: The U.S. Public Health Service does **not** recommend its use in children less than 15 kg or in pregnant women
**Treatment of Malaria**
*Adult:* **PO** 1250 mg (5 tablets) as single oral dose taken with at least 8 oz of water

*Child:* **PO** 20–25 mg/kg as single dose
**Prophylaxis for Malaria**
*Adult:* **PO** 250 mg once/wk × 4 wk (beginning 1 wk before travel), then 250 mg every other wk for duration of exposure and for 2 doses after leaving endemic area
*Child (weight 15–19 kg):* **PO** Given weekly: *15–19 kg:* ¼ tablet; *weight 20–30 kg:* ½ tablet; *weight 31–45 kg:* ¾ tablet

## ADMINISTRATION

### Oral

- Give with food and at least 8 oz water.
- Do not give concurrently with quinine or quinidine; wait at least 12 h beyond last dose of either drug before administering mefloquine
- Store at 15°–30° C (59°–86° F).

## ADVERSE EFFECTS (≥1%) **Body as a Whole:** Arthralgia, chills, fatigue, fever. **CNS:** Dizziness, nightmares, visual disturbances, headache, syncope, confusion, psychosis, aggression, suicide ideation (rare). **CV:** Bradycardia, ECG changes (including QT_c prolongation), first-degree AV block. **GI:** Nausea, vomiting, abdominal pain, anorexia, diarrhea. **Skin:** Rash, itching.

## DIAGNOSTIC TEST INTERFERENCE

Transient increase in *liver transaminases.*

## INTERACTIONS **Drug:** Mefloquine can prolong cardiac conduction in patients taking BETA-BLOCKERS, CALCIUM CHANNEL BLOCKERS, and possibly **digoxin. Quinine** may decrease plasma mefloquine concentrations. Mefloquine may decrease **valproic acid** serum concentrations by increasing its hepatic metabolism. Administration with **chloroquine**

may increase risk of seizures. Increased risk of cardiac arrest and seizures with **quinidine.**

## PHARMACOKINETICS **Absorption:** 85% absorbed, concentrates in red blood cells. **Onset:** 59 and 28 h for parasite and fever clearance times in patients with *P. vivax* infections, respectively; 166 and 93 h in patients with *P. malariae* infections. **Distribution:** Concentrated in red blood cells due to high-affinity binding to red blood cell membranes; 98% protein bound; distributed minimally into breast milk. **Metabolism:** In liver. **Elimination:** Primarily in bile and feces. **Half-Life:** 10–21 days (shorter in patients with acute malaria).

## NURSING IMPLICATIONS

### Black Box Warning

*Mefloquine has been associated with neuropsychiatric reactions that can persist after drug has been discontinued.*

### Assessment & Drug Effects

- Monitor carefully during prophylactic use for development of unexplained anxiety, depression, restlessness, or confusion; such manifestations may indicate a need to discontinue the drug.
- Evaluate cardiac and liver functions periodically with prolonged use.
- Monitor blood levels of anticonvulsants with concomitant therapy closely.
- Monitor lab tests: Periodic CBC with differential during prolonged use.

### Patient & Family Education

- Take drug on the same day each week when used for malaria prophylaxis.
- Do not perform potentially hazardous activities until response to drug is known.

- Report any of the following immediately: Fever, sore throat, muscle aches, visual problems, anxiety, confusion, mental depression, hallucinations.

# MEGESTROL ACETATE
(me-jess′trole)
**Megace, Megace ES**
**Classifications:** ANTINEOPLASTIC; PROGESTIN
**Therapeutic:** ANTINEOPLASTIC; APPETITE ENHANCER
**Prototype:** Progesterone

## AVAILABILITY Suspension; tablet

## ACTION & *THERAPEUTIC EFFECT*
Progestational hormone with antineoplastic properties for which an antiluteinizing effect mediated via the pituitary has been postulated. *Effective for treating breast, renal cell, or endometrial carcinoma. Also effective as an appetite enhancer. Has a local effect when instilled directly into the endometrial cavity.*

## USES Palliative agent for treatment of advanced carcinoma of breast or endometrium, AIDS-related wasting or cachexia.

## CONTRAINDICATIONS Diagnostic test for pregnancy; pregnancy (category X oral suspension, category D tablet); lactation.

## CAUTIOUS USE Older adults; severe hepatic disease; diabetes mellitus; renal impairment; thromboembolic disease.

## ROUTE & DOSAGE

### Palliative Treatment for Advanced Breast Cancer
*Adult:* **PO** 40 mg q.i.d.

**Palliative Treatment for Advanced Endometrial Cancer**

*Adult:* **PO** 40–320 mg/day in divided doses

**HIV-Related Cachexia/Anorexia**

*Adult:* **PO (suspension)** 800 mg daily or 625 mg of **Megace ES**

## ADMINISTRATION

### Oral

- Give with meals or food if GI distress occurs.
- Shake oral suspension well before use.
- Use appropriate handling and disposal precautions.
- Store at 15°–30° C (59°–86° F) in tightly closed container.

## ADVERSE EFFECTS (>1%) **Urogenital:** Vaginal bleeding, impotence. **Body as a Whole:** Breast tenderness, headache, increased appetite, weight gain, allergic-type reactions (including bronchial asthma), rash. **GI:** Abdominal pain, nausea, vomiting, diarrhea. **Hematologic:** DVT.

## INTERACTIONS **Drug:** May increase levels of **warfarin;** may decrease renal clearance of **dofetilide.** Do not use with **bosentan.**

## PHARMACOKINETICS **Absorption:** Appears to be well absorbed from GI tract. **Peak:** 1–3 h. **Duration:** 3–12 mo. **Metabolism:** Completely metabolized in liver. **Elimination:** 57–78% of dose excreted in urine within 10 days.

## NURSING IMPLICATIONS

### Assessment & Drug Effects

- Monitor weight periodically.
- Notify prescriber if abdominal pain, headache, nausea, vomiting, or breast tenderness become pronounced.
- Monitor for allergic reactions, including breathing distress characteristic of asthma, rash, urticaria, anaphylaxis, tachypnea, anxiety. Stop medication if they appear and notify prescriber.

### Patient & Family Education

- Use contraception measures to prevent pregnancy while taking this medication.
- Learn breast self-examination.
- Learn S&S of thrombophlebitis (see Appendix F).
- Review package insert to ensure understanding of megestrol therapy.
- Maintain adequate hydration while taking medication.

## MELOXICAM

(mel-ox′i-cam)

Mobic, Vivlodex

**Classification:** ANALGESIC, NONSTEROIDAL ANTI-INFLAMMATORY DRUG (NSAID)

**Therapeutic:** ANALGESIC, NSAID; ANTIPYRETIC; ANTIRHEUMATIC

**Prototype:** Ibuprofen

## AVAILABILITY Tablet; capsule

## ACTION & *THERAPEUTIC EFFECT*

A nonsteroidal anti-inflammatory drug (NSAID) that inhibits both COX-1 and COX-2 enzymes that are necessary for synthesis of prostaglandin, which is part of the inflammatory response. *Exhibits analgesic and anti-inflammatory actions. It improves the S&S of RA.*

## USES Relief of the signs and symptoms of osteoarthritis, rheumatoid arthritis; juvenile rheumatoid arthritis.

## CONTRAINDICATIONS Hypersensitivity to meloxicam, aspirin, salicylates, or NSAIDs; GI bleeding;

Common adverse effects in *italic;* life-threatening effects <u>underlined</u>; generic names in **bold;** classifications in SMALL CAPS; ✤ Canadian drug name; ⊘ Prototype drug

999

severe hepatic disease; perioperative pain with CABG surgery; lactation.

**CAUTIOUS USE** History of coagulation defects, liver dysfunction, gastrointestinal disease, anemia; asthma; bone marrow suppression; dehydration, edema, history of UGI bleeding; CV disease; jaundice; hepatic or renal impairment; hypertension, hypovolemia, immunosuppression; asthma; lactase deficiency, advanced renal dysfunction; hypertension or cardiac conditions aggravated by fluid retention and edema; older adults; females of childbearing age; pregnancy (category C); children.

## ROUTE & DOSAGE

### Osteoarthritis
*Adult:* **PO** 7.5–15 mg once daily; **Vivlodex** 5–10 mg once daily

### Rheumatoid Arthritis
*Adult:* **PO** 7.5 mg once daily ; may increase to 15 mg daily

### Juvenile Rheumatoid Arthritis
*Adolescent/Child (2–17 y):* **PO** 0.125 mg/kg/dose once daily (max: 7.5 mg/dose)

## ADMINISTRATION
### Oral
- Do not exceed the maximum recommended daily dose of 15 mg.
- Use the lowest effective dose for the shortest duration to minimize risk of serious adverse effects.
- May be taken with food to minimize gastrointestinal irritation.
- Store at 15°–30° C (59°–86° F).

**ADVERSE EFFECTS** (≥1%) **Body as a Whole:** Edema, fall, flu-like syndrome, pain. **GI:** Abdominal pain, diarrhea, dyspepsia, flatulence, nausea, constipation, ulceration, GI bleed. **Hematologic:** Anemia. **Musculoskeletal:** Arthralgia. **CNS:** Dizziness, headache, insomnia. **Respiratory:** Pharyngitis, upper respiratory tract infection, cough. **Skin:** Rash, pruritus. **Urogenital:** Micturition frequency, urinary tract infection.

**INTERACTIONS Drug:** Do not use with **cidofovir, ketorolac.** May decrease effectiveness of ACE INHIBITORS, DIURETICS; **aspirin, warfarin** may increase risk of bleed; may increase **lithium** levels and toxicity. **Herbal: Feverfew, garlic, ginger, ginkgo** may increase bleeding potential.

**PHARMACOKINETICS Absorption:** 89% bioavailable. **Peak:** 4–5 h. **Distribution:** Greater than 99% protein bound, distributes into synovial fluid. **Metabolism:** In liver (CYP2C9, CYP3A4). **Elimination:** Equally in urine and feces. **Half-Life:** 15–20 h.

## NURSING IMPLICATIONS

### Black Box Warning

*Meloxican has been associated with increased risk of serious, potentially fatal, GI bleeding and cardiovascular events (e.g., MI & CVA); risk may increase with duration of use and may be greater in the older adult and those with risk factors for CV disease.*

### Assessment & Drug Effects
- Monitor for and immediately report S&S of GI ulceration or bleeding, including black, tarry stool, abdominal or stomach pain; hepatotoxicity, including fatigue, lethargy, pruritus, jaundice, flu-like symptoms; skin rash; weight gain and edema.
- Withhold drug and notify prescriber if hepatotoxicity or GI bleeding is suspected.
- Monitor carefully patients with a history of CHF, HTN, or edema for fluid retention.

- Monitor for and report promptly S&S of CV thrombotic events (i.e., angina, MI, TIA, or stroke).
- Coadministered drugs: With warfarin, closely monitor INR when meloxicam is initiated or dose changed; monitor for lithium toxicity, especially during addition, withdrawal, or change in dose of meloxicam.
- Monitor lab tests: Hgb and Hct, CBC with differential, LFTs, serum electrolytes, BUN, and creatinine within 3 mo of initiating therapy and every 6–12 mo thereafter.

**Patient & Family Education**

- Report any of the following to the prescriber immediately: Nausea, black tarry stool, abdominal or stomach pain, unexplained fatigue or lethargy, itching, jaundice, flu-like symptoms, skin rash, weight gain, or edema.
- Discontinue drug if hepatotoxicity or GI bleeding is suspected. Note that GI bleeding may occur without forewarning and is more likely in older adults, in those with a history of ulcers or GI bleeding, and with alcohol consumption and cigarette smoking.
- Stop taking drug and report promptly to prescriber if you experience chest pain, shortness of breath, weakness, slurring of speech, or other signs of a cardiac or neurologic problem.

# MELPHALAN
(mel'fa-lan)
Alkeran
**Classifications:** ANTINEOPLASTIC; ALKYLATING AGENT
**Therapeutic:** ANTINEOPLASTIC
**Prototype:** Cyclophosphamide

**AVAILABILITY** Tablet; vial injection

## ACTION & *THERAPEUTIC EFFECT*
Forms a highly reactive carbonium ion that causes cross-linking and abnormal base-pairing in DNA, thereby interfering with DNA and RNA replication as well as protein synthesis. *Antineoplastic effects result from its activity against both resting and rapidly dividing tumor cells.*

**USES** Palliative treatment of multiple myeloma and other neoplasms, including Hodgkin's disease and carcinomas of breast and ovary.

**UNLABELED USES** Polycythemia vera.

**CONTRAINDICATIONS** Severe bone marrow suppression; pregnancy (category D); lactation.

**CAUTIOUS USE** Recent treatment with other chemotherapeutic agents; moderate to severe anemia, neutropenia, or thrombocytopenia; renal or hepatic impairment; men and women of child bearing age; older adults.

## ROUTE & DOSAGE

**Multiple Myeloma**
*Adult:* PO 6 mg/day for 2–3 wk, drug then withdrawn for 4–5 wk, restart at 2 mg/day when WBC and platelet counts start to rise; **IV** 16 mg/m² over 15 min q2wk for 4 doses

**Epithelial Ovarian Cancer**
*Adult:* PO 0.2 mg/kg/day for 5 days as single course, may repeat course q4–5wk

## ADMINISTRATION
**Oral**
- Give with meals to reduce nausea and vomiting. An antiemetic may be ordered.

M

---

Common adverse effects in *italic;* life-threatening effects underlined; generic names in **bold;** classifications in SMALL CAPS; ✦ Canadian drug name; ● Prototype drug

1001

**Intravenous**

This drug is a cytotoxic agent and caution should be used to prevent any contact with the drug. Follow institutional or standard guidelines for preparation, handling, and disposal of cytotoxic agents.

*PREPARE:* **IV Infusion:** Reconstitute melphalan powder by **rapidly** injecting 10 mL of the provided diluent into the vial to yield 5 mg/mL. Shake vigorously until clear. ▪ Immediately dilute further with NS to a concentration of 0.45 mg/mL or less. ▪ Note: 45 mg in 100 mL yields 0.45 mg/mL. ▪ Do not refrigerate reconstituted solution prior to infusion.

*ADMINISTER:* **IV Infusion:** Give over 15 min or longer. Administration **must be** completed within 60 min of reconstitution of drug because both reconstituted and diluted solutions are unstable. ▪ Ensure patency of IV site prior to infusion.

*INCOMPATIBILITIES:* **Solution/additive: D5W, lactated Ringer's. Y-site: Amphotericin B, chlorpromazine.**

▪ Store at 15°–30° C (59°–86° F) in light-resistant, airtight containers.

**ADVERSE EFFECTS** (≥1%) **Hematologic:** <u>Leukopenia, agranulocytosis, thrombocytopenia</u>, anemia, acute nonlymphatic leukemia. **Body as a Whole:** Uremia, angioneurotic peripheral edema. **GI:** Nausea, vomiting, stomatitis. **Skin:** Temporary alopecia. **Respiratory:** Pulmonary fibrosis.

**INTERACTIONS Drug:** Increases risk of nephrotoxicity with **cyclosporine, cimetidine** may decrease efficacy. **Food:** Food decreases absorption.

**PHARMACOKINETICS Absorption:** Incompletely and variably absorbed from GI tract. **Peak:** 2 h. **Distribution:** Widely distributed to all tissues. **Metabolism:** By spontaneous hydrolysis in plasma. **Elimination:** 25–50% in feces; 25–30% in urine. **Half-Life:** 1.5 h.

**NURSING IMPLICATIONS**

### Black Box Warning

*Melphalan has been associated with severe bone marrow suppression (with resulting infection and bleeding), development of leukemia, and with production of chromosomal aberrations thus making it potentially mutagenic in humans.*

**Assessment & Drug Effects**
▪ Monitor laboratory reports to anticipate leukopenic and thrombocytopenic periods.
▪ A degree of myelosuppression is maintained during therapy so as to keep leukocyte count in range of 3000–3500/mm³.
▪ Assess for flank and joint pains that may signal onset of hyperuricemia.
▪ Monitor lab tests: CBC with differential before each treatment and periodically as needed.

**Patient & Family Education**
▪ Be alert to onset of fever, profound weakness, chills, tachycardia, cough, sore throat, changes in kidney function, or prolonged infections and report to prescriber.
▪ Understand that reversible hair loss is an expected adverse effect.

## MEMANTINE
(me-man'teen)
Namenda, Namenda XR

Common adverse effects in *italic;* life-threatening effects <u>underlined;</u> generic names in **bold;** classifications in SMALL CAPS; ✤ Canadian drug name; ⊙ Prototype drug

**Classifications:** N-METHYL-
D-ASPARTATE (NMDA) RECEPTOR
ANTAGONIST; ANTIDEMENTIA
Therapeutic: ANTIDEMENTIA;
ANTI–ALZHEIMER'S

**AVAILABILITY** Tablet; solution; extended release capsule

**ACTION & THERAPEUTIC EFFECT**
Excess glutamate may play a role in Alzheimer's disease by overstimulating NMDA receptors. Blockade of NMDA receptors may slow intracellular calcium accumulation, preventing nerve damage without interfering with actions of glutamate that are required for memory and learning. *Improves cognitive functioning in moderate to severe Alzheimer's disease (AD) and in mild to moderate vascular dementia.*

**USES** Treatment of symptoms of moderate to severe Alzheimer's disease.

**UNLABELED USES** Treatment of moderate to severe vascular dementia, nystagmus.

**CONTRAINDICATIONS** Known memantine hypersensitivity; renal failure.

**CAUTIOUS USE** Severe renal impairment; severe hepatic impairment; cardiovascular disease; history of seizure disorder; older adults; pregnancy (category B); lactation; children.

## ROUTE & DOSAGE

**Alzheimer's Disease**
*Adult:* **PO Immediate release** Initiate with 5 mg once daily, increase dose by 5 mg/wk over a 3-wk period to target dose of 10 mg b.i.d.; **PO Extended release** 7 mg daily, increase at weekly intervals to 28 mg daily

**Severe Renal Impairment Dosage Adjustment**
Decrease to 5 mg b.i.d.

## ADMINISTRATION
**Oral**
- Ensure that extended-release capsule is swallowed whole. It should not be opened or chewed.
- Note: The recommended interval between dose increases is 1 wk.
- Dose reductions should be considered with moderate renal impairment.
- Store at 15°–30° C (59°–86° F).

**ADVERSE EFFECTS** (≥1%) **Body as a Whole:** Fatigue, pain, flu-like symptoms, peripheral edema. **CNS:** Dizziness, headache, confusion, somnolence, hallucinations, agitation, insomnia, abnormal gait, depression, anxiety, syncope, TIA, vertigo, ataxia, hypokinesia, aggressive reaction. **CV:** Hypertension, cardiac failure. **GI:** Constipation, vomiting, diarrhea, nausea, anorexia. **Hematologic:** Anemia **Metabolic:** Weight loss, increased alkaline phosphatase. **Musculoskeletal:** Back pain, arthralgia. **Respiratory:** Coughing, dyspnea, bronchitis, upper respiratory infections, pneumonia. **Skin:** Rash. **Special Senses:** Conjunctivitis. **Urogenital:** Urinary incontinence, UTI, frequent micturition.

**INTERACTIONS Drug:** Drugs that increase the pH of the urine (CARBONIC ANHYDRASE INIBITORS, **sodium bicarbonate**) may increase levels of memantine; may enhance the effects of **amantadine, dextromethorphan, ketamine, bromocriptine, pergolide, pramipexole,** and **ropinirole;** may enhance the adverse effects of **levodopa**-containing drugs.

Common adverse effects in *italic;* life-threatening effects underlined; generic names in **bold;** classifications in SMALL CAPS; ✤ Canadian drug name; ⊕ Prototype drug

1003

## PHARMACOKINETICS

**Absorption:** 100% from GI tract. **Duration:** 4–6 h. **Distribution:** Easily crosses the blood–brain barrier. **Metabolism:** Minimal. **Elmination:** Primarily excreted unchanged in urine. **Half-Life:** 60–80 h.

## NURSING IMPLICATIONS

### Assessment & Drug Effects

- Monitor respiratory and CV status, especially with preexisting heart disease.
- Assess for and report S&S of focal neurologic deficits (e.g., TIA, ataxia, vertigo).
- Monitor diabetics for loss of glycemic control.
- Monitor lab tests: Baseline LFTs and renal function tests; periodic urine pH.

### Patient & Family Education

- Report any of the following to the prescriber: Problems with vision, skin rash, shortness of breath, swelling in throat or tongue, agitation or restlessness, confusion, dizziness, or incontinence.
- Do not drive or engage in other hazardous activities until reaction to drug is known.

## MENINGOCOCCAL DIPHTHERIA TOXOID CONJUGATE

(me-nin'joe-kok-al)

**Menactra, Menveo**

**See Appendix J.**

## MEPERIDINE HYDROCHLORIDE

(me-per'i-deen)

**Demerol**

**Classification:** NARCOTIC (OPIATE AGONIST) ANALGESIC
**Therapeutic:** NARCOTIC ANALGESIC
**Prototype:** Morphine

## AVAILABILITY

Tablet; syrup; solution for injection

## ACTION & *THERAPEUTIC EFFECT*

Analgesia occurs through inhibition of ascending pain pathways, altering the perception of and response to pain; produces generalized CNS depression. *Control of moderate to severe pain. Does not alter pain threshold.*

## USES

Relief of moderate to severe acute pain, for preoperative medication, for support of anesthesia, and for obstetric analgesia.

## CONTRAINDICATIONS

Hypersensitivity to meperidine; convulsive disorders; acute abdominal conditions prior to diagnosis; chronic pain; MAOI therapy; pregnancy (category D at term).

## CAUTIOUS USE

Head injuries, increased intracranial pressure; asthma and other respiratory conditions; supraventricular tachycardia; prostatic hypertrophy; urethral stricture; glaucoma; older adult or debilitated patients; impaired kidney or liver function; hypothyroidism, Addison's disease; pregnancy (category B); children.

## ROUTE & DOSAGE

### Moderate to Severe Pain

Note: Should be titrated to pain response
*Adult:* **PO/Subcutaneous/IM/IV** 50–150 mg q3–4h prn
*Child:* **PO/Subcutaneous/IM/IV** 1–1.8 mg/kg q3–4h (max: 100 mg q4h) prn

### Preoperative

*Adult:* **IM/Subcutaneous** 50–100 mg 30–90 min before surgery
*Child:* **IM/Subcutaneous** 1.1–2.2 mg/kg 30–90 min before surgery

### Obstetric Analgesia during Labor/Delivery

*Adult:* **IM/Subcutaneous** 50–100 mg when pains become regular, may be repeated q1–3h

### Hepatic/Renal Impairment Dosage Adjustment

Metabolite accumulation can occur, adjust based on patient response

## ADMINISTRATION

### Oral

- Give syrup formulation in half a glass of water. Undiluted syrup may cause topical anesthesia of mucous membranes.
- May be administered with food or milk to minimize GI irritation.

### Subcutaneous/Intramuscular

- Be aware that subcutaneous route is painful and can cause local irritation. IM route is generally preferred when repeated doses are required.
- Aspirate carefully before giving IM injection to avoid inadvertent IV administration. IV injection of undiluted drug can cause a marked increase in heart rate and syncope.

### Intravenous

Note: Verify correct IV concentration and rate of infusion/injection for administration to infants or children with prescriber.

*PREPARE:* **Direct:** Dilute 50 mg in at least 5 mL of NS or sterile water to yield 10 mg/mL. **IV Infusion:** Dilute to a concentration of 1–10 mg/mL in NS, D5W, or other compatible solution.

*ADMINISTER:* **Direct:** Give slowly over 3–5 min at a rate not to exceed 25 mg/min. Slower injection preferred. **IV Infusion:** Usually given through a controlled infusion device at a rate not to exceed 25 mg/min.

*INCOMPATIBILITIES:* Solution/additive: **Aminophylline,** BARBITURATES, **furosemide, heparin, methicillin, morphine, phenytoin, sodium bicarbonate.** Y-site: **Allopurinol, amphotericin B cholesteryl complex, cefepime, doxorubicin liposome, furosemide, idarubicin, imipenem/cilastatin, lansoprazole, mezlocillin, minocycline, tetracycline.**

- Store at 15°–30° C (59°–86° F) in tightly closed, light-resistant containers unless otherwise directed by manufacturer.

## ADVERSE EFFECTS (≥1%) **Body as a Whole:** Allergic (*Pruritus,* urticaria, skin rashes, wheal and flare over IV site), profuse perspiration, physical dependence, psychological dependence. **CNS:** *Dizziness,* drowsiness, weakness, euphoria, dysphoria, *sedation,* headache, uncoordinated muscle movements, disorientation, decreased cough reflex, miosis, corneal anesthesia, <u>respiratory depression</u>. Toxic doses; Muscle twitching, tremors, hyperactive reflexes, excitement, hypersensitivity to external stimuli, agitation, confusion, hallucinations, dilated pupils, <u>convulsions</u>. **CV:** Facial flushing, light-headedness, hypotension, syncope, palpitation, bradycardia, tachycardia, <u>cardiovascular collapse, cardiac arrest (toxic doses)</u>. **GI:** Dry mouth, *nausea,* vomiting, *constipation,* biliary tract spasm. **Urogenital:** Oliguria, urinary retention. **Respiratory:** <u>Respiratory depression in newborn, bronchoconstriction</u> (large doses). **Skin:** Phlebitis (following IV use), pain, tissue irritation and induration, particularly following subcutaneous injection. **Metabolic:** Increased levels of serum amylase, BSP retention, bilirubin, AST, ALT.

**M**

---

Common adverse effects in *italic;* life-threatening effects <u>underlined</u>; generic names in **bold;** classifications in SMALL CAPS; ◆ Canadian drug name; ⊘ Prototype drug

## DIAGNOSTIC TEST INTERFERENCE

High doses of meperidine may interfere with **gastric emptying studies** by causing delay in gastric emptying.

## INTERACTIONS Drug: Alcohol

and other CNS DEPRESSANTS, **cimetidine** cause additive sedation and CNS depression; AMPHETAMINES may potentiate CNS stimulation; MAO INHIBITORS, **selegiline** may cause excessive and prolonged CNS depression, convulsions, cardiovascular collapse; **phenytoin** may increase toxic meperidine metabolites. Do not use with **ritonavir. Herbal: St. John's wort** may increase sedation.

## PHARMACOKINETICS Absorption: 50–60% from GI tract. Onset:

15 min PO; 10 min IM, Subcutaneous; 5 min IV. **Peak:** 1 h PO, IM, Subcutaneous. **Duration:** 2–4 h PO, IM, Subcutaneous; 2 h IV. **Distribution:** Crosses placenta; distributed into breast milk. **Metabolism:** In liver. **Elimination:** In urine. **Half-Life:** 3–5 h.

## NURSING IMPLICATIONS

### Assessment & Drug Effects

- Give narcotic analgesics in the smallest effective dose and for the least period of time compatible with patient's needs.
- Assess patient's need for prn medication. Record time of onset, duration, and quality of pain.
- Note respiratory rate, depth, and rhythm and size of pupils in patients receiving repeated doses. If respirations are 12/min or below and pupils are constricted or dilated (see ACTION and USES) or breathing is shallow, or if signs of CNS hyperactivity are present, consult prescriber before administering drug.
- Monitor vital signs closely. Heart rate may increase markedly, and

hypotension may occur. Meperidine may cause severe hypotension in postoperative patients and those with depleted blood volume.
- Schedule deep breathing, coughing (unless contraindicated), and changes in position at intervals to help to overcome respiratory depressant effects.
- Chart patient's response to drug and evaluate continued need.
- Repeated use can lead to tolerance as well as psychic and physical dependence of the morphine type.
- Be aware that abrupt discontinuation following repeated use results in morphine-like withdrawal symptoms. Symptoms develop more rapidly (within 3 h, peaking in 8–12 h) and are of shorter duration than with morphine. Nausea, vomiting, diarrhea, and pupillary dilatation are less prominent, but muscle twitching, restlessness, and nervousness are greater than produced by morphine.

### Patient & Family Education

- Exercise caution with ambulation and moving from a lying/sitting position to a standing position.
- Be aware that nausea, vomiting, dizziness, and faintness associated with fall in BP are more pronounced when walking than when lying down (these symptoms may also occur in patients without pain who are given meperidine). Symptoms are aggravated by the head-up position.
- Do not drive or engage in potentially hazardous activities until any drowsiness and dizziness have passed.
- Do not take other CNS depressants or drink alcohol because of their additive effects.

M

# MEPOLIZUMAB

(me-poe-liz'ue-mab)

Nucala

**Classifications:** MONOCLONAL ANTIBODY; INTERLEUKIN-5 ANTAGONIST; ANTIASTHMATIC

Therapeutic: ANTIASTHMATIC

**AVAILABILITY** Lyophilized powder for reconstitution and injection

**ACTION & *THERAPEUTIC EFFECT***
An antibody that acts as an interleukin 5 antagonist (IgG1 kappa). IL-5 is the major cytokine responsible for the growth and differentiation, recruitment, activation, and survival of eosinophils. Eosinophils are involved in the inflammation associated with the pathogenesis of asthma. *The inhibition of IL-5 signaling by mepolizumab, reduces the production and survival of eosinophils.*

**USES** Treatment of patients with severe asthma who are 12 y or older, and who exhibit an eosinophilic phenotype.

**CONTRAINDICATIONS** Hypersensitivity to mepolizumab.

**CAUTIOUS USE** Treat patients with a pre-existing helminth infection prior to starting therapy with mepolizumab. Clinical trials show no dosing differences with geriatric patients, but greater sensitivity cannot be ruled out and hepatic, renal, and cardiac function need to be considered. Pregnancy exposure data is insufficient to inform risk. Potential fetal effects are likely to be greater in the second and third trimesters. There is no information regarding transfer of mepolizumab to human milk and the effects on the breast-fed infant. The FDA approved product label recommends considering developmental and health benefits of breast-feeding and the mother's need for therapy.

## ROUTE & DOSAGE

### Asthma

*Adult:* **Subcutaneous** 100 mg q4wk

## ADMINISTRATION

Subcutaneous ONLY

- Visually inspect parenteral products for particulate matter. Solution can appear colorless, pale yellow, or pale brown and should be free of particles.
- Reconstitute mepolizumab in the vial with 1.2 mL sterile water for injection preferably using a 2–3 mL syringe and a 21-gauge needle, to result in a final concentration of 100mg/mL and should not be mixed with other medication.
- Direct the sterile water into the vial and then gently swirl the medication until the powder is dissolved (usually taking 5 min). Do not shake.
- If not used immediately, store below 30° C (86° F), but do not freeze. Discard if not used within 8 h of reconstitution.
- A 1-mL polypropylene syringe fitted with a disposable 21–27 gauge × 0.5 inch needle is preferable. Remove 1 mL of the reconstitute from the vial and administer subcutaneously into the upper arm, thigh or abdomen.
- Store unused vials below 25° C (77° F). Do not freeze and protect from light.

## ADVERSE EFFECTS (≥3%) **Body as a Whole:** Eczema, hypersensitivity reactions, influenza, *injection site reaction*, pruritus, pharyngitis,

M

Common adverse effects in *italic;* life-threatening effects underlined; generic names in **bold;** classifications in SMALL CAPS; ♣ Canadian drug name; ⓟ Prototype drug

1007

pyrexia, rash, toothache, viral infection. **CNS:** Asthenia, dizziness, fatigue, *headache*. **GI:** Abdominal pain, gastroenteritis, nausea, vomiting. **Musculoskeletal:** Back pain, muscle spasms, musculoskeletal pain. **Respiratory:** Allergic rhinitis, bronchitis, dyspnea, lower respiratory tract infection, nasal congestion, nasopharyngitis, viral respiratory tract infection. **Special Senses:** Ear infection. **Urogenital:** Cystitis, urinary tract infection.

**INTERACTIONS Drug:** Formal drug interaction trials have not been conducted.

**PHARMACOKINETICS Absorption:** 80% bioavailability. **Metabolism:** Degraded by proteolytic enzymes. **Half-Life:** 16–22 days.

## NURSING IMPLICATIONS

### Assessment & Drug Effects

- Patient may experience dizziness, headache, back pain, loss of strength and energy. Patient may need assistance when ambulating.
- Assess respiratory status and report any shortness of breath or abnormally low pulse oximetry readings.

### Patient & Family Education

- Notify prescriber if dizziness or fainting occurs.
- Seek out medical assistance with any signs of a significant drug reaction: Fever, itching, chest tightness, swelling of face, lips, tongue or throat.
- This is not a rescue medication for an asthma attack, it is a maintenance drug.
- Report urinary urgency or pain upon urination.
- Check with provider before taking additional prescription or over the counter medications.

# MEPROBAMATE ⓟ

(me-proe-ba'mate)

**Classifications:** CARBAMATE; ANXIOLYTIC; SEDATIVE-HYPNOTIC
**Therapeutic:** ANTIANXIETY; SEDATIVE-HYPNOTIC
**Controlled Substance:** Schedule IV

**AVAILABILITY** Tablet

## ACTION & *THERAPEUTIC EFFECT*

Carbamate derivative and CNS depressant. Acts on multiple sites in CNS and appears to block corticothalamic impulses. *Antianxiety agent. Hypnotic doses suppress REM sleep.*

## USES
Management of anxiety disorders or for the short-term relief of the symptoms of anxiety.

## CONTRAINDICATIONS
History of hypersensitivity to meprobamate or related carbamates; history of acute intermittent porphyria; pregnancy (category D); lactation.

## CAUTIOUS USE
Impaired kidney or liver function; convulsive disorders; history of alcoholism or drug abuse; patients with suicidal tendencies; children younger than 6 y.

## ROUTE & DOSAGE

### Anxiety

*Adult:* **PO** 1.2–1.6 g/day in 3–4 divided doses (max: 2.4 g/day)
*Child (6 y or older):* **PO** 100–200 mg b.i.d. or t.i.d.

### Renal Impairment Dosage Adjustment

*CrCl 10–50 mL/min:* Extend dosing interval to q9–12h
*CrCl less than 10 mL/min:* Extend dosing interval to q12–18h

## ADMINISTRATION

### Oral

- Give with food to minimize gastric distress.
- Treat physical dependence by gradual drug withdrawal over 1–2 wk to prevent onset of withdrawal symptoms.
- Store at 15°–30° C (59°–86° F) unless otherwise specified by manufacturer.

## ADVERSE EFFECTS (≥1%) Body as a Whole: Allergy or idiosyncratic reactions (itchy, urticarial, or erythematous maculopapular rash; exfoliative dermatitis, petechiae, purpura, ecchymoses, eosinophilia, peripheral edema, angioneurotic edema, adenopathy, fever, chills, proctitis, bronchospasm, oliguria, anuria, Stevens–Johnson syndrome), anaphylaxis. **CNS:** *Drowsiness* and *ataxia*, dizziness, vertigo, slurred speech, headache, weakness, paresthesias, impaired visual accommodation, paradoxic euphoria and rage reactions, seizures in epileptics, panic reaction, rapid EEG activity. **CV:** Hypotensive crisis, syncope, palpitation, tachycardia, arrhythmias, transient ECG changes, circulatory collapse (toxic doses). **GI:** Anorexia, nausea, vomiting, diarrhea. **Hematologic:** Aplastic anemia (rare); Leukopenia, agranulocytosis, thrombocytopenia, exacerbation of acute intermittent porphyria. **Respiratory:** Respiratory depression.

## DIAGNOSTIC TEST INTERFERENCE

Meprobamate may cause falsely high ***urinary steroid*** determinations. ***Phentolamine*** tests may be falsely positive; meprobamate should be withdrawn at least 24 h and preferably 48–72 h before the test.

## INTERACTIONS Drug: Alcohol, **entacapone,** TRICYCLIC ANTIDEPRESSANTS, ANTIPSYCHOTICS, OPIATES, SEDATING ANTIHISTAMINES, **pentazocine, tramadol,** MAOIS, SEDATIVE-HYPNOTICS, ANXIOLYTICS may potentiate CNS depression. Do not use with **perampanel** or **sodium oxybate. Herbal: Kava, valerian** may potentiate sedation.

## PHARMACOKINETICS Absorption: Well absorbed from GI tract. **Peak:** 1–3 h. **Onset:** 1 h. **Distribution:** Uniformly throughout body; crosses placenta. **Metabolism:** Rapidly in liver. **Elimination:** Renally excreted; excreted in breast milk. **Half-Life:** 10–11 h.

## NURSING IMPLICATIONS

### Assessment & Drug Effects

- Supervise ambulation, if necessary. Older adults and debilitated patients are prone to oversedation and to the hypotensive effects, especially during early therapy.
- Utilize safety precautions for hospitalized patients. Hypnotic doses may cause increased motor activity during sleep.
- Consult prescriber if daytime psychomotor function is impaired. A change in regimen or drug may be indicated.
- Withdraw gradually in physically dependent patients to prevent preexisting symptoms or withdrawal reactions within 12–48 h: Vomiting, ataxia, muscle twitching, mental confusion, hallucinations, convulsions, trembling, sleep disturbances, increased dreaming, nightmares, insomnia. Symptoms usually subside within 12–48 h.

### Patient & Family Education

- Take drug as prescribed. Psychic or physical dependence may occur with long-term use of high doses.
- Be aware that tolerance to alcohol will be lowered.

Common adverse effects in *italic;* life-threatening effects underlined; generic names in **bold;** classifications in SMALL CAPS; ♣ Canadian drug name; ⊙ Prototype drug

1009

- Make position changes slowly, especially from lying down to up-right; dangle legs for a few minutes before standing.
- Avoid driving or engaging in hazardous activities until response to drug is known.
- Report immediately onset of skin rash, sore throat, fever, bruising, unexplained bleeding.

# MEQUINOL/TRETINOIN
(me-qui'nol/tre-ti'noyn)
Solagé
**Classification:** RETINOID
**Therapeutic:** DEPIGMENTING AGENT; RETINOID
**Prototype:** Isotretinoin

## AVAILABILITY Solution

## ACTION & *THERAPEUTIC EFFECT*
Mequinol is a depigmenting agent and tretinoin is a retinoid used to improve dermatologic changes (e.g., fine wrinkling, mottled hyperpigmentation, roughness) associated with photo-damage and aging. Mequinol's mechanism of depigmentation is probably due to oxidation by tyrosine to cytotoxic products in melanocytes, and/or inhibition of melanin formation. Tretinoin, a retinoid, is used to improve photo-damage to the skin by acting via retinoic acid receptors (RARs). *Mequinol has depigmenting properties; tretinoin improves sun-damaged skin.*

## USES Treatment of solar lentigines (age spots).

## UNLABELED USES Facial wrinkles.

## CONTRAINDICATIONS Hypersensitivity to mequinol or tretinoin; pregnancy (category X); lactation.

## CAUTIOUS USE History of hypersensitivity to acitretin, isotretinoin, etretinate, or other vitamin A derivatives, or hydroquinone; patients with eczema, moderate to severe skin pigmentation, vitiligo; cold weather; children.

## ROUTE & DOSAGE

### Solar Lentigines
*Adult:* **Topical** Apply to solar lentigines b.i.d. at least 8 h apart

## ADMINISTRATION
**Topical**
- Apply doses at least 8 h apart; avoid application to unaffected areas.
- Avoid contact with eyes, lips, mucous membranes, or paranasal creases.
- Protect from light.

## ADVERSE EFFECTS (≥1%) **Skin:** *Erythema, burning, stinging, tingling, desquamation, pruritus,* skin irritation, temporary hypopigmentation, rash, dry skin, crusting, application site reaction.

## INTERACTIONS **Drug:** THIAZIDE DIURETICS, TETRACYCLINES, FLUOROQUINOLONES, PHENOTHIAZINES, SULFONAMIDES may augment phototoxicity.

## PHARMACOKINETICS **Absorption:** 4.4% through skin. **Peak:** 1–2 h.

## NURSING IMPLICATIONS
### Assessment & Drug Effects
- Monitor for and report peeling, erythema, or hypopigmentation.
- Monitor for signs of tretinoin toxicity: Headache, fever, weakness, and fatigue.

### Patient & Family Education
- Do not apply larger than recommended amounts.
- Do not wash affected area for at least 6 h after drug application; do not apply cosmetics to affected area for at least 30 min after drug application.

- Minimize exposure to sunlight or sunlamps. Use extra caution if also taking concurrently other drugs that are photosensitizing (e.g., thiazide diuretics, phenothiazines).
- Notify prescriber if vitiligo (hypopigmentation of skin) or S&S of tretinoin toxicity develop (see ASSESSMENT & DRUG EFFECTS).

# MERCAPTOPURINE (6-MP, 6-MERCAPTOPURINE) ℗

(mer-kap-toe-pyoor'een)

Purinethol

**Classifications:** ANTINEOPLASTIC; ANTIMETABOLITE, PURINE ANTAGONIST

Therapeutic: ANTINEOPLASTIC; IMMUNOSUPPRESSANT

## AVAILABILITY Tablet

## ACTION & THERAPEUTIC EFFECT

Antimetabolite and purine antagonist that inhibits purine metabolism. Blocks conversion of inosinic acid to adenine and xanthine ribotides within sensitive tumor cells. Also inhibits adenine-containing coenzymes, suggesting an influence over multiple cellular reactions. *Has delayed immunosuppressive properties and carcinogenic potential.*

**USES** Primarily for acute lymphocytic and myelogenous leukemia. Response in adults is less than in children, but mercaptopurine is initial drug of choice. In chronic granulocytic leukemia, produces temporary remission.

**UNLABELED USES** Prevention of transplant graft rejection; SLE; rheumatoid arthritis; Crohn's disease.

**CONTRAINDICATIONS** Prior resistance to mercaptopurine; infections; pregnancy (category D); lactation.

**CAUTIOUS USE** Impaired kidney or liver function.

## ROUTE & DOSAGE

### Leukemias

*Adult/Child:* **PO Loading Dose** 2.5 mg/kg/day, may increase up to 5 mg/kg/day after 4 wk if needed; **PO Maintenance Dose** 1.25–2.5 mg/kg/day

## ADMINISTRATION

### Oral

- Give total daily dose at one time
- Reduce dose of mercaptopurine usually by 1/3–1/4 when given concurrently with allopurinol.
- Store tablets in light- and air-resistant container.

## ADVERSE EFFECTS (≥1%) GI:
Stomatitis, esophagitis, anorexia, nausea, vomiting, diarrhea, intestinal ulcerations, impaired liver function, hepatic necrosis. **Hematologic:** Leukopenia, anemia, eosinophilia, pancytopenia, thrombocytopenia, abnormal bleeding, bone marrow hypoplasia. **Urogenital:** Hyperuricemia, oliguria, renal impairment. **Skin:** Rash. **Body as a Whole:** Drug fever.

## INTERACTIONS Drug: Allopurinol may inhibit metabolism and thus increase toxicity of mercaptopurine; may potentiate or antagonize anticoagulant effects of **warfarin.**

## PHARMACOKINETICS Absorption:
Approximately 50% absorbed from GI tract. **Peak:** 2 h. **Distribution:** Distributes into total body water. **Metabolism:** Rapidly by xanthine oxidase in liver. **Elimination:** 11% in urine within 6 h. **Half-Life:** 20–50 min.

## NURSING IMPLICATIONS

### Assessment & Drug Effects

- Monitor for S&S of liver damage. Hepatic toxicity occurs most often when dose exceeds 2.5 mg/kg/day.

M

Jaundice signals onset of hepatic toxicity and may necessitate terminating use.

- Withhold drug and notify prescriber at the first sign of an abnormally large or rapid fall in platelet and leukocyte counts.
- Record baseline data related to I&O ratio and pattern and body weight.
- Check vital signs daily. Report febrile states promptly.
- Protect patient from exposure to trauma, infections, or other stresses (restrict visitors and personnel who have colds) during periods of leukopenia.
- Report nausea, vomiting, or diarrhea. These may signal excessive dosage, especially in adults.
- Watch for signs of abnormal bleeding (ecchymoses, petechiae, melena, bleeding gums) if thrombocytopenia develops; report immediately.
- Monitor lab tests: Periodic CBC with differential, platelet count, Hgb, Hct, and LFTs.

### Patient & Family Education
- Report any signs of bleeding (e.g., hematuria, bruising, bleeding gums).
- Report signs of hepatic toxicity (see Appendix F).
- Increase hydration (10–12 glasses of fluid daily) to reduce risk of hyperuricemia. Consult prescriber about desirable volume.
- Notify prescriber of onset of chills, nausea, vomiting, flank or joint pain, swelling of legs or feet, or symptoms of anemia.

## MEROPENEM
(mer-o′pe-nem)
Merrem

**Classification:** CARBAPENEM ANTIBIOTIC
**Therapeutic:** ANTIBIOTIC
**Prototype:** Imipenem

**AVAILABILITY** Solution for injection

**ACTION & THERAPEUTIC EFFECT**
Broad-spectrum antibiotic that inhibits cell wall synthesis of bacteria by its strong affinity for penicillin-binding proteins of bacterial cell wall. *Effective against both gram-positive and gram-negative bacteria.*

**USES** Complicated appendicitis and peritonitis, bacterial meningitis caused by susceptible bacteria, complicated skin infections, intra-abdominal infections, skin/soft tissue infections.

**UNLABELED USES** Febrile neutropenia.

**CONTRAINDICATIONS** Hypersensitivity to meropenem, other carbapenem antibiotics or history of anaphylactic reactions to beta-lactams.

**CAUTIOUS USE** History of asthma or allergies, renal impairment, renal disease; epileptics, history of neurologic disorders, older adults, pregnancy (category B), lacatation; children younger than 3 mo.

**ROUTE & DOSAGE**

### Intra-Abdominal Infections
*Adult/Child (weight greater than 50 kg):* **IV** 1 g q8h
*Child (3 mo or older, weight less than 50 kg):* **IV** 20 mg/kg q8h (max: 1 g q8h)

### Bacterial Meningitis
*Adult/Child (weight greater than 50 kg):* **IV** 2 g q8h
*Child (3 mo or older, weight less than 50 kg):* **IV** 40 mg/kg q8h (max: 2 g q8h)

Common adverse effects in *italic*; life-threatening effects underlined; generic names in **bold**; classifications in SMALL CAPS; ✦ Canadian drug name; ☻ Prototype drug

### Complicated Skin Infection

*Adult/Child (weight greater than 50 kg):* **IV** 500 mg –1g q8h
*Child (3 mo or older, weight less than 50 kg):* **IV** 10 mg/kg q8h (max: 500 mg q8h)

### Renal Impairment Dosage Adjustment

*CrCl 26–50 mL/min:* q12h; *10–25 mL/min:* ½ dose q12h; *less than 10 mL/min:* ½ dose q24h

## ADMINISTRATION

### Intravenous

Note: Dosage reduction is recommended for older adults.

*PREPARE:* **Direct:** Reconstitute the 500-mg or 1-g vial, respectively, by adding 10 or 20 mL sterile water for injection to yield approximately 50 mg/mL. ▪ Shake to dissolve and let stand until clear. **IV Infusion:** Further dilute reconstituted solution in 50–250 mL of D5W, NS, or D5/NS.
*ADMINISTER:* **Direct:** Give doses of 5–20 mL over 3–5 min. **IV Infusion:** Give over 15–30 min.
*INCOMPATIBILITIES:* **Solution/additive: D5W, lactated Ringer's, amphotericin B, mannitol, multivitamins, potassium chloride, sodium bicarbonate.** **Y-site: Amiodarone, amphotericin B, ciprofloxacin, dacarbazine, daunorubicin, diazepam, dolasetron, doxorubicin, doxycycline, epirubicin, fenoldopam, garenoxacin, idarubicin, ketamine, metronidazole, mycophenolate, nicardipine, ondansetron, oritavancin, pantoprazole, quinupristin/dalfopristin, temocillin, topotecan, zidovudine.**

▪ Store undiluted at 15°–30° C (59°–86° F), diluted IV solutions should generally be used within 1 h of preparation.

## ADVERSE EFFECTS (≥1%) GI: Diarrhea, nausea, vomiting, constipation. **Other:** Inflammation at injection site, phlebitis, thrombophlebitis. **CNS:** Headache. **Skin:** Rash, pruritus, diaper rash. **Body as a Whole:** Apnea, oral moniliasis, sepsis, shock. **Hematologic:** Anemia. **Metabolic:** Hyperbilirubinemia.

## INTERACTIONS Drug: **Probenecid** delays meropenem excretion, may decrease **valproic acid** serum levels.

## PHARMACOKINETICS Distribution: Attains high concentrations in bile, bronchial secretions, cerebrospinal fluid. **Metabolism:** Renal and extrarenal metabolism via dipeptidases or nonspecific degradation. **Elimination:** In urine. **Half-Life:** 0.8–1 h.

## NURSING IMPLICATIONS

### Assessment & Drug Effects

▪ Determine history of hypersensitivity reactions to other beta-lactams, cephalosporins, penicillins, or other drugs.
▪ Discontinue drug and immediately report S&S of hypersensitivity (see Appendix F).
▪ Report S&S of superinfection or pseudomembranous colitis (see Appendix F).
▪ Monitor for seizures especially in older adults and those with renal insufficiency.
▪ Monitor lab tests: Baseline C&S; periodic LFTs and renal function tests.

### Patient & Family Education

▪ Learn S&S of hypersensitivity, superinfection, and pseudomembranous colitis; report any of these to prescriber promptly.

Common adverse effects in *italic;* life-threatening effects underlined; generic names in **bold;** classifications in SMALL CAPS; ♣ Canadian drug name; ⓟ Prototype drug

1013

## MESALAMINE ⊘

(me-sal′a-meen)

Apriso, Asacol, Canasa, Delzicol, Lialda, Pentasa, Rowasa, Salofalk ✦

**Classifications:** ANTI-INFLAMMATORY; PROSTAGLANDIN INHIBITOR

Therapeutic: GI; ANTI-INFLAMMATORY

**AVAILABILITY** Controlled release capsule; delayed release tablet; suppository; rectal suspension

**ACTION & THERAPEUTIC EFFECT** Thought to diminish inflammation by blocking cyclooxygenase and inhibiting prostaglandin synthesis in the colon. *Provides topical anti-inflammatory action in the colon of patients with ulcerative colitis.*

**USES** Indicated in active mild to moderate distal ulcerative colitis, proctosigmoiditis, or proctitis; maintenance of remission of ulcerative colitis.

**UNLABELED USES** Crohn's disease.

**CONTRAINDICATIONS** Hypersensitivity to mesalamine, salicylates (including aspirin); colitis exacerbation.

**CAUTIOUS USE** Sulfite hypersensitivity; predisposition to myocarditis or pericarditis; sensitivity to sulfasalazine; renal disease, renal impairment; asthmatic patients; older adults; pregnancy (category B or C depending on product); lactation; children younger than 12 y.

## ROUTE & DOSAGE

### Ulcerative Colitis

*Adult:* **Rectal (Rowasa)** 4 g once/day at bedtime, enema should be retained for about 8 h if possible or 1 suppository (500 mg) b.i.d.; **(Canasa)** 500 mg b.i.d., may increase up to 500 mg t.i.d. **PO (Asacol)** 800 mg t.i.d. × 6 wk; **(Pentasa)** 500 mg t.i.d. × 6 wk; **(Lialda)** 2.4 g daily or 4.8 mg daily **Maintenance Dose (Asacol)** 800 mg b.i.d. or 400 mg q.i.d.
*Adolescent/Child (weight 54–90 kg):* **PO** 27–44 mg/kg/day in divided doses; *weight 33 to less than 54 kg:* 37–61 mg/kg/day in divided doses; *weight 17 to less than 33 kg:* 36—71 mg/kg/day in divided doses

## ADMINISTRATION

### Oral

- Ensure that controlled-release and enteric forms of the drug are not crushed or chewed.
- Shake the bottle well to make sure the suspension is mixed.

### Rectal

- Use rectal suspension at bedtime with the objective of retaining it all night.
- Store at 15°–30° C (59°–86° F) away from heat and light.

**ADVERSE EFFECTS** (≥1%) **CNS:** *Headache,* fatigue, asthenia, malaise, weakness, dizziness. **GI:** *Abdominal pain, cramps,* or *discomfort,* flatulence, nausea, diarrhea, constipation, hemorrhoids, rectal pain, hepatitis (rare). **Skin:** Sensitivity reactions, rash, pruritus, alopecia. **Body as a Whole:** Fever. **Hematologic:** Thrombocytopenia (rare), eosinophilia. **Urogenital:** Interstitial nephritis.

**INTERACTIONS Drug:** May decrease the absorption of **digoxin.**

**PHARMACOKINETICS Absorption:** Rectal 5–35% absorbed from

colon depending on retention time of enema or suppository. **PO Asacol,** approximately 28% absorbed; 80% of drug is released in colon 12 h after ingestion. **PO Pentasa,** 50% of drug is released in colon at a pH less than 6. **Peak:** 3–6 h. **Distribution:** Rectal administration may reach as high as the ascending colon. **Asacol** is released in the ileum and colon; **Pentasa** is released in the jejunum, ileum, and colon. Low concentrations of mesalamine and higher concentrations of its metabolites are excreted in breast milk. **Metabolism:** Rapidly acetylated in the liver and colon wall. **Elimination:** Primarily in feces; absorbed drug excreted in urine. **Half-Life:** 2–15 h (depending on formulation).

## NURSING IMPLICATIONS

### Assessment & Drug Effects

- Assess for S&S of allergic-type reactions (e.g., hives, itching, wheezing, anaphylaxis). Suspension contains a sulfite that may cause reactions in asthmatics and some nonasthmatic persons.
- Expect response to therapy within 3–21 days; however, the usual course of therapy is from 3–6 wk depending on symptoms and sigmoidoscopic examinations.
- Monitor lab tests: Periodic urinalysis, BUN, and creatinine, especially with preexisting kidney disease.

### Patient & Family Education

- Report to prescriber promptly: Cramping, abdominal pain, bloody diarrhea, or other signs of rectal irritation.
- Check with prescriber before using any new medicine (prescription or OTC).
- Continue medication for full time of treatment even if you are feeling better.

# MESNA
(mes′na)

Mesnex

**Classifications:** CHEMOPROTECTANT; DETOXIFYING AGENT
**Therapeutic:** DETOXIFYING AGENT

## AVAILABILITY
Solution for injection; tablet

## ACTION & *THERAPEUTIC EFFECT*
Detoxifying agent used to inhibit hemorrhagic cystitis induced by ifosfamide. *Reacts chemically with urotoxic ifosfamide metabolites, resulting in their detoxification, and thus significantly decreases the incidence of hematuria.*

## USES
Prophylaxis for ifosfamide-induced hemorrhagic cystitis. Not effective in preventing hematuria due to other pathologic conditions such as thrombocytopenia.

## UNLABELED USES
Reduces the incidence of cyclophosphamide-induced hemorrhagic cystitis.

## CONTRAINDICATIONS
Hypersensitivity to mesna or other thiol compounds.

## CAUTIOUS USE
Autoimmune diseases; infants (injection); pregnancy (category B); lactation; neonates.

## ROUTE & DOSAGE

### Ifosfamide-Induced Hemorrhagic Cystitis

*Adult:* **IV** Dose = 20% of ifosfamide dose given 15 min before ifosfamide administration and 4 and 8 h after ifosfamide dose; **PO** 40% of ifosfamide dose 2 and 6 h after each ifosfamide dose

Common adverse effects in *italic;* life-threatening effects <u>underlined;</u> generic names in **bold;** classifications in SMALL CAPS; ◆ Canadian drug name; ⊙ Prototype drug

1015

## ADMINISTRATION

### Oral

- Give at 2 and 6 h after each dose of ifosfamide.

### Intravenous

**PREPARE: Direct:** Add 4 mL of D5W, NS, or LR for each 100 mg of mesna to yield 20 mg/mL.
**ADMINISTER: Direct:** Give a single dose by direct IV over 60 sec.
**INCOMPATIBILITIES: Solution/additive: Carboplatin, cisplatin, ifosfamide with epirubicin. Y-site: Amphotericin B cholesteryl complex, lansoprazole.**
- Inspect parenteral drug products visually for particulate matter and discoloration prior to administration. ■ Discard any unused portion of the ampul because drug oxidizes on contact with air.

- Refrigerate diluted solutions or use within 6 h of mixing even though diluted solutions are chemically and physically stable for 24 h at 25° C (77° F). ■ Store unopened ampul at 15°–30° C (59°–86° F) unless otherwise specified.

## ADVERSE EFFECTS (≥1%) GI: *Bad taste in mouth, soft stools,* nausea, vomiting.

## DIAGNOSTIC TEST INTERFERENCE

May produce a false-positive result in test for **urinary ketones.**

## INTERACTIONS Drug: May decrease the effect of **warfarin.**

## PHARMACOKINETICS Bioavailability: 45%–79% Metabolism: Rapidly oxidized in liver to active metabolite dimesna; dimesna is further metabolized in kidney. Elimination: 65% in urine within 24 h. Half-Life: Mesna 0.36 h, dimesna 1.17 h.

## NURSING IMPLICATIONS

### Assessment & Drug Effects

- Monitor urine for hematuria.
- About 6% of patients treated with mesna along with ifosfamide still develop hematuria.

### Patient & Family Education

- Mesna prevents ifosfamide-induced hemorrhagic cystitis; it will not prevent or alleviate other adverse reactions or toxicities associated with ifosfamide therapy.
- Report any unusual or allergic reactions to prescriber.
- Drink at least a quart of liquid a day when taking mesna.

## METAPROTERENOL SULFATE

(met-a-proe-ter′e-nole)

**Classifications:** BETA-ADRENERGIC AGONIST; BRONCHODILATOR
Therapeutic: BRONCHODILATOR
**Prototype:** Albuterol

## AVAILABILITY Tablet; syrup; solution for inhalation

## ACTION & *THERAPEUTIC EFFECT*

Potent synthetic beta-adrenergic agonist that acts selectively on beta$_2$-adrenergic receptors to relax smooth muscle of bronchi, uterus, and blood vessels supplying skeletal muscles. *Effective as a bronchodilator; additionally, it controls bronchospasm in asthmatics.*

## USES Bronchodilator in symptomatic relief of asthma and reversible bronchospasm associated with bronchitis and emphysema.

## UNLABELED USES Treatment and prophylaxis of heart block and to avert progress of premature labor (tocolytic action).

**CONTRAINDICATIONS** Sensitivity to metaproterenol or other sympathomimetic agents; seizure disorders; DM; hyperthyroidism.

**CAUTIOUS USE** Older adults; hypertension, cardiovascular disorders including coronary artery disease, cardiac arrhythmias, QT prolongation; MAOI therapy; pregnancy (category C); lactation; children. Not recommended for children younger than 6 y (**tablets**).

## ROUTE & DOSAGE

**Bronchospasm**
*Adult:* **PO** 20 mg q6–8h;
**Nebulizer** 5–10 inhalations of undiluted 5% solution; **IPPB** 2.5 mL of 0.4–0.6% solution q4–6h
*Geriatric:* **PO** 10 mg 3–4 × day, may increase to 20 mg 3–4 × day
*Child (younger than 2 y):* **PO** 0.4 mg/kg t.i.d.–q.i.d.; *2 to younger than 9 y:* 1.2–2.6 mg/kg/day in 3–4 divided doses; *6 to younger than 9 y:* 10 mg q6–8h; *9 y or older:* 20 mg q6–8h

## ADMINISTRATION

- Note: Patient may use tablets and aerosol concomitantly.

**Oral**
- Give with food to reduce GI distress.

**Inhalation**
- Instruct patient to shake metered dose aerosol container, exhale through nose as completely as possible, administer aerosol while inhaling deeply through mouth, and to hold breath about 10 sec before exhaling slowly. Administer second inhalation 10 min after first.
- Store all forms at 15°–30° C (59°–86° F); protect from light and heat.

**ADVERSE EFFECTS** (≥1%) **CNS:** Nervousness, weakness, drowsiness, *tremor (particularly after PO administration),* headache, fatigue. **CV:** *Tachycardia,* hypertension, cardiac arrest, palpitation. **GI:** Nausea, vomiting, bad taste. **Urogenital:** Occasional difficulty in micturition and muscle cramps. **Respiratory:** Throat irritation, cough, exacerbation of asthma.

**INTERACTIONS** **Drug:** **Epinephrine,** other SYMPATHOMIMETIC BRONCHODILATORS may compound effects of metaproterenol; MAO INHIBITORS, TRICYCLIC ANTIDEPRESSANTS potentiate action of metaproterenol on vascular system; the effects of both metaproterenol and BETA-ADRENERGIC BLOCKERS are antagonized.

**PHARMACOKINETICS** **Absorption:** 40% of PO doses reach systemic circulation. **Onset:** Inhaled: 1 min; PO 15 min. **Peak:** 1 h all routes. **Duration:** Inhaled: 1–5 h; PO 4 h. **Metabolism:** In liver. **Elimination:** In urine.

## NURSING IMPLICATIONS
### Assessment & Drug Effects
- Monitor respiratory status. Auscultate lungs before and after inhalation to determine efficacy of drug in decreasing airway resistance.
- Monitor cardiac status. Report tachycardia and hypotension.

### Patient & Family Education
- Report failure to respond to usual dose. Drug may have shorter duration of action after long-term use.
- Do not increase dose or frequency unless ordered by prescriber; there is the possibility of serious adverse effects.
- Anticipate tremor as a possible adverse effect.

M

# METFORMIN ℗

(met-for'min)

Fortamet, Glucophage, Glucophage XR, Glumetza, Riomet

**Classifications:** ANTIDIABETIC; BIGUANIDE

Therapeutic: ANTIHYPERGLYCEMIC

## AVAILABILITY

Tablet; sustained release tablet; oral solution

## ACTION & *THERAPEUTIC EFFECT*

Thought to both increase the binding of insulin to its receptors and potentiate insulin action. Improves tissue sensitivity to insulin, increases glucose transport into skeletal muscles and fat, and suppresses gluconeogenesis and hepatic production of glucose. *Effective in lowering serum glucose level and, ultimately, the HbA1C value.*

## USES

Treatment of type 2 diabetes mellitus as adjunct to diet and exercise.

## UNLABELED USES

Antipsychotic-induced weight gain, polycystic ovary syndrome.

## CONTRAINDICATIONS

Hypersensitivity to metformin; acute MI, cardiogenic shock; Type I DM; diabetic ketoacidosis; metabolic acidosis with or without coma; lactic acidosis; radiographic contrast administration; renal disease, renal failure, renal impairment with CrCl of 1.5 md/dL in men and 1.4 md/dL in women; sepsis; surgery.

## CAUTIOUS USE

Previous hypersensitivity to phenformin or buformin; anemia; coma; dehydration, diarrhea; impaired liver function; renal impairment; ethanol use; fever; gastroparesis, GI obstruction; CHF; hyperthyroidism, pituitary insufficiency; polycystic ovary syndrome; trauma, emesis; debilitated patients; older adults; pregnancy (category B); children younger than 10 y.

## ROUTE & DOSAGE

### Type 2 Diabetes Mellitus

*Adult:* **PO** Start with 500 mg daily to t.i.d. or 850 mg daily to b.i.d. with meals, may increase by 500–850 mg/day q1–3wk (max: 2550 mg/day); or start with 500 mg sustained release with p.m. meal, may increase by 500 mg/day at p.m. meal qwk (max: 2000 mg/day)

*Adolescent/Child (10 y or older):* **PO** Glucophage only: 500 mg b.i.d., may increase by 500 mg/day qwk (max: 2000 mg/day)

## ADMINISTRATION

### Oral

- Ensure that extended release tablets are not crushed or chewed. They **must be** swallowed whole.
- Use a calibrated oral syringe or container to measure the oral solution for accurate dosing.
- Give with or shortly after main meals.
- Withhold metformin 48 h before and 48 h after receiving IV contrast dye.
- Dose increments are usually made at 2- to 3-wk intervals.
- Store at 15°–30° C (59°–86° F).

## ADVERSE EFFECTS (≥1%)

**CNS:** Headache, dizziness, agitation, fatigue. **Metabolic:** Lactic acidosis. **GI:** *Nausea, vomiting, abdominal pain, bitter or metallic taste, diarrhea, bloatedness, anorexia;* malabsorption of amino acids, vitamin $B_{12}$, and folic acid possible. **Dermatologic:** Flushing, increased sweating.

---

Common adverse effects in *italic;* life-threatening effects underlined; generic names in **bold;** classifications in SMALL CAPS; ♣ Canadian drug name; ℗ Prototype drug

**INTERACTIONS Drug: Captopril, furosemide, nifedipine** may increase risk of hypoglycemia. **Cimetidine** reduces clearance of metformin. Concomitant therapy with AZOLE ANTIFUNGAL AGENTS (**fluconazole, ketoconazole, itraconazole**) and ORAL HYPOGLYCEMIC DRUGS has been reported in severe hypoglycemia. IODINATED RADIOCONTRAST DYES can cause lactic acidosis and acute kidney failure. **Amiloride, cimetidine, digoxin, dofetilide, midodrine, morphine, procainamide, quinidine, quinine, ranitidine, triamterene, trimethoprim,** or **vancomycin** may decrease metformin elimination by competing for common renal tubular transport systems. **Acarbose** may decrease metformin levels. **Iodinated contrast dyes** may cause lactic acidosis or acute kidney failure. **Herbal: Garlic, ginseng, glucomannan** may increase hypoglycemic effects. **Guar gum** decreases absorption.

**PHARMACOKINETICS Absorption:** 50–60% of dose reaches systemic circulation. **Peak:** 1–3 h. **Distribution:** Not bound to plasma proteins. **Metabolism:** Not metabolized. **Elimination:** In urine. **Half-Life:** 6.2–17.6 h.

## NURSING IMPLICATIONS

### Black Box Warning

*Metformin has been associated with potentially fatal lactic acidosis.*

### Assessment & Drug Effects

- Monitor vital signs and fasting and postprandial blood glucose values.
- Report promptly any of the following signs of lactic acidosis: Malaise, myalgia, somnolence, respiratory depression, abdominal distress.

- Monitor known or suspected alcoholics carefully for decreased liver function.
- Monitor cardiopulmonary status throughout course of therapy; cardiopulmonary insufficiency may predispose to lactic acidosis.
- Monitor lab tests: Periodic urine for glucose and ketones, fasting blood glucose, and HbA1C; baseline and periodic Hct & Hgb and RBC indices for anemia.

### Patient & Family Education

- Be aware that hypoglycemia is not a risk when drug is taken in recommended therapeutic doses unless combined with other drugs which lower blood glucose.
- Report to prescriber immediately S&S of infection, which increase the risk of lactic acidosis (e.g., abdominal pains, nausea, and vomiting, anorexia).
- Report promptly severe vomiting, diarrhea, fever, or any illness that causes limited fluid intake.
- Avoid drinking alcohol while taking this drug.

## METHADONE HYDROCHLORIDE

(meth'a-done)

Dolophine, Methadose

**Classifications:** NARCOTIC (OPIATE AGONIST); ANALGESIC

Therapeutic: NARCOTIC ANALGESIC; TOXICOLOGY AGENT

**Prototype:** Morphine

**Controlled Substance:** Schedule II

**AVAILABILITY** Tablet; oral solution; injection

## ACTION & *THERAPEUTIC EFFECT*

Synthetic narcotic that is a CNS depressant, which causes sedation and respiratory depression. Highly

**M**

Common adverse effects in *italic*; life-threatening effects <u>underlined</u>; generic names in **bold**; classifications in SMALL CAPS; ✦ Canadian drug name; ⓟ Prototype drug

1019

addictive, with abuse potential; abstinence syndrome develops more slowly, and withdrawal symptoms are less intense but more prolonged. *Relieves severe pain and manages withdrawal therapy from narcotics, especially heroin.*

**USES** To relieve severe pain; for detoxification and temporary maintenance treatment in hospital and in federally controlled maintenance programs for ambulatory patients with narcotic abstinence syndrome.

**CONTRAINDICATIONS** Hypersensitivity to methadone; significant respiratory depression; severe pulmonary disease; acute or severe bronchial asthma in absence of resuscitative equipment; hypercarpnia; known or suspected paralytic ileus; obstetric analgesia.

**CAUTIOUS USE** History of QT prolongation; liver, kidney, or cardiac dysfunction; COPD, acute or chronic asthma; preexisting respiratory depression, hypoxia, or hypercapnia; head injuries; severe hepatic or renal impairment; hypothyroidism; adrenal insufficiency; Addison's disease; patients at risk for hypotension; BPH; urethral stricture; older adults; pregnancy (category C); lactation. Safety and efficacy in children not established.

**ROUTE & DOSAGE**

**Pain**

*Adult:* **PO/Subcutaneous/IM**
2.5–10 mg q3–4h prn **IV** 2.5–10 mg q8–12h prn (opiate naïve patient)
*Child:* **PO/IV/Subcutaneous/IM**
0.1–0.2 mg/kg q4h × 2–3 doses, then q6–12h prn (max: 5–10 mg/dose)

**Detoxification Treatment**

*Adult:* **PO/Subcutaneous/IM**
(Doses are very patient specific and these are general ranges)
15–40 mg once/day, usually maintained at 20–120 mg/day

**Renal Impairment Dosage Adjustment**

*CrCl less than 10 mL/min:* Use 50–75% of dose

**ADMINISTRATION**

**Oral**

- Give for analgesic effect in the smallest effective dose to minimize the possible tolerance and physical and psychic dependence.
- Dilute dispersible tablets in 120 mL of water or fruit juice and allow at least 1 min for dispersion.

**Subcutaneous/Intramuscular**

- Note: IM route is preferred over subcutaneous when repeated parenteral administration is required (subcutaneous injections may cause local irritation and induration). Rotate injection sites.

**Intravenous**

*PREPARE:* **Direct/IV Infusion:** May be given undiluted or diluted with 1–5 mL of NS.
*ADMINISTER:* **Direct/IV Infusion:** Give over 5 or more minutes.
*INCOMPATIBILITIES:* **Y-site: Acyclovir, allopurinol, amphotericin B, dantrolene, daunorubicin, fluorouracil, ganciclovir, lansoprazole, lethohexital, pentobarbital, phenytoin pipercillin/tazobacatam, SMZ/TMP, thiopental.**

- Store at 15°–30° C (59°–86° F) in tight, light-resistant containers.

**ADVERSE EFFECTS** (≥1%) **CNS:** *Drowsiness,* light-headedness, dizziness, hallucinations. **GI:** Nausea, vomiting, dry mouth, *constipation.* **Body as a Whole:** Transient fall in BP, bone and muscle pain. **Urogenital:** Impotence. **Respiratory:** Respiratory depression.

**INTERACTIONS Drug: Alcohol** and other CNS DEPRESSANTS, **cimetidine** add to sedation and CNS depression; AMPHETAMINES may potentiate CNS stimulation; with MAO INHIBITORS, **selegiline, furazolidone** causes excessive and prolonged CNS depression, convulsions, cardiovascular collapse. **Food: Grapefruit juice** may increase serum levels and adverse effects. **Herbal: St. John's wort** decreases plasma levels.

**PHARMACOKINETICS Absorption:** Well absorbed from GI tract, variable IM absorption. **Onset:** 30–60 min PO; 10–20 min IM/Subcutaneous. **Peak:** 1–2 h. **Duration:** 6–8 h PO, IM, Subcutaneous; may last 22–48 h with chronic dosing. **Distribution:** Crosses placenta; distributed into breast milk. **Metabolism:** In liver (CYP3A4). **Elimination:** In urine. **Half-Life:** 15–25 h.

## NURSING IMPLICATIONS

### Black Box Warning

*Methadone has been associated with abuse potential, respiratory depression, and QT prolongation.*

### Assessment & Drug Effects

- Evaluate patient's continued need for methadone for pain. Adjustment of dosage and lengthening of between-dose intervals may be possible.
- Monitor respiratory status. Principal danger of overdosage, as with morphine, is extreme respiratory depression.
- Monitor closely for changes in cardiac status (e.g., QT interval prolongation) especially during drug initiation and titration.
- Be aware that because of the cumulative effects of methadone, abstinence symptoms may not appear for 36–72 h after last dose and may last 10–14 days. Symptoms are usually of mild intensity (e.g., anorexia, insomnia, anxiety, abdominal discomfort, weakness, headache, sweating, hot and cold flashes).
- Observe closely for recurrence of respiratory depression during use of narcotic antagonists such as naloxone.

### Patient & Family Education

- Be aware that orthostatic hypotension, sweating, constipation, drowsiness, GI symptoms, and other transient adverse effects of therapeutic doses appear to be more prominent in ambulatory patients. Most adverse effects disappear over a period of several weeks.
- Make position changes slowly, particularly from lying down to upright position; sit or lie down if you feel dizzy or faint.
- Do not drive or engage in potentially hazardous activities until response to drug is known.

## METHAMPHETAMINE HYDROCHLORIDE

(meth-am-fet′a-meen)

Desoxyn

**Classifications:** ADRENERGIC AGONIST; CEREBRAL STIMULANT; AMPHETAMINE
Therapeutic: CEREBRAL STIMULANT; ANOREXIANT
**Prototype:** Amphetamine sulfate
**Controlled Substance:** Schedule II

Common adverse effects in *italic;* life-threatening effects underlined; generic names in **bold;** classifications in SMALL CAPS; ♣ Canadian drug name; ◯ Prototype drug

1021

**AVAILABILITY** Tablet; long-acting tablet

**ACTION & *THERAPEUTIC EFFECT***
CNS stimulant actions approximately equal to those of amphetamine, but accompanied by less peripheral activity. *CNS stimulation results in increased motor activity, diminished sense of fatigue, alertness, increased focus, and mood elevation. Anorexigenic effect is due to direct inhibition of hypothalamic appetite center.*

**USES** Short-term adjunct in management of exogenous obesity, as adjunctive therapy in attention deficit disorder (ADD), narcolepsy, epilepsy, and postencephalitic parkinsonism, and in treatment of certain depressive reactions, especially when characterized by apathy and psychomotor retardation.

**CONTRAINDICATIONS** Hypersensitivity or idiosyncrasy to sympathomimetic amines; children with structural cardiac abnormalities; glaucoma; advanced arteriosclerosis; symptomatic cardiovascular disease; moderate to severe hypertension; hyperthyroidism; patients in agitated state or history of drug abuse; lactation.

**CAUTIOUS USE** Mild hypertension; psychopathic personalities; hyperexcitability states; history of suicide attempts; older adult or debilitated patients; pregnancy (category C); ADHD treatment in children younger than 6 y or for obesity treatment in children younger than 12 y; longer term use in children.

**ROUTE & DOSAGE**

**Attention Deficit Disorder**
*Child (6 y or older):* PO 2.5–5 mg 1–2 × day, may increase by 5 mg at weekly intervals up to 20–25 mg/day

**Obesity**
*Adult:* **PO** 5 mg 1–3 × day 30 min before meals or 5–15 mg of long-acting form once/day

**ADMINISTRATION**
**Oral**
- Give early in the day, if possible, to avoid insomnia.
- Ensure that long-acting tablets are not chewed or crushed; these need to be swallowed whole.
- Give 30 min before each meal when used for treatment of obesity. If insomnia results, advise patient to inform prescriber.
- Preserve in tight, light-resistant containers.

**ADVERSE EFFECTS** (≥1%) **CNS:** Restlessness, tremor, hyperreflexia, insomnia, headache, nervousness, anxiety, dizziness, euphoria, or dysphoria. **CV:** Palpitation, arrhythmias, hypertension, hypotension, circulatory collapse. **GI:** Dry mouth, unpleasant taste, nausea, vomiting, diarrhea, constipation. **Special Senses:** Increased intraocular pressure.

**INTERACTIONS Drug: Acetazolamide, sodium bicarbonate** decreases methamphetamine elimination; **ammonium chloride, ascorbic acid** increases methamphetamine elimination; effects of both methamphetamine and BARBITURATES may be antagonized; **furazolidone** may increase BP effects of AMPHETAMINES—interaction may persist for several weeks after discontinuing **furazolidone;** antagonizes antihypertensive effects of **guanethidine;** MAO INHIBITORS, **selegiline** can cause hypertensive crisis (fatalities reported)—do not administer AMPHETAMINES during or within 14 days of administration of these drugs; PHENOTHIAZINES may inhibit mood elevating effects of AMPHETAMINES; TRICYCLIC ANTIDEPRESSANTS enhance methamphetamine effects because they increase norepinephrine release; BETA-ADRENERGIC AGONISTS increase adverse cardiovascular effects of AMPHETAMINES.

## PHARMACOKINETICS Absorption: Readily absorbed from the GI tract. **Duration:** 6–12 h. **Distribution:** All tissues especially the CNS; excreted in breast milk. **Metabolism:** In liver. **Elimination:** Renal elimination.

## NURSING IMPLICATIONS

### Black Box Warning

*Methamphetamine has been associated with a high potential for abuse.*

### Assessment & Drug Effects
- Monitor weight throughout period of therapy.
- Be alert for a paradoxical increase in depression or agitation in depressed patients. Report immediately; drug should be withdrawn.

### Patient & Family Education
- Be alert for development of tolerance; happens readily, and prolonged use may lead to drug dependence. Abuse potential is high.
- Withdrawal after prolonged use is frequently followed by lethargy that may persist for several weeks.
- Weigh every other day under standard conditions and maintain a record of weight loss.

# METHAZOLAMIDE
(meth-a-zoe'la-mide)
**Classifications:** EYE PREPARATION; CARBONIC ANHYDRASE INHIBITOR; ANTIGLAUCOMA
Therapeutic: ANTIGLAUCOMA
**Prototype:** Acetazolamide

## AVAILABILITY Tablet

## ACTION & *THERAPEUTIC EFFECT*
Inhibits carbonic anhydrase activity in eye by reducing rate of aqueous humor formation with consequent lowering of intraocular pressure. *Effective in lowering intraocular pressure in glaucoma patients.*

## USES Adjunctive treatment in chronic simple (open-angle) glaucoma and secondary glaucoma and preoperatively in acute angle-closure glaucoma when delay of surgery is desired in order to lower intraocular pressure. May be used concomitantly with miotic and osmotic agents.

## CONTRAINDICATIONS Glaucoma due to severe peripheral anterior synechiae, severe or absolute glaucoma, hemorrhagic glaucoma; hypokalemia, hyponatremia; dialysis; hepatic disease; renal disease, anuria, renal failure.

## CAUTIOUS USE Pulmonary disease, COPD; diabetes mellitus; renal impairment; pregnancy (category C); lactation.

## ROUTE & DOSAGE

### Glaucoma
*Adult:* **PO** 50–100 mg b.i.d. or t.i.d.

Common adverse effects in *italic;* life-threatening effects underlined; generic names in **bold;** classifications in SMALL CAPS; ♣ Canadian drug name; ☉ Prototype drug

1023

## ADMINISTRATION

### Oral

- Give with meals to minimize GI distress.

## ADVERSE EFFECTS (≥1%) **Body as a Whole:** Malaise, drowsiness, fatigue, lethargy. **GI:** Mild GI disturbance, anorexia. **CNS:** Headache, vertigo, paresthesias, mental confusion, depression.

## INTERACTIONS **Drug:** Renal excretion of AMPHETAMINES, **ephedrine, flecainide, quinidine, procainamide,** TRICYCLIC ANTIDEPRESSANTS may be decreased, thereby enhancing or prolonging their effects; increases renal excretion of **lithium;** excretion of **phenobarbital** may be increased; **amphotericin B,** CORTICOSTEROIDS may add to potassium loss; hypokalemia caused by methazolamide may predispose patients on DIGITALIS GLYCOSIDES to **digitalis** toxicity; patients on high doses of SALICYLATES are at higher risk for SALICYLATE toxicity.

## PHARMACOKINETICS **Absorption:** Slowly from GI tract. **Onset:** 2–4 h. **Peak:** 6–8 h. **Duration:** 10–18 h. **Distribution:** Throughout body, concentrating in RBCs, plasma, and kidneys; crosses placenta. **Metabolism:** Partially in liver. **Elimination:** Primarily in urine.

## NURSING IMPLICATIONS

### Assessment & Drug Effects

- Supervise ambulation in older adult, since drug may cause vertigo.
- Assess patient's ability to perform ADL since drug may cause fatigue and lethargy.
- Monitor lab tests: Baseline and periodic CBC with platelet count; periodic serum electrolytes.

### Patient & Family Education

- Be aware that drug may cause drowsiness. Advise caution with hazardous activities until response to drug is known.

## METHENAMINE HIPPURATE

(meth-en′a-meen hip′yoo-rate)

Hiprex, Urex

## METHENAMINE MANDELATE

**Classification:** URINARY TRACT ANTI-INFECTIVE
**Therapeutic:** URINARY TRACT ANTI-INFECTIVE
**Prototype:** Trimethoprim

## AVAILABILITY **Methenamine Hippurate:** Tablet. **Methenamine Mandelate:** Tablet; suspension

## ACTION & *THERAPEUTIC EFFECT*

Tertiary amine that liberates formaldehyde in an acid medium, which is a nonspecific antibiotic agent with bactericidal activity. *Currently used only for suppression and prophylaxis of frequently recurring urinary tract infections such as in patients with neurogenic bladder or in those who require intermittent catheterization routinely.*

## USES Prophylactic treatment of recurrent urinary tract infections (UTIs). Also long-term prophylaxis when residual urine is present (e.g., neurogenic bladder).

## CONTRAINDICATIONS Renal insufficiency; liver disease; gout; severe dehydration; lactation.

## CAUTIOUS USE Oral suspension for patients susceptible to lipoid pneumonia (e.g., older adults, debilitated patients); gout; pregnancy (category C); children.

## ROUTE & DOSAGE

**UTI Prophylaxis**

*Adult:* **PO (Hippurate)** 1 g b.i.d.; **(Mandelate)** 1 g q.i.d.
*Child (6 y or younger):* **PO (Mandelate)** 18.4 mg/kg q.i.d.; *6–12 y:* **(Hippurate)** 0.5–1 g b.i.d.; **(Mandelate)** 500 mg q.i.d. or 50 mg/kg/day in 3 divided doses

## ADMINISTRATION

**Oral**

- Give after meals and at bedtime to minimize gastric distress.
- Give oral suspension with caution to older adult or debilitated patients because of the possibility of lipid (aspiration) pneumonia; it contains a vegetable oil base.
- Store at 15°–30° C (59°–86° F) in tightly closed container; protect from excessive heat.

**ADVERSE EFFECTS** (≥1%) **GI:** Nausea, vomiting, diarrhea, abdominal cramps, anorexia. **Renal:** Bladder irritation, dysuria, frequency, albuminuria, hematuria, crystalluria.

**DIAGNOSTIC TEST INTERFERENCE**
Methenamine (formaldehyde) may produce falsely elevated values for **urinary catecholamines** and **urinary steroids (17-hydroxycorticosteroids)** (by **Reddy method**). Possibility of false **urine glucose determinations** with **Benedict's** test. Methenamine interferes with **urobilinogen** and possibly **urinary VMA** determinations.

**INTERACTIONS Drug: Sulfamethoxazole** forms insoluble precipitate in acid urine; **acetazolamide, sodium bicarbonate** may prevent hydrolysis to formaldehyde.

**PHARMACOKINETICS Absorption:** Readily from GI tract, although 10–30% of dose is hydrolyzed to formaldehyde in stomach. **Peak:** 2 h. **Duration:** Up to 6 h or until patient voids. **Distribution:** Crosses placenta; distributed into breast milk. **Metabolism:** Hydrolyzed in acid pH to formaldehyde. **Elimination:** In urine. **Half-Life:** 4 h.

## NURSING IMPLICATIONS

### Assessment & Drug Effects

- Monitor urine pH; value of 5.5 or less is required for optimum drug action.
- Monitor I&O ratio and pattern; drug most effective when fluid intake is maintained at 1500 or 2000 mL/day.
- Consult prescriber about changing to enteric-coated tablet if patient complains of gastric distress.
- Supplemental acidification to maintain pH of 5.5 or below required for drug action may be necessary. Accomplish by drugs (ascorbic acid, ammonium chloride) or by foods.

### Patient & Family Education

- Do not self-medicate with OTC antacids containing sodium bicarbonate or sodium carbonate (to prevent raising urine pH).
- Achieve supplementary acidification by limiting intake of foods that can increase urine pH [e.g., vegetables, fruits, and fruit juice (except cranberry, plum, prune)] and increasing intake of foods that can decrease urine pH (e.g., proteins, cranberry juice, plums, prunes).

## METHIMAZOLE

(meth-im'a-zole)

Tapazole

**Classification:** ANTITHYROID HORMONE
**Therapeutic:** ANTITHYROID
**Prototype:** Propylthiouracil

M

---

Common adverse effects in *italic;* life-threatening effects <u>underlined</u>; generic names in **bold;** classifications in SMALL CAPS; ♣ Canadian drug name; ⊙ Prototype drug

1025

## AVAILABILITY Tablet

## ACTION & *THERAPEUTIC EFFECT*

Inhibits synthesis of thyroid hormones as the drug accumulates in the thyroid gland. Does not affect existing $T_3$ or $T_4$ levels. *Corrects hyperthyroidism by inhibiting synthesis of the thyroid hormone.*

## USES Hyperthyroidism and prior to surgery or radiotherapy of the thyroid; may be used cautiously to treat hyperthyroidism in pregnancy.

## CONTRAINDICATIONS Pregnancy (category D).

## CAUTIOUS USE Bone marrow suppression; older adults; hepatic disease.

## ROUTE & DOSAGE

### Hyperthyroidism
*Adult:* **PO** 5–15 mg q8h
*Child:* **PO** 0.2–0.4 mg/kg/day divided q8h

## ADMINISTRATION

### Oral
- Give at same time each day relative to meals.
- Store at 15°–30° C (59°–86° F) in light-resistant container.

## ADVERSE EFFECTS (≥1%) GI:
Hepatotoxicity (rare). **Endocrine:** Hypothyroidism. **Hematologic:** Leukopenia, agranulocytosis, granulocytopenia, thrombocytopenia, pancytopenia, and aplastic anemia. **Musculoskeletal:** Arthralgia. **CNS:** Peripheral neuropathy, drowsiness, neuritis, paresthesias, vertigo. **Skin:** Rash, alopecia, skin hyperpigmentation, urticaria, and pruritus. **Urogenital:** Nephrotic syndrome.

## INTERACTIONS Drug: Can reduce anticoagulant effects of **warfarin;** may increase serum levels of **digoxin;** may alter **theophylline** levels; may need to decrease dose of BETA-BLOCKERS.

## PHARMACOKINETICS Absorption: Readily absorbed from GI tract. **Onset:** 30–40 min. **Peak:** 1 h. **Duration:** 2–4 h. **Distribution:** Crosses placenta; distributed into breast milk. **Elimination:** 12% in urine within 24 h. **Half-Life:** 5–13 h.

## NURSING IMPLICATIONS

### Assessment & Drug Effects
- Closely monitor PT and INR in patients on oral anticoagulants. Anticoagulant activity may be potentiated.
- Monitor lab tests: Baseline and periodic thyroid function tests; periodic CBC with differential, prothrombin time, and LFTs.

### Patient & Family Education
- Be aware that skin rash or swelling of cervical lymph nodes may indicate need to discontinue drug and change to another antithyroid agent. Consult prescriber.
- Notify prescriber promptly if the following symptoms appear: Bruising, unexplained bleeding, sore throat, fever, jaundice.
- Methimazole does not induce hypothyroiditis.

## METHOCARBAMOL
(meth-oh-kar′ba-mole)
Robaxin
**Classifications:** CENTRALLY ACTING SKELETAL MUSCLE RELAXANT; CARBAMATE
Therapeutic: SKELETAL MUSCLE RELAXANT
**Prototype:** Cyclobenzaprine

Common adverse effects in *italic;* life-threatening effects underlined; generic names in **bold;** classifications in SMALL CAPS; ♣ Canadian drug name; ⊘ Prototype drug

**AVAILABILITY** Solution for injection; tablet

**ACTION & *THERAPEUTIC EFFECT***
Exerts skeletal muscle relaxant action by depressing multisynaptic pathways in the spinal cord and possibly by sedative effect. *Acts on multisynaptic pathways in spinal cord that control muscular spasms.*

**USES** Adjunct to physical therapy and other measures in management of discomfort associated with acute musculoskeletal disorders. Also used intravenously as adjunct in management of neuromuscular manifestations of tetanus.

**CONTRAINDICATIONS** Comatose states; CNS depression; acidosis, older adults; kidney dysfunction.

**CAUTIOUS USE** Epilepsy; renal disease, renal failure, renal impairment, seizure disorder; females of childbearing age; pregnancy (category C); lactation; children.

## ROUTE & DOSAGE

**Acute Musculoskeletal Disorders**
*Adult:* **PO** 1.5 g q.i.d. for 2–3 days, then 4–4.5 g/day in 3–6 divided doses; **IV/IM** 1 g q8h for up to 3 days

**Tetanus**
*Adult:* **IV** 1–3 g may be repeated q6h
*Child:* **PO** 15 mg/kg repeated q6h as needed up to 1.8 g/m²/day for 3 consecutive days if necessary

## ADMINISTRATION

**Oral**
- Tablets may be crushed, suspended in water, and given through an NG tube.

**Intramuscular**
- Do not exceed IM dose of 5 mL (0.5 g) into each gluteal region. Insert needle deep and carefully aspirate. Inject drug slowly. Rotate injection sites and observe daily for evidence of irritation.

**Intravenous**
*PREPARE:* **Direct:** May be given undiluted or diluted. **IV Infusion:** May dilute in up to 250 mL of NS or D5W.
*ADMINISTER:* **Direct:** Give at a rate of 300 mg or fraction thereof over 1 min or longer. **IV Infusion:** Infuse at a rate consistent with amount of fluid, but do not exceed direct rate. ▪ Keep patient recumbent during and for at least 15 min after IV injection in order to reduce possibility of orthostatic hypotension and other adverse reactions. ▪ Monitor vital signs and IV flow rate. ▪ Take care to avoid extravasation of IV solution, which may result in thrombophlebitis and sloughing.
*INCOMPATIBILITIES:* **Y-site: Furosemide.**

- Store at 15°–30° C (59°–86° F).

**ADVERSE EFFECTS** (≥1%) **Body as a Whole:** Fever, <u>anaphylactic reaction</u>, flushing, syncope, convulsions. **Skin:** Urticaria, pruritus, rash, thrombophlebitis, pain, sloughing (with extravasation). **Special Senses:** Conjunctivitis, blurred vision, nasal congestion. **CNS:** *Drowsiness, dizziness, lightheadedness,* headache. **CV:** Hypotension, bradycardia. **GI:** Nausea, metallic taste, dyspepsia. **Hematologic:** Slight reduction of white cell count with prolonged therapy. **Renal:** Polyethylene glycol in the injection may increase preexisting acidosis and urea retention in patients with renal impairment.

M

Common adverse effects in *italic;* life-threatening effects <u>underlined;</u> generic names in **bold;** classifications in SMALL CAPS; ♣ Canadian drug name; ☯ Prototype drug

1027

## DIAGNOSTIC TEST INTERFERENCE

Methocarbamol may cause false increases in *urinary 5-HIAA* (with *nitrosonaphthol reagent*) and *VMA (Gitlow method).*

## INTERACTIONS Drug: Alcohol

and other CNS DEPRESSANTS enhance CNS depression.

## PHARMACOKINETICS Absorption:

Readily absorbed from GI tract. **Onset:** 30 min. **Peak:** 1–2 h. **Metabolism:** In liver. **Elimination:** In urine. **Half-Life:** 1–2 h.

## NURSING IMPLICATIONS

### Assessment & Drug Effects

- Monitor vital signs closely during IV infusion.
- Supervise ambulation following parenteral administration.
- Monitor IV site closely to prevent extravasation.

### Patient & Family Education

- Make position changes slowly, particularly from lying down to upright position; dangle legs before standing.
- Be aware that adverse reactions after oral administration are usually mild and transient and subside with dosage reduction. Use caution regarding drowsiness and dizziness. Avoid activities requiring mental alertness and physical coordination until response to drug is known.

## METHOTREXATE SODIUM ℗

(meth-oh-trex′ate)

MTX, Otrexup, Rasuvo, Xatmep

**Classifications:** ANTINEOPLASTIC; ANTIMETABOLITE; IMMUNOSUPPRESSANT; DISEASE-MODIFYING ANTIRHEUMATIC DRUG (DMARD)
Therapeutic: ANTINEOPLASTIC; ANTIFOLATE; ANTIRHEUMATIC; ANTIPSORIATIC

## AVAILABILITY Tablet; solution for injection; oral solution

## ACTION & THERAPEUTIC EFFECT

Antimetabolite and folic acid antagonist that blocks folic acid participation in nucleic acid synthesis, thereby interfering with mitotic cell process. Rapidly proliferating tissues (malignant cells, bone marrow, and psoriasis) are sensitive to interference of the mitotic process by this drug. *Induces remission slowly; use often preceded by other antineoplastic therapies. Additionally has immunosuppressant effects, antipsoriatic, and antirheumatic effects.*

## USES Principally in combination

regimens to maintain induced remissions in neoplastic diseases. Effective in treatment of gestational choriocarcinoma and hydatidiform mole and as immunosuppressant in kidney transplantation, for acute and subacute leukemias and leukemic meningitis, especially in children. Used in lymphosarcoma, in certain inoperable tumors of head, neck, and pelvis, and in mycosis fungoides. Also used to treat severe psoriasis nonresponsive to other forms of therapy, rheumatoid arthritis.

## UNLABELED USES Psoriatic ar-

thritis, SLE, polymyositis.

## CONTRAINDICATIONS Hyper-

sensitivity to methotrexate; chronic liver disease; alcoholism or alcoholic liver disease; vaccination; ultraviolet exposure to psoriatic lesions; preexisting blood dyscrasias; rheumatoid arthritis; men and women of childbearing age; pregnancy (category X); lactation.

## CAUTIOUS USE Infections; peptic

ulcer, ulcerative colitis; renal impairment; very young or old patients; cancer patients with preexisting bone marrow impairment; poor nutritional status; children.

## ROUTE & DOSAGE

### Trophoblastic Neoplasm
*Adult:* **PO/IM** 15–30 mg/day for 5 days, repeat for 3–5 courses

### Acute Lymphocytic Leukemia
*Adult:* **IM/IV Loading Dose**
3.3 mg/m²/day × 4–6 wk
**PO/IM/IV Maintenance Dose**
30 mg/m² weekly in 2 doses
*Child/Adolescent:* **PO** (solution)
20 mg/m²/dose weekly

### Cutaneous T-Cell Lymphoma
*Adult:* **PO** 5–50 mg weekly; **IV/IM**
50 mg weekly

### Osteogenic Sarcoma
*Adult:* **IV** 12 g/m², (dose frequency differs based on chemotherapy regimen)

### Psoriasis/Rheumatoid Arthritis
*Adult:* **PO** 2.5 mg q12h for 3 doses each wk or 7.5 mg once/wk
*Child:* **PO/IM** 5–15 mg/m²/wk as single dose or in 3 divided doses 12 h apart

### Mycosis Fungoides
*Adult:* **PO/IM** 5–50 mg weekly

### Epidermoid Head/Neck Cancer
*Adult/Adolescent/Child:* **IV** 40 mg/m² on days 1 and 15 every 21 days
*Adult:* **PO** 25–50 mg/m² q7d
*Child:* **PO** 7.5–30 mg/m² q7–14days

## ADMINISTRATION

### Oral
- May be taken without respect to meals.

- Avoid skin exposure and inhalation of drug particles.

### Intramuscular
- Inject deeply into a large muscle.

### Intravenous
Note: Verify correct IV concentration and rate of infusion for administration to children with prescriber.

***PREPARE:*** **Direct:** Reconstitute powder vial by adding 2 mL of NS or D5W without preservatives to each 5 mg to yield 2.5 mg/mL. Reconstitute 1 g high-dose vial with 19.4 mL D5W or NS to yield 50 mg/mL. **IV Infusion:** Further dilute contents of the reconstituted 1 g high-dose vial in D5W or NS to a 25 mg/mL or less.

***ADMINISTER:*** **Direct:** Give at rate of 10 mg or fraction thereof over 60 sec. **IV Infusion:** Give over 1–4 h or as prescribed.

***INCOMPATIBILITIES:*** Solution/additive: **Bleomycin, metoclopramide, prednisolone, ranitidine.** Y-site: **Amiodarone, amphotericin B, capsofungin, chlorpromazine, codeine, daptomycin, dexrazone, diazepam, diltiazem, dobutamine, dopamine, doxycycline, droperidol, gemcitabine, gentamicin, idarubicin, ifosfamide, labetalol, levofloxacin, midazolam, mycphenolate, nalbuphine, nicardipine, pantoprazole, phenytoin, promethazine, propofol quinupristin/dalfopristin, ranacuronium, vancomycin.**

- Preserve drug in tight, light-resistant container.

## ADVERSE EFFECTS (≥1%) CNS:
*Headache,* drowsiness, blurred vision, dizziness, aphasia, hemiparesis; arachnoiditis, convulsions (after intrathecal administration); mental confusion, tremors, ataxia, coma. **GI:** <u>Hepatotoxicity</u>, GI ulcerations

---

Common adverse effects in *italic;* life-threatening effects <u>underlined</u>; generic names in **bold;** classifications in SMALL CAPS; ✤ Canadian drug name; ⊘ Prototype drug

1029

and hemorrhage, *ulcerative stomatitis, glossitis, gingivitis,* pharyngitis, nausea, vomiting, diarrhea, <u>hepatic cirrhosis</u>. **Urogenital:** <u>Defective oogenesis or spermatogenesis</u>, nephropathy, hematuria, menstrual dysfunction, infertility, abortion, fetal defects. **Hematologic:** *<u>Leukopenia, thrombocytopenia,</u>* anemia, <u>marked myelosuppression, aplastic bone marrow</u>, telangiectasia, thrombophlebitis at intra-arterial catheter site, hypogammaglobulinemia, and hyperuricemia. **Skin:** Erythematous rashes, pruritus, urticaria, folliculitis, vasculitis, photosensitivity, depigmentation, hyperpigmentation, alopecia. **Cardiovascular:** Arterial thrombosis, cerebral thrombosis, chest pain, deep vein thrombosis, hypotension, pericardial effusion, pericarditis. **Body as a Whole:** Malaise, undue fatigue, systemic toxicity (after intrathecal and intra-arterial administration), chills, fever, decreased resistance to infection, septicemia, osteoporosis, metabolic changes precipitating diabetes and <u>sudden death, pneumonitis, pulmonary fibrosis</u>.

## DIAGNOSTIC TEST INTERFERENCE

Severe reactions may occur when *live vaccines* are administered because of immunosuppressive activity of methotrexate.

## INTERACTIONS Drug:

Acitretin, **alcohol, azathioprine, sulfasalazine** increase risk of hepatotoxicity; **chloramphenicol, etretinate,** SALICYLATES, NSAIDS, SULFONAMIDES, SULFONYLUREAS, **phenylbutazone, phenytoin,** TETRACYCLINES, **PABA, penicillin, probenecid,** PROTON PUMP INHIBITORS may increase methotrexate levels with increased toxicity; **folic acid** may alter response to methotrexate. May increase **theophylline** levels; **cholestyramine** enhances methotrexate clearance. Avoid use with

**salicylates. Herbal:** Echinacea may increase risk of hepatotoxicity. **Food: Caffeine** greater than 180 mg/day (3–4 cups) may decrease effectiveness for rheumatoid arthritis.

## PHARMACOKINETICS
**Absorption:** Readily absorbed from GI tract. **Peak:** 0.5–2 h IM/IV; 1–4 h PO. **Distribution:** Widely distributed with highest concentrations in kidneys, gallbladder, spleen, liver, and skin; minimal passage across blood–brain barrier; crosses placenta; distributed into breast milk. **Metabolism:** In liver. **Elimination:** Primarily in urine. **Half-Life:** 2–4 h.

## NURSING IMPLICATIONS

### Black Box Warning

*Methotrexate has been associated with hepatotoxicity, lung damage, severe skin reactions, tumor lysis syndrome, and potentially fatal infections.*

### Assessment & Drug Effects

- Prolonged treatment with small frequent doses may lead to hepatotoxicity, which is best diagnosed by liver biopsy.
- Monitor for and report ulcerative stomatitis with glossitis and gingivitis, often the first signs of toxicity. Inspect mouth daily; report patchy necrotic areas, bleeding and discomfort, or overgrowth (black, furry tongue).
- Monitor I&O ratio and pattern. Keep patient well hydrated (about 2000 mL/24 h).
- Prevent exposure to infections or colds during periods of leukopenia. Be alert to onset of agranulocytosis (cough, extreme fatigue, sore throat, chills, fever) and report symptoms promptly.

- Be alert for and report symptoms of thrombocytopenia (e.g., ecchymoses, petechiae, epistaxis, melena, hematuria, vaginal bleeding, slow and protracted oozing following trauma).
- Monitor lab tests: Baseline and periodic LFTs, renal function tests, CBC with differential, and platelet count.

**Patient & Family Education**

- Report promptly any of the following: Diarrhea, mouth sores, fever, dehydration, cough, bleeding, shortness of breath, any signs of infection, or a skin rash.
- Use contraceptive measures during and for at least 3 mo (males) or 1 ovulatory cycle (females) after cessation of therapy.
- Avoid or moderate alcohol ingestion, which increases the incidence and severity of methotrexate hepatotoxicity.
- Do not use OTC proton pump inhibitors (e.g., omeprazole) without consulting prescriber.
- Practice fastidious mouth care to prevent infection, provide comfort, and maintain adequate nutritional status.
- Do not self-medicate with vitamins. Some OTC compounds may include folic acid (or its derivatives), which alters methotrexate response.
- Use contraceptive measures during and for at least 3 mo following therapy.
- Avoid exposure to sunlight and ultraviolet light. Wear sunglasses and sunscreen.

# METHOXSALEN ⊕

(meth-ox'a-len)

8-MOP, Oxsoralen, Uvadex

**Classifications:** PSORALEN; PIGMENTING AGENT
**Therapeutic:** PIGMENTING AGENT; ANTIPSORIATIC

**AVAILABILITY** Capsule; solution; lotion

**ACTION & *THERAPEUTIC EFFECT***
Plant derivative with strong photosensitizing effects: Used with ultraviolet-A light (UVA) in therapeutic regimens called PUVA (P-psoralen). After photoactivation by long wavelength, UVA, methoxsalen combines with epidermal cell DNA causing photo-damage (cytotoxic action). *Photo-damage inhibits rapid and uncontrolled epidermal cell turnover characteristic of psoriasis. Results in an inflammatory reaction with erythema. Strongly melanogenic.*

**USES** With controlled exposure to UVA to repigment vitiliginous skin and for symptomatic treatment of severe disabling psoriasis that is refractory to other forms of therapy.

**UNLABELED USES** (PUVA therapy) mycosis fungoides.

**CONTRAINDICATIONS** Sunburn, sensitivity (or its history) to psoralens, diseases associated with photosensitivity (e.g., SLE, albinism, melanoma or its history); invasive squamous cell cancer; cataract; aphakia; previous exposure to arsenic or ionizing radiation.

**CAUTIOUS USE** Hepatic insufficiency; GI disease; chronic infection; treatment with known photosensitizing agents; immunosuppressed patient; cardiovascular disease; pregnancy (category C); lactation. Safety **(lotion)** in children younger than 12 y not established. Safety **(oral)** in children not established.

**ROUTE & DOSAGE**

**Idiopathic Vitiligo**

*Adult:* **Topical** Apply lotion 1–2 h before exposure to UV light once/wk

---

Common adverse effects in *italic;* life-threatening effects underlined; generic names in **bold;** classifications in SMALL CAPS; ♣ Canadian drug name; ⊕ Prototype drug

M

## Psoriasis

*Adult:* **PO** Give 1.5–2 h before exposure to UV light 2–3 × wk: *weight less than 30 kg:* 10 mg; *weight 30–50 kg:* 20 mg; *weight 51–65 kg* 30 mg; *weight 66–80 kg:* 40 mg; *weight 81–90 kg:* 50 mg; *weight 91–115 kg:* 60 mg; *weight greater than 115 kg:* 70 mg

## ADMINISTRATION

- Note: Methoxsalen therapy with UV light (PUVA therapy) should be done under the complete control of a prescriber with special competence and experience in photochemotherapy.

### Oral

- Oxsoralen-Ultra soft gelatin capsules are **not** interchangeable with 8-MOP hard gelatin capsules.
- Give with milk or food to prevent GI distress.
- Maintain consistent time relationship between food–drug ingestion. Food digestion and absorption appear to affect drug serum levels.

### Topical

- Only small (less than 10 cm²), well-defined areas are treated with lotion. Systemic treatment is used for large areas.
- Apply lotion with cotton swabs, allow to dry 1–2 min, then reapply. Protect borders of the lesion with petrolatum and sunscreen lotion to prevent hyperpigmentation.
- Use finger cots or gloves to apply lotion and prevent photosensitization and burned skin.
- Apply sunscreen lotion to the skin for about one third of the initial exposure time during PUVA therapy until there is sufficient tanning. Do not apply to psoriatic areas before treatment.

- Store lotion and capsules at 15°–30° C (59°–86° F) in light-resistant containers unless otherwise directed by manufacturer.

## ADVERSE EFFECTS (≥1%) CNS:
Nervousness, dizziness, headache, mental depression or excitation, vertigo, insomnia. **Special Senses:** Cataract formation, ocular damage. **GI:** Cheilitis, *nausea* and other GI disturbances, toxic hepatitis. **Skin:** Phototoxic effects: <u>Severe edema and erythema</u>, *pruritus,* painful blisters; <u>burning</u>, peeling, thinning, freckling, and accelerated aging of skin; hyper- or hypopigmentation; severe skin pain (lasting 1–2 mo), photoallergic contact dermatitis (with topical use), exacerbation of latent photosensitive dermatoses, <u>malignant melanoma</u> (rare). **Body as a Whole:** Transient loss of muscular coordination, edema, leg cramps, systemic immune effects, drug fever.

## INTERACTIONS Drug: **Anthralin, coal tar, griseofulvin,** PHENOTHIAZINES, **nalidixic acid,** SULFONAMIDES, BACTERIOSTATIC SOAPS, TETRACYCLINES, THIAZIDES compound photosensitizing effects. **Food:** Food will increase peak and extent of absorption.

## PHARMACOKINETICS Absorption: Variably from GI tract. **Peak:** 2 h. **Duration:** 8–10 h. **Distribution:** Preferentially taken up by epidermal cells; distributes into lens of eye. **Elimination:** 80–90% in urine within 8 h. **Half-Life:** 0.75–2.4 h.

## NURSING IMPLICATIONS

### Assessment & Drug Effects

- Schedule a pretreatment ophthalmologic exam to rule out cataracts; repeat periodically during treatment and at yearly intervals thereafter.

Common adverse effects in *italic;* life-threatening effects <u>underlined;</u> generic names in **bold;** classifications in SMALL CAPS; ♣ Canadian drug name; ⊘ Prototype drug

- Fair-skinned patients appear to be at greatest risk for phototoxicity from PUVA therapy (see ADVERSE EFFECTS).
- Be aware that repigmentation is more rapid on fleshy areas (i.e., face, abdomen, buttocks) than on hands or feet.
- Monitor lab tests: Periodic CBC, LFT, renal function tests, and antinuclear antibody tests during oral therapy.

**Patient & Family Education**
- Expect that effective repigmentation may require 6–9 mo of treatment; periodic treatment usually is necessary to retain pigmentation. If, after 3 mo of treatment, there is no apparent response, drug is discontinued.
- Avoid additional exposure to UV light (direct or indirect) for at least 8 h after oral drug ingestion and UVA exposure.
- Understand intended treatment schedule: After topical application, the initial sunlight exposure is limited to 1 min, with subsequent gradual and incremental exposures by prescription.
- Avoid additional UV light for 24–48 h after topical application and UVA exposure.
- Wear sunscreen lotion (with SPF 15 or higher) and protective clothing (hat, gloves) to cover all exposed areas including lips, to prevent burning or blistering if sunlight cannot be avoided after the treatment.
- Do not sunbathe for at least 48 h after PUVA treatment. Sunburn and photochemotherapy are additive in the production of burning and erythema.
- Wear wraparound sunglasses with UVA-absorbing properties both indoors and outdoors during daylight hours for 24 h. Do not substitute prescription sunglasses or photosensitive darkening glasses; they may actually increase danger of cataract formation.
- Alert prescriber to appearance of new psoriatic areas, flares, or regressed cleared skin areas during treatment and maintenance periods.

## METHYCLOTHIAZIDE
(meth i-kloc-thye′a-zide)
**Classifications:** THIAZIDE DIURETIC; ANTIHYPERTENSIVE
**Therapeutic:** THIAZIDE DIURETIC; ANTIHYPERTENSIVE
**Prototype:** Hydrochlorothiazide

**AVAILABILITY** Tablet

**ACTION & THERAPEUTIC EFFECT**
Diuretic effect results from inhibition of the renal tubular reabsorption of electrolytes. Excretion of sodium and chloride is enhanced, along with a loss of potassium ions via the kidney. BP is lowered, probably by the loss of sodium, chloride and water, and, consequently, blood volume. Edema is also decreased in CHF patients by the same mechanism. *Antihypertensive effect as well as enhanced excretion of sodium and water.*

**USES** Antihypertensive treatment and adjunctively in the management of edema associated with CHF, renal pathology, and hepatic cirrhosis.

**CONTRAINDICATIONS** Hypersensitivity to thiazides, and sulfonamide derivatives; anuria; hypokalemia; lactation.

**CAUTIOUS USE** Renal disease; impaired kidney or liver function; older adults; gout; SLE; hypercalcemia; DM; moderate to high cholesterol, elevated triglyceride

**M**

Common adverse effects in *italic*; life-threatening effects underlined; generic names in **bold**; classifications in SMALL CAPS; ◆ Canadian drug name; ⦿ Prototype drug

1033

level; pregnancy (category B); children.

## ROUTE & DOSAGE

**Edema**

*Adult:* **PO** 2.5–5 mg once every other day

**Hypertension**

*Adult:* **PO** 2.5–10 mg/day

## ADMINISTRATION

### Oral

- Give early in the morning after eating (reduces gastric irritation) to prevent sleep interruption because of diuresis. If 2 doses are ordered, administer second dose no later than 3 p.m.
- Store at 15°–30° C (59°–86° F) unless otherwise instructed.

**ADVERSE EFFECTS** (≥1%) **Body as a Whole:** Postural hypotension, sialadenitis, unusual fatigue, dizziness, paresthesias. **Skin:** Photosensitivity. **Special Senses:** Yellow vision. **Metabolic:** *Hypokalemia.* **Hematologic:** <u>Agranulocytosis</u>.

**INTERACTIONS Drug:** **Amphotericin B,** CORTICOSTEROIDS increase hypokalemic effects; may antagonize hypoglycemic effects of **insulin,** SULFONYLUREAS; **cholestyramine, colestipol** decrease thiazide absorption; intensifies hypoglycemic and hypotensive effects of **diazoxide;** increased potassium and magnesium loss may cause **digoxin** toxicity; decreases **lithium** excretion, increasing its toxicity; NSAIDS may attenuate diuresis, and risk of NSAID-induced kidney failure increased.

**PHARMACOKINETICS Absorption:** Incompletely absorbed. **Onset:** 2 h. **Peak:** 6 h. **Duration:** Greater than 24 h. **Distribution:** Distributed throughout extracellular tissue; concentrates in kidney; crosses placenta; distributed in breast milk. **Metabolism:** Does not appear to be metabolized. **Elimination:** In urine.

## NURSING IMPLICATIONS

### Assessment & Drug Effects

- Expect antihypertensive effects in 3–4 days; maximal effects may require 3–4 wk.
- Monitor BP and I&O ratio during first phase of antihypertensive therapy. Report a sudden fall in BP, which may initiate severe postural hypotension and potentially dangerous perfusion problems, especially in the extremities.
- Monitor patient for S&S of hypokalemia (see Appendix F). Report promptly. Prescriber may change dose and institute replacement therapy.
- Monitor lab tests: Periodic serum electrolytes and CBC with differential.

### Patient & Family Education

- Eat a balanced diet to protect against hypokalemia; generally not severe even with long-term therapy. Prevent onset by eating potassium-rich foods including a banana (about 370 mg potassium) and at least 180 mL (6 oz) orange juice (about 330 mg potassium) every day.
- Watch carefully for loss of glycemic control (diabetics) and early signs of hyperglycemia (see Appendix F). Symptoms are slow to develop.
- Avoid OTC drugs unless the prescriber approves them. Many preparations contain both potassium and sodium, and may induce electrolyte imbalance adverse effects.
- Older adults are more responsive to excessive diuresis; orthostatic hypotension may be a problem.

Common adverse effects in *italic;* life-threatening effects <u>underlined</u>; generic names in **bold;** classifications in SMALL CAPS; ♣ Canadian drug name; ⊙ Prototype drug

- Change positions slowly and in stages from lying down to upright positions; avoid hot baths or showers, extended exposure to sunlight, and standing still. Accept assistance as necessary to prevent falling.
- Do not drive or engage in potentially hazardous activities until adjustment to the hypotensive effects of drug has been made.

## METHYLDOPA ⊕
(meth-ill-doe′pa)

## METHYLDOPATE HYDROCHLORIDE
(meth-ill-doe′pate)

**Classifications:** CENTRALLY ACTING ANTIHYPERTENSIVE; ALPHA-ADRENERGIC AGONIST
**Therapeutic:** CENTRALLY ACTING ANTIHYPERTENSIVE

**AVAILABILITY** Tablet; solution for injection

## ACTION & THERAPEUTIC EFFECT
Structurally related to catecholamines and their precursors. Inhibits decarboxylation of dopa, thereby reducing concentration of dopamine, a precursor of norepinephrine. It also inhibits the precursor of serotonin. Reduces renal vascular resistance; maintains cardiac output without acceleration, but may slow heart rate; tends to support sodium and water retention. *Lowers standing and supine BP.*

**USES** Hypertension, hypertensive urgency or emergency.

**CONTRAINDICATIONS** Hypersensitivity to methyldopa or methyldopate HCl; active liver disease (hepatitis, cirrhosis); pheochromocytoma; coadministration with MAOIs; blood dyscrasias.

**CAUTIOUS USE** History of impaired liver or kidney function or disease; renal failure; autoimmune disease; cardiac disease; angina pectoris; history of mental depression; Parkinson's disease; blood transfusion type and cross matching; young or older adults; pregnancy (category B); lactation; children.

## ROUTE & DOSAGE

### Hypertension
*Adult/Adolescent:* **PO** 250 mg b.i.d. or t.i.d., may be increased up to 3 g/day in divided doses, usual range 250–1000 mg total/day
*Geriatric:* **PO** lower doses may be needed
*Child:* **PO** 10 mg/kg/day in 2–4 divided doses (max: 3 g/day)

### Hypertensive Emergency/Urgency
*Adult:* **IV** 250–500 mg q6h
*Child:* **IV** 20–40 mg/kg/day

### Renal Impairment Dosage Adjustment
CrCl 10–50 mL/min: Dose q8–12h; *less than 10 mL/min:* Dose q12–24h

## ADMINISTRATION

### Oral
- Make dosage increases in evening to minimize daytime sedation.

### Intravenous
**PREPARE: Intermittent:** Dilute in 100 mL of D5W, as needed, to yield 10 mg/mL.
**ADMINISTER: Intermittent:** Give over 30–60 min.
**INCOMPATIBILITIES: Solution/additive: Amphotericin B, hydrocortisone, methohexital,**

M

Common adverse effects in *italic;* life-threatening effects underlined; generic names in **bold;** classifications in SMALL CAPS; ♣ Canadian drug name; ⊕ Prototype drug

1035

tetracycline. **Y-site: Acyclovir, amphotericin B, ampicillin, azathioprine, cefoperazone, dantrolene, diazepam, diazoxide, ganciclovir, gemtuzumab, haloperidol, hydralazine, imipenem, indomethacin, ketorolac, mitomycin, pentobarbital, phenytoin, piperacillin/tazobacam.**

**ADVERSE EFFECTS (≥1%) Body as a Whole:** Hypersensitivity (*fever,* skin eruptions, ulcerations of soles of feet, flu-like symptoms, lymphadenopathy, eosinophilia). **CNS:** *Sedation, drowsiness,* sluggishness, headache, weakness, fatigue, dizziness, vertigo, *decrease in mental acuity,* inability to concentrate, amnesia-like syndrome, parkinsonism, mild psychoses, depression, nightmares. **CV:** Orthostatic hypotension, syncope, bradycardia, myocarditis, edema, weight gain *(sodium and water retention),* paradoxic hypertensive reaction (especially with IV administration). **GI:** Diarrhea, constipation, abdominal distention, malabsorption syndrome, nausea, vomiting, dry mouth, sore or black tongue, sialadenitis, abnormal liver function tests, jaundice, hepatitis, hepatic necrosis (rare). **Hematologic:** *Positive direct Coombs' test* (common especially in African-Americans), granulocytopenia. **Special Senses:** *Nasal stuffiness.* **Endocrine:** Gynecomastia, lactation, *decreased libido, impotence,* hypothermia (large doses), positive tests for lupus and rheumatoid factors. **Skin:** Granulomatous skin lesions.

**DIAGNOSTIC TEST INTERFERENCE**
Methyldopa may interfere with **serum creatinine** measurements using **alkaline picrate method, AST** by **colorimetric methods,** and **uric acid** measurements by **phosphotungstate method** (with high methyldopa blood levels); it may produce false elevations of **urinary catecholamines** and increase in **serum amylase** in methyldopa-induced sialadenitis.

**INTERACTIONS Drug:** AMPHETAMINES, TRICYCLIC ANTIDEPRESSANTS, PHENOTHIAZINES, BARBITURATES may attenuate antihypertensive response; methyldopa may inhibit effectiveness of **ephedrine; haloperidol** may exacerbate psychiatric symptoms; with **levodopa** additive hypotension, increased CNS toxicity, especially psychosis; increases risk of **lithium** toxicity; **methotrimeprazine** causes excessive hypotension; MAO INHIBITORS may cause hallucinations; **phenoxybenzamine** may cause urinary incontinence. **Herbal: Licorice** may affect electrolyte levels; **ephedra, yohimbe, ginseng** may decrease efficacy.

**PHARMACOKINETICS Absorption:** About 50% absorbed from GI tract. **Peak:** 4–6 h. **Duration:** 24 h PO; 10–16 h IV. **Distribution:** Crosses placenta, distributed into breast milk. **Metabolism:** In liver and GI tract. **Elimination:** Primarily in urine. **Half-Life:** 1.7 h.

## NURSING IMPLICATIONS

### Assessment & Drug Effects

- Check BP and pulse at least q30min until stabilized during IV infusion and observe for adequacy of urinary output.
- Take BP at regular intervals in lying, sitting, and standing positions during period of dosage adjustment.
- Supervision of ambulation in older adults and patients with impaired

kidney function; both are particularly likely to manifest orthostatic hypotension with dizziness and light-headedness during period of dosage adjustment.

- Monitor fluid and electrolyte balance and I&O. Weigh patient daily, and check for edema because methyldopa favors sodium and water retention.
- Be alert that rising BP indicating tolerance to drug effect may occur during week 2 or 3 of therapy.
- Monitor lab tests: Baseline and periodic blood counts and LFTs especially during first 6–12 wk of therapy or if patient develops unexplained fever; periodic serum electrolytes.

### Patient & Family Education

- Exercise caution with hot baths and showers, prolonged standing in one position, and strenuous exercise that may enhance orthostatic hypotension. Make position changes slowly, particularly from lying down to upright posture; dangle legs a few minutes before standing.
- Be aware that transient sedation, drowsiness, mental depression, weakness, and headache commonly occur during first 24–72 h of therapy or whenever dosage is increased. Symptoms tend to disappear with continuation of therapy or dosage reduction.
- Avoid potentially hazardous tasks such as driving until response to drug is known; drug may affect ability to perform activities requiring concentrated mental effort, especially during first few days of therapy or whenever dosage is increased.
- Do not to take OTC medications unless approved by prescriber.

# METHYLERGONOVINE MALEATE

(meth-ill-er-goe-noe'veen)

Methergine

**Classifications:** ERGOT ALKALOID; OXYTOCIC
Therapeutic: OXYTOCIC
**Prototype:** OXYTOCIN

**AVAILABILITY** Tablet; solution for injection

## ACTION & *THERAPEUTIC EFFECT*

Ergot alkaloid that induces rapid, sustained tetanic uterine contraction that shortens third stage of labor and reduces blood loss. *Administered after delivery of the placenta to minimize the risk of postpartal hemorrhage.*

**USES** Routine management after delivery of placenta and for postpartum atony, subinvolution, and hemorrhage. With full obstetric supervision, may be used during second stage of labor.

**CONTRAINDICATIONS** Hypersensitivity to ergot preparations; induction of labor; use prior to delivery of placenta; threatened spontaneous abortion; prolonged use; uterine sepsis; hypertension; toxemia; angina; arteriosclerosis; CAD; dysfunctional uterine bleeding; eclampsia; hypertension; MI; neonates; PVD; preeclampsia; Raynaud's disease; sepsis; stroke; thromboangiitis obliterans; thrombophlebitis.

**CAUTIOUS USE** DM; hepatic disease; migraine headaches; renal impairment; pulmonary disease; pregnancy (category C); lactation.

M

Common adverse effects in *italic;* life-threatening effects <u>underlined;</u> generic names in **bold;** classifications in SMALL CAPS; ♣ Canadian drug name; ⑩ Prototype drug

1037

## ROUTE & DOSAGE

### Postpartum Hemorrhage

*Adult:* **PO** 0.2 q6–8h × 2–7 days; **IM/IV** 0.2 mg q2–4h (max: 5 doses)

## ADMINISTRATION

- Use parenteral routes only in emergencies.

### Oral

- Note: Dosing should not exceed 1 wk.

### Intramuscular

- Inject undiluted deep into a large muscle.

### Intravenous

*PREPARE:* **Direct:** Give undiluted or diluted in 5 mL of NS.
*ADMINISTER:* **Direct:** Give 0.2 mg or fraction thereof over 60 sec. ▪ Do not use ampules containing discolored solution or visible particles.

▪ Store at 15°–30° C (59°–86° F) unless otherwise directed. Protect from light.

## ADVERSE EFFECTS (≥1%) GI:
*Nausea, vomiting* (especially with IV doses). **CV:** Severe hypertensive episodes, bradycardia. **Body as a Whole:** Allergic phenomena including <u>shock</u>, ergotism.

## INTERACTIONS Drug: PARENTERAL SYMPATHOMIMETICS, other ERGOT ALKALOIDS, TRIPTANS add to pressor effects and carry risk of hypertension; PROTEASE INHIBITORS, **itraconazole** may increase the risk of toxicity.

## PHARMACOKINETICS Absorption: Readily from GI tract. **Onset:** 5–15 min PO; 2–5 min IM; immediate IV. **Duration:** 3 or more h PO; 3 h IM; 45 min IV. **Distribution:** Distributed into breast milk. **Metabolism:** Slowly in liver. **Elimination:** Mainly in feces, small amount in urine. **Half-Life:** 0.5–2 h.

## NURSING IMPLICATIONS

### Assessment & Drug Effects

- Monitor vital signs (particularly BP) and uterine response during and after parenteral administration of methylergonovine until partum period is stabilized (about 1–2 h).
- Notify prescriber if BP suddenly increases or if there are frequent periods of uterine relaxation.

### Patient & Family Education

- Report severe cramping or increased bleeding.
- Report any of the following: Cold or numb fingers or toes, nausea or vomiting, chest or muscle pain.

# METHYLNALTREXONE BROMIDE

(meth-yl-nal-trex'own bro'mide)

Relistor

**Classification:** NARCOTIC (OPIATE ANTAGONIST)
Therapeutic: GI STIMULANT (OPIOID INDUCED)

## AVAILABILITY Solution for injection

## ACTION & *THERAPEUTIC EFFECT*

A selective, peripherally acting antagonist of opioid binding to mu opioid receptors in tissues such as the GI tract. *Decreases constipating effects of opioids without interfering with analgesic effect of opioids in the CNS.*

## USES Treatment of opioid-induced constipation in patients with advanced illness who are receiving palliative care when response to laxative therapy has not been sufficient.

**UNLABELED USES** Management of nausea and vomiting related to morphine. Treatment of pruritus related to morphine. Management of urinary retention caused by opioids.

**CONTRAINDICATIONS** Known or suspected mechanical GI obstruction; severe or persistent diarrhea.

**CAUTIOUS USE** Renal impairment; history of GI tract lesions; pregnancy (category B); older adults; lactation. Safety and efficacy in children not established.

## ROUTE & DOSAGE

**Opioid-Induced Constipation**

*Adult (weight less than 38 kg):*
**Subcutaneous** Administer every other day *weight less than 38 kg:* 0.15 mg/kg; *weight 38 to less than 62 kg:* 8 mg; *weight 62 to less than 114 kg:* 12 mg; *weight greater than 114 kg:* 0.15 mg/kg

**Renal Impairment Dosage Adjustment**

*CrCl less than 30 mL/min:* Reduce normal adult dose by 50%

## ADMINISTRATION

**Subcutaneous**
- An 8 mg dose equals 0.4 mL and a 12 mg dose equals 0.6 mL.
- Insert needle at a 45-degree angle into a pinched fold of skin on the abdomen, thigh, or upper arm. Release skin and inject. Rotate injection sites.
- Store at 20°–25° C (68°–77° F) away from light. May store drawn up into syringe for 24 h at room temperature with ambient light.

## ADVERSE EFFECTS (≥1%) CNS:
Dizziness. **GI:** *Abdominal pain,* diarrhea, *flatulence, nausea.*

**PHARMACOKINETICS Peak:** 0.5 h. **Distribution:** 11–15% protein bound. **Metabolism:** Hepatic. **Elimination:** Primarily eliminated unchanged (85%) in urine and feces. **Half-Life:** 8 h.

## NURSING IMPLICATIONS
### Assessment & Drug Effects
- Monitor bowel pattern.
- Withhold drug and report promptly severe or persistent diarrhea.

### Patient & Family Education
- Ensure that patient/caregiver knows how to correctly inject subcutaneous medication.
- Stop methylnaltrexone and notify prescriber if severe or persistent diarrhea develops.

# METHYLPHENIDATE HYDROCHLORIDE
(meth-ill-fen'i date)

Aptensio XR, Concerta, Cotempla, Daytrana, Focalin XR, Metadate CD, Metadate ER, Methylin, Methylin ER, Quilivant XR, QuiliChew, Ritalin, Ritalin LA, Ritalin SR

**Classification:** CEREBRAL STIMULANT
**Therapeutic:** CEREBRAL STIMULANT
**Prototype:** Amphetamine
**Controlled Substance:** Schedule II

**AVAILABILITY** Tablet; chewable tablet; oral solution; sustained release capsule/tablet; transdermal patch; oral disintegrating tablet

## ACTION & *THERAPEUTIC EFFECT*
Acts mainly on cerebral cortex exerting a stimulant effect. Results in mild CNS and respiratory stimulation with potency intermediate between amphetamine and caffeine. *Effects are more prominent on mental rather than on motor activities. Also believed to have an anorexiant effect.*

---

**USES** Treatment of ADHD, narcolepsy.

**UNLABELED USES** Depression.

**CONTRAINDICATIONS** Hypersensitivity to drug; history of marked anxiety, tension, agitation; aortic stenosis; glaucoma; motor tics; family history or diagnosis of Tourette syndrome; glaucoma; concurrent use of MAOIs or within 14 days of their use; substance abuse; suicidal ideation. **Metadate CD, Metadate ER,** and **Methylin ER:** Patients with severe hypertension; angina pectoris, cardiac arrhythmias, heart failure; recent MI, hyperthyroidism or thyrotoxicosis.

**CAUTIOUS USE** History of drug dependency; alcoholism; emotionally unstable individual; personality disturbances; aggressive behavior or hostility; bipolar disorder, psychosis; abrupt discontinuation; anxiety, cardiac arrhythmias, cardiac disease, hypertension; dysphagia, esophageal stricture, GI obstruction, heart failure, hepatic disease, hyperthyroidism, history of paralytic ileus, CF; peripheral vasculopathy; mania; radiographic contrast administration; history of seizures; older adults; pregnancy (category C); lactation; children younger than 6 y of age.

**ROUTE & DOSAGE**

**Narcolepsy**

*Adult:* PO 10 mg b.i.d. or t.i.d. 30–45 min p.c. (range: 10–60 mg/day)

*Adolescent/Child (6 y or older):* PO 5 mg b.i.d., may increase weekly (max dose: 60 mg/day)

**Attention Deficit Disorder**

*Adult:* PO Immediate release

**products:** 20–30 mg daily in divided doses.; **Concerta extended release product:** 18–36 mg daily; (dose varies per previous methylphenidate use, see package insert for table) **Aptensio Extended release** 10 mg daily; **other extended release capsules:** corresponds to the previously titrated 8-h dosage of the IR tablets; in treatment naive patients initial dose of 20 mg each morning is appropriate.

*Adolescent/Child (6 y or older):* PO 5 mg before breakfast and lunch, with a gradual increase of 5–10 mg/wk as needed (max: 60 mg/day) or 20–40 mg sustained release daily before breakfast (max dose: 72 mg daily);. **Concerta Extended release** 18 mg daily (max: 54 mg/day); (dose varies per previous methylphenidate use, see package insert for table) **Transdermal patch** 10 mg patch worn for 9 hours × 1 wk then taper as needed. Increase no more than once weekly. Apply 2 h before desired effect. **Cotempla disintegrating tablet** 17.3 mg daily

**ADMINISTRATION**

**Oral**

- Give 30–45 min before meals. To avoid insomnia, give last dose before 6 p.m.
- Ensure that sustained release form is not chewed or crushed. It **must be** swallowed whole.
- May open Metadate CD capsules and sprinkle on food
- Store at 15°–30° C (59°–86° F).

**Transdermal**

- Apply patch to hip area 2 h before desired effect and remove not later than 9 h after application. Patch may be removed earlier than 9 h if a shorter duration of effect is desired.

- Alternate application site daily. Do not apply under tight clothing.

## ADVERSE EFFECTS (≥1%) CNS:

Dizziness, drowsiness, *nervousness, insomnia,* irritability, headache, emotional lability, anxiety, tremor. **CV:** Palpitations, changes in BP and pulse rate, angina, cardiac arrhythmias, exacerbation of underlying CV conditions. **Special Senses:** Difficulty with accommodation, blurred vision. **GI:** Dry throat, anorexia, nausea, vomiting, xerostomia, hepatotoxicity, abdominal pain, decreased appetite, xerostomia, weight loss. **Body as a Whole:** Hypersensitivity reactions (rash, fever, arthralgia, urticaria, ex foliative dermatitis, erythema multiforme), decreased libido, long-term growth suppression. **Respiratory:** Nasopharyngitis, cough, URI.

## INTERACTIONS Drug: MAO INHIBI-

TORS may cause hypertensive crisis; antagonizes effects of ANTIHYPERTENSIVES, potentiates action of CNS STIMULANTS (e.g., **amphetamine, caffeine**); may inhibit metabolism and increase serum levels of **fosphenytoin, phenytoin, phenobarbital,** and **primidone, warfarin,** TRICYCLIC ANTIDEPRESSANTS. Could cause serotonin syndrome with other serotenergic drugs (e.g., SSRIs).

## PHARMACOKINETICS Absorp-

**tion:** Readily from GI tract. Transdermal absorption increased with heat or inflamed skin. **Peak:** 1.9 h; 4–7 h sustained release, 2 h transdermal. **Duration:** 3–6 h; 8 h sustained release. **Elimination:** In urine.

## NURSING IMPLICATIONS

### Black Box Warning

*Methylphenidate has been associated with development of marked*

*tolerance, dependence, abnormal behavior, and psychotic episodes; and with severe depression following withdrawal from abusive use.*

### Assessment & Drug Effects

- Monitor BP and pulse at appropriate intervals.
- Monitor closely patient with a history of drug dependence or alcoholism. Chronic abusive use can lead to tolerance, psychic dependence, and psychoses.
- Supervise drug withdrawal carefully following prolonged use. Abrupt withdrawal may result in severe depression and psychotic behavior.
- Monitor lab tests: Periodic CBC with differential and platelet count; periodic LFTs during first 6–12 wk of therapy.

### Patient & Family Education

- Report adverse effects to prescriber, particularly nervousness and insomnia. These effects may diminish with time or require reduction of dosage or omission of afternoon or evening dose.
- Check weight at least 2 or 3 × weekly and report weight loss. Check height and weight in children; failure to gain in either should be reported to prescriber.
- Withhold patch from an ADHD child who exhibits anxiety, tension or agitation. Consult prescriber.
- Do not apply heat or heating pad over area where patch is located.

## METHYLPREDNISOLONE

(meth-ill-pred-niss'oh-lone)
Medrol

## METHYLPREDNISOLONE ACETATE

Depo-Medrol

---

## METHYLPREDNISOLONE SODIUM SUCCINATE
A-Methapred, Solu-Medrol

**Classifications:** BIOLOGICAL RESPONSE MODIFIER; ADRENAL CORTICOSTEROID; GLUCOCORTICOID
Therapeutic: GLUCOCORTICOID; ANTI-INFLAMMATORY
**Prototype:** Prednisone

## AVAILABILITY **Methylprednisolone:** Tablet. **Methylprednisolone Acetate:** Solution for injection. **Methylprednisolone Sodium Succinate:** Powder for injection

## ACTION & *THERAPEUTIC EFFECT*
Intermediate-acting synthetic adrenal corticosteroid with glucocorticoid activity. It inhibits phagocytosis, and release of allergic substances. It also modifies the immune response of the body to various stimuli. Sodium succinate form is characterized by rapid onset of action and is used for emergency therapy of short duration. *Has antiinflammatory and immunosuppressive properties.*

## USES
An anti-inflammatory agent in the management of acute and chronic inflammatory diseases, for palliative management of neoplastic diseases, and for control of severe acute and chronic allergic processes. *High-dose, short-term therapy:* Management of acute bronchial asthma, prevention of fat embolism in patient with long-bone fracture. Short-term management of rheumatic disorders.

## UNLABELED USES
Acetate form used as a long-acting contraceptive and for spinal cord injury, lupus nephritis, multiple sclerosis.

## CONTRAINDICATIONS
Hypersensitivity to corticosteroid drugs; Kaposi sarcoma; systemic fungal infections; use of solutions with benzyl alcohol preservative for premature infants or neonates.

## CAUTIOUS USE
Cushing's syndrome; GI disease, GI ulceration; hepatic disease; renal disease; hypertension; varicella, vaccinia; CHF; diabetes mellitus; ocular herpes simplex; glaucoma; coagulopathy; emotional instability or psychotic tendencies; pregnacy (category C); lactation.

## ROUTE & DOSAGE

### Inflammation
*Adult:* **PO** 2–60 mg/day in 1 or more divided doses; **IM** (Acetate) 10–80 mg/wk weekly or every other week; (Succinate) 10–80 mg daily; **IV** 10–40 mg prn or 30 mg/kg q4–6h × 48 h
*Child:* **PO/IM/IV** 0.5–1.7 mg/kg/day divided q6–12h

### Status Asthmaticus
*Adult/Child:* **IV** 2 mg/kg then 1–5 mg/kg qh

### Acute Spinal Cord Injury
*Adult/Child:* **IV** 30 mg/kg over 15 min, followed in 45 min by 5.4 mg/kg/h × 23 h

### *Obesity Dosage Adjustment*
Dose based on IBW if lower than actual weight

## ADMINISTRATION
### Oral
- Crush tablet before and give with fluid of patient's choice.
- Note: Preparation less irritating if given with food.
- Use alternate day therapy when given over long period.

Common adverse effects in *italic;* life-threatening effects <u>underlined</u>; generic names in **bold;** classifications in SMALL CAPS; ♣ Canadian drug name; ⊙ Prototype drug

### Intramuscular
- Use methylprednisolone acetate for IM injection.
- Give injection deep into large muscle (not deltoid).

### Intravenous
Use methylprednisolone sodium succinate for IV administration.

*PREPARE:* **Direct/Intermittent:** Available in ACT-O-Vial from which the desired dose may be withdrawn after initial dilution with supplied diluent. • May be further diluted according to prescriber's orders. Recommended dilution is 0.25 mg/mL.

*ADMINISTER:* **Direct:** Give each 500 mg or fraction thereof over 2–3 min. **Intermittent:** Give over 15–30 min.

*INCOMPATIBILITIES:* **Solution/additive: Dextrose 5%/sodium chlo-ride 0.45%, aminophylline, calcium gluconate, glycopyrrolate, metaraminol, nafcillin, penicillin G sodium. Y-site: Allopurinol, amsacrine, ciprofloxacin, cisatracurium** (2 mg/mL or greater concentration), **diltiazem, docetaxel, etoposide, filgrastim, fenoldopam, gemcitabine, ondansetron, paclitaxel, potassium chloride, propofol, sargramostim, vinorelbine.**

- Store at 15°–30° C (59°–86° F). Do not freeze.

## ADVERSE EFFECTS (≥1%) **CNS:** Euphoria, headache, insomnia, confusion, psychosis. **CV:** CHF, edema. **GI:** Nausea, vomiting, peptic ulcer. **Musculoskeletal:** Muscle weakness, delayed wound healing, muscle wasting, osteoporosis, aseptic necrosis of bone, spontaneous fractures. **Endocrine:** Cushingoid features, growth suppression in children, carbohydrate intolerance, hyperglycemia. **Special**

**Senses:** Cataracts. **Hematologic:** Leukocytosis. **Metabolic:** Hypokalemia.

## INTERACTIONS **Drug: Amphotericin B, furosemide,** THIAZIDE DIURETICS increase potassium loss; with ATTENUATED VIRUS VACCINES, may enhance virus replication or increase vaccine adverse effects; **isoniazid, phenytoin, phenobarbital, rifampin** decrease effectiveness of methylprednisolone because they increase metabolism of STEROIDS.

## PHARMACOKINETICS **Absorption:** Readily absorbed from GI tract. **Peak:** 1–2 h PO; 4–8 days IM. **Duration:** 1.25–1.5 days PO; 1–5 wk IM. **Metabolism:** In liver. **Half-Life:** Greater than 3.5 h; HPA suppression: 18–36 h.

## NURSING IMPLICATIONS

### Assessment & Drug Effects
- Monitor diabetics for loss of glycemic control.
- Monitor serum potassium and report S&S of hypokalemia (see Appendix F).
- Monitor for and report S&S of Cushing's syndrome (see Appendix F).
- Monitor lab tests: Periodic LFTs, renal function tests, thyroid function tests, CBC, serum electrolytes, and total cholesterol.

### Patient & Family Education
- Consult prescriber for any of the following: Slow wound healing, significant insomnia or confusion, or unexplained bone pain.
- Do not alter established dosage regimen (i.e., not to increase, decrease, or omit doses or change dose intervals). Withdrawal symptoms (rebound inflammation, fever) can be induced with sudden discontinuation of therapy.
- Report onset of signs of hypocorticism adrenal insufficiency immediately: Fatigue, nausea, anorexia, joint pain, muscular weakness, dizziness, fever.

M

---

Common adverse effects in *italic;* life-threatening effects underlined; generic names in **bold;** classifications in SMALL CAPS; ♣ Canadian drug name; ⊘ Prototype drug

1043

# METHYLTESTOSTERONE

(meth-ill-tess-toss'te-rone)

**Android, Metandren ✤, Testred, Virilon**

**Classification:** ANDROGEN/ANABOLIC STEROID

**Therapeutic:** ANABOLIC STEROID

**Prototype:** Testosterone

**Controlled Substance:** Schedule III

## AVAILABILITY Tablet

## ACTION & *THERAPEUTIC EFFECT*

Stimulates receptors in organs and tissues to promote growth and development of male sex organs and maintains secondary sex characteristics in androgen-deficient males. *Androgen activity is similar to testosterone; used in replacement therapy, and palliative treatment of postmenopausal female hormone responsive breast cancer.*

**USES** Androgen replacement therapy, delayed puberty (male), palliation of female mammary cancer (1–5 y postmenopausal), postpartum breast engorgement.

## CONTRAINDICATIONS Liver
dysfunction; prostate cancer; severe cardiac, renal, or hepatic disease; pregnancy (category X); lactation.

## CAUTIOUS USE Mild or moderate
liver, kidney, or cardiac dysfunction; heart failure, diabetes mellitus; prostatic hypertrophy.

## ROUTE & DOSAGE

**Replacement**

*Adult:* **PO** 10–50 mg/day in divided doses

**Breast Cancer**

*Adult:* **PO** 50–200 mg/day in divided doses for duration of therapeutic response or no longer than 3 mo if no remission

**Postpartum Breast Engorgement**

*Adult:* **PO** 80 mg/day for 3–5 days

## ADMINISTRATION

### Oral

- Place buccal tablets between cheek and gum. Ensure that tablet is absorbed, not chewed or swallowed; and eating or drinking avoided until absorption is complete.
- Store at 15°–30° C (59°–86° F). Avoid freezing.

## ADVERSE EFFECTS (≥1%) GI:
Cholestatic hepatitis with jaundice, irritation of oral mucosa with buccal administration. **Urogenital:** Renal calculi (especially in immobilized patient), priapism. **Endocrine:** *Acne, gynecomastia, edema,* oligospermia, menstrual irregularities.

## INTERACTIONS Drug: Increases
risk of bleeding associated with ORAL ANTICOAGULANTS; possibly increases risk of **cyclosporine** toxicity; may decrease glucose level, making adjustment of doses of **insulin,** SULFONYLUREAS necessary. **Herbal: Echinacea** may increase risk of hepatotoxicity.

## PHARMACOKINETICS Absorp-
**tion:** Readily from GI tract. **Metabolism:** In liver. **Elimination:** In urine.

## NURSING IMPLICATIONS

### Assessment & Drug Effects

- Report signs of hepatic toxicity (see Appendix F).
- Monitor for flank pain, abdominal pain radiating to groin, or other symptoms of renal calculi.
- Monitor lab tests: Periodic LFTs.

### Patient & Family Education

- Be prepared for distressing and undesirable adverse effects of virilization (women) since dosage sufficient to produce remission in breast cancer is quantitatively similar to that used for androgen replacement in the male.

- Report signs of virilism promptly. Voice change and hirsutism may be irreversible, even after drug is withdrawn.
- Report priapism (men) or other signs of excess sexual stimulation. The prescriber will terminate therapy.
- Report symptoms of jaundice with or without pruritus to prescriber; appears to be dose related. If liver function tests are altered at the same time, this drug will be withdrawn.

## METIPRANOLOL HYDROCHLORIDE

(me-ti-pran'ol-ol)

OptiPranolol

See Appendix A-1.

## METOCLOPRAMIDE HYDROCHLORIDE ℗

(met-oh-kloe-pra'mide)

Emex ♦, Maxeran ♦, Metozolv ODT, Octamide PFS, Reglan

**Classifications:** GI STIMULANT; PROKINETIC AGENT

Therapeutic: GI STIMULANT; ANTIEMETIC

AVAILABILITY Tablet; solution; injection; orally disintegrating tablet

## ACTION & THERAPEUTIC EFFECT

Potent central dopamine receptor antagonist that increases resting tone of esophageal sphincter, and tone and amplitude of upper GI contractions. Thus gastric emptying and intestinal transit are accelerated. Antiemetic action results from drug-induced elevation of CTZ threshold and enhanced gastric emptying. *Effective as an antiemetic agent as part of a chemotherapy regimen. In diabetic gastroparesis, it relieves anorexia, nausea, vomiting, or persistent fullness after meals.*

USES Management of diabetic gastric stasis (gastroparesis); to prevent nausea and vomiting associated with emetogenic cancer chemotherapy (e.g., cisplatin, dacarbazine) or surgery; to facilitate intubation of small bowel; symptomatic treatment of gastroesophageal reflux.

UNLABELED USES Tourette's syndrome, hiccups.

CONTRAINDICATIONS Sensitivity or intolerance to metoclopramide; uncontrolled seizures; allergy to sulfiting agents; pheochromocytoma; mechanical GI obstruction or perforation; ileus; symptomatic control of tardive dyskinesia; lactation.

CAUTIOUS USE CHF, cardiac disease; sulfite hypersensitivity, asthma, hypokalemia, hypertension; history of depression; hepatic disease, infertility, methemoglobin reductase deficiency, Parkinson's disease, kidney dysfunction; GI hemorrhage; G6PD deficiency, procainamide hypersensitivity, seizure disorder, seizures, tardive dyskinesia; history of intermittent porphyria; older adults; pregnancy (category B); longer than 12 wk; children.

## ROUTE & DOSAGE

| Gastroesophageal Reflux |
|---|
| *Adult:* **PO** 10–15 mg q.i.d. a.c. and at bedtime |
| *Child:* **PO** 0.1–0.2 mg/kg q.i.d. |

---

### Diabetic Gastroparesis

*Adult:* **PO/IV/IM** 10 mg q.i.d. a.c. and at bedtime for 2–8 wk
*Geriatric:* **PO** 5 mg a.c and at bedtime

### Small-Bowel Intubation, Radiologic Examination

*Adult:* **IM/IV** 10 mg administered over 1–2 min
*Child (younger than 6 y):* **IM/IV** 0.1 mg/kg over 1–2 min; *6–14 y:* 2.5–5 mg over 1–2 min

### Chemotherapy-Induced Emesis

*Adult:* **PO** 20–40 mg q4–6h, may repeat; **IM/IV** 2 mg/kg 30 min before antineoplastic administration, may repeat q2h for 2 doses, then q3h for 3 doses if needed

### Postoperative Nausea/Vomiting

*Adult:* **IM/IV** 10–20 mg near end of surgery

## ADMINISTRATION

### Oral

- Give 30 min before meals and at bedtime.
- Remove orally disintegrating tablet (ODT) from blister immediately before use. Place on tongue. ODT will melt and should then be swallowed.

### Intramuscular

- Give deep IM into a large muscle.

### Intravenous

Note: Verify correct IV concentration and rate of infusion for administration to infants or children with prescriber.

***PREPARE:*** **Direct:** Doses of 10 mg or less may be given undiluted. **IV Infusion:** Doses greater than 10 mg IV should be diluted in at least 50 mL of D5W, NS, D5/0.45% NaCl, LR or other compatible solution.

***ADMINISTER:*** **Direct:** Give over 1–2 min (or longer in pediatric patients). **IV Infusion:** Give over not less than 15 min.

***INCOMPATIBILITIES:*** **Solution/additive:** Calcium gluconate, chloramphenicol, cisplatin, dexamethasone, diphenhydramine, erythromycin, floxacillin, fluorouracil, furosemide, lorazepam, methotrexate, penicillin G potassium, sodium bicarbonate, TETRACYCLINES. **Y-site:** Allopurinol, amphotericin B cholesteryl complex, amsacrine, carmustine, cefepime, ceftobiprole, dantrolene, diazepam, diazoxide, doxorubicin liposome, furosemide, ganciclovir, gemtuzumab, milrinone acetate, lansoprazole, phenytoin, propofol, sulfamethoxazole/trimethoprim, TPN.

- Discard open ampules; do not store for future use. ■ Store at 15°–30° C (59°–86° F) in light-resistant bottle. Tablets are stable for 3 y; solutions and injections, for 5 y.

## ADVERSE EFFECTS (≥1%) CNS:

*Mild sedation, fatigue, restlessness,* agitation, headache, insomnia, disorientation, *extrapyramidal symptoms* (acute dystonic type), tardive dyskinesia, neurologic malignant syndrome with injection. **GI:** Nausea, constipation, *diarrhea,* dry mouth, altered drug absorption. **Skin:** Urticarial or maculopapular rash. **Body as a Whole:** Glossal or periorbital edema. **Hematologic:** Methemoglobinemia. **Endocrine:** Galactorrhea, gynecomastia, amenorrhea, impotence. **CV:** <u>Hypertensive crisis</u> (rare).

## DIAGNOSTIC TEST INTERFERENCE

Metoclopramide may interfere with gonadorelin test by increasing ***serum prolactin*** levels.

Common adverse effects in *italic;* life-threatening effects <u>underlined;</u> generic names in **bold;** classifications in SMALL CAPS; ♥ Canadian drug name; ⊕ Prototype drug

**INTERACTIONS Drug: Alcohol** and other CNS DEPRESSANTS add to sedation; ANTICHOLINERGICS, OPIATE ANALGESICS may antagonize effect on GI motility; PHENOTHIAZINES may potentiate extrapyramidal symptoms; may decrease absorption of **acetaminophen, aspirin, atovaquone, diazepam, digoxin, lithium, tetracycline;** may antagonize the effects of **amantadine, bromocriptine, levodopa, pergolide, ropinirole, pramipexole;** may cause increase in extrapyramidal and dystonic reactions with PHENOTHIAZINES, THIOANTHENES, **droperidol, haloperidol, loxapine, metyrosine;** may prolong neuromuscular blocking effects of **succinylcholine.**

**PHARMACOKINETICS Absorption:** Readily from GI tract. **Onset:** 30–60 min PO; 10–15 min IM; 1–3 min IV. **Peak:** 1–2 h. **Duration:** 1–3 h. **Distribution:** To most body tissues including CNS; crosses placenta; distributed into breast milk. **Metabolism:** Minimally in liver. **Elimination:** 95% in urine, 5% in feces. **Half-Life:** 2.5–6 h.

## NURSING IMPLICATIONS

### Black Box Warning

*Metoclopramide has been associated with tardive dyskinesia. Discontinue metoclopramide in patients who develop S&S of tardive dyskinesia.*

### Assessment & Drug Effects

▪ Report immediately the onset of restlessness, involuntary movements, facial grimacing, rigidity, or tremors. Extrapyramidal symptoms are most likely to occur in children, young adults, and the older adult and with high-dose treatment of vomiting associated with cancer chemotherapy. Symptoms can take months to regress.

▪ Monitor for possible hypernatremia and hypokalemia (see Appendix F), especially if patient has HF or cirrhosis.

▪ Monitor lab tests: Periodic serum electrolytes.

### Patient & Family Education

▪ Report S&S of acute dystonia, such as trembling hands and facial grimacing (see Appendix F), immediately.

▪ Avoid driving and other potentially hazardous activities for a few hours after drug administration.

▪ Avoid alcohol and other CNS depressants.

▪ Adverse reactions associated with increased serum prolactin concentration (galactorrhea, menstrual disorders, gynecomastia) usually disappear within a few weeks or months after drug treatment is stopped.

M

## METOLAZONE

(me-tole'a-zone)

Zaroxolyn ♦

**Classifications:** THIAZIDE DIURETIC; ANTIHYPERTENSIVE

**Therapeutic:** DIURETIC; ANTIHYPERTENSIVE

**Prototype:** Hydrochlorothiazide

### AVAILABILITY Tablet

### ACTION & *THERAPEUTIC EFFECT*

Diuretic action is associated with interference with transport of sodium ions across renal tubular epithelium. This enhances excretion of sodium, chloride, potassium, bicarbonate, and water. *Produces a decrease in the systolic and diastolic BPs, and reduces edema in CHF and kidney failure patients.*

---

Common adverse effects in *italic*; life-threatening effects underlined; generic names in **bold**; classifications in SMALL CAPS; ♦ Canadian drug name; ⊘ Prototype drug

**USES** Management of hypertension as sole agent or to enhance effectiveness of other antihypertensives in severe form of hypertension; also edema associated with CHF and kidney disease.

**CONTRAINDICATIONS** Hypersensitivity to metolazone and sulfonamides; anuria, hypokalemia; hepatic coma or precoma; SLE; pregnancy (category D); lactation.

**CAUTIOUS USE** History of gout; allergies; kidney and liver dysfunction; older adults; children.

## ROUTE & DOSAGE

**Edema**

*Adult:* **PO** 5–20 mg/day
*Child:* **PO** 0.2–0.4 mg/kg/day divided q12–24h

**Hypertension**

*Adult:* **PO** 2.5–5 mg/day

## ADMINISTRATION

**Oral**

- Do not interchange slow availability tablets and rapid availability tablets. They are not equivalent.
- Schedule doses to avoid nocturia and interrupted sleep. Give early in a.m. after eating to prevent gastric irritation (if given in 2 doses, schedule second dose no later than 3 p.m.).
- Store at 15°–30° C (59°–86° F) in tightly closed container.

**ADVERSE EFFECTS** (≥1%) **GI:** Cholestatic jaundice. **Body as a Whole:** Vertigo, orthostatic hypotension. **Hematologic:** Venous thrombosis, leukopenia. **Metabolic:** Dehydration, *hypokalemia, hyperuricemia, hyperglycemia.*

**INTERACTIONS Drug: Amphotericin B**, CORTICOSTEROIDS increase hypokalemic effects; may antagonize hypoglycemic effects of SULFONYLUREAS, **insulin; cholestyramine, colestipol** decrease thiazide absorption; intensifies hypoglycemic and hypotensive effects of **diazoxide;** because of increased potassium and magnesium loss, may cause **digoxin** toxicity; decreases **lithium** excretion, increasing its toxicity; NSAIDs may attenuate diuresis—increased risk of NSAID-induced kidney failure.

**PHARMACOKINETICS Absorption:** Incomplete. **Onset:** 1 h. **Peak:** 2–8 h. **Duration:** 12–24 h. **Distribution:** Distributed throughout extracellular tissue; concentrates in kidney; crosses placenta; distributed in breast milk. **Metabolism:** Does not appear to be metabolized. **Elimination:** In urine. **Half-Life:** 14 h.

## NURSING IMPLICATIONS

**Assessment & Drug Effects**

- Anticipate overdosage and adverse reactions in geriatric patients; may be more sensitive to effects of usual adult dose.
- Terminate therapy when adverse reactions are moderate to severe.
- Expect possible antihypertensive effects in 3 or 4 days, but 3–4 wk are required for maximum effect.
- Monitor lab tests: Periodic serum potassium, plasma glucose, and urinalysis.

**Patient & Family Education**

- Do not drink alcohol; it potentiates orthostatic hypotension.
- Antihypertensive therapy may require as adjunct a high-potassium, low-sodium, and low-calorie diet.
- Include potassium-rich foods in the diet.

- Be aware that if hypokalemia develops, dietary potassium supplement of 1000–2000 mg (25–50 mEq) is usually adequate treatment.

## METOPROLOL TARTRATE

(me-toe′proe-lole)

Apo-Metoprolol ♦, Betaloc ♦, Lopressor, Toprol XL

**Classifications:** CARDIOSELECTIVE; BETA-ADRENERGIC ANTAGONIST; ANTIHYPERTENSIVE; ANTIANGINAL
**Therapeutic:** ANTIHYPERTENSIVE; ANTIANGINAL
**Prototype:** Propranolol

**AVAILABILITY** Tablet; sustained release tablet; solution for injection

## ACTION & THERAPEUTIC EFFECT

Beta-adrenergic antagonist with preferential effect on beta$_1$ receptors located primarily on cardiac muscle. Antihypertensive action may be due to competitive antagonism of catecholamines at cardiac adrenergic neuron sites, drug-induced reduction of sympathetic outflow to the periphery, and to suppression of renin activity. *Reduces heart rate and cardiac output at rest and during exercise; lowers both supine and standing BP, slows sinus rate, and decreases myocardial automaticity. Antianginal effect is like that of propranolol.*

**USES** Management of mild to severe hypertension, treatment of heart failure, long-term treatment of angina pectoris and prophylactic management of stable angina pectoris reduce the risk of mortality after an MI.

**UNLABELED USES** CHF, migraine prophylaxis, arrythmias.

**CONTRAINDICATIONS** Hypersensitivity to metoprolol or other beta blockers; cardiogenic shock, severe bradycardia, advanced AV block without a pacemaker, bradycardia, sick sinus syndrome; pheochromocytoma, moderate to severe cardiac failure, right ventricular failure secondary to pulmonary hypertension; abrupt discontinuation; lactation.

**CAUTIOUS USE** Severe impairment of liver function; cardiomegaly, CHF controlled by digitalis and diuretics; major surgery; mental illness; bronchial asthma and other bronchospastic diseases; thyrotoxicosis, hyperthyroidism; moderate to severe cholesterol concentrations; elevated triglycerides; DM; PVD; MG; cerebrovascular insufficiency; pregnancy (category C), children younger than 6 y.

## ROUTE & DOSAGE

### Hypertension

*Adult:* **PO** 50–100 mg/day in 1–2 divided doses, may increase weekly up to 100–450 mg/day
*Geriatric:* **PO** 25 mg/day (range: 25–300 mg/day)
*Child (6 y or older):* **PO** 1 mg/kg daily (max: 200 mg)

### Angina Pectoris

*Adult:* **PO** 100 mg/day in 2 divided doses, may increase weekly up to 100–400 mg/day

### Heart Failure

*Adult:* **PO** 12.5–25 mg/day × 2 wk, then adjust dose

### Myocardial Infarction

*Adult:* **IV** 5 mg q2min for 3 doses, followed by PO therapy; **PO** 50 mg q6h for 48 h, then 100 mg b.i.d.

---

Common adverse effects in *italic;* life-threatening effects underlined; generic names in **bold;** classifications in SMALL CAPS; ♦ Canadian drug name; ⓟ Prototype drug

M

## ADMINISTRATION

### Oral

- Ensure that sustained-release form is not chewed or crushed. It **must be** swallowed whole.
- Give with food to slightly enhance absorption; however, administration with food not essential. It is important to give with or without food consistently to minimize possible variations in bioavailability.

### Intravenous

*PREPARE:* **Direct:** Give undiluted.
*ADMINISTER:* **Direct:** Give at a rate of 5 mg over 60 sec. ▪ Note conditions which are contraindications to drug administration.
*INCOMPATIBILITIES:* **Y-site: Allopurinol, amphotericin, B cholesteryl complex, dantrolene, diazepam, diazoxide, gemtuzumab, haloperidol, lepirudin, pantoprazole, phenytoin, SMZ/TMP.**

- Store at 15°–30° C (59°–86° F). Protect from heat, light, and moisture.

## ADVERSE EFFECTS (≥1%) **Body as a Whole:** Hypersensitivity (erythematous rash, fever, headache, muscle aches, sore throat, laryngospasm, respiratory distress). **CNS:** *Dizziness, fatigue, insomnia,* increased dreaming, mental depression. **CV:** *Bradycardia,* palpitation, cold extremities, Raynaud's phenomenon, intermittent claudication, angina pectoris, CHF, intensification of AV block, AV dissociation, complete heart block, cardiac arrest. **GI:** Nausea, *heartburn,* gastric pain, diarrhea or constipation, flatulence. **Hematologic:** Eosinophilia, thrombocytopenic and nonthrombocytopenic purpura, agranulocytosis (rare). **Skin:** Dry skin, pruritus, skin eruptions. **Special Senses:** Dry mouth and mucous membranes. **Metabolic:** Hypoglycemia. **Respiratory:** Bronchospasm (with high doses), *shortness of breath.*

## DIAGNOSTIC TEST INTERFERENCE

In common with other beta-blockers, metoprolol may cause elevated **BUN** or **serum creatinine levels** (patients with severe heart disease), elevated **serum transaminase, alkaline phosphatase, lactate dehydrogenase,** and **serum uric acid.**

## INTERACTIONS **Drug:** BARBITURATES, **rifampin** may decrease effects of metoprolol; **cimetidine, methimazole, propylthiouracil,** ORAL CONTRACEPTIVES may increase effects of metoprolol; additive bradycardia with **digoxin;** effects of both metoprolol and **hydralazine** may be increased; **indomethacin** may attenuate hypotensive response; BETA AGONISTS and metoprolol mutually antagonistic; **verapamil** may increase risk of heart block and bradycardia; increases **terbutaline** serum levels.

## PHARMACOKINETICS **Absorption:** Readily from GI tract; 50% of dose reaches systemic circulation. **Onset:** 15 min. **Peak:** 1.5 h; 20 min (IV). **Duration:** 13–19 h. **Distribution:** Crosses blood–brain barrier and placenta; distributed into breast milk. **Metabolism:** Extensively in liver (CYP2D6). **Elimination:** In urine. **Half-Life:** 3–4 h.

## NURSING IMPLICATIONS

### Black Box Warning

*Metoprolol has been associated with exacerbations of ischemic heart disease when stopped abruptly.*

---

Common adverse effects in *italic*; life-threatening effects underlined; generic names in **bold**; classifications in SMALL CAPS; ♣ Canadian drug name; ◐ Prototype drug

### Assessment & Drug Effects

- Take apical pulse and BP before administering drug. Report to prescriber significant changes in rate, rhythm, or quality of pulse or variations in BP prior to administration.
- Monitor BP, HR, and ECG carefully during IV administration.
- Expect maximal effect on BP after 1 wk of therapy.
- Observe hypertensive patients with CHF closely for impending heart failure: Dyspnea on exertion, orthopnea, night cough, edema, distended neck veins.
- Monitor I&O, daily weight; auscultate daily for pulmonary rales.
- Reduce dosage gradually over a period of 1–2 wk when drug is discontinued.
- Monitor lab tests: Baseline and periodic blood cell count, blood glucose, LFTs and renal function tests.

### Patient & Family Education

- Do not abruptly stop taking this drug. Sudden withdrawal can result in increase in anginal attacks and MI in patients with angina pectoris and thyroid storm in patients with hyperthyroidism.
- Learn how to take radial pulse before each dose. Report to prescriber if pulse is slower than base rate (e.g., 60 bpm) or becomes irregular. Consult prescriber for parameters.
- Reduce insomnia or increased dreaming by avoiding late evening doses.
- Monitor blood glucose (diabetics) for loss of glycemic control. Drug may mask some symptoms of hypoglycemia (e.g., BP and HR changes) and prolong hypoglycemia. Be alert to other possible signs of hypoglycemia not affected by metoprolol and report to prescriber if present: Sweating, fatigue, hunger, inability to concentrate.

- Report immediately to prescriber the onset of problems with vision.
- Relieve eye dryness by using sterile artificial tears available OTC.
- Do not drive or engage in potentially hazardous activities until response to drug is known.

## METRONIDAZOLE ⓟ
(me-troe-ni'da-zole)

Flagyl, Flagyl ER, Metro-Cream, MetroGel, MetroLotion, Nuvessa, Rosadan, Vandazole

**Classifications:** ANTITRICHOMONAL; AMEBICIDE

Therapeutic: AMEBICIDE; ANTIBACTERIAL

**AVAILABILITY** Tablet; capsule; sustained release tablet; vial; lotion; emulsion; cream; gel

### ACTION & THERAPEUTIC EFFECT

Interacts with DNA to cause loss of DNA structure and strand breakage resulting in inhibition of protein synthesis and cell death in susceptible organisms. *Has direct trichomonacidal and amebicidal activity; exhibits antibacterial activity against obligate anaerobic bacteria, gram-negative anaerobic bacilli, and* Clostridia.

### USES
Asymptomatic and symptomatic trichomoniasis in females and males; acute intestinal amebiasis and amebic liver abscess; preoperative prophylaxis in colorectal surgery, elective hysterectomy or vaginal repair, and emergency appendectomy. **IV:** Serious infections caused by susceptible anaerobic bacteria in intra-abdominal infections, skin

Common adverse effects in *italic;* life-threatening effects <u>underlined</u>; generic names in **bold;** classifications in SMALL CAPS; ◆ Canadian drug name; ⓟ Prototype drug

1051

infections, gynecologic infections, septicemia, and for both pre- and postoperative prophylaxis, bacterial vaginosis. **Topical:** Rosacea.

## UNLABELED USES
Treatment of pseudomembranous colitis, Crohn's disease, *H. pylori* eradication, bacterial vaginosis prophylaxis, gastric ulcer, pelvic inflammatory disease.

## CONTRAINDICATIONS
Hypersensitivity to metronidazole or other nitroimidazole drugs; use of disulfiram within 2 wk; use of alcohol within 24 h; development of abnormal neurologic signs; first trimester of pregnancy; lactation.

## CAUTIOUS USE
Coexistent candidiasis; CNS disorders; seizure disorders; heart failure; severe hepatic impairment; QT prolongation; severe renal impairment/failure; alcoholism; liver disease; older adults.

## ROUTE & DOSAGE

**Trichomoniasis**

*Adult:* **PO** 2 g once or 500 mg b.i.d. × 7 days

**Giardiasis, *Gardnerella***

*Adult:* **PO** 500 mg b.i.d. × 7 days or 750 ER tablet daily × 7 days
**Vaginal** Once or twice daily × 5 days

**Pelvic Inflammatory Disease (with other antibiotics)**

*Adult:* **PO** 500 mg b.i.d. x 14 days

**Amebiasis**

*Adult:* **PO** 500–750 mg t.i.d. × 5–10 days

*Child:* **PO** 35–50 mg/kg/day in 3 divided doses × 10 days

**Anaerobic Infections**

*Adult:* **PO** 7.5 mg/kg q6h (max: 4 g/day); **IV** 15 mg/kg; then 7.5 mg/kg q6h (max: 4 g/day)
*Child:* **PO** 30-50 mg/kg/day divided q6-8h (max: 4 g/day); **IV** 22.5–40 mg/kg/day divided q8h
*Neonate (weight less than 1.2 kg):* **IV**

**Rosacea**

*Adult:* **Topical** Apply 0.75% gel as a thin film to affected area b.i.d.; apply 1% gel as a thin film to affected area daily

## ADMINISTRATION

### Oral
- Crush tablets before ingestion if patient cannot swallow whole.
- Ensure that Flagyl ER (extended release form) is not chewed or crushed. It **must be** swallowed whole. Give on an empty stomach, 1 h before or 2 h after meals.
- Give immediately before, with, or immediately after meals or with food or milk to reduce GI distress.
- Give lower than normal doses in presence of liver disease.

### Topical
- Apply a thin film to affected area only.

### Intravenous
Note: Verify correct IV concentration and rate of infusion for administration to neonates, infants, or children with prescriber.

***PREPARE:*** **Intermittent:** Single-dose flexible containers (500 mg/100 mL) are ready for use without further dilution.

Common adverse effects in *italic;* life-threatening effects <u>underlined;</u> generic names in **bold;** classifications in SMALL CAPS; ♣ Canadian drug name; ⊙ Prototype drug

*ADMINISTER:* **Intermittent:** Give IV solution slowly over 30–60 min.
*INCOMPATIBILITIES:* **Solution/additive:** TPN, aztreonam. **Y-site: Amphotericin B cholesteryl complex, aztreonam, dantrolene, daptomycin, diazepam, drotecogin, filgrastim, ganciclovir, garenoxacin, lansoprazole, minocycline, pantoprazole, pemetrexed, phenytoin, procainamide, propofol, quinupristin/dalfopristin.**

▪ Note: Precipitation occurs if neutralized solution is refrigerated. ▪ Note: Use diluted and neutralized solution within 24 h of preparation.

▪ Store at 15°–30° C (59°–86° F); protect from light. ▪ Reconstituted Flagyl IV is chemically stable for 96 h when stored below 30° C (86° F) in room light. ▪ Diluted and neutralized IV solutions containing Flagyl IV should be used within 24 h of mixing.

**ADVERSE EFFECTS** (>1%) **Body as a Whole:** Hypersensitivity (rash, urticaria, pruritus, flushing), fever, fleeting joint pains, bacterial infection, overgrowth of *Candida*. **CNS:** Vertigo, headache, ataxia, confusion, irritability, depression, restlessness, weakness, fatigue, drowsiness, insomnia, paresthesias, sensory neuropathy (rare). **GI:** *Nausea,* vomiting, anorexia, epigastric distress, abdominal cramps, diarrhea, constipation, dry mouth, metallic taste, proctitis. **Urogenital:** Polyuria, dysuria, pyuria, incontinence, cystitis, decreased libido, dysmenorrhea, dryness of vagina and vulva, sense of pelvic pressure, vaginitis. **Special Senses:** Nasal congestion. **CV:** ECG changes (flattening of T wave).

## DIAGNOSTIC TEST INTERFERENCE

**Metronidazole** may interfere with certain chemical analyses for *AST,* resulting in decreased values.

## INTERACTIONS **Drug:** ORAL ANTICOAGULANTS potentiate hypoprothrombinemia; **alcohol** may elicit disulfiram reaction; oral solutions of **citalopram, ritonavir; lopinavir/ritonavir,** and IV formulations of **sulfamethoxazole; trimethoprim, nitroglycerin** may elicit disulfiram reaction due to the alcohol content of the dosage form; **disulfiram** causes acute psychosis; **phenobarbital** increases metronidazole metabolism; may increase **lithium** levels; **fluorouracil, azathioprine** may cause transient neutropenia. Use with **ziprasidone** could increase QT prolongation. **Warfarin** effects can be increased.

## PHARMACOKINETICS **Absorption:** 80% absorbed from GI tract. **Peak:** 1–3 h. **Distribution:** Widely distributed to most body tissues, including CSF, bone, cerebral and hepatic abscesses; crosses placenta; distributed in breast milk. **Metabolism:** 30–60% in liver. **Elimination:** 77% in urine; 14% in feces within 24 h. **Half-Life:** 6–8 h.

## NURSING IMPLICATIONS

### Assessment & Drug Effects

▪ Discontinue therapy immediately if symptoms of CNS toxicity (see Appendix F) develop. Monitor especially for seizures and peripheral neuropathy (e.g., numbness and paresthesia of extremities).

▪ Monitor for S&S of sodium retention, especially in patients on corticosteroid therapy or with a history of CHF.

▪ Monitor patients on lithium for elevated lithium levels.

**M**

---

- Report appearance of candidiasis or its becoming more prominent with therapy to prescriber promptly.
- Repeat feces examinations, usually up to 3 mo, to ensure that amebae have been eliminated.
- Monitor lab tests: Total and differential WBC counts before, during, and after therapy, especially if a second course is necessary.

**Patient & Family Education**
- Adhere closely to the established regimen without schedule interruption or changing the dose.
- Refrain from intercourse during therapy for trichomoniasis unless male partner wears a condom to prevent reinfection.
- Have sexual partners receive concurrent treatment. Asymptomatic trichomoniasis in the male is a frequent source of reinfection of the female.
- Do not drink alcohol during therapy; may induce a disulfiram-type reaction (see Appendix F). Avoid alcohol or alcohol-containing medications for at least 48 h after treatment is completed.
- Urine may appear dark or reddish brown (especially with higher than recommended doses). This appears to have no clinical significance.
- Report symptoms of candidal overgrowth: Furry tongue, color changes of tongue, glossitis, stomatitis; vaginitis, curd-like, milky vaginal discharge; proctitis. Treatment with a candidacidal agent may be indicated.

# MEXILETINE
(mex-il'e-teen)
Mexitil
**Classification:** CLASS IB ANTI-ARRHYTHMIC

Therapeutic: CLASS IB ANTIARRHYTHMIC
**Prototype:** Lidocaine

## AVAILABILITY Capsule

## ACTION & *THERAPEUTIC EFFECT*
Analog of lidocaine with class IB antiarrhythmic properties. Shortens action potential refractory period duration and improves resting potential. Produces modest suppression of sinus node automatically and AV nodal conduction. Prolongs the histo-ventricular interval only if patient has preexisting conduction disturbance. *Has antiarrhythmic properties for ventricular disturbances.*

**USES** Acute and chronic ventricular arrhythmias; prevention of recurrent cardiac arrests; suppression of PVCs due to ventricular tachyarrhythmias.

**UNLABELED USES** Wolff-Parkinson-White syndrome and supraventricular arrhythmias.

**CONTRAINDICATIONS** Severe left ventricular failure, cardiogenic shock, severe bradyarrhythmias. Preexisting second- or third-degree heart block without pacemaker; cardiogenic shock; lactation.

**CAUTIOUS USE** Patients with sinus node conduction irregularities, intraventricular conduction abnormalities; hypotension; severe congestive heart failure; renal failure; liver dysfunction; pregnancy (category C).

## ROUTE & DOSAGE

| Ventricular Arrhythmias |
| --- |
| *Adult:* **PO** 200–300 mg q8h (max: 1200 mg/day) |
| *Adult:* **PO** 1.4–5 mg/kg q8h |

Common adverse effects in *italic;* life-threatening effects <u>underlined</u>; generic names in **bold**; classifications in SMALL CAPS; ♣ Canadian drug name; ⊙ Prototype drug

## ADMINISTRATION

### Oral
- Give with food or milk to reduce gastric distress.

## ADVERSE EFFECTS (≥1%) CNS:
*Dizziness, tremor, nervousness, incoordination,* headache, blurred vision, paresthesias, numbness. **CV:** <u>Exacerbated arrhythmias</u>, palpitations, chest pain, syncope, hypotension. **GI:** *Nausea, vomiting, heartburn,* diarrhea, constipation, dry mouth, abdominal pain. **Skin:** Rash. **Body as a Whole:** Dyspnea, edema, arthralgia, fever, malaise, hiccups. **Urogenital:** Impotence, urinary retention.

## INTERACTIONS Drug: Phenytoin, phenobarbital, rifampin may decrease mexiletine levels; **cimetidine, fluvoxamine** may increase mexiletine levels; may increase **theophylline** levels; may increase proarrhythmic effects of **dofetilide** (separate administration by at least 1 wk).

## PHARMACOKINETICS Absorption: Readily from GI tract. **Peak:** 2–3 h **Distribution:** Distributed into breast milk. **Metabolism:** In liver. **Elimination:** In urine; renal elimination increases with urinary acidification. **Half-Life:** 10–12 h.

## NURSING IMPLICATIONS

### Black Box Warning

*Mexiletine has been associated with excessive mortality and non-fatal cardiac arrest; therefore, its use should be reserved for patients with life-threatening ventricular arrhythmias.*

### Assessment & Drug Effects
- Check pulse and BP before administration; make sure both are stabilized.
- Effective serum concentration range is 0.5–2 mcg/mL.

- Supervise ambulation in the weak, debilitated patient or the older adult during drug stabilization period. CNS adverse reactions predominate (e.g., intention tremors, nystagmus, blurred vision, dizziness, ataxia, confusion, nausea).
- Encourage drug compliance; affected particularly by the distressing adverse effects of tremor, ataxia, and eye symptoms.
- Check frequently with patient about adherence to drug regimen. If adverse effects are increasing, consult prescriber. Dose adjustment or discontinuation may be needed.
- Monitor lab tests: Baseline and periodic LFTs.

### Patient & Family Education
- Learn about pulse parameters to be reported: Changes in rhythm and rate (bradycardia = pulse below 60); symptomatic bradycardia (light-headedness, syncope, dizziness), and postural hypotension.

## MICAFUNGIN
(my-ca-fun'gin)
Mycamine
**Classification:** ANTIFUNGAL; ECHINOCANDIN
Therapeutic: ANTIFUNGAL
**Prototype:** Caspofungin

## AVAILABILITY Intravenous solution

## ACTION & *THERAPEUTIC EFFECT*
Micafungin is an antifungal agent that inhibits the synthesis of glucan, an essential component of fungal cell walls. Micafungin does not allow *Candida* fungi to replicate. *Has antifungal effects against various species of Candida.*

**USES** Treatment of patients with esophageal candidiasis, and for prophylaxis of *Candida* infections in patients undergoing hematopoietic stem cell transplantation. Susceptible organisms include *C. albicans, C. glabrata, C. krusei, C. parapsilosis,* and *C. tropicalis.*

**UNLABELED USES** Treatment of pulmonary *Aspergillus* infection.

**CONTRAINDICATIONS** Hypersensitivity to any component in micafungin.

**CAUTIOUS USE** Hepatic and renal dysfunction; older adult; pregnancy (category C); lactation; children younger than 4 mo.

## ROUTE & DOSAGE

### Esophageal Candidiasis
*Adult:* **IV** 150 mg/day over 1 h × 14 days

### Candidiasis Prophylaxis in Hematopoietic Stem Cell Transplantation Patients
*Adult:* **IV** 50 mg/day over 1 h × 18 days

### Disseminated Candidiasis
*Child/Infant (older than 4 mo):* **IV** 2 mg/kg daily

## ADMINISTRATION

### Intravenous

*PREPARE:* **IV Infusion:** Reconstitute the 50 or 100 mg vial with 5 mL NS (without a bacteriostatic agent) to yield 10 mg/mL or 20 mg/mL, respectively. ▪ Gently swirl, but do not shake, to dissolve. Solution should be clear. ▪ Add required dose to 100 mL NS.

*ADMINISTER:* **IV Infusion:** Give slowly over 1 h. ▪ Flush existing IV line with NS before/after infusion. ▪ Protect IV solution from light.

*INCOMPATIBILITIES:* Do not mix or infuse with any other medications.

▪ Store reconstituted vial and IV solution for up to 24 h at 25° C (77° F). ▪ Protect from light.

**ADVERSE EFFECTS** (≥1%) **CNS:** *Headache,* dizziness, somnolence. **CV:** Flushing, hypertension, phlebitis. **GI:** *Nausea, vomiting, diarrhea,* abdominal pain. **Hematologic/ Lymphatic:** Anemia, hemolytic anemia, leukemia, neutropenia, thrombocytopenia. **Hepatic:** Elevated liver enzymes, jaundice. **Metabolic:** Hypocalcemia, hypokalemia, hypomagnesemia. **Skin:** Pruritus, rash. **Body as a Whole:** Injection site pain, pyrexia, rigors.

**INTERACTIONS Drug:** Micafungin increases levels of **sirolimus** and **nifedipine.**

**PHARMACOKINETICS Distribution:** 99% protein bound. **Metabolism:** Biotransformation primarily in the liver. **Elimination:** Fecal (major) and renal. **Half-Life:** 14–17 h.

## NURSING IMPLICATIONS

### Assessment & Drug Effects
▪ Monitor for S&S of hypersensitivity during IV infusion; frequently monitor IV site for thrombophlebitis.
▪ Monitor for S&S of hemolytic anemia (i.e., jaundice).
▪ Monitor blood levels of sirolimus or nifedipine with concurrent therapy. If sirolimus or nifedipine toxicity occurs, dosages of these drugs should be reduced.
▪ Monitor lab tests: Periodic LFTs, renal function tests, serum electrolytes, and CBC.

### Patient & Family Education
▪ Report immediately any of the following: Facial swelling, wheezing,

M

difficulty breathing or swallowing, tightness in chest, rash, hives, itching, or sensation of warmth.

## MICONAZOLE NITRATE

(mi-kon'a-zole)

Desenex, Femizol-M, Fungoid, Lotrimin AF, Micatin, Monistat 3, Monistat 7, Monistat-Derm, M-Zole, Tetterine

**Classification:** AZOLE ANTIFUNGAL
**Therapeutic:** ANTIFUNGAL
**Prototype:** Fluconazole

**AVAILABILITY** Vaginal suppository; cream; ointment; powder; spray; solution

## ACTION & *THERAPEUTIC EFFECT*

Broad-spectrum agent with fungicidal activity. Appears to inhibit uptake of components essential for cell reproduction and growth as well as cell wall structure, thus promoting cell death of fungi. *Effective against* Candida albicans *and other species of this genus. Inhibits growth of common dermatophytes, and the organism responsible for tinea versicolor.*

**USES** Vulvovaginal candidiasis, tinea pedis (athlete's foot), tinea cruris, tinea corporis, and tinea versicolor caused by dermatophytes.

**CONTRAINDICATIONS** Hypersensitivity to miconazole.

**CAUTIOUS USE** Hypersensitivity to azole antifungals; diabetes mellitus; bone marrow suppression; pregnancy (category C); lactation; children younger than 2 y **(topical)** and children younger than 12 y **(vaginal).**

## ROUTE & DOSAGE

### Fungal Infection

*Adult:* **Topical** Apply cream sparingly to affected areas twice a day, and once daily for tinea versicolor, for 2 wk (improvement expected in 2–3 days, tinea pedis is treated for 1 mo to prevent recurrence); **Intravaginal** Insert suppository or vaginal cream each night × 7 days (100 mg) or 3 days (200 mg)

## ADMINISTRATION

### Topical

- Apply cream sparingly to intertriginous areas (between skin folds) to avoid maceration of skin.
- Massage affected area gently until cream disappears.
- Store at 15°–30° C (59°–86° F) unless otherwise directed.

**ADVERSE EFFECTS** (≥1%) **Urogenital:** Vulvovaginal burning, itching, or irritation; maceration, allergic contact dermatitis.

**INTERACTIONS Drug:** May increase INR with **warfarin;** may inactivate **nonoxynol-9** spermicides.

**PHARMACOKINETICS Absorption:** Small amount absorbed from vagina. **Metabolism:** Rapidly metabolized in liver. **Elimination:** In urine and feces. **Half-Life:** 2.1–24 h.

## NURSING IMPLICATIONS

### Assessment & Drug Effects

- Expect clinical improvement from topical application in 1 or 2 wk. If no improvement in 4 wk, diagnosis is reevaluated. Treat tinea pedis infection for 1 mo to assure permanent recovery.

**Patient & Family Education**

- Complete full course of treatment to ensure recovery.
- Do not interrupt vaginal application during menstrual period.
- Avoid contact of drug with eyes.

# MIDAZOLAM HYDROCHLORIDE

(mid'az-zoe-lam)

**Classifications:** ANESTHETIC; BENZODIAZEPINE; ANXIOLYTIC; SEDATIVE-HYPNOTIC
Therapeutic: ANESTHETIC; ANTIANXIETY; SEDATIVE-HYPNOTIC
**Prototype:** Lorazepam
**Controlled Substance:** Schedule IV

**AVAILABILITY** Syrup; solution for injection

**ACTION & *THERAPEUTIC EFFECT***
Short-acting benzodiazepine that intensifies activity of gammaaminobenzoic acid (GABA), a major inhibitory neurotransmitter of the brain, interfering with its reuptake and promoting its accumulation at neuronal synapses. Calms the patient, relaxes skeletal muscles, and in high doses produces sleep. *Is a CNS depressant with muscle relaxant, sedative-hypnotic, anticonvulsant, and amnestic properties.*

**USES** Sedation before general anesthesia, induction of general anesthesia; to impair memory of perioperative events (anterograde amnesia); for conscious sedation prior to short diagnostic and endoscopic procedures; and as the hypnotic supplement to nitrous oxide and oxygen (balanced anesthesia) for short surgical procedures.

**CONTRAINDICATIONS** Intolerance to benzodiazepines; acute narrow-angle glaucoma; shock, coma; acute alcohol intoxication; intra-arterial injection; status asthmaticus; pregnancy (category D), obstetric delivery; lactation.

**CAUTIOUS USE** COPD; chronic kidney failure; cardiac disease; pulmonary insufficiency; dementia; electrolyte imbalance; neuromuscular disease; Parkinson's disease; psychosis; CHF; bipolar disorder; older adults.

## ROUTE & DOSAGE

**Conscious Sedation**

*Adult:* **IM** 0.07–0.08 mg/kg 30–60 min before procedure; **IV** 1–2.5 mg, may repeat in 2 min prn; Intubated Patients, 0.05–0.2 mg/kg/h by continuous infusion
*Child:* **IM** 0.08 mg/kg × 1 dose; **PO** 0.3 mg/kg × 1 dose; Intubated Patients, 2 mcg/kg/min by continuous infusion, may increase by 1 mcg/kg/min q30min until light sleep is induced
*Neonate:* **IV** 0.5–1 mcg/kg/min

**IV Induction for General Anesthesia**

*Adult:* **IV** Premedicated, 0.15–0.25 mg/kg over 20–30 sec, allow 2 min for effect; **IV** Non-premedicated, 0.3–0.35 mg/kg over 20–30 sec, allow 2 min for effect
*Child:* **IV** 0.15 mg/kg followed by 0.05 mg/kg q2min × 1–3 doses

**Status Epilepticus**

*Child:* **IV Loading Dose** 2 mo or older: 0.15 mg/kg; **IV Maintenance Dose** 1 mcg/kg/min infusion, may titrate upward as needed q5min

Common adverse effects in *italic*; life-threatening effects underlined; generic names in **bold**; classifications in SMALL CAPS; ♣ Canadian drug name; ⊘ Prototype drug

## Preoperative Sedation

*Child (younger than 5 y):* **PO** 0.5 mg/kg; *5 y or older:* 0.4–0.5 mg/kg

## ADMINISTRATION

### Oral

- Oral route is reserved for children. Use supplied oral dispenser to dispense directly into mouth.
- Do not mix with any liquid prior to dispensing.

### Intramuscular

- Inject IM drug deep into a large muscle mass.

### Intravenous

*PREPARE:* **Direct:** Dilute in D5W or NS to a concentration of 0.25 mg/mL (e.g., 1 mg in 4 mL or 5 mg in 20 mL). **IV Infusion:** Add 5 mL of the 5 mg/mL concentration to 45 mL of D5W or NS to yield 0.5 mg/mL.

*ADMINISTER:* **Direct for Conscious Sedation:** Give over 2 min or longer. **Direct for Induction of Anesthesia:** Give over 20–30 sec. **Direct for Neonate: Do not** give bolus dose; give over at least 2 min. **IV Infusion:** Give at a rate based on weight.

*INCOMPATIBILITIES:* **Solution/additive:** Lactated Ringer's, pentobarbital, perphenazine, prochlorperazine. **Y-site:** Albumin, amoxicillin, amoxicillin/clavulanate, amphotericin B cholesteryl complex, ampicillin, bumetanide, butorphanol, ceftazidime, cefuroxime, clonidine, dexamethasone, foscarnet, fosphenytoin, furosemide, hydrocortisone, imipenem/cilastatin, methotrexate, nafcillin, omeprazole, sodium bicarbonate, TPN, trimethoprim/sulfamethoxazole.

- Store at 15°–30° C (59°–86° F), therapeutic activity is retained for 2 y from date of manufacture.

## ADVERSE EFFECTS (≥1%) CNS:

*Retrograde amnesia,* headache, euphoria, drowsiness, excessive sedation, confusion. **CV:** Hypotension. **Special Senses:** Blurred vision, diplopia, nystagmus, pinpoint pupils. **GI:** Nausea, vomiting. **Respiratory:** Coughing, laryngospasm (rare), respiratory arrest. **Skin:** Hives, swelling, burning, pain, induration at injection site, tachypnea. **Body as a Whole:** Hiccups, chills, weakness.

## INTERACTIONS Drug: Alcohol,

CNS DEPRESSANTS, ANTICONVULSANTS potentiate CNS depression; **cimetidine** increases midazolam plasma levels, increasing its toxicity; may decrease antiparkinsonism effects of **levodopa;** may increase **phenytoin** levels; **smoking** decreases sedative and antianxiety effects. **Food: Grapefruit juice** (greater than 1 qt/day) may increase risk of myopathy and rhabdomyolysis. **Herbal: Kava, valerian** may potentiate sedation. **Echinacea, St. John's wort** may reduce efficacy.

## PHARMACOKINETICS Onset:

1–5 min IV; 5–15 min IM, 20–30 min PO. **Peak:** 20–60 min. **Duration:** Less than 2 h IV; 1–6 h IM. **Distribution:** Crosses blood–brain barrier and placenta. **Metabolism:** In liver (CYP3A4). **Elimination:** In urine. **Half-Life:** 1–4 h.

## NURSING IMPLICATIONS

### Black Box Warning

*IV midazolam has been associated with respiratory depression and respiratory arrest. Rapid injection (less than 2 min) has been associated with seizures, and with*

---

Common adverse effects in *italic;* life-threatening effects underlined; generic names in **bold;** classifications in SMALL CAPS; ♣ Canadian drug name; ⊘ Prototype drug

1059

*severe hypotension in neonates, particularly when the patient has received fentanyl.*

### Assessment & Drug Effects

- Inspect insertion site for redness, pain, swelling, and other signs of extravasation during IV infusion.
- Monitor closely for indications of impending respiratory arrest. Resuscitative drugs and equipment should be immediately available.
- Monitor for hypotension, especially if the patient is premedicated with a narcotic agonist analgesic.
- Monitor vital signs for entire recovery period. In obese patient, half-life is prolonged during IV infusion; therefore, duration of effects is prolonged (i.e., amnesia, postoperative recovery).
- Be aware that overdose symptoms include somnolence, confusion, sedation, diminished reflexes, coma, and untoward effects on vital signs.

### Patient & Family Education

- Do not drive or engage in potentially hazardous activities until response to drug is known. You may feel drowsy, weak, or tired for 1–2 days after drug has been given.

## MIDODRINE HYDROCHLORIDE

(mid'o-dreen)

**Classification:** VASOPRESSOR
**Therapeutic:** ANTIHYPOTENSIVE
**Prototype:** Dexmedetomide

**AVAILABILITY** Tablet

### ACTION & *THERAPEUTIC EFFECT*

Vasopressor and alpha$_1$ agonist that activates the alpha-adrenergic receptors of the arteries and veins, resulting in increased vascular tone and elevation in blood pressure.

*Affects standing, sitting, and supine systolic and diastolic blood pressures. Effectiveness indicated by an increase in 1-min standing systolic BP and subjective feelings of clinical improvement.*

**USES** Orthostatic hypotension.

**CONTRAINDICATIONS** Severe organic heart disease; heart failure; kidney disease, renal failure; urinary retention; pheochromocytoma; thyrotoxicosis; MAOI therapy; persistent and excessive supine hypertension.

**CAUTIOUS USE** Renal impairment, hepatic impairment; history of visual problems; diabetes with hypotension or visual disorders; pregnancy (category C); lactation. Safety and efficacy in children not established.

### ROUTE & DOSAGE

**Orthostatic Hypotension**

*Adult:* **PO** 10 mg t.i.d. during the daytime hours, dosed not less than 3 h apart with last dose at least 4 h before bedtime (max: 20 mg/dose)

### ADMINISTRATION

**Oral**

- Do not give at bedtime or before napping (within 4 h of lying supine for any length of time).
- Give with caution in persons with pretreatment, supine systolic BP 170 mm Hg or higher.
- Store at 15°–30° C (59°–86° F).

**ADVERSE EFFECTS** (≥1%) **Body as a Whole:** *Paresthesia,* chills, pain, facial flushing. **CNS:** Confusion, nervousness, anxiety. **CV:** *Hypertension.* **GI:** Dry mouth. **Skin:** *Pruritus, piloerection,* rash. **Urogenital:** *Dysuria, urinary retention, urinary frequency.*

M

**INTERACTIONS Drug:** May antagonize effects of **doxazosin, prazosin, terazosin;** may potentiate vasoconstrictive effects of **ephedrine, phenylephrine, pseudoephedrine;** may cause hypertensive crisis with MAOIS.

**PHARMACOKINETICS Absorption:** Rapidly from GI tract. **Peak:** Midodrine 0.5 h; desglymidodrine 1–2 h. **Metabolism:** Rapidly metabolized to the active metabolite. **Elimination:** In urine. **Half-Life:** 25 min.

## NURSING IMPLICATIONS

### Assessment & Drug Effects
- Monitor supine and standing BP regularly. Withhold drug and notify prescriber if supine BP increases excessively; determine acceptable parameters.
- Monitor carefully effect of the drug in diabetics with orthostatic hypotension and those taking fludrocortisone acetate, which may increase intraocular pressure.
- Monitor lab tests. Baseline LFTs and renal function tests.

### Patient & Family Education
- Take last daily dose 4 h before bedtime.
- Report immediately to prescriber sensations associated with supine hypertension (e.g., pounding in ears, headache, blurred vision, awareness of heart beating).
- Discontinue drug and report to prescriber if S&S of bradycardia develop (e.g., dizziness, pulse slowing, fainting).
- Do not take allergy drugs, cold preparations, or diet pills without consulting prescriber.

## MIDOSTAURIN
(mye-doe-staw′rin)
Rydapt

**Classifications:** ANTINEOPLASTIC; TYROSINE KINASE INHIBITOR; FLT3 INHIBITOR
Therapeutic: ANTINEOPLASTIC

**AVAILABILITY** Capsule

## ACTION & *THERAPEUTIC EFFECT*
Inhibits multiple receptor tyrosine kinases. *Induces cell death in leukemic cells, resulting in decreased cell proliferation and cell survival.*

**USES** Treatment of mast cell leukemia; also used for the treatment of systemic mastocytosis and treatment of acute myeloid leukemia, if FLT3-positive, in combination with cytarabine and daunorubicin.

**CONTRAINDICATIONS** Pregnancy; lactation. Hypersensitivity to midostaurin or any components.

**CAUTIOUS USE** History of lung or gastrointestinal disease or hematological abnormalities. Concurrent use of products that impact QT interval. Safety and efficacy in children not established.

## ROUTE & DOSAGE

**Mast Cell Leukemia**
*Adult:* **PO** 100 mg b.i.d.

**Aggressive Systemic Mastocytosis (ASM)**
*Adult:* **PO** 100 mg b.i.d.

**Acute Myeloid Leukemia**
*Adult:* **PO** 50 mg b.i.d. on days 8–21 of each induction cycle (with cytarabine and daunorubicin), and on days 8–21 of each consolidation cycle (high-dose cytarabine)

**Hepatic and Renal Impairment Dosage Adjustment**
Unstudied in this population

*Toxicity Dosage Adjustment*
Specific adjustments available in the package insert

## ADMINISTRATION

### Oral
- Administer with food every 12 h.
- Do not crush/open capsules.
- Administer prophylactic antiemetics before therapy.
- Store at 25° C (77° F); excursions permitted to 15°–30° C (59°–86° F). Store in original package to protect from moisture.

## ADVERSE EFFECTS CV: *Edema*, QT changes, heart failure, myocardial infarction hypotension. **CNS:** *Headache, fatigue,* dizziness, insomnia, arthralgia, musculoskeletal pain. **Skin:** Hyperhidrosis, rash. **Metabolic:** *Hyperglycemia, hypocalemia, hyperuricemia,* hyponatremia, hypoalbuminemia, hypokalemia, hyperkalemia, hypophosphatemia. **GI:** Gastrointestinal hemorrhage, *nausea, vomiting, mucositis,* diarrhea, increased serum lipase, abdominal pain, constipation, hemorrhoids. **GU:** Urinary tract infection, renal failure. **Respiratory:** URTI, epistaxis, dyspnea, cough. **Hematologic:** *Febrile neutropenia, lymphocytopenia,* leukopenia, anemia, thrombobocytopenia, neutropenia, petechia. **OTHER:** Sepsis, mycosis.

## INTERACTIONS Major substrate of CYP3A4. Avoid combination with strong CYP3A4 inducers (e.g., **carbamazepine, phenytoin, rifampin**). Avoid use with other medications which may increase risk for QTc-prolongation (e.g., **hydroxychloroquine, ketoconazole, ziprasidone**).

## PHARMACOKINETICS Absorption: $C_{max}$ decreased if administered with food. **Distribution:** 99% protein bound. **Onset:** Peak in 1–3 h. **Metabolism:** Hepatic, primarily through CYP3A4, to active metabolites **Elimination:** 95% in feces, 5% in urine. **Half-Life:** 21 h.

## NURSING IMPLICATIONS

### Assessment & Drug Effects
- Monitor for potential pulmonary toxicity or signs of bone marrow supression.
- Verify pregnancy status within 7 days of initiating therapy in women with reproductive potential.
- Respiratory assessments for signs and symptoms of pulmonary toxicity.
- Assess EKG for QT interval if patient is on concurrent medication that may prolong the QT interval.
- Weekly CBC for the first 4 wk of treatment, every other week for the next 8 wk, and monthly thereafter during therapy.

### Patient and Family Education
- Report immediately to prescriber any signs of infection, high blood sugar, signs of bleeding, signs of kidney problems blood in the urine, difficulty urinating, prolonged nausea, vomiting and diarrhea, coffee ground emesis.
- May impair male fertility.
- Women and men should use effective means to avoid pregnancy while taking this drug for at least 4 mo after the last dose. Do not breast-feed for at least 4 mo after the last dose.

## MIGLITOL ✦
(mig'li-toll)
Glyset
**Classifications:** ANTIDIABETIC; ALPHA-GLUCOSIDASE INHIBITOR
**Therapeutic:** ANTIDIABETIC; GLYCEMIC CONTROL ENHANCER
**Prototype:** Acarbose

**AVAILABILITY** Tablet

**ACTION & *THERAPEUTIC EFFECT***
Enzyme inhibits intestinal glucosidases thus delaying the formation of glucose from saccharides in the small intestine resulting in a smaller rise in postprandial blood glucose concentration. *Helps control postprandial hyperglycemia, and reduces the levels of glysylated hemoglobin (HbA1C) in type 2 diabetics.*

**USES** Adjunct to diet for control of type 2 diabetes.

**UNLABELED USES** Type 1 diabetes.

**CONTRAINDICATIONS** Hypersensitivity to miglitol; diabetic ketoacidosis; digestive or absorptive disorders; history of or partial intestinal obstruction, IBD, lactation.

**CAUTIOUS USE** Hypersensitivity to acarbose; creatinine clearance greater than 2 mg/dL; high stress conditions (i.e., surgery, trauma); pregnancy (category B). Safety and efficacy in children younger than 18 y not established.

## ROUTE & DOSAGE

**Type 2 Diabetes Mellitis**

*Adult:* **PO** 25 mg t.i.d. at the start of each meal, may increase after 4–8 wk to 50 mg t.i.d. (max: 100 mg t.i.d.)

## ADMINISTRATION

**Oral**
- Give drug with first bite of each of the three main meals.
- Store at 15°–30° C (59°–86° F).

**ADVERSE EFFECTS** (≥1%) **GI:** *Abdominal pain, diarrhea, flatulence.* **Skin:** Rash. **Metabolic:** Hypoglycemia.

**INTERACTIONS Drug:** Miglitol may reduce bioavailability of **propranolol, ranitidine; charcoal, pancreatin, amylase, pancrelipase** may decrease effectiveness of miglitol. **Herbal: Garlic, ginseng** may potentiate hypoglycemic effects.

**PHARMACOKINETICS Absorption:** 25 mg dose is completely absorbed, amount absorbed decreases with increasing dose to where 100 mg dose is 50–70% absorbed. **Peak:** 2–3 h. **Distribution:** Minimal protein binding (less than 4%). **Metabolism:** Not metabolized. **Elimination:** Half-life 2 h; 95% excreted unchanged in urine, lower doses should be used in patients with renal impairment.

## NURSING IMPLICATIONS

**Assessment & Drug Effects**
- Monitor for therapeutic effectiveness: Indicated by improved blood glucose levels and decreased HbA1C.
- Monitor for S&S of hypoglycemia when used in combination with sulfonylureas, insulin, other hypoglycemic agents.
- Treat hypoglycemia with oral glucose (dextrose); miglitol interferes with the breakdown of sucrose (table sugar).
- Monitor lab tests: Daily postprandial blood glucose and HbA1C q3mo.

**Patient & Family Education**
- Keep a source of oral glucose available to treat low blood sugar; miglitol prevents digestive breakdown of table sugar.
- Abdominal discomfort, flatulence, and diarrhea tend to diminish with continued therapy.

Common adverse effects in *italic;* life-threatening effects underlined; generic names in **bold;** classifications in SMALL CAPS; ✤ Canadian drug name; ◯ Prototype drug

1063

# MILNACIPRAN

(mil-na-see'pran)

Savella

**Classifications:** ANTIDEPRESSANT; SEROTONIN NOREPINEPHRINE REUPTAKE INHIBITOR (SNRI); ANALGESIC

Therapeutic: ANALGESIC; SNRI

**Prototype:** Venlafaxine

## AVAILABILITY Tablet

## ACTION & *THERAPEUTIC EFFECT*

Exact mechanism of central pain inhibition is unknown. Is a potent inhibitor of both neuronal norepinephrine and serotonin reuptake without affecting uptake of other neurotransmitters. *Effective in reducing the pain associated with fibromyalgia.*

## USES Management of fibromyalgia.

## UNLABELED USES Treatment of depression.

## CONTRAINDICATIONS Within
14 days discontinued use of MAOIs; abrupt discontinuation of milnacipran; suicidal ideation; major depressive disorder; uncontrolled narrow-angle glaucoma; substantial alcohol use; chronic liver disease; ESRD; lactation.

## CAUTIOUS USE Suicidal tendencies; history of seizures or depression; history of cardiac disease or pre-existing tachyarrhythmias; male obstructive uropathies; history of GI bleeding; moderate and severe renal impairment; hepatic impairment; older adults; pregnancy (category C); children younger than 18 y.

## ROUTE & DOSAGE

### Fibromyalgia

*Adults/Adolescents (17 y or older):* **PO** Initial dose of 12.5 mg once daily on day 1, increase to 12.5 mg b.i.d. on days 2 and 3, 25 mg b.i.d. on days 4–7, and then 50 mg b.i.d. Dose can be increased to 100 mg b.i.d. if needed.

### *Renal Impairment Dosage Adjustment*

*CrCl 5–29 mL/min:* Decrease dose by 50% (i.e., 25–50 mg b.i.d.); *less than 5 mL/min:* Use not recommended

## ADMINISTRATION

### Oral

- Dose titration should occur over a period of 1 wk to the recommended dose.
- Give with food, if needed, to improve tolerability of drug.
- Do not give within 14 days of an MAOI.
- Store at 15°–30° C (59°–86° F).

## ADVERSE EFFECTS (≥2%) **Body as a Whole:** Chest pain and discomfort, chills. **CNS:** Anxiety, *dizziness, headache,* hypoesthesia, *insomnia,* migraine, paresthesia, tension headache, tremor. **CV:** *Hot flush,* increased blood pressure, increased heart rate, palpitations, tachycardia. **GI:** Abdominal pain, *constipation,* dry mouth, *nausea,* vomiting. **Metabolic:** Decreased appetite. **Respiratory:** Dyspnea, upper respiratory tract infection. **Skin:** Hyperhidrosis, pruritus, rash. **Special Senses:** Blurred vision. **Urogenital:** Decreased urine flow, dysuria, ejaculation disorder, erectile dysfunction, libido decreased, prostatitis, scrotal pain, testicular pain and

Common adverse effects in *italic;* life-threatening effects <u>underlined;</u> generic names in **bold;** classifications in SMALL CAPS; ✦ Canadian drug name; ◐ Prototype drug

swelling, urinary hesitation and retention, urethral pain.

**INTERACTIONS Drug: Lithium**
may increase risk of serotonin syndrome. Milnacipran may inhibit
antihypertensive effect of **clonidine** and other ALPHA₂ AGONISTS.
**Digoxin** may increase the risk of
postural hypotension and tachycardia. Milnacipran may increase
bleeding with **warfarin, aspirin**,
and NSAIDS; concurrent use with
**epinephrine** or **norepinephrine**
may cause paroxysmal hypertension and arrhythmia; concurrent
use with SELECTIVE SEROTONIN REUP-
TAKE INHIBITORS, SELECTIVE NOR-
EPINEPHRINE REUPTAKE INHIBITORS,
**tramadol**, OR 5-HT-2B/2D AGONISTS
(TRIPTANS) may cause additive serotonergic effects, hypertension, and
coronary vasoconstriction.

**PHARMACOKINETICS Absorp-
tion:** 85–90% bioavailability. **Distribution:** Minimal (13%) plasma protein binding. **Metabolism:** Less than
50% metabolized by liver. **Elimination:** Primarily renal. **Half-Life:** 6–8 h.

**NURSING IMPLICATIONS**

### Black Box Warning

*Milnacipan has been associated
with suicidal thinking and behavior in children, adolescents, and
young adults.*

**Assessment & Drug Effects**
- Monitor for and report promptly
  unusual changes in behavior
  (e.g., depression, anxiety, panic
  attack, insomnia, aggressiveness,
  mania) or suicidal ideation. Monitor closely during initial few
  months of therapy and during periods of dosage adjustment.
- Monitor HR and BP closely and
  report promptly sustained BP

elevations. Pre-existing hypertension should be controlled before
initiating this drug.
- Monitor for orthostatic hypotension and tachycardia with concurrent digoxin use.
- Monitor lab tests: Periodic serum
  sodium, especially with concurrent diuretic therapy.

**Patient & Family Education**
- Do not abruptly stop taking this
  drug. It should be tapered off
  gradually after extended use.
- Report prompt unusual changes
  in behavior or suicidal ideas.
- Do not engage in potentially hazardous activities until reaction to
  drug is known.
- Exercise care to take prescribed BP
  medications exactly as ordered.
- Concurrent use of aspirin or
  NSAIDs is not recommended due
  to increased risk of bleeding.
  Consult prescriber.
- Avoid consuming alcohol while
  taking this drug.

**M**

## MILRINONE LACTATE ⊕
(mil′ri-none)

**Classifications:** INOTROPIC AGENT;
VASODILATOR
**Therapeutic:** INOTROPIC AGENT
**Prototype:** Milrinone acetate

**AVAILABILITY** Solution for injection

**ACTION & *THERAPEUTIC EFFECT***
Has a positive inotropic action and
is a vasodilator with little chronotropic activity. Inhibitory action
against cyclic-AMP phosphodiesterase in cardiac and smooth
vascular muscle. Increases cardiac contractility and myocardial
contractility. *Therefore, increases
cardiac output and decreases pulmonary wedge pressure and*

*vascular resistance, without increasing myocardial oxygen demand or significantly increasing heart rate.*

**USES** Short-term management of CHF.

**UNLABELED USES** Short-term use to increase the cardiac index in patients with low cardiac output after surgery. To increase cardiac function prior to heart transplantation.

**CONTRAINDICATIONS** Hypersensitivity to milrinone; valvular heart disease; acute MI.

**CAUTIOUS USE** Atrial fibrillation, atrial flutter; renal disease; renal impairment, renal failure; older adults; pregnancy (category C); lactation; children.

## ROUTE & DOSAGE

**Heart Failure**

*Adult:* **IV Loading Dose** 50 mcg/kg IV over 10 min; **IV Maintenance Dose** 0.375–0.75 mcg/kg/min

## ADMINISTRATION

**Intravenous**

Note: Correct preexisting hypokalemia before administering milrinone. ▪See manufacturer's information for dosage reduction in the presence of renal impairment.

*PREPARE:* **IV Infusion Loading Dose:** Give undiluted or dilute each 1 mg in 1 mL NS or 0.45% NaCl. **IV Infusion Maintenance Dose:** Dilute 20 mg of milrinone in D5W, NS, or 0.45% NaCl to yield: 100 mcg/mL with 180 mL diluent; 150 mcg/mL with 113 mL diluent; 200 mcg/mL with 80 mL diluent.
*ADMINISTER:* **IV Infusion Loading Dose:** Give 50 mcg/kg over 10 min. **IV Infusion Maintenance**

**Dose:** Give at a rate based on weight. Use a microdrip set and infusion pump.
*INCOMPATIBILITIES:* Solution/additive: **Furosemide, procainamide.** Y-site: **Furosemide, imipenem/cilastatin, procainamide.**

▪Store according to manufacturer's directions.

**ADVERSE EFFECTS** (≥1%) **CV:** Increased ectopic activity, PVCs, *ventricular tachycardia,* ventricular fibrillation, supraventricular arrhythmias; possible increase in angina symptoms, hypotension. **CNS:** Headache. **Body as a Whole:** Hypokalemia.

**INTERACTIONS Drug: Disopyramide** may cause excessive hypotension.

**PHARMACOKINETICS** **Peak:** 2 min. **Duration:** 2 h. **Distribution:** 70% protein bound. **Elimination:** 80–85% excreted unchanged in urine within 24 h. Active renal tubular secretion is primary elimination pathway. **Half-Life:** 1.7–2.7 h.

## NURSING IMPLICATIONS

**Assessment & Drug Effects**

▪ Monitor cardiac status closely during and for several hours following infusion. Supraventricular and ventricular arrhythmias have occurred.
▪ Monitor BP and promptly slow or stop infusion in presence of significant hypotension. Closely monitor those with recent aggressive diuretic therapy for decreasing blood pressure.
▪ Monitor fluid and electrolyte status. Hypokalemia should be corrected whenever it occurs during administration.
▪ Monitor lab tests: Periodic serum electrolytes.

M

## Patient & Family Education

- Report immediately angina that occurs during infusion to prescriber.
- Be aware that drug may cause a headache, which can be treated with analgesics.

## MINOCYCLINE HYDROCHLORIDE

(mi-noe-sye′kleen)

Arestin, Minocin, Minolira, Solodyn, Ximino

**Classification:** TETRACYCLINE ANTIBIOTIC
**Therapeutic:** ANTIBIOTIC
**Prototype:** Tetracycline

**AVAILABILITY** Capsule; tablet; sustained release microsphere; solution for injection

## ACTION & *THERAPEUTIC EFFECT*

Bacteriostatic action that appears to be a result of reversible binding to ribosomal units of susceptible bacteria and inhibition of bacterial protein synthesis. *Effective against gram-positive and gram-negative bacteria, but usually used against gram-negative bacteria.*

## USES

Treatment of mucopurulent cervicitis, granuloma inguinale, lymphogranuloma venereum, proctitis, bronchitis, lower respiratory tract infections caused by *Mycoplasma pneumoniae,* Rickettsial infections, chlamydial infections, non-gonococcal urethritis, chlamydial conjunctivitis, plague, brucellosis, bartonellosis, tularemia, UTI, and prostatitis; acne vulgaris, gonorrhea, cholera, meningococcal carrier state, amebiasis, anthrax.

**CONTRAINDICATIONS** Hypersensitivity to minocyline or other tetracyclines; pregnancy (category D); lactation.

**CAUTIOUS USE** Renal and hepatic impairment; older adults; children younger than 8 y.

## ROUTE & DOSAGE

### Anti-Infective

*Adult:* **PO/IV** 200 mg followed by 100 mg q12h
*Child (8 y or older):* **PO/IV** 4 mg/kg (max: 200 mg) followed by 2 mg/kg q12h (max: 100 mg)

### Syphilis (when penicillin is contraindicated)

*Adult:* **PO/IV** 200 mg then 100 mg q12h × 10–15 days

### Acne

*Adult:* **PO** 200 mg × 1 then 100 mg q12h

### Moderate to Severe Acne (Solodyn, Minolira, Ximino only)

*Adult/Adolescent/Child (older than 12 y):* **PO** 1 mg/kg daily × 12 wk

### Meningococcal Infection Prophylaxis

*Adult:* **PO** 100 mg q12h × 5 days
*Child (8 y or older):* **PO** 4 mg/kg followed by 2 mg/kg q12h × 5 days (max: 100 mg/dose)

### Renal Impairment Dosage Adjustment

Do not exceed 200 mg/day in patients with renal impairment

## ADMINISTRATION

### Oral

- Shake suspension well before administration.

Common adverse effects in *italic;* life-threatening effects underlined; generic names in **bold;** classifications in SMALL CAPS; ♣ Canadian drug name; ⊘ Prototype drug

1067

- Ensure that sustained release tablets are swallowed whole.
- Administer with adequate fluid to decrease the risk of esophogeal irritation.
- Check expiration date. Outdated tetracycline can cause severe adverse effects.

### Intravenous

*PREPARE:* **IV Infusion:** Reconstitute with 5 mL of sterile water for injection and immediately further dilute in 100 to 1,000 mL of NS, D5W, D5NS, or 250 mL to 1,000 mL of LR.

*ADMINISTER:* Infuse over 60 min; avoid rapid administration. The injectable route should be used only if the oral route is not feasible or adequate. Prolonged intravenous therapy may be associated with thrombophlebitis.
*INCOMPATIBILITIES:* Solution/Additive: LR, TPN, TNA, **Doxapram hydrochloride, Rifampin**.

- Store intact vials at 20°–25° C (68°–77° F). Diluted solution in NS, D5W, D5NS, or LR is stable at room temperature for up to 4 h or at 2°–8° C (36°–46° F) for up to 24 h.

### ADVERSE EFFECTS (≥1%) **CNS:**
*Weakness, light-headedness, ataxia, dizziness, headache, fatigue, drowsiness, vertigo, tinnitus.* **GI:** *Nausea, vomiting,* anorexia, cramps, diarrhea, flatulence. **Hepatic:** Hepatitis, increased liver enzyme, hepatotoxicity. **Integumentary:** Pruritus. **Other:** Dental caries, dental pain.

### INTERACTIONS **Drug:** ANTACIDS, **iron, calcium, magnesium, zinc, kaolin and pectin,** sodium bicarbonate, bismuth subsalicylate can significantly decrease minocycline absorption; effects of both **desmopressin** and minocycline antagonized; increases **digoxin** absorption, increasing risk of **digoxin** toxicity; **methoxyflurane** increases risk of kidney failure. Do not use with **acitretin** or **isotretinoin**. **Food:** Dairy products significantly decrease minocycline absorption; food may also decrease its absorption.

### PHARMACOKINETICS **Absorption:** 90–100% from GI tract. **Peak:** 2–3 h. **Distribution:** Tends to accumulate in adipose tissue; crosses placenta; distributed into breast milk. **Metabolism:** Partially metabolized. **Elimination:** 20–30% in feces; ~12% in urine. **Half-Life:** 11–26 h.

### NURSING IMPLICATIONS
#### Assessment & Drug Effects
- Obtain history of hypersensitivity reactions prior to administration; drug is contraindicated with known tetracycline hypersensitivity.
- Monitor carefully for signs of hypersensitivity response (see Appendix F), particularly in patients with history of allergies, especially to drugs.
- Monitor at-risk patients for S&S of superinfection (see Appendix F).
- Assess risk of toxic effects carefully; increases with renal and hepatic impairment.
- Supervise ambulation, since light-headedness, dizziness, and vertigo occur frequently.
- Monitor lab tests: Baseline C&S, LFTs, BUN, renal function, serum magnesium with periodic testing for long-term therapy.

### Patient & Family Education

- Avoid hazardous activities or those requiring alertness while taking minocycline.
- Use sunscreen when outdoors and otherwise protect yourself from direct sunlight since photosensitivity reaction may occur.
- Report vestibular adverse effects (e.g., dizziness), which usually occur during first week of therapy. Effects are reversible if drug is withdrawn.
- Report loose stools or diarrhea or other signs of superinfection promptly to prescriber.
- Use or add barrier contraceptive while taking this drug if using hormonal contraceptive.
- Maintain adequate hydration while taking this drug.

## MINOXIDIL

(mi-nox'i-dill)

Rogaine

**Classifications:** NONNITRATE VASODILATOR; ANTIHYPERTENSIVE
**Therapeutic:** ANTIHYPERTENSIVE
**Prototype:** Hydralazine

**AVAILABILITY** Tablet; solution

**ACTION & THERAPEUTIC EFFECT**
Direct-acting vasodilator that appears to act by blocking calcium uptake through cell membranes. Reduces elevated systolic and diastolic blood pressures in supine and standing positions, by decreasing peripheral vascular resistance. *Effective as an antihypertensive. It increases heart rate and cardiac output.* **Topical:** *Reverses balding to some degree.*

**USES** Treat severe hypertension that is symptomatic or associated with damage to target organs and is not manageable with maximum therapeutic doses of a diuretic plus two other antihypertensive drugs. **Topical:** Treats alopecia areata and male pattern alopecia.

**CONTRAINDICATIONS** Hypersensitivity to minoxidil; pheochromocytoma; mild hypertension; recent acute MI, dissecting aortic aneurysm, valvular dysfunction; pulmonary hypertension; pericardial effusion; lactation.

**CAUTIOUS USE** Severe renal impairment; malignant hypertension; recent MI (within preceding month); CAD, chronic CHF; tachycardia; worsening of angina; older adults; pregnancy (category C); children younger than 12 y.

## ROUTE & DOSAGE

### Hypertension

*Adult:* **PO** 5–10 mg daily, titrate up as needed (max: 100 mg)
*Adolescent:* **PO** 5 mg/day titrate carefully (max. 100 mg/day)

### Alopecia

*Adult:* **Topical** Apply 1 mL of 2% solution to affected area b.i.d.

## ADMINISTRATION

### Oral

- Dose increments are usually made at 3–5 days intervals. If more rapid adjustment is necessary, adjustments can be made q6h with careful monitoring.

### Topical

- Do not apply topical product to an irritated scalp (e.g., sunburn, psoriasis).
- Store at 15°–30° C (59°–86° F) in tightly covered container unless otherwise directed.

**ADVERSE EFFECTS** (≥1%) **CV:** *Tachycardia,* angina pectoris, *ECG changes,* pericardial effusion and tamponade, rebound

Common adverse effects in *italic;* life-threatening effects <u>underlined;</u> generic names in **bold;** classifications in SMALL CAPS; ✦ Canadian drug name; ⊘ Prototype drug

1069

hypertension (following drug withdrawal); *edema,* including pulmonary edema; *CHF (salt and water retention).* **Skin:** *Hypertrichosis,* transient pruritus, darkening of skin, hypersensitivity rash, Stevens–Johnson syndrome. With topical use: Itching, flushing, scaling, dermatitis, folliculitis. **Body as a Whole:** Fatigue.

**INTERACTIONS Drug: Epinephrine, norepinephrine** cause excessive cardiac stimulation; **guanethidine** causes profound orthostatic hypotension.

**PHARMACOKINETICS Absorption:** Readily absorbed from GI tract. **Onset:** 30 min PO; at least 4 mo topical. **Peak:** 2–8 h PO. **Duration:** 2–5 days PO; new hair growth will remain 3–4 mo after withdrawal of topical. **Distribution:** Widely distributed including into breast milk. **Metabolism:** In liver. **Elimination:** 97% in urine and feces. **Half-Life:** 4.2 h.

## NURSING IMPLICATIONS

### Black Box Warning

*Minoxidil has been associated with pericardial effusion, occasionally progressing to tamponade, and it can exacerbate angina pectoris.*

### Assessment & Drug Effects

- Take BP and apical pulse before administering medication and report significant changes. Consult prescriber for parameters.
- Do not stop drug abruptly. Abrupt reduction in BP can result in CVA and MI. Keep prescriber informed.
- Monitor fluid and electrolyte balance closely throughout therapy. Sodium and water retention commonly occur. Monitor potassium intake and serum potassium levels in patient on diuretic therapy.
- Monitor I&O and daily weight. Report unusual changes in I&O ratio or daily weight gain, greater than 1 kg (2 lb).
- Observe patient daily for edema and auscultate lungs for rales. Be alert to signs and symptoms of CHF (see Appendix F).
- Observe for symptoms of pericardial effusion or tamponade. Symptoms are similar to those of CHF, but additionally patient may have paradoxical pulse (normal inspiratory reduction in systolic BP may fall as much as 10–20 mm Hg).
- Monitor lab tests: Periodic serum electrolytes.

### Patient & Family Education

- Learn about usual pulse rate and count radial pulse for one full minute before taking drug. Report an increase of 20 or more bpm.
- Notify prescriber promptly if the following S&S appear: Increase of 20 or more bpm in resting pulse; breathing difficulty; dizziness; light-headedness; fainting; edema (tight shoes or rings, puffiness, pitting); weight gain, chest pain, arm or shoulder pain; easy bruising or bleeding.
- Develops 3–9 wk after start of therapy and occurs in approximately 80% of patients; reversible within 1–6 mo after drug withdrawal.

## MIRABEGRON

(mir-a-be'gron)

**Myrbetriq**

**Classification:** GENITOURINARY AGENT; BETA-3 ADRENERGIC AGONIST, ANTISPASMOTIC

**Therapeutic:** ANTISPASMOTIC

**AVAILABILITY** Extended release tablet

## ACTION & *THERAPEUTIC EFFECT*

A beta adrenergic receptor agonist that relaxes the detrusor smooth muscle during the storage phase of the urinary bladder fill–void cycle thus increasing bladder capacity and tone. *Decreases episodes of urge incontinence and reduces urinary frequency.*

**USES** Treatment of overactive bladder and urinary incontinence.

**CONTRAINDICATIONS** Uncontrolled hypertension; ESRD; severe hepatic and renal impairment; lactation; hypersensitivity to mirabegron.

**CAUTIOUS USE** Hypertension, significant bladder outlet obstruction; moderate hepatic impairment, moderate renal impairment; pregnancy (category C). Safety and efficacy in children younger than 18 y not established.

## ROUTE & DOSAGE

### Overactive Bladder

*Adult:* **PO** 25 mg once daily; can be increased to 50 mg once daily

### Hepatic Impairment Dosage Adjustment

*Moderate hepatic impairment (Child Pugh class B):* Max: 25 mg once daily
*Severe hepatic impairment (Child Pugh class C):* Not recommended

### Renal Impairment Dosage Adjustment

*CrCl 15–29 mL/min:* Max: 25 mg once daily *CrCl less than 15 mL/min:* Not recommended

## ADMINISTRATION

### Oral

- May be given without regard to food.
- Ensure that tablet is swallowed whole. It should not be crushed, divided, or chewed.
- Store at 15°–30° C (59°–86° F).

**ADVERSE EFFECTS** (≥1%) **Body as a Whole:** Dry mouth, fatigue, influenza. **CNS:** Dizziness, anxiety, insomnia, *headache.* **CV:** *Hypertension*, tachycardia. **GI:** Abdominal pain, constipation, diarrhea. **Musculoskeletal:** Arthralgia, back pain. **Respiratory:** *Nasopharyngitis*, sinusitis, upper respiratory tract infection, influenza. **Urogenital:** Cystitis, *urinary tract infection.*

**INTERACTIONS Drug:** Mirabegron may increase the levels of other drugs requiring CYP2D6 for metabolism (e.g., **clozapine, doxorubicin, eliglustat, metoprolol**, other BETA-BLOCKERS, **desipramine**). Mirabegron increases the levels of **digoxin**. Do not use with MAOIS.

**PHARMACOKINETICS Absorption:** 29–35% bioavailable. **Peak:** 3.5 h. **Distribution:** 71% plasma protein bound. **Metabolism:** Extensive hepatic metabolism (CYP2D6, CYP3A4). **Elimination:** Renal (55%) and fecal (34%). **Half-Life:** 50 h.

## NURSING IMPLICATIONS

### Assessment & Drug Effects

- Monitor BP, especially in those with a history of hypertension.
- Monitor lab tests: Baseline and periodic LFTs and renal function tests.

### Patient & Family Education

- Report promptly signs of urinary tract infection, difficulty passing urine or urinary retention.
- Report to your prescriber if you are or plan to become pregnant.

M

Common adverse effects in *italic;* life-threatening effects underlined; generic names in **bold;** classifications in SMALL CAPS; ♣ Canadian drug name; ⦿ Prototype drug

1071

- Do not breast-feed without consulting prescriber.

# MIRTAZAPINE ℗
(mir-taz′a-peen)
Remeron, Remeron SolTab
**Classifications:** TETRACYCLIC ANTIDEPRESSANT; ANXIOLYTIC
Therapeutic: ANTIDEPRESSANT; ANTIANXIETY

**AVAILABILITY** Tablet; orally disintegrating tablet

## ACTION & *THERAPEUTIC EFFECT*
Tetracyclic antidepressant pharmacologically and therapeutically similar to tricyclic antidepressants. Tetracyclics enhance central non-adrenergic and serotonergic activity; mechanism of action thought to be due to normalization of neurotransmission efficacy. Mirtazapine is a potent antagonist of 5-HT$_2$ and 5-HT$_3$ serotonin receptors. *Acts as antidepressant. Effectiveness is indicated by mood elevation.*

**USES** Treatment of depression.

**UNLABELED USES** Pruritus, tremor.

**CONTRAINDICATIONS** Hypersensitivity to mirtazapine or mianserin; hypersensitivity to other antidepressants (e.g., tricyclic antidepressants and MAOI depressants), acute MI; fever, infection; agranulocytosis, suicidal ideation; jaundice, ethanol intoxication; lactation.

**CAUTIOUS USE** History of cardiovascular or GI disorders; BPH, urinary retention; preexisting hematological disease; thrombocytopenia; narrow-angle glaucoma, increased intraocular pressure; renal impairment, renal failure; moderate to severe hepatic impairment; hypercholesterolemia, hypertriglyceridemia, cardiac disease; angina, cardiac arrhythmias; bipolar disorder, mania, bone marrow suppression, PKU, history of MI; CVD; seizure disorder, seizures; depression; history of suicidal tendencies; hypovolemia, surgery; closed-angle glaucoma; ileus, GI obstruction, dehydration; diabetes mellitus, diabetic ketoacidosis; older adults; pregnancy (category C). Safety and efficacy in children not established.

## ROUTE & DOSAGE

**Depression**
*Adult:* **PO** 15 mg/day in single dose at bedtime, may increase q1–2wk (max: 45 mg/day)
*Geriatric:* **PO** Use lower doses

**Renal or Hepatic Impairment Dosage Adjustment**
Use lower doses

## ADMINISTRATION
**Oral**
- Give preferably prior to sleep to minimize injury potential.
- Begin drug no sooner than 14 days after discontinuation of an MAO inhibitor.
- Reduce dosage as warranted with severe renal or hepatic impairment and in older adults.
- Store at 20°–25° C (68°–77° F) in tight, light-resistant container.

**ADVERSE EFFECTS** (≥1%) **Body as a Whole:** Asthenia, flu syndrome, back pain, edema, malaise. **CNS:** *Somnolence,* dizziness, abnormal dreams, abnormal thinking, tremor, confusion, depression, agitation, vertigo, twitching. **CV:** Hypertension, vasodilation. **GI:** Nausea, vomiting, abdominal pain, *increased appetite/*

Common adverse effects in *italic;* life-threatening effects <u>underlined;</u> generic names in **bold;** classifications in SMALL CAPS; ♣ Canadian drug name; ℗ Prototype drug

weight gain, *dry mouth, constipation,* anorexia, cholecystitis, stomatitis, colitis, abnormal liver function tests. **Respiratory:** Dyspnea, cough, sinusitis. **Skin:** Pruritus, rash. **Urogenital:** Urinary frequency.

**INTERACTIONS Drug:** Additive cognitive and motor impairment with **alcohol** or BENZODIAZEPINES; increase risk of hypertensive crisis with MAOIS. **Herbal: Kava, valerian** may potentiate sedative effects.

**PHARMACOKINETICS Absorption:** Rapidly absorbed from GI tract, 50% reaches systemic circulation. **Peak:** 2 h. **Distribution:** 85% protein bound. **Metabolism:** In liver by cytochrome P450 system (CYP2D6, CYP1A2, CYP3A4). **Elimination:** 75% in urine, 15% in feces. **Half-Life:** 20–40 h.

## NURSING IMPLICATIONS

### Black Box Warning

*Mirtazapine has been associated with suicidal thinking and behavior in children, adolescents, and young adults*

### Assessment & Drug Effects

- Monitor for worsening of depression or suicidal ideation.
- Assess for weight gain and excessive somnolence or dizziness.
- Monitor for orthostatic hypotension with a history of cardiovascular or cerebrovascular disease. Periodically monitor ECG especially in those with known cardiovascular disease.
- Monitor those with history of seizures for lowering of the seizure threshold.
- Monitor lab tests: Periodic WBC with differential, lipid profile, and LFTs.

### Patient & Family Education

- Report immediately to prescriber signs of worsening mental status such as suicidal ideation, aggressiveness, agitation, anxiety, hostility, impulsivity, insomnia, irritability, panic attacks, and worsening of depression.
- Do not drive or engage in potentially hazardous activities until response to drug is known.
- Do not use alcohol while taking drug.
- Report immediately unexplained fever or S&S of infection, especially flu-like symptoms, to prescriber.
- Do not take other prescription or OTC drugs without consulting prescriber.
- Make position changes slowly especially from lying or sitting to standing. Report dizziness, palpitations, and fainting.
- Monitor weight periodically and report significant weight gains.

M

# MISOPROSTOL
(my-so-prost'ole)

Cytotec

**Classification:** PROSTAGLANDIN
**Therapeutic:** PROSTAGLANDIN

## AVAILABILITY Tablet

## ACTION & *THERAPEUTIC EFFECT*

Synthetic prostaglandin $E_1$ analog, with both antisecretory (inhibiting gastric acid secretion) and mucosal protective properties. Increases bicarbonate and mucosal protective properties. Inhibits basal and nocturnal gastric acid secretion and acid secretion in response to a variety of stimuli, including meals, histamine, pentagastrin, and coffee. Produces uterine contractions that may endanger pregnancy and cause a miscarriage. *Inhibits*

Common adverse effects in *italic;* life-threatening effects <u>underlined</u>; generic names in **bold;** classifications in SMALL CAPS; ♣ Canadian drug name; ⊚ Prototype drug

1073

*basal and nocturnal gastric acid secretion.*

**USES** Prevention of NSAID (including aspirin-induced) gastric ulcers in patients at high risk of complications from a gastric ulcer (e.g., the older adult and patients with a concomitant debilitating disease or a history of ulcers). Drug is taken for the duration of NSAID therapy and does not interfere with the efficacy of the NSAID.

**UNLABELED USES** Short-term treatment of duodenal ulcers; cervical ripening and induction of labor.

**CONTRAINDICATIONS** History of allergies to prostaglandins. **Topical:** Abnormal fetal position, caesarean section, ectopic pregnancy; fetal disease, incomplete abortion; multiparity, placenta previa, vaginal bleeding; pregnancy (category X).

**CAUTIOUS USE** Renal impairment; cardiovascular disease; IBD; lactation. Safety and efficacy in children not established.

## ROUTE & DOSAGE

### Prevention of NSAID-Induced Ulcers

*Adult:* **PO** 100–200 mcg q.i.d. p.c. and at bedtime

## ADMINISTRATION

### Oral
- Give with food to minimize GI adverse effects (manufacturer recommendation).
- Store away from heat, light, and moisture.

**ADVERSE EFFECTS** (≥1%) **CNS:** Headache. **GI:** *Diarrhea, abdominal pain,* nausea, flatulence, dyspepsia, vomiting, constipation. **Urogenital:** Spotting, cramps, dysmenorrhea, uterine contractions.

**INTERACTIONS Drug:** MAGNESIUM-CONTAINING ANTACIDS may increase diarrhea.

**PHARMACOKINETICS Absorption:** Readily from GI tract; extensive first pass metabolism. **Onset:** 30 min. **Peak:** 60–90 min. **Duration:** At least 3 h. **Metabolism:** In liver. **Elimination:** Primarily in urine; small amount in feces. **Half-Life:** 20–40 min.

## NURSING IMPLICATIONS

### Black Box Warning

*Misoprostol can cause abortion, premature birth, or birth defects.*

### Assessment & Drug Effects
- Monitor for diarrhea; may be minimized by giving drug after meals and at bedtime. Diarrhea is a common adverse effect that is dose related and usually self-limiting (often resolving in 8 days).

### Patient & Family Education
- Avoid pregnancy during misoprostol therapy; use an effective contraception method while taking drug.
- Avoid using concurrent magnesium-containing antacids because of increased incidence of diarrhea.
- Report postmenopausal bleeding to prescriber; it may be drug related.
- Drug has abortifacient property. Contact prescriber and immediately discontinue drug if you become pregnant.

## MITOMYCIN
(mye-toe-mye′sin)
Mutamycin, Mytozytrex
**Classifications:** ANTINEOPLASTIC (ANTIBIOTIC); ANTHRACYCLINE
**Therapeutic:** ANTINEOPLASTIC
**Prototype:** Doxorubicin

**AVAILABILITY** Solution for injection

## ACTION & *THERAPEUTIC EFFECT*

Potent antibiotic antineoplastic effective in certain tumors unresponsive to surgery, radiation, or other agents. It selectively inhibits synthesis of DNA. At high concentrations, cellular and enzymatic RNA as well as protein synthesis are suppressed. *Highly destructive to rapidly proliferating cells and slowly developing carcinomas.*

**USES** In combination with other chemotherapeutic agents in palliative, adjunctive treatment of disseminated adenocarcinoma of breast, pancreas, or stomach, squamous cell carcinoma of head, neck, lung, and cervix. Not recommended to replace surgery or radiotherapy or as a single primary therapeutic agent.

**CONTRAINDICATIONS** Hypersensitivity or idiosyncratic reaction; severe bone marrow suppression; coagulation disorders or bleeding tendencies; over-hydration; pregnancy (category D); lactation.

**CAUTIOUS USE** Renal impairment; myelosuppression; pulmonary disease or respiratory insufficiency; older adults; children.

## ROUTE & DOSAGE

**Cancer**

*Adult/Child:* **IV** 10–20 mg/m²/ day as a single dose q6–8wk, additional doses based on hematologic response

**Renal Impairment Dosage Adjustment**

*CrCl less than 10 mL/min:* Use 75% of dose

## ADMINISTRATION

**Intravenous**

Note: Verify correct IV concentration and rate of infusion/ injection for administration to children with prescriber.

**PREPARE: Direct:** Reconstitute each 5 mg vial with 10 mL sterile water for injection. Shake to dissolve. If product does not clear immediately, allow to stand at room temperature until solution is obtained. Reconstituted solution is purple. **IV Infusion:** Reconstituted solution may be further diluted to concentrations of 20–40 mcg in D5W, NS, or LR.
**ADMINISTER: Direct:** Give reconstituted solution over 5–10 min or longer. **IV Infusion:** Give over 10 min or longer as determined by total volume of solution. ▪ D5W IV solutions **must be** infused within 3 h of preparation (see storage, below). ▪ Monitor IV site closely. Avoid extravasation to prevent extreme tissue reaction (cellulitis) to the toxic drug.
**INCOMPATIBILITIES: Solution/additive:** DEXTROSE-CONTAINING SOLUTIONS, **bleomycin. Y-site: Aztreonam, cefepime, etoposide, filgrastim, gemcitabine, piperacillin/tazobactam, sargramostim, topotecan, vinorelbine.**

▪ Store drug reconstituted with sterile water for injection (0.5 mg/mL) for 14 days refrigerated or 7 days at room temperature. ▪ Drug diluted in D5W (20–40 mcg/mL) is stable at room temperature for 3 h.

**ADVERSE EFFECTS** (≥1%) **CNS:** Paresthesias. **GI:** Stomatitis, *nausea, vomiting,* anorexia, hematemesis, diarrhea. **Hematologic:** Bone marrow toxicity (*thrombocytopenia, leukopenia* occurring 4–8 wk after treatment onset),

M

Common adverse effects in *italic;* life-threatening effects underlined; generic names in **bold;** classifications in SMALL CAPS; ♣ Canadian drug name; ⊘ Prototype drug

1075

thrombophlebitis, anemia. **Respiratory:** <u>Acute bronchospasm,</u> hemoptysis, dyspnea, nonproductive cough, pneumonia, <u>interstitial pneumonitis.</u> **Skin:** Desquamation; induration, pain, necrosis, cellulitis at injection site; reversible alopecia, purple discoloration of nail beds. **Body as a Whole:** Pain, headache, fatigue, edema. **Urogenital:** <u>Hemolytic uremic syndrome,</u> renal toxicity.

## PHARMACOKINETICS **Metabolism:** Metabolized rapidly in liver. **Elimination:** In urine. **Half-Life:** 23–78 min.

## NURSING IMPLICATIONS

### Black Box Warning

*Mitomycin has been associated with severe bone marrow suppression, serious infections, hemorrhage, and irreversible renal failure.*

### Assessment & Drug Effects

- Withhold drug and notify prescriber if serum creatinine is greater than 1.7 mg/dL or if platelet count falls below 150,000/mm³ and WBC is down to 4000/mm³ or if prothrombin or bleeding times are prolonged.
- Monitor I&O ratio and pattern. Report any sign of impaired kidney function: Change in ratio, dysuria, hematuria, oliguria, frequency, urgency. Keep patient well hydrated (at least 2000–2500 mL orally daily if tolerated). Drug is nephrotoxic.
- Observe closely for signs of infection. Monitor body temperature frequently.
- Inspect oral cavity daily for signs of stomatitis or superinfection (see Appendix F).
- Monitor lab tests: Frequent CBC with differential, platelet count, Hgb, Hct, and serum creatinine

during and for at least 7 wk after treatment.

### Patient & Family Education

- Report to prescriber immediately if you have respiratory distress.
- Report signs of common cold to prescriber immediately.
- Understand that hair loss is reversible after cessation of treatment.

## MITOTANE
(mye′toe-tane)
Lysodren
**Classification:** ANTINEOPLASTIC
Therapeutic: ANTINEOPLASTIC

**AVAILABILITY** Tablet

## ACTION & *THERAPEUTIC EFFECT*
Cytotoxic agent with suppressant action on the adrenal cortex. Modifies peripheral metabolism of steroids and reduces production of adrenal steroids. Extra-adrenal metabolism of cortisol is altered, leading to reduction in 17-hydroxycorticosteroids (17-OHCS); however, plasma levels of corticosteroids do not fall. *Cytotoxic agent with suppressant action on the adrenal cortex.*

**USES** Inoperable adrenal cortical carcinoma (functional and nonfunctional).

**UNLABELED USES** Cushing's syndrome.

**CONTRAINDICATIONS** Shock, severe trauma; lactation.

**CAUTIOUS USE** Liver disease; infection; preexisting neurologic disease; pregnancy (category C); children.

Common adverse effects in *italic*; life-threatening effects <u>underlined</u>; generic names in **bold**; classifications in SMALL CAPS; ♣ Canadian drug name; ⊕ Prototype drug

## ROUTE & DOSAGE

**Adrenocortical Carcinoma**
*Adult:* **PO** Initially 1–6 g/day in divided doses t.i.d. or q.i.d. then increased to 9–10 g/day in divided doses (tolerated dose range: 2–16 g/day)

## ADMINISTRATION

### Oral

- Alert. Withhold temporarily and consult prescriber if shock or trauma occurs, since adrenal suppression is its prime action. Exogenous steroids may be required until the already depressed adrenal starts secreting steroids.
- Store at 15°–30° C (59°–86° F) in tight, light-resistant containers.

## ADVERSE EFFECTS (≥1%) CNS:
Vertigo, dizziness, drowsiness, tiredness, depression, *lethargy, sedation,* headache, confusion, tremors. **CV:** Hypertension, hypotension, flushing **GI:** *Anorexia, nausea, vomiting, diarrhea.* **Urogenital:** Hematuria, hemorrhagic cystitis, albuminuria. **Endocrine:** Adrenocortical insufficiency. **Special Senses:** Blurred vision, diplopia, lens opacity, toxic retinopathy. **Body as a Whole:** Generalized aching, fever, muscle twitching, hypersensitivity reactions, hyperpyrexia. **Skin:** *Rash,* cutaneous eruptions and pigmentation. **Metabolic:** *Hypouricemia, hypercholesterolemia.*

## DIAGNOSTIC TEST INTERFERENCE
Mitotane decreases ***protein-bound iodine (PBI)*** and ***urinary 17-OHCS levels.***

## INTERACTIONS **Drug:** Potentiates sedative effects of **alcohol** and other CNS DEPRESSANTS; may increase the metabolism of **phenytoin, phenobarbital, warfarin,** decreasing their effectiveness. POTASSIUM SPARING DIURETICS may decrease the effect.

## PHARMACOKINETICS **Absorption:** Approximately 40% absorbed from GI tract. **Onset:** 2–4 wk. **Peak:** 3–5 h. **Distribution:** Deposits in most body tissues, especially adipose tissue. **Metabolism:** In liver. **Elimination:** 10% in urine, 1–17% in feces. **Half-Life:** 18–159 days.

## NURSING IMPLICATIONS

### Assessment & Drug Effects

- Monitor pulse and BP for early signs of shock (adrenal insufficiency).
- Observe for symptoms of hepatotoxicity (see Appendix F). Report them promptly, since reduced hepatic capacity can increase toxicity of mitotane and because dose may have to be decreased.
- Notify prescriber if following persist and become more severe: Aching muscles, fever, flushing, and muscle twitching.
- Monitor obese patient for symptoms of adrenal hypofunction. Because a large portion of the drug deposits in fatty tissue, the obese are particularly susceptible to prolonged adverse effects.
- Make neurologic and behavioral assessments at regular intervals throughout therapy.

### Patient & Family Education

- Be aware that mitotane does not cure but does reduce tumor mass, pain, weakness, anorexia, and steroid symptoms.
- Report symptoms of adrenal insufficiency (weakness, fatigue, orthostatic hypotension, pigmentation, weight loss, dehydration, anorexia, nausea, vomiting, and diarrhea) to prescriber.
- Exercise caution when driving or performing potentially hazardous tasks requiring alertness because of drug-induced drowsiness, tiredness, dizziness. Symptoms tend to recede with continuation in therapy.

M

Common adverse effects in *italic;* life-threatening effects underlined; generic names in **bold;** classifications in SMALL CAPS; ♣ Canadian drug name; ⊘ Prototype drug

1077

# MITOXANTRONE HYDROCHLORIDE

(mi-tox'an-trone)

Novantrone

**Classification:** ANTINEOPLASTIC
**Therapeutic:** ANTINEOPLASTIC;
IMMUNOSUPPRESSANT
**Prototype:** Doxorubicin

**AVAILABILITY** Solution for injection

## ACTION & *THERAPEUTIC EFFECT*

Non-cell-cycle specific antitumor agent with less cardiotoxicity than doxorubicin. Interferes with DNA synthesis by intercalating with the DNA double helix, blocking effective DNA and RNA transcription. *Highly destructive to rapidly proliferating cells in all stages of cell division.*

**USES** In combination with other drugs for the treatment of acute nonlymphocytic leukemia (ANLL) in adults, bone pain in advanced prostate cancer. Reducing neurologic disability and/or frequency of clinical relapses in multiple sclerosis.

**UNLABELED USES** Breast cancer, non-Hodgkin's lymphomas, autologous bone marrow transplant.

**CONTRAINDICATIONS** Hypersensitivity to mitoxantrone; myelosuppression; baseline LVEF less than 50%; multiple sclerosis; pregnancy (category D); lactation.

**CAUTIOUS USE** Impaired cardiac function; impaired liver and kidney function; systemic infections; previous treatment with daunorubicin or doxorubicin due to increased possibility of decreased cardiac function; children.

## ROUTE & DOSAGE

### Combination Therapy (with Cytarabine) for ANLL

*Adult:* **IV Induction Therapy** 12 mg/m$^2$/day on days 1–3, may need to repeat induction course; **IV Consolidation Therapy** 12 mg/m$^2$ on days 1 and 2 (max lifetime dose: 80–120 mg/m$^2$)

### Prostate Cancer

*Adult:* **IV** 12–14 mg/m$^2$ q21days

### Multiple Sclerosis

*Adult:* **IV** 12 mg/m$^2$ q3mo (max lifetime dose: 140 mg/m$^2$) Discontinue drug in MS patients if LVEF drops below 50% or if there is a clinically significant reduction in LVEF.

## ADMINISTRATION

**Intravenous**

If mitoxantrone touches skin, wash immediately with copious amounts of warm water.

***PREPARE:* IV Infusion: Must be** diluted prior to use. Withdraw contents of vial and add to at least 50 mL of D5W or NS. ▪ May be diluted to larger volumes to extend infusion time. ▪ Use goggles, gloves, and protective gown during drug preparation and administration.

***ADMINISTER:* IV Infusion:** Administer into the tubing of a freely running IV of D5W or NS and infused over at least 3 min or longer (i.e., 30–60 min) depending on the total volume of IV solution. ▪ If extravasation occurs, stop infusion and immediately restart in another vein.

***INCOMPATIBILITIES:*** Solution/additive: **Heparin, hydrocortisone, paclitaxel.** Y-site: **Amphotericin**

Common adverse effects in *italic*; life-threatening effects <u>underlined</u>; generic names in **bold**; classifications in SMALL CAPS; ♣ Canadian drug name; ⊘ Prototype drug

B cholesteryl complex, ampicillin, ampicillin/sulbactam, atenolol, azithromycin, aztreonam, cefazolin, cefoperazone, cefotaxime, cefoxitin, ceftazidime, ceftriaxone, cefuroxime, clindamycin, dantrolene, dexamethasone, diazepam, digoxin, cefepime, doxorubicin liposome, ertapenem, foscarnet, fosphenytion, furosemide, gemtuzumab, heparin, idarubicin, lansoprazole, methylprednisolone, nafcillin, nitroprusside, paclitaxel, pantoprazole, pemetrexed, phenytoin, piperacillin/tazobactam, propofol, ticarcillin, voriconazole, TPN.

• Discard unused portions of diluted solution. • Once opened, multiple-use vials may be stored refrigerated at $2^\circ$–$8^\circ$ C ($35^\circ$–$46^\circ$ F) for 14 days.

## ADVERSE EFFECTS (≥1%) CV:
Arrhythmias, decreased left ventricular function, *CHF*, tachycardia, ECG changes, MI (occurs with cumulative doses of greater than 80–100 mg/m²), edema, increased risk of cardiotoxicity. GI: *Nausea, vomiting,* constipation, diarrhea, hepatotoxicity. Hematologic: Leukopenia, thrombocytopenia. Other: Discolors urine and sclera a blue-green color. Skin: Mild phlebitis, blue skin discoloration, alopecia.

## INTERACTIONS Drug: May impair immune response to VACCINES such as influenza and pneumococcal infections. May have increased risk of infection with yellow fever vaccine.

## PHARMACOKINETICS Distribution: Rapidly taken up by tissues and slowly released into plasma, 95% protein bound. Metabolism: In liver. Elimination: Primarily in bile. Half-Life: 37 h.

## NURSING IMPLICATIONS

### Black Box Warning

*Mitoxantrone has been associated with potentially fatal CHF that may occur during therapy or months to years after end of therapy; extravasation has been associated with severe, local tissue damage.*

### Assessment & Drug Effects
• Monitor IV insertion site. Transient blue skin discoloration may occur at site if extravasation has occurred.
• Monitor cardiac functioning throughout course of therapy including LVEF; report signs and symptoms of CHF or cardiac arrhythmias.
• Monitor lab tests: Baseline and periodic LFTs and CBC with differential.

### Patient & Family Education
• Understand potential adverse effects of mitoxantrone therapy.
• Expect urine to turn blue-green for 24 h after drug administration; sclera may also take on a bluish color.
• Be aware that stomatitis/mucositis may occur within 1 wk of therapy.
• Do not risk exposure to those with known infections during the periods of myelosuppression.

## MODAFINIL
(mod-a'fi-nil)
Provigil, Alertec ♦

## ARMODAFINIL
Nuvigil
Classification: CNS STIMULANT, ANALEPTIC
Therapeutic: CNS STIMULANT; ANTINARCOLEPTIC
Controlled Substance: Schedule IV

## AVAILABILITY Tablet

M

Common adverse effects in *italic*; life-threatening effects underlined; generic names in bold; classifications in SMALL CAPS; ♦ Canadian drug name; ⊚ Prototype drug

## ACTION & *THERAPEUTIC EFFECT*

Primary sites of CNS stimulant activity of modafinil appear to be in the hippocampus, the centrolateral nucleus of the thalamus, and the central nucleus of the amygdala. Modafinil may increase excitatory transmission in the thalamus and hippocampus. *Modafinil causes wakefulness, increased locomotor activity, and psychoactive and euphoric effects.*

**USES** Improve wakefulness in patients with narcolepsy or excessive sleepiness associated with shift work sleep disorder, obstructive sleep apnea/hypopnea syndrome.

**UNLABELED USES** Fatigue related to organic brain syndrome or multiple sclerosis, ADHD.

**CONTRAINDICATIONS** Hypersensitivity to modafinil.

**CAUTIOUS USE** Cardiovascular disease including left ventricular hypertrophy; cardiac disease, ischemic ECG changes, chest pain, arrhythmias, mitral valve prolapse, recent MI, unstable angina; history of drug or alcohol abuse; psychosis or emotional instability, depression, mania; neurologic disease, Tourette syndrome; severe hepatic impairment; renal impairment; sleep apnea; older adults; pregnancy (category C); lactation. Safety and efficacy in children under 18 y not established.

## ROUTE & DOSAGE

### Narcolepsy, Fatigue

Adult: **PO (Provigil)** 200 mg/each morning; **(Nuvigil)** 150 or 250 mg each morning

### Shift-Work Sleep Disorder

Adult: **PO (Provigil)** 200 mg 1 h prior to shift; **(Nuvigil)** 150 mg 1 h prior to shift

### Hepatic Impairment Dosage Adjustment

Reduce dose by 50%

## ADMINISTRATION

### Oral

- Give in the morning shortly after awakening.
- Store at 20°–25° C (68°–77° F).

**ADVERSE EFFECTS** (≥1%) **Body as a Whole:** Chest pain, neck pain, chills, back pain, eosinophilia. **CNS:** *Headache,* nervousness, dizziness, depression, anxiety, cataplexy, insomnia, paresthesia, dyskinesia, hypertonia. **CV:** Hypotension, hypertension, vasodilation, arrhythmia, syncope. **GI:** *Nausea,* diarrhea, dry mouth, *abdominal pain, anorexia,* abnormal LFTs, vomiting, mouth ulcer, gingivitis, thirst. **Respiratory:** Rhinitis, pharyngitis, lung disorder, dyspnea. **Skin:** Dry skin. **Special Senses:** Amblyopia, abnormal vision.

**INTERACTIONS Drug: Methylphenidate** may delay absorption of modafinil; modafinil may decrease levels of **cyclosporine,** ORAL CONTRACEPTIVES; modafinil may increase levels of **clomipramine, phenytoin, warfarin,** TRICYCLIC ANTIDEPRESSANTS. Do not take with **ritonavir.**

**PHARMACOKINETICS Absorption:** Rapidly absorbed. **Peak:** 2–4 h. **Distribution:** Approximately 60% protein bound. **Metabolism:** In liver to inactive metabolites. **Elimination:** In urine. **Half-Life:** 15 h.

## NURSING IMPLICATIONS

### Assessment & Drug Effects

- Therapeutic effectiveness: Indicated by improved daytime wakefulness.
- Monitor BP and cardiovascular status, especially with preexisting hypertension and mitral valve prolapse or other CV condition.

- Monitor for S&S of psychosis, especially when history of psychotic episodes exists.
- Coadministered drugs: Monitor INR with warfarin for first several months and when dosage is changed; monitor for toxicity with phenytoin.
- Monitor lab tests: CBC, periodic LFTs.

**Patient & Family Education**
- Use barrier contraceptive instead of/in addition to hormonal contraceptive.
- Inform prescriber of all prescription or OTC drugs in/added to your regimen.
- Notify prescriber if any S&S of an allergic reaction appear.

# MOEXIPRIL HYDROCHLORIDE
(mo-ex′i-pril)
Univasc
**Classifications:** ANGIOTENSIN-CONVERTING ENZYME (ACE) INHIBITOR; ANTIHYPERTENSIVE
**Therapeutic:** ANTIHYPERTENSIVE
**Prototype:** Enalapril

**AVAILABILITY** Tablet

**ACTION & *THERAPEUTIC EFFECT***
ACE inhibitor that results in decreased conversion of angiotensin I to angiotensin II. Results in decreased vasopressor activity and aldosterone secretion. Lowering angiotensin II plasma levels results in blood pressure decreases and plasma renin activity increases. *ACE inhibition and decreased aldosterone secretion are responsible for its antihypertensive effect.*

**USES** Hypertension.

**UNLABELED USES** CHF, left ventricular dysfunction.

**CONTRAINDICATIONS** Hypersensitivity to moexipril; history of angioedema related to an ACE inhibitor; pregnancy (category D second and third trimester).

**CAUTIOUS USE** Hypersensitivity to any other ACE inhibitor; renal impairment, renal artery stenosis, volume-depleted patients; hypertensive patient with CHF; history of autoimmune disease; severe liver dysfunction; immunosuppressed patients; hyperkalemia; patients undergoing surgery/anesthesia; preexisting neutropenia; pregnancy (category C first trimester); lactation. Safety and efficacy in children not established.

## ROUTE & DOSAGE

**Hypertension**

*Adult:* **PO** 7.5 mg once/day, may increase up to 30 mg/day in divided doses

***Renal Impairment Dosage Adjustment***

*CrCl 40 mL/min or less:* Start with 3.75 mg daily (max: Titrate up to 15 mg daily)

## ADMINISTRATION
**Oral**
- Give 1 h before or 2 h after meals. Food greatly reduces absorption of moexipril.
- May need to reduce starting dose 50% in patients with possible volume depletion or a history of renal insufficiency.
- Store at 15°–30° C (59°–86° F).

**ADVERSE EFFECTS** (≥1%) **CNS:** Headache, *dizziness,* drowsiness, sleep disturbances, nervousness, anxiety, mood changes. **CV:** Hypotension, chest pain, angina, peripheral edema, <u>MI</u>, palpitations,

Common adverse effects in *italic;* life-threatening effects <u>underlined;</u> generic names in **bold;** classifications in SMALL CAPS; ♣ Canadian drug name; ⊘ Prototype drug

1081

arrhythmias. **Endocrine:** Hyperkalemia. **GI:** Diarrhea, nausea, dyspepsia, abdominal pain, taste disturbances, constipation, vomiting, dry mouth, pancreatitis. **Urogenital:** Urinary frequency, increased BUN and serum creatinine. **Hematologic:** Neutropenia, hemolytic anemia. **Respiratory:** Cough, pharyngitis, rhinitis, flu-like symptoms. **Skin:** <u>Angioedema</u> (rare), rash, flushing.

**INTERACTIONS Drug:** Capsaicin may exacerbate cough. NSAIDS may reduce antihypertensive effects. May increase **lithium** levels and toxicity. POTASSIUM SUPPLEMENTS and POTASSIUM-SPARING DIURETICS may increase risk of hyperkalemia. **Food:** Food greatly reduces absorption of moexipril.

**PHARMACOKINETICS Absorption:** Readily absorbed from GI tract; approximately 13% of active metabolite reaches systemic circulation; absorption greatly reduced by food. **Onset:** 1 h. **Duration:** 24 h. **Distribution:** Approximately 50% protein bound. **Metabolism:** In liver to moexiprilat (active metabolite). **Elimination:** 13% in urine, 53% in feces. **Half-Life:** 2–9 h.

## NURSING IMPLICATIONS

### Black Box Warning

*Moexipril has been associated with fetal injury and death.*

### Assessment & Drug Effects

- Monitor closely for systematic hypotension that may occur within 1–3 h of first dose, especially in those with high blood pressure, on a diuretic or restricted salt intake, or otherwise volume depleted.
- Monitor BP and HR frequently during initiation of therapy, whenever a diuretic is added, and periodically throughout therapy.
- Determine trough BP (just before next dose) before dose adjustments are made.
- Monitor for and report promptly significant behavioral changes and/or neuropsychiatric events.
- Monitor lab tests: Periodic serum electrolytes, WBC with differential, Hct and Hgb, urinalysis, LFTs and renal function tests.

### Patient & Family Education

- Report to prescriber immediately if you suspect you are pregnant.
- Report to prescriber immediately swelling around face or neck or in extremities.
- Report S&S of hypotension (e.g., dizziness, weakness, syncope); nonproductive cough; skin rash; flu-like symptoms; jaundice; irregular heartbeat or chest pains; and dehydration from vomiting, diarrhea, or diaphoresis.
- Report promptly behavioral changes (e.g., aggression, anxiety, hostility, mood changes, insomnia, memory impairment).

## MOMETASONE FUROATE

(mo-met'a-sone)

Asmanex, Elocon, Nasonex

**See Appendix A-3.**

## MONTELUKAST

(mon-te-lu'cast)

Singulair

**Classifications:** BRONCHODILATOR (RESPIRATORY SMOOTH MUSCLE RELAXANT); LEUKOTRIENE RECEPTOR ANTAGONIST

**Therapeutic:** BRONCHODILATOR

**Prototype:** Zafirlukast

**AVAILABILITY** Tablet; chewable tablet; oral granules

**ACTION & *THERAPEUTIC EFFECT***
Selective receptor antagonist of leukotriene, thus inhibiting bronchoconstriction. Leukotrienes (inflammatory agents) induce bronchoconstriction and mucus production. Elevated sputum and blood levels of leukotrienes are present during acute asthma attacks. Montelukast controls asthmatic attacks by inhibiting leukotriene release as well as inflammatory action associated with the attack. *Effectiveness is indicated by improved pulmonary functions and better controlled asthmatic symptoms.*

**USES** Prophylaxis and chronic treatment of asthma or allergic rhinitis; exercise-induced bronchoconstriction (EIB).

**UNLABELED USES** Refractory urticaria, atopic dermatitis.

**CONTRAINDICATIONS** Hypersensitivity to montelukast; acute asthma attacks; bronchoconstriction due to acute asthma; status asthmaticus; suicidal ideation.

**CAUTIOUS USE** Hypersensitivity to other leukotriene receptor antagonists (e.g., zafirlukast, zileuton); history of mental illness; history of suicidal thoughts or behavior; severe liver disease; jaundice, PKU; severe asthma; pregnancy (category B); lactation; children younger than 6 mo.

**ROUTE & DOSAGE**

**Asthma**

*Adult:* **PO** 10 mg daily in evening
*Child (12 mo–5 y):* **PO** 4 mg daily in evening; *6–14 y:* 5 mg chewable tablet daily in evening

**EIB**

*Adult/Adolescent (15 y or older):* **PO** 10 mg 2 h before exercise (not more than 1/day)
*Child (6–14 y):* **PO** 5 mg 2 h before exercise

**Allergic Rhinitis**

*Adult/Adolescent:* **PO** 10 mg daily
*Child (6–14 y):* **PO** 5 mg daily; *6 mo–5 y:* 4 mg daily

**ADMINISTRATION**

**Oral**
- Give in the evening for maximum effectiveness.
- Ensure chewable tablets for children are not swallowed whole.
- Store at 15°–30° C (59°–86° F) in a tightly closed container and protect from light.

**ADVERSE EFFECTS** (≥1%) **Body as a Whole:** Asthenia, fever, trauma. **CNS:** Dizziness, *headache* <u>suicidal ideation</u>, hallucination, fatigue. **GI:** Abdominal pain, dyspepsia, gastroenteritis, dental pain, abnormal liver function tests (ALT, AST), diarrhea, nausea. **Respiratory:** Nasal congestion, cough, influenza, laryngitis, pharyngitis, sinusitis. **Skin:** Rash. **Urogenital:** Pyuria.

**PHARMACOKINETICS Absorption:** Rapidly absorbed from GI tract, bioavailability 64%. **Peak:** 3–4 h for oral tablet, 2–2.5 h for chewable tablet. **Distribution:** Greater than 99% protein bound. **Metabolism:** Extensively metabolized by CYP3A4 and 2C9. **Elimination:** In feces. **Half-Life:** 2.7–5.5 h.

M

## NURSING IMPLICATIONS

### Assessment & Drug Effects

- Monitor effectiveness carefully when used in combination with phenobarbital or other potent cytochrome P450 enzyme inducers.
- Lab test: Periodic liver function tests.

### Patient & Family Education

- Do not use for reversal of an acute asthmatic attack.
- Inform prescriber if short-acting inhaled bronchodilators are needed more often than usual with montelukast.
- Use chewable tablets (contain phenylalanine) with caution with PKU.

## MORPHINE SULFATE ⊕

(mor'feen)

Arymo, Astramorph, DepoDur, Duramorph, Infumorph, Kadian, MS Contin, MorphaBond ER, Statex ♣

**Classifications:** ANALGESIC; NARCOTIC (OPIATE AGONIST)
Therapeutic: NARCOTIC ANALGESIC
**Controlled Substance:** Schedule II

**AVAILABILITY** Tablet; controlled release tablet/capsule; oral solution; injection; extended release lysosomal injection; suppository

## ACTION & *THERAPEUTIC EFFECT*

Natural opium alkaloid with agonist activity that binds with the same receptors as endogenous opioid peptides. Narcotic agonist effects are identified with different locations of receptors: Analgesia at supraspinal level, euphoria, respiratory depression and physical dependence; analgesia at spinal level, sedation and miosis; and dysphoric, hallucinogenic, and cardiac stimulant effects. *Controls severe pain; also used as an adjunct to anesthesia.*

**USES** Symptomatic relief of severe acute and chronic pain.

**CONTRAINDICATIONS** Hypersensitivity to morphine or opiate agonists; convulsive disorders; acute or severe bronchial asthma with resuscitative equipment; severe respiratory depression; head injury; heart failure secondary to chronic lung disease; chemical-irritant-induced pulmonary edema; hypovolemia; undiagnosed acute abdominal conditions; following biliary tract surgery and surgical anastomosis; pancreatitis, known or suspected GI ileus; severe liver insufficiency; concomitant use of alcohol; hypothyroidism; within 14 days of use of MAOI; during labor for delivery of a premature infant, premature infants; pregnancy (category C all trimesters). **Release Oral Solution:** Hypersensitivity to morphine, respiratory insufficiency or depression; severe CNS depression; attack of bronchial asthma; heart failure secondary to chronic lung disease; cardiac arrhythmias; increased intracranial or cerebrospinal pressure; head injuries; brain tumor; acute alcoholism, DT; convulsive disorders; after biliary tract surgery; suspected surgical abdomen; surgical anastomosis; concomitantly with MAOIs or within 14 days of use. **ER:** Lactation.

**CAUTIOUS USE** Head trauma; increased cranial pressure; toxic psychosis; renal impairment; mild or moderate hepatic impairment; circulatory shock; CNS depression

Common adverse effects in *italic;* life-threatening effects <u>underlined;</u> generic names in **bold;** classifications in SMALL CAPS; ♣ Canadian drug name; ⊕ Prototype drug

or coma; seizure disorders; elevated ICP; GI obstruction; mild or moderate hepatic impairment; Addison's disease; hypothyroidism; BPH; urethra stricture; psychosis; history of orthostatic hypotension in ambulatory patients; cardiac arrhythmias, CVD; ulcerative colitis; constipation; emphysema; history of acute asthma attacks, COPD; pancreatitic or biliary tract disease; kyphoscoliosis; cor pulmonale; severe obesity; reduced blood volume; BPH; renal disease; history of substance abuse or alcoholism; older adults, young, or debilitated patients; children; labor, pregnancy (category C for low doses, short-term use, and not close to term); lactation.

## ROUTE & DOSAGE

### Pain Relief

**There is substantial interpatient variability in the relative potency of different opioid products. Opioid tolerance will impact dosing.**

*Adult:* **PO** 10–30 mg q4h prn or 15–30 mg sustained release q8–12h; **(Kadian)** dose q12–24h, increase dose prn for pain relief; **IV/IM/Subcutaneous** 2–10 mg/70 kg q3–4h; **Epidural** 5 mg given epidurally, may administer incremental doses of 1–2 mg with time between (max 10 mg q24h) **(DepoDur** only) 15 mg as single dose 30 min before surgery (max: 20 mg); **PR** 10–20 mg q4h prn *Child:* **IV/IM/Subcutaneous** 0.05–0.2 mg/kg q2–4h or 0.025–2.6 mg/kg/h by continuous infusion (max: 10 mg/dose)

### Renal Impairment Dosage Adjustment

Dose may need adjustment to prevent metabolite accumulation

## ADMINISTRATION

### Oral

- A fixed, individualized schedule is recommended when narcotic analgesic therapy is started to provide effective management; blood levels can be maintained and peaks of pain can be prevented (usually a 4-h interval is adequate).
- Lower dosages are recommended for older adult or debilitated patients.
- Do not break in half, crush, or allow sustained release tablet to be chewed.
- Do not give patient sustained release tablet within 24 h of surgery.
- Dilute oral solution in approximately 30 mL or more of fluid or semisolid food. A calibrated dropper comes with the bottle. Read labels carefully when using liquid preparation; available solutions: 20 mg/mL; 100 mg/mL.

### Intramuscular/Subcutaneous

- Give undiluted.

### Intravenous

Note: Verify correct IV concentration and rate of infusion/injection for administration to neonates, infants, or children with prescriber.

**PREPARE: Direct:** Dilute 2–10 mg in at least 5 mL of sterile water for injection. **Continuous:** Typically diluted to a range of 0.1–1 mg/mL. ■ More concentrated solutions may be required with fluid restriction.

**ADMINISTER: Direct:** Give a single dose over 4–5 min. Avoid rapid administration. **Continuous:** Infuse via a controlled infusion device at a rate determined by patient response as ordered.

**INCOMPATIBILITIES:** Solution/additive: **Aminophylline, amobarbital, chlorothiazide, floxacillin,**

Common adverse effects in *italic;* life-threatening effects underlined; generic names in **bold;** classifications in SMALL CAPS; ♣ Canadian drug name; ⊙ Prototype drug

1085

fluorouracil, haloperidol, heparin, meperidine, phenobarbital, phenytoin, sodium bicarbonate, thiopental sodium. **Y-site:** Alatarofloxacin mesylate, Alemtuzumab, amphotericin B cholesteryl complex, azathioprine, ceftobiprole, cloxacillin sodium dantrolene, diazoxide, daunorubicin citrate liposome, folic acid, ganciclovir sodium, garenoxacin mesylate, gemtuzumab, inamrinone lactate indomethacin, lansoprazole, micafungin, mitomycin, pentamidine, pentobarbital, phenytoin, sargramostim, trastuzumab.

▪ Store oral and parenteral medication at 15°–30° C (59°–86° F). Avoid freezing. Refrigerate suppositories. Protect all formulations from light.

## ADVERSE EFFECTS (≥1%) **Body as a Whole:** Hypersensitivity [*pruritus,* rash, urticaria, edema, hemorrhagic urticaria (rare), <u>anaphylactoid reaction</u> (rare)], sweating, skeletal muscle flaccidity; cold, clammy skin, hypothermia. **CNS:** Euphoria, insomnia, disorientation, visual disturbances, dysphoria, paradoxic CNS stimulation (restlessness, tremor, delirium, insomnia), convulsions (infants and children); decreased cough reflex, drowsiness, dizziness, deep sleep, coma, continuous intrathecal infusion may cause granulomas leading to paralysis, withdrawal syndrome. **Special Senses:** Miosis, visual disturbances, nystagmus. **CV:** Bradycardia, palpitations, syncope; flushing of face, neck, and upper thorax; orthostatic hypotension, peripheral edema, hypertension, tachycardia, <u>cardiac arrest</u>. **GI:** *Constipation,* anorexia,

flatulence, dry mouth, biliary colic, *nausea,* vomiting, elevated transaminase levels. **Urogenital:** Urinary retention or urgency, dysuria, oliguria, reduced libido or potency (prolonged use), amenorrhea, impotence. **Other:** Prolonged labor and respiratory depression of newborn. **Hematologic:** Precipitation of porphyria. **Respiratory:** <u>Severe respiratory depression</u> (as low as 2–4/min) or <u>arrest</u>; pulmonary edema.

## DIAGNOSTIC TEST INTERFERENCE
False-positive ***urine glucose*** determinations may occur using ***Benedict's solution. Plasma amylase*** and ***lipase*** determinations may be falsely positive for 24 h after use of morphine; ***transaminase levels*** may be elevated.

## INTERACTIONS **Drug:** CNS DEPRESSANTS, SEDATIVES, BARBITURATES, BENZODIAZEPINES, and TRICYCLIC ANTIDEPRESSANTS potentiate CNS depressant effects. Contraindicated with MAO INHIBITORS use in previous 14 days; they may precipitate hypertensive crisis. PHENOTHIAZINES may antagonize analgesia. Use with SSRIs can increase risk of serotonin syndrome. Use with **alcohol** may lead to potentially fatal overdoses (contraindicated with **Avinza**). **Herbal:** Kava, valerian, St. John's wort may increase sedation.

## PHARMACOKINETICS **Absorption:** Variably from GI tract. **Peak:** 60 min PO; 20–60 min PR; 50–90 min subcutaneous; 30–60 min IM; 20 min IV. **Duration:** Up to 7 h. **Distribution:** Crosses blood–brain barrier and placenta; distributed in breast milk. **Metabolism:** In liver. **Elimination:** 90% in urine in 24 h; 7–10% in bile.

Common adverse effects in *italic;* life-threatening effects <u>underlined</u>; generic names in **bold**; classifications in SMALL CAPS; ✦ Canadian drug name; 🅿 Prototype drug

## NURSING IMPLICATIONS

### Black Box Warning

*Morphine has been associated with potentially fatal respiratory depression, high abuse potential, risk with neuraxial administration.*

### Assessment & Drug Effects

- Obtain baseline respiratory rate, depth, and rhythm and size of pupils before administering the drug. Respirations of 12/min or below and miosis are signs of toxicity. Withhold drug and report to prescriber.
- Observe patient closely to be certain pain relief is achieved. Record relief of pain and duration of analgesia.
- Monitor carefully those at risk for severe respiratory depression after epidural or intrathecal injection: Older adult or debilitated patients or those with decreased respiratory reserve (e.g., emphysema, severe obesity, kyphoscoliosis).
- Continue monitoring for respiratory depression for at least 24 h after each epidural or intrathecal dose.
- Assess vital signs at regular intervals. Morphine-induced respiratory depression may occur even with small doses, and it increases progressively with higher doses (generally max: 90 min after subcutaneous, 30 min after IM, and 7 min after IV).
- Encourage changes in position, deep breathing, and coughing (unless contraindicated) at regularly scheduled intervals. Narcotic analgesics also depress cough and sigh reflexes and thus may induce atelectasis, especially in postoperative patients.
- Be alert for nausea and orthostatic hypotension (with light-headedness and dizziness) in ambulatory patients or when a supine patient assumes

the head-up position or in patients not experiencing severe pain.

- Monitor I&O ratio and pattern. Report oliguria or urinary retention. Morphine may dull perception of bladder stimuli; therefore, encourage the patient to void at least q4h. Palpate lower abdomen to detect bladder distention.
- Monitor bowel patterns; promote oral fluids and ambulation when able to aid in prevention of constipation. May need to contact provider for stool softeners and/or laxatives as needed.

### Patient & Family Education

- Avoid alcohol and other CNS depressants while receiving morphine.
- Do not use of any OTC drug unless approved by prescriber.
- Do not ambulate without assistance after receiving drug.
- Use caution or avoid tasks requiring alertness (e.g., driving a car) until response to drug is known since morphine may cause drowsiness, dizziness, or blurred vision

## MOXIFLOXACIN HYDROCHLORIDE

(mox-i-flox'a-sin)

Avelox, Moxeza, Vigamox

**Classifications:** QUINOLONE ANTIBIOTIC

Therapeutic: ANTIBIOTIC

**Prototype:** Ciprofloxacin

**AVAILABILITY** Tablet; ophthalmic solution; solution for injection

## ACTION & *THERAPEUTIC EFFECT*

It inhibits DNA gyrase, an enzyme required for DNA replication, transcription, repair, and recombination of bacterial DNA. *Broad spectrum antibiotic that is bactericidal against gram-positive and gram-negative organisms.*

Common adverse effects in *italic;* life-threatening effects underlined; generic names in **bold;** classifications in SMALL CAPS; ✦ Canadian drug name; ⓟ Prototype drug

1087

**USES** Treatment of acute bacterial sinusitis, acute bacterial exacerbation of chronic bronchitis, community-acquired pneumonia, skin and skin structure infections, plague, bacterial conjunctivitis, complicated skin infections.

**UNLABELED USES** Hospital-acquired pneumonia, infective endocarditis, tuberculosis, plague prophylaxis.

**CONTRAINDICATIONS** Hypersensitivity to moxifloxacin or other quinolones; moderate to severe hepatic insufficiency; syphilis; MG; tendon pain; viral infection; history of torsades de pointes; lactation.

**CAUTIOUS USE** CNS disorders; history of seizures; severe cerebral arteriosclerosis; peripheral neuropathy; cerebrovascular disease, history of ventricular arrhythmias, atrial fibrillation; hypokalemia; bradycardia, acute myocardial ischemia, acute MI; colitis, diarrhea, GI disease; DM; mild or moderate heart insufficiency; QT prolongation; seizure disorder; sunlight (UV) exposure; hepatic impairment; older adults; pregnancy (category C). Safety and efficacy in children younger than 18 y not established. **Ocular preparation:** Use in children younger than 4 mo.

## ROUTE & DOSAGE

**Acute Bacterial Sinusitis, Acute Bacterial Exacerbation of Chronic Bronchitis, Community-Acquired Pneumonia, Skin Infections, Plague**

*Adult:* **PO/IV** 400 mg daily × 5–14 days

**Complicated Skin Infection**

*Adult:* **PO/IV** 400 mg daily × 7–21 days

## ADMINISTRATION

### Oral

- Administer 4 h before or 8 h after multivitamins (containing iron or zinc), antacids (containing magnesium, calcium, or aluminum), sucralfate, or didanosine.

### Intravenous

*PREPARE:* **IV Infusion:** Avelox (400 mg) is supplied in ready-to-use 250 mL IV bags. No further dilution is necessary.

*ADMINISTER:* **IV Infusion:** Give over 60 min. AVOID RAPID OR BOLUS DOSE.

*INCOMPATIBILITIES:* **Allopurinol, aminophylline, amphotericin B (Abelcet), ceftobidprole, dantrolene, fluorouracil, fosphenytoin, furosemide, nitroprusside, pantoprazole, phenytoin, vancomycin, voriconazole.**

- Store at 15°–30° C (59°–86° F); protect from high humidity.

**ADVERSE EFFECTS** (≥1%) **CNS:** Dizziness, headache, insomnia, peripheral neuropathy. **GI:** Nausea, diarrhea, abdominal pain, vomiting, taste perversion, abnormal liver function tests, dyspepsia. **Metabolic:** Decreased amylase, decreased glucose, increased albumin, hyperchloremia. **Musculoskeletal:** Tendon rupture, cartilage erosion. **CV:** Arrythmia, heart failure, QT prolongation. **Optic:** Visual impairment, ocular hemorrhage.

**DIAGNOSTIC TEST INTERFERENCE** May cause false positive on *opiate screening tests.*

**INTERACTIONS Drug:** Iron, zinc, ANTACIDS, **aluminum, magnesium, calcium, sucralfate** decrease absorption; use cautiously with other agents that can prolong QT interval

Common adverse effects in *italic;* life-threatening effects underlined; generic names in **bold;** classifications in SMALL CAPS; ♣ Canadian drug name; ⊙ Prototype drug

(e.g., **erythromycin, amiodarone, bepridil, cisapride, doeftilide, procainamide, ziprasidone**).

## PHARMACOKINETICS
**Absorption:** 90% bioavailable. **Steady State:** 3 d. **Distribution:** 50% protein bound. **Metabolism:** In liver. **Elimination:** Unchanged drug: 20% in urine, 25% in feces; metabolites: 38% in feces, 14% in urine. **Half-Life:** 12 h.

## NURSING IMPLICATIONS

### Black Box Warning

*Moxifloxacin has been associated with increased risk of tendinitis and tendon rupture.*

### Assessment & Drug Effects
- Monitor for and notify prescriber immediately of adverse CNS effects.
- Notify prescriber immediately for S&S of hypersensitivity (see Appendix F).
- Monitor lab tests: Baseline C&S and serum potassium with history of hypokalemia, LFTs, serum creatinine/BUN.

### Patient & Family Education
- Notify prescriber immediately if you experience pain, swelling, or inflammation of a tendon, or weakness or inability to use one of your joints.
- Drink fluids liberally, unless directed otherwise.
- Increased seizure potential is possible, especially when history of seizure exists.
- Stop taking drug and notify prescriber if experiencing palpitations, fainting, skin rash, severe diarrhea, dizziness, light-headedness, vision disorders, agitation, insomnia.
- Avoid engaging in hazardous activities until reaction to drug is known.

# MUPIROCIN
(mu-pi-ro'sin)
**Bactroban, Bactroban Nasal, Centany**
**Classification:** PSEUDOMONIC ACID ANTIBIOTIC
**Therapeutic:** ANTIBIOTIC

## AVAILABILITY
Ointment; cream

## ACTION & *THERAPEUTIC EFFECT*
Inhibits bacterial protein synthesis by binding with the bacterial transfer RNA. *Susceptible bacteria are* Staphylococcus aureus *[including methicillin-resistant (MRSA) and beta-lactamase-producing strains] and other* Staphylococcus *and* Streptococcus pyogenes.

## USES
Impetigo due to *Staphylococcus aureus*, beta-hemolytic *Streptococci*, and *Streptococcus pyogenes*; nasal carriage of *S. aureus.*

## UNLABELED USES
Superficial skin infections; burns.

## CONTRAINDICATIONS
Hypersensitivity to any of its components and for ophthalmic use; lactation. **Topical:** Do not apply to breast.

## CAUTIOUS USE
Renal impairment; pregnancy (category B); lactation; children.

## ROUTE & DOSAGE

### Impetigo
*Adult/Child (2 mo or older):* **Topical** Apply to affected area t.i.d., if no response in 3–5 days, reevaluate (usually continue for 1–2 wk)

### Elimination of Staphylococcal Nasal Carriage
*Adult/Child:* **Intranasal** Apply intranasally b.i.d. for 5 days

M

Common adverse effects in *italic;* life-threatening effects <u>underlined;</u> generic names in **bold;** classifications in SMALL CAPS; ♣ Canadian drug name; ✪ Prototype drug

1089

## ADMINISTRATION

### Topical

- Apply thin layer of medication to affected area. Wash hands before and after application.
- Cover area being treated with a gauze dressing if desired.

## ADVERSE EFFECTS (≥1%) Skin:
Burning, stinging, pain, pruritus, rash, erythema, dry skin, tenderness, swelling. **Special Senses:** Intranasal, local stinging, soreness, dry skin, pruritus. **CNS:** Headache.

## INTERACTIONS Drug: Incompatible with **salicylic acid 2%;** do not mix in HYDROPHILIC VEHICLES (e.g., **Aquaphor**) or COAL TAR SOLUTIONS; **chloramphenicol** may interfere with bactericidal action of mupirocin.

## PHARMACOKINETICS Absorption: Not systemically absorbed.

## NURSING IMPLICATIONS

### Assessment & Drug Effects

- Watch for signs and symptoms of superinfection (see Appendix F). Prolonged or repeated therapy may result in superinfection by nonsusceptible organisms.
- Reevaluate drug use if patient does not show clinical response within 3–5 days.
- Discontinue the drug and notify prescriber if signs of contact dermatitis develop or if exudate production increases.

### Patient & Family Education

- Discontinue drug and contact prescriber if a sensitivity reaction or chemical irritation occurs (e.g., increased redness, itching, burning).

## NABILONE ⓟ

(nab′i-lone)

**Cesamet**

**Classifications:** SYNTHETIC CANNABINOID; ANTIEMETIC

**Therapeutic:** ANTIEMETIC
**Prototype:** Aprepitant
**Controlled Substance:** Schedule II

## AVAILABILITY Capsule

## ACTION & *THERAPEUTIC EFFECT*
Nabilone is a synthetic cannabinoid with multiple effects on the CNS. It is thought that the antiemetic effect results from its interaction with the cannabinoid receptor system (CB1-receptor) in neural tissues. In therapeutic doses, it produces relaxation, drowsiness, and euphoria. *It effectively controls emesis in patients receiving chemotherapy when other drugs have failed.*

## USES Prevention and treatment of nausea and vomiting in adult patients induced by cancer chemotherapy refractory to standard antiemetic therapy.

## CONTRAINDICATIONS Hypersensitivity to any cannabinoid; hypovolemia; lactation.

## CAUTIOUS USE History of psychosis; older adults; pregnancy (category C); children.

## ROUTE & DOSAGE

### Nausea and Vomiting
*Adult:* **PO** Initial dose of 1 or 2 mg b.i.d. 1–3 h before chemotherapy. May increase (max: 2 mg t.i.d.) May continue for 48 h after last dose of chemotherapy.

## ADMINISTRATION

### Oral

- Give 1–3 h before chemotherapy is begun. A dose of 1–2 mg the night before chemotherapy may be helpful in relieving nausea.
- Store at 15°–30° C (59°–86° F).

**ADVERSE EFFECTS** (≥1%) **CNS:** Asthenia, *ataxia, confusion difficulties,* depersonalization, *depression,* disorientation, *drowsiness, dysphoria, euphoria,* headache, sedation, *sleep disturbance, vertigo.* **CV:** Hypotension. **GI:** Anorexia, *dry mouth,* increased appetite, nausea. **Special Senses:** *Visual disturbances.*

**INTERACTIONS Drug:** SEDATIVES, HYPNOTICS, and other psychoactive substances can potentiate the CNS effects of nabilone. Coadministration of cannabinoids with **amphetamine, cocaine,** TRICYCLIC ANTIDEPRESSANTS, and/or SYMPATHOMIMETIC AGENTS can produce additive hypertension and tachycardia. Coadministration of cannabinoids with ANTIHISTAMINES or ANTICHOLINERGIC AGENTS can produce additive tachycardia and drowsiness. Coadministration of cannabinoids with BARBITURATES, BENZODIAZEPINES, **buspirone, ethanol, lithium,** MUSCLE RELAXANTS, OPIOIDS, and other CNS DEPRESSANTS can produce additive drowsiness and CNS depressant effects. **Food: Alcohol** can potentiate the CNS effects of nabilone.

**PHARMACOKINETICS Absorption:** Complete absorption from GI tract. **Peak:** 2 h. **Metabolism:** Extensive hepatic metabolism. **Elimination:** Fecal (major) and urine. **Half-Life:** 2 h.

**NURSING IMPLICATIONS**

**Assessment & Drug Effects**

- Monitor for and report S&S of adverse psychiatric reactions (e.g., disorientation, hallucinations, psychosis) for 48–72 h after last dose of nabilone.
- Monitor for S&S of tachycardia and postural hypotension, especially in the older adult and those with a history of heart disease or hypertension.

- Monitor lab tests: Periodic CBC with Hgb and Hct.

**Patient & Family Education**

- Do not use alcohol or other CNS depressants while using this medication.
- Do not drive or engage in potentially hazardous activities until response to drug is known.
- Report any of the following to a health care provider: Confusion, disorientation, hallucinations, or other bizarre behavior.

**NABUMETONE**

(na-bu-me'tone)

**Classification:** ANALGESIC, NONSTEROIDAL ANTI-INFLAMMATORY DRUG (NSAID)
**Therapeutic:** ANALGESIC, NSAID; ANTIRHEUMATIC; ANTIPYRETIC
**Prototype:** Ibuprofen

**AVAILABILITY** Tablet

**ACTION & THERAPEUTIC EFFECT** Blocks prostaglandin synthesis by inhibiting cyclooxygenase, an enzyme that converts arachidonic acid to precursors of prostaglandins. *Anti-inflammatory, analgesic, and antipyretic effects. Effective antirheumatic agent. Inhibits platelet aggregation and prolongs bleeding time.*

**USES** Rheumatoid arthritis and osteoarthritis.

**CONTRAINDICATIONS** Patients in whom urticaria, severe rhinitis, bronchospasm, angioedema, or nasal polyps are precipitated by aspirin or other NSAIDs; salicylate hypersensitivity; active peptic ulcer; bleeding abnormalities; CABG perioperative pain; lactation.

**CAUTIOUS USE** Hypertension, fluid retention, heart failure; history of GI ulceration, impaired liver or kidney

Common adverse effects in *italic;* life-threatening effects <u>underlined</u>; generic names in **bold;** classifications in SMALL CAPS; ♣ Canadian drug name; ⊕ Prototype drug

1091

function, chronic kidney failure, cardiac decompensation, bone marrow suppression; patients with SLE; elderly; pregnancy (category C). Safety and efficacy in children not established.

## ROUTE & DOSAGE

### Rheumatoid & Osteoarthritis

Adult: **PO** 1000 mg/day or 500 mg b.i.d. may increase (max: 2000 mg/day)

## ADMINISTRATION

### Oral

- Give with food, milk, or antacid (if prescribed) to reduce the possibility of GI upset.
- Store at 20° C–25° C (68° F–77° F). Protect from light.

**ADVERSE EFFECTS** (≥1%) **GI:** Diarrhea, abdominal pain, nausea, dyspepsia, flatulence, melena, ulcers, constipation, dry mouth, gastritis. **CNS:** Tinnitus, dizziness, headache, insomnia, vertigo, fatigue, diaphoresis, nervousness, somnolence. **Skin:** Rash, pruritus.

**INTERACTIONS Drug:** May attenuate the antihypertensive response to DIURETICS. Has additive bleeding risk with ANTICOAGULANTS. NSAIDS increase the risk of **methotrexate** toxicity. Do not use with **cidofovir** or **ketorolac. Food:** Food may increase the peak but not the overall absorption of nabumetone. Alcohol usage can increase risk of gastric irritation. **Herbal: Feverfew, garlic, ginger, ginkgo** may increase bleeding potential.

**PHARMACOKINETICS Absorption:** Readily absorbed from GI tract; approximately 35% is converted to its active metabolite on first pass through the liver. **Onset:** 1–3 wk for antirheumatic action. **Peak:** 3–6 h. **Distribution:** 99% pro-

tein bound; distributes into synovial fluid. **Metabolism:** In liver to its active metabolite, 6-methoxy-2-naphthylacetic acid (6MNA). **Elimination:** 80% of dose is excreted in urine as 6MNA; 10% excreted in feces. **Half-Life:** 24 h (6MNA).

## NURSING IMPLICATIONS

### Black Box Warning

*Nabumetone has been associated with increased risk of serious, potentially fatal, GI bleeding and cardiovascular events (e.g., MI & CVA); risk may increase with duration of use and may be greater in the older adult and those with risk factors for CV disease.*

### Assessment & Drug Effects

- Monitor for signs and symptoms of GI bleeding.
- Monitor for and report promptly S&S of CV thrombotic events (i.e., angina, MI, TIA, or stroke).
- Monitor lab tests: Baseline and periodic Hgb and Hct with prolonged or high-dose therapy; CBC, LFTs, serum creatinine/BUN, stool guaiac.

### Patient & Family Education

- Use caution with hazardous activities since nabumetone may cause dizziness, drowsiness, and blurred vision.
- Report abdominal pain, nausea, dyspepsia, or black tarry stools.
- Stop taking drug and report promptly to prescriber if you experience chest pain, shortness of breath, weakness, slurring of speech, or other signs of a cardiac or neurologic problem.
- Be aware that alcohol and aspirin will increase the risk of GI ulceration and bleeding.
- Notify your prescriber if any of the following occur: Persistent headache, skin rash or itching, visual disturbances, weight gain, or edema.

Common adverse effects in *italic;* life-threatening effects underlined; generic names in **bold;** classifications in SMALL CAPS; ✤ Canadian drug name; ✪ Prototype drug

# NADOLOL

(nay-doe'lole)

Corgard

**Classifications:** BETA-ADRENERGIC ANTAGONIST; ANTIHYPERTENSIVE
**Therapeutic:** ANTIHYPERTENSIVE
**Prototype:** Propranolol

**AVAILABILITY** Tablet

## ACTION & *THERAPEUTIC EFFECT*

Nonselective beta-adrenergic blocking agent that inhibits response to adrenergic stimuli by competitively blocking these receptors within the heart. Reduces heart rate and cardiac output at rest and during exercise, and also decreases conduction velocity through AV node and myocardial automaticity. *Decreases both systolic and diastolic BP at rest and during exercise.*

**USES** Hypertension, either alone or in combination with a diuretic. Also long-term prophylactic management of angina pectoris.

**CONTRAINDICATIONS** Bronchial asthma, severe COPD, inadequate myocardial function, sinus bradycardia, greater than first-degree conduction block, overt cardiac failure, cardiogenic shock; abrupt withdrawal; lactation.

**CAUTIOUS USE** CHF; DM; ischemic heart disease; hyperthyroidism; renal failure, renal impairment; pregnancy (category C); children younger than 18 y.

## ROUTE & DOSAGE

### Hypertension, Angina

*Adult:* **PO** 40 mg once/day, may increase up to 240–320 mg/day in 1–2 divided doses

## ADMINISTRATION

### Oral

- Do not discontinue abruptly; reduce dosage over a 1–2-wk period. Abrupt withdrawal can precipitate MI or thyroid storm in susceptible patients.
- Store at 15°–30° C (59°–86° F); protect drug from light.

**ADVERSE EFFECTS (≥1%) Body as a Whole:** Hypersensitivity (rash, pruritus, laryngospasm, respiratory disturbances). **CV:** *Bradycardia, peripheral vascular insufficiency (Raynaud's type),* palpitation, postural hypotension, conduction or rhythm disturbances, CHF. **GI:** Dry mouth, anorexia, flatulence. **CNS:** *Dizziness, fatigue,* sedation, headache, paresthesias; behavioral changes. **Special Senses:** Blurred vision, dry eyes. **Skin:** Dry skin. **Urogenital:** Impotence.

**INTERACTIONS Drug:** NSAIDS may decrease hypotensive effects; may mask symptoms of a hypoglycemic reaction to **insulin,** SULFONYLUREAS; **prazosin, terazosin** may increase severe hypotensive response to first dose. **Amiodarone** causes additive effects.

**PHARMACOKINETICS Absorption:** 30–40% of PO dose absorbed. **Peak:** 2–4 h. **Duration:** 17–24 h. **Distribution:** Widely distributed; crosses placenta; distributed in breast milk. **Elimination:** 70% in urine; also in feces. **Half-Life:** 10–24 h.

## NURSING IMPLICATIONS

### Black Box Warning

*Nadolol has been associated with exacerbations of ischemic heart disease following abrupt withdrawal.*

N

---

Common adverse effects in *italic;* life-threatening effects underlined; generic names in **bold;** classifications in SMALL CAPS; ✿ Canadian drug name; ☯ Prototype drug

**Assessment & Drug Effects**

- Assess heart rate and BP before administration of each dose. Withhold drug and notify prescriber if apical pulse drops below 60 bpm or systolic BP below 90 mm Hg.
- Do not abruptly stop this medication. It should be tapered off over 1–2 wk to prevent exacerbation of angina.
- Monitor for signs of CHF (e.g., cough, fatigue, dyspnea, rapid pulse, edema).
- Monitor patients with diabetes mellitus closely. Nadolol may prevent clinical manifestations of hypoglycemia (e.g., tachycardia, BP changes).
- Monitor I&O ratio and creatinine clearance in patients with impaired kidney function or with cardiac problems.

**Patient & Family Education**

- Check pulse before taking each dose. Do not take your medication if pulse rate drops below 60 (or other parameter set by prescriber) or becomes irregular. Consult your prescriber right away.
- Do not stop taking your medication or alter dosage without consulting your prescriber. Monitor weight. Report weight gain of 1–1.5 kg (2–3 lb) in a day and any other possible signs of CHF (e.g., cough, fatigue, dyspnea, rapid pulse, edema).
- Do not drive or engage in potentially hazardous activities until response to drug is known.

# NAFARELIN ACETATE

(na-fa're-lin)

Synarel

**Classification:** GONADOTROPIN-RELEASING HORMONE (GnRH) ANALOG
**Therapeutic:** GnRH ANALOG
**Prototype:** Leuprolide

**AVAILABILITY** Spray solution

**ACTION & *THERAPEUTIC EFFECT***
Inhibits pituitary gonadotropin secretion of LH and FSH resulting a temporary increase in ovarian steroid hormone production. *Decrease in serum estradiol concentrations results in the quiescence of tissues and functions that depend on LH and FSH.*

**USES** Endometriosis and precocious puberty.

**UNLABELED USES** Uterine leiomyomas, benign prostatic hyperplasia.

**CONTRAINDICATIONS** Hypersensitivity to GnRH or GnRH agonist analog; undiagnosed abnormal vaginal bleeding; women who may become pregnant; pregnancy (category X); lactation.

**CAUTIOUS USE** Polycystic ovarian disease; menstruation; osteoporosis; pituitary insufficiency; children.

## ROUTE & DOSAGE

**Endometriosis**

*Adult:* **Inhalation** 400 mcg in one nostril in morning and 200 mcg in other nostril in evening beginning between days 2 and 4 of menstrual cycle; if patient doesn't acheive amenorrhea after 2 mo of therapy, may increase to 200 mcg in each nostril b.i.d.; do not exceed 6 mo of treatment

**Precocious Puberty**

*Child:* **Inhalation** 400 mcg into each nostril every morning and evening. (total: 8 sprays)

## ADMINISTRATION

**Inhalation**

- Withhold any topical nasal decongestant, if being used, until at least 2 h after nafarelin administration.

- Store at 15°–30° C (59°–86° F); protect from light.

**ADVERSE EFFECTS** (≥1%) **GI:** *Bloating, abdominal cramps,* weight gain, nausea. **Endocrine:** *Hot flashes, anovulation, decreased libido, hypocalcemia, hyperphosphatemia, hypertriglyceridemia, amenorrhea, vaginal dryness,* galactorrhea. **Metabolic:** Decreased bone mineral content (reversible). **CNS:** Transient headache, inertia, mild depression, *moodiness,* fatigue. **Respiratory:** Nasal irritation. **Urogenital:** *Impotence, decreased libido,* dyspareunia. **Dermatologic:** Acne.

**DIAGNOSTIC TEST INTERFERENCE**
Increased *alkaline phosphatase;* marked increase in *estradiol* in first 2 wk, then decrease to below baseline; decreased *FSH* and *LH* levels; decreased *testosterone* levels.

**INTERACTIONS Drugs:** Do not use with ESTROGENS or ANDROGENS. **Herbal:** Do not use with black cohosh.

**PHARMACOKINETICS Absorption:** 21% absorbed from nasal mucosa. **Onset:** 4 wk. **Peak:** 12 wk. **Duration:** 30–50 days after discontinuing drug. **Distribution:** 78–84% bound to plasma proteins; crosses placenta. **Metabolism:** Hydrolyzed in kidney. **Elimination:** 44–55% in urine over 7 days, 19–44% in feces. **Half-Life:** 2.7 h.

**NURSING IMPLICATIONS**
**Assessment & Drug Effects**
- Make appropriate inquiries about breakthrough bleeding, which may indicate that patient has missed successive drug doses.
- Monitor for and report immediately S&S of thromboembolism, including signs of TIA, CVA, or MI.
- Monitor lab tests: Blood glucose, glycosylated hemoglobin A1C,

prostate-specific antigen, serum estradiol concentrations, serum gonadotropin concentrations, serum testosterone concentrations.

**Patient & Family Education**
- Read the information pamphlet provided with nafarelin.
- Inform prescriber if breakthrough bleeding occurs or menstruation persists.
- Use or add barrier contraceptive during treatment.

# NAFCILLIN SODIUM
(naf-sill'in)

**Classifications:** PENICILLIN ANTIBIOTIC; PENICILLINASE–RESISTANT PENICILLIN
**Therapeutic:** PENICILLIN ANTIBIOTIC
**Prototype:** Oxacillin sodium

**AVAILABILITY** Solution for injection

**ACTION & THERAPEUTIC EFFECT**
Interferes with synthesis of mucopeptides essential to formation and integrity of bacterial cell wall leading to bacterial cell lysis. *Effective against both penicillin-sensitive and penicillin-resistant strains of Staphylococcus aureus. Also active against pneumococci and group A betahemolytic streptococci.*

**USES** Primarily, infections caused by penicillinase-producing staphylococci. Serum concentrations are considerably enhanced by concurrent use of probenecid.

**CONTRAINDICATIONS** Hypersensitivity to penicillins, cephalosporins, and other allergens; use of oral drug in severe infections, gastric dilatation, cardiospasm, or intestinal hypermotility.

**CAUTIOUS USE** History of or suspected atopy or allergy (eczema, hives, hay fever, asthma); GI disease;

N

Common adverse effects in *italic;* life-threatening effects <u>underlined</u>; generic names in **bold;** classifications in SMALL CAPS; ✤ Canadian drug name; ⊘ Prototype drug

1095

hepatic disease or impairment; pregnancy (category B); lactation.

## ROUTE & DOSAGE

### Staphylococcal Infections

*Adult:* **IV** 500 mg–1 g q4h (max: 12 g/day); **IM** 500 mg q4–6h
*Child:* **IV** 50–200 mg/kg/day divided q4–6h (max: 12 g/day)
*Child (weight greater than 40 kg):* **IM** 500 mg q4–6h; *weight less than 40 kg:* 25 mg/kg b.i.d.
*Neonate:* **IV** 50–100 mg/kg/day divided q6–12h; **IM** 25–50 mg/kg b.i.d.

## ADMINISTRATION

### Intramuscular

- Reconstitute each 500 mg with 1.7 mL of sterile water for injection or NaCl injection to yield 250 mg/mL. Shake vigorously to dissolve.
- In adults: Make certain solution is clear. Select site carefully. Inject deeply into gluteal muscle. Rotate injection sites.
- In children: The preferred IM site in children younger than 3 y is the midlateral or anterolateral thigh. Check agency policy.
- Label and date vials of reconstituted solution. Remains stable for 7 days under refrigeration and for 3 days at 15°–30° C (59°–86° F).

### Intravenous

Note: Vials in the *ADD-Vantage Drug Delivery System* are to be used with *ADD-Vantage* diluent containers of NS 50 and 100 mL. See the manufacturer's instructions for reconstitution and administration.

*PREPARE:* **Intermittent:** Reconstitute powder as for IM injection. Dilute the required dose of reconstituted solution in 100–150 mL of compatible IV solution.

*ADMINISTER:* **Intermittent:** Give over 30–60 min.

*INCOMPATIBILITIES:* **Solution/additive: Aminophylline, ascorbic acid, aztreonam, bleomycin, chlorothiazide, cytarabine, gentamicin, hydrocortisone, methylprednisolone, norepinephrine, promazine. Y-site: Diltiazem, droperidol, insulin regular, labetalol, midazolam, nalbuphine, pentazocine, vancomycin, verapamil.**

- Note: Usually, limit IV therapy to 24–48 h because of the possibility of thrombophlebitis (see Appendix F), particularly in older adults.
- Discard unused portions 24 h after reconstitution.

## ADVERSE EFFECTS (≥1%) **Body as a Whole:** Drug fever, anaphylaxis (particularly following parenteral therapy). **GI:** Nausea, vomiting, *diarrhea,* increase in serum transaminase activity (following IM). **Hematologic:** Eosinophilia, thrombophlebitis following IV; neutropenia (long-term therapy). **Metabolic:** Hypokalemia (with high IV doses). **Skin:** Urticaria, pruritus, rash, pain and tissue irritation. **Urogenital:** Allergic interstitial nephritis.

## DIAGNOSTIC TEST INTERFERENCE

Can cause false-positive *urine protein* tests using *sulfosalicylic acid method* or serum protein tests.

## INTERACTIONS **Drug:** May antagonize hypoprothrombinemic effects of **warfarin. Probenecid** increases serum concentrations.

## PHARMACOKINETICS **Peak:** 30–120 min IM; 15 min IV. **Duration:** 4–6 h IM. **Distribution:** Distributes into CNS with inflamed meninges; crosses placenta; distributed into breast milk; 90% protein bound. **Metabolism:** Enters enterohepatic circulation. **Elimination:** Primarily in bile; 10–30% in urine. **Half-Life:** 1 h.

Common adverse effects in *italic;* life-threatening effects underlined; generic names in **bold;** classifications in SMALL CAPS; ✛ Canadian drug name; ○ Prototype drug

## NURSING IMPLICATIONS

### Assessment & Drug Effects

- Obtain a careful history before therapy to determine any prior allergic reactions to penicillins, cephalosporins, and other allergens.
- Inspect IV site for inflammatory reaction. Also check IV site for leakage; in the older adult patient especially, loss of tissue elasticity with aging may promote extravasation around the needle.
- Note: Allergic reactions, principally rash, occur most commonly.
- Monitor neutrophil count. Nafcillin-induced neutropenia (agranulocytosis) occurs commonly during third week of therapy. It may be associated with malaise, fever, sore mouth, or throat. Perform periodic assessments of liver and kidney functions during prolonged therapy.
- Be alert for signs of bacterial or fungal superinfections (see Appendix F) in patients on prolonged therapy.
- Determine IV sodium intake for patients with sodium restriction. Nafcillin sodium contains approximately 3 mEq of sodium per gram; periodic WBC with differential, renal function tests, LFTs.
- Monitor lab tests: Baseline and periodic WBC with differential; periodic LFTs, and renal function tests with nafcillin therapy longer than 2 wk.

### Patient & Family Education

- Report promptly S&S of neutropenia (see Assessment & Drug Effects), superinfection, or hypokalemia (see Appendix F).

## NAFTIFINE

(naf'ti-feen)

Naftin

**Classifications:** ANTIBIOTIC; ANTIFUNGAL
**Therapeutic:** ANTIFUNGAL
**Prototype:** Terbinafine

**AVAILABILITY** Cream; gel

## ACTION & *THERAPEUTIC EFFECT*

Synthetic broad-spectrum antifungal agent that may be fungicidal depending on the organism. Interferes in the synthesis of ergosterol, the principal sterol in the fungus cell membrane. Ergosterol becomes depleted and membrane function is affected. *Effective against topical infections caused by fungal organisms.*

**USES** Tinea pedis, tinea cruris, and tinea corporis.

**CONTRAINDICATIONS** Hypersensitivity to naftifine; occlusive dressing.

**CAUTIOUS USE** Pregnancy (category B); lactation. Safety and efficacy in children not established.

## ROUTE & DOSAGE

| Tinea Infections |
| --- |
| *Adult:* **Topical** Apply cream daily, or apply gel twice daily, up to 4 wk |

## ADMINISTRATION

### Topical

- Gently massage into affected area and surrounding skin. Wash hands before and after application.
- Do not apply occlusive dressing unless specifically directed to do so.
- Store at 15°–30° C (59°–86° F).

**ADVERSE EFFECTS** (≥1%) **Skin:** Burning or stinging, dryness, erythema, itching, local irritation.

**PHARMACOKINETICS Absorption:** 2.5–6% absorbed through intact skin. **Onset:** 7 days. **Metabolism:** In liver. **Elimination:** In urine and feces. **Half-Life:** 2–3 days.

N

Common adverse effects in *italic;* life-threatening effects <u>underlined</u>; generic names in **bold;** classifications in SMALL CAPS; ♣ Canadian drug name; ⊘ Prototype drug

1097

## NURSING IMPLICATIONS

### Assessment & Drug Effects

- Assess for irritation or sensitivity to cream; these are indications to discontinue use.
- Reevaluate use of drug if no improvement is noted after 4 wk.

### Patient & Family Education

- Learn correct application technique.
- Avoid contact with eyes or mucous membranes.

# NALBUPHINE HYDROCHLORIDE

(nal'byoo-feen)

Nubain

**Classifications:** ANALGESIC; NARCOTIC (OPIATE AGONIST-ANTAGONIST)
Therapeutic: NARCOTIC ANALGESIC
**Prototype:** Pentazocine

**AVAILABILITY** Solution for injection

## ACTION & *THERAPEUTIC EFFECT*

Synthetic narcotic analgesic with agonist and weak antagonist properties that is a potent analgesic. *Analgesic action that relieves moderate to severe pain with apparently low potential for dependence.*

**USES** Symptomatic relief of moderate to severe pain. Also preoperative sedation analgesia and as a supplement to surgical anesthesia.

**CONTRAINDICATIONS** History of hypersensitivity to nalbuphine, opiate agonists; pregnancy (category D in prolonged use or in high doses at term).

**CAUTIOUS USE** History of emotional instability or drug abuse; head injury, increased intracranial pressure; cardiac disease; impaired respirations, COPD; GI disorders;

impaired kidney or liver function; MI; biliary tract surgery; pregnancy (category B; see CONTRAINDICATIONS); lactation.

## ROUTE & DOSAGE

### Moderate to Severe Pain

*Adult:* **IV/IM/Subcutaneous** 10 mg/70 kg q3–6h prn (max: 160 mg/day)

### Surgery Anesthesia Supplement

*Adult:* **IV** 0.3–3 mg/kg, then 0.25–0.5 mg/kg as required

## ADMINISTRATION

### Intramuscular/Subcutaneous

- Inject undiluted.

### Intravenous

**PREPARE: Direct:** Give undiluted.
**ADMINISTER: Direct:** Give at a rate of 10 mg or fraction thereof over 3–5 min.

**INCOMPATIBILITIES:** Solution/additive: **Diazepam, dimenhydrinate, ketorolac, pentobarbital, promethazine, thi-ethylperazine. Y-site: Allopurinol, amphotericin B cholesteryl, cefepime, docetaxel, methotrexate, nafcillin, pemetrexed, piperacillin/tazobactam, sargramostim, sodium bicarbonate.**

- Store at 15°–30° C (59°–86° F), avoid freezing.

## ADVERSE EFFECTS (≥1%) **CV:**
Hypertension, hypotension, bradycardia, tachycardia, flushing. **GI:** Abdominal cramps, bitter taste, *nausea, vomiting,* dry mouth. **CNS:** *Sedation, dizziness,* nervousness, depression, restlessness, crying, euphoria, dysphoria, distortion of body image, unusual dreams, confusion, hallucinations; numbness

Common adverse effects in *italic;* life-threatening effects underlined; generic names in **bold;** classifications in SMALL CAPS; ♣ Canadian drug name; ⊙ Prototype drug

and tingling sensations, headache, vertigo. **Respiratory:** Dyspnea, asthma, respiratory depression. **Skin:** Pruritus, urticaria, burning sensation, *sweaty, clammy skin.* **Special Senses:** Miosis, blurred vision, speech difficulty. **Urogenital:** Urinary urgency.

### INTERACTIONS Drug: Alcohol
and other CNS DEPRESSANTS add to CNS depression.

### PHARMACOKINETICS Onset: 2–3
min IV; 15 min IM. **Peak:** 30 min IV. **Duration:** 3–6 h. **Distribution:** Crosses placenta. **Metabolism:** In liver. **Elimination:** In urine. **Half-Life:** 5 h.

### NURSING IMPLICATIONS

#### Assessment & Drug Effects

- Assess respiratory rate before drug administration. Withhold drug and notify prescriber if respiratory rate falls below 12.
- Watch for allergic response in persons with sulfite sensitivity.
- Administer with caution to patients with hepatic or renal impairment.
- Monitor ambulatory patients; nalbuphine may produce drowsiness.
- Watch for respiratory depression of newborn if drug is used during labor and delivery.
- Avoid abrupt termination of nalbuphine following prolonged use, which may result in symptoms similar to narcotic withdrawal: Nausea, vomiting, abdominal cramps, lacrimation, nasal congestion, piloerection, fever, restlessness, anxiety.

#### Patient & Family Education

- Do not drive or engage in potentially hazardous activities until response to drug is known.
- Avoid alcohol and other CNS depressants.

## NALDEMEDINE
(nal-dem′e-deen)

Symproic

**Classifications:** GI AGENT; PERIPHERALLY ACTING OPIOID ANTAGONIST
**Therapeutic:** GI AGENTS

### AVAILABILITY Tablet

### ACTION & *THERAPEUTIC EFFECT*
Blocks opioid binding at mu, delta, and kappa receptors; periperally blocks actions in GI tract. *It competitively blocks the effect of opioids on the GI tract, decreasing the constipating effects of opioids.*

### USES Treatment of opioid-induced
constipation in patients with chronic noncancer pain.

### CONTRAINDICATIONS Severe
hepatic impairment; known or suspected GI obstruction, or risk of recurrent obstruction. No well-controlled studies have been done on pregnant women. Naldemedine does cross the placenta and can cause opioid withdrawal in the fetus.

### CAUTIOUS USE History of peptic
ulcer disease, diverticular disease, peritoneal metastteses; disruption to blood-brain barrier; not known if safe in hepatic impairment; pregnancy; lactation (breast-feeding can resume 3 days after last dose). Efficacy has only been established in patients that have had 4 or more wk of opioid use; patients taking opioids for less than 4 wk may be less responsive. Safety and efficacy in children not established.

### ROUTE & DOSAGE

| **Opioid-Induced Constipation** |
| --- |
| *Adult:* **PO** 0.2 mg daily |

### ADMINISTRATION

#### Oral
- Administer without regard to meals.

N

Common adverse effects in *italic*; life-threatening effects underlined; generic names in **bold**; classifications in SMALL CAPS; ♣ Canadian drug name; ✪ Prototype drug

1099

- Discontinue if treatment with the opioid pain medication is also discontinued.
- Store at 20°–25° C (68°–77° F). Protect from light.

## ADVERSE EFFECTS GI: *Abdominal pain, diarrhea,* nausea, vomiting, gastroenteritis, gastrointestinal perforation. **Other:** Opioid withdrawal.

## INTERACTIONS Drug: Substrate of P-glycoprotein/ABCB1, CYP3A4, and UGT1A3. Avoid use with with strong CYP3A4 inducers (eg. **carbamazepine, phenytoin, rifampin**). Avoid use with OPIOID ANTAGONISTS. **Herbal:** Avoid use with **St. John's wort**.

## PHARMACOKINETICS Distribution: 93–94% protein bound. **Onset:** Peak concentration in 0.75 h. **Metabolism:** Primarily hepatic via CYP3A. **Elimination:** 35% in feces, 57% in urine. **Half-Life:** 11 h.

## NURSING IMPLICATIONS

### Assessment & Drug Effects
- Assess for symptoms of GI obstruction.
- Monitor for S&S of opioid withdrawal.
- Monitor for signs of GI perforation.

### Patient & Family Education
- Report to prescriber immediately any swelling or pain in stomach, peristent diarrhea, signs of allergic reaction.
- Report to prescriber any signs of withdrawal: Muscle aches, restlessness, anxiety that may progress to nausea, vomiting, abdominal cramping, goose bumps, and excessive yawning.
- Do not take with the following drugs: **Carvamazepine, phenytoin, rifampin,** or **St. John's wort.**
- Notify prescriber if discontinuing the opioid pain medication; naldemedine is only to be taken when a person is taking opioids.

- Notify prescriber if planning to get pregnant. If taken during pregnancy, it may cause withdrawal in the unborn baby.

# NALOXEGOL
(na-lox'i-gol)
**Movantik**
**Classifications:** NARCOTIC (OPIATE ANTAGONIST)
**Therapeutic:** NARCOTIC ANTAGONIST
**Prototype:** Naloxone
**Controlled Substance:** Schedule II

## AVAILABILITY Tablets

## ACTION & *THERAPEUTIC EFFECT*
A mu-opioid receptor antagonist with limited ability to cross the blood-brain barrier. *Functions peripherally in tissues such as the GI tract thereby decreasing the constipation associated with opioids.*

## USES Treatment of opioid-induced constipation (OIC) in adult patients with chronic non-cancer pain.

## CONTRAINDICATIONS Severe hypersensitivity to naloxegol; known or suspected GI obstruction; severe hepatic impairment; concurrent use of strong CYP3A4 inhibitors or inducers.

## CAUTIOUS USE Concurrent use of moderate CYP3A4 inhibitors; renal impairment; mild to moderate hepatic impairment; pregnancy (category C); lactation. Safety and efficacy in pediatric patients not established.

## ROUTE & DOSAGE

### Opioid-Induced Constipation
*Adult:* **PO** 25 mg once daily in the a.m.; if unable to tolerate, reduce to 12.5 mg

Common adverse effects in *italic*; life-threatening effects underlined; generic names in **bold**; classifications in SMALL CAPS; ♣ Canadian drug name; ⊙ Prototype drug

### Renal Impairment Dosage Adjustment

*CrCL less than 60 mL/min:* Initial dose is 12.5 mg once daily; may increase to 25 mg once daily if well tolerated
Co-Administered Drugs Dosage Adjustment
*Strong CYP3A4 inhibitors or inducers:* Not recommended
*Moderate CYP 3A4 inhibitors:* Reduce dose to 12.5 mg once daily

## ADMINISTRATION

### Oral

- Give on an empty stomach at least 1 h before or 2 h after the first meal of the day.
- Tablets **must be** swallowed whole, do not crush or chew.
- Laxative should be discontinued prior to administering this drug and may be resumed after 3 days if response to naloxegol is suboptimal.
- Drug should be discontinued if opioid pain medication is also discontinued.
- Store at 15°–30° C (59°–86°F).

## ADVERSE EFFECTS (≥ 3%) Body as a Whole: Hyperhidrosis. CNS: Headache. GI: *Abdominal pain*, *diarrhea*, *flatulence*, *nausea*, *vomiting*.

## INTERACTIONS Drug: Strong CYP3A4 inhibitors (e.g., **clarithromycin, itraconazole, ketoconazole**) and moderate CYP3A4 inhibitors (e.g., **diltiazem, erythromycin, verapamil**) will increase the levels of naloxegol and may increase the risk of adverse effects. Strong CYP3A4 inducers (e.g., **carbamazepine, rifampin**) may significantly decrease plasma levels of naloxegol. Food: Grapefruit or grapefruit juice may increase the levels of naloxegol. Herbal: St. John's Wort may significantly decrease plasma levels of naloxegol.

## PHARMACOKINETICS Peak: Less than 2h. Distribution: Readily distributed in peripheral tissue; not plasma protein bound. Metabolism: In liver to inactive metabolites. Elimination: Fecal (68%) and renal (16%). Half-Life: 6–11 h.

## NURSING IMPLICATIONS

### Assessment & Drug Effects

- Monitor for symptoms of GI obstruction (e.g., severe, persistent, or worsening abdominal pain).
- Monitor closely for GI perforation especially in those at risk (e.g., peptic ulcer disease, diverticular disease, GI tract malignancies, peritoneal metastases).
- Monitor vital signs and report symptoms of opioid withdrawal (e.g., chills, diaphoresis, anxiety, irritability, changes in BP or HR).

### Patient & Family Education

- Avoid consumption of grapefruit or grapefruit juice during treatment.
- Discontinue all maintenance laxative therapy prior to taking this drug. Laxative(s) can be used as needed if there is a poor response to naloxegol after 3 days.
- Do not breast-feed while taking this drug.

# NALOXONE HYDROCHLORIDE 🄿

(nal-ox'one)

**Narcan**

**Classification:** NARCOTIC (OPIATE ANTAGONIST)
**Therapeutic:** NARCOTIC ANTAGONIST

## AVAILABILITY Solution for injection

## ACTION & *THERAPEUTIC EFFECT*

A potent narcotic antagonist,

Common adverse effects in *italic;* life-threatening effects <u>underlined</u>; generic names in **bold;** classifications in SMALL CAPS; ♣ Canadian drug name; 🄿 Prototype drug

1101

essentially free of agonistic (morphine-like) properties. *Reverses the effects of opiates, including respiratory depression, sedation, and hypotension.*

## USES
Narcotic overdosage; complete or partial reversal of narcotic depression. Drug of choice when nature of depressant drug is not known and for diagnosis of suspected acute opioid overdosage. Challenge for opioid dependence.

## UNLABELED USES
Shock and to reverse alcohol-induced or clonidine-induced coma or respiratory depression.

## CONTRAINDICATIONS
Hypersensitivity to naloxone, naltrexone, nalmefene; respiratory depression due to nonopioid drugs; substance abuse.

## CAUTIOUS USE
Known or suspected narcotic dependence; brain tumor, head trauma, increased ICP; history of substance abuse; cardiac irritability; seizure disorders; pregnancy (category B); lactation.

## ROUTE & DOSAGE

### Opiate Overdose
*Adult:* **IV** 0.4–2 mg, may repeat q2–3min up to 10 mg if necessary
*Child (5 y or older and weight at least 20 kg):* **IV** 2 mg, may repeat q2–3min if needed
*Child/Infant (weight less than 20 kg):* **IV** 0.01–0.1 mg/kg, may repeat q2–3min up to 10 mg if necessary
*Neonate:* **IV/Subcutaneous/IM** 0.01 mg/kg, may repeat q2–3min

### Postoperative Opiate Depression
*Adult:* **IV** 0.1–0.2 mg, may repeat q2–3min for up to 3 doses if necessary

*Child:* **IV** 0.005–0.01 mg/kg, may repeat q2–3min up to 3 doses if necessary

### Challenge for Opioid Dependence
*Adult:* **IM** 0.2 mg, observe for 30 sec for signs/symptoms of withdrawal, if no signs/symptoms then 0.6 mg and observe for 20 min

## ADMINISTRATION
### Intramuscular/Subcutaneous
▪ Inject undiluted.

### Intravenous

*PREPARE:* **Direct:** May be given undiluted. **IV Infusion:** Dilute 2 mg in 500 mL of D5W or NS to yield 4 mcg/mL (0.004 mg/mL).
*ADMINISTER:* **Direct:** Give bolus dose over 30 sec. **IV Infusion:** Adjust rate according to patient response.
*INCOMPATIBILITIES:* **Y-site: Amphotericin B cholesteryl complex, lansoprazole.**

▪ Use IV solutions within 24 h.
▪ Store at 15°–30° C (59°–86° F), protect from excessive light.

## ADVERSE EFFECTS (≥1%)
**Body as a Whole:** Reversal of analgesia, tremors, hyperventilation, slight drowsiness, sweating. **CV:** Increased BP, tachycardia. **GI:** Nausea, vomiting. **Hematologic:** Elevated partial thromboplastin time.

## INTERACTIONS
**Drug:** Reverses analgesic effects of NARCOTIC (OPIATE) AGONISTS and NARCOTIC (OPIATE) AGONIST-ANTAGONISTS.

## PHARMACOKINETICS
**Onset:** 2 min. **Duration:** 45 min. **Distribution:** Crosses placenta. **Metabolism:** In liver. **Elimination:** In urine. **Half-Life:** 60–90 min.

## NURSING IMPLICATIONS

### Assessment & Drug Effects

- Observe patient closely; duration of action of some narcotics may exceed that of naloxone. Keep prescriber informed; repeat naloxone dose may be necessary.
- May precipitate opiate withdrawal if administered to a patient who is opiate dependent.
- Note: Effects of naloxone generally start to diminish 20–40 min after administration and usually disappear within 90 min.
- Monitor respirations and other vital signs.
- Monitor surgical and obstetric patients closely for bleeding. Naloxone has been associated with abnormal coagulation test results. Also observe for reversal of analgesia, which may be manifested by nausea, vomiting, sweating, tachycardia.

### Patient & Family Education

- Report postoperative pain that emerges after administration of this drug to prescriber.

## NALTREXONE HYDROCHLORIDE

(nal-trex'one)

Vivitrol, ReVia

## BROMIDE METHYLNALTREXONE

Relistor

**Classification:** NARCOTIC (OPIATE ANTAGONIST)
**Therapeutic:** NARCOTIC ANTAGONIST
**Prototype:** Naloxone HCl

**AVAILABILITY** Tablet; intramuscular injection. **Bromide Methylnaltrexone:** Solution for injection

## ACTION & *THERAPEUTIC EFFECT*

Opioid antagonist with a mechanism of action that appears to result from competitive binding at opioid receptor sites, thus it reduces euphoria and drug craving without supporting addiction. *Weakens or completely and reversibly blocks the subjective effects (the "high") of IV opioids and analgesics possessing both agonist and antagonist activity.*

**USES** Alcoholism, opiate agonist dependence. Opioid-related constipation in patients nonresponsive to laxatives (**relistor**).

**UNLABELED USES** Pruritus.

**CONTRAINDICATIONS** Hypersensitivity to naltrexone; patients receiving opioid analgesics; opiate agonist use within 7–10 days; acute opioid agonist withdrawal; opioid-dependent patient; acute hepatitis, liver failure, hepatic encephalopathy; suicidal ideation; any individual who (1) fails naloxone challenge, (2) has a positive urine screen for opioids, or (3) has a history of sensitivity to naltrexone; lactation.

**CAUTIOUS USE** Mild to moderate hepatic impairment (Child-Pugh class A or B); history of suicidal tendencies; renal impairment; pregnancy (category C). **IM form:** Special at-risk patients: Thrombocytopenia, coagulopathy (e.g., hemophilia), severe hepatic impairment; children younger than 18 y.

## ROUTE & DOSAGE

| Opioid Dependence |
| --- |
| *Adult:* **PO** 25 mg qd, if no response increase to 50 mg/day |
| *Adult:* **IM** 380 mg q4w |
| **Alcohol Dependence** |
| *Adult:* **PO** 50 mg once/day |
| **IM** 380 mg q 4 wk |

N

Common adverse effects in *italic;* life-threatening effects <u>underlined</u>; generic names in **bold**; classifications in SMALL CAPS; ♣ Canadian drug name; ⊘ Prototype drug

1103

**Opioid-Related Constipation (Relistor)**

*Adult (weight less than 38 kg or greater than 114 kg):* **Subcutaneous** 0.15 mg/kg every other day (max: 0.15 mg/kg in 24 h); *weight 38–62 kg:* 8 mg every other day (max: 8 mg/24 h); *weight 62–114 kg:* 12 mg every other day (max: 12 mg/24 h)

**Renal Impairment Dosage Adjustment (Relistor)**

*CrCl less than 30 mL/min:* Reduce dose by 50%

## ADMINISTRATION

### Oral
- Give with food to decrease nausea.

### Intramuscular
- Give IM into the gluteal muscle, alternating buttocks per injection. Aspirate before injection to ensure that drug is not injected IV.

### Subcutaneous (Methylnaltrexone Only)
- Give subcutaneously into upper arm, abdomen, or thigh.

## ADVERSE EFFECTS (≥1%) **GI:** Dry mouth, anorexia, *nausea, vomiting,* constipation, *abdominal cramps/pain,* <u>hepatotoxicity</u>. **Musculoskeletal:** *Muscle and joint pains.* **CNS:** *Difficulty sleeping, anxiety, headache, nervousness,* reduced or increased energy, irritability, dizziness, depression. **Skin:** Skin rash. **Hematologic: IM extended release form:** Hematoma formation at injection site. **Body as a Whole:** Chills.

## INTERACTIONS **Drug:** Increased somnolence and lethargy with PHENOTHIAZINES; reverses analgesic effects of NARCOTIC (OPIATE) AGONISTS and NARCOTIC (OPIATE) AGONIST-ANTAGONISTS.

## PHARMACOKINETICS **Absorption:** Rapidly from GI tract; 20% reaches systemic circulation (first pass effect). **Onset:** 15–30 min. **Peak:** 1 h; 30 min (Relistor). **Duration:** 24–72 h PO; 4 wk IM. **Metabolism:** In liver to active metabolite. **Elimination:** In urine. **Half-Life:** 10–13 h PO, 5–10 days IM.

## NURSING IMPLICATIONS

### Assessment & Drug Effects
- Monitor for development of depression or suicidal thinking.
- Monitor for and report promptly S&S of hepatotoxicity (see Appendix F).
- Monitor lab tests: LFTs before the treatment is started, at monthly intervals for 6 mo, and then periodically.

### Patient & Family Education
- Note: Naltrexone therapy may put you in danger of overdosing if you use opiates. Small doses even at frequent intervals will give no desired effects; however, a dose large enough to produce a high is dangerous and may be fatal.
- Do not self-dose with OTC drugs for treatment of cough, colds, diarrhea, or analgesia. Many available preparations contain small doses of an opioid. Consult prescriber for safe drugs if they are needed.

# NAPHAZOLINE HYDROCHLORIDE ℗

(naf-az'oh-leen)

Allerest, Clear Eyes, Comfort, Nafazair

**Classifications:** EYE AND EAR PREPARATION; VASOCONSTRICTOR; ALPHA-ADRENERGIC AGONIST; DECONGESTANT

Therapeutic: DECONGESTANT

## AVAILABILITY Ophthalmic solution

## ACTION & *THERAPEUTIC EFFECT*

Direct-acting alpha-adrenergic agonist that produces rapid and prolonged vasoconstriction of arterioles. *It decreases fluid exudation and mucosal engorgement.*

## USES Ocular vasoconstrictor.

## CONTRAINDICATIONS Narrow-angle glaucoma; concomitant use with MAO inhibitors or tricyclic antidepressants; lactation.

## CAUTIOUS USE Hypertension, cardiac irregularities, advanced arteriosclerosis; diabetes; hyperthyroidism; older adults; ocular infection or ocular trauma; pregnancy (category C); children.

## ROUTE & DOSAGE

**Conjunctival Hyperemia**

*Adult:* **Topical** 1–3 drops of 0.1% solution q3–4h prn or 1–2 drops of a 0.012–0.03% solution q4h prn

## ADMINISTRATION

### Optic

- Remove contact lenses before instilling ophthalmic drops.
- Do not touch the tip of the dropper to the eye, fingertips, or other surface to prevent contamination.
- Wash hands before and after use.
- Tilt the head back slightly and pull the lower eyelid down with the index finger to form a pouch. Squeeze the number of ordered drops in the pouch. Close eyes to spread drops.
- To avoid contamination or the spread of infection, do not use dropper for more than one person.

## ADVERSE EFFECTS (≥1%)

**Body as a Whole:** Hypersensitivity reactions, headache, nausea, weakness, sweating, drowsiness, hypothermia, <u>coma</u>. **CV:** Hypertension, bradycardia, <u>shock-like hypotension</u>. **Special Senses:** Transient nasal stinging or burning, dryness of nasal mucosa, pupillary dilation, increased intraocular pressure, blurred vision, rebound redness of the eye.

## PHARMACOKINETICS Onset: Within 10 min. **Duration:** 2–6 h.

## NURSING IMPLICATIONS

### Assessment & Drug Effects

- Watch for rebound congestion and chemical rhinitis with frequent and continued use.
- Monitor BP periodically for development or worsening of hypertension, especially with ophthalmic route.
- Overdose: Bradycardia and hypotension can result. Report promptly.

### Patient & Family Education

- Do not exceed prescribed regimen. Systemic effects can result from swallowing excessive medication.
- Discontinue medication and contact prescriber if nasal congestion is not relieved after 5 days.
- Prevent contamination of eye solution by taking care not to touch eyelid or surrounding area with dropper tip.

## NAPROXEN

(na-prox'en)

EC-Naprosyn, Naprosyn

## NAPROXEN SODIUM

Aleve, Anaprox, Anaprox DS

**Classifications:** ANALGESIC, NONSTEROIDAL ANTI-INFLAMMATORY DRUG (NSAID); ANTIPYRETIC
**Therapeutic:** NONNARCOTIC ANALGESIC, NSAID
**Prototype:** Ibuprofen

Common adverse effects in *italic;* life-threatening effects <u>underlined</u>; generic names in **bold;** classifications in SMALL CAPS; ♣ Canadian drug name; ☻ Prototype drug

1105

**AVAILABILITY** Tablet; sustained release tablet

**ACTION & *THERAPEUTIC EFFECT***
Propionic acid derivative that is an NSAID. Mechanism of action is related to inhibition of prostaglandin synthesis by inhibiting COX-1 and COX-2 isoenzymes. *Analgesic, anti-inflammatory, and antipyretic effects; also inhibits platelet aggregation and prolongs bleeding time.*

**USES** Anti-inflammatory and analgesic effects in symptomatic treatment of acute and chronic rheumatoid arthritis, juvenile arthritis (naproxen only), and for treatment of primary dysmenorrhea. Also management of ankylosing spondylitis, osteoarthritis, and gout.

**UNLABELED USES** Paget's disease of bone, Bartter's syndrome.

**CONTRAINDICATIONS** Hypersensitivity to naproxen or any other NSAIDs; active peptic ulcer; patients in whom asthma, rhinitis, urticaria, bronchospasm, or shock is precipitated by aspirin or other NSAIDs; perioperative pain associated with CABG; late pregnancy; lactation.

**CAUTIOUS USE** History of upper GI tract disorders; history of GI bleeding; impaired kidney, liver, or cardiac function; patients on sodium restriction **(naproxen sodium)**; low pretreatment Hgb concentration; fluid retention, hypertension, heart failure; coagulopathy; SLE; pregnancy (category C); children younger than 2 y. **OTC:** Children younger than 12 y.

**ROUTE & DOSAGE**

Note: 275 mg naproxen sodium = 250 mg naproxen

**Inflammatory Disease**
*Adult:* **PO** 250–500 mg b.i.d. (max: 1000 mg/day naproxen, 1100 mg/day naproxen sodium)
*Child (12 y or older):* **PO** 5 mg/kg b.i.d. (max: 1000 mg/day)

**Mild to Moderate Pain, Dysmenorrhea**
*Adult:* **PO** 500 mg followed by 200–250 mg q6–8h prn up to 1250 mg/day
*Child (12 y or older):* **PO** 440 mg q8–12h

**ADMINISTRATION**
**Oral**
- Ensure that extended release or enteric-coated form is not chewed or crushed. It **must be** swallowed whole. Administer with a full glass of water or other liquid.
- Give with food or an antacid (if prescribed) to reduce incidence of GI upset.
- Store at 15°–30° C (59°–86° F) in tightly closed container; protect from freezing and excessive heat.

**ADVERSE EFFECTS** (≥1%) **CNS:** *Headache, drowsiness, dizziness,* light-headedness, depression. **CV:** Palpitation, dyspnea, peripheral edema, CHF, tachycardia. **Special Senses:** Blurred vision, tinnitus, hearing loss. **GI:** *Anorexia, heartburn,* indigestion, *nausea,* vomiting, thirst, GI bleeding, elevated serum ALT, AST. **Hematologic:** Thrombocytopenia, leukopenia, eosinophilia, inhibited platelet aggregation, agranulocytosis (rare). **Skin:** Pruritus, rash, ecchymosis. **Urogenital:** Nephrotoxicity. **Respiratory:** Pulmonary edema.

**DIAGNOSTIC TEST INTERFERENCE**
Transient elevations in *BUN* and serum *alkaline phosphatase*

may occur. Naproxen may inter-fere with some urinary assays of **5-HIAA** and may cause falsely high **urinary 17-KGS** levels (using **m-dinitrobenzene reagent**). Nap-roxen should be withdrawn 72 h before adrenal function tests.

**INTERACTIONS Drug:** Bleeding time effects of ORAL ANTICOAGULANTS, **heparin** may be prolonged; may in-crease **lithium** toxicity. Do not use with **floctafenine** or with NSAIDs. **Herbal: Feverfew, garlic, ginger, ginkgo, evening primrose oil, glucosamine** may increase bleed-ing potential.

**PHARMACOKINETICS Absorp-tion:** Almost completely from GI tract when taken on empty stomach. **Peak:** 2 h naproxen; 1 h naproxen sodium. **Duration:** 7 h. **Metabolism:** In liver. **Elimination:** Primarily in urine; some biliary excretion (less than 1%). **Half-Life:** 12–15 h.

## NURSING IMPLICATIONS

### Black Box Warning

*Naproxen has been associated with increased risk of serious, po-tentially fatal, GI bleeding and cardiovascular events (e.g., MI & CVA); risk may increase with du-ration of use and may be greater in the older adult and those with risk factors for CV disease.*

### Assessment & Drug Effects

- Monitor for and report promptly S&S of GI ulceration or bleeding. Significant GI bleeding may occur without prior warning.
- Monitor for and report promptly S&S of CV thrombotic events (i.e., angina, MI, TIA, or stroke).
- Take detailed drug history prior to initiation of therapy. Observe for signs of allergic response in those with aspirin or other NSAID sensitivity.
- Baseline and periodic auditory and ophthalmic examinations are recommended in patients re-ceiving prolonged or high dose therapy.
- Monitor lab tests: Baseline and periodic CBC, LFTs, stool guaiac, and renal function tests with pro-longed or high dose therapy.

### Patient & Family Education

- Be aware that the therapeutic ef-fect of naproxen may not be ex-perienced for 3–4 wk.
- Stop taking drug and report promptly to prescriber if you ex-perience S&S of GI ulceration: Stomach pain, frequent indiges-tion and nausea, bloody or tarry stools, vomit with blood or coffee-ground appearance.
- Avoid alcohol and aspirin (as well as other NSAIDs) unless otherwise advised by a prescriber. Potential to increase risk of GI ulceration and bleeding.
- Stop taking drug and report promptly to prescriber if you ex-perience chest pain, shortness of breath, weakness, slurring of speech, or other signs of a cardiac or neurologic problem.

## NARATRIPTAN

(nar-a-trip′tan)

Amerge

**Classification:** SEROTONIN 5-HT$_1$ RECEPTOR AGONIST
**Therapeutic:** ANTIMIGRAINE
**Prototype:** Sumatriptan

### AVAILABILITY Tablet

### ACTION & *THERAPEUTIC EFFECT*

Binds to the serotonin receptors (5-HT$_{1D}$ and 5-HT$_{1B}$) on intracranial blood vessels, resulting in selective vasoconstriction of dilated vessels in the carotid circulation. It also inhibits the release of inflammatory neuropeptides associated with a migraine attack. *Inhibits vasoconstriction of dilated vessels selectively. This results in the relief of acute migraine headache attacks.*

**USES** Acute migraine headaches with or without aura.

**CONTRAINDICATIONS** Hypersensitivity to naratriptan; severe renal impairment (creatinine clearance less than 15 mL/min); severe hepatic impairment; history of ischemic heart disease (i.e., angina pectoris, MI), arteriosclerosis, cardiac arrhythmias; cardiac disease, CAD, peripheral vascular disease; cerebrovascular syndromes (i.e., strokes or TIA); uncontrolled hypertension; patients with hemiplegic or basilar migraine; older adults.

**CAUTIOUS USE** Cardiovascular disease; renal or hepatic insufficiency; elderly; pregnancy (category C); lactation. Safety and efficacy in children younger than 18 y not established.

## ROUTE & DOSAGE

### Acute Migraine

*Adult:* **PO** 1–2.5 mg; may repeat in 4 h if necessary (max: 5 mg/24 h); patients with mild or moderate renal or hepatic impairment should not exceed 2.5 mg/24 h

## ADMINISTRATION

### Oral

- Give any time after symptoms of migraine appear. If the first tablet was effective but symptoms return, a second tablet may be given, but no sooner than 4 h after the first. Do not exceed 5 mg in 24 h.
- If there is no response to the first tablet, contact prescriber before administering a second tablet.
- Do not give within 24 h of an ergot-containing drug or other 5-HT₁ agonist.
- Store at 2°–25° C (36°–77° F); protect from light.

**ADVERSE EFFECTS** (≥1%) **Body as a Whole:** Asthenia, fatigue, malaise, pain, pressure sensation, paresthesias, throat pressure, warm/cold sensations, hot flushes. **CNS:** Somnolence, dizziness, drowsiness, headache, hypesthesia, decreased mental acuity, euphoria, tremor. **CV:** Coronary artery vasospasm, transient myocardial ischemia, <u>MI</u>, ventricular tachycardia, ventricular fibrillation, chest pain/tightness/heaviness, palpitations. **GI:** Dry mouth, nausea, vomiting, diarrhea. **Respiratory:** Dyspnea. **Skin:** Flushing.

**INTERACTIONS Drug: Dihydroergotamine, methysergide,** and other 5-HT₁ AGONISTS may cause prolonged vasospastic reactions; SSRIs have rarely caused weakness, hyperreflexia, and incoordination; MAOIS should not be used with 5-HT₁ AGONISTS. **Herbal: Gingko, ginseng, echinacea, St. John's wort** may increase triptan toxicity.

**PHARMACOKINETICS Absorption:** Rapidly absorbed, 70% bioavailability. **Peak:** 2–4 h. **Distribution:** 28–31% protein bound. **Metabolism:** In liver. **Elimination:** Primarily in urine. **Half-Life:** 6 h.

## NURSING IMPLICATIONS

### Assessment & Drug Effects

- Monitor carefully cardiovascular status following first dose in patients at risk for CAD (e.g., postmenopausal women, men older than 40 y, persons with known CAD risk factors) or coronary artery vasospasms.

- Be aware that ECG is recommended following first administration of naratriptan to someone with known CAD risk factors and periodically with long-term use.
- Report immediately to the prescriber: Chest pain, nausea, or tightness in chest or throat that is severe or does not quickly resolve.
- Obtain periodic cardiovascular evaluation with continued use.

**Patient & Family Education**

- Carefully review patient information leaflet and guidelines for administration.
- Contact prescriber immediately for any of the following: Symptoms of angina (e.g., severe and/or persistent pain or tightness in chest or throat, severe nausea); hypersensitivity (e.g., wheezing, facial swelling, skin rash, or hives); or abdominal pain.
- Report any other adverse effects (e.g., tingling, flushing, dizziness) at next prescriber visit.

## NATALIZUMAB

(na-tal'-i-zu-mab)
Tysabri
**Classifications:** BIOLOGICAL RESPONSE MODIFIER; MONOCLONAL ANTIBODY; INTEGRIN INHIBITOR
**Therapeutic:** IMMUNOMODULATOR; MONOCLONAL ANTIBODY (IgG)
**Prototype:** Basiliximab

**AVAILABILITY** Solution for injection

## ACTION & *THERAPEUTIC EFFECT*

Natalizumab binds to integrins expressed on the surface of all leukocytes (except neutrophils) and inhibits adhesion of leukocytes to their counter-receptor(s) on activated vascular endothelial cells of the GI tract. Disruption of these interactions prevents transmigration of leukocytes across the endothelium into inflamed tissue. *Inhibition of T-cell infiltration into the brain is thought to impede the demyelinating process of MS. It reduces relapses and occurrence of brain lesions. Natalizumab is also thought to attenuate T lymphocyte–mediated intestinal inflammation in Crohn's disease and possibly ulcerative colitis.*

**USES** Treatment of relapsing forms of multiple sclerosis, treatment of Crohn's disease.

**CONTRAINDICATIONS** Prior hypersensitivity to natalizumab; murine protein hypersensitivity; have or have had progressive multifocal leukoencephalopathy (PML); active infection; S&S of PML; females of childbearing age; lactation.

**CAUTIOUS USE** Diabetes mellitus, immunocompromised patients; exposure to infection or tuberculosis; hepatic dysfunction; pregnancy (category C); children younger than 18 y.

## ROUTE & DOSAGE

| Multiple Sclerosis/Moderate to Severe Crohn's Disease |
|---|
| *Adult:* **IV** 300 mg infused over 1 h every 4 wk |

N

## ADMINISTRATION

**Intravenous**

*PREPARE:* **IV Infusion:** Before and after dilution, solution should be colorless and clear to slightly opaque. Do not use if the solution has visible particles, flakes, color, or is cloudy. ▪ Withdraw 300 mg (15 mL) from the vial and add to an IV bag with 100 mL of NS. Do not use with any other diluent. ▪ Gently invert the bag to mix; do not shake. ▪ The IV solution **must be** used within 8 h.
*ADMINISTER:* **IV Infusion:** Flush IV line before/after with NS. Infuse over 1 h. ▪ Do not give a bolus dose. ▪ Stop infusion immediately if S&S of hypersensitivity appear.
*INCOMPATIBILITIES:* **Solution/additive/Y-site:** Do not mix or infuse with other drugs.

▪ Store IV solution for up to 8 h at 2°–8° C (36°–46° F). ▪ Allow solution to warm to room temperature before administration. Protect from light.

## ADVERSE EFFECTS (≥1%) **Body as a Whole:** <u>Anaphylaxis</u> (rare, usually within 2 h of infusion), infections, fatigue, rigors, <u>risk of progressive multifocal leukoencephalopathy</u>. **CNS:** Depression, headache, syncope, tremor. **CV:** Chest discomfort. **GI:** Abdominal discomfort, abnormal liver function tests. **Hematologic:** Local bleeding from infusion site. **Musculoskeletal:** Arthralgia. **Respiratory:** Pneumonia. **Skin:** Acute urticaria. **Urogenital:** Urinary frequency, irregular menstruation, amenorrhea, dysmenorrhea. **Other:** Infusion-related reactions (headache, dizziness, fatigue, hypersensitivity reactions, urticaria, pruritus, and rigors).

## INTERACTIONS **Drug:** May reduce the effectiveness of VACCINES and TOXOIDS; may increase risk of infection with IMMUNOSUPPRESSANTS.

## PHARMACOKINETICS **Half-Life:** 11 days.

## NURSING IMPLICATIONS

### Black Box Warning

*Natalizumab has been associated with increased risk of progressive multifocal leukoencephalopathy (PML), an opportunistic viral infection of the brain that usually leads to death or severe disability.*

### Assessment & Drug Effects

▪ During IV infusion and for 1–2 h after, monitor closely for S&S of hypersensitivity (e.g., urticaria, dizziness, fever, rash, chills, pruritus, nausea, flushing, hypotension, dyspnea, and chest pain).
▪ Monitor neurologic status frequently. Report promptly any emerging S&S of dysfunction.
▪ Monitor lab tests: Baseline and periodic CBC with differential; periodic LFTs.

### Patient & Family Education

▪ Report immediately any of the following during/after IV infusion: Difficulty breathing, wheezing or shortness of breath, swelling or tightness about the neck and throat, chest pain, skin rash or hives.
▪ Report promptly S&S of infection (e.g., cough, fever, chills, or sore throat).

## NATAMYCIN
(na-ta-mye′sin)
Natacyn
**Classification:** ANTIFUNGAL ANTIBIOTIC
Therapeutic: ANTIFUNGAL
**Prototype:** Amphotericin B

**AVAILABILITY** Opthalmic suspension

Common adverse effects in *italic;* life-threatening effects <u>underlined</u>; generic names in **bold;** classifications in SMALL CAPS; ◆ Canadian drug name; ❷ Prototype drug

## ACTION & *THERAPEUTIC EFFECT*

Mechanism of action is by binding to sterols in the fungal cell membrane resulting in cell death of fungi. *Effective against many yeasts and filamentous fungi including* Candida, Aspergillus, Cephalosporium, Fusarium, *and* Penicillium.

## USES Ocular fungal infections.

## CONTRAINDICATIONS Hypersensitivity to natamycin or any of its components.

## CAUTIOUS USE Pregnancy (category C); lactation. Safety and efficacy in children not established.

## ROUTE & DOSAGE

### Fungal Keratitis

*Adult:* **Ophthalmic** 1 drop in conjunctival sac of infected eye q1–2h for 3–4 days, then decrease to 1 drop q6–8h, then gradually decrease to 1 drop q4–7days

## ADMINISTRATION

### Instillation

- Wash hands thoroughly before and after treatment. Infection is easily transferred from infected to noninfected eye and to other individuals.
- Shake well before using.
- Store at 2°–24° C (36°–75° F).

## ADVERSE EFFECTS (≥1%) **Special Senses:** Blurred vision, photophobia, eye pain. Uneven adherence of suspension to epithelial ulcerations or in fornices.

## PHARMACOKINETICS **Absorption:** Drug adheres to ulcerated surface of the cornea and is retained in conjunctival fornices. Does not appear to be systemically absorbed.

## NURSING IMPLICATIONS

### Assessment & Drug Effects

- Inspect eye for response and tolerance at least twice weekly.
- Note: Lack of improvement in keratitis within 7–10 days suggests that causative organisms may not be susceptible to natamycin. Reevaluation is indicated and possibly a change in therapy.

### Patient & Family Education

- Learn appropriate technique for application of eye drops.
- Expect temporary light sensitivity. Be prepared to wear sunglasses outdoors after drug administration and perhaps for a few hours indoors.
- Return to ophthalmologist for reevaluation of eye problem if you experience symptoms of conjunctivitis: Pain, discharge, itching, scratching "foreign body sensation," changes in vision.
- Do not share facecloths and hand towels; this will help prevent transmission of the fungal infection.

**N**

## NATEGLINIDE

(nat-e-gli'nide)

**Starlix**

**Classifications:** ANTIDIABETIC; MEGLITINIDE

**Therapeutic:** ANTIDIABETIC

**Prototype:** Repaglinide

## AVAILABILITY Tablet

## ACTION & *THERAPEUTIC EFFECT*

Lowers blood glucose levels by stimulating the release of insulin from the pancreatic cells of a type 2 diabetic. Significantly reduces postprandial blood glucose in type 2 diabetics and improves glycemic control when given before meals. *Effectiveness is indicated by preprandial blood glucose between 80 and 120 mg/dL and HbA1C 6.5% or less.*

---

Common adverse effects in *italic;* life-threatening effects underlined; generic names in **bold;** classifications in SMALL CAPS; ◆ Canadian drug name; ○ Prototype drug

**USES** Alone or in combination with metformin for the treatment of non-insulin-dependent diabetes mellitus.

**CONTRAINDICATIONS** Prior hypersensitivity to nateglinide. Type 1 (insulin-dependent) diabetes mellitus, diabetic ketoacidosis; hypoglycemia.

**CAUTIOUS USE** Renal impairment; liver dysfunction; adrenal or pituitary insufficiency; malnutrition; infection, trauma, surgery or unusual stress; surgery; trauma; pregnancy (category C); lactation.

## ROUTE & DOSAGE

**Diabetes Mellitus**
*Adult:* **PO** 60–120 mg t.i.d. 1–30 min prior to meals

## ADMINISTRATION

**Oral**
- Give, preferably, 1–30 min before meals. Omit the dose if the meal is skipped. Add a dose if an extra meal is eaten. Never double the dose.
- Store at 15°–30° C (59°–86° F).

**ADVERSE EFFECTS** (≥1%) **Body as a Whole:** Back pain, flu-like symptoms. **CV:** Dizziness. **GI:** Diarrhea. **Metabolic:** Hypoglycemia. **Musculoskeletal:** Arthropathy. **Respiratory:** Upper respiratory infection, bronchitis, cough.

**INTERACTIONS Drug:** NSAIDS, SALIYLATES, MAO INHIBITORS, BETA-ADRENERGIC BLOCKERS, may potentiate hypoglycemic effects; THIAZIDE DIURETICS, CORTICOSTEROIDS, THYROID PREPARATIONS, SYMPATHOMIMETIC AGENTS may attenuate hypoglycemic effects. **Herbal: Garlic, ginseng** may potentiate hypoglycemic effects.

**PHARMACOKINETICS Absorption:** Rapidly absorbed, 73% bioavailability. **Peak:** 1 h. **Distribution:** 98% protein bound. **Metabolism:** In liver by CYP2C9 (70%) and CYP3A4 (30%). **Elimination:** Primarily in urine. **Half-Life:** 1.5 h.

## NURSING IMPLICATIONS

### Assessment & Drug Effects
- Monitor carefully for S&S of hypoglycemia especially during the 1-wk period following transfer from a longer acting sulfonylurea.
- Monitor lab tests: Frequent 2 h postprandial blood glucose and FBS, and HbA1C q3mo.

### Patient & Family Education
- Take only before a meal to lessen the chance of hypoglycemia.
- When transferred to nateglinide from another oral hypoglycemia drug, start nateglinide the morning after the other agent is stopped, unless directed otherwise by prescriber.
- Watch for S&S of hyperglycemia or hypoglycemia (see Appendix F); report poor blood glucose control to prescriber.
- Report gastric upset or other bothersome GI symptoms to prescriber.

# NEBIVOLOL HYDROCHLORIDE
(ne-bi-vol'ol)
Bystolic
**Classifications:** BETA-ADRENERGIC ANTAGONIST; ANTIHYPERTENSIVE
**Therapeutic:** ANTIHYPERTENSIVE
**Prototype:** Propranolol

**AVAILABILITY** Tablet

## ACTION & *THERAPEUTIC EFFECT*
A beta-adrenergic receptor blocker that is a beta-1 selective antagonist in majority of individuals and a nonselective beta-blocker in poor metabolizers. At higher doses nebivolol blocks both beta-1 and

Common adverse effects in *italic;* life-threatening effects <u>underlined</u>; generic names in **bold;** classifications in SMALL CAPS; ♣ Canadian drug name; ⊘ Prototype drug

beta-2 receptors. *Effectiveness is measured by decreasing both systolic and diastolic pressures associated with hypertension*.

**USES** Management of hypertension either alone or in combination with other antihypertensive agents.

**UNLABELED USES** Management of heart failure.

**CONTRAINDICATIONS** Hypersensitivity to nebivolol; severe bradycardia; greater than first degree heart block; sick sinus syndrome without pacemaker; severe hepatic impairment (Child-Pugh greater than class C); decompensated HF; bronchospastic disease; abupt discontinuation; lactation.

**CAUTIOUS USE** Hypersensitivity to nebivolol or other beta-blockers; compensated CHF; history of angina or recent MI; PVD; bronchospastic disease; major surgery, anesthesia; moderate hepatic and moderate to severe renal impairment; pheochromocytoma; spontaneous hypoglycemia or DM; hyperthyroidism; pregnancy (category C). Safety and efficacy in children not established.

## ROUTE & DOSAGE

**Hypertension**

*Adult:* **PO** 5 mg daily; can increase q2wk up to 40 mg daily

*Hepatic Impairment Dosage Adjustment*

*Moderate hepatic impairment (Child-Pugh class B):* Decrease to 2.5 mg daily and increase cautiously as needed; *severe hepatic impairment:* Use is contraindicated

*Renal Impairment Dosage Adjustment*

*CrCl less than 30 mL/min:* Decrease to 2.5 mg daily and cautiously increase as needed

## ADMINISTRATION

**Oral**
- May give without regard to meals.
- Store at 20°–25° C (68°–77° F) in a tight, light-resistant container.

**ADVERSE EFFECTS** (≥1%) **Body as a Whole:** Chest pain, peripheral edema. **CNS:** Asthenia, dizziness, fatigue, *headache*, insomnia, paresthesia. **CV:** Bradycardia. **GI:** Abdominal pain, diarrhea, nausea. **Metabolic:** Decreased HDL levels, decreased platelet count, hypercholesterolemia, hypertriglyceridemia, hyperuricemia, increased blood urea nitrogen. **Respiratory:** Dyspnea. **Skin:** Rash.

**INTERACTIONS Drug:** Catecholamine-depleting agents (**reserpine, guanethidine**) may produce excessive reduction in sympathetic activity if used with nebivolol. Compounds that inhibit CYP2D6 (**fluoxetine, paroxetine, propafenone, quinidine**) may increase nebivolol levels. If used in combination with **clonidine,** simultaneous discontinuation of both drugs may cause life-threatening increases in blood pressure. Combination use with **digoxin** may increase the risk of bradycardia. **Cimetidine** increases the levels of nebivolol metabolites. **Verapamil** and **diltiazem** may increase the pharmacologic effects of nebivolol. Nebivolol may decrease the clearance of **disopyramide.** Nebivolol may decrease the AUC and $C_{max}$ of **sildenafil.** Do not use with **sotalol** or **tranylcypromine.**

**PHARMACOKINETICS Peak:** 1.5–4 h. **Distribution:** 98% plasma protein bound. **Metabolism:** Hepatic (via CYP2D6); extent depends on genetic profile. **Elimination:** In urine (38–67%) and feces (13–44%).

N

**Half-Life:** 12–19 h depending on genetic differences in metabolism.

## NURSING IMPLICATIONS

### Assessment & Drug Effects

- Monitor closely BP and HR. Report promptly significant bradycardia or S&S of heart failure.
- Monitor closely during the perioperative period for depressed cardiac functioning.
- Monitor diabetics for loss of glycemia control.
- Monitor respiratory status in those at risk for bronchospasm.
- Monitor lab tests: LFTs and serum creatinine.

### Patient & Family Education

- Use caution with dangerous activities until reaction to drug is known.
- Report promptly any of the following: Sudden weight gain, increasing shortness of breath, swelling in lower legs and feet; heart rate less than 60 beats per minute or other value established by prescriber.
- Diabetics may experience hypoglycemia without the usual signs and symptoms while on this drug.
- Do not abruptly stop taking this medication. It should be tapered off over 1–2 wk.

## NECITUMUMAB

(ne-si-toom'oo-mab)

**Portrazza**

**Classifications:** IMUNOMODULATOR; MONOCLONAL ANTIBODY; ANTINEOPLASTIC; EPIDERMAL GROWTH FACTOR RECEPTOR (EGFR) ANTAGONIST

**Therapeutic:** ANTINEOPLASTIC; EPIDERMAL GROWTH FACTOR RECEPTOR (EGFR) ANTAGONIST

**Prototype:** Trastuzumab

**AVAILABILITY** Solution for injection

## ACTION & THERAPEUTIC EFFECT

A recombinant human IgG1 monoclonal antibody that binds to the human epidermal growth factor receptor (EGFR) and blocks the binding of EGFR to its biological targets. *Expression and activation of EGFR has been correlated with malignant progression, induction of angiogenesis, and inhibition of apoptosis. The binding of necitumumab to EGFR induces its internalization and degradation.*

**USES** First-line treatment of patients with metastatic squamous non-small-cell lung cancer in combination with gemcitabine and cisplatin.

**CAUTIOUS USE** Cardiac arrest, cardiopulmonary arrest, venous and arterial thromboembolism (VTE and ATE), serious rash, and/or sudden death have occurred in patients treated with necitumumab in combination with gemcitabine and cisplatin. There are no adequate well-controlled studies in pregnant women; in animal data, it does cause fetal harm. It is not known whether necitumumab is present in human milk and the safest course is to advise women to discontinue breast-feeding during treatment and for 3 mo after the last dose.

## ROUTE & DOSAGE

### Non-Small-Cell Lung Cancer

*Adult:* **IV** 800 mg over 60 m on days 1 and 8 of 3wk cycle
*Previous Grade 1 or 2 infusion-related reaction:* Pre-medicate with diphenhydramine
*Additional Grade 1 or 2 infusion-related reaction:* Pre-medicated with diphenhydramine, acetaminophen, and dexamethasone

Common adverse effects in *italic;* life-threatening effects <u>underlined</u>; generic names in **bold;** classifications in SMALL CAPS; ♣ Canadian drug name; ● Prototype drug

### Infusion-Related Reactions (IRR) Dosage Adjustment

*Grade 1:* Decrease infusion rate by 50%
*Grade 2:* Stop infusion until resolution to Grade 0 or decrease infusion rate by 50%
*Grade 3 or 4:* Permanently discontinue

### Dermatologic Toxicity Dosage Adjustment

*Grade 3 or acneiform rash:* Withhold until symptoms resolve to less than or equal to Grade 2; resume at reduced dose of 400 mg for 1 cycle; may increase to 600 mg and 800 mg in subsequent cycles if symptom free. Permanently discontinue if rash does not resolve to less than or equal to Grade 2 within 6 wk or if symptoms worsen.

## ADMINISTRATION
Intravenous

*PREPARE:* **IV Infusion:** Withdraw the required volume of the drug and dilute with 0.9% sodium chloride injection in an IV infusion container to a final volume of 250 mL. Do not use solutions containing dextrose. Mix by gently inverting. Do not infuse with other electrolytes or medications.

*ADMINISTER:* **IV Infusion:** Administer via an infusion pump over 60 min through a separate infusion line. Flush the line with 0.9% sodium chloride injection at the end of the infusion.

*INCOMPATIBILITIES* Solution/additive: Do not mix with dextrose. Y-site: Administer through separate line.

- Store diluted solution at room temperature up to 25º C (77º F) for no more than 4 h, or under refrigeration 2º–8º C (36º–46º F) for no more than 24 h. Discard partially used or empty vials of necitumumab.

## ADVERSE EFFECTS (≥ 2%) **Body as a Whole:** Dysphagia, paronychia, phlebitis. **CNS:** *Headache.* **CV:** Cardiopulmonary arrest. **GI:** *Diarrhea,* stomatitis, *vomiting.* **Hematological:** *Hypocalcemia, hypokalemia, hypomagnesemia, hypophosphatemia.* **Metabolic:** Weight loss. **Musculoskeletal:** Muscle spasm. **Respiratory:** *Hemoptysis,* oropharyngeal pain, pulmonary embolism. **Skin:** Acne, *dermatitis acneiform,* dry skin, erythema, *generalized rash, maculopapular rash,* pruritus, skin fissures. **Special Senses:** Conjunctivitis.

## INTERACTIONS **Drug:** Necitumumab increases the levels of **gemcitabine.**

## PHARMACOKINETICS **Half-Life:** 14 days.

## NURSING IMPLICATIONS

### Assessment & Drug Effects
- Monitor electrolytes prior to administration of each dose and for 8 wk after the last dose.
- Most infusion-related reactions have been reported after the first or second administration.
- Monitor respiratory status and pulse oximetry in case of pulmonary embolism.
- Assess oral mucosa for sores and pain.
- Monitor daily weight.

### Patient & Family Education
- Use contraceptive measures during treatment.
- Report any shortness of breath, coughing up of blood, muscle spasms, or any eye infections.

Common adverse effects in *italic;* life-threatening effects underlined; generic names in **bold;** classifications in SMALL CAPS; ♣ Canadian drug name; ⊙ Prototype drug

1115

• Encourage family members to become CPR certified.

# NEFAZODONE
(nef-a-zo'done)

**Classifications:** ANTIDEPRESSANT; SEROTONIN NOREPINEPHRINE REUPTAKE INHIBITOR (SNRI)
Therapeutic: ANTIDEPRESSANT; SNRI
**Prototype:** Fluoxetine HCl

## AVAILABILITY Tablet

## ACTION & *THERAPEUTIC EFFECT*
Antidepressant with a dual mechanism of action. Inhibits neuronal serotonin ($5-HT_2$) and norepinephrine reuptake. *Effective in treating major depression without major cardiovascular adverse effects.*

## USES Treatment of depression.

## CONTRAINDICATIONS Hypersensitivity to nefazodone or alcohol; active hepatic disease, hepatitis, jaundice; elevated hepatic transaminase levels; MAOI therapy; mania; severe restlessness, suicidal ideation; surgery.

## CAUTIOUS USE History of seizure disorders, seizures; renal impairment; recent MI, unstable cardiac disease; hypotension; angina, stroke, hypovolemia, dehydration, bipolar disorder; history of mania; ECT therapy; older adults, women of childbearing age; pregnancy (category C); lactation. Safety and efficacy in children younger than 18 y not established.

## ROUTE & DOSAGE

### Depression
*Adult:* **PO** 100 mg b.i.d., may need to increase up to 300–600 mg/day in 2 divided doses
*Geriatric:* **PO** Start with 50 mg b.i.d.

## ADMINISTRATION
### Oral
• Do not give within 14 days of discontinuation of an MAO inhibitor.
• Can be given without regard to food.
• Store at 20° C–25° C (68°–77° F).

## ADVERSE EFFECTS (≥1%) **Body as a Whole:** Anaphylactic reactions, angioedema. **Cardiac:** Bradycardia, hypotension, peripheral edema. **CNS:** *Headache, dizziness, drowsiness,* asthenia, tremor, insomnia, agitation, anxiety. **GI:** Dry mouth, constipation, nausea, liver toxicity, liver failure. **Genitourinary:** Impotence, urinary frequency, and urinary retention. **Special Senses:** Visual disturbances, blurred vision, scotomata, tinnitus. **Endocrine:** Galactorrhea, gynecomastia, serotonin syndrome. **Respiratory:** Bronchitis, cough, dyspnea, pharyngitis. **Skin:** Stevens–Johnson syndrome.

## INTERACTIONS Drug: May cause serotonin syndrome (see Appendix F) with MAOIS or SSRIS; may increase plasma levels of some BENZODIAZEPINES, including **alprazolam** and **triazolam.** May decrease plasma levels and effects of **propranolol.** May increase levels and toxicity of **buspirone, carbamazepine, cilostazol, digoxin;** reports of $QT_c$ prolongation and ventricular arrhythmias with **pimozide;** increased risk of rhabdomyolysis with **lovastatin, simvastatin;** increased risk of **ergotamine** toxicity with **dihydroergotamine, ergotamine** or ERGOT ALKALOIDS. **Herbal:** St. **John's wort** may cause **serotonin** syndrome. Do not take **red yeast rice.**

## PHARMACOKINETICS Onset: 1 wk. **Distribution:** 99% protein bound. **Peak:** 3–5 wk. **Metabolism:** In liver via CYP3A4, CYP1A2,

CYP2D6, CYP2C to at least two active metabolites. **Half-Life:** Nefazodone 3.5 h, metabolites 2–33 h.

## NURSING IMPLICATIONS

### Black Box Warning

*Nefazodone has been associated with suicidal thinking and behavior in children, adolescents, and young adults, and with potentially fatal hepatotoxicity.*

### Assessment & Drug Effects

- Monitor for worsening of depression or emergence of suicidal ideation.
- Monitor patients with a history of seizures for increased activity.
- Monitor for and report promptly S&S of hepatotoxicity (see Appendix F).
- Assess safety, as dizziness and drowsiness are common adverse effects.
- Monitor lab tests: Periodic LFTs and CBC during long-term therapy.

### Patient & Family Education

- Report immediately to prescriber signs of worsening mental status such as suicidal ideation, aggressiveness, agitation, anxiety, hostility, impulsivity, insomnia, irritability, panic attacks, and worsening of depression.
- Be aware that significant improvement in mood may not occur for several weeks following initiation of therapy.
- Do not drive or engage in potentially hazardous activities until response to the drug is known.
- Report changes in visual acuity.
- Report signs of jaundice such as yellow coloration of the cornea of the eye or other S&S of liver dysfunction (anorexia, GI complaints, malaise, etc.).

## NELARABINE
### Arranon

**Classifications:** ANTINEOPLASTIC; PYRIMIDINE, ANTIMETABOLITE
**Therapeutic:** ANTINEOPLASTIC
**Prototype:** 5-Fluorouracil

### AVAILABILITY Solution

### ACTION & *THERAPEUTIC EFFECT*

Nelarabine inhibits DNA synthesis in lymphoblastic T-cells of acute leukemia and lymphoma. *The incorporation of a nelarabine metabolite in the leukemic blast cells halts DNA synthesis and causes cell death.*

### USES Treatment of patients with T-cell acute lymphoblastic leukemia lymphoma.

### CONTRAINDICATIONS Hepersensitivity to nelarabine; severe bone marrow suppression; older adults; pregnancy (category D); lactation.

### CAUTIOUS USE Severe renal impairment, severe renal failure; hepatic impairment; risk of infection, bleeding.

### ROUTE & DOSAGE

#### Adult T-Cell Leukemia/ Lymphoma

*Adult:* **IV** 1500 mg/m² on days 1, 3, and 5, repeated every 21 days
*Child:* **IV** 650 mg/m² over 1 h for 5 days, repeated every 21 days

#### *Toxicity Dosage Adjustment*

*Grade 2 or higher neurologic toxicity:* Discontinue therapy; *hematologic toxicities:* Delay therapy

N

Common adverse effects in *italic*; life-threatening effects <u>underlined</u>; generic names in **bold**; classifications in SMALL CAPS; ◆ Canadian drug name; ◯ Prototype drug

1117

## ADMINISTRATION

- Use gloves and protective clothing to prevent skin contact.

### Intravenous

This drug is a cytotoxic agent and caution should be used to prevent any contact with the drug. Follow institutional or standard guidelines for preparation, handling, and disposal of cytotoxic agents.

**PREPARE: IV Infusion:** Do not dilute. Transfer the required dose to a PVC or glass container for infusion. **ADMINISTER: IV Infusion for Adult:** Give over 2 h. **IV Infusion for Child:** Give over 1 h.

- Store vials at 15°–30° C (59°–86° F). Nelarabine is stable in PVC bags or glass infusion containers for 8 h up to 30° C.

## ADVERSE EFFECTS (≥1%) Body as a Whole:
Abnormal gait, *fatigue, pyrexia,* rigors. **CNS:** *Asthenia,* ataxia, *dizziness, headache, hypoesthesia, neuropathy, paresthesia, somnolence,* tremor. **CV:** Chest pain, *edema,* hypotension, *petechiae,* sinus tachycardia. **GI:** Abdominal pain, *constipation, diarrhea, nausea, vomiting,* stomatitis. **Hematologic/Lymphatic:** *Anemia, neutropenia, thrombocytopenia,* increased risk of infection. **Hepatic:** AST levels increased. **Metabolic:** Anorexia, dehydration, hyperglycemia. **Musculoskeletal:** Arthralgia, back pain, muscular weakness, *myalgia,* pain in extremities. **Respiratory:** *Cough, dyspnea, pleural effusion,* epistaxis, wheezing.

## PHARMACOKINETICS Distribution:
Extensive. **Metabolism:** Bioactivation to ara-GTP, oxidized to uric acid. **Elimination:** Renal. **Half-Life:** 3 h (active metabolite).

## NURSING IMPLICATIONS

### Black Box Warning

*Nelarabine has been associated with severe neurologic reactions.*

### Assessment & Drug Effects

- Monitor for and report immediately S&S of adverse CNS effects, including altered mental status (e.g., confusion, severe somnolence), seizures, and peripheral neuropathy (e.g., numbness, paresthesias, motor weakness, ataxia, paralysis). Note: Previous or concurrent treatment with intrathecal chemotherapy or previous craniospinal irradiation may increase risk of CNS toxicity.
- Discontinue IV and notify prescriber for neurologic adverse events of NCI Common Toxicity Criteria grade 2 or greater.
- Monitor for S&S of bleeding, especially with platelet counts less than 50,000/mm³.
- Monitor diabetics for loss of glycemic control.
- Monitor lab tests: Baseline and periodic CBC with differential and platelet count; periodic serum electrolytes, serum uric acid, LFTs, and renal function test.

### Patient & Family Education

- Do not drive or engage in potentially hazardous activities until response to drug is known.
- Report any of the following to a health care provider: Seizures; tingling or numbness in hands and feet; problems with fine motor coordination; unsteady gait and increased weakness with ambulating; fever or other signs of infections; black tarry stools,

blood tinged urine, or other signs of bleeding.

- Use effective contraceptive measures to avoid pregnancy while taking this drug.

## NELFINAVIR MESYLATE
(nel-fin'a-vir)

Viracept

**Classifications:** ANTIRETROVIRAL; PROTEASE INHIBITOR

**Therapeutic:** PROTEASE INHIBITOR

**Prototype:** Saquinavir

**AVAILABILITY** Tablet; powder for oral suspension

**ACTION & THERAPEUTIC EFFECT** Inhibits HIV-1 protease, which is responsible for the production of HIV-1 viral particles in an infected individual. This prevents the cleavage of viral polypeptide, resulting in the production of an immature, noninfectious virus. *Effectiveness is indicated by decreased viral load.*

**USES** Treatment of HIV infection in combination with other agents.

**CONTRAINDICATIONS** Hypersensitivity to nelfinavir; pancreatitis; Grade 2 or higher neurologic toxicity to drug; lactation.

**CAUTIOUS USE** Liver function impairment, hemophilia; diabetes mellitus, hyperglycemia; pregnancy (category B); children younger than 2 y.

## ROUTE & DOSAGE

### HIV Infection

*Adult/Adolescent:* **PO** 750 mg t.i.d. or 1250 mg b.i.d. with food

*Child (2–13 y):* **PO** 20–30 mg/kg t.i.d. with food (max: 750 mg/dose)

## ADMINISTRATION
### Oral

- Give with a meal or light snack.
- Oral powder may be mixed with a small amount of water, milk, soy milk, or dietary supplements; liquid should be consumed immediately. Do not mix oral powder in original container nor with acid food or juice (e.g., orange or apple juice, or apple sauce).
- Store at 15°–30° C (59°–86° F).

**ADVERSE EFFECTS (≥1%) Body as a Whole:** Allergic reactions, back pain, fever, malaise, pain, asthenia, myalgia, arthralgia. **CNS:** Headache, anxiety, depression, dizziness, insomnia, seizures. **GI:** Abdominal pain, *diarrhea,* nausea, flatulence, anorexia, dyspepsia, GI bleeding, hepatitis, vomiting, pancreatitis, increased liver function tests. **Hematologic:** Anemia, leukopenia, thrombocytopenia. **Respiratory:** Dyspnea, pharyngitis, rhinitis. **Skin:** Rash, pruritus, sweating, urticaria. **Endocrine:** Lipodystrophy, insulin resistance, dyslipidemia.

**INTERACTIONS Drug:** Other PROTEASE INHIBITORS, **ketoconazole** may increase nelfinavir levels; **rifabutin, rifampin,** PROTON PUMP INHIBITORS may decrease nelfinavir levels; nelfinavir will decrease ORAL CONTRACEPTIVE levels; may increase levels of **amiodarone, atorvastatin, simvastatin, sildenafil,** PDE 5 INHIBITORS; increase risk of **ergotamine** toxicity with **dihydroergotamine, ergotamine,** HMG-COA REDUCTASE INHIBITORS may have increased risk of rhabdomyolysis. BENZODIAZEPINES may increase risk of sedation. **Herbal: St. John's wort, garlic** may decrease antiretroviral activity. Use with **red**

**N**

Common adverse effects in *italic;* life-threatening effects <u>underlined</u>; generic names in **bold;** classifications in SMALL CAPS; ♣ Canadian drug name; ⊙ Prototype drug

1119

yeast rice may increase risk of rhabdomyolosis.

## PHARMACOKINETICS
**Absorption:** Food increases the amount of drug absorbed. **Distribution:** Greater than 98% protein bound. **Metabolism:** In the liver (CYP3A). **Elimination:** Primarily in feces. **Half-Life:** 3.5–5 h.

## NURSING IMPLICATIONS

### Assessment & Drug Effects
- Monitor hemophiliacs (type A or B) closely for spontaneous bleeding.
- Monitor carefully patients with hepatic impairment for toxic drug effects.

### Patient & Family Education
- Drug **must be** taken exactly as prescribed. Do not alter dose or discontinue drug without consulting prescriber.
- Use a barrier contraceptive even if using hormonal contraceptives.
- Be aware that diarrhea is a common adverse effect that can usually be controlled by OTC medications.

---

# NEOMYCIN SULFATE
(nee-oh-mye′sin)
**Mycifradin, Myciguent, Neo-Tabs, Neo-Fradin**
**Classification:** AMINOGLYCOSIDE ANTIBIOTIC
**Therapeutic:** ANTIBIOTIC
**Prototype:** Gentamicin

**AVAILABILITY** Tablet; oral solution; ointment, cream

## ACTION & THERAPEUTIC EFFECT
Inhibits bacterial protein synthesis through irreversible binding to the 30S ribosomal subunit within susceptible bacteria, thus causing bacteria not to replicate. *Active against a wide variety of gram-negative bacteria. Effective against certain gram-positive organisms, particularly penicillin-sensitive and some methicillin-resistant strains of Staphylococcus aureus (MRSA).*

## USES
Severe diarrhea caused by enteropathogenic *Escherichia coli;* preoperative intestinal antisepsis; to inhibit nitrogen-forming bacteria of GI tract in patients with cirrhosis or hepatic coma and for urinary tract infections caused by susceptible organisms. Also topically for short-term treatment of eye, ear, and skin infections.

## CONTRAINDICATIONS
Hypersensitivity to aminoglycosides; use of oral drug in patients with intestinal obstruction; ulcerative bowel lesions; IBD; topical applications over large skin areas; aminoglycosides; drug induced loss of hearing.

## CAUTIOUS USE
Dehydration; renal disease, renal impairment; hearing impairment; myasthenia gravis, parkinsonism; pregnancy (category C); lactation; children. **Topical otic applications:** Patients with perforated eardrum.

## ROUTE & DOSAGE

### Intestinal Antisepsis
*Adult:* **PO** 1 g q1h × 4 doses, then 1 g q4h × 5 doses
*Child:* **PO** 10.3 mg/kg q4–6h for 3 days

### Hepatic Coma

*Adult:* **PO** 4–12 g/day in 4 divided doses for 5–6 days
*Child:* **PO** 437.5–1225 mg/m² q6h for 5–6 days

### Diarrhea

*Adult:* **PO** 50 mg/kg in 4 divided doses for 2–3 days
*Child:* **PO** 8.75 mg/kg q6h for 2–3 days

### Cutaneous Infections

*Adult:* **Topical** Apply 1–3 × day

## ADMINISTRATION

### Oral

- Preoperative bowel preparation: Saline laxative is generally given immediately before neomycin therapy is initiated.

### Topical

- Consult prescriber about what to use for cleansing skin before each application.
- Make sure ear canal is clean and dry prior to instillation for topical therapy of external ear.

## ADVERSE EFFECTS (>1%) **Body as a Whole:** <u>Neuromuscular blockade</u> with muscular and <u>respiratory paralysis</u>, hypersensitivity reactions. **GI:** Mild laxative effect, diarrhea, nausea, vomiting; prolonged therapy: malabsorption-like syndrome including cyanocobalamin (vitamin B₁₂) deficiency, low serum cholesterol. **Urogenital:** <u>Nephrotoxicity</u>. **Special Senses:** <u>Ototoxicity</u>. **Skin:** *Redness,* scaling, pruritus, dermatitis.

## INTERACTIONS **Drug:** May decrease absorption of **cyanocobalamin.**

## PHARMACOKINETICS **Absorption:** 3% absorbed from GI tract in adults; up to 10% absorbed in

neonates. **Peak:** 1–4 h. **Elimination:** 97% excreted unchanged in feces. **Half-Life:** 3 h.

## NURSING IMPLICATIONS

### Black Box Warning

*Neomycin has been asssociated with neurotoxicity (including ototoxicity) and nephrotoxicity.*

### Assessment & Drug Effects

- Monitor closely for ototoxicity and nephrotoxicity. Risk is greatest in those with impaired renal function.
- Monitor I&O in patients receiving drug orally. Report oliguria or changes in I&O ratio. Inadequate neomycin excretion results in high serum drug levels and risk of nephrotoxicity.
- Monitor lab tests: Baseline and periodic serum renal function tests.

### Patient & Family Education

- Stop treatment and consult your prescriber if irritation occurs when you are using topical neomycin. Allergic dermatitis is common.
- Report any unusual symptom related to ears or hearing (e.g., tinnitus, roaring sounds, loss of hearing acuity, dizziness).
- Do not exceed prescribed dosage or duration of therapy.

## NEOSTIGMINE METHYLSULFATE ⊙
(nee-oh-stig′meen)
Bloxiverz
**Classifications:** CHOLINERGIC MUSCLE STIMULANT; CHOLINESTERASE INHIBITOR
**Therapeutic:** MUSCLE NERVE STIMULANT

Common adverse effects in *italic;* life-threatening effects <u>underlined;</u> generic names in **bold;** classifications in SMALL CAPS; ◆ Canadian drug name; ⊙ Prototype drug

1121

**AVAILABILITY** Solution for injection

## ACTION & *THERAPEUTIC EFFECT*

Produces reversible cholinesterase inhibition or inactivation with direct stimulant action on voluntary muscle fibers and possibly on autonomic ganglia and CNS neurons. Allows intensified and prolonged effect of acetylcholine at cholinergic synapses (basis for use in myasthenia gravis). *Produces generalized cholinergic response including miosis, increased tonus of intestinal and skeletal muscles, constriction of bronchi and ureters, slower pulse rate, and stimulation of salivary and sweat glands.*

**USES** To prevent and treat postoperative abdominal distention and urinary retention; for symptomatic control of and sometimes for differential diagnosis of myasthenia gravis; and to reverse the effects of nondepolarizing muscle relaxants (e.g., tubocurarine).

**CONTRAINDICATIONS** Hypersensitivity to neostigmine, cholinergics; bromides; ileus; mechanical obstruction of intestinal or urinary tract; peritonitis.

**CAUTIOUS USE** Recent ileorectal anastomoses; epilepsy; asthma; hepatic disease; bradycardia, CAD, recent coronary occlusion; vagotonia; cardiac arrhythmias; renal failure; renal impairment; renal disease; hyperthyroidism; MG; peptic ulcer; seizure disorder; older adults; pregnancy (category C); children; lactation.

## ROUTE & DOSAGE

**Diagnosis of Myasthenia Gravis**
*Adult:* **IM** 0.02 mg/kg

*Child:* **IM** 0.04 mg/kg

**Treatment of Myasthenia Gravis**
*Adult:* **IM/Subcutaneous** 0.5–2.5 mg q1–3h (max: 10 mg/day)
*Child:* **IM/Subcutaneous** 0.01–0.04 mg/kg q2–4h

**Reversal of Nondepolarizing Neuromuscular Blockade**
*Adult:* **IV** 0.5–2.5 mg slowly (max dose: 5 mg); may repeat
*Child:* **IV** 0.025–0.08 mg/kg
*Infant:* **IV** 0.025–0.1 mg/kg

**Postoperative Abdominal Distention and Urinary Retention**
*Adult:* **IM/Subcutaneous** 0.25 mg q4–6h for 2–3 days

**Myasthenia Gravis**
*Adult:* **IV** 0.5–2 mg q1–3h
*Child:* **IV** 0.01–0.04 mg/kg q2–4h

**Renal Impairment Dosage Adjustment**
*CrCl 10–50 mL/min:* Use 50% of dose; *less than 10 mL/min:* Use 25% of dose

## ADMINISTRATION

**Intramuscular/Subcutaneous**
- Give undiluted.

**Intravenous**

*PREPARE:* **Direct:** Give undiluted.
*ADMINISTER:* **Direct:** Give at a rate of 0.5 mg or a fraction thereof over 1 min.
*INCOMPATIBILITIES:* **Fluorescein.**

**ADVERSE EFFECTS** (≥1%) **Body as a Whole:** Muscle cramps, *fasciculations,* twitching, pallor, fatigability, generalized weakness, paralysis, agitation, fear,

Common adverse effects in *italic;* life-threatening effects underlined; generic names in **bold;** classifications in SMALL CAPS; ♣ Canadian drug name; ⊘ Prototype drug

<u>death</u>. **CV:** Tightness in chest, bradycardia, hypotension, elevated BP. **GI:** *Nausea,* vomiting, eructation, epigastric discomfort, abdominal cramps, diarrhea, involuntary or difficult defecation. **CNS:** CNS stimulation. **Respiratory:** *Increased salivation* and bronchial secretions, sneezing, cough, dyspnea, diaphoresis, respiratory depression. **Special Senses:** Lacrimation, miosis, blurred vision. **Urogenital:** Difficult micturition.

**INTERACTIONS Drug: Succinylcholine decamethonium** may prolong phase I block or reverse phase II block; neostigmine antagonizes effects of **tubocurarine; atracurium, vecuronium, pancuronium; procainamide, quinidine, atropine** antagonize effects of neostigmine.

**PHARMACOKINETICS Onset:** 10–30 min IM or IV. **Peak:** 20–30 min IM or IV. **Distribution:** Not reported to cross placenta or appear in breast milk. **Metabolism:** In liver. **Elimination:** 80% of drug and metabolites excreted in urine within 24 h. **Half-Life:** 50–90 min.

## NURSING IMPLICATIONS

### Assessment & Drug Effects

- Check pulse before giving drug to bradycardic patients. If below 60/min or other established parameter, consult prescriber. Atropine will be ordered to restore heart rate.
- Monitor respiration, maintain airway or assisted ventilation, and give oxygen as indicated when used as antidote for tubocurarine or other nondepolarizing neuromuscular blocking agents (usually preceded by atropine).

- Monitor pulse, respiration, and BP during period of dosage adjustment in treatment of myasthenia gravis.
- Report promptly and record accurately the onset of myasthenic symptoms and drug adverse effects in relation to last dose.
- Note carefully time of muscular weakness onset. It may indicate whether patient is in cholinergic or myasthenic crisis: Weakness that appears approximately 1 h after drug administration suggests cholinergic crisis (overdose) and is treated by prompt withdrawal of neostigmine and immediate administration of atropine. Weakness that occurs 3 h or more after drug administration is more likely due to myasthenic crisis (underdose or drug resistance) and is treated by more intensive anticholinesterase therapy.
- Record drug effect and duration of action. S&S of myasthenia gravis relieved by neostigmine include lid ptosis; diplopia; drooping facies; difficulty in chewing, swallowing, breathing, or coughing, and weakness of neck, limbs, and trunk muscles.
- Manifestations of neostigmine overdosage often appear first in muscles of neck and those involved in chewing and swallowing, with muscles of shoulder girdle and upper extremities affected next.
- Report to prescriber if patient does not urinate within 1 h after first dose when used to relieve urinary retention.

### Patient & Family Education

- Keep a diary of "peaks and valleys" of muscle strength.
- Keep an accurate record for prescriber of your response to drug. Learn how to recognize adverse effects, how to modify dosage

regimen according to your changing needs, or how to administer atropine if necessary.

- Be aware that certain factors may require an increase in size or frequency of dose (e.g., physical or emotional stress, infection, menstruation, surgery), whereas remission requires a decrease in dosage.

## NEPAFENAC

(nep′a-fe-nac)

Nevanac

**See Appendix A-1.**

## NERATINIB MALEATE

(neh-ra′tih-nib may′lee-ayt′)

Nerlynx

**Classifications:** ANTINEOPLASTIC; ANTI-HER2 AGENT; EGFR INHIBITOR; TYROSINE KINASE INHIBITOR
Therapeutic: ANTINEOPLASTIC

**AVAILABILITY** Tablet

## ACTION & *THERAPEUTIC EFFECT*

Neratinib is an irreversible inhibitor of epidermal growth factor receptor (EGFR), human epidermal growth factor receptor 2 (HER2), and HER4. *Approved as adjuvant treatment of breast cancer to help maintain remission.*

**USES** Treatment of early stage HER2-Positive breast cancer, post-trastuzumab treatment.

**CONTRAINDICATIONS** Pregnancy, lactation.

**CAUTIOUS USE** History of hepatic disease, geriatric patients.

## ROUTE & DOSAGE

**Breast Cancer**

*Adult:* **PO** 240 mg daily for 1 year

**Toxicity Dosage Adjustment**

*First dose reduction:* 200 mg once daily

*Second dose reduction:* 160 mg once daily

*First dose reduction:* 120 mg once daily

Specific toxicity and dose reduction strategies available in the package insert

## ADMINISTRATION

**Oral**

- Take dose with food at approximately the same time every day.
- Swallow tablets whole; do not chew, crush, or spit.
- Separate neratinib from antacids; may give 3 h after the antacid.
- Store at 20°–25° C (68°–77° F); excursions permitted at 15°–30° C (59°–86° F).

**ADVERSE EFFECTS** (≥ 2%) **GI:** *Abdominal pain*, anorexia, *diarrhea, nausea,* vomiting, stomatitis, swollen abdomen. **Skin:** Dry skin, rash, nail changes. **Metabolic:** Weight loss, elevated liver enzymes. **Musculoskeletal:** Spasm. **Renal:** UTI. **Other:** *Fatigue.*

**INTERACTIONS Drug:** Major substrate of CYP3A4, avoid use with CYP3A4 inducers (e.g., **carbamazepine, phenytoin, rifampin**) and inhibitors (e.g., **amiodarone, clarithromycin, erythromycin, itraconazole, verapamil**). Inhibits P-glycoprotein/ABCB1, avoid use with substrates of that glycoprotein (e.g., **topotecan, vincristine**). Avoid use with medications that reduce gastric acid, such as PROTON PUMP INHIBITORS and H-2 RECEPTOR ANTAGONISTS. **Herbal:** Avoid use with **St. John's wort.**

## PHARMACOKINETICS Distribution:
99% protein bound (primarily albumin). **Onset:** Peak in 2–8. **Metabolism:** Hepatic, primarily through CYP3A4. **Elimination:** 97% in feces, 1% in urine. **Half-Life:** 7–17 h.

## NURSING IMPLICATIONS

### Assessment & Drug Effects
- Antidiarrheal prophylaxis is recommended for the first 2 cycles.
- Monitor intake and output. Risk for fluid deficit related to diarrhea.
- Monitor lab tests: LFTs and pregnancy test prior to treatment.

### Patient & Family Education
- Many drugs and over the counter medications interact with this drug. Notify all prescribers that you are on this medication and check with prescriber before taking any other over the counter or natural products.
- Do not breast-feed while taking this medication. Resume breast-feeding 1 mo after taking the final dose.
- Call prescriber if diarrhea persists.
- Avoid grapefruit and grapefruit juice.
- If older than 65 y, more side effects may occur.
- Patients and spouses with reproductive potential should use effective birth control while taking the this medication and 3 mo after the last dose.
- If pregnancy occurs while taking this drug or within 1 mo of the final dose, call your prescriber right away.
- Report any confusion, mood changes, muscle pain/weakness, inability to pass urine, pass blood in the urine, if the urine is dark, loss of appetite, urinary urgency, more than 2 bowel movements in a day, or swelling of the belly.

- If a dose is missed, skip the dose and go back to the usual time. Do not take 2 doses at the same time or extra doses.

# NESIRITIDE
(nes-ir'i-tide)

Natrecor

**Classifications:** CARDIOVASCULAR; ATRIAL NATRIURETIC PEPTIDE HORMONE
Therapeutic: ATRIAL NATRIURETIC HORMONE (ANH)

## AVAILABILITY Vial

## ACTION & *THERAPEUTIC EFFECT*
Human atrial natriuretic hormone (ANH) is secreted by the right atrium when atrial blood pressure increases. Nesiritide, like ANH, inhibits antidiuretic hormone (ADH) by increasing urine sodium loss by the kidney and triggering the formation of a large volume of dilute urine. Nesiritide binds to a cyclic nucleic acid, which results in smooth muscle cell relaxation. *Effective in causing smooth muscle relaxation. The drug also causes dilation of veins and arteries. It is effective in managing dyspnea at rest in patients with acute CHF.*

## USES Acute treatment of decompensated CHF in patients who have dyspnea at rest or with minimal activity.

## CONTRAINDICATIONS Hypersensitivity to nesiritide, *Escherichia coli* protein, patients with a systolic blood pressure less than 90 mm Hg, cardiogenic shock, patients with low cardiac filling pressures, patients who should not receive vasodilators, such as those with significant valvular stenosis, restrictive or obstructive cardiomyopathy,

---

Common adverse effects in *italic;* life-threatening effects underlined; generic names in **bold;** classifications in SMALL CAPS; ♣ Canadian drug name; ⊘ Prototype drug

pericardial perfusion; constrictive pericarditis, pericardial tamponade.

**CAUTIOUS USE** Pregnancy (category C), lactation. Safety and efficacy in children not established.

## ROUTE & DOSAGE

### Acute Decompensated CHF

*Adult:* **IV** 2 mcg/kg bolus administered over 60 sec, followed by a continuous infusion of 0.01 mcg/kg/min (0.1 mL/kg/h) (max: 0.03 mcg/kg/min). Monitor blood pressure. If hypotension occurs, the dose should be reduced or discontinued. The infusion can subsequently be restarted at a dose that is reduced by 30% (with no bolus administration) after stabilization of hemodynamics.

## ADMINISTRATION

### Intravenous

*PREPARE:* **Direct and IV Infusion:** Reconstitute one 1.5 mg vial by adding 5 mL of IV solution removed from a 250 mL bag of selected diluent (i.e., D5W, NS, D5/0.45% NaCl, D5/0.2% NaCl). ▪ Rock the vial gently so that all surfaces, including the stopper, contact the diluent ensuring complete reconstitution. Do not shake the vial. ▪ Add the entire contents of the vial to the 250 mL IV bag to yield approximately 6 mcg/mL. Invert the bag several times to mix completely. ▪ Use within 24 h. ▪ Prime the IV tubing with 25 mL prior to connecting to the vascular access port.
*ADMINISTER:* **Direct:** Bolus dose **must be** withdrawn from the prepared infusion bag. Determine dose as follows: Bolus volume (mL) = (0.33) × (patient weight in kg). ▪ Give the bolus dose over

60 sec through an IV port in the tubing. **IV Infusion:** Infuse remainder of IV infusion immediately following the bolus dose. ▪ Determine the infusion rate as follows: Flow rate (mL/h) = (0.1) × (patient weight in kg).

*INCOMPATIBILITIES:* **Solution/additive: Promethazine. Y-site: Bumetanide, enalaprilat, ethacrynic acid, furosemide, heparin, hydralazine, regular insulin, micafungin.**

▪ Store at controlled room temperature at 20°–25° C (68°–77° F) or refrigerated.

## ADVERSE EFFECTS (≥1%) **Body as a Whole:** Headache, back pain, catheter pain, fever, injection site pain, leg cramps. **CNS:** Insomnia, dizziness, anxiety, confusion, paresthesia, somnolence, tremor. **CV:** *Hypotension,* ventricular tachycardia, ventricular extrasystoles, angina, bradycardia, tachycardia, atrial fibrillation, AV node conduction abnormalities. **GI:** Abdominal pain, nausea, vomiting. **Respiratory:** Cough, hemoptysis, apnea. **Skin:** Sweating, pruritus, rash. **Special Senses:** Amblyopia. **Renal:** Renal failure in acutely decompensated heart failure patients.

## INTERACTIONS **Drug:** Additive effects with ANTIHYPERTENSIVES.

## PHARMACOKINETICS **Onset:** 15 min. **Duration:** Greater than 60 min depending on dose. **Metabolism:** Proteolytic cleavage, proteolysis. **Half-Life:** 18 min.

## NURSING IMPLICATIONS

### Assessment & Drug Effects

▪ Monitor hemodynamic parameters (e.g., BP, PCWP, HR, ECG) throughout therapy.
▪ Establish hypotension parameters prior to initiating therapy. Notify

Common adverse effects in *italic;* life-threatening effects <u>underlined</u>; generic names in **bold**; classifications in SMALL CAPS; ✤ Canadian drug name; ⊘ Prototype drug prescriber immediately if systolic BP falls below 90 mm Hg.

- Reduce the dose or withhold the drug if hypotension occurs during administration. Reinitiate therapy infusion only after hypotension is corrected. Subsequent doses following a hypotensive episode are usually reduced by 30% and given without a prior bolus dose.
- **Monitor lab tests:** Baseline and periodic serum creatinine.

## NEVIRAPINE

(ne-vir′a-peen)

Viramune, Viramune XR

**Classifications:** ANTIRETROVIRAL; NONNUCLEOSIDE REVERSE TRANSCRIPTASE INHIBITOR (NNRTI)

**Therapeutic:** ANTIRETROVIRAL; NNRTI

**Prototype:** Efavirenz

**AVAILABILITY** Tablet; oral suspension; extended release tablet

### ACTION & *THERAPEUTIC EFFECT*

Nonnucleoside reverse transcriptase inhibitor (NNRTI) of HIV-1. Binds directly to reverse transcriptase and blocks RNA- and DNA-dependent polymerase activities, thus preventing replication of the virus. Does not inhibit HIV-2 RT. *Prevents replication of the HIV-1 virus. Resistant strains appear rapidly.*

**USES** Treatment of HIV with other agents.

**UNLABELED USES** Prevention of maternal-fetal HIV transmission.

**CONTRAINDICATIONS** Hypersensitivity to nevirapine; development of rash; severe skin reactions to the drug; hepatitis B or C; or early possible S&S of hepatitis; increased transaminases combined with rash or sign of hepatotoxicity; hepatic impairment of Child-Pugh class B or C use in post-exposure to HIV prophylaxis treatment; immune reconstitution complex; hormonal contraception; lactation.

**CAUTIOUS USE** Renal disease; hemodialysis; mild hepatic impairment, CNS disorders; pregnant women with CD4+ lymphocyte counts greater than 250/mm³; older adults; pregnancy (category B); neonates. **ER:** Children less than 6 y.

### ROUTE & DOSAGE

**HIV**

*Adult/Adolescent:* **PO Immediate release** 200 mg once daily for 14 days, then increase to 200 mg b.i.d.; or **Extended release** 400 mg daily

*Child/Infant (15 days or older):* **PO Immediate release** 150 mg/m² daily × 14 days, then 150 mg/m² twice daily (max: 400 mg) (max: 200 mg/dose)

*Adolescent/Child (6 y or older):* **Extended release** *0.58–0.83 m²:* 200 mg daily; *0.84–1.16 m²:* 300 mg daily; *1.17 m² or more:* 400 mg daily

**Hepatic Impairment Dosage Adjustment**

Do not use in Child-Pugh class B or C

### ADMINISTRATION

#### Oral

- Reinitiate with 200 mg/day for 14 days, then increase to b.i.d. dosing, when dosing is interrupted for more than 7 days.
- Ensure that extended release tablet is swallowed whole. It must not be crushed or chewed.
- Store at 15°–30° C (59°–86° F) in a tightly closed container.

---

Common adverse effects in *italic;* life-threatening effects underlined; generic names in **bold;** classifications in SMALL CAPS; ✦ Canadian drug name; ⊘ Prototype drug

**ADVERSE EFFECTS** (≥1%) **Body as a Whole:** Fever, paresthesia, myalgia. **CNS:** Headache. **GI:** Nausea, diarrhea, abdominal pain, hepatitis, increased liver function tests, <u>hepatotoxicity</u> (including <u>fulminant and cholestatic hepatitis, hepatic necrosis, and hepatic failure</u>, especially with long-term use). **Hematologic:** Anemia, neutropenia. **Skin:** *Rash,* <u>Stevens–Johnson syndrome</u>.

**INTERACTIONS Drug:** May decrease plasma concentrations of PROTEASE INHIBITORS, ORAL CONTRACEPTIVES; may decrease **methadone, dronedarone** levels. **Fluconazole** may increase adverse effects. **Herbal: St. John's wort, garlic** may decrease antiretroviral activity.

**PHARMACOKINETICS Absorption:** Rapidly from GI tract. **Peak:** 4h. **Distribution:** 60% protein bound, crosses placenta, distributed into breast milk. **Metabolism:** In liver (CYP3A). **Elimination:** Primarily in urine. **Half-Life:** 25–40 h.

**NURSING IMPLICATIONS**

**Black Box Warning**

*Nevirapine has been associated with severe, potentially fatal, hepatotoxicity and skin reactions.*

**Assessment & Drug Effects**
- Monitor carefully, especially during first 18 wk of therapy, for severe rash (with or without fever, blistering, oral lesions, conjunctivitis, swelling, joint aches, or general malaise) and for S&S of hepatotoxicity (see Appendix F).
- Withhold drug and notify prescriber if rash develops or liver function tests are abnormal.

- Monitor lab tests: Baseline and frequent LFTs.

**Patient & Family Education**
- Withhold drug and notify prescriber if severe rash appears or if you develop S&S of hepatitis.
- Do not drive or engage in potentially hazardous activities until response to drug is known. There is a high potential for drowsiness and fatigue.
- Use or add barrier contraceptive if using hormonal contraceptive.

# NIACIN (VITAMIN B₃, NICOTINIC ACID)

(nye'a-sin)

Niacor, Niaspan, Nicobid, Nico-400, Nicotinex, Novoniacin ♦, Slo-Niacin, Tri-B3 ♦

## NIACINAMIDE (NICOTINAMIDE)

**Classifications:** VITAMIN B₃; ANTILIPEMIC
**Therapeutic:** ANTILIPEMIC; LIPID-LOWERING AGENT

**AVAILABILITY** Tablet; sustained release tablet; capsule

## ACTION & *THERAPEUTIC EFFECT*

Water-soluble, heat-stable, B-complex vitamin (B₃) that functions with riboflavin as a control agent in coenzyme system that converts protein, carbohydrate, and fat to energy through oxidation-reduction. Niacinamide, an amide of niacin, is used as an alternative in the prevention and treatment of pellagra. *Produces vasodilation by direct action on vascular smooth muscles. Inhibits hepatic synthesis of VLDL, cholesterol,*

Common adverse effects in *italic;* life-threatening effects <u>underlined</u>; generic names in **bold**; classifications in SMALL CAPS; ♦ Canadian drug name; ☻ Prototype drug *and triglyceride, and, indirectly, LDL. Large doses effectively reduce elevated serum cholesterol and total lipid levels in hypercholesterolemia and hyperlipidemic states.*

**USES** In prophylaxis and treatment of pellagra, usually in combination with other B-complex vitamins, and in deficiency states accompanying carcinoid syndrome, isoniazid therapy, Hartnup's disease, and chronic alcoholism. Also in adjuvant treatment of hyperlipidemia (elevated cholesterol or triglycerides) in patients who do not respond adequately to diet or weight loss. Also as vasodilator in peripheral vascular disorders, Ménière's disease, and labyrinthine syndrome, as well as to counteract LSD toxicity and to distinguish between psychoses of dietary and nondietary origin.

**CONTRAINDICATIONS** Hypersensitivity to niacin or niacinamide; hepatic impairment; active hepatic disease, significant or unexplained elevations of hepatic transaminases two or three times ULN; hepatotoxicity, hemorrhaging or arterial bleeding; active peptic ulcer; persistent cutaneous reactions to niacin use; lactation.

**CAUTIOUS USE** History of gallbladder disease, liver disease, and peptic ulcer; excessive alcohol consumption; renal impairment; glaucoma; unstable angina or MI; new onset atrial fibrillation; coronary artery disease; diabetes mellitus; CAD; poorly controlled DM; predisposition to gout; allergy; thrombocytopenia; patients at risk for hypophosphatemia; pregnancy (category C). **ER:** Children younger than 18 y.

## ROUTE & DOSAGE

### Niacin Deficiency
*Adult:* **PO** 10–20 mg/day

### Pellagra
*Adult:* **PO** 50–100 mg 3–4 × day
*Child:* **PO** 50–100 mg t.i.d.

### Hyperlipidemia
*Adult:* **PO** 1.5–3 g/day in divided doses, may increase up to 6 g/day if necessary **(Niaspan product)** 1–2 g at bedtime
*Child:* **PO** 100–250 mg/day in 3 divided doses, may increase by 250 mg/day q2–3wk as tolerated

## ADMINISTRATION
### Oral
- Give with meals to decrease GI distress. Give with cold water (not hot beverage) to facilitate swallowing.
- Ensure that sustained release form is not chewed or crushed. It **must be** swallowed whole.
- Store at 15°–30° C (59°–86° F) in a light and moisture proof container.

## ADVERSE EFFECTS (≥1%) **CNS:** *Transient headache, tingling of extremities,* syncope. With chronic use: Nervousness, panic, toxic amblyopia, proptosis, blurred vision, loss of central vision. **CV:** *Generalized flushing with sensation of warmth,* postural hypotension, vasovagal attacks, arrhythmias (rare). **GI:** *Abnormalities of liver function tests; jaundice, bloating, flatulence, nausea,* vomiting, GI disorders, activation of peptic ulcer, xerostomia. **Skin:** *Increased sebaceous gland activity,* dry skin, skin rash, *pruritus,* keratitis nigricans. **Metabolic:** Hyperuricemia, hyperglycemia, glycosuria, hypoprothrombinemia, hypoalbuminemia.

---

Common adverse effects in *italic;* life-threatening effects underlined; generic names in **bold;** classifications in SMALL CAPS; ♣ Canadian drug name; ⊙ Prototype drug

1129

## DIAGNOSTIC TEST INTERFERENCE

Niacin causes elevated serum *bilirubin, uric acid, alkaline phosphatase, AST, ALT, LDH* levels and may cause *glucose intolerance.* Decreases *serum cholesterol* 15–30% and may cause false elevations with certain *fluorometric methods* of determining *urinary catecholamines.* Niacin may cause false-positive *urine glucose* tests using *copper sulfate reagents* (e.g., *Benedict's* solution).

## INTERACTIONS Drug: Potentiates

hypotensive effects of ANTIHYPERTENSIVE AGENTS.

## PHARMACOKINETICS Absorption: Readily from GI tract. Peak: 20–70 min. Distribution: Into breast milk. Metabolism: In liver. Elimination: Primarily in urine. Half-Life: 45 min.

## NURSING IMPLICATIONS

### Assessment & Drug Effects

- Monitor therapeutic effectiveness and record effect of therapy on clinical manifestations of deficiency (fiery red tongue, excessive saliva secretion and infection of oral membranes, nausea, vomiting, diarrhea, confusion). Therapeutic response usually begins within 24 h.
- Monitor diabetics and patients on high doses for decreased glucose tolerance and loss of glycemic control.
- Observe patients closely for evidence of liver dysfunction (jaundice, dark urine, light-colored stools, pruritus) and hyperuricemia in patients predisposed to gout (flank, joint, or stomach pain; altered urine excretion pattern).
- Monitor lab tests: Baseline and periodic blood glucose and

LFTs with prolonged high dose therapy.

### Patient & Family Education

- Be aware that you may feel warm and flushed in face, neck, and ears within first 2 h after oral ingestion and it may last several hours. Effects are usually transient and subside as therapy continues.
- Sit or lie down and avoid sudden posture changes if you feel weak or dizzy. Report these symptoms and persistent flushing to your prescriber.
- Be aware that alcohol and large doses of niacin cause increased flushing and sensation of warmth.
- Avoid exposure to direct sunlight until lesions have entirely cleared if you have skin manifestations.

# NICARDIPINE HYDROCHLORIDE

(ni-car'di-peen)

Cardene

**Classifications:** CALCIUM CHANNEL BLOCKER; ANTIHYPERTENSIVE
Therapeutic: ANTIHYPERTENSIVE; ANTIANGINAL
**Prototype:** Nifedipine

## AVAILABILITY Capsule; sustained release capsule; solution for injection

## ACTION & *THERAPEUTIC EFFECT*

Calcium channel entry blocker that inhibits the transmembrane influx of calcium ions into cardiac muscle and smooth muscle, thus affecting contractility. Selectively affects vascular smooth muscle more than cardiac muscle. *Significantly decreases systemic vascular resistance. It reduces BP at rest and during isometric and dynamic exercise.*

Common adverse effects in *italic;* life-threatening effects <u>underlined;</u> generic names in **bold;** classifications in SMALL CAPS; ✦ Canadian drug name; ☺ Prototype drug

**USES** Either alone or with beta-blockers for chronic, stable (effort-associated) angina; either alone or with other antihypertensives for essential hypertension.

**UNLABELED USES** CHF, cerebral ischemia, migraine.

**CONTRAINDICATIONS** Hypersensitivity to nicardipine; advanced aortic stenosis; cardiogenic shock; hypotension.

**CAUTIOUS USE** CHF; renal and hepatic impairment; severe bradycardia; older adult; GERD; hiatal hernia; renal disease; renal impairment; acute stroke; angina; CHF; acute myocardial infarction; older adults; pregnancy (category C); lactation. Safety and efficacy in children not established.

## ROUTE & DOSAGE

**Hypertension, Angina**

*Adult:* **PO** 20–40 mg t.i.d. or 30–60 mg SR b.i.d.; *Initiation of therapy in a drug-free patient:* **IV** 5 mg/h initially, increase dose by 2.5 mg/h q15min (or faster) (max: 15 mg/h); *for severe hypertension:* 4–7.5 mg/h; *for postop hypertension:* 10–15 mg/h initially, then 1–3 mg/h

## ADMINISTRATION

Note: To prevent symptoms of withdrawal, do not abruptly discontinue drug.

**Oral**

- Give on empty stomach. High-fat meals may decrease blood levels.
- Ensure that sustained release form is not chewed or crushed. **must be** swallowed whole.
- When converting from IV to oral dose, give first dose of t.i.d. regimen 1 h before discontinuing infusion.

**Intravenous**

*PREPARE:* **IV Infusion:** Dilute each 25 mg with 240 mL of D5W or NS to yield 0.1 mg/mL.

*ADMINISTER:* **IV Infusion:** Usually initiated at 50 mL/h (5 mg/h) with rate increases of 25 mL/h (2.5 mg/h) q5–15min up to a maximum of 150 mL/h. ▪ Infusion is usually slowed to 30 mL/h once the target BP is reached. *Substitute for oral doses:* Oral 20 mg q8h, IV equivalent is 0.5 mg/h; oral 30 mg q8h, IV equivalent is 1.2 mg/h; oral 40 mg q8h, IV equivalent is 2.2 mg/h.

*INCOMPATIBILITIES:* Solution/additive: **Sodium bicarbonate.** Y-site: **Acyclovir, aminocaproic acid, aminophylline, amphotericin B, ampicillin, ampicillin/sulbactam, atenolol, azithromycin, cefoperazone, ceftazidime, cefuroxime, clindamycin, dexamethasone, diazepam, ertapenem, fludarabine, fluorouracil, foscarnet, fosphenytoin, furosemide, ganciclovir, gemtuzumab, hydrocortisone, heparin, imipenem/cilastatin, ketorolac, lansoprazole, meropenem, mesna, methohexital, methotrexate, micafungin, pantoprazole, pemetrexed, pentobarbital, phenobarbital, phenytoin, piperacilin, potassium acetate, potassium phosphates.**

## ADVERSE EFFECTS (≥1%) CNS:

Dizziness or headache, fatigue, anxiety, depression, paresthesias, insomnia, somnolence, nervousness. **CV:** Pedal edema, hypotension, flushing, palpitations, tachycardia, increased angina. **GI:** Anorexia, nausea, vomiting, dry mouth, constipation, dyspepsia. **Skin:** Rash, pruritus. **Body as a Whole:** Arthralgia or arthritis.

N

**INTERACTIONS Drug: Adenosine** prolongs bradycardia. **Amiodarone** may cause sinus arrest and AV block. **Benazepril** blunts increase in heart rate and increase in plasma **norepinephrine** and **aldosterone** seen with nicardipine. BETA-BLOCKERS cause hypotension and bradycardia. **Cimetidine** increases levels of nicardipine, resulting in hypotension. Concomitant nicardipine and **cyclosporine** result in significant increase in **cyclosporine** serum concentrations 1–30 days after initiation of nicardipine therapy; following withdrawal of nicardipine, **cyclosporine** levels decrease. **Magnesium,** when used to retard premature labor, may cause severe hypotension and neuromuscular blockade. **Food: Grapefruit juice** (greater than 1 qt/ day) may increase plasma concentrations and adverse effects.

**PHARMACOKINETICS Absorption:** Immediately 35% of oral dose reaches systemic circulation. **Onset:** 1 min IV; 20 min PO. **Peak:** 0.5–2 h. **Duration:** 3 h IV. **Distribution:** 95% protein bound; distributed in breast milk. **Metabolism:** Rapidly and extensively in liver (CYP3A4); active metabolite has less than 1% activity of parent compound. **Elimination:** 35% in feces, 60% in urine; not affected by hemodialysis. **Half-Life:** 8.6 h.

## NURSING IMPLICATIONS

### Assessment & Drug Effects

- Establish baseline data before treatment is started including BP and pulse.
- Monitor closely BP values during initiation and titration of dosage. Hypotension with or without an increase in heart rate may occur.
- Avoid too rapid reduction in either systolic or diastolic pressure during parenteral administration.
- Discontinue IV infusion if hypotension or tachycardia develop.

- Observe for large peak and trough differences in BP. Initially, measure BP at peak effect (1–2 h after dosing) and at trough effect (8 h after dosing).

### Patient & Family Education

- Record and report any increase in frequency, duration, and severity of angina when initiating or increasing dosage. Keep a record of nitroglycerin use and promptly report any changes in previous anginal pattern.
- Do not change dosage regimen without consulting prescriber.
- Be aware that abrupt withdrawal may cause an increased frequency and duration of chest pain. This drug **must be** gradually tapered under medical supervision.
- Rise slowly from a recumbent position; avoid driving or operating potentially dangerous equipment until response to nicardipine is known.
- Notify prescriber if any of the following occur: Irregular heartbeat, shortness of breath, swelling of the feet, pronounced dizziness, nausea, or drop in BP.

# NICOTINE ⓟ
(nik'o-teen)

Nicotrol NS, Nicotrol Inhaler, Commit

# NICOTINE POLACRILEX
Nicorette Gum, Nicorette DS

# NICOTINE TRANSDERMAL SYSTEM
Habitrol, Nicoderm, Nicotrol, ProStep

**Classifications:** SMOKING DETERRENT; CHOLINERGIC RECEPTOR ANTAGONIST
**Therapeutic:** SMOKING DETERRENT

**AVAILABILITY** Gum; lozenges; spray; inhaler; transdermal patch

**ACTION & *THERAPEUTIC EFFECT***
Ganglionic cholinergic receptor antagonist that has both adrenergic and cholinergic effects. Includes stimulant and depressant effects on the peripheral nervous system and CNS; respiratory stimulation; peripheral vasoconstriction; increased heart rate, cardiac output, and stroke volume; increased tone and motor activity of GI smooth muscles; increased bronchial secretions (initially); antidiuretic activity. Heavy smokers are tolerant of these effects. *Rationale for use is to reduce withdrawal symptoms accompanying cessation of smoking. Success rate appears to be greatest in smokers with high "physical" type of nicotine dependence.*

**USES** In conjunction with a medically supervised behavior modification program, as a temporary and alternate source of nicotine by the nicotine-dependent smoker who is withdrawing from cigarette smoking.

**CONTRAINDICATIONS** Nonsmokers, immediate post-MI period; life-threatening arrhythmias; active temporomandibular joint disease; severe angina pectoris; women with childbearing potential (unless effective contraception is used). **Nicotine Transdermal** or **Inhaler System:** Pregnancy (category D).

**CAUTIOUS USE** Vasospastic disease (e.g., Buerger's disease, Prinzmetal's variant angina), cardiac arrhythmias, hyperthyroidism, type 1 diabetes, pheochromocytoma, esophagitis, oral and pharyngeal inflammation; denture use, denture caps, or partial bridges; hypertension and peptic ulcer disease (active or inactive); GERD. **Gum:** Pregnancy (category C). During lactation, only if benefit of a smoking cessation program outweighs risks; children younger than 18 y.

## ROUTE & DOSAGE

**Smoking Cessation**

*Adult:* **PO** Chew 1 piece of gum whenever having an urge to smoke, may be repeated as needed (max: 30 pieces of gum/day); **Intranasal** 1 dose = 2 sprays, 1 in each nostril, start with 1–2 doses (2–4 sprays) each hour (max: 5 doses/h, 40 doses/day), may continue for 3 mo; **Topical** Apply 1 transdermal patch q24h by the following schedule: **Habitrol, Nicoderm:** 21 mg/day × 6 wk, 14 mg/day × 2 wk, 7 mg/day × 2 wk; *weight less than 45 kg (100 lb), smoke less than ½ pack/day, or have cardiovascular disease:* 14 mg/day × 6 wk, 7 mg/day × 2–4 wk, **ProStep:** 22 mg/day × 4–8 wk, 11 mg/day × 2–4 wk; *weight less than 45 kg (100 lb), smoke less than ½ pack/day, or have cardiovascular disease:* 11 mg/day × 4–8 wk; **Nicotrol:** Apply 1 transdermal patch 16 h/day by the following schedule: 15 mg/day × 4–12 wk, 10 mg/day × 2–4 wk, 5 mg/day × 2–4 wk

## ADMINISTRATION
**Oral**
- Note: Most adverse local effects (irritation of tongue, mouth, and throat, jaw-muscle aches, dislike of taste) are transient and subside

**N**

Common adverse effects in *italic;* life-threatening effects <u>underlined;</u> generic names in **bold;** classifications in SMALL CAPS; ♣ Canadian drug name; ⊘ Prototype drug

1133

in a few days. Modification of the chewing technique may help.

**Transdermal**

- Remove the old patch before applying the next new patch.
- Apply patch to nonhairy, clean, dry skin site; immediately remove from protective container.
- Store at or below 30° C (86° F); patches are sensitive to heat.

## ADVERSE EFFECTS (≥1%) **CNS:**
*Headache, dizziness, light-headedness,* insomnia, irritability, dependence on nicotine. **CV:** Arrhythmias, tachycardia, palpitations, hypertension. **GI:** Air swallowing, *jaw ache, nausea,* belching, salivation, anorexia, dry mouth, laxative effects, constipation, *indigestion,* diarrhea, dyspepsia, vomiting, sialorrhea, abdominal pain, diarrhea. **Respiratory:** *Sore mouth or throat, cough, hiccups,* hoarseness; injury to mouth, teeth, temporomandibular joint pain, *irritation/tingling of tongue.* **Skin:** *Erythema, pruritus, local edema, rash;* skin reactions may be delayed, occurring after 3 wk of patch use. **Special Senses:** *Runny nose, nasal irritation, throat irritation, watering eyes,* minor epistaxis, nasal ulceration. **Body as a Whole:** Acute overdose/nicotine intoxication (perspiration; severe headache; dizziness; disturbed hearing and vision; mental confusion; severe weakness; fainting; hypotension; dyspnea; weak, rapid, irregular pulse; seizures); death (from respiratory failure secondary to drug-induced respiratory muscle paralysis).

## INTERACTIONS **Drug:** May increase metabolism of **caffeine, theophylline, acetaminophen, insulin, oxazepam, pentazocine propranolol. Food:** Coffee, cola may decrease nicotine absorption from nicotine gum.

## PHARMACOKINETICS **Absorption:** Approximately 90% of the nicotine in a piece of gum is released slowly over 15–30 min; rate of release is controlled by vigor and duration of chewing; readily absorbed from buccal mucosa; transdermal 75–90% absorbed through skin; 53–58% of nasal spray is absorbed. **Peak:** Transdermal 8–9 h; nasal spray 4–15 min. **Distribution:** Crosses placenta; distributed into breast milk. **Metabolism:** In liver, primarily to cotinine. **Elimination:** In urine. **Half-Life:** 30–120 min.

## NURSING IMPLICATIONS

### Assessment & Drug Effects

- Be aware that transient erythema, pruritus, or burning is common with transdermal patch and usually disappears 24 h after patch removal.
- Differentiate cutaneous hypersensitivity (contact sensitization) that does not resolve in 24 h from a transient local reaction. The former is an indication to discontinue the transdermal patch.

### Patient & Family Education

- Chew a piece of gum for approximately 30 min to get the full dose of nicotine.
- Chew only one piece of gum at a time. Chewing gum too rapidly can cause excessive buccal absorption and lead to adverse effects: Nausea, hiccups, throat irritation.
- Gradually decrease number of pieces of gum chewed in 24 h. Usually, a period of 3 mo is allowed before tapering use of gum.
- Promptly discontinue use of transdermal patch and notify prescriber if a severe or persistent local or generalized skin reaction occurs.

- Smoking while using the transdermal nicotine patch increases the risk of adverse reactions.

# NIFEDIPINE℗

(nye-fed'i-peen)

Adalat CC, Afeditab CR, Nifedical XL, Procardia, Procardia XL

**Classifications:** CALCIUM CHANNEL BLOCKER; ANTIANGINAL, ANTIHYPERTENSIVE

Therapeutic: ANTIHYPERTENSIVE, ANTIANGINAL

**AVAILABILITY** Capsule, sustained release tablet

**ACTION & THERAPEUTIC EFFECT**
Blocks calcium ion influx across cell membranes of cardiac muscle and vascular smooth muscle. Reduces myocardial oxygen utilization and supply and relaxes and prevents coronary artery spasm. Decreases peripheral vascular resistance and increases cardiac output. *The rise in peripheral blood flow is the basis for use in treatment of Raynaud's phenomenon as well as hypertension. Effective antianginal agent.*

**USES** Vasospastic "variant" or Prinzmetal's angina and chronic stable angina without vasospasm. Mild to moderate hypertension.

**UNLABELED USES** Vascular headaches; Raynaud's phenomenon; asthma; cardiomyopathy; primary pulmonary hypertension.

**CONTRAINDICATIONS** Known hypersensitivity to nifedipine; unstable angina; acute MI; cardiogenic shock; aortic stenosis; GI obstruction.

**CAUTIOUS USE** GERD; CHF; pregnancy (category C); lactation; children.

## ROUTE & DOSAGE

**Variant Angina**

*Adult:* **PO** 10 mg t.i.d. may titrate up to 180 mg/day; **Extended release** 30–60 mg daily; titrate up if necessary (max: 90 mg/day)

**Hypertension**

*Adult:* **PO Extended release** 30–60 mg once/day; titrate up if necessary (max: 90 mg/day)

## ADMINISTRATION

**Oral**

- Do not give within the first 1–2 wk following an MI.
- Do not give with grapefruit juice.
- Use only the sustained release form to treat chronic hypertension. Ensure that sustained release form is not chewed or crushed. It **must be** swallowed whole.
- Discontinue drug gradually, with close medical supervision to prevent severe hypertension and other adverse effects.
- Store intermediate release capsules at 15°–25° C (59°–77° F); protect from light and moisture.

**ADVERSE EFFECTS** (≥1%) **Body as a Whole:** Sore throat, weakness, fever, sweating, chills, febrile reaction. **CNS:** *Dizziness, light-headedness,* nervousness, mood changes, weakness, jitteriness, sleep disturbances, blurred vision, retinal ischemia, difficulty in balance, *headache.* **CV:** Hypotension, *facial flushing, heat sensation,* palpitations, *peripheral edema,* MI (rare), prolonged systemic hypotension with overdose. **GI:** Nausea, heartburn, *diarrhea,* constipation, cramps, flatulence, gingival hyperplasia, hepatotoxicity. **Musculoskeletal:** Inflammation, joint stiffness, muscle cramps. **Respiratory:** Nasal congestion, dyspnea, cough,

N

Common adverse effects in *italic;* life-threatening effects underlined; generic names in **bold;** classifications in SMALL CAPS; ♣ Canadian drug name; ℗ Prototype drug

1135

wheezing. **Skin:** Dermatitis, pruritus, urticaria. **Urogenital:** Sexual difficulties, possible male infertility.

## DIAGNOSTIC TEST INTERFERENCE

Nifedipine may cause mild to moderate increases of *alkaline phosphatase, CPK, LDH, AST, ALT.*

## INTERACTIONS Drug: BETA-BLOCK-ERS

may increase likelihood of CHF; may increase risk of **phenytoin** toxicity. Do not use with strong CYP3A4 inducers (e.g., BARBITUATES, **carbamazepine, phenobarbital, rifabutin, rifampin**). **Herbal: Melatonin** may increase blood pressure and heart rate. **Ginkgo, ginseng** may increase plasma concentrations. **St. John's wort** may decrease plasma concentrations. **Food: Grapefruit juice** (greater than 1 qt/day) may increase plasma concentrations and adverse effects.

## PHARMACOKINETICS

**Absorption:** Readily from GI tract; 45–75% reaches systemic circulation. **Onset:** 10–30 min. **Peak:** 30 min. **Distribution:** Distributed into breast milk; 92–98% protein bound. **Metabolism:** In liver via CYP3A4, P-glycoprotein. **Elimination:** 75–80% in urine, 15% in feces. **Half-Life:** 2–5 h.

## NURSING IMPLICATIONS

### Assessment & Drug Effects

- Monitor BP carefully during titration period. Patient may become severely hypotensive, especially if also taking other drugs known to lower BP. Withhold drug and notify prescriber if systolic BP less than 90.
- Monitor blood sugar in diabetic patients. Nifedipine has diabetogenic properties.
- Monitor for gingival hyperplasia and report promptly. This is a rare but serious adverse effect (similar to phenytoin-induced hyperplasia).

### Patient & Family Education

- Keep a record of nitroglycerin use and promptly report any changes in previous pattern. Occasionally, people develop increased frequency, duration, and severity of angina when they start treatment with this drug or when dosage is increased.
- Be aware that withdrawal symptoms may occur with abrupt discontinuation of the drug (chest pain, increase in anginal episodes, MI, dysrhythmias).
- Inspect gums visually every day. Changes in gingivae may be gradual, and bleeding may be exhibited only with probing.
- Seek prompt treatment for symptoms of gingival hyperplasia (easy bleeding of gingivae and gradual enlarging of gingival mass, especially on buccal side of lower anterior teeth). Drug will be discontinued if gingival hyperplasia occurs.
- Research shows that smoking decreases the efficacy of nifedipine and has direct and adverse effects on the heart in the patient on nifedipine treatment.

## NILOTINIB HYDROCHLORIDE

(ni-lot'i-nib hy-dro-chlor'ide)

Tasigna

**Classifications:** ANTINEOPLASTIC; KINASE INHIBITOR

Therapeutic: ANTINEOPLASTIC

**Prototype:** Erlotinib

### AVAILABILITY Capsule

### ACTION & *THERAPEUTIC EFFECT*

Nilotinib is a tyrosine kinase inhibitor designed to selectively inhibit the BCR-ABL tyrosine kinase on the Philadelphia chromosome found in chronic myelogenous leukemia (CML). It prevents tyrosine kinase enzyme from converting to its active conformation. Thus, it prevents proliferation of BCR-ABL cells and ultimately induces cell death in CML. Nilotinib enhances binding site affinity by offering alternate binding pathways for the ABL tyrosine kinases. *Increased kinase selectivity and binding site affinity makes nilotinib more potent than other similar drugs (imatinib) in preventing the proliferation of CML.*

**USES** Treatment of Philadelphia chromosome positive (Ph⁺) chronic myelogenous leukemia (CML) in patients resistant to or intolerant to prior therapy that included imatinib.

**CONTRAINDICATIONS** Hypoglycemia; hypomagnesemia; hypokalemia; long QT syndrome; drug-inducted QT prolongation; severe galactose or lactose intolerance; glucose-galactose malabsorption syndromes; pregnancy (category D); lactation.

**CAUTIOUS USE** History of pancreatitis; history of cardiac disease, recent MI, CHF, unstable angina; myelosuppression; total gastrectomy; hepatic impairment. Safety and efficacy in children younger than 18 y not established.

## ROUTE & DOSAGE

**Chronic Myelogenous Leukemia**
*Adult:* **PO** 300 or 400 mg b.i.d.

**QT Prolongation Dosage Adjustment**
See package insert.

**Myelosuppression Dosage Adjustment**
- If ANC less than 1 × 10⁹/L or platelet count less than 50 × 10⁹/L, discontinue nilotinib.

- If ANC greater than 1 × 10⁹/L and platelet count greater than 50 × 10⁹/L within 2 wk, resume previous dose.
- If ANC less than 1 × 10⁹/L or platelet count less than 50 × 10⁹/L for more than 2 wk, reduce to 400 mg PO daily

**Nonhematologic Abnormalities Dosage Adjustment**
*For grade 3 or higher serum lipase, amylase, bilirubin, or hepatic transaminases:* Withhold nilotinib and monitor abnormal level(s).
Resume nilotinib at 400 mg PO daily if toxicity resolves to grade 1 or lower.
*Other moderate/severe nonhematologic toxicities:* Withhold nilotinib until toxicity resolves, then resume at 400 mg PO daily. May increase to 400 mg b.i.d.

## ADMINISTRATION

**Oral**
- Give on an empty stomach, at least 2 h before or 1 h after eating.
- Ensure that capsules are swallowed whole with water.
- For those unable to swallow, contents of capsule may be added to 1 tsp of applesauce immediately before administration.
- Note: Hypokalemia and hypomagnesemia should be corrected prior to drug administration.
- Store at 15°–30° C (59°–86° F)

**ADVERSE EFFECTS** (≥1%) **Body as a Whole:** *Peripheral edema, pyrexia.* **CNS:** *Asthenia,* dizziness, *fatigue, headache,* insomnia, paresthesia. **CV:** Flushing, *hypertension,* palpitations, QT prolongation, pericardial

N

Common adverse effects in *italic;* life-threatening effects <u>underlined;</u> generic names in **bold;** classifications in SMALL CAPS; ✤ Canadian drug name; ⊕ Prototype drug

1137

effusion. **GI:** *Abdominal pain, constipation, diarrhea,* dyspepsia, flatulence, *nausea.* GI hemorrhage **Hematologic:** *Anemia, neutropenia,* pancytopenia, *thrombocytopenia.* **Metabolic:** Decreased albumin, elevated alkaline phosphatase, elevated ALT, elevated AST, elevated bilirubin, *elevated lipase, hyperglycemia,* hyperkalemia, hypocalcemia, hypokalemia, hyponatremia, *hypophosphatemia.* **Musculoskeletal:** *Arthralgia, back pain, bone pain,* chest pain, *muscle spasms, myalgia, pain in extremity.* **Respiratory:** *Cough,* dysphonia, *dyspnea, nasopharyngitis,* pleural effusion. **Skin:** Alopecia, dry skin, eczema, hyperhidrosis, night sweats, *pruritus, rash,* urticaria. **Special Senses:** Vertigo.

**INTERACTIONS** **Drug:** CYP3A4 Inducers **carbamazepine, dexamethasone, phenobarbital, phenytoin, rifabutin, rifampin, rifapentine**) decrease nilotinib levels. Inhibitors of CYP3A4 (**clarithromycin, indinavir, itraconazole, ketoconazole, nefazodone, nelfinavir, ritonavir, saquinavir, telithromycin, voriconazole**) increase nilotinib levels. Nilotinib increases the levels of **midazolam, warfarin. Food:** Food increases bioavailability. **Grapefruit** juice may increase nilotinib levels. **Herbal: St. John's wort** decreases nilotinib levels.

**PHARMACOKINETICS** **Peak:** 3 h. **Distribution:** 98% plasma protein bound. **Metabolism:** Hepatic to inactive metabolites. **Elimination:** 93% fecal. **Half-Life:** 17 h.

**NURSING IMPLICATIONS**

**Black Box Warning**

*Nilotinib has been associated with prolongation of the QT interval and sudden death.*

**Assessment & Drug Effects**
- Obtain a baseline ECG, then again 7 days after first drug dose, and periodically thereafter. Withhold drug and report immediately QT prolongation.
- Monitor closely patients with hepatic impairment for QT interval prolongation.
- Monitor diabetics for loss of glycemic control.
- Monitor lab tests: Baseline and periodic serum electrolytes, lipid profile, serum glucose, LFTs, serum lipase/amylase; CBC q2wk first 2 mo then monthly thereafter.

**Patient & Family Education**
- Women of childbearing age should use reliable forms of contraception, including a barrier type.
- Avoid grapefruit products while on nilotinib.

**NILUTAMIDE**
(ni-lu'ta-mide)
Nilandron
**Classifications:** ANTINEOPLASTIC; ANTIANDROGEN
Therapeutic ANTINEOPLASTIC; ANTIANDROGEN
**Prototype:** Flutamide

**AVAILABILITY** Tablet

**ACTION & THERAPEUTIC EFFECT**
Blocks the effects of testosterone at the androgen receptor sites, thus preventing the normal androgenic response. *Effective in blocking testosterone in treatment of metastatic prostate carcinoma.*

**USES** Use with surgical castration for metastatic prostate cancer.

**CONTRAINDICATIONS** Hypersensitivity to nalutamide; severe hepatic impairment, hepatitis; severe respiratory insufficiency;

drug-induced interstitial pneumonitis; lactation.

**CAUTIOUS USE** Asian patients relative to causing interstitial pneumonitis; alcoholics; pregnancy (category C). Safety and efficacy in children not established.

## ROUTE & DOSAGE

**Metastatic Prostate Cancer**
*Adult:* **PO** 300 mg daily × 30 days, then 150 mg daily

## ADMINISTRATION

**Oral**
- Give first dose on the day of or day after surgical castration.
- Store below 15° 30° C (59° 86° F) and protect from light.

**ADVERSE EFFECTS** (>1%) **Body as a Whole:** *Hot flushes, impotence, decreased libido, malaise,* edema, weight loss, arthritis. **CNS:** *Nervousness,* paresthesias. **CV:** Angina, heart failure, syncope. **GI:** Diarrhea, GI hemorrhage, melena, dry mouth. **Respiratory:** Cough, interstitial lung disease, rhinitis. **Skin:** Pruritus. **Other:** Alcohol intolerance. **Special Senses:** Cataracts, photophobia.

**INTERACTIONS Drug:** Carbamazepine, rifampin, phenytoin may decrease level; use caution in low therapeutic margin drugs. **Herbal: St. John's wort** may decrease levels. **Food:** Avoid alcohol (increased risk of ethanol intolerance).

**PHARMACOKINETICS Absorption:** Rapidly from GI tract. **Metabolism:** In the liver (CYP2C19). **Elimination:** In urine. **Half-Life:** 38–50 h.

## NURSING IMPLICATIONS

### Black Box Warning

*Nilutamide has been associated with development of interstitial pneumonitis.*

### Assessment & Drug Effects
- Obtain baseline chest x-ray before treatment and periodically thereafter.
- Closely monitor for S&S of pneumonitis; at the first sign of adverse pulmonary effects, withhold drug and notify prescriber. Abnormal ABGs may indicate need to discontinue drug.
- Monitor patients taking phenytoin, theophylline, or warfarin closely for toxic levels of these drugs.
- Monitor lab tests: Baseline LFTs, then regularly during first 4 mo, and periodically thereafter; LFTs with first sign of liver dysfunction.

### Patient & Family Education
- Report to prescriber immediately the following S&S of adverse effects on lungs: Development of chest pain, dyspnea, and cough with fever.
- Report S&S of liver injury to prescriber: Jaundice, dark urine, fatigue, or signs of GI distress including nausea, vomiting, abdominal pain.
- Use caution when moving from lighted to dark areas because the drug may slow visual adaptation to darkness. Tinted glasses may partially alleviate the problem.

## NIMODIPINE
(ni-mod'i-peen)
Nymalize
**Classifications:** CALCIUM CHANNEL BLOCKER; CEREBRAL ANTISPASMODIC

---

Common adverse effects in *italic;* life-threatening effects underlined; generic names in **bold;** classifications in SMALL CAPS; ♣ Canadian drug name; ☻ Prototype drug

**Therapeutic:** CEREBRAL ANTISPAS-
MODIC
**Prototype:** Nifedipine

**AVAILABILITY** Capsule; oral solution

## ACTION & *THERAPEUTIC EFFECT*
Calcium channel blocking agent
that is relatively selective for cerebral arteries compared with arteries
elsewhere in the body. *Reduces
vascular spasms in cerebral arteries
during a stroke.*

**USES** To improve neurologic deficits due to spasm following subarachnoid hemorrhage.

**UNLABELED USES** Migraine
prophylaxis.

**CONTRAINDICATIONS** Near-
fatal reaction to intravenous
administration; hypotension; cardiogenic shock.

**CAUTIOUS USE** Hepatic impairment or cirrhosis; acute MI; bradycardia, heart failure, ventricular dysfunction; older adults; pregnancy
(category C); lactation. Safety and
efficacy in children not established.

## ROUTE & DOSAGE

**Subarachnoid Hemorrhage**

*Adult:* **PO** 60 mg q4h for 21 days,
start therapy within 96 h of
subarachnoid hemorrhage

*Hepatic Impairment
Dosage Adjustment*

Decrease dose to 30 mg q4h

## ADMINISTRATION

**Oral**
- Administer 1 h before or 2 h after
  a meal

- Oral solution: Use the supplied oral
  syringe labeled "Oral Use Only."
  Following drug administration via
  enteral tube, fill syringe with 20 mL
  NS and flush the enteral tube.
- Capsule: If capsule cannot be
  swallowed whole, make a hole in
  both ends of the capsule with an
  18-gauge needle and extract the
  contents into a syringe. Remove
  needle and administer contents of
  syringe orally or via an enteral
  tube. NEVER administer capsule
  contents parenterally.
- Store below 40° C (104° F); protect from light.

**ADVERSE EFFECTS** (≥1%) **CNS:**
Headache. **CV:** *Hypotension*. **GI:**
Diarrhea, nausea.

**INTERACTIONS Drug:** Hypotensive effects increased when
combined with other CALCIUM
CHANNEL BLOCKERS. Effects could be
decreased when used with CYP
3A4 inhibitors (**clarithromycin,
voriconazole,** etc.). **Food:** Grapefruit juice (greater than 1 qt/day)
may increase plasma concentrations and adverse effects. **Herbal:**
Avoid use of melatonin.

**PHARMACOKINETICS Absorp-
tion:** Readily from GI tract; approximately 13% reaches systemic
circulation (first pass metabolism).
**Peak:** 1 h. **Distribution:** Crosses
blood–brain barrier; possibly
crosses placenta; distributed
into breast milk. **Metabolism:**
85% in liver; 15% in kidneys.
**Elimination:** Greater than 50% in
urine, 32% in feces. **Half-Life:**
8–9 h.

## NURSING IMPLICATIONS
**Assessment & Drug Effects**
- Take apical pulse prior to administering drug and hold it if pulse is
  below 60. Notify the prescriber.

---

Common adverse effects in *italic;* life-threatening effects <u>underlined;</u> generic names
in **bold;** classifications in SMALL CAPS; ✿ Canadian drug name; ⊙ Prototype drug
1140

- Establish baseline data before treatment is started: BP, pulse, and laboratory evaluations of liver and kidney function.
- Monitor frequently for adverse drug effects, including hypotension, peripheral edema, tachycardia, or skin rash.
- Monitor frequently for dizziness or light-headedness in older adult patients; risk of hypotension is increased.

**Patient & Family Education**
- Report gradual weight gain and evidence of edema (e.g., tight rings on fingers, ankle swelling).
- Keep follow-up appointments for monitoring of progress during therapy.

## NISOLDIPINE
(ni-sol′di-peen)
Sular
**Classifications:** CALCIUM CHANNEL BLOCKER; ANTIHYPERTENSIVE
**Therapeutic:** ANTIHYPERTENSIVE; ANTIANGINAL
**Prototype:** Nifedipine

**AVAILABILITY** Extended release tablet

### ACTION & *THERAPEUTIC EFFECT*
Inhibits calcium ion influx across cell membranes of cardiac muscle and vascular smooth muscle, which results in vasodilation, inotropism, and negative chronotropism. Inhibits vasoconstriction in the peripheral vasculature. *Significantly reduces total peripheral resistance, decreases blood pressure, and increases cardiac output. It is also a potent coronary vasodilator.*

**USES** Hypertension.

**UNLABELED USES** CHF, angina.

**CONTRAINDICATIONS** Hypersensitivity to nisoldipine or other calcium blockers; systolic BP less than 90 mm Hg, cardiogenic shock, severe hypotension, acute MI, sick sinus syndrome.

**CAUTIOUS USE** Severe hepatic impairment; severe obstructive coronary artery disease; class II to IV heart failure, especially with concurrent administration of a beta-blocker; severe aortic stenosis; hypertrophic cardiomyopathy with outflow tract obstruction; paroxysmal atrial fibrillation; GERD; CHF; digital ischemia, ulceration, or gangrene; nonobstructive hypertrophic cardiomyopathy; Duchenne muscular dystrophy; older adults; pregnancy (category C); lactation, children.

### ROUTE & DOSAGE

**Hypertension**
*Adult:* **PO** 17 mg daily may increase by 8.5 mg weekly as needed
*Geriatric:* **PO** 8.5 mg daily, may increase weekly as needed

### ADMINISTRATION
**Oral**
- Give drug with food to decrease GI distress, but do not give with grapefruit juice or a high-fat meal.
- Ensure that extended release form is not chewed or crushed. It **must be** swallowed whole.
- Drug is usually discontinued gradually to prevent adverse effects.
- Store at 15°–30° C (59°–86° F).

### ADVERSE EFFECTS (≥1%) **CNS:**
Dizziness, anxiety, tremor, weakness, fatigue, *headache*. **CV:** Hypotension, *peripheral edema*, palpitations, orthostatic hypotension. **GI:** Abdominal pain, cramps, constipation,

dry mouth, diarrhea, nausea. **Skin:** *Flushing,* rash, erythema, urticaria. **Urogenital:** Urinary frequency. **Respiratory:** Pulmonary edema (patients with CHF), wheezing, dyspnea, sinusitis. **Body as a Whole:** Myalgia.

**INTERACTIONS Drug:** May cause significant increase in **digoxin** level in patients with CHF. BETA-BLOCK-ERS may cause hypotension and bradycardia. **Phenytoin, carbamazepine, phenobarbital** may significantly decrease levels. Azole antifungals may affect metabolism; avoid combination. **Food:** High-fat food increases availability.

**PHARMACOKINETICS Absorption:** Rapidly from GI tract; 4–8% reaches systemic circulation. **Peak Effect:** 1–3 h. **Duration:** 8–12 h for hypertension, 7–8 h for angina. **Distribution:** 99% protein bound. **Metabolism:** Extensively in liver. **Elimination:** 70–75% in urine as metabolites. **Half-Life:** 2–14 h.

## NURSING IMPLICATIONS

### Assessment & Drug Effects

- Monitor blood pressure carefully during period of drug initiation and with dosage increments.
- Monitor cardiovascular status especially heart rate, frequency of angina attacks, or worsening heart failure.
- Assess for and report edematous weight gain.
- Monitor lab tests: Frequent digoxin levels with concurrent use.

### Patient & Family Education

- Do not discontinue the drug abruptly.
- Report symptoms of orthostatic hypotension or other bothersome adverse effects to prescriber.

- Do not drive or engage in potentially hazardous activities until response to drug is known.

# NITAZOXANIDE

(nit-a-zox′a-nide)
Alinia
**Classification:** ANTIPROTOZOAL
**Therapeutic:** ANTIPROTOZOAL
**Prototype:** Metronidazole

**AVAILABILITY** Oral suspension; tablet

## ACTION & *THERAPEUTIC EFFECT*
Antiprotozoal activity believed to be due to interference with an essential enzyme needed for anaerobic energy metabolism in protozoa. *Inhibits growth of sporozoites and oocysts of* Cryptosporidium parvum *and trophozoites of* Giardia lamblia.

**USES** Diarrhea caused by *Cryptosporidium parvum* and *Giardia lamblia.*

**UNLABELED USES** Rotavirus infection.

**CONTRAINDICATIONS** Prior hypersensitivity to nitazoxanide.

**CAUTIOUS USE** Hepatic and biliary disease, renal disease, renal impairment, renal failure, and combined renal and hepatic disease; pregnancy (category B); lactation. Safety and efficacy in children younger than 1 y not studied.

## ROUTE & DOSAGE

| Infectious Diarrhea |
| --- |
| *Adult/Adolescent:* **PO** 500 mg q12h × 3 days |
| *Child (1–3 y):* **PO** 100 mg q12h × 3 days; *4–11 y:* 200 mg q12h × 3 days |

## ADMINISTRATION

### Oral

- Prepare suspension as follows: Tap bottle until powder loosens. Draw up 48 mL of water, add half to bottle, shake to suspend powder, then add remaining 24 mL of water and shake vigorously.
- Give required dose (5 or 10 mL) with food.
- Keep container tightly closed, and shake well before each administration.
- Suspension may be stored for 7 days at 15°–30° C (59°–86° F), after which any unused portion **must be** discarded.

## ADVERSE EFFECTS (≥1%) CNS:
Headache. **Cardiac:** Flushing. **GI:** Abdominal pain, diarrhea, nausea, vomiting, heartburn.

## INTERACTIONS Food: Increases levels.

## PHARMACOKINETICS Peak:
1–4 h. **Distribution:** 99% protein bound. **Metabolism:** Rapidly hydrolyzed in liver to an active metabolite, tizoxanide (desacetyl-nitazoxanide). **Elimination:** In urine, bile, and feces.

## NURSING IMPLICATIONS

### Assessment & Drug Effects

- Monitor for therapeutic effectiveness: No watery stools and 2 or less soft stools with no hematochezia within the past 24 h or no symptoms and no unformed stools within the past 48 h.
- Monitor closely patients with pre-existing hepatic or biliary disease for adverse reactions.
- Assess appetite, level of abdominal discomfort and extent of bloating.
- Assess frequency and quantity of diarrhea and monitor total hydration status.
- Weigh daily to aid in assessment of possible fluid loss from diarrhea.

### Patient & Family Education

- Note that 5 mL of the oral suspension contains approximately 1.5 g of sucrose.
- Report either no improvement in or worsening of diarrhea and abdominal discomfort.

# NITROFURANTOIN
(nye-troe-fyoor'an-toyn)
**Furadantin, Novo-Furan ✦**

# NITROFURANTOIN MACROCRYSTALS
**Macrobid, Macrodantin**
**Classifications:** URINARY TRACT ANTI-INFECTIVE; NITROFURAN
Therapeutic: URINARY TRACT ANTIBIOTIC

## AVAILABILITY Suspension; capsule

## ACTION & *THERAPEUTIC EFFECT*
Synthetic nitrofuran derivative presumed to act by interfering with several bacterial enzyme systems. Highly soluble in urine and reportedly most active in acid urine. Antimicrobial concentrations in urine exceed those in blood. *Active against wide variety of gram-negative and gram-positive microorganisms*.

## USES Uncomplicated urinary tract infection, including cystitis.

## CONTRAINDICATIONS Hypersensitivity to nitrofurantoin including hepatic dysfunction; anuria, oliguria, significant impairment of kidney function (CrCl less than 60 mL/min); G6PD deficiency; history of cholestatic jaundice; pregnancy at term (38–42 wk), labor, or obstetric delivery; lactation.

## CAUTIOUS USE History of asthma, anemia, diabetes, vitamin B

Common adverse effects in *italic;* life-threatening effects <u>underlined</u>; generic names in **bold;** classifications in SMALL CAPS; ✦ Canadian drug name; ⊕ Prototype drug

1143

deficiency, hepatic disease; pulmonary disease; mild to moderate renal disease; electrolyte imbalance, debilitating disease; $B_{12}$ deficiency; pregnancy (category B); infants younger than 1 mo.

## ROUTE & DOSAGE

### UTI, Cystitis

*Adult:* **PO** 50–100 mg q.i.d. × 7 days, or 3 days after sterile urine sample
*Child/Infant (1 mo–12 y):* **PO** 1.25–1.75 mg/kg q6h (max: 400 mg/day)
*Adult/Adolescent (Macrobid only):* **PO** 100 mg q12h × 7 days

### Chronic Suppressive Therapy for UTI

*Adult:* **PO** 50–100 mg at bedtime
*Child (1 mo–12 y):* **PO** 1 mg/kg/day in 1–2 divided doses (max: 100 mg/day)

### Renal Impairment Dosage Adjustment

Avoid if CrCl less than 60 mL/min

## ADMINISTRATION

### Oral

- Give with food or milk to minimize gastric irritation.
- Avoid crushing tablets because of the possibility of tooth staining; dilute oral suspension in milk, water, or fruit juice, and rinse mouth thoroughly after taking drug.

## ADVERSE EFFECTS (≥1%) CNS:
Peripheral neuropathy, headache, nystagmus, drowsiness, vertigo. **GI:** *Anorexia, nausea, vomiting,* abdominal pain, diarrhea, cholestatic jaundice, <u>hepatic necrosis</u>. **Hematologic (rare):** Hemolytic or megaloblastic anemia (especially in patients with G6PD deficiency),

granulocytosis, eosinophilia. **Body as a Whole:** Angioedema, <u>anaphylaxis</u>, drug fever, arthralgia. **Respiratory:** Allergic pneumonitis, asthmatic attack (patients with history of asthma), pulmonary sensitivity reactions (<u>interstitial pneumonitis or fibrosis</u>). **Skin:** Skin eruptions, pruritus, urticaria, <u>exfoliative dermatitis</u>, transient alopecia. **Urogenital:** Genitourinary superinfections (especially with *Pseudomonas*), crystalluria (older adult patients), dark yellow or brown urine. **Other:** Tooth staining from direct contact with oral suspension and crushed tablets (infants).

## DIAGNOSTIC TEST INTERFERENCE
Nitrofurantoin metabolite may produce false-positive ***urine glucose*** test results with ***Benedict's reagent.***

## INTERACTIONS Drug: ANTACIDS may decrease absorption of nitrofurantoin; **nalidixic acid,** other QUINOLONES may antagonize antimicrobial effects; **probenecid, sulfinpyrazone** increase risk of nitrofurantoin toxicity.

## PHARMACOKINETICS Absorption: Readily from GI tract. **Peak:** Urine: 30 min. **Distribution:** Crosses placenta; distributed into breast milk. **Metabolism:** Partially in liver. **Elimination:** Primarily in urine. **Half-Life:** 20 min.

## NURSING IMPLICATIONS

### Assessment & Drug Effects

- Monitor I&O. Report oliguria and any change in I&O ratio.
- Be alert to signs of urinary tract superinfections (e.g., milky urine, foul-smelling urine, perineal irritation, dysuria).
- Assess for nausea (which occurs fairly frequently). May be relieved by using macrocrystalline preparation (Macrodantin).

Common adverse effects in *italic;* life-threatening effects <u>underlined</u>; generic names in **bold;** classifications in SMALL CAPS; ♣ Canadian drug name; ◉ Prototype drug

- Watch for acute pulmonary sensitivity reaction, usually within first week of therapy and apparently more common in older adults. May be manifested by mild to severe flu-like syndrome.
- With prolonged therapy, monitor for subacute or chronic pulmonary sensitivity reaction, commonly manifested by insidious onset of malaise, cough, dyspnea on exertion, altered ABGs.
- Monitor for S&S of peripheral neuropathy, which can be severe and irreversible. Withhold drug and notify prescriber immediately.
- Monitor lab tests: Baseline C&S, LFTs, PFTs, serum creatinine/BUN.

**Patient & Family Education**
- Report promptly muscle weakness, tingling, numbness.
- Nitrofurantoin may impart a harmless brown color to urine.
- Consult prescriber regarding fluid intake. Generally, fluids are not forced; however, intake should be adequate.

# NITROGLYCERIN ⊙
(nye-troe-gli'ser-in)

Minitran, Nitrocap, Nitrodisc, Nitro-Dur, Nitrogard, Nitrogard-SR, Nitrong SR, Nitrospan, Nitrostat, Nitrostat I.V., ProStakan

**Classification:** NITRATE VASODILATOR
Therapeutic: ANTIANGINAL; VASODILATOR

**AVAILABILITY** Solution for injection; sublingual tablet; sustained release tablet; capsule; transdermal patch; ointment

**ACTION & THERAPEUTIC EFFECT**
Organic nitrate and potent vasodilator that relaxes vascular smooth muscle. After conversion to nitric oxide, it leads to dose-related dilation of both venous and arterial blood vessels. Promotes peripheral pooling of blood, reduction of peripheral resistance, and decreased venous return to the heart. Both left ventricular preload and afterload are reduced and myocardial oxygen consumption or demand is decreased. *Produces antianginal, anti-ischemic, and antihypertensive effects.*

**USES** Prophylaxis, treatment, and management of angina pectoris. IV nitroglycerin is used to control BP in perioperative hypertension, CHF associated with acute MI; to produce controlled hypotension during surgical procedures, and to treat angina pectoris in patients who have not responded to nitrate or beta-blocker therapy. Treatment of pain associated with chronic anal fissure.

**UNLABELED USES** Sublingual and topical to reduce cardiac workload in patients with acute MI and in CHF. Ointment for adjunctive treatment of Raynaud's disease.

**CONTRAINDICATIONS** Hypersensitivity, idiosyncrasy, or tolerance to nitrates; severe anemia; head trauma, increased ICP. **Sublingual:** Early MI; severe anemia, increased ICP; hypersensitivity to nitroglycerin. **Sustained release form:** Glaucoma. **IV form:** Hypotension, uncorrected hypovolemia, constrictive pericarditis, pericardial tamponade; restrictive cardiomyopathy.

**CAUTIOUS USE** Severe liver or kidney disease, conditions that cause dry mouth, pregnancy (category C), lactation.

Common adverse effects in *italic*; life-threatening effects underlined; generic names in **bold**; classifications in SMALL CAPS; ♣ Canadian drug name; ⊙ Prototype drug

1145

## ROUTE & DOSAGE

### Angina

*Adult:* **Sublingual** 1–2 sprays (0.4–0.8 mg) or a 0.3–0.6-mg tablet q3–5min as needed (max: 3 doses in 15 min); **PO** 1.3–9 mg q8–12h **IV** Start with 5 mcg/min and titrate q3–5min until desired response (up to 200 mcg/min); **Transdermal Unit** Apply once q24h or leave on for 10–12 h, then remove and have a 10–12 h nitrate free interval;
**Topical** Apply 1.5–5 cm (½–2 in) of ointment q4–6h
*Child:* **IV** 0.25–0.5 mcg/kg/min, titrate by 0.5–1 mcg/kg/min q3–5min (max: 5 mg/kg/min)

### Anal Fissure

*Adult:* **Topical** 1 inch every 12 h for up to 3 wk

## ADMINISTRATION

### Sublingual Tablet

- Give 1 tablet and if pain is not relieved, give additional tablets at 5-min intervals, but not more than 3 tablets in a 15-min period.
- Typically available for self-administration in their original container. Instruct in correct use. Request patient to report all attacks.
- Instruct to sit or lie down upon first indication of oncoming anginal pain and to place tablet under tongue or in buccal pouch (hypotensive effect of drug is intensified in the upright position).

### Sustained Release Tablet or Capsule

- Give on an empty stomach (1 h before or 2 h after meals), with a full glass of water. Ensure it is swallowed whole.

- Be aware that sustained release form helps to prevent anginal attacks; it is not intended for immediate relief of angina.

### Transdermal Ointment

- Using dose-determining applicator (paper application patch) supplied with package, squeeze prescribed dose onto this applicator. Using applicator, spread ointment in a thin, uniform layer to premarked 5.5 by 9 cm (2¼ by 3½ in.) square. Place patch with ointment side down onto nonhairy skin surface (areas commonly used: Chest, abdomen, anterior thigh, forearm). Cover with transparent wrap and secure with tape. Avoid getting ointment on fingers.
- Rotate application sites to prevent dermal inflammation and sensitization. Remove ointment from previously used sites before reapplication.

### Transdermal Unit

- Apply transdermal unit (transdermal patch) at the same time each day, preferably to skin site free of hair and not subject to excessive movement. Avoid abraded, irritated, or scarred skin. Clip hair if necessary.
- Change application site each time to prevent skin irritation and sensitization.

### Intravenous

- Check to see if patient has transdermal patch or ointment in place before starting IV infusion. The patch (or ointment) is usually removed to prevent overdosage.

**PREPARE: IV Infusion:** Nitroglycerin is available undiluted and premixed in D5W IV solutions of varying concentrations. ▪ *IV Infusion from Concentrate:* Use only

Common adverse effects in *italic;* life-threatening effects underlined; generic names in **bold;** classifications in SMALL CAPS; ♣ Canadian drug name; ⊙ Prototype drug

non-PVC plastic or glass bottles and manufacturer-supplied IV tubing. ▪ Withdraw contents of one vial (25 or 50 mg) into syringe and inject immediately into 500 mL of IV solution to minimize contact with plastic; yields 50 mcg/mL or 100 mcg/mL. ▪ If less fluid is desired, add 5 mg to 100 mL to yield 50 mcg/mL. Other concentrations within the range of 25–400 mcg/mL may be used. ▪ Do not exceed 400 mcg/mL.

***ADMINISTER:* IV Infusion:** Give by continuous infusion regulated exactly by an infusion pump. ▪ IV dosage titration requires careful and continuous hemodynamic monitoring.

***INCOMPATIBILITIES:* Solution/additive: Caffeine, hydralazine, phenytoin. Y-site: Alteplase, levofloxacin.**

▪ Use only glass containers for storage of reconstituted IV solution. Polyvinyl chloride (PVC) plastic can absorb nitroglycerin and therefore should not be used. ▪ Non-polyvinyl-chloride (non-PVC) sets are recommended or provided by manufacturer.

## ADVERSE EFFECTS (≥1%) CNS:
*Headache,* apprehension, blurred vision, weakness, vertigo, dizziness, faintness. **CV:** *Postural hypotension,* palpitations, tachycardia (sometimes with paradoxical bradycardia), increase in angina, syncope, and circulatory collapse. **GI:** Nausea, vomiting, involuntary passing of urine and feces, abdominal pain, dry mouth. **Hematologic:** Methemoglobinemia (high doses). **Skin:** Cutaneous vasodilation with flushing, rash, exfoliative dermatitis, contact dermatitis with transdermal patch; topical allergic reactions with ointment: Pruritic

eczematous eruptions, anaphylactoid reaction characterized by oral mucosal and conjunctival edema. **Body as a Whole:** Muscle twitching, pallor, perspiration, cold sweat; local sensation in oral cavity at point of dissolution of sublingual forms.

## DIAGNOSTIC TEST INTERFERENCE
Nitroglycerin may cause increases in determinations of *urinary catecholamines* and *VMA;* may interfere with the *Zlatkis-Zak color reaction,* causing a false report of decreased *serum cholesterol.*

## INTERACTIONS Drug: Alcohol,
ANTIHYPERTENSIVE AGENTS compound hypotensive effects; IV nitroglycerin may antagonize **heparin** anticoagulation. Vasodilating effects may be enhanced by **sildenafil, vardenafil,** or **tadalafil,** so this combination should be avoided.

## PHARMACOKINETICS Absorption:
Significant loss to first pass metabolism after oral dosing. **Onset:** 2 min SL; 3 min PO; 30 min ointment. **Duration:** 30 min SL; 3–5 h PO; 3–6 h ointment. **Distribution:** Widely distributed; not known if distributes to breast milk. **Metabolism:** Extensively in liver. **Elimination:** Inactive metabolites in urine. **Half-Life:** 1–4 min.

## NURSING IMPLICATIONS
### Assessment & Drug Effects
▪ Administer IV nitroglycerin with extreme caution to patients with hypotension or hypovolemia since the IV drug may precipitate a severe hypotensive state.
▪ Monitor patient closely for change in levels of consciousness and for dysrhythmias.

Common adverse effects in *italic;* life-threatening effects underlined; generic names in **bold;** classifications in SMALL CAPS; ♣ Canadian drug name; ◉ Prototype drug

1147

- Be aware that moisture on sublingual tissue is required for dissolution of sublingual tablet. However, because chest pain typically leads to dry mouth, a patient may be unresponsive to sublingual nitroglycerin.
- Assess for headaches. Approximately 50% of all patients experience mild to severe headaches following nitroglycerin. Transient headache usually lasts about 5 min after sublingual administration and seldom longer than 20 min. Assess degree of severity and consult as needed with prescriber about analgesics and dosage adjustment.
- Supervise ambulation as needed, especially with older adult or debilitated patients. Postural hypotension may occur even with small doses of nitroglycerin. Patients may complain of dizziness or weakness due to postural hypotension.
- Take baseline BP and heart rate with patient in sitting position before initiation of treatment with transdermal preparations.
- One hour after transdermal (ointment or unit) medication has been applied, check BP and pulse again with patient in sitting position. Report measurements to prescriber.
- Assess for and report blurred vision or dry mouth.
- Assess for and report the following topical reactions: Contact dermatitis from the transdermal patch; pruritus and erythema from the ointment.

### Patient & Family Education

- Store tablet form in its original container.
- Sit or lie down upon first indication of oncoming anginal pain.
- Relax for 15–20 min after taking tablet to prevent dizziness or faintness.

- Be aware that pain not relieved by 3 sublingual tablets over a 15-min period may indicate acute MI or severe coronary insufficiency. Contact prescriber immediately or go directly to emergency room.
- Note: Sublingual tablets may be taken prophylactically 5–10 min prior to exercise or other stimulus known to trigger angina (drug effect lasts 30–60 min).
- Keep record for prescriber of number of angina attacks, amount of medication required for relief of each attack, and possible precipitating factors.
- Remove transdermal unit or ointment immediately from skin and notify prescriber if faintness, dizziness, or flushing occurs following application.
- You can use a sublingual formulation while transdermal unit or ointment is in place.
- Report blurred vision or dry mouth. Both warrant withdrawal of drug.
- Change position slowly and avoid prolonged standing. Dizziness, light-headedness, and syncope (due to postural hypotension) occur most frequently in older adults.
- Report any increase in frequency, duration, or severity of anginal attack.

## NITROPRUSSIDE SODIUM
(nye-troe-pruss′ide)

Nitropress

**Classifications:** NONNITRATE VASODILATOR; ANTIHYPERTENSIVE
Therapeutic: ANTIHYPERTENSIVE; VASODILATOR
**Prototype:** Hydralazine

**AVAILABILITY** Solution for injection

## ACTION & *THERAPEUTIC EFFECT*

Potent, rapid-acting hypotensive agent that acts directly on vascular smooth muscle to produce peripheral vasodilation, with consequently marked lowering of arterial BP, mild decrease in cardiac output, and moderate lowering of peripheral vascular resistance. *Effective antihypertensive agent used for rapid reduction of high blood pressure.*

## USES
Short-term, rapid reduction of BP in hypertensive crises and for producing controlled hypotension during anesthesia to reduce bleeding.

## UNLABELED USES
Refractory CHF or acute MI.

## CONTRAINDICATIONS
Compensatory hypertension, as in atriovenous shunt or coarctation of aorta, and for control of hypotension in patients with inadequate cerebral circulation; lactation.

## CAUTIOUS USE
Hepatic insufficiency, hypothyroidism, severe renal impairment, hyponatremia, older adult patients with low vitamin $B_{12}$ plasma levels or with Leber's optic atrophy; pregnancy (category C).

## ROUTE & DOSAGE

### Hypertensive Crisis

*Adult:* IV 0.3–0.5 mcg/kg/min (average 3 mcg/kg/min)
*Child:* IV 1 mcg/kg/min (average 3 mcg/kg/min) (max: 5 mcg/kg/min)

## ADMINISTRATION

Intravenous

*PREPARE:* **Continuous:** Dissolve each 50 mg in 2–3 mL of D5W.

Further dilute in 250 mL D5W to yield 200 mcg/mL or 500 mL D5W to yield 100 mcg/mL. ▪ Lower concentrations may be desirable depending on patient weight. ▪ Following reconstitution, solutions usually have faint brownish tint; if solution is highly colored, do not use it. ▪ Promptly wrap container with aluminum foil or other opaque material to protect drug from light.

*ADMINISTER:* **Continuous:** Administer by infusion pump or similar device that will allow precise measurement of flow rate required to lower BP. ▪ Give at the rate required to lower BP, usually between 0.5 and 10 mcg/kg/min. ▪ **Do not** exceed the maximum dose of 10 mcg/kg/min nor give this dose for longer than 10 min.

*INCOMPATIBILITIES:* Solution/additive: **Amiodarone, atracurium, dobutamine, nitroglycerin.** Y-site: **Acyclovir, amiodarone, amphotericin B conventional, ampicillin, ascorbic acid, atracurium, azathioprine, caspofungin, ceftazidime, chlorpromazine, cisatracurium, dantrolene, daunorubicin, diazepam, diazoxide, diphenhydramine, drotrecogin, erythromycin, haloperidol, hydralazine, hydroxyzine, imipenem/cilastatin, irinotecan, levofloxacin, mitomycin, mitoxantrone, moxifloxacin, mycophenolate, papaverine, pemetrexed, pentazocine, phenytoin, prochlorperazine, promethazine, quinidine, quinupristin/dalfopristin, sulfamethoxazole/trimethoprim, thiotepa, vinorelbine, voriconazole.**

▪ Store reconstituted solutions and IV solution at 15°–30° C (59°–86° F) protected from light; stable for 24 h.

Common adverse effects in *italic;* life-threatening effects <u>underlined</u>; generic names in **bold;** classifications in SMALL CAPS; ♣ Canadian drug name; ◑ Prototype drug

1149

**ADVERSE EFFECTS** (≥1%) **Body as a Whole:** Diaphoresis, apprehension, restlessness, muscle twitching, retrosternal discomfort. Thiocyanate toxicity (profound hypotension, tinnitus, blurred vision, fatigue, metabolic acidosis, pink skin color, absence of reflexes, faint heart sounds, loss of consciousness). **CV:** Profound hypotension, palpitation, increase or transient lowering of pulse rate, bradycardia, tachycardia, ECG changes. **GI:** Nausea, retching, abdominal pain. **Metabolic:** Increase in serum creatinine, fall or rise in total plasma cobalamins. **CNS:** Headache, dizziness. **Special Senses:** Nasal stuffiness. **Other:** Irritation at infusion site.

**PHARMACOKINETICS** **Onset:** Within 2 min. **Duration:** 1–10 min after infusion is terminated. **Metabolism:** Rapidly converted to cyanogen in erythrocytes and tissue, which is metabolized to thiocyanate in liver. **Elimination:** Excreted in urine primarily as thiocyanate. **Half-Life:** (Thiocyanate): 2.7–7 days.

## NURSING IMPLICATIONS

### Black Box Warning

*Nitroprusside has been associated with precipitous drops in BP that can lead to irreversible ischemic injuries or death.*

### Assessment & Drug Effects

- Monitor constantly to titrate IV infusion rate to BP response.
- Relieve adverse effects by slowing IV rate or by stopping drug; minimize them by keeping patient supine.
- Notify prescriber immediately if BP begins to rise after drug infusion rate is decreased or infusion is discontinued.
- Monitor I&O.

# NIVOLUMAB
(ni-vo'lu'mab)

Opdivo

**Classifications:** IMMUNOMODULATOR; MONOCLONAL ANTIBODY; PROGRAMMED DEATH RECEPTOR-1 BLOCKER; ANTINEOPLASTIC
**Therapeutic:** IMMUNOMODULATOR; ANTINEOPLASTIC
**Prototype:** Basiliximab

**AVAILABILITY** Solution for injection

**ACTION & THERAPEUTIC EFFECT**
Binds to the PD-1 (programmed cell death) receptor found on cytotoxic T-cells and prevents ligands produced by tumor cells from inhibiting the T-cell cytotoxic response, thus allowing tumor-specific cytotoxic T-cells to migrate into the tumor-inducing apoptosis. *Releases an immune pathway that restores the immune response to tumor cells causing tumor cell death.*

**USES** Treatment of patients with unresectable or metastatic melanoma and disease progression following ipilimumab and, if BRAF V600 mutation positive, a BRAF inhibitor; treatment of patients with metastatic squamous non-small-cell lung cancer (NSCLC) with progression on or after platinum-based chemotherapy; advanced renal cell cancer; Hodgkin's disease; hepatocellular cancer.

**CONTRAINDICATIONS** Grade 3 or 4 immune-mediated pneumonitis from drug use; immune related encephalopathy due to drug use; severe or life-threatening infusion reactions; pregnancy; lactation.

**CAUTIOUS USE** Immune-mediated pneumonitis (Grade 1 or 2), colitis, hepatitis, hepatic impairment; endocrinopathies, nephritis, rash, renal dysfunction; thyroid disorders; hyperglycemia, women of childbearing age. Safety and efficacy in children younger than 18 y not established.

## ROUTE & DOSAGE

### Metastatic Melanoma, Metastatic Squamous Non-Small-Cell Lung Cancer, Advanced Renal Cell Cancer, Hepatocellular Cancer

*Adult:* **IV** 240 mg over 60 min q2wk until disease progression or unacceptable toxicity

### Hodgkin's Disease

*Adult:* **IV** 3 mg/kg over 60 min once every 2 wk until disease progression or unacceptable toxicity

### *Toxicity Dosage Adjustment*

*Withhold treatment for any of the following:* Grade 2 pneumonitis, Grade 2 or 3 colitis, AST or ALT greater than 3 and up to 5 × ULN, total bilirubin greater than 1.5 and up to 3 × ULN, creatinine greater than 1.5 and up to 6 × ULN or greater than 1.5 times baseline, or any other severe or Grade 3 treatment related adverse reactions. Resume when toxicity decreases to Grade 0 or 1. See manufacturer's information for toxicities requiring drug discontinuation.

## ADMINISTRATION

### Intravenous

*PREPARE:* **IV Infusion:** Withdraw the required dose from the single use vial and add to an IV bag of NS or D5W to produce a final concentration of 1 mg/mL to 10 mg/

mL. Mix by gentle inversion but do not shake. IV infusion may be kept at room temperature for no more than 8 h including time of preparation and time for infusion.
*ADMINISTER:* **IV Infusion:** Give over 60 min through an IV line with a sterile, non-pyrogenic, low protein binding in-line filter (pore size of 0.2 micrometer to 1.2 micrometer). Flush at the end of infusion.
*INCOMPATIBILITIES:* **Y-site:** Do not coadminister other drugs through the same IV line.

■ Store under refrigeration at 2°–8° C (36°–46° F) for no more than 24 h from the time of infusion preparation. Protect from light.

## ADVERSE EFFECTS (≥1%) **Body as a Whole:** Asthenia, edema, *fatigue*, infusion-related reactions, peripheral edema, pain, pyrexia, sepsis. **CNS:** Dizziness, *headache*, peripheral neuropathy, sensory neuropathy. **CV:** Chest pain, <u>ventricular arrhythmia</u>. **GI:** Abdominal pain, anorexia, colitis, *constipation*, diarrhea, *nausea*, vomiting. **Hematological:** *Anemia, lymphopenia, thrombocytopenia*. **Metabolic:** *Decreased appetite*, hepatitis, *hypercalcemia, hyperglycemia*, diabetic ketoacidosis hyperkalemia, hyperthyroidism, hypocalcemia, *hypokalemia, hypomagnesemia, hyponatremia*, hypothyroidism, *increased ALT/AST*, hypercholesterolemia, *increased alkaline phosphatase*, increased amylase, *increased creatinine*, increased lipase, weight loss. **Musculoskeletal:** Arthralgia, *weakness, musculoskeletal pain.* **Respiratory:** *Cough, dyspnea*, <u>interstitial lung disease</u>, pneumonia, <u>pneumonitis</u>, upper respiratory tract infection. **Skin:** Exfoliative dermatitis, erythema multiforme, *rash*, pruritus, psoriasis, vitiligo. **Special Senses:** Iridocyclitis, eye redness, pain, or blurred vision.

---

## PHARMACOKINETICS Half-Life: 26.7 days.

## NURSING IMPLICATIONS

### Assessment & Drug Effects

- Monitor for and promptly report S&S of pneumonitis (e.g., fever, chills, coughing, shortness of breath, body aches, malaise).
- Monitor for and promptly report S&S of colitis (e.g., abdominal pain, blood or pus in stool, frequent diarrhea).
- Monitor for and promptly report S&S of pituitary, adrenal, and thyroid dysfunction.
- Monitor for and promptly report development of a rash.
- Monitor lab tests: Baseline and periodic LFT and renal function tests; periodic serum electrolytes, blood glucose levels, CBC with differential and platelet count, and thyroid function tests.

### Patient & Family Education

- Report promptly to prescriber any of the following: New or worsening cough, chest pain, shortness of breath, severe diarrhea or vomiting, severe abdominal pain, easy bruising, jaundice, unusual fatigue or agitation, decreased urine output, blood in urine, or swollen ankles, changes in vision.
- Use effective contraception during treatment and for at least 5 mo after the last dose.
- Do not breast-feed while receiving this drug.

## NIZATIDINE
(ni-za'ti-deen)
**Classifications:** H$_2$-RECEPTOR ANTAGONIST; ANTISECRETORY
Therapeutic: ANTIULCER; ANTISECRETORY
**Prototype:** Cimetidine

**AVAILABILITY** Capsule; oral solution

## ACTION & THERAPEUTIC EFFECT
Inhibits secretion of gastric acid by reversible, competitive blockage of histamine at the H$_2$ receptor, particularly those in the gastric parietal cells. *Significantly reduces nocturnal gastric acid secretion for up to 12 h.*

## USES Active duodenal ulcers; maintenance therapy for duodenal ulcers, GERD, benign gastric ulcer; *H. pylori* eradication.

## CONTRAINDICATIONS Hypersensitivity to nizatidine or other histamine H$_2$ antagonists.

## CAUTIOUS USE Hypersensitivity to other H$_2$-receptor antagonists; renal impairment or renal failure; older adults; pregnancy (category B); lactation; children 12 y or older; children and elderly with CrCl of less than 50 mL/min.

## ROUTE & DOSAGE

### Heartburn/Acid Dyspepsia
*Adult/Adolescent:* **PO** 75 mg immediately (acute relief); extended use 75 mg 1–2 times per day × 2 wk

### GERD
*Adult/Adolescent:* **PO** 150 mg b.i.d. × 12 wk

### Active Duodenal Ulcer/Benign Gastric Ulcer
*Adult:* **PO** 150 mg b.i.d. or 300 mg at bedtime

### Ulcer Maintenance Therapy
*Adult:* **PO** 150 mg at bedtime

### *H. Pylori* Eradication (in combination with other agents)
*Adult:* **PO** 150 mg b.i.d. or 300 mg at bedtime

### Renal Impairment Dosage Adjustment

*CrCl 20—50 mL/min:* **PO** Decrease the dose to 150 mg once daily
*CrCl less than 20 mL/min:* **PO** Decrease the dose to 150 mg every other day

## ADMINISTRATION

### Oral

- Give drug usually once daily at bedtime. Dose may be divided and given twice daily.
- Administer oral liquid drug using a calibrated measuring device.
- Be aware that antacids consisting of aluminum and magnesium hydroxides with simethicone decrease nizatidine absorption by about 10%. Administer the antacid 2 h after nizatidine.

## ADVERSE EFFECTS (≥1%) CNS:

Somnolence, fatigue headache, dizziness. **Skin:** Pruritus, sweating. **Metabolic:** Hyperuricemia, **Gastrointestinal:** Abdominal pain, anorexia, constipation, diarrhea, dry mouth, heart burn, nausea and vomiting.

## INTERACTIONS Drug: May de-

crease absorption of **delavirdine, didanosine, itraconazole, ketoconazole;** ANTACIDS may decrease absorption of nizatidine. Use caution with agents that may change acidity/solubility (e.g., **atazanavir, itraconazole, ketoconazole**) May increase **alcohol** levels. Do not use with **dasatinib.**

## PHARMACOKINETICS Absorp-

**tion:** Greater than 90% from GI tract. **Peak:** 0.5–3 h. **Metabolism:** In liver. **Elimination:** 60% in urine unchanged. **Half-Life:** 1–2 h.

## NURSING IMPLICATIONS

### Assessment & Drug Effects

- Monitor patient for alleviation of symptoms. Most ulcers should heal within 4 wk.
- Monitor for persistence of ulcer symptoms in patients who continue to smoke during therapy.
- Monitor lab tests: Periodic LFTs and renal function tests with long-term therapy, intragastric pH.

### Patient & Family Education

- Take medications for the full course of therapy even though symptoms may be relieved.
- Do not take other prescription or OTC medications without consulting prescriber.
- Stop smoking; smoking adversely affects healing of ulcers and effectiveness of the drug.

## NONOXYNOL-9

(noe-nox′ee-nole)

Conceptrol, Delfen, Emko, Gynol II, Koromex

**Classification:** SPERMICIDE CONTRACEPTIVE
**Therapeutic:** SPERMICIDE CONTRACEPTIVE

**AVAILABILITY** Gel; foam; suppositories

## ACTION & *THERAPEUTIC EFFECT*

Nonionic surfactant spermicidal incorporated into foams, gels, jelly, or suppositories. Immobilizes sperm by cell membrane disruption. *Applied over the cervix, blocks entrance to uterus by sperm, traps and absorbs seminal fluid, then releases the immediately available spermicide.*

---

Common adverse effects in *italic;* life-threatening effects <u>underlined</u>; generic names in **bold**; classifications in SMALL CAPS; ♣ Canadian drug name; ⊘ Prototype drug

1153

**USES** As barrier contraceptive alone or in conjunction with a vaginal diaphragm or with a condom.

**CONTRAINDICATIONS** Cystocele, prolapsed uterus, sensitivity or allergy to polyurethane or to nonoxynol-9; vaginitis; history of TSS; immediately after delivery or abortion.

**CAUTIOUS USE** HIV patients; menstruation; pregnancy (category C).

## ROUTE & DOSAGE

**Contraceptive**

*Adult:* **Topical** Apply or insert 30–60 min before intercourse. Repeat before each intercourse.

## ADMINISTRATION
**Topical**
- Apply foams, gels, jelly, cream: Fully load intravaginal applicator and insert about $2/3$ of its length [7.5–10 cm (3–4 in.)] into vagina.
- Use with diaphragm: Place 1–3 tsp spermicide formulation in dome prior to insertion. After diaphragm is in place, additional spermicide is recommended. Leave spermicide and diaphragm in place 6 h after intercourse.

## ADVERSE EFFECTS (≥1%) **Urogenital:** *Candidiasis;* vaginal irritation and dryness; increase in vaginal infections; menstrual and nonmenstrual <u>toxic shock syndrome (TSS)</u>.

## INTERACTIONS **Drug:** Intravaginal AZOLE ANTIFUNGALS may inactivate the spermicides.

## PHARMACOKINETICS **Onset:** Spermicidal action is prompt upon contact with sperm; minimal systemic absorption.

## NURSING IMPLICATIONS
**Patient & Family Education**
- Stop using nonoxynol-9 if pregnancy is suspected.
- Report symptoms of vaginal infection to prescriber: Burning, inflammation, intense vaginal and vulvar itching, cheesy, curd-like discharge, painful intercourse, dysuria. Nonoxynol-9 antifungal properties are weaker than its antibacterial potency, thus vulvovaginal candidiasis frequently occurs.
- Use spermicide before the first and every subsequent act of intercourse.

# NOREPINEPHRINE BITARTRATE
(nor-ep-i-nef′rin)
**Levophed, Noradrenaline**
**Classifications:** ADRENERGIC AGONIST; VASOPRESSOR
**Therapeutic:** VASOPRESSOR; CARDIAC INOTROPIC
**Prototype:** Epinephrine

**AVAILABILITY** Solution for injection

## ACTION & *THERAPEUTIC EFFECT*
Direct-acting sympathomimetic amine identical to natural catecholamine norepinephrine. Acts directly and predominantly on alpha-adrenergic receptors; little action on beta receptors except in heart (beta$_1$ receptors). Causes vasoconstriction and cardiac stimulation; also produces powerful constrictor action on resistance and capacitance blood vessels. *Peripheral vasoconstriction and moderate inotropic stimulation of heart result in increased systolic and diastolic blood pressure, myocardial oxygenation, coronary artery blood flow, and workload of the heart.*

**USES** To restore BP in certain acute hypotensive states. Also as adjunct in treatment of cardiac arrest.

**CONTRAINDICATIONS** Use as sole therapy in hypovolemic states, except as temporary emergency measure; mesenteric or peripheral vascular thrombosis; profound hypoxia or hypercarbia; use during cyclopropane or halothane anesthesia; hypertension; hyperthyroidism; lactation.

**CAUTIOUS USE** Severe heart disease; older adult patients; within 14 days of MAOI therapy; patients receiving tricyclic antidepressants; pregnancy (category C). Safe use in children not established.

## ROUTE & DOSAGE

**Hypotension**

*Adult:* IV Initial 8–12 mcg/min, titrate to response; maintenance dose usually 2–4 mcg/min

## ADMINISTRATION

Intravenous

**PREPARE:** **IV Infusion**: Dilute a 4 mL ampule in 1000 mL of D5W or D5/NS. ▪ More concentrated solutions (e.g., 4 mg in 500 mL to yield 8 mcg/mL) may be used based on fluid requirements.
▪ Do not use solution if discoloration or precipitate is present. Protect from light.
**ADMINISTER:** **IV Infusion:** Initial rate of infusion is 2–3 mL/min (8–12 mcg/min), then titrated to maintain BP, usually 0.5–1 mL/min (2–4 mcg/min). ▪ An infusion pump is used. Usually give

at the slowest rate possible required to maintain BP. Constantly monitor flow rate. ▪ Check infusion site frequently and immediately report any evidence of extravasation: Blanching along course of infused vein (may occur without obvious extravasation), cold, hard swelling around injection site. ▪ **Antidote for extravasation ischemia:** Phentolamine, 5–10 mg in 10–15 mL NS injection, is infiltrated throughout affected area (using syringe with fine hypodermic needle) as soon as possible. ▪ If therapy is to be prolonged, change infusion sites at intervals to allow effect of local vasoconstriction to subside. ▪ Avoid abrupt withdrawal; when therapy is discontinued, infusion rate is slowed gradually.

*INCOMPATIBILITIES:* Solution/additive: **Aminophylline, amobarbital, chlorothiazide, chlorphenir-amine, nafcillin, pentobarbital, phenobarbital, phenytoin, sodium bicarbonate, sodium iodide, streptomycin, warfarin.** Y-site: **Aminophylline, amiodarone, amphotericin B (conventional and lipid), ampicillin, azathioprine, dantrolene, diazepam, diazoxide, drotrecogin, folic acid, foscarnet, ganciclovir, gemtuzimab, haloperidol, hydralazine, indomethacin, insulin, mitomycin, nesiritide, pantoprazole, pentobarbital, phenobarbital, phenytoin, sodium bicarbonate, sulfamethoxazole.**

**ADVERSE EFFECTS** (≥1%) **Body as a Whole:** Restlessness, anxiety, *tremors,* dizziness, weakness, insomnia, pallor, plasma volume depletion, edema, hemorrhage, intestinal, <u>hepatic</u>, or renal <u>necrosis</u>,

Common adverse effects in *italic;* life-threatening effects <u>underlined</u>; generic names in **bold;** classifications in SMALL CAPS; ♣ Canadian drug name; ◌ Prototype drug

1155

retrosternal and pharyngeal pain, profuse sweating. **CV:** Palpitation, hypertension, reflex bradycardia, <u>fatal arrhythmias</u> (large doses), severe hypertension. **GI:** Vomiting. **Metabolic:** Hyperglycemia. **CNS:** Headache, violent headache, <u>cerebral hemorrhage</u>, convulsions. **Respiratory:** Respiratory difficulty. **Skin:** Tissue necrosis at injection site (with extravasation). **Special Senses:** Blurred vision, photophobia.

**INTERACTIONS Drug:** ALPHA- and BETA-BLOCKERS antagonize pressor effects; ERGOT ALKALOIDS, **furazolidone, guanethidine, methyldopa,** TRICYCLIC ANTIDEPRESSANTS may potentiate pressor effects; **halothane, cyclopropane** increase risk of arrhythmias.

**PHARMACOKINETICS Onset:** Very rapid. **Duration:** 1–2 min after infusion. **Distribution:** Localizes in sympathetic nerve endings; crosses placenta. **Metabolism:** In liver and other tissues by catecholamine O-methyltransferase and monoamine oxidase. **Elimination:** In urine.

## NURSING IMPLICATIONS

### Black Box Warning

*Antidote for extravasation ischemia: To prevent sloughing and necrosis from extravasation, infiltrate the area as soon as possible with 10–15 mL of NS containing 5–10 mg of phentolamine. Use a syringe with a fine needle and infiltrated liberally throughout the area (identified by its cold, hard, and pallid appearance). Phentolamine causes immediate and conspicuous local hyperemic changes if the area is infiltrated within 12 h.*

### Assessment & Drug Effects

- Monitor constantly while patient is receiving norepinephrine. Take baseline BP and pulse before start of therapy, then q2min from initiation of drug until stabilization occurs at desired level, then every 5 min during drug administration.
- Adjust flow rate to maintain BP at low normal (usually 80–100 mm Hg systolic) in normotensive patients. In previously hypertensive patients, systolic is generally maintained no higher than 40 mm Hg below pre-existing systolic level.
- Observe carefully and record mental status (index of cerebral circulation), skin temperature of extremities, and color (especially of earlobes, lips, nail beds) in addition to vital signs.
- Monitor I&O. Urinary retention and kidney shutdown are possibilities, especially in hypovolemic patients. Urinary output is a sensitive indicator of the degree of renal perfusion. Report decrease in urinary output or change in I&O ratio.
- Be alert to patient's complaints of headache, vomiting, palpitation, arrhythmias, chest pain, photophobia, and blurred vision as possible symptoms of overdosage. Reflex bradycardia may occur as a result of rise in BP.
- Continue to monitor vital signs and observe patient closely after cessation of therapy for clinical sign of circulatory inadequacy.

## NORETHINDRONE ◎
(nor-eth-in'drone)

Micronor, Norlutin, Nor-Q.D.

## NORETHINDRONE ACETATE

Aygestin ◆, Norlutate ◆

**Classification:** PROGESTIN
**Therapeutic:** PROGESTIN;
CONTRACEPTIVE

## AVAILABILITY Tablet

## ACTION & *THERAPEUTIC EFFECT*

Synthetic progestation hormone with androgenic, anabolic, and estrogenic properties. Progestin-only contraceptives alter cervical mucus, exert progestational effect on endometrium, interfere with implantation, and, in some cases, suppress ovulation. *Contraceptive that suppresses the midcycle surge of luteinizing hormone (LH).*

## USES Amenorrhea, abnormal uterine bleeding due to hormonal imbalance in absence of organic pathology; endometriosis. Also alone or in combination with an estrogen for birth control.

## CONTRAINDICATIONS Thromboembolic disorders, cerebral vascular or coronary vascular disease; carcinoma of breast, endometrium, or liver; abnormal vaginal bleeding; known or suspected pregnancy (category X).

## CAUTIOUS USE Cardiac disease; history of depression, seizure disorders, migraine; diabetes mellitus; CHF; history of thrombophlebitis or thromboembolic disease; lactation; children younger than 16 y.

## ROUTE & DOSAGE

### Amenorrhea

*Adult:* **PO Norethindrone** 5–20 mg on day 5 through day 25 of menstrual cycle; **Acetate** 2.5–10 mg on day 5 through day 25 of menstrual cycle

### Endometriosis

*Adult:* **PO Norethindrone** 10 mg/day for 2 wk; increase by 5 mg/day q2wk up to 30 mg/day, dose may remain at this level for 6–9 mo or until breakthrough bleeding; **Acetate** 5 mg/day for 2 wk, increase by 2.5 mg/day q2wk up to 15 mg/day, dose may remain at this level for 6–9 mo or until breakthrough bleeding

### Progestin-Only Contraception

*Adult:* **PO Norethindrone** 0.35 mg/day starting on day 1 of menstrual flow, then continuing indefinitely

## ADMINISTRATION

### Oral

- Note: Dosing schedule is based on a 28-day menstrual cycle.
- Use or add a barrier contraceptive when starting the minipill regimen (progestin-only contraception) for the first cycle or for 3 wk to ensure full protection.
- Protect drug from light and from freezing.

## ADVERSE EFFECTS (≥1%) CNS: Cerebral thrombosis or hemorrhage, depression. CV: Hypertension, pulmonary embolism, edema. GI: Nausea, vomiting, cholestatic jaundice, abdominal cramps. Urogenital: *Breakthrough bleeding,* cervical erosion, changes in menstrual flow, dysmenorrhea, vaginal candidiasis. Other: *Weight changes; breast tenderness,* enlargement or secretion.

## INTERACTIONS Drug: BARBITURATES, **carbamazepine, fosphenytoin,**

N

Common adverse effects in *italic;* life-threatening effects underlined; generic names in **bold;** classifications in SMALL CAPS; ♣ Canadian drug name; ● Prototype drug

1157

modafinil, phenytoin, primidone, pioglitazone, rifampin rifabutin, rifapentine, topiramate, troglitazone can decrease contraceptive effectiveness.

**PHARMACOKINETICS Absorption:** Readily absorbed from GI tract. **Metabolism:** In liver. **Elimination:** In urine and feces as metabolites.

## NURSING IMPLICATIONS

### Assessment & Drug Effects
- Monitor for S&S of thrombophlebitis (see Appendix F).
- Withhold drug and notify prescriber if any of the following occur: Sudden, complete, or partial loss of vision, proptosis, diplopia, or migraine headache.

### Patient & Family Education
- Wait at least 3 mo before becoming pregnant after stopping the minipill to prevent birth defects. Use a barrier or nonhormonal method of contraception until pregnancy is desired.
- If you have not taken all your pills and you miss a period, consider the possibility of pregnancy after 45 days from the last menstrual period; stop using this drug until pregnancy is ruled out.
- If you have taken all your pills and you miss 2 consecutive periods, rule out pregnancy and use a barrier or nonhormonal method of contraception before continuing the regimen.
- Promptly report prolonged vaginal bleeding or amenorrhea.
- Keep appointments for physical checkups (q6–12mo) while you are taking hormonal birth control.

## NORMAL SERUM ALBUMIN, HUMAN ⓟ
(al-byoo′min)

**Albuminar, Albutein, Buminate, Plasbumin**

**Classifications:** PLASMA DERIVATIVE; PLASMA VOLUME EXPANDER
**Therapeutic:** PLASMA VOLUME EXPANDER

**AVAILABILITY** Solution for injection

## ACTION & *THERAPEUTIC EFFECT*
Plasma volume expander that increases the osmotic pressure of plasma. *Expands volume of circulating blood by osmotically shifting tissue fluid into general circulation.*

**USES** To restore plasma volume and maintain cardiac output in hypovolemic shock; for prevention and treatment of cerebral edema; as adjunct in exchange transfusion for hyperbilirubinemia and erythroblastosis fetalis; to increase plasma protein level in treatment of hypoproteinemia; and to promote diuresis in refractory edema. Also used for blood dilution prior to or during cardiopulmonary bypass procedures. Has been used as adjunct in treatment of adult respiratory distress syndrome (ARDS).

**CONTRAINDICATIONS** Hypersensitivity to albumin; severe anemia; cardiac failure; within 24 h of severe burns; heart failure; patients with normal or increased intravascular volume.

**CAUTIOUS USE** Low cardiac reserve, pulmonary disease, absence of albumin deficiency; liver or kidney failure, dehydration, hypertension, hypernatremia; restricted sodium intake; pregnancy (category C).

## ROUTE & DOSAGE

**Emergency Volume Replacement**

*Adult:* **IV** 25 g, may repeat in 15–30 min if necessary (max: 250 g)

**Colloidal Volume Replacement (Nonemergency)**

*Child:* **IV** 12.5 g, may repeat in 15–30 min if necessary

**Hypoproteinemia**

*Adult:* **IV** 50–75 g (max: 2 mL/min)
*Child:* **IV** 25 g (max: 2 mL/min)

## ADMINISTRATION

### Intravenous

*PREPARE:* **IV Infusion:** Normal serum albumin, 5%, is infused without further dilution. ▪ Normal serum albumin, 20% and 25%, may be infused undiluted or diluted in NS or D5W (with sodium restriction).

*ADMINISTER:* **IV Infusion for Hypovolemic Shock:** Give initially as rapidly as necessary to restore blood volume. As blood volume approaches normal, rate should be reduced to avoid circulatory overload and pulmonary edema. ▪ Give 5% albumin at rate not exceeding 2–4 mL/min. Give 20% and 25% albumin at a rate not to exceed 1 mL/min. **IV Infusion with Normal Blood Volume:** Give 5% albumin human at a rate not to exceed 5–10 mL/min; give 20% and 25% albumin at a rate not to exceed 2 or 3 mL/min. **IV Infusion for Children:** Usual rate is 25%–50% of the adult rate.

*INCOMPATIBILITIES:* **Solution/additive: Amino acids, verapamil. Y-site: Fat emulsion, midazolam, vancomycin, verapamil.**

▪ Store at temperature not to exceed 37° C (98.6° F). ▪ Use solution within 4 h, once container is opened, because it contains no preservatives or antimicrobials. Discard unused portion.

## ADVERSE EFFECTS (≥1%) **Body as a Whole:** Fever, chills, flushing, increased salivation, headache, back pain. **Skin:** Urticaria, rash. **CV:** Circulatory overload, pulmonary edema (with rapid infusion); hypotension, hypertension, dyspnea, tachycardia. **GI:** Nausea, vomiting.

## DIAGNOSTIC TEST INTERFERENCE

False rise in *alkaline phosphatase* when albumin is obtained partially from pooled placental plasma (levels reportedly decline over period of weeks).

## NURSING IMPLICATIONS

### Assessment & Drug Effects

▪ Monitor BP, pulse and respiration, and IV albumin flow rate. Adjust flow rate as needed to avoid too rapid a rise in BP.
▪ Observe closely for S&S of circulatory overload and pulmonary edema (see Appendix F). If S&S appear, slow infusion rate just sufficiently to keep vein open, and report immediately to prescriber.
▪ Monitor I&O ratio and pattern. Report changes in urinary output. Increase in colloidal osmotic pressure usually causes diuresis, which may persist 3–20 h.
▪ Withhold fluids completely during succeeding 8 h, when albumin is given to patients with cerebral edema.

### Patient & Family Education

▪ Report chills, nausea, headache, or back pain to prescriber immediately.

## NORTRIPTYLINE HYDROCHLORIDE

(nor-trip'ti-leen)
Pamelor

Common adverse effects in *italic*; life-threatening effects <u>underlined</u>; generic names in **bold**; classifications in SMALL CAPS; ♣ Canadian drug name; ⊙ Prototype drug

1159

**Classification:** TRICYCLIC ANTIDEPRESSANT (TCA)
Therapeutic: ANTIDEPRESSANT
**Prototype:** Imipramine

**AVAILABILITY** Capsule; oral solution

**ACTION & *THERAPEUTIC EFFECT***
Mechanism of mood elevation is unknown. Studies suggest that it may interfere with the transport, release, and storage of catecholamines. *Effective in improving depressive moods.*

**USES** Treatment of major depression.

**UNLABELED USES** Nocturnal enuresis in children, ADHD, diabetic neuropathy.

**CONTRAINDICATIONS** Hypersensititivity to tricyclic antidepressants; acute recovery period after MI; AV block; history of QT prolongation; suicidal ideation; during or within 14 days of MAO inhibitor therapy; pregnancy (category D); lactation.

**CAUTIOUS USE** Narrow-angle glaucoma, cardiac disease; history of suicidal tendencies; hyperthyroidism, concurrent use with electroshock therapy; history of suicides; Parkinson's disease; asthma; bipolar disorder; older adults; children.

**ROUTE & DOSAGE**

**Antidepressant**
*Adult:* **PO** 25–50 mg per day, given in divided doses or once daily
*Geriatric:* **PO** Start with 10–25 mg at bedtime, increase by 25 mg q3days to 75 mg at bedtime (max: 150 mg/day)
*Adolescent:* **PO** 10–25 mg at bedtime; may increase (normal dose 30–50 mg daily)

***Pharmacogenetic Dosage Adjustment***
*Poor CYP2D6 metabolizers:* Start with 50% of dose

**ADMINISTRATION**
Oral
- Give with food to decrease gastric distress.
- In older adults, total daily dose may be given once a day at bedtime (preferred).
- Be aware that nortriptyline is a 4% alcohol solution.
- Supervise drug ingestion to be sure patient swallows medication.
- Store at 15°–30° C (59°–86° F) in tightly closed container.

**ADVERSE EFFECTS** (≥1%) **Body as a Whole:** Tremors, hyperhidrosis. **CV:** *Orthostatic hypotension.* **GI:** Paralytic ileus, anorexia, constipation, diarrhea, *dry mouth.* **Hematologic:** Agranulocytosis (rare). **CNS:** Drowsiness, confusional state (especially in older adults and with high dosage). **Skin:** Photosensitivity reaction. **Special Senses:** Blurred vision. **Urogenital:** *Urinary retention.*

**INTERACTIONS Drug:** May decrease response to ANTIHYPERTENSIVES; CNS DEPRESSANTS, **alcohol,** HYPNOTICS, BARBITURATES, SEDATIVES potentiate CNS depression; may increase hypoprothrombinemic effect of ORAL ANTICOAGULANTS; **levodopa,** SYMPATHOMIMETICS (e.g., **epinephrine, norepinephrine**) pose possibility of sympathetic hyperactivity with hypertension and hyperpyrexia; MAO INHIBITORS pose possibility of severe reactions: Toxic psychosis, cardiovascular instability; **methylphenidate** increases plasma TCA levels; THYROID DRUGS may increase possibility of arrhythmias; **cimetidine** may increase plasma TCA levels. Do not use with other agents that prolong QT interval (e.g., **bepridil, dofetilide, pimozide, ziprasidone**) **Herbal: Ginkgo** may decrease seizure threshold. **St. John's wort** may cause serotonin syndrome.

## PHARMACOKINETICS **Absorption:** Rapidly from GI tract. **Peak:** 7–8.5 h. **Duration:** Crosses placenta; distributed in breast milk. **Metabolism:** In liver (CYP2D6, CYP3A4). **Elimination:** Primarily in urine. **Half-Life:** 16–90 h.

## NURSING IMPLICATIONS

### Black Box Warning

*Nortriptyline hydrochloride has been associated with suicidal thinking and behavior in children, adolescents, and young adults.*

### Assessment & Drug Effects

- Monitor carefully for signs and symptoms of suicidality in children and adults.
- Monitor for S&S of serotonin syndrome (see Appendix F).
- Monitor BP and pulse rate during adjustment period of TCA therapy. If systolic BP falls more than 20 mm Hg or if there is a sudden increase in pulse rate, withhold medication and notify the prescriber.
- Monitor bowel elimination pattern and I&O ratio. Urinary retention and severe constipation are potential problems, especially in older adults.
- Observe patient with history of glaucoma. Symptoms that may signal acute attack (severe headache, eye pain, dilated pupils, halos of light, nausea, vomiting) should be reported promptly.

### Patient & Family Education

- Report immediately to prescriber signs of worsening mental status such as suicidal ideation, aggressiveness, agitation, anxiety, hostility, impulsivity, insomnia, irritability, panic attacks, and worsening of depression.
- Do not engage in hazardous activities until response to drug is known.
- Do not use OTC drugs unless prescriber approves.
- Consult prescriber about safe amount of alcohol, if any, that can be ingested.
- Nortriptyline enhances the effects of barbiturates and other CNS depressants are enhanced.

## NYSTATIN
(nye-stat'in)

Mycostatin, Nadostine ◆, Nilstat, Nyaderm ◆, Nystex, O-V Statin

**Classification:** ANTIFUNGAL ANTIBIOTIC
**Therapeutic:** ANTIFUNGAL
**Prototype:** Amphotericin B

**AVAILABILITY** Tablet; oral suspension; troche; vaginal tablet; cream; ointment; powder

## ACTION & THERAPEUTIC EFFECT
Nontoxic, nonsensitizing antifungal antibiotic that binds to sterols in fungal cell membrane, thereby changing membrane potential and allowing leakage of intracellular components that leads to fungi cell death. *Fungistatic and fungicidal activity against a variety of yeasts and fungi.*

**USES** Local infections of skin and mucous membranes caused by *Candida* sp. including *Candida albicans* (e.g., paronychia; cutaneous, oropharyngeal, vulvovaginal, and intestinal candidiasis).

**CONTRAINDICATIONS** Vaginal infections caused by *Gardnerella vaginalis* or *Trichomonas* sp.

**CAUTIOUS USE** Diabetes mellitus; pregnancy (category C); lactation.

Common adverse effects in *italic;* life-threatening effects <u>underlined</u>; generic names in **bold;** classifications in SMALL CAPS; ◆ Canadian drug name; ⊘ Prototype drug

1161

## ROUTE & DOSAGE

**Candida Infections**

*Adult:* **PO** 500,000–1,000,000 units t.i.d.; 1–4 troches 4–5 × day; Suspension: 400,000–600,000 units q.i.d. **Intravaginal** 1–2 tablets daily for 2 wk
*Child:* **PO** Suspension: 400,000–600,000 units q.i.d.
*Infant:* **PO** 100,000–200,000 units q.i.d.

## ADMINISTRATION

### Oral

- Give reconstituted powder for oral suspension immediately after mixing.
- Rinse mouth with 1–2 tsp oral suspension. Should be kept in mouth (swish) as long as possible (at least 2 min), then liquid should be spit out or swallowed (if "swish and swallow" is ordered).
- For children, infants: Apply drug with swab to each side of mouth. Avoid food or drink for 30 min after treatment.
- The troche dosage form should dissolve in mouth (about 30 min). Troches should not be chewed or swallowed. Food and drink should be avoided during period of dissolving and for 30 min after treatment.

### Topical

- Do not apply occlusive dressings over topical applications unless specifically directed to do so.

### Intravaginal

- Store vaginal tablets in refrigerator below 15° C (59° F).

## ADVERSE EFFECTS (≥1%) GI:
Nausea, vomiting, epigastric distress, diarrhea (especially with high oral doses).

## PHARMACOKINETICS Absorption: Poorly absorbed from GI tract. Elimination: In feces.

## NURSING IMPLICATIONS

### Assessment & Drug Effects

- Monitor oral cavity, especially the tongue, for signs of improvement.

### Patient & Family Education

- This drug may cause contact dermatitis. Stop using the drug and report to prescriber if redness, swelling, or irritation develops.
- Take for oral candidiasis (thrush) treatment after meals and at bedtime.
- Care of dentures: Remove dentures before each rinse with oral suspension and before use of troche. Remove dentures at night (infection occurs more frequently in person who wears dentures 24 h a day).
- Dust shoes and stockings, as well as feet, with nystatin dusting powder.
- Gently clean infected areas with tepid water before each application of topical preparation.
- Continue medication for vulvovaginal candidiasis during menstruation.
- Use vaginal tablets up to 6 wk before term to prevent thrush in the newborn.

## OBINUTUZUMAB
(o-bi-nu-tu′zu-mab)
Gazyva
**Classifications:** MONOCLONAL ANTIBODY; ANTINEOPLASTIC
Therapeutic: ANTINEOPLASTIC

## AVAILABILITY Solution for injection

## ACTION & *THERAPEUTIC EFFECT*
Type II anti-CD20 monoclonal antibody that binds to CD20 antigens on the surface

OBINUTUZUMAB

of B-lymphocytes and activates complement-dependent cytotoxicity, antibody-dependent cellular cytotoxicity, and antibody-dependent cellular phagocytosis. *Triggers immune responses that result in death of leukemic lymphocytic cells.*

**USES** Combination use with chlorambucil in the treatment of patients with previously untreated chronic lymphocytic leukemia (CLL); non-Hodgkin's lymphoma.

**CONTRAINDICATIONS** Grade 4 life-threatening infusion reactions; progressive multifocal leukoencephalopathy (PML); reactivation of latent Hepatitis B; lactation.

**CAUTIOUS USE** History of Hepatitis B virus infection; infusion reactions; tumor lysis syndrome; bone marrow suppression; pregnancy (category C). Safety and efficacy in children not established.

## ROUTE & DOSAGE

### Chronic Lymphocytic Leukemia

*Adult:* **IV** Six cycles every 28 days
*Cycle 1:* 100 mg on day 1; 900 mg on day 2; followed by 1000 weekly for 2 doses on days 8 and 15.
*Cycle 2–6:* 1000 mg on day 1 of each cycle, then every 28 days for 5 doses

### Non-Hodgkin's Lymphoma

*Adult:* **IV** 1000 mg on days 1, 8, and 15 on cycle 1; begin the next cycle of therapy on day 29. For cycles 2 to 6, give 1000 mg on day 1 repeated every 28 days

### Infusion Reaction Dosage Adjustment

*Grade 1–2 (mild or moderate):* Slow or interrupt infusion. Upon resolution of symptoms, continue therapy; if no further infusion reactions, rate escalation may resume
*Grade 3 (severe):* Interrupt infusion and manage symptoms. Upon resolution of symptoms, can restart at no more than ½ the previous rate; if no further infusion symptoms occur, rate escalation may resume. Permanently discontinue if patient experiences another Grade 3 reaction.
*Grade 4 (life threatening):* Permanently discontinue obinutuzumab

## ADMINISTRATION

### Intravenous

*PREPARE:* **Infusion: Cycle 1 (day 1 and day 2):** To prepare 100 mg dose for day 1, withdraw 4 mL (100 mg) of obinutuzumab from vial and inject into a 100 mL NS infusion bag. Use immediately. To prepare 900 mg dose for day 2, withdraw the remaining 36 mL (900 mg) from vial and inject into a 250 mL NS infusion bag. Gently invert to mix; do not shake or freeze. ▪**Cycle 1 (day 8 and 15) and cycles 2 to 6 (day 1):** To prepare 1000 mg dose, withdraw 40 mL of obinutuzumab from vial and inject into a 250 mL NS infusion bag. Gently invert to mix; do not shake or freeze. ▪**Note:** Final concentration should be 0.4 to 4 mg/mL. If not used immediately, may store at 2°–8 °C (36°–46° F) for up to 24 h; use immediately after reaching room temperature. Gently invert to mix; do not shake or freeze.
*ADMINISTER:* **Infusion:** Administer only as an infusion through a dedicated line. **Do not** give IV push or bolus. ▪ **Cycle 1 (day 1):** Infuse 100 mg dose at 25 mg/h

Common adverse effects in *italic;* life-threatening effects underlined; generic names in **bold;** classifications in SMALL CAPS; ♣ Canadian drug name; ◑ Prototype drug

1163

over 4 h. ▪ **Cycle 1 (day 2):** Infuse 900 mg dose at 50 mg/h; can increase q30 min by 50 mg/min, to max rate of 400 mg/h. ▪ **Cycle 1: (days 8 and 15) and Cycles 2–6 (day 1):** Infuse 1000 mg dose at 100 mg/h; can increase q30 min by 100 mg/h to max rate of 400 mg/h. Note: Patients are usually premedicated with acetaminophen, an antihistamine (e.g., diphenhydramine), and a glucocorticoid (e.g., dexamethasone or methylprednisolones).

*INCOMPATIBILITIES:* **Solution/additive:** Do not use with diluents other than **0.9% NaCl;** do not mix with other drugs. **Y-site:** Do not mix with any other drug.

**ADVERSE EFFECTS** (≥2%) **Body as a Whole:** *Infusion related reactions,* infections, pyrexia, tumor lysis syndrome. **Hematological:** Anemia, leukopenia, *neutropenia, thrombocytopenia.* **Gastrointestinal:** Constipation. **Metabolic:** Alkaline phosphatase increased, ALT/AST increased, creatinine increased, hyperkalemia, hypoalbuminemia, hypocalcemia, hypokalemia, hyponatremia. **Musculoskeletal:** Musculoskeletal pain. **Respiratory:** Cough.

**PHARMACOKINETICS** **Half-Life:** 28.4 d.

## NURSING IMPLICATIONS

### Black Box Warning

*Obinutuzumab has been associated with progressive multifocal leukoencephalopathy (PML) including fatal PML, and with Hepatitis B virus (HBV) reactivation, in some cases resulting in fulminant hepatitis, hepatic failure, and death.*

### Assessment & Drug Effects

▪ Monitor closely during entire infusion period for S&S of an infusion reaction: Bronchospasm, dyspnea, larynx and throat irritation, wheezing, laryngeal edema, tachycardia, flushing, hypertension, hypotension, fever, nausea, vomiting, diarrhea, headache, and/or chills. Immediately stop infusion if an infusion reaction is suspected and institute supportive measures.

▪ Monitor for and report promptly S&S of infection. Do not administer this drug if patient has an active infection. Note that infusion reactions are more frequent with first 1000 mg infused and may occur up to 24 h after infusion.

▪ Monitor for and report promptly signs of tumor lysis syndrome (e.g., nausea, vomiting, diarrhea, lethargy) during 72 h period after first infusion.

▪ Monitor lab tests: Prior to therapy, HBsAG and anti-HBc; periodic CBC with differential and platelet count, renal function tests, and serum uric acid, serum electrolytes.

### Patient & Family Education

▪ During infusion, immediately report signs of an infusion reaction such as wheezing, chest tightness, fever; itching, bad cough, or swelling of face, lips, tongue, or throat.

▪ Report promptly signs of tumor lysis syndrome (e.g., nausea, vomiting, diarrhea, lethargy) especially during 72 h period after first infusion.

▪ Report immediately to prescriber any of the following: Signs of infection, signs of liver toxicity (see Appendix F), tachycardia, severe headache, significant weakness, bruising, or unexplained bleeding.

▪ Do not accept vaccinations with live viral vaccines.

- Do not breast-feed without consulting prescriber.

## OCTREOTIDE ACETATE ℗ᵣ
(oc-tre′o-tide)
Sandostatin, Sandostatin LAR Depot
**Classification:** SOMATOSTATIN ANALOG
Therapeutic: HORMONE SUPPRESSANT; ACROMEGALY AGENT; ANTIDIARRHEAL

**AVAILABILITY** Solution for injection; depot injection

## ACTION & *THERAPEUTIC EFFECT*
A long-acting peptide that mimics natural hormone somatostatin. Suppresses secretion of serotonin, pancreatic peptides, gastrin, vasoactive intestinal peptide, insulin, glucagon, secretin, and motilin. *Stimulates fluid and electrolyte absorption from the GI tract and prolongs intestinal transit time; also inhibits the growth hormone.*

**USES** Symptomatic treatment of severe diarrhea and flushing episodes associated with metastatic carcinoid tumors. Also watery diarrhea associated with vasoactive intestinal peptide (VIP) tumors, acromegaly.

**UNLABELED USES** Acromegaly associated with pituitary tumors, fistula drainage, variceal bleeding, hepatorenal syndrome, orthostatic hypotension.

**CONTRAINDICATIONS** Hypersensitivity to octreotide.

**CAUTIOUS USE** Cholelithiasis, renal impairment; dialysis; hepatic disease, liver cirrhosis; cardiac disease, CHF; diabetes, TPN administration; hypothyroidism; older adults; pregnancy (category B); lactation.

## ROUTE & DOSAGE

### Carcinoid Syndrome
*Adult:* **Subcutaneous/IV** 100–600 mcg/day in 2–4 divided doses, titrate to response; **IM** May switch to depot injection after 2 wk at 20 mg q4wk × 3 mo

### VIPoma
*Adult:* **Subcutaneous/IV** 200–300 mcg/day in 2–4 divided doses, titrate to response; **IM** May switch to depot injection after 2 wk at 20 mg q4wk × 2 mo

### Acromegaly
*Adult:* **Subcutaneous** 50 mcg t.i.d., titrate up to 100 mcg–500 mcg t.i.d.; **IM** May switch to depot injection after 2 wk at 20 mg q4wk × at least 3 mo, then reassess

### *Renal Impairment Dosage Adjustment*
*Dialysis:* Reduce dose

## ADMINISTRATION
### Subcutaneous/Intramuscular
- **Sandostatin LAR Depot** should be given IM. Reconstitute according to manufacturer's directions.
- **Sandostatin** may be given subcutaneously or IV.
- Minimize GI side effects by giving injections between meals and at bedtime.
- Avoid multiple injections into the same site. Rotate subcutaneous sites on abdomen, hip, and thigh.
- Give deep IM into a large muscle. To reduce local irritation, allow solution to reach room temperature before injection and administer slowly.

**0**

---

## Intravenous

*PREPARE:* **Direct:** Give **Sandosta-tin** undiluted. **Intermittent:** Dilute in 50–200 mL D5W.
*ADMINISTER:* **Direct:** Give a single dose over 3–5 min. In emergency (e.g., carcinoid crisis), give rapid IV bolus over 60 sec. **Intermittent:** Give over 15–30 min.
*INCOMPATIBILITIES:* **Solution/additive: Fat emulsion, regular insulin. Y-site: Dantrolene, diazepam, micafungin, phenytoin, pantoprazole.**

**ADVERSE EFFECTS** (≥1%) **CNS:** Headache, fatigue, dizziness. **GI:** *Nausea, diarrhea, abdominal pain* and discomfort. **CV:** Bradycardia. **Metabolic:** Hypoglycemia, hyperglycemia, increased liver transaminases, hypothyroidism (after long-term use), cholelithiasis, pancreatitis. **Body as a Whole:** Flushing, edema, *injection site pain*, pruritus.

**INTERACTIONS Drug:** May decrease **cyclosporine** levels; may alter other drug and nutrient absorption because of alterations in GI motility.

**PHARMACOKINETICS Absorption:** Rapidly from subcutaneous injection. **Peak:** 0.4 h. **Duration:** Up to 12 h. **Metabolism:** In liver. **Elimination:** In urine. **Half-Life:** 1.5 h.

## NURSING IMPLICATIONS

### Assessment & Drug Effects

- Monitor for hypoglycemia and hyperglycemia (see Appendix F), because octreotide may alter the balance between insulin, glucagon, and growth hormone.
- Monitor fluid and electrolyte balance, as octreotide stimulates fluid and electrolyte absorption from GI tract.
- Monitor vitals signs, especially BP.
- Monitor bowel function, including bowel sounds and stool consistency.
- Monitor lab tests: Baseline and periodic thyroid function tests and vitamin $B_{12}$. As specific conditions indicate, periodic: Plasma serotonin levels with carcinoid tumors, plasma VIP levels with VIPoma, serum GH, serum IGF-1, and thyroid function tests.

### Patient & Family Education

- Learn proper technique for subcutaneous injection if self-medication is required.
- Note: Preferred sites for subcutaneous injections of octreotide are the hip, thigh, and abdomen. Multiple injections at the same subcutaneous injection site within short periods of time are not recommended. This is to avoid irritating the area.

## OFATUMUMAB

(o-fa-tu′mu-mab)

Arzerra

**Classifications:** BIOLOGIC RESPONSE MODIFIER; MONOCLONAL ANTIBODY; CD20 CYTOLYTIC ANTIBODY; ANTINEOPLASTIC
Therapeutic: ANTINEOPLASTIC

**AVAILABILITY** Solution for injection

**ACTION & THERAPEUTIC EFFECT**
A CD20 cytolytic IgG1 kappa monoclonal antibody. The CD20 molecule is present on normal B lymphocytes, both mature and immature lymphocytes, as well as on B-cells in chronic lymphocytic leukemia (CLL). Ofatumumab causes B-cell lysis possibly by complement-dependent cytotoxicity and by antibody-dependent, cell-mediated cytotoxicity. *Effectiveness*

*in treatment of CLL refractory to the standard drug regimen is based on the clinical improvement in response to ofatumumab.*

**USES** Chronic lymphocytic leukemia refractory.

**CONTRAINDICATIONS** Serious infusion reaction; leukoencephalopathy; hepatitis B reactivation; live vaccines; lactation.

**CAUTIOUS USE** History of hepatitis B; older adults; pregnancy (category C). Safety and efficacy in children not established.

## ROUTE & DOSAGE

**Chronic Lymphocytic Leukemia (CLL) - First Line or Refractory Dose**

Adult: **IV** Initial dose of 300 mg followed 1 wk later by 2000 mg qwk for 7 doses, followed by 2000 mg q4wk for 4 doses

## ADMINISTRATION

**Intravenous**

*PREPARE:* **Infusion:** Do not shake drug vials. ▪ Determine the volume of the required drug dose and withdraw an equal volume of NS from a 1000 mL polyolefin IV bag. Add ofatumumab to the IV bag and mix by gentle inversion.
*ADMINISTER:* **Infusion:** Infuse through an in-line filter and PVC administration set supplied with product. ▪ **Do not** give IV push or bolus. ▪ Do not mix or administer with any other drugs or solutions. *For doses 1 and 2:* Initiate infusion at 12 mL/h. If no infusion reaction occurs from 0–30 min, may increase

rate q30min as follows: 31–60 min, 25 mL/h; 61–90 min, 50 mL/h; 91–120 min, 100 mL/h; after 120 min, 200 mL/h. ▪ *For doses 3–12:* Initiate infusion at 25 mL/h. If no infusion reaction occurs from 0–30 min, may increase rate q30min as follows: 31–60 min, 50 mL/h; 61–90 min, 100 mL/h; 91–120 min, 200 mL/h; after 120 min, 400 mL/h.

▪ Store diluted solution at 2°–8° C (36°–46° F). ▪ Use within 12 h of preparation. Discard solution after 24 h.

**ADVERSE EFFECTS** (≥1%) **Body as a Whole:** Chills, *fatigue,* herpes zoster infection, *infusion reactions,* peripheral edema, *pyrexia,* sepsis. **CNS:** Headache, insomnia. **CV:** Hypertension, hypotension, tachycardia. **GI:** *Diarrhea, nausea.* **Hematologic:** Anemia, *neutropenia.* **Musculoskeletal:** Back pain, muscle spasms. **Respiratory:** *Bronchitis, cough, dyspnea,* nasopharyngitis, *pneumonia,* sinusitis, *upper respiratory tract infections.* **Skin:** Hyperhidrosis, *rash,* urticaria

**PHARMACOKINETICS** Half-Life: 14 days.

## NURSING IMPLICATIONS

**Black Box Warning**

Ofatumumab *has been associated with progressive multifocal leukoencephalopathy (PML) including fatal PML, and with Hepatitis B virus (HBV) reactivation, in some cases resulting in fulminant hepatitis, hepatic failure, and death.*

**Assessment & Drug Effects**

▪ Monitor for infusion reactions and stop infusion for any of the following:

**0**

Common adverse effects in *italic;* life-threatening effects underlined; generic names in **bold;** classifications in SMALL CAPS; ✦ Canadian drug name; ⊘ Prototype drug

1167

Bronchospasm, dyspnea, angioedema, flushing, significant changes in BP, tachycardia, back or abdominal pain, fever, rash, or urticaria.

- Monitor for and report promptly S&S of changes in neurologic status or suspected intestinal obstruction.
- Monitor lab tests: Baseline HBsAG, anti-HBc, and total anti-HBc (with both IgG and IgM) or anti-HBc IgG tests.

**Patient & Family Education**

- Report promptly any of the following: New or worsening abdominal pain or nausea, confusion, dizziness, loss of balance, difficulty talking or problems with vision, sore throat, fever, or other signs of infections.
- Avoid live vaccinations and close contact with those who have received live vaccines.

# OFLOXACIN

(o-flox′a-cin)

Ocuflox

**Classification:** QUINOLONE ANTIBIOTIC
Therapeutic: ANTIBIOTIC
**Prototype:** Ciprofloxacin

**AVAILABILITY** Tablet; ophthalmic solution; otic solution

## ACTION & *THERAPEUTIC EFFECT*

Inhibits DNA gyrase, an enzyme necessary for bacterial DNA replication and some aspects of its transcription, repair, recombination, and transposition. *Has a broad spectrum of activity against gram-positive and gram-negative bacteria. Most effective against aerobic and anaerobic gram-negative bacteria.*

**USES** Uncomplicated gonorrhea, prostatitis, respiratory tract infections, skin and skin structure infections, urinary tract infections, superficial ocular infections, pelvic inflammatory disease. Otic: Otitis externa, otitis media with perforated tympanic membranes.

**UNLABELED USES** EENT infections, *Helicobacter pylori* infections, *Salmonella* gastroenteritis, anthrax.

**CONTRAINDICATIONS** Hypersensitivity to ofloxacin or other quinolone antibacterial agents; tendon pain; sunlight (UV) exposure; QT prolongation; viral infection; tendinitis, tendon rupture; history of myasthenia gravis; syphilis.

**CAUTIOUS USE** Renal disease; patients with a history of epilepsy, psychosis, or increased intracranial pressure, cerebrovascular disease, CNS disorders such as seizures, epilepsy, myasthenia gravis; GI disease, colitis, dehydration; syphilis; atrial fibrillation; acute MI; CVA; pregnancy (category C); lactation; children and adolescents (except for **opthalmic** and **otic** preparation).

## ROUTE & DOSAGE

| **Uncomplicated Gonorrhea (Not CDC Recommended)** |
| --- |
| *Adult:* **PO** 400 mg for 1 dose |
| **Respiratory Tract and Skin and Skin Structure Infections** |
| *Adult:* **PO** 200–400 mg q12h × 10 days |
| **Urinary Tract Infection** |
| *Adult:* **PO** 200 mg q12h × 3–10 days |
| **Pelvic Inflammatory Disease** |
| *Adult:* **PO** 400 mg b.i.d. × 14 days |
| **Prostatitis** |
| *Adult:* **PO** 300 mg b.i.d. × 6 wk |

## Otitis Media with Perforation

*Adult:* **Otic** 10 drops (0.5 mL) q12h for 14 days

*Child (1 y or older):* **Otic** 5 drops (0.25 mL) q12h for 14 days

## Otitis Externa

*Adult:* **Otic** 10 drops (0.5 mL) q12h for 7 days

*Child (6 mo–13 y):* **Otic** 5 drops (0.25 mL) q12h for 7 days

### Renal Impairment Dosage Adjustment

*CrCl 20–50 mL/min:* Dose should be given q24h; *less than 20 mL/min:* ½ the dose q24h

### Hepatic Impairment Dosage Adjustment

*Severe impairment:* 400 mg daily

## ADMINISTRATION

### Oral

- Administer with our without food.
- Avoid administering mineral supplements or vitamins with iron or zinc within 2 h of drug.
- Do not give antacids with magnesium, aluminum, or sucralfate within 4 h before or 2 h after drug.

### Instillation

- **Do not** allow tip of dropper for ocular preparation to contact any surface.

## ADVERSE EFFECTS (≥1%) CNS: *Headache, dizziness, insomnia,* hallucinations. **GI:** Nausea, vomiting, diarrhea, GI discomfort. **Urogenital:** Pruritus, pain, irritation, burning, vaginitis, vaginal discharge, dysmenorrhea, menorrhagia, dysuria, urinary frequency. **Skin:** Pruritus, rash. **Other:** Cartilage erosion.

## DIAGNOSTIC TEST INTERFERENCE

May cause false positive on ***opiate screening tests.***

## INTERACTIONS Drug: Ofloxacin absorption decreased when it is administered with MAGNESIUM- or ALUMINUM-CONTAINING ANTACIDS. Other CATIONS, including **calcium, iron,** and **zinc,** also appear to interfere with ofloxacin absorption. May have additive effect with ANTIDIABETICS. Do not use with other agents that prolong QT interval (e.g., **dofetilide, dronedarone, thioridazine, ziprasidone**).

## PHARMACOKINETICS Absorption: 90–98% from GI tract. Peak: 1–2 h. Distribution: Distributes to most tissues; 50% crosses into CSF with inflamed meninges; 20–32% protein bound; crosses placenta; distributed into breast milk. Metabolism: Slightly in liver. Elimination: 72–98% in urine within 48 h. Half-Life: 5–7.5 h.

## NURSING IMPLICATIONS

### Black Box Warning

*Ofloxacin has been associated with an increased risk of tendinitis and tendon rupture, and increased muscle weakness in persons with MG.*

### Assessment & Drug Effects

- Withhold ofloxacin and notify prescriber at first sign of tendon pain, a skin rash, or other allergic reaction.
- Monitor for seizures, especially in patients with known or suspected CNS disorders. Discontinue ofloxacin and notify prescriber immediately if seizure occurs.
- Assess for signs and symptoms of superinfection (see Appendix F).
- Monitor lab tests: C&S tests prior to initial dose.

### Patient & Family Education

- Drink fluids liberally unless contraindicated.

Common adverse effects in *italic;* life-threatening effects <u>underlined</u>; generic names in **bold;** classifications in SMALL CAPS; ◆ Canadian drug name; ◌ Prototype drug

1169

- Be aware that dizziness or light-headedness may occur; use appropriate caution.
- Avoid excessive sunlight or artificial ultraviolet light because of the possibility of phototoxicity.

# OLANZAPINE

(olanz-a′peen)

Zyprexa, Zyprexa
Relprevv Zyprexa Zydis

**Classification:** ATYPICAL ANTIPSYCHOTIC
**Therapeutic:** ANTIPSYCHOTIC, ANTIMANIC
**Prototype:** Clozapine

**AVAILABILITY** Tablet; orally disintegrating tablet; powder for injection

## ACTION & *THERAPEUTIC EFFECT*

Antipsychotic activity is thought to be due to antagonism for both serotonin 5-HT$_{2A/2C}$ and dopamine D$_{1-4}$ receptors. May inhibit the CNS presynaptic neuronal reuptake of serotonin and dopamine. *Has effective antipsychotic activity.*

**USES** Management of schizophrenia, treatment of bipolar disorder and bipolar depression, acute agitation (IM); depression.

**UNLABELED USES** Alzheimer's dementia, acute psychosis.

**CONTRAINDICATIONS** Hypersensitivity to olanzapine; abrupt discontinuation, coma, severe CNS depression; dementia-related psychosis in older adults; lactation.

**CAUTIOUS USE** Known cardiovascular disease, stroke, MI, HF, CVD, neurologic disease, Parkinson's disease; history of seizures, conditions that lower seizure threshold (e.g., Alzheimer dementia); conditions that predispose to

hypotension; history of syncope; history of breast cancer; Japanese; DM; BPH; hepatic impairment, jaundice; predisposition to aspiration pneumonia; history of or high risk for suicide; elevated triglyceride levels; hyperlipedemia; older adults; pregnancy (category C); children. **IM form:** Older adults; debilitated or patients at risk for hypotension. Safety and efficacy in children not established.

## ROUTE & DOSAGE

### Psychotic Disorders

*Adult:* **PO** Start with 5–10 mg once/day, may increase by 2.5–5 mg qwk until desired response (usual range 10–15 mg/day, max: 20 mg/day); **IM Extended release** 150–300 mg q2wk or 405 mg q4wk
*Adolescent:* 2.5–5 mg daily (may increase to 10 mg daily)
*Geriatric:* **PO** Start with 5 mg once/day; **IM Extended release** varies depending on previous oral dose (see package insert for details)

### Treatment Resistant Depression

*Adult:* **PO** 5 mg daily may adjust per response (usual dose 5–20 mg/day)

### Acute Agitation

*Adult:* **IM** 10 mg, do not repeat more frequently than q2h (max: 30 mg/24h)
*Geriatric:* **IM** 2.5–5 mg once

## ADMINISTRATION

### Oral

- Do not push orally disintegrating tablet through blister foil. Peel foil back and remove tablet. Tablet will disintegrate with/without liquid.

### Intramuscular

- *Short-acting formulation:* Reconstitute with 2.1 mL of sterile water for injection to yield 5 mg/mL. Use within 1 h of reconstitution.
- *Extended-release formulation:* Reconstitute with supplied syringe and diluent. Use gloves and flush with water if skin contact is made. To produce a 150 mg/mL solution for injection add 1.3 mL of diluent to the 210 mg vial; or add 1.8 mL of diluent to the 300 mg vial; or add 2.3 mL of diluent to the 405 mg vial.
- Give deep IM into the gluteal muscle. Do not inject more than 5 mL into one site.

## ADVERSE EFFECTS (≥1%) Body as a Whole: *Weight gain,* fever, back and chest pain, peripheral and lower extremity edema, joint pain, twitching, premenstrual syndrome. CNS: *Somnolence, dizziness, headache, agitation, insomnia, nervousness, hostility,* anxiety, personality disorder, akathisia, hypertonia, tremor amnesia, euphoria, stuttering, *extrapyramidal symptoms* (dystonic events, *parkinsonism, akathisia*), tardive dyskinesia. CV: Postural hypotension, hypotension, tachycardia. Special Senses: Amblyopia, blepharitis. GI: Abdominal pain, constipation, dry mouth, increased appetite, increased salivation, nausea, vomiting, elevated liver function tests. Metabolic: Hyperglycemia, diabetes mellitus *increased prolactin.* Urogenital: Premenstrual syndrome, hematuria, urinary incontinence, metrorrhagia. Respiratory: Rhinitis, cough, pharyngitis, dyspnea. Skin: Rash.

## INTERACTIONS Drug: May enhance hypotensive effects of ANTIHYPERTENSIVES. May enhance effects of other CNS ACTIVE DRUGS, **alcohol. Carbamazepine, omeprazole, rifampin** may increase metabolism and clearance of olanzapine. **Fluvoxamine** may inhibit metabolism and clearance of olanzapine. Avoid medications prolong QT interval (e.g., **dofetilide, dronedarone, thioridazine, ziprasidone**).

## PHARMACOKINETICS Absorption: Rapidly from GI tract; 60% reaches systemic circulation. Onset: 15 min IM. Peak: 6 h. Distribution: 93% protein bound, secreted into breast milk of animals (human secretion unknown). Metabolism: In liver (CYP1A2). Elimination: Approximately 57% in urine, 30% in feces. Half-Life: 21–54 h.

## NURSING IMPLICATIONS

### Black Box Warning

*Olanzapine has been associated with increased mortality in older adults with dementia-related psychosis.*

#### Assessment & Drug Effects

- Monitor closely cerebrovascular status in elderly patients with dementia-related psychosis.
- Monitor diabetics for loss of glycemic control.
- Withhold drug and immediately report S&S of neuroleptic malignant syndrome (see Appendix F); assess for and report S&S of tardive dyskinesia (see Appendix F).
- Monitor BP and HR periodically. Monitor temperature, especially with other anticholinergic drugs.
- Monitor for and report orthostatic hypotension, especially during the initial dose-titration period.
- Monitor for seizures, especially in older adults and cognitively impaired persons.

- Monitor weight, BMI, and waist circumference at baseline and again at 4–8–12 wk, then periodically thereafter.
- Taper dosage slowly when discontinuing.
- Monitor lab tests: Periodic LFTs, lipid profile, serum electrolytes, HgA1C, and blood glucose.

**Patient & Family Education**

- Report immediately to prescriber behavioral changes, mood changes, or suicidal ideation.
- Report to prescriber difficulty with motor activity, change in balance, severe dizziness, difficulty speaking or swallowing, tremors, difficulty moving, rigidity.
- Carefully monitor blood glucose levels if diabetic.
- Do not drive or engage in potentially hazardous activities until response to drug is known; drug increases risk of orthostatic hypotension and cognitive impairment.
- Avoid alcohol and do not take additional medications without informing prescriber.
- Do not become overheated; avoid conditions leading to dehydration.

# OLMESARTAN MEDOXOMIL
(ol-me-sar'tan)

Benicar

**Classification:** ANGIOTENSIN II RECEPTOR (TYPE AT$_1$) ANTAGONIST, ANTIHYPERTENSIVE
**Therapeutic:** ANTIHYPERTENSIVE
**Prototype:** Losartan

## AVAILABILITY Tablet

## ACTION & *THERAPEUTIC EFFECT*

Angiotensin II receptor (type AT$_1$) antagonist acts as a potent vasodilator and primary vasoactive hormone of the renin-angiotensin-aldosterone system. Selectively blocks the binding of angiotensin II to the AT$_1$ receptors found in many tissues (e.g., vascular smooth muscle, adrenal glands). *Antihypertensive effect is due to its potent vasodilation effect.*

**USES** Treatment of hypertension.

**CONTRAINDICATIONS** Pregnancy (category D); lactation.

**CAUTIOUS USE** Renal artery stenosis; severe renal impairment; heart failure; hypovolemia; children younger than 6 y.

## ROUTE & DOSAGE

**Hypertension**

*Adult/Child (greater than 35 kg):*
**PO** 20 mg daily, may increase to 40 mg daily. Start with 5–10 mg daily if volume depleted.

*Child (6 y or older, weight 20–35 kg):* **PO** 10 mg daily; may increase to 20 mg daily

## ADMINISTRATION

**Oral**

- Determine if patient is volume depleted (e.g., patients treated with diuretics) prior to first administration of drug. If volume depletion is suspected, a lower starting dose is recommended.
- Store at 20°–25° C (68°–77° F).

**ADVERSE EFFECTS** (≥1%) **Body as a Whole:** Back pain, flu-like symptoms. **CNS:** Dizziness, headache. **CV:** Hypotension (especially if dehydrated) decreases in Hgb/Hct. **GI:** Diarrhea. **Metabolic:** Increased CPK, hyperglycemia, hypertriglyceridemia. **Respiratory:** Bronchitis, pharyngitis, rhinitis, sinusitis, upper respiratory infection. **Urogenital:** Hematuria, acute renal failure.

0

**INTERACTIONS Drug:** May increase hypotensive effect of other ANTIHYPERTENSIVES; may cause hyperkalemia with POTASSIUM-SPARING DIURETICS, POTASSIUM SUPPLEMENTS; increase risk of **lithium** toxicity. **Herbal: Ephedra, ma huang** may antagonize antihypertensive effects.

**PHARMACOKINETICS Absorption:** Rapidly absorbed, 26% reaches systemic circulation. **Peak:** 1–2 h. **Distribution:** 99% protein bound. **Metabolism:** Not metabolized by CYP 450 system. **Elimination:** 50% in urine, 50% in feces. **Half-Life:** 13 h.

## NURSING IMPLICATIONS

### Black Box Warning

*Olmesartan has been associated with fetal toxicity and death.*

### Assessment & Drug Effects

- Monitor closely any volume-depleted patient following initial drug doses. If serious hypotension occurs, place patient in supine position and notify prescriber immediately.
- Monitor BP and HR at drug trough (prior to a scheduled dose). Report hypotension or bradycardia.
- Monitor lab tests: Baseline and periodic renal function tests, and serum electrolytes.

### Patient & Family Education

- Report immediately to prescriber if a pregnancy is suspected.
- Discontinue drug immediately and notify prescriber if you experience swelling of the face, tongue, or throat, or if you believe you are pregnant.
- Notify prescriber of symptoms of hypotension (e.g., dizziness, fainting).

# OLODATEROL HYDROCHLORIDE
(o-lo-da′ter-ol)

Striverdi Respimat

**Classifications:** BRONCHODILATOR RESPIRATORY SMOOTH MUSCLE RELAXANT; BETA-2 ADRENERGIC AGONIST

Therapeutic: BRONCHODILATOR
**Prototype:** Albuterol

**AVAILABILITY** Inhaler

## ACTION & *THERAPEUTIC EFFECT*
Long-acting beta2-receptor agonist; activates beta2 airway receptors, resulting in the increase in the synthesis of cyclic 3′,5′ adenosine monophosphate (cAMP). *Elevated cAMP levels induce bronchodilation by relaxation of airway smooth muscle cells.*

**USES** Treatment of airflow obstruction in patients with chronic obstructive pulmonary disease (COPD), including chronic bronchitis and/or emphysema.

**CONTRAINDICATIONS** Asthma without a concomitant long term asthma control medication; acutely deteriorating COPD; olodaterol-induced bronchospasm; concurrent use of other long-acting beta₂-agonists; severe hypersensitivity reaction.

**CAUTIOUS USE** Hypersensitivity to other beta₂-agonist; cardiovascular disease; coronary insufficiency, cardiac arrhythmias, hypertrophic obstructive cardiomyopathy, known or suspected prolongation of QT interval, hypertension, hypokalemia; DM; seizure disorders; hyperthyroidism; pregnancy (category C); lactation.

0

---

Common adverse effects in *italic;* life-threatening effects underlined; generic names in **bold;** classifications in SMALL CAPS; ♣ Canadian drug name; ⊘ Prototype drug

## ROUTE & DOSAGE

### Chronic Obstructive Pulmonary Disease (COPD)

*Adult:* **Inhalation** Two inhalations once daily

## ADMINISTRATION

### Inhalation

- For oral inhalation only.
- Prime inhaler prior to initial use or if not used for longer than 21 days.
- Instruct to breathe in slowly through the mouth, then press the dose release button; patient should continue to breathe in slowly as long as possible, then hold breath for 10 seconds or for as long as comfortable.
- Store at 15°–30° C (59°–86° F). Protect from freezing. Discard 3 mo after cartridge is inserted into inhaler.

## ADVERSE EFFECTS (≥2%) **Body as a Whole:** Pyrexia. **CV:** Dizziness. **GI:** Constipation, diarrhea. **Musculoskeletal:** Arthralgia, back pain. **Respiratory:** Bronchitis, <u>cough increased risk of asthma-related deaths</u>, *nasopharyngitis,* pneumonia, upper respiratory tract infection. **Skin:** Rash. **Urogenital:** Urinary tract infection.

## INTERACTIONS **Drug:** Coadministration with other ADRENERGIC AGONISTS may cause a potentiation of sympathetic effects. Concomitant treatment with XANTINE DERIVATIVES (e.g., **caffeine, theophylline**), LOOP DIURETICS (e.g., **furosemide**), or THIAZIDE DIURETICS (e.g., **hydrochlorothiazide**) may potentiate hypokalemic effects. Olodaterol may have an additive QTc prolongation effect if used in combination with MONOAMINE OXIDASE INHIBITORS, TRICYCLIC ANTIDEPRESSANTS, or other drugs known to cause QTc prolongation.

BETA BLOCKERS (e.g., **atenolol, propranolol**) can interfere with the therapeutic actions of olodaterol.

## PHARMACOKINETICS **Peak:** Bioavailability via inhalation is 30%. **Peak:** 10-20 min. **Distribution:** 60% plasma protein bound. **Metabolism:** In liver. **Elimination:** Fecal (53%) and renal (38%) mostly as metabolites. **Half-Life:** 22 h.

## NURSING IMPLICATIONS

### Black Box Warning

*Long-acting beta2-adrenergic agonists (LABA), such as olodaterol, have been associated with increased risk of asthma-related death.*

### Assessment & Drug Effects

- Monitor FEV1, FVC, and/or other pulmonary function tests. Report immediately complaints of sudden shortness of breath.
- Monitor BP, HR, and level of CNS stimulation.
- Monitor cardiac status especially in those with preexisting cardiovascular disease.
- Monitor those with seizure disorders for increased seizure activity.
- Monitor for increased use of short-acting beta2-agonist inhaler; may be marker of a deteriorating condition.
- Diabetics should be monitored for loss of glycemic control.
- Monitor lab tests: Periodic serum potassium and serum glucose.

### Patient & Family Education

- Olodaterol should not be used to treat asthma or acute deteriorations of COPD.
- Report promptly to prescriber if you experience sudden shortness of breath, fast or irregular heartbeat or palpitations, or chest pain.
- Monitor blood glucose more frequently if diabetic.

Common adverse effects in *italic;* life-threatening effects <u>underlined;</u> generic names in **bold;** classifications in SMALL CAPS; ✦ Canadian drug name; ✪ Prototype drug

- Persons with seizures disorders should report promptly more frequent seizure activity.
- Do not breast-feed while using this drug.

## OLOPATADINE HYDROCHLORIDE

(o-lo-pa′ta-deen)

Patase, Pataday, Patanol

**See Appendix A-1.**

## OLSALAZINE SODIUM

(ol-sal′a-zeen)

Dipentum

**Classification:** ANTI-INFLAMMATORY
**Therapeutic:** GI ANTI-INFLAMMATORY
**Prototype:** Mesalamine

### AVAILABILITY Capsule

### ACTION & *THERAPEUTIC EFFECT*

Converted to 5-aminosalicylic acid (5-ASA) by colonic bacteria. 5-ASA inhibits prostaglandin production in the colon, thus leading to its anti-inflammatory properties. *5-ASA has anti-inflammatory activity in ulcerative colitis.*

### USES Maintenance therapy in patients with ulcerative colitis.

### CONTRAINDICATIONS Hypersensitivity to salicylates or olsalazine.

### CAUTIOUS USE Patients with preexisting kidney disease; elderly; colitis; pregnancy (category C); lactation. Safety and efficacy in children not established.

### ROUTE & DOSAGE

**Ulcerative Colitis**

*Adult:* **PO** 500 mg b.i.d., may increase up to 1.5–3 g/day in divided doses

## ADMINISTRATION

**Oral**
- Give with food in evenly divided doses.

### ADVERSE EFFECTS (≥1%) CNS:
Headache, drowsiness, depression, dizziness, vertigo. **GI:** *Diarrhea,* nausea, abdominal cramping, abdominal pain, anorexia, dyspepsia indigestion, vomiting, bloating, stomatitis. **Skin:** Rash, pruritis. **Body as a Whole:** Arthralgia, URI.

### PHARMACOKINETICS Absorption: 1–3% from GI tract; highly protein bound; high colonic concentrations are associated with efficacy. **Metabolism:** Prodrug metabolized to 2 molecules of 5-ASA; **Elimination:** Primarily in feces. **Half-Life:** 2–15 h.

## NURSING IMPLICATIONS

### Assessment & Drug Effects
- Monitor kidney function in patients with preexisting renal disease.
- Monitor for S&S of a hypersensitivity reaction (see Appendix F). Withhold olsalazine and notify prescriber at first sign of an allergic response.
- Obtain baseline CBC, LFTs, renal function tests and repeat at 6 and 12 months during treatment, then annually.

### Patient & Family Education
- Report diarrhea, a possible adverse effect, to the prescriber.

## OMACETAXINE MEPESUCCINATE

(o ma-ce-tax′een)

Synribo

**Classification:** ANTINEOPLASTIC; INHIBITOR OF ONCOGENIC PROTEINS; PROTEIN SYNTHESIS INHIBITOR
**Therapeutic:** ANTINEOPLASTIC

Common adverse effects in *italic;* life-threatening effects underlined; generic names in **bold;** classifications in SMALL CAPS; ♣ Canadian drug name; ⊘ Prototype drug

1175

**AVAILABILITY** Lyophilized powder for injection

**ACTION & *THERAPEUTIC EFFECT***
Mechanism of action not fully understood but believed to include inhibition of protein synthesis with possible reduction in levels of oncoproteins and anti-apoptotic proteins that stimulate CML cell growth. *May slow progression of CML with improvement in disease-related symptoms or increased survival.*

**USES** Treatment of chronic or accelerated phase chronic myeloid leukemia (CML) in adult patients who have resistance and/or intolerance to two or more tyrosine kinase inhibitors (TKI).

**CONTRAINDICATIONS** Poorly controlled diabetes (avoid use until controlled); pregnancy (category D); lactation.

**CAUTIOUS USE** History of GI bleeding; myelosuppression; thrombocytopenia; cerebral hemorrhage; DM or patients with risk factors for DM. Safety and efficacy in children younger than 18 y not established.

**ROUTE & DOSAGE**

**Chronic Myeloid Leukemia**

*Adult:* **Subcutaneous** 1.25 mg/m² b.i.d. for 14 consecutive days in a 28 day cycle; repeat until patient achieves hematological response; follow with 1.25 mg/m² b.i.d. for 7 consecutive days in a 28-day cycle; can repeat as necessary.

***Hematologic Toxicity Dosage Adjustment***

*Grade 4 neutropenia (ANC less than 0.5 × 10⁹/L) or Grade 3 thrombocytopenia (platelet count*

*less than 50 × 10⁹/L):* Delay next cycle until ANC is greater than or equal to 1.0 × 10⁹/L and platelet count is greater than or equal to 50 × 10⁹/L; then reduce the number of dosing days to 12 or 5.

**ADMINISTRATION**

**Subcutaneous**
- Reconstitute vial with 1 mL of NS for injection; swirl gently until clear. Yields 3.5 mg/mL.
- Avoid contact with the skin. If contact occurs, immediately and thoroughly wash affected area with soap and water.
- Rotate injection sites.
- May store reconstituted solution for 12 h at room temperature or 24 h if refrigerated. Protect from light.

**ADVERSE EFFECTS** (≥1%) **Body as a Whole:** *Asthenia,* catheter site pain, chest pain, chills, contusion, *fatigue,* general edema, hypersensitivity reaction, hyperthermia, *infection,* influenza-like illness, *infusion and injection site reactions,* malaise, mucosal inflammation, pain, peripheral edema, *pyrexia,* transfusion reaction. **CNS:** Agitation, anxiety, confusional state, depression, headache, insomnia, mental status change. **CV:** <u>Acute coronary syndrome</u>, angina pectoris, <u>arrhythmia</u>, bradycardia, hematoma, hot flush, hypertension, hypotension, palpitations, <u>tachycardia, ventricular extrasystoles</u>. **GI:** Abdominal distension, anal fissure, aphthous stomatitis, constipation, *diarrhea,* dry mouth, dyspepsia, dysphagia, gastritis, gastroesophageal reflux disease, gastrointestinal hemorrhage, gingival bleeding, gingival pain, gingivitis, hemorrhoids, melena, mouth hemorrhage, mouth ulceration, *nausea,* oral pain, stomatitis, upper abdominal pain, vomiting. **Hematological:** *Anemia,* bone marrow failure, febrile neutropenia, lymphopenia, *neutropenia, thrombocytopenia.* **Metabolic:** Alterations in glucose level, Anorexia, decreased appetitie, dehydration, increased ALT, increased bilirubin, increased creatinine, *increased uric acid.* **Musculoskeletal:** *Arthralgia,* back pain, bone pain, muscle spasms, musculoskeletal pain, stiffness, discomfort and/or weakness, myalgia, musculoskeletal chest pain, pain in extremity. **Respiratory:** Cough, dysphonia, dyspnea, epistaxis, hemoptysis, nasal congestion, pharyngolaryngeal pain, productive cough, rales, rhinorrhea, sinus congestion. **Skin:** Dry skin, ecchymosis, erythema, hyperhidrosis, night sweats, petechiae, pruritus, purpura, rash erythematous, rash papular, skin lesion, skin ulcer, skin exfoliation, skin hyperpigmentation. **Special Senses:** Blurred vision, cataract, conjunctival hemorrhage, conjunctivitis, diplopia, ear hemorrhage, ear pain, eyelid edema, eye pain, tinnitus. **Urogenital:** Dysuria.

### PHARMACOKINETICS **Peak:**
30 min. **Distribution:** Less than or equal to 50% plasma protein bound. **Metabolism:** Hydrolysis in plasma. **Elimination:** Primary route of elimination not determined. **Half-Life:** 6 h.

### NURSING IMPLICATIONS

#### Assessment & Drug Effects

- Monitor for and report promptly S&S of bleeding and infection.
- Evaluate neurologic status for S&S of cerebral hemorrhage.
- Monitor diabetics and prediabetics for loss of glycemic control.
- Lab test: Weekly CBC with differential during induction and initial

maintenance cycles, then q2wk as needed; periodic blood glucose.

#### Patient & Family Education

- Report promptly any S&S of hemorrhage including easy bruising, blood in urine or stool, slurred speech, confusion, or altered vision.
- Report S&S of infection such as fever of 101° F or greater.
- Report immediately severe or worsening skin rash.
- Monitor blood glucose closely if diabetic. Report immediately if good glycemic control is not maintained.
- Women should use effective means of contraception while taking this drug.
- Do not breast-feed while taking this drug.

---

# OMALIZUMAB
(o-mal-i-zoo'mab)

Xolair

**Classification:** BIOLOGIC RESPONSE MODIFIER; MONOCLONAL ANTIBODY; RESPIRATORY ANTI-INFLAMMATORY
**Therapeutic:** ANTIALLERGIC; ANTIASTHMATIC; ANTI-INFLAMMATORY

**AVAILABILITY** Solution for injection

### ACTION & *THERAPEUTIC EFFECT*
It inhibits binding of IgE to high-affinity IgE receptors on the surface of mast cells and basophils, limiting the release of inflammatory mediators. *Inhibits release of mediators of the allergic response and has an anti-inflammatory action on the respiratory system.*

### USES Control of moderate to
severe allergic asthma; chronic idiopathic urticaria.

### UNLABELED USES Seasonal allergic rhinitis, food allergies, chronic idiopathic urticaria.

---

Common adverse effects in *italic;* life-threatening effects underlined; generic names in **bold;** classifications in SMALL CAPS; ♥Canadian drug name; ⊙ Prototype drug

1177

**CONTRAINDICATIONS** Severe hypersensitivity to omalizumab; acute asthma, status asthmaticus.

**CAUTIOUS USE** Pregnancy (category B); lactation; children younger than 12 y.

## ROUTE & DOSAGE

### Allergic Asthma
*Adult/Adolescent:* **Subcutaneous** 150–375 mg q2–4wk. Dose is based on baseline IgE serum levels and body weight. (see package insert)

### Chronic Idiopathic Urticaria
*Adult/Adolescent:* **Subcutaneous** 150 or 300 mg q4w

## ADMINISTRATION

**Subcutaneous**
- To reconstitute: (1) Draw 1.4 mL of SW into 3-mL syringe with 1-inch, 18-gauge needle. (2) Keep vial upright and and inject SW, then gently swirl for about 1 min to wet powder. Do not shake. (3) Gently swirl vial q5min for 5–10 sec to dissolve remaining solids. Discard if not completely dissolved by 40 min. (4) Once dissolved invert vial for 15 sec to allow solution to drain toward stopper. (5) Insert new 3-mL syringe with a 1-inch, 18-gauge needle, into inverted vial with needle tip at the very bottom of solution, then withdraw all solution. (6) Replace 18-gauge with a 25-gauge needle for injection. (7) Expel any excess solution to obtain the 1.2 mL dose.
- Give subcutaneously and rotate injection sites. Doses more than 150 mg should be divided over more than one site. Solution is viscous and takes 5–10 sec to inject.

- Use within 8 h of reconstitution when stored in the vial at 2°–8° C (36°–46° F), or within 4 h of reconstitution when stored at room temperature.

**ADVERSE EFFECTS** (≥1%) **Body as a Whole:** <u>Anaphylaxis/anaphylactoid reactions</u>, *injection site reactions (bruising, erythema, warmth, burning, stinging, pruritus, hive formation, pain, induration, inflammation),* fatigue, generalized pain. **CNS:** Headache, dizziness. **GI:** *Nausea, vomiting, diarrhea, abdominal pain.* **Hematologic:** Epistaxis, menorrhagia, hematoma, anemia. **Musculoskeletal:** Arthralgia. **Respiratory:** Upper respiratory tract infections, sinusitis, pharyngitis. **Skin:** Rash, pruritus, urticaria, dermatitis. **Special Senses:** Earache.

**PHARMACOKINETICS Absorption:** Slowly absorbed from subcutaneous site; 53–71% reaches systemic circulation. **Peak:** 7–8 days. **Half-Life:** 22 days.

## NURSING IMPLICATIONS

### Black Box Warning

*Omalizumab has been associated with anaphylaxis as early as the first dose and as late as a year following initiation of treatment.*

### Assessment & Drug Effects
- Monitor closely for S&S of anaphylaxis, presenting as bronchospasm, hypotension, syncope, urticaria, and/or angioedema of the throat or tongue.
- Monitor for injection site reactions including bruising, redness, warmth, burning, stinging, itching, hive formation, pain, indurations, mass, and inflammation.

- Monitor lab tests: Platelet counts if signs of increased tendency to bleed appear. Obtain baseline serum total IgE and PFT.

**Patient & Family Education**

- Do not use this drug for relief of acute bronchospasm or status asthmaticus.
- Promptly report any of the following: Bleeding or unusual bruising, difficulty breathing or shortness of breath, skin rash or hives.
- Do not accept a live virus vaccine without consulting prescriber.

# OMEGA-3 FATTY ACIDS (EICOSAPENTAENOIC ACID AND DOCOSAHEXAENOIC ACID) EPA & DHA

(o-me'ga-3)

Dr. Sears OmegaRx, Eskimo-3, Fish Oil, Omega-3 Fatty Acids, ICAR Prenatal Essential Omega-3, Mega Twin EPA, Natrol DHA Neuromins, Natrol Omega-3, Natural Fish Oil, Oleomed Heart, Omacor, Omega-3 Fish Oil Concentrate, Sea Omega, ZonePerfect Omega 3

**Classifications:** NUTRITIONAL SUPPLEMENT; OMEGA-3 FATTY ACIDS

Therapeutic: OMEGA-3 FATTY ACIDS; ANTILIPEMIC

**AVAILABILITY** Capsule; oil for oral ingestion

## ACTION & *THERAPEUTIC EFFECT*

Mechanism of action of omega-3-acid ethyl esters is not completely understood. May include inhibition of acetyl-CoA and increased peroxisomal beta-oxidation in the liver. *Triglyceride lowering is the most consistent effect observed.*

**USES** Adjunct to diet to reduce hypertriglyceridemia.

**UNLABELED USES** Adjunct nutritional supplementation for hypertriglyceridemia, rheumatoid arthritis, or for the general purpose of maintaining a healthy heart.

**CONTRAINDICATIONS** Hypersensitivity to any component of the medication.

**CAUTIOUS USE** Known sensitivity or allergy to fish; pregnancy (category C); lactation; children.

## ROUTE & DOSAGE

**Hypertriglyceridemia (Lovaza Rx form)**

*Adult:* PO 4 g daily (as single or divided dose)

## ADMINISTRATION

**Oral**

- The daily dose may be given as one dose or divided b.i.d.
- Store 15°–30° C (59°–86° F).

**ADVERSE EFFECTS** (≥1%) **Body as a Whole:** Back pain, flu syndrome, unspecified pain. **GI:** Diarrhea, dyspepsia, eructation, nausea, vomiting. **Metabolic/Nutritional:** Increased total cholesterol and/or LDL levels, weight gain. **Skin:** Rash. **Special Senses:** Halitosis, taste disturbances.

**INTERACTIONS Drug:** ANTICOAGULANTS and THROMBOLYTICS are affected by inhibition of platelet aggregation with omega-3 fatty acids.

**PHARMACOKINETICS Metabolism:** Extensive liver metabolism.

Common adverse effects in *italic;* life-threatening effects <u>underlined</u>; generic names in **bold;** classifications in SMALL CAPS; ♣ Canadian drug name; ◐ Prototype drug

1179

## NURSING IMPLICATIONS

### Assessment & Drug Effects

- Monitor for S&S of hypersensitivity in those with known allergy to fish.
- Monitor diabetics for loss of glycemic control.
- Note: Poor therapeutic response after 2 mo is an indication to discontinue drug.
- Monitor blood levels of anticoagulants with concurrent therapy.
- Monitor lab tests: Baseline and periodic lipid profile.

### Patient & Family Education

- Do not take omega-3 fatty acids without consulting prescriber if you have a chronic medical disorder.

---

# OMEPRAZOLE ℗⁺

(o-me′pra-zole)

Losec ✦, Prilosec, Prilosec OTC, Zegerid

**Classifications:** PROTON PUMP INHIBITOR; ANTISECRETORY

Therapeutic: ANTIULCER

**AVAILABILITY** Capsule; powder for oral suspension; delayed release tablet

**ACTION & THERAPEUTIC EFFECT** An antisecretory compound that is a gastric acid pump inhibitor. Suppresses gastric acid secretion by inhibiting the $H^+$, $K^+$-ATPase enzyme system [the acid (proton $H^+$) pump] in the parietal cells. *Suppresses gastric acid secretion relieving gastrointestinal distress and promoting ulcer healing.*

**USES** Duodenal and gastric ulcer. Gastroesophageal reflux disease including severe erosive esophagitis (4 to 8 wk treatment). Long-term treatment of pathologic hypersecretory conditions such as Zollinger-Ellison syndrome, multiple endocrine adenomas, and systemic mastocytosis. In combination with clarithromycin to treat duodenal ulcers associated with *Helicobacter pylori.* Dyspepsia occurring more than twice weekly.

**UNLABELED USES** Healing or prevention of NSAID-related ulcers; stress gastritis prophylaxis.

**CONTRAINDICATIONS** Duodenal ulcers; proton pump inhibitors (PPIs), hypersensitivity; lactation; use of **Zegerid** in metabolic alkalosis, hypocalcemia, vomiting, GI bleeding.

**CAUTIOUS USE** Dysphagia; metabolic or respiratory alkalosis; hepatic disease; pregnancy (category C); use in GERD in children younger than 1 y. **OTC form:** Children younger than 18 y.

## ROUTE & DOSAGE

**Gastroesophageal Reflux, Erosive Esophagitis, Duodenal Ulcer**

*Adult/Adolescent/Child (weight over 20 kg):* **PO** 20–40 mg once/day for 4–8 wk
*Child (older than 1 y, weight 10–19 kg):* **PO** 10 mg once daily; *weight 5–9 kg:* 5 mg once daily

**Gastric Ulcer**

*Adult:* **PO** 40 mg daily for 4–8 wk

**Hypersecretory Disease**

*Adult:* **PO** 60 mg once/day up to 120 mg t.i.d.

**Duodenal Ulcer Associated with H. pylori**

*Adult:* **PO** 40 mg once/day for 14 days, then 20 mg/day for 14 days, in combination with clarithromycin 500 mg t.i.d. for 14 days

**Dyspepsia**

*Adult:* **PO** 20 mg daily × 14 days

Common adverse effects in *italic;* life-threatening effects <u>underlined;</u> generic names in **bold;** classifications in SMALL CAPS; ✦ Canadian drug name; ℗ Prototype drug

## ADMINISTRATION

### Oral

- Give before food, preferably breakfast; capsules **must be** swallowed whole (do not open, chew, or crush).
- Note: Antacids may be administered with omeprazole.
- *For NG tube administration:* Into a catheter-tipped syringe, empty a 2.5 mg packet of omeprazole spheres into 5 mL of water or a 10 mg packet into 15 mL of water. Immediately shake syringe, then allow to thicken for 2–3 min. Shake syringe again, then inject into NG tube.

## ADVERSE EFFECTS (≥1%) CNS:
Headache, dizziness, fatigue. GI: Diarrhea, abdominal pain, nausea, mild transient increases in liver function tests. Urogenital: Hematuria, proteinuria. Skin: Rash.

## DIAGNOSTIC TEST INTERFERENCE
Omeprazole has been reported to significantly impair peak cortisol response to exogenous ACTH. This finding is undergoing further investigation. May result in false-negative *13C-urea breath test.*

## INTERACTIONS   Drug:   May increase **diazepam, phenytoin, warfarin** levels. May affect levels of ANTIRETROVIRAL AGENTS. **Herbal: Ginkgo, St. John's wort** may decrease plasma concentrations. **Food:** Food decreases absorption by up to 35%.

## PHARMACOKINETICS   Absorption: Poorly from GI tract; 30–40% reaches systemic circulation. Onset: 0.5–3.5 h. Peak: Peak inhibition of gastric acid secretion: 5 days. Metabolism: In liver (CYP2C19). Elimination: 80% in urine, 20% in feces. Half-Life: 0.5–1.5 h.

## NURSING IMPLICATIONS

### Assessment & Drug Effects

- Monitor for and report lack of improvement or worsening GI symptoms.
- Monitor lab tests: Periodic B12 and LFTs with prolonged use.

### Patient & Family Education

- Bone density tests are advised with long-term use.
- Report any changes in urinary elimination such as pain or discomfort associated with urination, or blood in urine.
- Report severe diarrhea; drug may need to be discontinued.

## ONDANSETRON HYDROCHLORIDE ⊕
(on-dan'si-tron)
Zofran, Zofran ODT, Zuplenz
**Classifications:** 5-HT₃ ANTAGONIST; ANTIEMETIC
Therapeutic: ANTIEMETIC

**AVAILABILITY** Orally disintegrating tablet; oral solution; solution for injection; oral soluble film

## ACTION & *THERAPEUTIC EFFECT*
Selective serotonin (5-HT₃) receptor antagonist. Serotonin receptors are located centrally in the chemoreceptor trigger zone (CTZ) and peripherally on the vagal nerve terminals. Serotonin is released from the wall of the small intestine and stimulates the vagal efferent nerves through the serotonin receptors and initiates the vomiting reflex. *Prevents nausea and vomiting associated with cancer chemotherapy and anesthesia.*

## USES  Prevention of nausea and vomiting associated with chemotherapy or radiation; postoperative nausea and vomiting.

0

Common adverse effects in *italic;* life-threatening effects underlined; generic names in **bold**; classifications in SMALL CAPS; ♣ Canadian drug name; ⊕ Prototype drug

1181

**UNLABELED USES** Treatment of hyperemesis gravidarum; alcohol dependence; pruritus.

**CONTRAINDICATIONS** Hypersensitivity to ondansetron; or any component of the formulation; serotonin syndrome reaction to drug.

**CAUTIOUS USE** Hypersensitivity to other selective 5-HT₃ receptor antagonists; hepatic impairment; QT prolongation; abdominal surgery; PKU; older adults; pregnancy (category B); lactation. **PO:** Children younger than 4 y. **IV:** Infants.

## ROUTE & DOSAGE

### Prevention of Chemotherapy-Induced Nausea/Vomiting

*Adult/Adolescent:* **PO** 8–24 mg 30 min before chemotherapy, repeat at 8 h if needed
*Adult/Child/Infant (6 mo–18 y):* **IV** 0.15 mg/kg infused over 15 min beginning 30 min before chemotherapy, then repeat at 4 and 8 h
*Child (older than 4 y):* **PO** 4 mg 30 min before chemotherapy, then q8h × 2 more doses

### Prevention of Radiation-Induced Nausea/Vomiting

*Adult:* **PO** 8 mg 1–2 h before each daily fraction of radiotheraphy

### Nausea and Vomiting with Highly Emetogenic Chemotherapy

*Adult:* **PO** Single 24 mg dose 30 min before administration of single-day highly emetogenic chemotherapy

### Postoperative Nausea and Vomiting

*Adult:* **PO** 16 mg 1 h preoperatively
*Adult/Adolescent/Child (weight greater than 40 kg):* **IM/IV** 4 mg injected immediately prior to anesthesia induction or once postoperatively if patient experiences nausea/vomiting shortly after surgery
*Child/Infant: (weight less than 40 kg):* **IV** 0.05 mg–0.1 mg/kg immediately prior to or following anesthesia induction

### Hepatic Impairment Dosage Adjustment

*Child-Pugh class C:* Max: 8 mg/day

## ADMINISTRATION

### Oral

- Give tablets 30 min prior to chemotherapy and 1–2 h prior to radiation therapy.
- **Do not** push orally disintegrating tablet through blister foil. Peel foil back and remove tablet. Tablets will disintegrate with/without liquid.

### Intramuscular

- Give undiluted into a large muscle.

### Intravenous

*PREPARE:* **Direct for Postoperative Nausea and Vomiting:** May be given undiluted. **IV Infusion for Chemotherapy-Induced Nausea and Vomiting:** Dilute a single dose in 50 mL of D5W or NS. ▪ May be further diluted in selected IV solution.
*ADMINISTER:* **Direct for Postoperative Nausea and Vomiting:** Give over at least 30 sec, 2–5 min preferred. **IV Infusion for Chemotherapy-Induced Nausea and Vomiting:** Give over 15 min. ▪ When three separate doses are administered, infuse each over 15 min.
*INCOMPATIBILITIES:* **Solution/additive: Meropenem. Y-site: Acyclovir, allopurinol, aminophylline, amphotericin B,**

0

amphotericin B cholesteryl, ampicillin, ampicillin/sulbactam, amsacrine, azathioprine, cefmandole, cefepime, cefoperazone, ceftobiprole, chloramphenicol, dantrolene, diazoxide, ertapenem, foscarnet, fluorouracil, furosemide, ganciclovir, gemtuzumab, indomethacin, lansoprazole, lorazepam, meropenem, methohexital, methylprednisolone, micafungin, milrinone, pantoprazole, pemetrexed, pentobarbital, phenobarbital, phenytoin, rituximab, sargramostim, sodium bicarbonate, SMZ/TMP, thiopental, trastuzumab, TPN.

**ADVERSE EFFECTS** (≥1%) **CNS:** Dizziness, fatigue, light-headedness, *headache, sedation.* **GI:** *Diarrhea,* constipation, dry mouth, transient increases in liver aminotransferases and bilirubin. **Body as a Whole:** Hypersensitivity reactions.

**INTERACTIONS Drug:** Do not use with **apomorphine** due to risk of hypotension. Do not use with **hydroxychloroquine, mifepristone,** and other agents affecting QT interval due to risk of QT prolongation.

**PHARMACOKINETICS Peak:** 1–1.5 h. **Metabolism:** In liver (CYP3A4). **Elimination:** 44–60% in urine within 24 h; ~25% in feces. **Half-Life:** 3 h.

## NURSING IMPLICATIONS

### Assessment & Drug Effects

- Monitor fluid and electrolyte status. Diarrhea, which may cause fluid and electrolyte imbalance, is a potential adverse effect of the drug.
- Monitor cardiovascular status, especially in patients with a history of coronary artery disease. Rare cases of tachycardia and angina have been reported.

### Patient & Family Education

- Be aware that headache requiring an analgesic for relief is a common adverse effect.

# OPIUM, POWDERED OPIUM TINCTURE (LAUDANUM)
(oh'pee-um)

**Classifications:** NARCOTIC (OPIATE AGONIST) ANALGESIC; ANTI-DIARRHEAL
**Therapeutic:** NARCOTIC ANALGESIC; ANTIDIARRHEAL
**Prototype:** Morphine
**Controlled Substance:** Schedule II

**AVAILABILITY** Tincture

## ACTION & THERAPEUTIC EFFECT

Contains several natural alkaloids including morphine, codeine, papaverine. Antidiarrheal due to inhibition of GI motility and propulsion; leads to prolonged transit of intestinal contents, desiccation of feces, and constipation. *Antidiarrheal activity due to inhibition of GI motility.*

**USES** Diarrhea.

**CONTRAINDICATIONS** Diarrhea caused by poisoning (until poison is completely eliminated).

**CAUTIOUS USE** History of opiate agonist dependence; asthma; severe prostatic hypertrophy; hepatic disease; pregnancy (category C); lactation.

## ROUTE & DOSAGE

### Acute Diarrhea

*Adult:* **PO** 0.6 mL q.i.d. (max: 6 mL/day)

## ADMINISTRATION
### Oral
- Do not confuse this preparation with camphorated opium tincture (paregoric), which contains only 2 mg anhydrous morphine/5 mL, thus requiring a higher dose volume than that required for therapeutic dose of Deodorized Opium Tincture.
- Give drug diluted with about one third glass of water to ensure passage of entire dose into stomach.
- Store in tight, light-resistant containers.

## ADVERSE EFFECTS (≥1%) GI:
Nausea and other GI disturbances. **CNS:** Depression of CNS.

## INTERACTIONS Drug: Alcohol
and other CNS DEPRESSANTS add to CNS effects.

## PHARMACOKINETICS Absorption:
Variable absorption from GI tract. **Distribution:** Crosses placenta; distributed into breast milk. **Metabolism:** In liver. **Elimination:** In urine.

## NURSING IMPLICATIONS
### Assessment & Drug Effects
- Withhold medication and report to prescriber if respirations are 12/min or below or have changed in character and rate.
- Discontinue as soon as diarrhea is controlled; note character and frequency of stools.
- Offer small amounts of fluid frequently but attempt to maintain 3000–4000 mL fluid total in 24 h.
- Monitor body weight, I&O ratio and pattern, and temperature. If patient develops fever of 38.8° C (102° F) or above, electrolyte and hydration levels may need to be evaluated. Consult prescriber.

### Patient & Family Education
- Be aware that constipation may be a consequence of antidiarrheal therapy but that normal habit pattern usually is reestablished with resumption of normal dietary intake.
- Note: Addiction is possible with prolonged use or with drug abuse.

## OPRELVEKIN
(o-prel've-kin)
Neumega
**Classifications:** BLOOD FORMER; HEMATOPOIETIC GROWTH FACTOR
**Therapeutic:** HEMATOPOIETIC GROWTH FACTOR
**Prototype:** Epoetin alfa

## AVAILABILITY Solution for injection

## ACTION & THERAPEUTIC EFFECT
The primary hematopoietic activity of oprelvekin is stimulation of production of megakaryocytes (precursors of blood platelets) and thrombocytes by the bone marrow. *Effectiveness indicated by return of postnadir platelet count toward normal (50,000 or higher). Increases platelet count in a dose-dependent manner.*

## USES Prevention of severe thrombocytopenia following myelosuppressive chemotherapy (not effective after myeloablative chemotherapy).

## CONTRAINDICATIONS Hypersensitivity to oprelvekin; myeloablative chemotherapy; myeloid malignancies; lactation.

## CAUTIOUS USE Left ventricular dysfunction, cardiac disease, CHF, history of atrial arrhythmias, or other arrhythmias; electrolyte imbalance, hypokalemia; respiratory disease; papilledema; thromboembolic disorders; older adults; cerebrovascular disease, stroke, TIAs; pleural effusion,

pericardial effusion, ascites; ICP, brain tumor, visual disturbances; hepatic or renal dysfunction; pregnancy (category C); children.

## ROUTE & DOSAGE

### Thrombocytopenia

*Adult:* **Subcutaneous** 50 mcg/kg once daily starting 6–24 h after completing chemotherapy and continuing until platelet count is 50,000 cells/mcL or higher or up to 21 days

*Renal Impairment Dosage Adjustment*

*CrCl less than 30 mL/min:* 25 mcg/kg

## ADMINISTRATION

- Note: Do not use if solution is discolored or if it contains particulate matter.

**Subcutaneous**

- Reconstitute solution by gently injecting 1 mL of sterile water for injection (without preservative) toward the sides of the vial. Keep needle in vial and gently swirl to dissolve but do not shake solution. Without removing needle, withdraw specified amount of oprelvekin for injection.
- Give as single dose into the abdomen, thigh, hip, or upper arm.
- Discard any unused portion of the vial. It contains no preservatives.
- Use reconstituted solution within 3 h; store at 2°–8° C (36°–46° F) until used.
- Store unopened vials at 2°–8° C (36°–46° F). Do not freeze.

**ADVERSE EFFECTS** (≥1%) **Body as a Whole:** *Edema, neutropenic fever, fever,* asthenia, pain, chills, myalgia, bone pain, dehydration. **CNS:** *Headache, dizziness, insomnia,* nervousness. **CV:** *Tachycardia,* vaso-

dilation, palpitations, syncope, atrial fibrillation/flutter, peripheral edema, capillary leak syndrome. **GI:** *Nausea, vomiting, mucositis, diarrhea,* oral moniliasis, anorexia, constipation, dyspepsia. **Hematologic:** Ecchymosis. **Respiratory:** *Dyspnea, rhinitis, cough, pharyngitis,* pleural effusion, pulmonary edema, exacerbation of preexisting pleural effusion. **Skin:** Alopecia, *rash,* skin discoloration, exfoliative dermatitis. **Special Senses:** Conjunctival injection, amblyopia.

**INTERACTIONS Drug:** No clinically significant interactions established.

**PHARMACOKINETICS Absorption:** 80% from subcutaneous injection site. **Onset:** Days 5–9. **Duration:** 7 days after last dose. **Distribution:** Distributes to highly perfused organs. **Elimination:** In urine. **Half-Life:** 6.9 h.

## NURSING IMPLICATIONS

### Black Box Warning

*Oprelvekin has been associated with allergic or hypersensitivity reactions, including anaphylaxis. Oprelvekin should be discontinued if patient develops an allergic or hypersensitivity reaction.*

### Assessment & Drug Effects

- Monitor carefully for and immediately report S&S of fluid overload, hypokalemia, and cardiac arrhythmias.
- Monitor persons with preexisting fluid retention carefully (e.g., CHF, pleural effusion, ascites) for worsening of symptoms.
- Monitor lab tests: Baseline and periodic CBC; platelet count at nadir and until adequate recovery; periodic serum electrolytes.

### Patient & Family Education

- Review patient information leaflet with special attention to administration directions.

---

Common adverse effects in *italic;* life-threatening effects <u>underlined</u>; generic names in **bold;** classifications in SMALL CAPS; ♣ Canadian drug name; ● Prototype drug

- Report any of the following to the prescriber: Shortness of breath, edema of arms and/or legs, chest pain, unusual fatigue or weakness, irregular heartbeat, blurred vision.

# ORITAVANCIN
(or-ita-van′sin)
Orbactiv
**Classifications:** ANTIBIOTIC; LIPOGLYCOPROTEIN
Therapeutic: ANTIBIOTIC
**Prototype:** Vancomycin

**AVAILABILITY** Lyophilized powder

## ACTION & *THERAPEUTIC EFFECT*
Binds to components required for the bacterial cell wall preventing cell wall synthesis. *It is bactericidal against Staphylococcus aureus, Streptococcus pyogenes, and Enterococcus faecalis.*

## USES
Treatment of adult patients with acute bacterial skin and skin structure infections (ABSSSI) caused or suspected to be caused by susceptible isolates of designated gram-positive microorganisms.

## CONTRAINDICATIONS
Known hypersensitivity to oritavancin; IV unfractionated heparin sodium contraindicated for 48 h after receiving oritavancin; oritavancin induced *Clostridium difficile* associated diarrhea; oritavanicn induced osteomylitis.

## CAUTIOUS USE
Hypersensitivity to other antibiotics; concomitant warfarin use; colitis; severe renal or hepatic impairment; pregnancy (category C); lactation. Safety and efficacy in children younger than 18 y not established.

## ROUTE & DOSAGE

**Skin and Skin Structure Infections**
*Adult:* **IV** 1200 mg one time dose

## ADMINISTRATION
**Intravenous**

*PREPARE:* **IV Infusion:** Three 400 mg vials are need for a single 1200 mg dose. Reconstitute each 400 mg vial with 40 mL of SW for injection to yield 10 mg/mL. Swirl vials gently until completely dissolved. Do not shake. Must be further diluted as follows: Withdraw and discard 120 mL from a 1000 mL bag of D5W; then withdraw 40 mL from each reconstituted vial and add to the D5W bag to bring volume to 1000 mL with a concentration of 1.2 mg/mL.

*ADMINISTER:* **IV Infusion:** Infuse over 3 h. Flush line before/after with D5W if line used for other drugs or solutions.

*INCOMPATIBILITIES:* Do not mix or infuse with any other drugs or solutions.

- Storage: Bag for IV infusion should be used within 6 h when stored at room temperature, or within 12 h when refrigerated at 2-8°C (36-46°F). The combined storage time (reconstituted solution in the vial and diluted solution in the bag) and 3 h infusion time should not exceed 6 h at room temperature or 12 h if refrigerated.

## ADVERSE EFFECTS (≥ 1%) **Body as a Whole:** Hypersensitivity reaction, infusion site reaction, limb and subcutaneous abscess, osteomyelitis, peripheral edema, pruritus, rash. **CNS:** Dizziness, headache. **CV:** Tachycardia. **GI:** <u>Clostridium difficile-associated diarrhea</u>, diarrhea, *nausea,*

vomiting. **Hematological:** Anemia, eosinophilia. **Metabolic:** Hyperuricemia, hypoglycemia, increased ALT and AST, increased bilirubin. **Musculoskeletal:** Myalgia, tenosynovitis. **Respiratory:** Bronchospasm, wheezing. **Skin:** Angioedema, erythema multiforme, leucocytoclastic vasculitis, urticarial.

## DIAGNOSTIC TEST INTERFERENCE

**Drug:** Oritavancin has no effect on the coagulation system; however, prolongs *aPTT* for 48 h and *INR* for up to 24 h.

## INTERACTIONS **Drug:** Oritavancin
may increase the levels of other drugs requiring CYP2C9 or CYP2C19 for metabolism (e.g., **warfarin**) and may decrease the levels of other drugs requiring CYP2D6 or CYP3A4 for metabolism (e.g., **aripiprazole, axitinib, hydrocodone, ibrutinib, saxagliptin, simeprevir**).

## PHARMACOKINETICS **Distribution:**
Widely distributed with 85% plasma protein bound. **Metabolism:** Not significantly metabolized. **Elimination:** Slowly excreted unchanged via renal and fecal elimination. **Half-Life:** 245 h.

## NURSING IMPLICATIONS

### Assessment & Drug Effects

- Monitor patients for any infusion-related reactions.
- Monitor for S&S of superinfection, including *C. difficile*-associated diarrhea (CDAD) and pseudomembranous colitis, that may develop within days or up to several months after completion of therapy.
- If superinfection is suspected, withhold drug and contact prescriber.

### Patient & Family Education

- Report promptly to prescriber if you develop frequent watery or bloody diarrhea.
- Consult with prescriber if you are a female who is or plans to become pregnant.

- Do not breast-feed without consulting prescriber.

# ORLISTAT
(or'li-stat)

Alli, Xenical

**Classifications:** ANORECTANT; NONSYSTEMIC LIPASE INHIBITOR

**Therapeutic:** ANORECTANT

**Prototype:** Diethylpropion

## AVAILABILITY Capsule

## ACTION & *THERAPEUTIC EFFECT*

Nonsystemic inhibitor of gastrointestinal lipase. Reduces intestinal absorption of dietary fat by forming inactive enzymes with pancreatic and gastric lipase in the GI tract. *Indicated by weight loss/decreased body mass index (BMI). Reduces caloric intake in obese individuals.*

## USES Weight loss and weight
maintenance in conjunction with diet and exercise.

## CONTRAINDICATIONS Hyper-
sensitivity to orlistat; malabsorption syndrome; cholestasis; gallbladder disease; hypothyroidism; organic causes of obesity; anorexia nervosa, bulimia nervosa; pregnancy (category X).

## CAUTIOUS USE Gastrointestinal
diseases including frequent diarrhea; known dietary deficiencies in fat soluble vitamins (i.e., A, D, E); history of calcium oxalate nephrolithiasis or hyperoxaluria; older adults; lactation; children younger than 12 y.

## ROUTE & DOSAGE

### Weight Loss

*Adult/Adolescent (older than 12 y):* **PO** 60 or 120 mg t.i.d. with each main meal containing fat

## ADMINISTRATION

### Oral

- Give during or up to 1 h after a meal containing fat.
- Omit dose with nonfat-containing meal or if meal is skipped.
- Store at 15°–30° C (59°–86° F). Keep bottle tightly closed; **do not** use after the printed expiration date.

## ADVERSE EFFECTS (≥1%) **Body as a Whole:** Fatigue, back pain, infection. **CNS:** *Headache,* dizziness, anxiety. **CV:** Hypertension, stroke. **GI:** *Oily spotting, flatus with discharge, fecal urgency, fatty/oily stool, oily evacuation, increased defecation,* fecal incontinence, *abdominal pain/discomfort,* nausea, infectious diarrhea, rectal pain/discomfort, tooth disorder, gingival disorder, vomiting. **Skin:** Rash. **Urogenital:** Menstrual irregularity.

## DIAGNOSTIC TEST INTERFERENCE

Monitor PT/INR in patients on chronic stable doses of **warfarin.**

## INTERACTIONS **Drug:** **Orlistat** may increase absorption of **pravastatin;** may decrease absorption of fat soluble VITAMINS (A, D, E, K), **amiodarone,** THYROID HORMONES, **cyclosporine.** Taking **orlistat** with **atazanavir, ritonavir, tenofovir disoproxil fumarate, emtricitabine, lopinavir; ritonavir,** and **emtricitabine; efavirenz; tenofovir disoproxil fumarate** may decrease HIV control.

## PHARMACOKINETICS **Absorption:** Minimal. **Metabolism:** In gastrointestinal wall. **Elimination:** In feces. **Half-Life:** 1–2 h.

## NURSING IMPLICATIONS

### Assessment & Drug Effects

- Monitor weight and BMI; closely monitor diabetics for hypoglycemia.

- Monitor BP frequently, especially with preexisting hypertension.

### Patient & Family Education

- Take a daily multivitamin containing fat-soluble vitamins at least 2 h before/after orlistat.
- Remember common GI adverse effects typically resolve after 4 wk therapy.
- Avoid high-fat meals to minimize adverse GI effects. Distribute fat calories over three main meals daily.
- Monitor weight several times weekly. *Diabetics:* Monitor blood glucose carefully following any weight loss.

# ORPHENADRINE CITRATE

(or-fen′a-dreen)

**Classification:** CENTRAL ACTING SKELETAL MUSCLE RELAXANT
**Therapeutic:** SKELETAL MUSCLE RELAXANT
**Prototype:** Cyclobenzaprine

## AVAILABILITY Sustained release tablet; solution for injection

## ACTION & *THERAPEUTIC EFFECT*
Tertiary amine anticholinergic and central-acting skeletal muscle relaxant. Relaxes tense skeletal muscles indirectly, possibly by analgesic action or by atropine-like central action. *Relieves skeletal muscle spasm.*

## USES To relieve muscle spasm discomfort associated with acute musculoskeletal conditions.

## CONTRAINDICATIONS Narrow-angle glaucoma; achalasia; pyloric or duodenal obstruction, stenosing peptic ulcers; prostatic hypertrophy or bladder neck obstruction, urinary tract obstruction; myasthenia gravis; cardiospasm; tachycardia.

## CAUTIOUS USE History of cardiac disease, arrhythmias, coronary insufficiency; asthma; GERD; hepatic

disease; renal disease; renal impairment; older adults; pregnancy (category C); lactation; children.

## ROUTE & DOSAGE

### Muscle Spasm
*Adult:* **PO** 100 mg b.i.d.; **IM/IV** 60 mg q12h, convert to PO therapy as soon as possible

## ADMINISTRATION

### Oral
- Ensure that sustained release form is not chewed or crushed. It **must be** swallowed whole.

### Intramuscular
- Give undiluted deep into a large muscle.

### Intravenous
**PREPARE: Direct:** Give undiluted. Protect from light.
**ADMINISTER: Direct:** Give at a rate of 60 mg (2 mL) over 5 min with patient in supine position. ▪ Keep supine for 5–10 min post injection.

## ADVERSE EFFECTS (≥1%) CNS:
*Drowsiness,* weakness, headache, dizziness, mild CNS stimulation (high doses: restlessness, anxiety, tremors, confusion, hallucinations, agitation, tachycardia, palpitation, syncope). **Special Senses:** Increased ocular tension, dilated pupils, blurred vision. **GI:** *Dry mouth,* nausea, vomiting, abdominal cramps, constipation. **Urogenital:** *Urinary hesitancy* or *retention.* **Body as a Whole:** Hypersensitivity [pruritus, urticaria, rash, anaphylactic reaction (rare)].

## INTERACTIONS Drug: Propoxyphene may cause increased confusion, anxiety, and tremors; may worsen schizophrenic symptoms, or increase risk of tardive dyskinesia with

**haloperidol;** additive CNS depressant with ANXIOLYTICS, SEDATIVES, HYPNOTICS, **butorphanol, nalbuphine,** OPIATE AGONISTS, **pentazocine, tramadol, cyclobenzaprine** may increase anticholinergic effects. **Herbal: Valerian, kava** potentiate sedation.

## PHARMACOKINETICS Absorption:
Readily from GI tract. **Peak:** 2 h. **Duration:** 4–6 h. **Distribution:** Rapidly distributed in tissues; crosses placenta. **Metabolism:** In liver. **Elimination:** In urine. **Half-Life:** 14 h.

## NURSING IMPLICATIONS

### Assessment & Drug Effects
- Report complaints of mouth dryness, urinary hesitancy or retention, headache, tremors, GI problems, palpitation, or rapid pulse to prescriber. Dosage reduction or drug withdrawal is indicated.
- Monitor elimination patterns. Older adults are particularly sensitive to anticholinergic effects (urinary hesitancy, constipation); closely observe.
- Monitor therapeutic drug effect. In the patient with parkinsonism, orphenadrine reduces muscular rigidity but has little effect on tremors. Some reduction in excessive salivation and perspiration may occur, and patient may appear mildly euphoric.

### Patient & Family Education
- Relieve mouth dryness by frequent rinsing with clear tepid water, increasing noncaloric fluid intake, sugarless gum, or lemon drops. If these measures fail, a saliva substitute may help.
- Do not drive or engage in potentially hazardous activities until response to drug is known.
- Avoid concomitant use of alcohol and other CNS depressants; these may potentiate depressant effects.

# OSELTAMIVIR PHOSPHATE ⓟ

(o-sel′tam-i-vir)

**Tamiflu**

**Classification:** ANTIVIRAL;
NEURAMINDASE INHIBITOR;
ANTI-INFLUENZA

**Therapeutic:** ANTI-INFLUENZA

**AVAILABILITY** Capsule; oral suspension

**ACTION & *THERAPEUTIC EFFECT***
Inhibits influenza A and B viral neuraminidase enzyme, preventing the release of newly formed virus from the surface of the infected cells. Inhibits replication of the influenza A and B virus. *Effectiveness indicated by relief of flu symptoms. Prevents viral spread across the mucous lining of the respiratory tract.*

**USES** Treatment of uncomplicated acute influenza in adults symptomatic for no more than 2 days; prophylaxis of influenza.

**UNLABELED USES** $H_1N_1$ influenza.

**CONTRAINDICATIONS** Hypersensitivity to oseltamivir; development of allegic-like reaction(s) from drug including anapylaxis and serious skin reactions; severe hepatic impairment or severe hepatic disease; viral infections other than flu. Use within 2 wk of receiving a live vaccine; ESRD. Safety in immunosuppression not established.

**CAUTIOUS USE** Hereditary fructose intolerance; cardiac disease; COPD, children with asthma; mild or moderate hepatic impairment; psychiatric disorders; renal impairment; pregnancy (category C); lactation; infants younger than 1 y for propylaxis or neonates younger than 2 wk old for influenza treatment. Safety

and efficacy in chronic cardiac/respiratory disease not established.

## ROUTE & DOSAGE

### Influenza Treatment

*Adult/Adolescent/Child (over 40 kg):* **PO** 75 mg b.i.d. × 5 days
*Child (1–12 y, weight 20–40 kg):* **PO** 60 mg b.i.d. × 5 days; *weight 16–23 kg:* 45 mg b.i.d. × 5 days; *weight less than 15 kg:* 30 mg b.i.d. × 5 days
*Infant:* **PO** 3 mg/kg b.i.d. × 5 days

### Influenza Prevention

*Adult/Adolescent/Child (1 y or older and weight over 40 kg):* **PO** 75 mg daily × 10 days; begin within 2 days of contact with infected person
*Child (weight 23–40 kg):* **PO** 60 mg daily × 10 days; *weight 15–23 kg:* 45 mg daily × 10 days; *weight less than 15 kg:* 30 mg × 10 days

### Renal Impairment Dosage Adjustment

*CrCl 10–30 mL/min:* **Treatment:** 30 mg daily × 5 days; **Prophylaxis:** 30 mg every other day

## ADMINISTRATION

### Oral

- Give with food to decrease the risk of GI upset.
- Start within 48 h of onset of flu symptoms.
- Take missed dose as soon as possible unless next dose is due within 2 h.
- Store at 15°–30° C (59°–86° F); protect from moisture, keep dry.

**ADVERSE EFFECTS** (≥1%) **Body as a Whole:** Fatigue. **CNS:** Dizziness, headache, insomnia, vertigo. **GI:**

**O**

Nausea, vomiting, diarrhea, abdominal pain. **Respiratory:** Bronchitis, cough.

## PHARMACOKINETICS Absorption:
Readily absorbed, 75% bioavailable. **Distribution:** 42% protein bound. **Metabolism:** Extensively metabolized to active metabolite oseltamivir carboxylate by liver esterases **Elimination:** Primarily in urine. **Half-Life:** 1–2 h; oseltamivir carboxylate 6–10 h.

## NURSING IMPLICATIONS
### Assessment & Drug Effects
▪ Monitor ambulation in frail and older adult patients due to potential for dizziness and vertigo.
▪ Monitor children for abnormal behavior such as delirium or self-injury.

### Patient & Family Education
▪ Contact your prescriber regarding the use of this drug in children.

## OSIMERTINIB
(oh'si-mer'ti-nib)
Tagrisso

**Classifications:** ANTINEOPLASTIC; KINASE INHIBITOR; EPIDERMAL GROWTH FACTOR RECEPTOR INHIBITOR
**Therapeutic:** ANTINEOPLASTIC
**Prototype:** Erlotinib

## AVAILABILITY Tablets

## ACTION & THERAPEUTIC EFFECT
An irreversible epidermal growth factor receptor (EGFR) tyrosine kinase inhibitor. It preferentially binds to mutant forms of EGFR as compared to the normal wild-type EGFR. It also exhibits anti-tumor activity against cell lines with EGFR-mutations, such as the T790M resistance mutation. *This mutation can cause resistance to other EGFR tyrosine kinase inhibitors.*

## USES
Treatment of patients with metastatic EGFR T790M mutation-positive non-small-cell lung cancer (NSCLC) who have failed treatment with other EGFR tyrosine kinase inhibitor (TKI) therapy.

## CAUTIOUS USE
Interstitial pulmonary disease/interstitial lung disease (ILD) or pneumonitis, including fatalities, have been reported. Permanently discontinue use in patients with confirmed, treatment-related ILD or pneumonia. Use cautiously in patients with cardiac disease or other conditions that may increase the risk of QT prolongation including cardiac arrhythmias, congenital long QT syndrome, heart failure, bradycardia, myocardial infarction, hypertension, coronary artery disease, hypomagnesemia, hypokalemia, hypocalcemia or in patients receiving medications for long QT interval. Treatment should be held with an ejection fraction of less than 50% or with more than a 10% decrease from baseline. Geriatric patients (older than 65 y) are at a higher risk of adverse effects. There are no adequate well-controlled studies in pregnant women. It is not known if osimertinib is present in human milk. Recommendations are to discontinue breast-feeding during treatment and for 2 wk after the final dose.

## ROUTE & DOSAGE

### Non-Small Cell Lung Cancer
*Adult:* **PO** 80 mg once daily

### Adverse Reaction Dosage Adjustment
*Interstitial lung disease (ILD)/ pneumonitis:* Permanently discontinue

---

Common adverse effects in *italic;* life-threatening effects underlined; generic names in **bold;** classifications in SMALL CAPS; ♣ Canadian drug name; ⊕ Prototype drug

*QTc interval greater than 500 msec on at least 2 separate ECGs:*
Withhold until QTc interval is less than 481 msec; resume at 40 mg *QTc interval prolongation with signs or symptoms of life-threatening arrhythmia:* Permanently discontinue *Decrease in LVEF of 10% from baseline and below 50%:* Withhold up to 4 wk; resume if improved to baseline; if not, permanently discontinue *Symptomatic congestive heart failure:* Permanently discontinue *Other Grade 3 reaction:* Withhold for 3 wk; resume at 40–80 mg once daily if resolved to Grade 0–2; if not, permanently

## ADMINISTRATION

**Oral**
- Take without regard to food.

**Extemporaneous Compounding Oral**
- Disperse tablet in 15 mL of non-carbonated water only.
- Stir until tablet is in small pieces, it will not completely dissolve.
- Administer immediately.
- Rinse the container with 4–8 oz (120 mL–240 mL) of water and immediately drink.
- Store between 15°–30°F (59°–86°F).

## ADVERSE EFFECTS (≥2%) **Body as a Whole:** Fatigue, pneumonia. **CNS:** Headache. **CV:** Cardiomyopathy, deep vein thrombosis, increased QTc interval, jugular vein thrombosis, pulmonary embolism. **GI:** Constipation, decreased appetite, *diarrhea*, nausea, stomatitis. **Hematological:** *Anemia, lymphopenia, neutropenia, thrombocytopenia.* **Metabolic:** *Hypermagnesemia, hyponatremia.* **Musculoskeletal:** Back

pain. **Respiratory:** Cough, interstitial lung disease, pneumonitis. **Skin:** *Acne, acneform dermatitis, dermatitis, dry skin, erythema, erythematous, folliculitis, generalized rash, maculo-papular rash, nail toxicity, pruritis, pustular rash.*

## INTERACTIONS **Drug:** Strong CYP3A inhibitors (e.g., **itraconazole, nefazodone, ritonavir, telithromycin**) may increase the levels of osimertinib. Strong CYP3A inducers (e.g., **carbamazepine, phenytoin, rifampicin**) may decrease the levels of osimertinib. Osimertinib may alter the plasma levels of **carbamazepine, cyclosporine,** ERGOT ALKALOIDS, **fentanyl, quinidine,** and **phenytoin**. **Herbal:** **St. John's Wort** may decrease the levels of osimertinib.

## PHARMACOKINETICS **Peak:** 6 h. **Metabolism:** Hepatic oxidation by CYP enzymes. **Elimination:** Fecal (68%) and renal (14%). **Half-Life:** 48 h.

## NURSING IMPLCATIONS

**Assessment & Drug Effects**
- Hazardous agent (meets NIOSH 2016 criteria for handling and disposing)—double glove, wear a gown if there is a chance of vomit or spit up, eye/face protection for administration of a liquid. Crushed tablets should be prepared in a controlled device.
- Perform respiratory assessments being alert to complaints of shortness of breath and any pain in lower extremities or jugular veins that could be related to thrombosis. Hold drug and notify prescriber if symptoms develop.
- Perform oral exams for inspection of oral mucosa and complaints of pain.
- Monitor daily weight.

- Monitor lab tests: CBC with differential, monitor ECG, ejection fraction, and serum electrolytes.

**Patient & Family Education**
- Contact medical provider for shortness of breath, new or worsening cough, or pain, edema or warmth in extremities or neck.
- Women should use effective contraception during therapy and for 6 wk after the last dose. Males with female partners of reproductive potential should also use effective contraception during therapy and for 4 mo after the last dose.
- Report any changes in balance, confusion, weakness, severe dizziness or fainting.

# OSPEMIFENE
(os-pem'ih-feen)
Osphena
**Classifications:** ESTROGEN AGONIST/ANTAGONIST; SELECTIVE ESTROGEN RECEPTOR MODIFIER (SERM)
**Therapeutic:** ESTROGEN AGONIST/ANTAGONIST
**Prototype:** Tamoxifen

AVAILABILITY Tablet

ACTION & *THERAPEUTIC EFFECT*
A selective estrogen receptor agonist/antagonist that activates estrogenic pathways in some tissues (agonist) and blocks the pathways in other tissues (antagonist). *Exerts an estrogen-like effect on the vaginal epithelium thus reversing vulvovaginal atrophy and decreasing dyspareunia.*

USES Treatment of moderate to severe dyspareunia, a symptomatic estrogen-like effect on the vaginal epithelium of vulvar and vaginal atrophy, due to menopause.

CONTRAINDICATIONS Undiagnosed abnormal genital bleeding; known or suspected neoplasia; endometrial cancer; history of breast cancer; history or active VTE, pulmonary embolism (PE), or history of these conditions; active arterial thromboembolic disease (e.g., stroke, MI, or history of these conditions); severe hepatic impairment; known or suspected pregnancy (category X); lactation.

CAUTIOUS USE Risk for DVT, PE, or history of stroke; hypertension; smoking; DM, hypercholesterolemia; obesity, SLE, mild or moderate hepatic impairment.

## ROUTE & DOSAGE

**Dyspareunia**
*Adult:* PO 60 mg once daily
**Hepatic Impairment Dosage Adjustment**
*Severe hepatic impairment (Child-Pugh class C):* Do not administer

ADMINISTRATION
**Oral**
- Give with food.
- Store at 15°–30° C (59°–86° F).

ADVERSE EFFECTS (≥1%) **Musculoskeletal:** Muscle spasms. **Skin:** Hyperhidrosis. **Urogenital:** Genital discharge, vaginal discharge.

INTERACTIONS **Drug:** Coadministration of CYP2C9 and CYP3A4 Inhibitors (e.g., **fluconazole, ketoconazole**) may increase the levels of ospemifene. Coadministration of CYP2C9 and CYP3A4 inducers (e.g., **rifampin**) may decrease the levels of ospemifene. Coadministration with other drugs that are highly plasma protein bound may cause displacement reactions resulting in increased levels of either ospemifene

Common adverse effects in *italic;* life-threatening effects <u>underlined;</u> generic names in **bold;** classifications in SMALL CAPS; ♣ Canadian drug name; ⊘ Prototype drug

1193

or other drugs. **Food:** Food increases the bioavailability of ospemifene.

## PHARMACOKINETICS **Peak:** 2–2.5 h. **Distribution:** 99% plasma protein bound. **Metabolism:** Hepatic oxidation. **Elimination:** Fecal (75%) and renal (7%). **Half-Life:** 26 h.

## NURSING IMPLICATIONS

### Black Box Warning

*Ospemifene has been associated with increased risk of endometrial cancer in women who are not receiving a progestin, and with increased risk of DVT and CVA.*

### Assessment & Drug Effects

- Monitor for and report persistent or recurring genital bleeding.
- Monitor closely those with risk factors for cardiovascular disease and thromboembolism (e.g., hypertension, DM, tobacco use, hypercholesterolemia, obesity, history of SLE).

### Patient & Family Education

- Notify prescriber immediately if you become pregnant.
- Report promptly all instances of vaginal bleeding.
- This drug may cause or increase the occurrence of hot flashes.

## OXACILLIN SODIUM ℗

(ox-a-sill'in)

Bactocill

**Classifications:** PENICILLIN ANTIBIOTIC; PENICILLINASE-RESISTANT PENICILLIN

Therapeutic: ANTIBIOTIC

## AVAILABILITY Solution for injection

## ACTION & *THERAPEUTIC EFFECT*

Oxacillin inhibits final stage of bacterial cell wall synthesis by preferentially binding to specific penicil-lin-binding proteins (PBPs) located within the bacterial cell wall, leading to destruction of the cell wall of the organism. *It is highly active against most penicillinase-producing staphylococci, and is generally ineffective against gram-negative bacteria and methicillin-resistant staphylococci (MRSA).*

## USES Infections caused by staphylococci.

## UNLABELED USES Catheter-related infections.

## CONTRAINDICATIONS Hypersensitivity to oxacillin, penicillin, or any component of formulation.

## CAUTIOUS USE History of or suspected atopy or allergy (hives, eczema, hay fever, asthma); history of GI disease; hepatic or renal impairment; CHF; older adults; pregnancy (category B); lactation (may cause infant diarrhea); premature infants, neonates.

## ROUTE & DOSAGE

### Staphylococcal Infections

*Adult/Adolescent/Child (weight greater than 40 kg):* **IV** 250 mg–1 g q4–6h (max: 12 g/day)
*Child (weight less than 40 kg):* **IV** 50–100 mg/kg/day divided q4–6h (max: 12 g/day)
*Neonate:* **IV** 25 mg/kg/day

## ADMINISTRATION

Note: The total sodium content (including that contributed by buffer) in each gram of oxacillin is approximately 3.1 mEq or 71 mg.

### Intravascular

Note: Verify correct IV concentration and rate of infusion/injection with prescriber before IV administration to neonates, infants, and children.

*PREPARE:* **Direct:** Reconstitute each 1 g or fraction thereof with 10 mL with sterile water for injection or NS to yield 250 mg/1.5 mL. **Intermittent:** Dilute required dose of reconstituted solution in 50–100 mL of D5W, NS, D5/NS, or LR. **Continuous:** Dilute required dose of reconstituted solution in up to 1000 mL of compatible IV solutions.
*ADMINISTER:* **Direct:** Give at a rate of 1 g or fraction thereof over 10 min. **Intermittent:** Give over 15–30 min. **Continuous:** Give over 6 h.
*INCOMPATIBILITIES:* Solution/additive: **Cytarabine, verapamil.** Y-site: **Amphotericin B, calcium, dantrolene, diazepam, diazoxide, diphenhydramine, dobutamine, doxycycline, esmolol, ganciclovir, gentamicin, haloperidol, hydralazine, milrinone acetate, metaraminol, minocycline, netilmicin, pentazocine, phenytoin, polymyxin B, promethazine, protamine, pyridoxine, quinidine, succinylcholine, SMZ/TMP, tobramycin, verapamil.**

## ADVERSE EFFECTS (≥1%) **Body as a Whole:** Thrombophlebitis (IV therapy), superinfections, wheezing, sneezing, fever, anaphylaxis. **GI:** Nausea, vomiting, flatulence, *diarrhea,* hepatocellular dysfunction (elevated AST, ALT, hepatitis). **Hematologic:** Eosinophilia, leukopenia, thrombocytopenia, granulocytopenia, agranulocytosis; neutropenia (reported in children). **Skin:** Pruritus, rash, urticaria. **Urogenital:** Interstitial nephritis, transient hematuria, albuminuria, azotemia (newborns and infants on high doses).

## DIAGNOSTIC TEST INTERFERENCE

Oxacillin in large doses can cause false-positive *urine protein tests* using *sulfosalicylic acid methods.*

## PHARMACOKINETICS **Peak:** 30–120 min IM; 15 min IV. **Duration:** 4–6 h IM. **Distribution:** Distributes into CNS with inflamed meninges; crosses placenta; distributed into breast milk, 90% protein bound. **Metabolism:** Enters enterohepatic circulation. **Elimination:** Primarily in urine, some in bile. **Half-Life:** 0.5–1 h.

## NURSING IMPLICATIONS

### Assessment & Drug Effects

- Ask patient prior to first dose about hypersensitivity reactions to penicillins, cephalosporins, and other allergens.
- Hepatic dysfunction (possibly a hypersensitivity reaction) has been associated with IV oxacillin; it is reversible with discontinuation of drug. Symptoms may resemble viral hepatitis or general signs of hypersensitivity and should be reported promptly: Hives, rash, fever, nausea, vomiting, abdominal discomfort, anorexia, malaise, jaundice (with dark yellow to brown urine, light-colored or clay-colored stools, pruritus).
- Withhold next drug dose and report the onset of hypersensitivity reactions and superinfections (see Appendix F).
- Monitor lab tests: Periodic LFTs, CBC with differential, platelet count, and renal function tests.

### Patient & Family Education

- Take oral medication around the clock; do not miss a dose. Take all of the medication prescribed even if you feel better, unless otherwise directed by prescriber.

## OXALIPLATIN

(ox-a-li-pla′tin)

Eloxatin

**Classifications:** ANTINEOPLASTIC; ALKYLATING AGENT
Therapeutic: ANTINEOPLASTIC
**Prototype:** Cyclophosphamide

**AVAILABILITY** Solution for injection

## ACTION & *THERAPEUTIC EFFECT*
Oxaliplatin forms inter- and intra-strand DNA cross-links that inhibit DNA replication and transcription. The cytotoxicity of oxaliplatin is cell-cycle nonspecific. *Antitumor activity of oxaliplatin in combination with 5-fluorouracil (5-FU) has antiproliferative activity against colon carcinoma that is greater than either compound alone.*

**USES** Metastatic cancer of colon and rectum.

**UNLABELED USES** Non–small-cell lung cancer, non-Hodgkin's lymphoma, ovarian cancer.

**CONTRAINDICATIONS** History of known allergy to oxaliplatin or other platinum compounds; myelosuppression; pregnancy (category D); lactation.

**CAUTIOUS USE** Renal impairment, because clearance of ultrafilterable platinum is decreased in mild, moderate, and severe renal impairment; hepatic impairment; older adults; children.

## ROUTE & DOSAGE

**Metastatic Colon or Rectal Cancer**

*Adult:* **IV** 85 mg/m² once every 2 wk × 6 mo; adjust for toxicities (see package insert for adjustments)

**Renal Impairment Dosage Adjustment**

*CrCl less than 19 mL/min:* Omit dose or change therapy

## ADMINISTRATION

**Intravenous**

Premedication with an antiemetic is recommended.

*PREPARE:* **IV Infusion:** NEVER reconstitute with NS or any solution containing chloride. ▪ Reconstitute the 50 mg vial or the 100 mg vial by adding 10 mL or 20 mL, respectively, of sterile water for injection or D5W. ▪ MUST further dilute in 250–500 mL of D5W for infusion.

*ADMINISTER:* **IV Infusion: Do not** use needles or infusion sets containing aluminum parts. ▪ Flush infusion line with D5W before and after administration of any other concomitant medication. ▪ Give over 120 min with frequent monitoring of the IV insertion site. ▪ Discontinue at the first sign of extravasation and restart IV in a different site.

*INCOMPATIBILITIES:* **Solution/additive:** CHLORIDE-CONTAINING SOLUTIONS, ALKALINE SOLUTIONS, including **sodium bicarbonate, 5-fluorouracil (5-FU), dexamethasone.** **Y-site:** ALKALINE SOLUTIONS, including **sodium bicarbonate, diazepam, 5-fluorouracil (5-FU), cefepime, cefoperazone, dantrolene, diazepam.**

▪ Store reconstituted solution up to 24 h under refrigeration at 2°–8° C (36°–46° F). ▪ After final dilution, the IV solution may be stored for 6 h at room temperature [20°–25° C (68°–77° F)] or up to 24 h under refrigeration.

**ADVERSE EFFECTS** (≥1%) **Body as a Whole:** *Fever, edema, pain,* allergic reaction, arthralgia, rigors. **CNS:** *Fatigue, neuropathy, headache,* dizziness, insomnia. **CV:** Chest pain. **GI:** *Diarrhea, nausea, vomiting, anorexia, stomatitis, constipation,*

Common adverse effects in *italic;* life-threatening effects <u>underlined</u>; generic names in **bold;** classifications in SMALL CAPS; ✦Canadian drug name; ◐ Prototype drug *abdominal pain,* reflux, dyspepsia, taste perversion, mucositis, flatulence. **Hematologic:** *Anemia,* leukopenia, thrombocytopenia, neutropenia, thromboembolism. **Metabolic:** Hypokalemia, dehydration. **Respiratory:** *Dyspnea, cough,* rhinitis, pharyngitis, epistaxis, hiccup. **Skin:** Flushing, rash, alopecia, injection site reaction. **Urogenital:** Dysuria.

**INTERACTIONS Drug:** AMINOGLYCO-SIDES, **amphotericin B, vancomycin,** and other **nephrotoxic drugs** may increase risk of renal failure.

**PHARMACOKINETICS Distribution:** Greater than 90% protein bound. **Metabolism:** Rapid and extensive nonenzymatic biotransformation. **Elimination:** Primarily in urine. **Half-Life:** 391 h.

## NURSING IMPLICATIONS

### Black Box Warning

*Oxaliplatin has been associated with anaphylactic reactions within minutes of administration.*

### Assessment & Drug Effects

- Monitor for S&S of hypersensitivity (e.g., rash, urticaria, erythema, pruritus; rarely, bronchospasm and hypotension). Discontinue drug and notify prescriber if any of these occur.
- Monitor insertion site. Extravasation may cause local pain and inflammation that may be severe and lead to complications, including necrosis.
- Monitor for S&S of coagulation disorders including GI bleeding, hematuria, and epistaxis.
- Monitor for S&S of peripheral neuropathy (e.g., paresthesia, dysesthesia, hypoesthesia in the hands, feet, perioral area, or throat, jaw spasm, abnormal tongue sensation, dysar-

thria, eye pain, and chest pressure). Symptoms may be precipitated or exacerbated by exposure to cold temperature or cold objects.

- Do not apply ice to oral mucous membranes (e.g., mucositis prophylaxis) during the infusion of oxaliplatin as cold temperature can exacerbate acute neurological symptoms.
- Monitor lab tests: Before each administration cycle, WBC with differential, hemoglobin, platelet count, and blood chemistries (including ALT, AST, bilirubin, and creatinine). Baseline and periodic renal function tests.

### Patient & Family Education

- Use effective methods of contraception while receiving this drug.
- Avoid cold drinks, use of ice, and cover exposed skin prior to exposure to cold temperature or cold objects.
- Do not drive or engage in potentially hazardous activities until response to drug is known.
- Report any of the following to a health care provider: Difficulty writing, buttoning, swallowing, walking, numbness, tingling or other unusual sensations in extremities; non-productive cough or shortness of breath; fever, particularly if associated with persistent diarrhea or other evidence of infection.
- Report promptly S&S of a bleeding disorder such as black tarry stool, coke-colored or frankly bloody urine, bleeding from the nose or mucous membranes.

## OXANDROLONE
(ox-an′dro-lone)
Oxandrin
**Classification:** ANDROGEN/ANABOLIC STEROID

Common adverse effects in *italic;* life-threatening effects underlined; generic names in **bold;** classifications in SMALL CAPS; ♣ Canadian drug name; ☺ Prototype drug

1197

**Therapeutic:** ANABOLIC STEROID
**Prototype:** Testosterone
**Controlled Substance:** Schedule III

## AVAILABILITY Tablet

## ACTION & *THERAPEUTIC EFFECT*

A synthetic derivative of testosterone that promotes weight gain after weight loss following extensive surgery, chronic infections, or severe trauma. It offsets the protein catabolism associated with prolonged administration of corticosteroids, and relieves bone pain frequently accompanying osteoporosis. *Promotes weight gain and relieves bone pain caused by osteoporosis.*

## USES Adjunctive therapy to promote weight gain, offset protein catabolism associated with prolonged administration of corticosteroids, relieve bone pain accompanying osteoporosis.

## CONTRAINDICATIONS Hypersensitivity or toxic reactions to androgens; severe cardiac, hepatic, or renal disease; possibility of virilization of external genitalia of female fetus; polycythemia; hypercalcemia; known or suspected prostatic or breast cancer in males; benign prostatic hypertrophy with obstruction; patients easily stimulated sexually; asthenic males who may react adversely to androgenic overstimulation; conditions aggravated by fluid retention; hypertension; pregnancy (category X); lactation.

## CAUTIOUS USE Cardiac, hepatic, and mild to moderate renal disease, hypercholesterolemia, heart failure, peripheral edema, arteriosclerosis, coronary artery disease, MI; cholestasis; DM; BPH; prepubertal males, acute intermittent porphyria; older adults; children.

## ROUTE & DOSAGE

**Weight Gain**

*Adult:* **PO** 2.5 mg b.i.d. to q.i.d. (max: 20 mg/day) for 2–4 wk
*Child:* **PO** 0.1 mg/kg/day

**Bone Pain**

*Adult:* **PO** 2.5–20 mg b.i.d. to q.i.d. for 2–4 wk

## ADMINISTRATION

**Oral**
- Individualize doses; great variations in response exist.
- Store at 15°–30° C (59°–86° F).

## ADVERSE EFFECTS (≥1%) **CNS:** Habituation, excitation, insomnia, depression, changes in libido. **Urogenital:** *Males:* Phallic enlargement, increased frequency or persistence of erections, inhibition of testicular function, testicular atrophy, oligospermia, impotence, chronic priapism, epididymitis, bladder irritability; *Females:* Clitoral enlargement, menstrual irregularities. **Hepatic:** Cholestatic jaundice with or without hepatic necrosis and death, hepatocellular neoplasms, peliosis hepatitis (long-term use). **Skin:** Hirsutism and male pattern baldness in females, acne. **Endocrine:** Gynecomastia, deepening of voice in females, premature closure of epiphyses in children, edema, decreased glucose tolerance.

## DIAGNOSTIC TEST INTERFERENCE

May decrease levels of thyroxine-binding globulin (decreased total $T_4$ and increased $T_3$ RU and free $T_4$).

## INTERACTIONS **Drug:** May increase INR with **warfarin.** May inhibit metabolism of ORAL HYPOGLYCEMIC AGENTS. Concomitant STEROIDS

0

Common adverse effects in *italic;* life-threatening effects underlined; generic names in **bold;** classifications in SMALL CAPS; ♣ Canadian drug name; ⓞ Prototype drug may increase edema. **Herbal: Echinacea** may increase risk of hepatotoxicity.

## PHARMACOKINETICS    Half-Life:
10–13 h (increased in elderly patients).

## NURSING IMPLICATIONS

### Black Box Warning

*Oxandrolone has been associated with hepatic dysfunction, liver failure, liver cell tumors, and increased risk of atherosclerosis from blood lipid changes.*

### Assessment & Drug Effects
- Monitor weight closely throughout therapy.
- Assess for and report development of edema or S&S of jaundice (see Appendix F).
- Withhold and notify prescriber if hypercalcemia develops in breast cancer patient.
- Monitor growth in children closely.
- Monitor lab tests: Periodic LFTs, lipid profile, Hct and Hgb.

### Patient & Family Education
- Women: Report signs of virilization, including acne and changes in menstrual periods.
- Men: Report too frequent or prolonged erections or appearance/worsening of acne.
- Report S&S of jaundice (see Appendix F) or edema.
- Monitor blood glucose for loss of glycemic control if diabetic.

## OXAPROZIN
(ox-a-pro′zin)
Daypro
**Classification:** ANALGESIC, NON-STEROIDAL ANTI-INFLAMMATORY DRUG (NSAID)

Therapeutic: NONNARCOTIC ANALGESIC, NSAID; ANTIRHEUMATIC; ANTIPYRETIC
**Prototype:** Ibuprofen

## AVAILABILITY Tablet

## ACTION & *THERAPEUTIC EFFECT*
Long-acting NSAID agent, which is an effective prostaglandin synthetase inhibitor. It inhibits COX-1 and COX-2 enzymes needed for prostaglandin synthesis at the site of inflammation. *Has anti-inflammatory, antipyretic, and analgesic properties.*

**USES** Treatment of osteoarthritis and rheumatoid arthritis, juvenile rheumatoid arthritis.

**UNLABELED USES** Ankylosing spondylitis, chronic pain, gout, oral surgery pain, temporal arteritis, tendinitis.

**CONTRAINDICATIONS** Hypersensitivity to oxaprozin, salicylates, or any other NSAID; UGI bleeding; complete or partial syndrome of nasal polyps; angioedema; CABG perioperative pain; pregnancy (category D third trimester); lactation.

**CAUTIOUS USE** History of GI bleeding, alcoholism, smoking; history of severe hepatic dysfunction, renal insufficiency; cardiac disease; coagulopathy; photosensitivity; older adults; pregnancy (category C first and second trimester). Safety and efficacy in children younger than 6 y not established.

## ROUTE & DOSAGE

### Osteoarthritis, Rheumatoid Arthritis
*Adult:* **PO** 600–1200 mg daily (max: 1800 mg/day or 26 mg/kg, whichever is lower)

---

Common adverse effects in *italic;* life-threatening effects underlined; generic names in **bold;** classifications in SMALL CAPS; ♣Canadian drug name; ☻ Prototype drug

**Juvenile Rheumatoid Arthritis**

*Adolescent/Child (6 y or older, weight over 55 kg):* PO 1200 mg qd; *weight 32–54 kg:* 900 mg qd; *weight 22–31 kg:* 600 mg qd

## ADMINISTRATION

### Oral

- Give with meals or milk to decrease GI distress.
- Divide doses in those unable to tolerate once-daily dosing.
- Use lower starting doses for those with renal or hepatic dysfunction, advanced age, low body weight, or a predisposition to GI ulceration.

## ADVERSE EFFECTS (≥1%) CNS:

*Tinnitus, headache, insomnia, somnolence.* GI: *Diarrhea, abdominal pain, nausea, dyspepsia, flatulence, melena,* ulcers, *constipation, dry mouth,* gastritis. Skin: *Rash, pruritus.* Urogenital: *Dysuria, urinary frequency.*

## DIAGNOSTIC TEST INTERFERENCE

May cause false-positive reactions for BENZODIAZEPINES with *urine drug-screening* tests.

## INTERACTIONS Drug: May attenuate the antihypertensive response to DIURETICS. NSAIDs increase the risk of **methotrexate** or **lithium** toxicity. Use caution with ANTICOAGULANTS, PLATELET INHIBITORS. May increase **aspirin** toxicity. Do not use with **cidofovir** or **ketorolac.** Herbal: **Feverfew, garlic, ginger, ginkgo** may increase risk of bleeding.

## PHARMACOKINETICS Absorption: Readily from GI tract. Peak: 125 min. Onset: 1–6 wk for maximum therapeutic effect. Distribution: 99% protein bound. Distributes into synovial fluid, crosses placenta. Distributed into breast milk. Metabolism: In the liver. Elimination: 60% in urine, 30–35% in feces. Half-Life: 40 h.

## NURSING IMPLICATIONS

### Black Box Warning

*Oxaprozin has been associated with increased risk of serious, potentially fatal, GI bleeding and cardiovascular events (e.g., MI & CVA); risk may increase with duration of use and may be greater in the older adult and those with risk factors for CV disease.*

### Assessment & Drug Effects

- Monitor for S&S of GI bleeding, especially in patients with a history of inflammation or ulceration of upper GI tract, or those treated chronically with NSAIDs.
- Monitor for and report promptly S&S of CV thrombotic events (i.e., angina, MI, TIA, or stroke).
- Monitor patients with CHF for increased fluid retention and edema. Report rapid weight increases accompanied by edema.
- Auditory and ophthalmologic exams are recommended with prolonged or high-dose therapy.
- Monitor lab tests: Baseline and periodic Hgb, LFTs and renal function tests.

### Patient & Family Education

- Report immediately dark tarry stools, "coffee ground" or bloody emesis, or other GI distress.
- Avoid aspirin or other NSAIDs without explicit permission of prescriber.
- Stop taking drug and report promptly to prescriber if you experience chest pain, shortness of breath, weakness, slurring of speech, or other signs of a cardiac or neurologic problem.

- Be aware of the possibility of photosensitivity, which results in a rash on sun-exposed skin.
- Report immediately to prescriber ringing in ears, decreased hearing, or blurred vision.
- Do not exceed ordered dose. The goal of therapy is lowest effective dose.

## OXAZEPAM

(ox-a′ze-pam)

Ox-Pam ◆, Zapex ◆

**Classifications:** ANXIOLYTIC; SEDATIVE-HYPNOTIC; BENZODIAZEPINE
**Therapeutic:** ANTIANXIETY; SEDATIVE-HYPNOTIC
**Prototype:** Lorazepam
**Controlled Substance:** Schedule IV

**AVAILABILITY** Capsule; tablet

**ACTION & *THERAPEUTIC EFFECT***
Benzodiazepine derivative related to lorazepam. Effects are mediated by the inhibitory neurotransmitter GABA, and acts on the thalamic, hypothalamic, and limbic levels of CNS. *Has anxiolytic, sedative, hypnotic, and skeletal muscle relaxant effects*.

**USES** Management of anxiety; control acute withdrawal symptoms in chronic alcoholism.

**CONTRAINDICATIONS** Hypersensitivity to oxazepam and other benzodiazepines; respiratory depression; psychoses, suicidal ideation; acute alcohol intoxication; acute-angle glaucoma; pregnancy (category D); lactation.

**CAUTIOUS USE** Impaired kidney and liver function; alcoholism; addiction-prone patients; COPD; history of seizures; history of suicide; mental depression; bipolar disorder; older adults and debilitated patients; children younger than 6 y.

## ROUTE & DOSAGE

**Anxiety**
*Adult/Adolescent/Child (6 y or older):* **PO** 10–30 mg t.i.d. or q.i.d.
**Acute Alcohol Withdrawal**
*Adult:* **PO** 15–30 mg t.i.d. or q.i.d.

## ADMINISTRATION

**Oral**
- Give with food if GI upset occurs.
- Store in a tightly closed container at 15°–30° C (59°–86° F) unless otherwise specified.

**ADVERSE EFFECTS** (≥1%) **CNS:** *Drowsiness,* dizziness, mental confusion, vertigo, ataxia, headache, lethargy, syncope, tremor, slurred speech, paradoxic reaction (euphoria, excitement). **GI:** Nausea, xerostomia, jaundice. **Skin:** Skin rash, edema. **CV:** Hypotension, edema. **Hematologic:** Leukopenia. **Urogenital:** Altered libido.

**INTERACTIONS Drug: Alcohol,** CNS DEPRESSANTS, ANTICONVULSANTS potentiate CNS depression; **cimetidine** increases oxazepam plasma levels, increasing its toxicity; may decrease antiparkinsonism effects of **levodopa;** may increase **phenytoin** levels; smoking decreases sedative and antianxiety effects. **Herbal: Kava, valerian** may potentiate sedation.

**PHARMACOKINETICS Absorption:** Readily absorbed from GI tract. **Peak:** 2–3 h. **Distribution:** Crosses placenta; distributed into breast milk. **Metabolism:** In liver. **Elimination:** Primarily in urine, some in feces. **Half-Life:** 2–8 h.

Common adverse effects in *italic;* life-threatening effects underlined; generic names in **bold;** classifications in SMALL CAPS; ◆ Canadian drug name; ⊘ Prototype drug

1201

## NURSING IMPLICATIONS

### Assessment & Drug Effects

- Observe older adult patients closely for signs of overdosage. Report to prescriber if daytime psychomotor function is depressed.
- Monitor for increased signs and symptoms of suicidality.
- Note: Excessive and prolonged use may cause physical dependence.
- Monitor lab tests: Periodic LFTs and WBC count.

### Patient & Family Education

- Report promptly any mild paradoxic stimulation of affect and excitement with sleep disturbances that may occur within the first 2 wk of therapy. Dosage reduction is indicated.
- Consult prescriber before self-medicating with OTC drugs.
- Do not drive or engage in potentially hazardous activities until response to drug is known.
- Do not drink alcoholic beverages while taking oxazepam. The CNS depressant effects of each agent may be intensified.
- Contact prescriber if you intend to or do become pregnant during therapy about discontinuing the drug.
- Withdraw drug slowly following prolonged therapy to avoid precipitating withdrawal symptoms (seizures, mental confusion, nausea, vomiting, muscle and abdominal cramps, tremulousness, sleep disturbances, unusual irritability, hyperhidrosis).

## OXCARBAZEPINE

(ox-car′ba-ze-peen)
Oxtellar XR, Trileptal
**Classification:** ANTICONVULSANT
Therapeutic: ANTICONVULSANT
**Prototype:** Carbamazepine

**AVAILABILITY** Tablet; extended release tablet; oral suspension

## ACTION & *THERAPEUTIC EFFECT*

Anticonvulsant properties may result from blockage of voltage-sensitive sodium channels, which results in stabilization of hyperexcited neural membranes. *Inhibits repetitive neuronal firing, and decreased propagation of neuronal impulses.*

**USES** Monotherapy or adjunctive therapy in the treatment of partial seizures in adults and children age 4–16 y.

**CONTRAINDICATIONS** Hypersensitivity to oxcarbazepine including skin reactions; suicidal ideation or behavior; drug induced agranulocytosis, pancytopenia, leukopenia; lactation.

**CAUTIOUS USE** Renal impairment; renal failure; severe hepatic impairment; patients at risk for hyponatremia; Asian ancestry; infertility; suicidal tendencies; CNS effects including somnolence and gait changes; older adults; pregnancy (category C); children younger than 2 y. **Extended Release:** Use in children 6 y or older.

## ROUTE & DOSAGE

### Partial Seizures

*Adult:* **PO** Start with 300 mg b.i.d. and increase by 600 mg/day qwk to 1200–2400 mg/day in 2 divided doses for monotherapy or 1200 mg/day as adjunctive therapy
*Child (2–16 y):* **PO** Initiate with 8–10 mg/kg/day divided b.i.d. (max: 600 mg/day), gradually increase weekly to target dose

Common adverse effects in *italic;* life-threatening effects <u>underlined;</u> generic names in **bold;** classifications in SMALL CAPS; ♣ Canadian drug name; ⏺ Prototype drug (divided b.i.d.) based on weight: *Weight 20–29 kg:* 900 mg/day; *weight 29.1–39 kg:* 1200 mg/day; *weight greater than 39 kg:* 1800 mg/day

**Renal Impairment Dosage Adjustment**

*CrCl less than 30 mL/min:* Initiate at ½ usual starting dose (300 mg b.i.d.)

## ADMINISTRATION

### Oral

- Ensure that extended release tablet is swallowed whole. It should not be crushed or chewed.
- Initiate therapy at one-half the usual starting dose (300 mg/day) if creatinine clearance is less than 30 mL/min.
- Do not abruptly stop this medication; withdraw drug gradually when discontinued to minimize seizure potential.
- Store preferably at 25° C (77° F), but room temperature permitted. Keep container tightly closed.

## ADVERSE EFFECTS (≥1%) Body as a Whole: *Fatigue,* asthenia, peripheral edema, generalized edema, chest pain, weight gain. **CV:** Hypotension. **GI:** *Nausea, vomiting, abdominal pain,* diarrhea, dyspepsia, constipation, gastritis, anorexia, dry mouth. **Hematologic:** Lymphadenopathy. **Metabolic:** Hyponatremia. **Musculoskeletal:** Muscle weakness. **CNS:** *Headache, dizziness, somnolence, ataxia, nystagmus, abnormal gait, drowsiness,* insomnia, tremor, nervousness, agitation, abnormal coordination, speech disorder, confusion, abnormal thinking, aggravate convulsions, emotional lability. **Respiratory:** Rhinitis, cough, bronchitis,

pharyngitis. **Skin:** Acne, hot flushes, purpura, <u>Stevens–Johnson syndrome, toxic epidermal necrolysis</u>. **Special Senses:** *Diplopia, vertigo, abnormal vision,* abnormal accommodation, taste perversion, ear ache. **Urogenital:** Urinary tract infection, micturition frequency, vaginitis.

## INTERACTIONS Drug: **Carbamazepine, phenobarbital, phenytoin, valproic acid, verapamil;** CALCIUM CHANNEL BLOCKERS may decrease oxcarbazepine levels; may increase levels of **phenobarbital, phenytoin;** may decrease levels of **felodipine,** ORAL CONTRACEPTIVES. Do not use with transdermal **selegiline, cobicistat, elvitegravir, dasabuvir/ombitasvir/paritaprevir/ritonavir. Herbal: Ginkgo** may decrease anti-convulsant effectiveness. **Evening primrose oil** may decrease the seizure threshold.

## PHARMACOKINETICS Absorption: Rapidly and completely from GI tract. **Peak:** Steady-state levels reached in 2–3 days. **Distribution:** 40% protein bound. **Metabolism:** Extensively metabolized in liver to active 10-monohydroxy metabolite (MHD). **Elimination:** 95% in kidneys. **Half-Life:** 2 h, MHD 9 h.

## NURSING IMPLICATIONS

### Assessment & Drug Effects

- Monitor for and report S&S of: Hyponatremia (e.g., nausea, malaise, headache, lethargy, confusion); CNS impairment (e.g., somnolence, excessive fatigue, cognitive deficits, speech or language problems, incoordination, gait disturbances).
- Monitor phenytoin levels when administered concurrently.
- Monitor lab tests: Periodic serum sodium; plasma level of the

---

Common adverse effects in *italic;* life-threatening effects <u>underlined</u>; generic names in **bold**; classifications in SMALL CAPS; ✤ Canadian drug name; ❷ Prototype drug concomitant antiepileptic drug during titration of the oxcarbazepine dose.

**Patient & Family Education**

- Notify prescriber of the following: Dizziness, excess drowsiness, frequent headaches, malaise, double vision, lack of coordination, or persistent nausea.
- Exercise special caution with concurrent use of alcohol or CNS depressants.
- Use caution with potentially hazardous activities and driving until response to drug is known.
- Use or add barrier contraceptive since drug may render hormonal methods ineffective.

# OXICONAZOLE NITRATE

(ox-i-con′a-zole)

Oxistat

**Classification:** AZOLE ANTIFUNGAL
**Therapeutic:** ANTIFUNGAL
**Prototype:** Fluconazole

**AVAILABILITY** Cream; lotion

## ACTION & THERAPEUTIC EFFECT

Topical synthetic antifungal agent that presumably works by altering the cellular membrane of the fungi, resulting in increased membrane permeability, secondary metabolic effects, and growth inhibition. *Prevents growth of fungi that cause tinea pedis, tinea cruris, and tinea corporis.*

**USES** Topical treatment of tinea pedis, tinea cruris, and tinea corporis due to *Trichophyton rubrum* and *Trichophyton mentagrophytes;* also used for cutaneous candidiasis caused by *Candida albicans* and *Candida tropicalis.*

## CONTRAINDICATIONS Hypersensitivity to oxiconazole.

**CAUTIOUS USE** Hypersensitivity to other azole antifungals; pregnancy (category B); lactation.

## ROUTE & DOSAGE

**Tinea and Other Dermal Infections**

*Adult:* **Topical** Apply to affected area once daily in the evening

## ADMINISTRATION

**Topical**

- Apply cream to cover the affected areas once daily (in the evening).
- Treat tinea corporis and tinea cruris for 2 wk; tinea pedis for 1 mo to reduce the possibility of recurrence.
- Store at 15°–30° C (59°–86° F).

**ADVERSE EFFECTS** (≥1%) **Skin:** Transient burning and stinging, dryness, erythema, pruritus, and local irritation.

**PHARMACOKINETICS Absorption:** Less than 0.3% is absorbed systemically.

## NURSING IMPLICATIONS

**Patient & Family Education**

- Use only externally. Do not use intravaginally.
- Discontinue drug and contact prescriber if irritation or sensitivity develops.
- Avoid contact with eyes.
- Contact prescriber if no improvement is noted after the prescribed treatment period.

# OXYBUTYNIN CHLORIDE ℗

(ox-i-byoo′ti-nin)

Ditropan XL, Gelnique, Oxytrol

**Classifications:** ANTICHOLINERGIC; ANTIMUSCARINIC; GU ANTISPASMODIC
**Therapeutic:** GU ANTISPASMODIC

**AVAILABILITY** Tablet; extended release tablet; oral solution; transdermal patch; topical gel

## ACTION & *THERAPEUTIC EFFECT*

Exerts a direct antispasmodic effect on smooth muscle and inhibits the muscarinic action of acetylcholine on smooth muscle. *Relaxes bladder smooth muscle and increases bladder capacity.*

**USES** To relieve symptoms associated with voiding in patients with uninhibited neurogenic bladder and reflex neurogenic bladder. Also has been used to relieve pain of bladder spasm following transurethral surgical procedures.

**CONTRAINDICATIONS** Hypersensitivity of oxybutynin; narrow angle glaucoma, myasthenia gravis, partial or complete GI obstruction, gastric retention, paralytic ileus, intestinal atony (especially older adult or debilitated patients), megacolon, pyloric stenosis, severe colitis, GU obstruction, urinary retention, unstable cardiovascular status. **Extended Release:** With renal impairment.

**CAUTIOUS USE** Autonomic neuropathy, hiatus hernia with reflex esophagitis; hepatic or renal dysfunction; urinary infection; hyperthyroidism; CHF, coronary artery disease, hypertension; prostatic hypertrophy; older adults; pregnancy (category B); lactation; children 6 y and older.

## ROUTE & DOSAGE

**Overactive Bladder**

*Adult/Adolescent:* **PO** 5 mg 2–3 × day (max: 20 mg/day); **Sustained release** 5 mg daily, may increase up to 30 mg/day; **Topical** Apply 1 patch twice weekly; or apply contents of 1 10% gel package once daily
*Geriatric:* **PO** 2.5–5 mg b.i.d. (max: 15 mg/day) or; **Sustained release** 5 mg daily, may increase up to 30 mg/day, **Topical** Apply 1 patch twice weekly
*Child (6 y or older):* **PO** 5 mg daily

## ADMINISTRATION

### Oral

- Ensure that sustained release form is not chewed or crushed. It **must be** swallowed whole. May be given without regard to meals and should be given at the same time each day.

### Topical

- Ensure that old patch is removed prior to application of new patch.
- Gel may be applied to abdomen, upper arms/shoulder, and thigh. Squeeze entire contents of the gel packet onto application site. Wear gloves and gently rub into skin until dried. Avoid contact with eyes, nose, open sores, recently shaved skin, and skin with rashes.

**ADVERSE EFFECTS** (≥1%) **Body as a Whole:** Severe allergic reactions including urticaria, skin rashes, suppression of lactation, decreased sweating, fever. **CNS:** *Drowsiness, dizziness, weakness, insomnia, headache, restlessness, psychotic behavior (overdosage).* **CV:** Palpitations, tachycardia, flushing. **Special Senses:** Mydriasis, *blurred vision,* cycloplegia, increased ocular tension. **GI:** *Dry mouth,* nausea, vomiting, *constipation,* bloated feeling. **Skin:** *Pruritus at application site,* rash, application site reactions, erythema. **Urogenital:** Urinary hesitancy or retention, impotence.

**INTERACTIONS: Drugs:** Do not use with **alosetron, idelalisib, tegaserod.**

Common adverse effects in *italic*; life-threatening effects underlined; generic names in **bold**; classifications in SMALL CAPS; ♣ Canadian drug name; ⓟ Prototype drug

1205

**PHARMACOKINETICS Absorption:** Diffuses across intact skin. **Onset:** 0.5–1 h. **Peak:** 3–6 h. **Duration:** 6–10 h. **PO:** 96 h transdermal. **Metabolism:** In liver. **Elimination:** Primarily in urine. **Half-Life:** 2–5 h.

## NURSING IMPLICATIONS

### Assessment & Drug Effects

- Periodic interruptions of therapy are recommended to determine patient's need for continued treatment. Tolerance has occurred in some patients.
- Keep prescriber informed of expected responses to drug therapy (e.g., effect on urinary frequency, urgency, urge incontinence, nocturia, completeness of bladder emptying).
- Monitor patients with colostomy or ileostomy closely; abdominal distention and the onset of diarrhea in these patients may be early signs of intestinal obstruction or of toxic megacolon.

### Patient & Family Education

- Do not drive or engage in potentially hazardous activities until response to drug is known.
- Exercise caution in hot environments. By suppressing sweating, oxybutynin can cause fever and heat stroke.

# OXYCODONE HYDROCHLORIDE

(ox-i-koe′done)

Oxaydo, OxyContin, Roxicodone, Roxybond, Xtampza

**Classifications:** NARCOTIC (OPIATE AGONIST); ANALGESIC
**Therapeutic:** NARCOTIC ANALGESIC
**Prototype:** Morphine
**Controlled Substance:** Schedule II

**AVAILABILITY** Tablet. **OxyContin:** Sustained release tablet; oral solution

## ACTION & *THERAPEUTIC EFFECT*

Semisynthetic derivative of an opium agonist that binds with stereo-specific receptors in various sites of CNS to alter both perception of pain and emotional response to pain. *Active against moderate to moderately severe pain. Appears to be more effective in relief of acute than long-standing pain.*

**USES** Relief of moderate to moderately severe pain, neuralgia. Relieves postoperative, postextractional, postpartum pain.

**CONTRAINDICATIONS** Hypersensitivity to oxycodone and principle drugs with which it is combined; bronchial asthma; known gastrointestinal obstruction; significant respiratory depression. pregnancy (category D for prolonged use or high doses at term); lactation.

**CAUTIOUS USE** Alcoholism; renal or hepatic disease; viral infections; Addison's disease; cardiac arrhythmias; chronic ulcerative colitis; history of drug abuse or dependency; gallbladder disease, acute abdominal conditions; head injury, intracranial lesions; history of seizures, hypothyroidism; BPH; respiratory disease; urethral stricture; peptic ulcer or coagulation abnormalities (combination products containing aspirin); older adult or debilitated patients; children.

## ROUTE & DOSAGE

### Moderate to Severe Pain

*(Dose individualized per opioid tolerance and patient response)*

Adult: **PO** 5–15 mg q4–6h prn; **Controlled release** 10 mg q12h (reserved for opioid tolerant patients)

Common adverse effects in *italic*; life-threatening effects <u>underlined</u>; generic names in **bold**; classifications in SMALL CAPS; ♣ Canadian drug name; ⊘ Prototype drug

*Hepatic Impairment Dosage Adjustment*

Start initial therapy at ⅓ to ½ normal dose and titrate carefully

## ADMINISTRATION

### Oral

- Ensure that sustained release form is not chewed or crushed. It **must be** swallowed whole.
- Administer with approximately the same amount of food to ensure consistent plasma levels.
- May be administered via gastrostomy or nasogastric tube. Flush the tube with water, pour capsule contents into the tube with 15 mL of water; flush tube 2 more times with 10 mL of water per flush; milk or nutritional supplements may be used for flushing instead of water.
- Store at 15°–30° C (59°–86° F). Protect from light and moisture.

## ADVERSE EFFECTS (≥1%) CNS:

Euphoria, dysphoria, abnormal dreaming, agitation, abnormal thinking, anxiety, lightheadedness, *headache, dizziness, sedation.* **GI:** Anorexia, nausea, abdominal pain, vomiting, *constipation,* jaundice, hepatotoxicity (combinations containing acetaminophen). **Respiratory:** Shortness of breath, cough, respiratory depression. **Skin:** Pruritus, skin rash. **CV:** Bradycardia, flushing, edema, orthostatic hypotension. **Endrocrine and Metabolic:** Hyperglycemia, hyponatremia. **Body as a Whole:** Unusual bleeding or bruising, arthralgia, back pain, fever, blurred vision. **Urogenital:** Dysuria, frequency of urination, urinary retention. **Ocular:** Miosis.

## DIAGNOSTIC TEST INTERFERENCE

*Serum amylase* levels may be elevated because oxycodone causes spasm of sphincter of Oddi. *Blood glucose determinations:* False decrease (measured by *glucose oxidase-peroxidase method*). *5-HIAA determination:* False positive with use of *nitroisonaphthol reagent* (quantitative test is unaffected).

## INTERACTIONS Drug: Alcohol

and other CNS DEPRESSANTS add to CNS depressant activity. Monitor closely if used with **amiodarone.** Use caution with CYP3A4 INHIBITORS due to increased risk of toxicities. Serotonin syndrome could occur when used with TRIPTANS. Do not use with BENZODIAZEPINES due to increased risk of sedation. **Herbal: St. John's wort** may increase sedation. **Food:** Grapefruit juice can increase adverse effects.

## PHARMACOKINETICS Absorption: Readily from GI tract.

**Onset:** 10–15 min. **Peak:** 30–60 min. **Duration:** 4–5 h. **Distribution:** Crosses placenta; distributed into breast milk. **Metabolism:** In liver by CYP3A4, CYP2D6. **Elimination:** Primarily in urine. **Half-Life:** 3–5 h.

## NURSING IMPLICATIONS

### Black Box Warning

*Oxycodone has been associated with high abuse potential, and life-threatening respiratory depression, neonatal opioid withdrawal, Cytochrome P450 3A4 interaction.*

### Assessment & Drug Effects

- Monitor respiratory status. Withhold drug and notify prescriber if respiratory depression occurs.
- Monitor patient's response closely, especially to sustained-release preparations.

Common adverse effects in *italic;* life-threatening effects underlined; generic names in **bold;** classifications in SMALL CAPS; ♣ Canadian drug name; ● Prototype drug

1207

- Consult prescriber if nausea continues after first few days of therapy.
- Note: Lightheadedness, dizziness, sedation, or fainting appears to be more prominent in ambulatory than in nonambulatory patients and may be alleviated if patient lies down. Monitor blood pressure.
- Evaluate patient's continued need for oxycodone preparations. Monitor effectiveness of pain relief. Psychic and physical dependence and tolerance may develop with repeated use. The potential for drug abuse is high.
- Be aware that serious overdosage of any oxycodone preparation presents problems associated with a narcotic overdose (respiratory depression, circulatory collapse, extreme somnolence progressing to stupor, coma, or death.) After long term use, discontinuation should be tapered. Monitor for signs of opioid withdrawal.

**Patient & Family Education**

- Do not alter dosage regimen by increasing, decreasing, or shortening intervals between doses. Habit formation and liver damage may result.
- Avoid potentially hazardous activities such as driving a car or operating machinery while using oxycodone preparation.
- Do not drink large amounts of alcoholic beverages while using oxycodone preparations; risk of liver damage is increased.
- Check with prescriber before taking OTC drugs for colds, stomach distress, allergies, insomnia, or pain.
- Inform surgeon or dentist that you are taking an oxycodone preparation before any surgical procedure is undertaken.

# OXYMETAZOLINE HYDROCHLORIDE

(ox-i-met-az'oh-leen)

Afrin, Dristan, Nafrine ♥, Neo-Synephrine 12 Hour, Nostrilla, Rhofade

**Classifications:** NASAL PREPARATION; DECONGESTANT

Therapeutic: DECONGESTANT

**Prototype:** Naphazoline

**AVAILABILITY** Intranasal solution; cream; ophthalmic drop

## ACTION & *THERAPEUTIC EFFECT*

Sympathomimetic agent that acts directly on alpha receptors of sympathetic nervous system resulting in relief of nasal congestion. *Constricts smaller arterioles in nasal passages and has prolonged decongestant effect.*

**USES** Relief of nasal congestion in a variety of allergic and infectious disorders of the upper respiratory tract; ocular pruritis (ophthalmic drops); acne rosacea (cream).

**CONTRAINDICATIONS** Closed-angle glaucoma.

**CAUTIOUS USE** Within 14 days of MAO inhibitors, CAD, hypertension, hyperthyroidism, DM; lactation; children younger than 2 y.

## ROUTE & DOSAGE

### Nasal Congestion

*Adult /Adolescent/Child (6 y and older):* **Intranasal** 2–3 drops or 2–3 sprays of 0.05% solution into each nostril b.i.d. for up to 3–5 days

### Acne Rosacea (cream only)

*Adult:* **Topical** Apply thin layer once daily

Common adverse effects in *italic;* life-threatening effects <u>underlined</u>; generic names in **bold;** classifications in SMALL CAPS; ♣ Canadian drug name; ⊙ Prototype drug

## ADMINISTRATION

### Topical
▪ Prime the pump. Apply a smooth and even layer across entire face (forehead, each cheek, nose, and chin). Avoid eyes and lips. Do not apply to open wounds or irritated skin. Wash hands after application.

### Instillation of Nasal Spray
▪ Place spray nozzle in nostril without occluding it and tilt head slightly forward prior to instillation of spray; instruct patient to sniff briskly during administration.
▪ Rinse dropper or spray tip in hot water after each use to prevent contamination of solution by nasal secretions.
▪ Wash hands after administration.

## ADVERSE EFFECTS (≥1%) Special
**Senses:** *Burning,* stinging, dryness of nasal mucosa, *sneezing.* **Body as a Whole:** Headache, lightheadedness, drowsiness, insomnia, palpitations, *rebound congestion,* exacerbation of acne rosacea, application site erythema, and pain (topical).

## PHARMACOKINETICS Onset:
5–10 min. **Duration:** 6–10 h.

## NURSING IMPLICATIONS

### Assessment & Drug Effects
▪ Monitor for S&S of excess use. If noted, discuss possibility of rebound congestion (nasal).
▪ Monitor for improvement of facial erythema due to rosacea (topical).

### Patient & Family Education
▪ Wash hands carefully after handling oxymetazoline. Anisocoria (inequality of pupil size, blurred vision) can develop if eyes are rubbed with contaminated fingers.

▪ Do not to exceed recommended dosage. Rebound congestion (chemical rhinitis) may occur with prolonged or excessive use (nasal administration).
▪ Systemic effects can result from swallowing excessive medication (nasal administration).
▪ Report any development of facial acne.

## OXYMETHOLONE
(ox-i-meth'oh-lone)

Anadrol-50

**Classification:** ANDROGEN/ANABOLIC STEROID
**Therapeutic:** ANABOLIC STEROID
**Prototype:** Testosterone
**Controlled Substance:** Schedule III

## AVAILABILITY Tablet

## ACTION & *THERAPEUTIC EFFECT*
Mechanism of action in refractory anemias is unclear but may be due to direct stimulation of bone marrow, protein anabolic activity, or to androgenic stimulation of erythropoiesis. *Stimulates formation of red blood cells in the bone marrow. Stimulates bone growth, aids in bone matrix reconstitution.*

## USES Aplastic anemia.

## CONTRAINDICATIONS Hypersensitivity to oxymetholone; prostatic hypertrophy with obstruction; prostatic or male breast cancer; carcinoma of the breast in women with hypercalcemia; hepatic decompensation; hepatic carcinoma; nephrosis or nephrotic stage of nephritis; females of childbearing age; pregnancy (category X); lactation.

## CAUTIOUS USE Prepubertal males; older males; DM; history of cardiac, renal, or hepatic impairment; CAD; artherosclerosis; children.

0

## ROUTE & DOSAGE

### Aplastic Anemia
*Adult/Adolescent/Child:* **PO** 1–2 mg/kg/day (may require doses up to 5 mg/kg/day)

## ADMINISTRATION

**Oral**
- For treatment of anemias, a minimum trial period of 3–6 mo is recommended, since response tends to be slow.
- Store at 15°–30° C (59°–86° F). Protect from heat and light.

## ADVERSE EFFECTS (≥1%) **Endocrine:** Androgenic in women: Suppression of ovulation, lactation, or menstruation; *hoarseness or deepening of voice* (often irreversible); *hirsutism; oily skin; acne;* clitoral enlargement; regression of breasts; male-pattern baldness. Hypoestrogenic effects in women: Flushing, sweating; vaginitis with pruritus, drying, bleeding; menstrual irregularities. **Males:** Premature epiphyseal closure, phallic enlargement, priapism. Postpubertal: Testicular atrophy, decreased ejaculatory volume, azoospermia, oligospermia (after prolonged administration or excessive dosage), impotence, epididymitis, gynecomastia; increased risk of atherosclerosis. **CV:** *Edema,* skin flush. **GI:** *Nausea, vomiting, anorexia,* diarrhea, jaundice, hepatotoxicity. **Urogenital:** Bladder irritability. **Metabolic:** Hypercalcemia. **Hematologic:** Bleeding (with concurrent anticoagulant therapy), iron deficiency anemia, leukemia.

## INTERACTIONS **Drug:** May enhance hypoprothrombinemic effects of **warfarin. Herbal: Echinacea** may increase risk of hepatotoxicity.

## PHARMACOKINETICS **Absorption:** Readily from GI tract. **Metabolism:** In liver. **Elimination:** In urine. **Half-Life:** 9 h.

## NURSING IMPLICATIONS

### Black Box Warning

*Oxymetholone has been associated with hepatic dysfunction, liver failure, liver cell tumors, and increased risk of atherosclerosis from blood lipid changes.*

### Assessment & Drug Effects
- Monitor patient with a history of seizures closely because an increase in their frequency may be noted.
- Monitor periodically for edema that may develop with or without CHF.
- Monitor for and report jaundice or other S&S of hepatotoxicity (see Appendix F). Withhold drug at first sign of liver toxicity.
- Monitor for hypercalcemia (see Appendix F), especially in women with breast cancer.
- Monitor lab tests: Periodic Hgb and Hct, serum iron and iron binding capacity, and LFTs.

### Patient & Family Education
- Monitor blood glucose for loss of glycemic control if diabetic.
- Stop taking drug and notify prescriber if jaundice appears.
- Women: Notify prescriber of signs of virilization.

# OXYMORPHONE HYDROCHLORIDE
(ox-i-mor'fone)
Numorphan, Opana, Opana ER
**Classifications:** NARCOTIC (OPIATE AGONIST); ANALGESIC
Therapeutic: NARCOTIC ANALGESIC
**Prototype:** Morphine
**Controlled Substance:** Schedule II

## AVAILABILITY Solution for injection; suppository; extended release tablet; tablet

Common adverse effects in *italic;* life-threatening effects underlined; generic names in **bold;** classifications in SMALL CAPS; ♣ Canadian drug name; ⊘ Prototype drug

1210

### ACTION & *THERAPEUTIC EFFECT*

The precise mechanism of the action is unknown; however, specific CNS opioid receptors for endogenous compounds with opioid-like activity have been identified throughout the CNS and play a role in the analgesic effects of this drug. *Effective in relief of moderate to severe pain.*

**USES** Relief of moderate to severe pain, preoperative medication, support of anesthesia.

### CONTRAINDICATIONS

Hypersensitivity to oxymorphone; pulmonary edema resulting from chemical respiratory irritants; ileus; respiratory depression without appropriate monitoring; acute or severe bronchial asthma; upper airway obstruction; hypercapnia; moderate and severe hepatic function impairment; status asthmaticus.

### CAUTIOUS USE

Alcoholism; biliary tract disease; bladder obstruction; severe pulmonary disease, respiratory insufficiency, COPD; head injury; circulatory shock; history of seizures; renal impairment; depression; older adults and debilitated patients; pregnancy (category C); lactation; children younger than 18 y.

### ROUTE & DOSAGE

#### Moderate to Severe Pain

*Adult:* **PO** 10–20 mg q4–6h prn; **Extended release** 5–10 mg q12h; **Subcutaneous/IM** 1–1.5 mg q4–6h prn **IV** 0.5 mg q4–6h then switch to alternate route **PR** 5 mg q4–6h prn

### ADMINISTRATION

#### Oral

- Give on an empty stomach at least 1 h before or 2 h after eating.

- Extended-release tablets must be swallowed whole with enough water to ensure immediate, complete swallowing. Tablets must not be crushed or chewed.

#### Subcutaneous/Intramuscular

- Give undiluted.

#### Intravenous

*PREPARE:* **Direct:** May be given undiluted or diluted in 5 mL of sterile water or NS.
*ADMINISTER:* **Direct:** Give at a rate of 0.5 mg over 2–5 min.

- Protect drug from light. Store suppositories in refrigerator 2°–15° C (36°–59° F).

### ADVERSE EFFECTS (≥1%) GI:

*Nausea, vomiting, euphoria.* **CNS:** *Dizziness,* lightheadedness, sedation. **Respiratory:** Respiratory depression (see morphine), apnea, respiratory arrest. **Body as a Whole:** Sweating, coma, shock. **CV:** Cardiac arrest, circulatory depression.

### INTERACTIONS Drug: Alcohol

and other CNS DEPRESSANTS add to CNS depression; **propofol** increases risk of bradycardia.

### PHARMACOKINETICS Onset:

5–10 min IV; 10–15 min IM; 15–30 min PR. **Peak:** 1–1.5 h. **Duration:** 3–6 h. **Distribution:** Crosses placenta. **Metabolism:** In liver. **Elimination:** In urine. **Half-Life:** PO 7–9 h; extended release 9–11 h.

### NURSING IMPLICATIONS

#### Black Box Warning

*Oxymorphone has been associated with high abuse potential, respiratory depression, accidental overdose (especially in children), and death with coingestion of alcohol.*

Common adverse effects in *italic;* life-threatening effects underlined; generic names in **bold;** classifications in SMALL CAPS; ♣ Canadian drug name; ⊙ Prototype drug

1211

## Assessment & Drug Effects

- Monitor respiratory rate. Withhold drug and notify prescriber if rate falls below 12 breaths/min.
- Supervise ambulation and advise patient of possible lightheadedness. Older adult and debilitated patients are most susceptible to CNS depressant effects of drug.
- Evaluate patient's continued need for narcotic analgesic. Prolonged use can lead to dependence of morphine type.
- Medication contains sulfite and may precipitate a hypersensitivity reaction in susceptible patient.

## Patient & Family Education

- Use caution when walking because of potential for injury from dizziness.
- Do not consume alcohol while taking oxymorphone.

# OXYTOCIN INJECTION ℗ᵣ
(ox-i-toe'sin)

Pitocin

**Classification:** OXYTOCIC
Therapeutic: OXYTOCIC

**AVAILABILITY** Solution for injection

## ACTION & THERAPEUTIC EFFECT

Synthetic polypeptide identical pharmacologically to natural oxytocin released by posterior pituitary. By direct action on myofibrils, produces phasic contractions characteristic of normal delivery. Uterine sensitivity to oxytocin increases during gestational period and peaks sharply before parturition. *Effective in initiating or improving uterine contractions at term.*

**USES** To initiate or improve uterine contraction at term, management of inevitable, incomplete, or missed abortion; stimulation of uterine contractions during third stage of labor; stimulation to overcome uterine inertia; control of postpartum hemorrhage and promotion of postpartum uterine involution. Also used to induce labor in cases of maternal diabetes, preeclampsia, eclampsia, and erythroblastosis fetalis.

**CONTRAINDICATIONS** Hypersensitivity to oxytocin; significant cephalopelvic disproportion, unfavorable fetal position or presentations that are undeliverable without conversion before delivery, obstetric emergencies that favor surgical intervention, fetal distress in which delivery is not imminent, prematurity, placenta previa, prolonged use in severe toxemia or uterine inertia, hypertonic uterine patterns, conditions predisposing to thromboplastin or amniotic fluid embolism (dead fetus, abruptio placentae), grand multiparity, invasive cervical carcinoma, primipara older than 35 y, past history of uterine sepsis or of traumatic delivery; pregnancy (category X); lactation.

**CAUTIOUS USE** Preeclampsia; history of seizures; history of mental hypertension.

## ROUTE & DOSAGE

**Labor Induction**

*Adult:* **IV** 0.5–2 milliunits/min, may increase by 1–2 milliunits/min q15–60min (max: 20 milliunits/min); dose is decreased when labor is established; **High dose regimen** 6 milliunits/min, may increase by 6 milliunits/min q15–60min until contraction pattern established.

**Postpartum Bleeding**

*Adult:* **IM** 10 units total dose; **IV** Infuse a total of 10–40 units at a rate of 20–40 milliunits/min after delivery

Common adverse effects in *italic;* life-threatening effects <u>underlined;</u> generic names in **bold;** classifications in SMALL CAPS; ♦ Canadian drug name; ℗ Prototype drug

**Incomplete Abortion**
*Adult:* **IV** 10–20 milliunits/min

## ADMINISTRATION

### Intramuscular
- Give 10 units IM after delivery of the placenta.

### Intravenous

*PREPARE:* **IV Infusion:** When diluting oxytocin for IV infusion, rotate bottle gently to distribute medicine throughout solution. **IV Infusion for Inducing Labor:** Add 10 units (1 mL) to 1 L of D5W, NS, LR, or D5NS to yield 10 milliunits/mL. **IV Infusion for Postpartum Bleeding/Incomplete Abortion:** Add 10–40 units (1–4 mL) to 1 L of D5W, NS, LR, or D5NS to yield 10–40 milliunits/mL.

*ADMINISTER:* **IV Infusion:** Use an infusion pump for accurate control of infusion rate. **IV Infusion for Inducing Labor:** Initially infuse 0.5–2 milliunits/min; increase by 1–2 milliunits/min at 30–60 min intervals. **IV Infusion for Postpartum Bleeding:** Initially infuse 10–40 milliunits/min, then adjust to control uterine atony. **IV Infusion for Incomplete Abortion:** Infuse 10–20 milliunits/min. Do not exceed 30 units in 12 h.

*INCOMPATIBILITIES:* **Y-site:** Amphotericin B, ampicillin, chlorpromazine, dantrolene, diazepam, diazoxide, haloperidol, hydralazine, indomethacin, insulin, methohexital, pantoprazole, phenytoin, remifentanil, sulfamethoxazole/trimethoprim.

## ADVERSE EFFECTS (≥1%) **Body as a Whole:** Fetal trauma from too rapid propulsion through pelvis, fetal death, anaphylactic reactions, postpartum hemorrhage, precordial pain, edema, cyanosis or redness of skin. **CV:** Fetal bradycardia and arrhythmias, maternal cardiac arrhythmias, hypertensive episodes, subarachnoid hemorrhage, increased blood flow, fatal afibrinogenemia, ECG changes, PVCs, cardiovascular spasm and collapse. **GI:** Neonatal jaundice, maternal nausea, vomiting. **Endocrine:** ADH effects leading to severe water intoxication and hyponatremia, hypotension. **CNS:** Fetal intracranial hemorrhage, anxiety. **Respiratory:** Fetal hypoxia, maternal dyspnea. **Urogenital:** Uterine hypertonicity, tetanic contractions, uterine rupture, pelvic hematoma.

## INTERACTIONS **Drug:** VASOCONSTRICTORS cause severe hypertension; **cyclopropane anesthesia** causes hypotension, maternal bradycardia, arrhythmias. **Herbal:** **Ephedra, ma huang** may cause hypertension.

## PHARMACOKINETICS **Duration:** 1 h. **Distribution:** Distributed throughout extracellular fluid; small amount may cross placenta. **Metabolism:** Rapidly destroyed in liver and kidneys. **Elimination:** Small amounts excreted unchanged in urine. **Half-Life:** 3–5 min.

## NURSING IMPLICATIONS

### Assessment & Drug Effects
- Start flow charts to record maternal BP and other vital signs, I&O ratio, weight, strength, duration, and frequency of contractions, as well as fetal heart tone and rate, before instituting treatment.
- Monitor fetal heart rate and maternal BP and pulse at least

Common adverse effects in *italic;* life-threatening effects underlined; generic names in **bold;** classifications in SMALL CAPS; ✚ Canadian drug name; ⊙ Prototype drug

1213

q15min during infusion period; evaluate tonus of myometrium during and between contractions and record on flow chart. Report change in rate and rhythm immediately.

- Stop infusion to prevent fetal anoxia, turn patient on her side, and notify prescriber if contractions are prolonged (occurring at less than 2-min intervals) and if monitor records contractions about 50 mm Hg or if contractions last 90 sec or longer. Stimulation will wane rapidly within 2–3 min. Oxygen administration may be necessary.

- If local or regional (caudal, spinal) anesthesia is being given to the patient receiving oxytocin, be alert to the possibility of hypertensive crisis (sudden intense occipital headache, palpitation, marked hypertension, stiff neck, nausea, vomiting, sweating, fever, photophobia, dilated pupils, bradycardia or tachycardia, constricting chest pain).

- Monitor I&O during labor. If patient is receiving drug by prolonged IV infusion, watch for symptoms of water intoxication (drowsiness, listlessness, headache, confusion, anuria, weight gain). Report changes in alertness and orientation and changes in I&O ratio (i.e., marked decrease in output with excessive intake).

- Check fundus frequently during the first few postpartum hours and several times daily thereafter.

**Patient & Family Education**
- Be aware of purpose and anticipated effect of oxytocin.
- Report sudden, severe headache immediately to health care providers.

# PACLITAXEL
(pac-li-tax′el)
Abraxane, Taxol
**Classifications:** ANTINEOPLASTIC; TAXANE
Therapeutic: ANTINEOPLASTIC; ANTIMICROTUBULE

**AVAILABILITY** Solution for injection; powder for injection (with 900 mg human albumin)

**ACTION & THERAPEUTIC EFFECT** During cell division paclitaxel acts as an antimicrotubular agent that interferes with the microtubule network essential for interphase and mitosis. This results in abnormal spindle formation during mitosis. *Interferes with growth of rapidly dividing cells including cancer cells, and eventually causes cell death. Additionally, the breakup of the cytoskeleton within nondividing cells interrupts intracellular transport and communications.*

**USES** Ovarian cancer, breast cancer, Kaposi's sarcoma, non–small-cell lung cancer (NSCLC).

**UNLABELED USES** Squamous cell head and neck cancer, small-cell lung cancer, endometrial cancer, esophageal cancer, gastric cancer, testicular cancer, germ cell tumors, and other solid tumors, leukemia, melanoma.

**CONTRAINDICATIONS** Taxol: Hypersensitivity to paclitaxel, or taxanes; baseline neutrophil count less than 1500 cells/mm³; thrombocytopenia; with AIDS-related Kaposi's sarcoma baseline neutrophil count less than 1000 cells/mm³; pregnancy (category D); lactation. For **Abraxane:** Baseline neutrophil count less than 1500 cells/mm³.

Common adverse effects in *italic;* life-threatening effects underlined; generic names in **bold;** classifications in SMALL CAPS; ♦ Canadian drug name; ☻ Prototype drug

**CAUTIOUS USE** Cardiac arrhythmias, cardiac disease; impaired liver function; alcoholism; older adults; peripheral neuropathy. Safety and efficacy in children not established.

## ROUTE & DOSAGE

### Ovarian Cancer, NSCLC
*Adult:* **IV** 135 mg/m² 24 h infusion repeated q3wk

### Breast Cancer
*Adult:* **IV** 175–250 mg/m² over 3 h q3wk
*Abraxane:* **IV** 260 mg/m² over 30 min q3wk

### Kaposi's Sarcoma
*Adult:* **IV** 135 mg/m² infused over 3 h q3wk or 100 mg/m² infused over 3 h q2wk

## ADMINISTRATION

**Intravenous**

Note: Premedication is required (except with **Abraxane**) to avoid severe hypersensitivity. ▪ Follow institutional or standard guidelines for preparation, handling, and disposal of cytotoxic agents.

*PREPARE:* **IV Infusion: Dilution of Conventional Paclitaxel:** Do not use equipment or devices containing polyvinyl chloride (PVC) in preparation of infusion. ▪ Dilute to a final concentration of 0.3–1.2 mg/mL in any of the following: D5W, NS, D5/NS, or D5W in Ringer's injection. The prepared solution may be hazy, but this does not indicate a loss of potency.
**Abraxane Vial Reconstitution:** Slowly inject 20 mL NS over at least 1 min onto the inside wall of the vial to yield 5 mg/mL.

▪ **Do not** inject directly into the cake powder. Allow vial to sit for at least 5 min, then gently swirl for at least 2 min to completely dissolve. If foaming occurs, let stand for at least 15 min until foam subsides. ▪ If particulates or settling are visible, gently invert vial to ensure complete resuspension prior to use. ▪ Remove the required dose and inject into an empty sterile, PVC or non-PVC type IV bag.
*ADMINISTER:* **IV Infusion:** Because tissue necrosis occurs with extravasation, frequently assess patency of a peripheral IV site. ▪ **Conventional Paclitaxel:** Infuse over 1–24 h through IV tubing containing an in-line (0.22 micron or less) filter. Do not use equipment containing PVC. ▪ **Abraxane: Do not** use an in-line filter. Infuse over 30 min.
*INCOMPATIBILITIES:* **Solution/additive: PVC bags** and **infusion sets** should be avoided (except with Abraxane) due to leaching of DEHP (plasticizer). ▪ Do not mix with any other medications. **Y-site: Amphotericin B, amphotericin B cholesteryl sulfate complex, chlorpromazine, diazepam, digoxin, doxorubicin liposome, gemtuzumab, hydroxyzine, idarubicin, indomethacin, labetalol, methylprednisolone, mitoxantrone, phenytoin, propranolol.**

▪ **Conventional paclitaxel** solutions diluted for infusion are stable at room temperature (approximately 25° C/77° F) for up to 27 h. ▪ Reconstituted **Abraxane** should be used immediately but may be kept refrigerated for up to 8 h if needed.

## ADVERSE EFFECTS (≥1%) CV:
Ventricular tachycardia, ventricular

Common adverse effects in *italic;* life-threatening effects <u>underlined;</u> generic names in **bold;** classifications in SMALL CAPS; ♣ Canadian drug name; ⊙ Prototype drug

1215

ectopy, *transient bradycardia,* chest pain. **CNS:** Fatigue, headaches, *peripheral neuropathy,* weakness, seizures. **GI:** *Nausea, vomiting,* diarrhea, taste changes, *mucositis,* elevations in serum triglycerides. **Hematologic:** <u>Neutropenia</u>, *anemia,* <u>thrombocytopenia</u>. **Body as a Whole:** *Hypersensitivity reactions (hypotension, dyspnea with <u>bronchospasm</u>, urticaria, abdominal and extremity pain, diaphoresis, <u>angioedema</u>), myalgias, arthralgias, alopecia.* **Skin:** *Alopecia,* tissue necrosis with extravasation. **Urogenital:** Minor elevations in kidney and liver function tests.

**INTERACTIONS Drug:** Increased myelosuppression if **cisplatin, doxorubicin** is given before paclitaxel; **ketoconazole** can inhibit metabolism of paclitaxel; additive bradycardia with BETA-BLOCKERS, **digoxin, verapamil;** additive risk of bleeding with ANTICOAGULANTS, NSAIDS, PLATELET INHIBITORS (including **aspirin**), THROMBOLYTIC AGENTS.

**PHARMACOKINETICS Distribution:** Greater than 90% protein bound; does not cross CSF. **Metabolism:** In liver (CYP3A4, 2C8). **Elimination:** Feces 70%, urine 14%. **Half-Life:** 1–9 h.

## NURSING IMPLICATIONS

### Black Box Warning

*Paclitaxel has been associated with severe hypersensitivity, anaphylaxis, and neutropenia.*

### Assessment & Drug Effects

- Monitor for hypersensitivity reactions, especially during first and second administrations of the paclitaxel. S&S requiring treatment, but not necessarily discontinuation of the drug, include dyspnea, hypotension, and chest pain. Discontinue immediately and manage symptoms aggressively if angioedema and generalized urticaria develop.
- Monitor vital signs frequently, especially during the first hour of infusion. Bradycardia occurs in approximately 12% of patients, usually during infusion. It does not normally require treatment. Cardiac monitoring is indicated for those with severe conduction abnormalities.
- Monitor for anemia, neutropenia, and thrombocytopenia.
- Monitor for peripheral neuropathy, the severity of which is dose dependent. Severe symptoms occur primarily with higher than recommended doses.
- Monitor lab tests: Periodic CBC with differential and platelet count, and Hct & Hgb throughout course of treatment.

### Patient & Family Education

- Immediately report to prescriber S&S of paclitaxel hypersensitivity: Difficulty breathing, chest pain, palpitations, angioedema (subcutaneous swelling usually around face and neck), and skin rashes or itching.
- Be sure to have periodic blood work as prescribed.
- Avoid aspirin, NSAIDs, and alcohol to minimize GI distress.
- Be aware of high probability of developing hair loss (greater than 80%).

# PALBOCICLIB
(pal-bo-cyc′lib)

Ibrance

**Classifications:** ANTINEOPLASTIC; KINASE INHIBITOR; CYCLIN-DEPENDENT KINASE (CDK) INHIBITOR

Therapeutic: ANTINEOPLASTIC

## AVAILABILITY Capsules

## ACTION & *THERAPEUTIC EFFECT*

Inhibits an enzyme (cyclin-dependent kinase) that is essential for cancer cells to progress through the cell cycle at the G1/S phase. *Reduces proliferation of breast cancer cells by preventing progression through the cell cycle.*

**USES** Treatment of postmenopausal women with estrogen receptor (ER)-positive, human epidermal growth factor receptor 2 (HER2)-negative advanced breast cancer in combination with letrozole.

**CONTRAINDICATIONS** Pregnancy; lactation.

**CAUTIOUS USE** Concomitant use of moderate or strong CYP3A4 inhibitor; grapefruit products; bone marrow suppression; infection; thromboembolic events including pulmonary embolism.

## ROUTE & DOSAGE

### Breast Cancer

*Adult:* **PO** 125 mg once daily in combination with letrozole for 21 days, followed by 7 days with letrozole only; repeat cycle until progressive disease or unacceptable toxicity occur

#### Hematologic Toxicity Dosage Adjustment

*Grade 3:* Withhold initiation of next cycle until recovery to Grade 2 or less

*Grade 3 with ANC (less than 1000 to 500/mm³) and Fever 38.5° C (101.3° F) or greater and/or infection:* Withhold until recovery to Grade 2 or less (at least 1000/mm³); resume at 100 mg once daily if first occurrence or 75 mg once daily if second occurrence

*Grade 4:* Withhold until recovery to Grade 2 or less; resume at 100 mg once daily if first occurrence or 75 mg once daily if second occurrence

#### Non-Hematologic Toxicity Dosage Adjustment

*Grade 3 or higher:* Withhold until recovery to Grade 2 or less depending on toxicity; resume at 100 mg once daily if first occurrence or 75 mg once daily if second occurrence

#### Co-Administered Strong CYP3A Inhibitor Dosage Adjustment

Decrease dose to 75 mg once daily

## ADMINISTRATION

### Oral

- Give with food at approximately the same time each day.
- Capsules must be swallowed whole. They must not be crushed, chewed, or opened prior to swallowing (do not administer if capsules are broken, cracked, or not fully intact).
- Do not administer with grapefruit juice.
- Store at 20°–25° C (68°–77° F).

**ADVERSE EFFECTS** (≥5%) **Body as a Whole:** Asthenia, *fatigue,* peripheral neuropathy. **GI:** *Diarrhea, nausea, stomatitis,* vomiting. **Hematological:** *Anemia, leukopenia, neutropenia,* thrombocytopenia. **Metabolic:** Decreased appetite. **Respiratory:** Epistaxis, pulmonary embolism, *upper respiratory infection.* **Skin:** *Alopecia.*

**INTERACTIONS Drug:** Concomitant use of strong CYP3A inhibitors (e.g., **clarithromycin, indinavir, itraconazole, ketoconazole,**

Common adverse effects in *italic;* life-threatening effects underlined; generic names in **bold;** classifications in SMALL CAPS; ♣ Canadian drug name; ⊙ Prototype drug

1217

**lopinavir/ritonavir, nefazodone, nelfinavir, posaconazole, ritonavir, saquinavir, telaprevir, telithromycin, verapamil,** and **voriconazole**) increases the levels of palbociclib. Concomitant use of strong CYP3A inducers (e.g., **phenytoin, rifampin, carbamazepine**) decreases the levels of palbociclib. Concomitant use of moderate CYP3A inducers (e.g., **bosentan, efavirenz, etravirine, modafinil, nafcillin**) may decrease the levels of palbociclib. Palbociclib increases the levels of midazolam. Palbociclib may increase the levels of other drugs requiring CYP3A isozymes (e.g., **alfentanil, cyclosporine, dihydroergotamine, ergotamine, everolimus, fentanyl, pimozide, quinidine, sirolimus, tacrolimus**). **Food: Grapefruit** or **grapefruit juice** may increase the levels of palbociclib. **Herbal: St John's wort** decreases the levels of palbociclib.

## PHARMACOKINETICS **Absorption:** 46% bioavailable. **Peak:** 6–12 h. **Distribution:** 85% plasma protein bound. **Metabolism:** In liver. **Elimination:** Fecal (74.1%) and renal (17.5%). **Half-Life:** 29 h.

## NURSING IMPLICATIONS

### Assessment & Drug Effects

- Monitor for and report promptly S&S of infection; report fever of 101° F or greater.
- Monitor for S&S of pulmonary embolism (e.g., shortness of breath, anxiety, chest pain, hemoptysis, fainting, irregular or rapid HR).
- Monitor lab tests: Baseline CBC with differential, repeat q2wk for first 2 cycles, then prior to each cycle or more often if indicated.

### Patient & Family Education

- Report immediately to prescriber any of the following S&S: Fever, chills, dizziness, weakness, increased tendency to bleed and/or bruise, shortness of breath or rapid breathing, chest pain, or rapid heart rate.
- Do not consume grapefruit or grapefruit juice while taking this drug.
- Women should use effective contraception during treatment and for at least 2 wk after the last dose.
- Do not breast-feed while taking this drug.

# PALIFERMIN
(pal-i-fur'men)
Kepivance

**Classifications:** BIOLOGIC RESPONSE MODIFIER; KERATINOCYTE GROWTH FACTOR; CYTOKINE
Therapeutic: KERATINOCYTE GROWTH FACTOR (KGF)

## AVAILABILITY Powder for injection

## ACTION & *THERAPEUTIC EFFECT*
Naturally occurring keratinocyte growth factor (KGF) is produced and regulated in response to epithelial tissue injury. Binding of KGF to its receptors in epithelial cells results in proliferation, differentiation, and repair of injury to epithelial cells. Palifermin is a synthetic form of KGF; thus it enhances replacement of injured cells. *Reduces the incidence of severe oral mucositis that interferes with food consumption in the cancer patient.*

## USES Reduction of the incidence and duration of severe oral mucositis in patients with hematologic malignancies who are receiving myelotoxic therapy requiring hematopoietic stem cell support.

## CONTRAINDICATIONS Hypersensitivity to *Escherichia coli*-derived

protein, palifermin; nonhematologic malignancies; within 24 h of
chemotherapy; lactation.

**CAUTIOUS USE** Use contraception for females of childbearing age;
pregnancy (category C); children.

## ROUTE & DOSAGE

**Mucositis Prophylaxis**
*Adult:* **IV** 60 mcg/kg/day for
3 days before and 3 days after
myelotoxic therapy (total: 6 doses)

## ADMINISTRATION
**Intravenous**
Do not give within 24 h before/
after or during myelotoxic chemotherapy.

*PREPARE:* **Direct:** Use double
gloves and protective gown
while preparing and administering. If there is any chance
that the patient may resist, wear
eye/face protection. Reconstitute powder with 1.2 mL sterile
water **only** to yield 5 mg/mL.
Gently swirl to dissolve but do
not shake. ▪ Powder will dissolve in about 3 min. Should be
used immediately.
*ADMINISTER:* **Direct:** Give as a bolus dose. ▪ If heparin is used to
maintain the IV line, flush
before/after with NS. ▪ If diluted
solution was refrigerated (max
refrigeration time: 24 h), may
warm to room temperature for
up to 1 h but protect from light.
*INCOMPATIBILITIES:* **Y-site: Heparin.**

▪ Store powder vial at 2°–8° C
(36°–46° F). Protect from light. ▪ If
needed, may store reconstituted solution refrigerated for up to 24 h. ▪
Discard any reconstituted solution

left at room temperature for longer
than 1 h.

**ADVERSE EFFECTS** (≥1%)
**Body as a Whole:** *Edema, arthralgia, fever, pain.* **CNS:** *Dysesthesia.* **GI:** *Mouth/tongue
thickness or discoloration, taste alterations, abdominal pain, anorexia, vomiting.* **Metabolic:** *Elevated
serum amylase, elevated serum
lipase.* **Musculoskeletal:** *Arthralgia.*
**Skin:** *Erythema, pruritus, rash.*
**Urogenital:** Proteinuria.

**INTERACTIONS Drug:** Should not
be administered within 24 h before,
during infusion of or within 24 h
after administration of ANTINEO-
PLASTIC agents.

**PHARMACOKINETICS Distribu-
tion:** Extravascular distribution.
**Half-Life:** 4.5 h.

## NURSING IMPLICATIONS
**Assessment & Drug Effects**
▪ Monitor for improvement in mucositis.
▪ Monitor for S&S of oral toxicities
and skin toxicities
**Patient & Family Education**
▪ Report any of the following to a
health care provider: Alteration of
taste, discoloration or enlargement of the tongue, lack of sensation around the mouth, skin rash,
itching, or edema.

## PALIPERIDONE
(pa-li'per-i-done)
Invega

## PALIPERIDONE PALMITATE
Invega Sustenna
**Classification:** ATYPICAL
ANTIPSYCHOTIC
**Therapeutic:** ANTIPSYCHOTIC
**Prototype:** Clozapine

**AVAILABILITY** Extended release tablet; solution for injection

**ACTION & *THERAPEUTIC EFFECT*** Interferes with binding of dopamine to dopamine type 2 ($D_2$) receptors, serotonin ($5\text{-}HT_{2A}$) receptors, and alpha-adrenergic receptors. *Effective in controlling symptoms of schizophrenia as well as other psychotic symptoms.*

**USES** Treatment of schizophrenia, schizoaffective disorder.

**UNLABELED USES** Agitation, bipolar disorder, mania.

**CONTRAINDICATIONS** Hypersensitivity to paliperidone, risperidone; concurrent administration with drugs that produce $QT_c$ prolongation; severe GI narrowing (pathologic or iatrogenic); drug induced NMS; older adults with dementia-related psychosis; lactation.

**CAUTIOUS USE** History of cerebrovascular events; hypovolemia, dehydration; cardiovascular disease; QT prolongation; history of cardiac arrhythmias; risk factors for hypotension; renal impairment; CNS pathology; systemic infection; DM; hyperglycemia; obesity; Parkinson's disease; older adults; pregnancy (category C); children younger than 12 y.

**ROUTE & DOSAGE**

### Schizophrenia

*Adult:* **PO** Initially 6 mg/day; may adjust up/down in 3 mg increments; at least 5 day intervals needed for dosage increments (max: 12 mg/day); **IM** 234 mg on day 1, then 156 mg on day 8, then monthly dose of 117 mg (dose may vary based on patient response); **Converting PO to IM** 3 mg/day PO = 39–78 mg/mo IM; 60 mg/day PO = 117 mg/mo IM; 12 mg/day PO = 234 mg/mo IM
*Adolescent:* **PO** 3 mg daily

### Schizoaffective Disorder

*Adult:* **PO** 6 mg daily, dose adjusted at intervals of more than 4 days (max: 12 mg/day); **IM** 234 mg on day 1, then 156 mg on day 8, then monthly dose of 117 mg (dose may vary based on patient response)

### Renal Impairment Dosage Adjustment

*CrCl 50–79 mL/min:* Max: 6 mg/day; **IM** 156 mg on day 1 and 117 mg 1 wk later, then monthly 78 mg injections; *CrCl 10–49 mL/min:* Max: 3 mg/day; **IM** not recommended

**ADMINISTRATION**

**Oral**
- Extended release tablets **must be** swallowed whole. They should not be chewed or crushed.
- Give in the morning with or without food.

**Intramuscular**
- Give as a single injection; do not administer in divided doses.
- First 2 doses on day 1 and 1 wk later: Inject slowly, deep into the deltoid muscle.
- Monthly maintenance dose: Inject slowly, deep into the deltoid or gluteal muscle.
- Store at 15°–30° C (59°–86° F). Protect from moisture.

**ADVERSE EFFECTS** (≥1%) **Body as a Whole:** Back pain, cough, pain in extremity, pyrexia; injection site reaction. **CNS:** *Akathisia,* *anxiety,* asthenia, dizziness, dystonia, extrapyramidal disorder, fatigue, *headache,* hypertonia, parkinsonism, *somnolence,* tremor. **CV:** Atrioventricular block, bundle branch block, ECG T-wave abnormalities, hypertension, orthostatic hypotension, $QT_c$ prolongation, sinus arrhythmia, *tachycardia.* **GI:** Abdominal pain, dry mouth, dyspepsia, nausea, salivary hypersecretion. **Metabolic:** Increased insulin levels, weight gain. **Special Senses:** Blurred vision.

**INTERACTIONS Drug:** Enhanced CNS depression with **alcohol** or CNS DEPRESSANTS. Paliperidone may enhance the effects of ANTIHYPERTENSIVE AGENTS. Paliperidone can diminish the effects of DOPAMINE AGONISTS **(levodopa, bromocriptine, cabergoline, pergolide, pramipexole, ropinirole). Carbamazepine** decreases effectiveness. Avoid with agents that increase QT interval (e.g., **bepridil, cisapride, dofetilide, quinidine, ziprasidone**). Avoid CYP3A4 inhibitors (e.g., AZOLE ANTIFUNGALS). **Food:** High fat/high caloric meal increases paliperidone levels.

**PHARMACOKINETICS Absorption:** Bioavailability is 28%. **Peak:** 24 h. **Distribution:** 74% protein bound. **Metabolism:** In liver (26–41%). **Elimination:** Urine (major, 50–70% unchanged) and stool (minor). **Half-Life:** 23 h.

**NURSING IMPLICATIONS**

### Black Box Warning

*Paliperidone has been associated with increased mortality in older adults with dementia-related psychosis.*

**Assessment & Drug Effects**

- Baseline ECG recommended to rule out congenital, long-QT syndrome.
- Prior to initiating therapy, hypokalemia and hypomagnesemia should be corrected.
- Monitor weight.
- Monitor CV status and monitor BP especially in those prone to hypotension.
- Reassess patient periodically in order to maintain on the lowest effective drug dose.
- Monitor closely neurologic status of older adults.
- Supervise closely those with suicidal ideation.
- Monitor closely those at risk for seizures.
- Assess degree of cognitive and motor impairment, and assess for environmental hazards.
- Monitor diabetics for loss of glycemic control.
- Monitor lab tests: Baseline and periodic serum electrolytes; periodic renal function tests, LFTs, lipid profile, thyroid function tests, blood glucose, and CBC.

**Patient & Family Education**

- Exercise caution with hazardous activities until response to drug is known.
- Carefully monitor blood glucose levels if diabetic.
- Be aware of the risk of orthostatic hypotension.
- The shell of the tablet may be eliminated in the stool whole, but this does not mean the drug was not absorbed.
- Monitor for signs and symptoms of suicidal ideation.
- Be aware of the possibility of seizure activity.

P

Common adverse effects in *italic;* life-threatening effects underlined; generic names in **bold;** classifications in SMALL CAPS; ♣ Canadian drug name; ⊕ Prototype drug

1221

# PALIVIZUMAB
(pal-i-viz'u-mab)
Synagis
**Classifications:** IMMUNOMODULA-
TOR; MONOCLONAL ANTIBODY;
IMMUNOGLOBULIN
Therapeutic: IMMUNOGLOBULIN (IGG)

**AVAILABILITY** Solution for injection

## ACTION & *THERAPEUTIC EFFECT*
Exhibits neutralizing and fu-
sion-inhibitory activity against
the respiratory syncytial virus
(RSV). *Provides passive immunity
against respiratory syncytial virus.
Indicated by prevention of lower
respiratory tract infection.*

**USES** Prevention of serious lower
respiratory tract infections in children susceptible to RSV.

**CONTRAINDICATIONS** Hypersensitivity to palivizumab.

**CAUTIOUS USE** Hypersensitivity
to other immunoglobulin preparations, blood products, or other
medications; kidney or liver dysfunction; acute RSV infection;
pregnancy (category C).

## ROUTE & DOSAGE

**RSV**
*Child:* **IM** 15 mg/kg qmo during
RSV season

## ADMINISTRATION
**Intramuscular**
- Give IM only into the anterolateral aspect of the thigh. Volumes
greater than 1 mL should be divided and given in different sites.

**ADVERSE EFFECTS** (≥1%) **Body as
a Whole:** *Otitis media,* pain, hernia.
**GI:** Increased AST, diarrhea, nau-

sea, vomiting, gastroenteritis. **Respiratory:** *URI, rhinitis,* pharyngitis,
cough, wheeze, bronchiolitis, asthma, croup, dyspnea, sinusitis, apnea.
**Skin:** *Rash.*

**PHARMACOKINETICS Half-Life:**
20 days.

## NURSING IMPLICATIONS
### Assessment & Drug Effects
- Monitor carefully for and immediately report S&S of respiratory
illness including fever, cough,
wheezing, and chest retractions.
- Assess for and report erythema or
indurations at injection site.

### Patient & Family Education
- Contact prescriber for S&S of respiratory illness, vomiting, diarrhea, or if redness develops at
injection site.

# PALONOSETRON
(pal-o-no'si-tron)
Aloxi
**Classifications:** SEROTONIN 5-HT$_3$
RECEPTOR ANTAGONIST; ANTIEMETIC
Therapeutic: ANTIEMETIC
**Prototype:** Ondansetron

**AVAILABILITY** Solution for injection

## ACTION & *THERAPEUTIC EFFECT*
Selectively blocks serotonin
5-HT$_3$ receptors found centrally
in the chemoreceptor trigger zone
(CTZ) of the hypothalamus, and
peripherally at vagal nerve endings in the intestines. *Prevents
acute chemotherapy-induced
nausea and vomiting associated
with initial and repeat courses of
moderately or highly emetogenic
chemotherapy.*

**USES** Prevention of acute and
delayed nausea and vomiting

Common adverse effects in *italic;* life-threatening effects <u>underlined</u>; generic names
in **bold;** classifications in SMALL CAPS; ♣ Canadian drug name; ☻ Prototype drug

associated with highly emetogenic cancer chemotherapy; postoperative nausea/vomiting.

## CONTRAINDICATIONS
Hypersensitivity to palonosetron.

## CAUTIOUS USE
Dehydration; cardiac arrhythmias, QT prolongation; electrolyte imbalance; pregnancy (category B); lactation; children younger than 18 y.

## ROUTE & DOSAGE

### Prevention of Chemotherapy-Induced Nausea and Vomiting

*Adult:* **IV** 0.25 mg infused over 30 sec 30 min prior to chemotherapy; do not repeat for at least 7 days
*Child:* **IV** 20 mcg/kg infused over 15 min prior to chemotherapy

### Post-Operative Nausea/Vomiting

*Adult:* **IV** 0.075 mg single dose administered over 10 sec immediately before anesthesia

## ADMINISTRATION

### Intravenous

***PREPARE: Direct:*** Do not dilute and do not mix with other drugs.
***ADMINISTER:*** Prevention of chemotherapy-induced nausea and vomiting. **Direct:** Give 30 min prior to start of chemotherapy. Adults: Give over 30 sec. Children: Give over 15 min. Flush IV line with NS before and after administration. Prevention of nausea and vomiting; infuse over 10 sec prior to anesthesia induction.
***INCOMPATIBILITIES:*** Do not mix with other drugs.

■ Store at room temperature of 15°–30° C (59°–86° F). Protect from light.

## ADVERSE EFFECTS (≥1%)
**CNS:** Headache, anxiety, dizziness. **Cardiac:** Prolonged QT interval. **GI:** Constipation, diarrhea, abdominal pain. **Dermatologic:** Pruritus.

## INTERACTIONS
**Drug:** Can cause profound hypotension with **apomorphine**. May cause serotonin syndrome with other serotonergic drugs (e.g., SSRI).

## PHARMACOKINETICS
**Metabolism:** In liver (CYP2D6, 1A2, 3A4). **Elimination:** Primarily renal. **Half-Life:** 40 h.

## NURSING IMPLICATIONS

### Assessment & Drug Effects

■ Monitor closely cardiac status especially in those taking diuretics or otherwise at risk for hypokalemia or hypomagnesemia, with congenital QT syndrome, or patients taking antiarrhythmic or other drugs that lead to QT prolongation.

### Patient & Family Education

■ Report promptly any of the following: Difficulty breathing, wheezing, or shortness of breath; palpitations or chest tightness; skin rash or itching; swelling of the face, tongue, throat, hands, or feet.

---

## PAMIDRONATE DISODIUM
(pa-mi′dro-nate)

**Classification:** BISPHOSPHONATE (BONE METABOLISM REGULATORY)
**Therapeutic:** BONE METABOLISM REGULATORY
**Prototype:** Etidronate

## AVAILABILITY
Powder for injection; solution for injection

P

---

Common adverse effects in *italic;* life-threatening effects <u>underlined;</u> generic names in **bold;** classifications in SMALL CAPS; ♣ Canadian drug name; ⊘ Prototype drug

1223

## ACTION & *THERAPEUTIC EFFECT*

A bone-resorption inhibitor thought to absorb calcium phosphate crystals into bone. May also inhibit osteoclast activity, thus contributing to inhibition of bone resorption. *Reduces bone turnover and, when used in combination with adequate hydration, it increases renal excretion of calcium, thus reducing serum calcium concentrations.*

## USES Hypercalcemia of malignancy and Paget's disease, bone metastases in multiple myeloma or breast cancer.

## UNLABELED USES Primary hyperparathyroidism, osteoporosis prophylaxis.

## CONTRAINDICATIONS Hypersensitivity to pamidronate; breast cancer, severe renal disease, hypercalcemia, hypercholesterolemia, polycythemia, prostatic cancer; pregnancy (category D); lactation.

## CAUTIOUS USE Hypersensitivity to pamidronate or other bisphosphonates; heart failure, nephrosis or nephrotic syndrome, moderate renal disease, chronic kidney failure; hepatic disease, cholestasis; peripheral edema, prostate hypertrophy; cancer patients with stomatitis; older adults. Safe use in children not established.

## ROUTE & DOSAGE

**Moderate Hypercalcemia of Malignancy (corrected calcium 12–13.5 mg/dL)**

*Adult:* **IV** 60–90 mg infused over 4–24 h, may repeat in 7 days

**Severe Hypercalcemia of Malignancy (corrected calcium greater than 13.5 mg/dL)**

*Adult:* **IV** 90 mg infused over 4–24 h, may repeat in 7 days

**Paget's Disease**

*Adult:* **IV** 30 mg once daily for 3 days (90 mg total)

**Osteolytic Metastases**

*Adult:* **IV** 90 mg once/mo

## ADMINISTRATION

**Intravenous**

*PREPARE:* **IV Infusion:** Add 10 mL sterile water for injection to reconstitute the 30 or 90 mg vial to yield 3 or 9 mg/mL, respectively. Allow to completely dissolve. **IV Infusion for Hypercalcemia of Malignancy:** Withdraw the required dose and dilute in D5W, NS, or 1/2NS as follows: Use 1000 mL. **IV Infusion for Paget's Disease and Multiple Myeloma:** Withdraw the required dose and dilute in D5W, NS, or 1/2NS as follows: Use 500 mL. **IV Infusion for Breast Cancer Bone Metastases:** Withdraw the required dose and dilute in D5W, NS, or 1/2NS as follows: Use 250 mL.

*ADMINISTER:* **IV Infusion:** Regulate infusion rate carefully. Rapid infusion may cause renal damage. **IV Infusion for Hypercalcemia of Malignancy:** Infuse over 2–24 h. **IV Infusion for Paget's Disease and Multiple Myeloma:** Infuse over 4 h. **IV Infusion for Breast Cancer Bone Metastases:** Infuse over 2 h.

*INCOMPATIBILITIES:* Solution/additive: CALCIUM-CONTAINING SOLUTIONS (including **lactated Ringer's**). **Y-site: Amphotericin B, caspofungin, dantrolene, diazepam, gemtuzumab, leucovorin, phenytoin.**

▪ Refrigerate reconstituted pamidronate solution at 2°–8° C (36°–46° F); the IV solution may be stored at room temperature. Both are stable for 24 h.

## ADVERSE EFFECTS (≥1%) Body as a Whole: *Fever with or without rigors* generally occurs within 48 h and subsides within 48 h despite continued therapy; *thrombophlebitis at injection site;* general malaise lasting for several weeks; transient increase in bone pain; jaw osteonecrosis. **Metabolic:** *Hypocalcemia.* **GI:** Nausea, *abdominal pain, epigastric discomfort.* **CV:** Hypertension. **Skin:** Rash.

## INTERACTIONS Drug: Concurrent use of **foscarnet** may further decrease serum levels of ionized calcium.

## PHARMACOKINETICS Absorption: 50% of dose is retained in body. **Onset:** 24–48 h. **Peak:** 6 days. **Duration:** 2 wk–3 mo. **Distribution:** Accumulates in bone; once deposited, remains bound until bone is remodeled. **Metabolism:** Not metabolized. **Elimination:** 50% excreted in urine unchanged. **Half-Life:** 28 h.

## NURSING IMPLICATIONS

### Assessment & Drug Effects
▪ Assess IV injection site for thrombophlebitis.
▪ Monitor for S&S of hypocalcemia, hypokalemia, hypomagnesemia, and hypophosphatemia. Continue monitoring for hypocalcemia at least 2 wk after treatment completed.
▪ Monitor for seizures especially in those with a preexisting seizure disorder.
▪ Monitor vital signs. Be aware that drug fever, which may occur with pamidronate use, is self-limiting, usually subsiding in 48 h even with continued therapy.
▪ Monitor I&O and hydration status. Patient should be adequately hydrated, without fluid overload.
▪ Monitor lab tests: Baseline and prior to each treatment serum creatinine; frequent serum electrolytes; periodic CBC with differential.

### Patient & Family Education
▪ Be aware that transient, self-limiting fever with/without chills may develop.
▪ Generalized malaise, which may last for several weeks following treatment, is an anticipated adverse effect.
▪ Report to prescriber immediately perioral tingling, numbness, and paresthesia. These are signs of hypocalcemia.

## PANCRELIPASE ⊙

(pan-kre-li'pase)

Creon, Pancreaze, Pertzye, Ultresa, Viokace, Zenpep

**Classification:** ENZYME REPLACEMENT THERAPY
**Therapeutic:** PANCREATIC ENZYME REPLACEMENT THERAPY

## AVAILABILITY Tablet or capsule containing lipase, protease, and amylase

## ACTION & *THERAPEUTIC EFFECT*
Pancreatic enzyme concentrate similar to natural pancreatin but

Common adverse effects in *italic;* life-threatening effects underlined; generic names in **bold;** classifications in SMALL CAPS; ◆ Canadian drug name; ⊙ Prototype drug

1225

on a weight basis has 12 times the lipolytic activity and at least 4 × the trypsin and amylase content of pancreatin. *Facilitates hydrolysis of fats into glycerol and fatty acids, starches into dextrins and sugars, and proteins into peptides for easier absorption.*

**USES** Replacement therapy in symptomatic treatment of malabsorption syndrome due to cystic fibrosis; managment of exocrine pancreatic insufficiency due to pancreatectomy.

**CONTRAINDICATIONS** None listed in the manufacturer's labeling.

**CAUTIOUS USE** Hypersensitivity to pancrelipase or porcine; GI disease, gout; hyperuricemia; renal impairment; Crohn's disease, short bowel syndrome; pregnancy (category C); lactation.

## ROUTE & DOSAGE

**Pancreatic Insufficiency**

**Various brands are not interchangeable, see package insert for interchangeability**
*Adult/Adolescent/Child (4 y or older):* **PO** 500 lipase units/kg/meal; titrate based on symptoms
*Child (1–3 y):* **PO** 1000 lipase units/kg/meal; titrate based on symptoms
*Neonate/Infant (younger than 12 mo):* **PO** varies per brand, see package insert

## ADMINISTRATION

**Oral**
- Give capsules with food and sufficient liquid. Do not crush or chew capsules or capsule contents; capsules should be swallowed whole.

- May open capsule and sprinkle contents on soft acidic food, which should be swallowed without chewing. Follow with a full glass of water or juice.
- Determine dosage in relation to fat content in diet (suggested ratio: 300 mg pancrelipase for each 17 g dietary fat).

**ADVERSE EFFECTS** (≥1%) **GI:** Anorexia, *abdominal pain,* nausea, vomiting, abdominal pain, dyspepsia diarrhea. **Metabolic:** Hyperuricosuria. hyperglycemia. **CV:** Peripheral edema. **CNS:** Dizziness, headache, otalgia. **Hematologic:** Lymphadenopathy. **Otic:** *Ear pain.* **Respiratory:** Nasal congestion, cough.

**INTERACTIONS Drug:** Effectiveness can be decreased by concurrent ANTACID use.

**PHARMACOKINETICS Distribution:** Acts locally in GI tract. **Elimination:** Feces.

## NURSING IMPLICATIONS

**Assessment & Drug Effects**
- Monitor I&O and weight. Note appetite and quality of stools, weight loss, abdominal bloating, polyuria, thirst, hunger, itching. Pancreatic insufficiency is frequently associated with steatorrhea, bulky stools, and insulin-dependent diabetes.
- Monitor uric acid levels in patients with hyperuricemia, gout or renal impairment.
- S&S of colon stricture (cramping, abdominal pain, constipation, vomiting, inability to pass gas or stool).

**Patient & Family Education**
- Notify prescriber if breast-feeding or intending to breast-feed during treatment.

# PANCURONIUM BROMIDE
(pan-kyoo-roe′nee-um)

**Classification:** NONDEPOLARIZING SKELETAL MUSCLE RELAXANT
Therapeutic: SKELETAL MUSCLE RELAXANT
**Prototype:** Atracurium

**AVAILABILITY** Solution for injection

## ACTION & THERAPEUTIC EFFECT
Produces skeletal muscle relaxation or paralysis by competing with acetylcholine at cholinergic receptor sites on the skeletal muscle endplate and thus blocks nerve impulse transmission. *Induces skeletal muscle relaxation or paralysis.*

## USES
Adjunct to anesthesia to induce skeletal muscle relaxation. Also to facilitate management of patients undergoing mechanical ventilation.

## CONTRAINDICATIONS
Hypersensitivity to the drug or bromides.

## CAUTIOUS USE
History of severe anaphylactic reactions to other neuromuscular blocking agents requires appropriate emergency treatment. Debilitated patients; dehydration; MG; neuromuscular disease; pulmonary, liver, or kidney disease; fluid or electrolyte imbalance; pregnancy (category C); lactation; neonate less than 1 mo.

## ROUTE & DOSAGE

**Skeletal Muscle Relaxation**
*Adult/Child/Infant:* **IV** 0.04–0.1 mg/kg initial dose, may give additional doses of 0.01 mg/kg at 30–60 min intervals
*Neonate:* **IV** 0.02 mg/kg test dose

## ADMINISTRATION
**Intravenous**
Plastic syringe may be used for administration, but drug may adsorb to plastic with prolonged storage.

*PREPARE:* **Direct:** Give undiluted.
*ADMINISTER:* **Direct:** Give over 30–90 sec.
*INCOMPATIBILITIES:* **Solution/additive: Allopurinol, amphotericin B (conventional and lipid), caspofungin, dantrolene, diazepam, furosemide, gemtuzumab, lansoprazole, mitomycin, pantoprazole, phenytoin.**

▪ Refrigerate at 2°–8° C (36°–46° F). Do not freeze.

## ADVERSE EFFECTS (≥1%)
**CV:** *Increased pulse rate and BP,* ventricular extrasystoles. **Skin:** Transient acneiform rash, burning sensation along course of vein. **Body as a Whole:** Salivation, skeletal muscle weakness, <u>respiratory depression</u>.

## DIAGNOSTIC TEST INTERFERENCE
Pancuronium may decrease *serum cholinesterase* concentrations.

## INTERACTIONS
**Drug:** GENERAL ANESTHETICS increase neuromuscular blocking and duration of action; AMINOGLYCOSIDES, **bacitracin, polymyxin B, clindamycin, lidocaine,** parenteral **magnesium, quinidine, quinine, trimethaphan, verapamil** increase neuromuscular blockade; DIURETICS may increase or decrease neuromuscular blockade; **lithium** prolongs duration of neuromuscular blockade; NARCOTIC ANALGESICS possibly add to respiratory depression; **succinylcholine** increases onset and depth of neuromuscular blockade; **phenytoin** may cause resistance to or reversal of neuromuscular blockade.

P

---

Common adverse effects in *italic*; life-threatening effects <u>underlined</u>; generic names in **bold**; classifications in SMALL CAPS; ♣ Canadian drug name; ❷ Prototype drug

## PHARMACOKINETICS

**Onset:** 30–45 sec. **Peak:** 2–3 min. **Duration:** 60 min. **Distribution:** Well distributed to tissues and extracellular fluids; crosses placenta in small amounts. **Metabolism:** Small amount in liver. **Elimination:** Primarily in urine. **Half-Life:** 2 h.

## NURSING IMPLICATIONS

### Assessment & Drug Effects

- Assess cardiovascular and respiratory status continuously.
- Observe patient closely for residual muscle weakness and signs of respiratory distress during recovery period. Monitor BP and vital signs. Peripheral nerve stimulator may be used to assess the effects of pancuronium and to monitor restoration of neuromuscular function.
- Note: Consciousness is not affected by pancuronium. Patient will be awake and alert but unable to speak.

---

# PANITUMUMAB

(pan-i-tu-mu'mab)

*Vectibix*

**Classifications:** ANTINEOPLASTIC; BIOLOGIC RESPONSE MODIFIER; MONOCLONAL ANTIBODY; KINASE INHIBITOR

*Therapeutic:* ANTINEOPLASTIC

**Prototype:** Erlotinib

---

## AVAILABILITY Solution for injection

## ACTION & *THERAPEUTIC EFFECT*

Epidermal growth factor receptors (EGFRs) are overexpressed in many human cancers, including those of the colon and rectum. EGFRs control the activity of intracellular tyrosine kinases that regulate transcription of DNA molecules involved in cancer cell growth, survival, and proliferation. *Panitumumab inhibits overexpression of EGFRs in cancer cells, decreasing their proliferation, survival, and decreasing their invasive capacity and metastases.*

## USES Treatment of EGFR-expressing metastatic colorectal carcinoma in patients with disease progression on or following fluoropyrimidine-, oxaliplatin-, and irinotecan-containing chemotherapy regimens.

## CONTRAINDICATIONS Pulmonary fibrosis; interstitial lung disease; lactation.

## CAUTIOUS USE Photosensitivity with drug use; electrolyte imbalances, especially hypomagnesemia, and hypocalcemia; lung disorders; pregnancy (category C). Safe use in children not established.

## ROUTE & DOSAGE

### Metastatic Colorectal Carcinoma

*Adult:* **IV** 6 mg/kg q14days

### *Dosage Adjustments for Infusion Reactions and Dermatologic Reactions*

*Mild or moderate infusion reactions (Grade 1 or 2):* Reduce infusion rate by 50%

*Severe infusion reactions (Grade 3 or 4):* Discontinue permanently

*Intolerable or severe dermatologic toxicity (greater than Grade 3):* Withhold drug. If toxicity does not improve to at least Grade 2 within 1 mo, permanently discontinue. If toxicity improves to at least Grade 2 and patient is symptomatically improved after withholding no more than 2 doses, resume at 50% of original dose. If toxicities recur, discontinue permanently. If toxicities do not recur, subsequent doses may be increased by increments of 25% of original dose until 6 mg/kg is reached.

Common adverse effects in *italic*; life-threatening effects underlined; generic names in **bold**; classifications in SMALL CAPS; ✣ Canadian drug name; ⓟ Prototype drug

## ADMINISTRATION
### Intravenous

*PREPARE:* **IV Infusion:** Dilute doses up to 1000 mg with NS to a total volume of 100 mL. ▪ Dilute higher doses with NS to a total volume of 150 mL. ▪ Final concentration should not exceed 10 mg/mL. ▪ Mix by gentle inversion and do not shake. Solution will contain small translucent particles that will be removed by filtration during infusion.

*ADMINISTER:* **IV Infusion:** Infuse doses less than 1000 mg over 60 min. ▪ Infuse doses greater than 1000 mg over 90 min. ▪ Use an infusion pump and a 0.2 or 0.22 micron in line filter. ▪ Flush the line before/after infusion with NS. ▪ Discontinue infusion immediately if an anaphylactic reaction is suspected (i.e., bronchospasm, fever, chills, hypotension).

▪ Store unopened vials at 2°–8° C (36°–46° F). Protect vials from direct sunlight. ▪ Use diluted infusion solution within 6 h if stored at room temperature, or within 24 h if stored at 2°–8° C (36°–46° F).

## ADVERSE EFFECTS (≥1%) **Body as a Whole:** *Fatigue,* infectious sequelae and septic death, infusion reactions, peripheral edema. **GI:** *Abdominal pain, constipation, diarrhea,* mucosal inflammation, *nausea,* stomatitis, *vomiting.* **Metabolic:** *Hypomagnesemia.* **Respiratory:** *Cough,* pulmonary fibrosis. **Skin:** *Acneiform dermatitis, dry skin, erythema, pruritus, skin exfoliation, skin fissures, nail disorders, paronychia.* **Special Senses:** Conjunctivitis, eye/eyelid irritation, increased lacrimation, ocular hyperemia.

## PHARMACOKINETICS **Half-Life:** 7.5 days.

## NURSING IMPLICATIONS

### Black Box Warning

*Panitumumab has been associated with frequent, sometimes severe, dermatologic toxicities, and severe infusion reactions.*

### Assessment & Drug Effects
▪ Monitor for S&S of a severe infusion reaction; check vital signs q30min during infusion and 30 min postinfusion.
▪ Monitor for and report S&S of dermatologic toxicity such as acne-like dermatitis, pruritus, erythema, rash, skin exfoliation, dry skin, and skin fissures; inflammatory or infectious sequelae in those who experience severe dermatologic toxicities.
▪ Withhold drug and notify prescriber for any signs of drug toxicity.
▪ Monitor lab tests: Periodic serum electrolytes during and for 8 wk following completion of therapy.

### Patient & Family Education
▪ Immediately report any discomfort experienced during and shortly after drug infusion.
▪ Wear sunscreen and limit sun exposure while receiving panitumumab.
▪ Report any of the following to a health care provider: Any signs of irritation, inflammation, or infection of the skin, nails, or eyes; shortness of breath or any other breathing difficulty.
▪ Women of childbearing age should use reliable means of contraception during and for 6 mo after the last dose of panitumumab.

## PANTOPRAZOLE SODIUM
(pan-to′pra-zole)
Protonix

**Classifications:** GASTRIC PROTON PUMP INHIBITOR; ANTISECRETORY

---

Common adverse effects in *italic;* life-threatening effects underlined; generic names in **bold;** classifications in SMALL CAPS; ♣ Canadian drug name; ⊙ Prototype drug

Therapeutic: ANTIULCER
**Prototype:** Omeprazole

**AVAILABILITY** Delayed release tablet; solution for injection; delayed release oral suspension

**ACTION & *THERAPEUTIC EFFECT*** Gastric acid secretion is decreased by inhibiting the $H^+$, $K^+$-ATPase enzyme system responsible for acid production. *Suppresses gastric acid secretion by inhibiting the acid (proton $H^+$) pump in the parietal cells.*

**USES** Short-term treatment of erosive esophagitis associated with gastroesophageal reflux disease (GERD), hypersecretory disease.

**UNLABELED USES** Peptic ulcer disease, dyspepsia, stress ulcer prophylaxis, heartburn, duodenal ulcer.

**CONTRAINDICATIONS** Hypersensitivity to pantoprazole or other proton pump inhibitors (PPIs).

**CAUTIOUS USE** Mild to severe hepatic insufficiency, cirrhosis; concurrent administration of EDTA-containing products; elderly (avoid after 8 wk); history of lupus erythematosus, history of osteoporosis; pregnancy (category C); lactation. Safety and efficacy in children younger than 5 y not established for uses other than erosive esophagitis. There is no commercially available dosage formulation appropriate for children younger than 5 y.

**ROUTE & DOSAGE**

**Erosive Esophagitis**
*Adult:* **PO** 40 mg daily × 8 wks **IV** 40 mg daily × 7–10 days
*Adolescent/Child (5 y and older, weight 40 kg or more):* **PO** 40 mg daily x 8 wk; *weight 15–39 kg:* 20 mg daily x 8 wk

**Hypersecretory Disease**
*Adult:* **PO** 40 mg b.i.d. (doses up to 240 mg/day have been used) **IV** 80 mg b.i.d.; adjust based on acid output

**ADMINISTRATION**
**Oral**
- Do not crush or break in half. **Must be** swallowed whole with or without food.
- Granules for oral suspension should be given 30 min before meals. Granules should be put into apple juice or applesauce, not water and given within 10 min of preparation.
- *NG tube administration:* Add granules for suspension to a catheter tip syringe inserted into a 16 French catheter (or larger). Add 40 mL of apple juice in 10 mL increments to fully suspend granules and ensure that all of the drug is washed into the stomach.
- Store tablet and oral suspension at 20°–25° C (66°–77° F), but room temperature permitted. Excursions permitted to 15°–30° C (59°–86° F).

**Intravenous**

*PREPARE:* **IV 15 Min Infusion:** Reconstitute each 40 mg vial with 10 mL NS to yield 4 mg/mL. ▪ The required dose of 40 or 80 mg may be further diluted to a **total volume** of 100 mL in D5W, NS, or LR to yield 0.4 mg/mL or 0.8 mg/mL, respectively.
*ADMINISTER:* **IV Infusion:** Give through a dedicated line or flushed IV line before and after each dose with D5W, NS, or LR. ▪ Give the 4 mg/mL concentration over at least 2 min. ▪ Infuse the 0.4 or 0.8 mg/mL concentration over 15 min.
*INCOMPATIBILITIES:* Solution/additive: Solutions containing **zinc.**

Common adverse effects in *italic;* life-threatening effects <u>underlined;</u> generic names in **bold;** classifications in SMALL CAPS; ✦ Canadian drug name; ⊙ Prototype drug

# PANTOPRAZOLE SODIUM

**Y-site:** Alemtuzumab, alfentanil, amphotericin b, atneolol, atracurium, atropine, aztreonam, bertylium, buprenorphine, butorphanol, caffeine, calcium salts, cefepime, cefoperazone, cefotaxime, chloramphenical, chlorpromazine, cimetidine, ciprofloxacin, cisatracuirum, cisplatin, dacarbazine, dactinomycin, dantrolene, daptomycin, daunorubicin, dexamethasone sodium phosphate, dexmedetomidine hydrochloride, dexrazoxane, diazepam, diltiazem, diphenhydramine, dobutamine, dolasetron, doxorubicin, droperidol, ephedrine, epirubicin, esmolol, estrogens, etoposide, famotidine, fenoldopam, fentanyl, fluconazole, fludarabine, gatifloxacin, gemcitabine, gemtuzumab, glycopyrrolate, haloperidol, hydralazinc, hydroxyzine, idarubicin, ifosfamide, indomethacin, isavuconazonium, ketorolac, labetalol, leucovorin, levofloxacin, levophanol, lidocaine, linezolid, lorazepam, mechlprethamine, melphalan, meperidine, meropenem, methotrexate, methylprednisolone, metoprolol, metrondiazole, milrinone, minocycline, mitomycin, mitoxantrone hydrochloride, mivacurium chloride, moxifloxacin, multiple vitamin injections, mycophenolate, nalbuphine, naloxone, nesiritide, nicardipine, ondansetron, palonosetron, pancuronium, pemetrexed, pentamidine isethionate, phenytoin, polymyxin B, potassium acetate, potassium phosphate, prochlorperazine, promethazine, propranolol, quinideine, quinupristin/dalfopristin, ranitidine, remifentanil, rocuronium, salbutamol, sodium acetate, sodium phosphate, streptozocin, theotipa, tolazoline hydrochloride, topotecan, trimethobenzamide hydrochloride, vecuronium, verapamil, vinblastine, vincristine, vinorelbine, voriconazole.

▪ Reconstituted IV solutions may be stored for up to 6 h at 15°–30° C (59°–86° F) before further dilution. ▪ The diluted 100 mL solution should be infused within 24 h or infused within 24 h of reconstitution.

## ADVERSE EFFECTS (≥1%) CV: Edema GI: Diarrhea, flatulence, abdominal pain. CNS: *Headache,* insomnia, depression. Skin: Rash Body as a Whole: arthralgia, infection. Hematologic: Leukopenia, thrombocytopenia. Optic: Blurred vision.

## INTERACTIONS Drug: Contraindicated with **atazanavir** or **rilpivirine.** May decrease absorption of **ampicillin,** IRON SALTS, **itraconazole, ketoconazole;** increases INR with **warfarin. Herbal:** Ginkgo may decrease plasma levels. **Lab Test:** May cause false-positive urine tetrahydrocannabinol (THC) test

## PHARMACOKINETICS Absorption: Well absorbed with 77% bioavailability. Peak: 2.4 h. Distribution: 98% protein bound. Metabolism: In liver (CYP2C19). Elimination: 71% in urine, 18% in feces. Half-Life: 1 h.

## NURSING IMPLICATIONS
### Assessment & Drug Effects
▪ Monitor for and immediately report S&S of angioedema or a severe skin reaction.
▪ Monitor for improvement in gastroesophageal comfort.
▪ Monitor lab tests: Vitamin B$_{12}$ with long-term therapy.

### Patient & Family Education
▪ Contact prescriber promptly if any of the following occur: Peeling,

Common adverse effects in *italic;* life-threatening effects underlined; generic names in **bold;** classifications in SMALL CAPS; ♣ Canadian drug name; ⊘ Prototype drug

1231

blistering, or loosening of skin; skin rash, hives, or itching; swelling of the face, tongue, or lips; difficulty breathing or swallowing.

# PAPAVERINE HYDROCHLORIDE
(pa-pav′er-een)
**Classification:** NONNITRATE VASODILATOR
Therapeutic: VASODILATOR; SMOOTH MUSCLE RELAXANT
**Prototype:** Hydralazine

**AVAILABILITY** Solution for injection

## ACTION & *THERAPEUTIC EFFECT*
Exerts nonspecific direct spasmolytic effect on smooth muscles unrelated to innervation. Acts directly on myocardium, depresses conduction and irritability, and prolongs refractory period. *Relaxes the smooth muscle of the heart as well as produces relaxation of vascular smooth muscles.*

**USES** Smooth muscle spasms.

**UNLABELED USES** Impotence, cardiac bypass surgery.

## CONTRAINDICATIONS Parenteral use in complete AV block.

## CAUTIOUS USE Glaucoma; myocardial depression; QT prolongation, angina pectoris; recent stroke; pregnancy (category C); lactation.

## ROUTE & DOSAGE

**Smooth Muscle Spasm**
*Adult:* **IM/IV** 30–120 mg q3h as needed

## ADMINISTRATION
**Intramuscular**
- Aspirate carefully before injecting IM to avoid inadvertent entry into blood vessel, and administer slowly.

**Intravenous**
- IV administration to children: Verify correct IV concentration and rate of infusion with prescriber.

*PREPARE:* **Direct:** Give undiluted or diluted in an equal volume of sterile water for injection.
*ADMINISTER:* **Direct:** Give slowly over 1–2 min. Avoid rapid injection.
*INCOMPATIBILITIES:* **Solution/additive: Aminophylline, heparin, lactated Ringer's. Y site: aminophylline, amphotericin B, ampicillin, bumetidine, CEPHALOSPORINS, clindamycin, dantrolene, diazepam, diazoxide, furosemide, heparin, indomethacin, ketorolac, methylprednisolone, phenobarbital, phenytoin, piperacillin.**

**ADVERSE EFFECTS** (≥1%) **Body as a Whole:** General discomfort, facial flushing, sweating, weakness, coma. **CNS:** Dizziness, drowsiness, headache, sedation. **CV:** Slight rise in BP, paroxysmal tachycardia, transient ventricular ectopic rhythms, AV block, arrhythmias. **GI:** Nausea, anorexia, constipation, diarrhea, abdominal distress, dry mouth and throat, hepatotoxicity (jaundice, eosinophilia, abnormal liver function tests); with rapid IV administration. **Respiratory:** Increased depth of respiration, respiratory depression, fatal apnea. **Skin:** Pruritus, skin rash. **Special Senses:** Diplopia, nystagmus. **Urogenital:** Priapism.

**INTERACTIONS Drug:** May decrease **levodopa** effectiveness; **morphine** may antagonize smooth muscle relaxation effect of papaverine.

**PHARMACOKINETICS Absorption:** Readily from GI tract. **Peak:** 1–2 h. **Duration:** 12 h sustained release. **Metabolism:** In liver. **Elimination:** In urine chiefly as metabolites. **Half-Life:** 90 min.

## NURSING IMPLICATIONS

### Assessment & Drug Effects

- Monitor pulse, respiration, and BP in patients receiving drug parenterally. If significant changes are noted, withhold medication and report promptly to prescriber.

### Patient & Family Education

- Notify prescriber if any adverse effect persists or if GI symptoms, jaundice, or skin rash appears. Liver function tests may be indicated.
- Do not drive or engage in potentially hazardous activities until response to drug is known. Alcohol may increase drowsiness and dizziness.

# PAREGORIC (CAMPHORATED OPIUM TINCTURE)

(par-e-gor'ik)

**Classifications:** ANTIDIARRHEAL; NARCOTIC (OPIATE AGONIST) ANALGESIC
**Therapeutic:** ANTIDIARRHEAL
**Prototype:** Loperamide
**Controlled Substance:** Schedule III

## AVAILABILITY Liquid

## ACTION & THERAPEUTIC EFFECT

Decreases GI motility and effective propulsive peristalsis while diminishing digestive secretions. *Delayed transit of intestinal contents results in desiccation of feces and constipation.*

## USES Short-term treatment for symptomatic relief of acute diarrhea and abdominal cramps.

## CONTRAINDICATIONS Hypersensitivity to opium alkaloids; diarrhea caused by poisons (until eliminated); COPD.

## CAUTIOUS USE Asthma; liver disease; liver disease; GI disease; history of opiate agonist dependence; severe prostatic hypertrophy; pregnancy (category C); lactation; children.

## ROUTE & DOSAGE

### Acute Diarrhea

*Adult:* **PO** 5–10 mL after loose bowel movement, 1–4 × daily if needed
*Child:* **PO** 0.25–0.5 mL/kg 1–4 × day

## ADMINISTRATION

### Oral

- Give paregoric in sufficient water (2 or 3 swallows) to ensure its passage into the stomach (mixture will appear milky).

## ADVERSE EFFECTS (≥1%) GI: Anorexia, nausea, vomiting, *constipation,* abdominal pain. Body as a Whole: Dizziness, faintness, drowsiness, facial flushing, sweating, physical dependence.

## INTERACTIONS Drug: Alcohol and other CNS DEPRESSANTS add to CNS effects.

## PHARMACOKINETICS Absorption: Readily from GI tract. Duration: 4–5 h. Distribution: Crosses placenta; distributed into breast milk. Metabolism: In liver. Elimination: In urine. Half-Life: 2–3 h.

## NURSING IMPLICATIONS

### Assessment & Drug Effects

- Paregoric may worsen the course of infection-associated diarrhea by delaying the elimination of pathogens.
- Be aware that adverse effects are primarily due to morphine content. Paregoric abuse results because of the narcotic content of the drug.
- Assess for fluid and electrolyte imbalance until diarrhea has stopped.

### Patient & Family Education

- Adhere strictly to prescribed dosage schedule.

---

Common adverse effects in *italic;* life-threatening effects underlined; generic names in **bold;** classifications in SMALL CAPS; ♣ Canadian drug name; ⓟ Prototype drug

1233

- Maintain bed rest if diarrhea is severe with a high level of fluid loss.
- Replace fluids and electrolytes as needed for diarrhea. Drink warm clear liquids and avoid dairy products, concentrated sweets, and cold drinks until diarrhea stops.
- Observe character and frequency of stools. Discontinue drug as soon as diarrhea is controlled. Report promptly to prescriber if diarrhea persists more than 3 days, if fever is higher than 38.8° C (102° F), abdominal pain develops, or if mucus or blood is passed.
- Understand that constipation is often a consequence of antidiarrheal treatment and a normal elimination pattern is usually established as dietary intake increases.

## PARICALCITOL

(par-i-cal′ci-tol)
Zemplar
**Classification:** VITAMIN D ANALOG
Therapeutic: VITAMIN D ANALOG
**Prototype:** Calcitriol

**AVAILABILITY** Vial; capsule

### ACTION & *THERAPEUTIC EFFECT*

Synthetic vitamin D analog that reduces parathyroid hormone (PTH) activity levels in chronic kidney failure (CRF). Lowers serum levels of calcium and phosphate. Decreases parathyroid hormone release as well as bone resorption in some patients. *Effectiveness indicated by iPTH levels less than 1.5–3 × the upper limit of normal.*

**USES** Prevention and treatment of secondary hyperparathyroidism associated with CRF.

**CONTRAINDICATIONS** Hypersensitivity to paricalcitol; hypercalcemia; evidence of vitamin D toxicity; concurrent administration of phosphate preparations and vitamin D.

**CAUTIOUS USE** Severe liver disease; abnormally low levels of PTH; pregnancy (category C); lactation. Safety and efficacy in children not established.

### ROUTE & DOSAGE

**Secondary Hyperparathyroidism**

*Adult:* **IV** 0.04 mcg/kg–0.1 mcg/kg (max: 0.24 mcg/kg), no more than every other day during dialysis; **PO** iPTH less than 500 pg/mL, 1 mcg/day or 2 mcg 3 × wk; iPTH greater than 500 pg/mL, 2 mcg/day or 4 mcg 3 × wk

**Renal Impairment Dosage Adjustment**

*Stage 5 Chronic Kidney Disease (CKD):* See package insert

### ADMINISTRATION

**Oral**
- Give no more frequently than every other day when dosing 3 × wk.
- Store at 15°–30° C (59°–86° F).

**Intravenous**

**PREPARE: Direct:** Give undiluted.
**ADMINISTER: Direct:** Give IV bolus dose anytime during dialysis.

- Store at 25° C (77° F). Discard unused portion of a single dose vial.

**ADVERSE EFFECTS** (≥1%) **Body as a Whole:** Chills, feeling unwell, fever, flu-like symptoms, sepsis, edema. **CNS:** Lightheadedness. **CV:** Palpitations. **GI:** Dry mouth, GI bleeding, *nausea,* vomiting. **Respiratory:** Pneumonia. **Metabolic:** Hypercalcemia.

**INTERACTIONS Drug:** Hypercalcemia may increase risk of **digoxin** toxicity; may increase **magnesium**

Common adverse effects in *italic;* life-threatening effects underlined; generic names in **bold;** classifications in SMALL CAPS; ♣ Canadian drug name; ⊚ Prototype drug absorption and toxicity in renal failure. Do not use with **vitamin D analogs. Herbal:** Be cautious of **vitamin D** content in herbal and OTC products.

## PHARMACOKINETICS **Distribution:** Greater than 99% protein bound. **Metabolism:** Via CYP3A4. **Elimination:** In feces. **Half-Life:** 15 h.

### NURSING IMPLICATIONS

#### Assessment & Drug Effects

- Monitor for S&S of hypercalcemia (see Appendix F).
- Withhold drug and notify prescriber if hypercalcemia occurs.
- Coadministered drugs: Monitor for digoxin toxicity if serum calcium level is elevated.
- Monitor lab tests: Serum calcium, serum phosphorus, and serum or plasma intact PTH at least every 2 wk for 3 mo, then monthly for 3 mo, and every 3 mo thereafter. Increase frequency of lab tests with coadministration of strong CYP3A inhibitors.

#### Patient & Family Education

- Report immediately any of the following to the prescriber: Weakness, anorexia, nausea, vomiting, abdominal cramps, diarrhea, muscle or bone pain, or excessive thirst.
- Adhere strictly to dietary regimen of calcium supplementation and phosphorus restriction to ensure successful therapy.
- Avoid excessive use of aluminum-containing compounds such as antacids/vitamins.

## PAROMOMYCIN SULFATE ⓟ
(par-oh-moe-mye′sin)

**Classifications:** AMINOGLYCOSIDE ANTIBIOTIC; AMEBICIDE
Therapeutic: AMEBICIDE

**AVAILABILITY** Capsule

## ACTION & *THERAPEUTIC EFFECT*
Aminoglycoside antibiotic with broad-spectrum antibacterial activity. *Exerts direct bactericidal and amebicidal action, primarily in lumen of GI tract. Ineffective against extraintestinal amebiasis.*

## USES Acute and chronic intestinal amebiasis; adjunctive therapy for hepatic coma/encephalopathy.

## CONTRAINDICATIONS Aminoglycoside hypersensitivity; intestinal obstruction; impaired kidney function.

## CAUTIOUS USE GI ulceration; renal failure, renal impairment; older adults; myasthenia gravis; parkinsonism; pregnancy (category C); children.

## ROUTE & DOSAGE

| Intestinal Amebiasis |
| --- |
| *Adult/Child:* **PO** 25–35 mg/kg divided in 3 doses for 7–10 days |
| **Hepatic Coma** |
| *Adult:* **PO** 4 g/day in divided doses for 5–10 days |

## ADMINISTRATION

### Oral
- Administer with meals.

## ADVERSE EFFECTS (≥1%) **CNS:** Headache, vertigo. **GI:** *Diarrhea, abdominal cramps,* steatorrhea, *nausea, vomiting, heartburn,* secondary enterocolitis. **Skin:** Exanthema, rash, pruritus. **Special Senses:** Ototoxicity. **Urogenital:** Nephrotoxicity (in patients with GI inflammation or ulcerations) oliguria, proteinuria, pyuria. **Body as a Whole:** Eosinophilia, overgrowth of nonsusceptible organisms.

## DIAGNOSTIC TEST INTERFERENCE
Prolonged use of paromomycin

Common adverse effects in *italic;* life-threatening effects underlined; generic names in **bold;** classifications in SMALL CAPS; ♦ Canadian drug name; ⓟ Prototype drug

1235

may cause reduction in **serum cholesterol.**

**INTERACTIONS Drug:** May decrease absorption of **cyanocobalamin.** Do not use with **cidofovir** or **gallium.** Use caution with other AMINO-GLYCOSIDES or agents that may increase risk of nephrotoxicity.

**PHARMACOKINETICS** **Absorption:** Poorly from intact GI tract. **Elimination:** In feces. **Half-Life:** 2–3 h.

## NURSING IMPLICATIONS

### Assessment & Drug Effects

- Monitor therapeutic effectiveness. Criterion of cure is absence of amoebae in stool specimens examined at weekly intervals for 6 wk after completion of treatment, and thereafter at monthly intervals for 2 y.
- Monitor for appearance of a superinfection during therapy (see Appendix F).
- Monitor closely patients with history of GI ulceration for nephrotoxicity and ototoxicity (see Appendix F). Drug absorption can take place through diseased mucosa.

### Patient & Family Education

- Do not prepare, process, or serve food until treatment is complete when receiving drug for intestinal amebiasis. Isolation is not required.
- Practice strict personal hygiene, particularly hand washing after defecation and before eating food.

## PAROXETINE

(par-ox′e-teen)

Brisdelle, Pexeva, Paxil, Paxil CR

**Classifications:** ANTIDEPRESSANT; SELECTIVE SEROTONIN 5-HT REUPTAKE INHIBITOR (SSRI)

**Therapeutic:** ANTIDEPRESSANT; SSRI; ANTIANXIETY
**Prototype:** Fluoxetine

**AVAILABILITY** Tablet; sustained release tablet; suspension; capsule

## ACTION & THERAPEUTIC EFFECT

Antidepressant that is a serotonin 5-HT reuptake inhibitor. It is highly potent and a highly selective inhibitor of serotonin reuptake by neurons in CNS. *Efficacious in depression resistant to other antidepressants and in depression complicated by anxiety.*

**USES** Depression, obsessive-compulsive disorders, panic attacks, excessive social anxiety, generalized anxiety, post traumatic stress disorder (PTSD), premenstrual dysphoric disorder (PMDD), hot flashes.

**UNLABELED USES** Diabetic neuropathy, myoclonus, bipolar depression in conjunction with lithium, chronic headache, premature ejaculation, fibromyalgia.

**CONTRAINDICATIONS** Hypersensitivity to paroxetine; suicidal ideation; concomitant use of MAO inhibitors or within 14 days of stoppage; bipolar disorder; alcohol; pregnancy (category D and X for **Brisdelle**).

**CAUTIOUS USE** History of mania, suicidal tendencies; history of drug abuse; anorexia nervosa; ECT therapy; MDD; seizure disorder; renal/hepatic impairment; history of metabolic disorders; volume-depleted patients, recent MI, unstable cardiac disease; abrupt discontinuation; older adults; lactation. Not FDA approved for children and adolescents.

Common adverse effects in *italic;* life-threatening effects underlined; generic names in **bold;** classifications in SMALL CAPS; ◆ Canadian drug name; ⊘ Prototype drug

## ROUTE & DOSAGE

### Depression

*Adult:* **PO** 20 mg/day may increase by 10 mg weekly (max: 50 mg/day); 25 mg sustained release daily in morning, may increase by 12.5 mg (max: 62.5 mg/day); use lower starting doses for patients with renal or hepatic insufficiency

*Geriatric:* **PO** Start with 10 mg/day (12.5 mg/day sustained release), [max: 40 mg/day (50 mg/day sustained release)]

### Panic Disorder

*Adult:* **PO** 10 mg daily then increase to 40 mg/day; **Sustained release** 12.5 mg daily, may increase (max: 75 mg/day)

### Social Anxiety Disorder

*Adult:* **PO** 20–60 mg/day

### Generalized Anxiety, PTSD, OCD

*Adult:* **PO** Start with 20 mg once daily, may increase by 10 mg/day at weekly intervals if needed to target dose of 40 mg once daily (max: 60 mg/day)

*Geriatric:* **PO** Start with 10 mg once daily, may increase by 10 mg/day at weekly intervals if needed (max: 40 mg/day)

### Premenstrual Dysphoric Disorder

*Adult:* **PO** 12.5 mg once daily (up to 25 mg once daily) throughout the month or daily for 2 wk before menstrual period

### Hot Flashes

*Adult:* **PO** 7.5 mg daily (Brisdelle formulation); **Extended release** 12.5 mg daily may titrate up to 25 mg daily

### *Pharmacogenetic Dosage Adjustment*

*Poor CYP2D6 metabolizers:* Start with 65% of dose

## ADMINISTRATION

### Oral

- Ensure that sustained release form is not chewed or crushed. **Must be** swallowed whole.
- Usually administered every morning. Administering with food will decrease GI adverse effects. Do not administer concomitantly with antacids.
- Be aware that at least 14 days should elapse when switching a patient from/to an MAO inhibitor to/from paroxetine.

## ADVERSE EFFECTS (≥1%) **CV:**
Postural hypotension. **CNS:** *Headache,* tremor, agitation or nervousness, anxiety, paresthesias, dizziness, insomnia, *sedation.* **GI:** *Nausea,* constipation, *vomiting,* anorexia, diarrhea, dyspepsia, flatulence, increased appetite, taste aversion, *dry mouth.* **Urogenital:** Urinary hesitancy or frequency, change in male fertility, decrease in libido. **Hepatic:** Isolated reports of elevated liver enzymes. **Special Senses:** Blurred vision. **Skin:** Diaphoresis, rash, pruritus. **Metabolic:** Hyponatremia in older adults. **Body as a Whole:** Bone fracture (in older adults), weakness.

## INTERACTIONS **Drug:** Do not use with **pimozide. Activated charcoal** reduces absorption of paroxetine. **Cimetidine** increases paroxetine levels. MAO INHIBITORS, **selegiline** may cause an increased vasopressor response leading to hypertensive crisis or death. Use with other seretonergic agents (e.g., SSRIs) or MAOIs can cause serotonin syndrome. **Phenytoin** can cause liver enzyme induction resulting in

P

Common adverse effects in *italic;* life-threatening effects <u>underlined;</u> generic names in **bold;** classifications in SMALL CAPS; ♣ Canadian drug name; ⬤ Prototype drug

1237

lower paroxetine levels and shorter half-life. **Warfarin** may increase risk of bleeding and **thioridazine** levels, and prolong $QT_c$ interval leading to heart block; increase **ergotamine** toxicity with **dihydroergotamine, ergotamine.** May reduce the efficacy of **tamoxifen. Herbal: St. John's wort** may cause serotonin syndrome (headache, dizziness, sweating, agitation).

## PHARMACOKINETICS **Absorption:** 99% from GI tract. **Onset:** 2 wk. **Peak:** 5–8 h. **Distribution:** Very lipophilic. 95% protein bound. Distributes into breast milk. **Metabolism:** Extensively in the liver to inactive metabolites via CYP2D6. **Elimination:** Less than 2% is excreted unchanged in urine. 65% of dose appears in urine as metabolites. Metabolites of paroxetine are also excreted in feces, presumably via bile. **Half-Life:** 24 h.

## NURSING IMPLICATIONS

### Black Box Warning

*Paroxetine has been associated with suicidal ideation and behavior in children, adolescents, and young adults.*

### Assessment & Drug Effects

- Monitor for worsening of depression or emergence of suicidal ideation. Closely monitor those younger than 18 y for suicidal thinking and behavior.
- Monitor for adverse effects, which include headache, weakness, sedation, dizziness, insomnia; nausea, constipation, or diarrhea; dry mouth; sweating; male ejaculatory disturbance. These occur in more than 10% of all patients and may result in poor compliance with drug regimen.

- Monitor older adults for fluid and sodium imbalances.
- Monitor for significant weight loss.
- Monitor patients with history of mania for reactivation of condition.
- Monitor patients with preexisting cardiovascular disease carefully because paroxetine may adversely affect hemodynamic status.

### Patient & Family Education

- Monitor children, adolescents, and young adults for changes in behavior that may indicate suicidal ideation.
- Use caution when operating hazardous machinery or equipment until response to drug is known.
- Concurrent use of alcohol may increase risk of adverse CNS effects.
- Adaptation to some adverse effects (especially dizziness and nausea) may occur over a period of 4–6 wk.
- Do not stop drug therapy after improvement in emotional status occurs.
- Notify prescriber of any distressing adverse effects.

## PATIROMER
(pa-tir'oh-mer)

Veltassa

**Classifications:** CATIONIC EXCHANGE POLYMER; POTASSIUM BINDER

Therapeutic: POTASSIUM BINDER

**AVAILABILITY** Powder for oral suspension

## ACTION & *THERAPEUTIC EFFECT*

A nonabsorbed, cation exchange polymer that binds to potassium in the lumen of the gastrointestinal tract and increases its fecal elimination. *The binding of potassium reduces the concentration of free potassium in the gastrointestinal*

Common adverse effects in *italic;* life-threatening effects <u>underlined;</u> generic names in **bold;** classifications in SMALL CAPS; ✦ Canadian drug name; ⓟ Prototype drug *lumen, resulting in a reduction of serum potassium levels.*

**USES** Treatment of hyperkalemia. Due to its delayed onset of action, it should not be used in the emergency treatment of life-threatening hyperkalemia.

**CONTRAINDICATIONS** Hypersensitivity to patiromer. Avoid use in patients with severe constipation, GI obstruction, fecal impaction, including post-operative bowel motility disorders.

**CAUTIOUS USE** Use cautiously in patients with a history of hypomagnesemia. Maternal use during pregnancy is not expected to result in fetal risk. According to the manufacturer, breast feeding is not expected to result in risk to the infant. If an infant does experience adverse effects, it should be reported to the FDA.

## ROUTE & DOSAGE

| Hyperkalemia |
| --- |
| *Adult:* **PO** 8.4 grams once daily; may increase to 25.2 grams once daily |

## ADMINISTRATION

### Oral

- Administer patiromer 6 h before or 6 h after other orally administered medications to prevent patiromer from binding to other oral medications.
- Administer with food.
- Do not administer in its dry form.
- Do not heat or add to heated food or liquids.

### Oral Liquid Formulation

- Prepare each dose immediately before administration.
- Measure 1/3 cup of water. Pour half into the cup and then empty the entire contents of the packet into the glass. Stir thoroughly and add the remaining water. Stir again, the particles will not completely dissolve. The mixture will look cloudy. Add more water if needed for desired consistency.
- Drink immediately, rinse the glass with more water and drink again. Repeat as needed to ensure that the entire dose has been given.
- Store at 2°–8° C (36°–46° F). If stored at room temperature 25° C (77° F), use within 3 mo of being taken out of refrigeration. Avoid exposure to excessive heat above 40° C (104° F).

**ADVERSE EFFECTS** (≥2%) **CNS:** Nausea. **GI:** Abdominal discomfort, constipation, diarrhea, flatulence. **Metabolic:** Hypokalemia, hypomagnesemia.

**INTERACTIONS Drug:** Patiromer can bind to other coadministered oral drugs and reduce their absorption. Oral drugs should be taken at least 6 h before or 6 h after patiromer.

**PHARMACOKINETICS Absorption:** Not orally absorbed.

## NURSING IMPLICATIONS

### Assessment & Drug Effects

- Older adults may experience more gastrointestinal adverse reactions.
- Monitor lab tests: Serum magnesium and potassium levels.

### Patient & Family Education

- Immediately report to prescriber for any of the following: Mood changes, muscle pain, weakness, muscle cramps or spasms, seizures, lack of appetite, severe nausea or vomiting, or an abnormal heart beat.
- Report signs of a significant reaction: Wheezing, chest tightness, itching, swelling of face, lips, tongue, or throat.

Common adverse effects in *italic*; life-threatening effects underlined; generic names in **bold**; classifications in SMALL CAPS; ♣ Canadian drug name; ♆ Prototype drug

1239

# PAZOPANIB

(pas-o′pa-nib)

Votrient

**Classifications:** ANTINEOPLASTIC; KINASE INHIBITOR

Therapeutic: ANTINEOPLASTIC

**Prototype:** Erlotinib

## AVAILABILITY Tablet

## ACTION & *THERAPEUTIC EFFECT*

A multi-tyrosine kinase (i.e., multi-kinase) inhibitor that limits tumor growth by inhibiting cell surface vascular endothelial growth factor receptors and other receptors needed for tumor angiogenesis and growth. *Pazopanib inhibits growth of advanced renal cell carcinoma*.

## USES Treatment of advanced renal cell carcinoma; soft tissue sarcoma.

## CONTRAINDICATIONS Hepatotoxicity; severe hepatic impairment; ALT elevation greater than $3 \times$ ULN concurrently with bilirubin elevation of greater than $2 \times$ ULN; cerebral or GI bleeding within last 6 mo; GI perforation or fistula; uncontrolled hypertension; drug induced left ventricular ejection fraction (LVEF); wound dehiscence; stop drug 7 days before surgical procedures; patients who have had an arterial thrombotic event within 6 mo; reversible posterior leukoencephalopathy syndrome; nephrotic syndrome; pregnancy (category D); lactation.

## CAUTIOUS USE Risk for QT prolongation or history of QT prolongation; electrolyte imbalance; CHF; cardiac dysfuction; risk for or history of thrombotic event; risk for or history of GI perforation or fistula; moderate hepatic impairment; history of hypothyroidism; infection; older adults; children younger than 18 y.

## ROUTE & DOSAGE

### Renal Cell Carcinoma/Soft Tissue Sarcoma

*Adult:* **PO** 800 mg once daily reduce to 400 mg once daily if larger dose isn't tolerated or if patient is taking a strong CYP3A4 inhibitor

**Hepatic Impairment Dosage Adjustment**

See package insert for details

## ADMINISTRATION

### Oral

- Give without food at least 1 h before or 2 h after a meal.
- Ensure that the tablets are swallowed whole. They should not be crushed or chewed.

## ADVERSE EFFECTS (≥1%) **Body as a Whole:** Alopecia, *asthenia*, epistaxis, *fatigue, hair color changes*. **CNS:** *Headache*. **CV:** Chest pain, *hypertension*, myocardial infarction, QT elevation, transient ischemic attack. **GI:** *Abdominal pain, diarrhea*, dyspepsia, *nausea*, rectal hemorrhage, *vomiting*. **Hematologic:** Leukopenia, lymphocytopenia, neutropenia, thrombocytopenia. **Metabolic:** *Alterations in glucose, anorexia, AST and ALT elevation, decreased magnesium, decreased phosphorus, decreased sodium*, decreased weight, *elevated bilirubin*, hypothyroidism, lipase enzyme elevation, proteinuria. **Musculoskeletal:** Myalgia, pain, weakness. **Respiratory:** Hemoptysis, dyspnea, cough. **Skin:** Facial edema, palmar-plantar erythrodysesthesia, rash, skin depigmentation. **Special Senses:** Dysgeusia, blurred vision. **Urogenital:** Hematuria.

Common adverse effects in *italic;* life-threatening effects underlined; generic names in **bold;** classifications in SMALL CAPS; ♣ Canadian drug name; ⊙ Prototype drug

## INTERACTIONS Drug: Strong INHIBITORS OF CYP3A4 (e.g., **ketoconazole, ritonavir, clarithromycin**) may increase pazopanib levels. INDUCERS OF CYP3A4 (e.g., **rifampin**) may decrease pazopanib levels. Pazopanib may increase the levels of other drugs that require CYP3A4, CYP2D6, or CYP2C8 for their metabolism. Do not use with agents that prolong QT interval (e.g., **bepridil, cisapride, dofetilide, quinidine, ziprasidone**). **Food: Grapefruit juice** may increase pazopanib levels.

## PHARMACOKINETICS Peak: 2–4 h. **Distribution:** Greater than 99% plasma protein bound. **Metabolism:** Hepatic oxidation by CYP3A4. **Elimination:** Primarily fecal. **Half-Life:** 30.9 h.

## NURSING IMPLICATIONS

### Black Box Warning

*Pazopanib has been associated with severe, sometimes fatal, hepatotoxicity.*

### Assessment & Drug Effects

- Monitor BP closely. Consult prescriber for desired parameters and report promptly BP elevations above desired levels.
- Monitor cardiac status, especially in those at higher risk for QT interval prolongation. ECG monitoring as warranted.
- Withhold drug and notify prescriber immediately if ALT exceeds 3 × ULN and bilirubin exceeds 2 × ULN.
- Monitor lab tests: CBC with differential. Baseline LFTs, then q4wk for 4 mo, and periodically thereafter; periodic thyroid function tests, urinalysis for proteinuria; baseline and periodic serum electrolytes.

### Patient & Family Education

- Report promptly any of the following: Unexplained signs of bleeding, jaundice, unusually dark urine, unusual tiredness, or pain in the right upper abdomen.
- Do not take OTC drugs, herbs, vitamins or dietary supplements without consulting prescriber.
- Women of childbearing age should use adequate means of contraception to avoid pregnancy while on this drug.

# PEGFILGRASTIM
(peg-fil-gras'tim)
Neulasta

**Classifications:** HEMATOPOIETIC GROWTH FACTOR; GRANULOCYTE COLONY-STIMULATING FACTOR (G-CSF)
**Therapeutic:** HEMATOPOIETIC GROWTH FACTOR; G-CSF
**Prototype:** Filgrastim

**AVAILABILITY** Solution for injection

## ACTION & THERAPEUTIC EFFECT
Endogenous G-CSF regulates the production of neutrophils within the bone marrow; primarily affects neutrophil proliferation, differentiation, and selected end-cell functional activity (including enhanced phagocytic activity, antibody-dependent killing, and increased expression of some functions associated with cell-surface cellsurface antigens). *Increases neutrophil proliferation and differentiation within the bone marrow.*

## USES To decrease the incidence of infection, as manifested by febrile neutropenia, in patients with nonmyeloid malignancies receiving myelosuppressive anticancer drugs associated with a significant incidence of severe neutropenia with fever.

Common adverse effects in *italic;* life-threatening effects <u>underlined;</u> generic names in **bold;** classifications in SMALL CAPS; ♣ Canadian drug name; ⓟ Prototype drug

1241

## CONTRAINDICATIONS
Severe hypersensitivity to perfilgrastim, filgrastin, or any component of the formulation; myeloid cancers; splenomegaly; ARDS from drug.

## CAUTIOUS USE
Sickle cell disorders; neutropenic patients with sepsis; leukemia; pregnancy (category C); lactation. Safety and efficacy in children not established.

## ROUTE & DOSAGE

### Neutropenia
*Adult (weight greater than 45 kg):*
**Subcutaneous** 6 mg once/chemotherapy cycle at least 24 h after chemotherapy

## ADMINISTRATION
### Subcutaneous
- Do not administer pegfilgrastim in the period 14 days before or 24 h after cytotoxic chemotherapy.
- Use only one dose/vial; do not reenter the vial.
- Prior to injection, pegfilgrastim may be allowed to reach room temperature for a maximum of 6 h. Discard any vial left at room temperature for longer than 6 h.
- Aspirate prior to injection to avoid injection into a blood vessel. Inject subcutaneously; do not inject intradermally. Recommended injection sites include outer area of upper arms, abdomen (excluding 2-in. area around navel), front of middle thighs, and upper outer areas of the buttocks.
- Store refrigerated at 2°–8° C (36°–46° F). Do not freeze. Avoid shaking.

## ADVERSE EFFECTS (≥1%)
**Body as a Whole:** *Bone pain,* hyperuricemia, *fever.* **Hematologic:** Anemia. **GI:** Nausea, diarrhea, vomiting, anorexia, increased LFTs. **CNS:** *Asthenia,* *headache.* **Body as a Whole:** *Bone pain,* hyperuricemia, myalgia, *fever.*

## INTERACTIONS
**Drug:** Can interfere with activity of CYTOTOXIC AGENTS; do not use 14 days before or less than 24 h after CYTOTOXIC AGENTS; **lithium** may increase release of neutrophils.

## PHARMACOKINETICS
**Absorption:** Readily absorbed from subcutaneous site. **Half-Life:** 15–80 h.

## NURSING IMPLICATIONS
### Assessment & Drug Effects
- Discontinue pegfilgrastim if absolute neutrophil count exceeds 10,000/mm³ after the chemotherapy-induced nadir. Neutrophil counts should then return to normal.
- Monitor patients with preexisting cardiac conditions closely. MI and arrhythmias have been associated with a small percent of patients receiving pegfilgrastim.
- Monitor temperature q4h. Incidence of infection should be reduced after administration of pegfilgrastim.
- Assess degree of bone pain if present. Consult prescriber if nonnarcotic analgesics do not provide relief.
- Monitor lab tests: Baseline CBC with differential and platelet count; then CBC twice weekly during therapy; regular Hct and Hgb, and platelet count.

### Patient & Family Education
- Report bone pain and, if necessary, request analgesics to control pain.
- Note: Proper drug administration and disposal is important. A puncture-resistant container for the disposal of used syringes and needles should be utilized.

## PEGINTERFERON ALFA-2A Ⓟ
(peg-in-ter-fer′on)

Common adverse effects in *italic;* life-threatening effects <u>underlined;</u> generic names in **bold;** classifications in SMALL CAPS; ✦ Canadian drug name; Ⓟ Prototype drug

**Pegasys**

**Classifications:** BIOLOGIC
RESPONSE MODIFIER; IMMUNOMODU-
LATOR; ALPHA INTERFERON
Therapeutic: ANTIVIRAL;
ANTIHEPATITIS

**AVAILABILITY** Solution for injection

**ACTION & *THERAPEUTIC EFFECT***
Interferon-stimulated genes modulate processes leading to inhibition of
viral replication in infected cells, inhibition of cell proliferation, and im-
munomodulation. *Induces antiviral
effects by activation of macrophages,
natural killer cells, and T-cells, thus
boosting cellular immunity and suppressing hepatic inflammation and
replication of hepatitis C virus.*

**USES** Chronic hepatitis C or chronic hepatitis B.

**UNLABELED USES** Renal cell
carcinoma, chronic myelogenous
leukemia.

**CONTRAINDICATIONS** Hypersensitivity to peginterferon alfa-2a or
any of its components; drug induced
life-threatening neuromuscular, autoimmune, ischemic or infectious
disorder(s); severe immunosuppression; autoimmune thyroid diseases
(e.g., Graves' disease, thyroiditis);
autoimmune hepatitis; encephalopathy; history of significant or uncontrolled cardiac disease; pancreatitis;
dental work; sepsis; *E. coli* hypersensitivity, neonates and infants because it contains benzyl alcohol.

**CAUTIOUS USE** History of neuropsychiatric disorder; alcoholism,
substance abuse; risk of pulmonary
failure; bipolar disorder, mania,
psychosis, history of suicides; bone
marrow suppression; cardiac arrhythmias, history of MI, cardiac
disease, heart failure, uncontrolled

hypertension; pulmonary disease,
including COPD; thyroid dysfunction; DM; autoimmune disorders;
ulcerative and hemorrhagic colitis;
pancreatitis; pulmonary disorders;
liver impairment; HBV or HIV coinfection; retinal disease; renal impairment with creatinine clearance
less than 50 mL/min; organ transplant recipients; older adults; pregnancy (category C), lactation. Safe
use in children younger than 5 y
not established.

## ROUTE & DOSAGE

**Chronic Hepatitis B**

*Adult:* **Subcutaneous** 180 mcg
once weekly × 48 wk

**Chronic Hepatitis C**

*Adult:* **Subcutaneous** 180 mg
weekly plus sofosbuvir and
ribavirin × 12 wk (depending on
viral genotype)

*Child:* **Subcutaneous** 180
mcg/1.73 m$^2$ once weekly (max:
180 mcg/wk) plus ribavirin

***Hematologic Parameters,
Adverse Effects, Renal
Impairment, and Hepatic
Impairment Dosage Adjustments***
See package insert

## ADMINISTRATION

### Subcutaneous

- Give dose on the same day of
  each week. Consider night time
  administration to increase patient's tolerance. Administer subcutaneously in the abdomen or
  thigh and rotate injection sites.
- Warm refrigerated vial by rolling
  in hands for about 1 min. Do not
  use if particulate matter is visible
  in the vial or product is discolored. Discard any unused portion.
- Withhold drug and notify prescriber for any of the following: ANC

P

Common adverse effects in *italic;* life-threatening effects <u>underlined;</u> generic names
in **bold;** classifications in SMALL CAPS; ♣ Canadian drug name; ● Prototype drug

1243

less than 750/mm³ or platelet count less than 50,000/mm³.

- Store in the refrigerator at 36°–46° F (2°–8° C), do not freeze or shake. Protect from light. Vials are for single use only.

## ADVERSE EFFECTS (≥1%) Body as a Whole: *Musculoskeletal pain, myalgia, arthralgia, fatigue, inflammation at injection site, flu-like symptoms, rigors, fever,* pain, malaise, asthenia, exacerbation of autoimmune disease. **CNS:** *Headache, depression,* anxiety, *irritability, insomnia, dizziness,* impaired concentration, impaired memory, <u>suicidal ideation/attempts</u>. **GI:** *Nausea, diarrhea, abdominal pain, anorexia,* dry mouth. **Hematologic:** <u>Thrombocytopenia</u>, *neutropenia*. **Skin:** *Alopecia, pruritus,* dermatitis, sweating, rash.

## INTERACTIONS Drug: May increase **theophylline** levels; increased risk of fetal defects with **ribavirin;** additive myelosuppression with ANTINEOPLASTICS. Use with NNRTIS or PROTEASE INHIBITORS increases risk of hepatic damage. May require dosage adjustments of NRTIS. Do not administer LIVE VACCINES.

## PHARMACOKINETICS Peak: 72–96 h. **Elimination:** 30% in urine. **Half-Life:** 80 h.

## NURSING IMPLICATIONS

### Black Box Warning

*Peginterferon Alfa-2A has been associated with fatal or life-threatening neuropsychiatric, autoimmune, ischemic, and infectious disorders.*

### Assessment & Drug Effects

- Monitor for S&S of hypersensitivity (e.g., angioedema, bronchoconstriction) and, if noted, institute appropriate medical action immediately. Note that transient rashes are not an indication to discontinue treatment.
- Withhold drug and notify prescriber for any of the following: Severe neuropsychiatric events (e.g., psychosis, hallucinations, suicidal ideation, depression, bipolar disorders, and mania), severe neutropenia or thrombocytopenia, abdominal pain accompanied by bloody diarrhea and fever, S&S of pancreatitis, new or worsening ophthalmologic disorders, or any other severe adverse event (see CAUTIOUS USE).
- Monitor respiratory and cardiovascular status; report dyspnea, chest pain, and hypotension immediately; perform baseline and periodic ECG and chest X-ray.
- Baseline and periodic ophthalmology exams are recommended.
- Monitor lab tests: Baseline creatinine clearance, uric acid, CBC with differential, platelet count, Hct and Hgb, TSH, ALT, AST, bilirubin, blood glucose; CBC with differential, platelet count, Hct and Hgb after 2 wk and other blood chemistries after 4 wk. Serum HCV RNA level after 24 wk of treatment.

### Patient & Family Education

- If you miss a drug dose and remember within 2 days of the scheduled dose, take the dose and continue with your regular schedule. If more than 2 days have passed, contact prescriber for instructions.
- Notify prescriber immediately for any of the following: Severe depression or suicidal thoughts, severe chest pain, difficulty breathing, changes in vision, unusual bleeding or bruising, bloody diarrhea, high fever, severe stomach or lower back pain, severe chest pain, development of a new or worsening of a preexisting skin condition.

Common adverse effects in *italic;* life-threatening effects <u>underlined</u>; generic names in **bold;** classifications in SMALL CAPS; ♣ Canadian drug name; ⊘ Prototype drug

- Follow up with lab tests; compliance with lab testing is extremely important while taking this drug.
- Do not drive or engage in other potentially hazardous activities until reaction to drug is known.
- Women should use reliable means of contraception while taking this drug and notify prescriber immediately if they become pregnant.

# PEGINTERFERON ALFA-2B

(peg-in-ter-fer'on)
Peg-Intron, Sylatron
**Classifications:** BIOLOGIC RESPONSE MODIFIER; IMMUNOMODULATOR; ALPHA INTERFERON
Therapeutic: ANTIVIRAL; ANTIHEPATITIS
**Prototype:** Peginterferon alfa-2a

**AVAILABILITY** Powder for injection

## ACTION & *THERAPEUTIC EFFECT*
Binds to specific membrane receptors on the cell surface, thereby initiating suppression of cell proliferation, enhanced phagocytic activity of macrophages, augmentation of specific cytotoxic lymphocytes for target cells, and inhibition of viral replication in virus-infected cells. *Induces antiviral effects by activation of macrophages, natural killer cells, and T-cells, thus boosting cellular immunity and suppressing hepatic inflammation and replication of hepatitis C virus.*

**USES** Chronic hepatitis C, melanoma.

**UNLABELED USES** Renal carcinoma, hepatitis B.

## CONTRAINDICATIONS Hypersensitivity to peginterferon or interferon alfa; autoimmune hepatitis; decompensated liver disease {Child-Pugh (class B and C)} in cirrhotic chronic hepatitis C patients before or

during treatment; DM; pancreatitis; persistently severe or worsening S&S of life-threatening neuropsychiatric, autoimmune, ischemic, or infectious disorders; history of significant or unstable cardiac disease; uncontrollable DM or hypo- or hyperthyroidism. **Sylatron:** Hepatic decompensation. {Child-Pugh (class B and C)}.

**CAUTIOUS USE** History of neuropsychiatric disorder; suicidal tendencies; bone marrow suppression, ulcerative and hemorrhagic colitis; pulmonary disorders; HBV or HIV coinfection; thyroid dysfunction; DM; cardiovascular disease; autoimmune disorders; pulmonary disease, COPD; retinal disease; renal impairment with creatinine clearance less than 50 mL/min; older adults; pregnancy (category C). Safety and efficacy in children younger than 3 y not established.

## ROUTE & DOSAGE

### Chronic Hepatitis C
*Adult/Adolescent/Child:*
**Subcutaneous** Dose specific to patient weight and genotype, see package insert.

### Melanoma (Sylatron only)
*Adult:* **Subcutaneous** 6 mcg/kg/wk × 8 doses then 3 mcg/kg/wk for up to 5 y

## ADMINISTRATION
**Subcutaneous**
- Give dose on the same day of each week.
- *Vial reconstitution:* Be aware that two Safety Lok™ syringes are provided in the drug package: One for reconstitution and one for injection. Reconstitute with only 0.7 mL of supplied diluent and

Common adverse effects in *italic;* life-threatening effects underlined; generic names in **bold;** classifications in SMALL CAPS; ✦ Canadian drug name; ❂ Prototype drug

1245

discard remaining diluent. Enter the vial only once as it does not contain a preservative. Swirl gently to produce a clear, colorless solution. Use solution immediately.

- *Redipen use:* To reconstitute the lyophilized powder in the Redipen, hold the Redipen upright with dose button down and press the 2 halves of the pen together until there is an audible click. Gently invert the pen to mix but do not shake. Select the dose by pulling back on the dosing button until the dark bands are visible and turning the button until the dark band is aligned with the correct dose.
- Store dry vial at 15°–30° C (59°–86° F). If necessary, store reconstituted solution up to 24 h at 2°–8° C (36°–46° F).

**ADVERSE EFFECTS** (≥1%) **Body as a Whole:** *Musculoskeletal pain, fatigue, inflammation at injection site, flu-like symptoms, rigors, fever, weight loss, viral infection,* pain, malaise, hypertonia. **CNS:** *Headache, depression, anxiety, emotional lability, irritability, insomnia, dizziness.* **GI:** *Nausea, anorexia, diarrhea, abdominal pain,* vomiting, dyspepsia, hepatomegaly. **Endocrine:** Hypothyroidism, weight loss. **Hematologic:** <u>Thrombocytopenia</u>, neutropenia. **Respiratory:** *Pharyngitis,* sinusitis, cough. **Skin:** *Alopecia, pruritus, dry skin,* sweating, rash, flushing.

**INTERACTIONS Drug:** May increase **theophylline** levels; additive myelosuppression with ANTINEOPLASTICS; **zidovudine** may increase hematologic toxicity; increase **doxorubicin** toxicity, increase neurotoxicity with **vinblastine; aldesleukin (IL-2)** may potentiate the risk of kidney failure. Use with NNRTIS or PROTEASE INHIBITORS may increase risk of hepatic damage. May require dosage adjustments of NRTIS. Do not administer LIVE VACCINES.

**PHARMACOKINETICS Peak:** 15–44 h. **Duration:** 48–72 h. **Elimination:** 30% in urine. **Half-Life:** 40 h (22–60 h).

## NURSING IMPLICATIONS

### Black Box Warning

*Peg-Intron has been associated with fatal or life-threatening neuropsychiatric, autoimmune, ischemic, and infectious disorders. Sylatron has been associated with serious depression with suicidal ideation, completed suicides, and other serious neuropsychiatric disorders.*

### Assessment & Drug Effects

- Monitor for S&S of hypersensitivity (e.g., angioedema, bronchoconstriction) and, if noted, institute appropriate medical action immediately. Note that transient rashes are not an indication to discontinue treatment.
- Monitor for and report immediately S&S of neuropsychiatric disorders (e.g., psychosis, hallucinations, suicidal ideation, depression).
- Monitor respiratory and cardiovascular status; report dyspnea, chest pain, and hypotension immediately; baseline and periodic ECG and chest X-ray.
- Withhold drug and notify prescriber for any of the following: Severe neuropsychiatric events, severe neutropenia or thrombocytopenia, abdominal pain accompanied by bloody diarrhea and fever, S&S of pancreatitis, or any other severe adverse event (see CAUTIOUS USE).
- Baseline and periodic ophthalmology exams are recommended.
- Monitor lab tests: Baseline and periodic creatinine clearance,

serum uric acid, CBC with differential, platelet count, Hct and Hgb, TSH, ALT, AST, bilirubin, blood glucose; serum HCV RNA level after 24 wk of treatment.

**Patient & Family Education**
- Drink fluids liberally while taking this drug, especially during the initial stages of therapy.
- Learn reasons for withholding drug (see ASSESSMENT & DRUG EFFECTS).
- Use effective means of contraception while taking this drug. Women should not become pregnant.
- Follow up with lab tests; compliance with lab testing is extremely important while taking this drug.

# PEGINTERFERON BETA-1A

(peg-in-ter-fer'on)

Plegridy

**Classifications:** BIOLOGIC RESPONSE MODIFIER; IMMUNOMODULATOR; BETA INTERFERON
**Therapeutic:** IMMUNOMODULATOR
**Prototype:** Peginterferon alfa-2A

**AVAILABILITY** Prefilled solution for injection

**ACTION & THERAPEUTIC EFFECT**
Exact mechanism of action in the treatment of multiple sclerosis is unknown. Interferon beta-1A alters the expression and response to surface antigens and enhances immune cell activities. *Improves symptoms and functionality in patients with relapsing MS.*

**USES** Treatment of patients with relapsing forms of multiple sclerosis.

**CONTRAINDICATIONS** History of hypersensitivity to natural or recombinant interferon beta or peginterferon, or any other component of the formulation; suicidal ideation or other severe psychiatric symptoms.

**CAUTIOUS USE** Severe renal impairment; seizure disorder; hepatic impairment; depression, history of suicidal thoughts; seizure disorder; myelosuppression; CHF; cardiomyopathy; serious injections site reactions; older adults; pregnancy (category C); lactation. Safety and efficacy in children younger than 18 y not established.

## ROUTE & DOSAGE

| Multiple Sclerosis |
|---|
| *Adult:* **Subcutaneous** 63 mcg on day 1; 94 mcg on day 15; 125 mcg on day 29 and 125 mcg every 14 days thereafter |

## ADMINISTRATION

**Subcutaneous**
- Allow prefilled syringe or pen to warm to room temperature (approx. 30 min) prior to injection; do not use external heat sources (e.g., hot water) to warm.
- Inject into the abdomen, back of the upper arm, or thigh; rotate injection sites; do not inject into area where skin is red, irritated, bruised, or scarred.
- Store in the closed original carton to protect from light, at 2°–8° C (36°–46° F). Do not freeze; discard if frozen.

**ADVERSE EFFECTS** (≥ 2%) **Body as a Whole:** *Asthenia, chills,* hyperthermia, *influenza-like illness,* injection site edema, *injection site erythema,* injection site hematoma, *injection site illness, injection site pain, injection site pruritus,* injection site rash, injection site hematoma, pain, *pyrexia.* **CNS:** *Headache.* **GI:** Nausea, vomiting. **Hematological:**

P

Common adverse effects in *italic;* life-threatening effects underlined; generic names in **bold;** classifications in SMALL CAPS; ♣ Canadian drug name; ⊙ Prototype drug

1247

Decreased white cell counts. **Metabolic:** Increased ALT and AST, increased gamma-glutamyl transferase. **Musculoskeletal:** Arthralgia, *myalgia.* **Skin:** Pruritus.

**INTERACTIONS Drugs:** Use with NRTIS should be done with caution as it may impact antiviral clearance. Avoid use with **vigabatrin.**

**PHARMACOKINETICS Peak:** 1–1.5 days. **Distribution:** Well distributed to tissues. **Metabolism:** Not extensive. **Elimination:** Primarily renal. **Half-Life:** 78 h.

**NURSING IMPLICATIONS**

**Assessment & Drug Effects**
- Monitor for injection site reactions (e.g., erythema, pain, pruritus, edema, necrosis).
- Monitor for and report promptly any of the following: S&S of hypersensitivity or hepatic injury; S&S of myelosuppression (e.g., infections, bleeding, anemia); new onset or worsening signs of CV disease (i.e., CHF); mental status changes.
- Monitor for increased seizure activity with a preexisting seizure disorder.
- Monitor lab tests: Baseline and periodic CBC with differential and platelet count, LFTs, renal function tests; periodic thyroid function tests.

**Patient & Family Education**
- Report promptly to prescriber if you develop signs of infection or bleeding.
- Consult your prescriber if you experience mental status changes (e.g., depression, suicidal ideation, anxiety, emotional instability, illogical thinking).
- Notify prescriber immediately if you experience worsening symptoms of heart failure such as shortness of breath, swelling of your lower legs, or excessive weight gain.
- Notify your prescriber if you are pregnant or plan to become pregnant.
- Do not breast-feed without first consulting your prescriber.

# PEGLOTICASE
(peg-lo'ti-case)
Krystexxa
**Classifications:** ANTIGOUT; URIC ACID METABOLIZING ENZYME
Therapeutic: ANTIGOUT

**AVAILABILITY** Solution for injection

**ACTION & *THERAPEUTIC EFFECT***
Pegloticase is a recombinant uric acid specific enzyme that catalyzes the conversion of uric acid to a water soluble, inert metabolite readily eliminated by the kidney. *It lowers the serum uric acid, thus reducing uric acid-induced inflammation.*

**USES** Treatment of chronic gout.

**CONTRAINDICATIONS** Established G6PD deficiency; lactation.

**CAUTIOUS USE** African or Mediterranean ancestry; consider discontinuing if uric acid level above 6 mg/mL; retreatment with pegloticase following discontinuation of therapy for longer than 6 wk; CHF; pregnancy (category C); children younger than 18 y.

**ROUTE & DOSAGE**

| Chronic Gout |
| --- |
| *Adult:* **IV** 8 mg over 2 hrs q2wk |

Common adverse effects in *italic;* life-threatening effects <u>underlined;</u> generic names in **bold;** classifications in SMALL CAPS; ◆ Canadian drug name; ⊘ Prototype drug

## ADMINISTRATION

### Intravenous

▪ Note: Premedication with antihistamines and corticosteroids is required to minimize the risk of anaphylaxis and infusion reactions. ▪ Pegloticase should only be administered in a health care setting and by health care providers trained to manage anaphylaxis and infusion reactions.

*PREPARE: IV Infusion:* Do not shake vial. ▪ Withdraw 1 mL of pegloticase from the 2 mL vial and inject into 250 mL of NS. Do not mix or dilute with other drugs. ▪ Invert IV bag to mix but do not shake. ▪ Discard unused pegloticase remaining in vial.

*ADMINISTER: IV Infusion:* If refrigerated, bring to room temperature prior to infusion. **Do not** give IV push or bolus. Infuse over NO LESS THAN 120 min. ▪ Monitor closely throughout infusion and for 2 h postinfusion for S&S of anaphylaxis or an infusion reaction (e.g., urticarial, erythema, dyspnea, flushing, chest discomfort, chest pain, and rash). ▪ If S&S of anaphylaxis or an infusion reaction occur, stop infusion and immediately notify prescriber. ▪ If anaphylaxis is ruled out and infusion is restarted, it should be run at a slower rate. ▪ Infusion bags may be stored refrigerated for 4 h after dilution.

*INCOMPATIBILITIES: Solution/additive:* Do not mix with another drug. **Y-site:** Do not mix with another drug.

▪ Store unopened vials in refrigerator at (2°–8° C or 36°–46° F) and protect from light. Do not shake or freeze.

▪ Diluted solution may be stored up to 4 h at 2°–8° C (36°–46° F). Warm to room temperature before administration. Diluted solution is also stable at room temperature for up to 4 h, but should be protected from light.

## ADVERSE EFFECTS (≥5%) **Body as a Whole:** Anaphylaxis, contusion, ecchymosis, arthralgia, gout flare, infusion reaction, pruritus. **CV:** Chest pain. **GI:** *Nausea* vomiting, constipation **Respiratory:** Dyspnea, nasopharyngitis. **Skin:** Erythema, urticaria. **Metabolic:** Anemia. **CNS:** Headache.

## INTERACTIONS **Drug:** Potential interaction with other pegylated products (**pegfilgrastim, peginterferon alfa-2a**). Do not use with **allopurinol, febuxostat, probenecid, sulfinpyrazone.**

## NURSING IMPLICATIONS

### Black Box Warning

*Pegloticase has been associated with anaphylaxis and infusion reactions during and after administration. G6PD deficiency-associated hemolysis and methemoglobinemia.*

### Assessment & Drug Effects

▪ Monitor closely during infusion and for 2 h postinfusion for S&S of anaphylaxis (see Appendix F) or an infusion reaction (see IV ADMINISTRATION).
▪ Assess vital signs frequently during and for 2 h postinfusion.
▪ Monitor cardiac status, especially with preexisting congestive heart failure.
▪ Notify prescriber if uric acid level is 6 mg/mL or above. Two consecutive readings above 6

Common adverse effects in *italic;* life-threatening effects underlined; generic names in **bold;** classifications in SMALL CAPS; ♣ Canadian drug name; ⓟ Prototype drug

1249

mm/mL may indicate need to discontinue treatment.

- Monitor lab tests: Baseline and periodic serum uric acid level.

**Patient & Family Education**
- Report promptly any discomfort (e.g., wheezing, facial swelling, skin rash, redness of the skin, difficulty breathing, flushing, chest discomfort, chest pain, rash) during or following IV infusion.
- Gout flares may increase during the first 3 mo of therapy and are not a reason to discontinue pegloticase.

# PEMBROLIZUMAB

(pem-bro-li'zu-mab)

**Keytruda**

**Classifications:** IMMUNOMODULATOR; MONOCLONAL ANTIBODY; PROGRAMMED DEATH RECEPTOR-1 BLOCKER

**Therapeutic:** IMMUNOSUPPRESSANT

**Prototype:** Basiliximab

**AVAILABILITY** Lyophilized powder

**ACTION & *THERAPEUTIC EFFECT***
Activation of programmed cell death (PD-1) receptors found on T cells inhibits T cell proliferation and cytokine production. Increased activation of PD-1 receptors occurs in some tumors and can contribute to inhibition of active T-cell immune response to tumors. Pembrolizumab binds to the PD-1 receptor and blocks its activation thus removing inhibition of the immune response, including the anti-tumor immune response. *Blocking PD-1 activity results in decreased tumor growth.*

**USES** Treatment of patients with unresectable or metastatic melanoma and disease progression following ipilimumab and a BRAF inhibitor (for those patients who have a BRAF V600 mutation), metastatic non–small-cell lung cancer; head/neck cancer; colorectal cancer; Hogkin's disease, urothelial cancer.

**CONTRAINDICATIONS** Any life-threatening adverse reaction; drug induced Grade 3–4 renal failure, hepatitis, or infusion-related reactions; drug induced life-threatening immune-mediated colitis; pregnancy (category D); lactation.

**CAUTIOUS USE** Renal or hepatic impairment; drug induced pneumonitis; asthma; COPD; prior thoracic radiation; inflammation of the pituitary (hypophysitis); DM; thyroid disorders; colitis; organ donor recipients; women of child bearing age. Safety and efficacy in children younger than 18 y not established.

## ROUTE & DOSAGE

**Metastatic Melanoma**

*Adult:* **IV** 200 mg every 3 wk until disease progression or unacceptable toxicity

**Non–Small-Cell Lung Cancer/Head/Neck Cancer**

*Adult:* **IV** 200 mg q3w for up to 24 mo until disease progression or unacceptable toxicity

***Toxicity Dosage Adjustment***
See package insert

## ADMINISTRATION

**Intravenous**

*PREPARE:* **IV Infusion:** Reconstitute by adding 2.3 mL SW for injection along vial wall to yield

25 mg/mL. Slowly swirl vial; do not shake. Allow up to 5 min for bubbles to dissipate. Withdraw required volume from vial and dilute in IV NS to a final concentration of 1–10 mg/mL. Mix by gently inverting bag. Discard unused portion of the vial.

***ADMINISTER:*** **IV Infusion:** Infuse over 30 min through a 0.2–0.5 micron sterile, nonpyrogenic, low protein-binding inline or add-on filter.

***INCOMPATIBILITIES:*** Do not mix or infuse with any other medications.

- Store intact vials at 2°–8° C (36°–46° F). Reconstituted and solutions diluted for infusion may be stored at room temperature for up to 6 h (infusion must be completed within 6 h of reconstitution) or refrigerated at 2°–8° C (36°–46° F) for no more than 24 h from the time of reconstitution.

**ADVERSE EFFECTS** (≥ 10%) **Body as a Whole:** Cellulitis, chills, *fatigue,* immunogenic response, peripheral edema, pyrexia, sepsis. **Cardiovascular:** Peripheral edema. **CNS:** Dizziness, headache, insomnia. **GI:** Abdominal pain, *constipation, anorexia, diarrhea, nausea,* vomiting. **Hematological:** Anemia. **Metabolic:** *Decreased appetite,* hyperglycemia, hypercholesterolemia, hypertriglyceridemia, hypoalbuminemia, hypocalcemia, hyponatremia, increased AST. **Musculoskeletal:** *Arthralgia,* back pain, myalgia, pain in extremity. **Respiratory:** *Cough,* dyspnea, pneumonia, upper respiratory tract infection, pleural effusion. **Skin:** Pruritus, *rash,* vitiligo. **Urogenital:** Renal failure.

**INTERACTIONS Drug:** If used with **clozapine** monitor ANC.

**PHARMACOKINETICS Half-Life:** 26 days.

**NURSING IMPLICATIONS**

**Assessment & Drug Effects**

- Monitor for S&S of hypersensitivity or infusion-related reactions.
- Monitor for S&S of drug toxicity including pneumonitis, colitis, hepatitis, pituitary disorders, nephritis, thyroid dysfunction.
- Monitor lab tests: Baseline and periodic LFTs, renal function tests, thyroid function tests; periodic lipid profile and serum electrolytes, blood glucose levels.

**Patient & Family Education**

- Report promptly to prescriber if you experience signs of pulmonary toxicity such as new or worsening cough, chest pain, or shortness of breath.
- Report signs of colitis or liver damage such as diarrhea, severe abdominal pain, jaundice, severe nausea or vomiting, or easy bruising or bleeding.
- Report signs of endocrine dysfunction including persistent or unusual headache, extreme weakness, dizziness or fainting, or vision changes.
- Women of childbearing potential should use highly effective contraception during and for 4 mo after the last dose of this drug.
- Do not breast-feed while taking this drug.

**PEMETREXED**

(pe-me-trex'ed)

Alimta

**Classifications:** ANTINEOPLASTIC; ANTIMETABOLITE, ANTIFOLATE

Therapeutic: ANTINEOPLASTIC

**Prototype:** Methotrexate

---

Common adverse effects in *italic;* life-threatening effects underlined; generic names in **bold;** classifications in SMALL CAPS; ✦ Canadian drug name; ⊙ Prototype drug

1251

**AVAILABILITY** Powder for injection

## ACTION & *THERAPEUTIC EFFECT*
Suppresses tumor growth by inhibiting both DNA synthesis and folate metabolism at multiple target enzymes. *Appears to arrest the cell cycle, thus inhibiting tumor growth.*

**USES** Treatment of malignant pleural mesothelioma that is unresectable or in patients that are not surgery candidates in combination with cisplatin; treatment of locally advanced or metastatic non–small-cell lung cancer (NSCLC).

**UNLABELED USES** Solid tumors, including bladder, breast, colorectal, gastric, head and neck, pancreatic, and renal cell cancers.

**CONTRAINDICATIONS** Mannitol hypersensitivity; creatinine clearance is less than 45 mL/min, renal failure, active infection; vaccines; pregnancy (category D); lactation.

**CAUTIOUS USE** Anemia, thrombocytopenia, neutropenia, dental disease; older adults; hepatic disease, renal impairment; hypoalbuminemia, hypovolemia, dehydration, ascites, pleural effusion; children younger than 18 y.

## ROUTE & DOSAGE

### Malignant Mesothelioma, Non–Small-Cell Lung Cancer

*Adult:* **IV** 500 mg/m² on day 1 of each 21-day cycle

### Renal Impairment Dosage Adjustment

*CrCl less than 45 mL/min:*
Not recommended

## ADMINISTRATION

**Intravenous**
Pre-/posttreatment with folic acid, vitamin B₁₂, and dexamethasone are needed to reduce hematologic and gastrointestinal toxicity, and the possibility of severe cutaneous reactions from pemetrexed.

This drug is a cytotoxic agent and caution should be used to prevent any contact with the drug. Follow institutional or standard guidelines for preparation, handling, and disposal of cytotoxic agents.

*PREPARE:* **IV Infusion:** Reconstitute each 100 mg or 500 mg vial with 4.2 mL or 20 mL, respectively, of preservative-free NS. ▪ Do not use any other diluent. Swirl gently to dissolve. Each vial will contain 25 mg/mL. ▪ Withdraw the needed amount of reconstituted solution and add to 100 mL of preservative-free NS. ▪ Discard any unused portion.

*ADMINISTER:* **IV Infusion:** **Do not** give a bolus dose. ▪ Infuse over 10 min.

*INCOMPATIBILITIES:* Solution/additive: Solutions containing **calcium, lactated Ringer's.** Y-site: **Amphotericin B, calcium, cefazolin, cefotaxime, cefotetan, cefoxitin, ceftazidime, chlorpromazine, ciprofloxacin, dobutamine, doxorubicin, doxycycline, droperidol, gemcitabine, gentamicin, irinotecan, metronidazole, minocycline, mitoxantrone, nalbuphine, ondansetron, prochlorperazine, tobramycin, topotecan.**

▪ Store unopened single-use vials at room temperature at 15°–30° C (59°–86° F). ▪ The reconstituted

drug is stable for up to 24 h at 2°–8°
C (36°–46° F) or at 25° C (77° F).

**ADVERSE EFFECTS** (≥1%) **Body
as a Whole:** *Fatigue, fever,*
hypersensitivity reaction, edema,
myalgia, arthralgia. **CNS:** Neuropathy, *mood alteration, depression.*
**CV:** Chest pain, thromboembolism. **GI:** *Nausea, vomiting, constipation, anorexia, stomatitis,
diarrhea,* dehydration, dysphagia, esophagitis, odynophagia,
increased LFTs. **Hematologic:**
*Neutropenia,* leukopenia, anemia,
thrombocytopenia. **Respiratory:**
*Dyspnea.* **Skin:** *Rash, desquamation,* alopecia. **Urogenital:** *Increases serum creatinine,* renal
failure.

**INTERACTIONS Drug:** Increased risk of renal toxicity with
other nephrotoxic drugs (**acyclovir, adefovir, amphotericin B,**
AMINOGLYCOSIDES, **carboplatin,
cidofovir, cisplatin, cyclosporine, foscarnet, ganciclovir,
sirolimus, tacrolimus, vancomycin**); NSAIDS may increase risk
of renal toxicity in patients with
preexisting renal insufficiency;
may cause additive risk of bleeding with ANTICOAGULANTS, PLATELET
INHIBITORS, **aspirin,** THROMBOLYTIC
AGENTS.

**PHARMACOKINETICS Metabo-
lism:** Not extensively. **Elimination:**
Primarily in urine. **Half-Life:** 3.5 h.

**NURSING IMPLICATIONS**

**Assessment & Drug Effects**
▪ Withhold drug and notify prescriber if the absolute neutrophil
count (ANC) is less than 1500
cells/mm³ or the platelet count is
less than at least 100,000 cells/
mm³, or if the CrCl is less than
45 mL/min.

▪ Notify prescriber for S&S of neuropathy (paresthesia) or thromboembolism.
▪ Monitor lab tests: Baseline and periodic CBC with differential; monitor for nadir and recovery before
each dose (on days 8 and 15,
respectively, of each cycle); periodic LFTs, serum creatinine and BUN.

**Patient & Family Education**
▪ Report promptly any of the following to prescriber: Symptoms
of anemia (e.g., chest pain, unusual weakness or tiredness, fainting spells, lightheadedness,
shortness of breath); symptoms
of poor blood clotting (e.g.,
bruising; red spots on skin;
black, tarry stools; blood in
urine); symptoms of infection
(e.g., fever or chills, cough, sore
throat, pain or difficulty passing
urine); symptoms of liver problems (e.g., yellowing of skin).
▪ Do not take nonsteroidal antiinflammatory drugs (NSAIDs)
without first consulting the prescriber.

# PENBUTOLOL
(pen-bu′tol-ol)
Levatol
**Classifications:** BETA-ADRENERGIC
ANTAGONIST; ANTIHYPERTENSIVE
**Therapeutic:** ANTIHYPERTENSIVE
**Prototype:** Propranolol

**AVAILABILITY** Tablet

**ACTION & *THERAPEUTIC EFFECT***
Synthetic beta₁- and beta₂-adrener-
gic blocking agent that competes
with epinephrine and norepinephrine for available beta receptor
sites. Lowers both supine and
standing BP in hypertensive patients. Hypotensive effect is associated with decreased cardiac output,

---

Common adverse effects in *italic;* life-threatening effects <u>underlined;</u> generic names
in **bold;** classifications in SMALL CAPS; ◆ Canadian drug name; ⊘ Prototype drug

suppressed renin activity as well as beta blockage. *Effective in lowering mild to moderate blood pressure.*

**USES** Mild to moderate hypertension.

**CONTRAINDICATIONS** Hypersensitivity to penbutolol; cardiogenic shock, acute CHF, sinus bradycardia, second and third degree AV block; bronchial asthma, acute bronchospasm; Raynaund's disease; COPD; abrupt withdrawal.

**CAUTIOUS USE** Cardiac failure; PVD; chronic bronchitis; diabetes; mental depression; myasthenia gravis, cerebrovascular insufficiency, stroke; renal disease; major surgery; hyperthyroid; older adults; pregnancy (category C); lactation. Safety and efficacy in children not established.

## ROUTE & DOSAGE

### Hypertension
*Adult:* **PO** 20 mg daily, may increase to 40–80 mg/day

## ADMINISTRATION

### Oral
- Discontinue by reducing the dose gradually over 1 to 2 wk.

**ADVERSE EFFECTS** (≥1%) **CNS:** Dizziness, fatigue, *headache,* insomnia. **CV:** AV block, bradycardia. **GI:** Nausea, diarrhea, dyspepsia. **Respiratory:** Cough, dyspnea. **Urogenital:** Impotence.

**INTERACTIONS Drug:** DIURETICS and other HYPOTENSIVE AGENTS increase hypotensive effect; effects of **albuterol, metaproterenol, terbutaline, pirbuterol,** and **penbutolol** are antagonized; NSAIDS blunt hypotensive effect; decreases hypoglycemic effect of **glyburide; amiodarone** increases risk of bradycardia and sinus arrest.

**PHARMACOKINETICS Absorption:** Readily from GI tract. **Peak:** 2–3 h. **Duration:** 20 h. **Metabolism:** In liver. **Elimination:** In urine. **Half-Life:** 5 h.

## NURSING IMPLICATIONS

### Assessment & Drug Effects
- Take apical pulse before administering drug. If pulse is below 60, or other established parameter, hold the drug and contact prescriber.
- Take a BP reading before giving drug, if BP is not stabilized. If systolic pressure is 90 mm Hg or less, hold drug and contact prescriber.
- Check BP near end of dosage interval or before administration of next dose to evaluate effectiveness.
- Monitor therapeutic effectiveness. Full effectiveness of the drug may not be seen for 4–6 wk.
- Watch for S&S of bronchial constriction. Report promptly and withhold drug.
- Monitor diabetics for loss of glycemic control. Drug suppresses clinical signs of hypoglycemia (e.g., BP changes, increased pulse rate) and may prolong hypoglycemic state.
- Monitor carefully for exacerbation of angina during drug withdrawal.

### Patient & Family Education
- Do not discontinue the drug without prescriber's advice because of the possible exacerbation of ischemic heart disease.
- If diabetic, report persistent S&S of hypoglycemia (see Appendix F) to prescriber (diabetics).

P

- Avoid driving or other potentially hazardous activities until response to drug is known.
- Make position changes slowly and avoid prolonged standing. Notify prescriber if dizziness and lightheadedness persist.
- Comply with and do not alter established regimen (i.e., do not omit, increase, or decrease dosage or change dosage interval).
- Avoid prolonged exposure of extremities to cold.
- Avoid excesses of alcohol. Heavy alcohol consumption [i.e., greater than 60 mL (2 oz)/day] may elevate arterial pressure; therefore, to maintain treatment effectiveness, either avoid alcohol or drink moderately (less than 60 mL/day). Consult prescriber.

## PENCICLOVIR
(pen-cy'clo-vir)

Denavir

**Classification:** ANTIVIRAL
**Therapeutic:** TOPICAL ANTIVIRAL
**Prototype:** Acyclovir

**AVAILABILITY** Cream

## ACTION & *THERAPEUTIC EFFECT*
Antiviral agent active against herpes simplex virus type 1 (HSV-1) and type 2 (HSV-2). HSV-1 and HSV-2 infected cells phosphorylate penciclovir utilizing viral thymidine kinase. Competes with viral DNA, thus inhibiting both viral DNA synthesis and replication. *Effectiveness is measured in decreased viral load.*

**USES** Treatment of recurrent herpes labialis (cold sores).

**CONTRAINDICATIONS** Hypersensitivity to penciclovir or famciclovir; lactation.

**CAUTIOUS USE** Acyclovir, or related antiviral hypersensitivity; pregnancy (category B). Safety and efficacy in children younger than 12 y not established. Safety in immunocompromised patients not established.

## ROUTE & DOSAGE

**Cold Sores**

*Adult:* **Topical** Apply q2h while awake × 4 days

## ADMINISTRATION
**Topical**
- Apply as soon as possible after developing lesion.
- Do not apply to mucous membranes or near the eyes.
- Store at or below 30° C (86° F). Do not freeze.

**ADVERSE EFFECTS** (≥1%) **CNS:** Headache. **Skin:** Erythema.

**PHARMACOKINETICS Absorption:** Minimally absorbed from cold sore.

## NURSING IMPLICATIONS
**Assessment & Drug Effects**
- Monitor the extent of lesions and treatment effectiveness.

**Patient & Family Education**
- Wash hands before and after application. Avoid contact of drug with eyes.
- Apply sunscreen to lips; may minimize recurrence of lesions.

## PENICILLAMINE
(pen-i-sill'a-meen)

Cuprimine, Depen

**Classifications:** CHELATING AGENT; DISEASE-MODIFYING ANTIRHEUMATIC DRUG (DMARD)
**Therapeutic:** CHELATING AGENT; ANTIRHEUMATIC (DMARD)

---

Common adverse effects in *italic;* life-threatening effects underlined; generic names in **bold;** classifications in SMALL CAPS; ♣ Canadian drug name; ◐ Prototype drug

**AVAILABILITY** Capsule; tablet

**ACTION & *THERAPEUTIC EFFECT***
Combines chemically with cystine to form a soluble disulfide complex that prevents stone formation and may even dissolve existing cystic stones. Forms stable soluble chelate with copper, zinc, iron, lead, mercury, and possibly other heavy metals and promotes their excretion in urine. Mechanism of action in rheumatoid arthritis appears to be related to inhibition of collagen formation. *With Wilson's disease, therapeutic effectiveness is indicated by improvement in psychiatric and neurologic symptoms, visual symptoms, and liver function. With rheumatoid arthritis, therapeutic effectiveness is indicated by improvement in grip strength, decrease in stiffness following immobility, reduction of pain, decrease in sedimentation rate and rheumatoid factor.*

**USES** To promote renal excretion of excess copper in Wilson's disease (hepatolenticular degeneration); active rheumatoid arthritis in patients who have failed to respond to conventional therapy; cystinuria.

**UNLABELED USES** Scleroderma, primary biliary cirrhosis, porphyria cutanea tarda, lead poisoning.

**CONTRAINDICATIONS** Hypersensitivity to penicillamine or to any penicillin; history of penicillamine-related aplastic anemia or agranulocytosis; rheumatoid arthritis patients with renal insufficiency or who are pregnant; renal failure; concomitant administration with drugs that can cause severe hematologic or renal reactions (e.g., antimalarials, gold salts); pregnancy (category D); lactation.

**CAUTIOUS USE** Allergy-prone individuals; DM; renal disease, renal impairment; hepatic impairment, hepatic disease; history of hematologic disease; children.

## ROUTE & DOSAGE

### Wilson's Disease
*Adult:* **PO** 250 mg q.i.d., with 3 doses 1 h a.c. and the last dose at least 2 h after the last meal

### Cystinuria
*Adult:* **PO** 250–500 mg q.i.d., with doses adjusted to limit urinary excretion of cystine to 100–200 mg/day
*Child:* **PO** 30 mg/kg/day in 4 divided doses with doses adjusted to limit urinary excretion of cystine to 100–200 mg/day

### Rheumatoid Arthritis (RA)
*Adult:* **PO** 125–250 mg/day; may increase at 1–3 mo intervals up to 1–1.5 g/day
*Child:* **PO** 3 mg/kg/day (up to 250 mg/day) × 3 mo, then 6 mg/kg/day (up to 500 mg/day) in 2 divided doses × 3 mo [max: 10 mg/kg/day (up to 1.5 g/day) in 3–4 divided doses]

### Renal Impairment Dosage Adjustment
*CrCl less than 50 mL/min:* Avoid use

### Hemodialysis Dosage Adjustment
In RA patients dose may be decreased from 250 mg daily to 250 mg 3 × wk

## ADMINISTRATION
### Oral
- Give on empty stomach (60 min before or 2 h after meals) to avoid absorption of metals in foods by penicillamine.

- Give contents in 15–30 mL of chilled fruit juice or pureed fruit (e.g., applesauce) if patient cannot swallow capsules or tablets.

## ADVERSE EFFECTS (≥1%) Body as a Whole:
Fever, arthralgia, lymphadenopathy, thyroiditis, SLE-like syndrome, thrombophlebitis, hyperpyrexia, myasthenia gravis syndrome, tingling of feet, weakness. **GI:** *Anorexia, nausea, vomiting,* epigastric pain, diarrhea, oral lesions, *reduction or loss of taste perception (particularly salt and sweet), metallic taste,* activation of peptic ulcer, pancreatitis. **Urogenital:** Membranous glomerulopathy, *proteinuria,* hematuria. **Hematologic:** Thrombocytopenia, leukopenia, agranulocytosis, thrombotic thrombocytopenic purpura, hemolytic anemia, aplastic anemia. **Metabolic:** Pyridoxine deficiency. **Skin:** *Generalized pruritus, urticaria,* mammary hyperplasia, alveolitis, skin friability, excessive skin wrinkling, *early and late occurring rashes,* pemphigus-like rash, alopecia. **Special Senses:** Tinnitus, optic neuritis, ptosis.

## INTERACTIONS Drug:
ANTIMALARIALS, CYTOTOXICS, **gold** therapy may potentiate hematologic and renal adverse effects; **iron** may decrease penicillamine absorption.

## PHARMACOKINETICS Absorption:
Readily from GI tract. **Peak:** 1 h. **Distribution:** Crosses placenta. **Metabolism:** In liver. **Elimination:** In urine. **Half-Life:** 1–7 h.

## NURSING IMPLICATIONS

### Black Box Warning

*Penicillamine has been associated with serious hematological and renal adverse reactions.*

### Assessment & Drug Effects
- Monitor for and report promptly S&S of granulocytopenia and/or thrombocytopenia such as fever, sore throat, chills, bruising, or bleeding.
- Monitor skin, lymph nodes, and body temperature, during the first month of therapy, every 2 wk for the next 5 mo, and monthly thereafter.
- Withhold drug and contact prescriber if the patient with rheumatoid arthritis develops proteinuria greater than 1 g (some clinicians accept greater than 2 g) or if platelet count drops to less than 100,000/mm³, or platelet count falls below 3500–4000/mm³, or neutropenia occurs.
- Monitor lab tests: Baseline WBC with differential, direct platelet count, Hgb, and urinalyses prior to initiation of therapy and twice weekly during the first month of therapy, then every 2 wk for the next 5 mo, and monthly thereafter.

### Patient & Family Education
- Note. Clinical evidence of therapeutic effectiveness may not be apparent until 1–3 mo of drug therapy.
- Take exactly as prescribed. Allergic reactions occur in about one third of patients receiving penicillamine. Temporary interruptions of therapy increase possibility of sensitivity reactions.
- Take temperature nightly during first few months of therapy. Fever is a possible early sign of allergy.
- Observe skin over pressure sites: Knees, elbows, shoulder blades, toes, buttocks. Penicillamine increases risk of skin breakdown.
- Report unusual bruising or bleeding, sore mouth or throat, fever, skin rash, or any other unusual symptoms to prescriber.

P

Common adverse effects in *italic;* life-threatening effects underlined; generic names in **bold;** classifications in SMALL CAPS; ✤ Canadian drug name; ⊙ Prototype drug

1257

# PENICILLIN G BENZATHINE

(pen-i-sill'in)

Bicillin, Bicillin L-A, Permapen

**Classifications:** BETA-LACTAM ANTIBIOTIC; NATURAL PENICILLIN
Therapeutic: ANTIBIOTIC
**Prototype:** Penicillin G potassium

**AVAILABILITY** Solution for injection

**ACTION & *THERAPEUTIC EFFECT***
Acts by interfering with synthesis of mucopeptides essential to formation and integrity of the bacterial cell wall. *Effective against many strains of* Staphylococcus aureus, *gram-positive cocci, gram-negative cocci. Also effective against gram-positive bacilli and gram-negative bacilli as well as some strains of* Salmonella, Shigella, *and spirochetes.*

**USES** Infections highly susceptible to penicillin G, such as streptococcal, pneumococcal, and staphylococcal infections, venereal disease such as syphilis (including early, late, and congenital forms), and nonvenereal diseases (e.g., yaws, bejel, and pinta). Also used in prophylaxis of rheumatic fever.

**CONTRAINDICATIONS** Hypersensitivity to penicillins; IV administration.

**CAUTIOUS USE** History of or suspected allergy (eczema, hives, hay fever, asthma); hypersensitivity to cephalosporins or carbapenems; history of colitis; IBD; renal disease, renal impairment; GI disease; pregnancy (category B); lactation; infants, neonates.

## ROUTE & DOSAGE

### Mild to Moderate Infections
*Adult:* **IM** 1,200,000 units once/day
*Child (weight greater than 27 kg):* **IM** 900,000 units once/day; *weight less than 27 kg:* 300,000–600,000 units once/day

### Syphilis
*Adult:* **IM** Less than 1 y duration: 2,400,000 units as single dose; greater than 1 y duration: 2,400,000 units/wk for 3 wk
*Child (younger than 2 y):* **IM** 50,000 units/kg as single dose

### Prophylaxis for Rheumatic Fever
*Adult:* **IM** 1.2 million units q4wk
*Child:* **IM** 1.2 million units q3–4wk

## ADMINISTRATION

**Intramuscular**
- Do not confuse penicillin G benzathine with preparations containing procaine penicillin G (e.g., Bicillin C-R).
- Make IM injection deep into upper outer quadrant of buttock. In infants and small children, the preferred site is the midlateral aspect of the thigh.
- Shake multiple-dose vial vigorously before withdrawing desired IM dose. Shake prepared cartridge unit vigorously before injecting drug.
- Select IM site with care. Injection into or near a major peripheral nerve can result in nerve damage.
- Inadvertent IV administration has resulted in arterial occlusion and cardiac arrest.
- Make injections at a slow steady rate to prevent needle blockage.
- Store at 15°–30° C (59°–86° F).

P

Common adverse effects in *italic;* life-threatening effects underlined; generic names in **bold;** classifications in SMALL CAPS; ✚ Canadian drug name; ⊙ Prototype drug

## ADVERSE EFFECTS (≥1%) **Body as a Whole:** *Local pain,* tenderness, and fever associated with IM injection, chills, fever, wheezing, anaphylaxis, neuropathy, nephrotoxicity; superinfections, Jarisch-Herxheimer reaction in patients with syphilis. **Skin:** Pruritus, urticaria, and other skin eruptions. **Hematologic:** Eosinophilia, hemolytic anemia, and other blood abnormalities. Also see PENICILLIN G POTASSIUM.

## INTERACTIONS **Drug: Probenecid** decreases renal elimination; may decrease efficacy of ORAL CONTRACEPTIVES.

## PHARMACOKINETICS **Absorption:** Slowly absorbed from IM site. **Peak:** 12–24 h. **Duration:** 26 days. **Distribution:** Crosses placenta; distributed into breast milk. **Metabolism:** Hydrolyzed to penicillin in body. **Elimination:** Excreted slowly by kidneys.

## NURSING IMPLICATIONS

### Black Box Warning

*Penicillin G has been associated with serious adverse reaction due to inadvertent IV administration.*

Note: See penicillin G potassium for numerous additional clinical implications.

### Assessment & Drug Effects
- Determine history of hypersensitivity reactions to penicillins, cephalosporins, or other allergens prior to initiation of drug therapy.
- Monitor lab tests: Baseline C&S and repeat at completion of therapy.

### Patient & Family Education
- Report immediately to prescriber the onset of an allergic reaction. There is great risk of severe and prolonged reactions because drug is absorbed so slowly.

## PENICILLIN G POTASSIUM ℗
(pen-i-sill'in)
Megacillin ◆

## PENICILLIN G SODIUM
**Classifications:** BETA-LACTAM ANTIBIOTIC; NATURAL PENICILLIN
Therapeutic: ANTIBIOTIC

**AVAILABILITY** Vial; solution for injection

## ACTION & *THERAPEUTIC EFFECT*
Acid-labile, penicillinase-sensitive, natural penicillin that acts by interfering with synthesis of mucopeptides essential to formation and integrity of bacterial cell wall. Antimicrobial spectrum is narrow compared to that of semisynthetic penicillins. *Highly active against gram-positive cocci (e.g., non-penicillinase-producing* Staphylococcus, Streptococcus *groups) and gram-negative cocci. Also effective against gram-positive bacilli and gram-negative bacilli as well as some strains of salmonella and* Shigella *and spirochetes.*

**USES** Moderate to severe systemic infections caused by penicillin-sensitive microorganisms. Certain staphylococcal infections; streptococcal infections. Also used as prophylaxis in patients with rheumatic or congenital heart disease. Since oral preparations are absorbed erratically and thus **must be** given in comparatively high doses, this route is generally used only for mild or stabilized infections or long-term prophylaxis.

**UNLABELED USES** Skin/soft tissue infection.

**CONTRAINDICATIONS** Hypersensitivity to any of the penicillins or corn for dextrose solution prep; cardiospasm; viral infections; patients on sodium restriction.

**CAUTIOUS USE** History of or suspected allergy (asthma, eczema, hay fever, hives); history of allergy to cephalosporins; GI disorders; kidney or liver dysfunction, cardiac or vascular conditions; electrolyte imbalance; renal disease or renal impairment; MG; older adults; pregnancy (category B); lactation; young infants; neonates.

## ROUTE & DOSAGE

### Moderate to Severe Infections

*Adult:* **IV/IM** 2–24 million units divided q4h
*Child:* **IV/IM** 250,000–400,000 units/kg divided q4h

## ADMINISTRATION

Note: Check whether prescriber has prescribed penicillin G potassium or sodium.

### Intramuscular

- Do not use the 20,000,000 unit dosage form for IM injection.
- Reconstitute for IM: Loosen powder by shaking bottle before adding diluent (sterile water for injection or sterile NS). Keep the total volume to be injected small. Solutions containing up to 100,000 units/mL cause the least discomfort. Adding 10 mL diluent to the 1,000,000 unit vial = 100,000 units/mL. Shake well to dissolve.
- Select IM site carefully. IM injection is made deep into a large muscle mass. Inject slowly. Rotate injection sites.

### Intravenous

*PREPARE:* **Intermittent/Continuous:** Reconstitute as for IM injection then withdraw the required dose and add to 100–1000 mL of D5W or NS IV solution, depending on length of each infusion.
*ADMINISTER:* **Intermittent:** *Adults:* Give over at least 1 h; *Infants and Children:* Give over 15–30 min. **Continuous:** Give at a rate required to infuse the daily dose in 24 h. ▪ With high doses, IV penicillin G should be administered slowly (usually over 24 h) to prevent electrolyte imbalance from potassium or sodium content.▪ Prescriber will often prescribe specific flow rate.
*INCOMPATIBILITIES:* **Solution/additive: Dextran 40, fat emulsion, aminophylline, amphotericin B, cephalothin, chlorpromazine, dopamine, hydroxyzine, metaraminol, metoclopramide, pentobarbital, prochlorperazine, promazine, sodium bicarbonate,** TETRACYCLINES.

- Store dry powder (for parenteral use) at room temperature. After reconstitution (initial dilution), store solutions for 1 wk under refrigeration. ▪ Intravenous infusion solutions containing penicillin G are stable at room temperature for at least 24 h.

## ADVERSE EFFECTS (≥1%) Body as a Whole: Coughing, sneezing, feeling of uneasiness; <u>systemic anaphylaxis</u>, fever, widespread increase in capillary permeability and vasodilation with <u>resulting edema (mouth, tongue, pharynx, larynx), laryngospasm</u>, malaise, serum sickness (fever, malaise, pruritus, urticaria, lymphadenopathy, arthralgia, angioedema

of face and extremities, neuritis prostration, eosinophilia), SLE-like syndrome, injection site reactions (pain, inflammation, abscess, phlebitis), superinfections (especially with *Candida* and gramnegative bacteria), neuromuscular irritability (twitching, lethargy, confusion, stupor, hyperreflexia, multifocal myoclonus, localized or generalized seizures, coma). **CV:** Hypotension, circulatory collapse, cardiac arrhythmias, cardiac arrest. **GI:** Vomiting, diarrhea, severe abdominal cramps, nausea, epigastric distress, diarrhea, flatulence, dark discoloration of tongue, sore mouth or tongue. **Urogenital:** Interstitial nephritis, Loeffler's syndrome, vasculitis. **Hematologic:** Hemolytic anemia, thrombocytopenia. **Metabolic:** Hyperkalemia (penicillin G potassium); hypokalemia, alkalosis, hypernatremia, CHF (penicillin G sodium). **Respiratory:** Bronchospasm, asthma. **Skin:** Itchy palms or axilla, pruritus, *urticaria,* flushed skin, *delayed skin rashes* ranging from urticaria to exfoliative dermatitis, Stevens–Johnson syndrome, fixed-drug eruptions, contact dermatitis.

## DIAGNOSTIC TEST INTERFERENCE

*Blood grouping and compatibility tests:* Possible interference associated with penicillin doses greater than 20 million units daily. *Urine glucose:* Massive doses of penicillin may cause false-positive test results with *Benedict's solution* and possibly *Clinitest* but not with *glucose oxidase methods* (e.g., *Clinistix, Diastix, TesTape*). *Urine protein:* Massive doses of penicillin can produce false-positive results when turbidity measures are used (e.g., *acetic acid* and *heat, sulfosalicylic acid*); *Ames*

*reagent* reportedly not affected. *Urinary PSP excretion tests:* False decrease in urinary excretion of PSP. *Urinary steroids:* Large IV doses of penicillin may interfere with accurate measurement of *urinary 17-OHCS* (*Glenn–Nelson technique* not affected).

## INTERACTIONS

**Drug: Probenecid** decreases renal elimination; penicillin G may decrease efficacy of ORAL CONTRACEPTIVES; **colestipol** decreases penicillin absorption; POTASSIUM-SPARING DIURETICS may cause hyperkalemia with penicillin G potassium. **Food:** Food increases breakdown in stomach.

## PHARMACOKINETICS

**Peak:** 15–30 min IM. **Distribution:** Widely distributed; good CSF concentrations with inflamed meninges; crosses placenta; distributed in breast milk. **Metabolism:** 16–30% metabolized. **Elimination:** 60% in urine within 6 h. **Half-Life:** 0.4–0.9 h.

## NURSING IMPLICATIONS

### Assessment & Drug Effects

- Obtain an exact history of patient's previous exposure and sensitivity to penicillins and cephalosporins and other allergic reactions of any kind prior to treatment with penicillin.
- Hypersensitivity reactions are more likely to occur with parenteral penicillin than with the oral drug. Skin rash is the most common type allergic reaction and should be reported promptly to prescriber.
- Observe all patients closely for at least 30 min following administration of parenteral penicillin. The rapid appearance of a red flare or wheal at the IM or IV injection site is a possible sign of sensitivity.

P

Common adverse effects in *italic;* life-threatening effects underlined; generic names in **bold;** classifications in SMALL CAPS; ♣ Canadian drug name; ⊕ Prototype drug

1261

Also suspect an allergic reaction if patient becomes irritable, has nausea and vomiting, breathing difficulty, or sudden fever. Report any of the foregoing to prescriber immediately.

- Be aware that reactions to penicillin may be rapid in onset or may not appear for days or weeks. Symptoms usually disappear fairly quickly once drug is stopped, but in some patients may persist for 5 days or more.
- Allergy to penicillin is unpredictable. It has occurred in patients with a negative history of penicillin allergy and also in patients with no known prior contact with penicillin (sensitization may have occurred from penicillin used commercially in foods and beverages).
- Be alert for neuromuscular irritability in patients receiving parenteral penicillin in excess of 20 million units/day who have renal insufficiency, hyponatremia, or underlying CNS disease, notably myasthenia gravis or epilepsy. Seizure precautions are indicated. Symptoms usually begin with twitching, especially of face and extremities.
- Monitor I&O, particularly in patients receiving high parenteral doses. Report oliguria, hematuria, and changes in I&O ratio. Consult prescriber regarding optimum fluid intake. Dehydration increases the concentration of drug in kidneys and can cause renal irritation and damage.
- Observe closely for signs of toxicity, especially in neonates, young infants, older adults, and patients with impaired kidney function receiving high-dose penicillin therapy. Urinary excretion of penicillin is significantly delayed in these patients.

- Observe patients on high-dose therapy closely for evidence of bleeding, and bleeding time should be monitored. (In high doses, penicillin interferes with platelet aggregation.)
- Monitor lab tests: Baseline C&S; periodic LFTs, kidney function tests, and serum electrolytes with high-dose therapy.

**Patient & Family Education**

- Understand that hypersensitivity reaction may be delayed. Report skin rashes, itching, fever, malaise, and other signs of a delayed reaction to prescriber immediately (see ADVERSE EFFECTS).
- Notify prescriber if following symptoms appear when taking penicillin for treatment of syphilis: Headache, chills, fever, myalgia, arthralgia, malaise, and worsening of syphilitic skin lesions. Reaction is usually self-limiting. Check with prescriber if symptoms do not improve within a few days or get worse.
- Report S&S of superinfection (see Appendix F).

# PENICILLIN G PROCAINE
(pen-i-sill'in)

**Classifications:** BETA-LACTAM ANTIBIOTIC; NATURAL PENICILLIN
Therapeutic: ANTIBIOTIC
**Prototype:** Penicillin G potassium

**AVAILABILITY** Solution for injection

**ACTION & *THERAPEUTIC* EFFECT**
Long-acting form of penicillin G. The procaine salt has low solubility and thus creates a tissue depot from which penicillin is slowly absorbed. Slower onset of action than penicillin G potassium, but longer duration of action. It

inhibits the final stage of bacterial cell wall synthesis by binding to specific penicillin-binding proteins (PBPs) located in the bacterial cell wall. This results in cell death of bacteria. *Same actions and antibacterial activity as for penicillin G potassium and is similarly inactivated by penicillinase and gastric acid.*

**USES** Moderately severe infections due to penicillin G-sensitive microorganisms that are susceptible to low but prolonged serum penicillin concentrations. Commonly, uncomplicated pneumococcal pneumonia, uncomplicated gonorrheal infections, and all stages of syphilis. May be used concomitantly with penicillin G or probenecid when more rapid action and higher blood levels are indicated.

**CONTRAINDICATIONS** History of hypersensitivity to any of the penicillins.

**CAUTIOUS USE** History of or suspected allergy, hypersensitivity to cephalosporins, carbapenem; asthmatics; procaine; history of seizures; asthmatics; GI disease, renal disease; severe renal impairment; pregnancy (category B); lactation; children.

## ROUTE & DOSAGE

**Moderate to Severe Infections**
*Adult:* **IM** 600,000–1,200,000 units once/day
*Child:* **IM** 300,000 units once/day

**Pneumococcal Pneumonia**
*Adult:* **IM** 600,000 units q12h

**Uncomplicated Gonorrhea**
*Adult:* **IM** 4,800,000 units divided between 2 different injection sites

at one visit preceded by 1 g of probenecid 30 min before injections

**Syphilis**
*Adult:* **IM** Primary, secondary, latent: 600,000 units/day for 8 days; late latent, tertiary, neurosyphilis: 600,000 units/day for 10–15 days
*Child:* **IM** 500,000–1,000,000 units/m$^2$ once/day

## ADMINISTRATION

**Intramuscular**
- Shake multiple-dose vial thoroughly before withdrawing medication to ensure uniform suspension of drug.
- Use 20-gauge needle to avoid clogging.
- Give IM deep into upper outer quadrant of gluteus muscle; in infants and small children midlateral aspect of thigh is generally preferred. Select IM site carefully. Accidental injection into or near major peripheral nerves and blood vessels can cause neurovascular damage.
- Aspirate carefully before injecting drug to avoid entry into a blood vessel. Inadvertent IV administration reportedly has resulted in pulmonary infarcts and death.
- Inject drug at a slow, but steady rate to prevent needle blockage. Give in two sites if the dose is very large. Rotate injection sites.

**ADVERSE EFFECTS** (≥1%) **Body as a Whole:** Procaine toxicity [e.g., mental disturbances (anxiety, confusion, depression, combativeness, hallucinations), expressed fear of impending death, weakness,

Common adverse effects in *italic;* life-threatening effects underlined; generic names in **bold;** classifications in SMALL CAPS; ✦ Canadian drug name; ⊙ Prototype drug

1263

dizziness, headache, tinnitus, unusual tastes, palpitation, changes in pulse rate and BP, seizures. Also see PENICILLIN G POTASSIUM.

**INTERACTIONS Drug: Probenecid** decreases renal elimination; may decrease efficacy of ORAL CONTRACEPTIVES.

**PHARMACOKINETICS Absorption:** Slowly from IM site. **Peak:** 1–3 h. **Duration:** 15–20 h. **Distribution:** Crosses placenta; distributed into breast milk. **Metabolism:** Hydrolyzed to penicillin in body. **Elimination:** By kidneys within 24–36 h.

## NURSING IMPLICATIONS

### Assessment & Drug Effects

- Obtain an exact history of patient's previous exposure and sensitivity to penicillins, cephalosporins, and to procaine, and other allergic reactions of any kind prior to treatment.
- Test patient by injecting 0.1 mL of 1–2% procaine hydrochloride intradermally if sensitivity is suspected. Appearance of a wheal, flare, or eruption indicates procaine sensitivity.
- Be alert to the possibility of a transient toxic reaction to procaine, particularly when large single doses are administered. The reaction manifested by mental disturbance and other symptoms (see ADVERSE EFFECTS) occurs almost immediately and usually subsides after 15–30 min.

### Patient & Family Education

- Report any skin reaction at the site of injection.
- Report onset of rash, itching, fever, chills, or other symptoms of an allergic reaction to prescriber.

# PENICILLIN V
# PENICILLIN V POTASSIUM
(pen-i-sill'in)
Apo-Pen-VK ◆, Nadopen-V ◆, Novopen-VK ◆,

**Classifications:** BETA-LACTAM ANTIBIOTIC; NATURAL PENICILLIN
**Therapeutic:** ANTIBIOTIC
**Prototype:** Penicillin G potassium

**AVAILABILITY** Tablet; suspension

**ACTION & *THERAPEUTIC EFFECT***
Acid-stable analog of penicillin G with which it shares actions. It binds with the necessary penicillin-binding proteins (PBP) in cell wall of bacteria interfering with cell wall synthesis and resulting in cell lysis. *Penicillin V is bactericidal and is inactivated by penicillinase. Less active than penicillin G against gonococci and other gram-negative microorganisms.*

**USES** Mild to moderate infections caused by susceptible *Streptococci, Pneumococci,* and *Staphylococci.* Also Vincent's infection and as prophylaxis in rheumatic fever.

**UNLABELED USES** Bite wounds, cutaneous anthrax, pharyngitis.

**CONTRAINDICATIONS** Hypersensitivity to any penicillin.

**CAUTIOUS USE** History of or suspected allergy (hay fever, asthma, hives, eczema) reactions; hypersensitivity to cephalosporins, beta-lactamase inhibitors, or carbapenem; GI disease; cystic fibrosis; renal impairment, hepatic impairment; pregnancy (category B); lactation; children.

Common adverse effects in *italic;* life-threatening effects <u>underlined</u>; generic names in **bold;** classifications in SMALL CAPS; ♣ Canadian drug name; ◐ Prototype drug

## ROUTE & DOSAGE

### Mild to Moderate Infections

*Adult:* **PO** 250–500 mg q6h
*Child (younger than 12 y):* **PO**
15–50 mg/kg/day in 3–6
divided doses

### Rheumatic Fever Prophylaxis

*Adult:* **PO** 125–250 mg b.i.d.

### Endocarditis Prophylaxis

*Adult:* **PO** 2 g 30–60 min before
procedure, then 500 mg q6h for
8 doses
*Child (weight less than 30 kg):*
**PO** 1 g 30–60 min before
procedure, then 250 mg q6h for
8 doses

## ADMINISTRATION

### Oral

- Give after a meal rather than on
  an empty stomach; drug may be
  better absorbed and result in
  higher blood levels.
- Shake well before pouring. Following reconstitution, oral solution is stable for 14 days under
  refrigeration.

## ADVERSE EFFECTS (≥1%) **Body as a Whole:** Nausea, vomiting, *diarrhea,* epigastric distress. *Hypersensitivity reactions* (e.g., flushing, pruritus, urticaria, or other skin eruptions, eosinophilia, <u>anaphylaxis</u>; hemolytic anemia, <u>leukopenia</u>, <u>thrombocytopenia</u>, neuropathy, superinfections).

## INTERACTIONS **Drug: Probenecid** decreases renal elimination; may decrease efficacy of ORAL CONTRACEPTIVES; **colestipol** decreases absorption. **Food:** Food increases breakdown in stomach.

## PHARMACOKINETICS **Absorption:** 60–73% absorbed from GI tract. **Peak:** 30–60 min. **Duration:** 6 h. **Distribution:** Highest levels in kidneys; crosses placenta; distributed into breast milk. **Elimination:** In urine. **Half-Life:** 30 min.

## NURSING IMPLICATIONS

Note: See penicillin G potassium for numerous additional nursing implications.

### Assessment & Drug Effects

- Obtain careful history concern-
  ing hypersensitivity reactions to
  penicillins, cephalosporins, and
  other allergens before therapy
  begins.
- Monitor lab tests: Baseline C&S;
  LFTs, and hematologic studies at
  regular intervals in patients receiving prolonged therapy.

### Patient & Family Education

- Take penicillin V around the
  clock at specific intervals to maintain a constant blood level
- Do not miss any doses and continue taking medication until it is
  all gone unless otherwise directed
  by the prescriber.
- Discontinue medication and
  promptly report to prescriber
  the onset of hypersensitivity reactions and superinfections (see
  Appendix F).
- Use specially marked measuring
  device to ensure accurate doses
  of oral liquid preparation.

# PENTAMIDINE ISETHIONATE

(pen-tam'i-deen)
Nebupent, Pentacarinat ♦,
Pentam 300
**Classification:** ANTIPROTOZOAL
Therapeutic: ANTIPROTOZOAL

Common adverse effects in *italic;* life-threatening effects <u>underlined;</u> generic names in **bold;** classifications in SMALL CAPS; ♣ Canadian drug name; ♦ Prototype drug

1265

**AVAILABILITY** Solution for injection; aerosol

## ACTION & *THERAPEUTIC EFFECT*

Blocks parasite reproduction by interfering with nucleotide (DNA, RNA), phospholipid, and protein synthesis. *Effective against the protozoan parasite* Pneumocystis carinii *in AIDS patients.*

**USES** *P. carinii* pneumonia (PCP).

**UNLABELED USES** African trypanosomiasis and visceral leishmaniasis. (Drug supplied for latter uses is through the Centers for Disease Control and Prevention, Atlanta, GA.)

**CONTRAINDICATIONS** QT prolongation, history of torsades de pointes; lactation.

**CAUTIOUS USE** Hypertension, hypotension; hyperglycemia; pancreatitis; hypoglycemia; hypocalcemia; blood dyscrasias; liver or kidney dysfunction; diabetes mellitus; pancreatitis; asthma; cardiac arrhythmias; pregnancy (category C); children.

## ROUTE & DOSAGE

**Treatment of *Pneumocystis carinii* Pneumonia**

*Adult/Child:* **IM/IV** 4 mg/kg/day for 14–21 days; infuse IV over 60 min

**Prophylaxis of *Pneumocystis carinii* Pneumonia**

*Adult:* **Inhaled** 300 mg/nebulizer q3–4wk
*Child:* **IV/IM** 4 mg/kg monthly

## ADMINISTRATION

**Inhaled**

- Reconstitute contents of one vial in 6 mL sterile water (not saline) and administer using nebulizer.
- Do not mix with any other drug.

**Intramuscular**

- Dissolve contents of 1 vial (300 mg) in 3 mL sterile water for injection.
- Give deep IM into a large muscle.
- The IM injection is painful and frequently causes local reactions (pain, indurations, swelling). Select alternate sites for daily doses and institute local treatment if indicated.

**Intravenous**

*PREPARE:* **IV Infusion:** Dissolve contents of 1 vial in 3–5 mL sterile water for injection or D5W.
- Further dilute in 50–250 mL of D5W.
*ADMINISTER:* **IV Infusion:** Give over 60–120 min.
*INCOMPATIBILITIES:* Y-site: **Aldesleukin,** CEPHALOSPORINS, **fluconazole, foscarnet, linezolid.**

- Note: IV solutions are stable at room temperature for up to 24 h. Protect solution from light.

**ADVERSE EFFECTS** (≥1%) **CNS:** Confusion, hallucinations, neuralgia, dizziness, sweating. **CV:** Sudden, severe hypotension, cardiac arrhythmias, ventricular tachycardia, phlebitis. **GI:** Anorexia, nausea, vomiting, pancreatitis, unpleasant taste. **Urogenital:** Acute kidney failure. **Hematologic:** Leukopenia, thrombocytopenia, anemia. **Metabolic:** Hypoglycemia, hypocalcemia, *hyperkalemia.* **Respiratory:** *Cough, bronchospasm,* laryngitis, shortness of breath, chest pain, pneumothorax. **Skin:** Stevens–Johnson syndrome, facial flush (with IV injection), *local reactions at injection site.*

P

Common adverse effects in *italic;* life-threatening effects <u>underlined;</u> generic names in **bold;** classifications in SMALL CAPS; ♣ Canadian drug name; ◯ Prototype drug

**INTERACTIONS Drug:** AMINOGLYCO-SIDES, **amphotericin B, cidofovir, cisplatin, ganciclovir, cyclosporine, vancomycin,** other nephrotoxic drugs increase risk of nephrotoxicity.

**PHARMACOKINETICS Absorption:** Readily after IM injection. **Distribution:** Leaves bloodstream rapidly to bind extensively to body tissues. **Elimination:** 50–66% in urine within 6 h; small amounts found in urine for as long as 6–8 wk. **Half-Life:** 6.5–13.2 h.

## NURSING IMPLICATIONS

### Assessment & Drug Effects

- Monitor BP and HR continuously during the infusion, every half hour for 2 h thereafter, and then every 4 h until BP stablizes. Sudden severe hypotension may develop after a single dose. Place patient in supine position while receiving the drug.
- Measure and record I&O ratio and pattern.
- Be alert and report promptly S&S of impending kidney dysfunction (e.g., changed I&O ratio, oliguria, edema).
- Characteristics of pneumonia in the immunocompromised patient include constant fever, scanty (if any) sputum, dyspnea, tachypnea, and cyanosis.
- Monitor temperature changes and institute measures to lower the temperature as indicated. Fever is a constant symptom in *P. carinii* pneumonia, but may be rapidly elevated [as high as 40° C (104° F)] shortly after drug infusion.
- Monitor lab tests: Periodic serum electrolytes, renal function tests, LFTs, CBC with differential, platelet count, and blood glucose.

### Patient & Family Education

- Report promptly to prescriber increasing respiratory difficulty.
- Monitor blood glucose for loss of glycemic control if diabetic.
- Report any unusual bruising or bleeding. Avoid using aspirin or other NSAIDs.
- Increase fluid intake (if not contraindicated) to 2–3 qt (L)/day.

## PENTAZOCINE HYDROCHLORIDE ℗

(pen-taz'oh-seen)

Talwin

**Classifications:** NARCOTIC (OPIATE AGONIST–ANTAGONIST); ANALGESIC

**Therapeutic:** NARCOTIC ANALGESIC

**Controlled Substance:** Schedule IV

**AVAILABILITY** Solution for injection

## ACTION & *THERAPEUTIC EFFECT*

Synthetic analgesic with potency approximately one-third that of morphine. Opiates exert their effects by stimulating specific opiate receptors that produce analgesia, respiratory depression, and euphoria as well as physical dependence. *Effective for moderate to severe pain relief. Acts as weak narcotic antagonist and has sedative properties.*

**USES** Relief of moderate to severe pain; also used for preoperative analgesia or sedation, and as supplement to surgical anesthesia.

**CONTRAINDICATIONS** Hypersensitivity to sulfite; head injury, increased intracranial pressure; seizures; emotionally unstable

Common adverse effects in *italic;* life-threatening effects <u>underlined</u>; generic names in **bold;** classifications in SMALL CAPS; ✤ Canadian drug name; ℗ Prototype drug

1267

patients, respiratory depression, or history of drug abuse.

**CAUTIOUS USE** Impaired kidney or liver function; cardiac disease; COPD, asthmas, GI obstruction; biliary surgery; patients with MI who have nausea and vomiting; pregnancy (category C); lactation; children younger than 12 y.

## ROUTE & DOSAGE

**Moderate to Severe Pain (Excluding Patients in Labor)**

*Adult:* **IM/IV/Subcutaneous** 30 mg q3–4h (max: 360 mg/day)

**Anesthesia**

*Adult:* **IM/IV/Subcutaneous** 30 mg dose; may repeat q3–4h as needed (max: 360 mg daily)
*Adolescent/Child:* **IM** 0.5 mg/kg single dose (max: 30 mg)

**Pain during Labor**

*Adult:* **IM** 30 mg dose; **IV** 20 mg dose may repeat q2–3h (total: 2–3 doses)

**Renal Impairment Dosage Adjustment**

*CrCl 10–50 mL/min:* Give 75% of dose; *less than 10 mL/min:* Give 50% of dose

## ADMINISTRATION

### Subcutaneous/Intramuscular

- IM is preferred to subcutaneous route when frequent injections over an extended period are required.
- Observe injection sites daily for signs of irritation or inflammation.

### Intravenous

*PREPARE:* **Direct:** Give undiluted or diluted with 1 mL sterile water for injection for each 5 mg.

*ADMINISTER:* **Direct:** Give slowly at a rate of 5 mg over 60 sec.

*INCOMPATIBILITIES:* Solution/additive: **Alemtuzumab, aminophylline,** BARBITURATES, **sodium bicarbonate, glycopyrrolate, heparin, nafcillin. Y-site: Alemtuzumab, aminophylline, amphotericin B, ampicillin, atenolol, azathioprine, aztrenam, bivalirudin, cefmandole, cefazolin, cefoperazone, cefotaxime, cefotetan, cefoxitin, ceftizoxime, ceftriaxone, cefuroxime, chloramphenicol, dantrolene, daptomycin, diazepam, diazoxide, foscarnet, furosemide, gallium, ganciclovir, gemtuzumab, indomethacin, ketorolac, methylprednisolone, mitomycin, nafcillin, nitroprusside, oxacillin, pemetrexed, penicillin G, pentobarbital, phenobarbital, phenytoin, piperacillin, SMZ/TMP, ticarcillin, nafcillin.**

**ADVERSE EFFECTS** (≥1%) **Body as a Whole:** Flushing, allergic reactions, <u>shock</u>. **CNS:** *Drowsiness,* sweating, *dizziness, lightheadedness, euphoria,* psychotomimetic effects, confusion, anxiety, hallucinations, disturbed dreams, bizarre thoughts, euphoria and other mood alterations. **CV:** Hypertension, palpitation, tachycardia. **GI:** *Nausea, vomiting,* constipation, dry mouth, alterations of taste. **Urogenital:** Urinary retention. **Respiratory:** <u>Respiratory depression</u>. **Skin:** Injection-site reactions (induration, nodule formation, sloughing, sclerosis, cutaneous depression), rash, pruritus. **Special Senses:** Visual disturbances.

**INTERACTIONS Drug: Alcohol** and other CNS DEPRESSANTS add to CNS depression; NARCOTIC ANALGESICS may precipitate narcotic withdrawal syndrome.

**PHARMACOKINETICS Onset:** 15 min IM, Subcutaneous; 2–3 min IV. **Peak:** 1 h IM, 15 min IV. **Duration:** 3 h IM, 1 h IV. **Distribution:** Crosses placenta. **Metabolism:** Extensively in liver. **Elimination:** Primarily in urine; small amount in feces. **Half-Life:** 2–3 h.

## NURSING IMPLICATIONS

### Assessment & Drug Effects

- Monitor therapeutic effect. Tolerance to analgesic effect sometimes occurs. Psychologic and physical dependence have been reported in patients with history of drug abuse, but rarely in patients without such history. Addiction liability matches that of codeine.
- Monitor vital signs and assess for respiratory depression. Keep supine to minimize adverse efffects.
- Monitor drug-induced CNS depression.
- Be aware that pentazocine may produce acute withdrawal symptoms in some patients who have been receiving opioids on a regular basis.
- Monitor I&O as drug may cause urinary retention.

### Patient & Family Education

- Avoid driving and other potentially hazardous activities until response to drug is known.
- Do not discontinue drug abruptly following extended use; may result in chills, abdominal and muscle cramps, yawning, runny nose, tearing, itching, restlessness, anxiety, drug-seeking behavior.

# PENTOBARBITAL

(pen-toe-bar′bi-tal)

# PENTOBARBITAL SODIUM

Nembutal, Novopentobarb ◆

**Classifications:** ANXIOLYTIC; SEDATIVE-HYPNOTIC; BARBITURATE; ANTICONVULSANT

Therapeutic: ANTIANXIETY; SEDATIVE-HYPNOTIC; ANTICONVULSANT

**Prototype:** Secobarbital
**Controlled Substance:** Schedule II

**AVAILABILITY** Solution for injection

**ACTION & *THERAPEUTIC EFFECT*** Short-acting barbiturate with anticonvulsant properties. Potent respiratory depressant. Initially, barbiturates suppress REM sleep, but with chronic therapy REM sleep returns to normal. *Effective as a sedative and hypnotic and anticonvulsant.*

**USES** Sedative or hypnotic for preanesthetic medication, induction of general anesthesia, adjunct in manipulative or diagnostic procedures, and emergency control of acute convulsions.

**CONTRAINDICATIONS** History of sensitivity to barbiturates; parturition, fetal immaturity, uncontrolled pain; ethanol intoxication; hepatic encephalopathy; porphyria; suicidal ideation; pregnancy (category D); lactation.

**CAUTIOUS USE** COPD, sleep apnea; heart failure; hypertension, hypotension, pulmonary disease;

P

Common adverse effects in *italic;* life-threatening effects underlined; generic names in **bold;** classifications in SMALL CAPS; ◆ Canadian drug name; ❶ Prototype drug

1269

alcoholism; mental status changes, suicidality, major depression; neonates; renal impairment, renal failure; children.

## ROUTE & DOSAGE

### Preoperative Sedation

*Adult:* **IM** 150–200 mg in 2 divided doses
*Child:* **IV** 2–6 mg/kg (max: 100 mg)

### Hypnotic/Insomnia

*Adult:* **IM** 150–200 mg
*Child:* **IM** 2–6 mg/kg (max: 100 mg)

### Status Epilepticus

*Adult:* **IV** 5–15 mg/kg loading, then 0.5–3 mg/kg/h
*Child:* **IM** 5–15 mg/kg loading, then 0.5–5 mg/kg/h

## ADMINISTRATION

Note: Do not give within 14 days of starting/stopping an MAO inhibitor.

### Intramuscular

▪ Do not use parenteral solutions that appear cloudy or in which a precipitate has formed.
▪ Make IM injections deep into large muscle mass, preferably upper outer quadrant of buttock. Aspirate needle carefully before injecting it to prevent inadvertent entry into blood vessel. Inject no more than 5 mL (250 mg) in any one site because of possible tissue irritation.

### Intravenous

*PREPARE:* **Direct:** Give undiluted or diluted (preferred) with sterile water, D5W, NS, or other compatible IV solutions.
*ADMINISTER:* **Direct:** Give slowly. Do not exceed rate of 50 mg/min.
*INCOMPATIBILITIES:* **Solution/additive: Atropine, butorphanol, chlorpheniramine, chlorpromazine, cimetidine, codeine, dimenhydrinate, diphenhydramine, droperidol, ephedrine, fentanyl, glycopyrrolate, hydrocortisone, hydroxyzine, inulin, levorphanol, meperidine, methadone, midazolam, morphine, nalbuphine, norepinephrine,** TETRACYCLINES, **penicillin G, pentazocine, perphenazine, phenytoin, promazine, prochlorperazine, promethazine, ranitidine, sodium bicarbonate, streptomycin, succinylcholine, triflupromazine, vancomycin.** Y-site: **Amphotericin B cholesteryl, fenoldopam, TPN.**

▪ Take extreme care to avoid extravasation. Necrosis may result because parenteral solution is highly alkaline. ▪ Do not use cloudy or precipitated solution.

## ADVERSE EFFECTS (≥1%) Body as a Whole: Drowsiness, lethargy, hangover, paradoxical excitement in the older adult patient. CV: Hypotension with rapid IV. Respiratory: With rapid IV (respiratory depression, laryngospasm, bronchospasm, apnea).

## INTERACTIONS Drug: Phenmetrazine antagonizes effects of pentobarbital; CNS DEPRESSANTS, alcohol, SEDATIVES add to CNS depression; MAO INHIBITORS cause excessive CNS depression; methoxyflurane creates risk of nephrotoxicity. Herbal: Kava, valerian may potentiate sedation.

## PHARMACOKINETICS Onset: 10–15 min IM; 1 min IV. Duration: 15 min IV. Distribution: Crosses placenta. Metabolism: Primarily in liver. Elimination: In urine. Half-Life: 4–50 h.

Common adverse effects in *italic;* life-threatening effects underlined; generic names in **bold**; classifications in SMALL CAPS; ♣ Canadian drug name; ⊙ Prototype drug

## NURSING IMPLICATIONS
### Assessment & Drug Effects
- Monitor BP, pulse, and respiration q3–5min during IV administration. Observe patient closely; maintain airway. Have equipment for artificial respiration immediately available.
- Observe patient closely for adverse effects for at least 30 min after IM administration of hypnotic dose.
- Monitor for hypersensitivity reactions (see Appendix F) especially with a history of asthma or angioedema.
- Monitor for adverse CNS effects including exacerbation of depression and suicidal ideation.
- Monitor those in acute pain, children, the elderly, and debilitated patients for paradoxical excitement restlessness.
- Concurrent drug: Monitor warfarin and phenytoin levels frequently to ensure therapeutic range.
- Monitor lab tests: Periodic pentobarbital level. Note: Plasma level greater than 30 mcg/mL may be toxic and 65 mcg/mL and above may be lethal.

### Patient & Family Education
- Exercise caution when driving or operating machinery for the remainder of day after taking drug.
- Avoid alcohol and other CNS depressants for 24 h after receiving this drug.
- Women using oral contraceptives should use an additional, alternative form of contraception.

## PENTOXIFYLLINE
(pen-tox-i'fi-leen)

**Classifications:** HEMATOLOGIC; RED BLOOD CELL MODIFIER; BLOOD VISCOSITY REDUCER

**Therapeutic:** RED BLOOD CELL MODIFIER; BLOOD VISCOSITY IMPROVER

**AVAILABILITY** Sustained release tablet

## ACTION & *THERAPEUTIC EFFECT*
Maintains the flexibility of RBCs, increasing erythrocyte cAMP activity, thus allowing erythrocyte membranes to maintain their integrity and become more resistant to deformity. Improvement in blood viscosity results in increased blood flow to the microcirculation and enhanced tissue oxygenation. *Results in increased blood flow to the extremities, reduced pain and paresthesia of intermittent claudication.*

**USES** Intermittent claudication associated with occlusive peripheral vascular disease; diabetic angiopathies.

**UNLABELED USES** To improve psychopathologic symptoms in patient with cerebrovascular insufficiency and to reduce incidence of stroke in the patient with recurrent TIAs.

**CONTRAINDICATIONS** Intolerance to pentoxifylline or to methylxanthines (caffeine and theophylline); intracranial bleeding; retinal bleeding; lactation.

**CAUTIOUS USE** Angina, hypotension, arrhythmias, cerebrovascular disease; peptic ulcer disease; renal failure; renal impairment; risk of bleeding; pregnancy (category C); children younger than 18 y.

## ROUTE & DOSAGE

**Intermittent Claudication**
*Adult:* **PO** 400 mg t.i.d. with meals

## ADMINISTRATION
### Oral
- Give on an empty stomach or with food; be consistent with time of day and relationship to food in establishing the daily regimen.

---

Common adverse effects in *italic*; life-threatening effects <u>underlined</u>; generic names in **bold**; classifications in SMALL CAPS; ♣Canadian drug name; ☻ Prototype drug

- Store tablets at 15°–30° C (59°–86° F).

## ADVERSE EFFECTS (≥1%) Body as a Whole: Fever, flushing, convulsions, somnolence, loss of consciousness. CNS: Agitation, nervousness, *dizziness,* drowsiness, headache, insomnia, tremor, confusion. CV: Angina, chest pain, dyspnea, arrhythmias, palpitations, hypotension, edema, flushing. Eye: Blurred vision, conjunctivitis, scotomas. GI: Abdominal discomfort, belching, flatus, bloating, diarrhea, *dyspepsia, nausea, vomiting.* Skin: Brittle fingernails, pruritus, rash, urticaria. Other: Earache, unpleasant taste, excessive salivation, <u>leukopenia</u>, malaise, sore throat, swollen neck glands, weight change.

## INTERACTIONS Drug: **Ciprofloxacin, cimetidine** may increase levels and toxicity, **warfarin** may have additive effects. Do not use with **ketorolac**. Herbal: **Evening primrose oil, ginseng, ginkgo** may increase bleeding risk.

## PHARMACOKINETICS Absorption: Readily from GI tract; 10–50% reaches systemic circulation (first pass metabolism). Peak: 2–4 h. Distribution: Distributed into breast milk. Metabolism: In liver and erythrocytes. Elimination: Primarily in urine. Half-Life: 0.4–0.8 h.

## NURSING IMPLICATIONS
### Assessment & Drug Effects
- Monitor therapeutic effectiveness which is indicated by relief from pain and cramping in calf muscles, buttocks, thighs, and feet during exercise and improves walking performance (time and duration).
- Monitor BP if patient is also on antihypertensive treatment. Drug may slightly decrease an already stabilized BP, necessitating a reduced dose of the hypotensive drug.

### Patient & Family Education
- Consult prescriber to determine CV status and capacity before re-establishing walking as exercise.
- Pay particular attention to care of the feet because of arterial insufficiency (diminished perfusion to feet).
- Be aware that bleeding and prolonged PT/INR associated with this treatment have been reported. Report promptly unexplained bleeding, easy bruising, nose bleed, pinpoint rash to prescriber.
- Avoid driving or working with hazardous machinery until drug response has stabilized because of potential for tiredness, blurred vision, dizziness.

## PERAMIVIR
(per-a-mi′vir)
Rapivab
**Classifications:** ANTIVIRAL; NEURAMINIDASE INHIBITOR
Therapeutic: ANTI-INFLUENZA
**Prototype:** Oseltamivir

## AVAILABILITY Solution for injection

## ACTION & *THERAPEUTIC EFFECT*
Inhibits influenza A and B viral neuraminidase enzyme, preventing the release of newly formed viruses from the surface of the infected cells. Inhibits replication of the influenza A and B virus. *Relieves flu symptoms and prevents viral spread across the mucous lining of the respiratory tract.*

## USES Treatment of acute uncomplicated influenza in patients 18 y or older who have been symptomatic for no more than 2 days.

Common adverse effects in *italic*; life-threatening effects <u>underlined</u>; generic names in **bold**; classifications in SMALL CAPS; ✚ Canadian drug name; ⓟ Prototype drug

**CAUTIOUS USE** Serious skin reactions; abnormal behavior including hallucinations and delirium; renal impairment; pregnancy (category C); lactation. Safety and efficacy in patients younger than 18 y not established.

## ROUTE & DOSAGE

**Influenza**

*Adult:* **IV** Single 600 mg dose within 48 h of symptoms

**Renal Impairment Dosage Adjustment**

*CrCL 30–49 mL/min:* Reduce to 200 mg
*CrCL 10–29 mL/min:* Reduce to 100 mg

## ADMINISTRATION

**Intravenous**

*PREPARE:* **IV Infusion:** Dilute required dose in NS, 0.45% NaCl, D5W, or LR to a max volume of 100 mL.
*ADMINISTER:* **IV Infusion:** Give over 15–30 min.
*INCOMPATIBILITIES:* **Solution/additive:** Do not mix with other IV medications. **Y-site:** Do not coinfuse with other IV medications

▪ Store refrigerated at 2°–8° C (36°–46° F) for up to 24 h if not administered immediately. If refrigerated, allow solution to reach room temperature then administer immediately.

## ADVERSE EFFECTS (≥2%) **CNS:**
Insomnia. **CV:** Hypertension. **GI:** Constipation, *diarrhea*. **Hematological:** Neutropenia. **Metabolic:** Hyperglycemia, increased ALT/AST, increased creatine phosphokinase. **Skin:** Exfoliative dermatitis, rash, Stevens–Johnson syndrome.

## PHARMACOKINETICS **Distribution:** 30% plasma protein bound. **Metabolism:** Minimal. **Elimination:** Primarily renal (90%). **Half-Life:** 20 h.

## NURSING IMPLICATIONS

### Assessment and Drug Effects
▪ Monitor for and report promptly skin rash, dermatitis, erythema.
▪ Monitor for neuropsychiatric events, especially in children.
▪ Monitor lab tests: Baseline serum urea nitrogen and serum creatinine.

### Patient & Family Education
▪ Seek immediate medical attention if a skin reaction occurs.
▪ Contact prescriber for any signs of abnormal behavior including illogical thinking, altered speech, hallucinations, or delusions.

## PERINDOPRIL ERBUMINE
(per in'do-pril)
Aceon

**Classifications:** ANGIOTENSIN-CONVERTING ENZYME (ACE) INHIBITOR; ANTIHYPERTENSIVE
**Therapeutic:** ANTIHYPERTENSIVE
**Prototype:** Captopril

## AVAILABILITY Tablet

## ACTION & *THERAPEUTIC EFFECT*
Inhibits the renin angiotensin-converting enzyme (ACE) that catalyzes the conversion of angiotensin I to angiotensin II, a potent vasoconstrictor substance. Also reduces aldosterone production causing a potassium sparing effect. In addition, it decreases systemic vascular resistance (afterload) and pulmonary capillary wedge pressure (PCWP), a measure of preload, and improves cardiac output as well as activity tolerance. *Effective in lowering blood pressure by vasodilatation resulting from*

---

Common adverse effects in *italic*; life-threatening effects underlined; generic names in **bold**; classifications in SMALL CAPS; ♣Canadian drug name; ⊘ Prototype drug *inhibition of ACE. Improves cardiac output as well as activity tolerance in CAD.*

**USES** Hypertension, myocardial infarction prophylaxis, reduction of cardiovascular mortality.

**UNLABELED USES** Heart failure.

**CONTRAINDICATIONS** Hypersensitivity to perindopril or any other ACE inhibitor; history of angioedema induced by an ACE inhibitor, patients with hypertrophic cardiomyopathy, hepatoxicity; renal artery stenosis; pregnancy (category D); lactation.

**CAUTIOUS USE** Renal insufficiency, volume-depleted patients, severe liver dysfunction; autoimmune diseases, immunosuppressant drug therapy; hyperkalemia or potassium-sparing diuretics; surgery; neutropenia; febrile illness; older adults. Safety and efficacy in children not established.

## ROUTE & DOSAGE

**Hypertension, Stable Coronary Artery Disease**

*Adult:* **PO** 2–4 mg once daily, may be increased to 8 mg daily in 1 or 2 divided doses (max: 16 mg/day)

**Myocardial Infarction Prophylaxis**

*Adult:* **PO** 4 mg daily × 2 wk, then 8 mg daily

**Renal Impairment Dosage Adjustment**

*CrCl 30–59 mL/min:* Start 2 mg daily; *CrCl 16–29 mL/min:* Start 2 mg every other day; *CrCl less than 16 mL/min:* Give 2 mg on dialysis days only

## ADMINISTRATION

**Oral**

- Manufacturer recommends an initial dose of 2–4 mg in 1 or 2 divided doses if concurrently ordered diuretic cannot be discontinued 2–3 days before beginning perindopril. Consult prescriber.
- Give on an empty stomach 1 h before meals.
- Dosage adjustments are generally made at intervals of at least 1 wk.
- Store at 20°–25° C (68°–77° F) and protect from moisture.

**ADVERSE EFFECTS** (≥1%) **CNS:** Dizziness, light-headedness (in the absence of postural hypotension), headache, mood and sleep disorders, fatigue. **CV:** Palpitations. **Endocrine:** Hyperkalemia. **GI:** Nausea, vomiting, epigastric pain, diarrhea, taste disturbances, dyspepsia. **Urogenital:** Proteinuria, impotence, sexual dysfunction. **Special Senses:** Dry eyes, blurred vision. **Body as a Whole:** *Cough,* angioedema, pruritus, muscle cramps, sinusitis, hypertonia, fever. **Skin:** Rash.

**INTERACTIONS** **Drug:** POTASSIUM-SPARING DIURETICS (**amiloride, spironolactone, triamterene**) may increase the risk of hyperkalemia. POTASSIUM SUPPLEMENTS increase the risk of hyperkalemia; lithium levels can be increased. Use with **azathioprine** may cause anemia and leukopenia. **Pregabalin** may increase risk of angioedema. **Food:** Food can decrease drug absorption 35%.

**PHARMACOKINETICS** **Absorption:** Readily from GI tract, absorption significantly decreased when taken with food. **Peak:** **Perindopril:** 1 h; **perindoprilat:** 3–7 h. **Duration:** 24 h. **Metabolism:** Hydrolyzed in the liver to its active form, perindoprilat. **Elimination:** Primarily in urine. **Half-Life: Perindopril:** 0.8–1 h, **perindoprilat:** 30–120 h.

## NURSING IMPLICATIONS

### Black Box Warning

*Perindropril has been associated with fetal injury and death.*

### Assessment & Drug Effects

- Monitor BR and HR carefully following initial dose for several hours until stable, especially in patients using concurrent diuretics, on salt restriction, or volume depleted.
- Place patient immediately in a supine position if excess hypotension develops.
- Monitor closely kidney function in patients with CHF.
- Monitor serum lithium levels and assess for S&S of lithium toxicity when used concurrently; increased caution is needed when diuretic therapy is also used.
- Monitor lab tests: Periodic serum potassium, BUN, and creatinine.

### Patient & Family Education

- Discontinue drug and immediately report S&S of angioedema (i.e., swelling) of face or extremities to prescriber. Seek emergency help for swelling of the tongue or any other signs of potential airway obstruction.
- Contact prescriber immediately if you become pregnant.
- Be aware that light-headedness can occur, especially during early therapy; excess fluid loss of any kind (e.g., vomiting, diarrhea) will increase risk of hypotension and fainting.
- Avoid using potassium supplements unless specifically directed to do so by prescriber.
- Report S&S of infection (e.g., sore throat, fever) promptly to prescriber.

# PERMETHRIN ℗

(per-meth′rin)

Nix, Elimite, Acticin

**Classifications:** SCABICIDE; PEDICULICIDE
Therapeutic: SCABICIDE; PEDICULICIDE

## AVAILABILITY Cream; liquid

## ACTION & *THERAPEUTIC EFFECT*

Inhibits sodium ion influx through nerve cell membrane channels, resulting in delayed repolarization of the action potential and paralysis of the pest. *It prevents burrowing into host's skin. Since lice are completely dependent on blood for survival, they die within 24–48 h. Also active against ticks, mites, and fleas.*

## USES Pediculosis capitis.

## CONTRAINDICATIONS Hypersensitivity to pyrethrins, chrysanthemums, sulfites, or other preservatives or dyes; acute inflammation of the scalp; lactation.

## CAUTIOUS USE Children younger than 2 y **(liquid),** and less than 2 mo **(lotion);** asthma; pregnancy (category B).

## ROUTE & DOSAGE

### Head Lice

*Adult/Child (2 y or older):*
**Topical** Apply sufficient volume to clean wet hair to saturate the hair and scalp; leave on 10 min, then rinse hair thoroughly

## ADMINISTRATION

### Topical

- Saturate scalp as well as hair with the lotion; this is not a shampoo.

---

Common adverse effects in *italic*; life-threatening effects underlined; generic names in **bold**; classifications in SMALL CAPS; ♥Canadian drug name; ℗ Prototype drug

Shake lotion well before application.

- Hair should be washed with regular shampoo before treatment with permethrin, thoroughly rinsed and dried.
- Rinse hair and scalp thoroughly and dry with a clean towel following 10 min exposure to the medication. Head lice are usually eliminated with one treatment.
- Store drug away from heat at 15°–25° C (59°–77° F) and direct light. Avoid freezing.

## ADVERSE EFFECTS (≥1%) Skin:
*Pruritus, transient tingling,* burning, stinging, numbness; erythema, edema, rash.

## PHARMACOKINETICS Absorption:
Less than 2% of amount applied is absorbed through intact skin. **Metabolism:** Rapidly hydrolyzed to inactive metabolites. **Elimination:** Primarily in urine.

## NURSING IMPLICATIONS

### Assessment & Drug Effects
- Do not attempt therapy if patient is known to be sensitive to any pyrethrin or pyrethroid. Stop treatment if a reaction occurs.

### Patient & Family Education
- When hair is dry, comb with a fine-tooth comb (furnished with medication) to remove dead lice and remaining nits or nit shells.
- Be aware that drug remains on hair shaft up to 14 days; therefore, recurrence of infestation rarely occurs (less than 1%).
- Inspect hair shafts daily for at least 1 wk to determine drug effectiveness. Contact prescriber if live lice are observed after 7 days. Signs of inadequate treatment: Itching, redness of skin, skin abrasion, infected scalp areas.

- Resume regular shampooing after treatment; residual deposit of drug on hair is not reduced.
- Be aware that drug is usually irritating to the eyes and mucosa. Flush well with water if medicine accidentally gets into eyes.

# PERPHENAZINE
(per-fen'a-zeen)

**Classifications:** PHENOTHIAZINE ANTIPSYCHOTIC; ANTIEMETIC
**Therapeutic:** ANTIPSYCHOTIC; ANTIEMETIC
**Prototype:** Chlorpromazine

## AVAILABILITY Tablet

## ACTION & *THERAPEUTIC EFFECT*
Affects all parts of CNS, particularly the hypothalamus. Antipsychotic effect is due to its ability to antagonize neurotransmitter dopamine by acting on its receptors in the brain. Antiemetic action results from direct blockade of dopamine in the chemoreceptor trigger zone (CTZ) in the medulla. *Has antipsychotic and antiemetic properties.*

## USES Schizophrenia, symptomatic control of severe nausea and vomiting.

## CONTRAINDICATIONS Hypersensitivity to perphenazine and other phenothiazines; preexisting liver damage; suspected or established subcortical brain damage, comatose states, CNS depression; dementia-related psychosis; hepatic encephalopathy; QT prolongation; bone marrow depression; hematological disease; pregnancy (category undetermined); lactation.

## CAUTIOUS USE Previously diagnosed breast cancer; liver or kidney

dysfunction; renal impairment; cardiovascular disorders; drug or alcohol abuse; epilepsy; psychic depression, patients with suicidal tendency; cardiac and pulmonary disease; glaucoma; history of intestinal or GU obstruction; older adults or debilitated patients; children younger than 12 y.

## ROUTE & DOSAGE

### Psychotic Disorders
*Adult/Adolescent:* PO 4–8 mg t.i.d. (max: 64 mg/day)

### Nausea
*Adult:* PO 8–16 mg daily in divided doses (up to 24 mg/day)

### Hemodialysis Dosage Adjustment
Not dialyzable

### Pharmacogenetic Adjustment
*Poor CYP2D6 metabolizers:* Start with 30% of dose

## ADMINISTRATION

### Oral
- May be taken with or without food.
- Administer with food, milk, or full glass of water to minimize gastric irritation.

## ADVERSE EFFECTS (≥1%) CNS:
*Extrapyramidal effects (dystonic reactions, akathisia, parkinsonian syndrome, tardive dyskinesia), sedation,* convulsions. **CV:** *Orthostatic hypotension,* tachycardia, bradycardia. **Special Senses:** Mydriasis, blurred vision, corneal and lenticular deposits. **GI:** Constipation, *dry mouth,* increased appetite, <u>adynamic ileus,</u> abnormal liver function tests, cholestatic jaundice. **Urogenital:** *Urinary retention,* gynecomastia, menstrual irregularities, inhibited ejaculation. **Hematologic:** <u>Agranulocytosis,</u> thrombocytopenic purpura, <u>aplastic</u> or hemolytic

anemia. **Body as a Whole:** Photosensitivity, itching, erythema, urticaria, angioneurotic edema, drug fever, <u>anaphylactoid reaction,</u> sterile abscess. Nasal congestion, decreased sweating. **Metabolic:** Hyperprolactinemia, galactorrhea, weight gain.

## DIAGNOSTIC TEST INTERFERENCE
Perphenazine may cause falsely abnormal ***thyroid function*** tests because of elevations of ***thyroid globulin.***

## INTERACTIONS Drug: Alcohol
and other CNS DEPRESSANTS enhance CNS depression; ANTACIDS, ANTIDIARRHEALS may decrease absorption of phenothiazines; ANTICHOLINERGIC AGENTS add to anticholinergic effects including fecal impaction and paralytic ileus; BARBITURATES, ANESTHETICS increase hypotension, excitation and may increase risk of QT prolongation. **Herbal: Kava** increased risk and severity of dystonic reactions.

## PHARMACOKINETICS Absorption:
Poorly absorbed from GI tract; 20% reaches systemic circulation. **Peak:** 4–8 h PO. **Duration:** 6–12 h. **Distribution:** Crosses placenta. **Metabolism:** In liver (CYP2D6) with some metabolism in GI tract. **Elimination:** In urine and feces. **Half-Life:** 9.5 h.

## NURSING IMPLICATIONS

### Black Box Warning

*Perphenazine has been associated with increased mortality in older adults with dementia-related psychosis.*

### Assessment & Drug Effects
- Monitor mental status and report promptly suicidal ideation, significant changes in mood, behavior, or functional ability.

---

Common adverse effects in *italic*; life-threatening effects <u>underlined</u>; generic names in **bold**; classifications in SMALL CAPS; ♥ Canadian drug name; ⓟ Prototype drug

- Monitor vital signs periodically and report significant changes in HR or BP (especially with marked dosage increases).
- Report restlessness, weakness of extremities, dystonic reactions (spasms of neck and shoulder muscles, rigidity of back, difficulty swallowing or talking); motor restlessness (akathisia: inability to be still); and parkinsonian syndrome (tremors, shuffling gait, drooling, slow speech).
- Withhold medication and report immediately to prescriber S&S of tardive dyskinesia (i.e., fine, wormlike movements or rapid protrusions of the tongue, chewing motions, lip smacking).
- ECG and ophthalmologic examination are recommended prior to initiation and periodically during therapy.
- Suspect hypersensitivity, withhold drug, and report to prescriber if jaundice appears between weeks 2 and 4.
- Monitor urine and bowel elimination pattern especially with daily doses greater than 24 mg.
- Monitor ophthalmic screening at onset of therapy and periodically throughout.
- Monitor lab tests: Periodic CBC with differential, LFTs, renal function tests, serum electrolytes, fasting blood glucose and HgA1C.

### Patient & Family Education

- Make all position changes slowly and in stages, particularly from recumbent to upright posture, and to lie down or sit down if lightheadedness or dizziness occurs.
- Do not drive or engage in potentially hazardous activities until response to drug is known.
- Discontinue drug and report to prescriber immediately if jaundice appears between weeks 2 and 4.

- Avoid long exposure to sunlight and to sunlamps. Photosensitivity results in skin color changes from brown to blue-gray.
- Adhere strictly to dosage regimen. Contact prescriber before changing it for any reason.
- Drug should be discontinued gradually over a period of several weeks following prolonged therapy.
- Avoid OTC drugs unless prescriber prescribes them.
- Be aware that perphenazine may discolor urine reddish brown.

## PERTUZUMAB
(per-tu′zu-mab)
Perjeta
**Classification:** MONOCLONAL ANTIBODY; HUMAN EPIDERAL GROWTH FACTOR RECEPTOR 2 PROTEIN (HER2) ANTAGONIST; ANTINEOPLASTIC
Therapeutic: ANTINEOPLASTIC; HER2 ANTAGONIST
**Prototype:** Trastuzumab

**AVAILABILITY** Solution for injection

**ACTION & *THERAPEUTIC EFFECT***
Inhibits kinase-mediated intracellular signaling pathways by blocking HER2 receptors which results in cancer cell growth arrest and apoptosis; stimulates antibody-dependent cell-mediated cytotoxicity (ADCC) of cancer cells. *Inhibits proliferation of tumor cells with HER2 receptors.*

**USES** Indicated for the treatment of patients with HER2-positive metastatic breast cancer (with trastuzumab and docetaxel).

**CONTRAINDICATIONS** Hyersensitivity to pertuzumab; severe infusion reaction; clinical significant decrease in left ventricular function

Common adverse effects in *italic*; life-threatening effects underlined; generic names in **bold**; classifications in SMALL CAPS; ♣ Canadian drug name; ☺ Prototype drug due to drug; pregnancy (category D); lactation.

**CAUTIOUS USE** Hepatic impairment; severe renal impairment; prior use of anthracycline or radiation; uncontrolled hypertension; recent MI, serious cardiac arrhythmias; CHF. Safety and efficacy in children younger than 18 y not established.

## ROUTE & DOSAGE

### Metastatic Breast Cancer

*Adult:* IV Initial dose of 840 mg; follow q3wk with 420 mg in combination with trastuzumab and docetaxel. Withhold or discontinue if trastuzumab is withheld or discontinued.

### Dosing Interruption Due to Decreased Left Ventricular Ejection Fraction (LVEF)

*Decreased LVEF to less than 45% or LVEF between 45%–49% with a 10% or greater absolute decrease below pretreatment values:* Withhold pertuzumab and trastuzumab for at least 3 wk. *If the LVEF recovers to greater than 49% or to 45%–49% with less than 10% absolute decrease from baseline:* Resume pertuzumab therapy. *If the LVEF does not improve or declines further within approximately 3 wk:* Discontinue pertuzumab and trastuzumab.

## ADMINISTRATION

### Intravenous

This drug is a cytotoxic agent and caution should be used to prevent any contact with the drug. Follow institutional or standard guidelines for preparation, handling, and disposal of cytotoxic agents.

*PREPARE:* **IV Infusion:** Dilute required dose in 250 mL NS in a PVC or non-PVC polyolefin bag. Invert to mix but do not shake. Prepare just before use.
*ADMINISTER:* **IV Infusion:** Infuse initial dose of pertuzumab over 60 min; infuse subsequent doses of pertuzumab over 30–60 min. If trastuzumab is given concurrently with initial dose of pertuzumab, infuse trastuzumab over 90 min; give subsequent doses of trastuzumab over 30–90 min.
*INCOMPATIBILITIES:* **Solution/additive:** Do not mix with other drugs. Do not mix/dilute with dextrose (5%) solution. **Y-site:** Do not mix with other drugs.

▪ Observe closely during first 60 min after initial infusion and for 30 min after subsequent infusions. Slow or stop infusion for significant infusion-related reactions. Monitor vital signs and other parameters frequently until complete return to baseline. ▪ Store vials at 2°–8° C (36°–46° F). Store IV infusion refrigerated for up to 24 h.

## ADVERSE EFFECTS (≥10%) **Body as a Whole:** Hypersensitivity, increased lacrimation, mucosal inflammation, peripheral edema, pyrexia. **CNS:** Asthenia, dizziness, *fatigue*, headache, insomnia, *peripheral neuropathy*. **GI:** Constipation, decreased appetite, *diarrhea*, dyspepsia, dysgeusia, *nausea*, stomatitis, vomiting. **Hematological:** Anemia, febrile neutropenia, leukopenia, *neutropenia*. **Musculoskeletal:** Arthralgia, myalgia, weakness. **Respiratory:** Dyspnea, cough, nasopharyngitis, URI, epistaxis. **Skin:** Alopecia, dry skin, nail disorder, pruritus, *rash*. **Cardiac:** Decreased left ventricular ejection fraction.

## PHARMACOKINETICS **Half-Life:** 18 d.

Common adverse effects in *italic*; life-threatening effects <u>underlined</u>; generic names in **bold**; classifications in SMALL CAPS; ♣Canadian drug name; ◉ Prototype drug

1279

## NURSING IMPLICATIONS

### Black Box Warning

*Pertuzumab has been associated with a significant decrease in left ventricular function, and with fetal death and birth defects.*

### Assessment & Drug Effects

- Monitor vital signs and cardiac status closely during drug administration and for 60 min after initial infusion and 30 min after subsequent infusions.
- Assess frequently for infusion-related reactions. Slow or stop infusion for significant infusion-related reactions. Institute appropriate support therapies.
- Assess for and report S&S of peripheral neuropathy and infection.
- Monitor lab tests: Baseline and periodic CBC with differential.

### Patient & Family Education

- Report promptly S&S of infection.
- Use effective means of contraception during and for 6 mo following end of therapy.
- Report promptly to prescriber if you become pregnant.
- Do not breast-feed while taking this drug.
- Monitor weight daily and report greater than 2 lb weight gain in a day, swelling in the lower extremities, or shortness of breath.

## PHENAZOPYRIDINE HYDROCHLORIDE

(fen-az-oh-peer'i-deen)

Azo-Standard, Baridium, Geridium, Phenazo ✦, Phenazodine, Pyridiate, Pyridium, Pyronium ✦, Urodine, Urogesic

**Classification:** URINARY TRACT ANALGESIC

**Therapeutic:** URINARY TRACT ANALGESIC

**AVAILABILITY** Tablet

**ACTION & *THERAPEUTIC EFFECT***
Azo dye that has local anesthetic action on urinary tract mucosa, which imparts little or no antibacterial activity. *Effective as a urinary tract analgesic.*

**USES** Symptomatic relief of pain, burning, frequency, and urgency arising from irritation of urinary tract mucosa, as from infection, trauma, surgery, or instrumentation.

**CONTRAINDICATIONS** Renal insufficiency, renal disease including glomerulonephritis, pyelonephritis, renal failure, uremia; hepatic disease; glucose-6-phosphate dehydrogenase deficiency, severe hepatitis.

**CAUTIOUS USE** GI disturbances; older adults; pregnancy (category B); lactation; children.

### ROUTE & DOSAGE

#### Cystitis

*Adult:* **PO** 200 mg t.i.d.
*Child:* **PO** 12 mg/kg/day in 3 divided doses

### ADMINISTRATION

#### Oral
- Give with or after meals.

**ADVERSE EFFECTS** (≥1%) **Body as a Whole:** Headache, vertigo. **GI:** Mild GI disturbances. **Urogenital:** Kidney stones, transient acute kidney failure. **Metabolic:** Methemoglobinemia, hemolytic anemia. **Skin:** Skin pigmentation. **Special Senses:** May stain soft contact lenses.

**DIAGNOSTIC TEST INTERFERENCE**
Phenazopyridine may interfere with

Common adverse effects in *italic*; life-threatening effects underlined; generic names in **bold**; classifications in SMALL CAPS; ✦ Canadian drug name; ☻ Prototype drug any urinary test that is based on color reactions or spectrometry: **Bromsulphalein** and **phenolsulfonphthalein** excretion tests; urinary **glucose** test using **Clinistix** or **TesTape** (**copper-reduction methods** such as **Clinitest** and **Benedict's test** reportedly not affected); **bilirubin** using "foam test" or **Ictotest; ketones** using **nitroprusside** (e.g., **Acetest, Ketostix,** or **Gerhardt ferric chloride**); **urinary protein** using **Albustix, Albutest,** or **nitric acid ring test;** urinary **steroids; urobilinogen; assays** for **porphyrins.**

### PHARMACOKINETICS **Absorption:** Readily absorbed from GI tract. **Distribution:** Crosses placenta in trace amounts. **Metabolism:** In liver and other tissues. **Elimination:** Primarily in urine.

### NURSING IMPLICATIONS

#### Assessment & Drug Effects

▪ Monitor for therapeutic effectiveness as indicated by relief from pain and burning upon urination.

#### Patient & Family Education

▪ Drug will impart an orange to red color to urine and may stain clothing.

### PHENELZINE SULFATE ℗

(fen'el-zeen)

**Classifications:** ANTIDEPRESSANT; MONOAMINE OXIDASE (MAO) INHIBITOR

Therapeutic: ANTIDEPRESSANT; MAO INHIBITOR

### AVAILABILITY Tablet

### ACTION & *THERAPEUTIC EFFECT*

Antidepressant action believed to be due to irreversible inhibition of MAO, thereby permitting increased concentrations of endogenous epinephrine, norepinephrine, serotonin, and dopamine within presynaptic neurons and at receptor sites. *Antidepressant utilization is limited to individuals who do not respond well to other classes of antidepressants.*

### USES Atypical or nonendogenous depression.

### CONTRAINDICATIONS Hypersensitivity to MAO inhibitors; suicidal ideation; pheochromocytoma; untreated hyperthyroidism; cardiac arrhythmias, uncontrolled hypertension; increased intracranial pressure; intracranial bleeding; atonic colitis; glaucoma; frequent headaches; bipolar depression; accompanying alcoholism or drug addiction; paranoid schizophrenia; older adults or debilitated patients; lactation.

### CAUTIOUS USE Epilepsy, pyloric stenosis; DM; manic-depressive states; agitated patients; schizophrenia or psychosis; seizures; suicidal tendencies; chronic brain syndromes; pregnancy (category C); children and adolescents.

### ROUTE & DOSAGE

**Depression**
*Adult:* **PO** 15 mg t.i.d., rapidly increase to at least 60 mg/day, may need up to 90 mg/day

### ADMINISTRATION

#### Oral

▪ Avoid rapid discontinuation, particularly after high dosage, since a rebound effect may occur (e.g., headache, excitability, hallucinations, and possibly depression).
▪ Store in tightly covered containers away from heat and light.

### ADVERSE EFFECTS (≥1%) **Body as a Whole:** Dizziness or vertigo, headache, *orthostatic hypotension*, drowsiness

Common adverse effects in *italic*; life-threatening effects underlined; generic names in **bold**; classifications in SMALL CAPS; ✦ Canadian drug name; ℗ Prototype drug

1281

or *insomnia,* weakness, fatigue, edema, tremors, twitching, akathisia, ataxia, hyperreflexia, faintness, hyperactivity, marked agitation, anxiety, seizures, trismus, opisthotonos, <u>respiratory depression, coma</u>. **CNS:** Mania, hypomania, confusion, memory impairment, delirium, hallucinations, euphoria, acute anxiety reaction, toxic precipitation of schizophrenia, convulsions, peripheral neuropathy. **CV:** <u>Hypertensive crisis</u> (intense occipital headache, palpitation, marked hypertension, stiff neck, nausea, vomiting, sweating, fever, photophobia, dilated pupils, bradycardia or tachycardia, constricting chest pain, intracranial bleeding), hypotension or hypertension, <u>circulatory collapse</u>. **GI:** *Constipation, dry mouth, nausea,* vomiting, *anorexia,* weight gain. **Hematologic:** Normocytic and normochromic anemia, <u>leukopenia</u>. **Skin:** Hyperhidrosis, skin rash, photosensitivity. **Special Senses:** Blurred vision.

## DIAGNOSTIC TEST INTERFERENCE
Phenelzine may cause a slight false increase in ***serum bilirubin.***

## INTERACTIONS **Drug:** TRICYCLIC ANTIDEPRESSANTS may cause hyperpyrexia, seizures; **fluoxetine, sertraline, paroxetine** may cause serotonin syndrome (see Appendix F); SYMPATHOMIMETIC AGENTS (e.g., **amphetamine, phenylephrine, phenylpropanolamine**), **guanethidine** and **reserpine** may cause hypertensive crisis; CNS DEPRESSANTS have additive CNS depressive effects; OPIATE ANALGESICS (especially **meperidine**) may cause hypertensive crisis and circulatory collapse; **buspirone,** hypertension; GENERAL ANESTHETICS, prolonged hypotensive and CNS depressant effects; hypertension, headache, hyperexcitability reported with **dopamine, methyldopa,**

**levodopa, tryptophan; metrizamide** may increase risk of seizures; HYPOTENSIVE AGENTS and DIURETICS have additive hypotensive effects. **Food:** Aged meats or aged cheeses, protein extracts, sour cream, alcohol, anchovies, liver, sausages, overripe figs, bananas, avocados, chocolate, soy sauce, bean curd, natural yogurt, fava beans—**tyramine**-containing foods—may precipitate hypertensive crisis. Avoid **chocolate** or **caffeine.** Herbal: Ginseng, **ephedra, ma huang, St. John's wort** may cause hypertensive crisis.

## PHARMACOKINETICS **Absorption:** Readily absorbed from GI tract. **Onset:** 2 wk. **Metabolism:** Rapidly metabolized. **Elimination:** 79% of metabolites excreted in urine in 96 h.

## NURSING IMPLICATIONS

### Black Box Warning

*Phenelzine has been associated with increased risk of suicidal thinking and behavior (suicidality) in children, adolescents, and young adults.*

### Assessment & Drug Effects
- Monitor children, adolescents, and adults for changes in behavior that may indicate suicidality.
- Prior to initiation of treatment, evaluate patient's BP in standing and recumbent positions.
- Monitor BP and pulse between doses when titrating initial dosages. Observe closely for evidence of adverse drug effects. Thereafter, monitor at regular intervals throughout therapy.
- Report immediately if hypomania (exaggeration of motility, feelings, and ideas) occurs as depression improves. This reaction may also appear at higher than recommended doses or with long-term therapy.

P

- Observe for and report therapeutic effectiveness of drug: Improvement in sleep pattern, appetite, physical activity, interest in self and surroundings, as well as lessening of anxiety and bodily complaints.
- Observe patient with diabetes closely for S&S of hypoglycemia (see Appendix F).
- Patients on prolonged therapy should be checked periodically for altered color perception, changes in fundi or visual fields. Changes in red-green vision may be the first indication of eye damage.

### Patient & Family Education
- Maximum antidepressant effects generally appear in 2–6 wk and persist several weeks after drug withdrawal.
- Avoid self-medication. OTC preparations (e.g., cough, cold, hay fever remedies, and appetite suppressants) can precipitate severe hypertensive reactions if taken during therapy or within 2–3 wk after discontinuation of an MAO inhibitor.
- Report immediately to prescriber the onset of headache and palpitation, or any other unusual effects which may indicate need to discontinue therapy.
- Do not consume foods and beverages containing tyramine or tryptophan or drugs containing pressor agent. These can cause severe hypertensive reactions. Get a list from your care provider.
- Avoid drinking excessive caffeine and chocolate beverages (e.g., coffee, tea, cocoa, or cola).
- Make position changes slowly, especially from recumbent to upright posture, and dangle legs over bed a few minutes before rising to walk. Avoid standing still for prolonged periods. Also avoid hot showers and baths

(resulting vasodilatation may potentiate hypotension); lie down immediately if feeling light-headed or faint.
- Check weight 2 or 3 × wk and report unusual gain.
- Report jaundice. Hepatotoxicity is believed to be a hypersensitivity reaction unrelated to dosage or duration of therapy.

## PHENOBARBITAL ℗ℛ
(fee-noe-bar′bi-tal)
Solfoton

## PHENOBARBITAL SODIUM
Luminal

**Classifications:** ANTICONVULSANT; SEDATIVE-HYPNOTIC; BARBITURATE
**Therapeutic:** ANTICONVULSANT; SEDATIVE-HYPNOTIC
**Controlled Substance:** Schedule IV

**AVAILABILITY**  Tablet; capsule; liquid; solution for injection

### ACTION & *THERAPEUTIC EFFECT*
Sedative and hypnotic effects appear to be due primarily to interference with impulse transmission of cerebral cortex by inhibition of reticular activating system. Limiting spread of seizure activity results by increasing the threshold for motor cortex stimulation. *Effective as a sedative, hypnotic, and an anticonvulsant with no analgesic effect.*

**USES**  Long-term management of tonic-clonic (grand mal) seizures and partial seizures; status epilepticus, eclampsia, febrile convulsions in young children. Also used as a sedative in anxiety or tension states; in pediatrics as preoperative and postoperative sedation and to treat pylorospasm in infants.

**UNLABELED USES**  Treatment and prevention of hyperbilirubinemia

Common adverse effects in *italic*; life-threatening effects underlined; generic names in **bold**; classifications in SMALL CAPS; ✦Canadian drug name; ℗ℛ Prototype drug

1283

in neonates and in the management of chronic cholestasis; benzodiazepine withdrawal.

**CONTRAINDICATIONS** Hypersensitivity to barbiturates; manifest hepatic or familial history of porphyria; severe respiratory or kidney disease; history of previous addiction to sedative hypnotics; alcohol intoxication; uncontrolled pain; renal failure, anuria; pregnancy (category D).

**CAUTIOUS USE** Impaired liver, kidney, cardiac, or respiratory function; sleep apnea; COPD; history of allergies; patients with fever; hyperthyroidism; diabetes mellitus or severe anemia; seizure disorders; during labor and delivery; patient with borderline hypoadrenal function; older adult or debilitated patients; lactation; young children and neonates.

## ROUTE & DOSAGE

### Anticonvulsant

*Adult:* **PO/IV** 1–3 mg/kg/day in divided doses
*Child:* **PO/IV** 4–8 mg/kg/day in divided doses

### Status Epilepticus

*Adult:* **IV** 300–800 mg, then 120–240 mg q20min (total max: 1–2 g)
*Child:* **IV** 10–20 mg/kg in single or divided doses, then 5 mg/kg/dose q15–30min (total max: 40 mg/kg)
*Neonate:* **IV** 15–20 mg/kg in single or divided doses

### Sedative/Hypnotic

*Adult:* **PO** 30–120 mg/day; **IV/IM** 100–320 mg/day
*Child:* **PO** 2 mg/kg/day in 3 divided doses **IV/IM** 3–5 mg/kg

### Renal Impairment Dosage Adjustment

*CrCl less than 10 mL/min:* Dose q12–16h

### Hemodialysis Dosage Adjustment
20–50% dialyzed

## ADMINISTRATION

### Oral
- Give crushed and mixed with a fluid or with food if patient cannot swallow pill. Do not permit patient to swallow dry crushed drug.

### Intramuscular
- Give IM deep into large muscle mass; do not exceed 5 mL at any one site.

### Intravenous
Note: Verify correct IV concentration and rate of infusion for neonates, infants, children with prescriber. Use IV route ONLY if other routes are not feasible.

*PREPARE:* **Direct:** May be given undiluted or diluted in 10 mL of sterile water for injection.

*ADMINISTER:* **Direct:** Give no faster than 60 mg/min in adults and 30 mg/min in children. Give within 30 min after preparation.

*INCOMPATIBILITIES:* Solution/additive: **Ampicillin, cephalothin, chlorpromazine, cimetidine, clindamycin, dexamethasone, diphenhydramine, erythromycin, ephedrine, hydralazine, hydrocortisone sodium succinate, hydroxyzine, insulin, kanamycin, levorphanol, meperidine, methadone, methylphenidate, morphine, nitrofurantoin, norepinephrine, pentazocine, pentobarbital, phytonadione, procaine, prochlorperazine, promazine, promethazine, sodium bicarbonate, streptomycin,** TETRACYCLINES,

**vancomycin, warfarin. Y-site: Amphotericin B cholesteryl complex, hydromorphone, TPN with albumin.**

▪ Be aware that extravasation of IV phenobarbital may cause necrotic tissue changes that necessitate skin grafting. Check injection site frequently.

## ADVERSE EFFECTS (≥1%) **Body as a Whole:** Myalgia, neuralgia, <u>CNS depression, coma, and death</u>. **CNS:** *Somnolence,* nightmares, insomnia, "hangover," headache, anxiety, thinking abnormalities, dizziness, nystagmus, irritability, paradoxic excitement and exacerbation of hyperkinetic behavior (in children); confusion or depression or marked excitement (older adult or debilitated patients); ataxia. **CV:** Bradycardia, syncope, hypotension. **GI:** Nausea, vomiting, constipation, diarrhea, epigastric pain, liver damage. **Hematologic:** Megaloblastic anemia, <u>agranulocytosis</u>, <u>thrombocytopenia</u>. **Metabolic:** Hypocalcemia, osteomalacia, rickets. **Musculoskeletal:** Folic acid deficiency, vitamin D deficiency. **Respiratory:** <u>Respiratory depression</u>. **Skin:** Mild maculopapular, morbilliform rash; erythema multiforme, <u>Stevens–Johnson syndrome</u>, <u>exfoliative dermatitis (rare)</u>.

## DIAGNOSTIC TEST INTERFERENCE

BARBITURATES may affect ***bromsulphalein*** retention tests (by enhancing liver uptake and excretion of dye) and increase ***serum phosphatase.***

## INTERACTIONS **Drug: Alcohol,** CNS DEPRESSANTS compound CNS depression; phenobarbital may decrease absorption and increase metabolism of ORAL ANTICOAGULANTS; increases metabolism of CORTICOSTEROIDS, ORAL CONTRACEPTIVES, ANTICONVULSANTS, **digitoxin,** possibly

decreasing their effects; ANTIDEPRESSANTS potentiate adverse effects of phenobarbital; **griseofulvin** decreases absorption of phenobarbital; **quinine** increases plasma levels. **Herbal: Kava, valerian** may potentiate sedation.

## PHARMACOKINETICS **Absorption:** 70–90% slowly from GI tract. **Peak:** 8–12 h PO; 30 min IV. **Duration:** 4–6 h IV. **Distribution:** 20–45% protein bound; crosses placenta; enters breast milk. **Metabolism:** In liver (CYP2C19). **Elimination:** In urine. **Half-Life:** 2–6 days.

## NURSING IMPLICATIONS
### Assessment & Drug Effects
▪ Observe patients receiving large doses for at least 30 min to ensure that sedation is not excessive.
▪ Chronic use in children or infants requires continuous assessment related to normal cognitive and behavioral functioning.
▪ Keep patient under constant observation when drug is administered IV, and record vital signs at least every hour or more often if indicated.
▪ Check IV injection site very frequently to prevent extravasation of phenobarbital. It could result in tissue damage requiring skin grafting.
▪ Monitor serum drug levels. Serum concentrations greater than 50 mcg/mL may cause coma. Therapeutic serum concentrations of 15–40 mcg/mL produce anticonvulsant activity in most patients. These values are usually attained after 2 or 3 wk of therapy with a dose of 100–200 mg/day.
▪ Expect barbiturates to produce restlessness when given to patients in pain because these drugs do not have analgesic action.

P

---

Common adverse effects in *italic*; life-threatening effects <u>underlined</u>; generic names in **bold**; classifications in SMALL CAPS; ♣ Canadian drug name; ⊕ Prototype drug

- Be prepared for paradoxical responses and report promptly in older adult or debilitated patient and children [i.e., irritability, marked excitement (inappropriate tearfulness and aggression in children), depression, and confusion].
- Monitor for drug interactions. Barbiturates increase the metabolism of many drugs, leading to decreased pharmacologic effects of those drugs.
- Monitor for and report chronic toxicity symptoms (e.g., ataxia, slurred speech, irritability, poor judgment, slight dysarthria, nystagmus on vertical gaze, confusion, insomnia, somatic complaints).
- Monitor lab tests: Periodic LFTs, CBC with differential, Hct and Hgb, and renal function tests.

### Patient & Family Education

- Be aware that anticonvulsant therapy may cause drowsiness during first few weeks of treatment, but this usually diminishes with continued use.
- Avoid potentially hazardous activities requiring mental alertness until response to drug is known.
- Do not consume alcohol in any amount when taking a barbiturate; it may severely impair judgment and abilities.
- Increase vitamin D-fortified foods (e.g., milk products) because drug increases vitamin D metabolism. A vitamin D supplement may be prescribed.
- Maintain adequate dietary folate intake: Fresh vegetables (especially green leafy), fresh fruits, whole grains, liver. Long-term therapy may result in nutritional folate ($B_9$) deficiency. A supplement of folic acid may be prescribed.
- Adhere to drug regimen (i.e., do not change intervals between doses or

increase or decrease doses) without contacting prescriber.
- Do not stop taking drug abruptly because of danger of withdrawal symptoms (8–12 h after last dose), which can be fatal.
- Report to prescriber the onset of fever, sore throat or mouth, malaise, easy bruising or bleeding, petechiae, jaundice, rash when on prolonged therapy.
- Avoid pregnancy when receiving barbiturates. Use or add barrier device to hormonal contraceptive when taking prolonged therapy.

## PHENTERMINE HYDROCHLORIDE
(phen-ter'meen)

Adipex-P, Lomaira

**Classification:** ANOREXIANT
Therapeutic: APPETITE SUPPRESSANT
**Prototype:** Diethylpropion
**Controlled Substance:** Schedule IV

**AVAILABILITY** Tablet; capsule

## ACTION & *THERAPEUTIC EFFECT*
Sympathetic amine with actions that include CNS stimulation and blood pressure elevation. *Appetite suppression or metabolic effects along with diet adjustment result in weight loss in obese individuals.*

**USES** Short-term (8–12 wk) adjunct for weight loss.

**CONTRAINDICATIONS** Known hypersensitivity to sympathetic amines; glaucoma; moderate to severe uncontrolled hypertension, advanced arteriosclerosis, cardiovascular disease, cardiac arrhythmias, stroke; hyperthyroidism; agitated states; history of drug abuse; during or within 14 days of administration of MAO inhibitor; glaucoma; pregnancy (category X); lactation.

Common adverse effects in *italic*; life-threatening effects <u>underlined</u>; generic names in **bold**; classifications in SMALL CAPS; ✦ Canadian drug name; ❷ Prototype drug

**CAUTIOUS USE** Hypertension, DM; seizures; renal impairment; older adults; children younger than 16 y.

## ROUTE & DOSAGE

**Obesity**

*Adult/Adolescent:* **PO** 15–37.5 mg each morning; 8 mg t.i.d. (Lomaira)

## ADMINISTRATION

### Oral

- Ensure that at least 14 days have elapsed between the first dose of phentermine and the last dose of an MAO inhibitor.
- Give 30 min before meals.
- Do not administer if an SSRI is currently prescribed.
- Store in a tight container.

## ADVERSE EFFECTS (≥1%) **Body as a Whole:** Hypersensitivity (urticaria, rash, erythema, burning sensation), chest pain, excessive sweating, clamminess, chills, flushing, fever, myalgia. **CV:** Palpitations, tachycardia, arrhythmias, hypertension or hypotension, syncope, precordial pain, pulmonary hypertension. **GI:** Dry mouth, altered taste, nausea, vomiting, abdominal pain, diarrhea, constipation, stomach pain. **Endocrine:** Gynecomastia. **Hematologic:** Bone marrow suppression, agranulocytosis, leukopenia. **Musculoskeletal:** Muscle pain. **CNS:** Overstimulation, nervousness, restlessness, dizziness, insomnia, weakness, fatigue, malaise, anxiety, euphoria, drowsiness, depression, agitation, dysphoria, tremor, dyskinesia, dysarthria, confusion, incoordination, headache, change in libido. **Skin:** Hair loss, ecchymosis. **Special Senses:** Mydriasis, blurred vision. **Urogenital:** Dysuria, polyuria, urinary frequency, impotence, menstrual upset.

**INTERACTIONS Drug:** MAO INHIBITORS, **furazolidone** may increase pressor response resulting in hypertensive crisis. TRICYCLIC ANTIDEPRESSANTS may decrease anorectic response. May decrease hypotensive effects of **guanethidine.**

**PHARMACOKINETICS Absorption:** Absorbed from the small intestine. **Duration:** 4–14 h. **Elimination:** Primarily in urine. **Half-Life:** 19–24 h.

## NURSING IMPLICATIONS

### Assessment & Drug Effects

- Assess for tolerance to the anorectic effect of the drug. Withhold drug and report to prescriber when this occurs.
- Monitor periodic cardiovascular status, including BP, exercise tolerance, peripheral edema.
- Monitor weight at least 3 × wk.

### Patient & Family Education

- Do not take this drug late in the evening because it could cause insomnia.
- Report immediately any of the following: Shortness of breath, chest pains, dizziness or fainting, swelling of the extremities.
- Tolerance to the appetite suppression effects of the drug usually develops in a few weeks. Notify prescriber, but do not increase the drug dose.
- Weigh yourself at least 3 × wk at the same time of day with the same amount of clothing.

## PHENTOLAMINE MESYLATE

(fen-tole′a-meen)

Regitine

**Classifications:** ALPHA-ADRENERGIC RECEPTOR ANTAGONIST; VASODILATOR

**Therapeutic:** VASODILATOR; ANTIHYPERTENSIVE

**Prototype:** Prazosin

---

Common adverse effects in *italic*; life-threatening effects underlined; generic names in **bold**; classifications in SMALL CAPS; ♣ Canadian drug name; ⬤ Prototype drug

**AVAILABILITY** Solution for injection

**ACTION & *THERAPEUTIC EFFECT***
Alpha-adrenergic blocking agent that competitively blocks alpha-adrenergic receptors, but action is transient and incomplete. Causes vasodilation and decreases general vascular resistance as well as pulmonary arterial pressure, primarily by direct action on vascular smooth muscle. *Prevents hypertension resulting from elevated levels of circulating epinephrine or norepinephrine.*

**USES** Diagnosis of pheochromocytoma and to prevent or control hypertensive episodes prior to or during pheochromocytomectomy.

**UNLABELED USES** Prevention of dermal necrosis and sloughing following IV administration or extravasation of norepinephrine.

**CONTRAINDICATIONS** Hypersensitivity to phentolamine; MI (previous or present), CAD; peptic ulcer disease.

**CAUTIOUS USE** Gastritis; pregnancy (category C); lactation; children.

**ROUTE & DOSAGE**

**To Test for Pheochromocytoma**
*Adult:* **IV/IM** 5 mg
*Child:* **IV/IM** 0.05–0.1 mg/kg (max: 5 mg)

**To Treat Extravasation**
*Adult:* **Intradermal** 5–10 mg diluted in 10 mL of normal saline injected into affected area within 12 h of extravasation
*Child:* **Intradermal** 0.1–0.2 mg/kg diluted with normal saline injected into affected area within 12 h of extravasation

**ADMINISTRATION**
Note: Place patient in supine position when receiving drug parenterally. ▪ Monitor BP and pulse q2min until stabilized.

**Intradermal**
▪ Reconstitute 5 mg vial with 1 mL of sterile water for injection, then further dilute in 10–15 mL NS.

**Intramuscular**
▪ Reconstitute 5 mg vial with 1 mL of sterile water for injection.

**Intravenous**
***PREPARE:* Direct:** Reconstitute as for IM. May be further diluted with up to 10 mL of sterile water. ▪ Use immediately.
***ADMINISTER:* Direct:** Give a single dose over 60 sec.

**ADVERSE EFFECTS** (≥1%) **Body as a Whole:** Weakness, dizziness, flushing, *orthostatic hypotension.* **GI:** *Abdominal pain, nausea, vomiting, diarrhea, exacerbation of peptic ulcer.* **CV:** *Acute and prolonged hypotension, tachycardia, anginal pain,* cardiac arrhythmias, MI, cerebrovascular spasm, shock-like state. **Special Senses:** Nasal stuffiness, conjunctival infection.

**INTERACTIONS Drug:** May antagonize BP raising effects of **epinephrine, ephedrine.**

**PHARMACOKINETICS Peak:** 2 min IV; 15–20 min IM. **Duration:** 10–15 min IV; 3–4 h IM. **Elimination:** In urine. **Half-Life:** 19 min.

**NURSING IMPLICATIONS**
**Assessment & Drug Effects**
***Test for pheochromocytoma:***
▪ *IV administration:* Keep patient at rest in supine position throughout test, preferably in quiet darkened

room. ▪ Prior to drug administration, take BP q10min for at least 30 min to establish that BP has stabilized before IV injection. ▪ Record BP immediately after injection and at 30-sec intervals for first 3 min; then at 1-min intervals for next 7 min.

▪ *IM administration:* Post-injection, BP determinations at 5-min intervals for 30–45 min.

#### Patient & Family Education
▪ Avoid sudden changes in position, particularly from reclining to upright posture and dangle legs and exercise ankles and toes for a few minutes before standing to walk.
▪ Lie down or sit down in head-low position immediately if light-headed or dizzy.

## PHENYLEPHRINE HYDROCHLORIDE
(fen-ill-ef'rin)

AK-Dilate Ophthalmic, Alconefrin, Isopto Frin, Mydfrin, Nostril, Rhinall, Sinarest Nasal, Sinex

**Classifications:** EYE AND NOSE PREPARATION; ALPHA-ADRENERGIC AGONIST; MYDRIATIC; VASOPRESSOR; DECONGESTANT
Therapeutic: VASOCONSTRICTOR; DECONGESTANT; MYDRIATIC
**Prototype:** Dexmedetomide

**AVAILABILITY** Tablet; nasal solution; ophthalmic solution; solution for injection; suppository

#### ACTION & *THERAPEUTIC EFFECT*
Potent, synthetic, direct-acting sympathomimetic with strong alpha-adrenergic cardiac stimulant actions. Elevates systolic and diastolic pressures through arteriolar constriction. Reduces intraocular

pressure by increasing outflow and decreasing rate of aqueous humor secretion. *Effective antihypotensive agent. Topical applications to eye produce vasoconstriction and prompt mydriasis of short duration, usually without causing cycloplegia. Nasal decongestant action qualitatively similar to that of epinephrine but more potent.*

**USES** Parenterally to maintain BP during anesthesia, to treat vascular failure in shock, and to overcome paroxysmal supraventricular tachycardia. Used topically for rhinitis of common cold, allergic rhinitis, and sinusitis; in selected patients with wide-angle glaucoma; as mydriatic for ophthalmoscopic examination or surgery, and for relief of uveitis.

**CONTRAINDICATIONS** Severe CAD, severe hypertension, atrial fibrillation, atrial flutter, cardiac arrhythmias; severe organic cardiac disease, cardiomyopathy; uncontrolled hypertension; ventricular fibrillation or tachycardia; acute MI, angina, thyrotoxicosis; cerebral arteriosclerosis, MAOI; labor, delivery, infants, neonates. **Ophthalmic preparations:** Narrow-angle glaucoma.

**CAUTIOUS USE** Hyperthyroidism; DM; heart failure; thyroid disease; BPH; 21 days before or following termination of MAO inhibitor therapy; older adults; pregnancy (category C); children younger than 6 y. **Ophthalmic:** Lactation.

### ROUTE & DOSAGE

| Hypotension |
| --- |
| *Adult:* **IM/Subcutaneous** 2–5 mg (initial dose not to exceed 5 mg) q10–15min as needed; **IV** 0.2 mg (range: 0.1–0.5 mg) every 10–15 min as needed |

Common adverse effects in *italic*; life-threatening effects underlined; generic names in **bold**; classifications in SMALL CAPS; ♣Canadian drug name; ⊕ Prototype drug

1289

**Supraventricular Tachycardia**

*Adult:* IV 0.25–0.5 mg bolus, then 0.1–0.2 mg doses (total max: 1 mg)

**Vasoconstrictor**

*Adult:* **Ophthalmic** See Appendix A-1; **Intranasal** 2–3 drops or sprays of 0.25–0.5% solution q3–4h as needed

*Child (6–12 y):* **Intranasal** 2–3 drops or sprays of 0.25% solution q3–4h as needed

## ADMINISTRATION

### Instillation

- Nasal preparations: Instruct patient to blow nose gently (with both nostrils open) to clear nasal passages before administration of medication.
- Instillation (drops): Tilt head back while sitting or standing up, or lie on bed and hang head over side. Stay in position a few minutes to permit medication to spread through nose. (Spray): With head upright, squeeze bottle quickly and firmly to produce 1 or 2 sprays into each nostril; wait 3–5 min, blow nose, and repeat dose. (Jelly): Place in each nostril and sniff it well back into nose.
- Clean tips and droppers of nasal solution dispensers with hot water after use to prevent contamination of solution. Droppers of ophthalmic solution bottles should not touch any surface including the eye.
- Ophthalmic preparations: To avoid excessive systemic absorption, apply pressure to lacrimal sac during and for 1–2 min after instillation of drops.

### Subcutaneous/Intramuscular

- Give undiluted.

### Intravenous

Note: Ensure patency of IV site prior to administration.

*PREPARE:* **Direct:** Dilute each 10 mg (1 mL) of 1% solution in 9 mL of sterile water. **IV Infusion:** Dilute each 10 mg in 500 mL D5W or NS (concentration: 0.02 mg/mL).

*ADMINISTER:* **Direct:** Give a single dose over 30 sec. **IV Infusion:** Titrate to maintain BP.

*INCOMPATIBILITIES:* **Y-site: Acyclovir, amphotericin B (conventional and lipid), azathioprine, dantrolene, diazepam, diazoxide, ganciclovir, indomethacin, insulin, lansoprazole, minocycline, mitomycin, pentamidine, phenytoin, SMZ/TMP, propofol.**

- Protect from exposure to air, strong light, or heat, any of which can cause solutions to change color to brown, form a precipitate, and lose potency.

## ADVERSE EFFECTS (≥1%) **Special Senses:** *Transient stinging,* lacrimation, brow ache, headache, blurred vision, allergy (pigmentary deposits on lids, conjunctiva, and cornea with prolonged use), increased sensitivity to light. *Rebound nasal congestion* (hyperemia and edema of mucosa), *nasal burning,* stinging, dryness, *sneezing.* **CV:** Palpitation, tachycardia, bradycardia (overdosage), arrhythmia, hypertension. **GI:** Nausea. **Body as a Whole:** Trembling, sweating, pallor, sense of fullness in head, tingling of extremities, sleeplessness, dizziness, light-headedness, weakness, restlessness, anxiety, precordial pain, *tremor,* severe visceral or peripheral vasoconstriction, necrosis if IV infiltrates.

## INTERACTIONS Drug: ERGOT ALKA-LOIDS, **guanethidine, reserpine,** TRICYCLIC ANTIDEPRESSANTS increase pressor effects of phenylephrine; **halothane, digoxin** increase risk of arrhythmias; MAO INHIBITORS cause hypertensive crisis; **oxytocin** causes persistent hypertension;

P

ALPHA-BLOCKERS, BETA-BLOCKERS antagonize effects of phenylephrine.

## PHARMACOKINETICS    Onset:
Immediate IV; 10–15 min IM/Subcutaneous. **Duration:** 15–20 min IV; 30–120 min IM/Subcutaneous; 3–6 h topical. **Metabolism:** In liver and tissues by monoamine oxidase.

## NURSING IMPLICATIONS
### Assessment & Drug Effects
- Monitor infusion site closely as extravasation may cause tissue necrosis and gangrene. If extravasation does occur, area should be immediately injected with 5–10 mg of phentolamine (Regitine) diluted in 10–15 mL of NS.
- Monitor pulse, BP, and central venous pressure (q2–5min) during IV administration.
- Control flow rate and dosage to prevent excessive dosage. IV overdoses can induce ventricular dysrhythmias.
- Observe for congestion or rebound miosis after topical administration to eye.

### Patient & Family Education
- Be aware that instillation of 2.5–10% strength ophthalmic solution can cause burning and stinging.
- Do not exceed recommended dosage regardless of formulation.
- Inform the prescriber if no relief is experienced from preparation in 5 days.
- Wear sunglasses in bright light because after instillation of ophthalmic drops, pupils will be large and eyes may be more sensitive to light than usual. Stop medication and notify prescriber if sensitivity persists beyond 12 h after drug has been discontinued.
- Be aware that some ophthalmic solutions may stain contact lenses.

## PHENYTOIN ⓟ
(fen′i-toy-in)
Dilantin-125, Dilantin

## PHENYTOIN SODIUM EXTENDED
Dilantin, Phentek

## PHENYTOIN SODIUM PROMPT
Dilantin

**Classifications:** ANTICONVULSANT; HYDANTOIN
**Therapeutic:** ANTICONVULSANT

**AVAILABILITY** Capsule; sustained release capsule; chewable tablet; suspension; solution for injection

### ACTION & *THERAPEUTIC EFFECT*
Anticonvulsant action elevates the seizure threshold and/or limits the spread of seizure discharge. Phenytoin is accompanied by reduced voltage, frequency, and spread of electrical discharges within the motor cortex. *Inhibits seizure activity. Effective in treating arrhythmias associated with QT prolongation.*

**USES** To control tonic-clonic (grand mal) and complex partial seizures; treatment of status epilepticus; seizure prophylaxis due to specific neurologic conditions.

**UNLABELED USES** Treatment of trigeminal neuralgia (tic douloureux).

**CONTRAINDICATIONS** Hypersensitivity to hydantoin products; rash; seizures due to hypoglycemia; sinus bradycardia, complete or incomplete heart block; Adams-Stokes syndrome; pregnancy (category D).

**CAUTIOUS USE** Impaired liver or kidney function; alcoholism; blood dyscrasias; hypotension, severe myocardial insufficiency, impending or frank heart failure; pancreatic

P

adenoma; DM, hyperglycemia; respiratory depression; acute intermittent porphyria; older adult, debilitated, or gravely ill patients.

## ROUTE & DOSAGE

### Status Epilepticus

*Adult:* **IV** 15-20 mg/kg *Adolescent/Child/Infant:* **IV** 20 mg/kg
*Neonate:* **IV** 15–20 mg/kg

### Maintenance Dose of Tonic/Clonic or Partial Seizure

*Adult:* **PO/IV** 4-7 mg/kg/day
*Adolescent/Child:* **PO/IV** 5 mg/kg/day in divided doses (max: 300 mg/day)
*Infant/Neonate:* **PO/IV** 4-8 mg/kg/day divided into 2-3 doses/day

## ADMINISTRATION

### Oral

- Ensure that sustained release form is not chewed or crushed. **Must be** swallowed whole.
- Do not give within 2–3 h of antacid ingestion.
- Shake suspension vigorously before pouring to ensure uniform distribution of drug.
- Note: Chewable tablets are not intended for once-a-day dosage since drug is too quickly bioavailable and can therefore lead to toxic serum levels.
- Use sustained release capsules ONLY for once-a-day dosage regimens.

### Intravenous

Note: Verify correct rate of IV injection for administration to infants or children with prescriber.
- Inspect solution prior to use. May use a slightly yellowed injectable solution safely. Precipitation may be caused by refrigeration, but slow warming to room temperature restores clarity.

*PREPARE:* **Direct:** Give undiluted. Use only when clear without precipitate.

*ADMINISTER:* **Direct for Adult** Give 50 mg or fraction thereof over 1 min (25 mg/min in older adult or when used as antiarrhythmic). **Do not** give more rapidly. ▪ Follow with an injection of sterile saline through the same in-place catheter or needle. **Do not** use solutions containing dextrose.

**Direct for Child/Neonate:** Give 1 mg/kg/min. **Do not** give more rapidly. ▪ Follow with an injection of sterile saline through the same in-place catheter or needle. **Do not** use solutions containing dextrose.

*INCOMPATIBILITIES:* Solution/additive: **Do not administer with other medications.** Y-site: **Do not administer with other medications.**
- Observe injection site frequently during administration to prevent infiltration. Local soft tissue irritation may be serious, leading to erosion of tissues.

## ADVERSE EFFECTS (≥1%) CNS:
Usually dose-related: Nystagmus, *drowsiness,* ataxia, dizziness, mental confusion, tremors, insomnia, headache, seizures. **CV:** Bradycardia, hypotension, cardiovascular collapse, ventricular fibrillation, phlebitis. **Special Senses:** Photophobia, conjunctivitis, diplopia, blurred vision. **GI:** *Gingival hyperplasia,* nausea, vomiting, constipation, epigastric pain, dysphagia, loss of taste, weight loss, hepatitis, liver necrosis. **Hematologic:** *Thrombocytopenia, leukopenia,* leukocytosis, agranulocytosis, pancytopenia, eosinophilia; megaloblastic, hemolytic, or aplastic anemias. **Metabolic:** Fever, hyperglycemia, glycosuria, weight gain, edema, transient increase in serum thyrotropic (TSH) level, osteomalacia or

rickets associated with hypocalcemia and elevated alkaline phosphatase activity. **Skin:** Alopecia, hirsutism (especially in young female); rash: scarlatiniform, maculopapular, urticaria, morbilliform; <u>bullous, exfoliative, or purpuric dermatitis; Stevens–Johnson syndrome, toxic epidermal necrolysis,</u> keratosis, neonatal hemorrhage. **Urogenital:** Acute renal failure, Peyronie's disease. **Respiratory:** Acute pneumonitis, pulmonary fibrosis. **Body as a Whole:** Periarteritis nodosum, acute systemic lupus erythematosus, craniofacial abnormalities (with enlargement of lips); lymphadenopathy.

## DIAGNOSTIC TEST INTERFERENCE

Phenytoin (HYDANTOINS) may produce lower than normal values for *dexamethasone* or *metyrapone* tests; may increase serum levels of *glucose, BSP,* and *alkaline phosphatase* and may decrease *PBI* and *urinary steroid* levels.

## INTERACTIONS

**Drug: Alcohol** decreases phenytoin effects; OTHER ANTICONVULSANTS may increase or decrease phenytoin levels; phenytoin may decrease absorption and increase metabolism of ORAL ANTICOAGULANTS; phenytoin increases metabolism of CORTICOSTEROIDS, ORAL CONTRACEPTIVES, and **nisoldipine,** decreasing their effectiveness; **amiodarone, chloramphenicol, omeprazole,** and **ticlopidine** increase phenytoin levels; ANTITUBERCULOSIS AGENTS decrease phenytoin levels. Closely monitor if used with ANTIRETROVIRALS. **Food: Folic acid, calcium,** and **vitamin D** absorption may be decreased by phenytoin; phenytoin absorption may be decreased by enteral nutrition supplements. **Herbal: Ginkgo** may decrease anticonvulsant effectiveness.

## PHARMACOKINETICS

**Absorption:** Completely from GI tract. **Peak:** 1.5–3 h prompt release; 4–12 h sustained release. **Distribution:** 95% protein bound; crosses placenta; small amount in breast milk. **Metabolism:** Oxidized in liver to inactive metabolites. **Elimination:** By kidneys. **Half-Life:** 22 h.

## NURSING IMPLICATIONS

### Black Box Warning

*Phenytoin has been associated with severe adverse cardiovascular effects when administered too rapidly.*

### Assessment & Drug Effects

- Monitor infusion site closely as extravasation may cause tissue necrosis.
- Continuously monitor vital signs and symptoms during IV infusion and for an hour afterward. Watch for respiratory depression. Constant observation and a cardiac monitor are necessary with older adults or patients with cardiac disease. Margin between toxic and therapeutic IV doses is relatively small.
- Be aware of therapeutic serum concentration: 10–20 mcg/mL; toxic level: 30–50 mcg/mL; lethal level: 100 mcg/mL. Steady-state therapeutic levels are not achieved for at least 7–10 days.
- Observe patient closely for neurologic adverse effects following IV administration.
- Monitor for gingival hyperplasia, which appears most commonly in children and adolescents and never occurs in patients without teeth.
- Make sure patients on prolonged therapy have adequate intake of vitamin D-containing foods and sufficient exposure to sunlight.

Common adverse effects in *italic*; life-threatening effects <u>underlined</u>; generic names in **bold**; classifications in SMALL CAPS; ♦Canadian drug name; ⊘ Prototype drug

1293

- Monitor diabetics for loss of glycemic control.
- Monitor for S&S of hypocalcemia (see Appendix F), especially in patients receiving other anticonvulsants concurrently, as well as those who are inactive, have limited exposure to sun, or whose dietary intake is inadequate.
- Observe for symptoms of folic acid deficiency: Neuropathy, mental dysfunction.
- Be alert to symptoms of hypomagnesemia (see Appendix F); neuromuscular symptoms: Tetany, positive Chvostek's and Trousseau's signs, seizures, tremors, ataxia, vertigo, nystagmus, muscular fasciculations.
- Monitor lab tests: Periodic serum phenytoin concentration.

### Patient & Family Education
- Be aware that drug may make urine pink or red to red-brown.
- Report symptoms of fatigue, dry skin, deepening voice when receiving long-term therapy because phenytoin can unmask a low thyroid reserve.
- Do not alter prescribed drug regimen. Stopping drug abruptly may precipitate seizures and status epilepticus.
- Do not request/accept change in drug brand when refilling prescription without consulting prescriber.
- Understand the effects of alcohol: Alcohol intake may increase phenytoin serum levels, leading to phenytoin toxicity.
- Discontinue drug immediately if a measles-like skin rash or jaundice appears and notify prescriber.
- Be aware that influenza vaccine during phenytoin treatment may increase seizure activity. Consult prescriber.

# PHYSOSTIGMINE SALICYLATE
(fi-zoe-stig'meen)

**Classification:** CHOLINESTERASE INHIBITOR
**Therapeutic:** ANTICHOLINERGIC ANTIDOTE, CHOLINESTERASE INHIBITOR
**Prototype:** Neostigmine

## AVAILABILITY Solution for injection

## ACTION & THERAPEUTIC EFFECT
Inhibits the destructive action of acetylcholinesterase and thereby prolongs and exaggerates the effect of the acetylcholine on the skeletal muscle, GI tract and within the CNS. *Effective in reversing anticholinergic toxicity.*

## USES To reverse anticholinergic toxicity.

## CONTRAINDICATIONS Asthma; DM; gangrene, cardiovascular disease; mechanical obstruction of intestinal or urogenital tract; peptic ulcer disease; asthma; any vagotonic state; closed-angle glaucoma; secondary glaucoma; inflammatory disease of iris or ciliary body; lactation.

## CAUTIOUS USE Epilepsy; parkinsonism; bradycardia; hyperthyroidism; seizure disorders; hypotension; pregnancy (category C); children.

## ROUTE & DOSAGE

### Reversal of Anticholinergic Effects
*Adult:* **IM/IV** 0.5–2 mg (IV not faster than 1 mg/min), repeat as needed
*Child:* **IV** 0.02 mg/kg/dose, may repeat q5–10min (max total dose: 2 mg)

Common adverse effects in *italic*; life-threatening effects underlined; generic names in **bold**; classifications in SMALL CAPS; ✦ Canadian drug name; ⊘ Prototype drug

## ADMINISTRATION

- Use only clear, colorless solutions. Red-tinted solution indicates oxidation, and such solutions should be discarded.

**Intramuscular**
- Give undiluted.

**Intravenous**
Note: Verify correct rate of IV injection for infants or children with prescriber.

*PREPARE:* **Direct:** Give undiluted.
*ADMINISTER:* **Direct for Adult:** Give slowly at a rate of no more than 1 mg/min. ▪ Rapid administration and overdosage can cause a cholinergic crisis. **Direct for Child:** Give 0.5 mg or fraction thereof over at least 1 min. ▪ Rapid administration and overdosage can cause a cholinergic crisis.
*INCOMPATIBILITIES:* **Solution/additive: Phenytoin, ranitidine. Y-site: Dobutamine.**

**ADVERSE EFFECTS** (≥1%) **Body as a Whole:** *Sweating,* cholinergic crisis (acute toxicity), hyperactivity, respiratory distress, convulsions. **CNS:** Restlessness, hallucinations, twitching, tremors, *sweating,* weakness, ataxia, convulsions, collapse. **GI:** *Nausea, vomiting, epigastric pain, diarrhea, salivation.* **Urogenital:** Involuntary urination or defecation. **Special Senses:** Miosis, *lacrimation,* rhinorrhea. **Respiratory:** Dyspnea, bronchospasm, respiratory paralysis, pulmonary edema. **Cardiovascular:** Irregular pulse, palpitations, bradycardia, rise in BP.

**INTERACTIONS Drug:** Antagonizes effects of **echothiophate, isofluorphate.**

**PHARMACOKINETICS Absorption:** Readily from mucous membranes, muscle, subcutaneous tissue; 10–12% absorbed from GI tract. **Onset:** 3–8 min IM/IV. **Duration:** 0.5–5 h IM/IV. **Distribution:** Crosses blood–brain barrier. **Metabolism:** In plasma by cholinesterase. **Elimination:** Small amounts in urine. **Half-Life:** 15–40 min.

## NURSING IMPLICATIONS

**Assessment & Drug Effects**
- Monitor vital signs and state of consciousness closely in patients receiving drug for atropine poisoning. Since physostigmine is usually rapidly eliminated, patient can lapse into delirium and coma within 1 to 2 h; repeat doses may be required.
- Monitor closely for adverse effects related to CNS and for signs of sensitivity to physostigmine. Have atropine sulfate readily available for clinical emergency.
- Discontinue parenteral or oral drug if following symptoms arise: Excessive salivation, emesis, frequent urination, or diarrhea.
- Eliminate excessive sweating or nausea with dose reduction.

## PHYTONADIONE (VITAMIN K₁)

(fye-toe-na-dye′one)
Mephyton
**Classifications:** VITAMIN K; ANTIDOTE
**Therapeutic:** VITAMIN K; ANTIDOTE

**AVAILABILITY** Tablet; solution for injection

## ACTION & *THERAPEUTIC EFFECT*
Fat-soluble substance chemically identical to and with similar activity as naturally occurring vitamin K. Vitamin K is essential for hepatic biosynthesis of blood clotting Factors II, VII, IX, and X. *Promotes liver synthesis of clotting factors.*

P

---

Common adverse effects in *italic*; life-threatening effects underlined; generic names in **bold**; classifications in SMALL CAPS; ♣ Canadian drug name; ☯ Prototype drug

**USES** Drug of choice as antidote for overdosage of coumarin and indandione oral anticoagulants. Also reverses hypoprothrombinemia secondary to administration of oral antibiotics, quinidine, quinine, salicylates, sulfonamides, excessive vitamin A, and secondary to inadequate absorption and synthesis of vitamin K (as in obstructive jaundice, biliary fistula, ulcerative colitis, intestinal resection, prolonged hyperalimentation). Also prophylaxis of and therapy for neonatal hemorrhagic disease.

**CONTRAINDICATIONS** Hypersensitivity to phytonadione, benzyl alcohol, or castor oil; severe liver disease.

**CAUTIOUS USE** Biliary tract disease, obstructive jaundice, pregnancy (category C). **IV:** Older adults.

## ROUTE & DOSAGE

### Anticoagulant Overdose

*Adult:* **PO/Subcutaneous/IM** 2.5–10 mg; rarely up to 50 mg/day, may repeat parenteral dose after 6–8 h if needed or PO dose after 12–24 h; **IV** Emergency only: 10–15 mg at a rate of 1 mg/min or less, may be repeated in 4 h if bleeding continues

### Hemorrhagic Disease of Newborns

*Infant:* **IM/Subcutaneous** 0.5–1 mg immediately after delivery, may repeat in 6–8 h if necessary

### Other Prothrombin Deficiencies

*Adult:* **IM/Subcutaneous/IV** 2–25 mg
*Child/Infant:* **IM/Subcutaneous/IV** 0.5–5 mg

## ADMINISTRATION

### Oral
- Bile salts must be given with tablets if patient has deficient bile production.
- Store in tightly closed container and protect from light. Vitamin K is rapidly degraded by light.

### Intramuscular/Subcutaneous
- Subcutaneous route is preferred. IM route has been associated with severe reactions.
- Apply gentle pressure to site following injection. Swelling (internal bleeding) and pain sometimes occur with injection.

### Intravenous
Note: Reserve IV route only for emergencies.

*PREPARE:* **Direct:** Dilute a single dose in 10 mL D5W, NS, or D5/NS. ▪ Protect infusion solution from light.
*ADMINISTER:* **Direct:** Give solution immediately after dilution at a rate not to exceed 1 mg/min.
*INCOMPATIBILITIES:* **Solution/additive:** Ascorbic acid, cephalothin, dobutamine, doxycycline, magnesium sulfate, nitrofurantoin, phenobarbital, ranitidine, vancomycin, warfarin. **Y-site:** Dobutamine.

- Protect infusion solution from light by wrapping container with aluminum foil or other opaque material. ▪ Discard unused solution and contents in open ampule.

## ADVERSE EFFECTS (≥1%) **Body as a Whole:** Hypersensitivity or <u>anaphylaxis-like reaction:</u> Facial flushing, cramp-like pains, convulsive movements, chills, fever, diaphoresis, weakness, dizziness, shock,

**P**

cardiac arrest. **CNS:** Headache (after oral dose), brain damage, death. **GI:** Gastric upset. **Hematologic:** Paradoxic hypoprothrombinemia (patients with severe liver disease), severe hemolytic anemia. **Metabolic:** Hyperbilirubinemia, kernicterus. **Respiratory:** Bronchospasm, dyspnea, sensation of chest constriction, respiratory arrest. **Skin:** Pain at injection site, hematoma, and nodule formation, erythematous skin eruptions (with repeated injections). **Special Senses:** Peculiar taste sensation.

### DIAGNOSTIC TEST INTERFERENCE

Falsely elevated *urine steroids* (by modifications of *Reddy, Jenkins, Thorn procedure*).

### INTERACTIONS **Drug:** Antagonizes

effects of **warfarin; cholestyramine, colestipol, mineral oil** decrease absorption of oral phytonadione.

### PHARMACOKINETICS **Absorption:** Readily from intestinal lymph if bile is present. **Onset:** 6–12 h PO; 1–2 h IM/Subcutaneous; 15 min IV. **Peak:** Hemorrhage usually controlled within 3–8 h; normal prothrombin time may be obtained in 12–14 h after administration. **Distribution:** Concentrates briefly in liver after absorption; crosses placenta; distributed into breast milk. **Metabolism:** Rapidly in liver. **Elimination:** In urine and bile.

## NURSING IMPLICATIONS

### Black Box Warning

*Phytonadione has been associated with severe reactions (resembling hypersensitivity or anaphylaxis) during and immediately after IV and IM administration.*

### Assessment & Drug Effects

- Monitor patient constantly. Severe reactions, including fatalities, have occurred during and immediately after IV and IM injection (see ADVERSE EFFECTS).
- Frequency, dose, and therapy duration are guided by PT/INR clinical response.
- Monitor therapeutic effectiveness which is indicated by shortened PT, INR, bleeding, and clotting times, as well as decreased hemorrhagic tendencies.
- Be aware that patients on large doses may develop temporary resistance to coumarin-type anticoagulants. If oral anticoagulant is reinstituted, larger than former doses may be needed. Some patients may require change to heparin.
- Monitor lab tests: Baseline and frequent PT.

### Patient & Family Education

- Maintain consistency in diet and avoid significant increases in daily intake of vitamin K-rich foods when drug regimen is stabilized. Know sources rich in vitamin K: Asparagus, broccoli, cabbage, lettuce, turnip greens, pork or beef liver, green tea, spinach, watercress, and tomatoes.

## PILOCARPINE HYDROCHLORIDE ⊙

## PILOCARPINE NITRATE

(pye-loe-kar′peen)

Adsorbocarpine, Isopto Carpine, Minims Pilocarpine ♦, Miocarpine ♦, Ocusert, Pilo, Pilocar, Salagen

**Classifications:** EYE PREPARATION; MIOTIC (ANTIGLAUCOMA); DIRECT-ACTING CHOLINERGIC
**Therapeutic:** ANTIGLAUCOMA

Common adverse effects in *italic*; life-threatening effects underlined; generic names in **bold**; classifications in SMALL CAPS; ♦ Canadian drug name; ⊙ Prototype drug

1297

**AVAILABILITY** Ophthalmic solution; ophthalmic gel; ocular insert; tablet

**ACTION & *THERAPEUTIC EFFECT***
In open-angle glaucoma, pilocarpine causes contraction of the ciliary muscle, increasing the outflow of aqueous humor, which reduces intraocular pressure (IOP). In closed-angle glaucoma, it induces miosis by opening the angle of the anterior chamber of the eye, through which aqueous humor exits. *Decrease in IOP results from stimulation of ciliary and papillary sphincter muscles, thus facilitating outflow of aqueous humor.*

**USES** Open-angle and angle-closure glaucomas; to reduce IOP and to protect the lens during surgery and laser iridotomy; to counteract effects of mydriatics and cycloplegics following surgery or ophthalmoscopic examination; to treat xerostomia.

**CONTRAINDICATIONS** Secondary glaucoma, acute iritis, acute inflammatory disease of anterior segment of eye; uncontrolled asthma; lactation. **Ocular therapeutic system:** Not used in acute infectious conjunctivitis, keratitis, retinal detachment, or when intense miosis is required, or with contact lens use.

**CAUTIOUS USE** Bronchial asthma; biliary tract disease; COPD; hypertension; pregnancy (category C).

**ROUTE & DOSAGE**

### Acute Glaucoma

*Adult/Child:* **Ophthalmic** 1 drop of 1–2% solution in affected eye q5–10min for 3–6 doses, then 1 drop q1–3h until IOP is reduced

### Chronic Glaucoma

*Adult/Child:* **Ophthalmic** 1 drop of 0.5–4% solution in affected eye q4–12h or 1 ocular system **(Ocusert)** q7days

### Miotic

*Adult/Child:* **Ophthalmic** 1 drop of 1% solution in affected eye

### Xerostomia

*Adult:* **PO** 5 mg t.i.d., may increase up to 10 mg t.i.d.

**ADMINISTRATION**

**Oral**
- Give with a full glass of water, if not contraindicated.

**Instillation**
- Note: During acute phase, prescriber may prescribe instillation of drug into unaffected eye to prevent bilateral attack of acute glaucoma.
- Apply gentle digital pressure to periphery of nasolacrimal drainage system for 1–2 min immediately after instillation of drops to prevent delivery of drug to nasal mucosa and general circulation.

**ADVERSE EFFECTS** (≥1%) **CNS:** Oral (asthenia, headaches, dizziness, chills). **Special Senses:** Ciliary spasm with brow ache, twitching of eyelids, eye pain with change in eye focus, miosis, *diminished vision in poorly illuminated areas,* blurred vision, reduced visual acuity, sensitivity, contact allergy, lacrimation, follicular conjunctivitis, conjunctival irritation, cataract, retinal detachment. **GI:** *Nausea,* vomiting, abdominal cramps, diarrhea, epigastric distress, *salivation.* **Respiratory:** Bronchospasm, rhinitis. **CV:** Tachycardia. **Body as a Whole:** Tremors, *increased sweating,* urinary frequency.

P

**INTERACTIONS Drug:** The actions of pilocarpine and **carbachol** are additive when used concomitantly. Oral form may cause conduction disturbances with BETA-BLOCKERS. Antagonizes the effects of concurrent ANTICHOLINERGIC DRUGS (e.g., **atropine, ipratropium**). **Food:** High-fat meal decreases absorption of pilocarpine.

**PHARMACOKINETICS Absorption:** Topical penetrates cornea rapidly; readily absorbed from GI tract. **Onset:** Miosis 10–30 min, IOP reduction 60 min; salivary stimulation 20 min. **Peak:** Miosis 30 min; IOP reduction 75 min; salivary stimulation 60 min. **Duration:** Miosis 4–8 h; IOP reduction 4–14 h (7 days with Ocusert); salivary stimulation 3–5 h. **Metabolism:** Inactivated at neuronal synapses and in plasma. **Elimination:** In urine. **Half-Life:** 0.76–1.35 h.

## NURSING IMPLICATIONS

### Assessment & Drug Effects

- Be aware that hourly tonometric tests may be done during early treatment because drug may cause an initial transitory increase in IOP.
- Monitor changes in visual acuity.
- Monitor for adverse effects. Brow pain and myopia tend to be more prominent in younger patients and generally disappear with continued use of drug.

### Patient & Family Education

- Understand that therapy for glaucoma is prolonged and that adherence to established regimen is crucial to prevent blindness.
- Do not drive or engage in potentially hazardous activities until vision clears. Drug causes blurred vision and difficulty in focusing.
- Discontinue medication if symptoms of irritation or sensitization persist and report to prescriber.

# PIMAVANSERIN

(pim-a-van'ser-in)

Nuplazid

**Classifications:** ATYPICAL ANTIPSYCHOTIC

**Therapeutic:** ANTIPSYCHOTIC

**Prototype:** Clozapine

## AVAILABILITY Tablets

## ACTION & THERAPEUTIC EFFECT

An inverse agonist and antagonist with a high binding affinity for the serotonin 5-HT$_{2A}$ receptor and a lower binding affinity for the 5-HT$_{2C}$ receptor.

## USES Treatment of hallucinations and delusions associated with Parkinson's disease.

## CONTRAINDICATIONS Avoid use in patients with cardiac disease or other risk factors for prolonged QT intervals, torsade de pointes, and/or sudden death such as cardiac arrhythmias, congenital long QT syndrome, heart failure, bradycardia, myocardial infarction, hypertension, coronary artery disease, hypomagnesemia, hypokalemia, hypocalcemia, or in patients receiving medications known to prolong the QT interval. Females and elderly patients are also at risk for QT prolongation. Pimavanserin is not recommended for patients with severe renal impairment (CrCl less than 30 mL/min), including renal failure. Not recommended for patients with mild, moderate or severe hepatic disease or impairment. Drug has not been evaluated in this population. Not approved for patients with dementia, related psychosis and delusions associated with Parkinson's disease.

## CAUTIOUS USE Cautious use for older adults. No data on use in pregnant or lactating women.

Common adverse effects in *italic*; life-threatening effects underlined; generic names in **bold**; classifications in SMALL CAPS; ♣Canadian drug name; ⊘ Prototype drug

1299

## ROUTE & DOSAGE

### Hallucinations and Delusions

*Adult:* **PO** 34 mg once daily

### Hepatic Impairment Dosage Adjustment

Not recommended in patients with hepatic impairment

### Renal Impairment Dosage Adjustment

*CrCl less than 30 mL/min:* Not recommended

### Concomitant Use with CYP3A4 Inhibitors Dosage Adjustment

Decrease dose to 17 mg once daily if used with a strong CYP3A4 inhibitor

## ADMINISTRATION

### Oral

▪ May be administered without regard to food.
▪ Store at 15°–30° C (59°–86° F).

## ADVERSE EFFECTS (≥2%) **Body as a Whole:** Gait disturbance, peripheral edema. **CNS:** Confusional state, hallucinations. **CV:** QT interval prolongation. **GI:** Constipation, nausea.

## INTERACTIONS **Drug:** Concomitant use of drugs that prolong the QT interval (e.g., **amiodarone, chlorpromazine, disopyramide, gatifloxacin, moxifloxacin, procainamide, quinidine, sotalol, thioridazine, ziprasidone**) may be additive to the QT effects of pimavanserin and increase the risk of cardiac arrhythmia. Concomitant use with a strong CYP3A4 inhbitor (e.g., **clarithromycin, indinavir, itraconazole, ketoconazole**) increases the levels of primavanserin. Concomitant use

with a strong CYP3A4 inducer (e.g., **carbamazepine, phenytoin, rifampin**) may decrease the levels of primavanserin. **Herbal: St. John's wort** may decrease the levels of primavanserin.

**PHARMACOKINETICS Peak:** 6 h. **Distribution:** 95% plasma protein bound. **Metabolism:** Hepatic oxidation to active and inactive metabolites. **Elimination:** Renal and fecal. **Half-Life:** 57 h.

## NURSING IMPLICATIONS

### Assessment & Drug Effects

▪ Monitor ECG: Prolonged QT interval has been reported.
▪ Monitor vital signs.
▪ Assess for peripheral edema and perform daily weights.
▪ Assess cognition and gait, patient at risk for confusion, hallucinations, and altered gait that impact safety.
▪ Monitor lab tests: LFTs, serum creatinine, and electrolytes.

### Patient & Family Education

▪ No data on use in pregnant women; contraceptive measures should be taken.
▪ Check with provider before taking any over the counter medication and make sure to tell healthcare providers the patient is currently taking this medication.
▪ Avoid drinking alcohol while taking this medication.
▪ Report any swelling noted in hands or feet.
▪ Report a fast or pounding heartbeat, chest pain, confusion, or severe dizziness.

## PIMECROLIMUS

(pim-e-cro-lim'us)

**Elidel**

**Classifications:** BIOLOGIC RESPONSE MODIFIER; IMMUNOMODULATOR
Therapeutic: IMMUNOSUPPRESSANT; ANTI-INFLAMMATORY
**Prototype:** Cyclosporine

## AVAILABILITY Cream

## ACTION & THERAPEUTIC EFFECT

Selectively inhibits inflammatory action of skin cells by blocking T-cell activation and cytokine release. It appears to inhibit the production of IL-2, IL-4, IL-10, and interferon gamma in T-cells. *Produces significant anti-inflammatory activity without evidence of skin atrophy.*

**USES** Short-term intermittent treatment of mild to moderate atopic dermatitis, eczema.

**CONTRAINDICATIONS** Hypersensitivity to pimecrolimus or components in the cream; Netherton's syndrome; immunocompromised individuals; application to active cutaneous viral infection; occlusive dressing; artificial or natural sunlight (UV) exposure; continuous long-term use; lactation; children younger than 2 y.

**CAUTIOUS USE** Infection at topical treatment sites; history of untoward effects with topical cyclosporine or tacrolimus; skin papillomas; immunocompromised patients; pregnancy (category C).

## ROUTE & DOSAGE

**Atopic Dermatitis**
*Adult/Adolescent/Child (older than 2 y):* **Topical** Apply thin layer to affected skin b.i.d. (avoid continuous long-term use)

## ADMINISTRATION

**Topical**
- Do not apply to any skin surface that appears to be infected.
- Limit application to areas of involvement with atopic dermatitis.

## ADVERSE EFFECTS (≥1%) **Body as a Whole:** Flu-like symptoms, infections, fever, increased risk of cancer. **CNS:** Headache. **GI:** Gastroenteritis, abdominal pain, nausea, vomiting, diarrhea, constipation. **Respiratory:** Sore throat, *upper respiratory infection, cough,* nasal congestion, asthma exacerbation, rhinitis, epistaxis **Skin:** *Burning,* irritation, pruritus, skin infection, impetigo, folliculitis, skin papilloma, herpes simplex dermatitis, urticaria, acne. **Special Senses:** Ear infection, earache, conjunctivitis.

## PHARMACOKINETICS **Absorption:** Minimal through intact skin. **Metabolism:** No evidence of skin-mediated metabolism, metabolized in liver by CYP3A4. **Elimination:** Primarily in feces.

## NURSING IMPLICATIONS

### Assessment & Drug Effects
- Assess for and report persistent skin irritation that develops following application of the cream and lasts for more than 1 wk.

### Patient & Family Education
- Minimize exposure of treated area to natural or artificial sunlight.
- Immediately report a new or changed skin lesion to the prescriber.
- Stop topical application once signs of dermatitis have disappeared. Resume application at the first sign of recurrence.
- Continuous, long-term use of this cream is not recommended.

Common adverse effects in *italic*; life-threatening effects underlined; generic names in **bold**; classifications in SMALL CAPS; ♣ Canadian drug name; ☻ Prototype drug

1301

- Wash hands thoroughly after application if hands are not the treatment sites.
- Report any significant skin irritation that results from application of the cream.

# PIMOZIDE
(pi'moe-zide)

**Orap**

**Classification:** ANTIPSYCHOTIC
**Therapeutic:** ANTIPSYCHOTIC; CNS DOPAMINERGIC RECEPTOR ANTAGONIST
**Prototype:** Haloperidol

**AVAILABILITY** Tablet

## ACTION & *THERAPEUTIC EFFECT*
Potent central dopamine antagonist that alters release and turnover of central dopamine stores. Blockade of CNS dopaminergic receptors results in suppression of the motor and phonic tics that characterize Tourette's disorder. *Effective in suppressing motor and phonic tics associated with Tourette's disorder.*

**USES** Tourette's syndrome resistant to standard therapy.

**UNLABELED USES** Schizophrenia, delusions of parasitosis.

**CONTRAINDICATIONS** Treatment of simple tics other than those associated with Tourette's disorder; drug-induced tics; history of cardiac dysrhythmias and conditions marked by prolonged QT syndrome, patient taking drugs that may prolong QT interval (e.g., quinidine); congenital heart defects, cardiac arrhythmias; torsade de pointes; electrolyte imbalance; Parkinson's disease; NMS; severe toxic CNS depression or coma states; lactation.

**CAUTIOUS USE** Kidney and liver dysfunction; cardiac disease;

glaucoma; BPH; renal or hepatic impairment; urinary retention; low WBC; seizure disorders; older adults; pregnancy (category C). Safe use in children younger than 12 y is not known.

## ROUTE & DOSAGE

**Tourette's Disorder**
*Adult:* **PO** 1–2 mg/day in divided doses, gradually increase dose every other day up to 0.2 mg/kg/day or 10 mg/day in divided doses (max: 0.2 mg/kg/day or 10 mg/day)
*Adolescent:* **PO** 0.05 mg/kg/day at bedtime, gradually increase as needed (max: 0.2 mg/kg/day or 10 mg, whichever is less)

## ADMINISTRATION

**Oral**
- May be taken with or without food.
- Increase drug dose gradually, usually over 1–3 wk, until maintenance dose is reached.
- Follow regimen prescribed by prescriber for withdrawal: Usually slow, gradual changes over a period of days or weeks (drug has a long half-life). Sudden withdrawal may cause reemergence of original symptoms (motor and phonic tics) and of neuromuscular adverse effects of the drug.

**ADVERSE EFFECTS** (≥1%) **Body as a Whole:** *Akathisia,* speech disorder, *torticollis, tremor,* handwriting changes, *akinesia,* fainting, hyperpyrexia, tardive dyskinesia, *rigidity, oculogyric crisis,* hyperreflexia; seizures, <u>neuroleptic malignant syndrome</u>; *extrapyramidal dysfunction,* hyperthermia, autonomic dysfunction; diaphoresis, weight changes, asthenia, chest pain, periorbital edema.

Common adverse effects in *italic*; life-threatening effects <u>underlined</u>; generic names in **bold**; classifications in SMALL CAPS; ✦ Canadian drug name; ⊘ Prototype drug

**CNS:** Headache, *sedation, drowsiness,* insomnia, seizures, stupor, depression, akethesia, rigidity. **CV:** Prolongation of QT interval, inverted or flattened T wave, appearance of U wave, labile blood pressure. **Urogenital:** Loss of libido, impotence, nocturia, urinary frequency, amenorrhea, dysmenorrhea, mild galactorrhea, urinary retention, <u>acute renal failure</u>. **Respiratory:** Dyspnea, <u>respiratory failure</u>. **Skin:** Sweating, skin irritation. **Special Senses:** Visual disturbances, photosensitivity, decreased accommodation, blurred vision, cataracts. **GI:** Increased salivation, nausea, vomiting, diarrhea, anorexia, abdominal cramps, *dry mouth, constipation.*

## INTERACTIONS Drug: Alcohol
and other CNS DEPRESSANTS increase CNS depression; ANTICHOLINERGIC AGENTS (e.g., TRICYCLIC ANTIDEPRESSANTS, **atropine**) increase anticholinergic effects; PHENOTHIAZINES, TRICYCLIC ANTIDEPRESSANTS, ANTIARRHYTHMICS, MACROLIDE ANTIBIOTICS, AZOLE ANTIFUNGALS, PROTEASE INHIBITORS, **nefazodone, sertraline, zileuton** increase risk of arrhythmias and heart block; pimozide antagonizes effects of ANTICONVULSANTS—there is loss of seizure control. Avoid with medications that increase QT interval (e.g., **bepridil, dofetilide, procainamide, ziprasidone**) **Food: Grapefruit juice** (greater than 1 qt/day) may increase plasma concentrations and adverse effects.

## PHARMACOKINETICS Absorption:
Slowly and variably from GI tract (40–50% absorbed). **Peak:** 6–8 h. **Metabolism:** In liver (by CYP3A4, CYP2D6, CYP1A2). **Elimination:** 80–85% in urine, 15–20% in feces. **Half-Life:** 55 h.

## NURSING IMPLICATIONS

Note: See haloperidol for additional nursing implications.

### Assessment & Drug Effects
- Obtain ECG baseline data at beginning of therapy and check periodically, especially during dosage adjustments.
- Notify prescriber immediately for widening or prolongation of the QT interval, which suggests developing cardiotoxicity.
- Risk of tardive dyskinesia appears to be greatest in women, older adults, and those on high-dose therapy.
- Be aware that extrapyramidal reactions often appear within the first few days of therapy, are dose-related, and usually occur when dose is high.
- Be aware that anticholinergic effects (dry mouth, constipation) may increase as dose is increased.

### Patient & Family Education
- Adhere to established drug regimen (i.e., do not change dose or intervals and discontinue only with prescriber's guidance).
- Use measures to relieve dry mouth (frequent rinsing with water, saliva substitute, increased fluid intake) and constipation (increased dietary fiber, drink 6–8 glasses of water daily).
- Do not drive or engage in potentially hazardous activities because drug-caused hand tremors, drowsiness, and blurred vision may impair alertness and abilities.
- Pseudoparkinsonism symptoms are usually mild and reversible with dose adjustment.
- Be alert to the earliest symptom of tardive dyskinesia ("flycatching"— an involuntary movement of the tongue), and report promptly to the prescriber.
- Return to prescriber for periodic assessments of therapy benefit and cardiac status.
- Understand dangers of ingesting alcohol to prevent augmenting CNS depressant effects of pimozide.

P

---

Common adverse effects in *italic*; life-threatening effects <u>underlined</u>; generic names in **bold**; classifications in SMALL CAPS; ✦ Canadian drug name; ⊘ Prototype drug

1303

# PINDOLOL
(pin'doe-lole)

**Classifications:** BETA-ADRENERGIC RECEPTOR ANTAGONIST; ANTIHYPERTENSIVE
Therapeutic: ANTIHYPERTENSIVE; ANTIANGINAL
**Prototype:** Propranolol

## AVAILABILITY Tablet

## ACTION & *THERAPEUTIC EFFECT*
Competitively blocks beta-adrenergic receptors primarily in myocardium, and beta receptors within smooth muscle. *Lowers blood pressure by decreasing peripheral vascular resistance. Exerts vasodilation as well as hypotensive effects.*

## USES Management of hypertension.

## UNLABELED USES Angina, traumatic brain injury.

## CONTRAINDICATIONS Bronchospastic diseases, asthma; cardiogenic shock, AV block, second and third degree heart block; severe bradycardia; overt cardiac failure; pulmonary failure; abrupt withdrawal; lactation.

## CAUTIOUS USE Nonallergic bronchospasm; COPD; CHF; angina; history of cardiac failure that is well controlled; major surgery; DM; hyperthyroidism; MG; impaired liver and kidney function; pregnancy (category B). Safety and efficacy in children not established.

## ROUTE & DOSAGE

### Hypertension
*Adult:* **PO** 5 mg b.i.d., may increase by 10 mg/day q3–4wk if needed up (max: 60 mg/day in 2–3 divided doses)
*Geriatric:* **PO** Start with 5 mg daily

## ADMINISTRATION
### Oral
- Give drug at same time of day each day with respect to time of food intake for most predictable results.
- Withdraw or discontinue treatment gradually over a period of 1–2 wk.

## ADVERSE EFFECTS (≥1%) CNS:
*Fatigue,* dizziness, insomnia, drowsiness, confusion, fainting, decreased libido. **CV:** *Bradycardia,* hypotension, CHF. **GI:** Nausea, *diarrhea, constipation,* flatulence. **Respiratory:** Bronchospasm, pulmonary edema, dyspnea. **Body as a Whole:** Back or joint pain. Sensitivity reactions seen as antinuclear antibodies (ANA) (10–30% of patients). **Hematologic:** Agranulocytosis. **Urogenital:** Impotence. **Metabolic:** Hypoglycemia (may mask symptoms of a hypoglycemic reaction).

## INTERACTIONS Drug: DIURETICS and other HYPOTENSIVE AGENTS increase hypotensive effect; effects of **albuterol, metaproterenol, terbutaline, pirbuterol,** and **pindolol** antagonized; NSAIDS blunt hypotensive effect; decreases hypoglycemic effect of **glyburide; amiodarone** increases risk of bradycardia and sinus arrest.

## PHARMACOKINETICS Absorption: Rapidly from GI tract; 50–95% reaches systemic circulation (first pass metabolism). **Onset:** 3 h. **Peak:** 1–2 h. **Duration:** 24 h. **Distribution:** Distributed into breast milk. **Metabolism:** 40–60% in liver. **Elimination:** In urine. **Half-Life:** 3–4 h.

## NURSING IMPLICATIONS
### Assessment & Drug Effects
- Monitor HR and BP. Report bradycardia and hypotension. Dosage adjustment may be indicated.

P

Common adverse effects in *italic,* life-threatening effects underlined; generic names in **bold**; classifications in SMALL CAPS; ✦Canadian drug name; ⊕ Prototype drug

- Note: Hypotensive effect may begin within 7 days but is not at maximum therapeutically until about 2 wk after beginning of treatment.

**Patient & Family Education**
- Pindolol masks the dizziness and sweating symptoms of hypoglycemia. Monitor blood glucose for loss of glycemic control.
- Adhere to the prescribed drug regimen, if a change is desired, consult prescriber first. Abrupt withdrawal of drug might precipitate a thyroid crisis in a patient with hyperthyroidism, and angina in the patient with ischemic heart disease, leading to an MI.

# PIOGLITAZONE HYDROCHLORIDE
(pi-o-glit'a-zone)
Actos
**Classifications:** ANTIDIABETIC; THIAZOLIDINEDIONE (GLITAZONE)
**Therapeutic:** ANTIDIABETIC; INSULIN SENSITIZER
**Prototype:** Rosiglitazone maleate

**AVAILABILITY** Tablet

**ACTION & *THERAPEUTIC EFFECT***
Decreases hepatic glucose output and increases insulin-dependent muscle glucose uptake in skeletal muscle and adipose tissue. Improves glycemic control in noninsulin-dependent diabetics (type 2) by enhancing insulin sensitivity of cells without stimulating pancreatic insulin secretion. *Improves glycemic control as indicated by improved blood glucose levels and decreased HbA1C.*

**USES** Adjunct to diet in the treatment of type 2 diabetes mellitus.

**CONTRAINDICATIONS** Hypersensitivity to pioglitazone, rosiglitazone; type 1 diabetes, or treatment of DKA; New York Heart Association (NYHA) Class III or IV heart failure; active liver disease or ALT levels greater than 2.5 × NL; jaundice; fracture risk factors; lactation.

**CAUTIOUS USE** Liver dysfunction; cardiovascular disease; hypertension, CHF, anemia, edema; osteoporosis; history of bladder cancer; older adults, pregnancy (category C). Safety and efficacy in children younger than 18 y not recommended.

## ROUTE & DOSAGE

**Type 2 Diabetes Mellitus**
Adult: **PO** 15–30 mg once daily (max: 45 mg daily)
***Disease State Dosage Adjustment***
*Patients with NHYA Class I or II heart failure:* (max: 15 mg once daily)
***Drug Interaction Dosage Adjustment***
*If used with gemfibrozil* (max: 15 mg)

## ADMINISTRATION
**Oral**
- Give without regard to food.
- Do not initiate therapy if baseline serum ALT greater than 2.5 × normal.
- Store at 15°–30° C (59°–86° F) in tightly closed container; protect from humidity and moisture.

**ADVERSE EFFECTS** (≥1%) **Body as a Whole:** Headache, myalgia, edema, rhabdomyolysis. **CV:** Edema, fluid retention, exacerbation of heart failure. **GI:** Tooth disorder. **Respiratory:** *Upper respiratory tract infection,* sinusitis, pharyngitis. **Metabolic:** Hypoglycemia, mild anemia.

---

Common adverse effects in *italic*; life-threatening effects <u>underlined</u>; generic names in **bold**; classifications in SMALL CAPS; ✦Canadian drug name; ℗ Prototype drug

**INTERACTIONS Drug: Pioglitazone** may decrease serum levels of ORAL CONTRACEPTIVES; **ketoconazole, gemfibrozil, mifepristone** may increase serum levels of **pioglitazone.** BILE ACID SEQUESTRANTS, **bosentan** may decrease effect. **Herbal: Garlic, ginseng** may potentiate hypoglycemic effects.

**PHARMACOKINETICS Absorption:** Rapidly absorbed. **Peak:** 2 h; steady state concentrations within 7 days. **Duration:** 24 h. **Distribution:** Greater than 99% protein bound. **Metabolism:** In liver to active metabolites. **Elimination:** Primarily in bile and feces. **Half-Life:** 16–24 h.

## NURSING IMPLICATIONS

### Black Box Warning

*Pioglitazone has been associated with exacerbation of CHF.*

#### Assessment & Drug Effects

- Monitor for S&S hypoglycemia (possible when insulin/sulfonylureas are coadministered).
- Monitor closely for S&S of CHF or exacerbation of symptoms with preexisting CHF.
- Withhold drug and notify prescriber if ALT greater than 3 × ULN or patient has jaundice.
- Monitor weight and notify prescriber of development of edema.
- Monitor lab tests: Baseline and periodic LFTs; periodic fasting plasma glucose and HbA1C.

#### Patient & Family Education

- Be aware that resumed ovulation is possible in nonovulating premenopausal women.
- Use or add barrier contraceptive if using hormonal contraception.
- Report immediately to prescriber: Unexplained anorexia, nausea, vomiting, abdominal pain, fatigue, dark urine; or S&S of fluid retention such as weight gain, edema, or activity intolerance.
- Combination therapy: May need adjustment of other antidiabetic drugs to avoid hypoglycemia.
- Learn of and adhere strictly to guidelines for liver function tests. Be sure to have blood tests for liver function periodically.

## PIPERACILLIN/ TAZOBACTAM ℞

(pi-per′a-cil-lin/taz-o-bac′tam)

Zosyn

**Classifications:** ANTIBIOTIC; EXTENDED SPECTRUM PENICILLIN

Therapeutic: ANTIBIOTIC

**AVAILABILITY** Solution for injection

**ACTION & THERAPEUTIC EFFECT** Tazobactam has little antibacterial activity itself; however, in combination with piperacillin, it extends the spectrum of bacteria that are susceptible to piperacillin. *Two-drug combination has antibiotic activity against an extremely broad spectrum of gram-positive, gram-negative, and anaerobic bacteria.*

**USES** Treatment of moderate to severe appendicitis, uncomplicated and complicated skin and skin structure infections, endometritis, pelvic inflammatory disease, or nosocomial- or community-acquired pneumonia caused by beta-lactamase-producing bacteria.

**CONTRAINDICATIONS** Hypersensitivity to piperacillin, tazobactam, penicillins; coagulopathy.

**CAUTIOUS USE** Hypersensitivity to cephalosporins, carbapenem, or betalactamase inhibitors such as

Common adverse effects in *italic*; life-threatening effects <u>underlined</u>; generic names in **bold**; classifications in SMALL CAPS; ♣Canadian drug name; ☉ Prototype drug clavulanic acid and sulbactam; GI disease, colitis; CF; eczema; kidney failure; complicated urinary tract infections; pregnancy (category B); lactation.

## ROUTE & DOSAGE

### Moderate to Severe Infections
*Adult:* **IV** 3.375 g q6h, infused over 30 min, for 7–10 days
*Child (younger than 6 mo):* **IV** 150–300 mg piperacillin/kg/day divided q6–8h; *6 mo or older:* 240 mg piperacillin component/kg/day divided q8h

### Nosocomial Pneumonia
*Adult:* **IV** 4.5 g q6h, infused over 30 min, for 7–10 days

### Renal Insufficiency Dosage Adjustment
*CrCl 20–40 mL/min:* 2.25 g q6h; *less than 20 mL/min:* 2.25 g q8h

### Hemodialysis Dosage Adjustment
2.25 g q12h (for nosocomial pneumonia dose q8h); give additional 0.75 g after dialysis session

## ADMINISTRATION

Note: Verify correct IV concentration and rate of infusion for administration to infants or children with prescriber.

### Intravenous

*PREPARE:* **Intermittent:** Reconstitute powder with 5 mL of diluent (e.g., D5W, NS) for each 1 g or fraction thereof; shake well until dissolved. ▪ Further dilute to a total of 50 to 150 mL in selected diluent (e.g., NS, sterile water for injection, D5W, dextran 6% in NS, and LR only with solution containing EDTA).
*ADMINISTER:* **Intermittent:** Give over at least 30 min. ▪ **Do not**

administer through a line with another infusion.

*INCOMPATIBILITIES:* **Solution/additive: Aminoglycosides, lactated Ringer's, albumin, blood products, solutions containing sodium bicarbonate. Y-site: Acyclovir, aminoglycosides, amiodarone, amphotericin B, amphotericin B cholesteryl complex, azithromycin, chlorpromazine, cisatracurium, cisplatin, dacarbazine, daunorubicin, dobutamine, doxorubicin, doxorubicin liposome, doxycycline, droperidol, famotidine, ganciclovir, gatifloxacin, gemcitabine, haloperidol, hydroxyzine, idarubicin, miconazole, minocycline, mitomycin, mitoxantrone, nalbuphine, prochlorperazine, promethazine, streptozocin, vancomycin.**

## ADVERSE EFFECTS (≥1%) CNS:
Headache, insomnia, fever. **GI:** *Diarrhea, constipation, nausea, vomiting, dyspepsia,* pseudomembranous colitis. **Skin:** *Rash, pruritus,* hypersensitivity reactions.

## INTERACTIONS **Drug:** May increase risk of bleeding with ANTICOAGULANTS; **probenecid** decreases elimination of piperacillin.

## PHARMACOKINETICS **Distribution:** Distributes into many tissues, including lung, blister fluid, and bile; crosses placenta; distributed into breast milk. **Metabolism:** In liver. **Elimination:** In urine. **Half-Life:** 0.7–1.2 h.

## NURSING IMPLICATIONS
### Assessment & Drug Effects
▪ Obtain history of hypersensitivity to penicillins, cephalosporins, or other drugs prior to administration.

---

Common adverse effects in *italic*; life-threatening effects underlined; generic names in **bold**; classifications in SMALL CAPS; ♣Canadian drug name; ⊙ Prototype drug

P

- Monitor patient carefully during the first 30 min after initiation of the infusion for signs of hypersensitivity (see Appendix F).
- Monitor lab tests: Baseline C&S; periodic renal function tests, CBC with differential, PT and PTT, serum electrolytes, and LFTs.

**Patient & Family Education**

- Report rash, itching, or other signs of hypersensitivity immediately.
- Report loose stools or diarrhea as these may indicate pseudomembranous colitis.

# PIROXICAM

(peer-ox′i-kam)

Feldene

**Classifications:** NONNARCOTIC ANALGESIC; NONSTEROIDAL ANTI-INFLAMMATORY DRUG (NSAID)

Therapeutic: ANALGESIC; NSAID; ANTIPYRETIC

**Prototype:** Ibuprofen

## AVAILABILITY Capsule

## ACTION & *THERAPEUTIC EFFECT*

Nonsteroidal anti-inflammatory agent that strongly inhibits enzyme cyclooxygenase, both COX1 and COX2, the catalyst of prostaglandin synthesis. Decreased prostaglandin results in anti-inflammatory properties, analgesic and antipyretic effects. *Decreases inflammatory processes in bone-joint disease as well as has analgesic and antipyretic effects.*

## USES Acute and long-term relief of mild to moderate pain and for symptomatic treatment of osteoarthritis and rheumatoid arthritis; headache.

## CONTRAINDICATIONS Hypersensitivity to NSAIDs or salicylates; hemophilia; active peptic ulcer, GI bleeding; CABG perioperative pain; ST-elevated MI; lactation.

**CAUTIOUS USE** History of upper GI disease including ulcerative colitis; SLE; kidney dysfunction; hepatic disease; CHF; acute MI; compromised cardiac function; hypertension or other conditions predisposing to fluid retention; renal disease; alcoholism; coagulation disorders; older adults; pregnancy (category C). Safe use in children not established.

## ROUTE & DOSAGE

**Arthritis, Pain**
*Adult:* **PO** 10–20 mg 1–2 × day

## ADMINISTRATION

**Oral**

- Give at the same time every day.
- Give capsule with food or fluid to help reduce GI irritation.
- Dose adjustments should be made on basis of clinical response at intervals of weeks rather than days in order to prevent over dosage.
- Store in tightly closed container at 15°–30° C (59°–86° F) unless otherwise directed.

## ADVERSE EFFECTS (≥1%) **CNS:** Somnolence, dizziness, vertigo, depression, insomnia, nervousness. **CV:** Peripheral edema, hypertension, worsening of CHF, exacerbation of angina. **Special Senses:** Tinnitus, hearing loss, blurred vision, reduced visual acuity, changes in color vision, scotomas, corneal deposits, retinal disturbances. **GI:** *Nausea, vomiting, dyspepsia,* abdominal pain, <u>GI bleeding</u>, diarrhea, constipation, flatulence, dry mouth, <u>peptic ulceration</u>, anorexia, jaundice, hepatitis. **Hematologic:** Anemia, decreases in Hgb, Hct; <u>*leukopenia*</u>, eosinophilia, <u>aplastic anemia</u>; <u>*thrombocytopenia, prolonged bleeding time.*</u> **Skin:** Urticaria, erythema multiforme,

Common adverse effects in *italic*; life-threatening effects <u>underlined</u>; generic names in **bold**; classifications in SMALL CAPS; ♣ Canadian drug name; ◎ Prototype drug maculopapular, vesiculobullous rash; photosensitivity, sweating, Stevens-Johnson syndrome, bruising, dermatitis. **Body as a Whole:** Allergic rhinitis, angioedema, fever, palpitations, syncope, muscle cramps, fever, hypersensitivity reactions. **Metabolic:** Hypoglycemia, hyperglycemia, hyperkalemia, weight gain. **Urogenital:** Dysuria, acute kidney failure, papillary necrosis, hematuria, proteinuria, nephrotic syndrome. **Respiratory:** Bronchospasm, dyspnea.

**INTERACTIONS Drug:** ORAL ANTICO-AGULANTS, **heparin** may prolong bleeding time; may increase **lithium** toxicity; **alcohol,** NONSTEROIDAL ANTIINFLAMMATORIES increase risk of GI hemorrhage. Do not use with **cidofovir. Herbal: Feverfew, garlic, ginger, ginkgo** may increase bleeding potential.

**PHARMACOKINETICS Absorption:** Extensively from GI tract. **Onset:** 1 h analgesia; 7 days for rheumatoid arthritis. **Peak:** 3–5 h analgesia; 2–4 wk antirheumatic. **Duration:** 48–72 h analgesia. **Distribution:** Small amount distributed into breast milk. **Metabolism:** Extensively in liver by (CYP2C9). **Elimination:** Primarily in urine, some in bile (less than 5%). **Half-Life:** 50 h.

## NURSING IMPLICATIONS

### Black Box Warning

*Piroxican has been associated with increased risk of serious, potentially fatal, GI bleeding and cardiovascular events (e.g., MI and CVA); risk may increase with duration of use and may be greater in the older adult and those with risk factors for CV disease.*

### Assessment & Drug Effects

- Clinical evidence of benefits from drug therapy include pain relief in motion and in rest, reduction in night pain, stiffness, and swelling; increased ROM (range of motion) in all joints.
- Monitor for and report promptly S&S of GI ulceration or bleeding. Significant GI bleeding may occur without prior warning.
- Monitor for and report promptly S&S of CV thrombotic events (i.e., angina, MI, TIA, or stroke).
- Monitor lab tests: Periodic renal function tests, LFTs, CBC, Hgb, and Hct in the older adult and during long-term therapy.

### Patient & Family Education

- Do not self-dose with aspirin or other OTC drug without prescriber's advice.
- Do not increase dosage beyond prescribed regimen. Higher than recommended doses are associated with increased incidence of GI irritation and peptic ulcer.
- Incidence of GI bleeding with this drug is relatively high. Report symptoms of GI bleeding (e.g., dark, tarry stools, coffee-colored emesis) or severe gastric pain promptly to prescriber.
- Stop taking drug and report promptly to prescriber if you experience chest pain, shortness of breath, weakness, slurring of speech, or other signs of a cardiac or neurologic problem.
- Be alert to symptoms of drug-induced anemia: Profound fatigue, skin and mucous membrane pallor, lethargy.
- Avoid alcohol since it may increase the risk of GI bleeding.
- Be alert to signs of hypoprothrombinemia including bruises, pinpoint rash, unexplained bleeding, nose bleed, blood in urine, when piroxicam is taken concomitantly with an anticoagulant.

P

- Do not drive or engage in potentially hazardous activities until response to drug is known.
- Drink at least 6–8 full glasses of water daily and report signs of renal insufficiency (see Appendix F) to prescriber because most of drug is excreted by kidneys and impaired kidney function increases danger of toxicity.

# PITAVASTATIN CALCIUM

(pit-a-vah-stat'in)

Livalo, Zypitamag

**Classifications:** ANTIHYPERLIPIDEMIC; LIPID-LOWERING AGENT; HMG-COA REDUCTASE INHIBITOR (STATIN)

Therapeutic: ANTILIPEMIC; LIPID-LOWERING AGENT; STATIN

**Prototype:** Lovastatin

## AVAILABILITY Tablet

## ACTION & THERAPEUTIC EFFECT

Pitavastatin is a HMG-CoA reductase inhibitor that reduces plasma cholesterol levels by interfering with the production of cholesterol in the liver. It also promotes removal of LDL and VLDL from plasma. *Effectiveness is measured by decrease in blood level of total cholesterol, LDL cholesterol, and triglycerides and an increase in HDL cholesterol.*

## USES Treatment of hypercholesterolemia, hyperlipoproteinemia, and/or hypertriglyceridemia as an adjunct to dietary control.

## UNLABELED USES Regression of coronary atherosclerosis in patients with acute coronary syndrome (ACS).

## CONTRAINDICATIONS Hypersensitivity to pitavastatin; myopathy and rhabdomyolysis; acute renal failure; ESRD not on hemodialysis; active liver disease; large amounts of alcohol; pregnancy (category X); lactation.

**CAUTIOUS USE** Renal impairment; hepatic impairment; DM; older adults. Safety and efficacy in children not established.

## ROUTE & DOSAGE

**Hypercholesterolemia, Hyperlipoproteinemia, and/or Hypertriglyceridemia**

*Adult:* **PO** Initially 2 mg once daily; can be adjusted to 1–4 mg once daily

**Renal Impairment Dosage Adjustment**

*CrCl 30 to less than 60 mL/min:* Initially, 1 mg once daily; do not exceed 2 mg once daily

*hemodialysis:* Not recommended

## ADMINISTRATION

**Oral**

- May give without regard to meals any time of day.
- Store at 15°–30° C (59°–86° F).

**ADVERSE EFFECTS** (≥1%) **Body as a Whole:** Pain in extremity, influenza. **CNS:** Headache. **GI:** Constipation, diarrhea. **Hematologic:** Elevated creatine phosphokinase (CPK), elevated AST and ALT levels. **Musculoskeletal:** Arthralgia, back pain, myalgia. **Respiratory:** Nasopharyngitis. **Skin:** Pruritus, rash, urticaria.

**INTERACTIONS Drug: Cyclosporine, erythromycin,** HIV PROTEASE INHIBITORS, and **rifampin** increase pitavastatin levels. FIBRATES may increase the risk of myopathy and rhabdomyolysis. Combination use with **niacin** may increase the risk of skeletal muscle effects.

## PHARMACOKINETICS Absorption: 51% bioavailable. **Peak:** 1 h. **Distribution:** Greater than 99% plasma protein bound. **Metabolism:** In liver. **Elimination:** Primarily fecal (79%) with minor renal (15%) elimination. **Half-Life:** 12 h.

## NURSING IMPLICATIONS

### Assessment & Drug Effects
- Monitor for and report muscle pain, tenderness, or weakness.
- Withhold drug and notify prescriber for ALT/AST greater than 3 × ULN.
- Monitor lab tests: Lipid profile at baseline, at 4 wk, and periodically thereafter; LFTs at baseline, at 12 wk after initiation or elevation of dose, and periodically thereafter; creatine kinase levels if patient experiences muscle pain.

### Patient & Family Education
- Report promptly unexplained muscle pain, tenderness, or weakness.
- Avoid or minimize alcohol consumption while on this drug.
- Use effective contraceptive measures to avoid pregnancy while taking this drug.

## PLASMA PROTEIN FRACTION
(plas'ma)

Plasmanate

**Classification:** PLASMA VOLUME EXPANDER
**Therapeutic:** PLASMA VOLUME EXPANDER; ALBUMIN
**Prototype:** Normal serum albumin, human

**AVAILABILITY** Solution for injection

## ACTION & *THERAPEUTIC EFFECT*
Provides plasma proteins that increase colloidal osmotic pressure within the intravascular compartment equal to human plasma. It shifts water from the extravascular tissues back into the intravascular space, thus expanding plasma volume. *Used to maintain cardiac output by expanding plasma volume in the treatment of shock due to various causes.*

**USES** Emergency treatment of hypovolemic shock; temporary measure in treatment of blood loss when whole blood is not available.

**CONTRAINDICATIONS** Hypersensitivity to albumin; severe anemia; cardiac failure; patients undergoing cardiopulmonary bypass surgery

**CAUTIOUS USE** Patients with low cardiac reserve; absence of albumin deficiency; liver or kidney failure; pregnancy (category C); children.

## ROUTE & DOSAGE

**Plasma Volume Expansion**
*Adult:* IV 250–500 mL at a maximum rate of 10 mL/min

## ADMINISTRATION

**Intravenous**
Do not use solutions that show a sediment or appear turbid. Do not use solutions that have been frozen.

*PREPARE:* **IV Infusion:** Give undiluted. ▪ Once container is opened, solution should be used within 4 h because it contains no preservatives. ▪ Discard unused portions.
*ADMINISTER:* **IV Infusion:** Rate of infusion and volume of total

Common adverse effects in *italic*; life-threatening effects underlined; generic names in **bold**; classifications in SMALL CAPS; ◆ Canadian drug name; ⊘ Prototype drug

1311

dose will depend on patient's age, diagnosis, degree of venous and pulmonary congestion, Hct, and Hgb determinations. As with any oncotically active solution, infusion rate should be relatively slow. Range may vary from 1–10 mL/min. *INCOMPATIBILITIES:* PROTEIN HYDRO-LYSATES or solutions containing alcohol.

## ADVERSE EFFECTS (≥1%) GI:
Nausea, vomiting, hypersalivation, headache. **Body as a Whole:** Tingling, chills, fever, cyanosis, chest tightness, backache, urticaria, erythema, shock (systemic anaphylaxis), circulatory overload, pulmonary edema.

## NURSING IMPLICATIONS

### Assessment & Drug Effects
- Monitor vital signs (BP and pulse). Frequency depends on patient's condition. Flow rate adjustments are made according to clinical response and BP. Slow or stop infusion if patient suddenly becomes hypotensive.
- Report a widening pulse pressure (difference between systolic and diastolic); it correlates with increase in cardiac output.
- Report changes in I&O ratio and pattern.
- Observe patient closely during and after infusion for signs of hypervolemia or circulatory overload (see Appendix F). Report these symptoms immediately to prescriber.
- Make careful observations of patient who has had either injury or surgery in order to detect bleeding points that failed to bleed at lower BP.

## PLECANATIDE
(ple-kan'a-tide)

Trulance

**Classifications:** GUANYLATE CYCLASE-C AGONIST; ACCELERANT OF GI TRANSIT
Therapeutic: ACCELERANT OF GI TRANSIT

## AVAILABILITY Tablet

## ACTION & *THERAPEUTIC EFFECT*
Plecanatide increases the cyclic guanosine monophosphate (cGMP) levels by acting as an agonist of guanylate cyclase-C. This results in an increase of intestinal fluid and transit by stimulating chloride and bicarbonate excretion into the intestinal lumen. *Gastrointestinal time is accelerated which is helpful in combatting constipation.*

## USES Treatment of chronic idiopathic constipation.

## CONTRAINDICATIONS Known or suspected mechanical gastrointestinal obstruction. Patient currently has diarrhea; pediatric patients younger than 6 y.

## CAUTIOUS USE There are no adequate well-controlled studies of plecanatide used in pregnancy. Risk of birth defect or miscarriage cannot be determined. There are no data on the presence of plecanatide in animal or human milk, the effects on breast-feeding infants, or the effects of the milk production.

## ROUTE & DOSAGE

| Chronic Idiopathic Constipation |
|---|
| *Adult:* **PO** 3 mg daily |

## ADMINISTRATION

### Gastric or Nasogastric
- Tablets may be mixed with water and administered through a gastric feeding tube.

- Mix 30 mL of room temperature water into a cup with the tablet and swirl for at least 15 sec, flush the feeding tube with 30 mL of water, draw up the mixture with a syringe and adminster the mixture via the feeding tube immediately.
- Add additional 30 mL of water to the cup if any part of the tablet remains, swirl for at least 15 sec, and use the same syringe to administer via the feeding tube.
- Flush the feeding tube with at least 10 mL of water after administration.

**Oral**
- Swallow tablets whole.
- Take with or without food
- If patient has difficulty swallowing, tablets may be crushed and administered orally with water or applesauce.
- For administration with water, mix 30 mL of room temperature water into a cup with the tablet, swirl for at least 10 sec, and swallow entire amount immediately; add an additional 30 mL of water if any part of the tablet remains, swirl again, swallow immediately; do not store for later use.
- For administration with applesauce, crush the tablet into a powder and mix with 1 teaspoonful of applesauce at room temperature, consume the entire mixture immediately, do not store for later use.
- Store at 20°–25° C (68°–77° F); excursions permitted to 15°–30° C (59°–86° F). Do not subdivide or repackage; protect from moisture.

**ADVERSE EFFECTS** (≥2%) **GI:** Diarrhea.

**PHARMACOKINETICS Absorption:** Minimal systemic absorption. **Metabolism:** Metabolized within GI tract to active metabolite; degraded in intestinal lumen to small peptides and amino acids.

## NURSING IMPLICATIONS

### Black Box Warning

*Safety and efficacy of plecanatide not established in patients younger than 18 y. Diarrhea, sometimes severe, has been reported and dose interruption was required. Risk of serious dehydration in pediatric patients.*

**Assessment & Drug Effects**
- Monitor the frequency and consistency of bowel movements.
- Monitor for S&S of dehydration.
- Improvement of constipation is indicative of efficacy.

**Patient & Family Education**
- Notify all health care providers that this drug is being taken. This includes doctors, nurses, pharmacists and dentists.
- If this drug is taken by accident, get help right away.
- Notify prescriber if you become pregnant or plan on getting pregnant while taking this drug.
- Notify prescriber if you are breastfeeding.
- Notify prescriber right away if very loose stools persist.
- If a dose is missed, skip the dose and go back to normal administration time. Do not take 2 doses at the same time or extra doses.
- Consult with prescriber before taking any other prescription drugs, over the counter drugs, natural products or vitamins.

Common adverse effects in *italic*; life-threatening effects underlined; generic names in **bold**; classifications in SMALL CAPS; ✦Canadian drug name; ⊘ Prototype drug

1313

# PLERIXAFOR
(ple-rix′a-for)

**Mozobil**

**Classification:** BIOLOGICAL RESPONSE MODIFIER; INHIBITOR OF CXCR4 CHEMOKINE RECEPTOR

**Therapeutic:** CXCR4 CHEMOKINE RECEPTOR INHIBITOR; STEM CELL MOBILIZER

**AVAILABILITY** Solution for injection

## ACTION & *THERAPEUTIC EFFECT*
A hematopoietic stem cell mobilizer that induces leukocytosis and increases the number of circulating hematopoietic progenitor cells. *Plerixafor enables collection of peripheral blood stem cell (PBSC) for autologous transplantation.*

**USES** In combination with granulocyte colony-stimulating factor (G-CSF), used to mobilize peripheral blood stem cell (PBSC) for collection and subsequent autologous transplantation in patients with non-Hodgkin's lymphoma and multiple myeloma.

**CONTRAINDICATIONS** Leukemia; pregnancy (category D); lactation.

**CAUTIOUS USE** Neutrophil count greater than 50,000/mm$^3$; thrombocytopenia; splenomegaly; moderate-to-severe renal impairment; concurrent drugs that reduce renal function. Safety and efficacy in children not established.

## ROUTE & DOSAGE

### Peripheral Blood Stem Cell Mobilization
*Adult:* **Subcutaneous** 0.24 mg/kg once daily (max: 0.40 mg/day), 11 h prior to initiation of apheresis; administer with filgrastim for up to 4 consecutive days.

### Renal Impairment Dosage Adjustment
*CrCl less than or equal to 50 mL/min:* Reduce dose to 0.16 mg/kg (max: 27 mg/day)

### Obesity Dosage Adjustment
Dose based on actual body weight up to 175% of IBW

## ADMINISTRATION
**Subcutaneous**
- Give undiluted approximately 11 h prior to apheresis.
- Calculate the required dose as follows: 0.012 × actual weight in kg = mL to administer. Note that each vial contains 1.2 mL of 20 mg/mL solution. Discard unused solution.
- Store single-use vials at 15°–30° C (59°–86° F).

**ADVERSE EFFECTS** (≥5%) **Body as a Whole:** *Arthralgia, injection-site reactions.* **CNS:** *Dizziness, fatigue, headache,* insomnia. **GI:** *Diarrhea,* flatulence, *nausea, vomiting.*

**PHARMACOKINETICS** **Peak:** 30–60 min. **Distribution:** 58% plasma protein bound. **Metabolism:** Not significantly metabolized. **Elimination:** Primarily in urine. **Half-Life:** 3–5 h.

## NURSING IMPLICATIONS
**Assessment & Drug Effects**
- Monitor (during and for 1 h after administration) for and promptly report: Signs of a systemic reaction (e.g., urticaria, periorbital swelling, dyspnea, or hypoxia); signs of splenic enlargement (e.g., upper abdominal pain and/or scapular or shoulder pain).

- Monitor for orthostatic hypotension and syncope during or within 1 h of drug injection. Monitor ambulation or take other precautions as warranted.
- Monitor injection sites for skin reactions.
- Monitor lab tests: Baseline and periodic WBC with differential.

**Patient & Family Education**
- Report promptly any discomfort experienced during or shortly after drug injection.
- Exercise caution when changing position from lying or sitting to standing as rapid movement shortly after injection may trigger fainting.
- Report skin reactions at the injection site (e.g., itching, rash swelling, or pain).
- Females should use effective contraception while taking this drug.

# PNEUMOCOCCAL 13-VALENT VACCINE, DIPHTHERIA

(noo-moe'кок-al)
**Prevnar 13**
**See Appendix J.**

# PODOPHYLLUM RESIN (PODOPHYLLIN)

(pode-oh-fill'um)
Podoben, Podofin

# PODOFILOX

Condylox

**Classification:** KERATOLYTIC
**Therapeutic:** CYTOTOXIC; KERATOLYTIC

**AVAILABILITY** **Podophyllum:** Liquid. **Podofilox:** Gel; solution

**ACTION & THERAPEUTIC EFFECT**
Directly affects epithelial cell metabolism by arresting mitosis through binding to protein subunits of microtubules. *Slow disruption of cells and tissue erosion as a result of its caustic action. Selectively affects embryonic and tumor cells more than adult cells.*

**USES** Benign growths including external genital and perianal warts, papillomas, fibroids.

**CONTRAINDICATIONS** Birthmarks, moles, or warts with hair growth from them; cervical, urethral, oral warts; normal skin and mucous membranes peripheral to treated areas; DM; patient with poor circulation; concurrent use of steroids; irritated, or bleeding skin; application of drug over large area.

**CAUTIOUS USE** Pregnancy (category C); lactation. Safe use in children is not known.

**ROUTE & DOSAGE**

**Condylomata Acuminata**
*Adult:* Topical Use 10% solution and repeat 1–2 × wk for up to 4 applications

**Verruca Vulgaris (Common Wart)**
*Adult:* Topical Apply 0.5% solution q12h for up to 4 wk

**Genital/Perianal Warts**
*Adult:* Topical Apply b.i.d. X 3 days then withhold treatment X 4 days, may repeat cycle up to 4 X

**ADMINISTRATION**
Note: Use 10–25% solution for areas less than 10 cm² or 5% solution for areas of 10–20 cm², anal, or genital warts; apply drug to dry surface, allowing area to dry between drops, wash off after 1–4 h.

Common adverse effects in *italic*; life-threatening effects underlined; generic names in **bold**; classifications in SMALL CAPS; ♣ Canadian drug name; ⊕ Prototype drug

1315

### Topical

- Avoid podophyllum resin contact with eyes or similar mucosal surfaces; if it occurs, flush thoroughly with lukewarm water for 15 min and remove film precipitated by the water.
- Avoid application of drug to normal tissue. If it occurs, remove with alcohol. Protect surfaces surrounding area to be treated with a layer of petrolatum or flexible collodion.
- Remove drug thoroughly with soap and water after each treatment of accessible tissue surface.
- Apply a protective coat of talcum powder after treatment and drying of anogenital area.
- Remove drug with alcohol, if application causes extreme pain, pruritus, or swelling.
- Store in a tight, light-resistant container; avoid exposure to excessive heat.

### ADVERSE EFFECTS (≥1%) Body as a Whole: Severe systemic toxicity (sometimes fatal), sensorimotor neuropathy (reversible), symptomatic orthostatic hypotension, paresthesias and weakness of extremities, stocking-glove sensory loss, absent ankle reflexes, decreased response to painful stimuli, fever. CNS: Lethargy, mental confusion, disorientation, delirium, agitation, seizures, progressive stupor, polyneuritis, pyrexia, coma, visual and auditory hallucinations, acute psychotic reaction, ataxia, hypotonia, areflexia, increased CSF protein. CV: Sinus tachycardia. Hematologic: Bone marrow suppression similar to that caused by antineoplastic drug toxicity, leukopenia, thrombocytopenia. GI: Nausea, vomiting, diarrhea, abdominal pain, hepatotoxicity, paralytic ileus, increased serum concentrations of LDH, AST, and alkaline phosphatase. Urogenital: Renal failure, urinary retention. Respiratory: Decreased respirations, apnea, hyperventilation.

## NURSING IMPLICATIONS

### Assessment & Drug Effects

- Warts become blanched, then necrotic within 24–48 h. Sloughing begins after about 72 h with no scarring. Frequently, a mild topical anti-infective agent, with or without a dressing, is applied until the healing is complete.
- Monitor neurologic status. Sensorimotor polyneuropathy, if it occurs, appears about 2 wk after application of drug, worsens for 3 mo, and may persist for up to 9 mo. Cerebral effects may persist for 7–10 days; ataxia, hypotonia, and areflexia improve more slowly than effects on sensorium.

### Patient & Family Education

- Learn proper technique of treatment if self-administered as treatment of verruca vulgaris (common wart). Also be fully aware of the need to report treatment failure to prescriber.
- Be aware that as with any STD, the patient's sex partner should be examined.
- Systemic toxicity may be severe and serious and is associated with application of drug to large areas, to tissue that is friable, bleeding, or recently biopsied, or for prolonged time. Toxicity may occur within hours of application. There are significant dangers from overuse or misuse of this drug.
- Learn symptoms of toxicity and report any that appear promptly to prescriber (see ADVERSE EFFECTS).

## POLYCARBOPHIL
(pol-i-kar'boe-fil)
Equalactin, FiberNorm

**Classifications:** BULK-PRODUCING LAXATIVE; ANTIDIARRHEAL

Common adverse effects in *italic*; life-threatening effects underlined; generic names in **bold**; classifications in SMALL CAPS; ✦ Canadian drug name; ⓟ Prototype drug

Therapeutic: BULK LAXATIVE;
ANTI-DIARRHEAL
**Prototype:** Psyllium

**AVAILABILITY** Tablet; chewable tablet

**ACTION & THERAPEUTIC EFFECT**
Hydrophilic agent that absorbs free water in intestinal tract and opposes dehydrating forces of bowel by forming a gelatinous mass. *Restores more normal moisture level and motility in the lower GI tract; produces well-formed stool and reduces diarrhea.*

**USES** Constipation or diarrhea associated with acute bowel syndrome, diverticulosis, irritable bowel and in patients who should not strain during defecation. Also choleretic diarrhea, diarrhea caused by small-bowel surgery or vagotomy, and disease of terminal ileum.

**CONTRAINDICATIONS** Partial or complete GI obstruction; fecal impaction; dysphagia; acute abdominal pain; rectal bleeding; undiagnosed abdominal pain, or other symptoms symptomatic of appendicitis; poisonings; before radiologic bowel examination; bowel surgery.

**CAUTIOUS USE** Renal failure, renal impairment; pregnancy (category C); children younger than 3 y.

**ROUTE & DOSAGE**

**Constipation or Diarrhea**

*Adult:* **PO** 1 g q.i.d. prn (max: 6 g/day)
*Child:* **PO** 3–6 y, 500 mg b.i.d. prn (max: 1.5 g/day); 6–12 y: 500 mg t.i.d. prn (max: 3 g/day)

**ADMINISTRATION**
**Oral**
▪ Chewable tablets should be chewed well before swallowing.
▪ Give each dose with a full glass [240 mL (8 oz)] of water or other liquid.
▪ Repeat dose every 30 min up to the maximum dose in 24 h in severe diarrhea.
▪ Store at 15°–30° C (59°–86° F) in tightly closed container unless otherwise directed.

**ADVERSE EFFECTS** (≥1%) **GI:** Esophageal blockage, intestinal impaction, *abdominal fullness.* **Metabolic:** Low serum potassium, elevated blood glucose levels (with extended use). **Respiratory:** Asthma. **Skin:** Skin rash.

**INTERACTIONS Drug:** May decrease absorption and clinical effects of ANTIBIOTICS, **warfarin, digoxin, nitrofurantoin,** SALICYLATES.

**PHARMACOKINETICS Absorption:** Not absorbed from GI tract. **Onset:** 12–24 h. **Peak:** 1–3 days.

**NURSING IMPLICATIONS**
**Assessment & Drug Effects**
▪ Determine duration and severity of diarrhea in order to anticipate signs of fluid-electrolyte losses.
▪ Monitor and record number and consistency of stools/day, presence and location of abdominal discomfort (i.e., tenderness, distention), and bowel sounds.
▪ Monitor and record I&O ratio and pattern. Dehydration is indicated if output is less than 30 mL/h.
▪ Inspect oral cavity for dryness, and be alert to systemic signs of dehydration (e.g., thirst and fever). Dehydration from an episode of diarrhea appears rapidly in young children and older adults.

P

---

### Patient & Family Education

- Consult prescriber if sudden changes in bowel habit persist more than 1 wk, action is minimal or ineffective for 1 wk, or if there is no antidiarrheal action within 2 days.
- Be aware that extended use of this drug may cause dependence for normal bowel function.
- Do not discontinue polycarbophil unless prescriber advises if also taking an oral anticoagulant, digoxin, salicylates, or nitrofurantoin.

## POLYMYXIN B SULFATE

(pol-i-mix′in)

**Classifications:** ANTIBIOTIC; POLYMYXIN
**Therapeutic:** ANTIBIOTIC

**AVAILABILITY** Solution for injection

### ACTION & *THERAPEUTIC EFFECT*

Binds to lipid phosphates in bacterial membranes and changes permeability to permit leakage of cytoplasm from bacterial cells, resulting in cell death. *Bactericidal against susceptible gram-negative but not gram-positive organisms.*

**USES** Topically and in combination with other anti-infectives or corticosteroids for various superficial infections of eye, ear, mucous membrane, and skin. Concurrent systemic anti-infective therapy may be required for treatment of intraocular infection and severe progressive corneal ulcer. Used parenterally only in hospitalized patients for treatment of severe acute infections of urinary tract, bloodstream, and meninges; and in combination with Neosporin for continuous bladder irrigation to prevent bacteremia associated with use of indwelling catheter.

**CONTRAINDICATIONS** Hypersensitivity to polymyxin antibiotics; respiratory insufficiency; concurrent use of products that inhibit peristalsis, skeletal muscle relaxants, ether, or sodium citrate.

**CAUTIOUS USE** Impaired kidney function, renal failure; inflammatory bowel disease; myasthenia gravis; pulmonary disease. **IV/IM form:** Pregnancy (category C); lactation. **Topical form:** Pregnancy (category B). Safety and efficacy in children younger than 1 mo not established.

### ROUTE & DOSAGE

**Infections**

*Adult/Child:* **IV** 15,000–25,000 units/kg/day divided q12h; **IM** 25,000–30,000 units/kg/day divided q4–6h; **Intrathecal** 50,000 units × 3–4 days then every other day × 2 wk; *younger than 2 y:* 20,000 units × 3–4 days, then 25,000 units every other day
*Infant:* **IV** Up to 40,000 units/kg/day

**Renal Impairment Dosage Adjustment**

Reduce, specific dose unknown

### ADMINISTRATION

**Intramuscular**

- Routine administration by IM routes not recommended because it causes intense discomfort, along the peripheral nerve distribution, 40–60 min after IM injection.
- Make IM injection in adults deep into upper outer quadrant of buttock. Select IM site carefully to avoid injection into nerves or blood vessels. Rotate injection

P

sites. Follow agency policy for IM site used in children.

**Intravenous**

*PREPARE:* **Intermittent:** Reconstitute by dissolving 500,000 units in 5 mL sterile water for injection or NS to yield 100,000 units/mL. Withdraw a single dose and then further dilute in 300–500 mL of D5W.

*ADMINISTER:* **Intermittent:** Infuse over period of 60–90 min. ▪ Inspect injection site for signs of phlebitis and irritation.

*INCOMPATIBILITIES:* **Solution/additive: Amphotericin B, cefazolin, cephalothin, cephapirin, chloramphenicol, heparin, nitrofurantoin, prednisolone, tetracycline.**

▪ Protect unreconstituted product and reconstituted solution from light and freezing. Store in refrigerator at 2°–8° C (36°–46° F). ▪ Parenteral solutions are stable for 1 wk when refrigerated. Discard unused portion after 72 h.

**ADVERSE EFFECTS** (≥1%) **Body as a Whole:** Irritability, facial flushing, ataxia, circumoral, lingual, and peripheral paresthesias (stocking-glove distribution); severe pain (IM site), thrombophlebitis (IV site), superinfections, electrolyte disturbances (prolonged use; also reported in patients with acute leukemia); local irritation and burning (topical use), anaphylactoid reactions (rare). **CNS:** Drowsiness, dizziness, vertigo, convulsions, coma; neuromuscular blockade (generalized muscle weakness, respiratory depression or arrest); meningeal irritation, increased protein and cell count in cerebrospinal fluid, fever, headache, stiff neck (intrathecal use). **Special Senses:** Blurred vision, nystagmus, slurred speech, dysphagia, ototoxicity (vestibular and auditory) with high doses. **GI:** GI disturbances. **Urogenital:** Albuminuria, cylindruria, azotemia, hematuria; nephrotoxicity.

**INTERACTIONS Drug:** ANESTHETICS and NEUROMUSCULAR BLOCKING AGENTS may prolong skeletal muscle relaxation. AMINOGLYCOSIDES, LOOP DIURETICS, and **amphotericin B** have additive nephrotoxic potential.

**PHARMACOKINETICS Peak:** 2 h IM. **Distribution:** Widely distributed except to CSF, synovial fluid, and eye; does not cross placenta. **Metabolism:** Unknown. **Elimination:** 60% excreted unchanged in urine. **Half-Life:** 4.3–6 h.

## NURSING IMPLICATIONS

**Black Box Warning**

*Polymixin B has been associated with nephrotoxicity and neurotoxicity.*

### Assessment & Drug Effects

▪ Review electrolyte results. Patients with low serum calcium are particularly prone to develop neuromuscular blockade.
▪ Inspect tongue every day. Assess for S&S of superinfection (see Appendix F). Polymyxin therapy supports growth of opportunistic organisms. Report symptoms promptly.
▪ Monitor I&O. Maintain fluid intake sufficient to maintain daily urinary output of at least 1500 mL. Some degree of renal toxicity usually occurs within first 3 or 4 days of therapy even with therapeutic doses. Consult prescriber.
▪ Withhold drug and report findings to prescriber for any of the

P

Common adverse effects in *italic*; life-threatening effects underlined; generic names in **bold**; classifications in SMALL CAPS; ♣ Canadian drug name; ⊘ Prototype drug

1319

following: Decreases in urine output (change in I&O ratio), proteinuria, cellular casts, rising BUN, serum creatinine, or serum drug levels (not associated with dosage increase). All can be interpreted as signs of nephrotoxicity.

- Nephrotoxicity is generally reversible, but it may progress even after drug is discontinued. Therefore, close monitoring of kidney function is essential, even following termination of therapy.
- Be alert for respiratory arrest after the first dose and also as long as 45 days after initiation of therapy. It occurs most commonly in patients with kidney failure and high plasma drug levels and is often preceded by dyspnea and restlessness.
- Monitor lab tests: Baseline C&S and renal function tests; frequent serum drug levels during therapy.

**Patient & Family Education**
- Report to prescriber immediately any muscle weakness, shortness of breath, dyspnea, depressed respiration. These symptoms are rapidly reversible if drug is withdrawn.
- Report promptly to prescriber transient neurologic disturbances (burning or prickling sensations, numbness, dizziness). All occur commonly and usually respond to dosage reduction.
- Report promptly to prescriber the onset of stiff neck and headache (possible symptoms of neurotoxic reactions, including neuromuscular blockade). This response is usually associated with high serum drug levels or nephrotoxicity.
- Report promptly S&S of superinfection (see Appendix F).
- Report any S&S of colitis for up to 2 mo following discontinuation of drug.

# PONATINIB
(poe-na′ti-nib)
Iclusig

**Classifications:** ANTINEOPLASTIC; KINASE INHIBITOR
**Therapeutic:** ANTINEOPLASTIC
**Prototype:** Erlotinib

## AVAILABILITY Tablet

## ACTION & *THERAPEUTIC EFFECT*
Inhibits the action of certain tyrosine kinases (a family of enzymes needed for viability of leukemia cells) *thus inhibiting the growth and replication of mutant leukemic cells.*

## USES Treatment of chronic phase, accelerated phase, or blast phase chronic myeloid leukemia (CML) and Philadelphia chromosome-positive acute lymphocytic leukemia (Ph+ALL) that is resistant or intolerant to prior tyrosine kinase inhibitor therapy.

## CONTRAINDICATIONS Arterial thrombosis; stroke or MI, severe CHF, serious or severe hemorrhage induced by ponatinib; hepatotoxicity; tumor lysis syndrome; severe myelosuppression; compromised wound healing; GI perforation; pregnancy (category D); lactation.

## CAUTIOUS USE CHF, hypertension, cardiac arrhythmias, myelosuppression, DVT; pancreatitis; fluid retention; moderate to severe hepatic impairment.

## ROUTE & DOSAGE

**Chronic Myeloid Leukemia (CML)/Acute Lymphocyte Leukemia (ALL)**

*Adult:* **PO** 45 mg once daily

Common adverse effects in *italic*; life-threatening effects underlined; generic names in **bold**; classifications in SMALL CAPS; ♣ Canadian drug name; ⦿ Prototype drug

### Hepatic Impairment Dosage Adjustment

*Moderate or severe (Child-Pugh class B or C) impairment:*
Avoid use

### Myelosuppression Dosage Adjustment

*ANC less than $1 \times 10^9$/L or platelet less than $50 \times 10^9$/L*

*First occurrence:* Withhold until AMC is greater than or equal to $1.5 \times 10^9$/L and platelet is greater than or equal to $75 \times 10^9$/L, then resume at 45 mg
*Second occurrence:* Withhold until AMC is greater than or equal to $1.5 \times 10^9$/L and platelet is greater than or equal to $75 \times 10^9$/L, then resume at 30 mg
*Third occurrence:* Withhold until AMC is greater than or equal to $1.5 \times 10^9$/L and platelet is greater than or equal to $75 \times 10^9$/L, then resume at 15 mg

### Hepatotoxicity Dosage Adjustment

*Liver transaminase Grade 2 or higher (greater than $3 \times ULN$)*

*At 45 mg dose:* Withhold then resume at 30 mg when less than or equal to Grade 1 (less than $3 \times ULN$)

*At 30 mg dose:* Withhold then resume at 15 mg when less than or equal to Grade 1

*At 15 mg or with a concurrent elevation of bilirubin greater than $2 \times ULN$ and alkaline phosphatase less than $2 \times ULN$:*
Discontinue

### Pancreatitis and Lipase Elevations Dosage Adjustment

*Asymptomatic Grade 3 or 4 elevation of lipase (greater than $2 \times ULN$) or Grade 2 pancreatitis*

*At 45 mg dose:* Withhold then resume at 30 mg when less than or equal to Grade 1 (less than $1.5 \times ULN$)

*At 30 mg dose:* Withhold then resume at 15 mg when less than or equal to Grade 1

*At 15 mg:* Discontinue

### Symptomatic Grade 3 Pancreatitis

*At 45 mg dose:* Withhold then resume at 30 mg after complete resolution of symptoms and lipase elevation less than or equal to Grade 1

*At 30 mg dose:* Withhold then resume at 15 mg after complete resolution of symptoms and lipase elevation less than or equal to Grade 1

*At 15 mg:* Discontinue

### Strong CYP3A4 Inhibitors Dosage Adjustment

30 mg once daily

## ADMINISTRATION

**Oral**
- May give without regard to food.
- Tablets must be swallowed whole. They must not be crushed or chewed.
- Store at 15°–30° C (59°–86° F).

**ADVERSE EFFECTS (≥1%) Body as a Whole:** Chills, febrile neutropenia, peripheral edema, *pyrexia*, sepsis. **CNS:** Asthenia, dizziness, hemorrage, *fatigue*, *headache*,

Common adverse effects in *italic*; life-threatening effects underlined; generic names in **bold**; classifications in SMALL CAPS; ♣ Canadian drug name; ● Prototype drug

1321

insomnia, pain, peripheral neuropathy. **CV:** <u>Arterial fibrillation</u>, <u>ischemia</u>, <u>cardiac failure</u>, *hypertension*, <u>myocardial infarction</u>, pericardial effusion, peripheral arterial disease, <u>stroke</u> or TIA, <u>venous thromboembolism</u>. **GI:** *Abdominal pain and discomfort*, *constipation*, decreased appetite, diarrhea, <u>GI hemorrhage</u>, *nausea*, oral mucositis, pancreatitis, vomiting, weight loss. **Hematological:** Anemia, febrile neutropenia, leukopenia, lymphopenia, neutropenia, thrombocytopenia. **Metabolic:** Albumin decreased, alkaline phosphatase increased, ALT/AST increased, amylase increased, bicarbonate decreased, bilirubin increased, creatinine increased, hypercalcemia, hyperglycemia, hyperkalemia, hypernatremia, hypocalcemia, hypoglycemia, hypokalemia, hyponatremia, lipase increased, phosphorous decreased, triglycerides increased. **Musculoskeletal:** *Arthralgia*, back pain, bone pain, muscle spasms, myalgia, pain in extremity. **Respiratory:** Cough, dyspnea, nasopharyngitis, pleural effusion, pneumonia, upper respiratory tract infection. **Skin:** Cellulitis, *dry skin*, rash, and *related conditions*. **Urogenital:** Urinary tract infection.

**INTERACTIONS** **Drug:** Coadministration with strong CYP3A4 inducers (e.g., **carbamazepine, phenytoin, rifampin**) may decrease the levels of ponatinib. Coadministration with strong CYP3A4 inhibitors (e.g., **boceprevir, clarithromycin, conivaptan, indinavir, itraconazole, ketoconazole, lopinavir, nefazodone, nelfinavir, posaconazole, ritonavir, saquinavir, telaprenavir, telithromycin, voriconazole**) may increase the levels of ponatinib. Coadministration with drugs that elevate gastric pH (e.g., ANTACIDS, H$_2$ BLOCKERS, PROTON PUMP INHIBITORS) may decrease the levels of ponatinib. Studies have yet been done; however, since ponatinib inhibits the ABCG2 and P-gp transporter systems, it may alter the transport of drugs requiring either of these transporters. **Food:** Grapefruit juice may increase the levels of ponatinib. **Herbal: St. John's wort** may decrease the levels of ponatinib.

**PHARMACOKINETICS Peak:** 6 h. **Distribution:** Greater than 99% plasma protein bound. **Metabolism:** Hepatic oxidation and hydrolysis. **Elimination:** Fecal (87%) and renal (5%). **Half-Life:** 24 h.

## NURSING IMPLICATIONS

### Black Box Warning

*Ponatinib has been associated with cardiovascular, cerebrovascular, and peripheral vascular thrombosis, including fatal MI and stroke; and with hepatotoxicity and liver failure.*

### Assessment & Drug Effects

- Monitor cardiovascular status closely.
- Report bradycardia, development of edema, and S&S of CHF.
- Monitor I&O and daily weight. Report rapid weight gain.
- Monitor BP frequently. Be alert for S&S of hypertensive crisis (e.g., confusion, headache, chest pain, or shortness of breath).
- Monitor for and promptly report S&S of hepatotoxicity or pancreatitis.
- Monitor lab tests: Baseline and monthly LFTs; serum lipase q2wk for first month, and monthly thereafter or more often as indicated; CBC with differential and platelet count q2wk for the first 3 mo; periodic serum electrolytes and uric acid.

Common adverse effects in *italic*; life-threatening effects <u>underlined</u>; generic names in **bold**; classifications in SMALL CAPS; ✚ Canadian drug name; ⦿ Prototype drug

### Patient & Family Education

- Do not drink grapefruit juice while taking this drug.
- Report promptly signs of thrombosis (e.g., chest pain, shortness of breath, one-sided weakness, speech problems, leg pain or swelling).
- Report promptly signs of liver toxicity (e.g., jaundice, dark urine, clay-colored stool).
- Report promptly signs of heart failure (e.g., shortness of breath, chest pain, palpitations, dizziness, fainting, rapid weight gain, abdominal swelling).
- Women should use effective means of contraception to avoid pregnancy as ponatinib can cause severe fetal harm.

---

## PORACTANT ALFA ℗

(por·ac'tant)

Curosurf

**Classification:** LUNG SURFACTANT
**Therapeutic:** LUNG SURFACTANT

---

**AVAILABILITY** Suspension

**ACTION & THERAPEUTIC EFFECT**
Endogenous pulmonary surfactant lowers the surface tension on alveoli surfaces during respiration, and stabilizes the alveoli against collapse at resting pressures. *Alleviates respiratory distress syndrome (RDS) in premature infants caused by deficiency of surfactant.*

**USES** Treatment (rescue) of respiratory distress syndrome in premature infants.

**CONTRAINDICATIONS** Hypersensitivity to porcine products or poractant alpha.

**CAUTIOUS USE** Infants born more than 3 wk after ruptured membranes; intraventricular hemorrhage

of grade III or IV; major congenital malformations; nosocomial infection; pretreatment of hypothermia or acidosis due to increased risk of intracranial hemorrhage.

## ROUTE & DOSAGE

**Respiratory Distress Syndrome**

*Neonate:* **Intratracheal** 2.5 mL/kg birth weight, may repeat with 1.25 mL/kg q12h × 2 more doses if needed (max: 5 mL/kg)

## ADMINISTRATION

Note: Correction of acidosis, hypotension, anemia, hypoglycemia, and hypothermia is recommended prior to administration of poractant alfa.

**Intratracheal**

- Warm vial slowly to room temperature; gently turn upside down to form uniform suspension, but do not shake.
- Withdraw slowly the entire contents of a vial (concentration equals 80 mg/mL) into a 3 or 5 mL syringe through a large gauge (greater than 20 gauge) needle.
- Attach a 5 French catheter, precut to 8 cm, to the syringe.
- Fill the catheter with poractant alfa and discard excess through the catheter so that only the total dose to be given remains in the syringe.
- Refer to specific instruction provided by manufacturer for proper dosing technique. Follow instructions carefully regarding installation of drug and ventilation of infant. Note that catheter tip should not extend beyond distal tip of endotracheal tube.
- Store refrigerated at 2°–8° C (36°–46° F) and protect from light. Do not shake vials. Do not warm to room temperature and return to refrigeration more than once.

P

---

Common adverse effects in *italic*; life-threatening effects underlined; generic names in **bold**; classifications in SMALL CAPS; ✦Canadian drug name; ℗ Prototype drug

1323

**ADVERSE EFFECTS** (≥1%) **CV:** Bradycardia, hypotension. **Respiratory:** Intratracheal tube blockage, oxygen desaturation; pulmonary hemorrhage.

**PHARMACOKINETICS** Not studied.

## NURSING IMPLICATIONS

### Assessment & Drug Effects

- Stop administration of poractant alfa and take appropriate measures if any of the following occur: Transient episodes of bradycardia, decreased oxygen saturation, reflux of poractant alfa into endotracheal tube, or airway obstruction. Dosing may resume after stabilization.
- Do not suction airway for 1 h after poractant alfa instillation unless there is significant airway obstruction.

---

## POSACONAZOLE

(pos-a-con'a-zole)

Noxafil

**Classification:** AZOLE ANTIFUNGAL

Therapeutic: ANTIFUNGAL

**Prototype:** Fluconazole

**AVAILABILITY** Oral suspension; delayed release tablets

## ACTION & THERAPEUTIC EFFECT

Inhibits ergosterol synthesis, the principal sterol in the fungal cell membrane, thus interfering with the functions of fungal cell membrane. This results in increased membrane permeability causing leakage of cellular contents. *Has a broad spectrum of antifungal activity against common fungal pathogens.*

**USES** Prophylactic treatment of invasive *Aspergillus* and *Candida*, oropharyngeal candidiasis.

**UNLABELED USES** Treatment of febrile neutropenia or refractory invasive fungal infection; treatment of periorbital cellulitis due to *Rhizopus* sp.; treatment of refractory histoplasmosis; treatment of refractory coccidioidomycosis; treatment of fungal necrotizing fasciitis.

**CONTRAINDICATIONS** Hypersensitivity to posaconazole or other azole antifungals; coadministration with sirolimus, ergot alkaloids, or CYP3A4 substrates; history of QT prolongation; abnormal levels of potassium, magnesium, or calcium; liver disease caused by posaconazole; lactation.

**CAUTIOUS USE** Hypersensitivity to other azole antifungal antibiotics; hepatic disease or hepatitis; cardiac arrhythmias, hypokalemia; history of proarrhythmic conditions; CHF, myocardial ischemia, atrial fibrillation; AIDS; obesity; severe renal impairment; pregnancy (category C); children younger than 13 y.

## ROUTE & DOSAGE

| Prophylactic Treatment of Invasive *Aspergillus* and *Candida* Infections |
| --- |
| *Adult/Adolescent:* **PO** 200 mg t.i.d. |
| **Thrush** |
| *Adult/Adolescent:* **PO Oral Suspension** 100 mg b.i.d. × 1 day then 100 mg qd × 13 days; **PO Tablet** 300 mg b.i.d. for one day then 300 mg daily until recovery |

## ADMINISTRATION

### Oral Suspension

- Shake well before use. Give with a full meal or liquid nutritional supplement.

**Oral Tablet**
- Swallow whole, do not crush. Administer with food.
- Store at 15°–30° C (59°–86° F).

## ADVERSE EFFECTS (≥1%) Body as a Whole:
Anxiety, *bacteremia, dizziness, edema, fatigue, fever, headache, infection, insomnia, rigors,* weakness. **CNS:** QT/QT$_c$ prolongation, tremor. **CV:** *Hypertension, hypotension, tachycardia.* **GI:** *Abdominal pain, anorexia constipation, diarrhea, dyspepsia, mucositis, nausea,* vomiting. **Hematologic:** *Anemia, febrile neutropenia, neutropenia, petechiae,* thrombocytopenia. **Metabolic:** *Bilirubinemia,* creatinine levels increased, elevated liver enzymes, *hypocalcemia, hyperglycemia, hypokalemia, hypomagnesemia.* **Musculoskeletal:** *Arthralgia, back pain, musculoskeletal pain.* **Respiratory:** *Cough, dyspnea, epistaxis, pharyngitis,* upper respiratory tract infection. **Skin:** *Pruritus, rash.* **Special Senses:** Blurred vision, taste disturbances. **Urogenital:** *Vaginal hemorrhage.*

## INTERACTIONS Drug:
Posaconazole is known to increase the plasma levels of **cyclosporine, tacrolimus, rifabutin, midazolam,** and **phenytoin.** Coadministration with other drugs that cause QT prolongation (e.g., **quinidine**) can result in torsades de pointes. Posaconazole may increase the plasma levels of ERGOT ALKALOIDS, VINCA ALKALOIDS, HMG COA REDUCTASE INHIBITORS, and CALCIUM CHANNEL BLOCKERS. Avoid use with cimetidine, efavirenz, esomeprazole, phenytoin, due to decreases in efficacy. **Food:** Administration with food increases absorption of posaconazole.

## PHARMACOKINETICS Peak:
3–5 h. **Distribution:** 98% protein bound. **Metabolism:** Conjugated to inactive metabolites. **Elimination:** Primarily fecal elimination (71%) with minor renal elimination. **Half-Life:** 35 h.

## NURSING IMPLICATIONS
### Assessment & Drug Effects
- Monitor for and report S&S of breakthrough fungal infections, especially in those with severe renal impairment, or experiencing vomiting and diarrhea, or who cannot tolerate a full meal or supplement along with posaconazole.
- Monitor and report degree of improvement of oropharyngeal candidiasis.
- Monitor those with proarrhythmic conditions for development of arrhythmias.
- Withhold drug and notify prescriber of abnormal serum potassium, magnesium, or calcium levels.
- Monitor blood levels of phenytoin, cyclosporine, tacrolimus, and sirolimus with concurrent therapy. Monitor for adverse effects of concurrently administered statins or calcium channel blockers.
- Monitor lab tests: Baseline and periodic LFTs; periodic renal function tests, serum electrolytes, and CBC.

### Patient & Family Education
- Do not take any prescription or nonprescription drugs without informing your prescriber.
- Know parameters for withholding drug (i.e., inability to take with a full meal or nutritional supplement).
- Report immediately any of the following to your health care provider: Vomiting, diarrhea, inability to eat, jaundice of skin, yellowing of eyes, itching, or skin rash.

---

Common adverse effects in *italic*; life-threatening effects underlined; generic names in **bold**; classifications in SMALL CAPS; ♣Canadian drug name; ☻ Prototype drug

# POTASSIUM CHLORIDE
(poe-tass'ee-um)
Apo-K ♣, K-Dur, K-Long ♣,
KCl 5% and 20%, Klor,
Klor-10%, Klor-Con, Micro-K
Extentabs, Slo-Pot ♣

# POTASSIUM GLUCONATE
**Classification:** ELECTROLYTIC
REPLACEMENT SOLUTION
Therapeutic: ELECTROLYTE
REPLACEMENT

**AVAILABILITY** **Chloride:** Sustained release tablet; tablet; effervescent tablet; liquid; powder; solution for injection; vial. **Gluconate:** Liquid

## ACTION & *THERAPEUTIC EFFECT*
Principal intracellular cation that is essential for maintenance of intracellular isotonicity, transmission of nerve impulses, contraction of cardiac, skeletal, and smooth muscles, maintenance of normal kidney function, and for enzyme activity. *Effectiveness in hypokalemia is measured by serum potassium concentration greater than 3.5 mEq/L.*

**USES** To prevent and treat potassium deficit; effective in the treatment of hypokalemic alkalosis (chloride, not the gluconate).

**CONTRAINDICATIONS** Severe renal impairment; severe hemolytic reactions; untreated Addison's disease; crush syndrome; early postoperative oliguria (except during GI drainage); adynamic ileus; acute dehydration; heat cramps; hyperkalemia, patients receiving potassium-sparing diuretics; digitalis intoxication with AV conduction disturbance.

**CAUTIOUS USE** Cardiac or kidney disease; systemic acidosis;

slow-release potassium preparations in presence of delayed GI transit or Meckel's diverticulum; extensive tissue breakdown (such as severe burns); pregnancy (category C); lactation.

## ROUTE & DOSAGE

### Hypokalemia
*Adult:* **PO** 40–100 mEq/day in divided doses; **IV** Dose per package insert dependent on current serum potassium concentration
*Child:* **PO** 2–5 mEq/kg/day in divided doses; sustained release tablets not recommended; **IV** 0.25–0.5 mEq/kg/dose (max: 40 mEq/day)

### Prevention of Hypokalemia
*Adult:* **PO** 20 mEq/day in 1–2 doses
*Child:* **PO** 1–2 mEq/kg/day in 1–2 doses

## ADMINISTRATION
### Oral
- Give while patient is sitting up or standing (never in recumbent position) to prevent drug-induced esophagitis. Some patients find it difficult to swallow the large sized KCl tablet.
- Do not crush or allow to chew any potassium salt tablets. Observe to make sure patient does not suck tablet (oral ulcerations have been reported if tablet is allowed to dissolve in mouth).
- Swallow whole tablet with a large glass of water or fruit juice (if allowed) to wash drug down and to start esophageal peristalsis.
- Follow exactly directions for diluting various liquid forms of KCl. In general, dilute each 20 mEq potassium in at least 90 mL water or juice and allow to dissolve completely before administration.

P

- Dilute liquid forms as directed before giving it through nasogastric tube.

**Intravenous**

*PREPARE:* **IV Infusion:** Add desired amount to 100–1000 mL IV solution (compatible with all standard solutions). ▪ Usual maximum is 80 mEq/1000 mL, however, 40 mEq/L is preferred to lessen irritation to veins. Note: **NEVER** add KCl to an IV bag/bottle which is hanging. ▪ After adding KCl invert bag/bottle several times to ensure even distribution.

*ADMINISTER:* **IV Infusion for Adult/Child:** KCl is **never** given direct IV or in concentrated amounts by any route. ▪ Too rapid infusion may cause fatal hyperkalemia. **IV Infusion for Adult:** Infuse at rate not to exceed 10 mEq/h; in emergency situations, may infuse very cautiously up to 40 mEq/h with continuous cardiac monitoring. **IV Infusion for Child:** Infuse at a rate not to exceed 0.5–1.0 mEq/kg/h.

*INCOMPATIBILITIES:* Solution/additive: **Amoxicillin/clavulanate furosemide, imipenem-cilastin pentobarbital, phenobarbital, succinylcholine.** Y-site: **Amphotericin B cholesteryl complex, azithromycin, dantrolene, diazepam, ergotamine, lansoprazole, methylprednisolone, phenytoin, sulfamethoxazole/trimethoprim.**

▪ Take extreme care to prevent extravasation and infiltration. At first sign, discontinue infusion and select another site.

**ADVERSE EFFECTS** (≥1%) **GI:** *Nausea, vomiting,* diarrhea, abdominal distention, abdominal pain. **Body as a Whole:** Pain, mental confusion, irritability, listlessness, rash, phlebitis, paresthesias of extremities, muscle weakness and heaviness of limbs, difficulty in swallowing, <u>flaccid paralysis</u>. **Urogenital:** Oliguria, anuria. **Hematologic:** Hyperkalemia. **Respiratory:** <u>Respiratory distress</u>. **CV:** Hypotension, bradycardia; <u>cardiac depression, arrhythmias, or arrest;</u> altered sensitivity to digitalis glycosides. *ECG changes in hyperkalemia:* Tenting (peaking) of T wave (especially in right precordial leads), lowering of R with deepening of S waves and depression of RST; prolonged P-R interval, widened QRS complex, decreased amplitude and disappearance of P waves, prolonged QT interval, signs of right and left bundle block, <u>deterioration of QRS contour and finally ventricular fibrillation</u> and <u>death</u>.

**INTERACTIONS Drug:** POTASSIUM-SPARING DIURETICS, ANGIOTENSIN-CONVERTING ENZYME (ACE) INHIBITORS, ANTICHOLINERGIC AGENTS may cause hyperkalemia. Use with CALCIUM SALTS can cause metabolic acidosis. **Food:** Salty foods could increase the risk of hyperkalemia.

**PHARMACOKINETICS Absorption:** Readily from upper GI tract. **Elimination:** 90% in urine, 10% in feces.

## NURSING IMPLICATIONS
### Assessment & Drug Effects
- Monitor I&O ratio and pattern in patients receiving the parenteral drug. If oliguria occurs, stop infusion promptly and notify prescriber.
- Monitor for and report signs of GI ulceration (esophageal or epigastric pain or hematemesis).
- Monitor cardiac status of patients receiving parenteral potassium. Irregular heartbeat is usually the earliest clinical indication of hyperkalemia.

P

Common adverse effects in *italic*; life-threatening effects <u>underlined</u>; generic names in **bold**; classifications in SMALL CAPS; ♣Canadian drug name; ⊕ Prototype drug

1327

- Be alert for potassium intoxication (hyperkalemia, see S&S, Appendix F); may result from any therapeutic dosage, and the patient may be asymptomatic.
- The risk of hyperkalemia with potassium supplement increases (1) in older adults because of decremental changes in kidney function associated with aging, (2) when dietary intake of potassium suddenly increases, and (3) when kidney function is significantly compromised.
- Monitor lab tests: Baseline and periodic serum potassium.

**Patient & Family Education**

- Do not be alarmed when the tablet carcass appears in your stool. The sustained release tablet (e.g., Slow-K) utilizes a wax matrix as carrier for KCl crystals that passes through the digestive system.
- Learn about sources of potassium with special reference to foods and OTC drugs.
- Do not use any salt substitute unless it is specifically ordered by the prescriber. These contain a substantial amount of potassium and electrolytes other than sodium.
- Do not self-prescribe laxatives. Chronic laxative use has been associated with diarrhea-induced potassium loss.
- Notify prescriber of persistent vomiting because losses of potassium can occur.
- Report continuing signs of potassium deficit to prescriber: Weakness, fatigue, polyuria, polydipsia.
- Advise dentist or new prescriber that a potassium drug has been prescribed as long-term maintenance therapy.
- Do not open foil-wrapped powders and tablets before use.

# POTASSIUM IODIDE
(poe-tass'ee-um)

Pima, SSKI, Thyro-Block ◆

**Classifications:** ANTITHYROID; EXPECTORANT
Therapeutic: ANTITHYROID; EXPECTORANT
**Prototype:** Guaifenesin

## AVAILABILITY Syrup; solution

## ACTION & *THERAPEUTIC EFFECT*

Appears to increase secretion of respiratory fluids by direct action on bronchial tissue, thereby decreasing mucus viscosity. When the thyroid gland is hyperplastic, excess iodide ions temporarily inhibit secretion of thyroid hormone, foster accumulation in thyroid follicles, and decrease vascularity of gland. *Administration for hyperthyroidism is limited to short-term therapy. As an expectorant, the iodine ion increases mucous secretion formation in bronchi, and decreases viscosity of mucus.*

## USES To facilitate bronchial drainage and cough in emphysema, asthma, chronic bronchitis, bronchiectasis, and respiratory tract allergies characterized by difficult-to-raise sputum. Also used alone for hyperthyroidism or in conjunction with antithyroid drugs and propranolol in treatment of thyrotoxic crisis; in immediate preoperative period for thyroidectomy to decrease vascularity, fragility, and size of thyroid gland and for treatment of persistent or recurring hyperthyroidism that occurs in Graves' disease patients. Used as a radiation protectant in patients receiving radioactive iodine and to shield the thyroid gland from radiation in

P

the wake of a serious nuclear plant accident. (Use as an expectorant has been largely replaced by other agents.)

## CONTRAINDICATIONS
Hypersensitivity or idiosyncrasy to iodine; hyperthyroidism; hyperkalemia; acute bronchitis; pregnancy (category D); lactation.

## CAUTIOUS USE
Renal impairment; cardiac disease; pulmonary tuberculosis; Addison's disease.

## ROUTE & DOSAGE

**To Reduce Thyroid Vascularity**
*Adult/Child:* **PO** 50–250 mg t.i.d. for 10–14 days before surgery

**Expectorant**
*Adult:* **PO** 300–650 mg p.c. b.i.d. or t.i.d.
*Child:* **PO** 60–250 mg p.c. b.i.d. or t.i.d.

**Thyroid Blocking in Radiation Emergency**
*Adult:* **PO** 130 mg/day for 10 days
*Child (younger than 1 y):* **PO** 65 mg/day for 10 days; *1 y or older:* 130 mg/day for 10 days

## ADMINISTRATION
**Oral**
- Give with meals in a full glass (240 mL) of water or fruit juice and at bedtime with juice to disguise salty taste and minimize gastric distress.
- Avoid giving KI with milk; absorption of the drug may be decreased by dairy products.
- Adhere strictly to schedule and accurate dose measurements when iodide is administered to prepare thyroid gland for surgery, particularly at end of treatment period when possibility of "escape" (from iodide) effect on thyroid gland increases.
- Place container in warm water and gently agitate to dissolve if crystals are noted in the solution.
- Discard any solution that has turned a brownish yellow on standing, especially if exposed to light (caused by liberated trace of free iodine).
- Store in airtight, light-resistant container.

## ADVERSE EFFECTS (≥1%)
**GI:** Diarrhea, nausea, vomiting, stomach pain, nonspecific small bowel lesions (associated with enteric coated tablets). **Body as a Whole:** <u>Angioneurotic edema</u>, cutaneous and mucosal hemorrhage, fever, arthralgias, lymph node enlargement, eosinophilia, paresthesias, periorbital edema, weakness. *Iodine poisoning (iodism):* Metallic taste, stomatitis, salivation, coryza, sneezing; swollen and tender salivary glands (sialadenitis), frontal headache, vomiting (blue vomitus if stomach contained starches, otherwise yellow vomitus), bloody diarrhea. **Metabolic:** Hyperthyroid adenoma, goiter, hypothyroidism, collagen disease-like syndromes. **CV:** Irregular heartbeat. **CNS:** Mental confusion. **Skin:** Acneiform skin lesions (prolonged use), flare-up of adolescent acne. **Respiratory:** Productive cough, pulmonary edema.

## DIAGNOSTIC TEST INTERFERENCE
Potassium iodide may alter ***thyroid function*** test results and may interfere with ***urinary 17-OHCS*** determinations.

## INTERACTIONS
**Drug:** ANTITHYROID DRUGS, **lithium** may potentiate hypothyroid and goitrogenic

Common adverse effects in *italic*; life-threatening effects <u>underlined</u>; generic names in **bold**; classifications in SMALL CAPS; ♣Canadian drug name; ⊙ Prototype drug

1329

actions; POTASSIUM-SPARING DIURETICS, POTASSIUM SUPPLEMENTS, ACE INHIBITORS increase risk of hyperkalemia.

## PHARMACOKINETICS Absorption: Adequately absorbed from GI tract. **Distribution:** Crosses placenta. **Elimination:** Cleared from plasma by renal excretion or thyroid uptake.

## NURSING IMPLICATIONS

### Assessment & Drug Effects
- Keep prescriber informed about characteristics of sputum: Quantity, consistency, color.
- Monitor lab tests: Baseline and periodic serum potassium.

### Patient & Family Education
- Report to prescriber promptly the occurrence of abdominal pain, distension, nausea, or vomiting.
- Report clinical S&S of iodism (see ADVERSE EFFECTS). Usually, symptoms will subside with dose reduction and lengthened intervals between doses.
- Avoid foods rich in iodine if iodism develops: Seafood, fish liver oils, and iodized salt.
- Be aware that sudden withdrawal following prolonged use may precipitate thyroid storm.
- Do not use OTC drugs without consulting prescriber. Many preparations contain iodides and could augment prescribed dose [e.g., cough syrups, gargles, asthma medication, salt substitutes, cod liver oil, multiple vitamins (often suspended in iodide solutions)].
- Be aware that optimum hydration is the best expectorant when taking KI as an expectorant. Increase daily fluid intake.

## PRALATREXATE
(pra-la-trex′ate)
Folotyn
**Classifications:** ANTINEOPLASTIC; ANTIMETABOLITE, ANTIFOLATE
Therapeutic: ANTINEOPLASTIC
**Prototype:** Methotrexate

**AVAILABILITY** Solution for injection

## ACTION & *THERAPEUTIC EFFECT*
Blocks folic acid participation in nucleic acid synthesis, thereby interfering with cell division (mitosis). Rapidly dividing cells, including cancer cells, are sensitive to this interference in the mitotic process. *Effective in treatment of relapsed or refractory peripheral T-cell lymphoma (PTCL).*

**USES** Treatment of relapsed or refractory peripheral T-cell lymphoma (PTCL) and non-Hodgkin's lymphoma.

## CONTRAINDICATIONS Concomitant administration of hepatotoxity drugs; tumor lysis syndrome; pregnancy (category D); lactation.

## CAUTIOUS USE Thrombocytopenia, neutropenia, anemia; moderate to severe renal function impairment; liver function impairment; pancreatic problems due to drug use; ulcerative colitis; poor nutritional status; older adults. Safety and efficacy in children not established.

## ROUTE & DOSAGE

### Peripheral T-Cell Lymphoma
*Adult:* **IV** 30 mg/m² over 3–5 min. Repeat weekly for 6 wk in 7-wk cycles.

Common adverse effects in *italic*; life-threatening effects underlined; generic names in **bold**; classifications in SMALL CAPS; ✦Canadian drug name; ☺ Prototype drug

**Renal Impairment Dosage Adjustment**

*EGFR of 15-30 mL/min:* Reduce dose to 15 mg/m$^2$

**Toxicity and Organ Function Dosage Adjustments**

See package insert

## ADMINISTRATION

**Intravenous**

*PREPARE:* **Direct:** Withdraw from vial into syringe immediately before use. Do not dilute. Use gloves and other protective clothing during handling and preparation. ▪ Flush thoroughly if drug contacts skin or mucous membranes.

*ADMINISTER:* **Direct:** Give over 3–5 min via a side port of a free-flowing NS IV line. ▪ Withhold drug and notify prescriber for any of the following: Platelet count less than 100,000/mcL for first dose or less than 50,000/mcL for all subsequent doses, ANC less than 1000/mcL, or grade 2 or higher mucositis.

▪ Refrigerate at 2°–8° C (36°–46° F) until use and protect from light. ▪ Vials are stable at room temperature for up to 72 h if left in original carton.

## ADVERSE EFFECTS (≥10%) **Body as a Whole:** Abdominal pain, asthenia, *edema, fatigue,* night sweats, pain in extremity, *pyrexia,* sepsis. **CV:** Tachycardia. **GI:** *Constipation, diarrhea, mucositis, nausea, vomiting,* stomatitis. **Hematologic:** *Anemia,* leukopenia, *neutropenia,* thrombocytopenia. **Metabolic:** Anorexia, elevated AST and ALT, hypokalemia. **Musculoskeletal:** Back pain. **Respiratory:** *Cough, dyspnea, epistaxis,* pharyngolaryngeal pain,

upper respiratory tract infection. **Skin:** Pruritus, rash.

## INTERACTIONS **Drug:** **Probenecid** may increase pralatrexate levels. Drugs that are subject to substantial renal clearance (e.g., NSAIDS, **trimethoprim/sulfamethoxazole**) may delay the clearance of pralatrexate. Do not administer LIVE VACCINES.

## PHARMACOKINETICS **Distribution:** 67% bound to plasma proteins. **Metabolism:** Not extensively metabolized. **Elimination:** Primarily excreted in the urine. **Half-Life:** 12–18 h.

## NURSING IMPLICATIONS

### Assessment & Drug Effects

▪ Monitor vitals signs. Report immediately S&S of infection, especially fever of 100.5° F or greater.
▪ Monitor status of mucus membranes because mucositis is a dose-limiting toxicity.
▪ Monitor lab tests: Prior to each dose, CBC with differential and platelet count; baseline and periodic LFTs and renal function tests.

### Patient & Family Education

▪ Practice meticulous oral hygiene.
▪ Monitor for S&S of an infection. Contact the prescriber immediately if an infection is suspected or if your temperature is elevated.
▪ Report promptly unexplained bleeding or symptoms of anemia (e.g., excessive weakness, fatigue, intolerance to activity, pale skin).
▪ Folic acid and vitamin B$_{12}$ supplementation are recommended to reduce the risk of drug-related toxicities. Consult with prescriber.
▪ Use effective means of contraception to avoid pregnancy while taking this drug. If a pregnancy

Common adverse effects in *italic*; life-threatening effects underlined; generic names in **bold**; classifications in SMALL CAPS; ♣ Canadian drug name; ⊕ Prototype drug

1331

does occur, notify prescriber immediately.

- Do not take aspirin or NSAIDs without consulting prescriber.

# PRALIDOXIME CHLORIDE

(pra-li-dox'eem)

Protopam Chloride

**Classifications:** CHOLINESTERASE RECEPTOR AGONIST; DETOXIFICATION AGENT

Therapeutic: ANTIDOTE; CHOLINESTER-ASE ENHANCER

**AVAILABILITY** Solution for injection

## ACTION & THERAPEUTIC EFFECT

Reactivates cholinesterase by displacing the enzyme from its receptor sites; the free enzyme then can resume its function of degrading accumulated acetylcholine, thereby restoring normal neuromuscular transmission. *More active against effects of anticholinesterases at skeletal neuromuscular junction than at autonomic effector sites or in CNS respiratory center; therefore, atropine* **must be** *given concomitantly to block effects of acetylcholine and its accumulation in these sites.*

**USES** Antidote in treatment of poisoning by organophosphate insecticides and pesticides with anticholinesterase activity (e.g., parathion, TEPP, sarin) and to control overdosage by anticholinesterase drugs used in treatment of myasthenia gravis (cholinergic crisis).

**UNLABELED USES** To reverse toxicity of echothiophate ophthalmic solution.

**CONTRAINDICATIONS** Hypersensitivity to pralidoxime; use in poisoning by insecticide of the

carbonate class (Sevin), inorganic phosphates, or organophosphates having no anticholinesterase activity.

**CAUTIOUS USE** Myasthenia gravis; renal insufficiency; asthma; peptic ulcer; severe cardiac disease; pregnancy (category C); lactation.

## ROUTE & DOSAGE

### Organophosphate Poisoning

*Adult/Adolescent (17 y or older):* **IV** 1–2 g in 100 mL NS infused over 15–30 min; or 1–2 g as 5% solution in sterile water over not less than 5 min, may repeat after 1 h if muscle weakness not relieved.; **IM** 600 mg, may repeat in 15 min to total dose of 1800 mg if IV route is not feasible.
*Adolescent (younger than 17 y)/Child/Infant:* **IV** 20–50 mg/kg. May repeat in 1–2 h if needed (max dose: 2 g).

### Anticholinesterase Overdose in Myasthenia Gravis

*Adult:* **IV** 1–2 g in 100 mL NS infused over 15–30 min, followed by increments of 250 mg q5min prn

## ADMINISTRATION

### Intramuscular

- Give only if unable to give IV; **not** preferred route.
- Reconstitute as for direct IV injection (see below).

### Intravenous

**PREPARE: Direct:** Reconstitute 1-g vial by adding 20 mL sterile water for injection to yield 50 mg/mL (a

5% solution). ▪ If pulmonary edema is present, give without further dilution. **IV Infusion (preferred):** Further dilute reconstituted solution in 100 mL NS. ***ADMINISTER: Direct:*** In pulmonary edema, 1 g or fraction thereof over 5 min; do not exceed 200 mg/min. **IV Infusion (preferred):** Give over 15–30 min. ▪ Stop infusion or reduce rate if hypertension occurs.

**ADVERSE EFFECTS** (≥1%) **CNS:** Dizziness, headache, drowsiness. **GI:** Nausea. **Special Senses:** Blurred vision, diplopia, impaired accommodation. **CV:** Tachycardia, hypertension (dose related). **Body as a Whole:** Hyperventilation, muscular weakness, laryngospasm, muscle rigidity.

**INTERACTIONS Drug:** May potentiate the effects of BARBITURATES.

**PHARMACOKINETICS Peak:** 5–15 min IV; 10–20 min IM. **Distribution:** Distributed throughout extracellular fluids; crosses blood–brain barrier slowly if at all. **Metabolism:** Probably in liver. **Elimination:** Rapidly in urine. **Half-Life:** 0.8–2.7 h.

## NURSING IMPLICATIONS
### Assessment & Drug Effects
▪ Monitor BP, vital signs, and I&O. Report oliguria or changes in I&O ratio.
▪ Monitor closely. It is difficult to differentiate toxic effects of organophosphates or atropine from toxic effects of pralidoxime.
▪ Be alert for and report immediately: Reduction in muscle strength, onset of muscle twitching, changes in respiratory pattern, altered level of consciousness, increases or changes in heart rate and rhythm.

▪ Observe necessary safety precautions with unconscious patient because excitement and manic behavior reportedly may occur following recovery of consciousness.
▪ Keep patient under close observation for 48–72 h, particularly when poison was ingested, because of likelihood of continued absorption of organophosphate from lower bowel.
▪ In patients with myasthenia gravis, overdosage with pralidoxime may convert cholinergic crisis into myasthenic crisis.

# PRAMIPEXOLE DIHYDROCHLORIDE
(pra-mi-pex′ole)
**Mirapex, Mirapex ER**
**Classifications:** DOPAMINE RECEPTOR AGONIST; ANTIPARKINSON
**Therapeutic:** ANTIPARKINSON
**Prototype:** Levodopa

**AVAILABILITY** Tablet; extended release tablet

**ACTION & *THERAPEUTIC EFFECT***
Exhibits high affinity for the $D_2$ subfamily of dopamine receptors in the brain and higher binding affinity to $D_3$ than other dopamine receptor subtypes. *Effectiveness is indicated by improved control of neuromuscular functioning. Improves ADLs.*

**USES** Treatment of idiopathic Parkinson's disease and moderate to severe primary restless legs syndrome (RLS).

**CONTRAINDICATIONS** Hypersensitivity to pramipexole or ropinirole; abrupt withdrawal; lactation.

Common adverse effects in *italic*; life-threatening effects underlined; generic names in **bold**; classifications in SMALL CAPS; ♣Canadian drug name; ⊙ Prototype drug

1333

**CAUTIOUS USE** Renal impairment; impulse control/compulsive behavior symptoms; history of orthostatic hypotension; restless leg syndrome; older adults; pregnancy (category C). Safety and efficacy in children not established.

## ROUTE & DOSAGE

### Parkinson's Disease

*Adult:* **PO Immediate release** Start with 0.125 mg t.i.d. gradually increase every 5–7 days (max: 1.5 mg t.i.d.); **Extended release** 0.375 mg daily, may increase after 5 days (max: 4.5 mg/day)

### Restless Legs Syndrome

*Adult:* **PO** 0.125 mg taken 2–3 h before bed; dose can be increased every 4–7 days

### *Renal Impairment Dosage Adjustment*

*CrCl 35–59 mL/min:* **PO Immediate release** Start with 0.125 mg b.i.d.; *CrCl 15–34 mL/min:* Start 0.125 mg daily *CrCl 30–50 mL/min:* **PO Extended release** Start 0.375 mg every other day

## ADMINISTRATION

### Oral

- Ensure that extended release tablet is swallowed whole and not crushed or chewed.
- Give with food if nausea develops.

**ADVERSE EFFECTS** (≥1%) **Body as a Whole:** *Asthenia,* general edema, malaise, fever, decreased weight, accidental injury. **CNS:** *Dizziness, somnolence, sudden sleep attacks, insomnia, hallucinations, dyskinesia, extrapyramidal syndrome,* headache, confusion, amnesia, hypesthesia, dystonia, akathisia, myoclonus, peripheral edema. **CV:** *Postural hypotension,* chest pain. **GI:** *Nausea, constipation,* anorexia, dysphagia, dry mouth. **Respiratory:** Dyspnea, rhinitis. **Urogenital:** Decreased libido, impotence, urinary frequency or incontinence. **Special Senses:** Vision abnormalities.

**INTERACTIONS Drug: Cimetidine** decreases clearance; BUTYROPHE-NONES, **metoclopramide**, PHENO-THIAZINES, ANTIPSYCHOTICS may antagonize effects. Closely monitor use with other CNS DEPRESSANTS.

**PHARMACOKINETICS Absorption:** Rapidly from GI tract, greater than 90% bioavailability. **Peak:** 2 h. **Distribution:** 15% protein bound. **Metabolism:** Minimally in the liver. **Elimination:** Primarily in urine. **Half-Life:** 8–12 h.

## NURSING IMPLICATIONS

### Assessment & Drug Effects

- Monitor for S&S of orthostatic hypotension, especially when the dosage is increased.
- Monitor cardiac status, especially in those with significant orthostatic hypotension.
- Monitor for and report signs of tardive dyskinesia (see Appendix F).

### Patient & Family Education

- Do not abruptly stop taking this drug. It should be discontinued over a period of 1 wk.
- Hallucinations are an adverse effect of this drug and occur more often in older adults.
- Make position changes slowly especially from a lying or sitting to standing.
- Use caution with potentially dangerous activities until response to

Common adverse effects in *italic*; life-threatening effects underlined; generic names in **bold**; classifications in SMALL CAPS; ✤ Canadian drug name; ⊙ Prototype drug

drug is known; drowsiness is a common adverse effect.

- Avoid alcohol and use extra caution if taking other prescribed CNS depressants; both may exaggerate drowsiness, dizziness, and orthostatic hypotension.

## PRAMLINTIDE
Symlin

**Classifications:** ANTIDIABETIC; AMYLIN ANALOG
**Therapeutic:** ANTIHYPERGLYCEMIC

**AVAILABILITY** Solution for injection

## ACTION & THERAPEUTIC EFFECT
A synthetic analog of human amylin, a hormone secreted by pancreatic beta cells. Amylin reduces postmeal glucagon levels, thus lowering serum glucose level. *Pramlintide is an antihyperglycemic drug that controls postprandial blood glucose levels.*

**USES** Adjunct treatment of diabetes mellitus type 1 and type 2 in patients who use mealtime insulin therapy and who have failed to achieve desired glucose control despite optimal insulin therapy.

## CONTRAINDICATIONS
Hypersensitivity to pramlintide, metacresol; noncompliance with insulin regime or medical care; HbA1C greater than 9%; recurrent severe hypoglycemia; hypoglucemia unawareness; gastroparesis; dialysis.

## CAUTIOUS USE
Osteoporosis; alcohol; thyroid disease; older adults; pregnancy (category C); lactation. Safety and efficacy in children not established.

## ROUTE & DOSAGE

### Type 1 Diabetes Mellitus
*Adult:* **Subcutaneous** 15 mcg immediately before each major meal; may increase by 15 mcg increments if no clinically significant nausea for 3–7 days. If nausea or vomiting persists at 45 mcg or 60 mcg, reduce to 30 mcg.

### Type 2 Diabetes Mellitus
*Adult:* **Subcutaneous** 60 mcg immediately before each major meal; may increase to 120 mcg if no clinically significant nausea for 3–7 days. If nausea or vomiting persists at 120 mcg, reduce to 60 mcg.

## ADMINISTRATION
Subcutaneous
- Give subcutaneously into the abdomen or thigh (not the arm) immediately before each major meal. Rotate injection sites.
- Never mix pramlintide and insulin in the same syringe. Separate injection sites.
- Use a U100 insulin syringe to administer. One unit of pramlintide drawn from a 0.6 mg/mL vial contains 6 mcg of medication. Thus, a 30 mcg dose is equal to 5 units in a U100 syringe.
- Do not administer to patients with HbA1C greater than 9% or those taking drugs to stimulate GI motility.
- Note: When initiating pramlintide therapy, insulin dose reduction is required.
- Store at 2°–8° C (36°–46° F), and protect from light. Do not freeze. Discard vials that have been frozen or overheated. Discard open vials after 30 days.

P

Common adverse effects in *italic*; life-threatening effects <u>underlined</u>; generic names in **bold**; classifications in SMALL CAPS; ♦ Canadian drug name; ⊘ Prototype drug

1335

**ADVERSE EFFECTS (≥1%) CNS:** Dizziness, fatigue, *headache*. **GI:** Abdominal pain, *anorexia, nausea, vomiting*. **Musculoskeletal:** Arthralgia. **Respiratory:** *Coughing*, pharyngitis. **Body as a Whole:** *Allergic reaction, inflicted injury,* pancreatitis.

**INTERACTIONS Drugs:** Pramlintide can decrease rate and/or extent of GI absorption of other oral drugs. Significant slowing of gastric motility with ANTIMUSCARINICS.

**PHARMACOKINETICS Absorption:** 30–40% bioavailability. **Peak:** 20 min. **Distribution:** 60% protein bound. **Metabolism:** Extensive renal metabolism. **Half-Life:** 48 min.

## NURSING IMPLICATIONS

### Black Box Warning

*Pramlintide use with insulin increases the risk of severe hypoglycemia, particularly in type 1 diabetics. When severe hypoglycemia occurs, it is seen within 3 h following a pramlintide injection. Serious injuries may occur.*

### Assessment & Drug Effects

- Monitor for severe hypoglycemia, which usually occurs within 3 h of injection. Hypoglycemia is worse in type 1 diabetics.
- Monitor diabetics for loss of glycemic control.
- Withhold drug and notify prescriber for clinically significant nausea or increased frequency or severity of hypoglycemia.
- Monitor for and report promptly S&S of pancreatitis (e.g., upper abdominal plain that radiates to back, nausea and vomiting).

- Monitor lab tests: Baseline and periodic HbA1C; frequent pre/postmeal plasma glucose levels.

### Patient & Family Education

- Note: Patients should reduce a.c. rapid-acting or short-acting insulin dosages by 50% when pramlintide is initiated. Check with prescriber.
- Do not drive or engage in potentially hazardous activities until response to drug is known.
- Report any of the following to prescriber: Persistent, significant nausea; episodes of hypoglycemia (e.g., hunger, headache, sweating, tremor, irritability, or difficulty concentrating).

## PRAMOXINE HYDROCHLORIDE
(pra-mox'een)
Fleet Relief Anesthetic Hemorrhoidal, Prax, ProctoFoam, Tronolane, Tronothane ◆

**Classifications:** LOCAL ANESTHETIC (MUCOSAL); ANTIPRURITIC
**Therapeutic:** LOCAL ANESTHETIC; ANTIPRURITIC
**Prototype:** Procaine

**AVAILABILITY** Cream; gel; lotion; spray

## ACTION & *THERAPEUTIC EFFECT*
Produces anesthesia by blocking conduction and propagation of sensory nerve impulses in skin and mucous membranes. *Provides temporary relief from pain and itching on skin or mucous membrane.*

**USES** To relieve pain caused by minor burns and wounds; for temporary relief of pruritus secondary to dermatoses, hemorrhoids, and anal fissures; and to facilitate sigmoidoscopic examination.

**CONTRAINDICATIONS** Application to large areas of skin; prolonged use; preparation for laryngopharyngeal examination, bronchoscopy, or gastroscopy.

**CAUTIOUS USE** Extensive skin disorders; pregnancy (category C); lactation. Safety in children younger than 2 y not established.

### ROUTE & DOSAGE

**Relief of Minor Pain and Itching**
*Adult/Child (2 y or older):*
**Topical** Apply t.i.d. or q.i.d.

### ADMINISTRATION

**Topical**
- Clean thoroughly and dry rectal area before use for temporary relief of hemorrhoidal pain and itching.
- Administer rectal preparations in the morning and evening and after bowel movement or as directed by prescriber.
- Apply lotion or cream to affected surfaces with a gloved hand. Wash hands thoroughly before and after treatment.
- Do not apply to eyes or nasal membranes.

**ADVERSE EFFECTS** (≥1%) **Skin:** Burning, stinging, sensitization.

**PHARMACOKINETICS Onset:** 3–5 min. **Duration:** Up to 5 h.

### NURSING IMPLICATIONS

**Assessment & Drug Effects**
- Monitor for and report promptly significant tissue irritation or sloughing.

**Patient & Family Education**
- Drug is usually discontinued if condition being treated does not improve within 2–3 wk or if it worsens, or if rash or condition not present before treatment appears, or if treated area becomes inflamed or infected.
- Discontinue and consult prescriber if rectal bleeding and pain occur during hemorrhoid treatment.

## PRASUGREL
(pra-soo'grel)
**Effient**
**Classifications:** ANTIPLATELET; PLATELET INHIBITOR; ADP RECEPTOR ANTAGONIST
**Therapeutic:** PLATELET INHIBITOR
**Prototype:** Clopidogrel

**AVAILABILITY** Tablet

**ACTION & *THERAPEUTIC EFFECT***
An inhibitor of platelet activation and aggregation through irreversible binding to adenosine diphosphate (ADP) receptors on platelets. *Prasugrel prolongs bleeding time, thereby reducing atherosclerotic events in selected high risk patient managed with percutaneous coronary intervention (PCI).*

**USES** Prophylaxis of arterial thromboembolism in patients with acute coronary syndrome, including unstable angina, non–ST-elevation myocardial infarction (NSTEMI), or ST-elevation acute myocardial infarction (STEMI), who are being managed with percutaneous coronary intervention (PCI).

**CONTRAINDICATIONS** Active pathologic bleeding disorder; active bleeding; history of TIA or stroke; GI bleeding; within 7 days of CABG surgery or any surgery; adults over 75 y; concomitant use

Common adverse effects in *italic*; life-threatening effects <u>underlined</u>; generic names in **bold**; classifications in SMALL CAPS; ♣ Canadian drug name; ❻ Prototype drug

1337

of NSAIDs or other drugs that increase risk of bleeding.

**CAUTIOUS USE** Severe hepatic impairment (Child-Pugh class C, total score greater than 10); end-stage renal disease; pts less than 60 kg; pregnancy (category B); lactation.

## ROUTE & DOSAGE

### Thromboembolism Prophylaxis

*Adult (younger than 75 y, weight 60 kg or greater):* **PO** 60 mg loading dose, then 10 mg once daily; *younger than 75 y, weight less than 60 kg:* 60 mg loading dose, then 5 mg once daily

## ADMINISTRATION

### Oral
- Give without regard to food.
- Daily aspirin is recommended with prasugrel.
- Do not administer to patient with active bleeding or who is likely to undergo urgent CABG.
- Store at 15°–30° C (59°–86° F).

**ADVERSE EFFECTS** (≥1%) **Body as a Whole:** Fatigue, non-cardiac chest pain, pain in extremity, peripheral edema, pyrexia. **CNS:** Dizziness, headache. **CV:** <u>Artial fibrillation</u>, bradycardia, hypertension, hypotension. **GI:** Diarrhea, gastrointestinal hemorrhage, nausea. **Hematologic:** *Epistaxis, increased bleeding tendency, <u>leukopenia</u>*. **Metabolic:** Hypercholesterolemia, hyperlipidemia. **Musculoskeletal:** Back pain. **Respiratory:** Cough, dyspnea.

**INTERACTIONS Drug: Warfarin** or NSAIDS or ANTICOAGULANTS may increase the risk of bleeding. Do not use with PLATELET INHIBITOR or FIBRINOLYTICS.

**PHARMACOKINETICS Absorption:** 79% or higher. **Peak:** 30 min. **Metabolism:** Hydrolysis and oxidation to active metabolite. **Elimination:** Urine (68%) and feces (27%). **Half-Life:** 7 h.

## NURSING IMPLICATIONS

### Black Box Warning

*Prasugrel has been associated with severe, sometimes fatal, bleeding (especially in patients with active pathological bleeding, history of TIA or stroke, or those age 75 and older).*

### Assessment & Drug Effects
- Monitor vital signs. Suspect bleeding if patient is hypotensive and has recently undergone an invasive or surgical procedure.
- Monitor for and report promptly any S&S of active bleeding.
- Monitor lab tests: Periodic Hct and Hgb.

### Patient & Family Education
- Report promptly unexplained prolonged or excessive bleeding, or blood in urine or stool.
- Report immediately any of the following: Weakness, extremely pale skin, purple skin patches, jaundice, or fever.
- Inform all medical providers that you are taking prasugrel.
- Do not take OTC anti-inflammatory or pain medications without consulting prescriber.

## PRAVASTATIN
(pra-vah-stat'in)
Pravachol

**Classifications:** ANTIHYPERLIPEMIC; HMG-COA REDUCTASE INHIBITOR (STATIN)
**Therapeutic:** ANTILIPEMIC; STATIN
**Prototype:** Lovastatin

Common adverse effects in *italic*; life-threatening effects <u>underlined</u>; generic names in **bold**; classifications in SMALL CAPS; ♣Canadian drug name; ⦾ Prototype drug

**AVAILABILITY** Tablet

## ACTION & *THERAPEUTIC EFFECT*
Competitively inhibits HMG-CoA reductase, the enzyme that catalyzes cholesterol biosynthesis. HMG-CoA reductase inhibitors (statins) increase serum HDL cholesterol, decrease serum LDL cholesterol, VLDL cholesterol, and plasma triglyceride levels. *It is effective in reducing total and LDL cholesterol in various forms of hypercholesterolemia.*

**USES** Hypercholesterolemia (alone or in combination with bile acid sequestrants) and familial hypercholesterolemia; atherosclerosis.

**CONTRAINDICATIONS** Hypersensitivity to pravastatin; active liver disease or unexplained elevated serum transaminases; hepatic encephalopathy, hepatitis, jaundice, rhabdomyolysis; pregnancy (category X); lactation.

**CAUTIOUS USE** Alcoholics, history of liver disease; renal impairment; renal disease; women of child-bearing age who use contraceptive measures. Safe use in children younger than 8 y not established.

## ROUTE & DOSAGE

### Hyperlipidemia / Stroke Prophylaxis
*Adult:* **PO** Initially 40 mg daily then may increase up to 80 mg/day
*Adult (also taking immunosuppressive drug):* **PO** 10 mg daily may titrate up to 20 mg
*Adolescent:* **PO** 40 mg daily
*Child (8–13 y):* **PO** 20 mg daily

## ADMINISTRATION
**Oral**
- Give without regard to meals.
- Give in the evening.

**ADVERSE EFFECTS** (≥1%) **GI:** Nausea, diarrhea, abdominal pain, vomiting, constipation, flatulence, heartburn, transient elevations in serum liver transaminase levels. **CNS:** Dizziness, fatigue, headache. **Other:** Fatigue, rhinitis, cough, transient elevations in CPK, headache.

**DIAGNOSTIC TEST INTERFERENCE** May elevate CPK, blood glucose, and/or transaminase levels.

**INTERACTIONS Drug:** May increase PT when administered with **warfarin.** IMMUNOSPRESSANTS may increase risk of myopathy. **Herbal:** Do not use with red yeast rice.

**PHARMACOKINETICS Absorption:** Poorly from GI tract; 17% reaches systemic circulation. **Onset:** 2 wk. **Peak:** 4 wk. **Distribution:** 43–55% protein bound; does not cross blood–brain barrier, crosses placenta; distributed into breast milk. **Metabolism:** Extensive first-pass metabolism in liver; has no active metabolites. **Elimination:** 20% of dose excreted in urine, 71% in feces. **Half-Life:** 1.8–2.6 h.

## NURSING IMPLICATIONS
### Assessment & Drug Effects
- Monitor diabetics and prediabetics for loss of glycemic control.
- Monitor coagulation studies with patients receiving concurrent warfarin therapy. PT may be prolonged.
- Monitor lab tests: Baseline LFTs, repeat at 4–12 wk, then annually. LFTs and CPK if symptoms warrant testing.

Common adverse effects in *italic*; life-threatening effects underlined; generic names in **bold**; classifications in SMALL CAPS; ♣ Canadian drug name; ☻ Prototype drug

1339

## Patient & Family Education

- Report unexplained muscle pain, tenderness, or weakness, especially if accompanied by malaise or fever, to prescriber promptly.
- Report signs of bleeding to prescriber promptly when taking concomitant warfarin therapy.
- Monitor blood glucose for loss of glycemic control if diabetic or prediabetic.

# PRAZIQUANTEL ⊕

(pray-zi-kwon'tel)
Biltricide

**Classification:** ANTHELMINTIC
Therapeutic: ANTHELMINTIC

**AVAILABILITY** Tablet

## ACTION & *THERAPEUTIC EFFECT*

Increases permeability of parasite cell membrane to calcium. Leads to immobilization of their suckers and dislodgment from their residence in blood vessel walls. *Active against all developmental stages of schistosomes, including cercaria (free-swimming larvae). Also active against other trematodes (flukes) and cestodes (tapeworms).*

## USES
All stages of schistosomiasis (bilharziasis) caused by all *Schistosoma* species pathogenic to humans. Other trematode infections caused by Chinese liver fluke.

## UNLABELED USES
Lung, sheep liver, and intestinal flukes and tapeworm infections.

## CONTRAINDICATIONS
Hypersensitivity to praziquantel; ocular cysticercosis. Women should not breast-feed on day of praziquantel therapy or for 72 h after last dose of drug.

**CAUTIOUS USE** Hepatic disease; cardiac arrhythmias; pregnancy (category B); children younger than 4 y.

## ROUTE & DOSAGE

### Schistosomiasis

*Adult/Child (4 y or older):* **PO** 60 mg/kg in 3 equally divided doses at 4–6 h intervals on the same day, may repeat in 2–3 mo after exposure

### Other Trematodes

*Adult/Child (4 y or older):* **PO** 75 mg/kg in 3 equally divided doses at 4–6 h intervals on the same day

### Cestodiasis (Adult or Intestinal Stage)

*Adult:* **PO** 10–20 mg/kg as single dose

### Cestodiasis (Larval or Tissue Stage)

*Adult:* **PO** 50 mg/kg in 3 divided doses/day for 14 days

## ADMINISTRATION

### Oral

- Give dose with food and fluids. Tablets can be broken into quarters but should **not** be chewed.
- Advise patient to take sufficient fluid to wash down the medication. Tablets are soluble in water; gagging or vomiting because of bitter taste may result if tablets are retained in the mouth.
- Store tablets in tight containers at less than 30° C (86° F).

## ADVERSE EFFECTS (≥1%) CNS:
*Dizziness, headache, malaise,* drowsiness, lassitude, CSF reaction syndrome (exacerbation of

Common adverse effects in *italic*; life-threatening effects <u>underlined</u>; generic names in **bold**; classifications in SMALL CAPS; ✦Canadian drug name; ⊕ Prototype drug neurologic signs and symptoms such as seizures, increased CSF protein concentration, increased anticysticercal IgG levels, hyperthermia, intracranial hypertension) in patient treated for cerebral cysticercosis. **GI:** *Abdominal pain or discomfort with or without nausea;* vomiting, anorexia, diarrhea. **Hepatic:** *Increased AST, ALT (slight).* **Skin:** Pruritus, urticaria. **Body as a Whole:** Fever, sweating, symptoms of host-mediated immunologic response to antigen release from worms (fever, eosinophilia).

### DIAGNOSTIC TEST INTERFERENCE
Be mindful that selected drugs may interfere with stool studies for ova and parasites: ***Iron, bismuth, oil (mineral*** or ***castor), Metamucil*** (if ingested within 1 wk of test), ***barium, antibiotics, antiamebic*** and ***antimalarial drugs,*** and ***gallbladder dye*** (if administered within 3 wk of test).

### INTERACTIONS **Drug: Phenytoin** can lead to therapeutic failure. **Food: Grapefruit juice** (greater than 1 qt/day) may increase plasma concentrations and adverse effects.

### PHARMACOKINETICS **Absorption:** Rapidly, 80% reaches systemic circulation. **Peak:** 1–3 h. **Distribution:** Enters cerebrospinal fluid. **Metabolism:** Extensively to inactive metabolites. **Elimination:** Primarily in urine. **Half-Life:** 0.8–1.5 h.

### NURSING IMPLICATIONS
#### Assessment & Drug Effects
- Patient is reexamined in 2 or 3 mo to ensure complete eradication of the infections.

#### Patient & Family Education
- Do not drive or operate other hazardous machinery on day of treatment or the following day because

of potential drug-induced dizziness and drowsiness.
- Usually, all schistosomal worms are dead 7 days following treatment.
- Contact prescriber if you develop a sustained headache or high fever.

## PRAZOSIN HYDROCHLORIDE ℗
(pra′zoe-sin)
Minipress
**Classifications:** ALPHA-ADRENERGIC RECEPTOR ANTAGONIST; ANTIHYPERTENSIVE
**Therapeutic:** ANTIHYPERTENSIVE

### AVAILABILITY Capsule

### ACTION & *THERAPEUTIC EFFECT*
Causes selective inhibition of alpha$_1$ adrenoceptors that produces vasodilation in both resistance (arterioles) and capacitance (veins) vessels with the result that both peripheral vascular resistance and blood pressure are reduced. *Lowers blood pressure in supine and standing positions with most pronounced effect on diastolic pressure.*

### USES Treatment of hypertension.

### UNLABELED USES Severe refractory congestive heart failure, Raynaud's disease or phenomenon, ergotamine-induced peripheral ischemia, pheochromocytoma, benign prostatic hypertrophy.

### CONTRAINDICATIONS Hypersensitivity to prazosin; hypotension.

### CAUTIOUS USE Renal impairment; chronic kidney failure;

hypertensive patient with cerebral thrombosis; angina; men with sickle cell trait; older adults; pregnancy (category C); lactation; children.

## ROUTE & DOSAGE

### Hypertension

*Adult:* **PO** 1 mg b.i.d. or t.i.d., may increase to 20 mg/day in divided doses (average dose is 6–15 mg/day)

## ADMINISTRATION

### Oral

- Give initial dose at bedtime to reduce possibility of adverse effects such as postural hypotension and syncope. However, if first dose is taken during the day, advise patient not to drive a car for about 4 h after ingestion of drug.
- Give drug with food to reduce incidence of faintness and dizziness; food may delay absorption but does not affect extent of absorption.
- Store in tightly closed container away from strong light. Do not freeze.

## ADVERSE EFFECTS (≥1%) CNS:

*Dizziness, headache, drowsiness,* nervousness, vertigo, depression, paresthesia, insomnia. **CV:** Edema, dyspnea, syncope *first-dose phenomenon,* postural hypotension, *palpitations,* tachycardia, angina. **Special Senses:** Blurred vision, tinnitus, reddened sclerae. **GI:** Dry mouth, *nausea,* vomiting, diarrhea, constipation, abdominal discomfort, pain. **Urogenital:** Urinary frequency, incontinence, priapism (especially in men with sickle cell anemia), impotence. **Skin:** Rash, pruritus, alopecia, lichen planus. **Body as a Whole:** Diaphoresis, epistaxis, nasal congestion, arthralgia, transient *leukopenia,* increased serum uric acid, and BUN.

## INTERACTIONS **Drug:** DIURETICS, HYPOTENSIVE AGENTS and **alcohol** increase hypotensive effects. **Sildenafil, vardenafil,** and **tadalafil** may enhance hypotensive effects. Use with other ALPHA-BLOCKERS may increase adverse effects. Do not use with **tranylcypromine**.

## PHARMACOKINETICS **Absorption:** Approximately 60% of oral dose reaches the systemic circulation. **Onset:** 2 h. **Peak:** 2–4 h. **Duration:** Less than 24 h. **Distribution:** Widely distributed, including into breast milk. **Metabolism:** Extensively in liver. **Elimination:** 6–10% in urine, rest in bile and feces. **Half-Life:** 2–4 h.

## NURSING IMPLICATIONS

### Assessment & Drug Effects

- Be alert for first-dose phenomenon (rare adverse effect: 0.15% of patients); characterized by a precipitous decline in BP, bradycardia, and consciousness disturbances (syncope) within 90–120 min after the initial dose of prazosin. Recovery is usually within several hours. Preexisting low plasma volume (from diuretic therapy or salt restriction), beta-adrenergic therapy, and recent stroke appear to increase the risk of this phenomenon.
- Monitor blood pressure. If it falls precipitously with first dose, notify prescriber promptly.
- Full therapeutic effect may not be achieved until 4–6 wk of therapy.

### Patient & Family Education

- Avoid situations that would result in injury if you should faint, particularly during early phase of treatment. In most cases, effect does not recur after initial period of therapy; however, it may occur during acute febrile episodes, when drug dose is increased, or when another antihypertensive drug is added to the medication regimen.

- Make position and direction changes slowly and in stages. Dangle legs and move ankles a minute or so before standing when arising in the morning or after a nap.
- Lie down immediately if you experience light-headedness, dizziness, a sense of impending loss of consciousness, or blurred vision. Attempting to stand or walk may result in a fall.
- Do not drive or engage in other potentially hazardous activities until response to drug is known.
- Take drug at same time(s) each day.
- Report priapism or impotence. A change in the drug regimen usually reverses these difficulties.
- Do not take OTC medications, especially remedies for coughs, colds, and allergy, without consulting prescriber.
- Be aware that adverse effects usually disappear with continuation of therapy, but dosage reduction may be necessary.

# PREDNISOLONE
(pred-niss'oh-lone)
Prelone, Rayos

# PREDNISOLONE ACETATE
Flo-Pred, Pred Forte, Pred Mild

# PREDNISOLONE SODIUM PHOSPHATE
AK-Pred, Inflamase Forte, Inflamase Mild

**Classification:** ADRENAL CORTICOSTEROID

**Therapeutic:** ANTI-INFLAMMATORY; IMMUNOSUPPRESSANT
**Prototype:** Prednisone

**AVAILABILITY Prednisolone:** Tablet; delayed release tablet. **Acetate:** Ophthalmic suspension. **Sodium Phosphate:** Liquid; ophthalmic solution

## ACTION & THERAPEUTIC EFFECT
Has glucocorticoid activity similar to the naturally occurring hormone. It prevents or suppresses inflammation and immune responses. Its actions include inhibition of leukocyte infiltration at the site of inflammation, interference in the function of inflammatory mediators, and suppression of humoral immune responses. *Effective as an anti-inflammatory agent.*

**USES** Principally as an anti-inflammatory and immunosuppressant agent.

**CONTRAINDICATIONS** Hypersensitivity to prednisolone; systemic fungal infections; coadministration with live or attenuated virus vaccines; Kaposi sarcoma.

**CAUTIOUS USE** Cataracts; coagulopathy; elevated intraocular pressure; cataract; glaucoma; HF; hypertension; recent MI; TB; adrenal insufficiency; hyperthyroidism; DM; seizure disorders; hepatic impairment; renal impairment; psychosis; emotional instability; GI disorders/ bleeding; osteoporosis; older adults; pregnancy (category C); children.

## ROUTE & DOSAGE

**Anti-Inflammatory**
*Adult:* **PO** 5–60 mg/day in single or divided doses
*Child:* **PO** 0.1–2 mg/kg/day in divided doses

**Ophthalmic** See Appendix A-1

Common adverse effects in *italic;* life-threatening effects underlined; generic names in **bold;** classifications in SMALL CAPS; ♣ Canadian drug name; ⊘ Prototype drug

1343

## ADMINISTRATION

### Oral

- Give with meals to reduce gastric irritation. If distress continues, consult prescriber about possible adjunctive antacid therapy.
- Ensure that delayed release tablets are swallowed whole and not crushed or chewed.

### Alternate-Day Therapy (ADT) for Patient on Long-Term Therapy

- With ADT, the 48-h requirement for steroids is administered as a single dose every other morning.
- Be aware that ADT minimizes adverse effects associated with long-term treatment while maintaining the desired therapeutic effect.
- See PREDNISONE for numerous additional nursing implications.

## ADVERSE EFFECTS (≥1%) Endocrine: Hirsutism (occasional), adverse effects on growth and development of the individual and on sperm; Cushing's syndrome. Special Senses: Perforation of cornea (with topical drug). Body as a Whole: Sensitivity to heat; fat embolism, hypotension and shock-like reactions. CNS: Insomnia. GI: Gastric irritation or ulceration. Skin: Ecchymotic skin lesions; vasomotor symptoms. Also see PREDNISONE.

## INTERACTIONS Drug: BARBITURATES, phenytoin, rifampin increase steroid metabolism, therefore may need increased doses of prednisolone; amphotericin B, DIURETICS add to potassium loss; neostigmine, pyridostigmine may cause severe muscle weakness in patients with myasthenia gravis; VACCINES, TOXOIDS may inhibit antibody response. Food: Licorice may elevate plasma levels and adverse effects.

## PHARMACOKINETICS Absorption: Readily from GI tract. Peak: 1–2 h. Duration: 1–1.5 days. Distribution: Crosses placenta; distributed into breast milk. Metabolism: In liver. Elimination: HPA suppression: 24–36 h; in urine. Half-Life: 3.5 h.

## NURSING IMPLICATIONS

### Assessment & Drug Effects

- Be alert to subclinical signs of lack of improvement such as continued drainage, low-grade fever, and interrupted healing. In diseases caused by microorganisms, infection may be masked, activated, or enhanced by corticosteroids. Observe and report exacerbation of symptoms after short period of therapeutic response.
- Be aware that temporary local discomfort may follow injection of prednisolone into bursa or joint.

### Patient & Family Education

- Adhere to established dosage regimen (i.e., do not increase, decrease, or omit doses or change dose intervals).
- Report gastric distress or any sign of peptic ulcer.

## PREDNISONE ⊙

(pred'ni-sone)

Apo-Prednisone ♣, Deltasone, Meticorten, Orasone, Panasol, Prednicen-M, Sterapred, Winpred ♣

**Classification:** ADRENAL CORTICOSTEROID
Therapeutic: IMMUNOSUPPRESSANT; ANTI-INFLAMMATORY

## AVAILABILITY Tablet; solution

## ACTION & THERAPEUTIC EFFECT

Immediate-acting synthetic analog of hydrocortisone with predominantly corticosteroid properties. *Has anti-inflammatory and immunosuppressant properties.*

Common adverse effects in *italic*; life-threatening effects underlined; generic names in **bold**; classifications in SMALL CAPS; ♣ Canadian drug name; ⊙ Prototype drug

**USES** May be used as a single agent or conjunctively with antineoplastics in cancer therapy; also used in treatment of myasthenia gravis and inflammatory conditions as an immunosuppressant; acute respiratory distress syndrome, Addison's disease, adrenal hyperplasic, gout, gouty arthritis, headache, hemolytic anemia, sarcoidosis, Stevens–Johnson syndrome.

**UNLABELED USES** Absence seizures. COPD exacerbation, Bells palsy.

**CONTRAINDICATIONS** Known hypersensitivity to prednisone; systemic fungal infections; cerebral malaria; latent or active amebiasis; viral infections; live or attenuated vaccines, Kaposi sarcoma.

**CAUTIOUS USE** Patients with infections; nonspecific ulcerative colitis; diverticulitis; active or latent peptic ulcer; renal insufficiency; coagulopathy; psychosis; seizure disorders; adrenal insufficiency; TB; thromboembolic disease; CHF; hypertension; osteoporosis; MG; older adults; pregnancy (category C); lactation; children.

## ROUTE & DOSAGE

### Anti-Inflammatory

Doses are highly individualized (ranges are provided)
*Adult/Adolescent/Child:* **PO** 5–60 mg/day in single or divided doses

### Acute Asthma

*Child (younger than 12 y):* **PO** 1–2 mg/kg/day for 3–10 days

## ADMINISTRATION

### Oral

- Crush tablet and give with fluid of patient's choice if unable to swallow whole.

- Give at mealtimes or with a snack to reduce gastric irritation.
- Dose adjustment may be required if patient is subjected to severe stress (serious infection, surgery, or injury) or if a remission or disease exacerbation occurs.
- Do not abruptly stop drug. Reduce dose gradually by scheduled decrements (various regimens) to prevent withdrawal symptoms and permit adrenals to recover from drug-induced partial atrophy.

### Alternate-Day Therapy (ADT) for Patient on Long-Term Therapy

- With ADT, the 48 h requirement for steroids is administered as a single dose every other morning.
- Be aware that ADT minimizes adverse effects associated with long-term treatment while maintaining the desired therapeutic effect.

**ADVERSE EFFECTS** (≥1%) **CNS:** Euphoria, headache, insomnia, confusion, psychosis. **CV:** CHF, edema. **GI:** Nausea, vomiting, peptic ulcer. **Musculoskeletal:** Muscle weakness, delayed wound healing, muscle wasting, osteoporosis, aseptic necrosis of bone, spontaneous fractures. **Endocrine:** Cushing's syndrome, growth suppression in children, carbohydrate intolerance, hyperglycemia. **Special Senses:** Cataracts. **Hematologic:** Leukocytosis. **Metabolic:** Hypokalemia.

**INTERACTIONS Drug:** BARBITURATES, **phenytoin, rifampin** increase steroid metabolism—increased doses of prednisone may be needed; **amphotericin B,** DIURETICS increase **potassium** loss; **neostigmine, pyridostigmine** may cause severe muscle weakness in patients

Common adverse effects in *italic;* life-threatening effects underlined; generic names in **bold;** classifications in SMALL CAPS; ♣ Canadian drug name; ⊘ Prototype drug

1345

with myasthenia gravis; may inhibit antibody response to VACCINES, TOXOIDS.

## PHARMACOKINETICS Absorption: Readily from GI tract. **Peak:** 1–2 h. **Duration:** 1–1.5 days. **Distribution:** Crosses placenta; distributed into breast milk. **Metabolism:** In liver. **Elimination:** Hypothalamus-pituitary axis suppression: 24–36 h; in urine. **Half-Life:** 3.5 h.

## NURSING IMPLICATIONS

### Assessment & Drug Effects

- Establish baseline and continuing data regarding BP, I&O ratio and pattern, weight, fasting blood glucose level, and sleep pattern. Start flow chart as reference for planning individualized pharmacotherapeutic patient care.
- Check and record BP during dose stabilization period at least 2 × daily. Report an ascending pattern.
- Monitor patient for evidence of HPA axis suppression during long-term therapy by determining plasma cortisol levels at weekly intervals.
- Be aware that older adult patients and patients with low serum albumin are especially susceptible to adverse effects because of excess circulating free glucocorticoids.
- Be alert to signs of hypocalcemia (see Appendix F). Patients with hypocalcemia have increased requirements for pyridoxine (vitamin B$_6$), vitamins C and D, and folates.
- Be alert to possibility of masked infection and delayed healing (anti-inflammatory and immunosuppressive actions). Prednisone suppresses early classic signs of inflammation. When patient is on an extended therapy regimen, incidence of oral *Candida* infection is high. Inspect mouth daily

for symptoms: White patches, black furry tongue, painful membranes and tongue.
- Monitor bone density. Compression and spontaneous fractures of long bones and vertebrae present hazards, particularly in long-term corticosteroid treatment of rheumatoid arthritis or diabetes, in immobilized patients, and older adults.
- Be aware of previous history of psychotic tendencies. Watch for changes in mood and behavior, emotional stability, sleep pattern, or psychomotor activity, especially with long-term therapy, that may signal onset of recurrence. Report symptoms to prescriber.
- Monitor for withdrawal syndrome (e.g., myalgia, fever, arthralgia, malaise) and hypocorticism (e.g., anorexia, vomiting, nausea, fatigue, dizziness, hypotension, hypoglycemia, myalgia, arthralgia) with abrupt discontinuation of corticosteroids after long-term therapy.
- Monitor lab tests: Periodic fasting blood glucose and serum electrolytes during long-term use.

### Patient & Family Education

- Take drug as prescribed and do not alter dosing regimen or stop medication without consulting prescriber.
- Be aware that a slight weight gain with improved appetite is expected, but after dosage is stabilized, a sudden slow but steady weight increase [2 kg (5 lb)/wk] should be reported to prescriber.
- Avoid or minimize alcohol, which may contribute to steroid-ulcer development in long-term therapy.
- Report symptoms of GI distress to prescriber and do not self-medicate to find relief.
- Do not use aspirin or other OTC drugs unless they are prescribed specifically by the prescriber.

- Be fastidious about personal hygiene; give special attention to foot care, and be particularly cautious about bruising or abrading the skin.
- Report persistent backache or chest pain (possible symptoms of vertebral or rib fracture) that may occur with long-term therapy.
- Tell dentist or new prescriber about prednisone therapy.

# PREGABALIN
Lyrica

**Classifications:** ANTICONVULSANT; GABA-ANALOG; ANALGESIC/MISCELLANEOUS; ANXIOLYTIC
**Therapeutic:** ANTICONVULSANT; ANALGESIC; ANTI-ANXIETY
**Prototype:** Gabapentin
**Controlled Substance:** Schedule V

**AVAILABILITY** Capsule; oral solution

## ACTION & THERAPEUTIC EFFECT
An analog of gamma-aminobutyric acid (GABA) that increases neuronal GABA levels and reduces calcium currents in the calcium channels of neurons; this may account for its control of pain and anxiety. Its affinity for voltage-gated calcium channels may account for its antiseizure activity. *Has analgesic, anti-anxiety, and anticonvulsant properties.*

**USES** Management of neuropathic pain associated with diabetic peripheral neuropathy or spinal cord injury, adjunctive therapy for adult patients with partial-onset seizures, management of postherpetic neuralgia, fibromyalgia.

**UNLABELED USES** Treatment of generalized anxiety disorders, treatment of social anxiety disorder, treatment of moderate pain; myopathy related to drug use; restless leg syndrome, hot flashes.

**CONTRAINDICATIONS** Hypersensitivity to pregabalin or gabapentin.

**CAUTIOUS USE** History of angioedema; renal impairment or failure, hemodialysis; history of suicidal tendencies or depression; history of drug abuse or alcohol; history of PR interval prolongation; CHF, NYHA (Class III or IV) cardiac status; older adults; pregnancy (category C); lactation. Safe use in children younger than 18 y not established.

## ROUTE & DOSAGE

**Neuropathic Pain (Diabetic Peripheral Neuropathy)**
*Adult:* PO 50–100 mg t.i.d.

**Partial-Onset Seizures**
*Adult:* PO Initial dose 75 mg or less b.i.d or 50 mg t.i.d.; may increase to 300 mg b.i.d. or 200 mg t.i.d.

**Neuropathic Pain (Spinal Cord Injury)**
*Adult:* PO 75 mg b.i.d. may increase to 150–600 mg/day

**Fibromyalgia**
*Adult:* PO 75 mg b.i.d. may increase up to 150 b.i.d. within first week, then up to 300–450 mg daily (divided)

**Postherpetic Neuralgia**
*Adult:* PO Initial dose 75 mg b.i.d. or 50 mg t.i.d.; may increase to 150–300 mg b.i.d. or 100–200 mg t.i.d.

**Renal Impairment Dosage Adjustment**
*CrCl 30–60 mL/min:* 75–300 mg/day given in 2 or 3 divided doses; *15–30 mL/min:* 25–150 mg/day given in 1 or 2 divided doses; *less than 15 mL/min:* 25–75 mg once daily

**Hemodialysis Dosage Adjustment**
Dose based on renal function, give supplemental dose

## ADMINISTRATION
### Oral
- Dosage reduction is required with renal dysfunction.
- Drug should not be abruptly stopped; discontinue by tapering over a minimum of 1 wk.
- Give a supplemental dose immediately following dialysis.
- Store at 15°–30° C (59°– 86° F).

**ADVERSE EFFECTS** (≥1%) **Body as a Whole:** *Accidental injury,* flu syndrome, pain. **CNS:** Abnormal gait, amnesia, *ataxia,* confusion, *dizziness,* euphoria, headache, incoordination, myoclonus, nervousness, neuropathy, *somnolence,* speech disorder, abnormal thinking, tremor, twitching, vertigo. **CV:** Chest pain. **GI:** Constipation, dry mouth, flatulence, increased appetite, vomiting. **Urogenital:** Urinary incontinence. **Metabolic/Nutritional:** Edema, facial edema, hypoglycemia, *peripheral edema, weight gain.* **Musculoskeletal:** Back pain, myasthenia. **Respiratory:** Bronchitis, dyspnea. **Special Senses:** Abnormal vision, *blurry vision, diplopia.*

**INTERACTIONS Drug:** Concomitant use with THIAZOLIDINEDIONES may exacerbate weight gain and fluid retention.

## PHARMACOKINETICS **Absorption:** 90% bioavailability. **Peak:** 1.5 h. **Metabolism:** Negligible. **Elimination:** Primarily in the urine. **Half-Life:** 6 h.

## NURSING IMPLICATIONS
### Assessment & Drug Effects
- Monitor for and report promptly mental status or behavior changes (e.g., anxiety, panic attacks, restlessness, irritability, depression, suicidal thoughts).
- Monitor for weight gain, peripheral edema, and S&S of heart failure, especially with concurrent thiazolidinedione (e.g., rosiglitazone) therapy.
- Monitor diabetics for increased incidences of hypoglycemia.
- Supervise ambulation especially when other CNS drugs are used concurrently.
- Monitor lab tests: Baseline and periodic renal function tests; periodic platelet count.

### Patient & Family Education
- Do not drive or engage in potentially hazardous activities until response to drug is known.
- Report any of the following to a health care provider: Changes in vision (i.e., blurred vision); dizziness and incoordination; weight gain and swelling of the extremities, behavior or mood changes, especially suicidal thoughts.
- Avoid alcohol consumption while taking this drug.
- Inform your prescriber if you plan to become pregnant or father a child.

## PRIMAQUINE PHOSPHATE
(prim'a-kween)
**Classification:** ANTIMALARIAL
**Therapeutic:** ANTIMALARIAL
**Prototype:** Chloroquine

**AVAILABILITY** Tablet

## ACTION & *THERAPEUTIC EFFECT*
Acts on primary exoerythrocytic forms of *Plasmodium vivax* and *Plasmodium falciparum*. Destroys late tissue forms of *P. vivax* and thus effects radical cure (prevents relapse). *Gametocidal activity against all species of Plasmodia*

*that infect humans; interrupts transmission of malaria.*

**USES** To prevent relapse ("radical" or "clinical" cure) of *P. vivax.*

**UNLABELED USES** *P. ovale* malarias and to prevent treatment of *Pneumocystis carinii* pneumonia (PCP) in AIDS; malaria prophylaxis.

**CONTRAINDICATIONS** Hypersensitivity to primaquine or iodoquinol; rheumatoid arthritis; lupus erythematosus (SLE); hemolytic drugs, concomitant or recent use of agents capable of bone marrow depression (e.g., quinacrine; patients with G6PD deficiency), contraindicated in pregnancy.

**CAUTIOUS USE** Bone marrow depression; hematologic disease; methemoglobin reductase deficiency; cardiac disease or hypertension; children, lactation.

## ROUTE & DOSAGE

### Malaria Treatment
*Adult:* **PO** 52.6 mg (30 mg base) daily for 14 days in combination with chloroquine for chloroquine-susceptible infections or in combination with quinine plus doxycycline or tetracycline for chloroquine-resistant infections

## ADMINISTRATION
### Oral
- Give drug at mealtime or with an antacid (prescribed); may prevent or relieve gastric irritation. Notify prescriber if GI symptoms persist.
- Store in tight, light-resistant containers.

## ADVERSE EFFECTS (≥1%)
**Hematologic:** Hematologic reactions including granulocytopenia and acute hemolytic anemia in patients with G6PD deficiency, moderate leukocytosis or *leukopenia,* anemia, granulocytopenia, agranulocytosis. **GI:** Nausea, vomiting, epigastric distress, abdominal cramps. **Skin:** Pruritus. **Metabolic:** Methemoglobinemia (cyanosis). **Body as a Whole:** Headache, confusion, mental depression. **Special Senses:** Disturbances of visual accommodation. **CV:** Hypertension, arrhythmias (rare).

**INTERACTIONS Drug:** Toxicity of both **quinacrine** and primaquine increased. Increased toxicity with ANTIMALARIA agents. Avoid use with agents that prolong the QT interval (e.g., **dofetilide, dronedarone, pimozide, ziprasidone**) **Food:** avoid grapefruit juice.

**PHARMACOKINETICS Absorption:** Readily from GI tract. **Peak:** 1–2 h. **Metabolism:** Rapidly in liver to active metabolites. **Elimination:** In urine. **Half-Life:** 3.7–9.6 h.

## NURSING IMPLICATIONS
### Assessment & Drug Effects
- Be aware drug may precipitate acute hemolytic anemia in patients with G6PD deficiency, an inherited error of metabolism carried on the X chromosome, present in about 10% of American black males and certain white ethnic groups: Sardinians, Sephardic Jews, Greeks, and Iranians. Whites manifest more intense expression of hemolytic reaction than do blacks. Screen for prior to initiation of therapy.
- Monitor lab tests: Periodic CBC with differential, and Hct and Hgb.

### Patient & Family Education
- Examine urine after each voiding and to report to prescriber darkening of urine, red-tinged urine,

Common adverse effects in *italic;* life-threatening effects underlined; generic names in **bold;** classifications in SMALL CAPS; ♣ Canadian drug name; ⊙ Prototype drug

1349

PRIMAQUINE PHOSPHATE ♦ PRIMIDONE

and decrease in urine volume. Also report chills, fever, precordial pain, cyanosis (all suggest a hemolytic reaction). Sudden reductions in hemoglobin or erythrocyte count suggest an impending hemolytic reaction. Patient needs to stay hydrated through therapy.

# PRIMIDONE
(pri'mi-done)
Mysoline
**Classifications:** ANTICONVULSANT; BARBITURATE
Therapeutic: ANTICONVULSANT
**Prototype:** Phenobarbital

## AVAILABILITY Tablet

## ACTION & *THERAPEUTIC EFFECT*
Antiepileptic properties result from raising the seizure threshold and changing seizure patterns. *Effective as an anticonvulsant in all types of seizure disorders except absence seizures.*

## USES Alone or concomitantly with other anticonvulsant agents in the prophylactic management of complex partial (psychomotor) and generalized tonic-clonic (grand mal) seizures.

## UNLABELED USES Essential tremor.

## CONTRAINDICATIONS Hypersensitivity to barbiturates, porphyria; suicidal ideation; pregnancy (category D).

## CAUTIOUS USE Chronic lung disease, sleep apnea; liver or kidney disease, dialysis; hyperactive children; mental status changes, major depression, suicidal tendencies; lactation; children.

## ROUTE & DOSAGE

### Seizures
*Adult/Child (8 y or older):*
**PO** 125–250 mg/day, increased by 125–250 mg/wk (max: 2 g in 2–4 divided doses)
*Child (younger than 8 y):*
**PO** 50–125 mg/day, increased by 50–125 mg/wk (max: 2 g/day in 2–4 divided doses)
*Neonates:* **PO** 12–20 mg/kg/day in 2–4 divided doses

## ADMINISTRATION
### Oral
- Give whole or crush with fluid of patient's choice.
- Give with food if drug causes GI distress.

## ADVERSE EFFECTS (≥1%) CNS:
*Drowsiness, sedation, vertigo, ataxia, headache,* excitement (children), confusion, unusual fatigue, hyperirritability, emotional disturbances, acute psychoses (usually patients with psychomotor epilepsy). **Special Senses:** Diplopia, nystagmus, swelling of eyelids. **GI:** *Nausea, vomiting, anorexia.* **Hematologic:** <u>Leukopenia, thrombocytopenia,</u> eosinophilia, decreased serum folate levels, megaloblastic anemia (rare). **Skin:** Alopecia, maculopapular or morbilliform rash, edema, lupus erythematosus-like syndrome. **Urogenital:** Impotence. **Body as a Whole:** Lymphadenopathy, osteomalacia.

## INTERACTIONS Drug: Alcohol, CNS DEPRESSANTS compound CNS depression; **phenobarbital** may decrease absorption and increase metabolism of ORAL ANTICOAGULANTS; increases metabolism of CORTICOSTEROIDS, ORAL

CONTRACEPTIVES, ANTICONVULSANTS, **digitoxin,** possibly decreasing their effects; ANTIDEPRESSANTS potentiate adverse effects of primidone; **griseofulvin** decreases absorption of primidone. Do not use with **voriconazole.** Do not use with **voriconazole. Herbal: Kava, valerian** may potentiate sedation.

## PHARMACOKINETICS Absorption: Approximately 60–80% from GI tract. **Peak:** 4 h. **Distribution:** Distributed into breast milk. **Metabolism:** In liver to phenobarbital and PEMA. Affected cytochrome P450 isoenzymes and drug transporters: CYP2C9, CYP3A4, CYP1A2, CYP2C19, CYP2E1, UGT, and P-gp. **Elimination:** In urine. **Half-Life:** Primidone 3–24 h, PEMA 24–48 h; phenobarbital 72–144 h.

## NURSING IMPLICATIONS

### Assessment & Drug Effects

- Monitor primidone plasma levels (concentrations of primidone greater than 10 mcg/mL are usually associated with significant ataxia and lethargy). Therapeutic blood levels for primidone are 5–12 mcg/mL.
- Therapeutic response may not be evident for several weeks.
- Observe for S&S of folic acid deficiency: Mental dysfunction, psychiatric disorders, neuropathy, megaloblastic anemia. Determine serum folate levels if indicated.
- Monitor lab tests: Baseline CBC and complete metabolic panel, repeat q6mo; primidone blood level as needed.

### Patient & Family Education

- Avoid driving and other potentially hazardous activities during beginning of treatment because drowsiness, dizziness, and ataxia may be severe. Symptoms tend to disappear with continued therapy; if they persist, dosage reduction or drug withdrawal may be necessary.
- Avoid alcohol and other CNS depressants unless otherwise directed by prescriber.
- Do not take OTC medications unless approved by prescriber.
- Pregnant women should receive prophylactic vitamin K therapy for 1 mo prior to and during delivery to prevent neonatal hemorrhage.
- Withdraw primidone gradually to avoid precipitating status epilepticus.

# PROBENECID ⓟ
(proe-ben'c-sid)

Benuryl ♦, Probalan

**Classifications:** URICOSURIC; ANTIGOUT
**Therapeutic:** ANTIGOUT

## AVAILABILITY Tablet

## ACTION & *THERAPEUTIC EFFECT*
Competitively inhibits renal tubular reabsorption of uric acid, thereby promoting its excretion and reducing serum urate levels. *Prevents formation of new tophaceous deposits and uric acid build-up in the serum and tissues. As an additive to penicillin, it increases serum concentration of penicillins and prolongs their serum concentration.*

## USES Hyperuricemia in chronic gouty arthritis and tophaceous gout.

## UNLABELED USES Adjuvant to therapy with penicillin G and penicillin analogs to elevate and prolong plasma concentrations of these antibiotics; to promote uric acid excretion in hyperuricemia secondary to administration of thiazides and related diuretics, furosemide, ethacrynic acid, pyrazinamide.

Common adverse effects in *italic;* life-threatening effects underlined; generic names in **bold;** classifications in SMALL CAPS; ♦ Canadian drug name; ⓟ Prototype drug

1351

**CONTRAINDICATIONS** Blood dyscrasias; uric acid kidney stones; during or within 2–3 wk of acute gouty attack; overexcretion of uric acid (greater than 1000 mg/day); patients with creatinine clearance less than 50 mg/min; use with penicillin in presence of known renal impairment; use for hyperuricemia secondary to cancer chemotherapy.

**CAUTIOUS USE** History of peptic ulcer; pregnancy (category B); lactation; children older than 2 y.

## ROUTE & DOSAGE

**Gout**
*Adult:* **PO** 250 mg b.i.d. for 1 wk, then 500 mg b.i.d. (max: 3 g/day)

**Adjunct for Penicillin or Cephalosporin Therapy**
*Adult:* **PO** 500 mg q.i.d. or 1 g with single dose therapy (e.g., gonorrhea)
*Child (2–14 y or weight less than 50 kg):* **PO** 25–40 mg/kg/day in 4 divided doses

## ADMINISTRATION

### Oral
- Therapy is usually not initiated during an acute gouty attack. Consult prescriber.
- Minimize GI adverse effects by giving after meals, with food, milk, or antacid (prescribed). If symptoms persist, dosage reduction may be required.
- Give with a full glass of water if not contraindicated.
- Be aware that prescriber may prescribe concurrent prophylactic doses of colchicine for first 3–6 mo of therapy because frequency of acute gouty attacks may increase during first 6–12 mo of therapy.

**ADVERSE EFFECTS (≥1%) Body as a Whole:** Flushing, dizziness, fever, anaphylaxis. **CNS:** *Headache.* **GI:** *Nausea, vomiting, anorexia,* sore gums, hepatic necrosis (rare). **Urogenital:** Urinary frequency. **Hematologic:** Anemia, hemolytic anemia (possibly related to G6PD deficiency), aplastic anemia (rare). **Musculoskeletal:** Exacerbations of gout, uric acid kidney stones. **Skin:** Dermatitis, pruritus. **Respiratory:** Respiratory depression.

**DIAGNOSTIC TEST INTERFERENCE** False-positive *urine glucose* tests are possible with *Benedict's solution* or *Clinitest* [*glucose oxidase methods* not affected (e.g., *Clinistix, TesTape*)].

**INTERACTIONS Drug:** SALICYLATES may decrease uricosuric activity; may decrease **methotrexate** elimination, causing increased toxicity; decreases **nitrofurantoin** efficacy and increases its toxicity. Decreases clearance of PENICILLINS, CEPHALOSPORINS, and NSAIDS.

**PHARMACOKINETICS Absorption:** Readily from GI tract. **Onset:** 30 min. **Peak:** 2–4 h. **Duration:** 8 h. **Distribution:** Crosses placenta. **Metabolism:** In liver. **Elimination:** In urine. **Half-Life:** 4–17 h.

## NURSING IMPLICATIONS

### Assessment & Drug Effects
- Patients taking sulfonylureas may require dosage adjustment. Probenecid enhances hypoglycemic actions of these drugs (see DIAGNOSTIC TEST INTERFERENCES).
- Expect urate tophaceous deposits to decrease in size. Classic locations are in cartilage of ear pinna and big toe, but they can occur in bursae, tendons, skin, kidneys, and other tissues.

- Monitor lab tests: Periodic serum urate.

**Patient & Family Education**

- Drink fluid liberally (approximately 3000 mL/day) to maintain daily urinary output of at least 2000 mL or more. This is important because increased uric acid excretion promoted by drug predisposes to renal calculi.
- Prescriber may advise restriction of high-purine foods during early therapy until uric acid level stabilizes. Foods high in purine include organ meats (sweetbreads, liver, kidney), meat extracts, meat soups, gravy, anchovies, and sardines. Moderate amounts are present in other meats, fish, seafood, asparagus, spinach, peas, dried legumes, wild game.
- Avoid alcohol because it may increase serum urate levels.
- Do not stop taking drug without consulting prescriber. Irregular dosage schedule may sharply elevate serum urate level and precipitate acute gout.
- Report symptoms of hypersensitivity to prescriber. Discontinuation of drug is indicated.
- Do not take aspirin or other OTC medications without consulting prescriber. If a mild analgesic is required, acetaminophen is usually allowed.

---

# PROCAINAMIDE HYDROCHLORIDE ℗

(proe-kane-a′mide)

**Classification:** CLASS IA ANTIARRHYTHMIC
Therapeutic: CLASS IA ANTIARRHYTHMIC

**AVAILABILITY** Solution for injection

**ACTION & *THERAPEUTIC EFFECT***
Potent class IA antiarrhythmic that depresses excitability of myocardium to electrical stimulation, reduces conduction velocity in atria, ventricles, and His-Purkinje system. Produces peripheral vasodilation and hypotension, especially with IV use. *Effectively used for atrial arrhythmias; suppresses automaticity of His-Purkinje ventricular muscle.*

**USES** Prophylactically to maintain normal sinus rhythm following conversion of atrial flutter or fibrillation by other methods; to prevent recurrence of paroxysmal atrial fibrillation and tachycardia, paroxysmal AV junctional rhythm, ventricular tachycardia, ventricular and atrial premature contractions. Also cardiac arrhythmias associated with surgery and anesthesia.

**UNLABELED USES** Malignant hyperthermia; atrial fibrillation.

**CONTRAINDICATIONS** Hypersensitivity to procainamide or procaine, yellow dye 5 (tartrazine); blood dyscrasias; bundle branch block; complete AV block, second and third degree AV block unassisted by pacemaker; QT prolongation, torsades de pointes; non-life-threatening ventricular arrhythmias; leukopenia or agranulocytosis; SLE; concurrent use with other antiarrhythmic agents; myasthenia gravis.

**CAUTIOUS USE** Patient who has undergone electrical conversion to sinus rhythm; first-degree heart block; bone marrow suppression or cytopenia; hypotension, cardiac enlargement, CHF, MI, ischemic heart disease; coronary occlusion, ventricular dysrhythmia from digitalis intoxication, ventricular arrhythmias; hepatic or renal insufficiency; electrolyte imbalance; bronchial asthma; aspirin hypersensitivity; myasthenia

---

gravis; cytopenia; pregnancy (category C); lactation.

## ROUTE & DOSAGE

### Arrhythmias

*Adult:* **IV** 100 mg q5min at a rate of 25–50 mg/min until arrhythmia is controlled or 1 g given, then 2–6 mg/min; **IV** ACLS recommendation is 20–50 mg/min until either the arrhythmia is suppressed, hypotension occurs, the QRS complex is widened by 50%, or the max dose of 17 mg/kg is given
*Child:* **IV** PALS recommendation is 15 mg/kg over 30–60 min

### Renal Impairment Dosage Adjustment

*CrCl 35–59 mL/min:* Decrease initial maintenance dosage by approximately 30%.
*CrCl 15–34 mL/min:* Decrease initial maintenance dosage by 40–60%.
*CrCl less than 15 mL/min:* Individualize dosage

## ADMINISTRATION

### Intramuscular

▪ IM route should be used only when IV route is not feasible.

### Intravenous

Use IV route for emergency situations.

*PREPARE:* **Direct:** Dilute each 100 mg with 5–10 mL of D5W or sterile water for injection. **IV Infusion:** Add 1 g of procainamide to 250–500 mL of D5W solution to yield 4 mg/mL in 250 mL or 2 mg/mL in 500 mL.
*ADMINISTER:* **Direct:** Usual rate is 20 mg/min. Faster rates (up to 50 mg/min) should be used with caution. **IV Infusion for Adult:** 2–6 mg/min. **IV Infusion for Child:** 20–80 mcg/kg/min. ▪ Control IV administration over several hours by assessment of procainamide plasma levels. ▪ Use an infusion pump with constant monitoring. ▪ Keep patient in supine position. ▪ Be alert to signs of too rapid administration of drug (speed shock: Irregular pulse, tight feeling in chest, flushed face, headache, loss of consciousness, shock, cardiac arrest).

*INCOMPATIBILITIES:* **Solution/additive: Bretylium, esmolol, ethacrynate, milrinone, phenytoin. Y-site: Acyclovir sodium, azathioprine sodium, carboplatin, carmustine, cefamandole nafate, ceftizoxime, dantrolene sodium, diazepam, diazoxide, ganciclovir sodium, gemtuzumab ozogamicin, lansoprazole, metronidazole, milrinone acetate (amrinone), minocycline hydrochloride, phenytoin sodium, sulfamethoxazole-trimethoprim.**

▪ Store solution for up to 24 h at room temperature and for 7 days under refrigeration at 2°–8° C (36°–46° F). ▪ Slight yellowing does not alter drug potency, but discard solution if it is markedly discolored or precipitated.

## ADVERSE EFFECTS (≥1%) CNS:
Dizziness, psychosis. **CV:** Severe hypotension, pericarditis, <u>ventricular fibrillation</u>, AV block, tachycardia, flushing. **Gastrointestinal:** Diarrhea, nausea, taste disorder, vomiting. **Hematologic:** <u>Agranulocytosis with repeated use; *thrombocytopenia*</u>. **Body as a Whole:** Fever, muscle and joint pain, angioneurotic edema, myalgia, *SLE-like syndrome (50% of patients on*

Common adverse effects in *italic;* life-threatening effects <u>underlined;</u> generic names in **bold;** classifications in SMALL CAPS; ♣ Canadian drug name; ☻ Prototype drug *large doses for 1 y):* Polyarthralgias, pleuritic pain, pleural effusion. **Skin:** Maculopapular rash, pruritus, erythema, skin rash.

## DIAGNOSTIC TEST INTERFERENCE

It may alter results of the *edrophonium test.*

## INTERACTIONS

**Drug:** Other ANTI-ARRHYTHMICS add to therapeutic and toxic effects; ANTICHOLINERGIC AGENTS compound anticholinergic effects; ANTIHYPERTENSIVES add to hypotensive effects; **cimetidine** may increase levels with increase in toxicity; **fingolimod** increases antiarrhythmic effects.

## PHARMACOKINETICS

**Peak:** 15–60 min IM; **Duration:** 3 h; 8 h with sustained release. **Distribution:** Distributed to CSF, liver, spleen, kidney, brain, and heart; crosses placenta; distributed into breast milk. **Metabolism:** In liver to $N$-acetylprocainamide (NAPA), an active metabolite (30–60% metabolized to NAPA). **Elimination:** In urine. **Half-Life:** 3 h procainamide, 6 h NAPA.

## NURSING IMPLICATIONS

### Black Box Warning

*Procainamide has been associated with bone marrow depression.*

### Assessment & Drug Effects

- Check apical radial pulses before each dose during period of adjustment to the oral route.
- Patients with severe heart, liver, or kidney disease and hypotension are at particular risk for adverse effects.
- Monitor the patient's ECG and BP continuously during IV drug administration.
- Discontinue IV drug temporarily when (1) arrhythmia is interrupted, (2) severe toxic effects are present,

(3) QRS complex is excessively widened (greater than 50%), (4) PR interval is prolonged, or (5) BP drops 15 mm Hg or more. Obtain rhythm strip and notify prescriber.

- Ventricular dysrhythmias are usually abolished within a few minutes after IV dose and within an hour after IM administration.
- Report promptly complaints of chest pain, dyspnea, and anxiety. Digitalization may have preceded procainamide in patients with atrial arrhythmias. Cardiotonic glycosides may induce sufficient increase in atrial contraction to dislodge atrial mural emboli, with subsequent pulmonary embolism.

### Patient & Family Education

- Report to prescriber signs of reduced procainamide control: Weakness, irregular pulse, unexplained fatigability, anxiety.

# PROCAINE HYDROCHLORIDE ⊕

(proe'kane)

Novocain

**Classification:** LOCAL ANESTHETIC (ESTER-TYPE)
**Therapeutic:** LOCAL ANESTHETIC

## AVAILABILITY

Solution for injection

## ACTION & THERAPEUTIC EFFECT

Decreases sodium flux into nerve cell, thus depressing initial depolarization and preventing propagation and conduction of the nerve impulse. *Local anesthetic action produces loss of sensation and motor activity in circumscribed areas that are treated.*

## USES

Spinal anesthesia and epidural and peripheral nerve block by injection and infiltration methods.

## CONTRAINDICATIONS

Known hypersensitivity to procaine or to

Common adverse effects in *italic;* life-threatening effects underlined; generic names in **bold;** classifications in SMALL CAPS; ◆ Canadian drug name; ⊕ Prototype drug

1355

other drugs of similar chemical structure, to PABA, and to parabens; generalized septicemia, inflammation, or sepsis at proposed injection site; cerebrospinal diseases (e.g., meningitis, syphilis); heart block, hypotension, hypertension; bowel pathology, GI hemorrhage; coagulopathy, anticoagulants, *thrombocytopenia*.

## CAUTIOUS USE
Debilitated, acutely ill patients; obstetric delivery; increased intra-abdominal pressure; known drug allergies and sensitivities; impaired cardiac function, dysrhythmias; shock; older adults; pregnancy (category C); lactation; children.

## ROUTE & DOSAGE

### Spinal Anesthesia
*Adult:* **Intrathecal** 2 mL of 10% solution diluted with NS

### Infiltration Anesthesia/ Peripheral Nerve Block
*Adult/Adolescent/Child:* **Regional** Up to 200 mL of a 0.5% solution, up to 100 mL of a 1% solution

## ADMINISTRATION
- **0.5% Solution Preparation:** To prepare 60 mL of a 0.5% solution (5 mg/mL), dilute 30 mL of 1% solution with 30 mL of NS. Add 0.5–1 mL epinephrine 1:1000/100 mL anesthetic solution for vasoconstrictive effect (1:200,000–1:100,000).
- **0.25% Solution Preparation:** To prepare 60 mL of a 0.25% solution (2.5 mg/mL), dilute 45 mL of 1% solution with 45 mL of NS. Add 0.5–1 mL epinephrine 1:1000/100 mL anesthetic solution for vasoconstrictive effect (1:200,000–1:100,000).

- Do not use solutions that are cloudy, discolored, or that contain crystals. Discard unused portion of solutions not containing a preservative. Avoid use of solution with preservative for spinal, epidural, or caudal block.

***INCOMPATIBILITIES:*** **Solution/additive: Aminophylline, amobarbital, chlorothiazide, magnesium sulfate, phenobarbital, phenytoin, secobarbital, sodium bicarbonate.**

## ADVERSE EFFECTS (≥1%)
**CNS:** Anxiety, nervousness, dizziness, circumoral paresthesia, tremors, drowsiness, sedation, convulsions, <u>respiratory arrest</u>. With spinal anesthesia: Postspinal headache, arachnoiditis, palsies, spinal nerve paralysis, meningism. **Special Senses:** Tinnitus, blurred vision. **CV:** Myocardial depression, arrhythmias including bradycardia (also fetal bradycardia); hypotension. **GI:** Nausea, vomiting. **Skin:** Cutaneous lesions of delayed onset, urticaria, pruritus, angioneurotic edema, sweating, syncope, <u>anaphylactoid reaction</u>. **Urogenital:** Urinary retention, fecal or urinary incontinence, loss of perineal sensation and sexual function, slowing of labor and increased incidence of forceps delivery (all with caudal or epidural anesthesia).

## INTERACTIONS
**Drug:** May antagonize effects of SULFONAMIDES; increased risk of hypotension with MAOIS, ANTIHYPERTENSIVES.

## PHARMACOKINETICS
**Absorption:** Rapidly from injection site. **Onset:** 2–5 min. **Duration:** 1 h. **Metabolism:** Hydrolyzed by plasma pseudocholinesterases. **Elimination:** 80% of metabolites excreted in urine. **Half-Life:** 7.7 min.

## NURSING IMPLICATIONS

### Assessment & Drug Effects

- Be aware that reactions during dental procedure are usually mild, transient, and produced by epinephrine added to local anesthetic (e.g., headache, palpitation, tachycardia, hypertension, dizziness).
- Use procaine with epinephrine with caution in body areas with limited blood supply (e.g., fingers, toes, ears, nose). If used, inspect particular area for evidence of reduced perfusion (vasospasm): Pale, cold, sensitive skin.
- Hypotension is the most important complication of spinal anesthesia. Risk period is during first 30 min after induction and is intensified by changes in position that promote decreased venous return, or by preexisting hypertension, pregnancy, old age, or hypovolemia.

### Patient & Family Education

- Understand that there will be temporary loss of sensation in the area of the injection.
- Do not consume hot liquids or foods until sensation returns when drug used for dental procedure.

## PROCARBAZINE HYDROCHLORIDE

(proe-kar'ba-zeen)

Matulane

**Classifications:** ANTINEOPLASTIC; ALKYLATING AGENT
**Therapeutic:** ANTINEOPLASTIC
**Prototype:** Cyclophosphamide

## AVAILABILITY Capsule

## ACTION & *THERAPEUTIC EFFECT*

Hydrazine derivative with antimetabolite properties that is cell cycle–specific for the S phase of cell division. Suppresses mitosis at interphase and causes chromatin derangement. *Highly toxic to rapidly proliferating tissue.*

## USES Adjunct in palliative treatment of Hodgkin's disease.

## UNLABELED USES Solid tumors.

## CONTRAINDICATIONS Severe myelosuppression; pheochromocytoma; alcohol ingestion; foods high in tyramine content; sympathomimetic drugs. MAO inhibitors should be discontinued 14 days prior to therapy; tricyclic antidepressants discontinued 7 days before therapy; pregnancy (category D); lactation.

## CAUTIOUS USE Hepatic or renal impairment; cardiac disease; bipolar disorder, mania, paranoid schizophrenia; G6PD deficiency; parkinsonism; following radiation or chemotherapy before at least 1 mo has elapsed; alcoholism; infection; DM; children.

## ROUTE & DOSAGE

### Adjunct for Hodgkin's Disease

*Adult:* **PO** 2–4 mg/kg/day in single or divided doses for 1 wk, then 4–6 mg/kg/day until WBC less than 4000/mm$^3$ or platelets are less than 100,000/mm$^3$ or maximum response obtained; drug is then discontinued until bone marrow recovery is satisfactory; treatment is started again at 1–2 mg/kg/day
*Child/Adolescent:* **PO** 50 mg/m$^2$/day in single or divided doses for 1 wk, then 100 mg/m$^2$/day until WBC is less than 4000/mm$^3$ or platelets are less than 100,000/mm$^3$ or maximum response obtained; drug is then discontinued until bone marrow recovery is satisfactory; treatment is started again at 50 mg/m$^2$/day

---

Common adverse effects in *italic*; life-threatening effects <u>underlined</u>; generic names in **bold**; classifications in SMALL CAPS; ◆ Canadian drug name; Ⓟ Prototype drug

## ADMINISTRATION

### Oral

- Do not give if WBC count is less than 4000/mm³ or platelet count is less than 100,000/mm³. Consult prescriber.
- Store at 15°–30° C (59°–86° F). Protect from freezing, moisture, and light.

## ADVERSE EFFECTS (≥1%) CNS:

Myalgia, arthralgia, paresthesias, weakness, fatigue, lethargy, drowsiness, neuropathies, mental depression, acute psychosis, hallucinations, dizziness, headache, ataxia, nervousness, insomnia, coma, confusion, seizures. **GI:** *Severe nausea and vomiting,* anorexia, stomatitis, dry mouth, dysphagia, diarrhea, constipation, jaundice, ascites. **Hematologic:** Bone marrow suppression (*leukopenia,* anemia, *thrombocytopenia*), hemolysis, bleeding tendencies. **Skin:** Dermatitis, pruritus, herpes, hyperpigmentation, flushing, alopecia. **Respiratory:** *Pleural effusion, cough,* hoarseness. **CV:** Hypotension, tachycardia. **Body as a Whole:** Chills, fever, sweating, photosensitivity; intercurrent infections. **Urogenital:** Gynecomastia, depressed spermatogenesis, atrophy of testes.

## INTERACTIONS Drug: Alcohol,

PHENOTHIAZINES, and other CNS DEPRESSANTS add to CNS depression; TRICYCLIC ANTIDEPRESSANTS, MAO INHIBITORS, SYMPATHOMIMETICS, **ephedrine, phenylpropanolamine** may precipitate hypertensive crisis, hyperpyrexia; seizures or death. Procarbazine may enhance the effects of **CNS depressants.** A disulfiram-like reaction may occur following ingestion of **alcohol. Food:** Tyramine-containing foods may precipitate hypertensive crisis [see **phenelzine sulfate** (MAO INHIBITOR)].

## PHARMACOKINETICS Absorption:

Readily from GI tract. **Peak:** 1 h. **Distribution:** Widely distributed with high concentrations in liver, kidneys, intestinal wall, and skin. **Metabolism:** In liver. **Elimination:** In urine. **Half-Life:** 1 h.

## NURSING IMPLICATIONS

### Black Box Warning

*Procarbazine should be given only under supervision of a physician experienced in the use of potent antineoplastic drugs. Adequate clinical and laboratory facilities should be available to patients for proper monitoring of treatment.*

### Assessment & Drug Effects

- Monitor baseline and periodic BP, weight, temperature, pulse, and I&O ratio and pattern.
- Protect patient from exposure to infection and trauma when nadir of leukopenia is approached. Note and report changes in voiding pattern, hematuria, and dysuria (possible signs of urinary tract infection). Monitor I&O ratio and temperature closely.
- Withhold drug and notify prescriber of any of the following: CNS S&S (e.g., paresthesias, neuropathies, confusion); leukopenia [WBC count less than 4000/mm³; thrombocytopenia (platelet count less than 100,000/mm³)]; hypersensitivity reaction, the first small ulceration or persistent spot of soreness in oral cavity, diarrhea, and bleeding.
- Monitor for and report any of the following: Chills, fever, weakness, shortness of breath, productive cough. Drug will be discontinued.
- Assess for signs of liver dysfunction: Jaundice (yellow skin, sclerae, and soft palate), frothy or dark urine, clay-colored stools.

Common adverse effects in *italic;* life-threatening effects underlined; generic names in **bold;** classifications in SMALL CAPS; ♣ Canadian drug name; ⊙ Prototype drug

Tolerance to nausea and vomiting (most common adverse effects) usually develops by end of first week of treatment. Doses are kept at a minimum during this time. If vomiting persists, therapy will be interrupted.

Monitor lab tests: Baseline and q3-4days Hgb, Hct, WBC with differential, reticulocyte, and platelet count; baseline and weekly LFTs and renal function tests.

### Patient & Family Education

- Avoid OTC nose drops, cough medicines, and antiobesity preparations containing ephedrine, amphetamine, epinephrine, and tricyclic antidepressants because they may cause hypertensive crises. Do not use OTC preparations without prescriber's approval.
- Report to prescriber any sign of impending infection.
- Do not eat foods high in tyramine content (e.g., aged cheese, beer, wine).
- Avoid alcohol; ingestion of any form of alcohol may precipitate a disulfiram type reaction (see Appendix F).
- Report to prescriber immediately signs of hemorrhagic tendencies: Bleeding into skin and mucosa, easy bruising, nose bleeds, or blood in stool or urine. Bone marrow depression often occurs 2–8 wk after start of therapy.
- Avoid excessive exposure to the sun because of potential photosensitivity reaction: Cover as much skin area as possible with clothing, and use sunscreen lotion (SPF higher than 12) on all exposed skin surfaces.
- Use caution while driving or performing hazardous tasks until response to drug is known since drowsiness, dizziness, and blurred vision are possible adverse effects.

- Use contraceptive measures during procarbazine therapy.

# PROCHLORPERAZINE ℗
(proe-klor-per'a-zeen)
Compazine, Compro
# PROCHLORPERAZINE EDISYLATE
# PROCHLORPERAZINE MALEATE

**Classifications:** ANTIPSYCHOTIC; PHENOTHIAZINE; ANTIEMETIC
Therapeutic: ANTIPSYCHOTIC; ANTIEMETIC

**AVAILABILITY** Tablet; rectal suppositories; solution for injection. **Edisylate:** Solution for injection.

## ACTION & THERAPEUTIC EFFECT
Strong antipsychotic effects thought to be due to blockade of postsynaptic dopamine receptors in the brain. Antiemetic effect is produced by suppression of the chemoreceptor trigger zone (CTZ). *Effective antipsychotic and antiemetic properties.*

## USES Management of manifestations of psychotic disorders, of excessive anxiety, tension, and agitation, and to control severe nausea and vomiting.

## CONTRAINDICATIONS Hypersensitivity to prochlorperazine; blood dyscrasias, jaundice; comatose or severely depressed states; dementia-related psychosis in elderly; children weighing less than 9 kg (20 lb) or younger than 2 y of age; pediatric surgery; short-term vomiting in children or vomiting of unknown etiology; Reye's syndrome or other encephalopathies; lactation.

---

**CAUTIOUS USE** Parkinson's disease; decreased GI motility; paralytic ileus; GI obstruction; CVD; cerebrovascular disease, hypovolemia; hepatic impairment; renal impairment; Alzheimer disease; narrow angle glaucoma; seizure disorders; urinary retention, BPH; pregnancy (category C); children.

## ROUTE & DOSAGE

**Severe Nausea, Vomiting**

*Adult:* **PO** 5–10 mg 3–4 × day; **IM/IV** 5–10 mg q3–4h up to 40 mg/day; **PR** 25 mg b.i.d.

*Child (weight greater than 9 kg):* **PO/PR**

*Child (2–12 y, weight 18–39 kg):* **PO** 2.5 mg 3 × day; or 5 mg 2 × day (max: 15 mg/day); *(weight 14–17 kg):* **2.5 mg** 2–3 × day (max: 10 mg/day); *(weight 9–13 kg):* **2.5 mg** once/day or 2 × day (max: 7.5 mg/day).

*Child (2–12 y, weight 18–39 kg):* **IM** 0.132 mg/kg deep injection given 3–4 × day, not to exceed 10 mg/day on the first day of treatment (max: 15 mg/day on subsequent days); *weight 14–17 kg:* 0.132 mg/kg deep injection given 3–4 × day (max: 10 mg/day); *weight 9 to 13 kg:* 0.132 mg/kg deep injection given 3–4 × day; (max: 7.5 mg/day).

**Psychotic Disorders**

*Adult:* **PO** 5–10 mg 3–4 × day; titrate up q2–3days (up to 150 mg/day); **IM** 10–20 mg; may repeat q1–4h to gain control, then q4–6h

*Child (2–12 y):* **PO/PR** 2.5 mg 2–3 × day (max: 20 mg daily ages 2–5 and 25 mg daily ages 6–12); **IM** 0.132 mg/kg as a single dose

**Anxiety**

*Adult:* **PO** 5–10 mg 3–4 × day

## ADMINISTRATION

### Oral

- Administer with food, milk, or a glass of water to decrease gastric irritation.
- Dosages for older adults, emaciated patients, and children should be increased slowly.
- Do not give oral concentrate to children.
- Avoid skin contact with oral concentrate or injection solution because of possibility of contact dermatitis.

### Rectal

- Ensure that suppository is inserted beyond the anal sphincter.

### Intramuscular

- Do not inject drug subcutaneously.
- Make injection deep into the upper outer quadrant of the buttock in adults. Follow agency policy regarding IM injection site for children.
- Keep patient in recumbent position for at least 30 min following injection to minimize hypotensive effects.

### Intravenous

**PREPARE: Direct:** May be given undiluted or diluted in small amounts of NS. **IV Infusion:** Dilute in 50–100 mL of D5W, NS, D5/0.45% NaCl, LR, or other compatible solution.

Common adverse effects in *italic;* life-threatening effects <u>underlined</u>; generic names in **bold;** classifications in SMALL CAPS; ✦ Canadian drug name; ⦿ Prototype drug

**ADMINISTER: Direct: Do not** give a bolus dose. Give at a maximum rate of 5 mg/min. **IV Infusion:** Give over 15–30 min. Do not exceed direct IV rate.

**INCOMPATIBILITIES:** Solution/additive: **Aminophylline, calcium gluconate, cephalothin, chloramphenicol, chlorothiazide, epinephrine, furosemide, hydrocortisone, hydromorphone, methohexital, midazolam, morphine, penicillin G sodium, pentobarbital, phenobarbital, tetracycline, vancomycin, warfarin. Y-site: Acyclovir, aldesleukin, allopurinol, amifostine, aminocaproic acid, aminophylline, amphotericin B cholesteryl complex, ampicillin, azathioprine, aztreonam, bivalirudin, bretylium, cefmanadole, cefazolin, cefepime, cefoperazone, cefotaxime, cefotetan, cefoxitin, ceftazidime, ceftizoxime, ceftriaxone, cefuroxime, chloramphenicol, clindamycin, dantrolene, dexamethasone, diazepam, diazoxide, epoetin alfa, ertapenem, etoposide, fenoldopam, filgrastim, fluorouracil, folic acid, foscarnet, furosemide, gallium, ganciclovir, gemcitabine, gemtuzumab, imipenem-cilastatin, indomethacin, insulin, ketorolac, lansoprazole, levofloxacin, midazolam, minocycline, mitomycin, nitroprusside, pantoprazole, pemetrexed, pentamidine, pentobarbital, phenytoin, piperacillin-tazobactam, sodium bicarbonate, streptokinase, SMZ/TMP, urokinase.**

▪ Discard markedly discolored solutions; slight yellowing does not appear to alter potency.

**ADVERSE EFFECTS** (≥1%) **CNS:** *Drowsiness*, dizziness, *extrapyramidal reactions (akathisia, dystonia, or parkinsonism)*, persistent tardive dyskinesia, acute catatonia. **CV:** Hypotension. **GI:** Cholestatic jaundice, diarrhea, nausea, vomiting, taste disorder. **Skin:** Contact dermatitis, photosensitivity. **Endocrine:** Galactorrhea, amenorrhea. **Special Senses:** Blurred vision. **Hematologic:** *Leukopenia, agranulocytosis*.

**INTERACTIONS Drug: Alcohol,** CNS DEPRESSANTS increase CNS depression; ANTACIDS, ANTIDIARRHEALS decrease absorption, therefore, administer 2 h apart; **phenobarbital** increases metabolism of prochlorperazine; GENERAL ANESTHETICS increase excitation and hypotension; antagonizes antihypertensive action of **guanethidine; phenylpropanolamine** poses possibility of sudden death; TRICYCLIC ANTIDEPRESSANTS intensify hypotensive and anticholinergic effects; decreases seizure threshold—ANTICONVULSANT dosage may need to be increased. **Herbal: Kava** may increase risk and severity of dystonic reactions.

**PHARMACOKINETICS Absorption:** Readily from GI tract. **Onset:** 30–40 min PO; 60 min PR; 10–20 min IM. **Duration:** 3–4 h PO; 10–12 h sustained release PO; 3–4 h PR; up to 12 h IM. **Distribution:** Crosses placenta; distributed into breast milk. **Metabolism:** In liver. **Elimination:** In urine.

## NURSING IMPLICATIONS

**Black Box Warning**

*Prochlorperazine has been associated with increased mortality in older adults with dementia-related psychosis.*

**Assessment & Drug Effects**

- Position carefully to prevent aspiration of vomitus; may have depressed cough reflex.
- Most older adult and emaciated patients and children, especially those with dehydration or acute illness, appear to be particularly susceptible to extrapyramidal effects. Be alert to onset of symptoms: Early in therapy watch for pseudoparkinson's and acute dyskinesia. After 1–2 mo, be alert to akathisia.
- Monitor mental status and report significant changes in mood, behavior, or functional ability when used for long-term therapy.
- Be alert to signs of high core temperature: Red, dry, hot skin; full bounding pulse; dilated pupils; dyspnea; confusion; temperature over 40.6° C (105° F); elevated BP. Exposure to high environmental temperature places this patient at risk for heat stroke. Inform prescriber and institute measures to reduce body temperature rapidly.
- Monitor lab tests: Periodic CBC with differential, LFTs, fasting plasma glucose, HgbA1C, lipid profile with long-term therapy.

**Patient & Family Education**

- Take drug only as prescribed and do not alter dose or schedule. Consult prescriber before stopping the medication.
- Avoid hazardous activities such as driving a car until response to drug is known because drug may impair mental and physical abilities, especially during first few days of therapy.
- Be aware that drug may color urine reddish brown. It also may cause the sun-exposed skin to turn gray-blue.
- Protect skin from direct sun's rays and use a sunscreen lotion (SPF higher than 12) to prevent photosensitivity reaction.

- Withhold dose and report to the prescriber if the following symptoms persist more than a few hours: Tremor, involuntary twitching, exaggerated restlessness. Other reportable symptoms include light-colored stools, changes in vision, sore throat, fever, rash.

# PROGESTERONE ⊙

(proe-jess'ter-one)

Crinone Gel, Gesterol 50, Progestaject, Prometrium

**Classification:** PROGESTIN

Therapeutic: PROGESTIN

**AVAILABILITY** Capsule; solution for injection; gel; vaginal insert; vaginal suppository

**ACTION & *THERAPEUTIC EFFECT***
Has estrogenic, anabolic, and androgenic activity. Transforms endometrium from proliferative to secretory state; suppresses pituitary gonadotropin secretion, thereby blocking follicular maturation and ovulation. *Relaxes estrogen-primed myometrium and prohibits spontaneous contraction of uterus. Sudden drop in blood levels of progestin (and estradiol) causes "withdrawal bleeding" from endometrium. Intrauterine placement of progesterone hypothetically inhibits sperm survival, and suppresses endometrial proliferation (antiestrogenic effect).*

**USES** Secondary amenorrhea, functional uterine bleeding, endometriosis, and premenstrual syndrome. Largely supplanted by new progestins, which have longer action and oral effectiveness. Treatment of infertile women with progesterone deficiency.

**CONTRAINDICATIONS** Hypersensitivity to progestins, known

or suspected breast or genital malignancy; use as a pregnancy test; thrombophlebitis, thromboembolic disorders; ectopic pregnancy; cerebral apoplexy (or its history); severely impaired liver function or disease; undiagnosed vaginal bleeding, incomplete abortion; use during first 4 mo of pregnancy (category X); other than vaginal gel use for assisted reproductive technology (ART) in early pregnancy.

**CAUTIOUS USE** Anemia; diabetes mellitus; history of psychic depression; persons susceptible to acute intermittent porphyria or with conditions that may be aggravated by fluid retention (asthma, seizure disorders, cardiac or kidney function, migraine); impaired liver function; previous ectopic pregnancy; presence or history of salpingitis; venereal disease; unresolved abnormal Pap smear; genital bleeding of unknown etiology; previous pelvic surgery; lactation. **Vaginal gel:** In early first trimester (category B).

## ROUTE & DOSAGE

**Amenorrhea**
*Adult:* **IM** 5–10 mg for 6–8 consecutive days; **PO** 400 mg at bedtime × 10 days; **Vaginal gel** 45 mg every other day (up to 6 doses)

**Uterine Bleeding**
*Adult:* **IM** 5–10 mg/day for 6 days

**Premenstrual Syndrome**
*Adult:* **PR** 200–400 mg/day

**Assisted Reproductive Technology**
*Adult:* **Vaginal** 90 mg gel daily or b.i.d. until placental autonomy OR 10–12 wk; 100 mg insert 2–3 × daily up to 10 wk

## ADMINISTRATION

### Oral
- Give at bedtime and advise caution with ambulation because drug may cause drowsiness or dizziness.
- Do not give oral capsules, which contain peanut oil, to patients allergic to peanuts.

### Intramuscular
- Immerse vial in warm water momentarily to redissolve crystals (if present) and to facilitate aspiration of drug into syringe.
- Inject deeply IM. Injection site may be irritated. Inspect IM sites carefully and rotate areas systematically.

### Rectal
- Ensure that suppository is inserted beyond the anal sphincter.

### Vaginal
- A dosage increase from the 4% gel can only be accomplished by using the 8% gel. Increasing the volume of gel administered does not increase the amount of progesterone absorbed.
- Store drug at 15°–30° C (59°–86° F) unless otherwise specified by manufacturer. Protect from freezing and light.

## ADVERSE EFFECTS (≥1%) CNS:
Migraine headache, *dizziness,* lethargy, mental depression, somnolence, insomnia. **CV:** <u>Thromboembolic disorder, pulmonary embolism</u>. **Special Senses:** Change in vision, proptosis, diplopia, papilledema, retinal vascular lesions. **GI:** Hepatic disease, cholestatic jaundice; *nausea,* vomiting, *abdominal cramps.* **Urogenital:** Vaginal candidiasis, chloasma, cervical erosion and changes in secretions, *breakthrough bleeding,* dysmenorrhea, amenorrhea, pruritus vulvae. **Metabolic:** Hyperglycemia, decreased libido, transient increase in sodium and chloride

Common adverse effects in *italic;* life-threatening effects <u>underlined</u>; generic names in **bold**; classifications in SMALL CAPS; ♣ Canadian drug name; ☯ Prototype drug

1363

excretion, pyrexia. **Skin:** *Acne,* pruritus, allergic rash, photosensitivity, urticaria, hirsutism, alopecia. **Body as a Whole:** *Edema, weight changes;* pain at injection site; fatigue. **Endocrine:** Gynecomastia, galactorrhea.

## DIAGNOSTIC TEST INTERFERENCE

PROGESTINS may decrease levels of *urinary pregnanediol* and increase levels of *serum alkaline phosphatase, plasma amino acids, urinary nitrogen,* and *coagulation factors VII, VIII, IX,* and *X.* They also decrease *glucose tolerance* (may cause false-positive *urine glucose tests*) and lower *HDL* (high-density lipoprotein) levels.

## INTERACTIONS Drug: BARBITU-
RATES, **carbamazepine, phenytoin, rifampin** may alter contraceptive effectiveness; **ketoconazole** may inhibit progesterone metabolism; may antagonize effects of **bromocriptine.**

## PHARMACOKINETICS Absorption: Rapid from IM site; PO peaks at 3 h. **Metabolism:** Extensively in liver. **Elimination:** Primarily in urine; excreted in breast milk. **Half-Life:** 5 min.

## NURSING IMPLICATIONS

### Black Box Warning

*Progesterone in combination with estrogen has been associated with increased risk of invasive breast cancer.*

### Assessment & Drug Effects

- Record baseline data for comparative value about patient's weight, BP, and pulse at onset of progestin therapy. Report deviations promptly.

- Monitor lab tests: Periodic LFTs, blood glucose, and serum electrolytes.
- Monitor for and report immediately S&S of thrombophlebitis or thromboembolic disease.

### Patient & Family Education

- If other intravaginal therapy is being used concurrently, allow at least 6 h before/after progesterone vaginal gel insertion.
- Small, white globules may appear as a vaginal discharge, possibly caused by progesterone vaginal gel accumulation, even several days after usage.
- Inform prescriber promptly if any of the following occur: Sudden severe headache or vomiting, dizziness or fainting, numbness in an arm or leg, pain in calves accompanied by swelling, warmth, and redness; acute chest pain or dyspnea.
- Report to prescriber promptly unexplained sudden or gradual, partial or complete loss of vision, ptosis, or diplopia.
- Monitor for loss of glycemic control if diabetic.
- Notify prescriber if you become or suspect pregnancy. Learn the potential risk to the fetus from exposure to progestin.

# PROMETHAZINE HYDROCHLORIDE

(proe-meth'a-zeen)

Histantil ◆, Phenergan

**Classifications:** ANTIHISTAMINE; ANTIEMETIC; ANTIVERTIGO
**Therapeutic:** ANTIHISTAMINE; ANTIEMETIC; ANTIVERTIGO
**Prototype:** Prochlorperazine

**AVAILABILITY** Tablet; oral solution; rectal suppository; injection

## ACTION & *THERAPEUTIC EFFECT*

Exerts anti-serotonin, anticholinergic, and local anesthetic action. Antiemetic action thought to be due to depression of CTZ in medulla. *Long-acting derivative of phenothiazine with marked antihistamine activity and prominent sedative, amnesic, antiemetic, and anti-motion sickness actions.*

**USES** Motion sickness, nausea/vomiting, induction of sedation, pruritus.

**UNLABELED USES** Allergic rhinitis, hyperemesis gravidarum, nystagmus

**CONTRAINDICATIONS** Hypersensitivity to phenothiazines; acute MI; angina, atrial fibrillation, atrial flutter, cardiac arrhythmias, cardiomyopathy, uncontrolled hypertension; MAOI therapy; comatose or severely depressed states, hepatic encephalopathy, hepatic diseases; acutely ill or dehydrated children; children with Reye's syndrome; lactation; children younger than 2 y.

**CAUTIOUS USE** Impaired liver function; epilepsy; bone marrow depression; cardiovascular disease; peripheral vascular disease; asthma; acute or chronic respiratory impairment (particularly in children); hypertension; narrow angle glaucoma; stenosing peptic ulcer, pyloroduodenal obstruction; prostatic hypertrophy; bladder neck obstruction; older adult or debilitated patients; pregnancy (category C).

## ROUTE & DOSAGE

### Motion Sickness

*Adult:* **PO/PR** 25 mg q12h prn
*Child (2 y or older):* **PO/PR** 12.5–25 mg q12h prn (max: 25 mg/dose)

### Nausea

*Adult:* **PO/PR/IM/IV** 12.5–25 mg q4–6h prn
*Child (2 y or older):* **PO/PR/IM/IV** 0.25–1 mg/kg/dose q4–6h prn (max: 25 mg/dose)

### Pruritus

*Adult:* **PO/PR** 12.5 mg t.i.d. or 25 mg at bedtime; **IM/IV** 25 mg, repeat in 2 h if necessary, switch to PO
*Child (2 y or older):* **PO** 6.25–12.5 mg q.i.d.; **IV/IM** 0.5 mg/pound (max: 12.5 mg)

### Sedation

*Adult:* **PO/IM/IV** 25–50 mg/dose
*Child (2 y or older):* **PO/IM/IV** 0.5 mg/pound (max: 25 mg dose)

## ADMINISTRATION

### Oral

- Give with food, milk, or a full glass of water may minimize GI distress.
- Tablets may be crushed and mixed with water or food before swallowing.
- Oral doses for allergy are generally prescribed before meals and on retiring or as single dose at bedtime.

### Rectal

- Ensure that suppository is inserted beyond the rectal sphincter.

### Intramuscular

- Give IM injection deep into large muscle mass. Aspirate carefully before injecting drug. Intra-arterial injection can cause arterial or arteriolar spasm, with resultant gangrene.

### Intravenous

**PREPARE: Direct:** The 25 mg/mL concentration may be given undiluted. ▪ Dilute the 50 mg/mL concentration in NS to yield no more than 25 mg/mL (e.g., diluting the

P

Common adverse effects in *italic;* life-threatening effects <u>underlined;</u> generic names in **bold;** classifications in SMALL CAPS; ✚ Canadian drug name; ⦿ Prototype drug

1365

50 mg/mL concentration in 4 mL yields 10 mg/mL). ▪ Inspect parenteral drug before preparation. Discard if it is darkened or contains precipitate.

*ADMINISTER:* **Direct:** Give each 25 mg or fraction thereof over at least 1 min.

*INCOMPATIBILITIES:* **Solution/additive: Aminophylline, ampicillin, carbenicillin, cefazolin, cefotetan, ceftizoxime, chloramphenicol, chlordiazepoxide, chlorothiazide, dexamethasone, dimenhydrinate floxacillin, furosemide, heparin, hydrocortisone, ketorolac, methicillin, methohexital, nalbuphine, nitrofurantoin, penicillin G sodium, pentobarbital, phenobarbital. Y-site: Acyclovir, aldesleukin, allopurinol, aminophylline, amphotericin B asparaginase cholesteryl complex, ampicillin, azathioprine, bretylium, carmustine, cefamandole, cefepime, cefmetazole, cefonicid, cefoperazone, cefotaxime, cefotetan, cefoxitin, ceftazidime, ceftobiprole, ceftriaxone, cefuroxime, cephalothin, cephapirin, chloramphenicol, clindamycin, dantrolene, dexamethasone, diazepam, diazoxide, doxorubicin liposome, ertapenem, fluorouracil, foscarnet, furosemide, ganciclovir, gemtuzumab, heparin, indomethacin, ketorolac, lansoprazole, methicillin, methotrexate, methylprednisolone, mezlocillin, milrinone acetate, minocycline, nafcillin, nitroprusside, oxacillin, pantoprazole, penicillin G, pentobarbital, phenobarbital, phenytoin, piperacillin/tazobactam, streptokinase, TPN, urokinase.**

▪ Injection and oral: Store at 20°–25° C (68°–77° F) in tight, light-resistant container unless otherwise directed.

**ADVERSE EFFECTS** (≥1%) **Body as a Whole:** Deep sleep, coma, convulsions, cardiorespiratory symptoms, extrapyramidal reactions, nightmares (in children), CNS stimulation, abnormal movements. **Respiratory:** Irregular respirations, respiratory depression, apnea. **CNS:** *Sedation, drowsiness,* confusion, dizziness, disturbed coordination, restlessness, tremors. **CV:** Transient mild hypotension or hypertension. **GI:** Anorexia, nausea, vomiting, constipation. **Hematologic:** Leukopenia, agranulocytosis. **Special Senses:** *Blurred vision, dry mouth,* nose, or throat, tinnitus. **Skin:** Photosensitivity. **Urogenital:** Urinary retention.

**DIAGNOSTIC TEST INTERFERENCE**
May produce false results with *urinary pregnancy tests.* Promethazine can cause significant alterations of *flare response* in *intradermal allergen tests* if performed within 4 days of patient receiving promethazine.

**INTERACTIONS Drug: Alcohol** and other CNS DEPRESSANTS add to CNS depression and anticholinergic effects.

**PHARMACOKINETICS Absorption:** Readily from GI tract. **Onset:** 20 min PO/PR/IM; 5 min IV. **Duration:** 2–8 h. **Distribution:** Crosses placenta. **Metabolism:** In liver (CYP2D6, 2B6). **Elimination:** Slowly in urine and feces.

**NURSING IMPLICATIONS**

**Black Box Warning**

*Promethazine has been associated with severe respiratory depression*

Common adverse effects in *italic;* life-threatening effects underlined; generic names in **bold;** classifications in SMALL CAPS; ♣ Canadian drug name; ◯ Prototype drug

*and death in pediatric patients younger than 2 y.*

## Assessment & Drug Effects

- Monitor respiratory function in patients with respiratory problems, particularly children. Drug may suppress cough reflex and cause thickening of bronchial secretions.
- Supervise ambulation. Promethazine sometimes produces marked sedation and dizziness.
- Monitor for and report promptly S&S of neuroleptic malignant syndrome.
- Monitor for seizures in those with a history of seizure disorders.
- Patients in pain may develop involuntary (athetoid) movements of upper extremities following parenteral administration. These symptoms usually disappear after pain is controlled.

## Patient & Family Education

- For motion sickness: Take initial dose 30–60 min before anticipated travel and repeat at 8–12 h intervals if necessary. For duration of journey, repeat dose on arising and again at evening meal.
- Do not drive or engage in other potentially hazardous activities requiring mental alertness and normal reaction time until response to drug is known.
- Supervise children to avoid potential harm during play activities.
- Avoid sunlamps or prolonged exposure to sunlight.
- Avoid alcohol and other CNS depressants.

## PROPAFENONE
(pro-pa′fen-one)
Rythmol, Rythmol SR

**Classification:** CLASS IC ANTIARRHYTHMIC
**Therapeutic:** CLASS IC ANTIARRHYTHMIC
**Prototype:** Flecainide

**AVAILABILITY** Tablet; sustained release capsule

### ACTION & *THERAPEUTIC EFFECT*
Class IC antiarrhythmic drug with a direct stabilizing action on myocardial membranes. Reduces spontaneous automaticity. Exerts a negative inotropic effect on the myocardium. *Decreases rate of single and multiple PVCs and suppresses ventricular arrhythmias.*

**USES** Ventricular arrhythmias, atrial fibrillation, paroxysmal supraventricular tachycardia.

**UNLABELED USES** Wolff–Parkinson–White syndrome.

**CONTRAINDICATIONS** Hypersensitivity to propafenone; uncontrolled CHF, cardiogenic shock, sinoatrial, AV or intraventricular disorders (e.g., sick sinus node syndrome, AV block) without a pacemaker; cardiogenic shock; bradycardia, QT prolongation; marked hypotension; bronchospastic disorders; electrolyte imbalances; non-life-threatening arrhythmias.

**CAUTIOUS USE** CHF, COPD, chronic bronchitis; AV block; hepatic/renal impairment; older adult patients; pregnancy (category C); lactation. Safe use in children not established.

### ROUTE & DOSAGE

**Ventricular Arrhythmias**
*Adult:* **PO Immediate release**
Initiate with 150 mg q8h,

---

may be increased at 3–4 days intervals (max: 300 mg q8h)

**Atrial Fibrillation**

*Adult:* **PO Extended release** 225 mg q12h increase to response (max: 425 mg q12h).

## ADMINISTRATION

### Oral

- Dosage increments are usually made gradually with older adults or those with previous extensive myocardial damage.
- Significant dose reduction is warranted with severe liver dysfunction. Consult prescriber.
- Store at 15°–30° C (59°–86° F).

**ADVERSE EFFECTS** (≥1%) **CNS:** *Blurred vision, dizziness,* paresthesias, fatigue, somnolence, vertigo, headache. **CV:** Arrhythmias, ventricular tachycardia, hypotension, bundle branch block, AV block, complete heart block, sinus arrest, CHF. **Hematologic:** *Leukopenia,* granulocytopenia (both rare). **GI:** Nausea, abdominal discomfort, constipation, vomiting, dry mouth, *taste alterations,* cholestatic hepatitis. **Skin:** Rash.

**INTERACTIONS Drug: Amiodarone, quinidine** increases the levels and toxicity of propafenone. May increase levels and toxicity of TRICYCLIC ANTIDEPRESSANTS, **cyclosporine, digoxin,** BETA-BLOCKERS, **theophylline,** and **warfarin** may increase levels of both **propafenone** and **diltiazem. Phenobarbital** decreases levels of **propafenone.** Use with caution in drugs that prolong the QT interval.

## PHARMACOKINETICS

**Absorption:** Readily from GI tract. **Peak:** 3.5 h. **Distribution:** 97% protein bound, concentrates in the lung. Crosses placenta, distributed into breast milk.

**Metabolism:** Hepatic via CY2D6, CYPD3A4, CYP1A2. **Elimination:** 18.5–38% of dose excreted in urine as metabolites. **Half-Life:** 2–10 h in extensive metabolizers and 10–32 h in slow metabolizers.

## NURSING IMPLICATIONS

### Assessment & Drug Effects

- Monitor cardiovascular status frequently (e.g., ECG, Holter monitor) to determine effectiveness of drug and development of new or worsened arrhythmias.
- Monitor closely patients with preexisting CHF for worsening of this condition. Monitor for digoxin toxicity with concurrent use, because drug may increase serum digoxin levels.
- Report development of second- or third-degree AV block or significant widening of the QRS complex. Dosage adjustment may be warranted.

### Patient & Family Education

- Report to prescriber any of following: Chest pain, palpitations, blurred or abnormal vision, dyspnea, or signs and symptoms of infection.
- Be aware when taking concurrent warfarin of possible increase in plasma levels that increase bleeding risk. Report unusual bleeding or bruising.
- Monitor radial pulse daily and report decreased heart rate or development of an abnormal heartbeat.
- Be aware of possibility of dizziness and need for caution with walking, especially in older adult or debilitated patients.

## PROPANTHELINE BROMIDE

(proe-pan′the-leen)

Propanthel ◆

**Classifications:** ANTICHOLINERGIC; ANTIMUSCARINIC; ANTISPASMODIC
**Therapeutic:** ANTICHOLINERGIC
**Prototype:** Atropine

Common adverse effects in *italic;* life-threatening effects underlined; generic names in **bold;** classifications in SMALL CAPS; ◆ Canadian drug name; ⊘ Prototype drug

**AVAILABILITY** Tablet

**ACTION & *THERAPEUTIC EFFECT***
Has potent postganglionic nicotinic receptor blocking action and diminishes gastric acid secretion. *Decreases motility (smooth muscle tone) resulting in antispasmodic action and decreases gastric acid secretion.*

**USES** Adjunct in treatment of peptic ulcer disease.

**CONTRAINDICATIONS** Narrow-angle glaucoma; tachycardia, MI; paralytic ileus, GI obstructive disease; hemorrhagic shock; myasthenia gravis.

**CAUTIOUS USE** CAD, CHF, cardiac arrhythmias; liver disease, ulcerative colitis, hiatus hernia, esophagitis; kidney disease; BPH, glaucoma; debilitated patients; hyperthyroidism; autonomic neuropathy; brain damage; Down's syndrome; spastic disorders; pregnancy (category C); lactation. Safe use in children not established.

**ROUTE & DOSAGE**

**Peptic Ulcer Disease**
*Adult:* **PO** 15 mg before each meal and 30 mg at bedtime

**ADMINISTRATION**
**Oral**
- Give 30–60 min before meals and at bedtime. Advise not to chew tablet; drug is bitter.
- Give at least 1 h before or 1 h after an antacid (or antidiarrheal agent).
- Store dry powder and tablets at 20°–25° C (68°–77° F); protect from freezing and moisture.

**ADVERSE EFFECTS** (≥1%) **GI:** *Constipation, dry mouth.* **Special Senses:** Blurred vision, mydriasis, increased intraocular pressure. **CNS:** Drowsiness, confusion, headache, insomnia, nervousness. **Urogenital:** Decreased sexual activity, difficult urination. Neuromuscular and skeletal muscle weakness.

**INTERACTIONS Drug:** Decreased absorption of **ketoconazole;** ORAL POTASSIUM may increase risk of GI ulcers. Use with other ANTIMUSCARINIC agents can increase side effects. **Food:** Food significantly decreases absorption.

**PHARMACOKINETICS Absorption:** Incompletely from GI tract. **Onset:** 30–45 min. **Duration:** 4–6 h. **Metabolism:** 50% in GI tract before absorption; 50% in liver. **Elimination:** Primarily in urine; some in bile. **Half-Life:** 9 h.

**NURSING IMPLICATIONS**
**Assessment & Drug Effects**
- Assess bowel sounds, especially in presence of ulcerative colitis, since paralytic ileus may develop, predisposing to toxic megacolon.
- Be aware that older adult or debilitated patients may respond to a usual dose with agitation, excitement, confusion, drowsiness. Stop drug and report to prescriber if these symptoms are observed.
- Check BP, heart sounds and rhythm periodically in patients with cardiac disease.
- Monitor lab tests: Serum creatinine/BUN.

**Patient & Family Education**
- Void just prior to each dose to minimize risk of urinary hesitancy or retention. Record daily urinary volume and report problems to prescriber.
- Relieve dry mouth by rinsing with water frequently, chewing sugar-free gum, or sucking hard candy.

---

Common adverse effects in *italic;* life-threatening effects <u>underlined;</u> generic names in **bold;** classifications in SMALL CAPS; ♣ Canadian drug name; ⊙ Prototype drug

1369

- Maintain adequate fluid and high-fiber food intake to prevent constipation.
- Make all position changes slowly and lie down immediately if faintness, weakness, or palpitations occur. Report symptoms to prescriber.
- Do not drive or engage in potentially hazardous activities until response to drug is known.

# PROPOFOL
(pro'po-fol)
Diprivan

**Classifications:** GENERAL ANESTHESIA; SEDATIVE-HYPNOTIC
Therapeutic: SEDATIVE-HYPNOTIC; GENERAL ANESTHESIA

## AVAILABILITY Solution for injection

## ACTION & *THERAPEUTIC EFFECT*
Sedative-hypnotic used in the induction and maintenance of anesthesia or sedation. Rapid onset (40 sec) and minimal excitation during induction of anesthesia. *Effectively used for conscious sedation and maintenance of anesthesia.*

## USES Induction or maintenance of anesthesia as part of a balanced anesthesia technique; conscious sedation in mechanically ventilated patients.

## CONTRAINDICATIONS Hypersensitivity to propofol or propofol emulsion, which contain soybean and soy products, and egg phosphatide; patients with increased intracranial pressure or impaired cerebral circulation; patients whom general anesthesia or sedation is contraindicated; obstetrical procedures; lactation. Do not use for induction of anesthesia in children younger than 3 y and for maintenance of anesthesia in infants younger than 2 mo.

## CAUTIOUS USE Patients with severe cardiac or respiratory disorders, respiratory depression, hypoxemia, hypertension; history of epilepsy or seizures; hypovolemia; lipid metabolism disorders; older adults; pregnancy (category B).

## ROUTE & DOSAGE

### Induction of Anesthesia
*Adult:* **IV** 2–2.5 mg/kg as total dose; administered as approximately 40 mg q10 sec until onset of anesthesia
*Adult (55 y or older):* **IV** 1–1.5 mg/kg as total dose, administer approximately 20 mg q10sec until onset of anesthesia
*Adolescent/Child (3 y or older):* **IV** 2.5–3.5 mg/kg over 20–30 sec

### Maintenance of Anesthesia
*Adult:* **IV** 50–200 mcg/kg/min for 10–15 min
*Adult (55 y or older):* **IV** 50–100 mcg/kg/min
*Child/Infant (2 mo or older):* **IV** 125–300 mcg/kg/min

## ADMINISTRATION
- Use strict aseptic technique to prepare propofol for injection; drug emulsion supports rapid growth of microorganisms.
- Inspect for particulate matter and discoloration. Discard if either is noted.
- Shake well before use. Inspect for separation of the emulsion. Do not use if there is evidence of separation of phases of the emulsion.

### Intravenous
***PREPARE:*** **IV Infusion:** Give undiluted or diluted in D5W to a concentration not less than 2 mg/mL. Begin drug administration immediately after preparation and complete within 12 h.
***ADMINISTER:*** **IV Infusion:** Use syringe or volumetric pump to

Common adverse effects in *italic;* life-threatening effects <u>underlined;</u> generic names in **bold;** classifications in SMALL CAPS; ✦ Canadian drug name; ◉ Prototype drug control rate. ▪ Rate is determined by patient weight in kg. Depending on the form of the drug, indication, and patient's health status and age, drug may be given by variable rate infusion or intermittent IV bolus (usually over 3–5 min). ▪ Administer immediately after spiking the vial. Complete infusion within 12 h.

*INCOMPATIBILITIES:* Y-site: Amikacin, amphotericin B, ascorbic acid, atracurium, atropine, bretylium, calcium chloride, ceftolozane-tazobactam, ciprofloxacin, cisatracurium, diazepam, digoxin, doripenem, doxorubicin, hydrochloric acid, hydroxocobalamin, isavuconazonium sulfate, gentamicin, levofloxacin, methotrexate, methylprednisolone, metoclopramide, metronidazole, minocycline, mitoxantrone, netilmicin, nimodipine, phenytoin, remifentanil, temocillin sodium, tobramycin, verapamil.

▪ Store unopened between 4° C (40° F) and 22° C (72° F). Refrigeration is not recommended. Protect from light.

## ADVERSE EFFECTS (≥1%) CNS:
Headache, dizziness, *twitching, bucking, jerking, thrashing, clonic/myoclonic movements.* **Special Senses:** Decreased intraocular pressure. **CV:** *Hypotension,* bradycardia, ventricular asystole (rare). **GI:** Vomiting, abdominal cramping. **Respiratory:** Cough, hiccups, apnea. **Other:** Pain at injection site.

## DIAGNOSTIC TEST INTERFERENCE
Propofol produces a temporary reduction in *serum cortisol levels.* However, propofol does not seem to inhibit adrenal responsiveness to *ACTH.*

## INTERACTIONS Drug: Concurrent
continuous infusions of propofol and **alfentanil** produce higher plasma

levels of **alfentanil** than expected. CNS DEPRESSANTS cause additive CNS depression. **Amiodarone** use (current or recent) can increase risk of hypotension.

## PHARMACOKINETICS Onset:
9–36 sec. **Duration:** 6–10 min. **Distribution:** Highly lipophilic, crosses placenta, excreted in breast milk. **Metabolism:** Extensively in the liver (CYP2B6, 2C9). **Elimination:** Approximately 88% of the dose is recovered in the urine as metabolites. **Half-Life:** 5–12 h.

## NURSING IMPLICATIONS
### Assessment & Drug Effects
▪ Monitor hemodynamic status and assess for dose-related hypotension.
▪ Monitor vital signs.
▪ Take seizure precautions. Tonic-clonic seizures have occurred following general anesthesia with propofol.
▪ Be alert to the potential for drug-induced excitation (e.g., twitching, tremor, hyperclonus) and take appropriate safety measures.
▪ Provide comfort measures; pain at the injection site is quite common especially when small veins are used.
▪ Monitor lab tests: Urine zinc levels if administered for longer than 5 days or in patients experiencing burns, diarrhea, or major sepsis.

# PROPRANOLOL HYDROCHLORIDE ℗

(proe-pran'oh-lole)

Apo-Propranolol ♦, Inderal, Inderal LA, InnoPran XL, Novopranol ♦

**Classifications:** BETA-ADRENERGIC RECEPTOR ANTAGONIST; ANTIHYPERTENSIVE; CLASS II ANTIARRHYTHMIC
**Therapeutic:** ANTIHYPERTENSIVE; CLASS II ANTIARRHYTHMIC; ANTIANGINAL

Common adverse effects in *italic;* life-threatening effects underlined; generic names in **bold;** classifications in SMALL CAPS; ♦ Canadian drug name; ℗ Prototype drug

1371

**AVAILABILITY** Tablet; sustained release capsule; oral solution; solution for injection

**ACTION & *THERAPEUTIC EFFECT*** Nonselective beta-blocker of both cardiac and bronchial adreno-receptors that competes with epinephrine and norepinephrine for available beta receptor sites. In higher doses, it depresses cardiac function including contractility and arrhythmias. Lowers both supine and standing blood pressures in hypertensive patients. *Reduces heart rate, myocardial irritability (Class II antiarrhythmic), and force of contraction, depresses automaticity of sinus node and ectopic pacemaker, and decreases AV and intraventricular conduction velocity. Hypotensive effect is associated with decreased cardiac output. Has migraine prophylactic effects.*

**USES** Management of cardiac arrhythmias, myocardial infarction, tachyarrhythmias associated with digitalis intoxication, anesthesia, and thyrotoxicosis, hypertrophic subaortic stenosis, angina pectoris due to coronary atherosclerosis, pheochromocytoma, hereditary essential tremor; also treatment of hypertension alone, but generally with a thiazide or other antihypertensives.

**UNLABELED USES** Anxiety states, migraine prophylaxis, essential tremors, schizophrenia, tardive dyskinesia, acute panic symptoms (e.g., stage fright), recurrent GI bleeding in cirrhotic patients, treatment of aggression and rage, drug induced tremors.

**CONTRAINDICATIONS** Hypersensitivity to propranolol; greater than first-degree heart block; right ventricular failure secondary to pulmonary hypertension; ventricular dysfunction; sinus bradycardia, cardiogenic shock, significant aortic or mitral valvular disease; bronchial asthma or bronchospasm, severe COPD, pulmonary edema; major depression; PVD, Raynaud's disease; abrupt discontinuation.

**CAUTIOUS USE** History of anaphylactic reaction; peripheral arterial insufficiency; compensated heart failure; history of systemic insect sting reaction; history of psychiatric illness; patients prone to nonallergenic bronchospasm; major surgery; cerebrovascular disease, stroke; renal or hepatic impairment; pheochromocytoma, vasospastic angina; DM; patients prone to hypoglycemia; hyperthyroidism, cardiac arrhythmias; surgery; MG and other skeletal muscular diseases; Wolff-Parkinson-White syndrome; older adults; pregnancy (category C); lactation.

## ROUTE & DOSAGE

### Hypertension

*Adult:* **PO Immediate release** 40 mg b.i.d., usually need 160–480 mg/day in divided doses; **InnoPran XL** dose 80 mg each night, may increase to 120 mg at bedtime; **Other extended release forms:** 80 mg daily increase up to 120–160 mg

### Angina

*Adult:* **PO Immediate release** 10–20 mg/day in divided doses (increase up to 160–320 mg/day); **Extended release** 80 mg QD (increase to 160–320 mg/day)

### Arrhythmias

*Adult:* **PO** 10–30 mg q6–8h **IV** 1–3 mg q4h

### Post MI

*Adult:* **PO** 180–240 mg/day in divided doses

**Acute MI**

*Adult:* **IV** Total dose of 0.1 mg/kg given in 3 divided doses at 2–3 min intervals **PO Immediate release:** 180–320 mg/day in divided doses

**Migraine Prophylaxis**

*Adult:* **PO Immediate release** 80 mg/day in divided doses, may need 160–240 mg/day; **Extended release** 80 mg/day

**Essential Tremor**

*Adult:* **PO** 40 mg b.i.d. may increase to 120–320 mg/day in divided doses

## ADMINISTRATION

- Take apical pulse and BP before administering drug. Withhold drug if heart rate less than 60 bpm or systolic BP less than 90 mm Hg. Consult prescriber for parameters.

### Oral

- Do not give within 2 wk of an MAO inhibitor.
- Note that InnoPran XL should be given at bedtime.
- Be consistent with regard to giving with food or on an empty stomach to minimize variations in absorption.
- Ensure that sustained release form is not chewed or crushed. **Must be** swallowed whole.
- Reduce dosage gradually over a period of 1–2 wk and monitor patient closely when discontinued.

### Intravenous

Note: Verify correct IV concentration and rate of infusion for neonates with prescriber.

- Take apical pulse and BP before administering drug. Withhold drug if heart rate less than 60 bpm or

systolic BP less than 90 mm Hg.
- Consult prescriber for parameters.

**PREPARE: Direct:** May be given undiluted or dilute each 1 mg in 10 mL of D5W. **Intermittent:** Dilute a single dose in 50 mL of NS.

**ADMINISTER: Direct:** Give each 1 mg or fraction thereof over 1 min. **Intermittent:** Give each dose over 15–20 min.

**INCOMPATIBILITIES: Y-site: Amphotericin B (conventional and lipid), asparaginase, dantrolene, diazepam, diazoxide, indomethacin, insulin, lansoprazole, mitomycin, paclitaxel, pantoprazole, phenytoin, piperacillin/tazobactam, SMP/TMZ.**

- Store at 15°–30° C (59°–86° F) in tightly closed, light-resistant containers.

## ADVERSE EFFECTS (≥1%) **Body as a Whole:** Fever; pharyngitis; respiratory distress, weight gain, LE-like reaction, cold extremities, *fatigue*, arthralgia, anaphylactic/anaphylactoid reactions. **Urogenital:** Impotence or decreased libido. **Skin:** Erythematous, psoriasis-like eruptions; pruritus, Stevens–Johnson syndrome, toxic epidermal necrolysis, erythema multiforme, exfoliative dermatitis, urticaria. Reversible alopecia, hyperkeratoses of scalp, palms, feet; nail changes, dry skin. **CNS:** Drug-induced psychosis, *sleep disturbances*, depression, *confusion,* agitation, giddiness, *light-headedness, fatigue,* vertigo, *syncope,* weakness, *drowsiness,* insomnia, vivid dreams, visual hallucinations, delusions, reversible organic brain syndrome. **CV:** Palpitation, profound *bradycardia,* AV heart block, cardiac standstill, hypotension, angina pectoris, tachyarrhythmia, acute CHF, peripheral

Common adverse effects in *italic;* life-threatening effects <u>underlined</u>; generic names in **bold;** classifications in SMALL CAPS; ♣ Canadian drug name; ⊘ Prototype drug

1373

arterial insufficiency resembling Raynaud's disease, myotonia, paresthesia of *hands*. **Special Senses:** Dry eyes (gritty sensation), visual disturbances, conjunctivitis, tinnitus, hearing loss, nasal stuffiness. **GI:** Dry mouth, nausea, *vomiting*, heartburn, *diarrhea*, constipation, flatulence, abdominal cramps, mesenteric arterial thrombosis, ischemic colitis, pancreatitis. **Hematologic:** Transient eosinophilia, thrombocytopenic or nonthrombocytopenic purpura, agranulocytosis. **Metabolic:** Hypoglycemia, hyperglycemia, hypocalcemia (patients with hyperthyroidism). **Respiratory:** Dyspnea, laryngospasm, bronchospasm.

## DIAGNOSTIC TEST INTERFERENCE

BETA-ADRENERGIC BLOCKERS may produce false-negative test results in exercise tolerance ECG tests, and elevations in *serum potassium, peripheral platelet count, serum uric acid, serum transaminase, alkaline phosphatase, lactate dehydrogenase, serum creatinine, BUN,* and an increase or decrease in *blood glucose* levels in diabetic patients.

## INTERACTIONS  Drug: PHENO-

THIAZINES have additive hypotensive effects. BETA-ADRENERGIC AGONISTS (e.g., **albuterol**) antagonize effects. **Atropine** and TRICYCLIC ANTIDEPRESSANTS block bradycardia. DIURETICS and other HYPOTENSIVE AGENTS increase hypotension. High doses of **tubocurarine** may potentiate neuromuscular blockade. **Cimetidine** decreases clearance, increases effects. ANTACIDS, **ascorbic acid** may decrease absorption.

## PHARMACOKINETICS  Absorp-

**tion:** Completely from GI tract; undergoes extensive first-pass metabolism. **Peak:** 60–90 min immediate release; 6 h sustained release; 5 min IV. **Distribution:** Widely distributed including CNS, placenta, and breast milk. **Metabolism:** Almost completely in liver (CYP1A2, 2D6). **Elimination:** 90–95% in urine as metabolites; 1–4% in feces. **Half-Life:** 2.3 h.

## NURSING IMPLICATIONS

### Black Box Warning

*Propranolol has been associated with exacerbation of angina and MI following abrupt discontinuance.*

### Assessment & Drug Effects

- Obtain careful medical history to rule out allergies, asthma, and obstructive pulmonary disease. Propranolol can cause bronchiolar constriction even in normal subjects.
- Monitor apical pulse, respiration, BP for 2 h after initiation or dosage adjustment. Consult prescriber for acceptable parameters.
- Evaluate adequate control or dosage interval for patients being treated for hypertension by checking blood pressure near end of dosage interval or before administration of next dose.
- Monitor I&O ratio and daily weight as significant indexes for detecting fluid retention and developing heart failure.
- Monitor diabetics for loss of glycemic control.

### Patient & Family Education

- Do not discontinue abruptly; can precipitate withdrawal syndrome (e.g., tremulousness, sweating, severe headache, malaise, palpitation, rebound hypertension, MI, and life-threatening arrhythmias in patients with angina pectoris).

- Learn usual pulse rate and take radial pulse before each dose. Report to prescriber if pulse is below the established parameter or becomes irregular.
- Be aware that propranolol suppresses clinical signs of hypoglycemia (e.g., BP changes, increased pulse rate) and may prolong hypoglycemia.
- Understand importance of compliance. Do not alter established regimen (i.e., do not omit, increase, or decrease dosage or change dosage interval).
- Be aware that drug may cause mild hypotension (experienced as dizziness or light-headedness) in normotensive patients on prolonged therapy. Make position changes slowly and avoid prolonged standing. Notify prescriber if symptoms persist.
- Do not drive or engage in potentially hazardous activities until response to drug is known.
- Inform dentist, surgeon, or ophthalmologist that you are taking propranolol (drug lowers normal and elevated intraocular pressure).

# PROPYLTHIOURACIL (PTU) ⓟ
(proe-pill-thye-oh-yoor'a-sill)
Propyl-Thyracil ✦
**Classification:** ANTITHYROID
Therapeutic: ANTITHYROID

**AVAILABILITY** Tablet

## ACTION & *THERAPEUTIC EFFECT*
Interferes with use of iodine and blocks synthesis of thyroxine ($T_4$) and triiodothyronine ($T_3$). Antithyroid action is delayed days and weeks until preformed $T_3$ and $T_4$ are degraded. *Effective as an*

*antithyroid agent in various hyperthyroid conditions.*

**USES** Hyperthyroidism in patients with Graves' disease or toxic multinodular goiter; amelioration of hyperthyroid symptoms prior to surgery.

**CONTRAINDICATIONS** Hypersensitivity to propylthiouracil; concurrent administration of sulfonamides or coal tar derivatives such as aminopyrine or antipyrine; acute liver failure; exfoliative dermatitis; unexplained fever; pregnancy (category D).

**CAUTIOUS USE** Infection; bone marrow depression; impaired liver function; renal impairment; older adults; patients at risk for liver failure; lactation; children younger than 6 y.

## ROUTE & DOSAGE

**Hyperthyroidism**
*Adult:* **PO** 300–400 mg/day divided q8h, may need 600–1200 mg/day initially
*Child (6 y or older):* **PO** 50 mg daily in divided doses q8h

## ADMINISTRATION
### Oral
- Give at the same time each day with relation to meals. Food may alter drug response by changing absorption rate.
- If drug is being used to improve thyroid state before radioactive iodine (RAI) treatment, discontinue 3 or 4 days before treatment to prevent uptake interference. PTU therapy may be resumed if necessary 3–5 days after the RAI administration.

• Store drug at 15°–30° C (59°–86° F) in light-resistant container.

## ADVERSE EFFECTS (≥1%) CNS:
Paresthesias, headache, vertigo, drowsiness, neuritis. GI: Nausea, vomiting, diarrhea, dyspepsia, loss of taste, sialoadenitis, hepatitis. **Hematologic:** Myelosuppression, lymphadenopathy, periarteritis, hypoprothrombinemia, *thrombocytopenia*, *leukopenia*, agranulocytosis. **Metabolic:** Hypothyroidism (goitrogenic): Enlarged thyroid, reduced GI motility, periorbital edema, puffy hands and feet, bradycardia, cool and pale skin, worsening of ophthalmopathy, sleepiness, fatigue, mental depression, dizziness, vertigo, sensitivity to cold, paresthesias, nocturnal muscle cramps, changes in menstrual periods, unusual weight gain. **Skin:** Skin rash, urticaria, pruritus, hyperpigmentation, lightening of hair color, abnormal hair loss. **Body as a Whole:** Drug fever, lupus-like syndrome, arthralgia, myalgia, hypersensitivity vasculitis.

## DIAGNOSTIC TEST INTERFERENCE
Propylthiouracil may elevate *prothrombin time* and serum *alkaline phosphatase, AST, ALT* levels.

## INTERACTIONS Drug: Amiodarone, potassium iodide, sodium iodide, THYROID HORMONES can reverse efficacy.

## PHARMACOKINETICS Absorption: Rapidly from GI tract. Peak: 1–2 h. Distribution: Concentrates in thyroid gland; crosses placenta; some distribution into breast milk. Metabolism: Rapidly to inactive metabolites. Elimination: 35% in urine. Half-Life: 1–2 h.

## NURSING IMPLICATIONS

### Black Box Warning

*Propylthiouracil has been associated with acute, sometimes fatal, liver injury.*

### Assessment & Drug Effects
• Be aware that about 10% of patients with hyperthyroidism have leukopenia less than 4000 cells/mm$^3$ and relative granulocytopenia.
• Observe for signs of clinical response to PTU (usually within 2 or 3 wk): Significant weight gain, reduced pulse rate, reduced serum T$_4$.
• Satisfactory euthyroid state may be delayed for several months when thyroid gland is greatly enlarged.
• Be alert to signs of hypoprothrombinemia: Ecchymoses, purpura, petechiae, unexplained bleeding. Warn ambulatory patients to report these signs promptly.
• Be alert for important diagnostic signs of excess dosage: Contraction of a muscle bundle when pricked, mental depression, hard and nonpitting edema, and need for high thermostat setting and extra blankets in winter (cold intolerance).
• Monitor for urticaria (occurs in 3–7% of patients during weeks 2–8 of treatment). Report severe rash.
• Monitor lab tests: Baseline and periodic T$_3$ and T$_4$; periodic LFTs and CBC with differential and platelet count.

### Patient & Family Education
• Note that PTU treatment may be reinstituted if surgery fails to produce normal thyroid gland function.
• Report severe skin rash or swelling of cervical lymph nodes. Therapy may be discontinued.

- Report to prescriber sore throat, fever, and rash immediately (most apt to occur in first few months of treatment). Drug will be discontinued and hematologic studies initiated.
- Avoid use of OTC drugs for asthma, or cough treatment without checking with the prescriber. Iodides sometimes included in such preparations are contraindicated.
- Learn how to take pulse accurately and check daily. Report to prescriber continued tachycardia.
- Report diarrhea, fever, irritability, listlessness, vomiting, weakness; these are signs of inadequate therapy or thyrotoxicosis.
- Chart weight 2 or 3 × weekly; clinical response is monitored through changes in weight and pulse.
- Do not alter drug regimen (e.g., increase, decrease, omit doses, change dosage intervals).
- Check with prescriber about use of iodized salt and inclusion of seafood in the diet.

## PROTAMINE SULFATE

(proe′ta-meen)

**Classifications:** ANTIDOTE; HEPARIN ANTAGONIST
Therapeutic: ANTIHEMORRHAGIC

**AVAILABILITY** Solution for injection

**ACTION & THERAPEUTIC EFFECT**
Combines with heparin to produce a stable complex; thus it neutralizes the anticoagulant effect of heparin. *Effective antidote to heparin overdose.*

**USES** Antidote for heparin overdosage (after heparin has been discontinued).

**UNLABELED USES** Antidote for heparin administration during extracorporeal circulation.

**CONTRAINDICATIONS** Hemorrhage not induced by heparin overdosage; lactation.

**CAUTIOUS USE** Cardiovascular disease; history of allergy to fish; vasectomized or infertile males; diabetes mellitus; patients who have received protamine-containing insulin; pregnancy (category C); children.

## ROUTE & DOSAGE

**Antidote for Heparin Overdose**
*Adult/Child:* **IV** 1 mg for every 100 units of heparin to be neutralized (max: 100 mg in a 2 h period), give the first 25–50 mg by slow direct IV and the rest over 2–3 h

## ADMINISTRATION

Note: Titrate dose carefully to prevent excess anticoagulation because protamine has a longer half-life than heparin and also has some anticoagulant effect of its own.

**Intravenous**
Note: Verify correct IV concentration and rate of infusion for infants or children with prescriber.

*PREPARE:* **Direct:** May be given as supplied direct IV. **Continuous:** Dilute in 50 mL or more of NS or D5W.

*ADMINISTER:* **Direct** Give each 50 mg or fraction thereof slowly over 10–15 min. ▪ NEVER give more than 50 mg in any 10 min period or 100 mg in any 2 h period. **Continuous:** Do not exceed direct rate. Give over 2–3 h or longer as determined by coagulation studies.
*INCOMPATIBILITIES:* **Solution/additive:** RADIOCONTRAST MATERIALS, **furosemide.**

▪ Store protamine sulfate injection at 15°–30° C (59°–86° F). ▪ Solutions

Common adverse effects in *italic;* life-threatening effects <u>underlined</u>; generic names in **bold;** classifications in SMALL CAPS; ♣ Canadian drug name; ⦿ Prototype drug

1377

do not contain preservatives and should not be stored.

**ADVERSE EFFECTS** (≥1%) **CV:** *Abrupt drop in BP* (with rapid IV infusion), bradycardia. **Body as a Whole:** Urticaria, <u>angioedema</u>, pulmonary edema, <u>anaphylaxis</u>, dyspnea, lassitude; transient flushing and feeling of warmth. **GI:** Nausea, vomiting. **Hematologic:** Protamine overdose or "heparin rebound" (hyperheparinemia).

**PHARMACOKINETICS** **Onset:** 5 min. **Duration:** 2 h.

**NURSING IMPLICATIONS**

> **Black Box Warning**
>
> *Protamine can cause severe hypotension, cardiovascular collapse, noncardiogenic pulmonary edema, catastrophic pulmonary vasoconstriction, and pulmonary hypertension.*

**Assessment & Drug Effects**

- Monitor closely for a hypersensitivity reaction. Risk factors include high doses or overdose, repeated doses, and previous protamine administration (including protamine-containing drugs).
- Monitor BP, HR, and respiratory status q15–30min, or more often if indicated. Continue for at least 2–3 h after each dose, or longer as dictated by patient's condition.
- Observe closely patients who have had cardiac surgery for bleeding (heparin rebound). Even with apparent adequate neutralization of heparin by protamine, bleeding may occur 30 min to 18 h after surgery.
- Monitor lab tests: Activated clotting time or aPTT 5–15 min after administration of protamine, and again in 2–8 h if desirable.

# PROTEIN C CONCENTRATE (HUMAN)
(pro′teen)

Ceprotin

**Classifications:** HEMATOLOGIC; THROMBOLYTIC; PROTEIN SYNTHESIS INHIBITOR

Therapeutic: PROTEIN C REPLACEMENT THERAPY

**AVAILABILITY** Vial of lyophilized powder

**ACTION & *THERAPEUTIC EFFECT***
Protein C is a critical element in a pathway that provides a natural mechanism for control of the coagulation system. It prevents excess procoagulant responses to activating stimuli. *Protein C is necessary to decrease thrombin generation and intravascular clot formation.*

**USES** Treatment of patients with severe congenital protein C deficiency; protein C replacement therapy for the prevention and treatment of venous thrombosis and purpura fulminans in children and adults.

**CONTRAINDICATIONS** Hypersensitivity to human protein C; concurrent administration with tissue plasminogen activator (tPA); hypernatremia; lactation.

**CAUTIOUS USE** Concurrent administration of anticoagulants; heparin induced thrombocytopenia (HIT); renal impairment; hepatic impairment; older adults; pregnancy (category C); children.

**ROUTE & DOSAGE**

> **Acute Episodes of Venous Thrombosis and Purpura Fulminans and Short-Term Prophylaxis**

*Adult/Adolescent/Child/Infant:*
**IV** Initial dose 100–120 units/kg; then 60–80 units/kg q6h × 3; maintenance dose: 45–60 units/kg q6–12h.

## ADMINISTRATION

### Intravenous

*PREPARE:* **Direct/IV Infusion:** Bring powder and supplied diluent to room temperature. Insert supplied double-ended transfer needle into diluent vial, then invert and rapidly insert into protein C powder vial. (If vacuum does not draw diluent into vial, discard.) ▪ Remove transfer needle and gently swirl to dissolve. ▪ Resulting solution concentration is 100 units/mL and it should be colorless to slightly yellowish, clear to slightly opalescent and free from visible particles. ▪ Withdraw required dose with the supplied filter needle.

*ADMINISTER:* **Direct/IV Infusion:** Infuse at 2 mL/min. **Direct/IV Infusion for Child weighing greater than 10 kg:** Infuse at 0.2 mL/kg/min.

▪ Store at room temperature for no more than 3 h after reconstitution. ▪ Prior to reconstitution, protect from light.

## ADVERSE EFFECTS (≥1%) **Body as a Whole:** Fever, hyperhidrosis, hypersensitivity reactions (rash, pruritus), restlessness. **CNS:** Lightheadedness. **CV:** Hemothorax, hypotension.

## INTERACTIONS **Drug:** Protein C concentrate can increase bleeding caused by **alteplase, reteplase,** or **tenecteplase.**

## PHARMACOKINETICS **Peak:** 0.5–1 h. **Half-Life:** 9.9 h.

## NURSING IMPLICATIONS

### Assessment & Drug Effects

▪ Monitor for and promptly report S&S of bleeding or hypersensitivity reactions (see Appendix F).
▪ Monitor vital signs including BP and temperature.
▪ Monitor lab tests: Baseline and periodic protein C activity; periodic platelet count; frequent serum sodium with renal function impairment.

### Patient & Family Education

▪ Report immediately early signs of hypersensitivity reactions including hives, generalized itching, tightness in chest, wheezing, difficulty breathing.
▪ Report immediately any signs of bleeding including black tarry stools, pink/red-tinged urine, unusual bruising.

## PROTRIPTYLINE HYDROCHLORIDE

(proe-trip′te-leen)

**Classification:** TRICYCLIC ANTIDEPRESSANT
**Therapeutic:** ANTIDEPRESSANT
**Prototype:** Imipramine

**P**

## AVAILABILITY Tablet

## ACTION & *THERAPEUTIC EFFECT*

Believed to enhance actions of norepinephrine and serotonin by blocking their reuptake at the neuronal membrane. *Effective in the treatment of depressed individuals, particularly those who are withdrawn.*

## USES Treatment of major depression.

## UNLABELED USES Sleep apnea.

## CONTRAINDICATIONS Hypersensitivity to TCAs; concurrent use

Common adverse effects in *italic;* life-threatening effects underlined; generic names in **bold;** classifications in SMALL CAPS; ♣ Canadian drug name; ⦿ Prototype drug

1379

of MAOIs; acute recovery phase following MI or within 14 days of use; QT prolongation, bundle branch block; cardiac conduction defects; suicidal ideation.

**CAUTIOUS USE** Hepatic, cardiovascular, or kidney dysfunction; DM; hyperthyroidism; history of alcoholism; patients with insomnia; asthma; bipolar disorder; suicidal tendencies; children and adolescents; pregnancy (category C); lactation.

## ROUTE & DOSAGE

### Depression

*Adult:* **PO** 15–40 mg/day in 3–4 divided doses (max: 60 mg/day)
*Adolescent:* **PO** 5 mg t.i.d.

## ADMINISTRATION

### Oral

- Give whole or crush and mix with fluid or food.
- Give dosage increases in the morning dose to prevent sleep interference and because this TCA has psychic energizing action.
- Give last dose of day no later than mid-afternoon; insomnia rather than drowsiness is a frequent adverse effect.
- Store at 15°–30° C (59°–86° F) in tightly closed container.

## ADVERSE EFFECTS (≥1%) **Body as a Whole:** Photosensitivity, <u>edema</u> (general or of face and <u>tongue</u>). **GI:** *Xerostomia, constipation,* paralytic ileus, dyspepsia, nausea. **Special Senses:** Blurred vision. **Urogenital:** *Urinary retention,* ejaculation dysfunction. **CNS:** Insomnia, headache, confusion, tremor. **CV:** Change in heat or cold tolerance; *orthostatic hypotension, tachycardia,* arrhythmia.

## INTERACTIONS **Drug:** May decrease some response to ANTIHYPER-TENSIVES; CNS DEPRESSANTS, **alcohol,** HYPNOTICS, BARBITURATES, SEDATIVES potentiate CNS depression; ORAL ANTICOAGULANTS may increase hypoprothrombinemic effects; **ethchlorvynol** causes transient delirium; **levodopa** SYMPATHOMIMETICS (e.g., **epinephrine, norepinephrine**) increases possibility of sympathetic hyperactivity with hypertension and hyperpyrexia; MAO INHIBITORS present possibility of severe reactions—toxic psychosis, cardiovascular instability; **methylphenidate** increases plasma TCA levels; THYROID DRUGS may increase possibility of arrhythmias; **cimetidine** may increase plasma TCA levels. Do not use with agents that prolong the QT interval (e.g., **dofetilide, dronedarone, ziprasidone**). **Herbal: Ginkgo** may decrease seizure threshold; **St. John's wort** may cause serotonin syndrome (headache, dizziness, sweating, agitation).

## PHARMACOKINETICS **Absorption:** Rapidly from GI tract. **Peak levels:** 24–30 h. **Distribution:** Crosses placenta; distributed into breast milk. **Metabolism:** In liver. **Elimination:** Primarily in urine. **Half-Life:** 54–98 h.

## NURSING IMPLICATIONS

### Black Box Warning

*Protriptyline has been associated with increased risk of suicidal thinking and behavior in children, adolescents, and young adults.*

### Assessment & Drug Effects

- Monitor therapeutic effectiveness. Onset of initial effect characterized by increased activity and energy is fairly rapid, usually within 1 wk after therapy is initiated. Maximum effect may not occur for 2 wk or more.

- Monitor adolescents as well as adults for changes in behavior that may indicate suicidality. Suicide is an inherent risk with any depressed patient and may remain until there is significant improvement.
- Monitor vital signs closely and CV system responses during early therapy, particularly in patients with cardiovascular disorders and older adults receiving daily doses in excess of 20 mg. Withhold drug and inform prescriber if BP falls more than 20 mm Hg or if there is a sudden increase in pulse rate.
- Monitor I&O ratio and bowel pattern during early therapy and when patient is on large doses.
- Assess and advise prescriber as indicated for prominent anticholinergic effects (xerostomia, blurred vision, constipation, paralytic ileus, urinary retention, delayed micturition).
- Assess condition of oral membranes frequently; institute symptomatic treatment if necessary. Xerostomia can interfere with appetite, fluid intake, and integrity of tooth surfaces.

### Patient & Family Education

- Report promptly changes in mood or behavior indicative of suicidal thinking.
- Consult prescriber about safe amount of alcohol, if any, that can be taken. Actions of both alcohol and protriptyline are potentiated when used together for up to 2 wk after the TCA is discontinued.
- Consult prescriber before taking any OTC medications.
- Be aware that effects of barbiturates and other CNS depressants are enhanced by TCAs.
- Avoid potentially hazardous activities requiring alertness and skill until response to drug is known.
- Avoid exposure to the sun without protecting skin with sunscreen

lotion (SPF higher than 12). Photosensitivity reactions may occur.

## PSEUDOEPHEDRINE HYDROCHLORIDE

(soo-doe-e-fed'rin)

Cenafed, Decongestant Syrup, Dorcol Children's Decongestant, Eltor ◆, Eltor 120 ◆, Halofed, Novafed, PediaCare, Pseudofrin ◆, Robidrine ◆, Sudafed, Sudrin

**Classifications:** ALPHA- AND BETA-ADRENERGIC RECEPTOR AGONIST; DECONGESTANT
**Therapeutic:** NASAL DECONGESTANT
**Prototype:** Epinephrine

**AVAILABILITY** Tablet; sustained release tablet; liquid; drops

### ACTION & THERAPEUTIC EFFECT

Sympathomimetic amine that produces decongestion of respiratory tract mucosa by stimulating the sympathetic nerve endings including alpha-, beta$_1$-, and beta$_2$-receptors. *Effect is caused by vasoconstriction and thus increased nasal airway patency.*

**USES** Symptomatic relief of nasal congestion associated with rhinitis, coryza, and sinusitis and for eustachian tube congestion.

### CONTRAINDICATIONS

Hypersensitivity to sympathomimetic amines; severe hypertension; severe coronary artery disease; use within 14 days of MAOIS; hyperthyroidism; prostatic hypertrophy.

**CAUTIOUS USE** Hypertension, heart disease, renal impairment; acute MI, angina; closed-angle glaucoma; severe narrowing of bowel; concurrent use of ACE INHIBITOR; thryroid disease, DM, elevated IOP; PVD; BPH;

pregnancy (category C); lactation. Safe use in children younger than 2 y (**PO**), children younger than 12 y (**sustained release**) is not established.

## ROUTE & DOSAGE

### Nasal Congestion

*Adult:* **PO** 60 mg q4–6h or 120 mg sustained release q12h
*Geriatric:* **PO** 30–60 mg q6h prn
*Child (2–6 y):* **PO** 15 mg q4–6h (max: 60 mg/day); *6–11 y:* 30 mg q4–6h (max: 120 mg/day)

## ADMINISTRATION

### Oral
- Ensure that sustained release form is not chewed or crushed. **Must be** swallowed whole.

## ADVERSE EFFECTS (≥1%) Body
as a Whole: *Transient stimulation,* tremulousness, difficulty in voiding. **CV:** Arrhythmias, palpitation, *tachycardia.* **CNS:** *Nervousness,* dizziness, headache, sleeplessness, numbness of extremities. **GI:** Anorexia, dry mouth, nausea, vomiting.

## INTERACTIONS Drug: Other
SYMPATHOMIMETICS increase pressor effects and toxicity; MAO INHIBITORS may precipitate hypertensive crisis; BETA-BLOCKERS may increase pressor effects; may decrease antihypertensive effects of **guanethidine, methyldopa, reserpine.**

## PHARMACOKINETICS Absorption:
Readily from GI tract. **Onset:** 15–30 min. **Duration:** 4–6 h (8–12 h sustained release). **Distribution:** Crosses placenta; distributed into breast milk. **Metabolism:** Partially metabolized in liver. **Elimination:** In urine.

## NURSING IMPLICATIONS

### Assessment & Drug Effects
- Monitor HR and BP, especially in those with a history of cardiac disease. Report tachycardia or hypertension.

### Patient & Family Education
- Do not take drug within 2 h of bedtime because drug may act as a stimulant.
- Discontinue medication and consult prescriber if extreme restlessness or signs of sensitivity occur.
- Consult prescriber before concomitant use of OTC medications; many contain ephedrine or other sympathomimetic amines and might intensify action of pseudoephedrine.

## PSYLLIUM HYDROPHILIC MUCILLOID ⊕
(sill'i-um)

Hydrocil Instant, Karasil ✦, Konsyl, Metamucil, Modane Bulk, Perdiem Plain, Reguloid, Serutan, Siblin, V-Lax
**Classification:** BULK-PRODUCING LAXATIVE
Therapeutic: BULK LAXATIVE

## AVAILABILITY Powder; granules

## ACTION & *THERAPEUTIC EFFECT*
Bulk-producing laxative that absorbs liquid in the GI tract, facilitating peristalsis and bowel motility. *Bulk-producing laxative that promotes peristalsis and natural elimination.*

## USES Chronic atonic or spastic
constipation and constipation associated with rectal disorders or anorectal surgery.

Common adverse effects in *italic;* life-threatening effects <u>underlined;</u> generic names in **bold;** classifications in SMALL CAPS; ✦ Canadian drug name; ⊕ Prototype drug

**CONTRAINDICATIONS** Esophageal and intestinal obstruction, dysphagia; nausea, vomiting, fecal impaction, acute abdomen; undiagnosed abdominal pain, appendicitis.

**CAUTIOUS USE** Diabetics; pregnancy (category C); children younger than 6 y.

## ROUTE & DOSAGE

**Constipation or Diarrhea**

*Adult:* PO 1–2 rounded tsp or 1 packet 1–3 × day prn
*Child (younger than 6 y):* PO 1 tsp in water at bedtime

## ADMINISTRATION

### Oral

- Fill an 8-oz (240-mL) water glass with cool water, milk, fruit juice, or other liquid; sprinkle powder into liquid; stir briskly; and give immediately (if effervescent form is used, add liquid to powder). Granules should not be chewed.
- Follow each dose with an additional glass of liquid to obtain best results.
- Exercise caution with older adult patient who may aspirate the drug.

**ADVERSE EFFECTS** (≥1%) **Hematologic:** Eosinophilia. **GI:** Nausea and vomiting, diarrhea (with excessive use); GI tract strictures when drug used in dry form, abdominal cramps.

**INTERACTIONS Drug:** Psyllium may decrease absorption and clinical effects of ANTIBIOTICS, **warfarin, digoxin, nitrofurantoin,** SALICYLATES.

**PHARMACOKINETICS Absorption:** Not absorbed from GI tract. **Onset:** 12–24 h. **Peak:** 1–3 days.

## NURSING IMPLICATIONS

### Assessment & Drug Effects

- Report promptly to prescriber if patient complains of retrosternal pain after taking the drug. Drug may be lodged as a gelatinous mass (because of poor mixing) in the esophagus.
- Monitor therapeutic effectiveness. When psyllium is used as either a bulk laxative or to treat diarrhea, the expected effect is formed stools. Laxative effect usually occurs within 12–24 h. Administration for 2 or 3 days may be needed to establish regularity.
- Assess for complaints of abdominal fullness. Smaller, more frequent doses spaced throughout the day may be indicated to relieve discomfort of abdominal fullness.
- Monitor lab tests: Frequent warfarin and digoxin levels if either is given concurrently.

### Patient & Family Education

- Note sugar and sodium content of preparation if on low-sodium or low-calorie diet. Some preparations contain natural sugars, whereas others contain artificial sweeteners.
- Understand that drug works to relieve both diarrhea and constipation by restoring a more normal moisture level to stool.
- Be aware that drug may reduce appetite if it is taken before meals.

# PYRANTEL PAMOATE
(pi-ran'tel)
Pin-X
**Classification:** ANTHELMINTIC
**Therapeutic:** ANTHELMINTIC
**Prototype:** Praziquantel

**AVAILABILITY** Capsule; oral suspension

Common adverse effects in *italic*; life-threatening effects underlined; generic names in **bold;** classifications in SMALL CAPS; ♣ Canadian drug name; ⊘ Prototype drug

1383

**ACTION & *THERAPEUTIC EFFECT***
Exerts selective depolarizing neuromuscular blocking action that results in spastic paralysis of worm. *Causes evacuation of worms from intestines.*

**USES** *Enterobius vermicularis* (pinworm) and *Ascaris lumbricoides* (roundworm) infestations.

**UNLABELED USES** Hookworm infestations; trichostrongylosis.

**CONTRAINDICATIONS** Hypersensitivity to pyrantel.

**CAUTIOUS USE** Liver dysfunction; malnutrition; dehydration; anemia; pregnancy (category C).

**ROUTE & DOSAGE**

| Pinworm or Roundworm |
|---|
| *Adult/Child:* **PO** 11 mg/kg as a single dose (max: 1 g) |

**ADMINISTRATION**
Oral
- Shake suspension well before pouring it to ensure accurate dosage.
- Give with milk or fruit juices and without regard to prior ingestion of food or time of day.
- Store below 30° C (86° F). Protect from light.

**ADVERSE EFFECTS** (≥1%) **CNS:** Dizziness, headache, drowsiness, insomnia. **GI:** Anorexia, *nausea,* vomiting, abdominal distention, diarrhea, *tenesmus,* transient elevation of AST. **Skin:** Skin rashes.

**INTERACTIONS Drug: Piperazine** and pyrantel may be mutually antagonistic.

**PHARMACOKINETICS Absorption:** Poorly from GI tract. **Peak:** 1–3 h. **Metabolism:** In liver.

**Elimination:** Greater than 50% in feces, 7% in urine.

**NURSING IMPLICATIONS**
**Assessment & Drug Effects**
- Monitor stool for presence of eggs, worms, and occult blood.

**Patient & Family Education**
- Do not drive or engage in other potentially hazardous activities until response to drug is known.

## PYRAZINAMIDE
(peer-a-zin'a-mide)
PZA, Tebrazid ✦
**Classifications:** ANTIBIOTIC; ANTITUBERCULOSIS
Therapeutic: ANTITUBERCULOSIS

**AVAILABILITY** Tablet

**ACTION & *THERAPEUTIC EFFECT***
Mechanism of action is unknown. May be bacteriostatic or bactericidal. *Effective against* Mycobacterium tuberculosis. *Not used as sole agent against TB infection.*

**USES** Treatment of tuberculosis infection (with other agents).

**CONTRAINDICATIONS** Severe liver damage, acute gout.

**CAUTIOUS USE** History of gout or diabetes mellitus; impaired kidney function; alcoholism; history of peptic ulcer; acute intermittent porphyria; pregnancy (category C); lactation; children.

**ROUTE & DOSAGE**

| Tuberculosis |
|---|
| *Adult/Child:* **PO** 15–30 mg/kg/ day (max: 3 g/day) |

*Renal Impairment Dosage Adjustment*

*CrCl 10–50 mL/min:* Extend interval to q48–72 hours; *CrCl less than 10 mL/min:* Extend interval to q72h

## ADMINISTRATION

### Oral
- Discontinue drug if hepatic reactions (jaundice, pruritus, icteric sclerae, yellow skin) or hyperuricemia with acute gout (severe pain in great toe and other joints) occurs.
- Store at 15°–30° C (59°–86° F) in tightly closed container.

## ADVERSE EFFECTS (≥1%) Body as a Whole: *Active gout,* arthralgia, lymphadenopathy. **Urogenital:** Difficulty in urination. **CNS:** Headache. **Skin:** Urticaria. **Hematologic:** Hemolytic anemia, decreased plasma prothrombin. **GI:** Splenomegaly, <u>fatal hemoptysis</u>, aggravation of peptic ulcer, *hepatotoxicity, abnormal liver function tests.* **Metabolic:** *Rise in serum uric acid.*

## DIAGNOSTIC TEST INTERFERENCE
Pyrazinamide may produce a temporary decrease in *17-ketosteroids* and an increase in *protein-bound iodine.*

## INTERACTIONS Drug: Increase in liver toxicity (including fatal hepatoxicity in when treating latent TB) with **rifampin.**

## PHARMACOKINETICS Absorption: Readily from GI tract. **Peak:** 2 h. **Distribution:** Crosses blood–brain barrier. **Metabolism:** In liver. **Elimination:** Slowly in urine. **Half-Life:** 9–10 h.

## NURSING IMPLICATIONS

### Assessment & Drug Effects
- Observe and supervise closely. Patients should receive at least one other effective antituberculosis agent concurrently.
- Examine patients at regular intervals and question about possible signs of toxicity: Liver enlargement or tenderness, jaundice, fever, anorexia, malaise, impaired vascular integrity (ecchymoses, petechiae, abnormal bleeding).
- Hepatic reactions appear to occur more frequently in patients receiving high doses.
- Monitor lab tests: Baseline and periodic LFTs and uric acid level.

### Patient & Family Education
- Report to prescriber onset of difficulty in voiding. Keep fluid intake at 2000 mL/day if possible.
- Monitor blood glucose (diabetics) for possible loss of glycemic control.

# PYRETHRINS
(peer'e-thrins)

A-200 Pyrinate, Barc, Blue, Pyrinate, Pyrinyl, R&C, RID, TISIT, Triple X

**Classifications:** ANTIPARASITIC; PEDICULICIDE
**Therapeutic:** SCABICIDE
**Prototype:** Permethrin

## AVAILABILITY Liquid; gel; shampoo

## ACTION & *THERAPEUTIC EFFECT*
Acts as a contact poison affecting the parasite's nervous system, causing paralysis and death. *Controls head lice, pubic (crab) lice, and body lice and their eggs (nits).*

## USES External treatment of *Pediculus humanus* infestations.

Common adverse effects in *italic;* life-threatening effects <u>underlined</u>; generic names in **bold;** classifications in SMALL CAPS; ♣ Canadian drug name; ☯ Prototype drug

1385

**CONTRAINDICATIONS** Sensitivity to solution components; skin infections and abrasions.

**CAUTIOUS USE** Ragweed-sensitized patient; asthma; pregnancy (category C); lactation; infants; children.

## ROUTE & DOSAGE

### *Pediculus humanus* Infestations

Adult: **Topical** See ADMINISTRATION for appropriate application

## ADMINISTRATION

### Topical

- Apply enough solution to completely wet infested area, including hair. Allow to remain on area for 10 min.
- Wash and rinse with large amounts of warm water.
- Use fine-toothed comb to remove lice and eggs from hair.
- Shampoo hair to restore body and luster.
- Repeat treatment once in 24 h if necessary.
- Repeat treatment in 7–10 days to kill newly hatched lice.
- Do not apply to eyebrows or eyelashes without consulting prescriber.
- Flush eyes with copious amounts of warm water if accidental contact occurs.

**ADVERSE EFFECTS** (≥1%) **Body as a Whole:** Irritation with repeated use.

## NURSING IMPLICATIONS

### Patient & Family Education

- Do not swallow, inhale, or allow pyrethrins to contact mucosal surfaces or the eyes.
- Discontinue use and consult prescriber if treated area becomes irritated.
- Examine each family member carefully; if infested, treat immediately to prevent spread or reinfestation of previously treated patient.
- Dry clean, boil, or otherwise treat contaminated clothing. Sterilize (soak in pyrethrins) combs and brushes used by patient.
- Do not share combs, brushes, or other headgear with another person.

# PYRIDOSTIGMINE BROMIDE

(peer-id-oh-stig'meen)

Mestinon, Regonal

**Classifications:** CHOLINERGIC MUSCLE STIMULANT; ANTICHOLINESTERASE
Therapeutic: CHOLINESTERASE INHIBITOR; MUSCLE STIMULANT
**Prototype:** Neostigmine

**AVAILABILITY** Syrup; tablet; extended release tablet; solution for injection

## ACTION & *THERAPEUTIC EFFECT*

Indirect-acting cholinergic agent that inhibits cholinesterase activity. Facilitates transmission of impulses across myoneural junctions by blocking destruction of acetylcholine. *Has direct stimulant action on voluntary muscle fibers and possibly on autonomic ganglia and CNS neurons. Produces increased tone in skeletal muscles.*

**USES** Myasthenia gravis and as an antagonist to nondepolarizing skeletal muscle relaxants (e.g., curariform drugs).

**CONTRAINDICATIONS** Hypersensitivity to anticholinesterase agents; mechanical obstruction of urinary or intestinal tract; hypotension; lactation.

CAUTIOUS USE Hypersensitivity to bromides; bronchial asthma; epilepsy; recent cardiac occlusion; renal impairment; vagotonia; hyperthyroidism; peptic ulcer; cardiac dysrhythmias; bradycardia; pregnancy (category C).

## ROUTE & DOSAGE

### Myasthenia Gravis
Adult: **PO** 60 mg–1.5 g/day spaced according to response of individual patient; **Sustained release** 180–540 mg 1–2 × day at intervals of at least 6 h; **IM/IV** Approximately $1/30$ of PO dose
Child: **PO** 7 mg/kg/day divided into 5–6 doses
Neonates: **PO** 5 mg q4–6h; **IM/IV** 0.05–0.15 mg/kg q4–6h

### Reversal of Muscle Relaxants
Adult: **IV** 10–20 mg immediately preceded by IV atropine

## ADMINISTRATION
### Oral
- Give with food or fluid.
- Ensure that sustained release form is not chewed or crushed. **Must be** swallowed whole.
- Note: A syrup is available. Some patients may not like it because it is sweet; try to make it more palatable by giving it over ice chips. The syrup formulation contains 5% alcohol.

### Intramuscular
- Note: Parenteral dose is about $1/30$ the oral adult dose.
- Give deep IM into a large muscle.

### Intravenous
*PREPARE:* **Direct:** Give undiluted. **Do not** add to IV solutions.

*ADMINISTER:* **Direct:** Give at a rate of 0.5 mg over 1 min for myasthenia gravis; 5 mg over 1 min for reversal of muscle relaxants.

- Store at 15°–30° C (59°–86° F). Protect from light and moisture.

## ADVERSE EFFECTS (≥1%) **Skin:**
Acneiform rash. **Hematologic:** Thrombophlebitis (following IV administration). **GI:** *Nausea, vomiting, diarrhea.* **Special Senses:** *Miosis.* **Body as a Whole:** *Excessive salivation and sweating,* weakness, fasciculation. **Respiratory:** Increased bronchial secretion, bronchoconstriction. **CV:** Bradycardia, hypotension.

## INTERACTIONS **Drug:** Atropine
NONDEPOLARIZING MUSCLE RELAXANTS antagonize effects of pyridostigmine.

## PHARMACOKINETICS **Absorption:** Poorly from GI tract. **Onset:** 30–45 min PO; 15 min IM; 2–5 min IV. **Duration:** 3–6 h. **Distribution:** Crosses placenta. **Metabolism:** In liver and in serum and tissue by cholinesterases. **Elimination:** In urine.

P

## NURSING IMPLICATIONS
### Assessment & Drug Effects
- Report increasing muscular weakness, cramps, or fasciculations. Failure of patient to show improvement may reflect either underdosage or overdosage.
- Observe patient closely if atropine is used to abolish GI adverse effects or other muscarinic adverse effects because it may mask signs of overdosage (cholinergic crisis): Increasing muscle weakness, which through involvement of respiratory muscles can lead to death.
- Monitor vital signs frequently, especially respiratory rate.

Common adverse effects in *italic;* life-threatening effects <u>underlined;</u> generic names in **bold;** classifications in SMALL CAPS; ♣ Canadian drug name; ☺ Prototype drug

1387

- Observe for signs of cholinergic reactions (see Appendix F), particularly when drug is administered IV.
- Observe neonates of myasthenic mothers, who have received pyridostigmine, closely for difficulty in breathing, swallowing, or sucking.
- Observe patient continuously when used as muscle relaxant antagonist. Airway and respiratory assistance **must be** maintained until full recovery of voluntary respiration and neuromuscular transmission is assured. Complete recovery usually occurs within 30 min.

### Patient & Family Education

- Be aware that duration of drug action may vary with physical and emotional stress, as well as with severity of disease.
- Report onset of rash to prescriber. Drug may be discontinued.
- Sustained release tablets may become mottled in appearance; this does not affect their potency.

## PYRIDOXINE HYDROCHLORIDE (VITAMIN B₆)

(peer-i-dox′een)

**Classification:** VITAMIN
Therapeutic: VITAMIN B₆ REPLACEMENT

**AVAILABILITY** Tablet; solution for injection

## ACTION & *THERAPEUTIC EFFECT*

Water-soluble complex of three closely related compounds with B₆ activity. Converted in body to pyridoxal, a coenzyme that functions in protein, fat, and carbohydrate metabolism and in facilitating release of glycogen from liver and muscle. In protein metabolism, participates in enzymatic transformations of amino acids and conversion of tryptophan to niacin and serotonin. Aids in energy transformation in brain and nerve cells, and is thought to stimulate heme production. *Effectiveness is evaluated by improvement of B₆ deficiency manifestations: Nausea, vomiting, skin lesions resembling those of riboflavin and niacin deficiency, edema, CNS symptoms, hypochromic microcytic anemia.*

**USES** Prophylaxis and treatment of pyridoxine deficiency, as seen with inadequate dietary intake, drug-induced deficiency (e.g., isoniazid, oral contraceptives), and inborn errors of metabolism (vitamin B₆–dependent convulsions or anemia). Also to prevent chloramphenicol-induced optic neuritis, to treat acute toxicity caused by overdosage of cycloserine, hydralazine, isoniazid (INH); alcoholic polyneuritis; sideroblastic anemia associated with high serum iron concentration. Has been used for management of many other conditions ranging from nausea and vomiting in radiation sickness and pregnancy to suppression of postpartum lactation.

**CONTRAINDICATIONS IV:** Cardiac disease.

**CAUTIOUS USE** Renal impairment; neonatal prematurity with renal impairment; cardiac disease; pregnancy [category A or (C if greater than RDA)].

## ROUTE & DOSAGE

### Dietary Deficiency

*Adult:* **PO/IM/IV** 10–20 mg/day × 2–3 wk
*Child:* **PO** 5–25 mg/day × 3 wk, then 1.5–2.5 mg/day

P

**Pyridoxine Deficiency Syndrome**

*Adult:* **PO/IM/IV** Initial dose up to 600 mg/day may be required; then up to 50 mg/day

**Isoniazid-Induced Deficiency**

*Adult:* **PO/IM/IV** 100 mg/day × 3 wk, then 30 mg/day
*Child:* **PO** 10–50 mg/day × 3 wk, then 1–2 mg/kg/day

**Pyridoxine-Dependent Seizures**

*Neonate/Infant:* **PO/IM/IV** 50–100 mg/day

## ADMINISTRATION

### Oral

- Ensure that sustained release and enteric forms are not chewed or crushed. **Must be** swallowed whole.

### Intramuscular

- Give deep IM into a large muscle.

### Intravenous

*PREPARE:* **Direct:** Give undiluted. **Continuous:** May be added to most standard IV solutions.
*ADMINISTER:* **Direct:** Give at a rate of 50 mg or fraction thereof over 60 sec. **Continuous:** Give according to ordered rate for infusion.

- Store at 15°–30° C (59°–86° F) in tight, light-resistant containers. Avoid freezing.

## ADVERSE EFFECTS (≥1%) **Body as a Whole:** Paresthesias, slight flushing or feeling of warmth, temporary burning or stinging pain in injection site. **CNS:** Somnolence seizures (particularly following large parenteral doses). **Metabolic:** Low folic acid levels.

## INTERACTIONS **Drug:** Isoniazid, cycloserine, penicillamine, hydralazine, and ORAL CONTRACEPTIVES may increase pyridoxine requirements; may reverse or antagonize therapeutic effects of **levodopa.**

## PHARMACOKINETICS **Absorption:** Readily from GI tract. **Distribution:** Stored in liver; crosses placenta. **Metabolism:** In liver. **Elimination:** In urine.

## NURSING IMPLICATIONS

### Assessment & Drug Effects

- Monitor neurologic status to determine therapeutic effect in deficiency states.
- Record a complete dietary history so poor eating habits can be identified and corrected (a single vitamin deficiency is rare; patient can be expected to have multiple vitamin deficiencies).

### Patient & Family Education

- Learn rich dietary sources of vitamin B₆: Yeast, wheat germ, whole grain cereals, muscle and glandular meats (especially liver), legumes, green vegetables, bananas.
- Do not self-medicate with vitamin combinations (OTC) without first consulting prescriber.

# PYRIMETHAMINE

(peer-i-meth'a-meen)

Daraprim

**Classification:** FOLIC ACID ANTAGONIST
Therapeutic: ANTIMALARIAL
**Prototype:** Chloroquine

## AVAILABILITY Tablet

## ACTION & *THERAPEUTIC EFFECT*

Selectively inhibits action of dehydrofolic reductase in parasites

Common adverse effects in *italic;* life-threatening effects underlined; generic names in **bold**; classifications in SMALL CAPS; ♣ Canadian drug name; ⊙ Prototype drug

1389

with resulting blockade of folic acid metabolism. *Prevents development of fertilized gametes in the mosquito and thus helps to prevent transmission of malaria.*

**USES** Prophylaxis and treatment of malaria; toxoplasmosis.

**CONTRAINDICATIONS** Chloroguanide-resistant malaria; hypersensitivity to sulfonamides; megaloblastic anemia caused by folate deficiency; lactation.

**CAUTIOUS USE** Convulsive disorders; asthma; bone marrow suppression; folate deficiency; hepatic disease; renal disease; seizure disorder; pregnancy (category C); children.

## ROUTE & DOSAGE

### Malaria Treatment
*Adult/Adolescent/Child (4 y or older):* **PO** 25 mg daily × 2 days

### Malaria Chemoprophylaxis
*Adult/Adolescent/Child (10 y or older):* **PO** 25 mg once/wk; *4–10 y:* 12.5 mg once/wk; *younger than 4 y:* 6.25 mg once/wk

### Toxoplasmosis
*Adult:* **PO** 50–75 mg/day with a sulfonamide for 1–3 wk, then decrease dose by half and continue for 1 mo
*Child:* **PO** 1 mg/kg/day divided into 2 doses with a sulfonamide for 1–3 wk, then decrease to 0.5 mg/kg/day for 1 mo (max: 25 mg/day)

## ADMINISTRATION
### Oral
- Minimize GI distress by giving with meals. If symptoms persist, dosage reduction may be necessary.

- Give on same day each week for malaria prophylaxis. Begin when individual enters malarious area and continue for 10 wk after leaving the area.

**ADVERSE EFFECTS** (≥1%) **GI:** Anorexia, vomiting, atrophic glossitis, abdominal cramps, diarrhea. **Skin:** Skin rashes. **Hematologic:** *Folic acid deficiency (megaloblastic anemia, leukopenia, thrombocytopenia, pancytopenia,* diarrhea). **CNS:** CNS stimulation including convulsions, respiratory failure.

**INTERACTIONS Drug: Folic acid,** *para***-aminobenzoic acid (PABA)** may decrease effectiveness against toxoplasmosis.

**PHARMACOKINETICS Absorption:** Readily from GI tract. **Peak:** 2 h. **Distribution:** Concentrates in kidneys, lungs, liver, and spleen; distributed into breast milk. **Elimination:** Slowly in urine; excretion may extend over 30 days or longer. **Half-Life:** 54–148 h.

## NURSING IMPLICATIONS
### Assessment & Drug Effects
- Monitor patient response closely. Dosages required for treatment of toxoplasmosis approach toxic levels.
- Withhold drug and notify prescriber if hematologic abnormalities appear.
- Monitor lab tests: Twice weekly blood count, including platelets; LFTs and renal function tests as indicated.

### Patient & Family Education
- Be aware that folic acid deficiency may occur with long-term use of pyrimethamine. Report to prescriber weakness, and pallor (from anemia), ulcerations of oral mucosa, superinfections, glossitis; GI disturbances such as diarrhea and poor fat absorption, fever. Folate (folinic

Common adverse effects in *italic;* life-threatening effects <u>underlined;</u> generic names in **bold;** classifications in SMALL CAPS; ♣ Canadian drug name; ⦿ Prototype drug

acid) replacement may be prescribed. Increase food sources of folates (if allowed) in diet.

# QUAZEPAM
(qua'ze-pam)
Doral
**Classifications:** SEDATIVE-HYPNOTIC, NONBARBITUATE; BENZODIAZEPINE
Therapeutic: SEDATIVE
**Prototype:** Triazolam
**Controlled Substance:** Schedule IV

## AVAILABILITY Tablet

## ACTION & THERAPEUTIC EFFECT
Believed to potentiate gamma-aminobutyric acid (GABA) neuronal inhibition in the limbic, neocortical, and mesencephalic reticular systems. *Significantly decreases total wake time and significantly increases sleep time. REM sleep is essentially unchanged.*

## USES Insomnia characterized by difficulty in falling asleep, frequent nocturnal awakenings, or early morning awakenings.

## CONTRAINDICATIONS Hypersensitivity to quazepam or benzodiazepines; sleep apnea; respiratory depression or insufficiency; suicidal ideation; pregnancy (category X); lactation.

## CAUTIOUS USE Impaired liver and kidney function; history of seizures; depression; older adults; debilitated clients. Safety and efficacy in children younger than 18 y not established.

## ROUTE & DOSAGE

**Insomnia**
*Adult:* **PO** 7.5–15 mg at bedtime

## ADMINISTRATION
### Oral
- Initial dose is usually 15 mg but can often be effectively reduced after several nights of therapy.
- Use lowest effective dose in older adults as soon as possible.

## ADVERSE EFFECTS (≥1%) CNS:
*Drowsiness, headache,* fatigue, dizziness, dry mouth. **GI:** Dyspepsia. **Body as a Whole:** Physiological or psychological dependence.

## INTERACTIONS Drug: Alcohol,
CNS DEPRESSANTS, ANTICONVULSANTS potentiate CNS depression; **cimetidine** increases quazepam plasma levels, increasing its toxicity; may decrease antiparkinsonism effects of **levodopa;** may increase **phenytoin** levels; **smoking** decreases sedative effects of quazepam. **Sodium oxybate** is contraindicated with quazepam. **Herbal: Kava, valerian** may potentiate sedation.

## PHARMACOKINETICS Absorption: Readily from GI tract. Onset: 30 min. Peak: 2 h. Distribution: Crosses placenta; distributed into breast milk. Metabolism: In liver to active metabolites. Elimination: In urine and feces. Half-Life: 39 h.

## NURSING IMPLICATIONS
### Assessment & Drug Effects
- Monitor for respiratory depression in patients with chronic respiratory insufficiency.
- Monitor for suicidal tendencies in previously depressed clients.
- Daytime drowsiness is more likely to occur in older adult clients.
- For inpatient use, institute safety measures to prevent falls.

### Patient & Family Education
- Inform prescriber about any alcohol consumption and prescription or nonprescription medication that

---

Common adverse effects in *italic;* life-threatening effects underlined; generic names in **bold;** classifications in SMALL CAPS; ♥Canadian drug name; ❷ Prototype drug you take. Avoid alcohol use since it potentiates CNS depressant effects.

- Inform prescriber immediately if you become pregnant. This drug causes birth defects.
- Do not drive or engage in potentially hazardous activities until response to drug is known.
- Do not increase the dose of this drug; inform prescriber if the drug no longer works.
- This drug may cause daytime sedation, even for several days after drug is discontinued.

## QUETIAPINE FUMARATE

(ke-ti-a'peen)
Seroquel, Seroquel XR
**Classification:** ATYPICAL ANTIPSYCHOTIC
Therapeutic: ANTIPSYCHOTIC
**Prototype:** Clozapine

**AVAILABILITY** Tablet; extended release tablet

**ACTION & THERAPEUTIC EFFECT** Antagonizes multiple neurotransmitter receptors in the brain including serotonin ($5\text{-}HT_{1A}$ and $5\text{-}HT_2$) as well as dopamine $D_1$ and $D_2$ receptors. *Effectiveness indicated by a reduction in psychotic behavior.*

**USES** Management of schizophrenia, maintenance of acute bipolar disorder, and add-on therapy for major depressive disorder.

**UNLABELED USES** Management of agitation and dementia; generalized anxiety disorder; PTSD.

**CONTRAINDICATIONS** Hypersensitivity to quetiapine; alcohol use; suicidal ideation; dementia-related psychosis in older adults; NSM; lactation.

**CAUTIOUS USE** Liver function impairment; history of seizures or suicidical thoughts; or hepatic impairment; cardiovascular disease

(history of MI or ischemic heart disease, heart failure, arrhythmias, congenital QT prolongation; CVA, hypotension, dehydration, treatment with antihypertensives); MDD; risk factors for diabetes; DM; abnormal lipid profile; breast cancer; Alzheimer's, Parkinson's disease; patient at risk for aspiration pneumonia; debilitated patients; BPH; decreased GI motility; cerebrovascular disease; hypothyroidism; older adults; pregnancy (category C). Safe use in children younger than 10 y not established.

## ROUTE & DOSAGE

### Bipolar Disorder/Bipolar Depression

*Adult/Adolescent:* **PO Immediate release** 50 mg at bedtime on day 1; then increase in increments of up to 100 mg/day in divided doses as tolerated to 400 mg/day on day 4 or **Extended release** 400 mg daily at bedtime
*Child (older than 10 y):* **PO** 25 mg b.i.d. on day 1, 50 mg b.i.d. on day 2, 100 mg b.i.d. on day 3, 150 mg b.i.d. on day 4, and 200 mg b.i.d. beginning day 5

### Schizophrenia

*Adult:* **PO Immediate release** Start 25 mg b.i.d., may increase by 25–50 mg b.i.d. to t.i.d. on the second or third day as tolerated to a target dose of 300–400 mg/day divided b.i.d. to t.i.d., may adjust dose by 25–50 mg b.i.d. daily as needed (max: 800 mg/day); **Extended release** 300 mg daily at bedtime, titrate up to 400–800 mg daily (max: 800 mg/day)
*Adolescent:* **PO Immediate release** 25 mg b.i.d. then taper up by 50 mg daily up to 200 mg b.i.d.

### Manic Episodes in Bipolar Disorder Monotherapy or with

**Lithium/Divalproex (Immediate Release Only)**

*Adult:* **PO Immediate release** Start with total of 100 mg (in two doses) day 1, increase to 400 mg/day (in two doses) by day 4; or **Extended release** 300 mg on day 1, then 600 mg on day 2, may adjust by 400–800 mg/day based on response

*Geriatric:* Titrate more slowly due to risk of orthostatic hypotension

**Major Depressive Disorder (Adjunct)**

*Adult:* **PO** 50 mg once daily × day 1 and day 2, then increase to 150 mg daily

**Hepatic Impairment Dosage Adjustment**

**PO Immediate release** Start with 25 mg dose and increase by 25–50 mg/day; **Extended release** Start with 50 mg on day 1, then increase by 50 mg/day to the lowest effective and tolerable dose

## ADMINISTRATION

**Oral**

- Dose is usually retitrated over a period of several days when patient has been off the drug for longer than 1 wk.
- Follow recommended lower doses and slower titration for the older adults, the debilitated, and those with hepatic impairment or a predisposition to hypotension.
- May be administered with or without food. Swallow extended release tablets whole.
- Store at 15°–30° C (59°–86° F).

## ADVERSE EFFECTS (≥1%) **Body as a Whole:** Asthenia, fever, hypertonia, dysarthria, flu syndrome, *weight gain*, *fatigue*, peripheral edema, *increased risk of suicidal thinking.* **CNS:** *Dizziness, headache, somnolence,* agita-

tion. **CV:** *Increased arterial pressure* postural *hypotension, tachycardia,* palpitations, *systolic hypertension.* **GI:** *Dry mouth,* dyspepsia, abdominal pain, constipation, *increased appetite.* **Metabolic:** *Hypercholesterolemia,* hyperglycemia, diabetes mellitus. **Respiratory:** Rhinitis, *pharyngitis,* cough, dyspnea. **Skin:** Rash, sweating. **Hematologic:** <u>Leukopenia</u>.

## INTERACTIONS **Drug:** BARBITURATES, **carbamazepine, phenytoin, rifampin, thioridazine** may increase clearance of quetiapine. Quetiapine may potentiate the cognitive and motor effects of **alcohol,** enhance the effects of ANTIHYPERTENSIVE AGENTS, antagonize the effects of **levodopa** and DOPAMINE AGONISTS. **Ketoconazole, itraconazole, fluconazole, erythromycin** may decrease clearance of quetiapine. Drugs that increase the QT interval (e.g., **amiodarone, clarithromycin,** ANTIARRHYTHMICS, **haloperidol, ziprasodone**) increase risk of cardiac effects. Other ANTIPSYCHOTICS increase the risk of adverse effects. Do not use with **metoclopramide. Herbal: St. John's wort** may cause **serotonin** syndrome (see Appendix F).

## PHARMACOKINETICS **Absorption:** Rapidly and completely absorbed from GI tract. **Peak:** 1.5 h. **Distribution:** 83% protein bound. **Metabolism:** In liver (CYP3A4). **Elimination:** 73% in urine, 20% in feces. **Half-Life:** 6 h.

## NURSING IMPLICATIONS

### Black Box Warning

*Quetiapine has been associated with increased mortality in older adults with dementia-related psychosis, and with increased risk of suicidical thoughts and behavior in children, adolescents, and young adults.*

---

Common adverse effects in *italic;* life-threatening effects <u>underlined;</u> generic names in **bold;** classifications in SMALL CAPS; ✤Canadian drug name; ⊚ Prototype drug

## Assessment & Drug Effects
- Monitor diabetics for loss of glycemic control.
- Monitor for changes in behavior that may indicate suicidality.
- Reassess need for continued treatment periodically.
- Withhold the drug and immediately report S&S of tardive dyskinesia or neuroleptic malignant syndrome (see Appendix F).
- Monitor ECG periodically, especially in those with known cardiovascular disease.
- Baseline cataract exam is recommended when therapy is started and at 6 mo intervals thereafter.
- Monitor patients with a history of seizures for lowering of the seizure threshold.
- Monitor lab tests: Periodic LFTs, lipid profile, thyroid function, blood glucose, CBC with differential.

## Patient & Family Education
- Carefully monitor blood glucose levels if diabetic.
- Exercise caution with potentially dangerous activities requiring alertness, especially during the first week of drug therapy or during dose increments.
- Make position changes slowly, especially when changing from lying or sitting to standing to avoid dizziness, palpitations, and fainting.
- Avoid alcohol consumption and activities that may cause overheating and dehydration.

# QUINAPRIL HYDROCHLORIDE
(quin'a-pril)
Accupril
**Classifications:** ANGIOTENSIN-CONVERTING ENZYME (ACE) INHIBITOR; ANTIHYPERTENSIVE
Therapeutic: ANTIHYPERTENSIVE
**Prototype:** Enalapril

## AVAILABILITY Tablet

## ACTION & *THERAPEUTIC EFFECT*
Potent, long-acting ACE inhibitor that lowers BP by interrupting the conversion sequences initiated by renin to form angiotensin II, a vasoconstrictor. Also decreases circulating aldosterone. Reduces PCWP, systemic vascular resistance, and mean arterial pressure, with concurrent increases in cardiac output, cardiac index, and stroke volume. *Lowers BP by producing vasodilation. Effective in the treatment of CHF since it improves cardiac indicators*.

## USES
Mild to moderate hypertension, heart failure.

## CONTRAINDICATIONS
Hypersensitivity to quinapril or other ACE inhibitors (angioedema specifically); cholestatic jaundice; concomitant use with aliskiren in diabetic patients; pregnancy (category D).

## CAUTIOUS USE
History of angioedema; renal insufficiency; autoimmune disease, volume-depleted patients, aortic stenosis, hypertrophic cardiomyopathy; HF; renal artery stenosis, neutropenia; older adults; lactation. Safety and efficacy in children not established.

## ROUTE & DOSAGE

### Hypertension
*Adult:* **PO** 10–20 mg daily, may increase up to 80 mg/day in 1–2 divided doses
*Geriatric:* **PO** Start with 2.5–5 mg daily

### Heart Failure
*Adult:* **PO** 5 mg b.i.d. may increase to 10–20 mg b.i.d.

### Renal Impairment Dosage Adjustment
*CrCl 30–60 mL/min:* Start at 5 mg daily initially; *less than 10–30 mL/min:* 2.5 mg/day initially

## ADMINISTRATION

### Oral

- When patient has been treated with a diuretic, the diuretic is usually discontinued 2–3 days before beginning quinapril. If the diuretic cannot be discontinued, initial quinapril dose is usually lowered to 5 mg.
- Store at 15°–30° C (59°–86° F) and protect from moisture.

## ADVERSE EFFECTS (≥1%) CV: Edema, hypotension, chest pain. CNS: *Dizziness*, fatigue, headache. GI: Nausea, vomiting, diarrhea, <u>intestinal angioedema</u>. Hematologic: Eosinophilia, neutropenia. Metabolic: *Hyperkalemia*, proteinuria. Respiratory: *Cough*. Body as a Whole: <u>Angioedema</u>, myalgia.

## DIAGNOSTIC TEST INTERFERENCE

May increase *BUN* or *serum creatinine*.

## INTERACTIONS Drug: POTASSIUM-SPARING DIURETICS may increase risk of hyperkalemia. May elevate serum **lithium** levels, resulting in **lithium** toxicity. Do not use with **aliskiren**.

## PHARMACOKINETICS Absorption: Rapidly from GI tract. Onset: 1 h. Peak: 2–4 h. Duration: Up to 24 h. Distribution: 97% bound to plasma proteins; crosses placenta; not known if distributed into breast milk. Metabolism: Extensively metabolized in liver to its active metabolite, quinaprilat. Elimination: 50–60% in urine, primarily as quinaprilat; 30% in feces. Half-Life: 2 h.

## NURSING IMPLICATIONS

### Black Box Warning

*Quinapril has been associated with fetal toxicity and death.*

### Assessment & Drug Effects

- Following initial dose, monitor for several hours for first-dose hypotension, especially in salt- or volume-depleted patients (e.g., those pretreated with a diuretic).
- Monitor BP at time of peak effectiveness, 2–4 h after dosing, and at end of dosing interval just before next dose.
- Report diminished antihypertensive effect toward end of dosing interval. Inadequate trough response may indicate need to divide daily dose.
- Observe for S&S of hyperkalemia (see Appendix F)
- Monitor lab tests: Baseline and periodic renal function tests; periodic serum potassium; periodic WBC in those with collagen vascular disease or renal impairment.

### Patient & Family Education

- Discontinue quinapril and report S&S of angioedema (e.g., swelling of face or extremities, difficulty breathing or swallowing) to prescriber.
- Notify prescriber immediately if you become or suspect you are pregnant.
- Maintain adequate fluid intake and avoid potassium supplements or salt substitutes unless specifically prescribed by prescriber.
- Light-headedness and dizziness may occur, especially during the initial days of therapy. If fainting occurs, stop taking quinapril until the prescriber has been consulted.

## QUINIDINE SULFATE
(kwin′i-deen sul-fate)

## QUINIDINE GLUCONATE
**Classification:** CLASS IA ANTIARRHYTHMIC
**Therapeutic:** CLASS IA ANTIARRHYTHMIC
**Prototype:** Procainamide

Common adverse effects in *italic*; life-threatening effects <u>underlined</u>; generic names in **bold**; classifications in SMALL CAPS; ♣ Canadian drug name; ⊘ Prototype drug

1395

## AVAILABILITY Quinidine sulfate: Tablet. Quinidine gluconate: Sustained release tablet; solution for injection

## ACTION & *THERAPEUTIC EFFECT*
Depresses myocardial excitability, contractility, automaticity, and conduction velocity as well as prolongs refractory period. *Depresses myocardial excitability, conduction velocity, and irregularity of nerve impulse conduction.*

## USES Premature atrial, AV junctional, and ventricular contraction; paroxysmal atrial tachycardia, chronic ventricular tachycardia (when not associated with complete heart block); maintenance therapy after electrical conversion of atrial fibrillation or flutter; life-threatening malaria; Wolff-Parkinson-White syndrome.

## CONTRAINDICATIONS Hypersensitivity or idiosyncrasy to quinine or quinidine; thrombocytopenic purpura resulting from prior use of quinidine or quinine; myasthenia gravis; intraventricular conduction defects, complete AV block, AV conduction disorders; bundle branch block; marked QRS widening; thyrotoxicosis; extensive myocardial damage, frank CHF, hypotensive states; history of drug-induced torsades de pointes.

## CAUTIOUS USE Incomplete heart block; impaired kidney or liver function; sick sinus syndrome; bronchial asthma or other respiratory disorders; potassium imbalance; pregnancy (category C); lactation. Safe use for children as an antiarrhythmic agent is not known.

## ROUTE & DOSAGE

**Conversion to and/or Maintenance of Sinus Rhythm *Sulfate Immediate Release***

*Adult:* **PO** 200–300 mg q6–8h until sinus rhythm restored or toxicity occurs (max: 3–4 g)

**Sulfate Extended Release**

*Adult:* **PO** 300–600 mg q8–12h

**Gluconate**

*Adult:* **IM** 600 mg salt, then 400 mg salt; can repeat q2h if needed; **IV** 800 mg salt, monitor closely

**Malaria (Quinidine Gluconate)**

*Adult/Adolescent/Child:* **IV** 24 mg/kg loading dose, then 12 mg/kg q8h OR 10 mg/kg loading dose, then 0.02 mg/kg/min for 24 h

## ADMINISTRATION
### Oral
- Give with a full glass of water on an empty stomach for optimum absorption (i.e., 1 h before or 2 h after meals). Administer drug with food if GI symptoms occur (nausea, vomiting, diarrhea are most common). Do not administer with grapefruit juice.
- Ensure that extended release tablets are swallowed whole. They should not be crushed or chewed.
- Store in tight, light-resistant containers away from excessive heat.

### Intramuscular
- Aspirate carefully before injection to avoid inadvertent entry into blood vessel.

### Intravenous

***PREPARE:* IV Infusion:** Dilute 800 mg (10 mL) in 50 mL D5W to yield a maximum concentration of 16 mg/mL.
***ADMINISTER:* IV Infusion:** Give via infusion pump at a rate not to exceed 1 mL/min.

---

Common adverse effects in *italic*; life-threatening effects <u>underlined</u>; generic names in **bold**; classifications in SMALL CAPS; ♣ Canadian drug name; ⊘ Prototype drug

*INCOMPATIBILITIES:* Solution/additive: **Amiodarone, atracurium.** Y-site: **Acyclovir, aminophylline, amphotericin B, ampicillin, azathioprine, aztreonam, bivalirudin, bretylium, CEPHALOSPORINS, clindamycin, dantrolene, daptomycin, dexamethasone, diazoxide, ertapenem, foscarnet, furosemide, ganciclovir, gemtuzumab, heparin in dextrose, hydrocortisone, indomethacin, insulin, ketorolac, methicillin, methylprednisolone, mezlocillin, minocycline, nafcillin, nitroprusside, oxacillin, pantoprazole, premetrexed, penicillin, pentobarbital, phenobarbital, phenytoin, piperacillin, sodium bicarbonate, SMZ/TMP, ticarcillin.**

• Use supine position during drug administration; severe hypotension is most likely to occur in patients receiving drug via IV. • Protect IV solutions from light and heat to prevent brownish discoloration and possibly precipitation.

## ADVERSE EFFECTS (≥1%) CNS:
Headache, fever, tremors, apprehension, delirium, syncope with sudden loss of consciousness, seizures. **CV:** Hypotension, CHF, widened QRS complex, bradycardia, heart block, atrial flutter, ventricular flutter, fibrillation or tachycardia; quinidine syncope, torsades de pointes. **Special Senses:** Mydriasis, blurred vision, disturbed color perception, reduced visual field, photophobia, diplopia, night blindness, scotomas, optic neuritis, disturbed hearing (tinnitus, auditory acuity). **GI:** *Nausea, vomiting, diarrhea, esophagitis, abdominal pain,* hepatic dysfunction. **Hematologic:** Acute hemolytic anemia (especially in patients with G6PD deficiency), hypoprothrombinemia, leukopenia.

Thrombocytopenia, agranulocytosis (both rare). **Body as a Whole:** Cinchonism (nausea, vomiting, headache, dizziness, fever, tremors, vertigo, tinnitus, visual disturbances), angioedema, acute asthma, respiratory depression, vascular collapse. **Skin:** Rash, urticaria, cutaneous flushing with intense pruritus, photosensitivity. **Metabolic:** SLE, hypokalemia.

## INTERACTIONS Drug: Do not use with agents metabolized by CYP2D6. May increase **digoxin** levels by 50%; **amiodarone** may increase quinidine levels, increasing its risk of heart block; other ANTIARRHYTHMICS, PHENOTHIAZINES, **reserpine** add to cardiac depressant effects; ANTICHOLINERGIC AGENTS add to vagolytic effects; CHOLINERGIC AGENTS may antagonize cardiac effects; ANTICONVULSANTS, BARBITURATES, **rifampin** increase the metabolism of quinidine, thus decreasing its efficacy; CARBONIC ANHYDRASE INHIBITORS, **sodium bicarbonate,** CHRONIC ANTACIDS decrease renal elimination of quinidine, thus increasing its toxicity; **verapamil** causes significant hypotension; may increase hypoprothrombinemic effects of **warfarin.** Coadministration of other drug that prolongs the QT interval (e.g., **disopyramide, procainamide, amiodarone, bretylium, clarithromycin, levofloxacin**) may cause additive effects. **Diltiazem** may increase levels and decrease elimination of quinidine. **Food: Grapefruit juice** (greater than 1 qt/day) may decrease absorption.

## PHARMACOKINETICS Absorption: Almost completely from GI tract. **Onset:** 1–3 h. **Peak:** 0.5–1 h. **Duration:** 6–8 h. **Distribution:** Widely distributed to most body tissues except the brain; crosses placenta; distributed into breast milk. **Metabolism:** In liver (CYP3A4, P-gp).

Common adverse effects in *italic;* life-threatening effects underlined; generic names in **bold;** classifications in SMALL CAPS; ♣ Canadian drug name; ⊙ Prototype drug

1397

**Elimination:** Greater than 95% in urine, less than 5% in feces. **Half-Life:** 6–8 h.

## NURSING IMPLICATIONS

### Black Box Warning

*Quinidine as been associated with increased mortality (especially in those with structural heart disease) when used to treat non-life-threatening arrhythmias.*

### Assessment & Drug Effects

- Observe cardiac monitor and report immediately the following indications for stopping quinidine: (1) Sinus rhythm, (2) widening QRS complex in excess of 25% (i.e., longer than 0.12 sec), (3) changes in QT interval or refractory period, (4) disappearance of P waves, (5) sudden onset of or increase in ectopic ventricular beats (extrasystoles, PVCs), (6) decrease in heart rate to 120 bpm. Also report immediately any worsening of minor side effects.
- Continuous monitoring of ECG and BP is required. Observe patient closely (check sensorium and be alert for any sign of toxicity); determine plasma quinidine concentrations frequently when large doses (more than 2 g/day) are used or when quinidine is given parenterally (i.e., quinidine gluconate).
- Observe patient closely following each parenteral dose. Amount of subsequent dose is gauged by response to preceding dose.
- Monitor vital signs q1–2h or more often as needed during acute treatment. Count apical pulse for a full minute. Report any change in pulse rate, rhythm, or quality or any fall in BP.
- Severe hypotension is most likely to occur in patients receiving high oral doses or parenteral quinidine (i.e., quinidine gluconate).

- Monitor I&O. Diarrhea occurs commonly during early therapy; most patients become tolerant to this side effect. Evaluate serum electrolytes, acid-base, and fluid balance when symptoms become severe; dosage adjustment may be required.
- Monitor lab tests: Periodic blood count, serum electrolytes, LFTs, and renal function tests during long-term therapy. Periodic serum quinidine (target range 2–6 micrograms/mL or higher).

### Patient & Family Education

- Report feeling of faintness to prescriber. "Quinidine syncope" is caused by quinidine-induced changes in ventricular rhythm resulting in decreased cardiac output and syncope.
- Do not self-medicate with OTC drugs without advice from prescriber.
- Do not increase, decrease, skip, or discontinue doses without consulting prescriber.
- Notify prescriber immediately of disturbances in vision, ringing in ears, sense of breathlessness, onset of palpitations, and unpleasant sensation in chest. Be sure to note the time of occurrence and duration of chest symptoms.

## QUININE SULFATE

(kwye'nine)

Novoquinine ◆

**Classification:** ANTIMALARIAL
**Therapeutic:** ANTIMALARIAL
**Prototype:** Chloroquine

### AVAILABILITY Capsule

### ACTION & *THERAPEUTIC EFFECT*

Inhibits protein synthesis and depresses many enzyme systems in malaria parasite. *Effective against* Plasmodium vivax *and* Plasmodium malariae *but not* Plasmodium falciparum. *Generally replaced by less toxic and more effective agents in treatment of malaria.*

**USES** Chloroquine-resistant falciparum malaria and in combination with other antimalarials for radical cure of relapsing vivax malaria.

**UNLABELED USES** Restless leg syndrome.

**CONTRAINDICATIONS** Hypersensitivity to quinine or quinidine especially thrombocytopenia; tinnitus, optic neuritis; myasthenia gravis; G6PD deficiency; severe hepatic impairment (Child-Pugh class C).

**CAUTIOUS USE** Cardiac arrhythmias; restless leg syndrome. Same precautions as for quinidine sulfate when used in patients with cardiovascular conditions; chronic renal impairment; mild or moderate hepatic impairment; pregnancy (category C); lactation.

## ROUTE & DOSAGE

**Acute Malaria**
*Adult:* **PO** 650 mg q8h for 3 days
*Child:* **PO** 25 mg/kg/day in three divided doses q8h for 3 days
**Malaria Chemoprophylaxis**
*Adult:* **PO** 325 mg b.i.d. for 6 wk

## ADMINISTRATION
**Oral**
- Give with or after meals or a snack to minimize gastric irritation. Quinine has potent local irritant effect on gastric mucosa. Do not crush capsule; drug is not only irritating but also extremely bitter.
- Store in tight, light-resistant containers.

**ADVERSE EFFECTS** (≥1%) **Body as a Whole:** Cinchonism (tinnitus, decreased auditory acuity, dizziness, vertigo, headache, visual impairment, *nausea, vomiting, diarrhea,* fever); hypersensitivity (cutaneous flushing, visual impairment, pruritus, skin rash, fever, gastric distress, dyspnea, tinnitus); <u>hypothermia, coma</u>. **CNS:** Confusion, excitement, apprehension, syncope, delirium, convulsions, blackwater fever (extensive intravascular hemolysis with renal failure), <u>death</u>. **CV:** Angina, hypotension, tachycardia, <u>cardiovascular collapse</u>. **Hematologic:** <u>Leukopenia, thrombocytopenia, agranulocytosis</u>, hypoprothrombinemia, hemolytic anemia. **Respiratory:** Decreased respiration.

## DIAGNOSTIC TEST INTERFERENCE
Quinine may interfere with determinations of *urinary catecholamines* (*Sobel* and *Henry modification procedure*) and *urinary steroids (17-hydroxycorticosteroids)* (modification of *Roddy, Jenkins, Thorn* method). May cause false positive for OPIOIDS.

## INTERACTIONS **Drug:** May increase **digoxin** levels; ANTICHOLINERGIC AGENTS add to vagolytic effects; CHOLINERGIC AGENTS may antagonize cardiac effects; ANTICONVULSANTS, BARBITURATES, **rifampin** increase the metabolism of quinine, thus decreasing its efficacy; CARBONIC ANHYDRASE INHIBITORS, **sodium bicarbonate,** CHRONIC ANTACIDS decrease renal elimination of quinine, thus increasing its toxicity; **warfarin** may increase hypoprothrombinemic effects. **Amantadine, carbamazepine, phenobarbital** levels may be increased. Avoid use with **ritonavir. Food: Grapefruit juice** (greater than 1 qt/day) may increase plasma concentrations and adverse effects.

## PHARMACOKINETICS **Absorption:** Well from GI tract. **Peak:** 1–3 h.

Q

Common adverse effects in *italic;* life-threatening effects <u>underlined;</u> generic names in **bold;** classifications in SMALL CAPS; ♣Canadian drug name; ⓟ Prototype drug

1399

**Duration:** 6–8 h. **Distribution:** Widely distributed to most body tissues except the brain; crosses placenta; distributed into breast milk. **Metabolism:** In liver. **Elimination:** Greater than 95% in urine, less than 5% in feces. **Half-Life:** 8–21 h.

## NURSING IMPLICATIONS

### Black Box Warning

*Quinine use for treatment or prevention of nocturnal leg cramps has been associated with serious and life-threatening hematologic reactions and renal impairment.*

### Assessment & Drug Effects

- Be alert for S&S of rising plasma concentration of quinine marked by tinnitus and hearing impairment, which usually do not occur until concentration is 10 mcg/mL or more.
- Follow the same precautions with quinine as are used with quinidine in patients with atrial fibrillation; quinine may produce cardiotoxicity in these patients.

### Patient & Family Education

- Learn possible adverse reactions and report onset of any unusual symptom promptly to prescriber.

## QUINUPRISTIN/DALFOPRISTIN

(quin-u-pris'tin/dal'fo-pris-tin)

Synercid

**Classifications:** STREPTOGRAMIN ANTIBIOTIC; CYCLIC MACROLIDE

**Therapeutic:** ANTIBIOTIC

## AVAILABILITY Vial

## ACTION & *THERAPEUTIC EFFECT*

Dalfopristin inhibits the early phase of protein synthesis of bacteria, while quinupristin inhibits the late phase of protein synthesis of bacteria. Both actions lead to death of the bacteria organisms. *Effectiveness indicated by clinical improvement in S&S of life-threatening bacteremia. Active against gram-positive pathogens including vancomycin-resistant Enterococcus faecium (VREF), as well as some gram-negative anaerobes.*

**USES** Serious or life-threatening infections associated with VREF bacteremia; complicated skin and skin structure infections caused by *Staphylococcus aureus* or *Streptococcus pyogenes.*

**CONTRAINDICATIONS** Hypersensitivity to quinupristin/dalfopristin, pristinamycin, other streptogramins.

**CAUTIOUS USE** Renal or hepatic dysfunction; IBD; GI disease; pregnancy (category B); lactation. Safe use in children younger than 16 y not established.

## ROUTE & DOSAGE

**Vancomycin-Resistant**
***Enterococcus faecium***

*Adult:* **IV** 7.5 mg/kg infused over 60 min q8h

**Complicated Skin and Skin Structure Infections**

*Adult:* **IV** 7.5 mg/kg infused over 60 min q12h × 7 days

## ADMINISTRATION

### Intravenous

***PREPARE:* Intermittent:** Reconstitute a single 500 mg vial by slowly adding 5 mL D5W or sterile water for injection to yield 100 mg/mL. ▪ Gently swirl to dissolve but **do not** shake. Allow solution to clear. ▪ Withdraw the required dose and further dilute by adding to 100 mL (central line) or 250–500 mL (peripheral site) of D5W. ***ADMINISTER:* Intermittent:** Flush line before and after with D5W. **Do not** use saline. ▪ Administer over 1 h. ***INCOMPATIBILITIES:*** Solution/additive: **Saline solutions** and **lactated Ringer's** solution (flush lines with **D5W** before infusing other drugs). **Y-site:** Any drugs diluted in **saline.**

▪ Refrigerate unopened vials. After reconstitution solution is stable for 5 h at room temperature and 54 h refrigerated.

## ADVERSE EFFECTS (≥1%) **Body as a Whole:** Headache, pain, *myalgia, arthralgia.* **GI:** Nausea, diarrhea, vomiting. **Skin:** Rash, pruritus. **Other:** *Inflammation, pain, or edema at infusion site, other infusion site reactions,* thrombophlebitis.

## INTERACTIONS **Drug:** Inhibits CYP3A4 metabolism of **cyclosporine, midazolam, nifedipine,** PROTEASE INHIBITORS, **vincristine, vinblastine, docetaxel, paclitaxel, diazepam, tacrolimus, carbamazepine, quinidine, lidocaine, disopyramide.**

## PHARMACOKINETICS **Distribution:** Moderately protein bound. **Metabolism:** Metabolized to several active metabolites. **Elimination:** Primarily in feces (75–77%). **Half-Life:** 3 h quinupristin, 1 h dalfopristin.

## NURSING IMPLICATIONS

### Assessment & Drug Effects
▪ Monitor for S&S of infusion site irritation; change infusion site if irritation is apparent.
▪ Monitor for cutaneous reaction (e.g., pruritus/erythema of neck, face, upper body).
▪ Monitor lab tests: Baseline C&S and WBC with differential.

### Patient & Family Education
▪ Report burning, itching, or pain at infusion site to prescriber.
▪ Report any sensation of swelling of face and tongue; difficulty swallowing.

# RABEPRAZOLE SODIUM
(rab-e-pra′zole)

AcipHex

**Classification:** GASTRIC PROTON PUMP INHIBITOR
Therapeutic: ANTIULCER
**Prototype:** Omeprazole

## AVAILABILITY Delayed release tablet; delayed release capsule

## ACTION & THERAPEUTIC EFFECT
Suppresses gastric acid secretion by inhibiting the $H^+$, $K^+$ ATPase enzyme system [the acid (proton $H^+$) pump] in the parietal cells of the stomach. Produces an antisecretory effect on the hydrogen ion ($H^+$) in the parietal cells. *Effectiveness indicated by a negative for* H. pylori *with preexisting gastric ulcer; also by elimination of S&S of GERD or peptic ulcers.*

## USES Healing and maintenance of healing of erosive or ulcerative gastroesophageal reflux disease (GERD); healing of duodenal ulcers; treatment of hypersecretory conditions.

## CONTRAINDICATIONS Hypersensitivity to rabeprazole, or proton pump inhibitors (PPIs); concomitant use with rilpivirine-containing products; lactation.

## CAUTIOUS USE Severe hepatic impairment; mild to moderate hepatic disease; Japanese heritage; older adults; pregnancy (category B); children.

R

## ROUTE & DOSAGE

### Healing of Erosive GERD

*Adult:* **PO** 20 mg daily × 4–8 wk, may continue up to 16 wk if needed

### Symptomatic Therapy for GERD

*Adult/Adolescent:* **PO** 20 mg daily × 4–8 w
*Child (weight greater than 15 kg):* 10 mg daily × 12 wk; *weight less than 15 kg:* 5 mg daily × 12 wk

### Healing Duodenal Ulcer

*Adult:* **PO** 20 mg daily × 4 wk

### Hypersecretory Disease

*Adult:* **PO** 60 mg daily in 1–2 divided doses (max: 100 mg daily or 60 mg b.i.d.)

## ADMINISTRATION

### Oral

- Ensure that the tablet is swallowed whole. It should not be crushed or chewed. Capsule should be opened and sprinkled on a small amount of soft food 30 min before a meal. Do not chew or crush. May be administered with an antacid.
- Store at 15°–30° C (59°–86° F).

## ADVERSE EFFECTS (≥1%) **Body as a Whole:** *Headache,* increased susceptibility to infection. **Skin:** (Rare) <u>Stevens–Johnson syndrome, toxic epidermal necrolysis, erythema multiforme</u>. **GI:** Flatulence, constipation, abdominal pain, diarrhea, vomiting, <u>C. difficile diarrhea</u>. **Cardiovascular:** Peripheral edema. **CNS:** Headache, pain, dizziness. **Hepatic:** Increased liver enzymes, hepatic encephalopathy. **Muscular:** Arthralgia, myalgia. **Respiratory:** Pharyngitis.

## INTERACTIONS **Drug:** Contraindicated with **atazanavir** or **rilpivirine.** May decrease absorption of cefuroxime, ketoconazole; may increase **digoxin** levels; may decrease **nelfinavir** levels. **Herbal: Ginkgo** may decrease plasma levels.

## PHARMACOKINETICS **Absorption:** 52% bioavailability. **Distribution:** 96% protein bound. **Metabolism:** In liver by (CYP3A4, 2C19). **Elimination:** Primarily in urine. **Half-Life:** 1–2 h.

## NURSING IMPLICATIONS

### Assessment & Drug Effects

- Coadministered drugs: Monitor for changes in digoxin blood level.
- Monitor lab tests: Periodic magnesium level in patients on long-term treatment or those taking drugs that cause hypomagnesemia (e.g., digoxin, diuretics).

### Patient & Family Education

- Report diarrhea, skin rash, other bothersome adverse effects to prescriber.

# RALOXIFENE HYDROCHLORIDE

(ra-lox′i-feen)
*Evista*
**Classification:** SELECTIVE ESTROGEN RECEPTOR ANTAGONIST/AGONIST
**Therapeutic:** OSTEOPOROSIS PROPHYLACTIC
**Prototype:** Tamoxifen

## AVAILABILITY Tablet

## ACTION & *THERAPEUTIC EFFECT*

Exhibits selective estrogen receptor antagonist activity on uterus and breast tissue. Prevents tissue proliferation in both sites. Decreases bone resorption and increases bone density. *Effectiveness indicated by increased bone mineral density. Reduces the risk of invasive breast cancer in high risk postmenopausal women (e.g., breast cancer in situ, or atypical hyperplasia).*

R

Common adverse effects in *italic*; life-threatening effects <u>underlined</u>; generic names in **bold**; classifications in SMALL CAPS; ♣ Canadian drug name; ⊕ Prototype drug

USES Prevention and treatment of osteoporosis in postmenopausal women; breast cancer prophylaxis.

CONTRAINDICATIONS Active or past history of a thromboembolic event; drug induced venous thrombosis; hypersensitivity to raloxifene; severe hepatic impairment; pregnancy (category X); lactation.

CAUTIOUS USE Concurrent use of raloxifene and estrogen hormone replacement therapy and lipid-lowering agents; hyperlipidemia; hepatic impairment; moderate or severe renal impairment.

## ROUTE & DOSAGE

### Prevention/Treatment of Osteoporosis
*Adult:* PO 60 mg daily

### Breast Cancer Prophylaxis
*Postmenopausal Adult:* PO 60 mg daily

## ADMINISTRATION

### Oral
- Calcium and vitamin D supplementation are recommended with raloxifene: 1500 mg/day of elemental calcium and 400–800 units/day of vitamin D.
- Store at 15°–30° C (59°–86° F) in a tightly closed container and protect from light.

## ADVERSE EFFECTS (≥1%) Body
as a Whole: Infection, flu-like syndrome, leg cramps, fever, arthralgia, myalgia, arthritis. CNS: Migraine headache, depression, insomnia. CV: *Hot flashes,* chest pain, peripheral edema, decreased serum cholesterol. GI: Nausea, dyspepsia, vomiting, flatulence, GI disorder, gastroenteritis, weight gain. Respiratory: Sinusitis, pharyngitis, cough, pneumonia, laryngitis. Skin: Rash, sweating.

Urogenital: Vaginitis, UTI, cystitis, leukorrhea, endometrial disorder, breast pain, vaginal bleeding.

INTERACTIONS Drug: Use of ESTROGENS not recommended; absorption reduced by cholestyramine; use with warfarin may result in changes in prothrombin time (PT). Herbal: Soy isoflavones should be used with caution.

PHARMACOKINETICS Absorption: 60% absorbed, absolute bioavailability 2%. Metabolism: Extensive first-pass metabolism in liver. Elimination: Primarily in feces. Half-Life: 27.7–32.5 h.

## NURSING IMPLICATIONS

### Black Box Warning

*Raloxifene has been associated with increased risk of venous thromboembolism and death from stroke.*

### Assessment & Drug Effects
- Monitor carefully for and immediately report S&S of thromboembolic events.
- Do not give drug concurrently with cholestyramine; however, if unavoidable, space the two drugs as widely as possible.
- Monitor lab tests: Periodic LFTs.

### Patient & Family Education
- Contact prescriber immediately if unexplained calf pain or tenderness occurs.
- Avoid prolonged restriction of movement during travel.
- Drug does not prevent and may induce hot flashes.
- Do not take drug with other estrogen-containing drugs.
- Raloxifene is normally discontinued 72 h prior to prolonged immobilization (e.g., post-surgical recovery, prolonged bedrest). Consult prescriber.

R

Common adverse effects in *italic;* life-threatening effects <u>underlined</u>; generic names in **bold;** classifications in SMALL CAPS; ♣Canadian drug name; ⊙ Prototype drug

1403

# RALTEGRAVIR ⊕
(ral-te-gra′vir)
Isentress
**Classifications:** ANTIRETROVIRAL;
INTEGRASE INHIBITOR
Therapeutic: ANTIRETROVIRAL

**AVAILABILITY** Tablet; chewable tablet

## ACTION & *THERAPEUTIC EFFECT*
Inhibits HIV-1 integrase, an enzyme required for integration of proviral DNA into the helper T-cell genome, thus preventing formation of the HIV-1 provirus. *Inhibiting integration prevents replication and proliferation of the HIV-1 virus.*

## USES
In combination with other antiretroviral agents for the treatment of HIV-1 infection.

## CONTRAINDICATIONS
Treatment of naïve HIV-1 patients; lactation.

## CAUTIOUS USE
Hepatitis; mild to moderate hepatic impairment; individuals at increased risk of myopathy or rhabdomyolysis; lactase deficiency; PKU; history of psychiatric disease or suicidal ideation; older adults; pregnancy (category C); children younger than 2 y. Safety and efficacy in patients with severe hepatic impairment not established.

## ROUTE & DOSAGE

### HIV-1 Infection
*Adult/Adolescent:* **PO** 400 mg b.i.d.
*Child (2–12 y, weight 10–14 kg):* **PO**
75 mg b.i.d.; *weight 14–20 kg:*
100 mg b.i.d.; *weight 20–28 kg:* 150 b.i.d.; *weight 28–40 kg:* 200 mg b.i.d.; *weight over 40 kg:* 300 mg b.i.d.

### HIV Infection (with Concurrent Rifampin)
*Adult/Adolescent:* **PO** 800 mg b.i.d.

## ADMINISTRATION

### Oral
- May be given without regard to food.
- Film-coated tablets must be swallowed whole (400 mg). Chewable tablets (25 or 100 mg) may be chewed or swallowed whole.
- Give before dialysis.
- Store at 15–30° C (59–86° F).

## ADVERSE EFFECTS (≥1%) **Body as a Whole:** Asthenia, fatigue, pyrexia. **CNS:** Dizziness, headache. **GI:** Abdominal pain, *diarrhea*, nausea, vomiting. **Skin:** Lipodystrophy. **Hematologic:** Anemia, neutropenia.

## INTERACTIONS **Drug: Atazanavir** may increase plasma levels of raltegravir; **rifampin** and **tipranavir/ritonavir** may decrease plasma levels of raltegravir.

## PHARMACOKINETICS **Peak:** 3 h. **Distribution:** 83% protein bound. **Metabolism:** In the liver. **Elimination:** Stool and urine. **Half-Life:** 9 h.

## NURSING IMPLICATIONS

### Assessment & Drug Effects
- Monitor for and report S&S of immune reconstitution syndrome (inflammatory response to residual opportunistic infections such as MAC, CMV, PCP, or reactivation of varicella zoster).
- Monitor diabetics for loss of glycemic conrol.
- Monitor lab tests: Baseline and periodic CD4+ cell count and HIV RNA viral load; periodic CBC with differential, LFTs.

### Patient & Family Education
- Inform prescriber immediately if you plan to become or become pregnant during therapy.
- Report promptly unexplained leg pain or muscle cramping.

Common adverse effects in *italic;* life-threatening effects underlined; generic names in **bold;** classifications in SMALL CAPS; ✤ Canadian drug name; ⊕ Prototype drug

1404

# RAMELTEON ℗

(ra-mel'tee-on)

Rozerem

**Classifications:** MELATONIN RECEPTOR AGONIST; SEDATIVE-HYPNOTIC

Therapeutic: SEDATIVE

## AVAILABILITY Tablet

## ACTION & THERAPEUTIC EFFECT
A melatonin receptor agonist with high affinity for melatonin receptors in the brain. This activity is believed to promote sleep, as these receptors, in response to endogenous melatonin, are thought to be involved in maintaining the circadian rhythm underlying the normal sleep-wake cycle. *Effective in promoting onset of sleep.*

## USES Treatment of insomnia characterized by difficulty with sleep onset.

## CONTRAINDICATIONS Hypersensitivity to ramelteon; severe hepatic function impairment (Child-Pugh class C); severe sleep apnea or severe COPD; severe depression; suicidal ideation; lactation.

## CAUTIOUS USE Moderate hepatic function impairment (Child-Pugh class B); depression with suicidal tendencies; older adults; pregnancy (category C). Safety and efficacy in children younger than 18 y not established.

## ROUTE & DOSAGE

**Insomnia**
*Adult:* **PO** 8 mg within 30 min of bedtime

## ADMINISTRATION

**Oral**
- Give within 30 min of bedtime.
- Do not administer to anyone on concurrent fluvoxamine therapy without alerting prescriber. This

combination causes a dramatic increase in ramelteon blood level.
- Store at 15°–30° C (59°–86° F).

## ADVERSE EFFECTS (≥1%) CNS: Depression, dizziness, fatigue, headache, insomnia, somnolence. GI: Diarrhea, unpleasant taste, nausea. **Musculoskeletal:** Arthralgia, myalgia. **Respiratory:** Upper respiratory tract infection.

## INTERACTIONS Drug: Concurrent use with **ethanol** produces additive CNS depressant effects; **ketoconazole, itraconazole,** and **fluvoxamine** increase ramelteon levels; other CYP1A2 INHIBITORS (e.g., **ciprofloxacin, enoxacin, mexiletine, norfloxacin**) may also increase ramelteon levels; **rifampin** decreases ramelteon levels. **Food:** High-fat meal, **grapefruit** or **grapefruit juice** increase ramelteon levels.

## PHARMACOKINETICS Absorption: 84%. Peak: 45 min. Distribution: 82% protein bound. Metabolism: Rapid and extensive first pass hepatic metabolism; one metabolite, M-II, is active. Elimination: Primarily renal. Half-Life: 1–2.5 h.

## NURSING IMPLICATIONS

### Assessment & Drug Effects
- Monitor for and report worsening insomnia and cognitive or behavioral changes.
- Monitor for S&S of decreased testosterone levels (e.g., loss of libido) or increased prolactin levels (galactorrhea).
- Lab test: Baseline LFTs.

### Patient & Family Education
- Do not take with or immediately after a high fat meal.
- Do not drive or engage in potentially hazardous activities until response to drug is known.
- Do not consume alcohol while taking this drug.

R

- Report any of the following to prescriber: Worsening insomnia, cognitive or behavioral changes, problem with reproductive function.

# RAMIPRIL
(ram′i-pril)
Altace
**Classifications:** ANGIOTENSIN-CONVERTING ENZYME (ACE) INHIBITOR; ANTIHYPERTENSIVE
Therapeutic: ANTIHYPERTENSIVE
**Prototype:** Enalapril

**AVAILABILITY** Capsule

## ACTION & *THERAPEUTIC EFFECT*
Reduces peripheral vascular resistance by inhibiting the formation of angiotensin II, a potent vasoconstrictor. This also decreases serum aldosterone levels and reduces peripheral arterial resistance (afterload) as well as improves cardiac output and exercise tolerance. *Lowers BP, and improves cardiac output as well as exercise tolerance.*

**USES** Mild to moderate hypertension, CHF, stroke prophylaxis, myocardial infarction prophylaxis, post myocardial infarction.

**UNLABELED USES** Diabetic nephropathy, proteinuria.

**CONTRAINDICATIONS** Hypersensitivity to ramipril or any other ACE inhibitor, history of angioneurotic edema; intestinal angioedema; jaundice; elevated hepatic enzymes; hyperkalemia; concurrent use of aliskiren in diabetic patients; oliguria, or progressive azotemia; pregnancy (category D); lactation.

**CAUTIOUS USE** Impaired kidney or liver function, surgery or anesthesia; CHF; SLE, scleroderma. Safety and efficacy in children not established.

## ROUTE & DOSAGE

**Hypertension**
*Adult:* **PO** 2.5 mg daily, may increase up to 20 mg/day in 1–2 divided doses

**Stroke/MI Risk Reduction**
*Adult:* **PO** 2.5 mg daily × 1wk then 5 mg daily × 3wk, may increase up to 10 mg/day

**Post Myocardial Infarction**
*Adult:* **PO** 1.25–2.5 mg b.i.d. (may titrate up to 5 mg b.i.d.)

## ADMINISTRATION
**Oral**
- When patient has been treated with a diuretic, the diuretic is usually discontinued 2–3 days before beginning ramipril. If the diuretic cannot be discontinued, initial ramipril dose is usually lowered to 1.25 mg.
- Store at 15°–30° C (59°–86° F) and protect from moisture.

**ADVERSE EFFECTS** (≥1%) **CNS:** Dizziness, fatigue, headache. **GI:** Nausea, vomiting, diarrhea, eructation. **Metabolic:** Hyperkalemia, hyponatremia. **Skin:** Erythema, pruritus. **Body as a Whole:** Angioedema. **Respiratory:** *Cough.* **CV:** *Hypotension.* **Skin:** Stevens–Johnson syndrome.

**INTERACTIONS Drug:** POTASSIUM-SPARING DIURETICS may increase risk of hyperkalemia. May elevate serum **lithium** levels, resulting in lithium toxicity. NSAIDS may attenuate antihypertensive effects. Use with **azathioprine** increases risk of hematologic side effects. **Pregabalin** use increases the risk of angioedema. Use with ANGIOTENSION II RECEPTOR ANTAGONISTS does not offer additional benefit.

R

**PHARMACOKINETICS Absorption:** 60% from GI tract. **Onset:** 2 h. **Peak:** 6–8 h. **Duration:** Up to 24 h. **Distribution:** Crosses placenta; not known if distributed into breast milk. **Metabolism:** Rapidly metabolized in liver to active metabolite, ramiprilat. **Elimination:** 40–60% in urine, 40% in feces. **Half-Life:** 2–3 h.

## NURSING IMPLICATIONS

### Black Box Warning

*Ramipril has been associated with fetal injury and death.*

### Assessment & Drug Effects

- Monitor BP at time of peak effectiveness, 3–6 h after dosing and at end of dosing interval just before next dose.
- Report diminished antihypertensive effect.
- Monitor for first-dose hypotension, especially in salt- or volume-depleted persons.
- Observe for S&S of hyperkalemia (see Appendix F).
- Monitor lab tests: Periodic BUN, serum creatinine, and serum potassium.

### Patient & Family Education

- Notify prescriber immediately if you become or suspect you are pregnant.
- Discontinue drug and report S&S of angioedema to prescriber (e.g., swelling of face or extremities, difficulty breathing or swallowing).
- Maintain adequate fluid intake and avoid potassium supplements or salt substitutes unless specifically prescribed by the prescriber.
- Light-headedness and dizziness may occur, especially during the initial days of therapy. If fainting occurs, stop taking ramipril until the prescriber has been consulted.

# RAMUCIRUMAB

(ram-u-cir'u-mab)

Cyramza

**Classifications:** IMMUNOMODULATOR; MONOCLONAL ANTIBODY; VASCULAR ENDOTHELIAL GROWTH FACTOR RECEPTOR 2 (VEGFR2) ANTAGONIST

**Therapeutic:** IMMUNOMODULATOR

**AVAILABILITY** Solution for injection

## ACTION & *THERAPEUTIC EFFECT*

Inhibits vascular endothelial growth factor receptor 2 (VEGFR2) by binding to it and blocking its activation, thereby inhibiting proliferation and migration of endothelial cells. *VEGFR2 inhibition results in reduced tumor vascularity and growth.*

**USES** Treatment of advanced gastric cancer or gastroesophageal junction adenocarcinoma, as a single-agent after prior fluoropyrimidine- or platinum-containing chemotherapy.

## CONTRAINDICATIONS Uncontrolled severe hypertension; Grade 3–4 infusion-related reactions; urine protein greater than 3 mg/24 h; nephrotic syndrome; arterial thromboembolic events; GI perforation; Grade 3 or 4 bleeding; severe arterial thromboembolic event; Posterior Leukoencephalopathy Syndrome; lactation.

## CAUTIOUS USE Hypertension; protein urea; infusion related reactions; concurrent NSAIDs or drug that increase bleeding risk; impaired wound healing; hepatic impairment; pregnancy (category C). Safety and efficacy in children younger than 18 y not established.

R

## ROUTE & DOSAGE

### Gastric Cancer

*Adult:* **IV** 8 mg/kg every 2 wk

### Toxicity Dosage Adjustment

*Infusion related reactions:* Grade 1–2, decrease IV rate by 50%; Grade 3–4, permanently discontinue
*Severe hypertension:* Interrupt therapy until BP managed; permanently discontinue if BP cannot be controlled
*Proteinuria:* Urine protein levels 2g/24h or greater, interrupt therapy until levels are less than 2g/24h then reinitiate at 6 mg/kg q2wk (or 5 mg/kg q2wk in a recurrence); protein level is greater than 3mg/24h or nephrotic syndrome, permanently discontinue
*Arterial Thromboembolic Events, GI Perforation, or Grade 3 or 4 Bleeding:* Permanently discontinue

## ADMINISTRATION

### Intravenous

This drug is a cytotoxic agent and caution should be used to prevent any contact with the drug. Follow institutional or standard guidelines for preparation, handling, and disposal of cytotoxic agents.
*PREPARE:* **IV Infusion:** Dilute required dose in NS to a final volume of 250 mL. Invert gently to mix but do not shake. Discard unused portion of the vial.
*ADMINISTER:* **IV Infusion:** Give over 60 min through a 0.22 micron protein-sparing filter. **Do not** give IV push or bolus. Flush the line after infusion with NS. Reduce infusion rate (by 50%)

for Grade 1 or 2 infusion reaction. Stop infusion for Grade 3 or 4 infusion reaction.
*INCOMPATIBILITIES:* Do not mix or infuse with any other drugs or solutions.

- Store diluted solutions at 2°–8° C (36°–46° F) for no longer than 24 h (do not freeze) or may store for 4 h at room temperature [below 25° C (77° F)].

## ADVERSE EFFECTS (≥1%) **Body as a Whole:** Infusion related reactions, epistaxis. **CNS:** Headache. **CV:** *Hypertension.* **GI:** *Diarrhea,* intestinal obstruction. **Hematological:** Arterial thromboembolic events, hemorrhage, neutropenia. **Metabolic:** Hyponatremia, proteinuria. **Skin:** Rash.

## PHARMACOKINETICS **Half-Life:** Dose related (200–300 h).

## NURSING IMPLICATIONS

### Black Box Warning

*Ramucirumab has been associated with increased risk of hemorrhage, including severe and sometimes fatal hemorrhagic events. Permanently discontinue if severe bleeding occurs.*

### Assessment & Drug Effects

- Monitor closely for infusion related reactions.
- Monitor BP throughout therapy. Withhold drug and notify prescriber if severe hypertension occurs. Resume drug only after hypertension is medically controlled.
- If unexplained bleeding occurs, withhold drug and notify prescriber.
- Monitor for and report promptly S&S of liver dysfunction.
- Inspect wounds closely. If poor wound healing is suspected, withhold drug and notify prescriber.

Common adverse effects in *italic*; life-threatening effects underlined; generic names in **bold**; classifications in SMALL CAPS; ✥ Canadian drug name; ⊘ Prototype drug

- Monitor lab tests: Periodic LFTs, thyroid function, and urine protein.

**Patient & Family Education**

- Report promptly to prescriber if blood pressure is elevated or if symptoms of hypertension occur including severe headache, lightheadedness, or neurologic symptoms.
- Contact prescriber for bleeding or symptoms of bleeding including lightheadedness.
- Notify prescriber for severe diarrhea, vomiting, or severe abdominal pain.
- Monitor any wounds and report slow wound healing.
- Do not undergo surgery without first discussing the risk of poor wound healing with prescriber.

# RANITIDINE HYDROCHLORIDE
(ra-nye'te-deen)
*Zantac, Zantac-75*
**Classification:** ANTISECRETORY (H₂ RECEPTOR ANTAGONIST)
*Therapeutic:* ANTIULCER
**Prototype:** Cimetidine

**AVAILABILITY** Tablet; capsule; syrup; solution for injection

## ACTION & *THERAPEUTIC EFFECT*
Competitively inhibits histamine action at H₂-receptor sites on parietal cells, blocking gastric acid secretion. Indirectly reduces pepsin secretion. *Blocks daytime and nocturnal basal gastric acid secretion stimulated by histamine and reduces gastric acid release in response to food, caffeine, pentagastrin, and insulin.*

**USES** Short-term treatment of active duodenal ulcer; maintenance therapy for duodenal ulcer patient after healing of acute ulcer; treatment of gastroesophageal reflux disease; short-term treatment of active, benign gastric ulcer; treatment of pathologic GI hypersecretory conditions (e.g., Zollinger-Ellison syndrome, systemic mastocytosis, and postoperative hypersecretion); heartburn.

**CONTRAINDICATIONS** Hypersensitivity to ranitidine; acute porphyria.

**CAUTIOUS USE** Hypersensitivity to H₂-blockers; hepatic and renal dysfunction; renal failure; older adults; PKU; pregnancy (category B); lactation; infants younger than 2 wk. **OTC form:** Children younger than 12 y.

## ROUTE & DOSAGE

**Duodenal Ulcer, Gastric Ulcer, Gastroesophageal Reflux**
*Adult:* **PO** 150 mg b.i.d. or 300 mg at bedtime; **IV** 50 mg q6–8h; 150–300 mg/24 h by continuous infusion
*Child:* **PO** 4–5 mg/kg/day divided q8–12h (max: 300 mg/day); **IM/IV** 2–4 mg/kg/day divided q6–8h (max: 200 mg/day)
*Infant (younger than 2 wk):* **PO** 1.5–2 mg/kg/day divided q12h; **IV** 1.5 mg/kg/day divided q12h or 0.04 mg/kg/h by continuous infusion

**Duodenal Ulcer, Maintenance Therapy**
*Adult:* **PO** 150 mg at bedtime

**Pathologic Hypersecretory Conditions**
*Adult:* **PO** 150 mg b.i.d. up to 6 g/day; **IV** 1 mg/kg/h, adjusted for gastric output

**Heartburn**
*Adult:* **PO** 75–150 mg b.i.d.

**Renal Impairment Dosage Adjustment**
*CrCl less than 50 mL/min:*
**PO** q24h; **IV** q18–24h

**Hemodialysis Dosage Adjustment**
Time dose to administer at the end of dialysis

## ADMINISTRATION

### Oral
- May be given without regard to meals.
- Store tablets in light-resistant, tightly capped container at 15°–30° C (59°–86° F) in a dry place.

### Intramuscular
- Note: Does not need to be diluted.

### Intravenous
Note: Verify correct IV concentration and rate of infusion for infants and children with prescriber.

*PREPARE:* **Direct:** Dilute 50 mg NS, D5W, LR, or other compatible IV solution to a total volume of 20 mL. **Intermittent:** Dilute 50 mg in 100 mL of NS, D5W, LR, or other compatible IV solution. **Continuous:** Dilute total daily dose in 250 mL of NS, D5W, LR, or other compatible IV solution. Final concentration should be 2.5 mg/mL or less.

*ADMINISTER:* **Direct:** Give at a rate of 4 mL/min or 20 mL over not less than 5 min. **Intermittent:** Give over 15–30 min. **Continuous:** Give over 24 h. Do not exceed 6.25 mg/h.

*INCOMPATIBILITIES:* **Solution/additive: Amphotericin B, atracurium, cefamandole, cefazolin, cefoxitin, ceftazidime, cefuroxime, clindamycin, chlorpromazine, ethacrynic acid, insulin, hydroxyzine, pentobarbital, phenobarbital, phytonadione. Y-site: Amphotericin B cholesteryl, caspofungin, dantrolene, diazepam, diazoxide, drotrecogin, gemtuzumab, haloperidol, hetastarch in normal saline, insulin, lansoprazole, pantoprazole, phenytoin, quinupristin/dalfopristin, SMZ/TMP, temocillin.**

- Schedule dose to coincide with end of treatment if patient is having hemodialysis.

## ADVERSE EFFECTS (≥1%) CNS:
*Headache,* malaise, dizziness, somnolence, insomnia, vertigo, mental confusion, agitation, depression, hallucinations in older adults. **CV:** Bradycardia (with rapid IV push). **GI:** *Constipation,* nausea, *abdominal pain,* diarrhea. **Skin:** Rash. **Hematologic:** Reversible decrease in WBC count, thrombocytopenia. **Body as a Whole:** Hypersensitivity reactions, anaphylaxis (rare).

## DIAGNOSTIC TEST INTERFERENCE
Ranitidine may produce slight elevations in **serum creatinine** (without concurrent increase in **BUN**); (rare) increases in **AST, ALT, alkaline phosphatase, LDH,** and total **bilirubin.** Produces false-positive tests for **urine protein** with **Multistix** (use **sulfosalicylic acid** instead).

## INTERACTIONS Drug: May reduce absorption of **cefpodoxime, cefuroxime, delavirdine, ketoconazole, itraconazole.**

## PHARMACOKINETICS Absorption: Incompletely from GI tract

R

(50% reaches systemic circulation). **Peak:** 2–3 h PO. **Duration:** 8–12 h. **Distribution:** Distributed into breast milk. **Metabolism:** In liver. **Elimination:** In urine, with some excreted in feces. **Half-Life:** 2–3 h.

## NURSING IMPLICATIONS

### Assessment & Drug Effects

- Potential toxicity results from decreased clearance (elimination), which causes prolonged action; greatest risk for toxicity is in older adult patients or those with hepatic or renal dysfunction.
- Be alert for early signs of hepatotoxicity: Jaundice (dark urine, pruritus, yellow sclera and skin), elevated transaminases (especially ALT) and LDH.
- Long-term therapy may lead to vitamin B$_{12}$ deficiency.
- Monitor lab tests: Periodic LFTs. Periodic creatinine clearance if renal dysfunction is present or suspected.

### Patient & Family Education

- Note: Long duration of action provides ulcer pain relief that is maintained through the night as well as the day.
- Adhere to scheduled periodic laboratory checkups during ranitidine treatment.
- Do not supplement therapy with OTC remedies for gastric distress or pain without prescriber's advice.

## RANOLAZINE

(ra-no'la-zeen)

Ranexa

**Classifications:** ANTIANGINAL; PARTIAL FATTY ACID OXIDATION (PFOX) INHIBITOR

Therapeutic: ANTIANGINAL

**AVAILABILITY** Extended release tablet

## ACTION & *THERAPEUTIC EFFECT*

A partial fatty-acid oxidation inhibitor that shifts myocardial metabolism away from fatty acids to glucose. This shift requires less oxygen for oxidation and results in decreased oxygen demand. *Improves exercise tolerance and angina symptoms.*

**USES** Treatment of chronic stable angina in combination with calcium channel blockers, beta-blockers, or nitrates.

**CONTRAINDICATIONS** Severe hepatic impairment; severe renal impairment, renal failure, hypokalemia, hypomagnesemia; history of acute MI; lactation.

**CAUTIOUS USE** History of QT prolongation or torsades de pointes; renal impairment; older adult; pregnancy (category C); children.

## ROUTE & DOSAGE

### Chronic Stable Angina

*Adult:* **PO** 500 mg b.i.d. (max: 1000 mg b.i.d.) (patients taking concurrent CYP3A4 inhibitors have a max dose of 500 mg b.i.d.)

## ADMINISTRATION

### Oral

- **Must be** swallowed whole. Should not be crushed, broken, or chewed.
- Store at 15°–30° C (59°–86° F).

**ADVERSE EFFECTS** (≥1%) **Body as a Whole:** Peripheral edema. **CNS:** *Dizziness,* headache. **CV:** Palpitations. **GI:** Abdominal pain, *constipation,* dry mouth,

R

nausea, vomiting. **Respiratory:** Dyspnea. **Special Senses:** Tinnitus, vertigo.

## DIAGNOSTIC TEST INTERFERENCE

Ranolazine is not known to interfere with any diagnostic laboratory test.

## INTERACTIONS **Drug:** INHIBITORS OF P-GLYCOPROTEIN (e.g., **ritonavir, cyclosporine**) may increase ranolazine absorption. Ranolazine increases the plasma concentrations of **digoxin** and **simvastatin.** INHIBITORS OF CYP3A4 [e.g., **diltiazem, erythromycin, grapefruit juice,** HIV PROTEASE INHIBITORS, **ketoconazole,** MACROLIDE ANTIBIOTICS (especially **ketoconazole**), **verapamil**] can increase plasma levels and $QT_c$ elevation. **Paroxetine,** a CYP2D6 INHIBITOR, increases the plasma levels of ranolazine. CLASS I or III ANTIARRHYTHMICS (e.g., **quinidine, dofetilide, sotalol**), **thioridazine,** and **ziprasidone** can cause additive increases in $QT_c$ elevation. **Food: Grapefruit juice.**

## PHARMACOKINETICS **Absorption:** 73% of PO dose absorbed. **Peak:** 2–5 h. **Distribution:** 62% protein bound. **Metabolism:** Extensive hepatic metabolism. **Elimination:** 75% in urine; 25% in feces. **Half-Life:** 7 h.

## NURSING IMPLICATIONS

### Assessment & Drug Effects

- Monitor ECG at baseline and periodically for prolongation of the $QT_c$ interval.
- Monitor blood levels of digoxin with concurrent therapy.
- When coadministered with simvastatin, monitor for and report unexplained muscle weakness or pain.
- Monitor lab tests: Baseline and periodic renal function tests with moderate-to-severe renal impairment.

### Patient & Family Education

- Do not engage in hazardous activities until response to drug is known.
- Contact prescriber if you experience fainting while taking ranolazine.
- Do not drink grapefruit juice or eat grapefruit while taking this drug.

## RASAGILINE
(ras-a-gi'leen)
Azilect
**Classifications:** MONOAMINE OXIDASE-B (MAO-B) INHIBITOR; ANTIPARKINSON
Therapeutic: ANTIPARKINSON

## AVAILABILITY Tablet

## ACTION & *THERAPEUTIC EFFECT*
A potent monoamine oxidase B (MAO-B) inhibitor that prevents the enzyme monoamine oxidase B from breaking down dopamine in the brain. Rasagiline also interferes with dopamine reuptake at synapses in the brain. *Rasagiline helps to overcome dopaminergic motor dysfunction in Parkinson's disease.*

## USES Treatment of Parkinson's disease (monotherapy or adjunct).

## CONTRAINDICATIONS Moderate to severe hepatic impairment; alcoholism; biliary cirrhosis; major psychotic disorders; uncontrolled hypertension; within 14 days of use of other MAOIs.

## CAUTIOUS USE Mild hepatic dysfunction; cardiovascular disease; DM; asthma, bronchitis, hyperthyroidism; postural or orthostatic hypotension; migraine headaches; moderate to severe renal impairment, anuria; epilepsy or preexisting seizure disorders; pregnancy (category C); lactation. Safety and efficacy in children not established.

## ROUTE & DOSAGE

**Parkinson's Disease**
*Adult:* **PO** 1 mg/day as monotherapy; 0.5–1 mg/day if used with
levodopa as adjunctive therapy

**Hepatic Impairment**
**Dosage Adjustment**
*Mild Impairment:* 0.5 mg/day
**Concomitant Use of CYP1A2**
**Inhibitors Dosage Adjustment**
Max dose: 0.5 mg once daily

## ADMINISTRATION

**Oral**
▪ May be given without regard to
food.
▪ Store at 15°–30° C (59°–86° F).

## ADVERSE EFFECTS (≥1%) **Body as**
**a Whole:** Accidental injury, allergic
reaction, alopecia, gingivitis, hernia,
infection, neck pain, pruritus, peripheral edema. **CNS:** Abnormal dreams,
abnormal gait, amnesia, anxiety,
asthenia, ataxia, confusion, *depres-*
*sion,* dizziness, *dyskinesia,* dystonia,
*fall,* fever, flu-like syndrome, hallucinations, *headache,* hyperkinesias,
hypertonia, malaise, neuropathy,
neck pain, paresthesia, somnolence,
syncope, tremor, vertigo. **CV:** Angina
pectoris, <u>bundle branch block</u>, <u>cer-</u>
<u>ebrovascular accident</u>, chest pain,
postural hypotension. **GI:** Abdominal
pain, anorexia, *constipation,* diarrhea,
*dry mouth,* dyspepsia, dysphagia,
gastroenteritis, GI hemorrhage, *nau-*
*sea, vomiting.* **Hematologic:** Anemia,
hemorrhage. **Metabolic:** Abnormal liver function tests, albuminuria, *weight*
*loss.* **Musculoskeletal:** Arthralgia,
arthritis, bursitis, leg cramps, myasthenia, tenosynovitis. **Respiratory:**
Asthma, dyspnea, epistaxis, increased
cough, rhinitis. **Skin:** Ecchymosis,
eczema, skin carcinoma, skin ulcer,
sweating, urticaria, vesiculobullous
rash. **Special Senses:** Conjunctivitis.

**Urogenital:** Decreased libido, hematuria, impotence, urinary incontinence.

## INTERACTIONS **Drug:** INHIBITORS
OF CYP1A2 (e.g., **atazanavir, cipro-**
**floxacin, mexiletine**) may increase
rasagiline plasma levels. Rasagiline
increases the plasma levels of ANES-
THETICS; thus it **must** be discontinued 14 days prior to elective surgery.
Rasagiline can cause severe CNS
toxicity, including hyperpyrexia and
death, with ANTIDEPRESSANTS, SELECTIVE
SEROTONIN REUPTAKE INHIBITORS (SSRI),
SEROTONIN-NOREPINEPHRINE REUPTAKE
INHIBITORS (SNRI), NONSELECTIVE MAO IN-
HIBITORS, or SELECTIVE MAO-B INHIBITORS.
Rasagiline can increase the plasma
levels of **cyclobenzaprine** and SYM-
PATHOMIMETIC AMINES. Rasagiline and
**dextromethorphan** can cause brief
episodes of psychosis and bizarre behavior. Rasagiline can potentiate the
dopaminergic effects of **levodopa.**
Rasagiline can increase the plasma
levels of **meperidine, metha-**
**done, propoxyphene,** and **trama-**
**dol, acetaminophen,** resulting in
coma, severe hypertension or hypotension, severe respiratory depression, convulsions, and death. **Food:**
Caffeine or ethanol can cause significant side effects and caution should
be used. **Herbal:** Rasagiline increases
the plasma levels of **St. John's wort.**

## PHARMACOKINETICS **Absorp-**
**tion:** Rapidly absorbed with 36%
bioavailability. **Peak:** 1 h. **Distribution:**
88–94% protein bound. **Metabolism:**
Extensive hepatic metabolism
(CYP1A2, CYP2C8/9). **Elimination:**
Primarily renal (62%) with minor fecal elimination. **Half-Life:** 3 h.

## NURSING IMPLICATIONS

**Assessment & Drug Effects**
▪ Monitor BP for new onset hypertension or hypertension not adequately controlled.

---

R

- Monitor for orthostatic hypotension especially in combination with levodopa.
- Monitor for and report to prescriber any of the following: Symptoms of parkinsonism; new or worsening mental status and behavioral changes; somnolence and falling asleep during activities of daily living.
- Monitor for and report suspicious skin changes suggestive of melanoma or other skin cancers.

**Patient & Family Education**

- Do not take any prescription or nonprescription drug without consulting prescriber.
- Periodic skin examinations should be scheduled with a dermatologist. If you notice changes in a skin mole or new skin lesion, contact the dermatologist.
- Avoid foods and beverages containing tyramine (e.g., aged cheeses and meats, tap beer, red wine, soybean products).
- Make position changes slowly, especially when standing from a lying or sitting position.
- Do not drive or engage in potentially hazardous activities until response to drug is known.
- Report immediately any of the following to a health care provider: Palpitations, severe headache, blurred vision, difficulty thinking, seizures, chest pain, unexplained nausea or vomiting, or any sudden weakness or paralysis.

## RASBURICASE
(ras-bur'i-case)
Elitek, Fasturtec ✦
**Classifications:** ANTIGOUT;
ANTIMETABOLITE
Therapeutic: ANTIGOUT

**AVAILABILITY** Powder for injection

## ACTION & *THERAPEUTIC EFFECT*
A recombinant urate-oxidase enzyme produced by DNA technology. In humans, uric acid is the final step in the catabolic pathway of purines. Rasburicase catalyzes enzymatic oxidation of uric acid; thus it is only active at the end of the purine catabolic pathway. *Used to manage plasma uric acid levels in pediatric patients with leukemia, lymphoma, and solid tumor malignancies who are receiving anticancer therapy that results in tumor lysis, and therefore elevates plasma uric acid.*

## USES
Initial management of increased uric acid levels secondary to tumor lysis.

## CONTRAINDICATIONS
Severe hypersensitivity to rasburicase; deficiency in glucose-6-phosphate dehydrogenase (G6PD); history of anaphylaxis; hemolytic reactions or methemoglobinemia reactions to rasburicase; lactation.

## CAUTIOUS USE
Patients at risk for G6PD deficiency (e.g., African or Mediterranean ancestry); asthma; bone marrow suppression; pregnancy (category C); children younger than 1 mo.

## ROUTE & DOSAGE

**Hyperuricemia**

*Adult/Child (1 mo or older):* **IV** 0.2 mg/kg/day for up to 5 days

## ADMINISTRATION
**Intravenous**

*PREPARE:* **IV Infusion:** Reconstitute each 1.5 mg vial or 7.5 mg vial with 1 or 5 mL, respectively, of the provided diluent and mix by swirling very gently. **Do not shake.** Discard if particulate matter is visible or if product is

Common adverse effects in *italic*; life-threatening effects <u>underlined</u>; generic names in **bold**; classifications in SMALL CAPS; ✦ Canadian drug name; ◎ Prototype drug

discolored after reconstitution.
▪ Remove the predetermined dose from the reconstituted vials and inject into enough NS in an infusion bag to achieve a final total volume of 50 mL.
***ADMINISTER: IV Infusion:*** Give over 30 min. **Do not give bolus dose.** Infuse through an **unfiltered** line used for no other medications. ▪ If a separate line is not possible, flush the line with at least 15 mL of saline solution before/after infusion of rasburicase. ▪ Immediately discontinue IV infusion and institute emergency measures for S&S of anaphylaxis including chest pain, dyspnea, hypotension, and/or urticaria.
***INCOMPATIBILITIES:*** Do not mix or infuse with other drugs.

**ADVERSE EFFECTS** (≥1%) **Body as a Whole:** *Fever,* sepsis, severe hypersensitivity reactions including anaphylaxis at any time during treatment. **CNS:** *Headache,* anxiety. **GI:** *Mucositis, vomiting, nausea, diarrhea, abdominal pain.* **Hematologic:** Neutropenia. **Skin:** *Rash.*

**DIAGNOSTIC TEST INTERFERENCE** May give false elevations for ***uric acid*** if blood sample is left at room temperature.

**PHARMACOKINETICS    Half-Life:** 18 h.

**NURSING IMPLICATIONS**

### Black Box Warning

*Rasburicase has been associated with severe hypersensitivity reactions and with development of methemoglobinemia.*

**Assessment & Drug Effects**
▪ Patients at higher risk for G6PD deficiency (e.g., patients of African or Mediterranean ancestry) should be screened prior to starting therapy as this deficiency is a contraindication for this drug.
▪ Monitor closely for S&S of hypersensitivity and be prepared to institute emergency measures for anaphylaxis.
▪ Monitor cardiovascular, respiratory, neurologic, and renal status throughout therapy.
▪ Monitor lab tests: Plasma uric acid levels (4 h after rasburicase administration and q6–8h until tumor lysis syndrome resolution); CBC as needed; baseline G6PD deficiency screening (in patients at high risk for deficiency).

**Patient & Family Education**
▪ Report immediately any distressing S&S to prescriber.

## REGORAFENIB
(re-gor'a-fe-nib)
**Stivarga**
**Classification:** ANTINEOPLASTIC; KINASE INHIBITOR; MULTIKINASE INHIBITOR
**Therapeutic:** ANTINEOPLASTIC
**Prototype:** Erlotinib

**AVAILABILITY** Tablet

**ACTION & *THERAPEUTIC EFFECT***
Inhibits multiple kinase enzymes systems involved in normal cellular functions and in pathologic processes such as tumor development (oncogenesis), tumor angiogenesis, and maintenance of the tumor microenvironment. *Inhibits colorectal cancer tumor growth and metastasis.*

**USES** Metastatic colorectal cancer (CRC) in those previously treated with fluoropyrimidine-, oxaliplatin-, and irinotecan-based chemotherapy, an antivascular endothelial growth factor (VEGF) therapy, and, if cancer is a KRAS gene wild type, an anti-epidermal growth factor receptor (EGFR) therapy treatment of locally advanced, unresectable or metastatic gastrointestinal stromal tumors (GIST) in patients who have previously received imatinib and sunitinib.

**CONTRAINDICATIONS** Severe hepatic impairment (Child-Pugh class C); severe or life-threatening hemorrhage; severe or uncontrolled hypertension; posterior reversible encephalopathy syndrome; 2 wk before surgery; pregnancy (category D); lactation.

**CAUTIOUS USE** Mild to moderate hepatic impairment; moderate-to-severe renal impairment; hypertension; history of myocardial ischemia. Safety and efficacy in children younger than 18 y not established.

## ROUTE & DOSAGE

### Colorectal Cancer, GIST

*Adult:* **PO** 160 mg once daily for the first 21 days of a 28 day cycle; repeat until disease progression or unacceptable toxicity

#### Dosing Modifications

Withhold drug and consult prescriber for any Grade 2 or higher reaction according to the National Cancer Institute (NCI) Common Terminology Criteria for Adverse Events (CTCAE). See package insert for more specific details.

#### Permanently discontinue if:

- Unable to tolerate 80 mg dose
- AST or ALT levels greater than 20 × ULN
- Reversible posterior leukoencephalopathy syndrome occurs
- AST or ALT levels greater than 3 × ULN with concurrent bilirubin greater than 2 × ULN

- Previously elevated AST or ALT levels return to greater than 5 × ULN despite dose reduction to 120 mg
- Any Grade 4 adverse reaction occurs (resume only if the potential benefit outweighs the risks)
- Severe hemorrhage

## ADMINISTRATION

### Oral

- Give at same time each day.
- Swallow tablet whole with a low-fat breakfast that contains less than 30% fat.
- Store at 16°–30° C (56°–89° F). Keep tightly closed in original bottle and do not remove desiccant. Discard unused tablets 28 days after opening bottle.

**ADVERSE EFFECTS (≥1%) Body as a Whole:** Alopecia, *asthenia/fatigue*, fever, hepatotoxicity, *infection*, pain. **CNS:** Headache. **CV:** Gastroesophageal reflux, hemorrhage, *hypertension*, tremor. **GI:** *Diarrhea*, dry mouth, *mucositis*, anorexia. **Hematological:** Anemia, lymphopenia, neutropenia, bleeding, thrombocytopenia. **Metabolic:** *Decreased appetite and food intake*, hyperbilirubinemia, hypocalcemia, hypokalemia, hyponatremia, hypophosphatemia, hypothyroidism, increased ALT/AST, increased amylase, increased INR, increased lipase, *weight loss*. **Musculoskeletal:** Musculoskeletal stiffness. **Respiratory:** *Dysphonia*. **Skin:** *Palmar-plantar erythrodysesthesia*, rash. **Special Senses:** Taste disorder, dysphonia. **Urogenital:** Proteinuria.

**INTERACTIONS Drug:** Coadministration of strong CYP3A4 inhibitors (e.g., **clarithromycin, itraconazole, ketoconazole, posaconazole, telithromycin,**

R

**voriconazole**) increases the levels of regorafenib and decreases the levels of its active metabolites. Coadministration of strong CYP3A4 inducers (e.g., **carbamazepine, phenobarbital, phenytoin, rifampin**) decreases the levels of regorafenib and increases the levels of one of its active metabolites. Do not use with **topotecan. Food:** Grapefruit juice can increase the levels of regorafenib and decrease the levels of its active metabolites. **Herbal: St. John's wort** can decrease the levels of regorafenib and increase the levels of one of its active metabolites.

**PHARMACOKINETICS Absorption:** 69–83% bioavailable. **Peak:** 4 h. **Distribution:** Greater than 99% plasma protein bound. **Metabolism:** In liver to active metabolites. (CYP3A4 and UGT1A9). Also affects CYP2C9, CYP2B6, CYP2D6, UGT1A1, breast cancer resistance protein (BCRP). **Elimination:** Fecal (71%) and renal (19%). **Half-Life:** 28 h for parent drug, 25 h for one active metabolite, and 5 h for a second active metabolite.

## NURSING IMPLICATIONS

### Black Box Warning

*Regorafenib has been associated with severe and sometimes fatal hepatotoxicity.*

### Assessment & Drug Effects

- Monitor BP weekly for first 6 wk then once every cycle or more often as needed. Notify prescriber for recurrent or persistently elevated BP (e.g., greater than 150/100).
- Monitor cardiac status and assess for S&S of myocardial ischemia.
- Monitor for and report promptly S&S dermatological toxicity (i.e., hand–foot skin reaction) or hepatotoxicity (see Appendix F).

- Add for 2 wk prior to surgery to allow for proper wound healing.
- Monitor lab tests: Baseline and biweekly LFTs first 2 mo and monthly (or more frequently) thereafter; baseline and periodic CBC with differential, platelet count, and serum electrolytes, frequent INR with concurrent warfarin therapy.

### Patient & Family Education

- Seek medical attention immediately if you experience any of the following: Chest pain, shortness of breath, dizziness, fainting, severe abdominal pain, persistent abdominal swelling, high fever, chills, nausea, vomiting, severe diarrhea, or dehydration.
- Report promptly any of the following: Redness, pain, blisters, bleeding, or swelling on the palms of hands or soles of feet; signs of bleeding; signs of high BP including severe headaches, lightheadedness, or changes in vision.
- Women and men should use effective means of birth control during therapy and for at least 2 mo following completion of therapy.
- Contact your prescriber immediately if you become pregnant during treatment.
- Do not breast-feed while receiving this drug.

## REMIFENTANIL HYDROCHLORIDE

(rem-i-fent'a-nil)

**Ultiva**

**Classifications:** ANALGESIC, NARCOTIC (OPIATE AGONIST); GENERAL ANESTHESIA
**Therapeutic:** NARCOTIC ANALGESIC; GENERAL ANESTHESIA
**Prototype:** Morphine
**Controlled Substance:** Schedule II

**AVAILABILITY** Solution for injection

Common adverse effects in *italic;* life-threatening effects underlined; generic names in **bold;** classifications in SMALL CAPS; ♣ Canadian drug name; ⊘ Prototype drug

1417

## ACTION & *THERAPEUTIC EFFECT*

Synthetic, potent narcotic agonist analgesic that is rapidly metabolized; therefore respiratory depression is of shorter duration when discontinued. *Used as the analgesic component of an anesthesia regime.*

## USES

Analgesic during induction and maintenance of general anesthesia, as the analgesic component of monitored anesthesia care.

## CONTRAINDICATIONS

Hypersensitivity to fentanyl analogs, epidural or intrathecal administration.

## CAUTIOUS USE

Head injuries, increased intracranial pressure; debilitated, morbid obesity, poor-risk patients; COPD, other respiratory problems, bradyarrhythmia; older adults; pregnancy (category C); lactation. Safety in labor and delivery not established.

## ROUTE & DOSAGE

### Adjunct to Anesthesia

*Adult:* IV 0.5–1 mcg/kg/min or 1 mcg/kg bolus
*Child (birth–2 mo):* IV 0.4–1 mcg/kg/min; *1–12 y:* 0.5–1 mcg/kg/min or 1 mcg/kg bolus

### *Obesity Dosage Adjustment*

Dose based on IBW

## ADMINISTRATION

### Intravenous

IV administration to infants and children: Verify correct IV concentration and rate of infusion with prescriber.

*PREPARE:* **Direct/Continuous Infusion** Reconstitute by adding 1 mL of sterile water for injection, D5W, NS, D5NS, 1/2NS, or D5LR to each 1 mg of remifentanil to yield 1 mg/mL. Shake well to dissolve. ▪ Further dilute to a final concentration of 20, 25, 50, or 250 mcg/mL by adding the required dose to the appropriate amount of IV solution.

*ADMINISTER:* **Direct/Continuous Infusion** Give at the ordered rate according to patient's weight.
▪ Note that bolus doses should **not** be given during a continuous infusion of remifentanil.
▪ Flush IV tubing thoroughly following infusion.

*INCOMPATIBILITIES:* **Solution/additive:** Unknown. **Y-site: Amphotericin B, amphotericin B cholesteryl, chlorpromazine, diazepam.**
▪ Clear IV tubing completely of the drug following discontinuation of remifentanil infusion to ensure that inadvertent administration of the drug will not occur at a later time.
▪ Reconstituted solution is stable for 24 h at room temperature. Store vials of powder at 2°–25° C (36°–77° F).

## ADVERSE EFFECTS (≥1%)

**Body as a Whole:** Muscle rigidity, shivering. **CNS:** Dizziness, headache. **CV:** Hypotension, hypertension, bradycardia. **GI:** *Nausea,* vomiting. **Respiratory:** Respiratory depression, apnea. **Skin:** Pruritus.

## INTERACTIONS

**Drug: Alcohol** and other CNS DEPRESSANTS potentiate effects; MAO INHIBITORS may precipitate hypertensive crisis.

## PHARMACOKINETICS

**Duration:** 12 min. **Distribution:** 70% protein bound. **Metabolism:** Hydrolyzed by nonspecific esterases in the blood and tissues. **Elimination:** In urine. **Half-Life:** 3–10 min.

## NURSING IMPLICATIONS

### Assessment & Drug Effects

▪ Monitor vital signs during postoperative period; observe for and immediately report any S&S of respiratory distress or respiratory depression, or skeletal and thoracic muscle rigidity and weakness.

- Monitor for adequate postoperative analgesia.

## REPAGLINIDE ℗

(rep-a-gli'nide)

Prandin, GlucoNorm ◆

**Classifications:** ANTIDIABETIC; MEGLITINIDE

Therapeutic: ANTIHYPERGLYCEMIC

**AVAILABILITY** Tablet

### ACTION & *THERAPEUTIC EFFECT*

Hypoglycemic agent that lowers blood glucose levels by stimulating release of insulin from the pancreatic islets. *Significantly reduces postprandial blood glucose in type 2 diabetes. Minimal effects on fasting blood glucose.*

**USES** Adjunct to diet and exercise in type 2 diabetes.

### CONTRAINDICATIONS

Hypersensitivity to repaglinide; insulin-dependent diabetes, diabetic ketoacidosis; lactation.

### CAUTIOUS USE

Hypoglycemia; loss of glycemic control due to secondary failure; hepatic impairment; severe renal impairment; older adults, surgery, fever, systemic infection, trauma; pregnancy (category C); Safety and efficacy in children not established.

### ROUTE & DOSAGE

**Type 2 Diabetes**

*Adult (initial dose):* **PO** 0.5 mg 15–30 min a.c.; *initial dose for patients previously using glucose-lowering agents:* 1–2 mg 15–30 min a.c. (2–4 doses/day depending on meal pattern; max: 16 mg/day); *dosage range:* 0.5–4 mg 15–30 min a.c.

### ADMINISTRATION

**Oral**

- Give within 30 min of beginning a meal.
- Store at 15°–30° C (59°–86° F) in a tightly closed container and protect from moisture.

**ADVERSE EFFECTS** (≥1%) **Body as a Whole:** Arthralgia, back pain, paresthesia, allergy. **CNS:** Headache. **CV:** Chest pain, angina. **GI:** Nausea, diarrhea, constipation, vomiting, dyspepsia. **Respiratory:** URI, sinusitis, rhinitis, bronchitis. **Metabolic:** *Hypoglycemia.*

**INTERACTIONS Drug: Erythromycin, ketoconazole** may inhibit metabolism and potentiate hypoglycemia; BARBITURATES, **carbamazepine, rifabutin, rifampin, rifapentine, pioglitazone** may induce metabolism and cause hyperglycemia; **gemfibrozil** may increase risk of hypoglycemia and duration of action. Use with **deferasirox** requires a repaglinide dose reduction. **Herbal: Ginseng, garlic** may increase hypoglycemic effects. **Food: Grapefruit juice** (greater than 1 qt/day) may increase plasma concentrations and adverse effects.

**PHARMACOKINETICS Absorption:** Rapidly from GI tract, 56% bioavailability. **Peak:** 1 h. **Distribution:** 98% protein bound. **Metabolism:** In liver (CYP3A4). **Elimination:** 90% in feces. **Half-Life:** 1 h.

### NURSING IMPLICATIONS

**Assessment & Drug Effects**

- Monitor carefully for S&S of hypoglycemia especially during the 1-wk period following transfer from a longer-acting sulfonylurea.
- Monitor lab tests: Frequent FBS, postprandial blood glucose, and HbA1C q3mo.

R

Common adverse effects in *italic;* life-threatening effects underlined; generic names in **bold;** classifications in SMALL CAPS; ◆ Canadian drug name; ℗ Prototype drug

1419

**Patient & Family Education**

- Take only with meals to lessen the chance of hypoglycemia. If a meal is skipped, skip a dose; if a meal is added, add a dose.
- Start repaglinide the morning after the other agent is stopped when changing from another oral hypoglycemia drug.
- Be alert for S&S of hyperglycemia or hypoglycemia (see Appendix F); report poor blood glucose control to prescriber.

# RESERPINE ℗

(re-ser'peen)

**Classifications:** ALPHA-1 ADRENERGIC ANTAGONIST (PERIPHERAL ACTING); ANTIHYPERTENSIVE
Therapeutic: ANTIHYPERTENSIVE

## AVAILABILITY Tablet

## ACTION & *THERAPEUTIC EFFECT*

Interferes with binding of serotonin at receptor sites, decreases synthesis of norepinephrine by depleting dopamine (its precursor), and competitively inhibits their reuptake in storage granules. Depletes norepinephrine and serotonin in CNS, peripheral nervous system, heart, and other organs and tissues. *Sympathetic inhibition seen in small but persistent decrease in BP, frequently associated with bradycardia, and reduced cardiac output.*

## USES Hypertension.

## CONTRAINDICATIONS Hypersensitivity to reserpine; depression; acute peptic ulcer; ulcerative colitis; patients receiving electroconvulsive therapy; suicidal ideation; lactation.

## CAUTIOUS USE Renal insufficiency; history of mental depression; cerebrovascular accident; history of peptic ulcers, UC, gall stones; epilepsy; parkinsonism; older adults; pregnancy (category C); children.

## ROUTE & DOSAGE

**Hypertension**

*Adult:* **PO** 0.05 mg–0.1 mg once daily, then titrate to dose of 0.1 mg–0.25 mg once daily

## ADMINISTRATION

Oral

- Give with meals or with milk or other food to minimize possibility of gastric irritation (drug increases gastric secretions).
- Store in tight, light-resistant containers, preferably at 15°–30° C (59°–86° F), unless otherwise directed by manufacturer.

## ADVERSE EFFECTS (≥1%) CNS:

*Drowsiness,* sedation, *lethargy, depression,* nervousness, anxiety, nightmares, increased dreaming, headache, *dizziness,* increased appetite, dull sensorium; prolonged use of large doses: CNS stimulation (parkinsonian syndrome): Tremors, muscle rigidity; <u>respiratory depression</u>, convulsions, hypothermia. **CV:** <u>Bradycardia</u>, *edema,* orthostatic hypotension, increased AV conduction time (prolonged therapy); angina-like symptoms, arrhythmias, CHF (rare). **Special Senses:** *Nasal congestion,* epistaxis, lacrimation, blurred vision; miosis, ptosis, conjunctival congestion (acute toxicity). **GI:** Dry mouth or excessive salivation, *nausea, vomiting, abdominal cramps, diarrhea,* reactivation of peptic ulcer (hypersecretion), heartburn, biliary colic. **Hematologic:** Thrombocytopenic purpura, anemia, prolonged BT.

**Body as a Whole:** Hypersensitivity (pruritus, rash, asthma), muscle aches, dysuria, fixed-drug eruptions. **Urogenital:** Menstrual irregularities, breast engorgement, galactorrhea, gynecomastia, feminization (males), impaired sexual function, impotence.

## DIAGNOSTIC TEST INTERFERENCE

Possibility of elevated *blood glucose* values; however, it is also reported that reserpine may decrease thiazide-induced hyperglycemia. Increase in *serum prolactin* with chronic administration of *rauwolfia* alkaloids; overdoses may cause initial increase in excretion of *urinary catecholamines;* decreases with chronic administration. Large doses may cause initial rise in *urinary 5 HIAA* excretion. Initial IM doses may increase *urinary VMA* excretion followed by decrease by end of third day of therapy (with oral or parenteral administration). Possible interference with *urinary steroid* colorimetric determinations: *17-OHCS* and *17-KS.*

## INTERACTIONS **Drug: Diuretics,** other HYPOTENSIVE AGENTS compound hypotensive effects; CARDIAC GLYCOSIDES (**digoxin**) may increase risk of arrhythmias; MAO INHIBITORS may cause excitation and hypertension; CNS DEPRESSANTS compound depression; may decrease response to **levodopa. Herbal: St. John's wort** may antagonize hypotensive effects.

## PHARMACOKINETICS **Peak:** 2 h. **Distribution:** Widely distributed, especially to adipose tissue; crosses blood–brain barrier and placenta; distributed in breast milk. **Metabolism:** Extensively metabolized to inactive compounds. **Elimination:** Slowly excreted, 60% in feces within 96 h and 10% in urine. **Half-Life:** 4.5 and 11.3 h.

## NURSING IMPLICATIONS

### Assessment & Drug Effects

- Assess vital signs at frequent intervals. (Note: Drop in BP may be accompanied by bradycardia.)
- Supervise ambulation as indicated; postural hypotension occurs more frequently in elderly patients.
- Monitor I&O, especially in patients with impaired kidney function. Report changes in I&O ratio and pattern.
- Full therapeutic effect of oral drug for hypertension may not occur until 2–3 wk of therapy, and effects may persist for as long as 4–6 wk after drug is discontinued.
- Be aware that mental depression is a serious adverse effect and may be severe. It occurs most commonly in high dosage regimens (e.g., 0.5–1 mg/day or more) and may not appear until 2–8 mo of therapy and may last for several months after drug is withdrawn.

### Patient & Family Education

- Take drug at the same time each day, do not skip or double doses, and do not stop therapy without advice of prescriber.
- Do not drive or engage in potentially hazardous activities until response to drug is known.
- Learn about possible adverse effects and report promptly to prescriber.
- Report the following possible beginning symptoms of depression: Early morning insomnia, anorexia, inability to concentrate, despondency, self-deprecation, attitude of detachment, mood swings, or impotence.
- Make position changes slowly, particularly from recumbent to upright posture, and lie down or sit down (head-low position) if patient feels faint. Do not take hot showers or hot tub baths, and do not to stand still for prolonged periods. Report

**R**

---

Common adverse effects in *italic;* life-threatening effects underlined; generic names in **bold;** classifications in SMALL CAPS; ♣ Canadian drug name; ⊕ Prototype drug

1421

symptoms of dizziness or light-headedness to prescriber.

- Check for edema and record weight daily. Consult prescriber about gain of 1–2 kg (3–5 lb) in 1 wk.
- Do not take OTC medications without consulting prescriber or pharmacist (many preparations for coughs and colds contain agents that affect the actions of reserpine).

## RESLIZUMAB

(res-liz′ue-mab)

Cinqair

**Classifications:** INTERLEUKIN-5 ANTAGONIST; ANTIINFLAMMATORY; MONOCLONAL ANTIBODY
Therapeutic: ANTIINFLAMMATORY; ANTIASTHMATIC
**Prototype:** Basiliximab

**AVAILABILITY** Solution for injection

## ACTION & *THERAPEUTIC EFFECT*

An antibody that acts as an inter-leukin-5 antagonist (IgG1 kappa). IL-5 is the major cytokine responsible for the growth and differentiation, recruitment, activation, and survival of eosinophils. Eosinophils are involved in the inflammation associated with the pathogenesis of asthma. *The inhibition of IL-5 signaling by reslizumab, reduces the production and survival of eosinophils.*

**USES** Treatment of patients with severe asthma 18 y and older with an eosinophilic phenotype; reslizumab should not be used for treatment of other eosinophilic conditions or for the relief of acute broncho-spasm or status asthmaticus.

**CONTRAINDICATIONS** Hypersensitivity to reslizumab. Should not be used to treat acute asthma symptoms.

**CAUTIOUS USE** Use cautiously in patients with history of systemic neoplastic disease and in patients with a high risk of malignancy. Treat patients with pre-existing hel-minth infections prior to initiating treatment with reslizumab. Do not discontinue systemic or corticosteroids abruptly upon initiation of reslizumab. Pregnancy and lactation data are insufficient to determine risk. Safety and efficacy in children and adolescents younger than 18 y not established.

## ROUTE & DOSAGE

| Severe Asthma |
|---|
| *Adult:* IV 3 mg/kg once every 4 wk |

## ADMINISTRATION

### Intravenous

*PREPARE:* **IV Infusion:** Solution is clear to slightly hazy/opalescent, colorless to slightly yellow. Small particles may be translucent to white. Discard and do not use if discolored or other foreign particulate matter. ▪ Dilute in 50 mL of 0.9% sodium chloride. ▪ Reslizumab is compatible with poly-vinylchloride (PVC) or polyolefin infusion bags. Gently invert the bag to mix. Do not shake.

*ADMINISTER:* **IV Infusion:** ▪ **Do not** administer IV push or bolus. Administer immediately after preparation. ▪ Use an infusion set with an in-line, low protein-binding filter (pore size of 0.2 micron). Compatible with polyethersul-fone, polyvinylidene fluoride, nylon, cellulose acetate in-line filters. ▪ Infuse intravenously over 20–50 min. ▪ Do not infuse any other medication in the tubing. ▪ Stop infusion immediately if patient exhibits any signs of ana-

phylaxis and treat appropriately.
▪ Flush the intravenous administration set with 0.9% sodium chloride injection to ensure complete administration.

***INCOMPATIBILITIES*** **Solution/additive:** None listed (should be mixed with NS).

▪ Store intact vials in refrigerator at 2°–8° C (36°–46° F). Do not freeze or shake. Protect from light. If not used immediately, store in the refrigerator at 2°–8° C (36°–46° F) or at room temperature up to 25° C (77° F), protected from light for up to 16 h max. If refrigerated, warm to room temperature before administering. Single use vials; discard any unused portion.

### ADVERSE EFFECTS (≥1%) **Body as a Whole:** Elevated creatine phosphokinase, immunogenicity. **Musculoskeletal:** Myalgia. **Respiratory:** Oropharyngeal pain.

### PHARMACOKINETICS **Metabolism:** Proteolytic degradation. **Half-Life:** 24 days.

### NURSING IMPLICATIONS

#### Assessment & Drug Effects
▪ Assess for anaphylaxis has been noted to occur on the second dose, within 20 min after infusion is complete.
▪ Signs of anaphylaxis include dyspnea, decreased oxygen saturation, wheezing, and vomiting. If any symptoms occur, stop administration and notify prescriber.
▪ Assess respiratory status including pulse oximetry.
▪ Patients should be treated for parasitic helminth infections prior to administration of drug.

#### Patient & Family Education
▪ Women should use contraceptive measures.

▪ This is not a rescue drug and should not be used in an acute asthma attack.
▪ May experience sore throat and muscle pain.

# RETAPAMULIN
(re-te-pam′ue-lin)
**Altabax**
**Classifications:** ANTIBIOTIC; PLEUROMUTILIN
**Therapeutic:** TOPICAL ANTIBIOTIC

### AVAILABILITY Topical ointment

### ACTION & *THERAPEUTIC EFFECT*
Selectively inhibits bacterial protein synthesis at a site on the 50S subunit of the bacterial ribosome. *Effective against* Staphylococcus *(MRSA) and* Streptococcus *organisms.*

### USES Treatment of impetigo due to susceptible stains of *Staphylococcus aureus* (methicillin-sensitive strains only) or *Streptococcus pyogenes.*

### CONTRAINDICATIONS Severe hypersensitivity to retapamulin.

### CAUTIOUS USE Pregnancy (category B); lactation; children less than 9 mo.

### ROUTE & DOSAGE

| **Impetigo Infection** |
| --- |
| *Adult/Child/Infant (9 mo or older):* Apply in thin layer b.i.d. × 5 days |

### ADMINISTRATION
#### Topical
▪ Apply a thin layer to infected region. May cover with gauze dressing.
▪ Store at 15°–30° C (59°–86° F).

### ADVERSE EFFECTS (≥1%) **Body as a Whole:** Application-site irritation,

Common adverse effects in *italic;* life-threatening effects <u>underlined</u>; generic names in **bold;** classifications in SMALL CAPS; ✦Canadian drug name; ❍ Prototype drug

1423

pyrexia. **CNS:** Headache. **GI:** Diarrhea, nausea. **Metabolic:** Creatinine phosphokinase increased. **Respiratory:** Nasopharyngitis. **Skin:** Eczema, pruritus.

## PHARMACOKINETICS **Absorption:** Minimal systemic absorption. **Metabolism:** In liver.

## NURSING IMPLICATIONS

### Assessment & Drug Effects
- Monitor for excessive skin irritation. Report swelling, blistering, or oozing.

### Patient & Family Education
- Report any of the following at application site: Redness, itching, burning, swelling, blistering, or oozing.

## RETEPLASE RECOMBINANT
(re′te-plase)

Retavase

**Classification:** THROMBOLYTIC ENZYME, TISSUE PLASMINOGEN ACTIVATOR (T-PA)
Therapeutic: THROMBOLYTIC
**Prototype:** Alteplase

**AVAILABILITY** 10.4 international unit vials

## ACTION & *THERAPEUTIC EFFECT*
DNA recombinant human tissue-type plasminogen activator (t-PA) that acts as a catalyst in the cleavage of plasminogen to plasmin. Responsible for degrading the fibrin matrix of a clot. *Has antithrombolytic properties.*

**USES** Thrombolysis management of acute MI to reduce the incidence of CHF and mortality.

**CONTRAINDICATIONS** Active internal bleeding, history of CVA, recent neurologic surgery or trauma, intercranial neoplasm, or aneurysm, bleeding disorders, severe uncontrolled hypertension.

**CAUTIOUS USE** Any condition in which bleeding constitutes a significant hazard (i.e., severe hepatic or renal disease, CVA, hypertension, acute pancreatitis, septic thrombophlebitis); pregnancy (category C); lactation. Safety and efficacy in children not established.

## ROUTE & DOSAGE

**Thrombolysis during Acute MI**
*Adult:* **IV** 10 units injected over 2 min. Repeat dose in 30 min (20 units total).

## ADMINISTRATION

Intravenous

*PREPARE:* **Direct:** Reconstitute using only the diluent, syringe, needle, and dispensing pin provided with reteplase. ▪ Withdraw diluent with syringe provided. Remove needle from syringe, replace with dispensing pin and transfer diluent to vial of reteplase. Leave pin and syringe in place in vial and swirl to dissolve. **Do not** shake. ▪ When completely dissolved, remove 10 mL solution, replace dispensing pin with a 20-gauge needle.

*ADMINISTER:* **Direct:** Flush IV line before and after with 30 mL NS or D5W and **do not** give any other drug simultaneously through the same IV line. ▪ Give a single dose evenly over 2 min.

*INCOMPATIBILITIES:* **Solution/additive: Heparin. Y-site: Bivalirudin, heparin.**

▪ Store drug kit unopened at 2°–25° C (36°–77° F).

**ADVERSE EFFECTS** (≥1%) **Hematologic:** *Hemorrhage* (including *intracranial*, GI, genitourinary), anemia. **CV:** Reperfusion arrhythmias.

## DIAGNOSTIC TEST INTERFERENCE

Causes decreases in plasminogen and fibrinogen, making **coagulation** and **fibrinolytic** tests unreliable.

**INTERACTIONS Drug: Aspirin, abciximab, dipyridamole, heparin** may increase risk of bleeding.

**PHARMACOKINETICS Elimination:** In urine. **Half-Life:** 13–16 min.

## NURSING IMPLICATIONS

### Assessment & Drug Effects

- Discontinue concomitant heparin immediately if serious bleeding not controllable by local pressure occurs and, if not already given, withhold the second reteplase bolus.
- Monitor carefully all potential bleeding sites; monitor for S&S of internal hemorrhage (e.g., GI, GU, intracranial, retroperitoneal, pulmonary).
- Monitor carefully cardiac status for arrhythmias associated with reperfusion.
- Avoid invasive procedures, arterial and venous punctures, IM injections, and nonessential handling of the patient during reteplase therapy.

### Patient & Family Education

- Report changes in consciousness or signs of bleeding to prescriber immediately.

## RH₀(D) IMMUNE GLOBULIN

(row)

RhoGAM, Rhophylac, WinRho SDF

## RH₀(D) IMMUNE GLOBULIN MICRO-DOSE

BayRho-D Mini Dose, MICRho-GAM

**Classifications:** BIOLOGICAL RESPONSE MODIFIER; IMMUNOGLOBULIN (IgG)

Therapeutic: IMMUNOGLOBULIN

**Prototype:** Immune globulin

**AVAILABILITY RhoGAM, MICRho-GAM:** Solution in prefilled syringe. **Rhophylac:** Prefilled syringe; **WinRho SDF:** Vial

## ACTION & THERAPEUTIC EFFECT

Provides passive immunity by suppressing active antibody response and formation of anti-Rh₀(D) in Rh-negative [Rh₀(D)-negative] individuals previously exposed to Rh-positive [Rh₀(D)-positive, Dᵘ-positive] blood. *Effective against exposure to Rh-positive blood in Rh-negative individuals.*

**USES** To prevent isoimmunization in Rh-negative individuals exposed to Rh-positive RBC (see above). Rh₀(D) immune globulin microdose is for use only after spontaneous or induced abortion or termination of ectopic pregnancy up to and including 12 wk of gestation. Treatment of idiopathic thrombocytopenia purpura.

**CONTRAINDICATIONS** Rh₀(D)-positive patient; person previously immunized against Rh₀(D) factor, severe immune globulin hypersensitivity, bleeding disorders.

**CAUTIOUS USE** IgA deficiency; pregnancy (category C); neonates.

R

Common adverse effects in *italic*; life-threatening effects <u>underlined</u>; generic names in **bold**; classifications in SMALL CAPS; ♣ Canadian drug name; ● Prototype drug

1425

## ROUTE & DOSAGE

Note: Only **WinRho SDF** and **Rhophylac** can be given IV. **BayRho-D** and **RhoGAM** are available in regular and mini-dose vials.

### Antepartum Prophylaxis

*Adult:* **IM/IV** 300 mcg at approximately 28-wk gestation; followed by 1 vial of mini-dose or 120 mcg within 72 h of delivery if infant is Rh-positive

### Postpartum Prophylaxis

*Adult:* **IM/IV** 300 mcg preferably within 72 h of delivery if infant is Rh-positive

### Following Amniocentesis, Miscarriage, Abortion, Ectopic Pregnancy

*Adult:* **IM** If over 13-wk gestation, 300 mcg, preferably within 3 h but at least within 72 h; if less than 13 wk, give 50 mcg

### Transfusion Accident

*Adult:* **IM/IV** 300 mcg for each volume of RBCs infused divided by 15, given within at least 72 h of accident
*Child:* **IV** Administer 600 mcg q8h until total dose given. Exposure to positive whole blood 9 mcg/mL, exposure to positive RBCs 18 mcg/mL. **IM** Administer 1200 mcg q12h until total dose given. Exposure to positive whole blood 12 mcg/mL, exposure to positive RBCs 24 mcg/mL.

### Idiopathic Thrombocytopenia Purpura

*Adult/Child:* **IV** 50 mcg/kg, then 25–60 mcg/kg depending on response

## ADMINISTRATION

- BayRho-D (HyperRHO S/D), MIC-RhoGam, and RhoGAM are administered by IM route only. NEVER give IV.
- WinRho SDF and Rhophylac may be given IM or IV depending on the indication.

### Intramuscular

- Use the deltoid muscle. Give in divided doses at different sites, all at once or at intervals, as long as the entire dose is given within 72 h after delivery or termination of pregnancy.
- Observe patient closely for at least 20 min after administration. Keep epinephrine immediately available; systemic allergic reactions sometimes occur.

### Intravenous

**PREPARE: Direct:** No dilution is required for products supplied in liquid form. ▪ **WinRho SDF:** Remove entire contents of vial to obtain the labeled dosage. If partial vial is needed for dosage calculation, withdraw the entire contents to ensure accurate calculation of dosage requirement. ▪ **Rhophylac:** Bring to room temperature before use.

**ADMINISTER: Direct: Rhophylac:** Give at a rate of 2 mL/15–60 sec for ITP. ▪ **WinRho SDF:** Give over 3–5 min.

- Refrigerate commercially prepared solutions, although it may remain stable up to 30 days at room temperature according to manufacturer. ▪ Discard solutions that have been frozen. ▪ Store powder at 2°–8° C (36°–46° F) unless otherwise directed; avoid freezing.

## ADVERSE EFFECTS (≥1%) **Body as a Whole:** Injection site irritation, slight fever, myalgia, lethargy.

Common adverse effects in *italic;* life-threatening effects <u>underlined;</u> generic names in **bold;** classifications in SMALL CAPS; ♣ Canadian drug name; ⊕ Prototype drug

**INTERACTIONS Drug:** May interfere with immune response to LIVE VIRUS VACCINE; should delay use of LIVE VIRUS VACCINES for 3 mo after administration of Rh₀(D) immune globulin.

**PHARMACOKINETICS Peak:** 2 h IV, 5–10 days IM. **Half-Life:** 25 days.

## NURSING IMPLICATIONS

### Black Box Warning

*Rh₀(D) immune globulin has been associated with severe anemia, acute renal insufficiency, renal failure, DIC, and intravascular hemolysis leading to death.*

### Assessment & Drug Effects

- Obtain history of systemic allergic reactions to human immune globulin preparations prior to drug administration in patients with ITP.
- Monitor closely patients with ITP for at least 8 h after administration.
- Monitor for S&S of intravascular hemolysis, including back pain, shaking chills, fever, and discolored urine or hematuria.
- Monitor lab test: Dipstick urinalysis at baseline, 2 and 4 h after administration, and prior to the end of the monitoring period; periodic CBC, renal function tests, LFTs.

### Patient & Family Education

- Report promptly early signs of allergic or hypersensitivity reactions to Rh₀(D) immune globulin, including anaphylaxis, chest tightness, generalized urticaria, hives, and wheezing.
- When treated for ITP, immediately report symptoms of intravascular hemolysis (i.e., back pain, decreased urine output, discolored urine, fluid retention/edema, fever, shaking chills, shortness of breath, and/or sudden weight gain).
- Be aware that administration of Rh₀(D) immune globulin (antibody) prevents hemolytic disease of the newborn in a subsequent pregnancy.

## RIBAVIRIN
(rye-ba-vye′rin)

Copegus, Rebetol, RibaPak, Ribasphere, Virazole

**Classification:** ANTIVIRAL
**Therapeutic:** ANTIVIRAL
**Prototype:** Acyclovir

**AVAILABILITY** Inhalation solution; tablet; capsule; oral solution

## ACTION & THERAPEUTIC EFFECT

Synthetic nucleoside with broad-spectrum antiviral activity against DNA and RNA viruses. Mode is believed to involve multiple mechanisms including selective interference with viral ribonucleic protein synthesis. *Active against many RNA and DNA viruses.*

**USES** Aerosol product used for selected infants and young children with respiratory syncytial virus (RSV). Oral product used in combination with interferon-alfa-2b to treat hepatitis C or in combination with peginterferon alpha for treatment of hepatitis C.

**UNLABELED USES** Prophylaxis and treatment of influenza A and B, pneumonia caused by adenovirus; Lassa fever, measles, HSV-1, HSV-2, enterovirus 72 (formerly hepatitis A), SARS, cytomegalovirus.

**CONTRAINDICATIONS** Mild RSV infections of lower respiratory tract; infants requiring simultaneous

Common adverse effects in *italic;* life-threatening effects underlined; generic names in **bold;** classifications in SMALL CAPS; ♦ Canadian drug name; ⑩ Prototype drug

**1427**

assisted ventilation; unstable cardiac disease; pancreatitis; autoimmune hepatitis; HCV infection; renal failure; suicidal ideations; hemoglobinopathy; hepatic decompensation; women who are of child bearing age; pregnancy (category X); lactation.

**CAUTIOUS USE** COPD, asthma; risk for severe anemia; history of MI, cardiac arrhythmias, cardiac disease; decreased renal, hepatic, or cardiac function; respiratory depression; severe anemia; history of depression or suicidal tendencies; older adults; children younger than 3 y.

## ROUTE & DOSAGE

**RSV**

*Child:* **Inhalation** 20 mg via SPAG-2 nebulizer administered over 12–18 h/day for 3–7 days

**Hepatitis C (in combination with interferon-alfa 2b)** *adjust per genotype

*Adult (weight greater than 75 kg):* **PO** 600 mg b.i.d. for 24–48 wk; *weight less than 75 kg:* 400 mg in a.m., 600 mg in p.m. for 24–48 wk
*Child/Adolescent (weight greater than 73 kg):* **PO** 15 mg/kg/day or 1200 mg/day in divided doses; *weight 60–73 kg:* 15 mg/kg/day or 1000 mg/day in divided doses; *weight 47–59 kg:* 15 mg/kg/day or 800 mg/day in divided doses; *3 y or older, weight less than 47 kg:* 15 mg/kg/day in divided doses

**Chronic Hepatitis C (with Peginterferon Alfa-2b)**

*Adult:* **PO** 800–1400 mg daily in divided doses (see package insert for weight based dose)

*Adolescent/Child (3 y or older):* **PO** 400–1200 mg/day (see package insert for weight/age tables)

**Renal Impairment Dosage Adjustment**

*CrCl less than 50 mL/min:* Oral ribavirin should not be used

## ADMINISTRATION

### Oral
- Give tablets with food. Ensure that tablets and capsules are swallowed whole. They should not be opened, crushed, or chewed.

### Inhalation
- Administer only by SPAG-2 aerosol generator, following manufacturer's directions.
- Caution: Ribavirin has demonstrated teratogenicity in animals. Advise pregnant health care personnel of the potential teratogenic risks associated with exposure during ribavirin administration to patients.
- Do not give other aerosol medication concomitantly with ribavirin.
- Discard solution in the SPAG-2 reservoir at least q24h and whenever liquid level is low before fresh reconstituted solution is added.
- Store unopened vial in a dry place at 15°–25° C (59°–78° F) unless otherwise directed.
- Following reconstitution, store solution at 20°–30° C (68°–86° F) for 24 h.

**ADVERSE EFFECTS** (≥1%) **CV:** Hypotension (faintness, light-headedness, unusual fatigue), <u>MI, cardiac arrest</u>. **Special Senses:** Conjunctivitis, erythema of eyelids. **Hematologic:** *Neutropenia*, reticulocytosis, <u>hemolytic anemia</u> (especially in combination with interferon alpha). **Respiratory:** Deterioration of

Common adverse effects in *italic;* life-threatening effects <u>underlined;</u> generic names in **bold;** classifications in SMALL CAPS; ♣ Canadian drug name; ⊙ Prototype drug

respiratory function, dyspnea, <u>apnea</u>, chest soreness, bacterial pneumonia, ventilator dependence. **GI:** *Diarrhea, nausea, vomiting,* transient increases in AST, ALT, bilirubin; abdominal cramps, jaundice. **Metabolic:** *Weight loss.* **CNS:** *Asthenia, dizziness, headache, insomnia, fatigue.*

**INTERACTIONS Drug:** Ribavirin may antagonize the antiviral effects of **zidovudine** against HIV; increased risk of fetal defects with **peginterferon.** Use with **azathioprine** and **peginterferon alfa-2a** increases risk of pancytopenia.

**PHARMACOKINETICS Absorption:** Rapidly absorbed orally (44%) and systemically from lungs. **Peak:** Inhaled 60–90 min. PO 1.7–3 h. **Distribution:** Crosses placenta; distributed into breast milk. **Metabolism:** In cells to an active metabolite. **Elimination:** 85% in urine, 15% in feces. **Half-Life:** 24 h in plasma, 16–40 days in RBCs.

## NURSING IMPLICATIONS

### Black Box Warning

*Ribavirin has been associated with hemolytic anemia which may worsen cardiac disease and cause MI, and with fetal toxicity.*

### Assessment & Drug Effects

- Obtain specimens for rapid diagnosis of RSV infection before therapy is initiated or at least during the first 24 h of ribavirin therapy. Do not continue therapy without laboratory confirmation of RSV infection.
- Monitor respiratory function and fluid status closely during therapy. Note baseline rate and character of respirations and pulse. Observe for signs of labored breathing: Dyspnea,

apnea; rapid, shallow respirations, intercostal and substernal retraction, nasal flaring, limited excursion of lungs, cyanosis. Auscultate lungs for abnormal breath sounds.

- Observe patients requiring simultaneous assisted ventilation closely for S&S of worsening pulmonary function. Check equipment carefully every 2 h, including endotracheal tube, for malfunction. Precipitation of ribavirin and accumulation of fluid in tubing can obstruct the apparatus and cause inadequate ventilation and gas exchange.
- Monitor cardiac status, including ECG, especially in those with preexisiting cardiac dysfunction
- Monitor lab tests: Baseline CBC with differential and platelet count, repeat at 2 and 4 wk, and periodically thereafter; baseline and periodic serum electrolytes, LFTs, and renal function tests.

### Patient & Family Education

- Both male and female patients should take every precaution to prevent pregnancy during treatment and for 6 mo following the end of therapy.
- Inform prescriber immediately if a pregnancy occurs within 6 mo of completing therapy.
- Drink fluids liberally unless otherwise advised by prescriber.
- Use caution with hazardous activities until response to drug is known.

R

## RIBOFLAVIN (VITAMIN B₂)

(rye′bo-flay-vin)

**Classification:** VITAMIN
**Therapeutic:** VITAMIN REPLACEMENT

**AVAILABILITY** Tablet

## ACTION & *THERAPEUTIC EFFECT*

Works with a wide variety of proteins to catalyze many cellular respiratory

Common adverse effects in *italic;* life-threatening effects <u>underlined;</u> generic names in **bold;** classifications in SMALL CAPS; ◆ Canadian drug name; ⊕ Prototype drug

1429

reactions by which the body derives its energy. *Evaluated by improvement of clinical manifestations of deficiency: Digestive disturbances, headache, burning sensation of skin (especially "burning" feet), cracking at corners of mouth (cheilosis), glossitis, seborrheic dermatitis (and other skin lesions), mental depression, corneal vascularization (with photophobia, burning and itchy eyes, lacrimation, roughness of eyelids), anemia, neuropathy.*

**USES** To prevent and treat riboflavin deficiency, also to treat microcytic anemia.

**CAUTIOUS USE** Pregnancy (category A; category C if greater than RDA); lactation.

## ROUTE & DOSAGE

**Nutritional Deficiency Treatment**
*Adult:* **PO** 5–30 mg/day in divided doses
*Child:* **PO** 3–10 mg/day

**Microcytic Anemia**
*Adult:* **PO** 10 mg/day × 10 days

## ADMINISTRATION

**Oral**
- Give with food to enhance absorption.
- Store in airtight containers protected from light.

**ADVERSE EFFECTS** (≥1%)
**Urogenital:** May discolor urine bright yellow.

## DIAGNOSTIC TEST INTERFERENCE

In large doses, riboflavin may produce yellow-green fluorescence in *urine* and thus cause false elevations in certain *fluorometric determinations* of *urinary catecholamines.*

## PHARMACOKINETICS **Absorption:** Readily absorbed from GI

tract. **Distribution:** Little is stored; excess amounts are excreted in urine. **Elimination:** In urine. **Half-Life:** 66–84 min.

## NURSING IMPLICATIONS

### Assessment & Drug Effects
- Collaborate with prescriber, dietitian, patient, and responsible family member in planning for diet. A complete dietary history is an essential part of vitamin replacement so that poor eating habits can be identified and corrected. Deficiency in one vitamin is usually associated with other vitamin deficiencies.

### Patient & Family Education
- Be aware that large doses may cause an intense yellow discoloration of urine.
- Note: Rich dietary sources of riboflavin are found in liver, kidney, beef, pork, heart, eggs, milk and milk products, yeast, whole-grain cereals, vitamin B–enriched breakfast cereals, green vegetables, and mushrooms.

## RIFABUTIN
(rif-a-bu′tin)
Mycobutin
**Classifications:** ANTIBIOTIC; ANTITUBERCULOSIS
**Therapeutic:** ANTITUBERCULOSIS
**Prototype:** Rifampin

**AVAILABILITY** Capsule

## ACTION & *THERAPEUTIC EFFECT*

Semisynthetic bacteriostatic antibiotic. Mode of action may be to inhibit DNA-dependent RNA polymerase in susceptible bacterial cells but not in human cells. *Effective against* Mycobacterium avium complex (MAC) (or M. avium-intracellulare) *and many strains of* M. tuberculosis.

**USES** The prevention of disseminated *Mycobacterium avium* complex (MAC) disease in patients with advanced HIV infection.

**CONTRAINDICATIONS** Hypersensitivity to rifabutin or any other rifamycins; lactation.

**CAUTIOUS USE** Older adults, pregnancy (category B); children.

## ROUTE & DOSAGE

### Prevention of MAC
*Adult:* **PO** 300 mg daily, may give 150 mg b.i.d. if nausea is a problem
*Child:* **PO** 75 mg daily

## ADMINISTRATION

### Oral
- Give the usual dose of 300 mg/day or in two divided doses of 150 mg with food if needed to reduce GI upset.
- Store at room temperature, 15°–30° C (59°–86° F), unless otherwise directed.

**ADVERSE EFFECTS** (≥1%) **CNS:** *Headache.* **GI:** *Abdominal pain, dyspepsia, nausea, taste perversion, increased liver enzymes.* **Hematologic:** Thrombocytopenia, eosinophilia, leukopenia, neutropenia. **Skin:** Rash. **Other:** *Turns urine, feces, saliva, sputum, perspiration, and tears orange. Soft contact lenses may be permanently discolored.*

**INTERACTIONS Drug:** May decrease levels of BENZODIAZEPINES, BETA-BLOCKERS, **clofibrate, dapsone,** NARCOTICS, ANTICOAGULANTS, CORTICOSTEROIDS, **cyclosporine, quinidine,** ORAL CONTRACEPTIVES, PROGESTINS, SULFONYLUREAS, **ketoconazole, fluconazole,** BARBITURATES, **theophylline,** and ANTICONVULSANTS, resulting in therapeutic failure.

**PHARMACOKINETICS Absorption:** 12–20% of oral dose reaches the systemic circulation. **Peak:** 2–3 h. **Distribution:** 85% protein bound. Widely distributed, high concentrations in the lungs, liver, spleen, eyes, and kidney. Crosses placenta, distributed into breast milk. **Metabolism:** In the liver. Causes induction of hepatic enzymes. **Elimination:** Approximately 53% of dose is excreted in urine as metabolites, 30% is excreted in feces. **Half-Life:** 16–96 h (average 45 h).

## NURSING IMPLICATIONS

### Assessment & Drug Effects
- Monitor patients for S&S of active TB. Report immediately.
- Evaluate patients on concurrent oral hypoglycemic therapy for loss of glycemic control.
- Review patient's complete drug regimen because dosage adjustment of a significant number of drugs may be needed when rifabutin is added to regimen.
- Monitor lab tests: Periodic LFTs, CBC with differential and platelet count.

### Patient & Family Education
- Learn S&S of TB and MAC (e.g., persistent fever, progressive weight loss, anorexia, night sweats, diarrhea) and notify prescriber if any of these develop.
- Notify prescriber of following: Muscle or joint pain, eye pain or other discomfort, chest pain with dyspnea, rash, or a flu-like syndrome.
- Be aware that urine, feces, saliva, sputum, perspiration, tears, and skin may be colored brown-orange. Soft contact lens may be permanently discolored.

R

Common adverse effects in *italic;* life-threatening effects underlined; generic names in **bold;** classifications in SMALL CAPS; ♥ Canadian drug name; ⊘ Prototype drug

1431

- Rifabutin may reduce the activity of a wide variety of drugs. Provide a complete and accurate list of concurrent drugs to the prescriber for evaluation.

# RIFAMPIN ℗

(rif'am-pin)

**Rifadin, Rofact ♦**

**Classifications:** ANTIBIOTIC; ANTITUBERCULOSIS

**Therapeutic:** ANTITUBERCULOSIS

**AVAILABILITY** Capsule; solution for injection

## ACTION & *THERAPEUTIC EFFECT*

Inhibits DNA-dependent RNA polymerase activity in susceptible bacterial cells, thereby suppressing RNA synthesis. *Active against* Mycobacterium tuberculosis, M. leprae, Neisseria meningitidis, *and a wide range of gram-negative and gram-positive organisms.*

## USES Initial treatment and retreatment of tuberculosis; as short-term therapy to prevent meningococcal infection.

## UNLABELED USES Chemoprophylaxis in contacts of patients with *Haemophilus influenzae* type B infection; leprosy (especially dapsone-resistant leprosy); Legionnaire's disease, endocarditis, pruritus.

## CONTRAINDICATIONS Hypersensitivity to rifampin; obstructive biliary disease; meningococcal disease; intermittent rifampin therapy.

## CAUTIOUS USE Hepatic disease; history of alcoholism; IBD. Concomitant use of other hepatotoxic agents; pregnancy (category C).

# ROUTE & DOSAGE

## Pulmonary Tuberculosis

*Adult:* **PO/IV** 600 mg daily with other agents

*Adults (with HIV):* **PO/IV** 10 mg/kg (max: 600 mg) daily for 2 mo with other agents

*Child:* **PO/IV** 10–20 mg/kg/day (max: 600 mg/day) with other agents

*Infant/Child (with HIV):* **PO/IV** 10–20 mg/kg (max: 600 mg) daily for 2 mo with other agents

## Meningococcal Carriers

*Adult:* **PO/IV** 600 mg q12h for 2 consecutive days

*Adolescent/Child/Infant:* **PO/IV** 10–20 mg/kg q12h for 2 consecutive days (max: 600 mg/day)

*Neonate:* **PO/IV** 5 mg/kg b.i.d. for 2 days

## Hepatic Impairment Adjustment

Do not exceed 8 mg/kg/day

## Renal Impairment Adjustment

*CrCl less than 10 mL/min:* Reduce dose by 50%

# ADMINISTRATION

## Oral

- Give 1 h before or 2 h after a meal. Peak serum levels are delayed and may be slightly lower when given with food; capsule contents may be emptied into fluid or mixed with food.
- Note: An oral suspension can be prepared from capsules for use with pediatric patients. Consult pharmacist for directions.
- Keep a desiccant in bottle containing capsules to prevent moisture causing instability.

R

## Intravenous

*PREPARE:* **IV Infusion:** Reconstitute vial by adding 10 mL of sterile water for injection to each 600-mg to yield 60 mg/mL. Swirl to dissolve. ▪ Withdraw the ordered dose and further dilute in 500 mL of D5W (preferred) or NS. ▪ If absolutely necessary, 100 mL of D5W or NS may be used.
*ADMINISTER:* **IV Infusion:** Infuse 500 mL solution over 3 h and 100 mL solution over 30 min. ▪ Note: A less concentrated solution infused over a longer period is preferred.
*INCOMPATIBILITIES:* Solution/additive: **Minocycline.** Y-site: **Amiodarone, diltiazem, tramadol.**

▪ Use NS solutions within 24 h and D5W solutions within 4 h of preparation.

## ADVERSE EFFECTS (≥1%) CNS: Fatigue, drowsiness, headache, ataxia, confusion, dizziness, inability to concentrate, generalized numbness, pain in extremities, muscular weakness. **Special Senses:** Visual disturbances, transient low-frequency hearing loss, conjunctivitis. **GI:** *Heartburn, epigastric distress, nausea, vomiting, anorexia, flatulence, cramps, diarrhea,* pseudomembranous colitis, *transient elevations in liver function tests* (bilirubin, BSP, alkaline phosphatase, ALT, AST), pancreatitis. **Hematologic:** Thrombocytopenia, transient leukopenia, anemia, including hemolytic anemia. **Body as a Whole:** Hypersensitivity (fever, pruritus, urticaria, skin eruptions, soreness of mouth and tongue, eosinophilia, hemolysis), flu-like syndrome. **Urogenital:** Hemoglobinuria, hematuria, acute renal failure, light-chain proteinuria, menstrual disorders, hepatorenal syndrome (with

intermittent therapy). **Respiratory:** Hemoptysis. **Other:** Increasing lethargy, liver enlargement and tenderness, jaundice, brownish-red or orange discoloration of skin, sweat, saliva, tears, and feces; unconsciousness.

## DIAGNOSTIC TEST INTERFERENCE
Rifampin interferes with contrast media used for *gallbladder study;* therefore, test should precede daily dose of rifampin. May also cause retention of *BSP.* Inhibits standard assays for *serum folate* and *vitamin B₁₂,* may cause false positive opiate urine screen.

## INTERACTIONS Drug: Do not use with PROTEASE INHIBITORS and **nevirapine** as it may increase treatment failure rate. **Alcohol, isoniazid, pyrazinamide, ritonavir,** saquinavir increase risk of drug-induced hepatotoxicity decreases concentrations of **alfentanil, alosetron, alprazolam, amprenavir,** BARBITURATES, BENZODIAZEPINES, **carbamazepine, atovaquone, cevimeline, chloramphenicol, clofibrate,** CORTICOSTEROIDS, **cyclosporine, dapsone, delavirdine, diazepam, digoxin, diltiazem, disopyramide, estazolam, estramustine, fentanyl, fosphenytoin, fluconazole galantamine, indinavir, itraconazole, ketoconazole, lamotrigine, levobupivacaine, lopinavir, methadone, metoprolol, mexiletine, midazolam, nelfinavir,** ORAL SULFONYLUREAS, ORAL CONTRACEPTIVES, **phenytoin,** PROGESTINS, **propafenone, propranolol, quinidine, quinine, ritonavir, siro-limus, theophylline,** THYROID HORMONES, **tocainide, tramadol, verapamil, warfarin, zaleplon,** and **zonisamide,** leading to potential therapeutic failure. Do not use with **simvastatin.**

R

## PHARMACOKINETICS **Absorption:** Readily from GI tract. **Peak:** 2–4 h. **Distribution:** Widely distributed, including CSF; crosses placenta; distributed into breast milk. **Metabolism:** In liver to active and inactive metabolites; is enterohepatically cycled. **Elimination:** Up to 30% in urine, 60–65% in feces. **Half-Life:** 3 h.

## NURSING IMPLICATIONS

### Assessment & Drug Effects

- Monitor for extravasation during injection; local irritation and inflammation due to infiltration of the infusion may occur. If so, DC infusion and restart at another site.
- Check prothrombin time daily or as necessary to establish and maintain required anticoagulant activity when patient is also receiving an anticoagulant.
- Monitor lab tests: Periodic LFTs, CBC, and platelet count.

### Patient & Family Education

- Do not interrupt prescribed dosage regimen. Hepatorenal reaction with flu-like syndrome has occurred when therapy has been resumed following interruption.
- Be aware that drug may impart a harmless red-orange color to urine, feces, sputum, sweat, and tears. Soft contact lenses may be permanently stained.
- Report onset of jaundice, hypersensitivity reactions, and persistence of GI adverse effects to prescriber.
- Use or add barrier contraceptive if using hormonal contraception. Concomitant use of rifampin and oral contraceptives leads to decreased effectiveness of the contraceptive and to menstrual disturbances (spotting, breakthrough bleeding).
- Keep drug out of reach of children.

# RIFAPENTINE
(rif'a-pen-teen)
**Priftin**
**Classifications:** ANTIBIOTIC; ANTITUBERCULOSIS; MYCOBACTERIUM
**Therapeutic:** ANTITUBERCULOSIS
**Prototype:** Rifampin

## AVAILABILITY Tablet

## ACTION & *THERAPEUTIC EFFECT*
Inhibits DNA-dependent RNA polymerase activity in susceptible bacterial cells, thereby suppressing RNA synthesis. *Effective against* Mycobacterium tuberculosis, *indicated by improvement in clinical S&S (e.g., fever, cough, pleuritic pain, fatigue) and on chest X-ray.*

## USES Active or latent pulmonary tuberculosis in conjunction with at least one other agent.

## CONTRAINDICATIONS Hypersensitivity to any rifamycins (e.g., rifampin, rifabutin, rifapentine); porphyria; continuation phase of treatment in HIV-seropositive patients; soft contact lens; lactation.

## CAUTIOUS USE Patients with abnormal liver function tests or hepatic disease; HIV disease; cavitary pulmonary lesions, bilateral pulmonary disease; older adults; pregnancy (category C); children.

## ROUTE & DOSAGE

**Tuberculosis: Active**

*Adult/Adolescent:* **PO** 600 mg twice weekly (at least 72 h apart) × 2 mo, then 600 mg once weekly × 4 mo

### Latent Tuberculosis

*Adult/Adolescent/Child (weight greater than 50 kg):* **PO** 900 mg once weekly; *weight 32.1–50 kg:* 750 mg once weekly; *weight 25.1–32 kg:* 600 mg once weekly; *weight 14.1–25 kg:* 450 mg once weekly; *weight 10–14 kg:* 300 mg once weekly

## ADMINISTRATION

### Oral

- Give with an interval of NO LESS than 72 h between doses.
- Give with food to minimize GI upset.
- Store at 15°–30° C (59°–86° F) in a tightly closed container and protect from excess moisture.

## ADVERSE EFFECTS (≥1%) CNS:
Headache, dizziness. **CV:** Hypertension. **GI:** Increased liver function tests (ALT, AST), anorexia, nausea, vomiting, dyspepsia, diarrhea. **Urogenital:** *Hyperuricemia, pyuria, proteinuria, hematuria, urinary casts.* **Hematologic:** Neutropenia, lymphopenia, anemia, leukopenia, thrombocytosis. **Respiratory:** Hemoptysis. **Skin:** Rash, pruritus, acne. **Body as a Whole:** Arthralgia, pain.

## INTERACTIONS Drug: Decreased
activity of ORAL CONTRACEPTIVES, **phenytoin, disopyramide, mexiletine, quinidine, tocainide, warfarin, fluconazole, itraconazole, ketoconazole, diazepam,** BETA-BLOCKERS, CALCIUM CHANNEL BLOCKERS, CORTICOSTEROIDS, **haloperidol,** SULFONYLUREAS, **cyclosporine, tacrolimus, levothyroxine,** NARCOTIC ANALGESICS, **quinine,** REVERSE TRANSCRIPTASE INHIBITORS, TRICYCLIC ANTIDEPRESSANTS, **sildenafil, theophylline.**

## PHARMACOKINETICS Absorption: 70% absorbed. Peak: 5–6 h.
**Distribution:** 97.7% protein bound. **Metabolism:** Hydrolyzed by esterase enzyme to active metabolite in liver; inducer of cytochromes P450 3A4 and 2C8/9. **Elimination:** 70% in feces, 17% in urine. **Half-Life:** 13.3 h.

## NURSING IMPLICATIONS

### Assessment & Drug Effects

- Monitor carefully for S&S of toxicity with concurrent use of oral anticoagulants, digitalis preparations, or anticonvulsants.
- Monitor lab tests: Sputum smear and culture, baseline LFTs and repeat q4–6wk in those with preexisting hepatic impairment.

### Patient & Family Education

- Follow strict adherence to the prescribed dosing schedule to prevent emergence of resistant strains of tuberculosis.
- Be aware that food may be useful in preventing GI upset.
- Report immediately any of the following to the prescriber: Fever, weakness, nausea or vomiting, loss of appetite, dark urine or yellowing of eyes or skin, pain or swelling of the joints, severe or persistent diarrhea.
- Use or add barrier contraceptive if using hormonal contraception.

## RIFAXIMIN

(ri-fax′i-min)

Xifaxan

**Classifications:** RIFAMYCIN ANTIBIOTIC; MYCOBACTERIUM
**Therapeutic:** MYCOBACTERIUM
**Prototype:** Rifampin

## AVAILABILITY Tablet

## ACTION & *THERAPEUTIC EFFECT*

Inhibits bacterial RNA synthesis by

R

Common adverse effects in *italic;* life-threatening effects <u>underlined</u>; generic names in **bold;** classifications in SMALL CAPS; ♣ Canadian drug name; ⊕ Prototype drug

1435

binding to DNA-dependent RNA polymerase, thereby blocking RNA transcription. *Its spectrum of activity includes gram-positive and gram-negative aerobes and anaerobes.*

**USES** Treatment of traveler's diarrhea, hepatic encephalopathy.

**UNLABELED USES** Crohn's disease, diverticulitis, irritable bowel syndrome.

**CONTRAINDICATIONS** Hypersensitivity to rifaximin, other rifamycin antimicrobial agents or to any of its components; dysentery; lactation.

**CAUTIOUS USE** Diarrhea with fever and/or blood in the stool, or diarrhea due to organisms other than *E. coli;* IBD, worsening diarrhea or diarrhea persisting for longer than 24–48 h; pregnancy (category C); children younger than 12 y.

## ROUTE & DOSAGE

**Traveler's Diarrhea**
*Adult/Adolescent:* **PO** 200 mg t.i.d. for 3 days
*Reduce Risk of Hepatic Encephalopathy Recurrence*
*Adult:* **PO** 550 mg b.i.d.

## ADMINISTRATION

**Oral**
▪ May be given without regard to food.
▪ Store at 15°–30° C (59°–86° F).

**ADVERSE EFFECTS** (≥1%) **Body as a Whole:** Fever. **CNS:** Headache. **GI:** *Flatulence,* abdominal pain, rectal tenesmus, defecation urgency, nausea, constipation, vomiting.

**PHARMACOKINETICS Absorption:** Less than 0.4% absorbed

orally. **Peak:** 1.21 h. **Elimination:** In feces. **Half-Life:** 5.85 h.

## NURSING IMPLICATIONS

### Assessment & Drug Effects
▪ Withhold drug and notify prescriber if diarrhea worsens or lasts longer than 48 h after starting drug; an alternative treatment should be considered.
▪ Report promptly the appearance of blood in the stool.

### Patient & Family Education
▪ Report promptly any of the following: Fever; difficulty breathing; skin rash, itching, or hives; worsening diarrhea during or after treatment or blood in the stool.

## RILPIVIRINE
(ril-pi′vi-reen)
Edurant
**Classifications:** ANTIRETROVIRAL; NONNUCLEOSIDE REVERSE TRANSCRIPTASE INHIBITOR (NNRTI)
Therapeutic: ANTIRETROVIRAL; NNRTI
**Prototype:** Efavirenz

**AVAILABILITY** Tablet

## ACTION & THERAPEUTIC EFFECT
A nonnucleoside reverse transcriptase inhibitor (NNRTI) of human immunodeficiency virus type 1 (HIV-1). *Inhibits HIV-1 replication and slows/prevents disease progression.*

**USES** Treatment of HIV-1 infection in combination with other antiretroviral agents in adult patients who are treatment-naïve.

**CONTRAINDICATIONS** Concurrent drugs that significantly decrease rilpivirine plasma level such as anticonvulsants, antimycobacterials, proton pump inhibitors, systemic

R

dexamethasone, St. John's wort; lactation.

**CAUTIOUS USE** Congenital prolonged QT interval or concurrent drugs that prolong the QT interval; depressive disorders or suicidal ideation; older adult; severe renal impairment; hepatic impairment; pregnancy (category B). Safety and efficacy in children not established.

## ROUTE & DOSAGE

**HIV-1 Infection (with Other Agents)**
*Adult:* **PO** 25 mg once daily

## ADMINISTRATION

### Oral
- Give with a full meal.
- If antacids are prescribed, they must be given at least 2 h before or 4 h after rilpivirine.
- Store at 15–30° C (59–86° F) and protect from light.

**ADVERSE EFFECTS** (≥1%) **Body as a Whole:** Cholecystitis, cholelithiasis. **CNS:** Abnormal dreams, anxiety, *depressive disorders*, dizziness, fatigue, *headache, insomnia*, sleep disorders, somnolence, <u>suicidal thoughts</u>. **GI:** Abdominal pain, decreased appetite, diarrhea, nausea, vomiting. **Metabolic:** *Increase ALT and AST*, increased bilirubin, *increased cholesterol*, increased creatinine, increased triglycerides. **Skin:** *Rash.* **Urogenital:** Glomerulonephritis.

**INTERACTIONS Drug:** Strong CYP-3A4 inhibitors (e.g., **atazanavir, clarithromycin, delaviridine, indinavir, itraconazole, ketoconazole, nefazodone, nelfinavir, ritonavir, saquinavir,** and **telithromycin**) **voriconazole,** can increase rilpivirine levels, while strong CYP3A4 inducers (e.g., **rifampin, dexamethasone, phenytoin, carbamazepine, efavirenz,** and **phenobarbital**) can decrease rilpivirine levels. Antacids, GLUCOCORTICOIDS, H₂ RECEPTOR ANTAGONISTS, **methadone** can decrease rilpivirine. Rilpivirine can decrease the levels of **methadone.** Rilpivirine has been associated with QT prolongation. Coadministration of other drug that prolongs the QT interval (e.g., **disopyramide, procainamide, amiodarone, bretylium, clarithromycin, levofloxacin**) may cause additive effects. **Food:** Administration with a meal enhances absorption. **Herbal: St. John's wort** may decrease the levels of rilpivirine.

**PHARMACOKINETICS Peak:** 4–5 h. **Distribution:** 99.7% plasma protein bound. **Metabolism:** In liver. **Elimination:** Fecal (85%) and renal (6%). **Half-Life:** 50 h.

## NURSING IMPLICATIONS

### Assessment & Drug Effects
- Monitor closely for adverse effects in those with severe renal impairment.
- Monitor for and report promptly signs of depression or suicidal ideation.
- Monitor lab tests: Periodic plasma HIV RNA; baseline and periodic LFTs.

### Patient & Family Education
- Drug absorption is improved when taken with a full meal.
- Seek immediate medical assistance if you experience depression or thoughts of suicide.
- Do not self-treat depression with St. John's wort.
- Report to prescriber all prescription and nonprescription drugs and herbal products you use.

R

Common adverse effects in *italic*; life-threatening effects <u>underlined</u>; generic names in **bold**; classifications in SMALL CAPS; ♥Canadian drug name; ◑ Prototype drug

1437

- Do not use over-the-counter stomach medications without consent of your health care provider.
- If you use an antacid, take it at least 2 h before or 4 h after taking rilpivirine.

# RILUZOLE
(ri-lu'zole)
Rilutek
**Classifications:** AMYOTROPHIC LATERAL SCLEROSIS (ALS) AGENT; GLUTAMATE ANTAGONIST
Therapeutic: ALS AGENT

## AVAILABILITY Tablet

## ACTION & *THERAPEUTIC EFFECT*
Inhibits the presynaptic release of glutamic acid in the CNS. Effectiveness based on theory that pathogenesis of amyotrophic lateral sclerosis (ALS) is related to injury of motor neurons by glutamate. *Believed to reduce the degeneration of neurons in ALS.*

## USES Treatment of ALS.

## CONTRAINDICATIONS Hypersensitivity to riluzole; ALT levels are 5 × ULN or if clinical jaundice develops; lactation.

## CAUTIOUS USE Hepatic dysfunction, renal impairment; hypertension, history of other CNS disorders; older adults; pregnancy (category C). Safe use in children younger than 12 y is not established.

## ROUTE & DOSAGE

### ALS
*Adult:* **PO** 50 mg q12h

## ADMINISTRATION
### Oral
- Give at same time daily and at least 1 h before or 2 h after a meal. Do not give before/after a high-fat meal.
- Store at room temperature; protect from bright light.

## ADVERSE EFFECTS (≥1%) **Body as a Whole:** *Asthenia,* headache, back pain, malaise, arthralgia, weight loss, peripheral edema, flu-like syndrome. **CNS:** Hypertonia, depression, dizziness, dry mouth, insomnia, somnolence, circumoral paresthesia. **CV:** Hypertension, tachycardia, phlebitis, palpitation. **GI:** Abdominal pain, *nausea,* vomiting, dyspepsia, anorexia, diarrhea, flatulence, stomatitis. **Respiratory:** *Decreased lung function,* rhinitis, increased cough, apnea, bronchitis, dysphagia, dyspnea. **Skin:** Pruritus, eczema, alopecia, exfoliative dermatitis (rare). **Urogenital:** UTI.

## INTERACTIONS **Drug:** BARBITURATES, **carbamazepine** may increase risk of hepatotoxicity.

## PHARMACOKINETICS **Absorption:** Well absorbed from GI tract, 60% reaches systemic circulation. **Peak:** Steady-state levels by day 5. **Distribution:** 96% protein bound. **Metabolism:** In liver by CYP1A2. **Elimination:** 90% in urine. **Half-Life:** 12 h.

## NURSING IMPLICATIONS
### Assessment & Drug Effects
- Withhold drug and notify prescriber if liver enzymes are elevated.
- Monitor lab tests: Baseline LFTs, then monthly for 3 mo, then q3mo for remainder of first year, and periodically thereafter.

### Patient & Family Education
- Report any febrile illness to prescriber.
- Do not engage in potentially hazardous activities until response to drug is known.

R

- Learn common adverse effects and possible adverse interaction with alcohol.

# RIMANTADINE

(ri-man'ta-deen)

Flumadine

**Classifications:** ANTIVIRAL; ADMANTANE

**Therapeutic:** ANTIVIRAL

**Prototype:** Amantadine

## AVAILABILITY Tablet

## ACTION & THERAPEUTIC EFFECT

Believed to exert an inhibitory effect early in the viral replication cycle, probably by interfering with the viral uncoating procedure of the influenza A virus. Inhibits synthesis of both viral RNA and viral protein, thus causing viral destruction. *Prevents or interrupts influenza A infections.*

## USES Prophylaxis and treatment of influenza A.

## CONTRAINDICATIONS Hypersensitivity to rimantadine and amantadine; lactation; children younger than 1 y for prophylaxis treatment.

## CAUTIOUS USE History of seizures; renal or hepatic impairment; older adults; pregnancy (category C). Safe use in children younger than 17 y for treatment of Influenza A is not known.

## ROUTE & DOSAGE

### Prophylaxis of Influenza A

*Adult/Child (10 y or older):* **PO** 100 mg b.i.d.; *Child (1–9 y):* **PO** 5 mg/kg daily (max: 150 mg/day) in divided doses

*Geriatric:* **PO** 100 mg daily

### Treatment of Influenza A

*Adult/Adolescent (17 y or older):* **PO** 100 mg b.i.d. started within 48 h of symptoms and continued for 5–7 days from initial symptoms

*Geriatric:* **PO** 100 mg daily started within 48 h of symptoms and continued for 5–7 days from initial symptoms

### Hepatic Impairment Dosage Adjustment

100 mg daily with severe liver disease

### Renal Impairment Dosage Adjustment

*CrCl 10–30 mL/min:* Extend dosing interval to 24 h

## ADMINISTRATION

### Oral

- Store at 15°–30° C (59°–86° F).

## ADVERSE EFFECTS (≥1%) CNS: Nervousness, dizziness, headache, sleep disturbances, fatigue or malaise, drowsiness, anticholinergic effects. GI: Nausea, vomiting, diarrhea, dyspepsia, dry mouth, anorexia, abdominal pain.

## INTERACTIONS Drug: Intranasal influenza vaccine should not be used within 48 h.

## PHARMACOKINETICS Absorption: Readily absorbed from GI tract. Peak: Serum levels 3.2–4.3 h. Distribution: Concentrates in respiratory secretions. Metabolism: Extensively in liver. Elimination: By kidneys. Half-Life: 20–36 h.

## NURSING IMPLICATIONS

### Assessment & Drug Effects

- Monitor carefully for seizure activity in patients with a history of

R

Common adverse effects in *italic;* life-threatening effects <u>underlined</u>; generic names in **bold;** classifications in SMALL CAPS; ♣ Canadian drug name; ⊙ Prototype drug

1439

seizures. Seizures are an indication to discontinue the drug.
- Monitor cardiac, respiratory, and neurologic status while on drug. Report palpitations, hypertension, dyspnea, or pedal edema.

**Patient & Family Education**
- Report bothersome adverse effects to prescriber; especially hallucinations, palpitations, difficulty breathing, and swelling of legs.
- Use caution with hazardous activities until reaction to drug is known.

# RIMEXOLONE
(rim-ex′o-lone)
Vexol
**See Appendix A-1.**

# RISEDRONATE SODIUM
(ri-se-dron′ate)
Actonel, Atelvia
**Classifications:** BISPHOSPHONATE; BONE METABOLISM REGULATOR
**Therapeutic:** BONE RESORPTION INHIBITOR; OSTEOPOROSIS TREATMENT
**Prototype:** Etidronate disodium

**AVAILABILITY** Tablet; delayed release tablet

**ACTION & *THERAPEUTIC EFFECT***
Lowers serum alkaline phosphatase, presumably by decreasing release of phosphate from bone and increasing excretion of parathyroid hormone. Slows rate of bone resorption and new bone formation in pagetic bone lesions and in normal remodeling process. *Effectiveness indicated by decreased bone and joint pain and improved bone density.*

**USES** Paget's disease, prevention and treatment of osteoporosis.

**UNLABELED USES** Osteolytic metastases.

**CONTRAINDICATIONS** Hypersensitivity to risedronate or other bisphosphonates; hypocalcemia, vitamin D deficiency; severe renal impairment (CrCl less than 30 mL/min); esophageal stricture; lactation.

**CAUTIOUS USE** Renal impairment; CHF; hyperphosphatemia or vitamin D deficiency; hepatic disease; UGI disease; fever related to infection or other causes; pregnancy (category C). Safety and efficacy in children younger than 18 y not established.

## ROUTE & DOSAGE

**Paget's Disease**
*Adult:* **PO** 30 mg daily for 2 mo, may repeat after 2 mo rest if necessary
**Prevention and Treatment of Osteoporosis**
*Adult (female):* **PO** 5 mg daily OR 35 mg once weekly OR 150 mg once monthly OR 75 mg × 2 consecutive days once monthly
*Adult (male):* **PO** 35 mg weekly
*Adult (with chronic systemic glucocorticoid):* **PO** 5 mg daily

**Renal Impairment Dosage Adjustment**
*CrCl less than 30 mL/min:* Use not recommended

## ADMINISTRATION
**Oral**
- Give on an empty stomach (at least 30 min before first food or drink of the day) with at least 6–8 oz plain water. Ensure that tablet is swallowed whole. It should not be crushed or chewed.

R

- Note: Patient should be upright. Maintain upright position and empty stomach for at least 30 min after administration.
- Space calcium supplements and antacids as far as possible from risedronate.
- Store at 15°–30° C (59°–86° F) in a tightly closed container and protect from light.

**ADVERSE EFFECTS (≥1%) Body as a Whole:** Flu-like syndrome, asthenia, arthralgia, bone pain, back pain, leg cramps, myasthenia, infection. **CNS:** Headache, dizziness. **CV:** Chest pain, peripheral edema, hypertension. **GI:** *Diarrhea,* abdominal pain, nausea, vomiting, constipation, belching, colitis. **Respiratory:** Bronchitis, sinusitis. **Skin:** Rash. **Special Senses:** Amblyopia, tinnitus, dry eyes.

**DIAGNOSTIC TEST INTERFERENCE** May interfere with the use of *bone-imaging agents.*

**INTERACTIONS Drug:** Calcium, ANTACIDS significantly decrease absorption, use with NONSTEROIDAL ANTI-INFLAMMATORIES may increase risk of gastric ulcer. Use caution with PPIs due to changes in bioavailability. **Food:** Any food will decrease bioavailability. Take at least 30 min before first food or drink of the day.

**PHARMACOKINETICS Absorption:** Minimally absorbed from GI tract, bioavailability 0.63%. **Peak:** 1 h. **Distribution:** Approximately 60% of dose is distributed to bone. **Metabolism:** Not metabolized. **Elimination:** In urine; unabsorbed drug excreted in feces. **Half-Life:** 220 h.

**NURSING IMPLICATIONS**
**Assessment & Drug Effects**
- Monitor carefully for and immediately report S&S of GI bleeding and hypocalcemia.
- Monitor lab tests: Baseline and periodic electrolytes including serum calcium, phosphorus, and alkaline phosphatase.

**Patient & Family Education**
- Administration guidelines regarding upright position, empty stomach, and spacing relative to calcium supplements and antacids **must be** strictly followed.
- Report any of the following to prescriber: Eye irritation, significant GI upset, or flu-like symptoms.
- Preventive dental care important for at-risk populations.

## RISPERIDONE
(ris-per'i-done)
Risperdal, Risperdal M-TAB, Risperdal Consta
**Classification:** ATYPICAL ANTIPSYCHOTIC
**Therapeutic:** ANTIPSYCHOTIC
**Prototype:** Clozapine

**AVAILABILITY** Tablet; quick-dissolving tablet; oral solution; solution for injection

**ACTION & THERAPEUTIC EFFECT** Interferes with binding of dopamine to $D_2$-interlimbic region of the brain, serotonin (5-HT$_2$) receptors, and alpha-adrenergic receptors in the occipital cortex. It has low to moderate affinity for the other serotonin (5-HT) receptors. *Effective in controlling symptoms of schizophrenia as well as other psychotic symptoms.*

**USES** Treatment of schizophrenia; treatment of bipolar disorder; irritability associated with autism.

**UNLABELED USES** Insomnia in elderly patient, obsessive-compulsive disorder, stuttering, tardive dyskinesia, Tourette syndrome.

**CONTRAINDICATIONS** Hypersensitivity to risperidone; older adults with dementia-related psychosis; drug induced narcoleptic malignant syndrome (NMS); severe CNS depression, head trauma; lactation. **Risperdal Consta:** Lactation during use and for 12 wk after last injection.

**CAUTIOUS USE** Arrhythmias, hypotension, breast cancer, blood dyscrasia, cardiac disorders, cerebrovascular disease, hypotension, dehydration, DM; diabetic ketoacidosis, hyperglycemia, MI, obesity, orthostatic hypotension, mild or moderate CNS depression; GI obstruction, dysphagia; electrolyte imbalance, drug and alcohol abuse; heart failure, MI, ischemia; arrhythmias; renal or hepatic impairment; seizure disorder, suicidal tendencies; stroke, Parkinson's disease; Alzheimer dementia; risks for aspiration pneumonia; PKU; older adults; pregnancy (category C). Safe use in children younger than 13 y for schizophrenia; children younger than 10 y for bipolar disease and children younger than 5 y for autism not established.

## ROUTE & DOSAGE

### Schizophrenia
*Adult:* **PO** 2–4 mg/day in 1 or 2 doses, then titrate up (max: 16 mg/day); **IM** 25 mg once q2wk (max: 50 mg)
*Geriatric:* **PO** Start 0.5 mg b.i.d. and increase by 0.5 mg b.i.d. daily to an initial target of 1.5 mg b.i.d. (max: 4 mg/day); **IM** 25 mg once q2wk (max: 25 mg)
*Adolescent:* **PO** 0.5 mg once daily titrate up to target dose 3 mg/day

### Bipolar Disorder
*Adult:* **PO** 2–3 mg once daily for up to 3 wk (max: 6 mg/day); **IM** Initiate Risperdal Consta with 25 mg every 2 wk; may increase to 37.5–50 mg every 2 wk
*Geriatric:* **PO** Start with 0.5 mg b.i.d. and increase by 0.5 mg b.i.d. daily to an initial target of 1.5 mg b.i.d. (max: 6 mg/day). May convert to once daily dosing after stabilized.
*Adolescent (10 y or older):* **PO** 0.5 mg once daily titrate to recommended target dose range of 1–2.5 mg/day

### Irritability Associated with Autism
*Adolescent/Child (5 y or older, weight 20 kg or greater):* **PO** 0.5 mg daily; after 4 days, increase to 1 mg daily; can increase by 0.5 mg q2wk
*Child 5 y or older; weight 15–20 kg:* 0.25 mg daily; after 4 days, increase to 0.5 mg daily; can increase by 0.25 mg q2wk

### Renal Impairment Dosage Adjustment
*CrCl less than 30 mL/min:* Start with 0.5 mg b.i.d., increase by 0.5 mg b.i.d. daily to an initial target of 1.5 mg b.i.d., may increase by 0.5 mg b.i.d. at weekly intervals (max: 6 mg/day); lower **IM** dose may be required

### Hepatic Impairment Dosage Adjustment
**PO** start with dose of 0.5 mg b.i.d.

### Enzyme Inducer or CYP2D6 Inhibitor Dosage Adjustment
See package insert

## ADMINISTRATION
### Oral
- The oral solution may be mixed with water, orange juice, low-fat

milk, or coffee. It is not compatible with cola or tea.
- Orally disintegrating tablets should not be removed from the blister until immediately before administration. Tablets disintegrate immediately and may be swallowed with/without liquid.
- Store at 15°–30° C (59°–86° F).

**Intramuscular**
- Reconstitute using only in the diluent supplied in the dose pack. Shake vigorously for at least 10 sec to produce a uniform, thick, milky suspension. If 2 min or more pass before injection, shake vial again.
- Give deep IM into the upper-outer quadrant of the gluteal muscle with the supplied needle; do not substitute. Follow the manufacturer's instructions for use of the SmartSite Needle-Free Vial Access Device and Needle-Pro device.
- Store unopened vials at 2°–8° C (36°–46° F). Protect from light.

**ADVERSE EFFECTS** (≥1%) **Body as a Whole:** Orthostatic hypotension with initial doses, sweating, weakness, *fatigue.* **CNS:** *Sedation, drowsiness, headache,* transient blurred vision, *insomnia,* disinhibition, *agitation,* anxiety, increased dream activity, *dizziness,* catatonia, *extrapyramidal symptoms* (akathisia, dystonia, pseudoparkinsonism), especially with doses greater than 10 mg/day, neuroleptic malignant syndrome (rare), increased risk of stroke in elderly. **CV:** Prolonged QT$_c$ interval, tachycardia. **GI:** *Dry mouth,* dyspepsia, nausea, *vomiting, diarrhea, constipation,* abdominal pain, elevated liver function tests (AST, ALT). **Endocrine:** Galactorrhea. **Metabolic:** Hyperglycemia, diabetes mellitus, *hyperprolactinemia, weight gain.* **Respiratory:** Rhinitis, *cough,* dyspnea. **Skin:** Photosensitivity. **Urogenital:**

Urinary retention, menorrhagia, incontinence, decreased sexual desire, erectile dysfunction, sexual dysfunction male and female.

**DIAGNOSTIC TEST INTERFERENCE** *Liver function tests (AST, ALT)* are elevated.

**INTERACTIONS Drug:** Risperidone may enhance the effects of certain ANTIHYPERTENSIVE AGENTS. May antagonize the antiparkinson effects of **bromocriptine, cabergoline, levodopa, pergolide, pramipexole, ropinirole, carbamazepine, phenytoin, phenobarbital, rifampin** may decrease risperidone levels. Monitor closely when used with CYP3A4 substrates. **Clozapine** may increase risperidone levels. Do not use with nasal **azelastine, metoclopramide, orphenadrine, sulpiride, thalidomide, tiotropium.** Do not use with agents that prolong the QT interval (e.g., **dofetilide, dronedarone, procaine, ziprasidone**).

**PHARMACOKINETICS Absorption:** Rapidly; not affected by food. **Onset:** Therapeutic effect 1–2 wk. **Peak:** 1–2 h. **Distribution:** 0.7 L/kg; in animal studies, risperidone has been found in breast milk. **Metabolism:** Primarily in liver [CYP2D6, CYP3A4, P-glycoprotein (P-gp)]. **Elimination:** 70% in urine; 14% in feces. **Half-Life:** 20 h for slow metabolizers, 30 h for fast metabolizers.

## NURSING IMPLICATIONS

### Black Box Warning

*Risperidone has been associated with increased mortality in older adults with dementia-related psychosis.*

**Assessment & Drug Effects**
- Monitor diabetics for loss of glycemic control.

- Reassess patients periodically and maintain on the lowest effective drug dose.
- Monitor closely neurologic status of older adults.
- Monitor cardiovascular status closely; assess for orthostatic hypotension, especially during initial dosage titration.
- Monitor closely those at risk for seizures.
- Assess degree of cognitive and motor impairment, and assess for environmental hazards.
- Monitor lab tests: Periodic blood glucose, serum electrolytes, LFTs, and CBC.

**Patient & Family Education**
- Carefully monitor blood glucose levels if diabetic.
- Do not engage in potentially hazardous activities until the response to drug is known.
- Be aware of the risk of orthostatic hypotension.
- Avoid alcohol while taking this drug.

# RITONAVIR
(ri-ton′a-vir)
Norvir
**Classifications:** ANTIRETROVIRAL; PROTEASE INHIBITOR
Therapeutic: PROTEASE INHIBITOR
**Prototype:** Saquinavir

**AVAILABILITY** Tablet; capsule; oral solution; powder packets

**ACTION & THERAPEUTIC EFFECT**
HIV protease inhibitor that renders the enzyme incapable of processing the polyprotein precursor necessary for the production of mature HIV-1 particles. *Protease inhibitor of both HIV-1 and HIV-2 resulting in the formation of noninfectious viral particles.*

**USES** Alone or in combination with other antiretroviral agents or protease inhibitors for treatment of HIV infection. Often used to increase the effect of other antiretrovirals.

**CONTRAINDICATIONS** Hypersensitivity to ritonavir; severe hepatic impairment; concurrent use of saquinavir and ritonavir in patients with conditions that affect cardiac electrical activity; coadministration with sedative hypnotics, alpha 1 adrenoreceptor antagonists, anitanginal, anitarrhythmics, anti fungals, anti gout medications, GI motility agents, St. John's wort, HMG-CoA reductase inhibitors, phosphodiesterase type-5 inhibitor; ergot alkaloids; antimicrobial resistance to protease inhibitors; pancreatitis; toxic epidermal necrolysis, lactation for HIV patients..

**CAUTIOUS USE** Mild to moderate hepatic diseases, liver enzyme abnormalities, or hepatitis, jaundice; cardiac myopathy, ischemic heart diseaase or structural heart disease; diabetes mellitus, diabetic ketoacidosis, hyperlipidemia, hypertriglyceridemia; pancreatitis; hemophilia A or B, renal insufficiency; Graves' disease; Guillain-Barre syndrome; pregnancy (category B). Safe use in children younger than 1 mo not established.

## ROUTE & DOSAGE

**HIV**
*Adult:* **PO** 600 mg b.i.d.
*Child (1 mo or older):* **PO** start with 250 mg/m$^2$ b.i.d., then titrate up to 350–400 mg/m$^2$ b.i.d. (max: 600 mg b.i.d.), start with 250 mg/m$^2$ b.i.d., increase by 50 mg/m$^2$ q2–3days

## ADMINISTRATION
**Oral**
- Give preferably with food; oral solution may be mixed with chocolate

milk or nutritional therapy liquids within 1 h of dosing to improve taste.

- Capsules should be stored refrigerated at 2°–8° C (36°–46° F). Protect from light in tightly closed container. May be left at room temperature: Less than 25° C (77° F) if used within 30 days.
- Store oral powder at less than 30° C (86° F).
- Store solution at 20°–25° C (68°–77° F).

**ADVERSE EFFECTS** (≥1%) **Body as a Whole:** Myalgia, allergic reaction, bronchitis, arthralgia, rhinitis, taste alterations, visual disturbances, dysuria, hyperglycemia, diabetes. **CNS:** *Asthenia, fatigue,* headache, fever, malaise, circumoral or peripheral paresthesia, insomnia, dizziness, somnolence, abnormal thinking, amnesia, agitation, anxiety, confusion, convulsions, aphasia, ataxia, diplopia, emotional lability, euphoria, hallucinations, decreased libido, nervousness, neuralgia, neuropathy, peripheral neuropathy, paralysis, tremor, vertigo. **CV:** *Palpitations, vasodilation, flushing* hypotension, postural hypotension, syncope, tachycardia, prolonged QT interval. **Hematologic:** Anemia, thrombocytopenia, lymphadenopathy. **GI:** *Nausea, diarrhea, vomiting, abdominal pain,* dyspepsia, stomatitis, dysguesia, anorexia, dry mouth, constipation, flatulence, cholecystitis, cholestasis, abnormal liver function tests, hepatitis. **Respiratory:** *Cough, oropharyngeal pain.* **Skin:** Rash, sweating, acne, contact dermatitis, pruritus, urticaria, skin ulceration, dry skin **Metabolic:** *Hypercholesterolemia,* hypertriglyceridemia.

**INTERACTIONS Drug: Carbamazepine, dexamethasone, phenobarbital, phenytoin, rifabutin, rifampin,** smoking can decrease

ritonavir levels. **Ritonavir** may increase serum levels and toxicity of **clarithromycin,** especially in patients with renal insufficiency (reduce **clarithromycin** dose in patients with CrCl less than 60 mL/min); **alfuzosin, amiodarone, bepridil, bupropion, clozapine, desipramine; dihydroergotamine, flecainide, fluticasone, meperidine, pimozide, piroxicam, propoxyphene, quinidine, rifabutin, saquinavir, trazodone.** Ritonavir decreases levels of ORAL CONTRACEPTIVES, **theophylline;** may increase **ergotamine** toxicity with **dihydroergotamine, ergotamine;** may increase systemic steroid exposure with **fluticasone.** Liquid formulation may cause disulfiram-like reaction with **alcohol** or **metronidazole.** Can not be used with **lovastatin.** Concurrent use of **dasatinib** requires dose reduction. Use with **darunavir** may increase risk of hepatoxicity. Use with lowest possible dose of **atorvastatin.** See the complete prescribing information for a comprehensive table of potential, but not studied, drug interactions. **Herbal: St. John's wort, garlic** may decrease antiretroviral activity.

**PHARMACOKINETICS Absorption:** Rapidly from GI tract. **Peak:** 2–4 h. **Distribution:** 98–99% protein bound. **Metabolism:** In liver (CYP3A4). **Elimination:** Primarily in feces (greater than 80%).

**NURSING IMPLICATIONS**

### Black Box Warning

*Coadministration of ritonavir with sedative hypnotics, antiarrhythmics, or ergot alkaloids has been associated with potentially serious and/or life-threatening adverse reactions.*

**Assessment & Drug Effects**

- Withhold drug and notify prescriber in the presence of abnormal liver function.

Common adverse effects in *italic;* life-threatening effects <u>underlined</u>; generic names in **bold;** classifications in SMALL CAPS; ♣ Canadian drug name; ⊙ Prototype drug

1445

- Assess for S&S of GI distress, peripheral neuropathy, and other potential adverse effects.
- Monitor lab tests: Periodic LFTs, uric acid, lipid profile, CPK, blood glucose, urinalysis and HbA1C.

### Patient & Family Education

- Learn potential adverse reactions and drug interactions; report to prescriber use of any OTC or prescription drugs.
- Take this drug exactly as prescribed. Do not skip doses. Take at same time each day.
- Do not take ritonavir with any of the following drugs as fatal reactions may occur: **Amiodarone, astemizole, alfuzosin, bepridil, dihydroergotamine, ergotamine, flecainide, methylergonovine, midazolam, pimozide, propafenone, quinidine, triazolam, voriconazole.**

# RITUXIMAB

(ri-tux′i-mab)

Rituxan

**Classifications:** ANTINEOPLASTIC; BIOLOGIC RESPONSE MODIFIER; MONOCLONAL ANTIBODY; IMMUNOGLOBULIN (IGG); DISEASE-MODIFYING ANTIRHEUMATIC DRUG (DMARD)

Therapeutic: ANTINEOPLASTIC; ANTIRHEUMATIC; DMARD

**AVAILABILITY** Solution for injection

## ACTION & THERAPEUTIC EFFECT

A monoclonal antibody against the protein CD20, which is primarily found on the surface of immune system B cells. It destroys B cells by attaching to CD20 and is therefore used to treat diseases which are characterized by excessive numbers of B cells, overactive B cells, or dysfunctional B cells. CD20 antigen is expressed in more than 90% of B-cell non-Hodgkin lymphomas. B cells are also believed to play a role in the pathogenesis of RA and associated chronic synovitis as they may be acting at multiple sites in the autoimmune/inflammatory process. *Rituximab effectiveness in both rheumatoid arthritis and non-Hodgkin's lymphoma is measured by induced depletion of peripheral B-lymphocytes.*

**USES** Rheumatoid arthritis, CLL, non-Hodgkin's lymphoma, Wegener's granulomatosis, microscopic polyangiitis.

**UNLABELED USES** Acute lymphocytic leukemia, idiopathic thrombocytopenic purpura, multiple sclerosis, hemolytic anemia, mantle cell lymphoma.

**CONTRAINDICATIONS** Hypersensitivity to murine proteins, rituximab, or abciximab; serious infection; life-threatening cardiac arrhythmias; severe infusion reactions to rituximab; drug-induced activation of hepatitis B virus (HBV); drug-induced progressive multifocal leukoencephalopathy (PML); tumor lysis syndrome; severe mucocutaneous reaction to rituximab; oliguria, rising serum creatinine; live vaccines; lactation.

**CAUTIOUS USE** Prior exposure to murine-based monoclonal antibodies; history of allergies; asthma and other pulmonary disease (increased risk of bronchospasm); respiratory insufficiency; CAD; thrombocytopenia; history of cardiac arrhythmias; hypertension, renal impairment; older adults; pregnancy (category C). Safety and efficacy in children not established.

## ROUTE & DOSAGE

### Non-Hodgkin's Lymphoma

Adult: **IV** Varies based on disease-specific parameters, consult package insert

Common adverse effects in *italic;* life-threatening effects underlined; generic names in **bold;** classifications in SMALL CAPS; ✦ Canadian drug name; ⓟ Prototype drug

### Rheumatoid Arthritis

*Adult:* **IV** 1000 mg on days 1 and 15 (with methotrexate); repeat every 24 wk

### CLL

*Adult:* **IV** 375 mg/m² on day 1 of cycle 1 then 500 mg/m² (in combination with fludarabine/cyclophosphamide) on day 1 of cycles 2–6.

### Wegener's Granulomatosis/ Microscopic Polyangiitis

*Adult:* **IV** 375 mg/m² weekly × 4 wk

## ADMINISTRATION

### Intravenous ONLY

Premedicate before each infusion with acetaminophen and an antihistamine.

*PREPARE:* **IV Infusion:** Dilute ordered dose to 1–4 mg/mL by adding to an infusion bag of NS or D5W. ▪ Examples: 500 mg in 400 mL yields 1 mg/mL; 500 mg in 75 mL yields 4 mg/mL. ▪ Gently invert bag to mix. Discard unused portion left in vial.

*ADMINISTER:* **IV Infusion:** Infuse first dose at a rate of 50 mg/h; may increase rate at 50 mg/h increments q30min to maximum rate of 400 mg/h. ▪ For subsequent doses, infuse at a rate of 100 mg/h and increase by 100 mg/h increments q30min up to maximum rate of 400 mg/h. ▪ Slow or stop infusion if S&S of hypersensitivity appear (see Appendix F).

*INCOMPATIBILITES:* **Y-site:** aldesleukin, amphotericin B colloidal, ciprofloxacin, cyclosporine, daunorubicin, doxorubicin, furosemide, levofloxacin, minocycline, ofloxacin, ondansetron, quinupristin/dalfopristin, sodium bicarbonate, topotecan, vancomycin.

▪ Store unopened vials at 2°–8° C (36°–46° F) and protect from light. Solutions for infusion can be kept at room temperature for 24 h and an additional 24 h if refrigerated.

## ADVERSE EFFECTS (≥1%)

**Body as a Whole:** Angioedema, *fatigue,* night sweats, *fever, chills,* myalgia. **CNS:** Headache, dizziness, depression, insomnia. **CV:** Hypotension, hypertension, tachycardia, peripheral edema, *hypertension.* **Musculoskeletal:** Arthralgia, asthenia. **GI:** *Nausea,* diarrhea, vomiting, throat irritation, anorexia, abdominal pain, hepatitis B reactivation with fulminant hepatitis, <u>hepatic failure,</u> and <u>death.</u> **Hematologic:** <u>Leukopenia, thrombocytopenia, anemia, neutropenia.</u> **Respiratory:** Bronchospasm, dyspnea, rhinitis, epitaxis, cough. **Skin:** Pruritus, rash, urticaria. **Other: Infusion-related reactions:** *Fever, chills, rigors, pruritus, urticaria, pain, flushing,* chest pain, hypotension, hypertension, dyspnea; <u>fatal infusion-related reactions</u> have been reported.

## INTERACTIONS

**Drug:** Do not use with MONOCLONAL ANTIBODIES or TNF INHIBITORS. Avoid LIVE VACCINES. **Herbal:** Do not use with echinacea due to effect on immune system.

## PHARMACOKINETICS

**Duration:** 6–12 mo. **Half-Life:** 60–174 h (increases with multiple infusions).

## NURSING IMPLICATIONS

### Black Box Warning

*Rituximab has been associated with severe and sometimes fatal infusion reactions, severe mucocutaneous reactions, hepatitis B reactivation, and progressive multifocal leukoencephalopathy.*

### Assessment & Drug Effects

▪ Monitor carefully BP and ECG status during infusion and immediately

Common adverse effects in *italic*; life-threatening effects <u>underlined</u>; generic names in **bold**; classifications in SMALL CAPS; ✤ Canadian drug name; ◉ Prototype drug

1447

report S&S of hypersensitivity (e.g., fever, chills, urticaria, pruritus, hypotension, broncho-spasms; see Appendix F for others).

- Monitor for and report promptly S&S of progressive multifocal leukoencephalopathy (PML) (e.g., hemiparesis, visual field deficits, cognitive impairment, aphasia, ataxia, and/or cranial nerve deficits).

- Monitor lab tests: Baseline and periodic CBC with differential and platelet count, peripheral CD20+ B lymphocytes, LFTs, renal function tests, and serum uric acid.

### Patient & Family Education

- Do not take antihypertensive medication within 12 h of rituximab infusions.

- Note: Use effective contraception during and for up to 12 mo following rituximab therapy.

- Report any of the following experienced during infusion: Itching, difficulty breathing, tightness in throat, dizziness, headache, or nausea.

---

# RIVAROXABAN ℗ᵣ

(riv'a-rox'a-ban)

Xarelto

**Classifications:** ANTICOAGULANT; ANTITHROMBOTIC; SELECTIVE FACTOR XA INHIBITOR

Therapeutic: ANTICOAGULANT; ANTITHROMBOTIC

## AVAILABILITY Tablet

## ACTION & *THERAPEUTIC EFFECT*

A factor Xa inhibitor that selectively blocks the active site of factor Xa thus blocking activation of factor X to factor Xa (FXa) via the intrinsic and extrinsic pathways. *Inhibits the coagulation cascade thus preventing thrombosis formation.*

## USES Prevention or treatment of deep venous thrombosis (DVT); nonvalvular

atrial fibrillation; treatment or prevention of pulmonary embolism.

## CONTRAINDICATIONS Hypersensitivity to rivaroxaban; major active bleeding; severe renal impairment (CrCl less than 30 mL/min); moderate-to-severe hepatic impairment (Child-Pugh class B or C).

## CAUTIOUS USE Spinal/epidural anesthesia or spinal puncture; concurrent platelet aggregation inhibitors, other antithrombotic agents, fibrinolytic therapy, thienopyridines and chronic use of NSAIDs; mild hepatic impairment (Child-Pugh class A); moderate renal impairment (CrCl 49–30 mL/min); pregnancy (category C). Safety and efficacy in children younger than 18 y not established.

## ROUTE & DOSAGE

### Nonvalvular Atrial Fibrillation

*Adult:* **PO** 20 mg daily

### DVT Prevention

*Adult:* **PO** 10 mg once daily beginning 6–10 h after surgery once hemostasis has been established; continue for 12 days following knee replacement surgery or 35 days following hip replacement surgery; may increase to 20 mg if coadministered with a combined P-glycoprotein and strong CYP3A4 inducer

### DVT/PE Treatment

*Adult:* **PO** 15 mg b.i.d.

### Reduce Risk of Recurrent DVT/PE

*Adult:* **PO** 20 mg qd

### *Hepatic Impairment Dosage Adjustment*

*Mild impairment (Child-Pugh class A):* Avoid use if coagulopathy is present
*Moderate or severe impairment (Child-Pugh class B or C):* Avoid use

Common adverse effects in *italic*; life-threatening effects underlined; generic names in **bold**; classifications in SMALL CAPS; ✦ Canadian drug name; ℗ Prototype drug

### Renal Impairment Dosage Adjustment

CrCl 30 to less than 50 mL/min: Observe closely and evaluate any signs or symptoms of blood loss CrCl less than 30 mL/min: Avoid use. Discontinue use in patients who develop acute renal failure

## ADMINISTRATION

### Oral

- May be given without regard to food.
- *Following spinal/epidural anesthesia or spinal puncture:* Wait at least 18 h after the last dose of rivaroxaban to remove an epidural catheter. Do not give the next rivaroxaban dose earlier than 6 h after the removal of catheter. If traumatic puncture occurs, wait 24 h before giving rivaroxaban.
- Store at 15°–30° C (59°–86° F).

## ADVERSE EFFECTS (≥1%) Body as a Whole: Pain in extremity, wound secretion. CNS: Syncope. CV: Thrombocytopenia. Hematological: *Bleeding complications.* Metabolic: Elevated ALT and AST, elevated bilirubin, *elevated gamma glutamyltransferase.* Musculoskeletal: Muscle spasm. Skin: Blister, pruritus.

## INTERACTIONS Drug: Concomitant use with drugs that are combined P-gp and CYP3A4 inhibitors (**ketoconazole, ritonavir, clarithromycin, erythromycin, itraconazole, lopinavir, indinavir, conivaptan, azithromycin, diltiazem, verapamil, quinidine, ranolazine, dronedarone, amiodarone, felodipine**) may increase rivaroxaban exposure and increase bleeding risk. Concomitant use with drugs that are combined P-gp and CYP3A4 inducers (e.g., **rifampin, carbamazepine,**

**phenytoin**) may decrease rivaroxaban levels. Concomitant use with **clopidogrel** increases bleeding time and tendencies. **Herbal: St. John's wort** may decrease rivaroxaban levels.

## PHARMACOKINETICS Absorption: 80–100% bioavailable. **Peak:** 2–4 h. **Distribution:** 92–95% plasma protein bound. **Metabolism:** Approximately 50% metabolized to inactive compounds. **Elimination:** Renal (66%) and fecal (28%). **Half-Life:** 5–9 h.

## NURSING IMPLICATIONS

### Black Box Warning

*Rivaroxaban has been associated with epidural or spinal hematomas in those receiving neuraxial anesthesia or undergoing spinal puncture.*

### Assessment & Drug Effects

- Monitor vital signs closely and report immediately S&S of bleeding and internal hemorrhage (e.g., intracranial and epidural hematoma, retinal hemorrhage, GI bleeding).
- Monitor frequently and report immediately S&S of neurologic impairment such as tingling, numbness (especially in the lower limbs), and muscular weakness.
- Report immediately neurologic impairment or an unexplained drop in BP or falling Hgb & Hct values.
- Monitor lab tests: Baseline renal function tests, baseline and periodic Hgb & Hct.

### Patient & Family Education

- Report promptly any of the following: Unusual bleeding or bruising; blood in urine or tarry stools; tingling or numbness (especially in the lower limbs); and muscular weakness.
- Notify prescriber immediately if you become pregnant or intend to

R

Common adverse effects in *italic;* life-threatening effects <u>underlined</u>; generic names in **bold;** classifications in SMALL CAPS; ♣ Canadian drug name; ⊙ Prototype drug

1449

become pregnant, or if you are breast-feeding or intend to breast-feed.

- Confer with prescriber before using a nonsteroidal anti-inflammatory drug (NSAID), aspirin, or herbal products as these may increase risk of bleeding.

# RIVASTIGMINE TARTRATE

(ri-vas'tig-meen)

Exelon

**Classifications:** CHOLINESTERASE INHIBITOR; ANTIDEMENTIA

Therapeutic: ANTIALZHEIMER'S

**AVAILABILITY** Capsule; transdermal patch

**ACTION & *THERAPEUTIC EFFECT***
Inhibits acetylcholinesterase $G_1$ form of this enzyme in the cerebral cortex and the hippocampus. The $G_1$ form of acetylcholinesterase is found in higher levels in the brains of patients with Alzheimer's disease. *Inhibits acetylcholinesterase more specifically in the brain (hippocampus and cortex) than in the heart or skeletal muscle in Alzheimer's disease.*

**USES** Treatment of mild to moderate dementia of the Alzheimer's type, Parkinson's disease-related dementia.

**CONTRAINDICATIONS** Hypersensitivity to rivastigmine or carbamate derivatives; lactation.

**CAUTIOUS USE** History of toxicity to cholinesterase inhibitors; DM; sick sinus syndrome, bradycardia, or other supraventricular cardiac conduction conditions; asthma or obstructive pulmonary disease; GI disorders including intestinal obstruction; history of or at risk for PUD or GI bleeding; urogenital tract obstruction, BPH; history of seizures; smokers; hepatic or renal impairment; low body weight; pregnancy (category B).

## ROUTE & DOSAGE

### Alzheimer's/Parkinson's Related Dementia

*Adult/Geriatric:* **PO** Start with 1.5 mg b.i.d. may increase by 1.5 mg b.i.d. q2wk if tolerated, target dose 3–6 mg b.i.d. (max: 12 mg b.i.d.) (if discontinued for less than 3 days, restart at last dose or lower; if treatment is interrupted for several days, reinitiate with 1.5 mg b.i.d. and titrate q2wk as above)

### Transdermal

*Adult:* Apply 4.6 mg patch daily, after 4 wk, can increase to 9.5 mg patch if tolerated

## ADMINISTRATION

### Oral

- Give capsules with food.
- Withhold drug and notify prescriber if significant anorexia, nausea, or vomiting occur.
- Store capsules below 25° C (77° F).

### Transdermal

- Apply patch at same time each day to back, upper arm, or chest.
- Rotate application sites and do not reapply to same site for at least 14 days.
- Do not tape or otherwise cover the patch.
- If a patch falls off, do not reapply. Replace with a new patch and remove it following the original schedule for replacement.
- Store patch at 15°–30° C (59°–86° F) in sealed pouch until ready to use.

**ADVERSE EFFECTS** (≥1%) **Body as a Whole:** Asthenia, increased sweating, syncope, fatigue, malaise, flu-like syndrome. **CV:** Hypertension. **GI:** *Nausea, vomiting, anorexia*, dyspepsia, *diarrhea, abdominal pain*, constipation, flatulence, eructation.

Common adverse effects in *italic;* life-threatening effects <u>underlined;</u> generic names in **bold;** classifications in SMALL CAPS; ✦ Canadian drug name; ⦿ Prototype drug

**Metabolic:** Weight loss. **CNS:** *Dizziness, headache,* somnolence, tremor, insomnia, confusion, depression, anxiety, hallucination, aggressive reaction. **Respiratory:** Rhinitis.

**INTERACTIONS Drug:** May exaggerate muscle relations with **succinylcholine** and other NEUROMUSCULAR BLOCKING AGENTS, may attenuate effects of ANTICHOLINERGIC AGENTS.

**PHARMACOKINETICS Absorption:** Well absorbed. **Peak:** 1 h. **Duration:** 10 h. **Distribution:** Crosses blood–brain barrier with CSF peak concentrations in 1.4–2.6 h. **Metabolism:** By cholinesterase-mediated hydrolysis. **Elimination:** In urine. **Half-Life:** 1.5 h.

## NURSING IMPLICATIONS

### Assessment & Drug Effects

- Monitor cognitive function and ability to perform ADLs.
- Monitor for and report S&S of GI distress: Anorexia, weight loss, nausea, and vomiting.
- Monitor ambulation as dizziness is a common adverse effect.
- Monitor diabetics for loss of glycemic control.

### Patient & Family Education

- Review instruction sheet provided with liquid form of the drug.
- Monitor weight at least weekly.
- Report any of the following to the prescriber: Loss of appetite, weight loss, significant nausea and/or vomiting.
- Supervise activity since there is a high potential for dizziness.

# RIZATRIPTAN BENZOATE

(ri-za-trip'tan ben'zo-ate)

**Maxalt, Maxalt-MLT**

**Classification:** SEROTONIN 5-HT$_1$ RECEPTOR AGONIST (TRIPTANS)
**Therapeutic:** ANTIMIGRAINE
**Prototype:** Sumatriptan

**AVAILABILITY** Tablet; disintegrating tablets

**ACTION & *THERAPEUTIC EFFECT***
Selective (5-HT$_{1B/1D}$) receptor agonist that reverses the vasodilation of cranial blood vessels associated with a migraine. *Activation of the 5-HT$_{1B/1D}$ receptors reduces the pain pathways associated with the migraine headache as well as reversing vasodilation of cranial blood vessels.*

**USES** Acute migraine headaches with or without aura.

**CONTRAINDICATIONS** Hypersensitivity to rizatriptan; CAD; Prinzmetal's angina (potential for vasospasm); ischemic heart disease; risk factors for CAD such as hypertension, hypercholesterolemia, obesity, diabetes, smoking, and strong family history; hemiplegia; concurrent administration with ergotamine drugs or sumatriptan; concurrent administration with MAOIS; or within 14 days of use; basilar or hemiplegic migraine.

**CAUTIOUS USE** Hypersensitivity to sumatriptan; renal or hepatic impairment; hypertension; asthmatic patients; pregnancy (category C); lactation. Safety and efficacy in children younger than 18 y not established.

## ROUTE & DOSAGE

| Acute Migraine |
| --- |
| *Adult:* PO 5–10 mg, may repeat in 2 h if necessary (max: 30 mg/24 h); 5 mg with concurrent propranolol (max: 15 mg/24 h) |

## ADMINISTRATION

### Oral

- Give any time after symptoms of migraine appear. If symptoms

R

Common adverse effects in *italic*; life-threatening effects underlined; generic names in **bold**; classifications in SMALL CAPS; ♣ Canadian drug name; ⊘ Prototype drug

1451

return, a second tablet may be given but no sooner than 2 h after the first.
- Do not exceed 30 mg (three doses) in any 24 h period.
- Do not give within 24 h of an ergot-containing drug or another 5-HT$_1$ agonist.
- Store at 15°–30° C (59°–86° F) and protect from light and moisture.

**ADVERSE EFFECTS** (≥1%) **Body as a Whole:** Asthenia, fatigue, pain, pressure sensation, paresthesias, throat pressure, warm/cold sensations. **CNS:** Somnolence, dizziness, headache, hypesthesia, decreased mental acuity, euphoria, tremor. **CV:** Coronary artery vasospasm, transient myocardial ischemia, MI, ventricular tachycardia, ventricular fibrillation, chest pain/tightness/heaviness, palpitations. **GI:** Dry mouth, nausea, vomiting, diarrhea. **Respiratory:** Dyspnea. **Skin:** Flushing. **Endocrine:** Hot flashes.

**INTERACTIONS Drug: Propranolol** may increase concentrations of rizatriptan, use smaller rizatriptan doses; **dihydroergotamine, methysergide,** other 5-HT$_1$ AGONISTS may cause prolonged vasospastic reactions; SSRIS have rarely caused weakness, hyperreflexia, and incoordination; MAOIS should not be used with 5-HT$_1$ AGONISTS. **Herbal: St. John's wort** may increase triptan toxicity.

**PHARMACOKINETICS Absorption:** 45% of oral dose reaches systemic circulation. **Peak:** 1–1.5 h for oral tabs; 1.6–2.5 h for orally disintegrating tablets. **Metabolism:** Via oxidative deamination by monoamine oxidase A. **Elimination:** Primarily in urine (82%). **Half-Life:** 2–3 h.

**NURSING IMPLICATIONS**

**Assessment & Drug Effects**
- Monitor cardiovascular status carefully following first dose in patients at

risk for CAD (e.g., postmenopausal women, men older than 40 y, persons with known CAD risk factors) or coronary artery vasospasms.
- ECG is recommended following first administration of rizatriptan to someone with known CAD risk factors.
- Report immediately to prescriber: Chest pain or tightness in chest or throat that is severe or does not quickly resolve.
- Monitor periodically cardiovascular status with continued rizatriptan use.

**Patient & Family Education**
- Do not exceed 30 mg (three doses) in 24 h.
- Allow orally disintegrating tablets to dissolve on tongue; no liquid is needed.
- Contact prescriber immediately if any of the following develop following rizatriptan use: Symptoms of angina (e.g., severe and/or persistent pain or tightness in chest or throat), hypersensitivity (e.g., wheezing, facial swelling, skin rash, or hives), abdominal pain.
- Report any other adverse effects (e.g., tingling, flushing, dizziness) at next prescriber visit.

# ROFLUMILAST
(ro-flu'mi-last)
Daliresp

**Classifications:** RESPIRATORY AGENT; ANTI-INFLAMMATORY; PHOSPHODIESTERASE 4 (PDE4) INHIBITOR
Therapeutic: ANTI-INFLAMMATORY; PDE4 INHIBITOR

**AVAILABILITY** Tablet

**ACTION & THERAPEUTIC EFFECT**
Selectively inhibits phosphodiesterase 4 (PDE4), a major enzyme found in inflammatory and immune cells, thus indirectly suppressing

the release of cytokines and other products of inflammation. *Has an anti-inflammatory effect in pulmonary diseases*.

**USES** Reduction of the prevalence of chronic obstructive pulmonary disease (COPD) exacerbations.

**CONTRAINDICATIONS** Moderate-to-severe liver impairment (Child-Pugh class B or C); suicidal ideation; lactation

**CAUTIOUS USE** Mild hepatic impairment (Child-Pugh class A); history of psychiatric illness including anxiety, depression, or suicidal thoughts; clinically significant weight loss; pregnancy (category C). Safety and efficacy in children not established.

**ROUTE & DOSAGE**

**Chronic Obstructive Pulmonary Disease**
*Adult:* **PO** 500 mcg once daily

**ADMINISTRATION**

**Oral**
- May be given with or without food.
- Store at 15°–30° C (59°–86° F)

**ADVERSE EFFECTS** (≥1%) **Body as a Whole:** Influenza. **CNS:** Anxiety, depression, dizziness, headache, insomnia, tremor **GI:** Abdominal pain, decreased appetite, *diarrhea*, dyspepsia, gastritis, nausea, vomiting, *weight loss*. **Musculoskeletal:** Back pain, muscle spasms. **Respiratory:** Rhinitis, sinusitis. **Urogenital:** Urinary tract infection, <u>acute renal failure</u>.

**INTERACTIONS Drug:** Coadministration with strong CYP3A4 or CYP3A4/CYP1A2 inhibitors (e.g., **cimetidine,** **ketoconazole, ritonavir, erythromycin, fluvoxamine**) may increase the levels of roflumilast. Coadministration with strong CYP3A4 inducers (i.e., **carbamazepine, phenobarbital, phenytoin,** RIFAMYCINS) may decrease the levels of roflumilast. Coadministration **gestodene** may increase the levels of roflumilast. **Food:** None listed. **Herbal: St. John's wort** may decrease the levels of roflumilast.

**PHARMACOKINETICS Absorption:** 80% Bioavailable. **Peak:** 1 h. **Distribution:** 99% plasma protein bound. **Metabolism:** In liver to active and inactive metabolites. **Elimination:** Primarily renal. **Half-Life:** 17 h (30 h for active metabolite).

**NURSING IMPLICATIONS**

**Assessment & Drug Effects**
- Monitor for and report promptly new onset or worsening insomnia, anxiety, depression, suicidal thoughts, or other significant mood changes.
- Monitor weight at regular intervals. Report significant weight loss to prescriber.

**Patient & Family Education**
- Roflumilast is not a bronchodilator and does not provide relief of acute bronchospasm.
- Report to prescriber any of the following: Disturbing mood changes such as anxiety or depression; difficulty sleeping; suicidal thoughts; persistent nausea and/or diarrhea.
- Monitor your weight and report unexplained weight loss.
- Do not self-treat depression with St. John's wort.

**ROLAPITANT**
(ro-la'pi-tant)
Varubi

R

Common adverse effects in *italic;* life-threatening effects <u>underlined;</u> generic names in **bold;** classifications in SMALL CAPS; ◆ Canadian drug name; ⊘ Prototype drug

1453

**Classifications:** CENTRALLY ACT-ING ANTIEMETIC; SUBSTANCE P/NEU-ROKININ 1 (NK1) ANTAGONIST
Therapeutic: ANTIEMETIC
**Prototype** Arepitant

## AVAILABILITY Tablets

## ACTION & *THERAPEUTIC EFFECT*

Acts at neurokinin-1 (NK-1) receptors in vomiting centers within the CNS to block their activation by substance P which is released as an unwanted consequence of chemotherapy. *Prevents both acute and delayed chemotherapy-induced nausea and vomiting.*

## USES Used in adults, and in combination with other antiemetic agents, for the prevention of delayed nausea and vomiting associated with initial and repeat courses of emetogenic cancer chemotherapy.

## CONTRAINDICATIONS Hypersensitivity to rolapitant; concurrent use of thioridazine; severe hepatic impairment (Child-Pugh class C); lactation.

## CAUTIOUS USE CYP2D6 substrates with a narrow therapeutic index such as pimozide; mild or moderate hepatic impairment (Child-Pugh class A or B; prolonged QT interval; pregnancy. Safety and efficacy in children younger than 18 y not established.

## ROUTE & DOSAGE

### Chemotherapy-Induced Nausea/Vomiting Prophylaxis

*Adult:* PO 180 mg single dose 1–2 h prior to chemotherapy; repeat at intervals of at least 2 wk, prior to the start of each chemotherapy cycle

### *Hepatic Impairment Dosage Adjustment*
*Severe impairment (Child-Pugh class C):* Avoid use

## ADMINISTRATION

### Oral
- May give without regard to meals 1–2 h prior to chemotherapy.
- Capsule should be swallowed whole.
- Store at 15°–30° C (59°–86° F).

## ADVERSE EFFECTS (≥3%) **Body as a Whole:** Decreased appetite, dizziness, hiccups. **GI:** Abdominal pain, dyspepsia, stomatitis. **Hematological:** Anemia. **Metabolic:** Neutropenia. **Urogenital:** Urinary tract infection.

## INTERACTIONS **Drug:** Rolapitant may increase the levels of coadministered drugs that require CYP2D6 for metabolism (e.g., **dextromethorphan, pimozide, thioridazine**), are BCRP substrates (e.g., **irinotecan, methotrexate, topotecan**), or are P-glycoprotein substrates with a narrow therapeutic index (e.g., **digoxin**). Strong CYP3A4 inducers (e.g., **rifampin**) reduce the levels of rolapitant.

## PHARMACOKINETICS **Peak:** 4 h. **Distribution:** Highly plasma protein bound (>99.8%). **Metabolism:** In liver by CYP450 enzymes. **Elimination:** Fecal (73%) and renal (14%). **Half-Life:** Approx. 7 d.

## NURSING IMPLICATIONS

### Assessment & Drug Effects
- Monitor for degree of emetic control.
- Monitor cardiac status especially with preexisting CV disease or concurrent use of any CYP2D6 substrate such as pimozide.
- Monitor lab tests: Periodic CBC with differential, and Hct & Hgb.

### Patient & Family Education
- Report to prescriber if nausea and vomiting are not well controlled.

R

Common adverse effects in *italic;* life-threatening effects <u>underlined;</u> generic names in **bold;** classifications in SMALL CAPS; ♣ Canadian drug name; ⊘ Prototype drug

- Do not take rolapitant if taking thioridazine as the combination can cause serious or life-threatening heart rhythm changes.
- Do not take rolapitant more than once every 14 days.
- Inform prescriber when starting or stopping any concomitant medications.

## ROMIDEPSIN
(rom-i-dep′sin)
Istodax

**Classifications:** ANTINEOPLASTIC; HISTONE DEACETYLASE (HDAC) INHIBITOR
Therapeutic: ANTINEOPLASTIC

**AVAILABILITY** Powder for reconstitution for injection

**ACTION & THERAPEUTIC EFFECT**
Inhibits histone deacetylase, an enzyme required for completion of the cell cycle in certain cancers, thus inducing cell cycle arrest and apoptosis in these cancer cells. The mechanism of antineoplastic effect has not been fully characterized. *Effective as a cytotoxic agent against cutaneous T-cell lymphoma.*

**USES** Treatment of cutaneous or peripheral T-cell lymphoma.

**CONTRAINDICATIONS** Severe bone marrow depression; pregnancy (category D); lactation.

**CAUTIOUS USE** Risk factors for potassium or magnesium imbalance, thrombocytopenia, or leukopenia; congenital long QT syndrome, history of significant CV disease; moderate-to-severe hepatic impairment; end-stage renal disease. Safe use in children not established.

## ROUTE & DOSAGE

### Cutaneous or Peripheral T-Cell Lymphoma (CTCL)
*Adult:* **IV** 14 mg/m² over 4 h on days 1, 8, and 15, repeat every 28 days. Repeat cycle until disease progression has been treated or unacceptable toxicity occurs.

*Toxicity Dosage Adjustment (National Cancer Institute Common Toxicity Criteria, CTC)*

*For CTC grade 3 or 4 neutropenia or thrombocytopenia:* Hold romidepsin until ANC is 1,500/mm³ or higher and/or platelet count is 75,000/mm³ or higher, or parameters return to baseline values. Then, resume romidepsin 14 mg/m².

*For CTC grade 4 febrile neutropenia or thrombocytopenia requiring platelet transfusion:* Hold romidepsin until cytopenia is no greater than grade 1 and permanently reduce dose to 10 mg/m².

*For CTC grade 2 or 3 nonhematological toxicity:* Hold romidepsin until toxicity is no greater than grade 1 or returns to baseline. Resume romidepsin 14 mg/m².

*For recurrent CTC grade 3 nonhematological toxicity:* Hold romidepsin until toxicity is no greater than grade 1 or returns to baseline and permanently reduce dose to 10 mg/m².

*For CTC grade 4 nonhematological toxicity:* Hold romidepsin until toxicity is no greater than grade 1 or returns to baseline and permanently reduce dose to 10 mg/m².

R

Common adverse effects in *italic*; life-threatening effects <u>underlined</u>; generic names in **bold**; classifications in SMALL CAPS; ◆ Canadian drug name; ⊕ Prototype drug

1455

*For recurrent CTC grade 3 or 4 nonhematological toxicity after dose reduction:* Discontinue therapy.

## ADMINISTRATION
### Intravenous ONLY

This drug is a cytotoxic agent and caution should be used to prevent any contact with the drug. Follow institutional or standard guidelines for preparation, handling, and disposal of cytotoxic agents.

*PREPARE:* **IV Infusion:** Withdraw 2 mL of supplied diluent and inject slowly into the 10 mL powder vial to yield 5 mg/mL. Swirl to dissolve. ▪ Withdraw the required dose of reconstituted solution and add to 500 mL NS and invert container to dissolve. ▪ Should be administered as soon as possible after dilution.

*ADMINISTER:* **IV Infusion:** Give over 4 h. Note: Ensure that potassium and magnesium are within normal range before administration.

*INCOMPATIBILITIES:* **Solution/additive:** Do not mix with another drug. **Y-site:** Do not mix with another drug.

▪ Reconstituted vials are stable for 8 h and IV solutions are stable for 24 h at room temperature. Store unopened vials at 15°–30° C (59°–86° F).

## ADVERSE EFFECTS (≥20%) **Body as a Whole:** *Asthenia,* fatigue, hyperglycemia, *infections,* fever. **CV:** ECG ST-T wave changes, hypotension. **GI:** *Anorexia, constipation, diarrhea, dysgeusia, nausea, vomiting.* **Hematological:** *Anemia, neutropenia,* leukopenia, *lymphopenia, thrombocytopenia.* **Metabolic:** Elevated ALT, elevated AST, hypermagnesemia, hyperuricemia, hypoalbuminemia, hypocalcemia, hypokalemia, hypomagnesemia, hyponatremia, hypophosphatemia. **Skin:** Pruritus, dermatitis, exfoliative dermatitis.

## INTERACTIONS **Drug:** Coadministation of CYP3A4 inducers (e.g., **carbamazepine, phenobarbital, phenytoin, rifampin**) can decrease the levels of romidepsin. Coadministration of strong CYP3A4 inhibitors (e.g., **atazanavir, indinavir, itraconazole, ketoconazole, nefazodone, nelfinavir, ritonavir, saquinavir, telithromycin, voriconazole**) can increase the levels of romidepsin. Coadministration of drugs that prolong the QT interval (e.g., **amiodarone, bretylium, disopyramide, dofetilide, procainamide, quinidine, sotalol), arsenic trioxide, chlorpromazine, cisapride, dolasetron, droperidol, mefloquine, mesoridazine, moxifloxacin, pentamidine, pimozide, tacrolimus, thioridazine, and ziprasidone**) may produce life-threatening arrhythmias. **Food:** Grapefruit juice can increase the levels of romidepsin. **Herbal:** **St. John's wort** can decrease the levels of romidepsin.

## PHARMACOKINETICS **Distribution:** 92–94% plasma protein bound. **Metabolism:** Extensive hepatic metabolism by CYP3A4. **Elimination:** Primarily biliary excretion. **Half-Life:** 3 h.

## NURSING IMPLICATIONS
### Assessment & Drug Effects
▪ Monitor ECG at baseline and periodically throughout treatment.
▪ Report immediately electrolyte imbalances or QT prolongation.
▪ Monitor lab tests: Baseline and prior to each dose: Serum electrolytes, CBC with differential including platelet count, LFTs and serum albumin.

R

Common adverse effects in *italic;* life-threatening effects <u>underlined;</u> generic names in **bold;** classifications in SMALL CAPS; ♣ Canadian drug name; ◓ Prototype drug

## Patient & Family Education

- Report promptly any of the following: Excessive nausea, chest pain, shortness of breath, or abnormal heart beat.
- Seek medical attention if unusual bleeding occurs.
- Women of childbearing age who use an estrogen-containing contraceptive should add a barrier contraceptive to prevent pregnancy.

# ROPINIROLE HYDROCHLORIDE

(re-pin'i-role)

Requip, Requip XL

**Classifications:** DOPAMINE RECEPTOR AGONIST; ANTIPARKINSON
**Therapeutic:** ANTIPARKINSON
**Prototype:** Carbidopa

**AVAILABILITY** Tablet; extended release tablet

## ACTION & THERAPEUTIC EFFECT

Precise mechanism of action is unknown, but believed to be due to stimulation of postsynaptic dopamine $D_2$-type receptors within the caudate putamen in the brain. *Effectiveness indicated by improvement in idiopathic Parkinson's disease.*

**USES** Idiopathic Parkinson's disease, restless legs syndrome.

**CONTRAINDICATIONS** Hypersensitivity to ropinirole or pramipexole.

**CAUTIOUS USE** Hepatic impairment; severe renal impairment; mental instability; concomitant use of CNS depressants; pregnancy (category C); lactation. Safety and efficacy in children not established.

# ROUTE & DOSAGE

### Parkinson's Disease

*Adult:* **PO Immediate release** Start with 0.25 mg t.i.d., titrate up by 0.25 mg/dose t.i.d. qwk to a target dose of 1 mg t.i.d.; if response is still not satisfactory, may continue to increase by 1.5 mg/day qwk to a dose of 9 mg/day, and then by 3 mg/day or less weekly (max: 24 mg/day); **Extended release** 2 mg daily for 1–2 wk then increase by 2 mg/day at one week intervals (max: 24 mg/day)

### Restless Legs Syndrome

*Adult:* **PO** Take 0.25 mg 1–3 h before bed × 2 days, increase to 0.5 mg for the first wk, then increase by 0.5 mg qwk to a maximum of 4 mg

## ADMINISTRATION

### Oral

- Give with food to reduce occurrence of nausea.
- Do not crush extended release tablets. Ensure that they are swallowed whole.
- Drug should not be abruptly discontinued. Dose should be tapered over a period of days.
- Store at 15°–30° C (59°–86° F).

**ADVERSE EFFECTS (≥1%) Body as a Whole:** Increased sweating, dry mouth, flushing, asthenia, *fatigue,* pain, edema, malaise, *viral infection,* UTI, impotence. **CNS:** *Dizziness, somnolence, sudden sleep attacks,* hallucinations, confusion, amnesia, hypesthesia, yawning, hyperkinesia, impaired concentration, vertigo, hallucinations. **CV:** *Syncope,* chest pain, orthostatic symptoms, hypertension, palpitations, atrial fibrillation, extrasystoles, hypotension, tachycardia, peripheral edema, peripheral ischemia. **GI:** *Nausea, vomiting, dyspepsia,* abdominal pain, anorexia, flatulence. **Respiratory:** Pharyngitis, rhinitis, sinusitis, bronchitis, dyspnea. **Special Senses:** Abnormal vision, xerophthalmia, eye abnormality.

**INTERACTIONS Drug:** Ropinirole levels may be increased by ESTROGENS, QUINOLONE ANTIBIOTICS, **cimetidine, diltiazem, erythromycin, fluvoxamine, mexiletine;** effects may be antagonized by PHENOTHIAZINES, BUTYROPHENONES, **metoclopramide zileuton** may increase ropinerole levels.

**PHARMACOKINETICS Absorption:** Rapidly from GI tract; 55% bioavailability. **Peak:** 1–2 h. **Distribution:** 30–40% protein bound. **Metabolism:** In liver (CYP1A2). **Elimination:** Primarily in urine. **Half-Life:** 6 h.

## NURSING IMPLICATIONS

### Assessment & Drug Effects
- Monitor cardiac status. Report increases in BP and HR to prescriber.
- Monitor carefully for orthostatic hypotension, especially during dose escalation.
- Monitor level of alertness. Institute appropriate precautions to prevent injury due to dizziness or drowsiness.
- Monitor lab test: Periodic BUN and creatinine, and LFTs.

### Patient & Family Education
- Be aware that hallucinations are a possible adverse effect and occur more often in older adults.
- Make position changes slowly, especially after long periods of lying or sitting. Postural hypotension is common, especially during early treatment.
- Exercise caution with hazardous activities requiring alertness since drowsiness and sedation are common adverse effects. Effects are additive with alcohol or other CNS depressants.
- Report behavioral changes (e.g., impulsive behavior) to prescriber.

# ROPIVACAINE HYDROCHLORIDE
(ro-piv'i-cane)
Naropin
**Classification:** LOCAL ANESTHETIC (ESTER-TYPE)
**Therapeutic:** LOCAL ANESTHETIC
**Prototype:** Procaine HCl

**AVAILABILITY** Solution for injection

**ACTION & THERAPEUTIC EFFECT** Blocks the generation and conduction of nerve impulses, probably by increasing the threshold for electrical excitability. *Local anesthetic action produces loss of sensation and motor activity in areas of the body close to the injection site.*

**USES** Local and regional anesthesia, postoperative pain management, anesthesia/pain management for obstetric procedures.

**CONTRAINDICATIONS** Hypersensitivity to ropivacaine or any local anesthetic of the amide type; generalized septicemia, inflammation or sepsis at the proposed injection site; cerebral spinal diseases (e.g., meningitis); heart block, hypotension, hypertension, GI hemorrhage.

**CAUTIOUS USE** Debilitated, older adult, or acutely ill patients; arrhythmias, shock; pregnancy (category B); lactation.

R

Common adverse effects in *italic;* life-threatening effects <u>underlined</u>; generic names in **bold;** classifications in SMALL CAPS; ♣ Canadian drug name; ◎ Prototype drug

## ROUTE & DOSAGE

**Surgical Anesthesia**
*Adult:* **Epidural** 25–200 mg
(0.5–1% solution); **Nerve block**
5–250 mg (0.5%, 0.75% solution)

**Labor Pain**
*Adult:* **Epidural** 20–40 mg (0.2%
solution) then 12–28 mg/h

**Postoperative Pain Management**
*Adult:* **Epidural** 12–28 mg/h
(0.2% solution); **Infiltration**
2–200 mg (0.2–0.5% solution)

## ADMINISTRATION

**Intrathecal**
- Avoid rapid injection of large volumes of ropivacaine. Incremental doses should always be used to achieve the smallest effective dose and concentration.
- Use an infusion concentration of 2 mg/mL (0.2%) for postoperative analgesia.
- Do not use disinfecting agents containing heavy metal ions (e.g., mercury, copper, zinc, etc.) on skin insertion site or to clean the ropivacaine container top.
- Discard continuous infusions solution after 24 h; it contains no preservatives.
- Store unopened at 20°–25° C (68°–77° F).

## ADVERSE EFFECTS (≥1%) **Body as a Whole:** Pain, fever, rigors, hypoesthesia. **CNS:** Paresthesia, headache, dizziness, anxiety. **CV:** *Hypotension,* bradycardia, hypertension, tachycardia, chest pain, fetal bradycardia. **GI:** Nausea. **Skin:** Pruritus. **Urogenital:** Urinary retention, oliguria. **Hematologic:** Anemia.

## INTERACTIONS **Drug:** Additive adverse effects with other LOCAL ANESTHETICS.

## PHARMACOKINETICS **Onset:**
1–30 min (average 10–20 min) depending on dose/route of administration. **Duration:** 0.5–8 h depending on dose/route of administration. **Distribution:** 94% protein bound. **Metabolism:** In the liver by CYP1A. **Elimination:** In urine. **Half-Life:** 1.8–4.2 h.

## NURSING IMPLICATIONS

**Assessment & Drug Effects**
- Monitor carefully cardiovascular and respiratory status throughout treatment period. Assess for hypotension and bradycardia.
- Report immediately S&S of CNS stimulation or CNS depression.

**Patient & Family Education**
- Report any of the following to prescriber immediately: Restlessness, anxiety, tinnitus, blurred vision, tremors.

## ROSIGLITAZONE MALEATE ℗

(ros-i-glit'a-zone)
Avandia

**Classifications:** ANTIDIABETIC; THIAZOLIDINEDIONE (GLITAZONE)
**Therapeutic:** ANTIHYPERGLYCEMIC

## AVAILABILITY Tablet

## ACTION & *THERAPEUTIC EFFECT*

Lowers blood sugar levels by improving target cell response to insulin in Type 2 diabetics. It reduces cellular insulin resistance and decreases hepatic glucose output (gluconeogenesis). *Reduces hyperglycemia and hyperlipidemia, thus improving hyperinsulinemia without stimulating pancreatic insulin secretion. Effectiveness indicated by decreased HbA1C.*

R

Common adverse effects in *italic;* life-threatening effects underlined; generic names in **bold;** classifications in SMALL CAPS; ◆ Canadian drug name; ℗ Prototype drug

1459

**USES** Type 2 diabetes.

**UNLABELED USES** Polycystic ovary syndrome.

**CONTRAINDICATIONS** Hypersensitivity to rosiglitazone; patients with New York Heart Association Class III and IV cardiac status (e.g., CHF); symptomatic heart failure; initiation in patients with ischemic heart disease; active hepatic disease; ALT enzyme greater than 2.5 × ULN; high risk for bone fractures; Type I DM; lactation.

**CAUTIOUS USE** CHF or risk for CHF; angina; patients with ongoing edema; anemia; hepatic impairment; older adults; pregnancy (category C). Safety and efficacy in children younger than 18 y not established.

## ROUTE & DOSAGE

### Type 2 Diabetes Mellitus
*Adult:* **PO** Start at 4 mg daily or 2 mg b.i.d., may increase after 12 wk (max: 8 mg/day in 1–2 divided doses)

### Hepatic Impairment Dosage Adjustment
*If ALT is greater than 2.5 × ULN:* Do not use

## ADMINISTRATION

### Oral
- May be given without regard to meals.
- Store at 15°–30° C (59°–86° F) in tight, light-resistant container.

**ADVERSE EFFECTS** (≥1%) **Body as a Whole:** *Edema*, anemia, headache, back pain, fatigue. **CV:** Edema, fluid retention, exacerbation of heart failure, increased risk of heart attack. **GI:** Diarrhea. **Metabolic:** Hypoglycemia, increased cholesterol, weight gain. **Respiratory:** Upper respiratory tract infection, sinusitis. **Special Senses:** Macular edema. **Other:** Hyperglycemia. **CNS:** *Headache*.

**INTERACTIONS Drug: Insulin** may increase risk of heart failure or edema; enhance hypoglycemia with ORAL ANTIDIABETIC AGENTS, **ketoconazole, gemfibrozil** may increase effect. **Bosentan, rifampin** may reduce effect. **Herbal: Garlic, ginseng, green tea** may potentiate hypoglycemic effects.

**PHARMACOKINETICS Absorption:** 99% from GI tract. **Peak:** 1 h, food delays time to peak by 1.75 h. **Duration:** Greater than 24 h. **Distribution:** Greater than 99% protein bound. **Metabolism:** In liver (CYP2C8) to inactive metabolites. **Elimination:** 64% urine, 23% feces. **Half-Life:** 3–4 h. Liver disease increases serum concentrations and increases half-life by 2 h.

## NURSING IMPLICATIONS

### Assessment & Drug Effects
- Monitor for S&S of hypoglycemia (possible when insulin/sulfonylureas are coadministered).
- Monitor for S&S of CHF or exacerbation of symptoms with preexisting CHF.
- Withhold drug and notify prescriber if ALT greater than 2.5 × normal or patient jaundiced.
- Monitor weight and notify prescriber of development of edema.
- Monitor lab tests: Baseline LFTs, and periodically thereafter or more often when elevated; periodic fasting serum glucose and HbA1C.

## Patient & Family Education

- Report promptly any of the following: Rapid weight gain, edema, shortness of breath, or exercise intolerance.
- Be aware that resumed ovulation is possible in nonovulating premenopausal women.
- Use or add barrier contraceptive if using hormonal contraception.
- Report immediately to prescriber: S&S of liver dysfunction such as unexplained anorexia, nausea, vomiting, abdominal pain, fatigue, dark urine; or S&S of fluid retention such as weight gain, edema, or activity intolerance.
- Combination therapy: May need adjustment of other antidiabetic drugs to avoid hypoglycemia.

# ROSUVASTATIN

(ro-su-va-sta′ten)

Crestor

**Classifications:** ANTILIPEMIC; LIPID-LOWERING; HMG-COA REDUCTASE INHIBITOR (STATIN)

**Therapeutic:** ANTILIPEMIC; STATIN

**Prototype:** Lovastatin

## AVAILABILITY Tablet

## ACTION & *THERAPEUTIC EFFECT*

A potent inhibitor of HMG-CoA reductase, an enzyme that catalyzes the conversion of HMG-CoA to mevalonic acid, an early and rate-limiting step in cholesterol biosynthesis. This results in reducing the amount of mevalonic acid, a precursor of cholesterol. It increases the number of hepatic HDL receptors on the cell surface to enhance uptake and catabolism of LDL. It also inhibits hepatic synthesis of very low density lipoprotein (VLDL). *Reduces total cholesterol and LDL cholesterol; additionally, lowers plasma triglycerides and VLDL while increasing HDL.*

## USES

Adjunct to diet for the reduction of LDL cholesterol and triglycerides in patients with primary hypercholesterolemia, hypertriglyceridemia, and mixed dyslipidemia; prevention of cardiovascular disease.

## CONTRAINDICATIONS

Hypersensitivity to any component of the product, active liver disease or unexplained persistent elevations of serum transaminases; rhabdomyolysis; pregnancy (category X), women of childbearing potential not using appropriate contraceptive measures; lactation.

## CAUTIOUS USE

Concomitant use of cyclosporine and gemfibrozil; Asian descent; DM; excessive alcohol use or history of liver disease; renal impairment; older adults, hypothyroidism. Safe use in children younger than 10 y not established.

## ROUTE & DOSAGE

### Hyperlipidemia/Slowing Atherosclerosis Progression

*Adult/Adolescent/Child (10 y or older):* **PO** 10 mg once daily (5–40 mg/day (max: 40 mg/day); If taking cyclosporine, gemfibrozil, lopinavir/ritonavir, start with 5 mg/day

*Geriatric:* Initial dose of 5 mg/day

### Homozygous Familial Hypercholesterolemia

*Adult:* **PO** 20 mg daily (max: 40 mg/day)

R

**Prevention of Cardiovascular Disease**

*Adult:* **PO** 5–40 mg daily

***Renal Impairment Dosage Adjustment***

*CrCl less than 30 mL/min:*
5 mg once daily (max: 10 mg/day)

## ADMINISTRATION

### Oral

- Persons of Asian descent may be slow metabolizers and may require half the normal dose.
- May give any time of day without regard to food.
- Do not give within 2 h of an antacid.
- Store at or below 30° C (86° F).

**ADVERSE EFFECTS** (≥1%) **Body as a Whole:** Asthenia, back pain, flu-like syndrome, chest pain, infection, pain, peripheral edema. **CNS:** Headache, dizziness, insomnia, hypertonia, paresthesia, depression, anxiety, vertigo, neuralgia. **CV:** Hypertension, angina, vasodilatation, palpitations. **GI:** Diarrhea, dyspepsia, nausea, abdominal pain, constipation, gastroenteritis, vomiting, flatulence, gastritis. **Endocrine:** Diabetes. **Hematologic:** Anemia, ecchymosis. **Musculoskeletal:** Myalgia, arthritis, arthralgia, rhabdomyolysis (especially with dose greater than 40 mg). **Respiratory:** Pharyngitis, rhinitis, sinusitis, bronchitis, increased cough, dyspnea, pneumonia, asthma. **Skin:** Rash, pruritus. **Urogenital:** UTI.

**INTERACTIONS Drug: Atazanavir, cyclosporine, gemfibrozil, niacin** may increase risk of rhabdomyolysis; ANTACIDS may decrease rosuvastatin absorption; may cause increase in INR with **warfarin. Herbal: Red-yeast rice** increases rhabdomyolysis risk.

**PHARMACOKINETICS Absorption:** Well absorbed. **Peak:** 3–5 h. **Metabolism:** Limited metabolism in the liver (not CYP3A4). **Elimination:** Primarily in feces (90%). **Half-Life:** 20 h.

## NURSING IMPLICATIONS

### Assessment & Drug Effects

- Monitor for and report promptly S&S of myopathy (e.g., skeletal muscle pain, tenderness or weakness).
- Withhold drug and notify prescriber if CPK levels are markedly elevated (10 or more × ULN) or if myopathy is diagnosed or suspected.
- Monitor CV status, especially with a known history of hypertension or heart disease.
- Monitor diabetics for loss of glycemic control.
- Monitor lab tests: Baseline CPK and repeat with S&S of myopathy; periodic LFTs.

### Patient & Family Education

- Do not take antacids within 2 h of taking this drug.
- Women should use reliable means of contraception to prevent pregnancy while taking this drug.

## SACUBITRIL AND VALSARTAN
(sac'u-bi-tril and val-sar-tan)

Entresto

**Classifications:** CARDIOVASULAR AGENT; NEPRILYSIN INHIBITOR; ANGIOTENSIN II RECEPTOR BLOCKER

Therapeutic: HEART FAILURE AGENT

**AVAILABILITY** Tablets

## ACTIONS & *THERAPEUTIC EFFECT*

Sacubitril is a prodrug that, when converted to an active metabolite

(LBQ657), inhibits the enzyme, neprilysin, leading to increased levels of natriuretic peptides. Valsartan is an angiotensin receptor antagonist that selectively blocks the vasoconstriction and aldosterone-secreting effects of angiotensin II. *Decreases afterload thus facilitating increased cardiac output.*

**USES** Indicated for risk reduction of cardiovascular death and hospitalization from heart failure (HF) in patients with chronic HF (NYHA Class II-IV) and reduced ejection fraction.

**CONTRAINDICATIONS** Hypersensitivity to any component; history of angioedema related to previous ACE inhibitor or ARB therapy; concomitant use with ACE inhibitors; concomitant use with aliskiren in patients with diabetes; severe hepatic impairment; pregnancy; lactation.

**CAUTIOUS USE** Prior history of angioedema; African American ancestry; concomitant use of potassium-sparing diuretics, NSAIDs, or lithium; hypotension; renal impairment; mild to moderate hepatic impairment; potassium imbalance; risk factors for hyperkalemia including diabetes, hypoaldosteronism, or high potassium diet; older adults. Safety and efficacy in children 18 y or younger not established.

## ROUTE & DOSAGE

**Heart Failure**
*Adult:* **PO** Initial dose of 24/26 mg (sacubitril/valsartan) or 49/51 mg b.i.d.; double dose q2–4wk up to 97/103 mg b.i.d. as tolerated

*Hepatic Impairment Dosage Adjustment*
*Moderate impairment (Child-Pugh class B):* Initial dose of 24/26 mg

b.i.d., double dose q2–4wk up to 97/103 mg b.i.d. as tolerated
*Severe impairment (Child-Pugh class C):* Not recommended

*Renal Impairment Dosage Adjustment*
*Severe impairment:* Initial dose of 24/26 mg b.i.d., double dose q2–4wk up to 97/103 mg b.i.d. as tolerated

## ADMINISTRATION
**Oral**
- Correct volume or salt depletion prior to administration.
- May be given without regard to food.
- Store at 15°–30° C (59°–86° F). Protect from moisture.

**ADVERSE EFFECTS** (≥1%) **Body as a Whole:** Falls, renal failure. **CNS:** Dizziness. **CV:** *Hypotension*, orthostatic hypotension. **Hematological:** Decreased hemoglobin and hematocrit, increased serum creatinine. **Metabolic:** *Hyperkalemia*. **Respiratory:** Cough.

**INTERACTIONS Drug:** Concomitant use with an ANGIOTENSION CONVERTING ENZYME INHIBITOR increases the risk of angioedema. Concomitant use of POTASSIUM SPARING DIURETICS (e.g., **amiloride, spironolactone, triamterene**) may lead to increased potassium levels. Concomitant use with NSAIDs in older adults, patients who are volume-depleted, or patients with compromised renal function may result in worsening of renal function. Sacubitril/valsartan may increase the levels of **lithium.**

## PHARMACOKINETICS Absorption:
**Sacubitril** is greater than 60% bioavailable. **Peak:** Sacubitril 0.5 h.; LBQ657 2h.; valsartan 1.5 h. **Distribution:** Highly plasma protein bound (94–97%). **Metabolism:** Sacubitril is metabolized to an active metabolite, LBQ657; Valsartan minimal metabolism. **Elimination:** Sacubitril, 52–68% renal and 37–48% fecal; valsartan, 13% renal and 86% fecal. **Half-Life:** Sacubitril 1.4 h.; LBQ657 11.5 h.; valsartan 9.9 h.

## NURSING IMPLICATIONS

### Black Box Warning

*The valsartan component of the drug has been associated with fetal toxicity.*

### Assessment & Drug Effects
- Monitor cardiac status and BP frequently. Risk of hypotension increases with salt and/or volume depletion.
- Monitor activity tolerance and S&S of heart failure.
- Monitor for angioedema; if suspected, take measures necessary to ensure maintenance of a patent airway.
- Monitor for S&S of hyperkalemia (see Appendix F).
- Monitor for S&S of lithium toxicity with concurrent use.
- Monitor lab tests: Baseline and periodic LFTs and renal function tests; periodic serum potassium and Hct & Hgb.

### Patient & Family Education
- Seek medical care immediately if experiencing swelling of face, lips, tongue, and throat (angioedema). Persons of African heritage are at greater risk for angioedema.
- Make position changes slowly, especially when standing from a lying or sitting position.

- Do not use potassium supplements, salt substitutes, or OTC nonsteroidal anti-inflammatory drugs (NSAIDs) without consulting prescriber.
- Women should use effective means of contraception while taking this drug. If pregnancy is suspected, stop taking this drug and report immediately to prescriber.
- Do not breast-feed while taking this drug.

## SAFINAMIDE
(sa-fin'a-mide)
Xadago
**Classifications:** MONOAMINE OXIDASE (MAO) B INHIBITOR
**Therapeutic:** ANTI-PARKINSON AGENT

## AVAILABILITY Tablet

## ACTION & *THERAPEUTIC EFFECT*
Decreases dopamine catabolism via inhibition of type-B MAO which increases dopamine levels in the brain and subsequently increases dopaminergic activity. *Helpful adjunctive therapy in improving "off" episodes of Parkinson's disease.*

## CONTRAINDICATIONS Hypersensitivity to safinamide or any component of the formulation; severe hepatic impairment (Child-Pugh class C); concomitant use of other monomine oxidase inhibitors (MAOIs) or other drugs that are potent inhibitors of monoamine oxidase, opioids, serotonin-norepinephrine reuptake inhibitors (SNRIs) tricyclic or triazolopyridine antidepressants, cyclobenzaprine, methylphenidate, amphetamines, and their derivatives, St. John's wort, dextromethorphan; lactation.

## CAUTIOUS USE Hepatic impairment; ophthalmic disorders; psychotic disorders; pregnancy (category C).

S

Common adverse effects in *italic*; life-threatening effects underlined; generic names in **bold;** classifications in SMALL CAPS; ♣ Canadian drug name; ♦ Prototype drug

## ROUTE & DOSAGE

### Parkinson's Disease

*Adult:* **Initial PO** 50 mg daily; after 2 wk titrate to 100 mg daily

### Hepatic Impairment Dosage Adjustment

*Moderate impairment (Child-Pugh class B):* Max: 50 mg daily

*Severe impairment (Child-Pugh class C):* Do not use

## ADMINISTRATION
### Oral

- Administer without regard to meals at the same time every day. Always administer in association with levodopa/carbidopa.
- At doses 100 mg/day or less, Interaction with tyramine-containing foods and beverages is unlikely, however, patients should avoid foods and beverages with very high (greater than 150 mg) tyramine concentrations. Food's freshness is also a consideration; improperly stored or spoiled food can create an environment where tyramine concentrations may increase.
- Store at 25° C (77° F); excursions permitted between 15°–30° C (59° 86° F).

## ADVERSE EFFECTS (≥ 2%) GI:
Nausea. **CNS:** *Dyskinesia,* insomnia. **CV:** Hypertension. **Other:** Falls, hallucinations, impulse control disorder, serotonin syndrome.

## INTERACTIONS Drug: MAO-
INHIBITORS or similar acting drugs (e.g., **linezolid**) may increase risk of nonselective MAO inhibition, which may lead to a hypertensive crisis; 14 days washout is appropriate between discontinuing safinamide and initiating another MAOI. SYM-PATHOMIMETIC medications utilized with safinamide increases risk of hypertensive crisis (e.g., **methylphenidate, amphetamine,** and nasal or oral decongestants). Safinamide and **dextromethorphan** can cause brief episodes of psychosis and bizarre behavior. DOPAMINE AN-TAGONISTS may decrease effectiveness of safinamide. Safinamide can increase the plasma levels of **cyclobenzaprine** and other serotonergic medications increasing the risk of serotonin syndrome; therefore the combination should be avoided [e.g., SELECTIVE SEROTONIN REUPTAKE INHIBITORS (SSRI), SEROTONIN-NOREPHINEPHRINE REUPTAKE INHIBI-TORS (SNRI)]. Selective OPIODS such as **tramadol** and **methadone** may also increase risk of serotonin syndrome when taken with safinamide, so the combination is contraindicated. Safinamide and its major metabolite may inhibit the breast cancer resistance protein, increasing concentrations of BCRP substrates; monitor use with substrates of BCRP (e.g., **methotrexate, irrinotecan, topotecan**). **Food:** Tyramine containing foods (e.g., aged, fermented, cured, smoked, or pickled foods) may cause a release of norepinephrine resulting in a rise of blood pressure, and therefore should be avoided while on safinamide. **Herbal: St. John's wort** should be avoided.

## PHARMACOKINETICS Absorption:
95% bioavailability. **Distribution:** 88% protein binding, volume of distribution 165 L. **Onset:** Time to peak 2–3 h. **Metabolism:** Primarily by cytosolic amidases and MAOA. **Elimination:** 76% in urine. **Half-Life:** 20–26 h.

## NURSING IMPLICATIONS
### Assessment & Drug Effects

- Monitor for an increase of daily "on" time without troublesome

**S**

---

Common adverse effects in *italic;* life-threatening effects <u>underlined</u>; generic names in **bold**; classifications in SMALL CAPS; ♣ Canadian drug name; ⊘ Prototype drug

1465

dyskineisa associated with Parkinson's disease may indicate efficacy.
- Monitor blood pressure.
- Monitor for new or increased impulse control or compulsive behaviors such as gambling, sexual, or spending urges, which may be unrecognizable by the patient.
- Monitor for visual changes in patients with a history of retinal or macular degeneration, uveitis, inherited retinal conditions, family history of hereditary retinal disease, albinism, retinitis pigmentosa, or any active retinopathy (diabetic retinopathy).

**Patient & Family Education**
- Notify all health care providers that this drug is being taken. This includes prescribers, doctors, nurses, pharmacists, and dentists.
- Avoid driving and doing other tasks or actions that require alertness until drug affects are known; some people have fallen asleep during activities.
- Monitor blood pressure at home as directed by prescriber; this drug may cause high blood pressure.
- Avoid foods high in tyramine (e.g., cheese, and red wine).
- Do not stop this drug without calling prescriber.
- Notify prescriber before drinking alcohol or using drugs and natural products that may slow actions.
- Notify prescriber if pregnant or have plans to get pregnant to discuss drug risks during pregnancy.
- Notify prescriber right away with S&S of an allergic reaction: Rash, hives, wheezing, chest tightness, trouble breathing, swelling in the mouth, face or lips
- Notify prescriber if experiencing symptoms of high blood pressure: Very bad headache, dizziness, passing out, or change in eyesight.
- Notify prescriber regarding the following: Movement control difficulty,

hallucinations, confused or agitated feelings, strong urges that are hard to control, or experiencing falls.
- If this drug is taken along with drugs for depression, notify prescriber right away if experiencing the following: Agitation, change in balance, confusion, hallucinations, fast heart beat, muscle twitching or stiffness, seizure, shivering or shaking, profuse sweating, very bad diarrhea, upset stomach, vomiting or very bad headache.

## SALMETEROL XINAFOATE
(sal-me'ter-ol xin'a-fo-ate)
Serevent
**Classifications:** BETA$_2$-ADRENERGIC AGONIST; RESPIRATORY SMOOTH MUSCLE RELAXANT; BRONCHODILATOR
**Therapeutic:** BRONCHODILATOR
**Prototype:** Albuterol

**AVAILABILITY** Powder diskus for inhalation

**ACTION & THERAPEUTIC EFFECT**
Long-acting beta$_2$-adrenoreceptor agonist that stimulates beta$_2$-adrenoreceptors, relaxes bronchospasm, and increases ciliary motility, thus facilitating expectoration. *Relaxes bronchospasm and increases ciliary motility, thus facilitating expectoration of pulmonary secretions.*

**USES** Maintenance therapy for asthma or bronchospasm associated with COPD. Prevention of exercise-induced bronchospasm.

**CONTRAINDICATIONS** Hypersensitivity to salmeterol or milk proteins; primary treatment of status asthmaticus; acute asthma; acute bronchospasm; acutely deteriorating COPD; MAOI therapy.

Common adverse effects in *italic;* life-threatening effects underlined; generic names in **bold;** classifications in SMALL CAPS; ✚ Canadian drug name; ● Prototype drug

**CAUTIOUS USE** Cardiovascular disorders, cardiac arrhythmias, hypertension, QT prolongation, hypokalemia; history of seizures or thyrotoxicosis; hyperthyroidism; pheochromocytoma; liver and renal impairment; COPD; DM, sensitivity to other beta-adrenergic agonists; older adults; women in labor; pregnancy (category C); lactation. Safe use in children younger than 4 y not established.

## ROUTE & DOSAGE

### Asthma or Bronchospasm (COPD associated)
*Adult/Child (4 y or older):*
**Inhalation** 1 powder diskus (50 mcg) b.i.d. approximately 12 h apart

### Prevention of Exercise-Induced Bronchospasm
*Adult/Child (4 y or older):*
**Inhalation** 1 powder diskus (50 mcg) 30–60 min before exercise

## ADMINISTRATION

### Inhalation
- Do not use to relieve symptoms of acute asthma.
- Activate diskus by moving lever until it clicks. Patient should exhale fully (not into diskus), place diskus in mouth, and inhale quickly and deeply through the diskus. Diskus should be removed and breath held for 10 sec.
- Store at room temperature, 15°–30° C (59°–86° F).

**ADVERSE EFFECTS** (≥1%) **CNS:** Dizziness, *headache*, tremor. **CV:** Palpitations, sinus tachycardia. **Respiratory:** <u>Respiratory arrest</u> (rare), sinus congestion, rhinitis, bronchitis. **Skin:** Rash. **Body as a Whole:** Tolerance (tachyphylaxis), *musculoskeletal pain*.

**INTERACTIONS Drug:** Effects antagonized by BETA-BLOCKERS, MAOIs. Avoid use of strong CYP3A4 inhibitors. Do not use with **cobicistat** or **telaprevir**.

**PHARMACOKINETICS Onset:** 10–20 min. **Peak:** Effect 2 h. **Duration:** Up to 12 h. **Distribution:** 94–95% protein bound, excreted in breast milk. **Metabolism:** Salmeterol is extensively metabolized by hydroxylation. **Elimination:** Primarily in feces. **Half-Life:** 3–4 h.

## NURSING IMPLICATIONS

### Black Box Warning

*Salmeterol has been associated with increased risk of asthma-related hospitalization and death.*

### Assessment & Drug Effects
- Withhold drug and notify prescriber immediately if bronchospasms occur following its use.
- Monitor cardiovascular status; report tachycardia.
- Monitor lab tests: Periodic serum glucose and serum potassium.

### Patient & Family Education
- Never use a spacer device with the drug.
- Do not use this drug to treat an acute asthma attack.
- Notify prescriber immediately of worsening asthma or failure to respond to the usual dose of salmeterol.
- Do not use an additional dose prior to exercise if taking twice-daily doses of salmeterol.
- Take the preexercise dose 30–60 min before exercise and wait 12 h before an additional dose.

Common adverse effects in *italic*; life-threatening effects <u>underlined</u>; generic names in **bold**; classifications in SMALL CAPS; ♣ Canadian drug name; ◑ Prototype drug

1467

S

# SALSALATE
(sal′sa-late)

Mono-Gesic, Salsitab

**Classifications:** ANALGESIC
(SALICYLATE); NONSTEROIDAL
ANTI-INFLAMMATORY DRUG (NSAID)
Therapeutic: NONNARCOTIC ANALGESIC,
NSAID; DISEASE-MODIFYING
ANTIRHEUMATIC DRUG (DMARD)
**Prototype:** Aspirin

## AVAILABILITY Tablet

## ACTION & *THERAPEUTIC EFFECT*
Anti-inflammatory and analgesic activity of salsalate may be mediated through inhibition of the prostaglandin synthetase enzyme complex. *Has analgesic, anti-inflammatory, and antirheumatic effects.*

## USES Symptomatic treatment, rheumatoid arthritis, osteoarthritis, and related rheumatic disorders.

## CONTRAINDICATIONS Hypersensitivity to salicylates or NSAIDs; chronic renal insufficiency; peptic ulcer; children younger than 12 y; hemophilia; chickenpox, influenza, tinnitus.

## CAUTIOUS USE Liver function impairment; older adults; pregnancy (category C); lactation. Safety and efficacy in children not established.

## ROUTE & DOSAGE

**Arthritis**
*Adult:* **PO** 1500 mg b.i.d. or 1000 mg t.i.d. (max: 4 g/day)

## ADMINISTRATION
**Oral**
- Give with a full glass of water or food or milk to reduce GI adverse effects.

## ADVERSE EFFECTS (≥1%) **GI:**
Nausea, dyspepsia, heartburn, vomiting, diarrhea, risk of GI bleed. **Special Senses:** Tinnitus, hearing loss (reversible). **Body as a Whole:** Vertigo, flushing, headache, confusion, hyperventilation, sweating. **CNS:** Drowsiness.

## DIAGNOSTIC TEST INTERFERENCE
False-negative results for *Clinistix;* false-positives for *Clinitest*.

## INTERACTIONS **Drug: Aminosalicylic acid** increases risk of salicylate toxicity. **Ammonium chloride** and other ACIDIFYING AGENTS decrease renal elimination and increase risk of salicylate toxicity. ANTICOAGULANTS increase risk of bleeding. ORAL HYPOGLYCEMIC AGENTS increase hypoglycemic activity with salsalate doses greater than 2 g/day. CARBONIC ANHYDRASE INHIBITORS enhance salicylate toxicity. CORTICOSTEROIDS add to ulcerogenic effects. **Methotrexate** toxicity is increased. Low doses of salicylates may antagonize uricosuric effects of **probenecid** and **sulfinpyrazone. Herbal: Feverfew, garlic, ginger, ginkgo** may increase bleeding potential.

## PHARMACOKINETICS **Absorption:** Readily absorbed from small intestine. **Peak:** 1.5–4 h. **Metabolism:** Hydrolyzed in liver, GI mucosa, plasma, whole blood, and other tissues. **Elimination:** In urine. **Half-Life:** 1 h.

## NURSING IMPLICATIONS
**Assessment & Drug Effects**
- Symptom relief is gradual (may require 3–4 days to establish steady-state salicylate level).
- Monitor for adverse GI effects, especially in patient with a history of peptic ulcer disease.

Common adverse effects in *italic*; life-threatening effects underlined; generic names in **bold**; classifications in SMALL CAPS; ♣ Canadian drug name; ⊕ Prototype drug

## Patient & Family Education

- Do not take another salicylate (e.g., aspirin) while on salsalate therapy.
- Monitor blood glucose for loss of glycemic control in diabetes; drug may induce hypoglycemia when used with sulfonylureas.
- Report tinnitus, hearing loss, vertigo, rash, or nausea.

## SAQUINAVIR MESYLATE ⏻

(sa-quin'a-vir mes'y-late)

*Invirase*

**Classifications:** ANTIRETROVIRAL; PROTEASE INHIBITOR

**Therapeutic:** PROTEASE INHIBITOR

**AVAILABILITY** Gelatin capsule, tablet

## ACTION & THERAPEUTIC EFFECT

Inhibits the activity of HIV protease and prevents the cleavage of viral polyproteins essential for the maturation of HIV. *Effectiveness indicated by reduced viral load (decreased number of RNA copies), and increased number of T helper CD4 cells.*

**USES** HIV infection (used with other antiretroviral agents).

**CONTRAINDICATIONS** Significant hypersensitivity to saquinavir; congenital long QT syndrome; severe hepatic impairment; AV block; hypokalemia, or hypomagnesia; antimicrobial resistance to other protease inhibitors; monotherapy; lactation.

**CAUTIOUS USE** Hepatic insufficiency; severe renal impairment; hepatitis B or C; DM, diabetic ketoacidosis; CHF, bradyarrhythmias, electrolyte imbalances; hemophilia A or B; older adults; pregnancy (category B). Safety and efficacy

in HIV-infected children younger than 16 y not established.

## ROUTE & DOSAGE

### HIV

*Adult/Adolescent:* **PO** 1000 mg b.i.d. with ritonavir 100 mg b.i.d.

## ADMINISTRATION

### Oral

- Give with or up to 2 h after a full meal to ensure adequate absorption and bioavailability. Give with ritonavir.
- Do not administer to anyone taking rifampin or rifabutin because these drugs significantly decrease the plasma level of saquinavir.
- Store at 15°–30° C (59°–86° F) in a tightly closed bottle.

**ADVERSE EFFECTS** (≥1%) **CNS:** Headache, paresthesia, numbness, dizziness, peripheral neuropathy, ataxia, confusion, convulsions, hyperreflexia, hyporeflexia, tremor, agitation, amnesia, anxiety, depression, excessive dreaming, hallucinations, euphoria, irritability, lethargy, somnolence. **CV:** Chest pain, hypertension, hypotension, syncope. **Endocrine:** Dehydration, hyperglycemia, diabetes, weight changes, *lipodystrophy*. **Hematologic:** Anemia, splenomegaly, thrombocytopenia, pancytopenia. **GI:** *Nausea, diarrhea, abdominal discomfort,* dyspepsia, mucosal damage, change in appetite, dry mouth. **Skin:** Rash, pruritus, acne, erythema, seborrhea, hair changes, photosensitivity, skin ulceration, dry skin. **Body as a Whole:** Myalgia, allergic reaction. **Respiratory:** Bronchitis, cough, dyspnea, epistaxis, hemoptysis,

S

laryngitis, rhinitis. **Special Senses:** Xerophthalmia, earache, taste alterations, tinnitus, visual disturbances.

## INTERACTIONS Drug: Do not

use with **sildenafil, alfuzosin,** or **salmeterol.** Rifampin, **rifabutin** significantly decrease saquinavir levels. **Phenobarbital, phenytoin, dexamethasone, carbamazepine** may also reduce saquinavir levels. Saquinavir levels may be increased by **delavirdine, ketoconazole, ritonavir, clarithromycin, indinavir.** May increase serum levels of **triazolam, midazolam,** ERGOT DERIVATIVES, **nelfinavir, simvastatin.** May increase risk of **ergotamine** toxicity of **dihydroergotamine, ergotamine.** Dosage adjustments are needed when used with **bosentan, tadalafil,** or **colchicine. Herbal: St. John's wort, garlic** may decrease antiretroviral activity. **Food: Grapefruit juice** (greater than 1 qt/day) may increase plasma concentrations and adverse effects.

## PHARMACOKINETICS Absorp-

**tion:** Rapidly from GI tract; food significantly increases bioavailability. **Distribution:** 98% protein bound. **Metabolism:** In liver (CYP3A4), first-pass metabolism. **Elimination:** Primarily in feces (greater than 80%). **Half-Life:** 13 h.

## NURSING IMPLICATIONS

### Assessment & Drug Effects

- Assess for buccal mucosa ulceration or other distressing GI S&S.
- Monitor weight periodically.
- Monitor for toxicity if any of the following drugs is used concomitantly: Calcium channel blockers, clindamycin, dapsone, quinidine, triazolam, or simvastatin.

- Monitor for and report S&S of peripheral neuropathy.
- Monitor lab tests: Baseline and periodic $CD_4$ count, serum electrolytes, and lipid profile.

### Patient & Family Education

- Take drug within 2 h of a full meal.
- Be aware of all drugs which should not be taken concurrently with saquinavir.
- Be aware that saquinavir is not a cure for HIV infection and that its long-term effects are unknown.
- Report any distressing adverse effects to prescriber.

# SARGRAMOSTIM (GM-CSF)

(sar-gra'mos-tim)

Leukine

**Classifications:** HEMATOPOIETIC GROWTH FACTOR; GRANULOCYTE MACROPAHGE COLONY STIMULATING FACTOR (GM-CSF)

Therapeutic: HEMATPOIETIC GROWTH FACTOR; GM-CSF

**Prototype:** Filgrastim

## AVAILABILITY Solution for injection

## ACTION & THERAPEUTIC EFFECT

GM-CSF is a hematopoietic growth factor that stimulates proliferation and differentiation of progenitor cells in the granulocyte-macrophage pathways. *Effectiveness is measured by an increase in the number of mature white blood cells (i.e., neutrophil count).*

## USES Febrile neutropenia, neu-

tropenia caused by chemotherapy, peripheral blood stem cell (PBSC) mobilization.

## UNLABELED USES Neutropenia

secondary to other diseases; aplastic anemia, Crohn's disease, malignant melanoma.

S

## CONTRAINDICATIONS

Hypersensitivity to GM-CSF, yeast-derived products; excessive leukemic myeloid blasts in bone marrow or blood greater than or equal to 10%; within 24 h of chemotherapy or radiation treatment; if ANC exceeds 20,000 cells/mm³ discontinue drug or use half the dose; increased growth of tumor size; lactation.

## CAUTIOUS USE

Hypersensitivity to benzyl alcohol; history of cardiac arrhythmias, preexisting cardiac disease, renal or hepatic dysfunction, CHF, hypoxia, myelodysplastic syndromes; pulmonary infiltrates; fluid retention; kidney and liver dysfunction; use in AML for adults younger than 55 y; pregnancy (category C). Safety and efficacy in children not established.

## ROUTE & DOSAGE

### Neutropenia following Stem Cell Transplantation

*Adult:* **IV** 250 mcg/m²/day infused over 2 h for 21 days, begin 2–4 h after bone marrow transfusion and not less than 24 h after last dose of chemotherapy or 12 h after last radiation therapy

### Following PBSC

*Adult:* **IV/Subcutaneous** 250 mg/m²/day

### Neutropenia following Chemotherapy/Febrile Neutropenia

*Adult:* **IV/Subcutaneous** 250 mcg/m²/day starting ~day 11 or 4 days following induction chemotherapy

## ADMINISTRATION

- Note: Do not give within 24 h preceding or following chemotherapy or within 12 h preceding or following radiotherapy.

### Subcutaneous

- Reconstitute each 250 mcg powder vial with 1 mL of sterile water for injection (without preservative). Direct sterile water against side of vial and swirl gently. Avoid excessive or vigorous agitation. Do not shake. Use without further dilution for subcutaneous injection.

### Intravenous

*PREPARE:* **IV Infusion:** Reconstitute powder vial as for subcutaneous, then further dilute reconstituted solution with NS. If the final concentration is less than 1 mcg/mL, add albumin (human) to NS before addition of sargramostim. ▪Use 1 mg albumin/1 mL of NS to give a final concentration of 0.1% albumin. ▪ Administer as soon as possible and within 6 h of reconstitution or dilution for IV infusion. ▪Discard after 6 h. ▪ Sargramostim vials are single-dose vials, do not reenter or reuse. Discard unused portion.

*ADMINISTER:* **IV Infusion:** Give over 2, 4, or 24 h as ordered. ▪Do not use an in-line membrane filter. ▪ Interrupt administration and reduce the dose by 50% if absolute neutrophil count exceeds 20,000/mm³ or if platelet count exceeds 500,000/mm³. Notify prescriber. ▪Reduce the IV rate 50% if patient experiences dyspnea during administration. ▪Discontinue infusion if respiratory symptoms worsen. Notify prescriber.

*INCOMPATIBILITIES:* **Y-site: Acyclovir, amphotericin B, ampicillin, ampicillin/sulbactam,**

Common adverse effects in *italic*; life-threatening effects <u>underlined</u>; generic names in **bold**; classifications in SMALL CAPS; ✦ Canadian drug name; ⊙ Prototype drug

1471

amsacrine, cefonicid, ceftazidime, chlorpromazine, ganciclovir, haloperidol, hydrocortisone, hydromorphone, hydroxyzine, imipenem/cilastatin, lorazepam, methylprednisolone, mitomycin, morphine, nalbuphine, ondansetron, piperacillin, sodium bicarbonate, tobramycin.

▪ Refrigerate the sterile powder, the reconstituted solution, and store diluted solution at 2°–8° C (36°–46° F).
▪ Do not freeze or shake.

**ADVERSE EFFECTS** (≥1%) **CNS:** Lethargy, malaise, headache, fatigue. **CV:** Abnormal ST segment depression, supraventricular arrhythmias, edema, *hypotension, tachycardia,* pericardial effusion, pericarditis. **Hematologic:** Anemia, thrombocytopenia. **GI:** Nausea, vomiting, diarrhea, anorexia. **Body as a Whole:** *Bone pain, myalgia, arthralgias,* weight gain, hyperuricemia, *fever.* **Respiratory:** Pleural effusion. **Skin:** *Rash, pruritus.* **Other:** *First-dose reaction* (some or all of the following symptoms: hypotension, tachycardia, fever, rigors, flushing, nausea, vomiting, diaphoresis, back pain, leg spasms, and dyspnea).

**INTERACTIONS Drug:** CORTICO-STEROIDS and **lithium** should be used with caution because it may potentiate the myeloproliferative effects.

**PHARMACOKINETICS Absorption:** Readily from subcutaneous site. **Onset:** 3–6 h. **Peak:** 1–2 h. **Duration:** 5–10 days subcutaneous. **Elimination:** Probably in urine. **Half-Life:** 80–150 min.

**NURSING IMPLICATIONS**
**Assessment & Drug Effects**
▪ Discontinue treatment and notify prescriber if WBC 50,000/mm³.

▪ Monitor cardiac status. Occasional transient supraventricular arrhythmias have occurred during administration, particularly in those with a history of cardiac arrhythmias. Arrhythmias are reversed with discontinuation of drug.
▪ Give special attention to respiratory symptoms (dyspnea) during and immediately following IV infusion, especially in patients with preexisting pulmonary disease.
▪ Use drug with caution in patients with preexisting fluid retention, pulmonary infiltrates, or CHF. Peripheral edema, pleural or pericardial effusion has occurred after administration. It is reversible with dose reduction.
▪ Notify prescriber of any severe adverse reaction immediately.
▪ Monitor lab tests: Baseline and biweekly CBC with differential and platelet count; biweekly LFTs and renal function tests in patients with established kidney or liver dysfunction.

**Patient & Family Education**
▪ Notify nurse or prescriber immediately of any adverse effect (e.g., dyspnea, palpitations, peripheral edema, bone or muscle pain) during or after drug administration.

# SARILUMAB
(sar-il'ue-mab)
Kevzara
**Classifications:** DISEASE MODIFYING ANTIRHEUMATIC (DMARD); INTERLEUKIN-6 RECEPTOR ANTAGONIST; MONOCLONAL ANTIBODY
Therapeutic: DISEASE-MODIFYING ANTIRHEUMATIC (DMARD)

**AVAILABILITY** Subcutaneous injection

## ACTION & *THERAPEUTIC EFFECT*

Inhibits interleukin-6 (IL-6)-mediated signaling by binding to IL-6 receptors that are both soluble and membrane-bound. *Inhibition of the IL-6 receptors by sarilumab leads to a reduction in CRP levles, which can improve inflammatory processes such as rheumatoid arthritis.*

**USES** Treatment of rheumatoid arthritis that has failed or had insufficient response to other disease-modifying medications.

**CONTRAINDICATIONS** Hypersensitivity to sarilumab or excipients, live vaccines. Limited available data to determine if sarilumab during pregnancy is associated with risk for major birth defects or miscarriage. Monoclonal antibodies, like sarilumab, are transported across the placenta. There is no current data available on the presence of sarilumab in human milk or its effects on the breast-fed infant or milk production.

**CAUTIOUS USE** History of diverticulitis or concomitant use of NSAIDS or corticosteroid use, active hepatic disease, or impairment.

## ROUTE & DOSAGE

### Rheumatoid Arthritis

*Adult:* **Subcutaneous** 200 mg every 2 wk

### *Hepatic Impairment Dosage Adjustment*

*ALT/AST greater than 3–5 × ULN:* Hold therapy until ALT/ALT is less than 3 × ULN, then rzestart medication at 150 mg every 2 wk; increase to original dose as appropriate

*ALT/AST greater than 5 × ULN:* Discontinue therapy

## ADMINISTRATION

### Subcutaneous

- Allow to sit at room temperature for 30 min prior to administration; do not warm any other way.
- Solution should be clear and colorless to pale yellow.
- Do not shake.
- Not for IV administration.
- Rotate injection sites; do not inject where skin is tender, damaged, bruised, or scarred.
- Inject full amount of the prefilled syringe.
- If 3 days or less since missed dose, take as soon as possible; take next dose at regularly scheduled time.
- Store at 2°–8° C (36°–46° F) in the original carton to protect from light. Do not freeze or shake. May store at 25° C (77° F) or cooler for up to 14 days. After removal from the refrigerator, use within 14 days.

**ADVERSE EFFECTS** (≥ 2%) **Metabolic:** *Increased LFTs.* **Skin:** Injection site pruritis and erythema. **Genitourinary:** UTI **Hematologic:** Neutropenia, leukopenia.

**INTERACTIONS** Do not give live virus vaccines to patients on sarilumab; not studied with the use of JAK inhibitors or other biological DMARD agents (such as TNF antagonists). Potential interaction with CYP450 substrates, specifically those with narrow therapeutic index or specific desired effectiveness (e.g., **warfarin**, **theophylline**, oral contraceptives).

**PHARMACOKINETICS Absorption:** 34% bioavailability. **Onset:** Peak effect in 2–4 days. **Metabolism:** Similar to endogenous IgG, undergoes catabolic metabolism to small peptides and amino acids.

S

---

Common adverse effects in *italic;* life-threatening effects <u>underlined</u>; generic names in **bold;** classifications in SMALL CAPS; ♣ Canadian drug name; ⊘ Prototype drug

1473

**Elimination:** Through proteolytic pathway. **Half-Life:** 8–10 days, dependent on dose.

## NURSING IMPLICATIONS

### Black Box Warning

*Serious infections (e.g., bacterial, mycobacterial, invasive fungal, viral and opportunistic infections) which have led to hospitalization or death. Do not administer during active infections. Monitor patients for infection during use. Use caution in patients with TB exposure or history of serious opportunistic, chronic, or recurrent infection. Stop sarilumab if serious opportunistic infection develops.*

### Assessment & Drug Effects

- Monitor for improvement of signs or symptoms of rheumatoid arthritis.
- Monitor neutrophils and platelets: 4–8 wk after treatment initiation and approximately every 3 mo thereafter.
- Monitor for latent TB prior to initiation.
- Monitor for active TB in all patients, even if initial latent TB was negative.
- Monitor for S&S of infection during and after therapy.
- Monitor for gastrointestinal perforation.
- Monitor lab tests: ALT and AST levels 4–8 wk after treatment initiation and approximately every 3 mo thereafter. Other LFTs may be ordered if clinically indicated.

### Patient & Family Education

- Do not take this drug if infection is present.
- TB has been seen in patients that take this drug.
- Notify health care provider right away of signs of infection such as fever, flu-like symptoms, chills, very bad sore throat, ear or sinus pain, cough, pain while urinating, mouth sores or sores that will not heal.
- Notify all health care providers that this drug is being taken. This includes prescribers, doctors, nurses, pharmacists, and dentists
- Talk to prescriber before getting any vaccines.
- Birth control pills and other hormone-based birth control may not work to prevent pregnancy. Use another effective method for birth control while taking this drug.
- Notify prescriber if pregnant or plan to get pregnant.
- If pregnancy occurs while using this drug, notify your prescriber right away.
- Discuss possible breast-feeding risks with prescriber.
- Notify prescriber right away with S&S of an allergic reaction: Rash, hives, blistered skin, wheezing, chest tightness, unusual hoarseness, swelling of the mouth, face, lips, tongue or throat; very bad belly pain; vomiting dark brown coffee ground emesis, black tarry stools, shortness of breath, chest pain, dizziness, muscle pain or weakness, coughing up blood.

## SAXAGLIPTIN

(sax-a-glip'tin)

Onglyza

**Classifications:** INCRETIN MODIFIER; DIPEPTIDYL PEPTIDASE-4 (DPP-4) INHIBITOR; ANTIDIABETIC

Therapeutic: ANTIDIABETIC; HORMONE MODIFIER; DDP-4 INHIBITOR

**Prototype:** Sitagliptin

## AVAILABILITY Tablet

## ACTION & *THERAPEUTIC EFFECT*

Slows inactivation of incretin hormones [e.g., glucagon-like peptide-1 (GLP-1) and glucose-dependent insulinotropic polypeptide (GIP)]. As plasma glucose rises, incretin hormones stimulate release of insulin from the pancreas and GLP-1 also lowers glucagon secretion, resulting in reduced hepatic glucose production. *In type 2 diabetics, saxagliptin elevates the level of incretin hormones, thus increasing insulin secretion and reducing glucagon secretion. It lowers both fasting and postprandial plasma glucose levels.*

**USES** Treatment of type 2 diabetes mellitus.

## CONTRAINDICATIONS Hypersensitivity to saxagliptin; exfoliative skin condition; type 1 DM, concurrent administration with insulin.

**CAUTIOUS USE** Moderate to severe renal impairment; acute pancreatitis; history of angioedema with use of another DDP4 inhibitor; HF; lactose intolerance; older adults; pregnancy (category B); lactation. Safe use in children younger than 18 y not established.

## ROUTE & DOSAGE

### Type 2 Diabetes Mellitus

*Adult:* **PO** 2.5–5 mg daily. Limited to 2.5 mg daily when used with a strong CYP3A4/5 inhibitor.

### Renal Impairment Dosage Adjustment

*CrCl less than or equal to 50 mL/ min:* 2.5 mg once daily

## ADMINISTRATION

### Oral

- May be taken without regard to meals.
- Ensure that tablets are taken whole; they must not be cut or split.
- Dosing in the older adults should be based on creatinine clearance.
- Store at 15°–30° C (59°–86° F).

**ADVERSE EFFECTS (≥1%) Body as a Whole:** Peripheral edema. **CNS:** *Headache.* **GI:** Abdominal pain, gasteroenteritis, vomiting. **Metabolic:** Hypoglycemia. **Respiratory:** *Nasopharyngitis, upper respiratory tract infection.* **Skin:** Facial edema, urticaria. **Special Senses:** Sinusitis. **Urogenital:** *Urinary tract infection.*

**DIAGNOSTIC TEST INTERFERENCE** Dose-related decrease in ***absolute lymphocyte*** count.

**INTERACTIONS Drug: Rifampin** and other inducers of CYP3A4/5 enzymes decrease saxagliptin levels. Moderate (e.g., **amprenavir, aprepitant, erythromycin, fluconazole, fosamprenavir, verapamil**) and strong (e.g., **atazanavir, clarithromycin, indinavir, itraconazole, ketoconazole, nefazodone, nelfinavir, ritonavir, saquinavir, telithromycin**) inhibitors of CYP3A4/5 increase saxagliptin levels. Decrease saxagliptin dose when used with INSULIN or ANTIDIABETIC drug to minimize risk of hypoglycemia. **Food: Grapefruit juice** increases saxagliptin levels.

**PHARMACOKINETICS Peak:** 2 h. **Distribution:** Negligible plasma protein binding. **Metabolism:** Hepatic metabolism to active and inactive compounds. **Elimination:** Renal (75%) and fecal (22%). **Half-Life:** 2.5–3.1 h.

Common adverse effects in *italic;* life-threatening effects underlined; generic names in **bold;** classifications in SMALL CAPS; ✤ Canadian drug name; ⊙ Prototype drug

1475

## NURSING IMPLICATIONS

### Assessment & Drug Effects

- Monitor for and report S&S of significant GI distress including NV&D.
- Monitor for S&S of hypoglycemia when used in combination with a sulfonylurea or insulin.
- Monitor lab tests: Baseline and periodic creatinine clearance; periodic fasting and postprandial plasma glucose and HbA1C.

### Patient & Family Education

- Carry out blood glucose monitoring as directed by prescriber.
- Consult prescriber during periods of stress and illness as dosage adjustments may be required.
- When taken alone to control diabetes, saxagliptin is unlikely to cause hypoglycemia because it only works when the blood sugar is rising after food intake.
- Stop taking drug immediately if you experience symptoms of a serious allergic reaction such as swelling about the face or throat, or difficulty breathing or swallowing.

## SCOPOLAMINE
(skoe-pol'a-meen)
Transderm Scop

## SCOPOLAMINE HYDROBROMIDE

**Classifications:** ANTICHOLINERGIC; ANTIMUSCARINIC; ANTISPASMODIC; ANTIVERTIGO
**Therapeutic:** ANTISPASMODIC; ANTIEMETIC; ANTIVERTIGO
**Prototype:** Atropine

### AVAILABILITY
**Scopolamine:** Transdermal patch. **Scopolamine HBr:** Injection

### ACTION & *THERAPEUTIC EFFECT*

Inhibits the action on acetylcholine (ACh) on postganglionic cholinergic nerves as well as on smooth muscles that lack cholinergic innervation. *Produces CNS depression with marked sedative and tranquilizing effects for use in anesthesia. Effective as a preanesthetic agent to control bronchial, nasal, pharyngeal, and salivary secretions. Additionally, it prevents nausea and vomiting associated with motion sickness.*

**USES** In obstetrics with morphine to produce amnesia and sedation ("twilight sleep") and as preanesthetic medication. To control spasticity (and drooling) in postencephalitic parkinsonism, paralysis agitans, and other spastic states, as prophylactic agent for motion sickness and as mydriatic and cycloplegic in ophthalmology to prevent nausea and vomiting associated with motion sickness.

**CONTRAINDICATIONS** Hypersensitivity to anticholinergic drugs; narrow angle glaucoma; severe ulcerative colitis, GI obstruction; urinary tract obstruction diseases; toxemia of pregnancy.

**CAUTIOUS USE** Remove patch before undergoing MRI to prevent burns at the patch site. Hypertension; patients older than 40 y, pyloric obstruction, autonomic neuropathy, myasthenia gravis; thyrotoxicosis, liver disease; CAD; CHF; tachycardia, or other tachyarrhythmias; paralytic ileus; hiatal hernia, mild or moderate ulcerative colitis, gastric ulcer, GERD; renal impairment; parkinsonism; COPD, asthma or allergies; hyperthyroidism; brain damage, spastic paralysis; Down syndrome; older adults; pregnancy (category C); lactation; children, infants.

Common adverse effects in *italic;* life-threatening effects underlined; generic names in **bold**; classifications in SMALL CAPS; ♣ Canadian drug name; ⊘ Prototype drug

## ROUTE & DOSAGE

**Nausea/Vomiting**
*Adult:* **Subcutaneous** 0.6–1 mg
*Child:* **Subcutaneous** 6 mcg/kg
**Motion Sickness**
*Adult:* **Topical** 1 patch q72h starting
4 h before anticipated travel
**Refraction**
*Adult:* **Ophthalmic** 1–2 drops in
eye 1 h before refraction

## ADMINISTRATION

### Ophthalmic Instillation
- Minimize possibility of systemic absorption by applying pressure against lacrimal sac during and for 1 or 2 min following instillation of eye drops.

### Transdermal
- Apply transdermal disc system (Transderm Scōp, a controlled-release system) to dry surface behind the ear. Wear gloves or wash hands thoroughly before and after application.
- Replace with another disc on another site behind the ear if disc system becomes dislodged.

### Subcutaneous or Intramuscular
- Give undiluted.

### Intravenous

*PREPARE:* **Direct:** Dilute required dose with an equal volume of sterile water for injection.
*ADMINISTER:* **Direct:** Give a single dose slowly over 2–3 min.

- Preserve in tight, light-resistant containers and away from heat.

## ADVERSE EFFECTS (≥1%) **Body as a Whole:** Fatigue, dizziness, *drowsiness,* disorientation, restlessness, hallucinations, toxic psychosis. **GI:** *Dry mouth and throat, thirst,*

*constipation.* **Urogenital:** Urinary retention. **CV:** Decreased heart rate, orthostatic hypotension, tachycardia. **Special Senses:** Dilated pupils, photophobia, blurred vision, *local irritation,* follicular conjunctivitis. **Neuromuscular and Skeletal:** Tremor and weakness. **Respiratory:** Depressed respiration. **Skin:** Local irritation from patch adhesive, rash.

## INTERACTIONS **Drug: Amantadine,** ANTIHISTAMINES, TRICYCLIC ANTIDEPRESSANTS, **quinidine, disopyramide, procainamide** add to anticholinergic effects; decreases **levodopa** effects; **methotrimeprazine** may precipitate extrapyramidal effects; decreases antipsychotic effects (decreased absorption) of PHENOTHIAZINES. **Food: Grapefruit juice** (greater than 1 qt/day) may increase plasma concentrations and adverse effects.

## DIAGNOSTIC TEST INTERFERENCE
**Lab Test:** Interferes with *gastric secretion test.*

## PHARMACOKINETICS **Absorption:** Readily from GI tract and percutaneously. **Peak:** 20–60 min. **Duration:** 5–7 days. **Distribution:** Crosses placenta; distributed to CNS. **Metabolism:** In liver. **Elimination:** In urine.

## NURSING IMPLICATIONS
### Assessment & Drug Effects
- Observe patient closely; some patients manifest excitement, delirium, and disorientation shortly after drug is administered until sedative effect takes hold.
- Use of side rails is advisable, particularly for older adults, because of amnesic effect of scopolamine.
- In the presence of pain, scopolamine may cause delirium,

**S**

restlessness, and excitement unless given with an analgesic.

- Be aware that tolerance may develop with prolonged use.
- Terminate ophthalmic use if local irritation, edema, or conjunctivitis occur.

**Patient & Family Education**

- Vision may blur when used as mydriatic or cycloplegic; do not drive or engage in potentially hazardous activities until vision clears.
- Place disc on skin site the night before an expected trip or anticipated motion for best therapeutic effect.
- Wash hands carefully after handling scopolamine. Anisocoria (unequal size of pupils, blurred vision can develop by rubbing eye with drug-contaminated finger).

# SECNIDAZOLE
(sek-nid'a-zole)
Solosec
**Classifications:** ANTIBIOTIC; ANTIPROTOZOAL; NITROMIDAZOLE
Therapeutic: ANTIBIOTIC
**Prototype:** Metronidazole

**AVAILABILITY** Oral granules

**ACTION & *THERAPEUTIC EFFECT***
Secnidazole is a 5-nitroimidazole antimicrobial agent, which is a prodrug upon entering the bacterial cell. *Enzymes in the bacterial cell then reduce the nitro group to radical anions which are believed to interfere with DNA synthesis of the susceptible organism which stops replication of the bacterial cell.*

**USES** Treatment of bacterial vaginosis.

**CONTRAINDICATIONS** Hypersensitivity to secnidazole, any

component of the product, or other nitroimidazole derivatives. Limited available date with secnidazole use in human pregnancy are sufficient to inform a drug-associated risk of adverse developmental outcomes for the fetus; lactation.

**CAUTIOUS USE** Only use when active bacterial infections is identified to prevent drug-resistance; current candidiasis infection.

## ROUTE & DOSAGE

| Bacterial Vaginosis |
|---|
| *Adult:* **PO** 2 g 1 time single dose |

## ADMINISTRATION
**Oral**

- Administer without regard to timing of meals. Sprinkle entire contents of one packet onto applesauce, yogurt, or pudding; granules will not dissolve.
- Consume entire mixture within 30 min; do not chew or crunch granules.
- May consume water after administration to aid in swallowing.
- Store at 20°–25° C (68°–77° F); excursions permitted to 15°–30° C (59°–86° F).

**ADVERSE EFFECTS** (≥ 2%) **GI:** Nausea, diarrhea. **CNS:** Headache. **Reproductive:** Candida vaginitis, vulvo-vaginal.

**PHARMACOKINETICS Distribution:** 5% protein bound. **Onset:** Time to peak 4 h. **Metabolism:** Hepatic via CYP450. **Elimination:** 15% in urine. **Half-Life:** 17 h.

## NURSING IMPLICATIONS
**Assessment & Drug Effects**

- Monitor for improvement of S&S of bacterial vaginosis.

S

Common adverse effects in *italic*; life-threatening effects <u>underlined</u>; generic names in **bold**; classifications in SMALL CAPS; ♣ Canadian drug name; ⊘ Prototype drug

### Patient & Family Education

- Notify all health care providers that this drug is being taken. This includes prescribers, doctors, nurses, pharmacists, and dentists.
- Only take this medication as prescribed.
- Notify prescriber of pregnancy or plan to get pregnant.
- Do not breast-feed while taking this medication and wait at least 96 h after administration of the last dose before breast-feeding. Milk should be pumped and dumped during this time.
- Notify prescriber right away with S&S of an allergic reaction: Rash, hives, itching, blistered skin, wheezing, chest tightness, tightness in the throat, trouble breathing, unusual hoarseness, swelling of the mouth, face, lips, tongue, or throat.
- Notify prescriber of persistent belly pain, vomiting, diarrhea, headache, or change in taste.

## SECOBARBITAL SODIUM ⓟ

(see-koe-bar'bi-tal)

Seconal

**Classifications:** SEDATIVE-HYPNOTIC; BARBITURATE; ANXIOLYTIC
**Therapeutic:** SEDATIVE-HYPNOTIC
**Controlled Substance:** Schedule II

### AVAILABILITY Capsule

### ACTION & *THERAPEUTIC EFFECT*

Short-acting barbiturate with CNS depressant effects as well as mood alteration from excitation to mild sedation, hypnosis, and deep coma. Depresses the sensory cortex, decreases motor activity, alters cerebellar function and produces drowsiness, sedation, and hypnosis. *Alters cerebellar function and produces drowsiness, sedation, and hypnosis.*

### USES
Preoperatively to provide basal hypnosis for general, spinal, or regional anesthesia; management of insomnia.

### CONTRAINDICATIONS
History of sensitivity to barbiturates; porphyria; hepatic coma; severe respiratory disease; parturition, fetal immaturity; uncontrolled pain; pregnancy (category D).

### CAUTIOUS USE
Pregnant women with toxemia or history of bleeding; labor and delivery; seizure disorders; aspirin hypersensitivity; liver function impairment; renal impairment; hyperthyroidism, diabetes mellitus; depression; history of suicidal tendencies or drug abuse; acute or chronic pain; severe anemia; older adults (short term use only), debilitated individuals; lactation; children younger than 6 y.

### ROUTE & DOSAGE

| Preoperative Sedative |
| --- |
| *Adult:* **PO** 200–300 mg 1–2 h before surgery |
| *Child:* **PO** 2–6 mg/kg 1–2 h before surgery |
| **Insomnia** |
| *Adult:* **PO** 100 mg at bedtime |

### ADMINISTRATION

#### Oral
- Give hypnotic dose only after patient retires for the evening.
- Crush and mix with a fluid or with food if patient cannot swallow pill.

**ADVERSE EFFECTS** (≥1%) **CNS:** Drowsiness, lethargy, hangover, paradoxical excitement in older adults. **Respiratory:** <u>Respiratory depression, laryngospasm</u>.

**INTERACTIONS Drug: Phenmetrazine** antagonizes effects of secobarbital; CNS DEPRESSANTS, **alcohol,** SEDATIVES compound CNS depression; MAO INHIBITORS cause excessive CNS depression; **methoxyflurane** increases risk of nephrotoxicity. Do not use **nifedipine** concurrently. **Herbal: Kava, valerian** may potentiate sedation.

**PHARMACOKINETICS Absorption:** 90% from GI tract. **Onset:** 15–30 min. **Duration:** 1–4 h. **Distribution:** Crosses placenta; distributed into breast milk. **Metabolism:** In liver (CYP2C9, CYP2C19, CYP2E1, CYP3A, CYP1A2, UGT). **Elimination:** In urine. **Half-Life:** 30 h.

**NURSING IMPLICATIONS**

**Assessment & Drug Effects**

- Be alert to unexpected responses and report promptly. Older adults or debilitated patients and children sometimes have paradoxical response to barbiturate therapy (i.e., irritability, marked excitement as inappropriate tearfulness and aggression in children, depression, and confusion).
- Be aware that barbiturates do not have analgesic action, and may produce restlessness when given to patients in pain.
- Be alert for acute toxicity (intoxication) characterized by profound CNS depression, respiratory depression, hypoventilation, cyanosis, cold clammy skin, hypo-thermia, constricted pupils (but may be dilated in severe intoxication), shock, oliguria, tachycardia, hypotension, respiration arrest, circulatory collapse, and death.
- Monitor lab tests: Periodic LFTs, renal function tests and hematology tests during prolonged therapy.

**Patient & Family Education**

- Instances of sleep driving and sleep walking with no memory of the occurrence have been reported. Do not drive or engage in potentially hazardous activities until response to drug is established.
- Store barbiturates in a safe place; not on the bedside table or other readily accessible places. It is possible to forget having taken the drug, and in half-wakened conditions take more and accidentally overdose.
- Do not become pregnant. Use or add barrier contraception if using hormonal contraceptives.
- Report onset of fever, sore throat or mouth, malaise, easy bruising or bleeding, petechiae, or jaundice, rash to prescriber during prolonged therapy.
- Do not consume alcohol in any amount when taking a barbiturate. It may severely impair judgment and abilities.

**SECUKINUMAB**
(se-cu-kin'u-mab)
Cosentyx
**Classifications:** MONOCLONAL ANTIBODY; INTERLEUKIN INHIBITOR; ANTIPSORIATIC
Therapeutic: ANTIPSORIATIC
**Prototype:** Basilixumab

**AVAILABILITY** Solution in prefilled pens for injection

**ACTION & THERAPEUTIC EFFECT**
Selectively binds to interleukin-17A

(IL-17A) and inhibits its interaction with the IL-17 receptor. IL-17A is a naturally occurring cytokine involved in normal inflammatory and immune responses. *Inhibits the release of proinflammatory cytokines and chemokines, thus reducing psoriatic skin inflammation.*

**USES** Treatment of moderate to severe plaque psoriasis in adult patients who are candidates for systemic therapy or phototherapy; ankylosing spondylitis.

**CONTRAINDICATIONS** Serious hypersensitivity to secukinumab or any component of the formulation; active TB. Avoid live virus vaccines and understand that non live vaccines may not elicit sufficient immune response.

**CAUTIOUS USE** Concurrent infectious disease; history of chronic or recurrent infection; Crohn's disease; latex allergy when using *Sensoready®* pen or prefilled syringe; pregnancy (category B); lactation. Safety and efficacy in children younger than 18 y not established.

## ROUTE & DOSAGE

**Psoriasis**
*Adult:* **Subcutaneous** 300 mg at wk 0, 1, 2, 3, and 4; then 300 mg q4wk
**Ankylosing Spondylitis**
*Adult:* **Subcutaneous** 150 mg at wk 0, 1, 2, 3, and 4; then 150 mg q4wk

## ADMINISTRATION

**Subcutaneous ONLY**
- Remove *Sensoready®* pen, prefilled syringe, or vial from refrigerator and allow to stand for 15–30 min to reach room temperature.
- Vial reconstitution: Slowly inject 1 mL of SW onto the powder.

Tilt vial 45° and gently rotate for about 1 min; do not shake or invert. Let vial stand at room temperature for approx. 10 min for powder to dissolve. Once again, tilt vial 45° and gently rotate for about 1 min; do not shake or invert. Allow vial to stand undisturbed at room temperature for about 5 min. Use immediately or store refrigerated for up to 24 h.
- Inject into outer thigh, lower abdomen (2 inches or greater away from the navel) or outer upper arm; rotate injection sites and avoid areas where the skin is tender, bruised, erythematous, indurated, or affected by psoriasis.
- Store intact vials, *Sensoready®* pens, and prefilled syringes refrigerated at 2°–8° C (36° 46° F).

**ADVERSE EFFECTS** (≥1%) **CNS:** Headache. **GI:** Diarrhea. **Respiratory:** Mucocutaneous infections, *nasopharyngitis*, oral herpes, pharyngitis, rhinitis, rhinorrhea, upper respiratory tract infection. **Endocrine:** Hypercholesterolemia. **Skin:** Urticaria.

**INTERACTIONS Drugs:** Do not give LIVE VACCINES.

**PHARMACOKINETICS Absorption:** 55–77% bioavailable. **Peak:** 6 days. **Metabolism:** Peptide degradation. **Half-Life:** 22–31 days.

## NURSING IMPLICATIONS

### Assessment & Drug Effects
- Monitor for and report development of infection (e.g., nasopharyngitis, upper respiratory tract infection, and mucocutaneous candida infection).
- Monitor patients with Crohn's disease for exacerbations.

Common adverse effects in *italic;* life-threatening effects <u>underlined</u>; generic names in **bold;** classifications in SMALL CAPS; ♣ Canadian drug name; ⊕ Prototype drug

1481

**Patient & Family Education**

- Minimize exposure to persons with known, active infections as this drug may lower the ability of your immune system to fight infections.
- Immediately report to prescriber if you develop S&S of an infection.
- Do not accept immunizations/vaccines while receiving this drug.
- Do not breast-feed while taking this drug without consulting prescriber.

# SELEGILINE HYDROCHLORIDE (L-DEPRENYL)

(se-leg'i-leen)

Eldepryl, Emsam, Zelapar

**Classifications:** ANTIPARKINSON; ANTIDEPRESSANT (MAOI)

Therapeutic: ANTIPARKINSON; ANTIDEPRESSANT

**AVAILABILITY** Tablet, capsule; orally disintegrating tablet; transdermal patch

**ACTION & *THERAPEUTIC EFFECT***

Effectiveness in parkinsonism is thought to be due to increased dopaminergic activity. It interferes with dopamine reuptake at the synapse of neurons as well as its inhibition of MAO type B dopaminergic activity in the brain. Interference with dopamine reuptake at the MAO type A dopaminergic receptors in the brain is thought to be the mechanism for antidepression. *Effectiveness is measured in decreased tremors, reduced akinesia, improved speech and motor abilities as well as improved walking. At slightly higher doses it is an effective antidepressant.*

**USES** Adjunctive therapy of Parkinson's disease for patients being treated with levodopa and carbidopa who exhibit deterioration in the quality of their response to therapy, major depressive disorder.

**UNLABELED USES** Attention deficit/hyperactivity disorder, extrapyramidal symptoms.

**CONTRAINDICATIONS** Hypersensitivity to selegiline; uncontrolled hypertension; use with dextromethorphan, other MAO inhibitors (MAOIs), meperidine, methadone, propoxyphene, and tramadol; suidical ideation; lactation.

**CAUTIOUS USE** Hypertension; hepatic or renal impairment; history of suicidal tendencies, bipolar disorder; restless leg disorder; impulse control disorder; psychosis; older adults; pregnancy (category C). Safety and efficacy and children younger than 16 y not established.

## ROUTE & DOSAGE

**Parkinson's Disease**

*Adult:* **PO** 5 mg b.i.d. with breakfast and lunch (do not exceed 10 mg/day); **PO (Zelapar)** 1.25 mg daily × 6 wk (max: 2.5 mg daily)
*Geriatric:* **PO** Start with 5 mg qa.m.

**Depression**

*Adult:* **Transdermal** 6 mg/day, may increase by 3 mg/day q2wk up to 12 mg/day

## ADMINISTRATION

**Oral**

- Give orally disintegrating tablets before breakfast, without liquid. Do not push tablets through the foil backing; peel back the backing of blister with dry hands

S

# SELEGILINE HYDROCHLORIDE (L-DEPRENYL)

and gently remove tablet. Immediately place tablet on top of the tongue. Neither food nor liquids should be ingested for 5 min before/after administration.

- Store at 15°–30° C (59°–86° F).

## Transdermal

- Do not cut or trim patch.
- Before application wash the area with soap and warm water. Dry thoroughly.
- Apply to upper torso, upper thigh, or outer surface of upper arm. Do not apply to hairy, oily, irritated, broken, or calloused skin.
- Rotate sites.
- Wash hands after application.

## ADVERSE EFFECTS (≥1%) CNS:
*Sleep disturbances*, psychosis, agitation, confusion, dyskinesia, dizziness, hallucinations, dystonia, akathisia, *headache*. **CV:** *Hypotension*. **GI:** Anorexia, *nausea*, vomiting, abdominal pain, constipation, *diarrhea*, *xerostomia*.

## INTERACTIONS Drug: TRICYCLIC ANTIDEPRESSANTS may cause hyperpyrexia, seizures; **fluoxetine, sertraline, paroxetine** may cause serotonin syndrome or hyperthermia, diaphoresis, tremors, seizures, delirium; SYMPATHOMIMETIC AGENTS (e.g., **amphetamine, phenylephrine, phenylpropanolamine**), **guanethidine,** and **reserpine** may cause hypertensive crisis; CNS DEPRESSANTS have additive CNS depressive effects; OPIATE ANALGESICS (especially **meperidine**) may cause hypertensive crisis and circulatory collapse; **buspirone,** hypertension; GENERAL ANESTHETICS: Prolonged hypotensive and CNS depressant effects; hypertension, headache, hyperexcitability reported with **dopamine, methyldopa, levodopa,**

**tryptophan; metrizamide** may increase risk of seizures; HYPOTENSIVE AGENTS and DIURETICS have additive hypotensive effects. **Food:** Aged meats or aged cheeses, protein extracts, sour cream, alcohol, anchovies, liver, sausages, overripe figs, bananas, avocados, chocolate, soy sauce, bean curd, natural yogurt, fava beans—**tyramine**-containing foods may precipitate hypertensive crisis (less frequent with usual doses of **selegiline** than with other MAOIS). **Herbal: Ginseng, ephedra, ma huang, St. John's wort** may cause hypertensive crisis.

## PHARMACOKINETICS Absorption: Rapid; 73% reaches systemic circulation. **Onset:** 1 h. **Duration:** 1–3 days. **Distribution:** Crosses placenta; not known if distributed in breast milk. **Metabolism:** In liver to *N*-desmethyldeprenyl-amphetamine and methamphetamine. **Elimination:** In urine. **Half-Life:** 15 min (metabolites 2–20 h).

## NURSING IMPLICATIONS

### Black Box Warning

*Selegiline transdermal patch for depression has been associated with increased risk of suicidal thinking and behavior in children, adolescents, and young adults.*

### Assessment & Drug Effects

- Monitor vital signs, particularly during period of dosage adjustment. Report alterations in BP or pulse. Indications for discontinuation of the drug include orthostatic hypotension, hypertension, and arrhythmias.
- Monitor for changes in behavior that may indicate increased suicidality, especially in adolescents

Common adverse effects in *italic;* life-threatening effects underlined; generic names in **bold;** classifications in SMALL CAPS; ♣ Canadian drug name; ⊙ Prototype drug

1483

or children being treated for depression.

- Monitor all patients closely for behavior changes (e.g., hallucinations, confusion, depression, delusions).

### Patient & Family Education

- Do not exceed the prescribed drug dose.
- Report symptoms of MAO inhibitor-induced hypertension (e.g., severe headache, palpitations, neck stiffness, nausea, vomiting) immediately to prescriber.
- Do not drive or engage in potentially hazardous activities until response to drug is known.
- Make positional changes slowly and in stages. Orthostatic hypotension is possible as well as dizziness, light-headedness, and fainting.
- If the transdermal patch falls off, apply a new patch to a new area, and resume previous schedule.
- Only one should be worn at a given time. Remove the old transdermal patch.

## SELEXIPAG
(se-lex'i-pag)
Uptravi

**Classifications:** PROSTAGLANDIN; PULMONARY ANTIHYPERTENSIVE
**Therapeutic:** PULMONARY ANTIHYPERTENSIVE
**Prototype:** Epoprostenol

### AVAILABILITY Tablets

### ACTION & THERAPEUTIC EFFECT

Hydrolyzed in vivo to produce an active metabolite that acts as an agonist at the prostacyclin IP receptor. *Agonist action at the IP receptor produces inhibition of platelet function, a reduction in pulmonary vascular resistance, and* *relaxation of pulmonary vascular smooth muscle.*

**USES** Treatment of pulmonary arterial hypertension (PAH) in order to delay disease progression and reduce the risk of hospitalization.

**CONTRAINDICATIONS** Concomitant use with strong CYP2C8 inhibitors.

**CAUTIOUS USE** Avoid use in patients with severe hepatic impairment or pulmonary veno-occlusive disease (PVOD). There are no adequate and well-controlled studies in pregnancy or lactation.

### ROUTE & DOSAGE

**Pulmonary Arterial Hypertension**

*Adult:* **PO** 200 mcg b.i.d.; may increase weekly in 200 mcg increments (max dose: 1600 mcg)

**Hepatic Impairment Dosage Adjustment**

*Moderate impairment (Child-Pugh class B):* Reduce dosing interval to once daily
*Severe impairment (Child-Pugh class C):* Avoid use

### ADMINISTRATION

**Oral**
- Administer without regard to food. Administering with food may improve tolerability.
- Do not split, crush, or chew tablets.
- Store at 15°–30° C (59°–86° F).

**ADVERSE EFFECTS** (≥1%) **Body as a Whole:** Anemia, decreased appetite, flushing, *jaw pain*, pain in extremity, rash. **CNS:** *Headache.* **Endocrine:** Hyperthyroidism. **GI:** *Diarrhea, nausea,* anorexia, vomiting. **Metabolic:** Decreased hemoglobin. **Musculoskeletal:** Arthralgia, jaw pain, limb pain, *myalgia*. **Skin:** Rash.

## DIAGNOSTIC TEST INTERFERENCE

Causes a reduction in thyroid function test results.

## INTERACTIONS Drug: Do not use with strong CYP2C8 inhibitors (e.g., **gemfibrozil**), may increase the levels of selexipag and its active metabolite. **Rifampin** may decrease serum concentrations.

## PHARMACOKINETICS Peak:

3–4 h. **Distribution:** 99% plasma protein bound. **Metabolism:** Hydrolyzed to active metabolite; hepatic metabolism to inactive metabolites. Metabolized via CYP3A4, CYP2C8, UGT1A3. **Elimination:** Primarily fecal (93%). **Half-Life:** 6.2–13.5 h (active metabolite).

## NURSING IMPLICATIONS

### Assessment & Drug Effects

- Skin assessment for flushing and rash.
- Respiratory assessment, including pulse oximetry.
- Complaint of jaw, limb, muscle, or joint pain.
- Monitor lab tests: Thyroid function tests, LFTs.

### Patient & Family Education

- Women need to use appropriate contraceptive measures.
- Report any signs of significant reaction: Wheezing, chest tightness, fever, itching, swelling of face, lips, tongue, or throat.
- Patients may have decreased appetite.
- Report any shortness of breath, severe loss of strength or energy.

# SENNA (SENNOSIDES)

(sen'na)

Black-Draught, Gentlax B, Senexon, Senokot, Senolax

**Classification:** STIMULANT LAXATIVE
**Therapeutic:** STIMULANT LAXATIVE
**Prototype:** Bisacodyl

## AVAILABILITY Tablet; syrup

## ACTION & THERAPEUTIC EFFECT

Senna glycosides are converted in colon to active aglycone, which stimulates peristalsis. Concentrate is purified and standardized for uniform action and is claimed to produce less colic than crude form. *Peristalsis stimulated by conversion of drug to active chemical.*

## USES Acute constipation and preoperative and preradiographic bowel evacuation.

## CONTRAINDICATIONS Hypersensitivity; appendicitis, fecal impaction; fluid and electrolyte imbalances; irritable colon, nausea, vomiting, undiagnosed abdominal pain, intestinal obstruction.

## CAUTIOUS USE Diabetes mellitus; fluid and electrolyte imbalances; pregnancy (category C). Safe use in children younger than 1 mo not established.

## ROUTE & DOSAGE

### Constipation

*Adult:* **PO Standard Senna Concentrate** 1–2 tablets or ½–1 tsp at bedtime (max: 4 tablets or 2 tsp b.i.d.); **Syrup, Liquid** 10–15 mL at bedtime
*Child (weight greater than 27 kg):* **PO Standard Senna Concentrate** 1 tablet or ½ tsp at bedtime;

---

Common adverse effects in *italic;* life-threatening effects underlined; generic names in **bold;** classifications in SMALL CAPS; ♣ Canadian drug name; ⓟ Prototype drug

1485

*Child (1 mo–1 y):* **Syrup, Liquid** 1.25–2.5 mL at bedtime; *1–5 y:* 2.5–5 mL at bedtime; *5–15 y:* 5–10 mL at bedtime

## ADMINISTRATION

### Oral
- Give at bedtime, generally.
- Avoid exposing drug to excessive heat; protect fluid extracts from light.

## ADVERSE EFFECTS (≥1%)

**GI:** Abdominal cramps, flatulence, nausea, watery diarrhea, excessive loss of water and electrolytes, weight loss, melanotic segmentation of colonic mucosa (reversible).

## PHARMACOKINETICS

**Onset:** 6–10 h; may take up to 24 h. **Metabolism:** In liver. **Elimination:** In feces.

## NURSING IMPLICATIONS

### Assessment & Drug Effects
- Reduce dose in patients who experience considerable abdominal cramping.

### Patient & Family Education
- Be aware that drug may alter urine and feces color; yellowish brown (acid), reddish brown (alkaline).
- Continued use may lead to dependence. Consult prescriber if constipation persists.
- See bisacodyl for additional nursing implications.

# SERTACONAZOLE NITRATE

(ser-ta-con'a-zole)

**Ertaczo**

**Classifications:** ANTIBIOTIC; AZOLE ANTIFUNGAL
**Therapeutic:** ANTIFUNGAL
**Prototype:** Fluconazole

## AVAILABILITY
Cream

## ACTION & *THERAPEUTIC EFFECT*
Believed to act primarily by inhibiting cytochrome P450–dependent synthesis of ergosterol, a key component of the cell membrane of fungi resulting in fungal cell injury. *Has a broad spectrum of activity against common fungal pathogens.*

## USES
Treatment of tinea pedis in immunocompetent patients.

## CONTRAINDICATIONS
Hypersensitivity to imidazoles.

## CAUTIOUS USE
History of hypersensitivity to azole antifungals; pregnancy (category C); lactation; children younger than 12 y.

## ROUTE & DOSAGE

**Tinea Pedis**

*Adult/Child (12 y or older):*
**Topical** Apply thin layer to affected area twice daily for 4 wk

## ADMINISTRATION

### Topical
- Cleanse the affected area and dry thoroughly before application.
- Apply a thin layer of the cream to affected area between the toes and the immediately surrounding healthy skin. Gently rub into the skin.
- Store at 15°–30° C (57°–86° F).

## ADVERSE EFFECTS (≥1%)
**Skin:** Contact dermatitis, dry skin, burning, application site reaction, skin tenderness.

## PHARMACOKINETICS
**Absorption:** Negligible through intact skin.

## NURSING IMPLICATIONS

### Assessment & Drug Effects
- Monitor for clinical improvement, which should be seen about 2 wk after initiating treatment.

S

**Patient & Family Education**

- Report any of the following: Severe skin irritation, redness, burning, blistering, or itching.
- Do not stop using this medication prematurely. Athlete's foot takes about 4 wk to clear completely.
- Nursing mothers should ensure that this topical cream does not accidentally get on the breast.

# SERTRALINE HYDROCHLORIDE

(ser'tra-leen)
Zoloft
**Classifications:** ANTIDEPRESSANT; SELECTIVE SEROTONIN REUPTAKE INHIBITOR (SSRI)
**Therapeutic:** ANTIDEPRESSANT; SSRI
**Prototype:** Fluoxetine

**AVAILABILITY** Tablet; oral solution

## ACTION & THERAPEUTIC EFFECT

Potent inhibitor of serotonin (5-HT) reuptake in the brain. Chronic administration results in downregulation of norepinephrine, a reaction found with other effective antidepressants. *Effective in controlling depression, obsessive-compulsive disorder, anxiety, and panic disorder.*

**USES** Major depression, obsessive-compulsive disorder, panic disorder, social anxiety disorder, premenstrual dysphoric disorder, post-traumatic stress disorder.

**UNLABELED USES** Eating disorders, generalized anxiety disorder.

**CONTRAINDICATIONS** Patients taking MAO inhibitors or within 14 days of discontinuing MAO inhibitor; concurrent use of Antabuse; suicidal ideation, hyponatremia; mania or hypomania; children with MDD.

**CAUTIOUS USE** Seizure disorders, major affective disorders, bipolar disorder, history of suicide; liver dysfunction, renal impairment; abrupt discontinuation; anorexia nervosa, recent history of MI or unstable cardiac disease, dehydration; DM; risk factor for QT prolongation; ECT therapy, older adults; pregnancy (category C); lactation. Safe use for OCD in children younger than 6 y is not established.

## ROUTE & DOSAGE

| **Depression, Panic Disorder, PTSD** |
| --- |
| *Adult:* **PO** Begin with 50 mg/day, gradually increase every few weeks according to response (range: 50–200 mg) |
| *Geriatric:* **PO** Start with 25 mg/day |
| **Premenstrual Dysphoric Disorder** |
| *Adult:* **PO** Begin with 50 mg/day for first cycle, may titrate up to 150 mg/day |
| **Obsessive-Compulsive Disorder** |
| *Adult / Adolescent:* **PO** Begin with 50 mg/day, may titrate at weekly intervals up to 200 mg/day |
| *Child (6–12 y):* **PO** Begin with 25 mg/day, may increase by 50 mg/wk, as tolerated and needed, up to 200 mg/day |

## ADMINISTRATION

### Oral

- Give in the morning or evening.
- Do not give concurrently with an MAO inhibitor or within 14 days of discontinuing an MAO inhibitor.
- Oral solution: Dilute concentrate before use with 4 oz of water, ginger ale, lemon/lime soda, lemonade, or orange juice ONLY. Give immediately after mixing. Caution with latex sensitivity, as the dropper contains dry natural rubber.

S

---

## ADVERSE EFFECTS (≥1%)

**CV:** Palpitations, chest pain, hypertension, hypotension, edema, syncope, tachycardia. **CNS:** *Agitation, insomnia, headache, dizziness, somnolence, fatigue,* ataxia, incoordination, vertigo, abnormal dreams, aggressive behavior, delusions, hallucinations, emotional lability, paranoia, <u>suicidal ideation, seizure</u>, depersonalization. **Endocrine:** Gynecomastia, *male sexual dysfunction.* **GI:** *Nausea, vomiting, diarrhea, constipation,* indigestion, anorexia, flatulence, abdominal pain, dry mouth. **Special Senses:** Exophthalmos, blurred vision, dry eyes, diplopia, photophobia, tearing, conjunctivitis, mydriasis, tinnitus. **Skin:** Rash, urticaria, acne, alopecia. **Respiratory:** Rhinitis, pharyngitis, cough, dyspnea, bronchospasm. **Body as a Whole:** Myalgia, arthralgia, muscle weakness, bone fracture (older adults). **Metabolic:** Hyponatremia in older adults.

## DIAGNOSTIC TEST INTERFERENCE

May cause asymptomatic elevations in *liver function tests.* Slight decrease in *uric acid.*

## INTERACTIONS

**Drug:** MAOIS (e.g., **selegiline, phenelzine**) should be stopped 14 days before sertraline is started because of serious problems with other SEROTONIN REUPTAKE INHIBITORS (shivering, nausea, diplopia, confusion, anxiety). **Sertraline** may increase levels and toxicity of **diazepam, pimozide, tolbutamide.** Use cautiously with other centrally acting CNS drugs; increase risk of **ergotamine** toxicity with **dihydroergotamine, ergotamine.** Avoid with agents that prolong the QT interval (e.g., **bepridil, dronedarone, ziprasidone**). Concentrate interacts with **disulfiram. Herbal:** **St. John's wort** may cause **serotonin** syndrome (headache, dizziness, sweating, agitation). **Food: Grapefruit juice** (greater than 1 qt/day) may increase plasma concentrations and adverse effects.

## PHARMACOKINETICS

**Absorption:** Slowly from GI tract. **Onset:** 2–4 wk. **Distribution:** 99% protein bound; distribution into breast milk unknown. **Metabolism:** Extensive first-pass metabolism in liver to inactive metabolites (substrate of CYP2B6, CYP2C9, CYP2D6, CYP3A4, and CYP2C19). **Elimination:** 40–45% in urine, 40–45% in feces. **Half-Life:** 24 h.

## NURSING IMPLICATIONS

### Black Box Warning

*Sertraline has been associated with increased risk of suicidal thinking and behavior in children, adolescents, and young adults.*

### Assessment & Drug Effects

- Supervise patients at risk for suicide closely during initial therapy.
- Monitor for worsening of depression or emergence of suicidal ideation.
- Monitor older adults for fluid and sodium imbalances.
- Monitor patients with a history of a seizure disorder closely.
- Monitor lab tests: Thyroid function tests.

### Patient & Family Education

- Report diarrhea, nausea, dyspepsia, insomnia, drowsiness, dizziness, or persistent headache to prescriber.
- Report emergence of agitation, irritability, hostility or aggression, mania.
- Report signs of bleeding promptly to prescriber when taking concomitant warfarin.

## SEVELAMER HYDROCHLORIDE ⓟ

(se-vel′a-mer)

Renagel, Renvela

**Classifications:** ELECTROLYTE
AND WATER BALANCE AGENT;
PHOSPHATE BINDER
Therapeutic: PHOSPHATE BINDER

**AVAILABILITY** Tablet; oral powder
for suspension

## ACTION & *THERAPEUTIC EFFECT*

Polymer that binds intestinal phosphate; interacts with phosphate by
way of ion exchange and hydrogen
binding. *Effectiveness indicated by
a serum phosphate level 6.0 mg/dL
or less*

**USES** Hyperphosphatemia.

**CONTRAINDICATIONS** Hypersensitivity to sevelamer HCl; hypophosphatemia; fecal impaction;
bowel obstruction; appendicitis;
dysphagia, GI bleeding, major GI
surgery; lactation.

**CAUTIOUS USE** GI motility disorders; vitamin deficiencies (especially vitamins D, E, and K and folic
acid); pregnancy (category C); children younger than 18 y.

## ROUTE & DOSAGE

**Hyperphosphatemia**
*Adult:* **PO** 800–1600 mg t.i.d.
based on severity of hyperphosphatemia

## ADMINISTRATION

**Oral**
- Give with meals.
- Give other oral medications 1 h
  before or 3 h after Renagel.
- Store at 15°–30° C (59°–86° F);
  protect from moisture.

**ADVERSE EFFECTS** (≥1%) **Body
as a Whole:** Headache, infection,
pain. **CV:** Hypertension, hypotension, thrombosis. **GI:** Diarrhea,
dyspepsia, vomiting, nausea,
constipation, flatulence. **Respiratory:** Increased cough.

## NURSING IMPLICATIONS

### Assessment & Drug Effects
- Monitor lab tests: Periodic 24-hour
  urinary calcium and phosphorus,
  and serum magnesium; alkaline
  phosphatase q12mo or more often
  with elevated PTH; iPTH q3–12 mo
  depending on CKD severity.

### Patient & Family Education
- Take daily multivitamin supplement approved by prescriber.

## SILDENAFIL CITRATE ⓟ

(sil-den′a-fil ci′trate)

Revatio, Viagra

**Classifications:** PHOSPHODIESTER-
ASE (PDE) INHIBITOR; IMPOTENCE;
PULMONARY ANTIHYPERTENSIVE
Therapeutic: PULMONARY ANTIHY-
PERTENSIVE; IMPOTENCE

**AVAILABILITY** Tablet; solution for
injection; powder for oral suspension

## ACTION & *THERAPEUTIC EFFECT*

Enhances vasodilation effect of
nitric oxide in the corpus caverno-
sus of the penis, thus sustaining an
erection. PDE-5 inhibitors increase
pulmonary vasodilation by sustaining levels of cyclic guanosine
monophosphate (cGMP). Additionally, sildenafil produces a reduction
in the pulmonary to systemic vascular resistance ratio. *Effective for
treatment of erectile dysfunction,
whether organic or psychogenic in
origin. Sildenafil produces a significant improvement in arterial
oxygenation in pulmonary arterial
hypertension (PAH).*

S

**USES** Erectile dysfunction, pulmonary arterial hypertension.

**UNLABELED USES** Altitude sickness, Raynaud's phenomenon, sexual dysfunction, anorgasmy.

**CONTRAINDICATIONS** Hypersensitivity to sildenafil. Patients with pulmonary veno-occlusive disease (PVOD) and patients taking nitrate/nitrite therapy.

**CAUTIOUS USE** CAD with unstable angina, heart failure, MI, cardiac arrhythmias, stroke within 6 mo of starting drug; hypotension and hypertension; risk factors for CVA; aortic stenosis; anatomic deformity of the penis; sickle cell anemia, polycythemia; multiple myeloma; leukemia; active bleeding or a peptic ulcer, GERD, hiatal hernia; coagulopathy; retinitis pigmentosa; visual disturbances; hepatic disease, hepatitis, cirrhosis; severe renal impairment; older adults; pregnancy (category B); lactation; children and infants.

## ROUTE & DOSAGE

**Erectile Dysfunction**
*Adult:* **PO** 50 mg 0.5–4 h before sexual activity (dose range: 25 to 100 mg once/day)
*Geriatric:* **PO** 25 mg approximately 1 h before sexual activity
**Pulmonary Arterial Hypertension**
*Adult:* **PO** 5 mg or 20 mg t.i.d. (4–6 h apart); **IV** 2.5 mg or 10 mg t.i.d.
*Hepatic Impairment Dosage Adjustment*
*Child-Pugh class A or B:* Starting dose of 25 mg
*Renal Impairment Dosage Adjustment*
*CrCl less than 30 mL/min:* Starting dose of 25 mg

## ADMINISTRATION
**Oral**
- For erectile dysfunction: Dose 1 h prior to sexual activity (effective range is 0.5–4 h).

**Intravenous**

*PREPARE:* **Direct:** Give undiluted.
*ADMINISTER:* **Direct:** Give as a bolus dose.

- Store at 15°–30° C (59°–86° F) in a tightly closed container; protect from light.

**ADVERSE EFFECTS** (≥1%) **Body as a Whole:** Face edema, photosensitivity, shock, asthenia, pain, chills, fall, allergic reaction, arthritis, myalgia. **CNS:** *Headache,* dizziness, migraine, syncope, cerebral thrombosis, ataxia, neuralgia, paresthesias, tremor, vertigo, depression, insomnia, somnolence, abnormal dreams. **CV:** Flushing, chest pain, <u>MI</u>, angina, AV block, tachycardia, palpitation, hypotension, postural hypotension, <u>cardiac arrest</u>, <u>sudden cardiac death</u>, heart failure, cardiomyopathy, abnormal ECG, edema. **GI:** Dyspepsia, diarrhea, abdominal pain, vomiting, colitis, dysphagia, gastritis, gastroenteritis, esophagitis, stomatitis, dry mouth, abnormal liver function tests, thirst. **Respiratory:** Nasal congestion, asthma, dyspnea, epistaxis, laryngitis, pharyngitis, sinusitis, bronchitis, cough. **Skin:** Rash, urticaria, pruritus, sweating, <u>exfoliative dermatitis</u>. **Urogenital:** UTI. **Special Senses:** Abnormal vision (color changes, photosensitivity, blurred vision, sudden vision loss). **Hematologic:** Anemia, <u>leukopenia</u>. **Metabolic:** Gout, hyperglycemia, hyperuricemia, hypoglycemia, hypernatremia.

**INTERACTIONS Drug:** NITRATES increase risk of serious hypotension; if used within 4 h of **doxazosin,**

prazosin, terazosin, **tamsulosin**; cimetidine, **erythromycin**, ketoconazole, itraconazole, PROTEASE INHIBITORS increase sildenafil levels; **rifampin** can decrease sildenafil levels. Do not use with **telaprevir.** **Food: Grapefruit juice** (greater than 1 qt/day) may increase plasma concentrations and adverse effects.

**PHARMACOKINETICS Absorption:** Rapidly from GI tract. **Peak:** 30–120 min. **Distribution:** 96% protein bound. **Metabolism:** In liver (CYP3A4 and 2C9). **Elimination:** 80% in feces, 12% in urine. **Half-Life:** 4 h.

## NURSING IMPLICATIONS

### Assessment & Drug Effects
- Monitor carefully for and immediately report S&S of cardiac distress.

### Patient & Family Education
- Do not take sildenafil within 4 h of taking doxazosin, prazosin, terazosin, or tamsulosin.
- Consuming a high-fat meal before taking drug may cause delay in drug action.
- Report to prescriber: Headaches, flushing, chest pain, indigestion, blurred vision, sensitivity to light, changes in color vision.
- Seek medical attention if erection lasts for more than 4 h.

---

# SILODOSIN
(sil'o-do-sin)
Rapaflo
**Classifications:** ALPHA-1 ADRENERGIC RECEPTOR ANTAGONIST; GENITOURINARY SMOOTH MUSCLE RELAXANT
**Therapeutic:** GENITOURINARY SMOOTH MUSCLE RELAXANT
**Prototype:** Tamsulosin

**AVAILABILITY** Capsule

## ACTION & *THERAPEUTIC EFFECT*
Selective antagonist of post-synaptic alpha-1 adrenoreceptors located in the prostate, bladder base, bladder neck, prostatic capsule, and prostatic urethra. *Blockade of these alpha-1 adrenoreceptors causes the smooth muscle in these tissues to relax, resulting in improvement in urine flow and reduction in signs and symptoms of benign prostatic hyperplasia (BPH).*

**USES** Treatment of the signs and symptoms of BPH.

## CONTRAINDICATIONS
Severe renal impairment (CrCl less than 30 mL/min); severe hepatic impairment (Child-Pugh score greater than or equal to 10).

**CAUTIOUS USE** Moderate renal impairment; history of hypotension; cataract surgery; older adults; pregnancy (category B); lactation. Safe use in children not established.

## ROUTE & DOSAGE

| Benign Prostatic Hyperplasia |
| --- |
| *Adult:* **PO** 8 mg once daily with a meal |
| ***Renal Impairment Dosage Adjustment*** |
| *CrCl 30–49 mL/min:* **4 mg once daily;** *less than 30 mL/min:* Contraindicated |

## ADMINISTRATION

### Oral
- Give with meals.
- Store at 15°–30° C (59°–86° F). Protect from light and moisture.

**ADVERSE EFFECTS** (≥1%) **Body as a Whole:** Abdominal pain, asthenia. **CNS:** Dizziness, headache, insomnia. **CV:** Orthostatic hypotension. **GI:** Diarrhea. **Respiratory:** Nasal congestion, nasopharyngitis,

S

Common adverse effects in *italic;* life-threatening effects underlined; generic names in **bold**; classifications in SMALL CAPS; ♣ Canadian drug name; ⊘ Prototype drug

1491

rhinorrhea, sinusitis. **Urogenital:** *Retrograde ejaculation.*

## DIAGNOSTIC TEST INTERFERENCE
Increased *prostate specific antigen (PSA).*

## INTERACTIONS Drug:
Strong CYP3A4 inhibitors (e.g., **idelalisib, itraconazole, ritonavir**) or strong P-GLYCOPROTEIN INHIBITORS (e.g., **ketoconazole**) greatly increases silodosin levels. Moderate CYP3A4 inhibitors (e.g., **clarithromycin, diltiazem, erythromycin, verapamil**) may increase silodosin levels. Other ALPHA-BLOCKERS can cause additive pharmacodynamic effects. INHIBITORS OF UDP-GLUCURONOSYLTRANSFERASE 2B7 (e.g., **probenecid, valproic acid, fluconazole**) may increase silodosin levels. Do not use with **boceprevir.**

## PHARMACOKINETICS Absorption:
32% bioavailable. **Distribution:** Approximately 97% plasma protein bound. **Metabolism:** By CYP3A4 hepatic enzymes and is a P-glycoprotein (P-gp) substrate. **Elimination:** Renal and fecal. **Half-Life:** 13.3 h.

## NURSING IMPLICATIONS
### Assessment & Drug Effects
- Monitor I&O and ease of voiding.
- Monitor orthostatic vital signs (lying and then standing) at the beginning of therapy. Report a systolic pressure drop of 15 mm Hg or greater and HR increase of 15 beats or greater upon standing.
- Monitor for orthostatic hypotension, especially at the beginning of therapy and in those taking concurrent antihypertensive drugs.

### Patient & Family Education
- Make position changes slowly and in stages to minimize risk of dizziness and fainting.

- Avoid hazardous activities until reaction to drug is known.
- Report unexplained skin eruptions or purple skin patches.
- If cataract surgery is planned, inform ophthalmologist that you are taking silodosin.

## SILVER SULFADIAZINE ℗
(sul-fa-dye'a-zeen)
Silvadene, SSD
**Classification:** SULFONAMIDE
Therapeutic: TOPICAL ANTI-INFECTIVE

## AVAILABILITY Cream

## ACTION & *THERAPEUTIC EFFECT*
Silver salt is released slowly and exerts bactericidal effect only on bacterial cell membrane and wall. *Broad antimicrobial activity including many gram-negative and gram-positive bacteria and yeast.*

## USES
Prevention and treatment of sepsis in second- and third-degree burns.

## CONTRAINDICATIONS
Hypersensitivity to other sulfonamides; pregnant women at term.

## CAUTIOUS USE
Impaired kidney or liver function; porphyria; impaired respiratory function; G6PD deficiency; thrombocytopenia, leukopenia, hematological disease; pregnancy (category B); lactation; preterm infants; neonates younger than 2 mo.

## ROUTE & DOSAGE

### Burn Wound Treatment
*Adult/Child:* **Topical** Apply 1% cream 1–2 × day to thickness of approximately 1.5 mm (¹⁄₁₆ in.)

Common adverse effects in *italic;* life-threatening effects <u>underlined;</u> generic names in **bold;** classifications in SMALL CAPS; ♣ Canadian drug name; ℗ Prototype drug

## ADMINISTRATION

### Topical
- Do not use if cream darkens; it is water soluble and white.
- Apply with sterile, gloved hands to cleansed, debrided burned areas. Reapply cream to areas where it has been removed by patient activity; cover burn wounds with medication at all times.
- Bathe patient daily (in whirlpool or shower or in bed) as aid to debridement. Reapply drug.
- Note: Dressings are not required but may be used if necessary. Drug does not stain clothing.
- Store at room temperature away from heat.

**ADVERSE EFFECTS (≥1%) Body as a Whole:** Pain (occasionally), burning, itching, rash, reversible leukopenia. Potential for toxicity as for other SULFONAMIDES if applied to extensive areas of the body surface.

**INTERACTIONS Drug:** PROTEOLYTIC ENZYMES are inactivated by silver in cream.

**PHARMACOKINETICS Absorption:** Not absorbed through intact skin, however, approximately 10% could be absorbed when applied to second- or third-degree burns. **Distribution:** Distributed into most body tissues. **Metabolism:** In the liver. **Elimination:** In urine.

## NURSING IMPLICATIONS

### Assessment & Drug Effects
- Observe for and report hypersensitivity reaction: Rash, itching, or burning sensation in unburned areas.
- Observe patient for reactions attributed to sulfonamides.

- Note: Analgesic may be required. Occasionally, pain is experienced on application; intensity and duration depend on depth of burn.
- Continue treatment until satisfactory healing or burn site is ready for grafting, unless adverse reactions occur.

## SIMEPREVIR
(sim-e-pre'vir)
Olysio

**Classifications:** ANTIVIRAL; VIRAL PROTEIN INHIBTOR; DIRECT-ACTING ANTI-VIRUS; ANTIHEPATITIS
**Therapeutic:** ANTIHEPATITIS
**Prototype:** Boceprevir

**AVAILABILITY** Capsules

### ACTION & THERAPEUTIC EFFECT
A direct-acting antiviral agent (DAA) that inhibits viral enzymes needed for critical steps in HCV replication; prevents HCV replication.

**USES** Treatment of chronic hepatitis C (CHC) infection in combination with other agents, in HCV genotype 1 infection.

**CONTRAINDICATIONS** Severe hepatic impairment (Child-Pugh class C); autoimmune hepatitis; decompensated liver disease; lactation.

**CAUTIOUS USE** Renal impairment; mild or moderate hepatic impairment; sulfa allergy; individuals of eastern Asian ancestry; older adults; pregnancy (category C). Safety and efficacy in children younger than 18 y not established.

### ROUTE & DOSAGE

**Hepatitis C Infection**
Adult: **PO** 150 mg once a day for 12 wk in combination with other agents

> **Discontinuation Based on Inadequate Virologic Response**
>
> If HCV RNA 25 IU/mL or greater at wk 4: Discontinue all therapy

## ADMINISTRATION

### Oral

- Give with food and concurrently with peginterferon alfa and ribavirin.
- Capsules **must be** swallowed whole. They should not be cut or chewed.
- If peginterferon alfa or ribavirin is discontinued for any reason, simeprevir also **must be** discontinued.
- The dose of simeprevir **must not be** reduced or interrupted. If discontinued because of adverse reactions or inadequate response, treatment **must not be** reinitiated.
- Store at room temperature below 30° C (86° F). Protect from light.

## ADVERSE EFFECTS (≥ 1%) Body as a Whole: *Pruritus*. GI: *Nausea*. Hematological: *Increased serum bilirubin*, increased serum alkaline phosphatase. Musculoskeletal: *Myalgia*. Respiratory: *Dyspnea*. Skin: Grade 3 photosensitivity, pruritus, *rash* (includes: Cutaneous vasculitis, dermatitis exfoliative, eczema, erythema, maculopapular rash, photosensitivity reaction, toxic skin eruption, urticaria). CNS: Dizziness, fatigue, headache, insomnia.

## INTERACTIONS Drug: Simeprevir may increase the levels of drugs that are substrates for OATP1B1/3 and P-gp transport (e.g., **digoxin,** HMG COA REDUCTASE INHIBITORS). Simeprevir may increase the levels of drugs requiring intestinal CYP3A4 for metabolism (e.g., CALCIUM CHANNEL BLOCKERS, **cisapride, midazolam, sildenafil, tadalafil, triazolam, vardenafil**). Co-administration of simeprevir with moderate or strong inhibitors of CYP3A4 (e.g., AZOLE ANTIFUNGALS, HIV PROTEASE INHIBITORS, MACROLDES), may increase the levels of simeprevir. Co-administration with moderate or strong inducers of CYP3A4 (e.g., **carbamazepine, dexamethasone, efavirenz, phenobarbital, phenytoin**) may decrease the levels of simeprevir. **Food: Grapefruit** and **grapefruit juice** may increase the levels of simeprevir. **Herbal: Milk thistle** may increase the levels of simeprevir. **St. John's wort** may decrease the levels of simeprevir.

## PHARMACOKINETICS Absorption: Orally bioavailable. **Peak:** 4–6 h. **Distribution:** 99.9% plasma protein bound, extensively distributed to gut and liver. **Metabolism:** In liver. **Elimination:** Primarily unchanged in feces. **Half-Life:** 10–13 h.

## NURSING IMPLICATIONS

### Assessment & Drug Effects

- Monitor for adverse dermatologic effects (e.g., including erythema, eczema, maculopapular rash, urticaria, toxic skin eruption, exfoliative dermatitis) and follow for progression and/or development of mucosal signs (e.g., oral lesions, conjunctivitis) or systemic symptoms. If rash becomes severe, report promptly to prescriber.
- Monitor lab tests: Baseline and periodic LFTs, uric acid; serum HCV-RNA at baseline and at wk 4, 12, 24, and end of treatment, and during treatment follow-up; pretreatment and monthly pregnancy tests and up to 6 mo after therapy is discontinued.

### Patient & Family Education

- **Do not** reduce or interrupt the dose of simeprevir.

Common adverse effects in *italic;* life-threatening effects <u>underlined</u>; generic names in **bold;** classifications in SMALL CAPS; ♣ Canadian drug name; ◎ Prototype drug

- Avoid excessive sunlight and tanning devices, and take precautions to limit exposure as drug (e.g., sunscreen) may cause moderate to severe phototoxicity reaction.
- Women of childbearing potential and male partners of pregnant women should use effective means of contraception while taking this drug and for at least 6 mo following discontinuation of therapy.

## SIMVASTATIN
(sim-vah-sta′tin)
Zocor
**Classifications:** HMG-COA REDUCTASE INHIBITOR (STATIN); ANTIHYPERLIPEMIC
**Therapeutic:** ANTILIPEMIC; STATIN
**Prototype:** Lovastatin

### AVAILABILITY Tablet

### ACTION & *THERAPEUTIC EFFECT*
Inhibitor of HMG-CoA reductase. HMG-CoA reductase inhibitors increase HDL cholesterol, and decrease LDL cholesterol, and total cholesterol synthesis. *Effectiveness indicated by decreased serum triglycerides, decreased LDL, cholesterol, and modest increases in HDL cholesterol.*

### USES Hypercholesterolemia (alone or in combination with other agents), familial hypercholesterolemia. Reduces risk of CHD death and nonfatal MI and stroke.

### CONTRAINDICATIONS Hypersensitivity to simvastatin; active liver disease or unexplained elevation of serum transaminase, hepatic encephalopathy, hepatitis, jaundice, AST or ALT of 3 × ULN; rhabdomyolysis, acute renal failure; cholestasis; myopathy; MS; pregnancy (category X); lactation.

### CAUTIOUS USE Homozygous familial hypercholesterolemia, history of liver disease, alcoholics; renal disease, renal impairment; DM; seizure disorder; children younger than 10 y.

### ROUTE & DOSAGE

**Hypercholesterolemia, Hyperlipidemia, CV Prevention**
*Adult:* PO 10–20 mg each evening; usual dose 5–40 mg daily (max: 80 mg daily).
*Adolescent/Child (10 y or older and in females at least 1 y post-menarche):* PO 10 mg each night (may increase to 40 mg each night)

**Homozygous Familial Hypercholesterolemia**
*Adult:* PO 40 mg each evening

*Renal Impairment Dosage Adjustment*
*CrCl less than 20 mL/min:* Start with 5 mg each night

### ADMINISTRATION
Oral
- Adjust dosage usually at 4-wk intervals.
- Give in the evening.
- Store at 15°–30° C (59°–86° F).

### ADVERSE EFFECTS (≥1%) CV: Angina. CNS: Dizziness, headache, vertigo, asthenia, fatigue, insomnia. GI: Nausea, diarrhea, vomiting, abdominal pain, constipation, flatulence, heartburn, transient elevations in liver transaminases, transient elevations in CPK. Body as a Whole: Fatigue. Respiratory: Upper respiratory infection, rhinitis, cough. Endocrine: Increased risk of diabetes mellitus.

### INTERACTIONS Drug: Avoid use with **itraconazole, ketoconazole,**

S

Common adverse effects in *italic;* life-threatening effects <u>underlined;</u> generic names in **bold;** classifications in SMALL CAPS; ◆ Canadian drug name; ⊕ Prototype drug

1495

erythromycin, clarithromycin, telithromycin, PROTEASE INHIBITORS, nefazodone. Simvastatin dose will need to be decreased when given with **gemfibrozil, cyclosporine, danazole, amiodarone, verapamil, diltiazem.** May increase PT when administered with **warfarin; cyclosporine, gemfibrozil, fenofibrate, clofibrate,** antilipemic doses of **niacin, fluconazole, miconazole, sildenafil, tacrolimus,** may increase serum levels and increase risk of myopathy, rhabdomyolysis and acute kidney failure. Avoid use with **rifampin.** Use with **amiodarone** increases risk of rhabdomyolysis. Use with **amlodipine** increases risk of myopathy. **Food: Grapefruit juice** (greater than 1 qt/day) may increase risk of myopathy, rhabdomyolysis. **Herbal: St. John's wort** may decrease efficacy.

## LAB TEST INTERFERENCE May elevate *blood glucose* of *HbAlC* levels.

## PHARMACOKINETICS Absorption: Rapidly from GI tract. **Onset:** 2 wk. **Peak:** 4–6 wk. **Distribution:** 95% protein bound; achieves high liver concentrations; crosses placenta. **Metabolism:** Extensive first-pass metabolism to its active metabolite. **Elimination:** 60% in bile and feces.

## NURSING IMPLICATIONS

### Assessment & Drug Effects

- Assess for and report unexplained muscle pain. Determine CPK level at onset of muscle pain.
- Monitor coagulation studies with patients receiving concurrent warfarin therapy. PT may be prolonged.
- Monitor lab tests: Baseline and periodic lipid profile.

### Patient & Family Education

- Report unexplained muscle pain, tenderness, or weakness, especially if accompanied by malaise or fever, to prescriber.
- Report signs of bleeding to prescriber promptly when taking concurrent warfarin.
- Moderate intake of grapefruit juice while taking this medication.

## SIPULEUCEL-T
(sip-u-lew'cel)

Provenge

**Classifications:** BIOLOGIC RESPONSE MODIFIER; ACTIVE CELL IMMUNOTHERAPEUTIC; ANTINEOPLASTIC

Therapeutic: ANTINEOPLASTIC

**AVAILABILITY** Intravenous suspension

**ACTION & *THERAPEUTIC EFFECT*** While the mechanism of action is unknown, sipuleucel-T is designed to induce an immune response against prostatic acid phosphatase (PAP), an antigen expressed on most prostate cancer cells. *Stimulation of humoral and T-cell mediated responses are thought to slow tumor progression and improve survival.*

**USES** Prostate cancer.

**CONTRAINDICATIONS** Pregnancy category undetermined; not for use in women.

**CAUTIOUS USE** Concomitant use of chemotherapy; history of infusion reactions.

## ROUTE & DOSAGE

### Prostate Cancer

*Adult:* **IV** 250 mL infusion q2wk for a total of 3 doses

Common adverse effects in *italic*; life-threatening effects underlined; generic names in **bold**; classifications in SMALL CAPS; ✦ Canadian drug name; ⊙ Prototype drug

## ADMINISTRATION

### Intravenous

- Use universal precautions when handling sipuleucel-T. • Note: Premedication is recommended with oral acetaminophen and an antihistamine (e.g., diphenhydramine) approximately 30 min prior to administration.

*PREPARE:* **IV Infusion:** • Product is intended only for autologous use (i.e., patient donates to self). • Open the outer cardboard shipping box to verify the product and patient-specific labels located on the top of the insulated container. • **Do not** remove the insulated container from the shipping box, or open the lid of the insulated container, until the patient is ready for infusion. Inspect for leakage. • Contents of bag will be slightly cloudy, with a cream-to-pink color. Gently tilt bag to resuspend contents; inspect for clumps and clots that should disperse with gentle manual mixing. • Do not administer if the bag leaks during handling or if clumps remain in the bag.

*ADMINISTER:* **IV Infusion:** • Infusion must be started prior to the expiration date and time on *Cell Product Disposition Form* and label. Give over 60 min. • Administer through a dedicated line and **do not** use a cell filter. Ensure that entire contents of bag are infused. • Monitor closely during and for 1 h after infusion for an infusion reaction (e.g., dyspnea, hypertension, tachycardia, chills, fever, nausea). Infusion may be stopped or slowed depending on severity of reaction. • Do not reinitiate infusion with a bag held at room temperature for more than 3 h. *INCOMPATIBILITIES:* **Solution/additive:** Do not mix with another drug. **Y-site:** Do not mix with another drug.

## ADVERSE EFFECTS (≥5%) **Body as a Whole:** *Chills, citrate toxicity, fever,* hot flush, influenza-like illness, *pain,* peripheral edema. **CNS:** *Asthenia, dizziness, fatigue, headache,* insomnia, *paresthesia,* tremor. **GI:** Anorexia, *constipation,* diarrhea, *nausea, vomiting,* weight loss. **Hematologic:** *Anemia.* **Musculoskeletal:** *Back pain,* bone pain, *joint ache,* neck pain, *muscle ache,* muscle spasms, musculoskeletal chest pain, musculoskeletal pain, *pain in extremity.* **Respiratory:** Cough, dyspnea, upper respiratory infection. **Skin:** Rash, sweating. **Urogenital:** Hematuria, urinary tract infection.

## INTERACTIONS **Drug:** Due to the ability of sipuleucel-T to stimulate the immune system, concomitant use of immunosuppressive agents (e.g., **corticosteroids**) may alter the efficacy and/or safety of sipuleucel-T.

## NURSING IMPLICATIONS

### Assessment & Drug Effects

- Observe closely during infusion and for at least 1 h following for an infusion reaction (see Administration). Monitor vital signs throughout observation period. Note that an acute infusion reaction is more likely after the second infusion.
- Report immediately to prescriber if an infusion reaction occurs.

### Patient & Family Education

- Report immediately any of the following: Fever, chills, fatigue, breathing problems, dizziness, high blood pressure, palpitations, nausea, vomiting, headache, or muscle aches.

Common adverse effects in *italic;* life-threatening effects underlined; generic names in **bold;** classifications in SMALL CAPS; ♣ Canadian drug name; ⊙ Prototype drug

1497

# SIROLIMUS
(sir-o-li'mus)
**Rapamune**
**Classifications:** IMMUNOMODULA-
TOR; IMMUNOSUPPRESSANT
**Therapeutic:** IMMUNOSUPPRESSANT
**Prototype:** Cyclosporine

**AVAILABILITY** Tablet; oral solution

## ACTION & *THERAPEUTIC EFFECT*
Active in reducing a transplant rejection by inhibiting the response of helper T-lymphocytes and B-lymphocytes to cytokines [(interleukin) IL-2, IL-4, and IL-5]. *Inhibits antibody production and acute transplant rejection reaction in autoimmune disorders [e.g., systemic lupus erythematosus (SLE)]. Indicated by nonrejection of transplanted organ.*

**USES** Prophylaxis of kidney transplant rejection; treatment of lymphangioleiomyomatosis.

**CONTRAINDICATIONS** Hypersensitivity to sirolimus; lung or liver transplant patients; soya lecithin (soy fatty acids) hypersensitivity; PML; lactation.

**CAUTIOUS USE** Hypersensitivity to tacrolimus; impaired renal function; renal transplant patients; dialysis patients; hepatic impairment; UV exposure, retransplant patients, multiorgan transplant recipients, African American transplant patients; interstitial lung disease; viral or bacterial infection; hyperlipidemia, DM, atrial fibrillation, CHF, hypervolemia, palpitations; hepatic disease; CAD; myelosuppression; older adults; pregnancy (category C); children younger than 13 y.

## ROUTE & DOSAGE

**Kidney Transplant**
*Adult/Adolescent (over 40 kg):*
**PO** 6 mg loading dose immedi-ately after transplant, then 2 mg/day. Doses will need to be much higher if using cyclosporine or corticosteroids.
*Adolescent (13 y or older, weight less than 40 kg):* **PO** 3 mg/m² loading dose immediately after transplant, then 1 mg/m²/day.

**Lymphangioleiomyomatosis**
*Adult:* **PO** 2 mg daily, then adjust to target concentration of 5–15 mg/mL

### *Hepatic Impairment Dosage Adjustment*

Loading dose does not need to be modified.
*Mild to moderate:* Reduce maintenance does by 33%
*Severe impairment:* Reduce maintenance by 50%

## ADMINISTRATION
**Oral**
- Give 4 h after oral cyclosporine.
- Tablets should be swallowed whole. They should not be crushed or chewed.
- Add prescribed amount of sirolimus oral solution to a glass containing 2 oz (60 mL) or more of water or orange juice (do not use any other type of liquid). Stir vigorously and administer immediately. Refill glass with 4 oz (120 mL) or more of water or orange juice. Stir vigorously and administer immediately.
- Give consistently with respect to amount and type of food.
- Refrigerate; protect from light; use multidose bottles within 1 mo of opening.

**ADVERSE EFFECTS** (≥1%) **Body as a Whole:** *Asthenia, back pain, chest pain, fever, pain, arthralgia;* flu-like syndrome; generalized edema; infection; lymphocele; <u>malaise, sepsis,</u> arthrosis, bone necrosis, leg cramps,

Common adverse effects in *italic;* life-threatening effects <u>underlined;</u> generic names in **bold;** classifications in SMALL CAPS; ♣ Canadian drug name; ⦾ Prototype drug myalgia, osteoporosis, tetany, abscess, ascites, cellulitis, chills, face edema, hernia, pelvic pain, peritonitis. **CNS:** *Insomnia, tremor, headache,* anxiety, confusion, depression, dizziness, emotional lability, hypertonia, hyperesthesia, hypotonia, neuropathy, paresthesia, somnolence. **CV:** *Hypertension,* atrial fibrillation, CHF, hypervolemia, hypotension, palpitation, peripheral vascular disorder, postural hypotension, syncope, tachycardia, thrombophlebitis, thrombosis, vasodilation. **GI:** *Constipation, diarrhea, dyspepsia, nausea, vomiting, abdominal pain,* anorexia, dysphagia, eructation, esophagitis, flatulence, gastritis, gastroenteritis, gingivitis, gum hyperplasia, ileus, mouth ulceration, oral moniliasis, stomatitis, abnormal liver function tests. **Hematologic:** *Anemia,* thrombocytopenia, leukopenia, hemorrhage, ecchymosis, leukocytosis, lymphadenopathy, polycythemia, thrombotic, thrombocytopenic purpura. **Metabolic:** *Edema, hypercholesterolemia, hyperkalemia, hyperlipidemia, hypokalemia, hypophosphatemia, peripheral edema, weight gain,* Cushing's syndrome, diabetes, acidosis, hypercalcemia, hyperglycemia, hyperphosphatemia, hypomagnesemia, hypoglycemia, hypomagnesemia, hyponatremia; increased LDH, alkaline phosphatase, BUN, creatine phosphokinase, ALT, or AST; weight loss. **Respiratory:** *Dyspnea, pharyngitis, upper respiratory tract infection,* asthma, atelectasis, bronchitis, cough, epistaxis, hypoxia, lung edema, pleural effusion, pneumonia, rhinitis, sinusitis. **Skin:** *Acne, rash,* fungal dermatitis, hirsutism, pruritus, skin hypertrophy, skin ulcer, sweating. **Urogenital:** *UTI,* albuminuria, bladder pain, dysuria, hematuria, hydronephrosis, impotence, kidney pain, nocturia, renal tubular necrosis, oliguria, pyuria, scrotal edema, incontinence, urinary retention, glycosuria. **Special Senses:** Abnormal vision, cataract, conjunctivitis, deafness, ear pain, otitis media, tinnitus.

**INTERACTIONS Drug:** Sirolimus concentrations increased by **clarithromycin, cyclosporine, diltiazem, erythromycin, ketoconazole, itraconazole, telithromycin;** sirolimus concentrations decreased by **rifabutin, rifampin;** VACCINES may be less effective with sirolimus; **tacrolimus** increases mortality, hepatic artery thrombosis, and graft loss. **Food: Grapefruit juice** significantly increases plasma levels. High fat meals increase levels. **Herbal: St. John's wort** decreases efficacy.

**PHARMACOKINETICS Absorption:** Rapidly with 14% bioavailability. **Peak:** 2 h. **Distribution:** 92% protein bound, distributes in high concentrations to heart, intestines, kidneys, liver, lungs, muscle, spleen, and testes. **Metabolism:** In liver (CYP3A4). **Elimination:** 91% in feces, 2.2% in urine. **Half-Life:** 62 h.

## NURSING IMPLICATIONS

### Black Box Warning

*Sirolimus has been associated with increased susceptibility to infection and development of lymphoma.*

### Assessment & Drug Effects
- Monitor for S&S of graft rejection.
- Control hyperlipidemia prior to initiating drug.
- Monitor for and report promptly S&S of infection.
- Draw trough whole-blood sirolimus levels 1 h before a scheduled dose.
- Monitor lab tests: Periodic lipid profile, CBC with differential, LFTs, urinary protein, and creatinine, and serum sirolimus as indicated.

### Patient & Family Education
- Avoid grapefruit juice within 2 h of taking sirolimus.
- Limit exposure to sunlight (UV exposure).

**S**

- Note: Decreased effectiveness possible for vaccines during therapy.
- Use or add barrier contraceptive before, during, and for 12 wk after discontinuing therapy.

## SITAGLIPTIN ℗

(sit-a-glip'tin)

*Januvia*

**Classifications:** INCRETIN MODIFIER; DIPEPTIDYL PEPTIDASE-4 (DPP-4) INHIBITOR; ANTIDIABETIC

**Therapeutic:** ANTIDIABETIC; INCRETIN MODIFIER; DDP-4 INHIBITOR

**AVAILABILITY** Tablet

**ACTION & *THERAPEUTIC EFFECT***
Slows inactivation of incretin hormones [e.g., glucagon-like peptide-1 (GLP-1) and glucose-dependent insulinotropic polypeptide (GIP)] that are released by the intestine. As plasma glucose rises following food intake, incretin hormones stimulate release of insulin from the pancreas, and GLP-1 also lowers glucagon secretion, resulting in reduced hepatic glucose production. *Sitagliptin lowers both fasting and postprandial plasma glucose levels.*

**USES** Adjunct treatment of type 2 diabetes mellitus.

**CONTRAINDICATIONS** Serious hypersensitivity to sitagliptin; type I DM; diabetic ketoacidosis.

**CAUTIOUS USE** Moderate to severe renal impairment, renal failure, hemodialysis; older adults; history of pancreatitis; pregnancy (category C); lactation. Safe use in children younger than 18 y not established.

## ROUTE & DOSAGE

**Type 2 Diabetes Mellitus**
*Adult:* **PO** 100 mg/day

**Renal Impairment Dosage Adjustment**
*CrCl between 30 mL/min and 50 mL/min:* 50 mg/day; *less than 30 mL/min:* 25 mg/day

## ADMINISTRATION

**Oral**
- May be given without regard to meals.
- Note that dosage adjustment is recommended for moderate to severe renal impairment.
- Store at 20°–25° C (68°–77° F).

**ADVERSE EFFECTS** (≥1%) **CNS:** Headache. **Respiratory:** Nasopharyngitis, upper respiratory tract infection. **Endocrine:** Acute pancreatitis, hypoglycemia. **GI:** Acute pancreatitis, constipation.

**INTERACTIONS Drug:** Sitagliptin may increase **digoxin** levels. QUINOLONES may increase blood glucose. Monitor closely with **insulin** or SULFONYLUREAS.

**PHARMACOKINETICS Absorption:** 87% absorbed. **Peak:** 1–4 h. **Distribution:** 38% protein bound. **Metabolism:** 20% metabolized in the liver. **Elimination:** Primarily renal (87%) with minor elimination in the kidneys. **Half-Life:** 12.4 h.

## NURSING IMPLICATIONS

**Assessment & Drug Effects**
- Monitor for and report S&S of significant GI distress, including NV&D.
- Monitor for S&S of hypoglycemia when used in combination with a sulfonylurea drug or insulin.
- Monitor blood levels of digoxin with concurrent therapy.
- Monitor lab tests: Baseline and periodic CrCl; periodic fasting and postprandial plasma glucose and HbA1C.

## Patient & Family Education

- Taking this drug with another drug that can lower your blood sugar, such as a sulfonylurea or insulin, increases your risk of hypoglycemia.
- Stop taking this drug and notify prescriber immediately if you have an allergic reaction (e.g., swelling of your face, lips, throat; difficulty swallowing or breathing; raised, red areas on your skin (hives); skin rash, itching, flaking or peeling.
- Contact prescriber if you experience unexplained symptoms of liver problems (e.g., nausea or vomiting, abdominal pain, unusual tiredness, loss of appetite, dark urine, yellowing of your skin or the whites of your eyes).

# SODIUM BICARBONATE NA(HCO₃)

(sod'i-um bi-car'bon-ate)

Sodium Bicarbonate

**Classifications:** FLUID AND ELECTROLYTE BALANCE AGENT; ANTACID

**Therapeutic:** ANTACID

**AVAILABILITY** Tablet; solution for injection

## ACTION & *THERAPEUTIC EFFECT*

Rapidly neutralizes gastric acid to form sodium chloride, carbon dioxide, and water. After absorption of sodium bicarbonate, plasma alkali reserve is increased and excess sodium and bicarbonate ions are excreted in urine, thus rendering urine less acid. *Short-acting, potent systemic antacid; rapidly neutralizes gastric acid or systemic acidosis.*

**USES** Systemic alkalinizer to correct metabolic acidosis (as occurs in diabetes mellitus, shock, cardiac arrest, or vascular collapse), to minimize uric acid crystallization associated with uricosuric agents, to increase the solubility of sulfonamides, and to enhance renal excretion of barbiturate and salicylate overdosage. Commonly used as home remedy for relief of occasional heartburn, indigestion, or sour stomach. Used topically as paste, bath, or soak to relieve itching and minor skin irritations such as sunburn, insect bites, prickly heat, poison ivy, sumac, or oak. Sterile solutions are used to buffer acidic parenteral solutions to prevent acidosis. Also as a buffering agent in many commercial products (e.g., mouthwashes, douches, enemas, ophthalmic solutions).

**CONTRAINDICATIONS** Prolonged therapy with sodium bicarbonate; patients losing chloride (as from vomiting, GI suction, diuresis); hypocalcemia; metabolic alkalosis; respiratory alkalosis; peptic ulcer.

**CAUTIOUS USE** Edema, sodium-retaining disorders; heart disease, hypertension; preexisting respiratory acidosis; renal disease, renal insufficiency; hyperkalemia, hypokalemia; older adults; pregnancy (category C); children.

## ROUTE & DOSAGE

**Antacid**

*Adult:* **PO** 0.3–2 g 1–4 × day or ½ tsp of powder in glass of water

**Urinary Alkalinizer**

*Adult:* **PO** 4 g initially, then 1–2 g q4h

*Child:* **PO** 84–840 mg/kg/day in divided doses

**Cardiac Arrest**

*Adult:* **IV** 1 mEq/kg initially, then 0.5 mEq/kg q10min depending

Common adverse effects in *italic;* life-threatening effects <u>underlined</u>; generic names in **bold;** classifications in SMALL CAPS; ◆ Canadian drug name; ⊘ Prototype drug

1501

on arterial blood gas determinations (8.4% solutions contain 50 mEq/50 mL), give over 1–2 min *Child:* **IV** 0.5–1 mEq/kg q10min depending on arterial blood gas determinations, give over 1–2 min

**Metabolic Acidosis**

*Adult/Child:* **IV** Dose adjusted according to pH, base deficit, $Paco_2$, fluid limits, and patient response

## ADMINISTRATION

### Oral
▪ Do not add oral preparation to calcium-containing solutions.

### Intravenous

*PREPARE:* **Direct/IV Infusion** May give 4.2% (0.5 mEq/mL) and 5% (0.595 mEq/mL) $NaHCO_3$ solutions undiluted. ▪ Dilute 7.5% (0.892 mEq/mL) and 8.4% (1 mEq/mL) solutions with compatible IV solutions to a maximum concentration of 0.5 mEq/mL. ▪ For infants and children, dilute to at least 4.2%.

*ADMINISTER:* **Direct:** Give a bolus dose over 1–2 min only in emergency situations. ▪ For neonates or infants younger than 2 y, use only 4.2% solution for direct IV injection. **IV Infusion:** Usual rate is 2–5 mEq/kg over 4–8 h; do not exceed 50 mEq/h. ▪ Flush line before/after with NS. ▪ Stop infusion immediately if extravasation occurs. Severe tissue damage has followed tissue infiltration.

*INCOMPATIBILITIES:* **Solution/additive: Alcohol 5%, lactated Ringer's, amoxicillin, ascorbic acid, bupivacaine, carboplatin, carmustine, ciprofloxacin, cisplatin, codeine, corticotropin, dobutamine, dopamine, epinephrine, glycopyrrolate, hydromorphone, imipenem-cilastatin, insulin, isoproter-enol, labetalol, levorphanol, magnesium sulfate, meperidine, meropenem, methadone, metoclopramide, morphine, norepinephrine, oxytetracycline, penicillin G, pentazocine, pentobarbital, phenobarbital, procaine, promazine, streptomycin, succinylcholine, tetracycline, vancomycin, vitamin B complex with C. Y-site: Allopurinol, amiodarone, amphotericin B cholesteryl complex, calcium chloride, ciprofloxacin, cisatracurium, diltiazem, doxorubicin liposome, fenoldopam, hetastarch, idarubicin, imipenem/cilastatin, leucovorin, lidocaine, midazolam, milrinone acetate, nalbuphine, ondansetron, oxacillin, sargramostim, verapamil, vincristine, vindesine, vinorelbine.**

▪ Store in airtight containers. ▪ Note expiration date.

## ADVERSE EFFECTS (≥1%) **GI:**
*Belching, gastric distention,* flatulence. **Metabolic:** Metabolic alkalosis; electrolyte imbalance: Sodium overload (pulmonary edema), hypocalcemia (tetany), hypokalemia, milk-alkali syndrome, dehydration. **Other:** Rapid IV in neonates (hypernatremia, reduction in CSF pressure, intracranial hemorrhage). **Skin:** Severe tissue damage following extravasation of IV solution. **Urogenital:** Renal calculi or crystals, impaired kidney function.

## DIAGNOSTIC TEST INTERFERENCE

Small increase in *blood lactate* levels (following IV infusion of sodium bicarbonate); false-positive *urinary protein* determinations (using *ames reagent, sulfacetic acid,* heat and *acetic acid* or *nitric acid ring method*); elevated *urinary urobilinogen* levels (*urobilinogen* excretion increases in alkaline urine).

**INTERACTIONS Drug:** May decrease absorption of **ketoconazole;** may decrease elimination of **dextroamphetamine, ephedrine, pseudoephedrine, quinidine;** may increase elimination of **chlorpropamide, lithium,** SALICYLATES, TETRACYCLINES.

## PHARMACOKINETICS Absorption:
Readily from GI tract. **Onset:** 15 min. **Duration:** 1–2 h. **Elimination:** In urine within 3–4 h.

## NURSING IMPLICATIONS

### Assessment & Drug Effects

- Be aware that long-term use of oral preparation with milk or calcium can cause milk-alkali syndrome: Anorexia, nausea, vomiting, headache, mental confusion, hypercalcemia, hypophosphatemia, soft tissue calcification, renal and ureteral calculi, renal insufficiency, metabolic alkalosis.
- Observe for and report S&S of improvement or reversal of metabolic acidosis (see Appendix F).
- Monitor lab tests: Periodic measurements of acid-base status (blood pH, $PO_2$, $PCO_2$, $HCO_3^-$, and other electrolytes), usually several times daily during acute period.

### Patient & Family Education

- Do not use sodium bicarbonate as antacid. A nonabsorbable OTC alternative for repeated use is safer.
- Do not take antacids longer than 2 wk except under advice and supervision of a prescriber. Self-medication with routine doses of sodium bicarbonate or soda mints may cause sodium retention and alkalosis, especially when kidney function is impaired.
- Be aware that commonly used OTC antacid products contain sodium bicarbonate (e.g., Alka-Seltzer).

## SODIUM FERRIC GLUCONATE COMPLEX
(so'di-um fer'ric glu'co-nate)

**Ferrlecit**

**Classifications:** NUTRITIONAL SUPPLEMENT; IRON PREPARATION
**Therapeutic:** ANTIANEMIC; IRON REPLACEMENT
**Prototype:** Ferrous sulfate

**AVAILABILITY** Intravenous solution

## ACTION & *THERAPEUTIC EFFECT*
Stable iron complex used to restore iron loss in chronic kidney failure patients. The use of erythropoietin therapy and blood loss through hemodialysis require iron replacement. The ferric ion combines with transferrin and is transported to bone marrow where it is incorporated into hemoglobin. *Effectiveness indicated by improved Hgb and Hct, iron saturation, and serum ferritin levels.*

## USES Treatment of iron deficiency anemia.

## CONTRAINDICATIONS Any anemia not related to iron deficiency; hypersensitivity to sodium ferric gluconate complex; hemochromatosis, hemosiderosis; hemolytic anemia; thalassemia; neonates.

## CAUTIOUS USE Hypersensitivity to benzyl alcohol; active or suspected infection; cardiac disease; hepatic disease; older adults; pregnancy (category B); lactation. Safety and efficacy in children younger than 6 y not established.

## ROUTE & DOSAGE

### Iron Deficiency in Dialysis Patients
*Adult/Adolescent:* **IV** 125 mg infused over 1 h

S

Common adverse effects in *italic;* life-threatening effects <u>underlined</u>; generic names in **bold;** classifications in SMALL CAPS; ♣ Canadian drug name; ☻ Prototype drug

1503

*Child (6–15 y):* **IV** 1.5 mg/kg infused over 1 h (max:125 mg/dose)

## ADMINISTRATION

### Intravenous ONLY

*PREPARE:* **Direct for Adult:** May be given undiluted. **Direct for Child:** Dilute required doses in 25 mL NS. **IV Infusion for Adult/Child:** Dilute 125 mg in 100 mL of NS.
▪ Use immediately after dilution.
*ADMINISTER:* **Direct for Adult:** Give no faster than 12.5 mg/min. **IV Infusion for Adult/Child:** Give over **not** less than 60 min.
*INCOMPATIBILITIES:* **Solution/additive:** Do not mix with any other medications or add to parenteral nutrition solutions.

▪ Store unopened ampules at 20°–25° C (68°–77° F).

## ADVERSE EFFECTS (≥1%) **Body as a Whole:** <u>Hypersensitivity reaction (cardiovascular collapse, cardiac arrest, bronchospasm, oral/pharyngeal edema,</u> dyspnea, <u>angioedema,</u> urticaria, pruritus). **CV:** Flushing, hypotension, hypertension, tachycardia. **GI:** Vomiting, nausea, diarrhea. **Neuromuscular and Skeletal:** Muscle cramps. **Respiratory:** Dyspnea.

## PHARMACOKINETICS  **Half-life Elimination:** 1 h (bound iron).

## NURSING IMPLICATIONS

### Assessment & Drug Effects
▪ Monitor closely for S&S of severe hypersensitivity (see Appendix F) during IV administration.
▪ Monitor vital signs periodically during IV administration (transient hypotension possible especially during dialysis).
▪ Stop infusion immediately and notify prescriber if hypersensitivity is suspected.

▪ Monitor lab tests: Periodic Hgb, Hct, Fe saturation, and serum ferritin.

### Patient & Family Education
▪ Report to prescriber immediately: Difficulty breathing, itching, flushing, rash, weakness, lightheadedness, pain, or any other discomfort during infusion.

# SODIUM POLYSTYRENE SULFONATE
(pol-ee-stye'reen)
Kayexalate, SPS Suspension
**Classifications:** ELECTROLYTE AND WATER BALANCE; CATION EXCHANGE
Therapeutic: CATION EXCHANGE

**AVAILABILITY** Suspension; powder

## ACTION & *THERAPEUTIC EFFECT*
Sulfonic cation-exchange resin that removes potassium by exchanging sodium ion for potassium, particularly in large intestine; potassium-containing resin is then excreted through the bowel. *Removes potassium by exchanging sodium ion for potassium through the large intestine.*

**USES** Hyperkalemia.

## CONTRAINDICATIONS  Hypersensitivity to Kayexalate; GI obstruction; hypokalemia; lactation.

## CAUTIOUS USE Acute or chronic kidney failure; low birth weight infants; neonates with reduced gut; patients receiving digitalis preparations; patients who cannot tolerate even a small increase in sodium load (e.g., CHF, severe hypertension, and marked edema); patients with constipation or bowel obstruction; renal insufficiency. older adults; pregnancy (category C); children.

S

Common adverse effects in *italic;* life-threatening effects <u>underlined;</u> generic names in **bold;** classifications in SMALL CAPS; ♣ Canadian drug name; ● Prototype drug

## ROUTE & DOSAGE

### Hyperkalemia

*Adult:* **PO** 15 g 1–4 × per day
**Rectal** 30–50 g q6h as warm emulsion high into sigmoid colon
*Child:* **PO** 1 g/kg q6h; **Rectal** 1 g/kg q2–6h

## ADMINISTRATION

### Oral

- Give as a suspension in a small quantity of water or in syrup. Usual amount of fluid ranges from 20–100 mL or approximately 3–4 mL/g of drug.

### Rectal

- Use warm fluid (as prescribed) to prepare the emulsion for enema.
- Administer a cleansing enema (non-sodium-containing fluid) before and after rectal administration.
- Administer at body temperature and introduce by gravity, keeping suspension particles in solution by stirring. Flush suspension with 50–100 mL of fluid; then clamp tube and leave it in place.
- Urge patient to retain enema at least 30–60 min but as long as several hours if possible.
- Irrigate colon (after enema solution has been expelled) with 1 or 2 qt flushing solution (non-sodium containing). Drain returns constantly through a Y-tube connection.
- Store remainder of prepared solution for 24 h; then discard.

## ADVERSE EFFECTS (≥1%) GI:

*Constipation, fecal impaction (in older adults);* anorexia, gastric irritation, nausea, vomiting, diarrhea (with sorbitol emulsions), <u>gastrointestinal hemorrhage</u>. **Respiratory:** Bronchitis, bronchopneumonia. **Metabolic:** Sodium retention, hypocalcemia, hypokalemia, hypomagnesemia, hypervolemia.

## INTERACTIONS Drug: ANTACIDS, LAXATIVES containing **calcium** or **magnesium** may decrease potassium exchange capability of the resin. Do not use with products containing sorbitol.

## PHARMACOKINETICS Absorption: Not absorbed systemically. Onset: Several hours to days. Metabolism: Not metabolized. Elimination: In feces.

## NURSING IMPLICATIONS

### Assessment & Drug Effects

- Serum potassium levels do not always reflect intracellular potassium deficiency. Observe patient closely for early clinical signs of severe hypokalemia (see Appendix F). ECGs are also recommended.
- Consult prescriber about restricting sodium content from dietary and other sources since drug contains approximately 100 mg (4.1 mEq) of sodium/g (1 tsp, 15 mEq sodium).
- Monitor lab tests: Daily serum potassium; periodic acid–base balance, and serum electrolytes

### Patient & Family Education

- Check bowel function daily. Usually, a mild laxative is prescribed to prevent constipation (common adverse effect). Older adult patients are particularly prone to fecal impaction.

## SOFOSBUVIR

(so-fos'bu-vir)

Sovaldi

**Classifications:** ANTIVIRAL; NUCLEOTIDE ANALOG; VIRAL POLYMERASE INHIBITOR
Therapeutic: ANTIHEPATITIS

**AVAILABILITY** Film-coated tablets

## ACTION & *THERAPEUTIC EFFECT*

A direct-acting antiviral agent against HCV; is a prodrug converted to its active form via intracellular

Common adverse effects in *italic;* life-threatening effects <u>underlined</u>; generic names in **bold;** classifications in SMALL CAPS; ◆ Canadian drug name; ⊘ Prototype drug

1505

metabolism. *It inhibits HCV NS5B RNA-dependent RNA polymerase thus inhibiting viral replication.*

**USES** Treatment of chronic hepatitis C (CHC) infection in combination with either ribavirin or ledipasvir alone or with pegylated interferon and ribavirin.

**UNLABLED USES** Chronic hepatitis.

**CONTRAINDICATIONS** Inability to take concurrent peginterferon alfa/ribavirin or ribavirin alone; concomitant potent P-gp inducers (e.g., rifampin and St. John's wort); pregnancy (category X in combination with ritonavir or peginterferon alfa/ribavirin), women of childbearing age or their male partners without using two forms of contraception, and for 6 mo after use of ribavir by either partner; suicidal ideation; hepatic decompensation; lactation.

**CAUTIOUS USE** Concomitant drugs that are P-gp inducers; post-liver transplant; chronic depression; history of suicide; severe renal impairment; ESRD; liver transplant. Safety and efficacy in children younger than 18 y not established.

## ROUTE & DOSAGE

### Hepatitis C Infection

*Adult:* **PO** 400 mg once daily in combination with ribavirin (with/without peginterferon alfa) for 12 or 24 wk (see manufacturer's guidelines for dosing by genotype)

## ADMINISTRATION
### Oral

- Give without regard to food.
- Do not use as monotherapy; use only in combination with ribavirin (with or without peginterferon alfa).
- If the other agents used in combination with sofosbuvir are

permanently discontinued, sofosbuvir should also be discontinued.
- Store at room temperature below 30° C (86° F).

**ADVERSE EFFECTS** (≥ 1%) **Body as a Whole:** Asthenia, pyrexia. **CNS:** Chills, *fatigue, headache, insomnia,* irritability. **GI:** Decreased appetite, diarrhea, *nausea.* **Hematological:** Anemia, decreased hemoglobin, decreased neutrophils, neutropenia. **Metabolic:** Increased bilirubin, increased CPK, increased serum lipase, thrombocytopenia. **Musculoskeletal:** Myalgia. **Respiratory:** Influenza-like illness. **Skin:** Pruritus, rash.

**INTERACTIONS Drug:** Co-administration with drugs that are potent P-gp inducers in the intestine (e.g., RIFAMYCINS) may decrease the levels of sofosbuvir. Co-administration with drugs that inhibit P-gp may increase the levels of sofosbuvir. Co-administration of sofosbuvir with **carbamazepine, phenytoin, phenobarbital,** or **oxcarbazepine** may decrease the levels of sofosbuvir. **Herbal: St. John's wort must not** be used with sofosbuvir because it is a potent P-gp inducer.

**PHARMACOKINETICS Peak:** 0.5–2 h. **Distribution:** 61–65% plasma protein bound. **Metabolism:** Converted to active metabolite. **Elimination:** Primarily renal. **Half-Life:** 27 h (active metabolite).

## NURSING IMPLICATIONS
### Assessment & Drug Effects

- Monitor for and report promptly changes in mental status such as depression or suicidal ideation.
- Monitor for S&S of infection or anemia.
- Monitor lab tests: Baseline and periodic LFTs, serum creatinine; serum HCV-RNA at baseline during treatment, end of treatment, and during

S

treatment follow-up; pretreatment and monthly pregnancy tests and up to 6 mo after therapy discontinued; periodic CBC with differential.

**Patient & Family Education**

- Report immediately to prescriber if patient experiences mental status changes such as depression, thoughts of suicide, anxiety, emotional instability, or illogical thinking.
- Women of childbearing potential and male partners of pregnant women should use effective means of contraception while taking this drug and for at least 6 mo following discontinuation of therapy.

## SOFOSBUVIR AND VELPATASVIR

(soe-fos'bue-vir and vel-pat'as vir)

Epclusa

**Classifications:** ANTIVIRAL; VIRAL POLYMERASE INHIBITOR; ANTIHEPATITIS
Therapeutic: ANTIHEPATITIS

**AVAILABILITY** Tablets

**ACTION & THERAPEUTIC EFFECT**
Sofosbuvir is a prodrug that is metabolized to its active form (GS-461203) which then inhibits hepatitis C viral (HCV) NS5B RNA-dependent RNA polymerase, an enzyme required for viral replication. Velpatasvir inhibits HCV NS5A protein which is required for viral replication. *Inhibits replication of the HCV virus.*

**USES** Treatment of chronic hepatitis C virus (HCV) genotype 1, 2, 3, 4, 5, or 6 infection in adult patients without cirrhosis, or with compensated cirrhosis, or in combination with ribavirin, with decompensated cirrhosis.

**CONTRAINDICATIONS** Combination with ribavirin is contraindicated in patients for whom ribavirin is contraindicated.

**CAUTIOUS USE** No adequate human-controlled trials have been done to determine safety in pregnancy or lactation. No data is available to establish safety and efficacy in patients with severe renal impairment or end stage renal disease. Use with caution with patients previously infected with hepatitis B virus (HBV).

## ROUTE & DOSAGE

**Hepatitis C Viral Infection**

*Adult:* **PO** One tablet (400 mg sofosbuvir and 100 mg velpatasvir) once daily for 12 wk

*Hepatic Impairment Dosage Adjustment*

*Patients with decompensated cirrhosis (Child-Pugh class B or C):* Add ribavirin, maintain dose and duration

*Renal Impairment Dosage Adjustment*

*Severe impairment (eGFR less than 30 mL/min/1.73 m²) or with end stage renal disease:* Safety and efficacy not established

## ADMINISTRATION

**Oral**

- Take without regard to food.
- If administered with ribavirin, take ribavirin with food.
- Store below 30° C (86° F). Dispense only in original container.

**ADVERSE EFFECTS** (≥1%) **Body as a Whole:** Asthenia, *fatigue*, insomnia. **CNS:** Depression, *headache*. **GI:** Diarrhea, *nausea*. **Hematological:** *Anemia, decreased hemoglobin*, elevated lipase enzymes, elevated serum creatinine levels. **Skin:** Rash.

**INTERACTIONS Drug:** Coadministration of inducers of P-gp and/or

Common adverse effects in *italic;* life-threatening effects underlined; generic names in **bold;** classifications in SMALL CAPS; ♣ Canadian drug name; ⊙ Prototype drug

**1507**

CYP2B6, CYP2C8, or CYP3A4 (e.g., **carbamazepine, phenobarbital, phenytoin, rifabutin, rifampin, rifapentine**) may decrease the levels of sofosbuvir and/or velpatasvir. ACID REDUCING AGENTS (e.g., ANTACIDS, **famotidine, omeprazole**) may decrease the levels of velpatasvir. Coadministration of **aminodarone** may result in serious symptomatic bradycardia. Sofosbuvir and/or velpatasvir may increase the levels of **digoxin, topotecan,** HMG-COA REDUCTASE INHIBITORS, and **tenofovir disoproxil fumarate.** Efavirenz, **ritonavir,** and **tipranavir** can decrease the levels of sofosbuvir and/or velpatasvir. **Herbal: St. John's wort** may decrease the levels of sofosbuvir and/or velpatasvir.

**PHARMACOKINETICS Peak:** Sofosbuvir, 0.5–1 h; velpatasvir, 3 h. **Distribution:** Sofosbuvir, 61–65% plasma protein bound; velpatsavir, greater than 99.5% plasma protein bound. **Metabolism:** Hydrolytic and oxidative metabolism. **Elimination:** Sofosbuvir, renal (80%) and fecal (14%); velpatasvir, primarily fecal (95%). **Half-Life:** Sofosbuvir, 0.5 h; GS-r61203, 25 h; velpatasvir, 15 h.

## NURSING IMPLICATIONS

### Assessment & Drug Effects
- Monitor vital signs, as bradycardia and arrhythmias have been reported.
- Monitor cognition: Irritability, insomnia, and depression have been reported.
- Monitor lab tests: LFTs, plasma hepatitis, pregnancy testing, serum creatinine/BUN.

### Patient & Family Education
- Seek medical attention immediately if fainting or near fainting, fatigue, dizziness, shortness of breath, chest pain, and confusion or memory problems.
- Make sure to keep a list of all medications that the patient is taking and share that information with all prescribers.
- Do not take any other over-the-counter medications, herbals, vitamins, or other prescription drugs without first checking with your health care provider.

# SOLIFENACIN SUCCINATE
(sol-i-fen′a-sin)
VESIcare

**Classifications:** ANTICHOLINERGIC; ANTIMUSCARINIC; ANTISPASMODIC
**Therapeutic:** URINARY ANTISPASMODIC
**Prototype:** Oxybutynin

**AVAILABILITY** Tablet

## ACTION & *THERAPEUTIC EFFECT*
A selective muscarinic antagonist that depresses both voluntary and involuntary bladder contractions caused by detrusor overactivity. *Solifenacin improves the volume of urine/void and reduces the frequency of incontinent and urgency episodes.*

**USES** Treatment of overactive bladder (OAB).

**CONTRAINDICATIONS** Hypersensitivity to solifenacin; severe hepatic impairment (Child-Pugh class C); gastric retention; uncontrolled narrow-angle glaucoma; urinary retention; toxic megacolon; GI obstruction; ileus.

**CAUTIOUS USE** Bladder outflow obstruction; concurrent use of ketoconazole or other potent CYP3A4 inhibitors; obstructive disorders; decreased GI motility; history of

Common adverse effects in *italic;* life-threatening effects underlined; generic names in **bold;** classifications in SMALL CAPS; ♣ Canadian drug name; ⊕ Prototype drug

QT prolongation; controlled narrow-angle glaucoma; renal impairment; renal disease; mild to moderate hepatic impairment; older adults; myasthenia gravis; pregnancy (category C); lactation. Safety and efficacy in children not established.

## ROUTE & DOSAGE

### Overactive Bladder

*Adult:* PO 5 mg once daily; may be increased to 10 mg once daily if tolerated (max: 5 mg/day if taking drugs that inhibit CYP3A4—see INTERACTIONS, Drug)

### Hepatic Impairment Dosage Adjustment

*Child-Pugh class B:* Do not exceed 5 mg/day. *Child-Pugh class C:* Do not use

### Renal Impairment Dosage Adjustment

*CrCl less than 30 mL/min:* Max dose 5 mg/day

## ADMINISTRATION

### Oral

- Tablets should be swallowed whole.
- Store at 15°–30° C (59°–86° F).

**ADVERSE EFFECTS** (≥1%) **Body as a Whole:** Edema, fatigue. **CNS:** Fatigue. **GI:** *Dry mouth, constipation,* nausea, vomiting, dyspepsia, upper abdominal pain. **Special Senses:** Blurred vision, dry eyes. **Urogenital:** Urinary tract infection.

**INTERACTIONS Drug:** CYP3A4 inhibitors (e.g., **clarithromycin, delavirdine, diltiazem, efavirenz, erythromycin, fluconazole, fluvoxamine, itraconazole, nefazodone, norfloxacin, omeprazole,** PROTEASE INHIBITORS, **quinine, verapamil, troleandomycin, voriconazole, zafirlukast**) may increase levels and toxicity (max: 5 mg/day); **amantadine, amoxapine, bupropion, clozapine, cyclobenzaprine, diphenhydramine, disopyramide, maprotiline, olanzapine, orphenadrine,** PHENOTHIAZINES, TRICYCLIC ANTIDEPRESSANTS have additive anticholinergic adverse effects. Do not use with agents that increase QT interval (e.g., **dofetilide, dronedarone, posaconazole, ziprasidone**). **Food: Grapefruit juice** may increase solifenacin levels and toxicity.

**PHARMACOKINETICS Absorption:** 90% absorbed from GI tract. **Peak:** 3–8 h. **Metabolism:** Extensively metabolized in the liver by CYP3A4. **Elimination:** Primarily in urine, 22% in feces. **Half-Life:** 45–68 h.

## NURSING IMPLICATIONS

### Assessment & Drug Effects

- Monitor bladder function and report promptly urinary retention.
- Monitor ECG in patients with a known history of QT prolongation or patients taking medications that prolong the QT interval.

### Patient & Family Education

- Stop taking this drug and report to prescriber if urinary retention occurs.
- Report promptly any of the following: Blurred vision or difficulty focusing vision, palpitations, confusion, or severe dizziness.
- Report to prescriber problems with bowel elimination, especially constipation lasting 3 days or longer.
- Exercise caution in hot environments, as the risk of heat prostration increases with this drug.

Common adverse effects in *italic;* life-threatening effects underlined; generic names in **bold;** classifications in SMALL CAPS; ♣ Canadian drug name; ⊕ Prototype drug

1509

## SOMATROPIN ℗
(soe-ma-troe'pin)

Genotropin, Genotropin
MiniQuick, Humatrope,
Norditropin, NuSpin,
Omnitrope, Saizen, Serostim,
Zomacton, Zorbtive

**Classification:** GROWTH
HORMONE
Therapeutic: GROWTH HORMONE

**AVAILABILITY** Solution for injection

**ACTION & *THERAPEUTIC EFFECT***
Recombinant growth hormone
with the natural sequence of 191
amino acids characteristic of endogenous growth hormone (GH),
of pituitary origin. *Induces growth
responses in children.*

**USES** Growth failure due to GH deficiency; replacement therapy prior
to epiphyseal closure in patients
with idiopathic GH deficiency; GH
deficiency secondary to intracranial
tumors or panhypopituitarism; inadequate GH secretion; short stature in girls with Turner's syndrome;
AIDS wasting syndrome; short bowel
syndrome; small for gestational age.

**UNLABELED USES** Growth deficiency in children with rheumatoid arthritis.

**CONTRAINDICATIONS** Hypersensitivity to somatropin or any
ingredient; pediatric patient with
closed epiphyses; underlying intracranial lesion or growing cranial tumor; acute critical illness
caused by complications following
open heart surgery or abdominal
surgery, acute respiratory failure;
acute diabetic retinopathy; during
chemotherapy, radiation therapy,
active neoplastic disease; selective

cases of Prader-Willi syndrome
who are severely obese or have severe respiratory impairment; children with an intracranial tumor;
drug-induced acute pancreatitis.

**CAUTIOUS USE** Diabetes mellitus
or family history of the disease, history of glucose intolerance; Prader-
Willi syndrome with a diagnosis of
growth hormone deficiency (GHD);
skeletal abnormalities; Turner syndrome; HIV patients; history of upper airway obstruction, sleep apnea,
or unidentified URI; concomitant or
prior use of thyroid or androgens
in prepubertal male; hypothyroidism; chronic renal failure; obesity;
older adults; pregnancy (category
B or category C depending on the
brand); lactation; children.

## ROUTE & DOSAGE

Note: Dosing will vary based on
specific brand of product
**Growth Hormone Deficiency (GHD)**
*Adult:* **Subcutaneous Humatrope**
Not more than 0.006 mg/kg
once daily; dose may be
increased (max: 0.0125 mg/kg/
day); **Genotropin, Omnitrope**
0.04 mg/kg qwk divided into
daily doses (max: 0.08 mg/kg/
wk); **Norditropin** Initially 0.004
mg/kg/day (max: 0.016 mg/kg)
*Child:* **Subcutaneous Genotropin**
0.16–0.24 mg/kg/wk divided
into 6–7 daily doses; **Humatrope**
0.18–0.3 mg/kg/wk (0.54
international unit/kg/wk) divided
into equal doses given on either
3 alternate days or 6 × wk;
**Norditropin** 0.024–0.034 mg/
kg/day 6–7 × wk; **Omnitrope**
0.16–0.24 mg/kg/week divided
into 6–7 injections

Common adverse effects in *italic;* life-threatening effects <u>underlined</u>; generic names
in **bold;** classifications in SMALL CAPS; ♣ Canadian drug name; ℗ Prototype drug

## Small for Gestational Age

*Child:* **Subcutaneous Genotropin/Omnitrope** 0.48 mg/kg/week in divided doses; **Humatrope** 0.47 mg/kg divided into daily doses

## AIDS Wasting or Cachexia

*Adult (weight greater than 55 kg):* **Subcutaneous Serostim** 6 mg each night; *weight 45–55 kg:* 5 mg each night; *weight 35–45 kg:* 4 mg each night; *weight less than 35 kg:* 0.1 mg/kg each night

## Short Bowel Syndrome

*Adult:* **Subcutaneous Zorbtive** 0.1 mg/kg once daily for 4 wk (max: 8 mg/day)

## ADMINISTRATION

### Subcutaneous

- Reconstitute each brand following its manufacturer's instructions (vary from brand to brand).
- Read and carefully follow directions for use supplied with the Nutropin AQ Pen™ cartridge if this is the product being used.
- Rotate injection sites; abdomen and thighs are preferred sites. Do not use buttocks until the child has been walking for a year or more and the muscle is adequately developed.
- Store lyophilized powder at 2°–8° C (36°–46° F). After reconstitution, most preparations are stable for at least 14 days under refrigeration. **Do not freeze.**

## ADVERSE EFFECTS (≥1%) **Body as a Whole:** Pain, swelling at injection site; peripheral edema, myalgia. Fatalities reported in patients with Prader-Willi syndrome and one or more of the following: Severe obesity, history of respiratory impairment or sleep apnea, or unidentified respiratory infection, especially male patients. **Metabolic:** *Hypercalciuria;* oversaturation of bile with cholesterol, hyperglycemia, ketosis. **GI:** Nausea, flatulence, abdominal pain, vomiting. **Musculoskeletal:** Arthralgia, limb pain, myalgia. **Endocrine:** High circulating GH antibodies with resulting treatment failure, accelerated growth of intracranial tumor, pancreatitis. **CV:** Chest pain, edema. **CNS:** Pain, headache, malaise, paresthesia, dizziness.

## INTERACTIONS **Drug:** ANABOLIC STEROIDS, **thyroid hormone,** ANDROGENS, ESTROGENS may accelerate epiphyseal closure; **ACTH,** CORTICOSTEROIDS may inhibit growth response to somatropin.

## PHARMACOKINETICS **Metabolism:** In liver. **Elimination:** In urine. **Half-Life:** 15–50 min.

## NURSING IMPLICATIONS

### Assessment & Drug Effects

- Monitor growth at designated intervals.
- Hypercalciuria, a frequent adverse effect in the first 2–3 mo of therapy, may be symptomless; however, it may be accompanied by renal calculi, with these reportable symptoms: Flank pain and colic, GI symptoms, urinary frequency, chills, fever, and hematuria.
- Observe diabetics or those with family history of diabetes closely. Obtain regular fasting blood glucose and HbA1C.
- Examine patients with GH deficiency secondary to intracranial lesion frequently for progression

S

Common adverse effects in *italic;* life-threatening effects <u>underlined;</u> generic names in **bold;** classifications in SMALL CAPS; ✦ Canadian drug name; ⊘ Prototype drug

1511

or recurrence of underlying disease.

- Monitor lab test: Periodic serum and urine calcium and plasma glucose. Test for circulating GH antibodies (antisomatropin antibodies) in patients who respond initially but later fail to respond to therapy, thyroid function tests.

**Patient & Family Education**

- Be aware that during first 6 mo of successful treatment, linear growth rates may be increased 8–16 cm or more/year (average about 7 cm/y or approximately 3 in.). Additionally, subcutaneous fat diminishes but returns to pretreatment value later.
- Record accurate height measurements at regular intervals and report to prescriber if rate is less than expected.
- In general, growth response to somatropin is inversely proportional to duration of treatment.
- Bone age is typically assessed annually in all patients and especially those also receiving concurrent thyroid or androgen treatment, since these drugs may precipitate early epiphyseal closure. Take child for bone age assessment on appointed annual dates.

## SONIDEGIB
(son-i-de′gib)
Odomzo

**Classifications:** ANTINEOPLASTIC; BIOLOGICAL RESPONSE MODIFIER; SIGNAL TRANSDUCTION INHIBITOR; HEDGEHOG PATHWAY INHIBITOR
**Therapeutic:** ANTINEOPLASTIC
**Prototype:** Vismodegib

**AVAILABILITY** Capsules

## ACTION & *THERAPEUTIC EFFECT*

Hedgehog mutations associated with basal cell cancer can activate cell growth pathways resulting in unrestricted proliferation of skin basal cells. Sonidegib inhibits the Hedgehog pathway by binding to smoothened homologue (SMO), a transmembrane protein involved in Hedgehog signal transduction. Hedgehog regulates cell growth and differentiation in embryogenesis but is generally not active in adult tissue. Hedgehog regulates cell growth and differentiation in embryogenesis, but is generally not active in adult tissue. Hedgehog mutations associated with basal cell cancer can activate the pathway resulting in unrestricted proliferation of skin basal cells. *Inhibits the growth and differential of basal carcinoma cells.*

**USES** Treatment of adult patients with locally advanced basal cell carcinoma (BCC) that has recurred following surgery or radiation therapy, or those who are not candidates for surgery or radiation therapy.

**CONTRAINDICATION** Active TB infection; recurrent serum CK greater than 5 × ULN; recurrent severe musculoskeletal reactions.

**CAUTIOUS USE** History of rhabdomyolysis with other drugs which inhibit the Hedgehog pathway; Crohn's disease. Concomitant use of CYP3A4 inhibitors; grapefruit consumption; pregnancy (category B); lactation. Safety and efficacy in children not established.

## ROUTE & DOSAGE

| Advanced BCC |
| --- |
| *Adult:* **PO** 200 mg once daily |
| *Toxicity Dosage Adjustment* |

S

*Severe musculoskeletal reactions, first occurrence of serum CK 2.5–10 × ULN, or recurrent serum CK 2.5–5 × ULN:* Temporarily discontinue, then resume at 200 mg upon resolution
*Serum CK greater than 2.5 × ULN with worsening renal function:* Permanently discontinue
*Serum CK greater than 10 × ULN:* Permanently discontinue
*Recurrent severe serum CK greater than .5 × ULN:* Permanently discontinue
*Recurrent severe musculoskeletal reactions:* Permanently discontinue

## ADMINISTRATION
### Oral
- Give on an empty stomach at least 1 h before or 2 h after a meal.
- Capsules should be swallowed whole.

## ADVERSE EFFECTS (≥10%) Body as a Whole: *Fatigue, pain.* CNS: *Dysgeusia, headache.* GI: *Abdominal pain, diarrhea, nausea, vomiting.* Hematological: Anemia, lymphopenia. Metabolic: *Decreased appetite,* hyperglycemia, increased ALT/AST, increased amylase, increased lipase, increased serum creatinine, increased serum creatine kinase (CK), *weight loss.* Musculoskeletal: *Muscle spasm, musculoskeletal pain, myalgia.* Skin: *Alopecia, pruritus.*

## INTERACTIONS Drug: Concomitant use with strong CYP3A4 inhibitors (e.g., **itraconazole, ketoconazole, nefazodone, posaconazole, saquinavir, telithromycin, voriconazole**) or moderate CYP3A4 inhibitors (e.g., **atanzavir, diltiazem, fluconazole**) increases the levels of sonidegib.

Concomitant use with strong and moderate inhibitors (e.g., **carbamazepine, efavirenz, modafinil, phenobarbital, phenytoin, rifabutin, rifampin**) decreases the levels of sonidegib. **Food: Grapefruit** or **grapefruit juice** may increase the levels of sonidegib. **Herbal: St. John's wort** decreases the levels of sonidegib.

## PHARMACOKINETICS Absorption: Less than 10% absorbed. Peak: 2–4 h. Distribution: Greater than 97% plasma protein binding. Metabolism: In liver by CYP450 enzymes. Elimination: Fecal (70%) and renal (30%). Half-Life: 28 days.

## NURSING IMPLICATIONS

### Black Box Warning

*Sonidegib can cause embryo-fetal death or severe birth defects. Pregnancy status must be verified prior to initiating therapy. (See Patient & Family Education.)*

### Assessment & Drug Effects
- Monitor for and report to prescriber development of musculoskeletal pain, myalgia, dark urine, decreased urine output, or the inability to urinate.
- Monitor lab tests: Baseline pregnancy test; baseline and periodic serum creatine kinase (CK) and creatinine levels.

### Patient & Family Education
- Women of childbearing age should discuss potential risks of this drug to fetal development.
- Women should use effective means of contraception while taking this drug and for at least 20 mo after the last dose.
- Women taking this drug or partners of males taking this drug should immediately report to prescriber if a pregnancy is suspected.

Common adverse effects in *italic;* life-threatening effects underlined; generic names in **bold;** classifications in SMALL CAPS; ♣ Canadian drug name; ⊕ Prototype drug

1513

- Do not breast-feed while taking this drug.
- Males should use condoms (even after a vasectomy) during treatment and for at least 8 mo after the last dose to prevent exposure of females of childbearing age to this drug.
- Males should not donate semen during treatment and for at least 8 mo after the last dose.
- Report promptly any new unexplained muscle pain, tenderness or weakness occurring during treatment or that persists after discontinuing this drug.
- Report promptly dark urine, decreased urine output, or the inability to urinate.
- Avoid grapefruit products while taking this drug.

---

# SORAFENIB
(sor-a-fe'nib)
Nexavar

**Classifications:** ANTINEOPLASTIC; KINASE INHIBITOR; KINASE INHIBITOR
Therapeutic: ANTINEOPLASTIC
**Prototype:** Erlotinib

## AVAILABILITY Tablet

## ACTION & *THERAPEUTIC EFFECT*
A multi-kinase inhibitor targeting enzyme systems in both tumor cells and tumor vasculature. It appears to be cytostatic, requiring continued drug exposure for tumor growth inhibition. *Sorafenib inhibits enzymes responsible for uncontrolled tumor cellular proliferation and angiogenesis.*

## USES Treatment of advanced renal cell cancer.

## UNLABELED USES Treatment of advanced malignant melanoma. Treatment of metastatic hepatocellular cancer.

## CONTRAINDICATIONS Active infection; severe renal impairment (less

than 30 mL/min), or hemodialysis; pregnancy (category D); lactation.

**CAUTIOUS USE** Previous myelosuppressive therapy, either radiation or chemotherapy; mild or moderate renal disease; hepatic disease; heart failure, ventricular dysfunction, cardiac disease, peripheral edema; females of childbearing age. Safe use in children younger than 18 y not established.

## ROUTE & DOSAGE

### Renal Cell Cancer
*Adult:* **PO** 400 mg b.i.d.

#### Dosage Adjustments for Skin Toxicity
*Grade 2 (1st episode):* Continue therapy and treat symptoms. If no improvement in 7 days, discontinue until toxicity resolves to at least grade 1, then resume with 400 mg/day or 400 mg every other day
*Grade 2 (2nd or 3rd episode):* Discontinue until toxicity resolves to at least grade 1, then resume with 400 mg/day or 400 mg every other day
*Grade 2 (4th episode):* Discontinue therapy
*Grade 3 (1st or 2nd episode):* Discontinue until toxicity resolves to at least grade 1, then resume with 400 mg/day or 400 mg every other day
*Grade 3 (3rd episode):* Discontinue therapy

## ADMINISTRATION
### Oral
- Tablets **must be** swallowed whole. They should not be crushed, broken, or chewed.
- Give on an empty stomach 1 h before or 2 h after eating.
- Store at 15°–30° C (59°–86° F). Protect from moisture.

Common adverse effects in *italic;* life-threatening effects underlined; generic names in **bold;** classifications in SMALL CAPS; ♣ Canadian drug name; ◑ Prototype drug

**ADVERSE EFFECTS** (≥1%) **Body as a Whole:** Asthenia, bone pain, decreased appetite, *fatigue,* influenza-like illness, *joint pain,* mouth pain, muscle pain, pyrexia. **CNS:** Depression, *headache, sensory neuropathy.* **CV:** *Hypertension.* **GI:** *Abdominal pain, anorexia, constipation, diarrhea,* dyspepsia, dysphagia, mucositis, *nausea,* stomatitis, *vomiting.* **Hematologic:** *Anemia,* hemorrhage, leukopenia, *lymphopenia,* neutropenia, thrombocytopenia, thrombotic events. **Metabolic:** *Amylase elevation, hypophosphatemia, lipase elevation, weight loss.* **Musculoskeletal:** Arthralgia, myalgia. **Respiratory:** *Cough, dyspnea,* hoarseness. **Skin:** Acne, *alopecia, desquamation, dry skin,* erythema, exfoliative dermatitis, flushing, *hand-foot skin reaction, rash.* **Urogenital:** Erectile dysfunction.

**INTERACTIONS Drug:** Sorafenib may increase levels of drugs requiring glucuronidation by the UGT1A1 and UGT1A9 pathways (e.g., **irinotecan**). Due to thrombocytopenic effects, sorafenib can contribute to increased bleeding from NONSTEROIDAL ANTI-INFLAMMATORY DRUGS, PLATELET INHIBITORS (e.g., **aspirin, clopidogrel**), THROMBOLYTIC AGENTS, and **warfarin.** Inducers of CYP3A4 (e.g., **carbamazepine, phenobarbital, phenytoin, rifampin**) may decrease the levels of sorafenib. **Food:** Food decreases the absorption of sorafenib. **Herbal: St. John's wort** may decrease the levels of sorafenib.

**PHARMACOKINETICS Absorption:** 38–49% absorbed. **Peak:** 3 h. **Distribution:** 99.5% protein bound. **Metabolism:** In the liver. **Elimination:** Primarily fecal (77%) with minor elimination in the urine (19%). **Half-Life:** 25–48 h.

## NURSING IMPLICATIONS
### Assessment & Drug Effects
- Monitor for and report S&S of skin toxicity (e.g., rash, erythema, dermatitis, paresthesia, swelling, or pain in hands or feet). Severe reactions may require temporary suspension of therapy or dose reduction.
- Monitor for S&S of bleeding, especially in those on anticoagulation therapy.
- Monitor BP weekly for the first 6 wk of therapy and periodically thereafter. New-onset hypertension has been associated with sorafenib.
- Monitor blood levels of warfarin with concurrent therapy.
- Monitor lab tests: Periodic CBC with differential and platelet count, serum electrolytes, LFTs, lipase, amylase, and alkaline phosphatase.

### Patient & Family Education
- Report any of the following to a health care provider: Skin rash; redness, blisters, pain, or swelling of the palms or hands or soles of feet; signs of bleeding; unexplained chest, shoulder, neck and jaw, or back pain.
- Do not take any prescription or nonprescription drugs without consulting the prescriber.
- Male and female patients should use effective birth control during treatment and for at least 2 wk following completion of treatment.

## SOTALOL
(so-ta′lol)

Betapace, Betapace AF, Sorine, Sotylize

**Classifications:** BETA-ADRENERGIC ANTAGONIST; CLASS II AND III ANTIARRHYTHMIC
**Therapeutic:** CLASS II AND III ANTIARRHYTHMIC
**Prototype:** Amiodarone

Common adverse effects in *italic;* life-threatening effects underlined; generic names in **bold;** classifications in SMALL CAPS; ◆ Canadian drug name; ⊘ Prototype drug

1515

**AVAILABILITY** Tablet; solution for injection

**ACTION & *THERAPEUTIC EFFECT***
Has both class II and class III antiarrhythmic properties. Slows heart rate, decreases AV nodal conduction, and increases AV nodal refractoriness. Produces significant reduction in both systolic and diastolic blood pressure. *Antiarrhythmic properties are effective in controlling ventricular arrhythmias as well as atrial fibrillation/flutter.*

**USES** Treatment of life-threatening ventricular arrhythmias (sustained ventricular tachycardia) and maintenance of normal sinus rhythm in patients with atrial fibrillation/flutter.

**CONTRAINDICATIONS** Hypersensitivity to sotalol; bronchial asthma, acute bronchospasm; sinus bradycardia, second and third degree AV block without a functioning pacemaker, uncontrolled HF; cardiogenic shock; emphysema; major disease; congenital or acquired long QT prolongation; hypokalemia less than 4 mEq/L creatinine clearance of less than 40 mL/min; lactation.

**CAUTIOUS USE** CHF, electrolyte disturbances, within 14 days of MI; DM; sick sinus rhythm, PVD; untreated pheochromocytoma; MG; thyroid disease; history of psychiatric disease; hyperthyroidism; renal impairment; excessive diarrhea, or profuse sweating; older adults; pregnancy (category B).

## ROUTE & DOSAGE

**Ventricular Arrhythmias**
**(Betapace, Sorine, Sotylize)**
*Adult:* **PO** Initial dose of 80 mg b.i.d. or 160 mg daily taken prior to meals, may increase every 3–4 days (most patients respond to 240–320 mg/day in 2 or 3 divided doses, doses greater than 640 mg/day have not been studied)

***Renal Impairment Dosage Adjustment***
*CrCl greater than 60 mL/min:* q12h; *30–60 mL/min:* q24h; *10–30 mL/min:* q36–48h; *less than 10 mL/min:* Individualize carefully

**Atrial Fibrillation/Flutter**
**(Betapace AF, Sotylize)**
*Adult:* **PO** Initial dose of 80 mg b.i.d., may increase every 3–4 days (max: 240 mg/day in 1–2 divided doses); **IV** 75 mg b.i.d. may increase after 3 days depending on patient response

***Renal Impairment Dosage Adjustment***
*CrCl 40–60 mL/min:* Dose q24h; *less than 40 mL/min contraindicated*

## ADMINISTRATION

### Oral

- Sotalol and sotalol AF are **not** interchangable because of significant differences in labeling (i.e., patient package insert, dosing administration, safety information).
- Give without regard to meals.
- Drug should be initiated and doses increased only under close supervision, preferably in a hospital with cardiac rhythm monitoring and frequent assessment.
- Use smallest effective dose for patients with nonallergic bronchospasms.
- Do not discontinue drug abruptly. Gradually reduce dose over 1–2 wk.
- Store at room temperature, 15°–30° C (59°–86° F).

### Intravenous

*PREPARE:* **IV Infusion: Sotalol** infusion must be prepared to compensate for dead space in the infusion set. The directions that follow will yield 120 mL of prepared volume, but only 100 mL will be infused when using a volumetric infusion pump. Possible diluents include NS, D5W, and LR. For a target dose of 75 mg, use 6 mL sotalol injection and 114 mL diluent; for a target dose of 112.5 mg, use 9 mL sotalol injection and 111 mL diluent; for a target dose of 150 mg, use 12 mL sotalol injection and 108 mL diluent.

*ADMINISTER:* **IV Infusion:** Give at a constant rate over 5 h.

*INCOMPATIBILITIES:* Do not infuse with any other drugs or solutions.

### ADVERSE EFFECTS (≥1%) CV: AV

block, hypotension, aggravation of CHF, although the incidence of heart failure may be lower than for other beta-blockers, <u>life-threatening ventricular arrhythmias, including polymorphous ventricular tachycardia or torsades de pointes</u>, *bradycardia, dyspnea, chest pain, palpitation,* bleeding (less than 2%). **CNS:** Headache, *fatigue, dizziness,* weakness, lethargy, depression, lassitude. **GI:** Nausea, vomiting, diarrhea, dyspepsia, dry mouth. **Urogenital:** Impotence, decreased libido. **Metabolic:** Hyperglycemia. **Special Senses:** Visual disturbances. **Respiratory:** Respiratory complaints. **Skin:** Rash.

### INTERACTIONS Drug: Antagonizes

the effects of BETA AGONISTS. **Amiodarone** may lead to symptomatic bradycardia and sinus arrest. The hypoglycemic effects of ORAL HYPOGLYCEMIC AGENTS may be potentiated. May cause resistance to **epinephrine** in anaphylactic reactions. Should be used with caution with other ANTIARRHYTHMIC AGENTS, withhold Class I (e.g., **disopyramide, procainamide, quinidine**) or Class III ANTIARRHYTHMICS (e.g., **amiodarone, dofetilide**) for at least three half-lives prior to initiating sotalol. **Food:** Absorption may be reduced by food, especially **milk** and MILK PRODUCTS.

### PHARMACOKINETICS Absorption: Slowly and completely from GI

tract. Negligible first-pass metabolism. Reduced by food, especially milk and milk products. **Peak:** 2–3 h. **Duration:** 24 h. **Distribution:** Drug is hydrophilic and will enter the CSF slowly (about 10%). Crosses placental barrier. Distributed in breast milk. Not appreciably protein bound. **Metabolism:** Does not undergo significant hepatic enzyme metabolism and no active metabolites have been identified. **Elimination:** In urine with 75% of the drug excreted unchanged within 72 h. **Half-Life:** 7–18 h.

## NURSING IMPLICATIONS

### Black Box Warning

*Sotalol initiation, reinitiation, and dosage adjustment have been associated with serious, life-threatening arrhythmias; thus patients should be in a facility that can provide continuous ECG monitoring, calculation of creatinine clearance, and cardiac resuscitation.*

### Assessment & Drug Effects

- Monitor ECG at baseline and periodically thereafter (especially when doses are increased) because proarrhythmic events most often occur within 7 days of initiating therapy or increasing dose.
- Monitor cardiac status throughout therapy. Exercise special caution when sotalol is used concurrently with other antiarrhythmics, digoxin, or calcium channel blockers.

S

Common adverse effects in *italic;* life-threatening effects <u>underlined;</u> generic names in **bold;** classifications in SMALL CAPS; ✢ Canadian drug name; ⊕ Prototype drug

1517

- Monitor patients with broncho-spastic disease (e.g., bronchitis, emphysema) carefully for inhibition of bronchodilation.
- Monitor diabetics for loss of glycemic control. Beta blockage reduces the release of endogenous insulin in response to hyperglycemia and may blunt symptoms of acute hypoglycemia (e.g., tachycardia, BP changes).
- Monitor lab test: Baseline and periodic creatinine clearance, and serum electrolytes. Correct electrolyte imbalances of hypokalemia or hypomagnesemia prior to initiating therapy.

**Patient & Family Education**
- Be aware of risk for hypotension and syncope, especially with concurrent treatment with catecholamine-depleting drugs (e.g., reserpine, guanethidine).
- Take radial pulse daily and report marked bradycardia (pulse below 60 or other established parameter) hold the dose and notify the prescriber.
- Type 2 diabetics are at increased risk for hyperglycemia. All diabetics are at risk of possible masking of symptoms of hypoglycemia.
- Do not abruptly discontinue drug because of the risk of exacerbation of angina, arrhythmias, and possible myocardial infarction.

# SPINOSAD
(spin′oh-sad)
**Natroba**
**Classifications:** SCABICIDE; PEDICULICIDE
**Therapeutic:** SCABICIDE; PEDICULICIDE
**Prototype:** Permethrin

**AVAILABILITY** Topical suspension

## ACTION & *THERAPEUTIC EFFECT*
Kills lice directly without measurable absorption into the human body. *Eliminates lice infestation in humans.*

**USES** Topical treatment of head lice infestations caused by *Pediculus capitis* in patients 4 y or older.

**CONTRAINDICATIONS** Contains benzyl alcohol and is not recommended for use in neonates and infants below the age of 6 months.

**CAUTIOUS USE** Inflammatory skin conditions (e.g., psoriasis, eczema); pregnancy (category B); lactation; children 4 y or older.

## ROUTE & DOSAGE

**Head Lice Infestation**
*Adult/Child (4 y or older):* **Topical** May apply up to 120 mL to cover scalp/hair; may repeat in 7 d if necessary.

## ADMINISTRATION
**Topical**
- Shake well immediately prior to use.
- Apply sufficient amount (up to one bottle) to cover dry scalp, then apply to dry hair; leave on 10 min, then rinse hair and scalp thoroughly with warm water.
- Store at 15°–30° C (59°–86° F).

**ADVERSE EFFECTS** (≥1%) **Body as a Whole:** Application-site erythema and irritation. **Special Senses:** Ocular erythema.

## NURSING IMPLICATIONS
**Assessment & Drug Effects**
- Assess hair and scalp for presence of lice. If still present after 7 days of treatment, a second treatment should be applied.

## Patient & Family Education

- Avoid contact with eyes. If spinosad gets in or near the eyes, rinse thoroughly with water.
- Wash hands after applying spinosad.
- Use on children only under direct supervision of an adult.

# SPIRONOLACTONE ℗

(speer-on-oh-lak'tone)

Aldactone, CaroSpir

**Classifications:** ELECTROLYTIC AND WATER BALANCE; ALDOSTERONE ANTAGONIST; POTASSIUM-SPARING DIURETIC

Therapeutic: POTASSIUM-SPARING DIURETIC; ANTIHYPERTENSIVE

**AVAILABILITY** Tablet; suspension

## ACTION & THERAPEUTIC EFFECT

Competes with aldosterone for cellular receptor sites in distal renal tubules. Promotes sodium and chloride excretion without loss of potassium. *A diuretic agent that promotes sodium and chloride excretion without concomitant loss of potassium. Lowers systolic and diastolic pressures in hypertensive patients. Effective in treatment of primary aldosteronism.*

**USES** Essential hypertension, refractory edema due to CHF, hepatic cirrhosis, nephrotic syndrome, hypokalemia, and idiopathic edema. May be used to potentiate actions of other diuretics and antihypertensive agents or for its potassium-sparing effect. Also used for treatment of (and as presumptive test for) primary aldosteronism; severe heart failure.

**UNLABELED USES** Hirsutism in women with polycystic ovary syndrome or idiopathic hirsutism; adjunct in treatment of myasthenia gravis and familial periodic paralysis.

**CONTRAINDICATIONS** Anuria, acute renal insufficiency; renal failure; diabetic nephropathy; progressive impairment of kidney function, or worsening of liver disease; hyperkalemia; lactic acidosis; Addison disease; Concomitant eplerenone; pregnancy (category D, if used in gestational hypertension); lactation.

**CAUTIOUS USE** BUN of 40 mg/dL or greater, mild renal impairment; fluid and electrolyte imbalance; liver disease; severe heart failure; natremia; older adults; pregnancy (category C, if not used in gestational hypertension); children.

## ROUTE & DOSAGE

### Edema

Note: Tablet and suspension are not interchangable

*Adult:* **PO Tablet** 25–200 mg daily in single or divided dose; **CaroSpir Suspension** 75 mg daily in single or divided dose

*Child:* **PO Tablet** 1 mg/kg/day divided every 12–24 h

### Hypertension

*Adult:* **PO Tablet** 50–100 mg/day in single or divided doses, may titrate at 2 wk intervals; **CaroSpir Suspension** 20–75 mg daily may titrate at 2 wk intervals

### Primary Aldosteronism: Diagnosis

*Adult:* **PO Tablet** 400 mg/day for 4 days;

### Hypokalemia

*Adult:* **PO Tablet** 25–100 mg daily or in divided doses

S

Common adverse effects in *italic;* life-threatening effects underlined; generic names in **bold;** classifications in SMALL CAPS; ♣ Canadian drug name; ℗ Prototype drug

1519

**Severe Heart Failure**
*Adult:* **PO Tablet** 12.5–25 mg qd (if serum K+ 5 mEq/L or less); may increase dose to 50 mg qd if needed

## ADMINISTRATION
### Oral
- Use single gloves when handling intact tablets or capsules or administering from unit package. If cutting or crushing or handling uncoated tablets, use double gloves and a protective gown.
- Give with food to enhance absorption.
- Crush tablets and give with fluid of patient's choice if unable to swallow whole.
- Store in tight, light-resistant containers. Store suspension at 20°–25° C (68°–77° F); stable for 1 mo under refrigeration. Store tablets below 25° C (77° F).

## ADVERSE EFFECTS (≥1%) CNS:
Lethargy, mental confusion, fatigue (with rapid weight loss), headache, *drowsiness*, ataxia. **Endocrine:** *Gynecomastia* (both sexes), *erectile dysfunction, androgenic effects (hirsutism, irregular menses,* deepening of voice); parathyroid changes, decreased glucose tolerance, amenorrhea, decreased libido, SLE. **GI:** Abdominal cramps, *nausea, vomiting,* anorexia, *diarrhea.* **Skin:** Maculopapular or erythematous rash, urticaria, alopecia. **Metabolic:** Fluid and electrolyte imbalance (particularly hyperkalemia and hyponatremia); elevated BUN, mild acidosis, hyperuricemia, gout. **Body as a Whole:** Drug fever, vasculitis, leg cramps. **Hematologic:** Agranulocytosis. **CV:** Hypertension (post-sympathectomy patient).

## DIAGNOSTIC TEST INTERFERENCE
May produce marked increases in *plasma cortisol* determinations by *Mattingly fluorometric* method; these may persist for several days after termination of drug (spironolactone metabolite produces fluorescence). There is the possibility of false elevations in measurements of *digoxin serum levels* by *RIA* procedures.

## INTERACTIONS Drug:
Combinations of spironolactone and acidifying doses of **ammonium chloride** may produce systemic acidosis; use these combinations with caution. Diuretic effect of spironolactone may be antagonized by **aspirin** and other SALICYLATES. **Digoxin** should be monitored for decreased effect of CARDIAC GLYCOSIDES. Hyperkalemia may result with POTASSIUM SUPPLEMENTS, ACE INHIBITORS, ARBS, **heparin** may decrease **lithium** clearance resulting in increased tenacity; may alter anticoagulant response in **warfarin.** Do not use with **eplerenone, darifenacin,** or **tranylcypromine.** Avoid **amiloride, cyclosporine. Food:** Salt substitutes may increase risk of hyperkalemia.

## PHARMACOKINETICS Absorption:
~73% from GI tract. **Onset:** Gradual. **Peak:** 2–3 days; maximum effect may take up to 2 wk. **Duration:** 2–3 days or longer. **Distribution:** Crosses placenta, distributed into breast milk. **Metabolism:** In liver and kidneys to active metabolites; potent inhibitor of P-gp. **Elimination:** 40–57% in urine, 35–40% in bile. **Half-Life:** 1.3–2.4 h parent compound, 18–23 h metabolites.

## NURSING IMPLICATIONS

### Black Box Warning

*Spironolactone has been associated with tumor development in laboratory animals. Unnecessary use of this drug should be avoided.*

### Assessment & Drug Effects

- Check blood pressure before initiation of therapy and at regular intervals throughout therapy.
- Assess for signs of fluid and electrolyte imbalance, and signs of digoxin toxicity.
- Monitor daily I&O and check for edema. Report lack of diuretic response or development of edema, both may indicate tolerance to drug.
- Weigh patient under standard conditions before therapy begins and daily throughout therapy. Weight is a useful index of need for dosage adjustment. For patients with ascites, prescriber may want measurements of abdominal girth.
- Observe for and report immediately the onset of mental changes, lethargy, or stupor in patients with liver disease.
- Adverse reactions are generally reversible with discontinuation of drug. Gynecomastia appears to be related to dosage level and duration of therapy; it may persist in some after drug is stopped.
- Monitor lab tests: Periodic serum electrolytes especially during early therapy, blood glucose, BUN/creatinine.

### Patient & Family Education

- Be aware that the maximal diuretic effect may not occur until third day of therapy and that diuresis may continue for 2–3 days after drug is withdrawn.
- Report signs of hyponatremia or hyperkalemia (see Appendix F),

most likely to occur in patients with severe cirrhosis.
- Avoid replacing fluid losses with large amounts of free water (can result in dilutional hyponatremia).
- Weigh 2–3 × each wk. Report gains/loss of 5 lb or more.
- Do not drive or engage in potentially hazardous activities until response to the drug is known.
- Avoid excessive intake of high-potassium foods and salt substitutes.

## STAVUDINE (D4T)

(sta'vu deen)

**Zerit**

**Classifications:** ANTIRETROVIRAL; NUCLEOSIDE REVERSE TRANSCRIPTASE INHIBITOR (NRTI)

**Therapeutic:** ANTIRETROVIRAL; NRTI

**Prototype:** Lamivudine

**AVAILABILITY** Capsule; oral solution

**ACTION & THERAPEUTIC EFFECT**
Appears to act by being incorporated into growing DNA chains by viral transcriptase, thus terminating viral replication. *Inhibits the replication of HIV in human cells and decreases viral load.*

**USES** HIV treatment.

**UNLABELED USES** HIV prophylaxis.

**CONTRAINDICATIONS** Hypersensitivity to stavudine; lactic acidosis; lactation.

**CAUTIOUS USE** Previous hypersensitivity to zidovudine, didanosine, or zalcitabine; folic acid or $B_{12}$ deficiency; liver and renal insufficiency; alcoholism; peripheral neuropathy; history of pancreatitis; pregnancy (category C).

**S**

Common adverse effects in *italic;* life-threatening effects underlined; generic names in **bold;** classifications in SMALL CAPS; ✦ Canadian drug name; ◉ Prototype drug

1521

## ROUTE & DOSAGE

### HIV Infection

*Adult/Adolescent/Child /Infant (weight less than 30 kg):* PO 1 mg/kg q12h; *weight 30–59 kg:* 30 mg q12h; *weight 60 kg or greater:* 40 mg q12h
*Neonate (younger than 13 days):* PO 0.5 mg/kg q12h

### Renal Impairment Dosage Adjustment

*CrCl 25–50 mL/min:* Reduce dose by 50%; *less than 25 mL/min:* Reduce dose by 50% and extend interval to q24h

## ADMINISTRATION

### Oral

- Adhere strictly to 12-h interval between doses.
- Reconstitute powder by adding water to the container (amounts of water will vary according to manufacturer). Shake vigorously.
- Capsules and powder for reconstitution may be stored at a controlled room temperature of 25° C (77° F).

## ADVERSE EFFECTS (≥1%) CNS: *Peripheral neuropathy,* paresthesias, *headache.* GI: *Anorexia, nausea, vomiting, diarrhea,* cramping, pancreatitis, abdominal pain, <u>elevated liver function tests</u>, abdominal pain. Body as a Whole: *Headache,* chills/fever, *myalgia.* Hematologic: <u>Anemia, neutropenia.</u> Skin: *Rash.* Metabolic: <u>Lactic acidosis</u> in pregnant women; hyperglycemia, lipodystrophy.

## INTERACTIONS Drug: Didanosine may increase risk of pancreatitis and hepatotoxicity; **probenecid** can decrease elimination; **zalcitabine** increases risk of neuropathy; **zidovudine** may impact metabolism, avoid concurrent use. Use INTERFERONS, **ribavirin** cautiously. Herbal: Avoid use with echinacea.

## PHARMACOKINETICS Absorption: Readily absorbed from GI tract; 82% reaches systemic circulation. Peak: Effect 6 wk. Distribution: Distributes into CSF; excreted in breast milk of animals. Metabolism: Unknown. Elimination: In urine. Half-Life: 1–1.6 h.

## NURSING IMPLICATIONS

### Black Box Warning

*Stavudine has been associated with lactic acidosis and severe, sometimes fatal, hepatomegaly with steatosis.*

### Assessment & Drug Effects

- Monitor for peripheral neuropathy and report numbness, tingling, or pain, which may indicate a need to interrupt stavudine.
- Monitor for development of opportunistic infection.
- Monitor lab tests: Periodic measurement of acid–base balance, LFTs with preexisting hepatic impairment, renal function tests in the older adult. CBC with differential and serum lipid profile.

### Patient & Family Education

- Take drug exactly as prescribed.
- Report to prescriber any adverse drug effects that are bothersome.
- Report symptoms of peripheral neuropathy to prescriber immediately.

## STREPTOMYCIN SULFATE

(strep-toe-mye′sin)

**Classifications:** AMINOGLYCOSIDE ANTIBIOTIC; ANTITUBERCULOSIS
Therapeutic: ANTIBIOTIC; ANTITUBERCULOSIS
**Prototype:** Gentamicin

S

Common adverse effects in *italic;* life-threatening effects <u>underlined</u>; generic names in **bold;** classifications in SMALL CAPS; ♣ Canadian drug name; ◐ Prototype drug

## AVAILABILITY IM solution

## ACTION & *THERAPEUTIC EFFECT*
Inhibits bacterial protein synthesis through irreversible binding to the 30S ribosomal subunit of susceptible bacteria. *Active against a variety of gram-positive, gram-negative, and acid-fast organisms.*

**USES** In combination with other antitubercular drugs in treatment of all forms of active tuberculosis. Used alone or in conjunction with tetracycline for tularemia, plague, and brucellosis. Also used with other antibiotics in treatment of subacute bacterial endocarditis and in treatment of peritonitis, respiratory tract infections, granuloma inguinale, and chancroid when other drugs have failed.

**CONTRAINDICATIONS** History of toxic reaction or severe hypersensitivity to streptomycin; clinically significant reaction to other aminoglycosides; labyrinthine disease; concurrent or sequential use of neurotoxic and/or nephrotoxic drugs; myasthenia gravis; pregnancy (category D).

**CAUTIOUS USE** Impaired renal function; prerenal azotemia; auditory dysfunction; older adults; lactation prematures; neonates; and children.

## ROUTE & DOSAGE

**Endocarditis**
*Adult:* **IM** 1g b.i.d. × 2 wk then 500 mg b.i.d. × 4 wk
*Geriatric:* 500 mg bid for entire therapy

**Tuberculosis**
*Adult:* **IM** 15 mg/kg up to 1 g/day as single dose
*Child:* **IM** 20–40 mg/kg/day up to 1 g/day as single dose

**Tularemia**
*Adult:* **IM** 1–2 g/day in 1–2 divided doses for 7–10 days

**Plague**
*Adult:* **IM** 2 g/day in 2–4 divided doses

**Other Infection**
*Adult:* **IM** 1–2 g in divided doses q6–12h (max: 2 g/day)
*Child:* **IM** 20–240 mg/kg/day in divided doses q6–12h

## ADMINISTRATION

**Intramuscular**
- Give IM deep into large muscle mass to minimize possibility of irritation. Injections are painful.
- Avoid direct contact with drug; sensitization can occur. Use gloves during preparation of drug.
- Use commercially prepared IM solution undiluted; intended only for IM injection (contains a preservative, and therefore is not suitable for other routes).
- Store ampules at room temperature. Protect from light; exposure to light may slightly darken solution, with no apparent loss of potency.

**ADVERSE EFFECTS** (>1%) **CNS:** Paresthesias (peripheral, facial). **Body as a Whole:** Hypersensitivity angioedema, drug fever, enlarged lymph nodes, anaphylactic shock, headache, inability to concentrate, lassitude, muscular weakness, *pain and irritation at IM site,* superinfections, neuromuscular blockade, arachnoiditis. **GI:** Stomatitis, hepatotoxicity. **Hematologic:** Blood dyscrasias (leukopenia, neutropenia, pancytopenia, hemolytic or aplastic anemia, eosinophilia). **Special Senses:** *Labyrinthine damage,* auditory damage, optic nerve toxicity (scotomas). **Urogenital:** Nephrotoxicity.

S

**CNS:** Encephalopathy, <u>CNS depression syndrome in infants (stupor, flaccidity, coma, paralysis, cardiac arrest)</u>. **Respiratory:** <u>Respiratory depression</u>. **Skin:** Skin rashes, pruritus, <u>exfoliative dermatitis</u>.

## DIAGNOSTIC TEST INTERFERENCE

Streptomycin reportedly produces false-positive *urinary glucose* tests using *copper sulfate methods (Benedict's solution, Clinitest)* but not with *glucose oxidase methods* (e.g., *Clinistix, TesTape*). False increases in protein content in *urine* and *CSF* using *Folin-Ciocalteau reaction* and decreased *BUN* readings with *Berthelot reaction* may occur from test interferences.

## INTERACTIONS Drug:

May potentiate anticoagulant effects of **warfarin;** additive nephrotoxicity with **acyclovir, amphotericin B,** AMINOGLYCOSIDES, **carboplatin, cidofovir, cisplatin, cyclosporine, foscarnet, ganciclovir,** SALICYLATES, **tacrolimus, vancomycin.** Use with DIURETIC increases risk of ototoxic effects.

## PHARMACOKINETICS Peak:

1–2 h. **Distribution:** Diffuses into most body tissues and extracellular fluids; crosses placenta; distributed into breast milk. **Elimination:** In urine. **Half-Life:** 2–3 h adults, 4–10 h newborns.

## NURSING IMPLICATIONS

### Black Box Warning

*Streptomycin has been associated with increased risk of severe neurotoxic reactions, especially in those with impaired renal function.*

### Assessment & Drug Effects

- Be alert for and report immediately symptoms of ototoxicity (see Appendix F). Symptoms are most likely to occur in patients with impaired kidney function, patients receiving high doses (1.8–2 g/day) or other ototoxic or neurotoxic drugs, and older adults. Irreversible damage may occur if drug is not discontinued promptly.
- Early damage to vestibular portion of eighth cranial nerve (higher incidence than auditory toxicity) is initially manifested by moderately severe headache, nausea, vomiting, vertigo in upright position, difficulty in reading, unsteadiness, and positive Romberg sign.
- Be aware that auditory nerve damage is usually preceded by vestibular symptoms and high-pitched tinnitus, roaring noises, impaired hearing (especially to high-pitched sounds), sense of fullness in ears. Audiometric test should be done if these symptoms appear, and drug should be discontinued. Hearing loss can be permanent if damage is extensive. Tinnitus may persist several days to weeks after drug is stopped.
- Monitor I&O. Report oliguria or changes in I&O ratio (possible signs of diminishing kidney function). Sufficient fluids to maintain urinary output of 1500 mL/24 h are generally advised. Consult prescriber.
- Monitor lab tests: Baseline C&S; periodic BUN and creatinine; serum drug concentration as indicated.

### Patient & Family Education

- Report any unusual symptoms. Review adverse reactions with prescriber periodically, especially with prolonged therapy.
- Be aware of possibility of ototoxicity and its symptoms (see Appendix F).
- Report to prescriber immediately any of the following: Nausea, vomiting, vertigo, incoordination, tinnitus, fullness in ears, impaired hearing.

# STREPTOZOCIN

(strep-toe-zoe'sin)

Zanosar

**Classification:** ANTINEOPLASTIC, ALKYLATING; NITROSOUREA

Therapeutic: ANTINEOPLASTIC

**Prototype:** Cyclophosphamide

**AVAILABILITY** Solution for injection

**ACTION & THERAPEUTIC EFFECT**
Inhibits DNA synthesis in cells and prevents progression of cells into mitosis, affecting all phases of the cell cycle (cell-cycle nonspecific). *Successful therapy with streptozocin (alone or in combination) produces a biochemical response evidenced by decreased secretion of hormones as well as measurable tumor regression. Thus, serial fasting insulin levels during treatment indicate response to this drug.*

**USES** Pancreatic cancer.

**UNLABELED USES** Hodgkin disease, palliative treatment of metastatic carcinoid tumor.

**CONTRAINDICATIONS** Concurrent use with nephrotoxic drugs; pregnancy (category D); lactation.

**CAUTIOUS USE** Renal impairment; hepatic disease, hepatic impairment; patients with history of hypoglycemia; DM; children.

## ROUTE & DOSAGE

**Islet Cell Carcinoma of Pancreas**

*Adult/Adolescent/Child:* **IV** 500 mg/m²/day for 5 consecutive days q4– 6wk or 1 g/m²/wk for 2 wk, then increase to 1.5 g/m²/wk × 4–6 wk

**Renal Impairment Dosage Adjustment**

*CrCl 10–50 mL/min:* Give 75% of dose; *CrCl less than 10 mL/min:* Give 50% of dose

## ADMINISTRATION

**Intravenous**

This drug is a cytotoxic agent and caution should be used to prevent any contact with the drug. Follow institutional or standard guidelines for preparation, handling, and disposal of cytotoxic agents.

Use only under constant supervision by prescriber experienced in therapy with cytotoxic agents and only when the benefit to risk ratio is fully and thoroughly understood by patient and family

**PREPARE: IV Infusion:** Reconstitute with 9.5 mL D5W or NS, to yield 100 mg/mL. Solution will be pale gold. ▪ May be further diluted with up to 250 mL of the original diluent. ▪ Protect reconstituted solution and vials of drug from light.
**ADMINISTER: IV Infusion:** Give over 15–60 min. ▪ Inspect injection site frequently for signs of extravasation (patient complaints of stinging or burning at site, swelling around site, no blood return or questionable blood return). ▪ If extravasation occurs, area requires immediate attention to prevent necrosis. Remove needle, apply ice, and contact prescriber regarding further treatment to infiltrated tissue.
**INCOMPATIBILITIES: Y-site: Acyclovir, allopurinol, amphotericin, aztreonam, cefepime, daptomycin, levofloxacin, pantoprazole, piperacillin/tazobactam, trastuzumab.**
▪ Note: An antiemetic given routinely every 4 or 6 h and prophylactically 30 min before a treatment may provide sufficient control to maintain the treatment regimen (even if

Common adverse effects in *italic;* life-threatening effects underlined; generic names in **bold;** classifications in SMALL CAPS; ♣ Canadian drug name; ⊙ Prototype drug

1525

it reduces but does not completely eliminate nausea and vomiting).

- Discard reconstituted solutions after 12 h (contains no preservative and not intended for multidose use).

**ADVERSE EFFECTS (≥1%) CNS:** Confusion, lethargy, depression. **GI:** *Nausea, vomiting,* diarrhea, transient increase in AST, ALT, or alkaline phosphatase; hypoalbuminemia. **Hematologic:** *Mild* to moderate myelosuppression (leukopenia, thrombocytopenia, *anemia*). **Metabolic:** Glucose tolerance abnormalities (moderate and reversible); glycosuria without hyperglycemia, insulin shock (rare). **Urogenital:** Nephrotoxicity: Azotemia, anuria, proteinuria, hypophosphatemia, hyperchloremia; *Fanconi-like syndrome* (proximal renal tubular reabsorption defects, alkaline pH of urine, glucosuria, acetonuria, aminoaciduria); hypokalemia, hypocalcemia. **Other:** Local necrosis following extravasation.

**INTERACTIONS Drug:** MYELOSUPPRESSIVE AGENTS add to hematologic toxicity; nephrotoxic agents (e.g., AMINOGLYCOSIDES, **vancomycin, amphotericin B, cisplatin**) increase risk of nephrotoxicity; **phenytoin** may reduce cytotoxic effect on pancreatic beta cells.

**PHARMACOKINETICS Absorption:** Undetectable in plasma within 3 h. **Distribution:** Metabolite enters CSF. **Metabolism:** In liver and kidneys. **Elimination:** 70–80% of dose in urine, 1% in feces, and 5% in expired air. **Half-Life:** 35–40 min.

## NURSING IMPLICATIONS

### Black Box Warning

*Streptozocin has been associated with severe, sometimes fatal, renal toxicity, and with severe GI, hepatic, and hematologic toxicities.*

### Assessment & Drug Effects

- Ensure that repeat courses of streptozocin treatment are not given until patient's liver, kidney, and hematologic functions are within acceptable limits.
- Be alert to and report promptly early laboratory evidence of kidney dysfunction: Hypophosphatemia, mild proteinuria, and changes in I&O ratio and pattern.
- Mild adverse renal effects may be reversible following discontinuation of streptozocin, but nephrotoxicity may be irreversible, severe, or fatal.
- Be alert to symptoms of sepsis and superinfections or increased tendency to bleed (thrombocytopenia). Myelosuppression is severe in 10–20% of patients and may be cumulative and more severe if patient has had prior exposure to radiation or to other antineoplastics.
- Monitor and record temperature pattern to promptly recognize impending sepsis.
- Monitor lab tests: Weekly CBC; LFTs prior to each course of therapy; serial urinalyses and kidney function tests; baseline and weekly serum electrolytes, then for 4 wk after termination of therapy.

### Patient & Family Education

- Inspect site at weekly intervals and report changes in tissue appearance if extravasation occurred during IV infusion.
- Report symptoms of hypoglycemia (see Appendix F) even though this drug has minimal, if any, diabetogenic action.
- Drink fluids liberally (2000–3000 mL/day). Hydration may protect against drug toxicity effects.
- Report S&S of nephrotoxicity (see Appendix F).
- Do not take aspirin or NSAIDs without consulting prescriber.

S

- Report to prescriber promptly any signs of bleeding: Hematuria, epistaxis, ecchymoses, petechiae.
- Report symptoms that suggest anemia: Shortness of breath, pale mucous membranes and nail beds, exhaustion, rapid pulse.

## SUCCINYLCHOLINE CHLORIDE ℗

(suk-sin-ill-koe'leen)

Anectine, Quelicin

**Classification:** DEPOLARIZING SKELETAL MUSCLE RELAXANT
Therapeutic: SKELETAL MUSCLE RELAXANT

**AVAILABILITY** Solution for injection

## ACTION & *THERAPEUTIC EFFECT*
Synthetic, ultrashort-acting depolarizing neuromuscular blocking agent with high affinity for acetylcholine (ACh) receptor sites. *Initial transient contractions and fasciculations are followed by sustained flaccid skeletal muscle paralysis produced by state of accommodation that develops in adjacent excitable muscle membranes.*

**USES** To produce skeletal muscle relaxation as adjunct to anesthesia; to facilitate intubation and endoscopy, to increase pulmonary compliance in assisted or controlled respiration, and to reduce intensity of muscle contractions in pharmacologically induced or electroshock convulsions.

**CONTRAINDICATIONS** Hypersensitivity to succinylcholine; family history of malignant hyperthermia; burns; trauma.

**CAUTIOUS USE** Kidney, liver, pulmonary, metabolic, or cardiovascular disorders; myasthenia gravis; dehydration, electrolyte imbalance, patients taking digitalis, severe burns or trauma, fractures, spinal cord injuries, degenerative or dystrophic neuromuscular diseases, low plasma pseudocholinesterase levels (recessive genetic trait, but often associated with severe liver disease, severe anemia, dehydration, marked changes in body temperature, exposure to neurotoxic insecticides, certain drugs); collagen diseases, porphyria, intraocular surgery, glaucoma; during delivery with cesarean section; pregnancy (category C), lactation; children.

## ROUTE & DOSAGE

**Surgical and Anesthetic Procedures**

*Adult:* **IV** 0.3–1.1 mg/kg administered over 10–30 sec, may give additional doses prn; **IM** 2.5–4 mg/kg up to 150 mg
*Child:* **IV** 1–2 mg/kg administered over 10–30 sec, may give additional doses prn; **IM** 2.5–4 mg/kg up to 150 mg

**Prolonged Muscle Relaxation**

*Adult:* **IV** 0.5–10 mg/min by continuous infusion

***Obesity Dosage Adjustment***

Dose based on IBW

## ADMINISTRATION

**Intramuscular**
- Give IM injections deeply, preferably high into deltoid muscle.

**Intravenous**
Use only freshly prepared solutions; succinylcholine hydrolyzes rapidly with consequent loss of potency.

S

Common adverse effects in *italic;* life-threatening effects <u>underlined</u>; generic names in **bold;** classifications in SMALL CAPS; ◆ Canadian drug name; ℗ Prototype drug

1527

- Give initial small test dose (0.1 mg/kg) to determine individual drug sensitivity and recovery time.

*PREPARE:* **Direct:** Give undiluted. **Intermittent/Continuous:** Dilute 1 g in 500–1000 mL of D5W or NS. *ADMINISTER:* **Direct:** Give a bolus dose over 10–30 sec. **Intermittent/Continuous (Preferred):** Give at a rate of 0.5–10 mg/min. Do not exceed 10 mg/min.

*INCOMPATIBILITIES:* Solution/additive: Pentobarbital, sodium bicarbonate. Y-site: Amphotericin B conventional, azathioprine, dantrolene, diazepam, diazoxide, ganciclovir, gemtuzumab, indomethacin, mitomycin, nafcillin, PENICILLINS, pentobarbital, phenobarbital, phenytoin, sodium bicarbonate.

- Note: Expiration date and storage before and after reconstitution; varies with the manufacturer.

## ADVERSE EFFECTS (≥1%) CNS:

*Muscle fasciculations,* profound and prolonged muscle relaxation, muscle pain. **CV:** *Bradycardia,* tachycardia, hypotension, hypertension, arrhythmias, sinus arrest. **Respiratory:** *Respiratory depression,* bronchospasm, hypoxia, apnea. **Body as a Whole:** Malignant hyperthermia, increased IOP, excessive salivation, enlarged salivary glands. **Metabolic:** Myoglobinemia, hyperkalemia. **GI:** Decreased tone and motility of GI tract (large doses).

## INTERACTIONS Drug: Aminoglycosides, colistin, cyclophosphamide, cyclopropane, echothiophate iodide, halothane, lidocaine, MAGNESIUM SALTS, methotrimeprazine, NARCOTIC ANALGESICS, ORGANOPHOSPHAMIDE INSECTICIDES, MAO INHIBITORS, PHENOTHIAZINES, procaine, procainamide, quinidine, quinine, propranolol may prolong neuromuscular blockade; DIGITALIS GLYCOSIDES may increase risk of cardiac arrhythmias.

## PHARMACOKINETICS Onset: 0.5–1 min IV; 2–3 min IM. Duration: 2–3 min IV; 10–30 min IM. Distribution: Crosses placenta in small amounts. Metabolism: In plasma by pseudocholinesterases. Elimination: In urine.

## NURSING IMPLICATIONS

### Black Box Warning

*Succinylcholine has been associated with rare cases of acute rhabdomyolysis with hyperkalemia followed by ventricular arrhythmias, cardiac arrest, and death in children and adolescents.*

### Assessment & Drug Effects

- Be aware that transient apnea usually occurs at time of maximal drug effect (1–2 min); spontaneous respiration should return in a few seconds or, at most, 3 or 4 min.
- Have immediately available: Facilities for emergency endotracheal intubation, artificial respiration, and assisted or controlled respiration with oxygen.
- Monitor vital signs and keep airway clear of secretions.

### Patient & Family Education

- Patient may experience postprocedural muscle stiffness and pain (caused by initial fasciculations following injection) for as long as 24–30 h.
- Be aware that hoarseness and sore throat are common even when pharyngeal airway has not been used.
- Report residual muscle weakness to prescriber.

# SUCRALFATE
(soo-kral'fate)

**Carafate, Sulcrate ✦**

**Classifications:** ANTIULCER; GASTROADHESIVE

**Therapeutic:** ANTIULCER; GASTRO-PROTECTANT

**AVAILABILITY** Tablet; suspension

## ACTION & THERAPEUTIC EFFECT

Sucralfate and gastric acid react to form a viscous, adhesive, paste-like substance that resists further reaction with gastric acid. This "paste" adheres to the GI mucosa with a major portion binding electrostatically to the positively charged protein molecules in the damaged mucosa of an ulcer crater or an acute gastric erosion. *Absorbs bile, inhibits the enzyme pepsin, and blocks back diffusion of H+ ions. These actions plus adherence of the paste-like complex protect damaged mucosa against further destruction from ulcerogenic secretions and drugs.*

**USES** Duodenal ulcer.

## UNLABELED USES
Aspirin-induced erosions, stress ulcer prophylaxis, suspension for chemotherapy-induced mucositis.

## CONTRAINDICATION
Hypersensitivity to sucralfate.

## CAUTIOUS USE
Chronic kidney failure or dialysis due to aluminum accumulation; pregnancy (category B); lactation. Safe use in children not established.

## ROUTE & DOSAGE

**Duodenal Ulcer (Active disease)**
*Adult:* PO 1 g q.i.d. × 4–8 wk
**Duodenal Ulcer (Maintenance)**
*Adult:* PO 1 g b.i.d.

## ADMINISTRATION

### Oral
- Use drug solubilized in an appropriate diluent by a pharmacist when given through nasogastric tube.
- Administer antacids prescribed for pain relief 30 min before or after sucralfate.
- Separate administration of quinolones, digoxin, phenytoin, tetracycline from that of sucralfate by 2 h to prevent sucralfate from binding to these compounds in the intestinal tract and reducing their bioavailability.
- Store in tight container at room temperature, 15°–30° C (59°–86° F). Stable for 2 y after manufacture.

## ADVERSE EFFECTS (≥1%) GI:
Nausea, gastric discomfort, *constipation,* diarrhea.

## INTERACTIONS Drug:
May decrease absorption of QUINOLONES (e.g., **ciprofloxacin, norfloxacin**), **digoxin, phenytoin, tetracycline.**

## PHARMACOKINETICS Absorption:
Minimally absorbed from GI tract (less than 5%). **Duration:** Up to 6 h (depends on contact time with ulcer crater). **Elimination:** 90% in feces.

## NURSING IMPLICATIONS

### Assessment & Drug Effects
- Be aware of drug interactions and schedule other medications accordingly.

### Patient & Family Education
- Although healing has occurred within the first 2 wk of therapy, treatment is usually continued 4–8 wk.
- Be aware that constipation is a drug-related problem. Follow

S

---

Common adverse effects in *italic;* life-threatening effects <u>underlined;</u> generic names in **bold;** classifications in SMALL CAPS; ✦ Canadian drug name; ⊙ Prototype drug

1529

these measures unless contraindicated: Increase water intake to 8–10 glasses/day; increase physical exercise, increase dietary bulk. Consult prescriber: A suppository or bulk laxative (e.g., Metamucil) may be prescribed.

# SULFACETAMIDE SODIUM

(sul-fa-see'ta-mide)

Bleph 10, Cetamide, Ophthacet, Ovace, Sebizon, Sodium Sulamyd, Sulf-10

# SULFACETAMIDE SODIUM/ SULFUR

Sulfacet, Rosula

**Classification:** SULFONAMIDE ANTIBIOTIC
Therapeutic: ANTIBIOTIC
**Prototype:** Silver sulfadiazine

## AVAILABILITY  **Sulfacetamide:** Lotion; solution; ointment; **Sulfacetamide/Sulfur:** Gel, lotion

## ACTION & *THERAPEUTIC EFFECT*
Exerts bacteriostatic effect by interfering with bacterial utilization of PABA, thereby inhibiting folic acid biosynthesis required for bacterial growth. *Effective against a wide range of gram-positive and gram-negative microorganisms.*

## USES  Ophthalmic preparations are used for conjunctivitis, corneal ulcers, and other superficial ocular infections and as adjunct to systemic sulfonamide therapy for trachoma. The topical lotion is used for scaly dermatoses, seborrheic dermatitis, seborrhea sicca, and other bacterial skin infections.

## CONTRAINDICATIONS  Hypersensitivity to sulfonamides; neonates, pregnancy (category D near term).

## CAUTIOUS USE  Application of lotion to denuded or debrided skin; pregnancy (category C except near term); lactation. Safe use in children is not established.

## ROUTE & DOSAGE

### Conjunctivitis
*Adult:* **Ophthalmic** 1–3 drops of 10%, 15%, or 30% solution into lower conjunctival sac q2–3h, may increase interval as patient responds or use 1.5–2.5 cm (½–1 in.) of 10% ointment q6h and at bedtime

### Seborrhea, Rosacea
*Adult:* **Topical** Apply thin film to affected area 1–3 × day

## ADMINISTRATION
### Instillation
- Be aware that ophthalmic preparations and skin lotion are not interchangeable.
- Check strength of medication prescribed.
- See patient instructions for instilling eye drops.
- Discard darkened solutions; results when left standing for a long time.
- Store at 8°–15° C (46°–59° F) in tightly closed containers unless otherwise directed.

## ADVERSE EFFECTS (≥1%) **Special Senses:** *Temporary stinging or burning sensation,* retardation of corneal healing associated with long-term use of ophthalmic

**S**

ointment. **Body as a Whole:** Hypersensitivity reactions (<u>Stevens–Johnson syndrome</u>, lupus-like syndrome), superinfections with nonsusceptible organisms.

### INTERACTIONS **Drug:** **Tetracaine** and other LOCAL ANESTHETICS DERIVED FROM PABA may antagonize the antibacterial effects of SULFONAMIDES; SILVER PREPARATIONS may precipitate sulfacetamide from solution.

### PHARMACOKINETICS **Absorption:** Minimal systemic absorption, but may be enough to cause sensitization. **Metabolism:** In liver to inactive metabolites. **Elimination:** In urine.

### NURSING IMPLICATIONS
#### Assessment & Drug Effects
- Discontinue if symptoms of hypersensitivity appear (erythema, skin rash, pruritus, urticaria).

#### Patient & Family Education
- Wash hands thoroughly with soap and running water (before and after instillation).
- Examine eye medication; discard if cloudy or dark in color.
- Avoid contaminating any part of eye dropper that is inserted in bottle.
- Tilt head back, pull down lower lid. At the same time, look up while drop is being instilled into conjunctival sac. Immediately apply gentle pressure just below the eyelid and next to nose for 1 min. Close eyes gently, so as not to squeeze out medication.
- Report purulent eye discharge to prescriber. Sulfacetamide sodium is inactivated by purulent exudates.

## SULFADIAZINE
(sul-fa-dye′a-zeen)
**Classification:** SULFONAMIDE ANTIBIOTIC
**Therapeutic:** ANTIBIOTIC
**Prototype:** Silver sulfadiazide

### AVAILABILITY Tablet

### ACTION & THERAPEUTIC EFFECT
Exerts bacteriostatic effect by interfering with bacterial utilization of PABA, thereby inhibiting folic acid biosynthesis required for bacterial growth. *Effective against a wide range of gram-positive and gram-negative microorganisms.*

### USES Used in combination with pyrimethamine for treatment of cerebral toxoplasmosis and chloroquine-resistant malaria.

### CONTRAINDICATIONS Hypersensitivity to sulfonamides or to any ingredients in the formulation; porphyria; pregnancy (category D near term); lactation.

### CAUTIOUS USE Application of lotion to denuded or debrided skin; dehydration; hepatic disease; impaired renal function; pregnancy (category C except near term).

### ROUTE & DOSAGE

| Mild to Moderate Infections |
|---|
| *Adult:* **PO Loading Dose** 2–4 g loading dose; **PO Maintenance Dose** 2–4 g/day in 4–6 divided doses |
| *Child (2 mo or older):* **PO Loading Dose** 75 mg/kg; **PO Maintenance Dose** 150 mg/kg/day in 4–6 divided doses (max: 6 g/day) |

S

Common adverse effects in *italic;* life-threatening effects <u>underlined;</u> generic names in **bold;** classifications in SMALL CAPS; ♣ Canadian drug name; ⊙ Prototype drug

1531

**Rheumatic Fever Prophylaxis**

*Adult (weight less than 30 kg):* **PO** 500 mg/day; *weight greater than 30 kg:* 1 g/day

**Toxoplasmosis**

*Adult:* **PO** 2–8 g/day divided q6h
*Child (2 mo or older):* **PO** 100–200 mg/kg/day divided q6h
*Neonate:* **PO** 50 mg/kg q12h × 12 mo

## ADMINISTRATION

### Oral

- Maintain sufficient fluid intake to produce urinary output of at least 1500 mL/24 h for children between 3000 and 4000 mL/24 h for adults. Concomitant administration of urinary alkalinizer may be prescribed to reduce possibility of crystalluria and stone formation.
- Store in tight, light-resistant containers.

## ADVERSE EFFECTS (≥1%) CNS:
Headache, peripheral neuritis, peripheral neuropathy, tinnitus, hearing loss, vertigo, insomnia, drowsiness, mental depression, acute psychosis, ataxia, convulsions, kernicterus (newborns). **GI:** *Nausea, vomiting, diarrhea,* abdominal pains, hepatitis, jaundice, pancreatitis, stomatitis. **Hematologic:** Acute hemolytic anemia (especially in patients with G6PD deficiency), aplastic anemia, methemoglobinemia, agranulocytosis, thrombocytopenia, leukopenia, eosinophilia, hypoprothrombinemia. **Body as a Whole:** Headache, *fever,* chills, arthralgia, malaise, allergic myocarditis, serum sickness, anaphylactoid reactions, lymphadenopathy, local reaction following IM injection, fixed drug eruptions, diuresis, overgrowth of nonsusceptible organisms, LE phenomenon. **Skin:** Pruritus, urticaria, rash, erythema multiforme including *Stevens–Johnson syndrome, exfoliative dermatitis,* alopecia, photosensitivity, vascular lesions. **Urogenital:** *Crystalluria,* hematuria, proteinuria, anuria, toxic nephrosis, reduction in sperm count. **Metabolic:** Goiter, hypoglycemia. **Special Senses:** Conjunctivitis, conjunctival or scleral infection, retardation of corneal healing (ophthalmic ointment).

## INTERACTIONS Drug: PABA-CONTAINING LOCAL ANESTHETICS may antagonize sulfa's effects; ORAL ANTICOAGULANTS potentiate hypoprothrombinemia; may potentiate SULFONYLUREA-induced hypoglycemia. May decrease concentrations of **cyclosporine;** may increase levels of **phenytoin.**

## PHARMACOKINETICS Absorption: Readily absorbed from GI tract. **Peak:** 3–6 h. **Distribution:** Distributed to most tissues, including CSF; crosses placenta. **Metabolism:** In liver. **Elimination:** In urine.

## NURSING IMPLICATIONS

### Assessment & Drug Effects

- Monitor hydration status.
- Monitor lab tests: Baseline and periodic urine C&S; frequent CBC and urinalysis; sulfadiazone blood levels with serious infections.

### Patient & Family Education

- Take drug exactly as prescribed. Do not alter schedule or dose; take total amount prescribed unless prescriber changes the regimen.
- Drink fluids liberally unless otherwise directed.

S

- Report early signs of blood dyscrasias (sore throat, pallor, fever) promptly to the prescriber.

# SULFAMETHOXAZOLE-TRIMETHOPRIM (SMZ-TMP)

(sul-fa-meth'ox-a-zole-tri-meth'o-prim)

Bactrim, Bactrim DS, Co-Trim, Septra, Septra DS, Sulfatrom

**Classifications:** URINARY TRACT ANTI-INFECTIVE; SULFONAMIDE
Therapeutic: URINARY TRACT ANTI-INFECTIVE
**Prototype:** Trimethoprim

**AVAILABILITY** Tablet; suspension; solution for injection

## ACTION & *THERAPEUTIC* EFFECT
Both components of the combination are synthetic folate antagonist anti-infectives. Principal action is by enzyme inhibition that prevents bacterial synthesis of essential nucleic acids and proteins. *Effective against Pneumocystis jiroveci pneumonitis (formerly PCP), Shigellosis enteritis, and severely complicated UTIs due to most strains of the Enterobacteriaceae.*

**USES** *Pneumocystis jiroveci* pneumonitis (formerly PCP), shigellosis enteritis, and severe complicated UTIs. Also children with acute otitis media due to susceptible strains of *Haemophilus influenzae*, and acute episodes of chronic bronchitis or traveler's diarrhea in adults.

**UNLABELED USES** Isosporiasis; cholera; genital ulcers caused by *Haemophilus ducreyi;* prophylaxis for *P. jiroveci* pneumonia (formerly PCP) in neutropenic patients.

**CONTRAINDICATIONS** Hypersensitivity to SMZ, TMP, sulfonamides, or bisulfites, carbonic anhydrase inhibitors; group A beta-hemolytic streptococcal pharyngitis; megaloblastic anemia due to folate deficiency; G6PD deficiency; hyperkalemia; porphyria; pregnancy (category D near term); lactation.

**CAUTIOUS USE** Impaired kidney or liver function; bone marrow depression; possible folate deficiency; severe allergy or bronchial asthma; hypersensitivity to sulfonamide derivative drugs (e.g., acetazolamide, thiazides, tolbutamide); pregnancy (category C except near term). Safe use in infants younger than 2 mo not established.

## ROUTE & DOSAGE

**(Weight-based doses are calculated on TMP component)**
**Systemic Infections**

Adult: **PO** 160 mg TMP/800 mg SMZ q12h; **IV** 8–10 mg/kg/day TMP divided q6–12h
*Child (2 mo or older, weight less than 40 kg):* **PO** 4 mg/kg/day TMP q12h; *weight greater than 40 kg:* 160 mg TMP/800 mg SMZ q12h
*Child/Infant (2 mo or older):* **IV** 6–10 mg/kg/day TMP divided q6–12h

***Pneumocystis jiroveci* Pneumonia (formerly PCP)**

*Adult:* **PO** 15–20 mg/kg/day TMP divided q6h
*Adult/Adolescent/Child:* **IV** 15–20 mg/kg/day TMP divided q6h

S

Common adverse effects in *italic;* life-threatening effects <u>underlined</u>; generic names in **bold;** classifications in SMALL CAPS; ♣ Canadian drug name; 🅟 Prototype drug

1533

**Prophylaxis for *Pneumocystis jiroveci* Pneumonia (formerly PCP)**

*Adult:* PO 160 mg TMP/800 mg SMZ q24h
*Child:* PO 150 mg/m² TMP/750 mg/m² SMZ b.i.d. 3 consecutive days/wk (max: 320 mg TMP/day)

***Renal Impairment Dosage Adjustment***

*CrCl 10–30 mL/min:* Reduce dose by 50%; *less than 10 mL/min:* Reduce dose by 50–75%

## ADMINISTRATION

### Oral
- Give with a full glass of desired fluid.
- Maintain adequate fluid intake (at least 1500 mL/day) during therapy.
- Store at 15°–30° C (59°–86° F) in dry place protected from light. Avoid freezing.

### Intravenous

***PREPARE:* Intermittent:** Add contents of the 5 mL vial to 125 mL D5W. ▪ Use within 6 h. ▪ If less fluid is desired, dilute in 75 of 100 mL and use within 2 or 4 h, respectively.

***ADMINISTER:* Intermittent:** Infuse over 60–90 min. ▪ Avoid rapid infusion.

***INCOMPATIBILITIES:* Solution/additive:** Stability in **dextrose** and **normal saline** is concentration dependent, **fluconazole, linezolid, verapamil.** **Y-site:** Alfentanil, amikacin, aminophylline, amphotericin B, ampicillin, ampicillin/sulbactam, atropine, azathioprine, benztropine, bumetanide, buprenorphine, butaorphanol, calcium, capsofungin, cefamandol, cefazolin, cefmetazole, cefonicid, cefotaxime, cefotetan, cefoxitin, ceftazidime, ceftizoxime, ceftriaxone, cefuroxime, cephalothin, chloramphenicol, chlorpromazine, cimetidine, cisatracurium, clindamycin, codeiene, cyanocobalamine, cyclosporine, dantrolene, dexamethasone, dexmedetomide, diazepam, diazoxide, digoxin, diphenhydramine, dobutamine, dopamine, doxorubicin, doxycycline, ephedrine, epinephrine, epirubicin, epoetin alfa, erythromycin, famotidine, fentanyl, fluconazole, foscarnet, furosemide, ganciclovir, gentamicin, haloperidol, heparin, hydralazine, hydrocortisone, hydroxyzine, idarubicin, imipenem-cilastain, indomethacin, isoproterenol, ketorolac, lidocaine, mannitol, metaraminol, methicillin, methyldopate, methylprednisolone, metoclopramide, mezlocillin, miconazole, milrinone acetate, minocycline, midazolam, nafcillin, nalbuphine, naloxone, netilmicin, nitroglycerin, nitroprusside, norepinephrine, ondansetron, oxacillin, oxytocin, papaverine, penicillin, pentamidine, pentazocine, pentobarbital, phenobarbital, phentolamine, phenylephrine, phenytoin, phytonadione, piperacillin, potassium, prochlorperazine, promethazine, propranolol, protamine, pyridoxine, quinidine, quinupristin/dalfopristin, ranitidine, ritodrine, succinylcholine, sufentanil, theophylline, ticarcillin, tobramycin, tolazoline, vancomycin, verapamil, vinorelbine.

S

- Store unopened ampule at 15°–30° C (50°–86° F).

## ADVERSE EFFECTS (≥1%) Skin:
*Mild to moderate rashes (including fixed drug eruptions),* toxic epidermal necrolysis. **GI:** *Nausea, vomiting,* diarrhea, *anorexia,* hepatitis, pseudomembranous enterocolitis, stomatitis, glossitis, abdominal pain. **Urogenital:** Kidney failure, oliguria, anuria, crystalluria. **Hematologic:** Agranulocytosis (rare), aplastic anemia (rare), megaloblastic anemia, hypoprothrombinemia, thrombocytopenia (rare). **Body as a Whole:** Weakness, arthralgia, myalgia, photosensitivity, allergic myocarditis.

## DIAGNOSTIC TEST INTERFERENCE
May elevate levels of *serum creatinine, transaminase, bilirubin, alkaline phosphatase.*

## INTERACTIONS Drug: May enhance hypoprothrombinemic effects of ORAL ANTICOAGULANTS; may increase **methotrexate** toxicity. **Alcohol** may cause disulfiram reaction.

## PHARMACOKINETICS Absorption: Readily from GI tract. Peak: 1–4 h (oral). Distribution: Widely distributed, including CNS; crosses placenta; distributed into breast milk. Metabolism: In liver. Elimination: In urine. Half-Life: 8–10 h TMP, 10–13 h SMZ.

## NURSING IMPLICATIONS
### Assessment & Drug Effects
- Be aware that IV forms of the drug may contain sodium metabisulfite, which produces allergic-type reactions in susceptible patients: Hives, itching, wheezing, anaphylaxis. Susceptibility (low in general population) is seen most frequently in asthmatics or atopic nonasthmatic persons.
- Monitor coagulation tests and prothrombin times in patient also receiving warfarin. Change in warfarin dosage may be indicated.
- Monitor I&O volume and pattern. Report significant changes to forestall renal calculi formation. Also report failure of treatment (i.e., continued UTI symptoms).
- Older adult patients are at risk for severe adverse reactions, especially if liver or kidney function is compromised or if certain other drugs are given. Most frequently observed: Thrombocytopenia (with concurrent thiazide diuretics); severe decrease in platelets (with or without purpura); bone marrow suppression; severe skin reactions.
- Be alert for overdose symptoms (no extensive experience has been reported): Nausea, vomiting, anorexia, headache, dizziness, mental depression, confusion, and bone marrow depression.
- Monitor lab tests: Baseline and periodic urinalysis; CBC with differential, platelet count, BUN and creatinine clearance with prolonged therapy.

### Patient & Family Education
- Report immediately to prescriber if rash appears. Other reportable symptoms are sore throat, fever, purpura, jaundice; all are early signs of serious reactions.
- Monitor for and report fixed eruptions to prescriber. This drug can cause fixed eruptions at the same sites each time the drug is administered. Every contact with drug may not result in eruptions; therefore, patient may overlook the relationship.
- Drink 2.5–3 L (1 L is approximately equal to 1 qt) daily, unless otherwise directed.

S

---

Common adverse effects in *italic;* life-threatening effects underlined; generic names in **bold;** classifications in SMALL CAPS; ✦ Canadian drug name; ⊙ Prototype drug

## SULFASALAZINE
(sul-fa-sal'a-zeen)

Azulfidine, PMS Sulfasala-
zine ✦, PMS Sulfasalazine
E.C. ✦, Salazopyrin ✦, SAS
Enteric-500 ✦, S.A.S.-500 ✦

**Classifications:** ANTI-INFLAMMA-
TORY; SULFONAMIDE
**Therapeutic:** GI ANTI-INFLAMMATORY;
IMMUNOMODULATOR; DISEASE-MODI-
FYING ANTIRHEUMATIC DRUG
(DMARD)
**Prototype:** Mesalamine

**AVAILABILITY** Tablet; sustained release tablet

**ACTION & *THERAPEUTIC EFFECT***
Exerts antibacterial and anti-inflammatory effects. Inhibits prostaglandins known to cause diarrhea
and affect mucosal transport as
well as interference with absorption of fluids and electrolytes from
colon. Reduces *Clostridium* and
*Escherichia coli* in the stools. *Anti-
inflammatory and immunomodulatory properties are effective in
controlling the S&S of ulcerative
colitis and rheumatoid arthritis.*

**USES** Ulcerative colitis and relatively mild regional enteritis; rheumatoid arthritis.

**UNLABELED USES** Granulomatous
colitis, Crohn's disease, scleroderma.

**CONTRAINDICATIONS** Sensitivity to sulfasalazine, other
sulfonamides and salicylates,
trimethoprim; folate deficiency;
megaloblastic anemia; renal failure,
renal impairment; agranulocytosis;
intestinal and urinary tract obstruction; porphyria; pregnancy
(category D near term); lactation.

**CAUTIOUS USE** Severe allergy, or
bronchial asthma; blood dyscrasias;
hepatic or renal impairment; G6PD
deficiency; older adults; pregnancy
(category C except near term). Safe
use in children younger than 6 y not
established.

## ROUTE & DOSAGE

### Ulcerative Colitis, Rheumatoid Arthritis
*Adult:* **PO** 1–2 g/day in 4 divided
doses, may increase up to 8 g/
day if needed
*Child:* **PO** 40–50 mg/kg/day in
4 divided doses (max: 75 mg/kg/
day)

### Juvenile Rheumatoid Arthritis
*Child:* **PO** 10 mg/kg/day,
increase weekly by 10 mg/kg/
day [usual dose: 15–25 mg/kg
q12h (max: 2 g/day)]

## ADMINISTRATION
### Oral
- Give after eating to provide longer
intestine transit time.
- Do not crush or chew sustained
release tablets; **must be** swallowed whole.
- Use evenly divided doses over
each 24-h period; do not exceed
8-h intervals between doses.
- Consult prescriber if GI intolerance occurs after first few doses.
Symptoms are probably due to irritation of stomach mucosa and
may be relieved by spacing total
daily dose more evenly over 24 h
or by administration of enteric-
coated tablets.
- Store at 15°–30° C (59°–86° F) in
tight, light-resistant containers.

**ADVERSE EFFECTS** (≥1%) **Body as
a Whole:** *Nausea, vomiting, bloody*

S

*diarrhea; anorexia,* arthralgia, rash, anemia, oligospermia (reversible), blood dyscrasias, liver injury, infectious mononucleosis–like reaction, *allergic reactions.*

**INTERACTIONS Drug: Iron,** ANTIBIOTICS may alter absorption of sulfasalazine.

**PHARMACOKINETICS Absorption:** 10–15% from GI tract unchanged; remaining drug is hydrolyzed in colon to sulfapyridine (most of which is absorbed) and 5-aminosalicylic acid (30% of which is absorbed). **Peak:** 1.5–6 h sulfasalazine; 6–24 h sulfapyridine. **Distribution:** Crosses placenta; distributed into breast milk. **Metabolism:** In intestines and liver. **Elimination:** All metabolites are excreted in urine. **Half-Life:** 5–10 h.

**NURSING IMPLICATIONS**

**Assessment & Drug Effects**
- Monitor for GI distress. GI symptoms that develop after a few days of therapy may indicate need for dosage adjustment. If symptoms persist, prescriber may withhold drug for 5–7 days and restart it at a lower dosage level.
- Be aware that adverse reactions generally occur within a few days to 12 wk after start of therapy; most likely to occur in patients receiving high doses (4 g or more).
- Monitor lab tests: Periodic RBC and folate in patients on high doses (more than 2 g/day).

**Patient & Family Education**
- Examine stools and report to prescriber if enteric-coated tablets have passed intact in feces. Some patients lack enzymes capable of dissolving coating; conventional tablet will be ordered.

- Be aware that drug may color alkaline urine and skin orange-yellow.
- Remain under close medical supervision. Relapses occur in about 40% of patients after initial satisfactory response. Response to therapy and duration of treatment are governed by endoscopic examinations.

**SULINDAC**
(sul-in'dak)
Clinoril
**Classifications:** ANALGESIC, NONSTEROIDAL ANTI-INFLAMMATORY DRUG (NSAID); ANTIPYRETIC
**Therapeutic:** NONNARCOTIC ANALGESIC; NSAID
**Prototype:** Ibuprofen

**AVAILABILITY** Tablet

**ACTION & THERAPEUTIC EFFECT**
Anti-inflammatory action thought to result from inhibition of prostaglandin synthesis. *Exhibits anti-inflammatory, analgesic, and anti-pyretic properties.*

**USES** Acute and long-term symptomatic treatment of osteoarthritis, rheumatoid arthritis, ankylosing spondylitis; acute painful shoulder (acute subacromial bursitis or supraspinatus tendinitis); acute gouty arthritis.

**CONTRAINDICATIONS** Hypersensitivity to sulindac; hypersensitivity to aspirin (patients with "aspirin triad": Acute asthma, rhinitis, nasal polyps), other NSAIDs, or salicylates; significant kidney or liver dysfunction; CABG perioperative pain; GI bleeding; drug-induced CV event; pancreatitis; pregnancy (category D third trimester); lactation.

**CAUTIOUS USE** History of upper GI tract disorders; anticoagulant

S

Common adverse effects in *italic;* life-threatening effects underlined; generic names in **bold;** classifications in SMALL CAPS; ♣ Canadian drug name; ⊘ Prototype drug

1537

therapy; CHF; moderate or mild renal impairment; hepatic impairment; infection; preexisting asthma; SLE; compromised cardiac function, hypertension, pregnancy (category C first and second trimesters). Safety and efficacy in children not established.

## ROUTE & DOSAGE

**Arthritis, Ankylosing Spondylitis, Acute Gouty Arthritis**

*Adult:* **PO** 150–200 mg b.i.d. (max: 400 mg/day)

## ADMINISTRATION

### Oral

- Crush and give mixed with liquid or food if patient cannot swallow tablet.
- Administer with food, milk, or antacid (if prescribed) to reduce possibility of GI upset. Note: Food retards absorption and delays and lowers peak concentrations.

## ADVERSE EFFECTS (≥1%) **CNS:**
Drowsiness, *dizziness, headache,* anxiety, nervousness. **CV:** Palpitation, peripheral edema, CHF, (patients with marginal cardiac function). **Special Senses:** Blurred vision, amblyopia, vertigo, tinnitus, decreased hearing. **GI:** *Abdominal pain, dyspepsia, nausea, vomiting, constipation,* diarrhea, ulceration, flatulence, anorexia; stomatitis, sore or dry mucous membranes, dry mouth; GI bleeding, gastritis. **Hematologic:** Prolonged bleeding time, aplastic anemia, thrombocytopenia, leukopenia, eosinophilia. **Body as a Whole:** Angioneurotic edema, fever, chills, anaphylaxis. **Skin:** Stevens–Johnson syndrome, toxic epidermal necrolysis syndrome, rash, pruritus. **Urogenital:** Renal impairment.

## DIAGNOSTIC TEST INTERFERENCE
Abnormalities in *liver function tests* may occur.

## INTERACTIONS **Drug:** Do not use with **ketorolac** or **cidofovir. Heparin,** ORAL ANTICOAGULANTS may prolong bleeding time; may increase **lithium** or **methotrexate** toxicity; **aspirin,** other NSAIDs add to ulcerogenic effects; **dimethylsulfoxide (DMSO)** may decrease effects of sulindac; **altretamine** may cause hypoprothrombinemia. **Herbal: Feverfew, garlic, ginger, ginkgo** may increase bleeding potential.

## PHARMACOKINETICS **Absorption:** 90% from GI tract. **Peak:** 2 h without food, 3–4 h with food. **Duration:** 10–12 h. **Distribution:** Minimal passage across placenta; distributed into breast milk. **Metabolism:** In liver to active metabolite. **Elimination:** 75% in urine, 25% in feces. **Half-Life:** 7.8 h sulindac, 16.4 h sulfide metabolite.

## NURSING IMPLICATIONS

### Black Box Warning

*Sulindac has been associated with increased risk of serious, potentially fatal, GI bleeding and cardiovascular events (e.g., MI and CVA); risk may increase with duration of use and may be greater in the older adult and those with risk factors for CV disease.*

### Assessment & Drug Effects

- Assess for and report promptly unexplained GI distress.
- Monitor for and report promptly S&S of CV thrombotic events (i.e., angina, MI, TIA, or stroke).
- Schedule auditory and ophthalmic examinations in patients receiving prolonged or high-dose therapy.
- Monitor lab tests: Baseline and periodic CBC and metabolic panel.

Common adverse effects in *italic;* life-threatening effects underlined; generic names in **bold**; classifications in SMALL CAPS; ✦ Canadian drug name; ⊙ Prototype drug

### Patient & Family Education

- Do not drive or engage in potentially hazardous activities until response to drug is known.
- Report any incidence of unexplained bleeding or bruising immediately to prescriber (e.g., bleeding gums, black and tarry stools, coffee-colored emesis).
- Report onset of skin rash, itching, hives, jaundice, swelling of feet or hands, sore throat or mouth, shortness of breath, or night cough to prescriber.
- Be aware that adverse GI effects are relatively common. Report abdominal pain, nausea, dyspepsia, diarrhea, or constipation.
- Avoid alcohol and aspirin as they may increase risk of GI ulceration and bleeding tendencies.
- Monitor for and report promptly S&S of CV thrombotic events (i.e., angina, MI, TIA, or stroke)

---

## SUMATRIPTAN ⓟ

(sum-a-trip'tan)

Imitrex ALSUMA, Sumavel DosePro, Zecuity

**Classification:** SEROTONIN 5-HT$_1$ RECEPTOR AGONIST
Therapeutic: ANTIMIGRAINE

**AVAILABILITY** Tablet; solution for injection; nasal spray; transdermal patch

### ACTION & *THERAPEUTIC EFFECT*

Selective agonist for a serotonin receptor (probably 5-HT$_{1D}$) that causes vasoconstriction of cranial carotid arteries. *Relieves migraine headache. Also relieves photophobia, phonophobia, nausea and vomiting associated with migraine attacks.*

**USES** Treatment of acute migraine attacks with or without aura, cluster headache.

### CONTRAINDICATIONS

Hypersensitivity to sumatriptan; ischemic CAD; acute MI, angina, arteriosclerosis; cerebrovascular disease; colitis; concurrent use with MAO inhibitors; uncontrolled hypertension; intracranial bleeding; PVD; Raynaud's disease; stroke; severe hepatic disease; Wolff-Parkinson-White syndrome; basilar or hemiplegic migraine.

### CAUTIOUS USE

Impaired liver or kidney function; MAO inhibitors; older adults; pregnancy (category C). Safety and efficacy in children not established.

### ROUTE & DOSAGE

---

#### Migraine or Cluster Headache

*Adult:* **Subcutaneous** 6 mg any time after onset of migraine, if headache returns, may repeat with 6 mg subcutaneously at least 1 h after first injection (max: 12 mg/24 h); **PO** 25 mg × 1 dose, if headache returns may repeat once after 2 h (max: 100 mg); **Intranasal** 5, 10, or 20 mg in one nostril, if headache returns, may repeat once after 2 h (max: 40 mg/24 h); **Transdermal** Apply one patch, drug is released for 4 h, if needed a second patch can be applied after 2 h (max: 2 patches in 24 h)

---

### ADMINISTRATION

Note: Do not give within 24 h of an ergot-containing drug.

#### Oral

- Give any time after symptoms of migraine appear.
- A second tablet may be given if symptoms return but no sooner than 2 h after the first tablet.
- Do not exceed 100 mg in a single oral dose or 300 mg/day.

---

Common adverse effects in *italic;* life-threatening effects underlined; generic names in **bold;** classifications in SMALL CAPS; ♣ Canadian drug name; ⓟ Prototype drug

1539

**S**

### Intranasal

- Note: A single dose is one spray into ONE nostril.

### Transdermal System

- Apply patch to dry intact, nonirritated skin on upper arm or thigh; area should be relatively hair free and without scars, tattoos, abrasions, or other skin conditions.
- Within 15 min of applying patch, push button and the red LED light will turn on. Patch will stop operating when dosing is completed, then the red light will turn off and patch may be removed.

### Subcutaneous

- A second injection may be given 1 h or longer following first injection if initial relief is not obtained or if migraine returns.
- Be aware that if adverse effects are dose limiting, a lower dose may be effective.
- Store all forms at room temperature, 15°–30° C (59°–86° F). Protect from light.

### ADVERSE EFFECTS (≥1%) CV:

Chest pressure and tightness, hypotension or hypertension, hypertensive crisis, syncope, peripheral cyanosis, thromboembolism, heart block, sinus bradycardia, atrial fibrillation, ventricular fibrillation, ventricular tachycardia, coronary artery vasospasm, angina, transient myocardial ischemia, MI, cardiac arrest. **CNS:** *Tingling, warming sensation, pressure, numbness,* headache, *dizziness, vertigo,* drowsiness, sedation, seizure, CNS hemorrhage, subarachnoid hemorrhage, stroke. **Body as a Whole:** Dizziness, lightheadedness, myalgia, or muscle cramps, *pain on injection,* weakness, flushing, and a sensation of warmth or burning after injection. **GI:** Abdominal pain, cramping, diarrhea, nausea, vomiting.

### INTERACTIONS Drug: Dihydroergotamine,

ERGOT ALKALOIDS may cause vasospasm and a slight elevation in blood pressure. MAO INHIBITORS increase sumatriptan levels and toxicity (especially the oral form); do not use concurrently or within 2 wk of stopping MAO INHIBITORS; use with other serotonin altering drugs increases risk of serotonin syndrome (see Appendix F). **Herbal: St. John's wort** may increase triptan toxicity.

### PHARMACOKINETICS Onset:

10–30 min after subcutaneous administration. **Duration:** 1–2 h. **Distribution:** Widely distributed, 10–20% protein bound. May be excreted in breast milk. **Metabolism:** Hepatically to inactive metabolite. **Elimination:** 57% in urine, 38% in feces. **Half-Life:** 2 h.

## NURSING IMPLICATIONS

### Black Box Warning

*Sumatriptan has been associated with increased risk of serious, sometimes fatal, cardiovascular thrombotic reactions, MI, and CVA.*

### Assessment & Drug Effects

- Monitor cardiovascular status carefully following first dose in patients at relatively high risk for coronary artery disease (e.g., postmenopausal women, men over 40 years old, persons with known CAD risk factors) or who have coronary artery vasospasms.
- Report to prescriber immediately chest pain or tightness in chest or throat that is severe or does not quickly resolve following a dose of sumatriptan.
- Monitor therapeutic effectiveness. Pain relief usually begins within 10 min of injection, with complete relief in approximately 65% of all patients within 2 h.

Common adverse effects in *italic*; life-threatening effects <u>underlined</u>; generic names in **bold**; classifications in SMALL CAPS; ✛ Canadian drug name; ⊘ Prototype drug

## Patient & Family Education

- Review patient information leaflet provided by the manufacturer carefully.
- Learn correct use of autoinjector for self-administration of subcutaneous dose.
- Pain or redness at injection site is common but usually disappears in less than 1 h.
- Notify prescriber immediately if symptoms of severe angina (e.g., severe or persistent pain or tightness in chest, back, neck, or throat) or hypersensitivity (e.g., wheezing, facial swelling, skin rash, or hives) occur.
- Do not take any other serotonin receptor agonist (Axert, Maxalt, Zomig, Amerge) within 24 h of taking sumatriptan.
- Check with prescriber before taking any new OTC or prescription drugs.
- Report any other adverse effects (e.g., tingling, flushing, dizziness) at next prescriber visit.

---

# SUNITINIB
(sun i-ti′nib)
Sutent

**Classifications:** ANTINEOPLASTIC; KINASE INHIBITOR
**Therapeutic:** ANTINEOPLASTIC
**Prototype:** Erlotinib

## AVAILABILITY Capsule

## ACTION & *THERAPEUTIC EFFECT*

An antineoplastic agent that is a selective inhibitor of receptors for tyrosine kinases (RTKs) in solid tumors. Carcinogenic activity within these tumors is a result of tumor angiogenesis and proliferation. *Sunitinib causes tumor regression and decreased tumor growth.*

## USES Treatment of advanced renal cell cancer; treatment of gastrointestinal stromal tumors (GIST), pancreatic neuroendocrine tumor.

## CONTRAINDICATIONS Hypersensitivity to sunitinib; acute MI; fever, hepatotoxicity; tumor lysis syndrome; pancreatitis; urine protein of at least 3 g per 24 h; RPLS; pregnancy (category D); lactation.

## CAUTIOUS USE Cardiac dysfunction, CHF, poorly controlled hypertension, history of MI; history of $QT_c$ prolongation; thyroid dysfunction; DM; CVA; hepatic impairment; renal insufficiency (CrCl of 60 mL/min or less); females of childbearing age; children.

## ROUTE & DOSAGE

| **Advanced Renal Cell Cancer** |
| --- |
| *Adult:* **PO** 50 mg/day for 4 wk, followed by 2 wk off treatment. |
| **GIST Tumor** |
| *Adult:* **PO** 50 mg daily × 4 wk then 2 wk off |
| **Pancreatic Neuroendocrine Tumor** |
| *Adult:* **PO** 37.5 mg daily |
| *Dosage Adjustments with Concurrent Hepatic CYP3A4 Modifiers* |
| *CYP3A4 Inducers:* Increase to maximum of 87.5 mg/day<br>*CYP3A4 Inhibitors:* Decrease to minimum of 37.5 mg/day |

## ADMINISTRATION

### Oral

- Incremental dosage changes of 12.5 mg are recommended.
- Store at 15°–30° C (59°–86° F).

## ADVERSE EFFECTS (≥1%) Body as a Whole: *Alopecia, asthenia, dizziness, fatigue, fever,* hair color

---

Common adverse effects in *italic*; life-threatening effects <u>underlined</u>; generic names in **bold**; classifications in SMALL CAPS; ♣ Canadian drug name; ⊘ Prototype drug

1541

change, *headache, peripheral edema.* **CV:** Chest pain, hypertension, myocardial ischemia. **GI:** *Abdominal pain, altered taste, anorexia, constipation, diarrhea, dyspepsia, flatulence, glossodynia, nausea, mucositis, stomatitis, vomiting.* **Hematologic:** *Anemia, bleeding, neutropenia, lymphopenia,* thrombocytopenia. **Metabolic:** *Dehydration, elevated hepatic enzymes,* hepatotoxicity, *hypothyroidism, hyperbilirubinemia.* **Musculoskeletal:** *Arthralgia, back pain, myalgia/limb pain.* **Respiratory:** *Cough, dyspnea.* **Skin:** *Dry skin, hand-foot syndrome, rash, skin discoloration.*

**INTERACTIONS Drug:** Coadministration of CYP3A4 INDUCERS (e.g., **carbamazepine, dexamethasone, phenobarbital, phenytoin, rifabutin, rifampin, rifapentine**) may decrease plasma levels of sunitinib. Coadministration of CYP3A4 INHIBITORS (e.g., **atazanavir, clarithromycin, erythromycin, indinavir, itraconazole, ketoconazole, nefazodone, nelfinavir, ritonavir, saquinavir, telithromycin, voriconazole**) may increase plasma levels of sunitinib. **Food:** **Grapefruit** and **grapefruit juice** may increase the plasma levels of sunitinib. **Herbal:** **St. John's wort** may decrease the plasma levels of sunitinib.

**PHARMACOKINETICS** **Peak:** 6–12 h. **Distribution:** 95–98% protein bound. **Metabolism:** Extensive hepatic metabolism. **Elimination:** Primarily fecal (61%). **Half-Life:** 40–60 h.

**NURSING IMPLICATIONS**

### Black Box Warning

*Sunitinib has been associated with severe, sometimes fatal, hepatotoxicity.*

**Assessment & Drug Effects**
- Monitor for and report S&S of bleeding (e.g., GI, GU, gingival).
- Monitor BP regularly and assess regularly for S&S of congestive heart failure. Withhold drug and notify prescriber if severe hypertension or signs of heart failure develop.
- Monitor for and report S&S of hepatotoxicity (see Appendix F).
- Monitor lab tests: At the beginning of each treatment cycle, urinalysis for proteinuria, CBC with differential and platelet count; periodic LFTs and serum electrolytes; thyroid function tests as indicated.

**Patient & Family Education**
- Do not use any prescription or nonprescription drugs without consulting a prescriber.
- Skin discoloration (yellow color) and/or loss of skin and hair pigmentation may occur with this drug.
- Report any of the following to a health care provider: Painful redness of palms and soles of feet; severe abdominal pain, vomiting, and diarrhea; signs of bleeding; chest pain or discomfort; shortness of breath; swelling of feet, legs, or hands; rapid weight gain.
- Women of childbearing age are advised not to become pregnant while taking sunitinib.

# SUVOREXANT
(su-vor'ex-ant)

Belsomra

**Classifications:** SEDATIVE-HYPNOTIC; OXERIN RECEPTOR ANTAGONIST

Therapeutic: SEDATIVE-HYPNOTIC

**AVAILABILITY** Tablets

**ACTIONS & *THERAPEUTIC EFFECT***
Promotes the natural transition from wakefulness to sleep by inhibiting

---

Common adverse effects in *italic;* life-threatening effects underlined; generic names in **bold;** classifications in SMALL CAPS; ✦ Canadian drug name; ⓟ Prototype drug the wakefulness-promoting orexin neurons of the arousal system. *Suvorexant improves sleep onset and sleep maintenance.*

**USES** Treatment of insomnia characterized by difficulties with sleep onset and/or sleep maintenance.

**CONTRAINDICATIONS** Narcolepsy; severe hepatic impairment; suicidal ideation.

**CAUTIOUS USE** Daytime somnolence; persistent insomnia after 7–10 days of treatment; complex nighttime behaviors while out of bed and not fully awake; concurrent CNS depressants or CYP3A4 inhibitors; alcohol use; history of drug abuse; depression; history of suicidal thoughts; behavioral changes; compromised respiratory function; obese individuals especially females; pregnancy (category C); lactation. Safety and efficacy in children younger than 18 y not established.

## ROUTE & DOSAGE

**Insomnia**
*Adult:* **PO** 10 mg no more than once per night and within 30 min of bedtime; dose can be increased to 20 mg if tolerated

*CYP3A4 Inhibitors Dosage Adjustment*
*Moderate inhibitors:* Decrease dose to 5 mg (max: 10 mg)
*Strong inhibitors:* Not recommended

*Hepatic Impairment Dosage Adjustment*
*Severe impairment:* Not recommended

## ADMINISTRATION

### Oral
▪ Give within 30 min of bedtime, with at least 7 h before the planned time of awakening.
▪ Effect may be delayed if taken with or soon after a meal.
▪ Store at 20°–25° C (66°–77° F).

**ADVERSE EFFECTS** (>2%) **CNS:** Abnormal dreams, dizziness, headache, somnolence. **GI:** Diarrhea, dry mouth. **Respiratory:** Cough, upper respiratory tract infection.

**INTERACTIONS Drug:** Concomitant use with strong CYP3A4 inhibitors (e.g., **boceprevir, clarithromycin, conivaptan, indinavir, itraconazole, ketoconazole, nefazodone, nelfinavir, posaconazole, ritonavir, saquinavir, telaprevir, telithromycin**) or moderate CYP3A4 inhibitors (e.g., **amprenavir, aprepitant, atazanavir, ciprofloxacin, diltiazem, erythromycin, fluconazole, fosamprenavir, imatinib, verapamil**) will increase the levels of suvorexant. Concomitant use with strong CYP3A4 inducers (e.g., **carbamazepine, phenytoin, rifampin**) will decrease the levels of suvorexant. **Food: Grapefruit juice** will increase the levels of suvorexant. **Herbal: St. John's wort** may decrease the levels of suvorexant.

**PHARMACOKINETICS Absorption:** 82% bioavailable. **Peak:** 2 h. **Distribution:** Greater than 99% plasma protein bound. **Metabolism:** In liver by CYP3A4. **Elimination:** Fecal (66%) and renal (23%). **Half-Life:** 12 h.

## NURSING IMPLICATIONS
### Assessment & Drug Effects
▪ Monitor for adverse effects. Note that dose reduction may be required in obese women due to

S

Common adverse effects in *italic;* life-threatening effects <u>underlined;</u> generic names in **bold;** classifications in SMALL CAPS; ♣ Canadian drug name; ⊕ Prototype drug

1543

adverse effects, and in those using other CNS depressant drugs due to potential additive effects.

- Monitor respiratory status and level of daytime alertness.
- Monitor for and report promptly signs of abnormal thinking, worsening of depression, suicidal thoughts, or other abnormal behaviors.

### Patient & Family Education

- Do not take this drug if a full night of sleep is not anticipated.
- Report to prescriber if insomnia does not improve within 7–10 days.
- Avoid alcohol while taking this drug.
- Do not engage in potentially dangerous activities (e.g., driving) until response to drug is known.
- Report immediately to prescriber if experiencing any of the following: More outgoing or aggressive behavior than normal, confusion, agitation, memory loss, hallucinations, worsening depression or suicidal thoughts.
- Contact prescriber immediately if experiencing "sleep-walking" or doing other activities when asleep (e.g., eating, talking, driving a car).

## TACROLIMUS
(tac-rol'i-mus)

Astagraf XL, Hecoria, Prograf, Protopic

**Classifications:** BIOLOGIC RESPONSE MODIFIER; IMMUNOSUPPRESSANT
Therapeutic: IMMUNOSUPPRESSANT
**Prototype:** Cyclosporine

**AVAILABILITY** Capsule; injection; ointment; extended release capsule

**ACTION & *THERAPEUTIC EFFECT***
Inhibits helper T-lymphocytes by selectively inhibiting secretion of interleukin-2, interleukin-3, and interleukin-gamma, thus reducing transplant rejection. *Inhibits antibody production (thus subduing immune response) by creating an imbalance in favor of suppressor T-lymphocytes.*

**USES** Prophylaxis for organ transplant rejection, moderate to severe atopic dermatitis (e.g., eczema).

**UNLABELED USES** Acute organ transplant rejection, severe plaque-type psoriasis, ulcerative colitis, nephrotic syndrome.

**CONTRAINDICATIONS** Hypersensitivity to tacrolimus or castor oil; postoperative oliguria or renal failure with CrCl greater than or equal to 4 mg/dL; potassium sparing diretics; lactation.

**CAUTIOUS USE** Renal or hepatic insufficiency, liver transplants; hyperkalemia, QT prolongation; CHF; serious infections; polyoma virus infections; CMV disease diabetes mellitus, gout, history of seizures, hypertension; cardiomyopathy, left ventricular dysfunction (e.g., heart failure); neoplastic disease, especially lymphoproliferative disorders; pregnancy (category C). **Ointment:** Children younger than 2 y.

## ROUTE & DOSAGE

**Rejection Prophylaxis (Dose Varies Based on Concurrent Meds)**
*Adult:* **PO** 0.075–0.2 mg/kg/day in divided doses q12h, start no sooner than 6 h after transplant; give first oral dose 8–12 h after discontinuing IV therapy; **IV** 0.01–0.05 mg/kg/day as

continuous IV infusion, start no sooner than 6 h after transplant, continue until patient can take oral therapy
*Child:* **PO** 0.15–0.2 mg/kg/day **IV** 0.03–0.05 mg/kg/day

**Atopic Dermatitis**

*Adult:* **Topical** Apply thin layer to affected area b.i.d., continue until clearing of symptoms
*Child (2–15 y):* **Topical** Apply thin layer of 0.03% ointment to affected area b.i.d., continue until clearing of symptoms

**Renal Impairment Dosage Adjustment**

Start with lower dose

**Hemodialysis Dosage Adjustment**

Supplementation not necessary

## ADMINISTRATION

### Oral

- Patient should be converted from IV to oral therapy as soon as possible.
- Give first oral dose 8–12 h after discontinuing IV infusion.

### Topical

- Ensure that skin is clean and completely dry before application.
- Apply a thin layer to the affected area and rub in gently and completely.
- Do not apply occlusive dressing over the site.

### Intravenous

*PREPARE:* **IV Infusion:** Dilute 5 mg/mL ampules with NS or D5W to a concentration of 0.004–0.02 mg/mL (4–20 mcg/mL). ▪ Lower concentrations are preferred for children.

*ADMINISTER:* **IV Infusion:** Give as continuous IV. ▪ PVC-free tubing is recommended, especially at lower concentrations.

*INCOMPATIBILITIES:* **Y-site: Acyclovir, allopurinol, azathioprine, cefepime, dantrolene, diazepam, diazoxide, esomeprazole, ganciclovir, gemtuzumab, iron sucrose, lansoprazole, levothyroxine, omeprazole, phenytoin.**

- Store ampules at 5°–25° C (41°—77° F); store capsules at room temperature, 15°–30° C (59°–86° F). ▪ Store the diluted infusion in glass or polyethylene containers and discard after 24 h.

## ADVERSE EFFECTS: (≥1%) CNS:
*Headache, tremors, insomnia, paresthesia, hyperesthesia* and/or sensations of warmth, circumoral numbness **CV:** *Mild to moderate hypertension.* **Endocrine:** Hirsutism, *hyperglycemia, hyperkalemia, hypokalemia, hypomagnesemia,* hyperuricemia, decreased serum cholesterol. **GI:** *Nausea, abdominal pain, gas,* appetite changes, *vomiting, anorexia, constipation,* diarrhea, ascites. **Hematologic:** *Anemia, leukocytosis,* thrombocytopenic *purpura.* **Urogenital:** UTI, oliguria, nephrotoxicity, nephropathy. **Respiratory:** *Pleural effusion, atelectasis, dyspnea.* **Special Senses:** Blurred vision, photophobia. **Skin:** *Flushing, rash, pruritus, skin irritation,* alopecia, erythema, folliculitis, hyperesthesia, exfoliative dermatitis, hirsutism, photosensitivity, skin discoloration, skin ulcer, sweating. **Body as a Whole:** *Pain, fever, peripheral edema, increased risk of cancer.*

## INTERACTIONS Drug: Use with **cyclosporine** increases risk of nephrotoxicity. **Metoclopramide,**

T

Common adverse effects in *italic;* life-threatening effects underlined; generic names in **bold;** classifications in SMALL CAPS; ♣ Canadian drug name; ⊕ Prototype drug

1545

**lansoprazole,** CALCIUM CHANNEL BLOCKER, ANTIFUNGAL AGENTS, MACROLIDE ANTIBIOTICS, **bromocriptine, cimetidine, cyclosporine, methylprednisolone, omeprazole** may increase levels; **caspofungin, rifampin** may decrease levels. NSAIDS may lead to oliguria or anuria. **Herbal: St. John's wort** decreases efficacy. **Food: Grapefruit juice** (greater than 1 qt/day) may increase plasma concentrations and adverse effects.

## PHARMACOKINETICS **Absorption:** Erratic and incompletely from GI tract; absolute bioavailability approximately 14–25%; absorption reduced by food. **Peak:** PO 1–4 h. **Duration:** IV 12 h. **Distribution:** Within plasma, tacrolimus is found primarily in lipoprotein-deficient fraction; 75–97% protein bound; distributed into red blood cells; blood:plasma ratio reported greater than 4; animal studies have demonstrated high concentrations of tacrolimus in lung, kidney, heart, and spleen; distributed into breast milk. **Metabolism:** Extensively in liver (CYP3A4). **Elimination:** Metabolites primarily in bile. **Half-Life:** 8.7–11.3 h.

## NURSING IMPLICATIONS

### Black Box Warning

*Tacrolimus has been associated with increased susceptibility to bacterial, viral, fungal, and protozoal infections and possible development of lymphoma and skin cancer.*

### Assessment & Drug Effects
- Monitor for and promptly report S&S of infection.

- Monitor kidney function closely; report elevated serum creatinine or decreased urinary output.
- Monitor for neurotoxicity, and report tremors, changes in mental status, or other signs of toxicity.
- Monitor cardiovascular status and report hypertension.
- Monitor for ECG for QT prolongation especially in those with renal or hepatic impairment.
- Monitor lab tests: Periodic serum tacrolimus, serum electrolytes, blood glucose, LFTs, and renal function tests.

### Patient & Family Education
- Do not eat grapefruit or drink grapefruit juice while taking this drug.
- Report promptly unexplained hunger, thirst, and frequent urination.
- Be aware of potential adverse effects including increased risk for infection.
- Minimize exposure to natural or artificial sunlight while using the ointment.
- Notify prescriber of S&S of neurotoxicity.

## TADALAFIL
(ta-dal′a-fil)
**Adcirca, Cialis**
**Classifications:** IMPOTENCE; PHOSPHODIESTERASE (PDE) INHIBITOR; VASODILATOR
**Therapeutic:** IMPOTENCE; PULMONARY ANTIHYPERTENSIVE
**Prototype:** Sildenafil

## AVAILABILITY Tablet

## ACTION & *THERAPEUTIC EFFECT*
PDE is responsible for degradation of cyclic GMP in the corpus cavernosum of the penis. Cyclic GMP causes smooth muscle relaxation

in lung tissue and the corpus cavernosum, thereby allowing inflow of blood into the penis. PDE-5 inhibitors reduce pulmonary vasodilation by sustaining levels of cyclic guanosine monophosphate (cGMP). Additionally, tadalafil produces a reduction in the pulmonary-to-systemic vascular resistance ratio. *Tadalafil promotes sustained erection only in the presence of sexual stimulation. It also produces a significant improvement in arterial oxygenation in pulmonary hypertension.*

**USES** Treatment of erectile dysfunction, BPH, pulmonary hypertension.

**CONTRAINDICATIONS** Hypersensitivity to tadalafil, vardenafil, or sildenafil; MI within last 90 days; Class 2 or greater heart failure within last 6 mo; unstable angina or angina during intercourse; uncontrolled cardiac arrhythmias; nitrate/nitrite therapy; hypotension, uncontrolled hypertension; retinitis pigmentosa; CVA within last 6 mo; left ventricular outflow obstruction, aortic stenosis; severe (Child-Pugh class C) hepatic cirrhosis; women; lactation.

**CAUTIOUS USE** CAD, risk factors for CVA; renal insufficiency; mild to moderate (Child-Pugh class A or B) hepatic disease; anatomic deformity of the penis; sickle cell anemia; multiple myeloma; leukemia; active bleeding or a peptic ulcer; hiatal hernia, GERD; sickle cell disease; retinitis pigmentosa; severe renal impairment; concurrent use with other medicines for penile dysfunction; older adults; pregnancy (category B). Safety and efficacy for PAH in children younger than 18 y not established.

## ROUTE & DOSAGE

### Erectile Dysfunction
*Adult:* **PO** 2.5 mg daily OR 10 mg prior to anticipated sexual activity. May increase (max: 20 mg/day or reduce to 5 mg/day if needed)

### Pulmonary Hypertension
*Adult:* **PO** 40 mg daily

### BPH
*Adult:* **PO** 5 mg daily

### Hepatic Impairment Dosage Adjustment
*Mild to moderate impairment (Child-Pugh class A and B):* Max 10 mg/day; not recommended with severe hepatic impairment
*Severe hepatic impairment (Child-Pugh class C):* Not recommended

### Renal Impairment Dosage Adjustment
CrCl 30–50 mL/min: Start at half normal dose; less than 30 mL/min: Max dose 5 mg and once daily dosing is not recommended

## ADMINISTRATION
### Oral
- If not on the daily dose regimen, tadalafil is taken approximately 30 min before expected intercourse, but preferably not after a heavy or high-fat meal.
- Store at 15°–30° C (59°–86° F).

**ADVERSE EFFECTS (≥1%) Body as a Whole:** Flushing, back pain, asthenia, facial edema, fatigue, pain, transient global amnesia. **CNS:** *Head-ache,* dizziness, insomnia, somnolence, vertigo, hypesthesia, paresthesia. **CV:** Angina, chest pain, hyper-tension, hypotension, MI, orthostatic hypotension, palpitations, syncope, sinus tachycardia. **GI:** Dyspepsia, nausea, vomiting, abdominal pain, abnormal liver function tests, diarrhea, loose stools, dysphagia, esophagitis, gastritis, GERD, xerostomia. **Metabolic:** Increased GGTP. **Musculoskeletal:** Arthralgia, myalgia, neck pain. **Respiratory:** Nasal congestion, dyspnea, epistaxis, pharyngitis. **Skin:** Rash, pruritus, sweating. **Special Senses:** Blurred vision, changes in color vision, conjunctivitis, eye pain, lacrimation, swelling of eyelids, sudden vision loss. **Urogenital:** Spontaneous penile erection.

**INTERACTIONS Drug:** Do not use with any form of NITRATES or **riociguat** due to increased risk of hypotension. Do not use with **telaprevir.** May potentiate hypotensive effects of ETHANOL, **alfuzosin, doxazosin, prazosin, tamsulosin** (doses greater than 0.4 mg/day), **terazosin; erythromycin** (and other MACROLIDES), **indinavir,** PROTEASE INHIBITORS, **saquinavir,** may increase levels and toxicity of tadalafil; **barbiturates, bosentan, carbamazepine, dexamethasone, fosphenytoin, nevirapine, phenytoin, rifabutin, rifampin, troglitazone** may reduce level and effectiveness of tadalafil. If taking **ritonavir, itraconazole, ketoconazole,** or **voriconazole** (max dose: 10 mg q72h). **Food: Grapefruit juice** may increase levels and toxicity of tadalafil.

**PHARMACOKINETICS Absorption:** Rapidly absorbed, 15% reaches systemic circulation. **Onset:** 30–45 min. **Peak:** 2 h. **Duration:** Up to 36 h. **Metabolism:** In liver by CYP3A4. **Elimination:** In feces (61%) and urine (39%). **Half-Life:** 17.5 h.

**NURSING IMPLICATIONS**

**Assessment & Drug Effects**

- Monitor CV status and report angina or other S&S of cardiac dysfunction.

- Monitor for orthostatic hypotension.
- Monitor lab tests: Baseline and periodic PSA.

**Patient & Family Education**

- Do not take more than once/day.
- Note: With moderate renal insufficiency, the maximum recommended dose is 10 mg not more than once in every 48 h.
- Moderate use of alcohol when taking this drug.
- Do not take this drug without consulting prescriber if you are taking drugs called "alpha-blockers" or "nitrates" or any other drugs for high blood pressure, chest pain, or enlarged prostate.
- Report promptly any of the following: Palpitations, chest pain, back pain, difficulty breathing, or shortness of breath; dizziness or fainting; changes in vision; swollen eyelids; muscle aches; painful or prolonged erection (lasting longer than 4 h); skin rash, or itching.

# TAMOXIFEN CITRATE ⊕

(ta-mox′i-fen)

Nolvadex, Nolvadex-D ✦, Tamofen ✦

**Classifications:** ANTINEOPLASTIC; SELECTIVE ESTROGEN RECEPTOR MODIFIER (SERM)

Therapeutic: ANTINEOPLASTIC; ANTIESTROGEN

**AVAILABILITY** Tablet

**ACTION & THERAPEUTIC EFFECT**

Competes with estradiol at estrogen receptor (ER-positive) sites in target tissues such as breast, uterus, vagina, anterior pituitary. Estrogen is thought to increase breast cancer cell proliferation in ER-positive tumors. *Has effects on tumor with high concentration of estrogen receptors. Tamoxifen-receptor*

Common adverse effects in *italic;* life-threatening effects <u>underlined;</u> generic names in **bold;** classifications in SMALL CAPS; ✦ Canadian drug name; ⊕ Prototype drug *complexes move into the cell nucleus, decreasing DNA synthesis and estrogen responses.*

**USES** Palliative treatment of advanced with metastatic estrogen receptors (ER)-positive breast cancer in postmenopausal women, adjunctively with surgery in the treatment of breast carcinoma with positive lymph nodes; reduce risk of breast cancer in high risk patient.

**UNLABELED USES** Gynecomastia, oligospermia.

**CONTRAINDICATIONS** Anticoagulant therapy including coumadin; preexisting endometrial hyperplasia; intramuscular injections if platelets less than 50,000/mm³; history of thromboembolic disease; pregnancy (category D), especially during first trimester; lactation; children

**CAUTIOUS USE** Vision disturbances; cataracts, visual disturbance, leukopenia, bone marrow suppression; thrombocytopenia; hypercalcemia; hypercholesterolemia, lipid protein abnormalities; women with ductal carcinoma in situ (DCIS).

## ROUTE & DOSAGE

**Breast Carcinoma**
*Adult:* **PO** 20–40 mg 1–2 × day (morning and evening)

**Breast Cancer Prophylaxis**
*Adult:* **PO** 20 mg daily × 5 y

## ADMINISTRATION

**Oral**
- Doses greater than 20 mg/day should be given in divided doses a.m. and p.m.

- Store at 20°–25° C (68°–77° F); protect from light. Oral solution should be used within 3 mo of opening.

**ADVERSE EFFECTS** (≥1%) **Body as a Whole:** Increased bone pain, and transient local disease flair; loss of hair, weight loss, shortness of breath, photosensitivity, *hot flashes*. **CNS:** Depression, lightheadedness, dizziness, headache, mental confusion, sleepiness. **CV:** Thrombosis, pulmonary embolism, increased risk of stroke. **GI:** *Nausea and vomiting (about 25% of patients)*, distaste for food, anorexia. **Hematologic:** Leukopenia, thrombocytopenia. **Metabolic:** Hypercalcemia, increased bilirubin. **Skin:** Skin rash or dryness. **Special Senses:** Retinopathy, decreased visual acuity, blurred vision. **Urogenital:** Changes in menstrual period, milk production and leaking from breasts, vaginal discharge and bleeding, pruritus vulvae, risk of uterine malignancies.

**DIAGNOSTIC TEST INTERFERENCE** Tamoxifen may produce transient increase in *serum calcium*.

**INTERACTIONS Drug:** May enhance hypoprothrombinemic effects of **warfarin;** may increase risk of thromboembolic events with CYTOTOXIC AGENTS; **bromocriptine** may elevate tamoxifen levels, SSRI ANTIDEPRESSANTS may decrease effectiveness of tamoxifen.

**PHARMACOKINETICS Absorption:** Slowly from GI tract. **Peak:** 3–6 h. **Metabolism:** In liver (CYP2D6), enterohepatically cycled. **Elimination:** Primarily in feces. **Half-Life:** 7 days.

T

Common adverse effects in *italic;* life-threatening effects <u>underlined;</u> generic names in **bold;** classifications in SMALL CAPS; ✦ Canadian drug name; ◉ Prototype drug

1549

## NURSING IMPLICATIONS

### Black Box Warning

*Tamoxifen has been associated with increased risk of uterine malignancies, stroke, and pulmonary embolism.*

#### Assessment & Drug Effects

- Be aware that local swelling and marked erythema over preexisting lesions or the development of new lesions may signal soft-tissue disease response to tamoxifen. These symptoms rapidly subside.
- Monitor lab tests: Periodic CBC, including platelet count, LFTs, and lipid profile.

#### Patient & Family Education

- Do not change established dose schedule.
- Report to prescriber any of the following: Marked weakness or numbness in face or leg, especially on one side of the body; difficulty walking or loss of balance; unexplained sleepiness or mental confusion; edema; shortness of breath; or blurred vision.
- Report promptly any unexpected vaginal discharge or pain or pressure in your pelvis.
- Avoid OTC drugs unless specifically prescribed by the prescriber; particularly OTC pain medicines.
- Report onset of tenderness or redness in an extremity.

## TAMSULOSIN HYDROCHLORIDE ℗

(tam′su-lo-sin)

*Flomax*

**Classification:** ALPHA-ADRENERGIC RECEPTOR ANTAGONIST

**Therapeutic:** SMOOTH MUSCLE RELAXANT OF BLADDER OUTLET & PROSTATE GLAND

**AVAILABILITY** Capsule

**ACTION & *THERAPEUTIC EFFECT***
Antagonist of the alpha$_{1A}$-adrenergic receptors located in the prostate. This blockage can cause smooth muscles in the bladder outlet and the prostate gland to relax, resulting in improvement in urinary flow and a reduction in symptoms of BPH. *Effectiveness is indicated by improved voiding. Improves symptoms related to benign prostatic hypertrophy (BPH) related to bladder outlet obstruction.*

**USES** Benign prostatic hypertrophy.

**CONTRAINDICATIONS** Hypersensitivity to tamsulosin; women; lactation; children.

**CAUTIOUS USE** History of syncope, hypersensitivity to sulfonamides; hypotension; renal impairment, renal failure, renal disease; older adults; pregnancy (category B).

## ROUTE & DOSAGE

### Benign Prostatic Hypertrophy

*Adult:* **PO** 0.4 mg daily 30 min after a meal, may increase up to 0.8 mg daily

## ADMINISTRATION

#### Oral

- Give 30 min after the same meal each day.
- Instruct to swallow capsules whole; not to crush, chew, or open.
- If dose is interrupted for several days, reinitiate at the lowest dose, 0.4 mg.
- Store at 20°–25° C (68°–77° F).

T

Common adverse effects in *italic;* life-threatening effects <u>underlined</u>; generic names in **bold;** classifications in SMALL CAPS; ♣ Canadian drug name; ℗ Prototype drug

**ADVERSE EFFECTS** (≥1%) **Body as a Whole:** Asthenia, back or chest pain. **CNS:** *Headache, dizziness,* insomnia. **CV:** *Orthostatic hypotension (especially with first dose).* **GI:** Diarrhea, nausea. **Respiratory:** *Rhinitis,* pharyngitis, increased cough, sinusitis. **Urogenital:** Decreased libido, *abnormal ejaculation.* **Special Senses:** Amblyopia.

**INTERACTIONS Drug: Cimetidine** may decrease clearance of tamsulosin. **Sildenafil, vardenafil,** and **tadalafil,** and alcohol may enhance hypotensive effects.

**PHARMACOKINETICS Absorption:** Rapidly from GI tract. Greater than 90% bioavailability. **Peak:** 4–5 h fasting, 6–7 h fed. **Distribution:** Widely distributed in body tissues, including kidney and prostate. **Metabolism:** In the liver. **Elimination:** 76% in urine. **Half-Life:** 14–15 h.

**NURSING IMPLICATIONS**

**Assessment & Drug Effects**

▪ Monitor for signs of orthostatic hypotension; take BP lying down, then upon standing. Report a systolic pressure drop of 15 mm Hg or more or a HR 15 beats or more upon standing.
▪ Monitor patients on warfarin therapy closely.

**Patient & Family Education**

▪ Make position changes slowly to minimize orthostatic hypotension.
▪ Report dizziness, vertigo, or fainting to prescriber. Exercise caution with hazardous activities until response to drug is known.
▪ Be aware that concurrent use of cimetidine may increase the orthostatic hypotension adverse effect.

## TAPENTADOL
(ta-pent'a-dol)
**Nucynta, Nucynta ER**
**Classifications:** CENTRALLY ACTING NARCOTIC ANALGESIC; MU-OPIOID RECEPTOR AGONIST; INHIBITOR OF NOREPINEPHRINE REUPTAKE
**Therapeutic:** CENTRALLY ACTING NARCOTIC ANALGESIC
**Controlled Substance:** Schedule II

**AVAILABILITY** Tablet; extended release tablet

**ACTION & *THERAPEUTIC EFFECT***
Tapentadol is a centrally acting synthetic analgesic that is a mu-opioid agonist and also thought to inhibit norepinephrine reuptake. There is potential for opioid agonist abuse or addiction. *Effective in treatment of moderate to severe acute pain.*

**USES** Relief of acute moderate to severe pain, chronic pain (ER form only).

**CONTRAINDICATIONS** Hypersensitivity to tapentadol (e.g., anaphylaxis, angioedema); impaired pulmonary function (e.g., significant respiratory depression, acute or severe bronchial asthma, hypercapnia without monitoring or the absence of resuscitative equipment), known or suspected paralytic ileus; concomitant use of MAOI or use within 14 days; head injury, intracranial pressure (ICP); severe hepatic or renal impairment (CrCl less than 30 mL/min); alcohol consumption especially with tapentadol ER; labor and delivery; lactation.

**CAUTIOUS USE** Debilitated patients; upper airway obstruction; COPD; cor pulmonale; patients with decreased respiratory reserve;

Common adverse effects in *italic;* life-threatening effects <u>underlined;</u> generic names in **bold;** classifications in SMALL CAPS; ◆ Canadian drug name; ⊙ Prototype drug

1551

# TAPENTADOL

history of low blood pressure; cranial lesions without increased ICP; history of drug or alcohol abuse; history of seizures; mild or moderate renal or hepatic impairment; older adults; pregnancy (category C). Safe use in children younger than 18 y not established.

## ROUTE & DOSAGE

### Acute Moderate to Severe Pain
*Adult:* **PO** 50–100 mg q 4–6 h. On first day of dosing a second dose may be given 1 h later if initial dose ineffective (may titrate to max total daily dose: 700 mg day 1 and 600 mg thereafter).

### Chronic Pain (ER Form Only)
*Adult:* **PO** 100–250 mg b.i.d.

### Hepatic Impairment Dosage Adjustment
*Moderate impairment:* Reduce initial dose to 50 mg q 8 h. *Severe impairment (Child-Pugh class C):* Not recommended for use.

## ADMINISTRATION
### Oral
- Extended release (ER) tablets must be swallowed whole. They must not be cut, chewed, dissolved, or crushed due to risk of rapid release of a potentially fatal dose.
- On day 1 of therapy, a second dose may be given as soon as 1 h after the initial dose if pain relief is inadequate. All subsequent doses should be at 4–6 h intervals.
- Do not exceed a total daily dose of 700 mg on day 1 or 600 mg on subsequent days.
- When extended-release (ER) tablets are discontinued, a gradual downward titration of the dose should be used to prevent S&S of drug withdrawal.

- Do not administer if a paralytic ileus is suspected.
- Do not give within 14 days of an MAOI.
- Store at 15°–30° C (59°–86° F).

## ADVERSE EFFECTS (≥1%) **Body as a Whole:** Fatigue. **CNS:** *Headache,* abnormal dreams, anxiety, confusional state, *dizziness,* insomnia, lethargy, *somnolence,* tremor. **CV:** Hot flush. **GI:** *Constipation,* dry mouth, dyspepsia, *nausea, vomiting.* **Metabolic:** Decreased appetite. **Musculoskeletal:** Arthralgia. **Respiratory:** Nasopharyngitis, <u>respiratory depression</u>, upper respiratory tract infection. **Skin:** Hyperhidrosis, pruritus, rash. **Urogenital:** Urinary tract infection.

## INTERACTIONS **Drug:** Other OPIOID AGONISTS, GENERAL ANESTHETICS, PHENOTHIAZINES, ANTIEMETICS, other TRANQUILIZERS, SEDATIVES, HYPNOTICS, or other CNS DEPRESSANTS may cause additive CNS depression. MAO INHIBITORS can raise **norepinephrine** levels resulting in adverse cardiovascular events.

## PHARMACOKINETICS **Absorption:** 32% bioavailability. **Peak:** 1.25 h. **Metabolism:** In liver. **Elimination:** Primarily renal. **Half-Life:** 4 h.

## NURSING IMPLICATIONS

### Black Box Warning

*Tapentadol ER has been associated with serious, sometimes fatal, respiratory depression and with neonatal withdrawal syndrome.*

### Assessment & Drug Effects
- Monitor degree of pain relief, mental status, and level of alertness.
- Monitor vital signs. Withhold drug and notify prescriber for a respiratory rate of 12/min or less.

- If an opioid antagonist is required to reverse the action of tapentadol, continue to monitor respiratory status since respiratory depression may outlast duration of action of the opioid antagonists.
- Monitor for signs of misuse, abuse, and addiction.
- Withhold drug and report promptly S&S of serotonin syndrome (see Appendix F).
- Monitor ambulation. Fall precautions may be warranted.

**Patient & Family Education**
- Avoid engaging in hazardous activities until reaction to drug is known.
- Avoid alcohol while taking the extended release (ER) form of this drug.
- Consult prescriber before taking OTC drugs.

---

# TASIMELTEON
(tas-i-mel'tee-on)
Hetlioz
**Classifications:** SEDATIVE-HYPNOTIC; MELATONIN RECEPTOR AGONIST
Therapeutic: SEDATIVE
**Prototype:** Ramelteon

**AVAILABILITY** Gelatin capsules

**ACTION & THERAPEUTIC EFFECT**
Agonist of melatonin receptors MT1 and MT2. Activation of MT1 is thought to induce sleepiness, and MT2 activation is thought to help regulate circadian rhythms. *Improves insomnia or excessive sleepiness related to abnormal synchronization between the 24-h light–dark cycle and endogenous circadian rhythms.*

**USES** Treatment of non-24 h sleep–wake disorder (non-24).

**CONTRAINDICATIONS** Severe hepatic impairment.

**CAUTIOUS USE** Concomitant drugs (including alcohol) that cause CNS depression; mild-to-moderate hepatic impairment; older adults; pregnancy (category C); lactation. Safety and efficacy in children younger than 18 y not established.

**ROUTE & DOSAGE**

**Sleep-Wake Disorder (Non-24)**
*Adult:* **PO** 20 mg once daily at the same time before bedtime

**ADMINISTRATION**
- Give with food at approximately same time every night before bedtime.
- Capsules **must be** swallowed whole. They should not be opened or chewed.
- Store at 15°–30° C (59°–86° F). Protect from light and moisture.

**ADVERSE EFFECTS** (≥5%) **CNS:** Headache, nightmare/abnormal dreams. **Metabolic:** Increased ALT. **Respiratory:** Upper respiratory tract infection. **Urogenital:** Urinary tract infection.

**INTERACTIONS Drug:** Tasimelteon may enhance the effects of other CNS depressants. Co-administration with strong CYP1A2 inhibitors (e.g., **fluvoxamine**) or strong CYP3A4 inhibitors (e.g., **ketoconazole**) may increase the levels of tasimelteon. Co-administration with strong CYP3A4 inducers (e.g., **carbamazepine, phenytoin, rifampin**) may decrease the levels of tasimelteon. **Food: Grapefruit** and **grapefruit juice** may increase the levels of tasimelteon. **Herbal: St. John's wort** decreases the levels of tasimelteon.

---

Common adverse effects in *italic*; life-threatening effects <u>underlined</u>; generic names in **bold**; classifications in SMALL CAPS; ✤ Canadian drug name; ❂ Prototype drug

1553

## PHARMACOKINETICS **Peak:** 0.5–3 h. **Distribution:** 90% plasma protein bound. **Metabolism:** Extensive metabolism in liver. **Elimination:** Primarily renal. **Half-Life:** 1.3 h.

## NURSING IMPLICATIONS

### Assessment & Drug Effects

- Monitor for and report worsening insomnia and cognitive or behavioral changes.
- Monitor urinary output and report immediately dysuria or difficulty urinating.
- Assess risk for falls in older adults and otherwise frail persons.
- Monitor lab test: Baseline LFTs.

### Patient & Family Education

- If drug cannot be taken at approximately the same time on a given night, that dose should be skipped.
- Do not drive or engage in potentially hazardous activities until response to drug is known.
- Do not consume alcohol while taking this drug.
- Report any of the following to prescriber: Worsening insomnia, cognitive or behavioral changes, difficulty with urination.

## TAZAROTENE
(ta-zar′o-teen)
Avage, Tazorac
**Classifications:** RETINOID; ANTIACNE
Therapeutic: ANTIACNE
**Prototype:** Isotretinoin

**AVAILABILITY** Gel; cream

## ACTION & *THERAPEUTIC EFFECT*
Retinoid prodrug that blocks epidermal cell proliferation and hyperplasia. Suppresses inflammation present in the epidermis of psoriasis. *Effectiveness indicated by improvement in acne or psoriasis.*

**USES** Topical treatment of plaque psoriasis on up to 20% of the body, mild to moderate acne, facial fine wrinkling, mottled hypo- and hyperpigmentation (blotchy skin discoloration), and benign facial lentigines.

**CONTRAINDICATIONS** Hypersensitivity to tazarotene; pregnancy (category X), women who are or may become pregnant; lactation.

**CAUTIOUS USE** Concurrent administration with drugs that are photosensitizers (e.g., thiazide diuretics, tetracyclines); retinoid hypersensitivity. Safety and efficacy in children younger than 12 y not established.

## ROUTE & DOSAGE

### Plaque Psoriasis
*Adult:* **Topical** Apply thin film to affected area once daily in evening

### Acne
*Adult:* **Topical** After cleansing and drying face, apply thin film to acne lesions once daily in evening

### Fine Wrinkles
*Adult:* **Topical** Apply thin film of cream to affected area once daily

## ADMINISTRATION

### Topical
- Dry skin completely before application of a thin film of medication.
- Apply medication to no more than 20% of body surface in those with psoriasis.
- Apply only to affected areas; avoid contact with eyes and mucous membranes.

**ADVERSE EFFECTS** (≥1%) **Skin:** *Pruritus, burning/stinging, erythema,* *worsening of psoriasis, irritation, skin pain,* rash, desquamation of skin, irritant contact dermatitis, inflammation, fissuring, bleeding, dry skin, sunburn.

**INTERACTIONS Drug:** Increased risk of photosensitivity reactions with QUINOLONES (especially **sparfloxacin**), PHENOTHIAZINES, SULFONAMIDES, SULFONYLUREAS, TETRACYCLINES, THIAZIDE DIURETICS.

**PHARMACOKINETICS Absorption:** Rapidly absorbed through skin. **Distribution:** Active metabolite greater than 99% protein bound; crosses placenta, distributed into breast milk. **Metabolism:** Undergoes esterase hydrolysis to active metabolite AGN 190299. **Elimination:** In both urine and feces. **Half-Life:** 18 h.

**NURSING IMPLICATIONS**
**Assessment & Drug Effects**
▪ Monitor for photosensitivity in those concurrently using any of the following: Thiazides, tetracyclines, fluoroquinolones, phenothiazines, sulfonamides.

**Patient & Family Education**
▪ Understand fully the risk of serious fetal harm. Use reliable forms of effective contraception. Discontinue treatment and notify prescriber if pregnancy occurs.
▪ Alert: Immediately rinse thoroughly with water if contact with eyes occurs.
▪ Avoid all unnecessary exposure to sunlight or artificial UV light. If brief exposure is necessary, cover as much skin surface as possible and use sunscreens (minimum SPF 15).
▪ Do not apply to sunburned skin.
▪ Discontinue medication and notify prescriber if any of the following occur: Pruritus, burning, skin

redness, excessive peeling, worsening of psoriasis.
▪ Limit application of topicals with strong skin-drying effects to skin areas being treated with tazarotene.

## TEDIZOLID PHOSPHATE
(ted-i-zo'lid)
Sivextro
**Classifications:** OXAZOLIDINONE ANTIBIOTIC
**Therapeutic:** ANTIBIOTIC
**Prototype:** Linezolid

**AVAILABILITY** Tablets, lyophilized power for injection

**ACTION & THERAPEUTIC EFFECT**
Prevents formation of a functional 70S essential for the bacterial translation process, thus inhibiting protein synthesis and cell proliferation. *Bacteriostatic against enterococci, staphylococci, and streptococci.*

**USES** Treatment of acute bacterial skin and skin structure infections (ABSSSI) caused by designated susceptible bacteria.

**CONTRAINDICATIONS** *Clostridium difficile*-associated diarrhea, except of treatment thereof; neutrophil counts less than 1,000 cells/mm³.

**CAUTIOUS USE** Colitis; cardiac arrhythmia; history of anemia; pregnancy (category C); lactation. Safety and efficacy in children younger than 18 y not established.

## ROUTE & DOSAGE

**Skin and Skin Structure Infection**
*Adult:* **PO or IV** 200 mg once daily for 6 days

## ADMINISTRATION

### Oral

- Give without regard to food.
- Store at 15°–30° C (59°–86° F).

### Intravenous

*PREPARE:* **IV Infusion:** Reconstitute vial with 4 mL SW. **Do not** shake. Swirl gently and let stand until dissolved and foam disperses. If needed, invert vial to completely dissolve and swirl gently to prevent foaming. Place vial upright, tilt, and insert a syringe into bottom corner to remove 4 mL. **Do not** invert the vial during extraction. Further dilute in 250 mL of NS. Invert bag gently to mix but do not shake.

*ADMINISTER:* **IV Infusion:** Give over 1 h. **Do not** give IV push or bolus. Flush line before/after with NS if used for other drugs or solutions.

*INCOMPATIBILITIES:* **Solution/additive:** Solutions containing divalent cations (e.g., $Ca^{+2}$, $Mg^{+2}$), Lactated Ringer's, Hartmann's Solution.

- Store reconstituted solution for up to 24 h at room temperature or under refrigeration at 2°–8° C (36°–46° F).

## ADVERSE EFFECTS (≥1%) **Body as a Whole:** Flushing, hypersensitivity reactions, phlebitis, oral candidiasis. **CNS:** Dizziness, headache, hypoesthesia, insomnia, paresthesia, nerve paralysis, peripheral neuropathy. **CV:** Hypertension, palpitations, *tachycardia*. **GI:** *Clostridium difficile* colitis, diarrhea, nausea, vomiting. **Hematological:** Anemia. **Metabolic:** Decreased hemoglobin, decreased white blood cell count, increased ALT and AST, decreased platelet count, thrombocytopenia. **Skin:** Dermatitis, pruritus, urticarial. **Special Senses:** Asthenopia, blurred vision, visual impairment,

vitreous floaters. **Urogenital:** Vulvovaginal mycotic infection.

## INTERACTIONS **Drug:** Tedizolid may increase the levels of other drugs (e.g., **aproclonidine, benzafibrate, bupropion, carbamazepine, levodopa,** SEROTONIN 5-HT1D RECEPTOR AGONISTS) that require MAO for metabolism. Do not use with LIVE VACCINES. Use with **fentanyl** or other OPIOIDS could cause serotonin syndrome.

## PHARMACOKINETICS **Absorption:** 91% Bioavailable. **Peak:** 3 h. **Distribution:** 70–90% plasma protein bound; distributes into adipose and skeletal muscle tissue. **Elimination:** Fecal (82%) and renal (18%). **Half-Life:** 12 h.

## NURSING IMPLICATIONS

### Assessment & Drug Effects

- Monitor for S&S of superinfection, including *C. difficile*-associated diarrhea (CDAD) and pseudomembranous colitis that may develop months after treatment.
- Monitor lab tests: Baseline CBC with differential.

### Patient & Family Education

- Report promptly to prescriber if you develop frequent watery or bloody diarrhea even 2 mo or more after last dose of antibiotic.
- Consult with prescriber if you are a female who is or plans to become pregnant.
- Do not breast-feed without consulting prescriber.

## TELAVANCIN HYDROCHLORIDE
(tel-a-van'sin)

Vibativ

**Classifications:** ANTIBIOTIC; GLYCOPROTEIN

Therapeutic: ANTIBIOTIC

**Prototype:** Vancomycin

Common adverse effects in *italic*; life threatening effects underlined; generic names in **bold**; classifications in SMALL CAPS; ♣ Canadian drug name; ⊙ Prototype drug

**AVAILABILITY** Powder for reconstitution and injection

## ACTION & *THERAPEUTIC EFFECT*
Inhibits cell wall synthesis of bacteria. It binds to the bacterial membrane and disrupts the barrier function of the cell membrane of gram-positive bacteria. *Effective against a broad range of gram-positive bacteria.*

**USES** Treatment of complicated skin and skin structure infections hospital-acquired and ventilator-associated pneumonia.

**CONTRAINDICATIONS** End-stage renal disease or hemodialysis; uncompensated heart failure; QT prolongation.

**CAUTIOUS USE** Moderate or severe renal impairment, renal disease; elderly; ulcerative colitis; severe hepatic impairment; women of childbearing potential; pregnancy (category C); lactation. Safe use in children younger than 18 y has not been established.

## ROUTE & DOSAGE

**Complicated Skin and Skin Structure Infections**
*Adult:* **IV** 10 mg/kg q24h for 7–14 days

**Hospital-Acquired and Ventilator-Associated Bacterial Pneumonia**
*Adult:* **IV** 10 mg/kg q24h × 7–21 days

**Renal Impairment Dosage Adjustment**
*CrCl 30–50 mL/min:* Decrease to 7.5 mg/kg q 24 h; *10–29 mL/min:* Decrease to 10 mg/kg q 48 h

## ADMINISTRATION
**Intravenous**

*PREPARE:* **Infusion:** Reconstitute each 250 mg with 15 mL or each 750 mg vial with 45 mL of D5W or NS to yield 15 mg/mL. Mix thoroughly to dissolve. For doses of 150–800 mg, must further dilute in 100–250 mL of IV solution. For doses less than 100 mg or greater than 800 mg, should be further diluted in D5W, NS, or LR to a final concentration in the range of 0.6–8 mg/mL.
*ADMINISTER:* **Infusion:** Infuse over 60 min or longer to minimize infusion-related reactions. ▪ Do not infuse through the same line with any other drugs or additives.

▪ Storage: Reconstituted vials or infusion solution should be used within 4 h if at room temperature or 72 h if refrigerated. **Important note:** The total time holding time for reconstituted vials plus infusion solution cannot exceed 4 h at room temperature or 72 h refrigerated.

**ADVERSE EFFECTS** (≥1%) **Body as a Whole:** Generalized pruritus, rigors, infusion site erythema and pain. **CNS:** Dizziness, *taste disturbance.* **GI:** Abdominal pain, *Clostridium difficile*-associated diarrhea, diarrhea, *nausea, vomiting.* **Metabolic:** Decreased appetite, *increased serum creatinine.* **Skin:** Pruritus, rash. **Urogenital:** *Foamy urine.*

## DIAGNOSTIC TEST INTERFERENCE
Telavancin may cause increases in *PT, INR, aPTT,* and *ACT.* Telavancin interferes with *urine qualitative dipstick protein assays,* as well as quantitative *dye methods* (e.g., *pyrogallol red-molybdate*).

T

## PHARMACOKINETICS Distribution: 93% bound to albumin. **Metabolism:** Metabolized to 3-hydroxylated metabolites. **Elimination:** Primarily via the urine. **Half-Life:** 8–9 h.

## NURSING IMPLICATIONS

### Black Box Warning

*Telavancin has been associated with new-onset or worsening renal impairment and fetal toxicity.*

### Assessment & Drug Effects

- Monitor for red man syndrome (i.e., flushing of upper body, urticaria, pruritus, or rash) during infusion. If syndrome develops, slow infusion immediately. If reaction does not cease, stop infusion and notify prescriber.
- Withhold drug and notify prescriber for CrCl of 50 mL/min or less.
- Monitor for and report promptly the onset of watery diarrhea with or without fever, passage of tarry or bloody stools, pus, or mucus.
- Monitor ECG with concurrent use of drugs known to prolong the QT interval.
- Monitor lab tests: Baseline C&S. Baseline and frequent (q48–72h) renal function tests throughout therapy.

### Patient & Family Education

- Report promptly appearance of rash or itching during drug infusion.
- Report promptly loose stools or diarrhea even after completion of drug.
- Women should use effective means of contraception while on this drug. Notify prescriber if pregnancy occurs during treatment.

## TELBIVUDINE

(tel-bi'vu-deen)

Tyzeka

**Classifications:** ANTIRETROVIRAL; NUCLEOSIDE REVERSE TRANSCRIPTASE INHIBITOR (NRTI)
**Therapeutic:** ANTIRETROVIRAL; NRTI
**Prototype:** Lamivudine

## AVAILABILITY Tablet

## ACTION & *THERAPEUTIC EFFECT*

Its metabolite inhibits HBV DNA polymerase (reverse transcriptase) by competing with the natural nucleoside substrate. Incorporation into HBV viral DNA causes DNA chain termination, resulting in inhibition of HBV replication. *Effectiveness is measured by reducing the viral load and preventing infection of new hepatocytes.*

## USES Chronic hepatitis B infection.

## CONTRAINDICATIONS Hypersensitivity to telbivudine; concurrent use with peginterferon alfa-2a; lactic acidosis; severe hepatomegaly with steatosis; peripheral neuropathy; lactation.

## CAUTIOUS USE Moderate to severe renal impairment, hemodialysis; alcoholism; obesity in females; risk of hepatic disease; individuals with organ transplants; older adults; pregnancy (category B). Safe use in children younger than 16 y has not been established.

## ROUTE & DOSAGE

### Chronic Hepatitis B

*Adults/Adolescents (16 y or older):* **PO** 600 mg/day

### Renal Impairment Dosage Adjustment

*CrCl 30–49 mL/min:* 600 mg q48h; *CrCl less than 30 mL/min (not requiring dialysis):* 600 mg q72h; *CrCl less than 5–10 mL/min (ESRD):* 600 mg q96h

Common adverse effects in *italic;* life-threatening effects underlined; generic names in **bold;** classifications in SMALL CAPS; ◆ Canadian drug name; ◯ Prototype drug

## ADMINISTRATION

### Oral

- May be given without regard to food.
- Store at 15°–30° C (59°–86° F).

## ADVERSE EFFECTS (≥1%) Body as a Whole: *Fatigue and malaise, headache, influenza-like syndrome, post-procedural pain,* fever, neutropenia. **CNS:** Dizziness, insomnia. **GI:** *Abdominal pain, diarrhea, abdominal distension,* dyspepsia, *nausea, vomiting.* **Metabolic:** *Increased CPK levels,* increased serum lipase, increased ALT and AST, <u>lactic acidosis and severe hepatomegaly with steatosis</u>. **Musculoskeletal:** Arthralgia, back pain, myalgia. **Respiratory:** *Cough, nasopharyngitis,* pharyngolaryngeal pain, *upper respiratory tract infection.* **Skin:** Rash, pruritis.

## INTERACTIONS Drug: Coadministration with drugs that alter renal function may alter plasma concentrations of telbivudine. Do not use with **pegylated interferon alfa-2a** or interferon alfa-2b because of increased risk of peripheral neuropathy.

## PHARMACOKINETICS Peak: 1–4 h. **Distribution:** Minimal protein binding; widely distributed in tissues. **Elimination:** Primarily unchanged in urine. **Half-Life:** 40–49 h.

## NURSING IMPLICATIONS

### Black Box Warning

*Telbivudine has been associated with lactic acidosis and severe hepatomegaly with steatosis.*

### Assessment & Drug Effects

- Monitor for and report S&S of lactic acidosis (e.g., anorexia, nausea, vomiting, bloating, abdominal pain, malaise, tachycardia or other arrhythmia, and difficulty in breathing).
- Withhold drug and notify prescriber of any of the following: Suspected lactic acidosis, steatosis, or markedly elevated liver enzymes.
- Monitor lab tests: Periodic LFTs during and for several months after discontinuation of telbivudine; periodic renal function tests in the older adult and those taking drugs that may impair renal function.

### Patient & Family Education

- Avoid all alcohol consumption while taking this drug.
- Report any of the following to a health care provider: Loss of appetite, nausea and vomiting, abdominal pain, palpitations, or difficulty breathing.

## TELITHROMYCIN
(tel-i-thro-my'sin)
Ketek
**Classifications:** ANTIBIOTIC; KETOLIDE
**Therapeutic:** ANTIBIOTIC
**Prototype:** Erythromycin

## AVAILABILITY Tablet

## ACTION & *THERAPEUTIC EFFECT*
Results in inhibition of RNA-dependent protein synthesis of bacteria, thus resulting in cell death. Telithromycin concentrates in phagocytes where it works against intracellular respiratory pathogens. *Its broad spectrum of activity is effective against respiratory pathogens, including erythromycin- and penicillin-resistant pneumococci.*

## USES Treatment of community-acquired pneumonia.

## UNLABELED USES Sinusitis.

Common adverse effects in *italic;* life-threatening effects <u>underlined</u>; generic names in **bold;** classifications in SMALL CAPS; ♣ Canadian drug name; ⊘ Prototype drug

1559

**CONTRAINDICATIONS** Macrolide antibiotic hypersensitivity; QT prolongation; ongoing proarrhythmic conditions such as hypokalemia, hypomagnesemia, significant bradycardia, myasthenia gravis; severe renal impairment or renal failure; viral infections.

**CAUTIOUS USE** History of GI disease; hepatic disease; history of hepatitis or jaundice; pregnancy (category C); lactation. Safety and efficacy in children not established.

## ROUTE & DOSAGE

**Community-Acquired Pneumonia**
*Adult:* **PO** 800 mg daily for 7–10 days

**Renal Impairment Dosage Adjustment**
*CrCl less than 30 mL/min:* 600 mg daily (400 mg daily with concomitant hepatic impairment)

## ADMINISTRATION

**Oral**
- May be administered with or without food.
- Do not administer concurrently with simvastatin, lovastatin, atorvastatin, Class 1A (e.g., quinidine, procainamide) or Class III (e.g., dofetilide) antiarrhythmic agents.
- Store at 15°–30° C (59°–86° F). Keep container tightly closed. Protect from light.

**ADVERSE EFFECTS** (≥1%) **CNS:** Headache, dizziness. **CV:** Potential to cause QT$_c$ prolongation. **GI:** *Diarrhea,* nausea, vomiting, loose stools, dysgeusia. **Metabolic:** Elevated LFTs, liver failure. **Musculoskeletal:** May exacerbate myasthenia gravis. **Special Senses:** Blurred vision, diplopia, difficulty focusing.

**INTERACTIONS Drug: Pimozide** or CLASS IA or CLASS III ANTIARRHYTHMICS may cause life-threatening arrhythmias; may increase concentrations of **atorvastatin, lovastatin, simvastatin,** BENZODIAZEPINES; **rifampin** decreases telithromycin levels; ERGOT DERIVATIVES (**ergotamine, dihydroergotamine**) may cause severe peripheral vasospasm; **theophylline** may exacerbate adverse GI effects. **Food: Grapefruit juice** (greater than 1 qt/day) may increase plasma concentrations and adverse effects.

**PHARMACOKINETICS Absorption:** 57% bioavailable. **Peak:** 1 h. **Metabolism:** 50% in liver (CYP3A4), 50% by CYP-independent mechanisms. **Elimination:** In urine and feces. **Half-Life:** 10 h.

## NURSING IMPLICATIONS

**Black Box Warning**

*Telithromycin has been associated with fatal respiratory failure in patients with myasthenia gravis and is contraindicated in these patients.*

**Assessment & Drug Effects**
- Monitor ECG in patients at risk for QT$_c$ interval prolongation (i.e., bradycardia).
- Withhold drug and notify prescriber for S&S of QT$_c$ interval prolongation such as dizziness or fainting.
- Monitor for and report promptly S&S of liver dysfunction: Fatigue, anorexia, nausea, clay-colored stools, etc.
- Monitor lab tests: Baseline and periodic LFTs.

**Patient & Family Education**
- Stop taking drug and notify prescriber for episodes of dizziness or fainting; report signs of jaundice (yellow color of the skin and/or eyes), unexplained

Common adverse effects in *italic;* life-threatening effects <u>underlined</u>; generic names in **bold;** classifications in SMALL CAPS; ♣ Canadian drug name; ⊙ Prototype drug

fatigue, loss of appetite, nausea, dark urine, or clay-colored stool.
- Exercise caution when engaging in potentially hazardous activities; visual disturbances (e.g., blurred vision, difficulty focusing, double vision) are potential side effects of this drug. If visual problems occur, avoid quick changes in viewing between close and distant objects.

## TELMISARTAN

(tel-mi-sar'tan)

*Micardis*

**Classifications:** ANGIOTENSIN II RECEPTOR ANTAGONIST; ANTIHYPERTENSIVE

Therapeutic: ANTIHYPERTENSIVE
**Prototype:** Losartan potassium

**AVAILABILITY** Tablet

**ACTION & *THERAPEUTIC EFFECT***
Selectively blocks the binding of angiotensin II to the $AT_1$ receptors in many tissues (e.g., vascular smooth muscles, adrenal glands). Blocks the vasoconstricting and aldosterone-secreting effects of angiotensin II, thus resulting in an antihypertensive effect. *Effectiveness is indicated by a reduction in BP.*

**USES** Treatment of hypertension, cardiovascular risk reduction.

**CONTRAINDICATIONS** Hypersensitivity to telmisartan; development of angioedema due to use of telmisartan; women of child bearing age; concurrent use of aliskiren in diabetics; pregnancy (category D); lactation.

**CAUTIOUS USE** CAD; hypertropic cardiomyopathy; CHF; oliguria; hypotension in volume depleted patients; renal artery stenosis; advanced renal impairment; biliary

obstruction; liver dysfunction; renal impairment; older adults; pregnancy (category C first trimester, discontinue use as soon as detected). Safety and efficacy in children younger than 18 y not established.

## ROUTE & DOSAGE

**Hypertension**
*Adult:* **PO** 40 mg daily, may increase to 80 mg/day

**CV Risk Reduction**
*Adult:* **PO** 80 mg/day

## ADMINISTRATION

### Oral
- Do not remove tablets from blister pack until immediately before administration.
- Correct volume depletion prior to initial dose.
- Store at 15°–30° C (59°–86° F).

**ADVERSE EFFECTS** (≥1%) **Body as a Whole:** Back pain, flu-like syndrome, myalgia, fatigue. **CNS:** Dizziness, headache. **CV:** Hypotension, hypertension, chest pain, peripheral edema. **GI:** Diarrhea, dyspepsia, abdominal pain, nausea. **Respiratory:** Sinusitis, pharyngitis.

**INTERACTIONS Drug:** Telmisartan may increase **digoxin** or **lithium** levels. Increased risk of hyptension with ACE INHIBITORS or other ANTIHYPERTENSIVES.

**PHARMACOKINETICS Absorption:** Dose dependent, 42% of 40 mg dose is absorbed. **Peak:** 0.5–1 h. **Distribution:** Greater than 99% protein bound. **Metabolism:** Minimally metabolized. **Elimination:** Primarily in feces. **Half-Life:** 24 h.

## NURSING IMPLICATIONS

### Black Box Warning

*Telmisartan has been associated with fetal toxicity and death.*

### Assessment & Drug Effects

- Monitor BP carefully after initial dose; and periodically thereafter. Monitor more frequently with preexisting biliary obstructive disorders or hepatic insufficiency.
- Monitor dialysis patients closely for orthostatic hypotension.
- Monitor concomitant digoxin levels throughout therapy.
- Monitor lab tests: Periodic serum electrolytes, creatinine clearance, and LFTs.

### Patient & Family Education

- Report pregnancy to prescriber immediately.
- Allow between 2 and 4 wk for maximum therapeutic response.

## TEMAZEPAM
(te-maz′e-pam)
Restoril
**Classifications:** BENZODIAZEPINE; SEDATIVE-HYPNOTIC
Therapeutic: SEDATIVE
**Prototype:** Triazolam
**Controlled Substance:** Schedule IV

**AVAILABILITY** Capsule

## ACTION & *THERAPEUTIC EFFECT*
Believed to potentiate gamma-aminobutyric acid (GABA) neuronal inhibition. The sedative and anticonvulsant actions involve GABA receptors located in the limbic, neocortical, and mesencephalic reticular systems. *Reduces night awakenings and early morning awakenings; increases total sleep times, absence of rebound effects.*

**USES** To relieve insomnia.

**CONTRAINDICATIONS** Hypersensitivity reaction including angioedema; ethanol intoxication; drug abuse; narrow-angle glaucoma; psychoses; women of child-bearing age; abrupt discontinuation of temazepam; pregnancy (category X); lactation.

**CAUTIOUS USE** Severely depressed patient or one with suicidal thinking; history of drug abuse or dependence, acute intoxication; alcoholism; chronic pulmonary insufficiency; COPD; liver or kidney dysfunction; sleep apnea; debilitated individuals; older adults. Safe use in children younger than 18 y not established.

## ROUTE & DOSAGE

### Insomnia
*Adult:* **PO** 15–30 mg at bedtime
*Geriatric:* **PO** 7.5 mg at bedtime

## ADMINISTRATION

### Oral
- Give 20–30 min before bedtime.
- Store at 15°–30° C (59°–86° F) in tight container unless otherwise specified by manufacturer.

**ADVERSE EFFECTS** (≥1%) **CNS:** *Drowsiness,* dizziness, lethargy, confusion, headache, euphoria, relaxed feeling, weakness. **GI:** Anorexia, diarrhea. **CV:** Palpitations, *hypotension.* **Body as a Whole:** Physiological and psychological dependence.

**INTERACTIONS Drug: Alcohol,** CNS DEPRESSANTS, ANTICONVULSANTS potentiate CNS depression; **cimetidine** increases temazepam plasma levels, thus increasing its toxicity; may decrease antiparkinsonism effects of **levodopa;** may increase **phenytoin** levels; smoking decreases sedative effects. Do not use with **sodium oxybate. Herbal: Kava, valerian** may potentiate sedation.

Common adverse effects in *italic;* life-threatening effects <u>underlined;</u> generic names in **bold;** classifications in SMALL CAPS; ♣ Canadian drug name; ⊕ Prototype drug

T

**PHARMACOKINETICS** **Absorption:** Readily from GI tract; 98% protein bound. **Onset:** 30–50 min. **Peak:** 2–3 h. **Duration:** 10–12 h. **Distribution:** Crosses placenta; distributed into breast milk. **Metabolism:** In liver to oxazepam. **Elimination:** In urine. **Half-Life:** 8–24 h.

## NURSING IMPLICATIONS

### Assessment & Drug Effects

- Be alert to signs of paradoxical reaction (excitement, hyperactivity, and disorientation) in older adults. Psychoactive drugs are the most frequent cause of acute confusion in this age group.
- CNS adverse effects are more apt to occur in the patient with hypoalbuminemia, liver disease, and in older adults. Report promptly incidence of bradycardia, drowsiness, dizziness, clumsiness, lack of coordination. Supervise ambulation, especially at night.
- Be alert to S&S of overdose: Weakness, bradycardia, somnolence, confusion, slurred speech, ataxia, coma with reduced or absent reflexes, hypertension, and respiratory depression.

### Patient & Family Education

- Be aware that improvement in sleep will not occur until after 2–3 doses of drug.
- Notify prescriber if dreams or nightmares interfere with rest. An alternate drug or reduced dose may be prescribed.
- Be aware that difficulty getting to sleep may continue. Drug effect is evidenced by the increased amount of rest once asleep.
- Consult prescriber if insomnia continues in spite of medication.
- Do not smoke after medication is taken.

- Do not use OTC drugs (especially for insomnia) without advice of prescriber.
- Consult prescriber before discontinuing drug especially after long-term use. Gradual reduction of dose may be necessary to avoid withdrawal symptoms.
- Avoid use of alcohol and other CNS depressants.
- Do not drive or engage in other potentially hazardous activities until response to drug is known. This drug may depress psychomotor skills and cause sedation.

## TEMOZOLOMIDE
(tem-o-zol′o-mide)
Temodar
**Classifications:** ANTINEOPLASTIC; IMIDAZOTETRAZINE DERIVATIVE
Therapeutic: ANTINEOPLASTIC

**AVAILABILITY** Capsule; solution for injection

**ACTION & THERAPEUTIC EFFECT**
Cytotoxic agent with alkylating properties that are cell cycle nonspecific. Interferes with purine (e.g., guanine) metabolism and thus protein synthesis in rapidly proliferating cells. *Effectiveness is indicated by objective evidence of tumor regression.*

**USES** Adult patients with refractory anaplastic astrocytoma, glioblastoma multiforme with radiotherapy.

**UNLABELED USES** Malignant melanoma.

**CONTRAINDICATIONS** Hypersensitivity to temozolomide, or dacarbazine; severe bone marrow suppression; pregnancy (category D); lactation.

**CAUTIOUS USE** Bacterial or viral infection; severe hepatic or renal impairment; myelosuppression; prior

T

Common adverse effects in *italic;* life-threatening effects <u>underlined;</u> generic names in **bold;** classifications in SMALL CAPS; ♦ Canadian drug name; ⊘ Prototype drug

1563

radiotherapy or chemotherapy; older adults; children younger than 3 y.

## ROUTE & DOSAGE

### Astrocytoma

*Adult:* **PO/IV** 150 mg/m² daily days 1–5/28-day treatment cycle (may increase to 200 mg/m²/ day); subsequent doses are based on absolute neutrophil count on day 21 or at least 48 h before next scheduled cycle (see prescribing information for dosage adjustments based on neutrophil count)

### Glioblastoma Multiforme

*Adult:* **PO** 75 mg/m² daily for 42 days with focal radiotherapy; after 4 wk, maintenance phase of 150–200 mg/m² on days 1–5 of 28-day cycle

## ADMINISTRATION

### Oral

- Give consistently with regard to food.
- Do not administer unless absolute neutrophil count greater than 1500/microliter and platelet count greater than 100,000/microliter.
- Do not open capsules. Avoid inhalation or contact with skin or mucous membranes, if accidentally opened/damaged.
- Store at room temperature, 15°–30° C (59°–86° F).

### Intravenous

*PREPARE:* **Infusion:** Bring the 100 mg vial to room temperature, then reconstitute with 41 mL sterile water to yield 2.5 mg/mL. Gently swirl to dissolve but do not shake, and do not further dilute. Must use within 14 h of reconstitution, including infusion time.

*ADMINISTER:* **Infusion:** Infuse over 90 min. Flush line before and after with NS. Note: May be administered in the same line with NS but not with any other IV solution.

## ADVERSE EFFECTS (≥1%) **Body as a Whole:** *Headache, fatigue, asthenia, fever,* back pain, myalgia, weight gain; viral infection. **CNS:** *Convulsions, hemiparesis, dizziness, abnormal coordination, amnesia, insomnia,* paresthesia, somnolence, paresis, ataxia, dysphasia, abnormal gait, confusion, anxiety, depression. **CV:** *Peripheral edema.* **GI:** *Nausea, vomiting, constipation, diarrhea,* abdominal pain, anorexia. **Hematologic:** Anemia, <u>neutropenia</u>, <u>thrombocytopenia</u>, <u>leukopenia</u>, lymphopenia. **Respiratory:** Upper respiratory tract infection, pharyngitis, sinusitis, cough. **Skin:** Rash, pruritus. **Metabolic:** Adrenal hypercorticism. **Urogenital:** Urinary incontinence. **Special Senses:** Diplopia, abnormal vision.

## INTERACTIONS **Drug:** Valproic acid may decrease **temozolomide** levels.

## PHARMACOKINETICS **Absorption:** Rapidly. **Peak:** 1 h. **Metabolism:** Spontaneously metabolized to active metabolite MTIC. **Elimination:** Primarily in urine. **Half-Life:** 1.8 h.

## NURSING IMPLICATIONS

### Assessment & Drug Effects

- Monitor for S&S of toxicity: Infection, bleeding episodes, jaundice, rash, CNS disturbances.
- Monitor lab tests: Periodic CBC with differential and platelet count; periodic LFTs and routine serum chemistry, including serum calcium.

**Patient & Family Education**

- Take consistently with respect to meals.
- Report to prescriber signs of infection, bleeding, discoloration of skin or skin rash, dizziness, lack of balance, or other bothersome side effects promptly.
- Exercise caution with hazardous activities until response to drug is known.
- Use effective methods of contraception; avoid pregnancy.

# TEMSIROLIMUS

(tem-si-ro-li′mus)

Torisel

**Classifications:** BIOLOGIC RESPONSE MODIFIER; ANTINEO-PLASTIC; KINASE INHIBITOR; mTOR INHIBITOR
**Therapeutic:** ANTINEOPLASTIC
**Prototype:** Erlotinib

**AVAILABILITY** Injectable

**ACTION & *THERAPEUTIC EFFECT***

Inhibits an intracellular protein that controls cell division in renal carcinoma and other tumor cells. *Results in arrest of growth in tumor cells.*

**USES** Treatment of advanced renal cell carcinoma.

**UNLABELED USES** Astrocytoma, mantle cell lymphoma (MCL).

**CONTRAINDICATIONS** Hypersensitivity reaction including anaphylaxis; live vaccines; intracranial bleeding; bilirubin greater than 1.5 X ULN; interstitial lung disease; bowel perforation; acute renal failure; pregnancy (category D); lactation.

**CAUTIOUS USE** Hypersensitivity to temsirolimus, sirolimus, or polysorbate 80; renal impairment; DM; hyperlipemia; respiratory disorders; perioperative period due to potential for abnormal wound healing; CNS tumors (primary or by metastasis); hepatic impairment; older adults; children.

## ROUTE & DOSAGE

**Renal Cell Carcinoma**

*Adult:* **IV** 25 mg qwk

**Dosage Adjustment**

*Regimen with a strong CYP3A4 inhibitor:* 12.5 mg/wk
*Regimen with a strong CYP3A4 inducer:* 50 mg based on tolerability

**Hepatic Impairment Adjustment**

Dose reduction required

## ADMINISTRATION

**Intravenous**

Patients should receive prophylactic IV diphenhydramine 25–50 mg (or similar antihistamine) 30 min before each dose.

***PREPARE:* IV Infusion:** Inject 1.8 mL of supplied diluent into the 25 mg/mL vial to yield 10 mg/mL. ▪ Withdraw the required dose and inject rapidly into a 250 mL DEHP-free container of NS. Invert to mix.

***ADMINISTER:* IV Infusion:** Use DEHP-free infusion line with a 5 micron or less in-line filter. ▪ Infuse over 30–60 min. ▪ Complete infusion within 6 h of preparation.

***INCOMPATIBILITIES:* Solution/additive:** Do not add other drugs or agents to temsirolimus IV solutions.

---

Common adverse effects in *italic;* life-threatening effects underlined; generic names in **bold;** classifications in SMALL CAPS; ♣ Canadian drug name; ⊘ Prototype drug

T

■ Store at 2°–8° C (36°–46° F). Protect from light. The 10 mg/mL drug solution is stable for up to 24 h at 15°–30° C (59°–86° F).

## ADVERSE EFFECTS (≥1%) Body as a Whole: Allergic/hypersensitivity reactions, *asthenia,* chest pain, chills, *edema,* impaired wound healing, infections, pain, pyrexia. CNS: Depression, dysgeusia, headache, insomnia. CV: Hypertension, thrombophlebitis, venous thromboembolism. GI: Abdominal pain, *anorexia,* constipation, diarrhea, fatal bowel perforation, *mucositis, nausea,* vomiting. Hematologic: Decrease hemoglobin, *leukocytopenia, lymphopenia,* neutropenia, <u>thrombocytopenia</u>. Metabolic: *Elevated alkaline phosphatase, elevated AST, elevated serum creatinine,* hypokalemia, *hypophosphatemia,* hyperbilirubinemia, *hypercholesterolemia, hyperglycemia, hypertriglyceridemia,* weight loss. Musculoskeletal: Arthralgia, back pain, myalgia. Respiratory: Cough, dyspnea, epistaxis, interstitial lung disease, pharyngitis, pneumonia, rhinitis, upper respiratory tract infection. Skin: Acne, dry skin, nail disorder, pruritus, *rash*. Special Senses: Conjunctivitis. Urogenital: Urinary tract infection.

## INTERACTIONS Drug: AZOLE ANTIFUNGAL AGENTS (fluconazole, itraconazole, ketoconazole, posaconazole, voriconazole), cyclosporine, INHIBITORS OF CYP3A4 (HIV PROTEASE INHIBITORS, clarithromycin, diltiazem), mycophenolate mofetil, and sunitinib increase the plasma levels of temsirolimus. INDUCERS OF CYP3A4 (dexamethasone, rifampin, rifabutin, phenytoin) decrease the plasma level of temsirolimus. Food: Grapefruit and grapefruit juice increase the plasma level of temsirolimus. Herbal: St. John's wort decreases the plasma level of temsirolimus.

## PHARMACOKINETICS Peak: 0.5–2 h. Metabolism: In liver. Elimination: Primarily in stool. Half-Life: 17.3 h.

## NURSING IMPLICATIONS

### Assessment & Drug Effects
■ Withhold drug and notify prescriber for absolute neutrophil count less than 1000/mm³ or platelet count less than 75,000/mm³.
■ Monitor for infusion-related reactions during and for at least 1 h after completion of infusion.
■ Slow or stop infusion for infusion-related reactions. If infusion is restarted after 30–60 min of observation, slow rate to up to 60 min and continue observation.
■ Monitor respiratory status and report promptly dyspnea, cough, S&S of hypoxia, fever.
■ Monitor diabetics for loss of glycemic control.
■ Monitor lab tests: Baseline and periodic CBC with differential and platelet count, lipid profile, LFTs, alkaline phosphatase, renal function tests, serum electrolytes, plasma glucose, and ABGs.

### Patient & Family Education
■ Avoid live vaccines and close contact with those who have received live vaccines.
■ Use effective contraceptive measures to prevent pregnancy.
■ Men with partners of childbearing age should use reliable contraception throughout treatment and for 3 mo after the last dose of temsirolimus.
■ Report promptly any of the following: S&S of infection, difficulty

breathing, abdominal pain, blood in stools, abnormal wound healing, S&S of hypersensitivity (see Appendix F).

# TENECTEPLASE RECOMBINANT

(ten-ect′e-plase)

TNKase

**Classification:** THROMBOLYTIC ENZYME, TISSUE PLASMINOGEN ACTIVATOR (t PA)
Therapeutic: THROMBOLYTIC ENZYME
**Prototype:** Alteplase

## AVAILABILITY Vial

## ACTION & *THERAPEUTIC EFFECT*
Activates plasminogen, a substance created by endothelial cells in response to arterial wall injury that contributes to clot formation. Plasminogen is converted to plasmin which breaks down the fibrin mesh that binds the clot together, thus dissolving the clot. *Effective in producing thrombolysis of a clot involved in a myocardial infarction.*

## USES Reduction of mortality associated with acute myocardial infarction (AMI).

## CONTRAINDICATIONS Active internal bleeding; history of CVA; intracranial or intraspinal surgery with 2 mo; intracranial neoplasm; arteriovenous malformation, or aneurysm; known bleeding diathesis; brain tumor; increased intracranial pressure; coagulopathy; head trauma; stroke; surgery; severe uncontrolled hypertension; lactation.

## CAUTIOUS USE Recent major surgery, previous puncture of compressible vessels, CVA, recent GI or GU bleeding, recent trauma; hypertension, mitral valve stenosis, acute pericarditis, bacterial endocarditis; severe liver or kidney disease; hemorrhagic ophthalmic conditions; septic thrombophlebitis or occluded, infected AV cannula; advanced age; pregnancy (category C). Safety and efficacy in children not established.

## ROUTE & DOSAGE

**Acute Myocardial Infarction**

*Adult (weight less than 60 kg):* **IV** Infuse dose over 5 sec 30 mg; *weight 60–70 kg:* 35 mg; *weight 70–80 kg:* 40 mg; *weight 80–90 kg:* 45 mg; *weight greater than 90 kg:* 50 mg

## ADMINISTRATION

Intravenous

*PREPARE:* **Direct:** Read and follow instructions supplied with TwinPak™ Dual Cannula Device. ▪ Withdraw 10 mL of sterile water for injection from the supplied vial; inject entire contents into the TNKase vial directing the diluent stream into the powder. ▪ Gently swirl until dissolved but do not shake. The resulting solution contains 5 mg/mL. ▪ Withdraw the appropriate dose and discard any unused solution. ▪ Follow directions supplied with TwinPak™ for proper handling of syringe.
*ADMINISTER:* **Direct:** Dextrose-containing IV line **must be** flushed before and after bolus with NS. ▪ Give as a single bolus dose over 5 sec. ▪ The total dose given should not exceed 50 mg.
*INCOMPATIBILITIES:* **Solution/additive: Dextrose** solutions.

Common adverse effects in *italic;* life-threatening effects underlined; generic names in **bold;** classifications in SMALL CAPS; ♣ Canadian drug name; ⊕ Prototype drug

1567

▪ Store unopened TwinPak™ at or below 30° C (86° F) or under refrigeration at 2°–8° C (36°–46° F).

## ADVERSE EFFECTS (≥1%) Hematologic: <u>Major bleeding</u>, *hematoma*, GI bleed, bleeding at puncture site, hematuria, pharyngeal, epistaxis.

## DIAGNOSTIC TEST INTERFERENCE
Unreliable results for *coagulation test I* and measures of *fibrinolytic activity.*

## PHARMACOKINETICS Metabolism: In liver. Half-Life: 90–130 min.

## NURSING IMPLICATIONS
### Assessment & Drug Effects
▪ Avoid IM injections and unnecessary handling or invasive procedures for the first few hours after treatment.
▪ Monitor for S&S of bleeding. Should bleeding occur, withhold concomitant heparin and antiplatelet therapy; notify prescriber.
▪ Monitor cardiovascular and neurologic status closely. Persons at increased risk for life-threatening cardiac events include those with: A high potential for bleeding, recent surgery, severe hypertension, mitral stenosis and atrial fibrillation, anticoagulant therapy, and advanced age.
▪ Coagulation parameters may not predict bleeding episodes.

### Patient & Family Education
▪ Notify prescriber of the following immediately: A sudden, severe headache; any sign of bleeding; signs or symptoms of hypersensitivity (see Appendix F).
▪ Stay as still as possible and do not attempt to get out of bed until directed to do so.

# TENOFOVIR DISOPROXIL FUMARATE
(ten-o-fo'vir dy-so-prox'il fum'a-rate)
Viread
**Classifications:** ANTIRETROVIRAL; NUCLEOSIDE REVERSE TRANSCRIPTASE INHIBITOR (NRTI)
Therapeutic: ANTIRETROVIRAL; NRTI
**Prototype:** Zidovudine

## AVAILABILITY Tablet; oral powder

## ACTION & *THERAPEUTIC EFFECT*
A potent inhibitor of retroviruses, including HIV-1. The active form of tenofovir persists in HIV-infected cells for prolonged periods, thus, it results in sustained inhibition of HIV replication. *It reduces the viral load (plasma HIV-RNA), and CD4 counts.*

## USES In combination with other antiretrovirals for the treatment of HIV; chronic hepatitis B infection.

## CONTRAINDICATIONS Hypersensitivity to tenofovir; lactic acidosis, severe hepatomegaly, concurrent administration of nephrotoxic agents, acute renal failure; immune reconstitution syndrome; lactation.

## CAUTIOUS USE Hepatic dysfunction, alcoholism; renal impairment; obesity; low body weight; pathologic bone fractures; older adults; pregnancy (category B); children.

## ROUTE & DOSAGE

### HIV Infection
*Adult/Adolescent:* **PO** 300 mg once daily with meal

*Child:* **PO** See package insert for weight based dose (approx. 8 mg/kg daily)

**Chronic Hepatitis B**

*Adult/Child (12 y or older, weight 35 kg):* **PO** 300 mg daily

**Renal Impairment Dosage Adjustment**

*CrCl 30–49 mL/min:* Dose q48h; *10–29 mL/min:* Dose twice weekly

**Hemodialysis Dosage Adjustment** Dose weekly or after 12 h of dialysis

## ADMINISTRATION

### Oral

▪ Give at the same time each day with a meal.

▪ Measure powder form only with supplied dosing scoop. One level scoop contains 40 mg of tenofovir. Mix powder in 2–4 oz of soft food such as applesauce or yogurt (do not mix with liquid). Give immediately after mixing to avoid bitter taste.

▪ Give 2 h before or 1 h after didanosine (if ordered concurrently).

▪ Store at room temperature; excursions to 15°–30° C (59°–80° F) are permitted.

## ADVERSE EFFECTS (≥1%) **Body as a Whole:** Asthenia, *pruritus.* **CNS:** Headache. **GI:** *Nausea,* vomiting, diarrhea, flatulence, abdominal pain, anorexia. **Hematologic:** Neutropenia. **Metabolic:** Increased *creatine kinase,* AST, ALT, serum amylase, triglycerides, serum glucose.

## INTERACTIONS **Drug:** May increase **didanosine** toxicity; **acyclovir, amphotericin B, cidofovir, foscarnet, ganciclovir, probenecid, valacyclovir,** **valganciclovir** may increase tenofovir toxicity by decreasing its renal elimination. **Food:** Food increases absorption.

## PHARMACOKINETICS **Absorption:** Bioavailability 25% fasting, 40% with high fat meal. **Peak:** 1 h. **Distribution:** Less than 7% protein bound. **Metabolism:** Not metabolized by CYP450 enzyme system. **Elimination:** Renally eliminated. **Half-Life:** 11–14 h.

## NURSING IMPLICATIONS

### Black Box Warning

*Tenofovir has been associated with lactic acidosis and severe, sometimes fatal, hepatomegaly with steatosis, and with posttreatment exacerbation of hepatitis.*

### Assessment & Drug Effects

▪ Withhold drug and notify prescriber if patient develops clinical or lab findings suggestive of lactic acidosis or pronounced hepatotoxicity (e.g., hepatomegaly and steatosis even in the absence of marked transaminase elevations).

▪ Monitor for S&S of bone abnormalities (e.g., bone pain, stress fractures).

▪ Monitor closely patients receiving other nephrotoxic agents for changes in serum creatinine and phosphorus. Withhold drug and notify prescriber for creatinine clearance less than 60 mL/min.

▪ Monitor lab tests: Baseline and periodic renal function tests and LFTs; periodic serum electrolytes, and ABGs if lactic acidosis is suspected.

### Patient & Family Education

▪ Take this drug exactly as prescribed. Do not miss any doses. If you miss a dose, take it as soon as possible and then take your next

**T**

---

Common adverse effects in *italic;* life-threatening effects <u>underlined</u>; generic names in **bold**; classifications in SMALL CAPS; ✦ Canadian drug name; ◕ Prototype drug dose at its regular time. If it is almost time for your next dose, do not take the missed dose. Wait and take the next dose at the regular time. Do not double the next dose.

- Report any of the following to prescriber: Unexplained anorexia, nausea, vomiting, abdominal pain, fatigue, dark urine.

# TERAZOSIN

(ter-ay′zoe-sin)

**Classifications:** ALPHA-ADRENERGIC RECEPTOR ANTAGONIST; ANTIHYPERTENSIVE

Therapeutic: ANTIHYPERTENSIVE; BPH AGENT

**Prototype:** Prazosin

## AVAILABILITY Capsule

## ACTION & *THERAPEUTIC EFFECT*

Selectively blocks alpha$_1$-adrenergic receptors in vascular smooth muscle in many tissues, including the bladder neck and the prostate. Promotes vasodilation, thus producing relaxation that leads to reduction of peripheral vascular resistance and lowered BP as well as increased urine flow. *Effectiveness is measured in lowering of blood pressure values and controlling the symptoms of benign prostate hypertrophy.*

## USES To treat hypertension alone or in combination with other antihypertensive agents. To treat benign prostatic hypertrophy (BPH) and urinary flow obstruction.

## CONTRAINDICATIONS Hypersensitivity to terazosin.

## CAUTIOUS USE Prostate cancer; history of hypotensive episodes; angina; renal impairment, renal disease, renal failure; older adults; pregnancy (category C);

lactation. Safe use in children is not established.

## ROUTE & DOSAGE

**Hypertension**

*Adult:* **PO** Start with 1 mg at bedtime then increase to 1–5 mg once daily

**Benign Prostatic Hypertrophy**

*Adult:* **PO** Start with 1 mg at bedtime, then 1–10 mg/day (max: 20 mg/day)

## ADMINISTRATION

### Oral

- Give initial dose at bedtime to reduce the potential for severe hypotensive effect. After the initial dose, give any time of day.
- Store at 15°–30° C (59°–86° F) in tightly closed container away from heat and strong light. Do not freeze.

## ADVERSE EFFECTS (≥1%) CNS: *Asthenia (weakness), dizziness, headache,* drowsiness, weakness. **CV:** Postural hypotension, palpitation, *first-dose phenomenon (syncope).* **Special Senses:** Blurred vision. **GI:** *Nausea.* **Body as a Whole:** Weight gain, pain in extremities, peripheral edema. **Respiratory:** *Nasal congestion,* sinusitis, dyspnea. **Urogenital:** Impotence.

## INTERACTIONS Drug: Antihypertensive effects may be attenuated by NSAIDs. **Sildenafil, vardenafil,** and **tadalafil** may enhance hypotensive effects. Avoid use of **alfuzosin** or **tranylcypromine** due to increased hypotension.

## PHARMACOKINETICS Absorption: Readily from GI tract (90–94% protein bound). **Peak:** 1–2 h. **Metabolism:** In liver. **Elimination:**

Common adverse effects in *italic*; life-threatening effects <u>underlined</u>; generic names in **bold**; classifications in SMALL CAPS; ♣ Canadian drug name; ⊘ Prototype drug

60% in feces, 40% in urine. **Half-Life:** 9–12 h.

## NURSING IMPLICATIONS

### Assessment & Drug Effects

- Be alert for possible first-dose phenomenon (precipitous decline in BP with consciousness disturbance). This is rare; occurs within 90–120 min of initial dose.
- Monitor BP at end of dosing interval (just before next dose) to determine level of antihypertensive control.
- Be aware that drug-induced decrease in BP appears to be more position dependent (i.e., greater in the erect position) during the first few hours after dosing than at end of 24 h.
- A greatly diminished hypotensive response at end of 24 h indicates need for change in dosage (increased dose or twice daily regimen). Report to prescriber.

### Patient & Family Education

- Avoid situations that would result in injury should syncope (loss of consciousness) occur after first dose. If faintness develops, lie down promptly.
- Make position changes slowly (i.e., change in direction or from recumbent to upright posture). Dangle legs and move ankles a minute or so before standing when arising. Orthostatic hypotension (greatest shortly after dosing) can pose a problem with ambulation.
- Do not drive or engage in potentially hazardous activities for at least 12 h after first dose, after dosage increase, or when treatment is resumed after interruption of therapy.
- Monitor weight: Report sudden gain of more than 0.5–1 kg (1–2 lb) accompanied by edema in extremities to prescriber. Dose adjustment may be indicated.

- Do not alter established drug regimen. Consult prescriber if drug is omitted for several days. Drug will be started with the initial dosing regimen.
- Keep scheduled appointments for assessment of BP control and other clinically significant tests.
- Do not take OTC medications, particularly those that may contain an adrenergic agent (e.g., remedies for coughs, colds, allergy) without first consulting prescriber.

## TERBINAFINE HYDROCHLORIDE ⓟ

(ter-bin'a-feen)

**Lamisil, Lamisil DermaGel**

**Classifications:** ANTIBIOTIC; ANTIFUNGAL

**Therapeutic:** ANTIFUNGAL

**AVAILABILITY** Tablet; cream; gel

### ACTION & *THERAPEUTIC EFFECT*

Synthetic antifungal agent that inhibits sterol biosynthesis in fungi and ultimately causes fungal cell death. *Effective as an antifungal.*

**USES** Topical treatment of superficial mycoses such as interdigital tinea pedis, tinea cruris, and tinea corporis; oral treatment of onychomycosis due to tinea unguium.

**CONTRAINDICATIONS** Hypersensitivity to terbinafine; alcoholism; hepatic disease; hepatitis; jaundice; renal impairment; renal failure; lactation.

**CAUTIOUS USE** History of depression; pregnancy (category B). Safety and efficacy in children younger than 12 y not established.

Common adverse effects in *italic;* life-threatening effects <u>underlined</u>; generic names in **bold;** classifications in SMALL CAPS; ◆ Canadian drug name; ⓟ Prototype drug

1571

## ROUTE & DOSAGE

### Tinea Pedis, Tinea Cruris, or Tinea Corporis

*Adult:* **Topical** Apply daily or b.i.d. to affected and immediately surrounding areas until clinical signs and symptoms are significantly improved (1–7 wk)

### Onychomycosis

*Adult:* **PO** 250 mg daily × 6 wk for fingernails or × 12 wk for toenails

## ADMINISTRATION

### Oral

- Give tablets without regard to meals.
- Granules should be given with food. Sprinkle on a spoonful of soft, nonacidic food; do not mix granules with applesauce or other fruit-based foods. Entire spoonful should be swallowed without chewing.

### Topical

- Apply externally. Avoid application to mucous membranes and avoid contact with eyes.
- Do not use occlusive dressings unless specifically directed to do so by prescriber.
- Store at 15°–30° C (59°–86° F).

## ADVERSE EFFECTS (≥1%) **Skin:**
Pruritus, local burning, dryness, rash, vesiculation, redness, contact dermatitis at application site. **CNS:** *Headache.* **GI:** Diarrhea, dyspepsia, abdominal pain, liver test abnormalities, liver failure (rare). **Hematologic:** Neutropenia (rare). **Special Senses:** Taste disturbances, vision impairment.

## INTERACTIONS **Drug:** May increase **theophylline** levels; may decrease **cyclosporine** levels; **rifampin** may decrease **terbinafine** levels.

## PHARMACOKINETICS **Absorption:** 70% PO; approximately 3.5% of topical dose is absorbed systemically. **Elimination:** In urine. **Half-Life:** 36 h.

## NURSING IMPLICATIONS

### Assessment & Drug Effects

- Monitor for and report increased skin irritation.

### Patient & Family Education

- Learn correct technique for application of cream.
- Notify prescriber if drug causes increased skin irritation or sensitivity.
- Be aware that medication **must be** used for full treatment time to be effective.

# TERBUTALINE SULFATE
(ter-byoo′te-leen)
**Classifications:** BETA-ADRENERGIC RECEPTOR AGONIST; BRONCHO-DILATOR
Therapeutic: RESPIRATORY SMOOTH MUSCLE RELAXANT; BRONCHODILATOR
**Prototype:** Albuterol

## AVAILABILITY Tablet; solution for injection

## ACTION & *THERAPEUTIC EFFECT*
Synthetic adrenergic stimulant with selective beta$_2$-receptor activity in bronchial smooth muscles, inhibits histamine release from mast cells, and increases ciliary motility. *Relieves bronchospasm in chronic obstructive pulmonary disease (COPD) and significantly increases vital capacity. Increases uterine relaxation (thereby preventing or abolishing high intrauterine pressure).*

Common adverse effects in *italic;* life-threatening effects <u>underlined;</u> generic names in **bold;** classifications in SMALL CAPS; ◆ Canadian drug name; ● Prototype drug

**USES** Asthma, prevention and reversal of bronchospasm.

**UNLABELED USES** To delay delivery in preterm labor (FDA warns avoid use for this purpose).

**CONTRAINDICATIONS** Known hypersensitivity to sympathomimetic amines; severe hypertension and coronary artery disease; tachycardia with digitalis intoxication; within 14 days of MAO inhibitor therapy; angle-closure glaucoma; acute or maintenance tocolysis; prolonged use during preterm labor.

**CAUTIOUS USE** Angina, stroke, hypertension; DM; thyrotoxicosis; history of seizure disorders; MAOI therapy; cardiac arrhythmias; QT prolongation; thyroid disease; older adults; kidney and liver dysfunction; pregnancy (category C). Use caution in second and third trimester (may inhibit uterine contractions and labor). Children younger than 12 y.

## ROUTE & DOSAGE

### Bronchodilator

*Adult/Adolescent (15 y or older):*
**PO** 5 mg t.i.d. at 6 h intervals (max: 15 mg/day); **Subcutaneous** 0.25 mg q15–30min up to 0.5 mg in 4 h
*Adolescent (12–15 y):* **PO** 2.5 mg t.i.d. at 6 h intervals (max: 7.5 mg/day); **Subcutaneous** 0.25 mg q15–30min up to 0.5 mg in 4 h

## ADMINISTRATION

### Oral

- Give with fluid of patient's choice; tablets may be crushed.
- Be certain about recommended doses: PO preparation, 2.5 mg;

subcutaneous, 0.25 mg. A decimal point error can be fatal.
- Give with food if GI symptoms occur.

### Subcutaneous

- Give subcutaneous injection into lateral deltoid area.
- Store all forms at 15°–30° C (59°–86° F); protect from light. Do not freeze.

**ADVERSE EFFECTS** (≥1%) **CNS:** *Nervousness, tremor,* headache, *light-headedness,* drowsiness, fatigue, seizures. **CV:** *Tachycardia,* hypotension or hypertension, *palpitation,* maternal and fetal tachycardia. **GI:** Nausea, vomiting. **Body as a Whole:** Sweating, muscle cramps.

**DIAGNOSTIC TEST INTERFERENCE** Terbutaline may increase *blood glucose* and free *fatty acids.*

**INTERACTIONS Drug:** Epinephrine, other SYMPATHOMIMETIC BRONCHODILATORS may add to effects; MAO INHIBITORS, TRICYCLIC ANTIDEPRESSANTS potentiate action on vascular system, effects of both BETA-ADRENERGIC BLOCKERS and terbutaline antagonized.

**PHARMACOKINETICS Absorption:** 33–50% from GI tract. **Onset:** 30 min PO; less than 15 min subcutaneous; 5–30 min inhaled. **Peak:** 2–3 h PO; 30–60 min subcutaneous; 1–2 h inhaled. **Duration:** 4–8 h PO; 1.5–4 h subcutaneous; 3–4 h inhaled. **Distribution:** Into breast milk. **Metabolism:** In liver. **Elimination:** Primarily in urine, 3% in feces. **Half-Life:** 3–4 h.

## NURSING IMPLICATIONS

### Black Box Warning

*Terbutaline has been associated with serious, sometimes fatal, adverse reactions in pregnant women*

Common adverse effects in *italic;* life-threatening effects underlined; generic names in **bold;** classifications in SMALL CAPS; ♣ Canadian drug name; ● Prototype drug

1573

*including cardiac arrhythmias, myocardial ischemia, hypokalemia, and pulmonary edema.*

## Assessment & Drug Effects

- Assess vital signs: Baseline pulse and BP and before each dose. If significantly altered from baseline level, consult prescriber. Cardiovascular adverse effects are more apt to occur when drug is given by subcutaneous route or it is used by a patient with cardiac arrhythmia.
- Most adverse effects are transient, however, rapid heart rate may persist for a relatively long time.
- Aerosolized drug produces minimal cardiac stimulation or tremors.
- Be aware that muscle tremor is a fairly common adverse effect that appears to subside with continued use.
- Monitor patient being treated for premature labor for CV S&S for 12 h after drug is discontinued. Report tachycardia promptly.
- Monitor I&O ratio. Fluid restriction may be necessary. Consult prescriber.

## Patient & Family Education

- Inhalator therapy: Review instructions for use of inhalator (included in the package).
- Learn how to take your own pulse and the limits of change that indicate need to notify the prescriber.
- Consult prescriber if breathing difficulty is not relieved or if it becomes worse within 30 min after an oral dose.
- Consult prescriber if symptomatic relief wanes; tolerance can develop with chronic use.
- Do not self-dose this drug, particularly during long-term therapy. In the face of waning response, increasing the dose will not improve the clinical condition and may cause overdosage.

Understand that decreasing relief with continued treatment indicates need for another bronchodilator, not an increase in dose.

- Do not puncture container, use or store it near heat or open flame, or expose to temperatures above 49° C (120° F), which may cause bursting. Contents of the aerosol (inhalator) are under pressure.
- Do not use any other aerosol bronchodilator while being treated with aerosol terbutaline. Do not self-medicate with an OTC aerosol.
- Do not use OTC drugs without prescriber approval. Many cold and allergy remedies, for example, contain a sympathomimetic agent that when combined with terbutaline may cause harmful adverse effects.

# TERCONAZOLE

(ter-con'a-zole)
Terazol 7, Terazol 3
**Classification:** AZOLE ANTIFUNGAL
Therapeutic: VAGINAL ANTIFUNGAL
**Prototype:** Fluconazole

## AVAILABILITY Vaginal cream; vaginal suppository

## ACTION & *THERAPEUTIC EFFECT*

Thought to exert antifungal activity by disruption of normal fungal cell membrane permeability. *Exhibits fungicidal activity against Candida albicans.*

## USES Local treatment of vulvovaginal candidiasis.

## CONTRAINDICATIONS Hypersensitivity to terconazole or azole antifungals; use of tampons; lactation.

## CAUTIOUS USE Pregnancy (category C). Safety and efficacy in

children younger than 18 y not established.

## ROUTE & DOSAGE

### Candidiasis

*Adult:* **Intravaginal** One suppository (2.5 g) each night × 3 days; one applicator full of 0.4% cream each night × 7 days; one applicator full of 0.8% cream each night × 3 days

## ADMINISTRATION

### Intravaginal

- Insert applicator high into the vagina (except during pregnancy).
- Wash applicator before and after each use.
- Store away from direct heat and light.

## ADVERSE EFFECTS (≥1%) CNS:
*Headache.* **Urogenital:** Vaginal itching, burning, irritation. **Body as a Whole:** Rash, flu-like syndrome (fever, chills, headache, hypotension).

## INTERACTIONS Drug: May inactivate **nonoxynol-9** spermicides.

## PHARMACOKINETICS Absorption: Slow minimal absorption from vagina. **Onset:** Within 3 days. **Metabolism:** In liver. **Elimination:** Half in urine, half in feces. **Half-Life:** 4–11 h.

## NURSING IMPLICATIONS

### Assessment & Drug Effects

- Do not use if patient has a history of allergic reaction to other antifungal agents, such as miconazole.
- Monitor for sensitization and irritation; these may indicate need to discontinue drug.

### Patient & Family Education

- Use correct application technique.
- Do not use tampons concurrently with terconazole.

- Learn potential adverse reactions, including sensitization and allergic response.
- Be aware that terconazole may interact with diaphragms and latex condoms; avoid concurrent use within 72 h.
- Refrain from sexual intercourse while using terconazole.
- Wear only cotton underwear; change daily.

## TERIFLUNOMIDE
(ter-i-flu'no-mide)

Aubagio

**Classification:** IMMUNOMODULATOR; PYRIMIDINE SYNTHESIS INHIBITOR; ANTI-INFLAMMATORY
**Therapeutic:** IMMUNOMODULATOR; ANTI-INFLAMMATORY

## AVAILABILITY Tablet

## ACTION & *THERAPEUTIC EFFECT*
An immunomodulatory agent with anti-inflammatory properties; exact mechanism of action unknown, but may involve a reduction in the number of activated lymphocytes in the CNS. *Reduces the number of MS relapses.*

## USES Treatment of patients with relapsing forms of multiple sclerosis.

## CONTRAINDICATIONS Severe liver impairment; coadministration with leflunomide; acute renal failure; pregnancy (category X); lactation.

## CAUTIOUS USE Pre-existing liver disease; myelosuppression; serious infections; DM; history of peripheral neuropathy; hypertension. Safety and efficacy in children younger than 18 y not established.

**T**

Common adverse effects in *italic;* life-threatening effects underlined; generic names in **bold;** classifications in SMALL CAPS; ◆ Canadian drug name; ❷ Prototype drug

1575

## ROUTE & DOSAGE

**Multiple Sclerosis**
*Adult:* **PO** 7 or 14 mg once daily

## ADMINISTRATION

**Oral**
- May give with or without food.
- Store at 15°–30° C (59°–86° F).

**ADVERSE EFFECTS** (≥2%) **Body as a Whole:** *Influenza*, oral herpes, seasonal allergy. **CNS:** Anxiety, burning sensation, carpal tunnel syndrome, headache, *paraesthesia*, sciatica. **CV:** Palpitations. **GI:** Abdominal distension, *diarrhea*, *nausea*, toothache, upper abdominal pain, viral gastroenteritis. **Hematological:** <u>Leukopenia, neutropenia.</u> **Metabolic:** ALT and AST increased, gamma-glutamyltransferase increased, hypophosphatemia, neutrophil count decreased, white blood cell count decreased <u>hepatotoxicity.</u> **Musculoskeletal:** Musculoskeletal pain, myalgia. **Respiratory:** Bronchitis, sinusitis, upper respiratory tract infection. **Skin:** Acne, *alopecia*, pruritus. **Special Senses:** Blurred vision, conjunctivitis. **Urogenital:** Cystitis.

**INTERACTIONS Drug:** Teriflunomide may increase the levels of other drugs requiring CYP2C8 for metabolism (e.g., **paclitaxel, pioglitazone, repaglinide, rosiglitazone**) and may decrease the levels of other drugs requiring CYP1A2 for metabolism (e.g., **alosetron, duloxetine, theophylline, tizanidine**). Teriflunomide may decrease the effectiveness of **warfarin.** Teriflunomide can increase the levels of **ethinylestradiol** and **levonorgestrel.**

**PHARMACOKINETICS Peak:** 1–4 h. **Distribution:** Greater than 99% plasma protein bound. **Metabolism:** Primarily unchanged in liver. **Elimination:** Fecal (61%) and renal (23%). **Half-Life:** 18–19 d.

## NURSING IMPLICATIONS

### Black Box Warning

*Teriflunomide has been associated with severe liver injury, including fatal liver failure; it has also been associated with major birth defects.*

### Assessment & Drug Effects
- Monitor BP especially in those with a history of hypertension.
- Monitor for and report promptly S&S of hepatotoxicity (see Appendix F). Withhold drug until prescriber consulted if hepatotoxicity suspected.
- Assess for peripheral neuropathy (e.g., bilateral numbness or tingling of hands or feet) and S&S of hypokalemia (see Appendix F).
- Monitor lab tests: Baseline (within last 6 mo before beginning therapy) CBC with differential and LFTs; monthly LFTs for next 6 mo or more often when given with other potentially hepatotoxic drugs.

### Patient & Family Education
- Report promptly any of the following: Numbness or tingling of hands or feet; unexplained nausea, vomiting, or abdominal pain; fatigue; anorexia; jaundice and/or dark urine; fever.
- Consult with prescriber before accepting a vaccination during and for 6 mo following termination of therapy.
- Women should use effective contraception during treatment and until completion of an accelerated, drug-elimination procedure.

▪ Men should instruct their female partners to use reliable contraception. Those who wish to father a child should discontinue the drug and request an accelerated drug-elimination procedure.

# TERIPARATIDE
(ter-i-par'a-tide)
Forteo
**Classification:** PARATHYROID HORMONE AGONIST
**Therapeutic:** PARATHYROID HORMONE AGONIST

**AVAILABILITY** Solution for injection

## ACTION & *THERAPEUTIC EFFECT*
Parathyroid hormone (PTH) is the primary regulator of calcium and phosphate metabolism in bone and kidney. Biological actions of PTH and teriparatide are similar in bone and kidneys. *Stimulates new bone formation by preferential stimulation of osteoblastic activity over osteoclastic activity; improves bone microarchitecture, and increases bone mass and strength by stimulating new bone formation.*

**USES** Treatment of osteoporosis.

## CONTRAINDICATIONS Hypersensitivity to teriparatide; osteosarcoma; Paget's disease; unexplained elevations of alkaline phosphatase; bone metastases or a history of skeletal malignancies; metabolic bone diseases other than osteoporosis; preexisting hypercalcemia; prior history of radiation therapy involving the skeleton; pediatric patients or young adults with open epiphyses; lactation.

**CAUTIOUS USE** Active or recent urolithiasis, hypercalciuria; hypotension; concurrent use of digitalis; hepatic, renal, and cardiac disease; pregnancy (category C); children younger than 18 y.

## ROUTE & DOSAGE

**Osteoporosis**
*Adult:* **Subcutaneous** 20 mcg daily

## ADMINISTRATION
**Subcutaneous**
▪ Do not administer to anyone with hypercalcemia. Consult prescriber.
▪ Rotate subcutaneous injection sites.

## ADVERSE EFFECTS (≥1%) **Body as a Whole:** *Pain, asthenia, neck pain.* **CNS:** Headache, dizziness, depression, insomnia, vertigo. **CV:** Hypertension, angina, syncope. **GI:** Nausea, constipation, dyspepsia, vomiting. **Metabolic:** *Transient increase in calcium levels,* increase in serum uric acid, antibodies to teriparatide after 12 mo therapy. **Musculoskeletal:** *Arthralgia,* leg cramps. **Respiratory:** Rhinitis, cough, pharyngitis, dyspnea, pneumonia. **Skin:** Rash, sweating.

## INTERACTIONS **Drug:** May increase risk of **digoxin** toxicity.

## PHARMACOKINETICS **Absorption:** Extensively absorbed from subcutaneous site. **Onset:** 2 h for calcium concentration increase. **Peak:** Max calcium concentrations 4–6 h. **Duration:** 16–24 h. **Metabolism:** Parathyroid hormone is metabolized by nonspecific enzymes. **Elimination:** Primarily in urine. **Half-Life:** 1 h subcutaneous.

T

Common adverse effects in *italic*; life-threatening effects underlined; generic names in **bold**; classifications in SMALL CAPS; ♣ Canadian drug name; ⊘ Prototype drug

1577

## NURSING IMPLICATIONS

### Black Box Warning

*Teriparatide has been associated with development of osteosarcoma in laboratory animals, and it should not be prescribed for those at increased baseline risk for osteosarcoma.*

### Assessment & Drug Effects

- Monitor cardiovascular status including BP and subjective reports of angina.
- Concurrent drugs: Monitor closely for digoxin toxicity with concurrent use.
- Monitor lab tests: Periodic serum calcium, alkaline phosphatase, and uric acid.

### Patient & Family Education

- Report unexplained leg cramps and bone pain.
- Learn correct technique for subcutaneous injection.

## TESAMORELIN ACETATE

(tes'a-moe-rel'in as'e-tate)

Egrifta

**Classifications:** GROWTH HORMONE RELEASING FACTOR ANALOG; GROWTH HORMONE MODIFIER

Therapeutic: GROWTH HORMONE MODIFIER

**AVAILABILITY** Powder for reconstitution and injection

## ACTION & THERAPEUTIC EFFECT

Binds to pituitary growth hormone-releasing factor receptors and stimulates the secretion of endogenous growth hormone which has anabolic and lipolytic properties. *Reduces fat deposition in those with HIV-associated lipodystrophy.*

**USES** Reduction of excess abdominal fat in HIV-infected patients with lipodystrophy.

**CONTRAINDICATIONS** Active malignancy; hypersensitivity to tesamorelin and/or mannitol; suppression of the hypothalamic-pituitary from hypophysectomy, hypopituitarism, pituitary tumor/surgery, head irradiation or trauma; pregnancy (category X); lactation.

**CAUTIOUS USE** Acute illness or trauma; injection site reactions; nonmalignant neoplasms; renal or hepatic impairment; conditions resulting in or associated with fluid retention (e.g., edema, carpal tunnel syndrome); glucose intolerance or diabetes; retinopathy; age 65 y and older. Safety and efficacy in children not established.

## ROUTE & DOSAGE

### Lipodystrophy in HIV Patients

*Adult:* **Subcutaneous** 2 mg once daily

## ADMINISTRATION

### Subcutaneous

- Use provided diluent only.
- Reconstitute 2 mg vial with 2.1 mL diluent; gently roll vial for 30 sec to mix; do not shake.
- When using 1 mg vials, to produce a 2 mg dose, reconstitute the first 1 mg vial with 2.2 mL diluent; gently roll vial (do not shake) for 30 sec to mix; reconstitute the second 1 mg vial with the entire solution from first vial; gently roll vial (do not shake) for 30 sec to mix.
- Use immediately after prepreparation. Rotate injection sites.
- Store dry vials at 2°–8° C (36°–46° F). Protect from light. Reconstituted solution should be discarded if not used immediately.

Common adverse effects in *italic;* life-threatening effects underlined; generic names in **bold;** classifications in SMALL CAPS; ♣ Canadian drug name; ⊙ Prototype drug

**ADVERSE EFFECTS** (≥1%) **Body as a Whole:** Chest pain, pain, peripheral edema. **CNS:** Depression, hypesthesia, insomnia, pareshesia, peripheral neuropathy. **CV:** Hypertension, palpitations. **GI:** Dyspepsia, nausea, upper abdominal pain, vomiting. **Injection site:** *Erythema*, hemorrhage, irritation, pain, pruritus, rash, reaction, swelling, urticaria. **Metabolic:** Increased blood creatine phosphate. **Musculoskeletal:** *Arthralgia*, carpal tunnel syndrome, joint stiffness and swelling, muscle spasm, muscle pain, musculoskeletal pain, musculoskeletal stiffness, *myalgia, pain in extremity*. **Skin:** Hot flush, night sweats, pruritus, rash, urticarial.

**INTERACTIONS Drug:** Tesamorelin may decrease the enzymatic activation of **cortisone** and **prednisone**. Tesamorelin may alter the metabolism of compounds requiring CYP450 enzymes; careful monitoring is suggested.

**PHARMACOKINETICS Peak:** 15 min. **Half-Life:** 26–38 min.

## NURSING IMPLICATIONS

### Assessment & Drug Effects

- Evaluate abdominal girth with periodic measurements at the level of the umbilicus.
- Assess for injections site reactions (i.e., erythema, pruritus, pain, irritation, and bruising).
- Monitor prediabetics and diabetics for loss of glycemic control.
- Monitor lab tests: Baseline and frequent IGF-1 level baseline and periodic FBG and HbA1C.

### Patient & Family Education

- Seek immediate medical attention for any of the following: Rash or hives; swelling of face or throat; shortness of breath or trouble breathing; rapid heartbeat; feeling of faintness or fainting.
- Notify your prescriber if you experience swelling, an increase in joint pain, or pain or numbness in your hands or wrist (carpal tunnel syndrome).
- Women should discontinue tesamorelin and notify prescriber if pregnancy occurs.
- If diabetic, monitor fasting and postprandial blood glucose as directed.

## TESTOSTERONE ⊙

(tess-toss'ter-one)

Androderm, AndroGel, Axiron, Foresta, Natesto, STRIANT, Testim, Testopel, Vogelxo

## TESTOSTERONE CYPIONATE

Depo-Testosterone

## TESTOSTERONE ENANTHATE

Delatestryl, Malogex ♦

**Classifications:** ANDROGEN/ANABOLIC STEROID; ANTINEOPLASTIC
**Therapeutic:** ANTINEOPLASTIC; ANABOLIC STEROID
**Controlled Substance:** Schedule III

**AVAILABILITY Testosterone:** Implantable pellet; transdermal patch; transdermal gel; intranasal gel; buccal tablet. **Testosterone Cypionate:** IM injection. **Testosterone Enanthate:** IM injection

## ACTION & *THERAPEUTIC EFFECT*

Synthetic steroid compound with both androgenic and anabolic activity. Controls development and maintenance of secondary sexual characteristics. **Androgenic activity:** Responsible for the growth spurt of the adolescent, onset of puberty, and

---

Common adverse effects in *italic;* life-threatening effects underlined; generic names in **bold**; classifications in SMALL CAPS; ♦ Canadian drug name; ⊙ Prototype drug for growth termination by epiphyseal closure. **Anabolic activity:** Increases protein metabolism and decreases its catabolism. Large doses suppress spermatogenesis, thereby causing testicular atrophy. *Antagonizes effects of estrogen excess on female breast and endometrium. Responsible for the growth spurt of the adolescent male and onset of puberty.*

USES Androgen replacement therapy, delayed puberty (male), hypogonadism, palliation of female mammary cancer (1–5 y postmenopausal), palliative treatment of breast cancer, and to treat postpartum breast engorgement. Available in fixed combination with estrogens in many preparations.

CONTRAINDICATIONS Hypersensitivity or toxic reactions to androgens; benzoic acid or benzyl alcohol hypersensitvity; serious cardiac, liver, or kidney disease; hypercalcemia; known or suspected prostatic or breast cancer in male; BPH with obstruction; asthenic males who may react adversely to androgenic overstimulation; conditions aggravated by fluid retention; hypertension; DVT; hepatic dysfunction as a result of use of testosterone; older adults; pregnancy (category X); possibility of virilization of external genitalia of female fetus; lactation.

CAUTIOUS USE Cardiac, liver, and kidney disease; prepubertal males; DM; history of MI; CAD; BPH; older adults; acute intermittent porphyria.

ROUTE & DOSAGE

**Male Hypogonadism**
*Adult:* **IM Cypionate, Enanthate** 50–400 mg q2–4wk; **IM Propionate** 10–25 mg 2–3/wk; **Topical** Start with 6 mg/day

system applied daily, if scrotal area inadequate, use 4 mg/day system; **Androderm** Apply to torso; **AndroGel** Apply one packet to upper arms, shoulders, or abdomen once daily; **Striant** Apply one patch to the gum region just above the incisor tooth q12h

**Delayed Puberty**
*Adult:* **IM Cypionate, Enanthate** 50–200 mg q2–4wk; **Subcutaneous** 2–6 pellets inserted q3–6mo; **IM Propionate** up to 100 mg per mo

**Metastatic Breast Cancer**
*Adult:* **IM Cypionate, Enanthate** 200–400 mg q2–4wk; **IM Propionate** 50–100 mg 3 × wk

ADMINISTRATION
**Buccal**
- Apply buccal patch to gum just above the incisor tooth.

**Nasal**
- Instruct not to blow nose or sniff for 1 h after receiving Natesto.

**Transdermal**
- Apply transdermal system on clean, dry scrotal skin. Dry shave scrotal hair for optimal skin contact. Do not use chemical depilatories. Wear patch for 22–24 h.
- Topical gel preparations may be applied to shoulders and upper arms.
- Store at 15°–30° C (59°–86° F).

**Intramuscular**
- Give IM injections deep into gluteal musculature.
- Store IM formulations prepared in oil at room temperature. Warming and shaking vial will redisperse precipitated crystals.

ADVERSE EFFECTS (≥1%) **CNS:** Excitation, insomnia. **CV:** Skin flushing and vascularization. **GI:** Nausea, vomiting, anorexia, diarrhea, gastric pain, jaundice. **Hematologic:** <u>Leukopenia</u>. **Metabolic:** Hypercalcemia, hypercholesterolemia, *sodium and water retention (especially in older adults) with edema*. **Renal:** Renal calculi (especially in the immobilized patient), bladder irritability. **Urogenital:** *Increased libido*. **Skin:** *Acne*, injection site irritation and sloughing, pruritus. **Body as a Whole:** Hypersensitivity to testosterone, anaphylactoid reactions (rare). **Hematologic:** Precipitation of acute intermittent porphyria. **Endocrine:** Female—suppression of ovulation, lactation, or menstruation; hoarseness or deepening of voice (often irreversible); hirsutism; oily skin; clitoral enlargement; regression of breasts; male-pattern baldness (in disseminated breast cancer); flushing, sweating; vaginitis with pruritus, drying, bleeding; menstrual irregularities. Male—prepubertal-premature epiphyseal closure, phallic enlargement, priapism. Postpubertal—testicular atrophy, decreased ejaculatory volume, azoospermia, oligospermia (after prolonged administration or excessive dosage), Impotence, epididymitis, priapism, *gynecomastia*.

## DIAGNOSTIC TEST INTERFERENCE

Testosterone alters *glucose tolerance* tests; decreases *thyroxine-binding globulin concentration* (resulting in decreased *total T₄* serum levels and increased *resin of T₃* and *T₄*). Increases *creatinine* and *creatinine* excretion (lasting up to 2 wk after therapy is discontinued) and alters response to *metyrapone test*. It suppresses *clotting factors II, V, VII, X* and decreases excretion of *17-ketosteroids*. May increase or decrease *serum cholesterol*.

## INTERACTIONS **Drug:** ORAL ANTICOAGULANTS may potentiate

hypoprothrombinemia. May decrease **insulin** requirements. May have increased concentration if used with **ceritinib, conivaptan, topotecan**.

## PHARMACOKINETICS **Absorption: Cypionate** and **enanthate** are slowly absorbed from lipid tissue. **Duration:** 2–4 wk **cypionate** and **enanthate**. **Distribution:** 98% bound to sex hormone-binding globulin. **Metabolism:** Primarily in liver. **Elimination:** 90% in urine, 6% in feces. **Half-Life:** 10–100 min.

## NURSING IMPLICATIONS

### Assessment & Drug Effects

- Check I&O and weigh patient daily during dose adjustment period. Weight gain (due to sodium and water retention) suggests need for decreased dosage. When dosage is stabilized, urge patient to check weight at least twice weekly and to report increases, particularly if accompanied by edema in dependent areas. Dose adjustment and diuretic therapy may be started.
- Monitor serum calcium closely. Androgenic therapy is usually terminated if serum calcium rises above 14 mg/dL.
- Report S&S of hypercalcemia (see Appendix F) promptly. The immobilized patient is particularly prone to develop hypercalcemia, which indicates progression of bone metastasis in patients with metastatic breast cancer. Treatment includes withdrawing testosterone and checking calcium, phosphate, and BUN levels daily.
- Instruct diabetic to report sweating, tremor, anxiety, vertigo. Testosterone-induced anabolic action enhances hypoglycemia (hyperinsulinism). Dosage adjustment of antidiabetic agent may be required.

Common adverse effects in *italic;* life-threatening effects <u>underlined</u>; generic names in **bold;** classifications in SMALL CAPS; ♣ Canadian drug name; ⊘ Prototype drug

1581

- Observe patients on concomitant anticoagulant treatment for signs of overdosage (e.g., ecchymoses, petechiae). Report promptly to prescriber; anticoagulant dose may need to be reduced.
- Monitor prepubertal or adolescent males throughout therapy to avoid precocious sexual development and premature epiphyseal closure. Skeletal stimulation may continue 6 mo beyond termination of therapy.
- Monitor lab tests: Periodic serum cholesterol, serum electrolytes, and LFTs.

### Patient & Family Education

- Review directions for application of transdermal patches.
- Report soreness at injection site, because a postinjection site boil may be an associated adverse reaction.
- Report priapism (sustained and often painful erections occurring especially in early replacement therapy), reduced ejaculatory volume, and gynecomastia to prescriber. Symptoms indicate necessity for temporary withdrawal or discontinuation of testosterone therapy.
- Notify prescriber promptly if pregnancy is suspected or planned. Masculinization of the fetus is most likely to occur if testosterone (androgen) therapy is provided during first trimester of pregnancy.
- Androgens may cause virilism in women at dosage required to treat carcinoma. Report increase in libido (early sign of toxicity), growth of facial hair, deepening of voice, male-pattern baldness. The onset of hoarseness can easily be overlooked unless its significance as an early and possibly irreversible sign of virilism is appreciated. Reevaluation of treatment plan is indicated.

## TETRACAINE HYDROCHLORIDE

(tet'ra-kane)

**Pontocaine**

**Classification:** LOCAL ANESTHETIC (ESTER TYPE)
**Therapeutic:** LOCAL ANESTHETIC
**Prototype:** Procaine HCl

**AVAILABILITY** Solution for injection; powder; solution; cream; gel; ointment; ophthalmic solution

## ACTION & THERAPEUTIC EFFECT

A potent and toxic local anesthetic that depresses initial depolarization phase of the action potential, thus preventing propagation and conduction of the nerve impulse. *Effectiveness indicated by loss of sensation and motor activity in circumscribed body areas close to injection or application site.*

**USES** Spinal anesthesia (high, low, saddle block) and topically to produce surface anesthesia. **Eye:** To anesthetize conjunctiva and cornea prior to superficial procedures (including tonometry, gonioscopy, removal of foreign bodies or sutures, corneal scraping). **Nose and Throat:** To abolish laryngeal and esophageal reflexes prior to bronchoscopy, esophagoscopy. **Skin:** To relieve pruritus, pain, burning.

**CONTRAINDICATIONS** Debilitated patients; prolonged use of ophthalmic preparations; known hypersensitivity to tetracaine or other local anesthetics of ester type (e.g., procaine, chloroprocaine, cocaine), sulfite, or to PABA or its derivatives; coagulopathy; anticoagulant therapy; thrombocytopenia; increased bleeding time; infection at application or injection site.

Common adverse effects in *italic;* life-threatening effects underlined; generic names in **bold;** classifications in SMALL CAPS; ♣ Canadian drug name; ⊘ Prototype drug

**CAUTIOUS USE** Shock; cachexia, cardiac decompensation; QT prolongation; older adults; pregnancy (category C); lactation; children younger than 16 y.

## ROUTE & DOSAGE

**Local Anesthesia**

*Adult:* **Topical** Before procedure, 1–2 drops of 0.5% solution or 1.25–2.5 cm of ointment in lower conjunctival fornix or 0.5% solution or ointment to nose or throat; **Spinal** 1% solution diluted with equal volume of 10% dextrose injected in subarachnoid space

## ADMINISTRATION

**Topical**

- Avoid use of solutions that are cloudy, discolored, or crystallized.
- When tetracaine is used on mucosa of larynx, trachea, or esophagus, the manufacturer recommends adding 0.06 mL of a 0.1% epinephrine solution to each mL tetracaine solution to slow absorption of the anesthetic.
- Store ophthalmic solution and ointment at 15°–30° C (59°–86° F); refrigerate topical. Avoid freezing. Use tight, light-resistant containers.

**ADVERSE EFFECTS** (≥1%) **Body as a Whole:** <u>Anaphylactic reactions</u>, convulsions, faintness, syncope. **CNS:** Postspinal headache, headache, spinal nerve paralysis, anxiety, nervousness, seizures. **CV:** Bradycardia, arrhythmias, hypotension. **Special Senses:** Stinging; corneal erosion, retardation or prevention of healing of corneal abrasion, transient pitting and sloughing of corneal surface, dry corneal epithelium; dry mucous membranes, prolonged depression of cough reflex.

**INTERACTIONS Drug:** May antagonize effects of SULFONAMIDES.

**PHARMACOKINETICS** **Onset:** 1 min eye; 3 min mucosal surface; 3 min spinal. **Duration:** Up to 15 min eye; 30–60 min mucosal surface; 1.5–3 h spinal. **Metabolism:** In liver and plasma. **Elimination:** In urine.

## NURSING IMPLICATIONS

**Assessment & Drug Effects**

- Recovery from anesthesia to the pharyngeal area is complete when patient has feeling in the hard and soft palates and when muscles in the faucial (tonsillar) pillars contract with stimulation.
- Do not give food or liquids until these normal pharyngeal responses are present (usually about 1 h after anesthetic administration). The first small amount of liquid (water) should be given under supervision of care provider.
- Be aware that increased blood concentration of the drug may result from excess application of tetracaine to the skin (to relieve pruritus or burning), application to debrided or infected skin surfaces, or too rapid injection rate.
- High blood concentrations of tetracaine can lead to adverse systemic effects involving CNS and CV systems: Convulsions, respiratory arrest, dysrhythmias, cardiac arrest.

**Patient & Family Education**

- Do not use ophthalmic drug longer than prescribed period. Prolonged use to eye surface may cause corneal epithelial erosions and retard healing of corneal surface.
- Natural barriers to eye infection and injury are removed by the anesthesia. Do not rub eye after drug

T

Common adverse effects in *italic*; life-threatening effects <u>underlined</u>; generic names in **bold**; classifications in SMALL CAPS; ✢ Canadian drug name; Ⓟ Prototype drug

1583

instillation until anesthetic effect has dissipated (evidenced by return of blink reflex). Patching for temporary protection of the corneal epithelium may be ordered.

▪ Wash or disinfect hands before and after self-administration of solutions or ointment.

## TETRACYCLINE HYDROCHLORIDE 🅿️

(tet-ra-sye′kleen)

Novotetra ✦, Sumycin

**Classifications:** ANTIBIOTIC; TETRACYCLINE

**Therapeutic:** ANTIBIOTIC

**AVAILABILITY** Capsule; suspension

## ACTION & *THERAPEUTIC EFFECT*

Tetracyclines exert antiacne action by suppressing growth of *Propionibacterium acnes* within sebaceous follicles. *Effective against a variety of gram-positive and gram-negative bacteria and against most chlamydiae, mycoplasmas, rickettsiae, and certain protozoa (e.g., amebae). Exerts antiacne action against* Propionibacterium acnes.

**USES** Chlamydial infections (e.g., lymphogranuloma venereum, psittacosis, trachoma, inclusion conjunctivitis, nongonococcal urethritis); mycoplasmal infections (e.g., *Mycoplasma pneumoniae*); rickettsial infections (e.g., Q fever, Rocky Mountain spotted fever, typhus); spirochetal infections: Relapsing fever *(Borrelia),* leptospirosis, syphilis (penicillin-hypersensitive patients); amebiases; uncommon gram-negative bacterial infections [e.g., brucellosis, shigellosis, cholera, gonorrhea (penicillin-hypersensitive patients), granuloma inguinale, tularemia]; gram-positive infections

(e.g., tetanus). Also used orally (solution) for inflammatory acne vulgaris.

**UNLABELED USES** Actinomycosis, acute exacerbations of chronic bronchitis; Lyme disease; pericardial effusion (metastatic); acute PID; sexually transmitted epididymo orchitis; with quinine for multi-drug-resistant strains of *Plasmodium falciparum* malaria; anti-infective prophylaxis for rape victims; recurrent cystic thyroid nodules; melioidosis; and as fluorescence test for malignancy.

**CONTRAINDICATIONS** Hypersensitivity to tetracyclines; severe renal or hepatic impairment, common bile duct obstruction; UV exposure; pregnancy (category D); lactation.

**CAUTIOUS USE** History of kidney or liver dysfunction; myasthenia gravis; history of allergy, asthma, hay fever, urticaria; undernourished patients; infants, children younger than 8 y.

## ROUTE & DOSAGE

**Systemic Infection**

*Adult:* **PO** 250–500 mg b.i.d.–q.i.d. (1–2 g/day)
*Child (8 y or older):* **PO** 25–50 mg/kg/day in 2–4 divided doses

**Acne**

*Adult/Child (8 y or older):* **PO** 500–1000 mg/day in 4 divided doses

## ADMINISTRATION

### Oral

▪ Give with a full glass of water on an empty stomach at least 1 h before or 2 h after meals (food, milk, and milk products can reduce absorption by 50% or more).

- Do not give immediately before bed.
- Give with food if patient is having GI symptoms (e.g., nausea, vomiting, anorexia); do not give with foods high in calcium such as milk or milk products.
- Shake suspension well before pouring to ensure uniform distribution of drug. Use calibrated liquid measure to dispense.
- Check expiration date for all tetracyclines. Fanconi-like syndrome (renal tubular dysfunction) and also an LE-like syndrome have been attributed to outdated tetracycline preparations.
- Tetracycline decomposes with age, exposure to light, and when improperly stored under conditions of extreme humidity, heat, or cold. The resultant product may be toxic.
- Store at 15°–30° C (59°–86° F) in tightly covered container in dry place. Protect from light.

## ADVERSE EFFECTS (≥1%) CNS:
Headache, intracranial hypertension (rare). **Special Senses:** Pigmentation of conjunctiva due to drug deposit. **GI:** Reported mostly for oral administration, but also may occur with parenteral tetracycline (*nausea, vomiting,* epigastric distress, heartburn, *diarrhea,* bulky loose stools, steatorrhea, *abdominal discomfort, flatulence,* dry mouth); dysphagia, retrosternal pain, esophagitis, esophageal ulceration with oral administration, abnormally high liver function test values, decrease in serum cholesterol, fatty degeneration of liver [jaundice, increasing nitrogen retention (azotemia), hyperphosphatemia, acidosis, irreversible shock]; foul-smelling stools or vaginal discharge, stomatitis, glossitis; black hairy tongue (lingua nigra), diarrhea: Staphylococcal enterocolitis. **Body as a Whole:** Drug fever, angioedema, serum sickness, anaphylaxis. **Urogenital:** Particularly in patients with kidney disease; increase in BUN/serum creatinine, renal impairment even with therapeutic doses; Fanconi-like syndrome (outdated tetracycline) (characterized by polyuria, polydipsia, nausea, vomiting, glycosuria, proteinuria acidosis, aminoaciduria); vulvovaginitis, pruritus vulvae or ani (possibly hypersensitivity). **Skin:** Dermatitis, *phototoxicity:* Discoloration of nails, onycholysis (loosening of nails); cheilosis; fixed drug eruptions particularly on genitalia; thrombocytopenic purpura; urticaria, rash, exfoliative dermatitis; with topical applications: Skin irritation, dry scaly skin, transient stinging or burning sensation, slight yellowing of skin at application site, acute contact dermatitis. **Other:** Pancreatitis, local reactions: Pain and irritation (IM site), Jarisch-Herxheimer reaction.

## DIAGNOSTIC TEST INTERFERENCE
TETRACYCLINES may cause false increases in **urinary catecholamines** (by **fluorometric methods**), and false decreases in **urinary urobilinogen.** Parenteral TETRACYCLINES containing **ascorbic acid** reportedly may produce false-positive **urinary glucose** determinations by **copper reduction methods** (e.g., **Benedict's reagent, Clinitest**); TETRACYCLINES may cause false-negative results with **glucose oxidase methods** (e.g., **Clinistix, TesTape**).

## INTERACTIONS Drug: ANTACIDS,
**calcium**, and **magnesium** bind tetracycline in gut and decrease absorption. ORAL ANTICOAGULANTS potentiate

**T**

Common adverse effects in *italic;* life-threatening effects underlined; generic names in **bold;** classifications in SMALL CAPS; ♣ Canadian drug name; ⊙ Prototype drug

1585

hypoprothrombinemia. ANTIDIARRHEAL AGENTS with **kaolin** and pectin may decrease absorption. Effectiveness of ORAL CONTRACEPTIVES decreased. **Methoxyflurane** may produce fatal nephrotoxicity. **Food:** Dairy products and **iron, zinc** supplements decrease tetracycline absorption.

## PHARMACOKINETICS **Absorption:** 75–80% of dose absorbed. **Peak:** 2–4 h. **Distribution:** Widely distributed, preferentially binds to rapid growing tissues; crosses placenta; enters breast milk. **Metabolism:** Not metabolized; enterohepatic cycling. **Elimination:** 50–60% in urine within 72 h. **Half-Life:** 6–12 h.

## NURSING IMPLICATIONS

### Assessment & Drug Effects

- Report GI symptoms (e.g., nausea, vomiting, diarrhea) to prescriber. These are generally dose-dependent, occurring mostly in patients receiving 2 g/day or more and during prolonged therapy. Frequently, symptoms are controlled by reducing dosage or administering with compatible foods.
- Be alert to evidence of superinfections (see Appendix F). Regularly inspect tongue and mucous membrane of mouth for candidiasis (thrush). Suspect superinfection if patient complains of irritation or soreness of mouth, tongue, throat, vagina, or anus, or persistent itching of any area, diarrhea, or foul-smelling excreta or discharge.
- Withhold drug and notify prescriber if superinfection develops. Superinfections occur most frequently in patients receiving prolonged therapy, the debilitated, or those who have diabetes.
- Monitor I&O in patients receiving parenteral tetracycline. Report

oliguria or any changes in appearance of urine or in I&O.
- Monitor lab tests: Periodic renal function tests, LFTs, and hematopoietic function tests, particularly during high-dose, long-term therapy.

### Patient & Family Education

- Report onset of diarrhea to prescriber. It is important to determine whether diarrhea is due to irritating drug effect or superinfections or pseudomembranous colitis (caused by overgrowth of toxin-producing bacteria: *Clostridium difficile*) (see Appendix F). The latter two conditions can be life threatening and require immediate withdrawal of tetracycline and prompt initiation of symptomatic and supportive therapy.
- Reduce incidence of superinfection (see Appendix F) by meticulous care of mouth, skin, and perineal area. Rinse mouth of food debris after eating; floss daily and use a soft-bristled toothbrush.
- Avoid direct exposure to sunlight during and for several days after therapy is terminated to reduce possibility of photosensitivity reaction (appearing like an exaggerated sunburn).
- Exercise caution with potentially hazardous activities until reaction to drug is known.
- Report immediately sudden onset of painful or difficult swallowing (dysphagia) to prescriber. Esophagitis and esophageal ulceration have been associated with bedtime administration of tetracycline capsules or tablets with insufficient fluid, particularly to patients with hiatal hernia or esophageal problems.
- Response to acne therapy usually requires 2–8 wk, maximal results may not be apparent for up to 12 wk.

# TETRAHYDROZOLINE HYDROCHLORIDE

(tet-ra-hye-drozz'a-leen)

Mallazine, Murine Plus, Optigene, Soothe, Tyzine, Visine

**Classifications:** EYE AND NOSE PREPARATION; VASOCONSTRICTOR; DECONGESTANT

Therapeutic: NASAL DECONGESTANT; OCULAR VASOCONSTRICTOR

**Prototype:** Naphazoline

**AVAILABILITY** Ophthalmic solution; nasal solution

## ACTION & *THERAPEUTIC EFFECT*

Alpha-adrenergic agonist that causes intense vasoconstriction when applied topically to mucous membranes, and when applied as eyedrops. *Ophthalmic solution is effective for allergic reactions of the eye, nasal solution is antiinflammatory and also decreases allergic congestion.*

**USES** Symptomatic relief of minor eye irritation and allergies and for nasopharyngeal congestion of allergic or inflammatory origin.

**CONTRAINDICATIONS** Hypersensitivity to tetrahydrozoline; use of ophthalmic preparation in glaucoma or other serious eye diseases; use within 14 days of MAO inhibitor therapy.

**CAUTIOUS USE** Hypertension; cardiovascular disease; hyperthyroidism; DM; pregnancy (category C); lactation. Use in children younger than 2 y; use of 0.1% or higher strengths in children younger than 6 y.

## ROUTE & DOSAGE

**Decongestant**

*Adult:* **Ophthalmic** See Appendix A-1; **Nasal** 2–4 drops of 0.1% solution or spray in each nostril q3h prn
*Child (2–6 y):* **Nasal** 2–4 drops of 0.05% solution or spray in each nostril q3h prn; *6 y or older:* Same as adult

## ADMINISTRATION

**Instillation**

- Make sure interval between doses is at least 4–6 h since drug action lasts 4–8 h.
- Place patient in upright position when using nasal spray. (If patient is reclining, a stream rather than a spray may be ejected, with consequent overdosage.)
- Use lateral, head-low position to administer nasal drops.

**ADVERSE EFFECTS** (≥1%) **Special Senses:** *Transient stinging, irritation, sneezing,* dryness, headache, tremors, drowsiness, light-headedness, insomnia, palpitation. **Body as a Whole:** With overdose: Marked drowsiness, sweating, <u>coma</u>, hypotension, <u>shock</u>, bradycardia.

**PHARMACOKINETICS Absorption:** May be absorbed from nasal mucosa. **Duration:** 4–8 h.

## NURSING IMPLICATIONS

**Patient & Family Education**

- Discontinue medication and consult prescriber if relief is not obtained within 48 h or if symptoms persist or increase.
- Do not exceed recommended dosage. Rebound congestion and rhinitis may occur with frequent or prolonged use of nasal preparation.

**T**

---

# THEOPHYLLINE

## THEOPHYLLINE ℗ℝ
(thee-off'i-lin)

Elixophyllin, PMS Theophylline ♣, Pulmophylline ♣, Thea-24, Theochron, Theophylline Ethylenediamine, Theospan-SR, Uniphyl

**Classifications:** BRONCHODILATOR (RESPIRATORY SMOOTH MUSCLE RELAXANT); XANTHINE
Therapeutic: BRONCHODILATOR

**AVAILABILITY** Liquid; sustained release tablet; sustained release capsule; solution for injection

**ACTION & THERAPEUTIC EFFECT**
Xanthine derivative that relaxes smooth muscle by direct action, particularly of bronchi and pulmonary vessels, and stimulates medullary respiratory center with resulting increase in vital capacity. *Effective for relief of bronchospasm in asthmatics, chronic bronchitis, and emphysema.*

**USES** Prophylaxis and symptomatic relief of bronchial asthma, as well as bronchospasm associated with chronic bronchitis and emphysema. Also used for emergency treatment of paroxysmal cardiac dyspnea and edema of CHF.

**UNLABELED USES** Treatment of apnea and bradycardia of premature infants and to reduce severe bronchospasm associated with cystic fibrosis and acute descending respiratory infection.

**CONTRAINDICATIONS** Hypersensitivity to theophylline; CAD or angina pectoris when myocardial stimulation might be harmful; severe renal or hepatic impairment.

**CAUTIOUS USE** Compromised cardiac or circulatory function, cardiac arrhythmias; hypertension; acute pulmonary edema; multiple organ failure; CHF; seizure disorders; hyperthyroidism; active peptic ulcer; prostatic hypertrophy; glaucoma; DM; older adults; pregnancy (category C); lactation; children; and neonates.

## ROUTE & DOSAGE

**Bronchospasm**

*Adult/Child:* **PO/IV Loading Dose** 5 mg/kg
*Adult (nonsmoker):* **IV** by continuous infusion; **PO Immediate release** divided q6h; or **PO Sustained release** q8–12h: 0.4 mg/kg/h; *smoker:* 0.6 mg/kg/h; *with CHF or cirrhosis:* 0.2 mg/kg/h
*Child (1–9 y):* **IV** by continuous infusion; **PO Immediate release** divided q6h; or **PO Sustained release** q8–12h: 0.8 mg/kg/h; *10–12 y,* 0.6 mg/kg/h; *infant:* 0.5–0.7 mg/kg/h; *neonate:* 0.13 mg/kg/h

***Obesity Dosage Adjustment***
Dose based on IBW

## ADMINISTRATION
Note: All doses based on ideal body weight.

**Oral**
- Wait 4–6 h after the last IV dose, when switching from IV to oral dosing.
- Give with a full glass of water and after meals to minimize gastric irritation.
- Give sustained release forms and enteric-coated tablets whole. Chewable tablets **must be**

T

chewed thoroughly before swallowing. Sustained release granules from capsules can be taken on an empty stomach or mixed with applesauce or water.

- Note: Timing of dose is critical. Be certain patient understands necessity to adhere to the correct intervals between doses.

**Intravenous**

*PREPARE:* Use as supplied with no further preparation.
*ADMINISTER:* **IV Infusion:** Infuse at a rate based on patient's weight.
*INCOMPATIBILITIES:* **Solution/additive: Ascorbic acid, ceftriaxone, cimetidine, hetastarch. Y-site: Hetastarch, phenytoin.**

**ADVERSE EFFECTS** (>1%) **CNS:** Stimulation (irritability, restlessness, insomnia, dizziness, headache, tremor, hyperexcitability, muscle twitching, drug-induced seizures). **CV:** Palpitation, *tachycardia,* extrasystoles, flushing, marked hypotension, circulatory failure. **GI:** *Nausea,* vomiting, anorexia, epigastric or abdominal pain, diarrhea, activation of peptic ulcer. **Urogenital.** Transient urinary frequency, albuminuria, kidney irritation. **Respiratory:** Tachypnea, respiratory arrest. **Body as a Whole:** Fever, dehydration.

**DIAGNOSTIC TEST INTERFERENCE**
False-positive elevations of *serum uric acid* (*Bittner* or **colorimetric** methods). *Probenecid* may cause false high *serum theophylline* readings, and spectrophotometric methods of determining *serum theophylline* are affected by a furosemide, sulfathiazole, phenylbutazone, probenecid, theobromine.

**INTERACTIONS Drug:** Increases **lithium** excretion, lowering lithium levels; **cimetidine,** high-dose **allopurinol** (600 mg/day), QUINOLONES,

MACROLIDE ANTIBIOTICS, and **zileuton** can significantly increase theophylline levels; **tobacco** use significantly decreases levels. **Herbal: St. John's wort** may decrease theophylline efficacy. **Daidzein** (in soy), **black pepper** increase serum concentrations and adverse effects.

**PHARMACOKINETICS Absorption:** Most products are 100% absorbed from GI tract. **Peak:** IV 30 min; uncoated tablet 1 h; sustained release 4–6 h. **Duration:** 4–8 h; varies with age, smoking, and liver function. **Distribution:** Crosses placenta. **Metabolism:** Extensively in liver. **Elimination:** Parent drug and metabolites excreted by kidneys; excreted in breast milk.

**NURSING IMPLICATIONS**
**Assessment & Drug Effects**
- Monitor vital signs. Improvement in respiratory status is the expected outcome.
- Observe and report early signs of possible toxicity: Anorexia, nausea, vomiting, dizziness, shakiness, restlessness, abdominal discomfort, irritability, palpitation, tachycardia, marked hypotension, cardiac arrhythmias, seizures.
- Monitor for tachycardia, which may be worse in patients with severe cardiac disease. Conversely, theophylline toxicity may be masked in patients with tachycardia.
- Monitor drug levels closely in heavy smokers. Cigarette smoking induces hepatic microsomal enzyme activity, decreasing serum half-life and increasing body clearance of theophylline. An increase of dosage from 50–100% is usual in heavy smokers.
- Monitor plasma drug level closely in patients with heart failure, kidney or liver dysfunction, alcoholism,

Common adverse effects in *italic;* life-threatening effects underlined; generic names in **bold;** classifications in SMALL CAPS; ✤ Canadian drug name; ⊘ Prototype drug

1589

high fever. Plasma clearance of xanthines may be reduced.

- Take necessary safety precautions and forewarn older adult patients of possible dizziness during early therapy.
- Monitor patients on sustained release preparations for S&S of overdosage. Continued slow absorption leads to high plasma concentrations for a prolonged period.
- Note: Neonates of mothers using this drug have exhibited slight tachycardia, jitteriness, and apnea.
- Monitor **closely** for adverse effects in infants younger than 6 mo and prematures; theophylline metabolism is prolonged as is the half-life in this age group.
- Monitor lab tests: Theophylline plasma level when initiating therapy and with dosage increases.

**Patient & Family Education**

- Take medication at the same time every day.
- Avoid charcoal-broiled foods (high in polycyclic carbon content); may increase theophylline elimination and reduce the half-life as much as 50%.
- Limit caffeine intake because it may increase incidence of adverse effects.
- Cigarette smoking may significantly lower theophylline plasma concentration.
- Be aware that a low-carbohydrate, high-protein diet increases theophylline elimination, and a high-carbohydrate, low-protein diet decreases it.
- Drink fluids liberally (2000–3000 mL/day) if not contraindicated to decrease viscosity of airway secretions.
- Avoid self-dosing with OTC medications, especially cough suppressants, which may cause retention of secretions and CNS depression.

# THIAMINE HYDROCHLORIDE (VITAMIN B₁)

(thye'a-min)

**Classification:** VITAMIN B₁
**Therapeutic:** VITAMIN B₁ REPLACEMENT THERAPY

**AVAILABILITY** Tablet; capsule; solution for injection

## ACTION & *THERAPEUTIC EFFECT*

Water-soluble B₁ vitamin and member of B-complex group used for thiamine replacement therapy. Functions as an essential coenzyme in carbohydrate metabolism and has a role in conversion of tryptophan to nicotinamide. *Effectiveness is evidenced by improvement of clinical manifestations of thiamine deficiency (e.g., anorexia, depression, loss of memory).*

**USES** Treatment and prophylaxis of thiamine deficiency.

**CONTRAIDINDICATION** Hypersensitivity to thiamine.

**CAUTIOUS USE** Pregnancy (category A; category C if above RDA).

## ROUTE & DOSAGE

**Thiamine Deficiency**

*Adult:* **IV/IM/PO** 30–50 mg daily
*Child:* **IV/IM/PO** 10–25 mg daily × 2 wk then 5–10 **PO** × 1 mo

**Wernicke's Encephalopathy**

*Adult:* **IV/IM** 100 mg/day then 50–100 mg/day until on normal diet

**Dietary Supplement**

*Adult:* **PO** 15–30 mg/day
*Child:* **PO** 10–50 mg/day

## ADMINISTRATION

### Oral
- Do not crush or chew enteric-coated tablets. These **must be** swallowed whole.

### Intramuscular
- Give deep IM into a large muscle; may be painful. Rotate sites and apply cold compresses to area if necessary for relief of discomfort.

### Intravenous
Note: Intradermal test dose is recommended prior to administration in suspected thiamine sensitivity. Deaths have occurred following IV use.

*PREPARE:* **Direct:** Give undiluted. **IV Infusion:** Diluted in 1000 mL of most IV solutions.

*ADMINISTER:* **Direct:** Give at a rate of 100 mg over 5 min. **IV Infusion:** Give at the ordered rate.

*INCOMPATIBILITIES:* **Y-site: aminophylline, amphotericin B, azathioprine, cefoperazone, ceftazidime, ceftizoxime, chloramphenicol, dantrolene, diazepam, diazoxide, folic acid, furosemide, ganciclovir, hydrocortisone, imipenem/cilastatin, iamrinone, indomethacin, methylprednisolone, pentobarbital, phenobarbital, phenytoin, sodium bicarbonate, SMZ/TMP.**

- Preserve in tight, light-resistant, nonmetallic containers. Thiamine is unstable in alkaline solutions (e.g., solutions of acetates, barbiturates, bicarbonates, carbonates, citrates) and neutral solutions.

## ADVERSE EFFECTS (≥1%) **Body as a Whole:** Feeling of warmth, weakness, sweating, restlessness, tightness of throat, angioneurotic edema, <u>anaphylaxis</u>. **Respiratory:** Cyanosis, pulmonary edema. **CV:** <u>Cardiovascular collapse</u>, slight fall in BP following rapid IV administration. **GI:** GI hemorrhage, nausea. **Skin:** Urticaria, pruritus.

## INTERACTIONS **Drug:** No clinically significant interactions established.

## PHARMACOKINETICS **Absorption:** Limited from GI tract. **Distribution:** Widely distributed, including into breast milk. **Elimination:** In urine.

## NURSING IMPLICATIONS

### Assessment & Drug Effects
- Record patient's dietary history carefully as an essential part of vitamin replacement therapy. Collaborate with prescriber, dietitian, patient, and responsible family member in developing a diet teaching plan that can be sustained by patient.

### Patient & Family Education
- Food–drug relationships: Learn about rich dietary sources of thiamine (e.g., yeast, pork, beef, liver, wheat and other whole grains, nutrient-added breakfast cereals, fresh vegetables, especially peas and dried beans).
- Body requirement of thiamine is directly proportional to carbohydrate intake and metabolic rate; requirement increases when diet consists predominantly of carbohydrates.

# THIOGUANINE (TG, 6-THIOGUANINE)
(thye-oh-gwah′neen)

Lanvis ◆, Tabloid

**Classifications:** ANTINEOPLASTIC; ANTIMETABOLITE; PURINE ANTAGONIST
**Therapeutic:** ANTINEOPLASTIC
**Prototype:** Mercaptopurine

Common adverse effects in *italic;* life-threatening effects <u>underlined</u>; generic names in **bold;** classifications in SMALL CAPS; ◆ Canadian drug name; ☯ Prototype drug

1591

**AVAILABILITY** Tablet

**ACTION & *THERAPEUTIC EFFECT***
Tumor inhibitory properties may be caused by a sequential blockade of the synthesis and utilization of the purine nucleotides in DNA and DNA. *Interferes with nucleic acid biosynthesis, and has been found active against selected human neoplastic diseases*.

**USES** In combination with other antineoplastics for remission induction in acute myelogenous leukemia and as treatment of chronic myelogenous leukemia.

**CONTRAINDICATIONS** Patients with prior resistance to this drug; severe bone marrow depression; liver toxicity caused by drug; pregnancy (category D); lactation.

**CAUTIOUS USE** Resistance to mercaptopurine; hepatic disease; children.

**ROUTE & DOSAGE**

**Leukemia**
*Adult:* **PO** 2 mg/kg/day, may increase to 3 mg/kg/day if no response after 4 wk

**ADMINISTRATION**
**Oral**
- Withhold drug and notify prescriber if toxicity develops. There is no known antagonist; prompt discontinuation of the drug is essential to avoid irreversible myelosuppression from toxicity.
- Store at 15°–30° C (59°–86° F) in airtight container.

**ADVERSE EFFECTS** (≥1%) **Hematologic:** Leukopenia, thrombocytopenia, anemia. **GI:** Jaundice, nausea, vomiting, anorexia, stomatitis, diarrhea. **Urogenital:** *Hyperuricemia.* **Other:**
Hepatotoxicity (risk increased with long-term use).

**INTERACTIONS Drug:** Severe hepatotoxicity with **busulfan;** may decrease immune response to VACCINES; increase risk of bleeding with ANTICOAGULANTS; NSAIDS, SALICYLATES; PLATELET INHIBITORS, THROMBOLYTIC AGENTS; effects may be reversed by **filgrastim, sargramostim.**

**PHARMACOKINETICS Absorption:** Variable and incomplete absorption from GI tract. **Peak:** 8 h. **Distribution:** Crosses placenta. **Metabolism:** In liver. **Elimination:** In urine. **Half-Life:** 11 h.

**NURSING IMPLICATIONS**
**Assessment & Drug Effects**
- Determine hematologic parameters for withholding drug.
- Monitor I&O ratio and report oliguria.
- Observe patient's skin and sclera for jaundice. It should be reported promptly as a symptom of toxicity; drug will be discontinued promptly.
- Expect that the drop in leukocyte count may be slow over a period of 2–4 wk. Treatment is interrupted if there is a rapid fall within a few days.
- Monitor lab tests: Frequent CBC with differential and platelet count; weekly LFTs early in therapy and monthly thereafter.

**Patient & Family Education**
- Report promptly to prescriber any of the following: Fever, sore throat, jaundice, nausea, vomiting, signs of infection, bleeding from any site, or symptoms of anemia.
- Women should use effective means of contraception while taking this drug.

T

# THIORIDAZINE HYDROCHLORIDE

(thye-o-rid'a-zeen)

**Classification:** ANTIPSYCHOTIC; PHENOTHIAZINE
Therapeutic: ANTIPSYCHOTIC
**Prototype:** Chlorpromazine

**AVAILABILITY** Tablet

## ACTION & THERAPEUTIC EFFECT

Blocks postsynaptic dopamine receptors in the mesolimbic system of the brain. The decrease in dopamine neurotransmission has been found to correlate to antipsychotic effects. *Effective in reducing excitement, hypermotility, abnormal initiative, affective tension, and agitation by inhibiting psychomotor functions. Also effective as an antipsychotic agent, and for behavioral disorders in children.*

**USES** Treatment of schizophrenia in patients who fail to respond adequately to treatment with other antipsychotics.

**CONTRAINDICATIONS** Hypersensitivity to phenothiazines; severe CNS depression; CV disease; family history of QT prolongation or cardiac arrhythmias; coadministration of drug that is known to prolong the QTc interval; suicidal ideation; older adults with dementia related psychosis; lactation.

**CAUTIOUS USE** Premature ventricular contractions; previously diagnosed breast cancer; patients exposed to extremes in heat or to organophosphorus insecticides; history of suicidal tendencies; Parkinson's disease; seizure disorders; closed-angle glaucoma; respiratory disorders; pregnancy (category undetermined). Safe use in children younger than 2 y not established.

## ROUTE & DOSAGE

### Schizophrenia

*Adult:* **PO** 50–100 mg t.i.d., may increase up to 800 mg/day as needed or tolerated
*Child (2 y or older):* **PO** 0.5 mg/kg/day in divided doses; (max: 3 mg/kg/day) if hospitalized, may start at 25 mg t.i.d.

**Pharmacogenetic Dosage Adjustment**

*Poor CYP2D6 metabolizers:* Start with 40% of dose

## ADMINISTRATION

**Oral**

- Give with fluid of patient's choice; tablet may be crushed.
- Schedule phenothiazine at least 1 h before or 1 h after an antacid or antidiarrheal medication.
- Add increases in dose to the first dose of the day to prevent sleep disturbance.
- Store at 15°–30° C (59°–86° F) in tightly covered, light-resistant containers unless otherwise indicated.

## ADVERSE EFFECTS (≥1%) **CNS:**
*Sedation,* dizziness, drowsiness, lethargy, extrapyramidal syndrome, nocturnal confusion, hyperactivity. **Special Senses:** Nasal congestion, blurred vision, pigmentary retinopathy. **GI:** Xerostomia, *constipation, paralytic ileus,* increased appetite, weight gain. **Urogenital:** Amenorrhea, breast engorgement, gynecomastia, galactorrhea, *urinary retention.*

Common adverse effects in *italic;* life-threatening effects underlined; generic names in **bold;** classifications in SMALL CAPS; ♣ Canadian drug name; ⊙ Prototype drug

1593

**CV:** Ventricular dysrhythmias, hypotension, prolonged QT$_c$ interval.

## INTERACTIONS Drug: Alcohol, ANXIOLYTICS, SEDATIVE-HYPNOTICS, other CNS DEPRESSANTS add to CNS depression; additive adverse effects with other PHENOTHIAZINES; **amiodarone, amoxapine, arsenic trioxide, bepridil, clarithromycin, daunorubicin, diltiazem, disopyramide, dofetilide, dolasetron, doxorubicin, encainide, erythromycin, flecainide, fluoxetine, fluvoxamine gatifloxacin, grepafloxacin, haloperidol, ibutilide, indapamide, local anesthetics, maprotiline, moxifloxacin, octreotide, paroxetine, pentamidine, pimozide, procainamide, probucol, quinidine, risperidone, sotalol, sertraline, sparfloxacin, terodiline, tocainide, tricyclic antidepressants, venlafaxine, verapamil, ziprasidone** can prolong QT$_c$ interval resulting in arrhythmias. **Herbal: Kava** may increase risk and severity of dystonic reactions.

## PHARMACOKINETICS Absorption: Well absorbed from GI tract. **Onset:** Days to weeks. **Distribution:** Crosses placenta; distributed into breast milk. **Metabolism:** In liver (CYP2D6). **Elimination:** In urine. **Half-Life:** 26–36 h.

## NURSING IMPLICATIONS

### Black Box Warning

*Thioridazine has been associated with prolongation of the QTc interval, development of torsades de pointes–type arrhythmias and sudden death; and with increased mortality in older adults with dementia-related psychosis.*

### Assessment & Drug Effects

- Monitor for changes in behavior that may indicate increased possibility of suicide ideation.
- Orthostatic hypotension may occur in early therapy. Monitor ambulation.
- Monitor ECG periodically throughout therapy, especially during a period of dose adjustment.
- Report promptly S&S of torsades de pointes (e.g., dizziness, palpitations, syncope).
- Monitor I&O ratio and bowel elimination pattern. Check for abdominal distention and pain. Encourage adequate fluid intake as prophylaxis for constipation and xerostomia. The depressed patient may not seek help for either symptom or for urinary retention.
- Obtain baseline and periodic ophthalmic exam.
- Monitor lab tests: Periodic CBC, serum electrolytes, lipid profile, fasting plasma glucose level, HbA1C, and LFTs.

### Patient & Family Education

- Avoid alcohol during phenothiazine therapy. Concomitant use enhances CNS depression effects.
- Be aware that marked drowsiness generally subsides with continued therapy or reduction in dosage.
- Do not drive or engage in potentially hazardous activities until response to drug is known.
- Make position changes slowly, particularly from lying down to upright posture; dangle legs a few minutes before standing.
- Vasodilation produced by hot showers or baths or by long exposure to environmental heat may accentuate hypotensive effect.
- Note: Thioridazine may color urine pink-red to reddish brown.
- Do not use any OTC drugs unless approved by the prescriber.

Common adverse effects in *italic*; life-threatening effects underlined; generic names in **bold**; classifications in SMALL CAPS; ♣ Canadian drug name; ⊘ Prototype drug

# THIOTEPA

(thye-oh-tep′a)

Tepadina

**Classifications:** ANTINEOPLASTIC; ALKYLATING AGENT

Therapeutic: ANTINEOPLASTIC

**Prototype:** Cyclophosphamide

**AVAILABILITY** Solution for injection

## ACTION & *THERAPEUTIC EFFECT*

Cell-cycle nonspecific alkylating agent that selectively reacts with DNA phosphate groups to produce chromosome cross-linkage and consequent blocking of nucleoprotein synthesis. Highly toxic hematopoietic agent. *Myelosuppression is cumulative and unpredictable and may be delayed.*

## USES
To produce remissions in malignant lymphomas, including Hodgkin's disease, and adenocarcinoma of breast and ovary. Also in chronic granulocytic and lymphocytic leukemia, superficial papillary carcinoma of urinary bladder, bronchogenic carcinoma, and in malignant effusions secondary to neoplastic disease of serosal cavities.

## UNLABELED USES
Prevention of pterygium recurrences following postoperative beta-irradiation; leukemia, malignant meningeal neoplasms.

## CONTRAINDICATIONS
Hypersensitivity to thiotepa; acute leukemia; acute infection; concomitant use with live or attenuated vaccines; pregnancy (category D); lactation.

## CAUTIOUS USE
Chronic lymphocytic leukemia; myelosuppression produced by radiation; bone marrow invasion by tumor cells; impaired kidney or liver function; children.

## ROUTE & DOSAGE

### Malignant Lymphomas
*Adult:* **IV** 0.3–0.4 mg/kg q1–4wk

### Malignant Pleural Effusion
*Adult:* **Intracavitary** 0.6–0.8 mg/kg instilled through same tubing used for paracentesis at intervals of at least 1 wk

### Bladder Cancer
*Adult:* **Intravesicular** 60 mg in 30–60 mL of distilled water instilled into bladder to be retained for 2 h once/wk for 4 wk

### Non-Hodgkin's Lymphoma
*Adult:* **IV** 20–40 mg/m$^2$ q3–4 wk (in combinations) or 0.3–0.4 mg/kg q1–4 wk

## ADMINISTRATION

**Intravenous**

Use only under constant supervision by prescribers experienced in therapy with cytotoxic agents. ▪Avoid exposure of skin and respiratory tract to particles of thiotepa during solution preparation.

***PREPARE:* Direct:** Reconstitute each 15 mg or 30 mg vial with 1.5 mL or 3 mL sterile water for injection (supplied), respectively, to yield 10 mg/mL. ▪ Filter solution through a 0.22 micron filter to eliminate haze. Use immediately.

***ADMINISTER:* Direct:** Give 60 mg or fraction thereof over 1 min. Flush with 5 mL NS before and after infusion.

***INCOMPATIBILITIES:* Solution/additive: Cisplatin. Y-site: Cisplatin, filgrastim, minocycline, vinorelbine.**

▪ Store powder for injection and reconstituted solutions at 2°–8° C (35°–46° F); protect from light. ▪ Solutions reconstituted with sterile water only are stable for 8 h under refrigeration.

---

Common adverse effects in *italic;* life-threatening effects <u>underlined</u>; generic names in **bold**; classifications in SMALL CAPS; ♣ Canadian drug name; ⊕ Prototype drug

T

**ADVERSE EFFECTS** (≥1%) **GI:** Anorexia, nausea, vomiting, stomatitis, ulceration of intestinal mucosa. **Hematologic:** <u>Leukopenia, thrombocytopenia, anemia, pancytopenia</u>. **Skin:** Hives, rash, pruritus. **Urogenital:** Amenorrhea, interference with spermatogenesis. **Body as a Whole:** Headache, febrile reactions, pain and weeping of injection site, hyperuricemia, slowed or lessened response in heavily irradiated area, sensation of throat tightness. **Other:** Reported with intravesical administration (lower abdominal pain, hematuria, hemorrhagic chemical cystitis, vesical irritability).

**INTERACTIONS Drug:** May prolong muscle paralysis with **mivacurium;** ANTICOAGULANTS, NSAIDS, SALICYLATES, ANTIPLATELET AGENTS may increase risk of bleeding. Do not administer with LIVE VACCINES.

**PHARMACOKINETICS Absorption:** Rapidly cleared from plasma. **Onset:** Gradual response over several weeks. **Metabolism:** In liver. **Elimination:** 60% in urine within 24–72 h.

**NURSING IMPLICATIONS**

**Assessment & Drug Effects**

- Monitor closely because most patients will manifest some evidence of toxicity.
- Be aware that because of cumulative effects, maximum myelosuppression may be delayed 3–4 wk after termination of therapy.
- Withhold drug and notify prescriber if leukocyte count falls to 3000/mm³ or below or if platelet count falls below 150,000/mm³.
- Monitor lab tests: CBC with differential, LFTs, renal function tests, and platelet count at least weekly during therapy and for at least 3 wk after therapy is discontinued.

**Patient & Family Education**

- Be aware of possibility of amenorrhea (usually reversible in 6–8 mo).
- Report onset of fever, bleeding, a cold or illness, no matter how mild to prescriber; medical supervision may be necessary.

# THIOTHIXENE HYDROCHLORIDE

(thye-oh-thix′een)

**Classification:** ANTIPSYCHOTIC; PHENOTHIAZINE
**Therapeutic:** ANTIPSYCHOTIC
**Prototype:** Chlorpromazine

**AVAILABILITY** Capsule

**ACTION & *THERAPEUTIC EFFECT*** Mechanism of action is related to blockade of postsynaptic dopamine receptors in the mesolimbic region of the brain. Additionally, blockade of alpha₁-adrenergic receptors in the CNS produces sedation and muscle relaxation. *Possesses antipsychotic, sedative, adrenolytic, and antiemetic activity.*

**USES** Manifestations of psychotic disorders.

**CONTRAINDICATIONS** Hypersensitivity to thiothixene; comatose states; CNS depression; older adults with dementia related psychosis; circulatory collapse; blood dyscrasias; NMS; lactation.

**CAUTIOUS USE** History of convulsive disorders; alcohol withdrawal; glaucoma; prostatic hypertrophy; cardiovascular disease; older adults; patients who might be exposed to organophosphorus insecticides or to extreme heat; previously diagnosed breast cancer; pregnancy (category C). Safe use in children younger than 12 y not established.

Common adverse effects in *italic;* life-threatening effects <u>underlined;</u> generic names in **bold;** classifications in SMALL CAPS; ◆ Canadian drug name; ⊙ Prototype drug

## ROUTE & DOSAGE

### Psychotic Disorders

*Adult/Adolescent:* **PO** 2 mg t.i.d., may increase up to 15 mg/day as needed or tolerated (max: 60 mg/day)

## ADMINISTRATION

### Oral

- Capsules may be opened and mixed with food or water for ease of administration.

## ADVERSE EFFECTS (≥1%) CNS:

*Drowsiness,* insomnia, dizziness, cerebral edema, convulsions, *extrapyramidal symptoms (dose related),* paradoxical exaggeration of psychotic symptoms; <u>sudden death, neuroleptic malignant syndrome</u>, tardive dyskinesia, depressed cough reflex **GI:** Xerostomia, constipation. **CV:** Tachycardia, *orthostatic hypotension.* **Urogenital:** Impotence, gynecomastia, galactorrhea, amenorrhea. **Skin:** Rash, photosensitivity. **Special Senses:** Blurred vision, pigmentary retinopathy. **Metabolic:** Decreased serum uric acid levels.

## INTERACTIONS Drug: Alcohol,

ANXIOLYTICS, SEDATIVE-HYPNOTICS, other CNS DEPRESSANTS add to CNS depression; additive adverse effects with other PHENOTHIAZINES; **Herbal: Kava** may increase risk and severity of dystonic reactions.

## PHARMACOKINETICS Absorption:

Slowly absorbed from GI tract. **Onset:** Days to weeks PO; 1–6 h IM. **Duration:** Up to 12 h. **Distribution:** May remain in body for several weeks; crosses placenta. **Metabolism:** In liver. **Elimination:** In bile and feces. **Half-Life:** 34 h.

## NURSING IMPLICATIONS

### Black Box Warning

*Thiothixene has been associated with increased mortality in older adults with dementia-related psychosis.*

### Assessment & Drug Effects

- Monitor BP for excessive hypotensive response when thiothixene is added to drug regimen of patient on hypertensive treatment until therapy is stabilized.
- Report extrapyramidal effects (pseudoparkinsonism, akathisia, dystonia) to prescriber; dose adjustment or short-term therapy with an antiparkinsonism agent may provide relief.
- Be alert to first symptoms of tardive dyskinesia (see Appendix F). Withhold drug and notify prescriber.
- Monitor lab tests: Periodic complete metabolic panel, lipid profile, and LFTs.

### Patient & Family Education

- Make position changes slowly, particularly from lying down to upright because of danger of lightheadedness; sit a few minutes before walking.
- Do not drive or engage in potentially hazardous activities until response to drug is known.
- Avoid alcohol and other depressants during therapy.
- Take drug as prescribed; do not alter dosing regimen or stop medication without consulting prescriber. Abrupt discontinuation can cause delirium.
- Do not use any OTC drugs without approval of prescriber.
- Avoid excessive exposure to sunlight to prevent a photosensitivity reaction. If sun exposure is expected, protect skin with sunscreen lotion (SPF 12 or above).

T

---

Common adverse effects in *italic;* life-threatening effects <u>underlined;</u> generic names in **bold;** classifications in SMALL CAPS; ♣ Canadian drug name; ⊘ Prototype drug

- Schedule periodic eye exams and report blurred vision to prescriber.

# THROMBIN
(throm'bin)

Recothrom, Thrombinar, Thrombostat

**Classification:** COAGULATOR; TOPICAL HEMOSTATIC
**Therapeutic:** COAGULATOR; HEMOSTATIC

**AVAILABILITY** Topical application

## ACTION & *THERAPEUTIC EFFECT*
Plasma protein prepared from prothrombin of bovine origin. Induces clotting of whole blood or fibrinogen solution without addition of other substances. *Facilitates conversion of fibrinogen to fibrin resulting in clotting of whole blood.*

**USES** Hemostasis aid.

## CONTRAINDICATIONS
Known hypersensitivity to any of thrombin components or to material of bovine origin; parenteral use; entry or infiltration into large blood vessels.

## CAUTIOUS USE
Older adults; pregnancy (category C). Safety and efficacy in children and infants not established.

## ROUTE & DOSAGE

### Hemostasis
*Adult:* **Topical** 100–2000 NIH units/mL, depending on extent of bleeding, may be used as solution, in dry form, by mixing thrombin with blood plasma to form a fibrin "glue," or in conjunction with absorbable gelatin sponge

## ADMINISTRATION
**Topical**
- Ensure that sponge recipient area is free of blood before applying thrombin.
- Prepare solutions in sterile distilled water or isotonic saline.
- Use solutions within a few hours of preparation. If several hours are to elapse between time of preparation and use, solution should be refrigerated, or preferably frozen, and used within 48 h.
- Store lyophilized preparation at 2°–8° C (36°–46° F).

## ADVERSE EFFECTS (≥1%) **Body as a Whole:** Sensitivity, allergic and febrile reactions, <u>intravascular clotting and death when thrombin is allowed to enter large blood vessels.</u>

# THYROID DESSICATED
(thye'roid)

Armour Thyroid, Nature-Thyroid, NP Thyroid, Westhroid, WP Thyroid

**Classification:** THYROID HORMONE
**Therapeutic:** THYROID HORMONE REPLACEMENT
**Prototype:** Levothyroxine sodium

**AVAILABILITY** Tablet

## ACTION & *THERAPEUTIC EFFECT*
The mechanisms by which thyroid hormones exert their effects are not well understood. They enhance oxygen consumption, increase the basal metabolic rate and the metabolism of carbohydrates,

Common adverse effects in *italic;* life-threatening effects <u>underlined;</u> generic names in **bold;** classifications in SMALL CAPS; ✦ Canadian drug name; ⊙ Prototype drug

lipids, and proteins. They exert a profound influence on every organ system and are of particular importance in the development of the CNS. *Effectiveness indicated by diuresis, followed by sense of well-being, increased pulse rate, increased pulse pressure, increased appetite, increased psychomotor activity, loss of constipation, normalization of skin texture and hair, and increased $T_3$ and $T_4$ serum levels.*

**USES** Treatment of hypothyroidism of any etiology, and for the treatment or prevention of various types of euthyroid (non-toxic) goiter.

**CONTRAINDICATIONS** Thyrotoxicosis; acute MI not associated with hypothyroidism, cardiovascular disease; morphologic hypogonadism; nephrosis; uncorrected hypoadrenalism.

**CAUTIOUS USE** Angina pectoris, hypertension, older adults who may have occult cardiac disease; renal insufficiency; DM; history of hyperthyroidism, malabsorption states; pregnancy (category A).

## ROUTE & DOSAGE

**Hypothyroidism**

*Adult/Adolescent:* **PO** 30 mg/day, may increase by 15 mg q2–3 wk to 60–180mg/day
*Infant/Child:* See package insert for weight-based dosing.

## ADMINISTRATION

**Oral**
- Give preferably on an empty stomach.
- Initiate dosage generally at low level and systematically increase in small increments to desired maintenance dose.
- Store in dark bottle to minimize spontaneous deiodination. Keep desiccated thyroid dry.

**ADVERSE EFFECTS** (≥1%) **Endocrine:** Hyperthyroidism, thyroid storm [high temperature (as high as 41° C [106° F]), tachycardia, vomiting, <u>shock, coma</u>. **Special Senses:** Staring expression in eyes. **CV:** CHF, angina, cardiac arrhythmias, palpitation, tachycardia. **Body as a Whole:** Weight loss, tremors, headache, nervousness, fever, insomnia, warm and moist skin, heat intolerance, leg cramps, menstrual irregularities, <u>shock</u>, changes in appetite. **GI:** Diarrhea or abdominal cramps. **Metabolic:** Hyperglycemia (usually offset by increased tissue oxidation of sugar).

**DIAGNOSTIC TEST INTERFERENCE** Thyroid increases *basal metabolic rate;* may increase *blood glucose levels, creatine phosphokinase, AST, LDH, PBI.* It may decrease *serum uric acid, cholesterol, thyroid-stimulating hormone (TSH), iodine 131* uptake. Many medications may produce false results in *thyroid function tests.*

**INTERACTIONS Drug:** ORAL ANTICOAGULANTS potentiate hypoprothrombinemia; may increase requirements for **insulin,** SULFONYLUREAS; **epinephrine** may precipitate coronary insufficiency; **cholestyramine,** aluminum, or calcium-containing products may decrease thyroid absorption. **Food:** Certain foods, beverages, and enteral feedings can inhibit the absorption of thyroid hormones.

**PHARMACOKINETICS Absorption:** Variably absorbed from GI tract. **Peak:** 1–3 wk. **Distribution:**

Common adverse effects in *italic*; life-threatening effects <u>underlined</u>; generic names in **bold**; classifications in SMALL CAPS; ✦ Canadian drug name; ⓟ Prototype drug

1599

Does not readily cross placenta; minimal amounts in breast milk. **Metabolism:** Deiodination in thyroid gland. **Elimination:** In urine and feces. **Half-Life:** $T_3$, 1–2 days; $T_4$, 6–7 days.

## NURSING IMPLICATIONS

### Assessment & Drug Effects

- Observe patient carefully during initial treatment for untoward reactions such as angina, palpitations, cardiac pain.
- Be alert for symptoms of overdosage (see ADVERSE EFFECTS) that may occur 1–3 wk after therapy is started.
- Monitor response until regimen is stabilized to prevent iatrogenic hyperthyroidism. In drug-induced hyperthyroidism, there may also be increased bone loss. Such a patient is vulnerable to pathologic fractures.
- Monitor vital signs: Assess pulse before each dose during period of dosage adjustment. Consult prescriber if rate is 100 or more or if there has been a marked change in rate or rhythm.
- TSH 4–8 wk after initiation or dose change, repeat at 6 mo, then q12mo thereafter.

### Patient & Family Education

- Be aware that replacement therapy for hypothyroidism is life-long; continued follow-up care is important.
- Monitor pulse rate and report increases greater than parameter set by prescriber.
- Report to prescriber onset of chest pain or other signs of aggravated CV disease (dyspnea, tachycardia).
- Report evidence of any unexplained bleeding to prescriber when taking concomitant anticoagulant.
- Use monthly height and weight measurement to monitor growth in juvenile undergoing treatment.

# TIAGABINE HYDROCHLORIDE

(ti-a′ga-been)

Gabitril

**Classifications:** ANTICONVULSANT; GABA INHIBITOR

Therapeutic: ANTICONVULSANT

**Prototype:** Valproic acid sodium (sodium valproate)

## AVAILABILITY Tablet

## ACTION & *THERAPEUTIC EFFECT*

Potent and selective inhibitor of GABA uptake into presynaptic neurons; allows more GABA to bind to the surfaces of postsynaptic neurons in the CNS. *Effectiveness indicated by reduction in seizure activity.*

## USES Adjunctive therapy for partial seizures.

## CONTRAINDICATIONS Hypersensitivity to tiagabine; lactation.

## CAUTIOUS USE Liver function impairment; history of spike and wave discharge on EEG; status epilepticus; pregnancy (category C). Safe use in children younger than 12 y not established.

## ROUTE & DOSAGE

### Seizures

*Adult:* **PO** Start with 4 mg daily, may increase dose by 4–8 mg/day qwk (max: 56 mg/day in 2–4 divided doses)

*Adolescent (12–18 y):* **PO** Start with 4 mg daily, after 2 wk may increase dose by 4–8 mg/day qwk (max: 32 mg/day in 2–4 divided doses)

## ADMINISTRATION

### Oral

- Give with food.

Common adverse effects in *italic;* life-threatening effects <u>underlined;</u> generic names in **bold;** classifications in SMALL CAPS; ◆ Canadian drug name; ⊘ Prototype drug

- Make dosage increases, when needed, at weekly intervals.
- Store at 20°–25° C (68°–77° F) in a tightly closed container and protect from light.

**ADVERSE EFFECTS** (≥1%) **Body as a Whole:** Infection, flu-like syndrome, pain, myasthenia, allergic reactions, chills, malaise, arthralgia. **CNS:** *Dizziness, asthenia, tremor, somnolence, nervousness,* difficulty concentrating, ataxia, depression, insomnia, abnormal gait, hostility, confusion, speech disorder, difficulty with memory, paresthesias, emotional lability, agitation, dysarthria, euphoria, hallucinations, paranoia, hyperkinesia, hypertonia, hypotonia, myoclonus, twitching, vertigo. Risk of new-onset seizures. **CV:** Vasodilation, hypertension, palpitations, tachycardia, syncope, edema, peripheral edema. **GI:** Abdominal pain, diarrhea, nausea, vomiting, increased appetite, mouth ulcers. **Respiratory:** Pharyngitis, cough, bronchitis, dyspnea, epistaxis, pneumonia. **Skin:** Rash, pruritus, alopecia, dry skin, sweating, ecchymoses. **Special Senses:** Amblyopia, nystagmus, tinnitus. **Urogenital:** Dysmenorrhea, dysuria, metrorrhagia, incontinence, vaginitis, UTI.

**INTERACTIONS Drug: Carbamazepine, mitotane, phenytoin, phenobarbital** decrease levels of tiagabine. Use with ANTIDEPRESSANTS, ANTIPSYCHOTICS, STIMULANTS, AMPHETAMINES, and NARCOTICS may increase seizure risk. Avoid use of **ceritinib, idelalisib, posaconazole,** as it may increase toxicity risk. **Herbal: Ginkgo, kava** may decrease anticonvulsant effectiveness. **Evening primrose oil** may affect seizure threshold. **Food:** Use of ethanol regularly may require lower tiagabine dose.

**PHARMACOKINETICS Absorption:** Rapidly absorbed; 90% bioavailability. **Peak:** 45 min. **Distribution:** 96% protein bound. **Metabolism:** In liver (CYP3A4). **Elimination:** 25% in urine, 63% in feces. **Half-Life:** 7–9 h (4–7 h with other enzyme-inducing drugs).

## NURSING IMPLICATIONS
### Assessment & Drug Effects
- Be aware that concurrent use of other anticonvulsants may decrease effectiveness of tiagabine or increase the potential for adverse effects.
- Monitor carefully for S&S of CNS depression and suicidal ideation.
- Monitor lab tests: Plasma tiagabine before and after changes are made in the drug regimen, LFTs.

### Patient & Family Education
- Do not stop taking drug abruptly; may cause sudden onset of seizures.
- Exercise caution while engaging in potentially hazardous activities because drug may cause dizziness.
- Use caution when taking other prescription or OTC drugs that can cause drowsiness.
- Report any of the following to the prescriber: Rash or hives; red, peeling skin; dizziness; drowsiness; depression; GI distress; nervousness or tremors, difficulty concentrating or talking.

# TICAGRELOR
(tye'ka-gre-lor)

Brilinta

**Classifications:** ANTIPLATELET; PLATELET ADP RECEPTOR ANTAGONIST; PLATELET AGGREGATION INHIBITOR; ANTITHROMBOTIC
**Therapeutic:** PLATELET AGGREGATION INHIBITOR; ANTITHROMBOTIC
**Prototype:** Clopidogrel

**AVAILABILITY** Tablet

## ACTION & *THERAPEUTIC EFFECT*
Ticagrelor and its major metabolite reversibly interact with the platelet

ADP receptor to prevent signal transduction and platelet activation. *Prevents platelet activation and clot formation.*

**USES** Prophylaxis to prevent arterial thromboembolism in patients with acute coronary syndrome (ACS).

**UNLABELED USES** Unstable angina/non-ST elevation MI.

**CONTRAINDICATIONS** Hypersensitivity (e.g., angioedema) to ticagrelor; severe hepatic impairment; history of intracranial hemorrhage; active bleeding (e.g., peptic ulcer); use within 24 h.

**CAUTIOUS USE** Mild-to-moderate hepatic impairment; second or third AV block, sick sinus syndrome; history of bleeding disorders, percutaneous invasive procedures, and use of drugs that increase risk of bleeding (e.g., anticoagulant and fibrinolytic therapy, high dose aspirin, long-term NSAIDs); older adults; pregnancy (category C); lactation. Safety and efficacy in children not established.

## ROUTE & DOSAGE

### Arterial Thromboembolism Prophylaxis

*Adult:* **PO** 180 mg loading dose (plus aspirin) followed by 90 mg b.i.d. (with 75–100 mg aspirin once daily) for 1 y; after 1 y 60 mg b.i.d.

## ADMINISTRATION

### Oral
▪ May be given without regard to food.
▪ Store at 15°–30° C (59°–86° F).

**ADVERSE EFFECTS** (≥3%) **Body as a Whole:** Fatigue, noncardiac chest pain. **CNS:** Dizziness, headache.

**CV:** Atrial fibrillation, bradycardia, chest pain, hypertension, hypotension, *increased bleeding*. **GI:** Diarrhea, nausea. **Metabolic:** Increased serum creatinine, increased uric acid levels. **Urogenital:** Hematuria, UTI. **Musculoskeletal:** Back pain. **Respiratory:** Cough, *dyspnea.*

**INTERACTIONS Drug:** Strong CYP3A4 inhibitors (e.g., **ketoconazole, itraconazole, voriconazole, clarithromycin, nefazodone, ritonavir, saquinavir, nelfinavir, indinavir, atazanavir,** and **telithromycin**) can increase ticagrelor levels, while potent CYP3A4 inducers (e.g., **rifampin, dexamethasone, phenytoin, carbamazepine,** and **phenobarbital**) can decrease ticagrelor levels. Ticagrelor can increase the levels of **simvastatin** and **lovastatin.** Do not use with **avanafil, defibrotide.**

**PHARMACOKINETICS Absorption:** 30–42% Bioavailable. **Onset:** 1.5–5 h. **Distribution:** Greater than 99% plasma protein bound. **Metabolism:** CYP3A4, CYP3A5, P-gp metabolism to active compound. **Elimination:** Fecal (58%) and renal (26%). **Half-Life:** 7 h (ticagrelor); 9 h (active metabolite).

## NURSING IMPLICATIONS

### Black Box Warning

*Ticagrelor has been associated with serious, sometimes fatal, bleeding.*

### Assessment & Drug Effects
▪ Monitor cardiac status with ECG and frequent BP measurements. Report immediately development of hypotension in any one who has recently undergone coronary angiography, PCI, CABG, or other surgical procedures.

Common adverse effects in *italic;* life-threatening effects underlined; generic names in **bold;** classifications in SMALL CAPS; ♣ Canadian drug name; ☯ Prototype drug

- Monitor for and report promptly S&S of bleeding or dyspnea. Monitor lab tests: CBC and LFTs.

**Patient & Family Education**

- Report promptly to prescriber any of the following: Unexplained, prolonged, or excessive bleeding; blood in stool or urine; shortness of breath.
- Daily doses of aspirin **should not** exceed 100 mg. Do not take any other drugs that contain aspirin. Consult prescriber if taking a nonsteroidal anti-inflammatory drug (NSAID).
- Inform all health care providers that you are taking ticagrelor.

# TICARCILLIN DISODIUM/ CLAVULANATE POTASSIUM

(tye-kar-sill'in/clav-yoo'la-nate)

Timentin

**Classifications:** ANTIBIOTIC; EXTENDED-SPECTRUM PENICILLIN

Therapeutic: ANTIBIOTIC

**Prototype:** Piperacillin/ tazobactam

**AVAILABILITY** Solution for injection

## ACTION & THERAPEUTIC EFFECT

Used alone, clavulanic acid antibacterial activity is weak, but in combination with ticarcillin prevents degradation by beta-lactamase and extends ticarcillin spectrum of activity. *Combination drug extends ticarcillin spectrum of activity against many strains of beta-lactamase-producing bacteria (synergistic effect).*

## USES
Infections of lower respiratory tract and urinary tract and skin and skin structures, infections of bone and joint, and septicemia caused by susceptible organisms. Also mixed infections and as presumptive therapy before identification of causative organism.

**CONTRAINDICATIONS** Hypersensitivity to ticarcillin/clavulanate or penicillins or to cephalosporins, coagulopathy.

**CAUTIOUS USE** DM; GI disease; asthma; history of allergies; renal impairment; pregnancy (category B); lactation.

## ROUTE & DOSAGE

### Moderate to Severe Infections

*Adult/Adolescent/Child (weight greater than 60 kg):* **IV** 3.1 g q4–6h

*Child/Infant (3 mo or older and weight less than 60 kg):* **IV** 200–300 mg/kg/day divided q4–6h (based on ticarcillin)

*Infant (younger than 3 mo and weight less than 60 kg):* **IV** 200–300 mg/kg/day divided q6–8h (based on ticarcillin)

### Renal Impairment Dosage Adjustment

*CrCl 30–60 mL/min:* Give 2 g q4h; *10–30 mL/min:* Give 2 g q8h; *less than 10 mL/min:* Give 2 g q12h

### Hemodialysis Dosage Adjustment

2 g q12h, supplement with 3.1 g after dialysis

## ADMINISTRATION

**Intravenous**

Note: Verify correct IV concentration and rate of infusion for administration to infants and children with prescriber.

*PREPARE:* **Intermittent:** Reconstitute by adding 13 mL sterile

T

Common adverse effects in *italic;* life-threatening effects <u>underlined;</u> generic names in **bold;** classifications in SMALL CAPS; ♣ Canadian drug name; ⊙ Prototype drug

1603

water for injection or NS injection to the 3.1 g vial to yield 200 mg/mL ticarcillin with 6.7 mg/mL clavulanic acid. Shake until dissolved. ▪ Further dilute the required does in NS, D5W, or LR to concentrations between 10–100 mg/mL. ▪ **Do not** use if discoloration or particulate matter is present.

*ADMINISTER:* **Intermittent:** Give over 30 min.

*INCOMPATIBILITIES:* Solution/additive: AMINOGLYCOSIDES, **sodium bicarbonate. Y-site:** acyclovir, alatrofloxacin, amphotericin B cholesteryl complex, azathioprine, azithromycin, caspofunging, cefamandole, chlorpormazine, dantrolene, daunorubicin, diazepam, diazoxide, dobutamine, dolasetron, drotrecogin alfa, epirubicin, erythromycin, ganciclovir, gemtuzumab, haloperidol, hydroxyzine, idarubicin, inamrinone, lansoprazole, minocycline, mitomycin, mitoxantrone, mycophenolate, papervine, pentamidine, pentazocine, phenytoin, promethazine, protamine, quinidine, quinupristin/dalfopristin, SMZ/TMP, vancomycin.

▪ Store vial with sterile powder at 21°–24° C (69°–75° F) or colder. ▪ If exposed to higher temperature, powder will darken, indicating degradation of clavulanate potassium and loss of potency. Discard vial. ▪ See package insert for information about storage and stability of reconstituted and diluted IV solutions of drug.

## ADVERSE EFFECTS (≥1%) **Body as a Whole:** Hypersensitivity reactions, pain, burning, swelling at injection site; phlebitis, thrombophlebitis; superinfections. **CNS:**

Headache, blurred vision, mental deterioration, convulsions, hallucinations, seizures, giddiness, neuromuscular hyperirritability. **GI:** *Diarrhea, nausea,* vomiting, disturbances of taste or smell, stomatitis, flatulence. **Hematologic:** Eosinophilia, <u>thrombocytopenia</u>, <u>leukopenia</u>, neutropenia, hemolytic anemia. **Metabolic:** Hypernatremia, transient increases in serum AST, ALT, BUN, and alkaline phosphatase; increases in serum LDH, bilirubin, and creatinine and decreased serum uric acid.

## DIAGNOSTIC TEST INTERFERENCE
May interfere with test methods used to determine *urinary proteins* except for tests for urinary protein that use *bromphenol blue. Positive direct antiglobulin (Coombs') test* results, apparently caused by clavulanic acid, have been reported. This test may interfere with *transfusion cross-matching procedures.*

## INTERACTIONS **Drugs:** May increase risk of bleeding with ANTICOAGULANTS; **probenecid** decreases elimination of ticarcillin.

## PHARMACOKINETICS **Distribution:** Widely distributed with highest concentrations in urine and bile; crosses placenta; distributed into breast milk. **Metabolism:** In liver. **Elimination:** In urine. **Half-Life:** 1.1–1.2 h ticarcillin, 1.1–1.5 h clavulanate.

## NURSING IMPLICATIONS
### Assessment & Drug Effects
▪ Be aware that serious and sometimes fatal anaphylactoid reactions have been reported in patients with penicillin hypersensitivity or history of sensitivity

T

to multiple allergens. Reported incidence is low with this combination drug.

- Monitor cardiac status because of high sodium content of drug.
- Overdose symptoms: This drug may cause neuromuscular hyperirritability or seizures.
- Monitor lab tests: Baseline C&S; periodic LFTs and renal function tests, CBC, platelet count, and serum electrolytes.

**Patient & Family Education**
- Report urticaria, rashes, or pruritus to prescriber immediately.
- Report frequent loose stools, diarrhea, or other possible signs of pseudomembranous colitis (see Appendix F) to prescriber.

# TICLOPIDINE HYDROCHLORIDE

(ti-clo'pi-deen)

**Classifications:** ANTICOAGULANT; PLATELET AGGREGATION INHIBITOR; ADP RECEPTOR ANTAGONIST
**Therapeutic:** PLATELET AGGREGATION INHIBITOR
**Prototype:** Clopidogrel

## AVAILABILITY Tablet

## ACTION & *THERAPEUTIC EFFECT*

Platelet aggregation inhibitor that interferes with platelet membrane functioning and therefore platelet interactions. Ticlopidine interferes with ADP-induced binding of fibrinogen to the platelet membrane at specific receptor sites. *Platelet adhesion and platelet aggregation are inhibited and prolong bleeding time.*

## USES Reduction of the risk of thrombotic stroke; adjunctive therapy for stent thrombosis prophylaxis.

**UNLABELED USES** Prevention of venous thromboembolic disorders; maintenance of bypass graft patency and of vascular access sites in hemodialysis patients; improvement of exercise performance in patients with ischemic heart disease and intermittent claudication; prevention of postoperative deep venous thrombosis (DVT).

**CONTRAINDICATIONS** Hypersensitivity to ticlopidine; hematopoietic disease, coagulopathy; neutropenia thrombotic thrombocytopenic purpura (TTP) leukemia; pathologic bleeding; severe liver impairment; lactation.

**CAUTIOUS USE** Hepatic function impairment, renal impairment; patients at risk for bleeding from trauma, surgery, or a bleeding disorder; GI bleeding in patients with history of thienopyridine hypersensitivity; allergic cross-reactivity; pregnancy (category B). Safe use in children younger than 18 y not established.

## ROUTE & DOSAGE

**Prevention of Stroke/Stent Thrombosis**
*Adult:* **PO** 250 mg b.i.d. with food

## ADMINISTRATION

**Oral**
- Hold medication and notify provider if neutrophil count falls below 1200/mm³.
- Give with food or just after eating to minimize GI irritation.
- Do not give within 2 h of an antacid.
- Store at 15°–30° C (59°–86° F).

**ADVERSE EFFECTS** (≥1%) **CNS:** Dizziness. **GI:** Nausea, vomiting, diarrhea, abdominal cramps; dyspepsia, flatulence, anorexia; hypercholesterolemia, abnormal liver function tests (few cases of hepatotoxicity reported). **Endocrine:** Hypercholesterolemia.

Common adverse effects in *italic;* life-threatening effects underlined; generic names in **bold;** classifications in SMALL CAPS; ♦ Canadian drug name; ⊙ Prototype drug

1605

**Hematologic:** Neutropenia (resolves in 1–3 wk), thrombocytopenia, leukopenia, agranulocytosis (usually within first 3 mo), and pancytopenia; hemorrhage (ecchymosis, epistaxis, menorrhagia, GI bleeding), thrombotic thrombocytopenic purpura (usually within first month). **Skin:** Urticaria, maculopapular rash, erythema nodosum (generally occur within the first 3 mo of therapy, with most occurring within the first 3–6 wk).

## DIAGNOSTIC TEST INTERFERENCE

Increases *total serum cholesterol* by 8–10% within 4 wk of beginning therapy. *Lipoprotein ratios* remain unchanged. Elevates *alkaline phosphatase* and *serum transaminases.*

## INTERACTIONS Drug: ANTACIDS

decrease bioavailability of ticlopidine. ANTICOAGULANTS increase risk of bleeding. **Cimetidine** decreases clearance of ticlopidine. CORTICOSTEROIDS counteract increased bleeding time associated with ticlopidine. May decrease **cyclosporine** levels. Increases **theophylline** serum levels. May increase levels of **citalopram, metoprolol, lomitapide, pimoxide, phenytoin, tizanidine**. Can decrease levels of **clopidogrel.** Do not use with **defibrotide. Food:** Food may increase bioavailability of **ticlopidine. Herbal: Evening primrose oil** increases bleeding risk.

## PHARMACOKINETICS Absorption: 90% from GI tract; increased absorption when taken with food. **Onset:** Antiplatelet activity, 6 h; maximal effect at 3–5 days. **Peak:** Peak serum levels at 2h. **Duration:** Bleeding times return to baseline within 4–10 days. **Distribution:** 90% bound to plasma proteins. **Metabolism:** Rapidly and extensively metabolized in liver (CYP1A2, CYP2B6, CYP2C19). **Elimination:** 60% of metabolites excreted in urine, 23% in

feces. **Half-Life:** 12.6 h; terminal half-life is 4–5 days with repeated dosing.

## NURSING IMPLICATIONS

### Black Box Warning

*Ticlopidine has been associated with life-threatening neutropenia, agranulocytosis, thrombotic thrombocytopenic purpura (TTP), and aplastic anemia.*

### Assessment & Drug Effects

- Report promptly laboratory values indicative of neutropenia, thrombocytopenia, or agranulocytosis.
- Monitor for signs of bleeding (e.g., ecchymosis, epistaxis, hematuria, GI bleeding).
- Monitor lab tests: Baseline CBC with differentials and platelet count, repeat q2wk from second week to end of third month of therapy, repeat as indicated thereafter if S&S of infection develop, and LFTs.

### Patient & Family Education

- Stop taking this drug and report promptly to prescriber any of the following: Nausea, diarrhea, rash, sore throat, or other signs of infection, signs of bleeding, or signs of liver damage (e.g., yellow skin or sclera, dark urine or clay-colored stools).
- Understand risk of GI bleeding; do not take aspirin along with ticlopidine.
- Do not take antacids within 2 h of ticlopidine.
- Keep appointments for regularly scheduled blood tests.

## TIGECYCLINE

(ti-ge-cy′cline)

Tygacil

**Classifications:** ANTIBIOTIC; GLYCYLCYCLINE

Therapeutic: ANTIBIOTIC

**Prototype:** Tetracycline

Common adverse effects in *italic;* life-threatening effects underlined; generic names in **bold;** classifications in SMALL CAPS; ♦ Canadian drug name; ⓟ Prototype drug

**AVAILABILITY** Solution for injection

## ACTION & *THERAPEUTIC EFFECT*

Inhibits protein production in bacteria by binding to the 30S ribosomal subunit and blocking entry of transfer RNA molecules into ribosome of bacteria. This prevents formation of peptide chains within bacteria, thus interfering with their growth. *Tigecycline is active against a broad spectrum of bacterial pathogens and is bacteriostatic.*

**USES** Treatment of complicated skin and skin structure infections, community acquired pneumonia, and complicated intra-abdominal infections.

**CONTRAINDICATIONS** Hypersensitivity to tigecycline; viral infections; pregnancy (category D); and during tooth development of the fetus.

**CAUTIOUS USE** Severe hepatic impairment (Child-Pugh class C); hypersensitivity to tetracycline, intestinal perforations, intra-abdominal infections; GI disorders; lactation. Safe use in children younger than 8 y not established.

## ROUTE & DOSAGE

**Community Acquired Pneumonia, Complicated Skin/ Intra-abdominal Infections**
*Adult:* **IV** 100 mg initially, followed by 50 mg q12h over 30–60 min × 5–14 days

**Hepatic Impairment Dosage Adjustment**
*Child-Pugh class C:* Initial dose 100 mg, followed by 25 mg q12h

## ADMINISTRATION

▪ Note that dosage adjustment is required with severe hepatic impairment.

**Intravenous**

*PREPARE:* **Intermittent:** Reconstitute each 50 mg with 5.3 mL of NS or D5W to yield 10 mg/mL. ▪ Swirl gently to dissolve; reconstituted solution should be yellow to orange in color. ▪ After reconstitution, immediately withdraw exactly 5 mL from each vial and add to 100 mL of NS or D5W for infusion. ▪ The maximum concentration in the IV bag should be 1 mg/mL (two 50 mg doses).

*ADMINISTER:* **Intermittent:** Give over 30–60 min through a dedicated line or Y site; when using Y-site, flush IV line with NS or D5W before/after infusion.

*INCOMPATIBILITIES:* **Y-site: Amiodarone, amphotericin B, bleomycin, chloramphenicol, chlorpromazine, dantrolene, daunorubicin, diazepam, epirubicin, esmoprazole, idarubicin, methylprednisolone, nicardapine, omeprazole, phenytoin, quinuprustin/dalfopristin, verapamil, voriconazole.**

▪ Store in the IV bag at room temperature for up to 6 h, or refrigerated at 2°–8° C (36°–46° F) for up to 24 h.

## ADVERSE EFFECTS (≥1%) **CNS:** Asthenia, dizziness, headache, insomnia. **CV:** Hypertension, hypotension, peripheral edema, phlebitis. **GI:** Abdominal pain, constipation, diarrhea, dyspepsia, *nausea, vomiting.* **Hematologic/ Lymphatic:** Abnormal healing, anemia, infection, leukocytosis, thrombocythemia. **Metabolic/Nutritional:** Alkaline phosphatase increased, ALT increased, amylase

**T**

Common adverse effects in *italic;* life-threatening effects <u>underlined;</u> generic names in **bold;** classifications in SMALL CAPS; ✦ Canadian drug name; ⊕ Prototype drug

1607

increased, AST increased, bilirubin-emia, BUN increased, hyperglyce-mia, hypokalemia, hypoproteinemia, lactic dehydrogenase increased. **Musculoskeletal:** Back pain. **Respiratory:** Dyspnea, increased cough, pulmonary physical findings. **Skin:** Pruritus, rash, sweating. **Body as a Whole:** Abscess, fever, local reaction to injection, pain.

**INTERACTIONS Drug:** Increased concentrations of **warfarin** required close monitoring of INR. Efficacy of ORAL CONTRACEPTIVES may be decreased when used in combination with tigecycline.

**PHARMACOKINETICS Distribution:** 71–89% protein bound. **Metabolism:** Negligible. **Elimination:** Fecal (major) and renal. **Half-Life:** 27 h (single dose); 42 h (multiple doses).

## NURSING IMPLICATIONS

### Black Box Warning

*Tigecycline has been associated with increased mortality, thus its use should be reserved for situations where alternative treatments are not suitable.*

### Assessment & Drug Effects

- Monitor for hypersensitivity reaction in those with reported tetra-cycline allergy.
- Monitor for and report S&S of superinfection (see Appendix F) or pseudomembranous enterocolitis (see Appendix F).
- Monitor diabetics for loss of glycemic control.
- Monitor lab tests: Baseline C&S, and periodic LFTs.

### Patient & Family Education

- Avoid direct exposure to sunlight during and for several days after

therapy is terminated to reduce risk of photosensitivity reaction.
- Report to prescriber loose stools or diarrhea either during or shortly after termination of therapy.
- Use a barrier contraceptive in addition to oral contraceptives if trying to avoid pregnancy.

## TILUDRONATE DISODIUM
(til-u′dro-nate)
Skelid
**Classification:** BONE METABOLISM REGULATOR (BISPHOSPHONATE)
**Therapeutic:** BONE METABOLISM REGULATOR
**Prototype:** Etidronate disodium

**AVAILABILITY** Tablet

**ACTION & *THERAPEUTIC EFFECT***
Inhibits osteoclastic activity that leads to resorption of the bone matrix. Acts primarily by inhibiting normal or abnormal bone resorption, thus reducing bone formation. *Effectiveness indicated by decreasing levels of alkaline phosphatase.*

**USES** Treatment of Paget's disease.

**CONTRAINDICATIONS** Hypersensitivity to bisphosphonates (e.g., alendronate, etidronate, pamidronate, tiludronate); hypocalcemia; severe kidney failure (CrCl less than 30 mL/min); lactation.

**CAUTIOUS USE** Hypercalcemia, renal impairment; active UGI problems (e.g., gastritis, dysphagia, ulcer, esophageal disease); hypoparathyoidism; vitamin D deficiency; CHF; older adults; pregnancy (category C). Safety and efficacy in children not established.

## ROUTE & DOSAGE

**Paget's Disease**
*Adult:* **PO** 400 mg/day with 6–8 oz of water × 3 mo

## ADMINISTRATION
### Oral
- Give with 6–8 oz of plain water 2 h before or after food.
- Do not give within 2 h of drugs containing calcium, aspirin, or indomethacin. Give aluminum- or magnesium-containing antacids no sooner than 2 h after tiludronate.
- Store in manufacturer's packaging at 15°–30° C (59°–86° F).

## ADVERSE EFFECTS (≥1%) **Body as a Whole:** *Pain,* flu-like syndrome, edema. **CNS:** Headache, dizziness, paresthesias. **CV:** Chest pain. **GI:** *Nausea, diarrhea,* dyspepsia, vomiting, flatulence. **Special Senses:** Cataract, conjunctivitis, glaucoma. **Respiratory:** Rhinitis, sinusitis, coughing, pharyngitis. **Skin:** Rash. **Metabolic:** Hyperparathyroidism, vitamin D deficiency. **Musculoskeletal:** Arthralgia, arthrosis.

## INTERACTIONS **Drug:** Absorption decreased by CALCIUM-, ALUMINUM-, or MAGNESIUM-CONTAINING ANTACIDS, **aspirin.** Absorption increased by **indomethacin.**

## PHARMACOKINETICS **Absorption:** Poorly absorbed from GI tract. **Steady-State:** 30 days. **Metabolism:** Not metabolized. **Elimination:** Primarily in urine. **Half-Life:** 150 h.

## NURSING IMPLICATIONS
### Assessment & Drug Effects
- Monitor for S&S of upper GI dysfunction or ulceration.
- Monitor lab tests: Periodic serum calcium and serum phosphate.

### Patient & Family Education
- Do not remove tablets from foil strips until time to be taken.
- Wait at least 2 h after taking tiludronate to take aluminum- and magnesium-containing antacids.
- Consult prescriber to determine appropriate daily intake of vitamin D and calcium.

## TIMOLOL MALEATE
(tye'moe-lole)
Betimol, Istalol, Timoptic, Timoptic XE
**Classifications:** BETA-ADRENERGIC ANTAGONIST; EYE PREPARATION; MIOTIC; ANTIHYPERTENSIVE; ANTIANGINAL
**Therapeutic:** ANTIGLAUCOMA; ANTIHYPERTENSIVE; ANTIANGINAL
**Prototype:** Propranolol

**AVAILABILITY** Tablet; ophthalmic solution; opthalmic gel

## ACTION & THERAPEUTIC EFFECT
Exhibits antihypertensive, antiarrhythmic, and antianginal properties, and suppresses plasma renin activity. When applied topically, lowers elevated and normal intraocular pressure (IOP) by reducing formation of aqueous humor and possibly by increasing outflow. *Topically, lowers elevated and normal intraocular pressure (IOP). Orally, useful for mild hypertension, angina, and migraine headaches.*

**USES** Topically (ophthalmic solution) to reduce elevated IOP in chronic, open-angle glaucoma, aphakic glaucoma, secondary glaucoma, and ocular hypertension. Oral product is used as monotherapy or in combination with a thiazide diuretic to prevent reinfarction after MI and to treat mild hypertension; migraine prophylaxis.

Common adverse effects in *italic;* life-threatening effects underlined; generic names in **bold;** classifications in SMALL CAPS; ◆ Canadian drug name; ⊙ Prototype drug

1609

**UNLABELED USES** Prophylactic management of stable, uncomplicated angina pectoris.

**CONTRAINDICATIONS** Bronchospasm; severe COPD; bronchial asthma or history there of; HF; abrupt discontinuation, acute bronchospasm, second and third degree AV block, sinus bradycardia, cardiogenic shock, acute pulmonary edema, Raynaud's disease.

**CAUTIOUS USE** Bronchitis, patients subject to bronchospasm, asthma; first-degree heart block, HF; renal impairment; hepatic disease; vasospastic angina; PVD; pheochromocytoma; thyrotoxicosis, hyperthyroidism; COPD; cerebrovascular insufficiency; stroke, CVD; depression; psoriasis; MG, DM, history of spontaneous hypoglycemia; older adults; pregnancy (category C). Safe use in children not established.

## ROUTE & DOSAGE

**Glaucoma**
See Appendix A-1.

**Hypertension**
*Adult:* **PO** 10 mg b.i.d. (may increase to 20 mg b.i.d.)

**Post-MI Reinfarction**
*Adult:* **PO** 10 mg b.i.d.

**Migraine Prophylaxis**
*Adult:* **PO** 10 mg b.i.d. or up to 30 mg daily

## ADMINISTRATION

**Oral**
- Give with fluid of patient's choice; tablet may be crushed.
- Dosage increases for hypertension should be made at weekly intervals.

**ADVERSE EFFECTS** (≥1%) **CNS:** *Fatigue*, lethargy, weakness, somnolence, anxiety, *headache*, dizziness, *confusion*, psychic dissociation, *depression*. **CV:** Palpitation, *bradycardia, hypotension*, syncope, AV conduction disturbances, CHF, aggravation of peripheral vascular insufficiency. **Special Senses:** *Eye irritation* including conjunctivitis, blepharitis, keratitis, superficial punctate keratopathy. **GI:** Anorexia, *dyspepsia, nausea*. **Skin:** Rash, urticaria. **Respiratory:** Difficulty in breathing, bronchospasm. **Body as a Whole:** Fever. **Metabolic:** Hypoglycemia, hypokalemia.

**INTERACTIONS** **Drug:** ANTIHYPERTENSIVE AGENTS, DIURETICS, SELECTIVE SEROTONIN REUPTAKE INHIBITORS potentiate hypotensive effects; NSAIDS may antagonize hypotensive effects.

**PHARMACOKINETICS** **Absorption:** 90% from GI tract; some systemic absorption from topical application. **Peak:** 1–2 h PO; 1–5 h topical. **Distribution:** Distributed into breast milk. **Metabolism:** 80% metabolized in liver to inactive metabolites. **Elimination:** In urine.

## NURSING IMPLICATIONS

### Black Box Warning

*Timolol has been associated with exacerbation of angina and MI when abruptly discontinued following chronic administration.*

### Assessment & Drug Effects
- Check pulse before administering timolol, topical or oral. If there are extremes (rate or rhythm), withhold medication and notify prescriber.
- Assess pulse rate and BP at regular intervals and more often in patients with severe heart disease.

- Note: Some patients develop tolerance during long-term therapy.

**Patient & Family Education**
- Be aware that drug may cause slight reduction in resting heart rate. Learn how to assess pulse rate and report significant changes. Consult prescriber for parameters.
- Do not stop drug abruptly; angina may be exacerbated. Dosage is reduced over a period of 1–2 wk.
- Report promptly to prescriber difficulty breathing. Drug withdrawal may be indicated.

# TINIDAZOLE
(tin'i-da-zole)
Tindamax
**Classification:** AZOLE ANTIBIOTIC
**Therapeutic:** ANTIBIOTIC;
ANTIPROTOZOAL, AMEBICIDE
**Prototype:** Metronidazole

## AVAILABILITY Tablet

## ACTION & *THERAPEUTIC EFFECT*
Effective against dividing and nondividing cells of targeted bacteria and protozoa. It inhibits formation of their DNA helix and thus inhibits DNA synthesis of these organisms. This leads to bacterial and protozoal cell death. *Demonstrates activity against infections caused by protozoa and anaerobic bacteria.*

## USES Treatment of trichomoniasis, giardiasis, amebiasis, bacterial vaginosis, and amebic liver abscess.

## CONTRAINDICATIONS Hypersensitivity to tinidazole or other azole antibiotics; pregnancy (category X first trimester); lactation within 72 h of tinidazole use.

## CAUTIOUS USE CNS diseases, liver dysfunction, alcoholism, ethanol intoxication; hematologic disease;

neurologic disease; bone marrow depression; dialysis; candidiasis; pregnancy (category C second and third trimester); children younger than 3 y.

## ROUTE & DOSAGE

### Giardiasis
*Adult:* **PO** 2 g as single dose
*Child (3 y or older):* **PO** 50 mg/kg (up to 2 g) as single dose

### Intestinal Amebiasis
*Adult:* **PO** 2 g once daily for 3 days
*Child (3 y or older):* **PO** 50 mg/kg/day (up to 2 g/day) once daily for 3 days

### Amebic Liver Abscess
*Adult:* **PO** 2 g once daily for 3–5 days
*Child (3 y or older):* **PO** 50 mg/kg/day (up to 2 g/day) once daily for 3–5 days

### Trichomoniasis
*Adult:* **PO** 2 g as single dose

### Bacterial Vaginosis
*Adult:* **PO** 2 g daily × 2 days OR 1 g daily × 5 days

### *Hemodialysis Dosage Adjustment*
If dose given on dialysis day, give supplemental dose (½ regular dose) post-dialysis

## ADMINISTRATION
### Oral
- Give with food to minimize GI distress; may be crushed in artificial cherry syrup if tablets cannot be swallowed whole.
- If given on a dialysis day, add a 50% dose of tinidazole at the end of hemodialysis.
- Separate the dosing of cholestyramine and tinidazole by 2–4 h when used concurrently.

Common adverse effects in *italic*; life-threatening effects underlined; generic names in **bold**; classifications in SMALL CAPS; ♣ Canadian drug name; ☺ Prototype drug

1611

▪ Do not give within 2 wk of the last dose of disulfiram.
▪ Store at 15°–30° C (59°–86° F). Protect from light.

## ADVERSE EFFECTS (≥1%) Body as a Whole: Weakness, fatigue, malaise. CNS: Dizziness, headache. GI: Metallic/bitter taste, nausea, anorexia, dyspepsia, cramps, epigastric discomfort, vomiting, constipation.

## INTERACTIONS Drug: May increase INR with **warfarin; alcohol** may cause **disulfiram**-like reaction; may increase the half-life of **fosphenytoin, phenytoin;** may increase levels and toxicity of **lithium, fluorouracil, cyclosporine, tacrolimus; cholestyramine** may decrease absorption of tinidazole; **cimetidine** or **ketoconazole** may increase levels.

## PHARMACOKINETICS Peak: 2 h. Distribution: Crosses blood–brain barrier and placenta and is excreted in breast milk. Metabolism: In the liver by CYP3A4. Elimination: Primarily in urine. Half-Life: 12–14 h.

## NURSING IMPLICATIONS

### Assessment & Drug Effects
▪ Withhold drug and notify prescriber for S&S of CNS dysfunction (e.g., seizures, numbness or paresthesia of extremities). Drug should be discontinued if abnormal neurologic signs appear.
▪ Monitor INR/PT frequently with concomitant oral anticoagulants. Continue monitoring for at least 8 days after discontinuation of tinidazole.
▪ Monitor serum lithium levels with concurrent use.
▪ Monitor for phenytoin toxicity with concurrent IV phenytoin.

▪ Monitor lab tests: CBC with differential if retreatment is required.

### Patient & Family Education
▪ Stop taking the drug and report promptly: Convulsions, numbness, tingling, pain, or weakness in the hands or feet; dizziness or unsteadiness; fever.
▪ Harmless urine discoloration may occur while taking this drug.

## TIOCONAZOLE
(ti-o-con'a-zole)
Vagistat-1
**Classifications:** AZOLE ANTIFUNGAL
Therapeutic: ANTIFUNGAL
**Prototype:** Fluconazole

## AVAILABILITY Vaginal ointment

## ACTION & *THERAPEUTIC EFFECT*
Broad-spectrum antifungal agent that inhibits growth of human pathogenic yeasts by disrupting normal fungal cell membrane permeability. *Effective against* Candida albicans, *other species of* Candida, *and* Torulopsis glabrata.

## USES Local treatment of vulvovaginal candidiasis.

## CONTRAINDICATIONS Hypersensitivity to tioconazole or other imidazole antifungal agents; lactation.

## CAUTIOUS USE Diabetes mellitus; HIV infections; immunosuppression; pregnancy (category C); children younger than 12 y.

## ROUTE & DOSAGE

### Candidiasis
*Adult:* **Intravaginal** One applicator full at bedtime × 1 day

TIOCONAZOLE ♦ TIOTROPIUM BROMIDE

## ADMINISTRATION

### Instillation
- Insert applicator high into the vagina (except during pregnancy).
- Wash applicator before and after each use.
- Store away from direct heat and light.

### ADVERSE EFFECTS (≥1%) Urogenital: Mild erythema, burning, discomfort, rash, itching.

### INTERACTIONS Drug: May inactivate spermicidal effects of nonoxynol-9.

### PHARMACOKINETICS Absorption: Minimal absorption from vagina.

## NURSING IMPLICATIONS

### Assessment & Drug Effects
- Do not use for patient with a history of allergic reaction to other antifungal agents, such as miconazole.
- Monitor for sensitization and irritation; these may be an indication to discontinue drug.

### Patient & Family Education
- Learn correct application technique.
- Understand potential adverse reactions, including sensitization and allergic response.
- Tioconazole may interact with diaphragms and latex condoms; avoid concurrent use within 72 h.
- Refrain from sexual intercourse while using tioconazole.
- Wear only cotton underwear; change daily.

---

# TIOTROPIUM BROMIDE

(ti-o-tro'pi-um)

Spiriva HandiHaler, Spiriva Respimat

**Classifications:** ANTICHOLINERGIC; ANTIMUSCARINIC; ANTISPASMODIC; BRONCHODILATOR

Therapeutic: BRONCHODILATOR; ANTISPASMODIC
**Prototype:** Atropine

### AVAILABILITY Capsule with powder for inhalation; respiratory spray

### ACTION & THERAPEUTIC EFFECT
A long-acting, antispasmodic agent. In the bronchial airways, it exhibits inhibition of muscarinic receptors of the smooth muscle resulting in bronchodilation. *Bronchodilation after inhalation of tiotropium is predominantly a site-specific effect.*

### USES Maintenance treatment of bronchospasm associated with chronic obstructive pulmonary disease (COPD); reducing COPD exacerbations; long-term maintenance treatment of asthma.

### CONTRAINDICATIONS Hypersensitivity to tiotropium, atropine, or ipratropium; acute bronchospasm.

### CAUTIOUS USE Decreased renal function; BPH, urinary bladder neck obstruction; narrow-angle glaucoma; older adults; pregnancy (category C); lactation. Safe use in children younger than 18 y not established.

## ROUTE & DOSAGE

| COPD |
|---|
| *Adult:* **Inhaled Spiriva HandiHaler** 18 mcg OR **Spiriva Respimat** once daily using inhaler device provided |
| **Asthma** |
| *Adult:* **Inhaled Spiriva Respimat** 2.5 mcg daily |

T

---

Common adverse effects in *italic;* life-threatening effects <u>underlined</u>; generic names in **bold**; classifications in SMALL CAPS; ♣ Canadian drug name; ❷ Prototype drug

1613

## ADMINISTRATION

**Inhalation ONLY**

- Place capsule in HandiHaler® and press button to puncture. Instruct patient to exhale deeply, then put the mouthpiece to the lips and breathe in the dose deeply and slowly; remove HandiHaler® and hold breath for at least 10 sec, and then exhale slowly; rinse mouth with water to minimize dry mouth.
- Ensure that drug does not contact the eyes.
- Store at 15°–30° C (59°–86° F).

## ADVERSE EFFECTS (≥1%) Body as a Whole: Nonspecific chest pain, dependent edema, infection, moniliasis, flu-like syndrome, cough, allergic reactions. **CNS:** Dysphonia, paresthesia, depression. **GI:** Abdominal pain, constipation, *dry mouth, dyspepsia,* vomiting, reflux, stomatitis. **Metabolic:** Hypercholesterolemia, hyperglycemia. **Musculoskeletal:** Myalgia, skeletal pain. **Respiratory:** Epistaxis, *pharyngitis, rhinitis,* laryngitis, *sinusitis, upper respiratory tract infection.* **Skin:** Rash. **Special Senses:** Cataract. **Urogenital:** Urinary tract infection.

## INTERACTIONS Drug: May cause additive anticholinergic effects with other ANTICHOLINERGIC AGENTS.

## PHARMACOKINETICS Absorption: 19.5% absorbed from the lungs. **Peak:** 5 min. **Metabolism:** Less than 25% of dose is metabolized in liver by CYP2D6 and 3A4. **Elimination:** 14% of dose excreted in urine; remaining is excreted in feces as nonabsorbed drug. **Half-Life:** 5–6 days.

## NURSING IMPLICATIONS

**Assessment & Drug Effects**

- Withhold drug and notify prescriber if S&S of angioedema occurs.
- Monitor for anticholinergic effects (e.g., tachycardia, urinary retention).

- Monitor lab tests: Pulmonary function tests.

**Patient & Family Education**

- Do not allow powdered medication to contact the eyes, as this may cause blurring of vision and pupil dilation.
- Tiotropium bromide is intended as a once-daily maintenance treatment. It is not useful for treatment of acute episodes of bronchospasm (i.e., rescue therapy).
- Withhold drug and notify prescriber if swelling around the face, mouth, or neck occurs.
- Report any of the following: Constipation, increased heart rate, blurred vision, urinary difficulty.

# TIPRANAVIR

(ti-pra'na-vir)

Aptivus

**Classifications:** ANTIRETROVIRAL; PROTEASE INHIBITOR

Therapeutic: ANTIRETROVIRAL

**Prototype:** Saquinavir

## AVAILABILITY Capsule; oral solution

## ACTION & *THERAPEUTIC EFFECT*

Inhibits virus-specific processing of the viral polyproteins in HIV-1 infected cells, thus preventing the formation of mature viral particles. *Helps decrease viral load of HIV-1 strains resistant to other protease inhibitors.*

## USES Treatment of HIV-1 infection in combination with other agents.

## CONTRAINDICATIONS Known hypersensitivity to tipranavir; moderate to severe (Child-Pugh class B and C, respectively) hepatic impairment; drug induced hepatic decomposition or intracranial hemorrhage; pancreatitis; lactation.

## CAUTIOUS USE Hypersensitivity to sulfonamides; patients with

chronic hepatitis B or hepatitis C co-infection; hemophilia; coagulopathy; elevated liver enzymes; diabetes mellitus or hyperglycemia; hyperlipidemia; pregnancy (category C); children younger than 2 y.

## ROUTE & DOSAGE

### HIV-1 Infection

*Adult:* **PO** 500 mg (with 200 mg ritonavir) b.i.d.
*Adolescent/Child (older than 2 y):* **PO** 14 mg/kg b.i.d. OR 375 mg/m² b.i.d. (with ritonavir)

## ADMINISTRATION

### Oral

- Coadminister with ritonavir. Give with food.
- Store solution at 15°–30° C (59°–86° F). Once opened, use contents of bottle within 60 days.
- Store capsules prior to opening bottle at 2°–8° C (36°–46° F). After bottle is opened, may be stored at 25° C (77° F) for up to 60 days.

## ADVERSE EFFECTS (≥1%) **Body as a Whole:** Fatigue, pyrexia, muscle cramps. **CNS:** Asthenia, depression, headache, dizziness, drowsiness, <u>intracranial hemorrhage</u>, insomnia. **GI:** Abdominal pain, *diarrhea*, nausea, vomiting, gastroesophageal reflux, pancreatitis. **Hematologic:** Decreased white blood cell levels, risk of hemorrhage. **Hepatic:** *Elevated liver enzymes (amylase, ALT, AST).* **Metabolic:** *Increased cholesterol, increased triglycerides.* **Respiratory:** Bronchitis, cough, epistaxis. **Skin:** Rash, pruritis.

## INTERACTIONS **Drug:** Do not use with **sildenafil, alfuzosin, salmeterol.** Do not use with ERGOT ALKALOIDS. Do not use with other PROTEASE INHIBITORS. Adjust **tipranavir** dosing when used with **bosentan, tadalafil, colchicine. Aluminum-** and

**magnesium-**based ANTACIDS may decrease tipranavir absorption. AZOLE ANTIFUNGAL AGENTS, **clarithromycin, erythromycin,** and other inhibitors of CYP3A4 may increase tipranavir levels. **Efavirenz, loperamide,** NRTIS, and RIFAMYCINS (e.g., **rifampin**) may decrease tipranavir levels. Tipranavir increases **rifabutin** levels. Coadministration of tipranavir and **tenofovir** decreases the levels of both compounds. Tipranavir increases the concentration of BENZODIAZEPINES, **desipramine,** and numerous ANTIARRHYTHMIC AGENTS **(amiodarone, flecainide, propafenone, quinidine).** Combination use of tipranavir and HMG COA REDUCTASE INHIBITORS increases the risk of myopathy. Tipranavir capsules contain **alcohol** that can produce disulfiram-like reactions with **metronidazole** and **disulfiram.** Adjust **midazolam** dose. **Food:** Food enhances the bioavailability of tipranavir, avoid large doses of vitamin E. **Herbal: St. John's wort** decreases the levels of tipranavir.

## PHARMACOKINETICS **Peak:** 3 h. **Distribution:** Greater than 99.9% protein bound. **Metabolism:** Extensive hepatic oxidation to inactive metabolites (when given alone); minimal metabolism (when given with ritonavir). **Elimination:** Fecal (primary) and renal (minimal). **Half-Life:** 6 h.

## NURSING IMPLICATIONS

### Black Box Warning

*Tipranavir has been associated with hepatitis, hepatic decompensation, and intracranial hemorrhage.*

### Assessment & Drug Effects

- Monitor for and report immediately S&S of liver toxicity (see Appendix F).
- Monitor for S&S of adverse drug reactions and toxicity from

concurrently administered drugs. Many drugs interact with tipranavir.

- Monitor diabetics for loss of glycemic control: Hyperglycemia.
- Use barrier contraceptive if using hormonal contraceptive.
- Monitor blood levels of anticoagulants with concurrent therapy.
- Monitor lab tests: Baseline and frequent LFTs and lipid profile; viral load, CD4 count, and fasting plasma glucose as indicated.

### Patient & Family Education

- If a dose is missed, take it as soon as possible and then return to the normal schedule. Never double a dose.
- Inform prescriber of all medications and herbal products you are taking.
- Protect against sunlight exposure to minimize risk of photosensitivity.
- Report any of the following to prescriber: Fatigue, weakness, loss of appetite, nausea, jaundice, dark urine, or clay colored stools.

## TIROFIBAN HYDROCHLORIDE

(tir-o-fi'ban)

Aggrastat

**Classifications:** ANTICOAGULANT; ANTIPLATELET; GLYCOPROTEIN (GP) IIB/IIIA RECEPTOR INHIBITOR

Therapeutic: ANTIPLATELET

**Prototype:** Abciximab

**AVAILABILITY** Solution for injection

## ACTION & *THERAPEUTIC EFFECT*

Binds to the glycoprotein IIb/IIIa receptor on platelets thus inhibiting platelet aggregation. *Effectiveness indicated by minimizing thrombotic events during treatment of acute coronary syndrome.*

## USES Acute coronary syndromes (unstable angina, MI).

## CONTRAINDICATIONS Hypersensitivity to tirofiban; active internal bleeding within 30 days; acute pericarditis; aortic dissection; intracranial aneurysm, intracranial mass, coagulopathy; history of aneurysm or AV malformation; history of intracranial hemorrhage or neoplasm; active abnormal bleeding; retinal bleeding; hemorrhagic retinopathy; major surgery or trauma within 3 days; stroke within 30 days; history of hemorrhagic stroke; thrombocytopenia following administration of tirofiban; history of thrombopenia due to prior exposure to tirofiban; severe rash during use of tirofiban; within 4 h of PCI; lactation.

## CAUTIOUS USE Platelet count less than 150,000 mm³; severe renal insufficiency; pregnancy (category B). Safety and efficacy in children younger than 18 y not established.

## ROUTE & DOSAGE

### Acute Coronary Syndromes

*Adult:* **IV** 25 mcg/kg over 3 min and then 0.15 mcg/kg/min for up to 18 h; specific weight based dosing in package insert

### *Renal Impairment Dosage Adjustment*

*CrCl less than or equal to 60 mL/ min:* Give 25 mcg/kg over 3 min and then 0.075 mcg/kg/min

## ADMINISTRATION

### Intravenous

*PREPARE:* **IV Infusion:** Use as supplied with no further preparation.
*ADMINISTER:* **IV Infusion:** Give an initial loading dose of 25 mcg/kg over 3 min and then 0.15 mcg/kg/min for up to 18 h.
*INCOMPATIBILITIES:* **Y-site:** Amphotericin B, dantrolene,

Common adverse effects in *italic;* life-threatening effects underlined; generic names in **bold**; classifications in SMALL CAPS; ♦ Canadian drug name; ⓟ Prototype drug

**diasepam, lansoprazole, phenytoin, tenecteplase.**

▪ Discard unused IV solution 24 h following start of infusion. ▪ Store unopened containers at 15°–30° C (59°–86° F). ▪ Do not freeze and protect from light.

**ADVERSE EFFECTS** (≥1%) **Body as a Whole:** Edema, swelling, pelvic pain, vasovagal reaction, leg pain. **CNS:** Dizziness. **CV:** Bradycardia, coronary artery dissection. **GI:** GI bleeding. **Hematologic:** *Bleeding* (major bleeding), anemia, thrombocytopenia. **Skin:** Sweating.

**INTERACTIONS Drug:** Increased risk of bleeding with ANTICOAGULANTS, NSAIDS, SALICYLATES, ANTIPLATELET AGENTS **Herbal: Feverfew, garlic, ginger, ginkgo, horse chestnut** may increase risk of bleeding.

**PHARMACOKINETICS Duration:** 4–8 h after stopping infusion. **Distribution:** 65% protein bound. **Metabolism:** Minimally metabolized. **Elimination:** 65% in urine, 25% in feces. **Half-Life:** 2 h.

## NURSING IMPLICATIONS

### Assessment & Drug Effects

▪ Withhold drug and notify prescriber if thrombocytopenia (platelets less than 100,000) is confirmed.
▪ Monitor carefully for and immediately report S&S of internal or external bleeding.
▪ Minimize unnecessary invasive procedures and devices to reduce the risk of bleeding.
▪ Monitor lab tests: Platelet count, Hgb and Hct before treatment, (within 6 h of infusing loading dose), and frequently throughout treatment; periodic APTT and ACT.

### Patient & Family Education

▪ Report unexplained pelvic or abdominal pain.

# TIZANIDINE HYDROCHLORIDE

(ti-zan′i-deen)

Zanaflex

**Classification:** CENTRAL ACTING SKELETAL MUSCLE RELAXANT
**Therapeutic:** SKELETAL MUSCLE RELAXANT; ANTISPASMODIC
**Prototype:** Cyclobenzaprine

**AVAILABILITY** Tablet; capsule

**ACTION & THERAPEUTIC EFFECT**
Reduces spasticity by increasing presynaptic inhibition of motor neurons. Greatest effect on polysynaptic afferent reflex activity at the spinal cord level. *Site of action is the spinal cord; reduces skeletal muscle spasms. Effectiveness indicated by decreased muscle tone.*

**USES** Acute and intermittent management of increased muscle tone associated with spasticity including spasticity related to multiple sclerosis or spinal cord injury.

**CONTRAINDICATIONS** Hypersensitivity to tizanidine; concomitant therapy with **ciprofloxacin** or **fluvoxamine** (potent CYP1A2 inhibitors); lactation. Effect of tizanidine on labor and delivery is unknown.

**CAUTIOUS USE** Patients with hepatic impairment, hepatic disease; renal insufficiency (CrCl less than 25 mL/min), or renal failure; history of hypotension; psychosis; women taking oral contraceptives; history of QT prolongation; history of narcotic abuse; older adults because of renal impairment and orthostatic hypotension; pregnancy (category C). Safety and efficacy in children not established.

T

## ROUTE & DOSAGE

### Spasticity

*Adult:* **PO** Start with 2 mg can be repeated at 6–8 h intervals (max: 3 doses/24 h) and may gradually increase up to 8 mg q6–8h prn (max: 3 doses or 36 mg/24 h)

### Renal Impairment Dosage Adjustment

*CrCl less than 25 mL/min:* Use lower dose

## ADMINISTRATION

### Oral

- Can be given without regard to food, but patient should choose with food or without food and administer medication consistently.
- Dose increases are usually made gradually in 2- to 4-mg increments.
- Store at 15°–30° C (59°–86° F).

**ADVERSE EFFECTS** (≥1%) **Body as a Whole:** *Asthenia (tiredness),* flu-like syndrome, fever, myasthenia, back pain, infection. **CNS:** *Somnolence, dizziness,* dyskinesia, nervousness, depression, anxiety, paresthesia. **CV:** *Hypotension, bradycardia.* **GI:** *Dry mouth,* constipation, abnormal liver function tests, vomiting, abdominal pain, diarrhea, dyspepsia. **Respiratory:** Pharyngitis, rhinitis. **Skin:** Rash, sweating, skin ulcer. **Urogenital:** *UTI,* urinary frequency. **Special Senses:** Speech disorder, blurred vision.

**INTERACTIONS Drug:** ORAL CONTRACEPTIVES decrease clearance of **tizanidine. Alcohol** and other CNS DEPRESSANTS increase CNS depression. **Fluvoxamine, ciprofloxacin** increase tizanidine levels and toxicity. Avoid use of agents that can prolong the QT interval (e.g., **dofetilide, dronedarone, pimozide, thioridazine, ziprasidone**).

**Herbal: Kava, valerian** may potentiate sedation.

**PHARMACOKINETICS Absorption:** Rapidly from GI tract; 40% bioavailability. **Peak:** 1–2 h. **Duration:** 3–6 h. **Distribution:** Crosses placenta, distributed into breast milk. **Metabolism:** In the liver (CYP1A2). **Elimination:** 60% in urine, 20% in feces. **Half-Life:** 2.5 h.

## NURSING IMPLICATIONS

### Assessment & Drug Effects

- Monitor cardiovascular status and report orthostatic hypotension or bradycardia.
- Monitor closely older adults, those with renal impairment, and women taking oral contraceptives for adverse effects because drug clearance is reduced.
- Monitor lab tests: Baseline LFTs and 1 mo after max dose is achieved or if hepatic injury suspected.

### Patient & Family Education

- Exercise caution with potentially hazardous activities requiring alertness since sedation is a common adverse effect. Effects are additive with alcohol or other CNS depressants.
- Make position changes slowly because of the risk of orthostatic hypotension.
- Report unusual sensory experiences; hallucinations and delusions have occurred with tizanidine use.

## TOBRAMYCIN SULFATE

(toe-bra-mye'sin)

AKTob, Bethkis,TobraDex, Tobrex, Tobi Podhaler, Tobrasol

**Classification:** AMINOGLYCOSIDE ANTIBIOTIC
**Therapeutic:** ANTIBIOTIC
**Prototype:** Gentamicin sulfate

**AVAILABILITY** Solution for injection; nebulizer solution; capsule for inhalation; ophthalmic solution; ophthalmic ointment

## ACTION & *THERAPEUTIC EFFECT*

Binds irreversibly to one of two aminoglycoside binding sites on the 30S ribosomal subunit of the bacteria, thus inhibiting protein synthesis, resulting in bacterial cell death. *Effective in treatment of gram-negative bacteria. Exhibits greater antibiotic activity against* Pseudomonas aeruginosa *than other aminoglycosides.*

**USES** Treatment of severe infections caused by susceptible organisms.

**CONTRAINDICATIONS** History of hypersensitivity to tobramycin and other aminoglycoside; pregnancy (category D).

**CAUTIOUS USE** Impaired kidney function; renal disease; dehydration; hearing impairment; myasthenia gravis; parkinsonism; older adults; lactation; premature, neonatal infants.

## ROUTE & DOSAGE

### Moderate to Severe Infections

*Adult:* **IV/IM** 3–6 mg/kg/day in 2–3 divided doses OR 4–7 mg/kg/day single dose
*Adolescent/Child/Infant:* **IM/IV** 2.5 mg/kg/dose q8h
*Neonate:* **IM/IV** 2.5 mg/kg q12–24h
*Premature Neonate:* **IV/IM** See package insert for dosage by weight and gestational age

### Cystic Fibrosis

*Adult: Child:* **IM/IV** 10 mg/kg/dose q24h; **Nebulized** 300 mg inhaled b.i.d. × 28 days, may repeat after 28-day drug-free period

*Podhaler:* 112 mg (4 caps) q12h × 28 days may repeat after 28 drug-free days

### Ocular Infection

*Adults/Adolescents/Children/Infants 2 mo or older:* **Topical**
Apply a thin strip to the conjunctiva (about 1 cm) q8–12h; **Drops** 1–2 drops into the infected eye q4h

### Renal Impairment Dosage Adjustment

Increase interval.

### Hemodialysis Dosage Adjustment

Administer dose after dialysis and monitor levels

### Obesity Dosage Adjustment

Dose based on IBW; in morbid obesity, use dosing weight of IBW + 0.4 (Weight – IBW)

## ADMINISTRATION

Note: Doses should be based on ideal body weight.

### Inhalation

- Administer over 10–15 min using a handheld reusable nebulizer with a compressor (use only those supplied). Patient should sit upright and breathe normally through the nebulizer mouthpiece.

### Intramuscular

- Give deep IM into a large muscle. Rotate injection sites.

### Intravenous

Note: Verify correct IV concentration and rate of infusion to neonates, infants, or children with prescriber.

**PREPARE: Intermittent** ▪ Dilute each dose in 50–100 mL or more of D5W, NS or D5/NS. ▪ Final concentration should not exceed 5 mg/mL.
**ADMINISTER: Intermittent:** Infuse diluted solution over 20–60 min.

Common adverse effects in *italic;* life-threatening effects underlined; generic names in **bold;** classifications in SMALL CAPS; ✦ Canadian drug name; ◉ Prototype drug

1619

▪ Avoid rapid infusion.
***INCOMPATIBILITIES:*** Solution/additive: Alcohol 5% in dextrose, cefamandole, cefe-pime. **Y-site: Allopurinol, amphotericin B cholesteryl complex, azathioprine sodium, azathioprine, azithromycin, cangrelor, cefazolin, cefoperazone, cefotetan, ceftobiprole, ceftriaxone, cloxacillin sodium, dacarbazine, dantrolene, defibrotide, dexamethasone, diazepam, diazoxide, drotrecogin, folic acid, ganciclovir, garenoxacin mesylate, gemtuzumab, heparin, hetastarch, indomethacin, lansoprazole, oxacillin, pemetrexed, pentamidine, pentobarbital, phenytoin, piperacillin/tazobactam, propofol, sargramostim, SMZ/TMP.**

▪ Store at 15°–30° C (59°–86° F) prior to reconstitution. After reconstitution, solution may be refrigerated and used within 96 h. ▪ If kept at room temperature, use within 24 h.

## ADVERSE EFFECTS (≥1%) **CNS:**
Neurotoxicity (including ototoxicity), *nephrotoxicity,* increased AST, ALT, LDH, serum bilirubin; anemia, fever, rash, pruritus, urticaria, nausea, vomiting, headache, lethargy, superinfections; hypersensitivity. **Genitourinary:** Oliguria, proteinuria. **Special Senses:** *Burning, stinging of eye after drug instillation;* eyelid itching and edema.

## INTERACTIONS **Drug:** ANESTHETICS, SKELETAL MUSCLE RELAXANTS add to neuromuscular blocking effects; **acyclovir, amphotericin B, bacitracin, capreomycin,** CEPHALOSPORINS, **colistin, cisplatin, carboplatin, foscarnet, methoxyflurane, polymyxin B, vancomycin, furosemide, ethacrynic acid** increase risk of ototoxicity, nephrotoxicity. Do not use with **cidofovir** or **gallium.**

## PHARMACOKINETICS **Peak:**
30–90 min IM. **Duration:** Up to 8 h. **Distribution:** Crosses placenta; accumulates in renal cortex. **Elimination:** In urine. **Half-Life:** 2–3 h in adults.

## NURSING IMPLICATIONS

### Black Box Warning

*Tobramycin has been associated with ototoxicity and nephrotoxicity.*

### Assessment & Drug Effects
▪ Weigh patient before treatment for calculation of dosage.
▪ Observe patient receiving tobramycin closely because of the high potential for toxicity, even in conventional doses.
▪ Monitor auditory, and vestibular functions closely, particularly in patients with known or suspected renal impairment and patients receiving high doses.
▪ Be aware that drug-induced auditory changes are irreversible (partial or total); usually bilateral. Partial or bilateral deafness may continue to develop even after therapy discontinued.
▪ Monitor I&O. Report oliguria, changes in I&O ratio, and cloudy or frothy urine (may indicate proteinuria). Keep patient well hydrated to prevent chemical irritation in renal tubules; older adults are especially susceptible to renal toxicity.
▪ Be aware that prolonged use of ophthalmic solution may encourage superinfection with nonsusceptible organisms including fungi.
▪ Report overdose symptoms for eye medication: Increased lacrimation, keratitis, edema and itching of eyelids.
▪ Monitor lab tests: Baseline C&S; baseline and periodic renal function tests; periodic peak and trough drug levels.

### Patient & Family Education

- Report symptoms of superinfections (see Appendix F) to prescriber. Prompt treatment with an antibiotic or antifungal medication may be necessary.
- Report S&S of hearing loss, tinnitus, or vertigo to prescriber.

## TOCILIZUMAB

(to-si-ly′zu-mab)

Actemra

**Classification:** BIOLOGIC RESPONSE MODIFIER; INTERLEUKIN-6 INHIBITOR; DISEASE-MODIFYING ANTIRHEUMATIC DRUG (DMARD)

**Therapeutic:** DISEASE-MODIFYING ANTIRHEUMATIC DRUG (DMARD)

**AVAILABILITY** Solution for injection

### ACTION & *THERAPEUTIC EFFECT*

Binds to interleukin 6 (IL-6) receptors inhibiting IL-6 mediated signaling and suppressing systemic inflammatory responses; also reduces IL-6 production in joints affected by inflammatory processes such as rheumatoid arthritis. *Reduction of joint inflammation reduces joint pain and improves joint function.*

**USES** Treatment of moderate to severe rheumatoid arthritis or juvenile idiopathic arthritis; cytokine release syndrome.

**CONTRAINDICATIONS** History of anaphylaxis reaction with tocilizumab; severe neutropenia, severe thrombocytopenia; live vaccines; severe hepatic impairment; positive hepatitis B or hepatitis C virus serology; active hepatic disease.

**CAUTIOUS USE** History of chronic or recurring infections; history of hypersensitivity; mild hepatic impairment; thrombocytopenia or neutropenia; risk for GI perforation; demyelinating disorders; preexisting or recent-onset demyelinating disorders; history of hyperlipidemia; older adults; pregnancy (category C); lactation. Safety and efficacy in children younger than 2 y not established.

## ROUTE & DOSAGE

### Rheumatoid Arthritis

*Adult:* **IV** 4 mg/kg q4wk. May increase up to 8 mg/kg q4wk

### Polyarticular Juvenile Idiopathic Arthritis

*Child/Adolescent (older than 2 y and weight greater than 30 kg):* **IV** 8 mg/kg q4wk; *older than 2 y and weight less than 30 kg:* **IV** 10 mg/kg q4wk

### Systematic Juvenile Idiopathic Arthritis

*Child/Adolescent (older than 2 y and weight greater than 30 kg):* **IV** 8 mg/kg q2wk; *older than 2 y and weight less than 30 kg:* **IV** 12 mg/kg q2wks

### Cytokine Release Syndrome

*Adult (30 kg or more):* **IV** 8 mg/kg (max: 800 mg/dose), may repeat for 3 additional doses (at least 8 h apart) *Adult/Adolescent/Child (weight less than 30 kg)* **IV** 12 mg/kg (max: 800 mg/dose), may repeat for 3 additional doses (at least 8 h apart)

### *Absolute Neutrophil Count (ANC) Adjustment*

*ANC = 500–1000/mm³:* Stop tocilizumab and restart at 4 mg/kg with an increase to 8 mg/kg as appropriate when ANC is greater than 1000 cells/mm³. *ANC less than 500/mm³:* Discontinue tocilizumab.

### *Platelet Count Dosage Adjustment*

*Platelet count 50,000–100,000/mm³:* Stop tocilizumab and restart at

Common adverse effects in *italic*; life-threatening effects underlined; generic names in **bold**; classifications in SMALL CAPS; ♣ Canadian drug name; ⊕ Prototype drug

1621

4 mg/kg with an increase to 8 mg/kg as appropriate when platelet count is greater than 100,000/mm³. *Platelet count less than 50,000/mm³:* Discontinue tocilizumab.

### Hepatic Impairment Dosage Adjustment

*Do not initiate tocilizumab if AST/ALT is greater than 1.5 × ULN. Mild impairment (AST and/or ALT 1–3 × ULN):* Modify dose of concomitant DMARDs, if appropriate. For persistent increases in this range, reduce tocilizumab dose to 4 mg/kg or interrupt tocilizumab until AST/ALT have normalized. *Moderate impairment (AST and/or ALT greater than 3–5 × ULN confirmed by repeat testing):* Interrupt tocilizumab until AST/ALT is less than 3 × ULN, then follow recommendations for 1–3 × ULN. *For persistent increases greater than 3 × ULN:* Discontinue tocilizumab. *Severe impairment (AST and/or ALT greater than 5 × ULN):* Discontinue tocilizumab.

## ADMINISTRATION

### Subcutaneous

▪ When transitioning from IV to subcutaneous route, give the first subcutaneous dose at the time of the next scheduled IV dose. Administer the full amount in the pre-filled syringe. Allow to reach room temperature prior to use.

### Intravenous

*PREPARE:* **IV Infusion:** For children weighing less than 30 kg, start with 50 mL of NS. For adults or children weighing 30 kg or more, start with 100 mL NS. From the bag of NS remove a volume of solution equal to the volume of tocilizumab necessary to deliver the required dose. Slowly add the required dose of tocilizumab to the IV bag, then gently invert to mix. Solution should reach room temperature prior to infusion. Discard unused drug remaining in vial.
*ADMINISTER:* **IV Infusion:** Give over 60 min. **Do not** give IV push or a bolus dose.
*INCOMPATIBILITIES:* **Solution/additive:** Do not mix with another drug. **Y-site:** Do not infuse tocilizumab concurrently with any drug in the same IV line.

▪ Store IV solution refrigerated for up to 24 h or at room temperature for up to 4 h. Protect from light. Store unopened vials refrigerated in original packaging to protect from light.

## ADVERSE EFFECTS (≥1%) **Body as a Whole:** Infusion reactions, serious infections (includes invasive fungal infections, tuberculosis, and bacterial, viral, and other infections caused by opportunistic pathogens), upper abdominal pain. **CV:** Hypertension. **CNS:** dizziness, headache. **GI:** Gastritis, diarrhea mouth ulceration. **Hematological:** Neutropenia, thrombocytopenia. **Metabolic:** *Elevations of ALT and AST levels,* increased LDL/cholesterol levels. **Respiratory:** Bronchitis, nasopharyngitis, upper respiratory tract infection. **Skin:** Rash.

## INTERACTIONS **Drug:** Do not use with other biological DMARDs. Caution should be used when tocilizumab is combined with CYP3A4 substrate drugs (like **cyclosporine**) that have a narrow therapeutic index. Use with other IMMUNE MODULATORS can increase risk of infection. Do not administer LIVE VACCINES.

## PHARMACOKINETICS Half-Life:
11–13 days.

## NURSING IMPLICATIONS

### Black Box Warning

*Tocilizumab has been associated with increased risk of serious infections that may lead to hospitalization or death.*

### Assessment & Drug Effects

- Monitor for signs of serious allergic reactions during and shortly following each infusion.
- Monitor for and promptly report S&S of infection, including TB or hepatitis B infection in carriers of HBV.
- Monitor for S&S of polyneuropathy.
- Monitor lab tests. Baseline latent TB screening; baseline and frequent (q4–8wk) WBC with differential and platelet count; baseline and periodic LFTs; periodic lipid profile.

### Patient & Family Education

- Do not accept vaccinations with live vaccines while taking this drug.
- You should be tested for TB prior to taking this drug.
- Promptly report S&S of infection including: Chills, fever, cough, shortness of breath, diarrhea, stomach or abdominal pain, burning on urination, sores anywhere on your body, unexplained or excessive fatigue.
- Carriers of hepatitis B should report promptly signs of activation of the virus (e.g., clay-colored stools, dark urine, jaundice, unexplained fatigue).
- Report promptly if you become pregnant.

## TOFACITINIB

(toe'fa-sye'ti-nib)

Xeljanz

**Classifications:** BIOLOGICAL RESPONSE MODIFIER; JANUS KINASE (JAK) INHIBITOR; DISEASE-MODIFYING ANTIRHEUMATIC DRUG (DMARD)

Therapeutic: DISEASE-MODIFYING ANTIRHEUMATIC DRUG (DMARD)

## AVAILABILITY Tablet

## ACTION & *THERAPEUTIC EFFECT*

Inhibits a specific tyrosine kinase enzyme and interferes with a signaling pathway that transmits extracellular information to the cell nucleus, influencing DNA transcription. *It improves rheumatoid arthritis by inhibiting the production of inflammatory mediators.*

## USES Treatment of moderately to severely active rheumatoid arthritis in patients who have had an inadequate response or intolerance to methotrexate. It may be used as monotherapy or in combination with methotrexate or other nonbiologic disease-modifying antirheumatic drugs (DMARDs).

## CONTRAINDICATIONS Serious uncontrolled infection, opportunistic infection or sepsis; live vaccines; severe hepatic impairment, hepatitis B or C; lactation.

## CAUTIOUS USE Renal transplant patients; active TB or history of latent or active TB; history of herpes virus infection; history of chronic or recurrent infections; history or risk of GI perforation; DM; bradycardia, prolonged PR interval, conduction abnormalities; ischemic heart disease; patients at risk for interstitial lung disease; moderate or severe renal impairment; moderate hepatic impairment; Asian patients; malignancy; older adults; pregnancy (category C). Safety and efficacy in children not established.

## ROUTE & DOSAGE

### Rheumatoid Arthritis
*Adult:* **PO** 5 mg b.i.d.

---

Common adverse effects in *italic;* life-threatening effects <u>underlined</u>; generic names in **bold**; classifications in SMALL CAPS; ♣ Canadian drug name; ☯ Prototype drug

### Hepatic Impairment Dosage Adjustment

*Moderate impairment (Child-Pugh class B):* 5 mg once daily
*Severe impairment (Child-Pugh class C):* Not recommended

### Renal Impairment Dosage Adjustment

*Moderate to severe impairment:* 5 mg once daily

### Lymphopenia Dosage Adjustment

*If less than 500 cells/m³:* Discontinue

### Neutropenia Dosage Adjustment

*If ANC = 500–1000 cells/m³:* Withhold until ANC is greater than 1000 cells/m³ then resume at normal dose
*If ANC less than 500–1000 cells/m³:* Discontinue

### Anemia Dosage Adjustment

*If hemoglobin is less than 8 g/dL or if decreased by greater than 2 g/dL:* Withhold until hemoglobin levels normalize

## ADMINISTRATION

### Oral

- May be given without regard to food.
- Store at 15°–30° C (59°–86° F).

**ADVERSE EFFECTS (≥1%) Body as a Whole:** Dehydration, hepatic steatosis, herpes zoster, peripheral edema, pyrexia. **CNS:** Fatigue, insomnia, paresthesia. **CV:** hypertension. **GI:** Abdominal pain, diarrhea, dyspepsia, gastritis, headache, nausea, vomiting. **Hematological:** Anemia. **Metabolic:** Increased ALT, increased HDL and LDL, increased serum creatinine. **Musculoskeletal:** Arthralgia, joint swelling, musculoskeletal pain, tendonitis. **Respiratory:** Cough, dyspnea, nasopharyngitis, pneumo-nia, sinus congestion, tuberculosis, upper respiratory infections. **Skin:** Cellulitis, erythema, pruritus, rash. **Urogenital:** Urinary tract infection.

**INTERACTIONS Drug:** Coadministration with potent inhibitors of CYP3A4 (e.g., **ketonazole**) may increase the levels of tofacitinib. Coadministration with drugs that are moderate inhibitors of CYP3A4 and potent inhibitors of CYP2C19 (e.g., **fluconazole**) may increase the levels of tofacitinib. Coadministration with potent CYP3A4 inducers (e.g., **phenobarbital, phenytoin, rifampin**) may decrease the levels of tofacitinib. Coadministration with other potent immunosuppressive drugs (e.g., **azathioprine, tacrolimus, cyclosporine**) increases the risk of added immunosuppression. **Food: Grapefruit juice** may increase the levels of tofacitinib. **Herbal: St. John's wort** may decrease the levels of tofacitinib.

**PHARMACOKINETICS Absorption:** 74% bioavailable. **Peak:** 0.5–1 h. **Distribution:** 40% plasma protein bound. **Metabolism:** Hepatic oxidation. **Elimination:** Hepatic (70%) and renal (30%). **Half-Life:** 3 h.

## NURSING IMPLICATIONS

### Black Box Warning

*Tofacitinib has been associated with increased risk of developing serious infections that may lead to hospitalization or death.*

### Assessment & Drug Effects

- Evaluate for latent or active infection prior to administration of tofacitinib.
- Monitor closely for S&S of TB, including those who tested negative for latent TB prior to initiating therapy.
- Monitor for reactivation of viral infection (herpes zoster).

Common adverse effects in *italic;* life-threatening effects <u>underlined</u>; generic names in **bold;** classifications in SMALL CAPS; ♣ Canadian drug name; ⊙ Prototype drug

- Monitor closely for S&S of other infections during and after treatment. Withhold therapy and notify prescriber if an infection is suspected.
- Monitor lab tests: Baseline lymphocyte count and q3mo thereafter; baseline neutrophil count and Hgb, then q3mo after 4–8 wk of treatment; periodic LFTs; lipid profile 4–8 wk after initiation of therapy.

**Patient & Family Education**
- Report promptly to prescriber any new-onset abdominal symptoms, S&S of respiratory tract infection or any other type of infection.

# TOLAZAMIDE

(tole-az'a-mide)

Tolinase

**Classification:** ANTIDIABETIC, SULFONYLUREA
**Therapeutic:** ANTIDIABETIC
**Prototype:** Glyburide

**AVAILABILITY** Tablet

## ACTION & *THERAPEUTIC EFFECT*
Lowers blood glucose primarily by stimulating pancreatic beta cells to secrete insulin. Antidiabetic action is a result of stimulation of the pancreas to secrete more insulin in the presence of blood sugar; it requires functioning beta cells. *Effectiveness is measured in decreasing the serum blood level to within normal limits and decreasing HbA1C value to 6.5 or lower.*

**USES** Type 2 diabetes mellitus

## CONTRAINDICATIONS
Known sensitivity to sulfonylureas and to sulfonamides; type 1 diabetes complicated by ketoacidosis; infection; trauma; lactation.

## CAUTIOUS USE
Renal disease; renal failure, renal impairment; older adults; pregnancy (category C). Safety in children not established.

# ROUTE & DOSAGE

**Type 2 Diabetes Mellitus**
*Adult:* **PO** 100 mg–250 mg daily or b.i.d. a.c., may adjust dose by 100–250 mg/day at weekly intervals (max: 1 g/day)

## ADMINISTRATION
**Oral**
- Give in the morning with or before meals.
- Divide dose of more than 500 mg and give b.i.d.
- Store at 15°–30° C (59°–86° F) in a tightly closed container unless otherwise directed. Keep drug out of the reach of children.

**ADVERSE EFFECTS** (≥1%) **GI:** Nausea, vomiting, cholestatic jaundice. **Metabolic:** Hypoglycemia. **CNS:** Vertigo. **Skin:** Photosensitivity. **Hematologic:** Agranulocytosis.

**INTERACTIONS Drug: Alcohol** elicits disulfiram-type reaction in some patients; ORAL ANTICOAGULANTS, **chloramphenicol, clofibrate, phenylbutazone,** MAO INHIBITORS, SALICYLATES, **probenecid,** SULFONAMIDES may potentiate hypoglycemic actions; THIAZIDES may antagonize hypoglycemic effects; **cimetidine** may increase tolazamide levels, causing hypoglycemia. **Herbal: Ginseng, karela** may potentiate hypoglycemic effects.

**PHARMACOKINETICS Absorption:** Slowly from GI tract. **Onset:** 60 min. **Peak:** 4–6 h. **Duration:** 10–15 h (up to 20 h in some patients). **Distribution:** Distributed in highest concentrations in liver, kidneys, and intestines; crosses placenta; distributed into breast milk. **Metabolism:** Extensively in liver. **Elimination:** 85% in urine, 15% in feces. **Half-Life:** 7 h.

**T**

---

Common adverse effects in *italic;* life-threatening effects <u>underlined;</u> generic names in **bold;** classifications in SMALL CAPS; ♣ Canadian drug name; ⊘ Prototype drug

## NURSING IMPLICATIONS

### Assessment & Drug Effects

- Monitor closely for daytime and nighttime hypoglycemia since tolazamide is long acting.
- Monitor for and report signs of an allergic reaction (e.g., rash, urticaria, pruritus).
- Monitor lab tests: Periodic HbA1C and frequent FBS; periodic CBC.

### Patient & Family Education

- Check blood glucose daily or as ordered by prescriber. Important to continue close medical supervision for first 6 wk of treatment.
- Learn the S&S of hypoglycemia and hyperglycemia and check blood glucose level when either is suspected.
- Report to prescriber if you experience frequent and/or severe episodes of hypoglycemia.
- Do not take OTC preparations unless approved or prescribed by prescriber.
- Understand that alcohol can precipitate a disulfiram-type reaction.
- Many drugs interact with tolazamide. Monitor blood glucose more frequently whenever a new drug is added to your regimen.

## TOLBUTAMIDE

(tole-byoo′ta-mide)

Mobenol ◆, Novobutamide ◆, Orinase

## TOLBUTAMIDE SODIUM

Orinase Diagnostic

**Classification:** ANTIDIABETIC, SULFONYLUREA
**Therapeutic:** ANTIDIABETIC
**Prototype:** Glyburide

**AVAILABILITY** Tablet; vial

## ACTION & *THERAPEUTIC EFFECT*

Lowers blood glucose concentration by stimulating pancreatic beta cells to synthesize and release insulin. No action demonstrated if functional beta cells are absent. *Lowers blood glucose concentration by stimulating pancreatic beta cells to synthesize and release insulin.*

**USES** Management of mild to moderately severe, stable type 2 diabetes that is not controlled by diet and weight reduction alone. Also used in treatment of patients who are unresponsive to other sulfonylureas and adjunctively with insulin to stabilize certain cases of labile diabetes. Used as diagnostic agent to rule out pancreatic islet cell adenoma or diabetes.

**CONTRAINDICATIONS** Hypersensitivity to sulfonylureas or to sulfonamides; history of repeated episodes of diabetic ketoacidosis; type 1 diabetes as sole therapy; diabetic coma; severe stress, infection, trauma, or major surgery; severe renal insufficiency, liver or endocrine disease; lactation.

**CAUTIOUS USE** Cardiac, thyroid, pituitary, or adrenal dysfunction; severe hepatic disease, renal disease, renal impairment, renal failure; history of peptic ulcer; alcoholism; infection; debilitated, malnourished, or uncooperative patient, older adults; pregnancy (category C). Safe use in children not established.

## ROUTE & DOSAGE

| Type 2 Diabetes |
| --- |
| *Adult:* **PO** 250 mg to 3 g/day in 1–2 divided doses |

## ADMINISTRATION
### Oral

- Tablets may be crushed and given with full glass of water if patient desires.
- Do not give at bedtime because of danger of nocturnal hypoglycemia, unless specifically prescribed.
- Store below 40° C (104° F), preferably at 15°–30° C (59°–86° F) in well-closed container. Avoid freezing.

## ADVERSE EFFECTS (≥1%) GI:
Nausea, epigastric fullness, heartburn, anorexia, constipation, diarrhea, cholestatic jaundice (rare). **Hematologic:** Agranulocytosis, thrombocytopenia, leukopenia, hemolytic anemia, aplastic anemia, pancytopenia. **Metabolic:** Hepatic porphyria, disulfiram-like reactions, SIADH, hypoglycemia without loss of consciousness or neurologic symptoms (unusual fatigue, tremulousness, hunger, drowsiness, GI distress, sweating, anxiety, headache) severe hypoglycemia (visual disturbances, ataxia, paresthesias, confusion, tachycardia, seizures, coma). **Skin:** Allergic skin reactions: Pruritus, erythema, urticaria, morbilliform or maculopapular eruptions; porphyria cutanea tarda, photosensitivity. **Special Senses:** Taste alterations. **CNS:** Headache.

## DIAGNOSTIC TEST INTERFERENCE
The SULFONYLUREAS may produce abnormal *thyroid function test* results and reduced *RAI uptake* (after long-term administration). A tolbutamide metabolite may cause false-positive *urinary protein* values when turbidity procedures are used (such as heat and *acetic acid* or *sulfosalicylic acid*); *Ames reagent* strips reportedly not affected.

## INTERACTIONS Drug: **Phenylbutazone** increases hypoglycemic effects; THIAZIDE DIURETICS may attenuate hypoglycemic effects; **alcohol** may produce disulfiram reaction; BETA-BLOCKERS may mask symptoms of a hypoglycemic reaction. **Herbal: Ginseng, karela** may potentiate hypoglycemic effects.

## PHARMACOKINETICS Absorption: Readily from GI tract. **Peak:** 3–5 h. **Distribution:** Into extracellular fluids. **Metabolism:** Principally in liver. **Elimination:** 75–85% in urine; some in feces. **Half-Life:** 7 h.

## NURSING IMPLICATIONS
### Assessment & Drug Effects

- Supervise closely during initial period of therapy until dosage is established. One or 2 wk of therapy may be required before full therapeutic effect is achieved.
- Monitor closely during adjustment period, watching for S&S of impending hypoglycemia (see Appendix F). Detection of a hypoglycemic reaction in a diabetic patient also receiving a beta-blocker, especially older adults, is difficult.
- Evaluate nondefinitive vague complaints; hypoglycemic symptoms may be especially vague in older adults. Observe patient carefully, especially 2–3 h after eating, check urine for sugar and ketone bodies and capillary blood glucose.
- Report repetitive complaints of headache and weakness a few hours after eating; may signal incipient hypoglycemia.
- Be aware that pruritus and rash, frequently reported adverse effects, may clear spontaneously; if these persist, drug will be discontinued.
- Monitor lab tests: Periodic HbA1C, fasting serum glucose and urine glucose.

Common adverse effects in *italic*; life-threatening effects <u>underlined</u>; generic names in **bold**; classifications in SMALL CAPS; ♣ Canadian drug name; ⊙ Prototype drug

1627

## Patient & Family Education

- Learn the S&S of hyperglycemia (see Appendix A) and check blood glucose level when hyperglycemia is suspected.
- Hypoglycemia is frequently caused by overdosage of hypoglycemic drug, inadequate or irregular food intake, nausea, vomiting, diarrhea, and added exercise without caloric supplement or dose adjustment. Learn the S&S of hypoglycemia (see Appendix F) and check blood glucose level whenever hypoglycemia is suspected.
- Report any illness promptly. Prescriber may want to evaluate need for insulin.
- Do not self-medicate with OTC drugs unless approved or prescribed by prescriber.
- Be aware that alcohol, even in moderate amounts, can precipitate a disulfiram-type reaction (see Appendix F). A hypoglycemic response after ingesting alcohol requires emergency treatment.
- Protect exposed skin areas from the sun with a sunscreen lotion (SPF 12–15) because of potential photosensitivity (especially in the alcoholic).
- Monitor blood glucose daily or as directed by prescriber.
- Be alert to added danger of loss of control (hyperglycemia) when a drug that affects the hypoglycemic action of sulfonylureas (see DRUG INTERACTIONS) is withdrawn or added to the tolbutamide regimen. Monitor blood glucose carefully.
- Use or add barrier contraceptive if using hormonal contraceptives.

# TOLCAPONE ℗

(tol′ca-pone)

Tasmar

**Classification:** ANTICHOLINERGIC; CATECHOLAMINE-O-METHYL-TRANSFERASE (COMT) INHIBITOR

Therapeutic: ANTIPARKINSON

## AVAILABILITY Tablet

## ACTION & *THERAPEUTIC EFFECT*

Selective and reversible inhibitor of catecholamine-O-methyltransferase (COMT). COMT is the enzyme responsible for metabolizing catecholamines and, therefore, levodopa. *Concurrent administration of tolcapone and levodopa increases the amount of levodopa available to control Parkinson's disease by increasing dopaminergic brain stimulation.*

## USES Idiopathic Parkinson's disease as adjunct to levodopa/carbidopa.

## CONTRAINDICATIONS Hypersensitivity to tolcapone; liver disease; drug-induced signs of liver decompensation; MAOI therapy.

## CAUTIOUS USE History of hypersensitivity to other COMT inhibitors (e.g., entacapone; nitecapone); anorexia nervosa; hematuria; hypotension; syncopy; renal disease; renal impairment; pregnancy (category C); lactation.

## ROUTE & DOSAGE

### Parkinson's Disease

*Adult:* **PO** 100 mg t.i.d. (max: 200 mg t.i.d.)

## ADMINISTRATION

### Oral

- Give with food if GI upset occurs.
- Give only in conjunction with levodopa/carbidopa therapy.
- Therapy with tolcapone **should not** be initiated if patient has ALT/AST greater than 2 × ULN or has known liver disease.
- Store at 20°–25° C (68°–77° F) in a tightly closed container.

**ADVERSE EFFECTS** (≥1%) **Body as a Whole:** Muscle cramps, orthostatic complaints, fatigue, falling, balance difficulties, hyperkinesia, stiffness, arthritis, hypokinesia. **CNS:** *Dyskinesia, sleep disorder, dystonia, excessive dreaming,* somnolence, confusion, dizziness, headache, hallucination, syncope, paresthesias. **CV:** Chest pain, hypotension. **GI:** *Nausea,* anorexia, diarrhea, vomiting, constipation, <u>fulminant liver failure, severe hepatocellular injury,</u> dry mouth, abdominal pain, dyspepsia, flatulence. **Respiratory:** URI, dyspnea, sinus congestion. **Skin:** Sweating. **Urogenital:** UTI, urine discoloration, micturition disorder

**INTERACTIONS Drug:** Will increase **levodopa** levels when taken simultaneously; CNS DEPRESSANTS may cause additive sedation; do not give with non-selective MAOIS **(isocarboxazid, phenelzine, or tranylcypromine furazolidone, linezolid, procarbazine).** Avoid concurrent use of azelastine, paraldehyde. **Food:** Decreases levels. **Herbal:** Avoid use of valerian, **St. John's wort,** kava, gota kola.

**PHARMACOKINETICS Absorption:** Rapidly from GI tract, bioavailability 65%. **Peak:** 2 h. **Distribution:** Over 99% protein bound. **Metabolism:** Extensively metabolized by COMT and glucuronidation. **Elimination:** 60% in urine, 40% in feces; clearance reduced by 50% in patients with liver disease. **Half-Life:** 2–3 h.

## NURSING IMPLICATIONS

### Black Box Warning

*Tolcapone has been associated with risk of potentially fatal, acute fulminant liver failure.*

### Assessment & Drug Effects

- More frequent PT and INR when given concurrently with warfarin.
- Withhold drug and notify prescriber if liver dysfunction is suspected.
- Monitor carefully for and immediately report S&S of hepatic impairment (e.g., jaundice, dark urine).
- Monitor lab tests: Monthly LFTs for first 3 mo, every 6 wk for the next 3 mo, and periodically thereafter.

### Patient & Family Education

- Notify prescriber promptly about any of following: Increased loss of muscle control, fainting, yellowing of skin or eyes, darkening of urine, severe diarrhea, hallucinations.
- Do not engage in hazardous activities until response to drug is known. Avoid use of alcohol or sedative drugs while on tolcapone.
- Rise slowly from a sitting or lying position to avoid a rapid drop in BP with possible weakness or fainting.
- Nausea is a common possible adverse effect especially at the beginning of therapy.
- Do not suddenly stop taking this drug. Doses **must be** gradually reduced over time.

# TOLMETIN SODIUM
(tole′met-in)

**Classification:** ANALGESIC, NONSTEROIDAL ANTI-INFLAMMATORY (NSAID); ANTIPYRETIC
**Therapeutic:** NONNARCOTIC ANALGESIC, NSAID; DISEASE-MODIFYING ANTIRHEUMATIC DRUG (DMARD)
**Prototype:** Ibuprofen

**AVAILABILITY** Tablet; capsule

## ACTION & *THERAPEUTIC EFFECT*
Competitively inhibits both cyclooxygenase (COX) isoenzymes, COX-1 and COX-2, by blocking

T

---

Common adverse effects in *italic;* life-threatening effects <u>underlined;</u> generic names in **bold;** classifications in SMALL CAPS; ♣ Canadian drug name; ⊘ Prototype drug

1629

arachidonate binding to prostaglandin sites, and thus inhibits prostaglandin synthesis. *Possesses analgesic, antiinflammatory, antipyretic, and antirheumatic activity.*

**USES** In treatment of rheumatoid arthritis, juvenile rheumatoid arthritis, juvenile idiopathic arthritis.

**CONTRAINDICATIONS** History of intolerance or hypersensitivity to tolmetin, aspirin, and other NSAIDs; active peptic ulcer, CABG perioperative pain; in patients with active GI disease including peptic ulcer and ulcerative colitis; in patients with functional class IV rheumatoid arthritis (severely incapacitated, bedridden, or confined to a wheelchair). Safety during pregnancy (category D third trimester); lactation.

**CAUTIOUS USE** History of PUD or GI bleeding; impaired kidney function; SLE; hypertension; patients with fluid retention; CHF; compromised cardiac function; liver dysfunction; coagulation disorders; older adults; pregnancy (category C first and second trimester). Safe use in children younger than 2 y not established.

## ROUTE & DOSAGE

**Arthritis**

*Adult:* **PO** 400 mg t.i.d. (max: 2 g/day)

**Juvenile Rhematoid Arthritis**

*Child (2 y or older):* **PO** 20 mg/kg/day in 3–4 divided doses (max: 30 mg/kg/day)

## ADMINISTRATION

**Oral**

- Schedule to include a morning dose (on arising) and a bedtime dose.
- May be administered with magnesium or aluminum hydroxide containing antacids to minimize GI irritation. Administration with food or milk reduces bioavailability of the drug by 16%.
- Give with fluid of patient's choice; crush tablet or empty capsule to mix with water or food if patient cannot swallow tablet/capsule.
- Store at 20°–25°C (68°–77° F) in tightly capped and light-resistant container unless otherwise instructed.

**ADVERSE EFFECTS** (≥1%) **CNS:** *Headache, dizziness, vertigo, lightheadedness,* mood elevation or depression, tension, nervousness, weakness, drowsiness, insomnia, tinnitus. **CV:** Mild edema, sodium and water retention, mild to moderate hypertension thrombotic event/MI/stroke. **GI:** Epigastric or abdominal pain, dyspepsia, *nausea,* vomiting, flatulence heartburn, constipation, peptic ulcer, GI bleeding. **Hematologic:** Transient and small decreases in hemoglobin and hematocrit, purpura, petechiae, granulocytopenia, leukopenia. **Respiratory:** Brochospasm. **Urogenital:** Hematuria, proteinuria, increased BUN. **Skin:** Toxic epidermal necrolysis, morbilliform eruptions, urticaria, pruritus. **Body as a Whole:** Anaphylaxis (especially after drug is discontinued and then reinstituted).

**DIAGNOSTIC TEST INTERFERENCE** Tolmetin prolongs *bleeding time,* inhibits *platelet aggregation,* elevates *BUN, alkaline phosphatase,* and *AST* levels; may decrease *hemoglobin* and *hematocrit* values. Metabolites may produce false-positive results for *proteinuria* [with tests that rely on acid precipitation (e.g., *sulfosalicylic acid*)].

**INTERACTIONS Drug:** ORAL ANTICOAGULANTS, **heparin** may prolong bleeding time; may increase **lithium** toxicity; **aspirin,** other NSAIDs add to ulcerogenic effects; may increase

Common adverse effects in *italic;* life-threatening effects underlined; generic names in **bold;** classifications in SMALL CAPS; ✦ Canadian drug name; ⊙ Prototype drug

**methotrexate** toxicity. Do not use with **ketorolac** due to increased risk of toxicities. **Herbal: Feverfew,** cat's claw, **garlic, ginger, ginkgo** may increase bleeding potential.

## PHARMACOKINETICS

**Absorption:** Rapidly from GI tract. **Peak:** 30–60 min; therapeutic effect in 3–7 days. **Distribution:** Crosses blood–brain barrier and placenta; distributed into breast milk. **Metabolism:** In liver. **Elimination:** In urine. **Half-Life:** 60–90 min.

## NURSING IMPLICATIONS

### Black Box Warning

*Tolmetin sodium has been associated with increased risk of serious, potentially fatal, GI bleeding and cardiovascular events (e.g., MI and CVA); risk may increase with duration of use and may be greater in the older adult and those with risk factors for CV disease.*

### Assessment & Drug Effects

- Monitor for and report promptly S&S of GI ulceration or bleeding. Significant GI bleeding may occur without prior warning.
- Monitor for and report promptly S&S of CV thrombotic events (i.e., angina, MI, TIA, or stroke).
- Monitor BP throughout the course of therapy.
- Monitor patients with kidney damage closely. Evaluate I&O ratio and encourage patient to increase fluid intake to at least 8 full glasses/day.
- Monitor lab tests: Periodic renal function tests with long-term therapy; CBC; Hct & Hgb if symptoms of anemia appear; LFTs, serum creatinine/BUN, and stool guaiac.

### Patient & Family Education

- Stop taking drug and report promptly to prescriber if you experience S&S of GI ulceration: Stomach pain, frequent indigestion and nausea, bloody or tarry stools, vomit with blood or coffee-ground appearance.
- Monitor weight and report an increase greater than 2 kg (4 lb)/wk with impaired kidney or cardiac function; check for swelling in ankles, tibiae, hands, and feet.
- Report promptly signs of abnormal bleeding (ecchymosis, epistaxis, melena, petechiae), itching, skin rash, persistent headache, edema.
- Stop taking drug and report promptly to prescriber if you experience chest pain, shortness of breath, weakness, slurring of speech, or other signs of a cardiac or neurologic problem.
- Avoid potentially hazardous activities until response to drug is known because dizziness and drowsiness are common adverse effects.

## TOLNAFTATE
(tole-naf'tate)

Aftate, Pitrex ♣, Tinactin

**Classification:** ANTIFUNGAL ANTIBIOTIC
**Therapeutic:** ANTIFUNGAL

**AVAILABILITY** Cream; solution; gel; powder; spray

## ACTION & *THERAPEUTIC EFFECT*

Distorts hyphae and stunts mycelial growth on susceptible fungi. *Fungistatic or fungicidal as well as anti-infective against bacteria, protozoa, and viruses.*

**USES** Tinea pedis (athlete's foot), tinea cruris (jock itch), tinea corporis (body ringworm); also tinea capitis and tinea unguium if infection is superficial, plantar or palmar lesions adjunctively with keratolytic agents, and tinea versicolor (caused by *Malassezia furfur*).

**CONTRAINDICATIONS** Skin irritations prior to therapy, nail and scalp infections; immunosuppressed patients, diabetes mellitus, peripheral vascular disease.

**CAUTIOUS USE** Excoriated skin; pregnancy (category C); lactation. Safe use in children younger than 2 y is not established.

## ROUTE & DOSAGE

**Tinea Infestations**

*Adult/Child:* **Topical** Apply 0.5–1 cm (¼–½ in.) of cream or 3 drops of solution b.i.d. in morning and evening; powder may be used prophylactically in normally moist areas

## ADMINISTRATION

**Topical**
- Cleanse site thoroughly with water and dry completely before applying. Massage thin layer gently into skin. Make sure area is not wet from excess drug after application.
- Shake aerosol powder container well before use.
- Note: Cream and powder are not recommended for nail or scalp infection.
- Use liquids (solutions) for scalp infection or to treat hairy areas.
- Store cream, gel, powder, and topical solution in light-resistant containers at 15°–30° C (59°–86° F); store aerosol container at 2°–30° C (38°–86° F). Avoid freezing and exposure to light.

**ADVERSE EFFECTS** (≥1%) **Skin:** Local irritation, stinging of skin from aerosol formulation.

## NURSING IMPLICATIONS

**Patient & Family Education**
- Expect relief from pruritus, soreness, and burning within 24–72 h after start of treatment.

- Continue treatment for 2–3 wk after disappearance of all symptoms to prevent recurrence.
- Return to prescriber for reevaluation in absence of improvement within 4 wk.
- Note: If skin has thickened as a result of the infection, desired clinical response may be delayed for 4–6 wk.
- Avoid contact with eyes of all drug forms.
- Place container in warm water to liquify contents if solution solidifies. Potency is unaffected.

## TOLTERODINE TARTRATE
(tol-ter′o-deen tar′trate)

**Detrol, Detrol LA**

**Classifications:** ANTICHOLINERGIC; MUSCARINIC RECEPTOR ANTAGONIST

**Therapeutic:** ANTIMUSCARINIC; BLADDER ANTISPASMODIC

**Prototype:** Oxybutynin

**AVAILABILITY** Tablet; sustained release capsule

**ACTION & *THERAPEUTIC* EFFECT** Selective muscarinic urinary bladder receptor antagonist. Reduces urinary incontinence, urgency, and frequency. *Controls urinary bladder incontinence by controlling contractions.*

**USES** Overactive bladder, urinary incontinence, urinary urgency.

**CONTRAINDICATIONS** Hypersensitivity to tolterodine or fesoterodine; uncontrolled narrow-angle glaucoma; gastric retention, obstruction, or pyloric stenosis; urinary retention; lactation. **Extended release:** Severe hepatic impairment (Child-Pugh class C).

**CAUTIOUS USE** Cardiovascular disease; liver disease; controlled narrow-angle glaucoma; significant urinary retention; severe hepatic impairment; obstructive GI disease; obstructive uropathy; MG; history of QT prolongation; paralytic ileus or intestinal atony; renal impairment; ulcerative colitis; older adults; pregnancy (category C). Safety and efficacy in children not established.

## ROUTE & DOSAGE

### Overactive Bladder

*Adult:* **PO** 2 mg b.i.d. or **Sustained release:** 4 mg daily

*Hepatic Impairment Dosage Adjustment*

Reduce dose by 50%

*Renal Impairment Dosage Adjustment*

*CrCl less than 30 ml/min:* Reduce dose 50%

*Concurrent Medication Dosage Adjustment*

*Concurrent CYP3A4 inhibiting drugs.* Reduce dose by 50%

## ADMINISTRATION

### Oral

- Do not crush or chew sustained release tablets. These **must be** swallowed whole.
- Doses greater than 1 mg b.i.d. are not recommended for those with significantly reduced liver function or kidney function or concurrently receiving macrolide antibiotics, azole antifungal agents, or other cytochrome P450 3A4 inhibitors.
- Store at 15°–30° C (59°–86°F) in a tightly closed container.

## ADVERSE EFFECTS (≥1%) **Body as a Whole:** Back pain, fatigue, flu-like syndrome, falls, arthralgia, weight gain. **CNS:** Headache, paresthesias, vertigo, dizziness, nervousness, somnolence. **CV:** Chest pain, hypertension. **GI:** *Dry mouth,* dyspepsia, constipation, abdominal pain, diarrhea, flatulence, nausea, vomiting, weight gain. **Urogenital:** Dysuria, micturition frequency, urinary retention,

UTI. **Respiratory:** Bronchitis, cough, pharyngitis, rhinitis, sinusitis, URI. **Skin:** Pruritus, rash, erythema, dry skin. **Special Senses:** Dry eyes, vision abnormalities.

## INTERACTIONS Drug: Additive anticholinergic effects with **amantadine, amoxapine, bupropion, clozapine, cyclobenzaprine, disopyramide, maprotiline, olanzapine, orphenadrine,** SEDATING H₁-BLOCKERS, PHENOTHIAZINES, TRICYCLIC ANTIDEPRESSANTS. Increased effects with CYP3A4 inhibitors (e.g., **clarithromycin, cyclosporine, erythromycin, itraconazole,** or **ketoconazole**). Do not use with agents that prolong QT interval (e.g., **dotetilide, dronedarone, voriconazole, ziprasidone**). **Food:** Grapefruit juice may increase **tolterodine** levels in some patients.

## PHARMACOKINETICS Absorption: 77% absorbed, decreased with food. **Peak:** 1–2 h. **Distribution:** 96% protein bound. **Metabolism:** In liver by CYP2D6 and CYP3A4. **Elimination:** 77% in urine, 17% in feces. **Half-Life:** 1.9–3.7 h.

## NURSING IMPLICATIONS

### Assessment & Drug Effects

- Monitor voiding pattern and report promptly urinary retention.
- Monitor vital signs carefully (HR and BP), especially in those with cardiovascular disease.
- Monitor lab tests: LFTs.

### Patient & Family Education

- Notify prescriber promptly if you experience eye pain, rapid heartbeat, difficulty breathing, skin rash or hives, confusion, or incoordination.
- Report blurred vision, sensitivity to light, and dry mouth (all common adverse effects) to prescriber if bothersome.
- Avoid the use of alcohol or OTC antihistamines.

Common adverse effects in *italic;* life-threatening effects <u>underlined</u>; generic names in **bold;** classifications in SMALL CAPS; ♣ Canadian drug name; ⊚ Prototype drug

1633

# TOLVAPTAN

· (tol-vap′tan)

Samsca

**Classification:** ELECTROLYTE & WATER BALANCE AGENT; DIURETIC; VASOPRESSIN ANTAGONIST

Therapeutic: VASOPRESSIN ANTAGONIST; DIURETIC

**Prototype:** Conivaptan

## AVAILABILITY Tablet

## ACTION & *THERAPEUTIC EFFECT*

Selective vasopressin $V_2$-receptor antagonist; antagonizes the effect of vasopressin and causes an increase in urine water excretion, decrease in urine osmolality, and increase in serum sodium concentrations. *Effectiveness is measured by increase in serum sodium level toward lower limit of normal, and/ or decrease in sign and symptoms of hyponatremia.*

## USES Treatment of hypervolemic and euvolemic hyponatremia.

## CONTRAINDICATIONS Rapid correction of serum sodium (e.g., greater than 12 mEq/L/24 h); cognitively impaired; serious neurologic symptoms; hypovolemic hyponatremia; hypertonic saline; concurrent administration with strong CYP3A inhibitors; lactation.

## CAUTIOUS USE Must be initiated or reinitiated in a hospital setting; cirrhosis; pregnancy (category C). Safe use in children younger than 18 y not established.

## ROUTE & DOSAGE

### Hyponatremia

*Adult:* **PO** Initially 15 mg once daily; may be adjusted up to 60 mg once daily

## ADMINISTRATION

### Oral

- Administer ONLY in setting where serum sodium can be closely monitored.
- Doses may be increased at 24 h intervals or greater.
- Do not administer if patient is unable to sense or respond to thirst.
- Store at 15°–30°C (59°–86°F).

## ADVERSE EFFECTS (≥1%) **Body as a Whole:** *Asthenia,* pyrexia, *thirst.* **GI:** *Constipation, dry mouth, nausea.* **Metabolic:** Anorexia, *hyperglycemia.* **Urogenital:** *Pollakiuria, polyuria.*

## INTERACTIONS **Drug:** Strong CYP3A4 INHIBITORS (e.g., **clarithromycin, ketoconazole, itraconazole, telithromycin, saquinavir, nelfinavir, ritonavir, nefazodone**) may increase tolvaptan levels. Moderate CYP3A INHIBITORS (e.g., **erythromycin, fluconazole, aprepitant, diltiazem, verapamil**) may increase tolvaptan levels. P-GLYCOPROTEIN INHIBITORS (e.g., **cyclosporine**) may require tolvaptan dosage reduction. CYP3A INDUCERS (e.g., **rifabutin, rifapentine, rifampin, barbiturates, phenytoin, carbamazepine**) decrease the levels of tolvaptan. Tolvaptan increases the levels of **digoxin**. BETA-BLOCKERS, ANGIOTENSIN RECEPTOR BLOCKERS, ANGIOTENSIN-CONVERTING ENZYME INHIBITORS and POTASSIUM-SPARING DIURETICS may cause hyperkalemia. **Food:** Administration with **grapefruit juice** may increase tolvaptan levels. **Herbal: St. John's wort** may decrease the levels of tolvaptan.

## PHARMACOKINETICS **Absorption:** Approximately 40% absorbed. **Peak:** 2–4 h. **Distribution:** 99% plasma protein bound. **Metabolism:** In liver through CYP3A4. **Elimination:** Eliminated entirely by non-renal routes. **Half-Life:** 12 h.

Common adverse effects in *italic;* life-threatening effects underlined; generic names in **bold;** classifications in SMALL CAPS; ✤ Canadian drug name; ⊘ Prototype drug

## NURSING IMPLICATIONS

### Black Box Warning

*Tolvaptan has been associated with serious, sometime fatal, adverse events when hyponatremia is corrected too rapidly (e.g., more than 12 mEq/L per 24 h).*

### Assessment & Drug Effects

- Monitor vital signs frequently throughout therapy. Monitor ECG as warranted.
- Monitor weight and I&O closely as copious diuresis is expected.
- Fluid restriction should be avoided during the first 24 h of therapy.
- Monitor mental status throughout treatment. Report promptly changes in mental status (e.g., lethargy, confusion, disorientation, hallucinations, seizures).
- Report promptly symptoms of osmotic demyelination syndrome (ODS): Dysarthria, mutism, dysphagia, lethargy, affective changes, spasticity, seizures, or coma.
- Monitor digoxin levels closely with concurrent administration.
- Monitor lab tests: Baseline and frequent serum electrolytes; frequent serum sodium during initiation and titration.

### Patient & Family Education

- Continue to drink fluid in response to thirst until otherwise directed. Fluid restrictions are usually required after the first 24 h of therapy.
- Report promptly any of the following: Trouble speaking or swallowing, drowsiness, mood changes, confusion, involuntary body movements, or muscle weakness in arms or legs.

## TOPIRAMATE
(to-pir'a-mate)

**Topamax, Qudexy XR, Trokendi XR**

**Classifications:** ANTICONVULSANT; GAMMA-AMINOBUTYRATE (GABA) ENHANCER

**Therapeutic:** ANTICONVULSANT; ANTIEPILEPTIC

**AVAILABILITY** Tablet; extended release capsule; sprinkle capsule

### ACTION & *THERAPEUTIC EFFECT*

Exhibits sodium channel-blocking action, as well as enhances the ability of GABA to induce a flux of chloride ions into the neurons, thus potentiating the activity of this inhibitory neurotransmitter (GABA). *Effectiveness indicated by a decrease in seizure activity.*

**USES** Adjunctive therapy for partial-onset seizures; generalized tonic-clonic seizures; migraine prophylaxis.

**UNLABELED USES** Cluster headache, bulimia nervosa, neuropathic pain, infantile spasms, bipolar disorder, obesity.

**CONTRAINDICATIONS** Hypersensitivity to topiramate; suicidal ideation; visual field defects, or persistent or severe metabolic acidosis due to drug; abrupt withdrawal; pregnancy (category D); lactation. Effect on labor and delivery is unknown. **Extended release:** Recent alcohol use (i.e., within 6 h prior to and 6 h after administration).

**CAUTIOUS USE** Moderate and severe renal impairment, hepatic impairment; COPD; chronic acidosis; history of suicidal thoughts or psychiatric disturbances; severe pulmonary disease; older adults. **Immediate release:** Children younger than 2 y.

T

Common adverse effects in *italic;* life-threatening effects <u>underlined</u>; generic names in **bold;** classifications in SMALL CAPS; ♣ Canadian drug name; ⊙ Prototype drug

1635

## ROUTE & DOSAGE

### Partial-Onset Seizures (Monotherapy)

*Adult/Adolescent/Child (older than 10 y):* **PO Immediate release** Initiate with 25 mg b.i.d., increase by 25 mg/wk to efficacy; **PO Maintenance dose** 200–400 mg/day divided b.i.d. (max: 1600 mg/day); **PO Extended release** 50 mg daily then increase by 50 mg/wk to reach 400 mg daily
*Child (2–16 y):* **PO** Initiate with 1–3 mg/kg at bedtime × 1 wk, then increase by 1–3 mg/kg/day in 2 divided doses q1–2wk to a target range of 5–9 mg/kg/day

### Epilepsy (Adjunctive Therapy)

*Adult:* **PO Immediate release** Start at 25 mg daily then titrate to 100–200 mg b.i.d.;
**Extended Release** Start with 25 mg daily then titrate to 200–400 mg daily

### Generalized Tonic-Clonic Monotherapy

*Adults/Adolescents/Children (older than 10 y):* **PO Immediate release** 50 mg/day in 2 daily divided doses, taper up dose by 50 mg per wk up to 400 mg/day
*Child (2–10 y):* **PO** Weight-based dosing in package insert

### Migraine Prophylaxis

*Adult:* **PO Immediate release** Initiate with 25 mg b.i.d., increase by 25 mg/wk to 100 mg/day or max tolerated dose

### Renal Impairment Dosage Adjustment

*CrCl less than 70 mL/min:* Decrease dose by 50%

## ADMINISTRATION

### Oral

- Make dosage increments of 50 mg at weekly intervals to the recommended dose, usually 400 mg/day.
- Do not break tablets unless absolutely necessary because of bitter taste.
- Store at 15°–30° C (59°–86° F) in a tightly closed container. Protect from light and moisture.

## ADVERSE EFFECTS (≥1%) **Body as a Whole:** *Fatigue, speech problems, weight loss;* decreased sweating and hyperthermia in children; metabolic acidosis, upper respiratory infection. **CNS:** *Somnolence, dizziness, ataxia, psychomotor slowing, confusion, nystagmus, paresthesia, memory difficulty, difficulty concentrating, nervousness,* depression, anxiety, tremor. **GI:** *Anorexia,* nausea. **Endocrine:** *Abnormal bicarbonate level.* **Special Senses:** Angle closure glaucoma (rare).

## INTERACTIONS **Drug:** Increased CNS depression with **alcohol** and other CNS DEPRESSANTS; may increase **phenytoin** concentrations; may decrease ORAL CONTRACEPTIVE, **valproate** concentrations; may increase risk of kidney stone formation with other CARBONIC ANHYDRASE INHIBITORS. **Carbamazepine, phenytoin, valproate** may decrease topiramate concentrations. Use cautiously with **metformin. Herbal: Ginkgo** may decrease anticonvulsant effectiveness.

## PHARMACOKINETICS **Absorption:** Rapidly absorbed from GI tract; 80% bioavailability. **Peak:** 2 h. **Distribution:** 13–17% protein bound. **Metabolism:** Minimally metabolized in the liver. **Elimination:** Primarily in urine. **Half-Life:** 21 h.

## NURSING IMPLICATIONS

### Assessment & Drug Effects

- Monitor mental status and report significant cognitive impairment.

Common adverse effects in *italic;* life-threatening effects <u>underlined</u>, generic names in **bold;** classifications in SMALL CAPS; ♣ Canadian drug name; ⦿ Prototype drug

- Monitor lab tests: Periodic electrolytes and serum creatinine.

**Patient & Family Education**
- Do not stop drug abruptly; discontinue gradually to minimize seizures.
- To minimize risk of kidney stones, drink at least 6–8 full glasses of water each day.
- Exercise caution with potentially hazardous activities. Sedation is common, especially with concurrent use of alcohol or other CNS depressants.
- Use or add barrier contraceptive if using hormonal contraceptives.
- Be aware that psychomotor slowing and speech/language problems may develop while on topiramate therapy.
- Report adverse effects that interfere with activities of daily living.

# TOPOTECAN HYDROCHLORIDE ◑

(toe-po-tee'can)

**Hycamtin**

**Classifications:** ANTINEOPLASTIC; CAMPTOTHECIN; DNA TOPOISOMERASE I INHIBITOR
**Therapeutic:** ANTINEOPLASTIC

**AVAILABILITY** Solution for injection; oral capsule

## ACTION & *THERAPEUTIC EFFECT*

Antitumor mechanism is related to inhibition of the activity of topoisomerase I, an enzyme required for DNA replication. Topoisomerase I is essential for the relaxation of supercoiled double-stranded DNA that enables replication and transcription to proceed. *Topotecan permits uncoiling of DNA strands but prevents recoiling of the two strands of DNA, resulting in a permanent break in the DNA strands.*

**USES** Metastatic ovarian cancer, cervical cancer, small cell lung cancer.

**CONTRAINDICATIONS** Previous hypersensitivity to topotecan, irinotecan, or other camptothecin analogs; acute infection; severe bone marrow depression; severe thrombocytopenia; neutropenic colitis; interstitial lung disease; pregnancy (category D); lactation.

**CAUTIOUS USE** Myelosuppression; mild to moderate renal impairment; history of bleeding disorders; previous cytotoxic or radiation therapy; older adults.

## ROUTE & DOSAGE

**Metastatic Ovarian Cancer and Small Cell Lung Cancer**

*Adult:* **IV** 1.5 mg/m$^2$ daily for 5 days starting on day 1 of a 21-day course. Four courses of therapy recommended. Subsequent doses can be adjusted by 0.25 mg/m$^2$ depending on toxicity. **PO** 2.3 mg/m$^2$ × 5 days, repeat q21days

**Cervial Cancer**

*Adult:* 0.75 mg/m$^2$ days 1–3 every 3 weeks

**Renal Impairment Dosage Adjustment**

*CrCl 20–39 mL/min:* **IV** Use 0.75 mg/m$^2$ **PO** Reduce to 1.8 mg/m$^2$

**Toxicity Dosage Adjustment**

In severe neutropenia reduce dose by 0.4 mg/m$^2$ for subsequent courses

## ADMINISTRATION

**Oral**
- Capsules must be swallowed whole. They must not be crushed, chewed, or opened.

---

Common adverse effects in *italic*; life-threatening effects underlined; generic names in **bold**; classifications in SMALL CAPS; ♣ Canadian drug name; ◑ Prototype drug

1637

T

- Avoid direct contact of the capsule contents with the skin or mucous membranes. If contact occurs, wash thoroughly with soap and water or wash eyes immediately with gently flowing water for at least 15 min.

### Intravenous

- Initiate therapy only if baseline neutrophil count 1500/mm³ or higher and platelet count 100,000/mm³ or higher. ▪ Do not give subsequent doses until neutrophils 1000/mm³ or higher, platelets 100,000/mm³ or higher, and Hgb greater than 9.0 mg/dL.

This drug is a cytotoxic agent and caution should be used to prevent any contact with the drug. Follow institutional or standard guidelines for preparation, handling, and disposal of cytotoxic agents.

PREPARE: IV Infusion: Reconstitute each 4-mg vial with 4 mL sterile water for injection to yield 1 mg/mL. ▪ Withdraw the required dose and inject into 50–100 mL of NS or D5W.

ADMINISTER: IV Infusion: Give over 30 min immediately after preparation.

INCOMPATIBILITIES: Y-site: Acyclovir, allopurinol, amifostine, aminophylline, amphotericin B, ampicillin/sulbactam, atenolol, bumetanide, calcium gluconate, cefepime, ceftazidime, clindamycin, dantrolene, dexamethasone, diazepam, digoxin, ertapenem, fluorouracil, foscarnet, fosphenytoin, ganciclovir, hydrocortisone, imipenem/cilastatin, ketorolac, meropenem, methohexital, mitomycin, nafcillin, pantoprazole, pemetrexed, pentobarbital, phenobarbital, phenytoin, piperacillin, piperacillin/tazobactam, potassium acetate, potassium phosphate, rituximab, sodium bicarbonate, sodium phosphate, SMZ/TMP, thiopental, ticarcillin, trastuzumab.

- Store vials at 20°–25° C (68°–77° F); protect from light. Reconstituted vials are stable for 24 h.

## ADVERSE EFFECTS (≥1%) Body as a Whole: *Asthenia, fever, fatigue.* GI: *Nausea, vomiting, diarrhea, constipation, abdominal pain, stomatitis, anorexia,* transient elevations in liver function tests. Hematologic: Leukopenia, *neutropenia, anemia,* thrombocytopenia. Respiratory: *Dyspnea,* cough. Skin: *Alopecia, rash.* CNS: *Headache, asthenia, pain.*

## INTERACTIONS Drug: Increased risk of bleeding with ANTICOAGULANTS, NSAIDS, SALICYLATES, ANTIPLATELET AGENTS. Avoid use with **clozapine, filgrastim, phenytoin, lefunomide, natalizumab, pimecrolimus, tacrolimus, tofacitinib,** and LIVE VACCINES.

## PHARMACOKINETICS Distribution: 35% bound to plasma proteins. Metabolism: Undergoes pH-dependent hydrolysis. Elimination: ~30% in urine. Half-Life: 2–3 h.

## NURSING IMPLICATIONS

### Black Box Warning

*Topotecan has been associated with severe bone marrow suppression.*

### Assessment & Drug Effects

- Assess for GI distress, respiratory distress, neurosensory symptoms, and S&S of infection throughout therapy.
- Monitor lab tests: Baseline and periodic CBC with differential; periodic renal function tests and LFTs.

### Patient & Family Education

- Learn common adverse effects and measures to control or minimize

Common adverse effects in *italic;* life-threatening effects underlined, generic names in **bold;** classifications in SMALL CAPS; ♣ Canadian drug name; ⊘ Prototype drug

when possible. Immediately report any distressing adverse effects to prescriber.
▪ Avoid pregnancy during therapy.

# TORSEMIDE

(tor'se-mide)

Demadex

**Classification:** ELECTROLYTE AND
WATER BALANCE; LOOP DIURETIC
Therapeutic: DIURETIC;
ANTIHYPERTENSIVE
**Prototype:** Furosemide

**AVAILABILITY** Tablet; solution for
injection

## ACTION & *THERAPEUTIC EFFECT*
Inhibits reabsorption of sodium and
chloride primarily in the loop of
Henle and renal tubules. Binds to the
sodium/potassium/chloride carrier
in the loop of Henle and in the renal
tubules. *Long acting potent "loop"
diuretic and antihypertensive agent.*

**USES** Management of edema, hypertension.

**CONTRAINDICATIONS** Hypersensitivity to torsemide or sulfonamides;
anuria.

**CAUTIOUS USE** Renal impairment;
CVD; ventricular arrhythmias; gout
or hyperuricemia; DM or history of
pancreatitis; liver disease with cirrhosis and ascites; fluid and electrolyte depletion; hearing impairment;
older adults; pregnancy (category
B); lactation. Safety and efficacy in
children not established.

## ROUTE & DOSAGE

### Edema of HF or Chronic Renal Failure
*Adult:* **PO/IV** 10–20 mg once
daily, may increase up to
200 mg/day as needed

### Edema with Hepatic Cirrhosis
*Adult:* **PO/IV** 5–10 mg once daily
administered with an aldosterone
antagonist or potassium-sparing
diuretic, may increase up to
40 mg/day as needed

### Hypertension
*Adult:* **PO** 5 mg once daily, may
increase to 10 mg/day if no
response after 4–6 wk

## ADMINISTRATION
▪ Note: With hepatic cirrhosis, use an
aldosterone antagonist concomitantly to prevent hypokalemia
and metabolic alkalosis.

### Oral
▪ Be aware that oral and IV doses are
therapeutically equivalent; patients
may be switched between the two
forms with no change in dosage.

### Intravenous
*PREPARE:* **Direct:** Given undiluted.
*ADMINISTER:* **Direct:** Give slowly
over 2 min.
▪ Store at 15°–30° C (59°–86° F).

**ADVERSE EFFECTS** (>1%) **CNS:**
Headache, dizziness, fatigue,
insomnia. **CV:** Orthostatic hypotension, chest pain, ECG abnormality.
**Endocrine:** *Hypokalemia,* hyponatremia, hyperuricemia. **GI:** Nausea,
diarrhea. **Skin:** Rash, pruritus. **Body
as a Whole:** Muscle cramps, rhinitis.
**Urogenital:** Polyuria. **Special Senses:**
Ototoxicity.

**INTERACTIONS Drug:** NSAIDs may
reduce diuretic effects. Also see
furosemide for potential drug interactions such as increased risk of **digoxin** toxicity due to hypokalemia,
prolonged neuromuscular blockade
with NEUROMUSCULAR BLOCKING AGENTS,
and decreased **lithium** elimination
with increased toxicity. **Herbal: Ginseng** may decrease efficacy.

T

Common adverse effects in *italic;* life-threatening effects underlined; generic names
in **bold;** classifications in SMALL CAPS; ♣ Canadian drug name; ⊕ Prototype drug

1639

**PHARMACOKINETICS Absorption:** Readily from GI tract. **Onset:** IV 10 min; PO 60 min. **Peak:** IV within 60 min; PO 60–120 min. **Duration:** 6–8 h. **Metabolism:** In liver (CYP system). **Elimination:** 80% in bile; 20% in urine. **Half-Life:** 210 min.

## NURSING IMPLICATIONS

### Assessment & Drug Effects
- Monitor BP often and assess for orthostatic hypotension; assess respiratory status for S&S of pulmonary edema.
- Monitor ECG, as electrolyte imbalances predispose to cardiac arrhythmias.
- Monitor I&O with daily weights. Assess for improvement in edema.
- Monitor diabetics for loss of glycemic control.
- Monitor coagulation parameters and lithium levels in patients on concurrent anticoagulant and/or lithium therapy.
- Monitor lab tests: Periodic serum electrolytes.

### Patient & Family Education
- Check weight at least weekly and report abrupt gains or losses to prescriber.
- Understand the risk of orthostatic hypotension.
- Report symptoms of hypokalemia (see Appendix F) or hearing loss immediately to prescriber.
- Monitor blood glucose for loss of glycemic control if diabetic.

## TRAMADOL HYDROCHLORIDE
(tra'mad-ol)
ConZip, Rybix, Ryzolt, Ultram, Ultram ER, Zydol ♦
**Classifications:** ANALGESIC; NARCOTIC (OPIATE AGONIST)
**Therapeutic:** NARCOTIC ANALGESIC
**Prototype:** Morphine sulfate
**Controlled Substance:** Schedule IV

**AVAILABILITY** Tablet; orally disintegrating tablet; extended release tablet; extended release capsule

## ACTION & *THERAPEUTIC EFFECT*
Centrally acting opiate receptor agonist that inhibits the uptake of norepinephrine and serotonin, suggesting both opioid and nonopioid mechanisms of pain relief. May produce opioid-like effects, but causes less respiratory depression than morphine. *Effective agent for control of moderate to moderately severe pain.*

**USES** Management of moderate or moderately severe pain.

**CONTRAINDICATIONS** Hypersensitivity to tramadol or other opioid analgesics including anaphylactoid reaction; severe respiratory depression; severe or acute asthmas; patients on MAO Inhibitors; substance abuse; suicidal; alcohol intoxication; lactation. **Extended release:** Do not administer to patients with severe hepatic impairment.

**CAUTIOUS USE** Debilitated patients; chronic respiratory disorders; respiratory depression; liver disease; renal impairment; myxedema, hypothyroidism, or hypoadrenalism; GI disease; acute abdominal conditions; increased ICP or head injury, increased intracranial pressure; history of seizures; older adults: pregnancy (category C); children younger than 16 y. **Extended release:** Do not use in children younger than 18 y.

## ROUTE & DOSAGE

| Pain |
|---|
| *Adult:* **PO Immediate release** 25 mg daily, titrated up to dose of 100 mg/day (max: 400 mg/day); **PO Extended release** 100 mg qd may titrate up q5d (max dose: 300 mg/day) |

**PO Disintegrating tablet:** 50 mg q4–6h may increase q3d to 200 mg/day

**Renal Impairment Dosage Adjustment**

*CrCl less than 30 mL/min:* Decrease to 50–100 mg q12h

**Hepatic Impairment Dosage Adjustment**

*Cirrhosis:* Decrease to 50–100 mg q12h

## ADMINISTRATION

### Oral

- Extended release tablets should be swallowed whole. They should not be crushed or chewed.
- Store at 15°–30° C (59°–86° F).

## ADVERSE EFFECTS (≥1%) CNS:

Drowsiness, *dizziness, vertigo, fatigue, headache, somnolence,* restlessness, euphoria, confusion, anxiety, coordination disturbance, sleep disturbances, seizures. **CV:** Palpitations, vasodilation, orthostatic hypotension. **GI:** *Nausea, constipation,* vomiting, xerostomia, dyspepsia, diarrhea, abdominal pain, anorexia, flatulence. **Body as a Whole:** Sweating, anaphylactic reaction (even with first dose), withdrawal syndrome (anxiety, sweating, nausea, tremors, diarrhea, piloerection, panic attacks, paresthesia, hallucinations) with abrupt discontinuation, flushing. **Skin:** Rash. **Special Senses:** Visual disturbances. **Urogenital:** Urinary retention/frequency, menopausal symptoms.

## DIAGNOSTIC TEST INTERFERENCE

Increased *creatinine, liver enzymes;* decreased *hemoglobin; proteinuria.*

## INTERACTIONS Drug: Carbamazepine

significantly decreases tramadol levels (may need up to twice usual dose). Tramadol may increase adverse effects of MAO INHIBITORS. TRICYCLIC ANTIDEPRESSANTS, **cyclobenzaprine,** PHENOTHIAZINES, SELECTIVE SEROTONIN-REUPTAKE INHIBITORS (SSRIS), MAO INHIBITORS may enhance seizure risk with tramadol. May increase CNS adverse effects when used with other CNS DEPRESSANTS. **Herbal: St. John's wort** may increase sedation.

## PHARMACOKINETICS Absorption:

Rapidly absorbed from GI tract; 75% reaches systemic circulation. **Onset:** 30–60 min. **Peak:** 2 h. **Duration:** 3–7 h. **Distribution:** Approximately 20% bound to plasma proteins; probably crosses blood–brain barrier; crosses placenta; 0.1% excreted into breast milk. **Metabolism:** Extensively in liver by cytochrome P450 system. **Elimination:** Primarily in urine. **Half-Life:** 6–7 h.

## NURSING IMPLICATIONS

### Assessment & Drug Effects

- Assess for level of pain relief and administer prn dose as needed but not to exceed the recommended total daily dose.
- Monitor vital signs and assess for orthostatic hypotension or signs of CNS depression.
- Withhold drug and notify prescriber if S&S of hypersensitivity occur.
- Assess bowel and bladder function; report urinary frequency or retention.
- Use seizure precautions for patients who have a history of seizures or who are concurrently using drugs that lower the seizure threshold.
- Monitor ambulation and take appropriate safety precautions.

### Patient & Family Education

- Exercise caution with potentially hazardous activities until response to drug is known.

T

Common adverse effects in *italic;* life-threatening effects underlined; generic names in **bold;** classifications in SMALL CAPS; ♣ Canadian drug name; ⊙ Prototype drug

1641

- Do not exceed the total number of mg prescribed for a 24 h period.
- Understand potential adverse effects and report problems with bowel and bladder function, CNS impairment, and any other bothersome adverse effects to prescriber.

# TRAMETINIB
(tra-me'ti-nib)
Mekinist
**Classifications:** ANTINEOPLASTIC; MITOGEN-ACTIVATED EXTRACELLULAR KINASE (MEK) INHIBITOR
Therapeutic: ANTINEOPLASTIC
**Prototype:** Erlotinib

## AVAILABILITY Tablet

## ACTION & *THERAPEUTIC EFFECT*
A reversible inhibitor of certain kinases that transmit signals and promote cellular proliferation and cancer growth. *Trametinib inhibits BRAF V600 mutation-positive melanoma cell growth in vitro and in vivo.*

## USES Treatment of unresectable or metastatic melanoma in patients with BRAF V600E or V600K mutations, as detected by an FDA-approved test.

## CONTRAINDICATIONS Symptomatic cardiomyopathy or LVEF decreases by 10% below pretreatment level and less than the LLN; drug-related loss of vision or other visual disturbances; drug-induced interstitial lung disease or pneumonitis; pregnancy (category D); lactation.

## CAUTIOUS USE Severe renal impairment; moderate or severe hepatic impairment; cardiac disorders; CHF; respiratory disorders; ocular disorders; hypertension. Safety and efficacy in children not established.

## ROUTE & DOSAGE

### Malignant Melenoma
*Adult:* **PO** 2 mg once daily

### Toxicity Dosage Adjustment
For specific toxicities see manufacturer guidelines.

## ADMINISTRATION
### Oral
- Give at least 1 h before or 2 h after a meal.
- Store at 2°–8° C (36°–46° F) and protect from moisture and light. Keep in original bottle and do not remove desiccant.

## ADVERSE EFFECTS (≥1%) CNS: Dizziness, dysgeusia. CV: Bradycardia, cardiomyopathy, hypertension. GI: Abdominal pain and tenderness, aphthous stomatitis, *diarrhea*, mouth ulceration, mucosal inflammation, and stomatitis. Hematological: Conjunctival hemorrhage, *edema*, epistaxis, gingival bleeding, hematochezia, hematuria, hemorrhoidal hemorrhage, *lymphedema*, melena, *peripheral edema*, rectal hemorrhage, and vaginal hemorrhage. Metabolic: *Anemia, hypoalbuminemia, increased alkaline phosphatase, increased ALT/AST.* Musculoskeletal: Rhabdomyolysis. Skin: *Dermatitis acneiform*, cellulitis, dry skin, folliculitis, paronychia, pruritus, *rash.* Special Senses: Dry eye, blurred vision.

## PHARMACOKINETICS Absorption: 72% bioavailable. Peak: 1.5 h. Distribution: 97.4% plasma protein bound. Metabolism: In liver. Elimination: Fecal (80%) and renal (20%). Half-Life: 3.9–4.8 d.

Common adverse effects in *italic;* life-threatening effects underlined; generic names in **bold;** classifications in SMALL CAPS; ♣ Canadian drug name; ⊕ Prototype drug

# NURSING IMPLICATIONS

## Assessment & Drug Effects

- Monitor cardiovascular status throughout therapy. Report promptly new-onset or worsening hypertension and S&S of heart failure.
- Monitor pulmonary status throughout therapy. Report promptly signs of interstitial lung disease including cough, dyspnea, and signs of hypoxia or pleural effusion.
- Monitor for and report promptly S&S of retinal detachment.
- Evaluate for signs of skin toxicity. Report to prescriber development of progressive rash or signs of skin infection.
- Monitor lab tests: Prior to therapy the presence of BRAF V600E or V600K mutation in tumor specimens must be confirmed.

## Patient & Family Education

- Report to prescriber if you experience any of the following S&S of heart failure or lung problems: Rapid heart rate, shortness of breath, unproductive cough, swelling of ankles and feet, excessive fatigue.
- Report to prescriber if you experience blurred vision, see colored dots or halo around objects.
- Report promptly signs of skin toxicity such as skin rash, acne, redness, swelling, peeling, or tenderness of hands or feet.
- Women should use highly effective contraception during treatment due to potential for serious fetal harm.
- Contact prescriber immediately if a pregnancy is suspected.

# TRANDOLAPRIL

(tran-do′la-pril)

**Mavik**

**Classifications:** ANGIOTENSIN-CONVERTING ENZYME (ACE) INHIBITOR; ANTIHYPERTENSIVE

**Therapeutic:** ANTIHYPERTENSIVE; ACE INHIBITOR
**Prototype:** Enalapril

## AVAILABILITY Tablet

## ACTION & *THERAPEUTIC EFFECT*

Inhibits ACE and interrupts conversion by renin which leads to the formation of angiotensin II from angiotensin I. Inhibition of ACE leads to vasodilation as well as to decreased aldosterone. Decreased aldosterone leads to diuresis and a slight increase in serum potassium. *Lowers blood pressure by specific inhibition of ACE. Unlike other ACE inhibitors, all racial groups respond to trandolapril, including low-renin hypertensives.*

## USES
Treatment of hypertension, reduction of CV morbidity/mortality post MI in patients with heart failure.

## CONTRAINDICATIONS
Hypersensitivity to trandolapril or ACE inhibitors; history of angioedema related to previous treatment with an ACE inhibitor; idiopathic angioedema; jaundice due to trandolapril; pregnancy (category D).

## CAUTIOUS USE
Renal impairment, hepatic insufficiency; patients prone to hypotension (e.g., CHF, ischemic heart disease, aortic stenosis, CVA, dehydration); SLE, scleroderma; lactation. Safety and efficacy in children younger than 18 y not established.

## ROUTE & DOSAGE

### Hypertension

*Adult:* **PO** 1 mg (2 mg in black patients) once daily, may increase weekly to 2–4 mg once daily (max: 8 mg/day). Lower dose

---

Common adverse effects in *italic;* life-threatening effects underlined; generic names in **bold;** classifications in SMALL CAPS; ◆ Canadian drug name; ● Prototype drug used in patients also taking a diuretic.

**Post MI**

*Adult:* **PO** 1 mg daily for 2 days then increase to 4 mg daily for 2–4 years

**Renal Impairment Dosage Adjustment**

*CrCl less than 30 mL/min:* Start with 0.5 mg once daily

**Hepatic Impairment Dosage Adjustment**

*Hepatic cirrhosis:* Start with 0.5 mg once daily

## ADMINISTRATION

**Oral**
- Note: If concurrently ordered diuretic cannot be discontinued 2–3 days before beginning trandolapril therapy, initial dose is usually reduced to 0.5 mg.
- Dosage adjustments are typically made at intervals of at least 1 wk.
- Store at 15°–30° C (59°–86° F).

## ADVERSE EFFECTS (≥1%) **Body as a Whole:** Fatigue, angioedema, fever, malaise. **CNS:** *Dizziness*, drowsiness. **CV:** *Hypotension*, syncope bradycardia, edema, palpitations. **GI:** Nausea, diarrhea. **Respiratory:** *Cough*. **Skin:** Rash, pruritus. **Metabolic:** Hyperkalemia, increased liver enzymes.

## INTERACTIONS **Drug:** DIURETICS, **rituximab** may enhance hypotensive effects. POTASSIUM-SPARING DIURETICS (**amiloride, spironolactone, triamterene**), POTASSIUM SUPPLEMENTS, POTASSIUM-CONTAINING SALT SUBSTITUTES, **aliskiren,** may increase risk of hyperkalemia. May increase serum levels and toxicity of **lithium.** NSAIDs may reduce the therapeutic response. Avoid use with **cyclosporine.**

## PHARMACOKINETICS **Absorption:** Rapidly absorbed from GI tract and converted to active form, trandolaprilat, in liver; 70% of dose reaches systemic circulation as trandolaprilat. **Peak:** 4–10 h. **Distribution:** 80% protein bound; crosses placenta, secreted into breast milk of animals (human secretion unknown). **Metabolism:** In liver to trandolaprilat. **Elimination:** 33% in urine, 66% in feces. **Half-Life:** 6 h trandolapril, 22.5 h trandolaprilat.

## NURSING IMPLICATIONS

### Black Box Warning

*Trandolapril has been associated with fetal toxicity.*

### Assessment & Drug Effects
- Monitor BP carefully for 1–3 h following initial dose, especially in patients using concurrent diuretics, on salt restriction, or volume depleted.
- Monitor serum lithium levels frequently with concurrent lithium therapy and assess for S&S of lithium toxicity; increase caution when diuretic therapy is also used.
- Monitor lab tests: Baseline LFTs and renal function tests; periodic serum potassium and sodium.

### Patient & Family Education
- Discontinue drug and immediately report S&S of angioedema of face or extremities to prescriber. Seek emergency help for swelling of the tongue or any other sign of potential airway obstruction.
- Be aware that lightheadedness can occur, especially during early therapy. Excess fluid loss of any kind will increase risk of hypotension and syncope.

Common adverse effects in *italic*; life-threatening effects underlined; generic names in **bold**; classifications in SMALL CAPS; ✦ Canadian drug name; ⦿ Prototype drug

- Report promptly if you are or suspect you are pregnant.

# TRANYLCYPROMINE SULFATE
(tran-ill-sip'roe-meen)
**Parnate**
**Classification:** ANTIDEPRESSANT; MONOAMINE OXIDASE INHIBITOR (MAOI)
**Therapeutic:** ANTIDEPRESSANT; MAOI
**Prototype:** Phenelzine

## AVAILABILITY Tablet

## ACTION & *THERAPEUTIC EFFECT*
Potent MAO with a antidepressant activity that arises from the increased availability of monoamines resulting from the inhibition of the enzyme MAO. This leads to increased concentration of neurotransmitters, such as epinephrine, norepinephrine, and dopamine in the CNS. *Drug of last choice for severe depression unresponsive to other MAO inhibitors.*

## USES Major depression.

## UNLABELED USES Orthostatic hypotension, panic disorder, social anxiety disorder.

## CONTRAINDICATIONS Confirmed or suspected cerebrovascular defect, cardiovascular disease; hepatic disease or abnormal LFT; hypertension, pheochromocytoma history of severe or recurrent headaches; recent acute MI; angina; renal failure; suicidal ideation; anuria; lactation.

## CAUTIOUS USE Bipolar disorder; Parkinson's disease; psychosis; schizophrenia, anxiety/agitation; CHF; DM; seizure disorders; hyperthyroidism; history of suicidal attempts; renal impairment; older adults; pregnancy

(category C); children and adolescents with major depressive disorder or other psychiatric disorders.

## ROUTE & DOSAGE

### Major Depression
*Adult:* PO 30 mg/day in 2 divided doses, may increase by 10 mg/day at 2–3 wk intervals (max: 60 mg/day)

## ADMINISTRATION
### Oral
- Contraindicated drugs should be discontinued 1–2 wk before starting therapy.
- Crush tablet and give with fluid or mix with food if patient cannot swallow pill.
- Note: Doses given in the late evening may cause insomnia.

## ADVERSE EFFECTS (≥1%) CNS:
Vertigo, dizziness, tremors, muscle twitching, headache, blurred vision suicidality. **CV:** *Orthostatic hypotension,* arrhythmias, hypertensive crisis. **GI:** Dry mouth, anorexia, constipation, diarrhea, abdominal discomfort. **Skin:** Rash. **Urogenital:** Impotence. **Body as a Whole:** Peripheral edema, sweating.

## INTERACTIONS Drug: TRICYCLIC ANTIDEPRESSANTS, SSRIS, AMPHETAMINES, **ephedrine, reserpine, guanethidine, buspirone, methyldopa, dopamine, levodopa, tryptophan** may precipitate hypertensive crisis, and must be discontinued before **tranylcypromine** treatment. **Alcohol** and other CNS DEPRESSANTS add to CNS depressant effects; **meperidine** can cause fatal cardiovascular collapse; ANESTHETICS exaggerate hypotensive and CNS depressant effects; **metrizamide** increases risk of seizures; DIURETICS and other ANTIHYPERTENSIVE AGENTS

---

Common adverse effects in *italic;* life-threatening effects underlined; generic names in **bold;** classifications in SMALL CAPS; ✦ Canadian drug name; ◉ Prototype drug

1645

add to hypotensive effects. **Food: Tyramine-**containing foods may precipitate hypertensive crisis (e.g., aged or matured cheese, air-dried or cured meats including sausages and salamis; fava or broad bean pods, tap/draft beers, sauerkraut, soy sauce, and other soybean condiments). **Herbal: Ginseng, ephedra, ma huang, St. John's wort** may lead to hypertensive crisis; **ginseng** may lead to manic episodes.

## PHARMACOKINETICS **Absorption:** Completely from GI tract. **Onset:** 10 days. **Metabolism:** Rapidly in liver to active metabolite. **Elimination:** Primarily in urine. **Half-Life:** 90–190 min.

## NURSING IMPLICATIONS

### Black Box Warning

*Tranylcypromine sulfate has been associated with suicidal thinking and behavior in children, adolescents, and young adults.*

### Assessment & Drug Effects

- Monitor BP closely. Severe hypertensive reactions are known to occur with MAO inhibitors.
- Report immediately to prescriber signs of worsening mental status such as suicidal ideation, aggressiveness, agitation, anxiety, hostility, impulsivity, insomnia, irritability, panic attacks, and worsening of depression.
- Expect therapeutic response within 3 days, but full antidepressant effects may not be obtained until 2–3 wk of drug therapy.

### Patient & Family Education

- Do not eat tyramine-containing foods (see FOOD–DRUG INTERACTIONS).
- Be aware that excessive use of caffeine-containing beverages

(chocolate, coffee, tea, cola) can contribute to development of rapid heartbeat, arrhythmias, and hypertension.
- Report promptly emergence of anxiety, agitation, panic attacks, insomnia, irritability, hostility, aggressiveness, impulsivity, mania, worsening depression, suicidal ideation, or other unusual changes in behavior.
- Make position changes slowly, particularly from recumbent to upright posture.
- Avoid potentially hazardous activities until response to drug is known.
- Avoid alcohol or other CNS depressants because of their possible additive effects.

## TRASTUZUMAB ⓟ

(tra-stu′zu-mab)

**Herceptin**

**Classifications:** IMMUNOMODULATOR; MONOCLONAL ANTIBODY; ANTINEOPLASTIC; ANTI–HUMAN EPIDERMAL GROWTH FACTOR (ANTI–HER)

**Therapeutic:** ANTINEOPLASTIC; IMMUNOMODULATOR; ANTI–HER

**AVAILABILITY** Solution for injection

**ACTION & *THERAPEUTIC EFFECT*** Recombinant DNA monoclonal antibody ($IgG_1$ kappa) that selectively binds to the human epidermal growth factor receptor-2 protein ($HER_2$). *Inhibits growth of human tumor cells that overexpress $HER_2$ proteins.*

**USES** Metastatic breast cancer in those whose tumors overexpress the $HER_2$ protein. $HER_2$-positive breast cancer after surgery.

**CONTRAINDICATIONS** Concurrent administration of anthracycline

Common adverse effects in *italic;* life-threatening effects underlined; generic names in **bold;** classifications in SMALL CAPS; ♣ Canadian drug name; ⓟ Prototype drug

or radiation; anaphylaxis; angioedema; interstitial pneumonitis; acute respiratory distress syndrome; drug induced nephrotic syndrome; pregnancy (category D); lactation during and for 6 mo following administration of trastuzumab.

**CAUTIOUS USE** Preexisting cardiac dysfunction; pulmonary disease; previous administration of cardiotoxic therapy (e.g., anthracycline or radiation); hypersensitivity to benzyl alcohol; older adults.

## ROUTE & DOSAGE

**Metastatic Breast Cancer**
*Adult:* **IV** 4 mg/kg, then 2 mg/kg qwk

## ADMINISTRATION

Note: Trastuzumab and ado-trastuzumab emtansine are different products and are **not** interchangeable.

### Intravenous

*PREPARE:* **IV Infusion:** Reconstitute each vial with 20 mL of supplied diluent (bacteriostatic water) to produce a multidose vial containing 21 mg/mL. ▪ Note: For patients with a hypersensitivity to benzyl alcohol, reconstitute with sterile water for injection; this solution **must be** used immediately with any unused portion discarded. ▪ Withdraw the ordered dose and add to a 250 mL of NS and invert bag to mix. ▪ Do not give or mix with dextrose solutions.
*ADMINISTER:* **IV Infusion:** Infuse loading dose (4 mg/kg) over 90 min; infuse subsequent doses (2 mg/kg) over 30 min. ▪ Do not give IV push or as a bolus dose.
*INCOMPATIBILITIES:* Solution/additive: **Dextrose** solution; do not

mix or coadminister with other drugs. Y-site: **Aldesleukin, amikacin, amphotericin B, aztreonam, cefoperazone, cefotaxime, cefotetan, cefoxitin, chlorpromazine, clindamycin, cyclosporine, fludarabine, furosemide, idarubicin, irinotecan, levofloxacin, levorphanol, morphine, nalbuphine, netilmicin, ofloxacin, ondansetron, piperacillin, piperacillin/tazobactam, streptozocin, ticarcillin, topotecan.**

▪ Store unopened vials and reconstituted vials at 2°–8° C (36°–46° F).
▪ Discard reconstituted vials 28 days after reconstitution.

**ADVERSE EFFECTS (≥1%) Body as a Whole:** *Pain, asthenia, fever, chills,* flu syndrome, allergic reaction, *fatigue* bone pain, *arthralgia,* hypersensitivity (anaphylaxis, urticaria, bronchospasm, angioedema, or hypotension), *increased incidence of infections,* infusion reaction (*chills, fever,* nausea, vomiting, pain, rigors, headache, dizziness, dyspnea, hypotension, rash). **CNS:** *Headache, insomnia, dizziness, paresthesias,* depression, peripheral neuritis, neuropathy myalgia. **CV:** CHF, cardiac dysfunction (dyspnea, cough, paroxysmal nocturnal dyspnea, peripheral edema, S3 gallop, reduced ejection fraction), tachycardia, *edema,* cardiotoxicity. **GI:** *Diarrhea, abdominal pain, nausea, vomiting,* anorexia. **Hematologic:** *Anemia,* leukopenia, *thrombocytopenia, neutropenia.* **Respiratory:** *Cough, dyspnea,* rhinitis, pharyngitis, sinusitis. **Skin:** *Rash,* herpes simplex, acne.

**INTERACTIONS Drug: Paclitaxel** may increase trastuzumab levels and toxicity.

**PHARMACOKINETICS Half-Life:** 5.8 days.

**T**

---

## NURSING IMPLICATIONS

### Black Box Warning

*Trastuzumab has been associated with cardiomyopathy, infusion reactions, pulmonary toxicity, and embryo-fetal toxicity.*

### Assessment & Drug Effects

- Monitor for infusion reactions within 24 h of infusion. Stop infusion and notify prescriber if patients develop dyspnea, significant hypotension, or any other sign of infusion reaction. Monitor closely until symptoms resolve. chills and fever during the first IV infusion; these adverse events usually respond to prompt treatment without the need to discontinue the infusion. Notify prescriber immediately.
- Monitor carefully cardiovascular status at baseline and throughout course of therapy, assessing for S&S of heart failure (e.g., dyspnea, increased cough, PND, edema, S3 gallop). Those with preexisting cardiac dysfunction are at high risk for cardiotoxicity.
- Monitor lab tests: Periodic CBC with differential, platelet count, and Hgb and Hct.

### Patient & Family Education

- Report promptly any unusual symptoms (e.g., chills, nausea, fever) during infusion.
- Report promptly any of the following: Shortness of breath, swelling of feet or legs, persistent cough, difficulty sleeping, loss of appetite, abdominal bloating.

## TRAVOPROST

(tra′vo-prost)

Travatan

**See Appendix A-1**.

## TRAZODONE HYDROCHLORIDE

(tray′zoe-done)

Oleptro

**Classifications:** ANTIDEPRESSANT
**Therapeutic:** ANTIDEPRESSANT
**Prototype:** Imipramine

**AVAILABILITY** Tablet; extended release tablet

**ACTION & *THERAPEUTIC EFFECT***
Potentiates serotonin effects by selectively blocking its reuptake at presynaptic membranes in CNS. Produces varying degrees of sedation in normal and mentally depressed patients. *Increases total sleep time, decreases number and duration of awakenings in depressed patient, and decreases REM sleep. Has antianxiety effect in severely depressed patient.*

**USES** Major depressive disorder.

**UNLABELED USES** Adjunctive treatment of alcohol dependence, anxiety, panic disorder, insomnia.

**CONTRAINDICATIONS** Initial recovery phase of MI; ventricular ectopy; electroshock therapy; within 14 days of MAOIs use; initiation in patients treated with linezolid or methylene blue IV; suicidal ideation.

**CAUTIOUS USE** Bipolar disorder, MDD; older adults; history of suicidal tendencies; cardiac arrhythmias or disease; patients at risk for QT prolongation; volume depleted individuals; hepatic disease, renal impairment; history of GI bleeding; older adults; pregnancy (category C); lactation. Safe use in children not established.

## ROUTE & DOSAGE

### Depression

*Adult:* **PO Immediate release** 150 mg/day in divided doses, may increase by 50 mg/day q3–4days (max: 400–600 mg/day); **PO Extended release** 150 mg daily may increase by 75 mg/day at 3 day intervals (max: 375 mg/day)

### Pharmacogenetic Dosage Adjustment

*Poor CYP2D6 metabolizer:* Start with 80% of normal dose

## ADMINISTRATION

### Oral

- Ensure that extended release tablets are swallowed whole. They should not be crushed or chewed.
- Give drug with food; increases amount of absorption by 20% and appears to decrease incidence of dizziness or light-headedness. Maintain the same schedule for food-drug intake throughout treatment period to prevent variations in serum concentration.
- Store in tightly closed, light-resistant container at 15°–30° C (59°–86° F).

## ADVERSE EFFECTS (≥1%) **CNS:**
*Drowsiness,* light headedness, tiredness, dizziness, insomnia, *nervousness,* headache, agitation, impaired memory and speech, disorientation. **CV:** Hypotension (including orthostatic hypotension), hypertension, syncope, shortness of breath, chest pain, tachycardia, palpitations, bradycardia, PVCs, ventricular tachycardia (short episodes of 3–4 beats). **Special Senses:** Nasal and sinus congestion, blurred vision, eye irritation, sweating or clamminess, tinnitus. **GI:** *Dry mouth,* anorexia, constipation, abdominal distress, nausea, vomiting, dysgeusia, flatulence, diarrhea. **Urogenital:** Hematuria, increased frequency, delayed urine flow, male priapism, ejaculation inhibition. **Hematologic:** Anemia. **Musculoskeletal:** Skeletal aches and pains, muscle twitches. **Skin:** Skin eruptions, rash, pruritus, acne, photosensitivity. **Body as a Whole:** Weight change.

## INTERACTIONS **Drug:** ANTIHYPERTENSIVE AGENTS may potentiate hypotensive effects; **alcohol** and other CNS DEPRESSANTS add to depressant effects; may increase **digoxin** or **phenytoin** levels; MAO INHIBITORS may precipitate hypertensive crisis; **ketoconazole, indinavir, ritonavir, saquinavir** may increase levels and toxicity. Use of other serotonergic agents may increase risk of serotonin syndrome. Do not use with **conivaptan, ivabradine, linezolid, mifepristone, saquinavir.** **Herbal: Ginkgo** may increase sedation.

## PHARMACOKINETICS **Absorption:** Readily from GI tract. **Onset:** 1–2 wk. **Peak:** 1–2 h. **Distribution:** Distributed into breast milk. **Metabolism:** In liver (CYP2D6). **Elimination:** 75% in urine, 25% in feces. **Half-Life:** 5–9 h.

## NURSING IMPLICATIONS

### Black Box Warning

*Trazodone hydrochloride has been associated with suicidal thinking and behavior in children, adolescents, and young adults.*

### Assessment & Drug Effects

- Monitor BP and heart rate and rhythm. Report to prescriber

Common adverse effects in *italic;* life-threatening effects <u>underlined</u>; generic names in **bold;** classifications in SMALL CAPS; ✦ Canadian drug name; ● Prototype drug

1649

development of tachycardia, bradycardia, or palpitations.

- Monitor for orthostatic hypotension, especially in the elderly or those taking concurrent antihypertensive drugs.
- Monitor children and adolescents for changes in behavior that indicate increased suicidality.
- Observe patient's level of activity. If it appears to be increasing toward sleeplessness and agitation with changes in reality orientation, report to prescriber. Manic episodes have been reported.
- Be aware that overdose is characterized by an extension of common adverse effects: Vomiting, lethargy, drowsiness, and exaggerated anticholinergic effects.

**Patient & Family Education**

- Report immediately to prescriber signs of worsening mental status such as suicidal ideation, aggressiveness, agitation, anxiety, hostility, impulsivity, insomnia, irritability, panic attacks, and worsening of depression.
- Consult prescriber if drowsiness becomes a distressing adverse effect. Dose regimen may be changed so that largest dose is at bedtime.
- Limit or abstain from alcohol use. The depressant effects of CNS depressants and alcohol may be potentiated by this drug.
- Do not self-medicate with OTC drugs for colds, allergy, or insomnia treatment without advice of prescriber. Many of these drugs contain CNS depressants.
- Male patient should report inappropriate or prolonged penile erections. The drug may be discontinued.

# TRETINOIN

(tret'i-noyn)

Atralin, Avita, Refissa, Renova, Retin-A, Retin-A Micro, Retinoic Acid, Tretin-X Vesanoid

**Classifications:** ANTINEOPLASTIC; ANTIACNE (RETINOID); ANTIPSORIATIC
**Therapeutic:** ANTINEOPLASTIC; ANTIACNE; ANTIPSORIATIC
**Prototype:** Isotretinoin

**AVAILABILITY** Cream; gel; capsule

**ACTION & *THERAPEUTIC EFFECT***
**Antiacne activity:** Reverses retention hyperkeratosis and micro comedo formation in acne pathology. **Antineoplastic activity:** Induces cellular differentiation in malignant cells. Its exact mechanism of action is unknown. *Effective in early treatment and control of acne vulgaris grades I–III. Effective in treatment of (Acute Promyelocytic Leukemia) APL.*

**USES** Topical treatment of acne vulgaris grades I–III, especially during early stages when number of comedones is greatest; adjunctively in management of associated comedones and in treatment of flat warts; oral for remission induction treatment of acute promyelocytic leukemia; cream as adjunctive therapy for mitigation of fine wrinkles.

**UNLABELED USES** Psoriasis, senile keratosis, ichthyosis vulgaris, keratosis palmaris and plantaris, basal cell carcinoma, photodamaged skin (photoaging), and other skin conditions. **Orphan drug:** For squamous metaplasia of conjunctiva or cornea with mucous deficiency and keratinization.

**CONTRAINDICATIONS** Hypersensitivity to retinoid; eczema; exposure to sunlight or ultraviolet rays, sunburn; pregnancy (**oral:** category D).

**CAUTIOUS USE** Patient in an occupation necessitating considerable sun exposure or weather extremes; hepatic disease; pregnancy (**topical:** category C); lactation; children younger than 18 y.

## ROUTE & DOSAGE

**Acne**

*Adult:* **Topical** Apply once/day at bedtime

**Acute Promyelocytic Leukemia**

*Adult:* **PO** 45 mg/m²/day

**Antiwrinkle Cream**

*Adult:* **Topical** (0.05% cream) Apply to face once daily at bedtime

## ADMINISTRATION

**Oral**
- Give with food.
- Capsules must be swallowed whole; they cannot be opened, crushed, or chewed.

**Topical**
- Cleanse using a mild bland soap, and thoroughly dry areas being treated before applying drug. Avoid use of medicated, drying, or abrasive soaps and cleansers.
- Wash hands before and after treatment. Apply lightly over affected areas. Do not apply to non-affected skin area.
- Avoid contact of drug with eyes, mouth, angles of nose, open wounds, mucous membranes.
- Store gel and liquid formulations below 30° C (86° F) and solution below 27° C (80° F).

**ADVERSE EFFECTS** (≥1%) **Body as a Whole:** Note: Listed adverse effects occur primarily with oral administration; only skin effects with topical administration. *Bone pain, malaise, shivering, hemorrhage, peripheral edema, pain, chest discomfort, weight gain or loss,* DIC. **CNS:** *Dizziness, paresthesias, anxiety, insomnia, depression, headache, fever, weakness, fatigue,* cerebral hemorrhage, intracranial hypertension, hallucinations. **CV:** *Arrhythmias, flushing, hypotension, hypertension,* CHF. **Special Senses:** Visual disturbances, ocular disturbances, change in visual acuity, earache. **GI:** *Nausea, vomiting, abdominal pain, diarrhea, constipation, dyspepsia,* GI hemorrhage. **Respiratory:** *Dyspnea, respiratory insufficiency, pneumonia, rales, pleural effusion, wheezing.* **Skin:** Local inflammatory reactions, transient stinging or warmth on site, *redness, scaling, severe erythema,* blistering, crusting and peeling, temporary hypopigmentation or hyperpigmentation, *increased sweating.* **Urogenital:** Renal insufficiency, dysuria, acute kidney failure.

**INTERACTIONS** **Drug:** TOPICAL ACNE MEDICATIONS (including **sulfur, resorcinol, benzoyl peroxide,** and **salicylic acid**) may increase inflammation and peeling; topical products containing **alcohol** or **menthol** may cause stinging.

**PHARMACOKINETICS** **Absorption:** Minimally absorbed from intact skin, topical; 60% absorbed, PO. **Elimination:** About 0.1% of topical dose is excreted in urine within 24 h; 63% excreted in urine and 31% in feces, PO. **Half-Life:** 45 min, topical; 2–2.5 h, PO.

## NURSING IMPLICATIONS

### Assessment & Drug Effects

**Topical**
- Be aware that topical treatment to dark-skinned individuals may cause unsightly postinflammatory hyperpigmentation; that is reversible with termination of drug treatment.

- Clinical response to topical treatment should be evident in 2–3 wk; complete and satisfactory response (in 75% of the patients) may require 3–4 mo.
- Be aware that erythema and desquamation during the first 1–3 wk of topical treatment do not represent exacerbation of the skin problem but a probable response to the drug from deep previously unseen lesions.

**Patient & Family Education**
**Topical**
- As treatment is continued, lesions gradually disappear, leaving an inflammatory background; scaling and redness decrease after 8–10 wk of therapy.
- Wash face no more often than 2–3 × daily.
- Be aware that drug is not curative; relapses commonly occur within 3–6 wk after treatment has been discontinued.
- Avoid exposure to sun; when cannot be avoided, use a SPF 15 or higher sunscreen.
- Do not self-medicate with additional acne treatment because of danger of drug interactions.

# TRIAMCINOLONE
(trye-am-sin'oh-lone)
Atolone, Kenacort, Kenalog-E

# TRIAMCINOLONE ACETONIDE
Azmacort, Cenocort A₂, Kenalog, Nasacort HFA, Triam-A, Triamonide, Trikort, Trilog, Tri-Nasal

# TRIAMCINOLONE DIACETATE
Kenacort

# TRIAMCINOLONE HEXACETONIDE
Aristospan

**Classification:** ADRENAL CORTICOSTEROID; GLUCOCORTICOID
**Therapeutic:** ANTI-INFLAMMATORY; IMMUNOSUPPRESSANT
**Prototype:** Prednisone

**AVAILABILITY** **Triamcinolone:** Tablet; syrup. **Triamcinolone acetonide:** Solution for injection; aerosol; inhaler; spray; nasal spray; cream, ointment, lotion; topical spray. **Triamcinolone diacetate:** Tablet. **Triamcinolone hexacetonide:** Solution for injection.

**ACTION & *THERAPEUTIC EFFECT***
Immediate-acting synthetic fluorinated adrenal corticosteroid with glucocorticoid properties. Possesses minimal sodium and water retention properties in therapeutic doses. *Anti-inflammatory and immunosuppressant drug that is effective in the treatment of bronchial asthma.*

**USES** An anti-inflammatory or immunosuppressant agent. Orally inhaled: Bronchial asthma in patient who has not responded to conventional inhalation treatment. Therapeutic doses do not appear to suppress HPA (hypothalamic-pituitary-adrenal) axis.

**CONTRAINDICATIONS** Hypersensitivity to corticosteroids or benzyl alcohol; kidney dysfunction; glaucoma; acute bronchospasm; fungal infection.

**CAUTIOUS USE** Coagulopathy, hemophilia, diabetes mellitus, GI disease; CHF; herpes infection; infection; IBD; myasthenia gravis; MI; ocular exposure, ocular infection; osteoporosis; peptic ulcer disease; PVD; skin abrasion; pregnancy (category C);

Common adverse effects in *italic*; life-threatening effects underlined; generic names in **bold;** classifications in SMALL CAPS; ◆ Canadian drug name; ⊙ Prototype drug lactation. Safe use in children younger than 6 y not established.

## ROUTE & DOSAGE

### Inflammation, Immunosuppression

*Adult:* **IM/Subcutaneous** 4–48 mg/day in divided doses; **Intra-articular/Intradermal** 4–48 mg/day; **Inhaled** 2–4 inhalations q.i.d. **Topical** See Appendix A
*Child:* **IM/Subcutaneous** 3.3–50 mg/m$^2$/day in divided doses; **Intra-articular/Intradermal** 3.3–50 mg/m$^2$/day

### Acetonide

*Adult:* **IM** 60 mg, may repeat with 20–100 mg q6wk; **Intradermal** 1 mg/injection site (max: 30 mg total); **Intra-articular** 2.5–4.0 mg; **Inhalation** See Appendix A
*Child (6–12 y):* **IM** 0.03–0.2 mg q1–7days; **Inhalation** See Appendix A

### Hexacetonide

*Adult:* **Intralesional** Up to 0.5 mg/in$^2$ of skin; **Intra-articular** 2–20 mg q3–4wk

## ADMINISTRATION

### Inhalation

- Follow manufacturer's directions for specific oral or nasal inhaler and instruct patient on proper administration technique.

### Subcutaneous/Intramuscular

- Do not give triamcinolone injection IV.
- IM injections should only be given into a large, well developed muscle such as the gluteal muscle.
- Store at 15°–30° C (59°–86° F). Protect from light.

## ADVERSE EFFECTS (≥1%) CNS:
Euphoria, headache, insomnia, confusion, psychosis. **CV:** CHF, edema. **GI:** Nausea, vomiting, peptic ulcer. **Musculoskeletal:** Muscle weakness, delayed wound healing, muscle wasting, osteoporosis, aseptic necrosis of bone, spontaneous fractures. **Endocrine:** Cushingoid features, growth suppression in children, carbohydrate intolerance, hyperglycemia. **Special Senses:** Cataracts. **Hematologic:** Leukocytosis. **Metabolic:** Hypokalemia. **Skin:** Burning, itching, folliculitis, hypertrichosis, hypopigmentation.

## INTERACTIONS Drug: BARBITURATES,
**phenytoin, rifampin** increase steroid metabolism—may need increased doses of triamcinolone; **amphotericin B,** DIURETICS add to potassium loss; **neostigmine, pyridostigmine** may cause severe muscle weakness in patients with myasthenia gravis; may inhibit antibody response to VACCINES, TOXOIDS.

## PHARMACOKINETICS Absorption:
Readily absorbed from all routes. **Onset:** 24–48 h PO, IM. **Peak:** 1–2 h PO; 8–10 h IM. **Duration:** 2.25 days PO; 1–6 wk IM. **Metabolism:** In liver. **Elimination:** In urine. **Half-Life:** 2–5 h; HPA suppression, 18–36 h.

## NURSING IMPLICATIONS

### Assessment & Drug Effects

- Notify prescriber if wheezing occurs immediately following a dose of inhaled triamcinolone.
- Do not use occlusive dressing over topical application unless specifically ordered to do so.
- Monitor growth in children receiving prolonged, systemic triamcinolone therapy.
- Monitor for signs of negative nitrogen balance (e.g., muscle atro-

T

---

Common adverse effects in *italic*; life-threatening effects underlined; generic names in **bold**; classifications in SMALL CAPS; ✤ Canadian drug name; ⊙ Prototype drug

1653

phy), especially in older or debilitated patients receiving prolonged therapy.
- Report to prescriber immediately if a local infection develops at site of topical application.
- Report symptoms of hypercortisolism or Cushing's syndrome (see Appendix F), hyperglycemia (see Appendix F), and glucosuria (e.g., polyuria). These may arise from systemic absorption after topical application, especially in children and if used over extensive areas for prolonged periods or if occlusive dressings are used.

**Patient & Family Education**
- Report promptly any of the following: Sore throat, fever, swelling of feet or ankles, or muscle weakness.
- Adhere to drug regimen; do not increase or decrease established regimen and do not discontinue abruptly.
- Asthmatics should report promptly worsening of asthma symptoms following oral inhalation.

# TRIAMTERENE
(trye-am'ter-een)
Dyrenium
**Classification:** POTASSIUM-SPARING DIURETIC
Therapeutic: POTASSIUM-SPARING DIURETIC
**Prototype:** Spironolactone

## AVAILABILITY Capsule

## ACTION & *THERAPEUTIC EFFECT*
Has weak diuretic action with a potassium-sparing effect. Promotes excretion of sodium, chloride, and carbonate. Blocks potassium excretion by direct action on distal renal tubule rather than by inhibiting aldosterone. *Has a diuretic action and a potassium-sparing effect.*

## USES Treatment of edema.

## CONTRAINDICATIONS Hypersensitivity to triamterene; anuria, severe or progressive kidney disease or dysfunction with possible exception of nephrosis; severe liver disease; diabetic neuropathy; elevated serum potassium; severe electrolyte or acid-base imbalance; coadministration of other potassium-sparing agents.

## CAUTIOUS USE Impaired kidney or liver function; gout; history of gouty arthritis; CHF; arrhythmias; DM; history of kidney stones; older adults; pregnancy (category C). Safety and efficacy in children not established.

## ROUTE & DOSAGE

**Edema**
*Adult:* **PO** 100 mg b.i.d. (max: 300 mg/day)
***Renal Impairment Dosage Adjustment***
*CrCl less than 10 mL/min:* Avoid use

## ADMINISTRATION
**Oral**
- Empty capsule and give with fluid or mix with food, if patient cannot swallow capsule.
- Give drug with or after meals to prevent or minimize nausea.
- Schedule doses to prevent interruption of sleep from diuresis (e.g., with or after breakfast if a single dose is taken, or no later than 6 p.m. if more than one dose is prescribed). Consult prescriber.
- Withdraw drug gradually in patients on prolonged or high-dose

Common adverse effects in *italic*; life-threatening effects underlined; generic names in **bold**; classifications in SMALL CAPS; ✤ Canadian drug name; ⊘ Prototype drug therapy in order to prevent rebound increased urinary excretion of potassium.

- Store in tight, light-resistant containers at 15°–30° C (59°–86° F) unless otherwise directed.

## ADVERSE EFFECTS (≥1%) GI: Diarrhea, nausea, vomiting, and other GI disturbances. CNS: Dizziness, headache, dry mouth, anaphylaxis, weakness, muscle cramps. Skin: Pruritus, rash, photosensitivity. CV: Hypotension (large doses). Metabolic: *Hyperkalemia and other electrolyte imbalances, elevated BUN, elevated uric acid* (patients predisposed to gouty arthritis), hyperchloremic acidosis. Hematologic: Blood dyscrasias: Granulocytopenia, eosinophilia, megaloblastic anemia in patients with reduced folic acid stores (e.g., hepatic cirrhosis).

## DIAGNOSTIC TEST INTERFERENCE
Pale blue fluorescence in urine interferes with *fluorometric assay* of *quinidine* and *lactic dehydrogenase activity*. Treatment of edema, ascites, hypokalemia, hyperaldosteronism.

## INTERACTIONS Drug: May increase lithium levels, thus increasing its toxicity, indomethacin may decrease renal elimination of triamterene; ANGIOTENSIN-CONVERTING ENZYME (ACE) INHIBITORS, other POTASSIUM-SPARING DIURETICS may cause hyperkalemia. Food: High potassium foods may increase risk of hyperkalemia.

## PHARMACOKINETICS Absorption: Rapidly but variably from GI tract. Onset: 2–4 h. Duration: 7–9 h. Metabolism: In liver to active and inactive metabolites. Elimination: In urine. Half-Life: 100–150 min.

## NURSING IMPLICATIONS

### Black Box Warning

*Triamterene has been associated with increased risk of hyperkalemia.*

### Assessment & Drug Effects
- Monitor BP during periods of dosage adjustment. Hypotensive reactions, although rare, have been reported. Take care with ambulation, particularly for older adults.
- Weigh patient under standard conditions, prior to drug initiation and daily during therapy.
- Diuretic response usually occurs on first day of therapy; maximum effect may not occur for several days.
- Monitor and report oliguria and unusual changes in I&O ratio. Consult prescriber regarding allowable fluid intake.
- Be alert for S&S of kidney stone formation; reported in patients taking high doses or who have low urine volume and increased urine acidity.
- Observe for S&S of hyperkalemia (see Appendix F), particularly in patients with renal insufficiency, on high-dose or prolonged therapy, older adults, and those with diabetes.
- Monitor diabetics closely for loss of glycemic control.
- Monitor lab tests: Baseline and periodic serum potassium; periodic renal function tests with known or suspected renal insufficiency.

### Patient & Family Education
- Do not use salt substitutes; unlike most diuretics, triamterene promotes potassium retention.
- Do not restrict salt; there is a possibility of low-salt syndrome (hyponatremia). Consult prescriber.

T

---

- Report significant fatigue or weakness, malaise, fever, sore throat, or mouth and unusual bleeding or bruising to prescriber.
- Be aware that drug may cause photosensitivity; avoid exposure to sun and sunlamps.
- Drug may impart a harmless pale blue fluorescence to urine.

## TRIAZOLAM ©

(trye-ay'zoe-lam)

Halcion

**Classifications:** SEDATIVE-HYPNOTIC; BENZODIAZEPINE
**Therapeutic:** SEDATIVE
**Controlled Substance:** Schedule IV

## AVAILABILITY Tablet

## ACTION & *THERAPEUTIC EFFECT*

Blockade of cortical and limbic arousal results in hypnotic activity. *Decreases sleep latency and number of nocturnal awakenings, decreases total nocturnal wake time, and increases duration of sleep.*

## USES Short-term management of insomnia.

## CONTRAINDICATIONS Hypersensitivity to triazolam and benzodiazepines; ethanol intoxication; suicidal ideations; pregnancy (category X); lactation.

## CAUTIOUS USE Depression; bipolar disorder; dementia; psychosis; myasthenia gravis; Parkinson's disease; debilitated patients; patients with suicidal tendency; impaired kidney or liver function; chronic pulmonary insufficiency; sleep apnea; older adults.

## ROUTE & DOSAGE

**Insomnia**
*Adult:* **PO** 0.25 mg at bedtime (max: 0.5 mg/day)
*Geriatric:* **PO** 0.125 mg at bedtime

## ADMINISTRATION

### Oral
- Give immediately before bed; onset of drug action is rapid.
- Do not exceed recommended doses.
- Store at 15°–30° C (59°–86° F).

## ADVERSE EFFECTS (≥1%) CNS:
*Drowsiness,* lightheadedness, headache, dizziness, ataxia, visual disturbances, confusional states, *memory impairment, "rebound insomnia," anterograde amnesia,* paradoxical reactions, minor changes in EEG patterns. **GI:** Nausea, vomiting, constipation. **Body as a Whole:** Physiological dependence, psychological dependence, tolerance, withdrawal.

## INTERACTIONS Drug: Alcohol, CNS DEPRESSANTS, ANTICONVULSANTS, **nefazodone,** BENZODIAZEPINES potentiate CNS depression; **cimetidine** increases triazolam plasma levels, thus increasing its toxicity; may decrease antiparkinsonism effects of **levodopa.** Contraindicated with **boceprevir, cobicistat, delavirdine,** systemic AZOLE ANTIFUNGALS, PROTEASE INHIBITORS. **Herbal: Kava, valerian** may potentiate sedation. **St. John's wort** may decrease efficacy. **Food: Grapefruit juice** (greater than 1 qt/day) may increase plasma concentrations and adverse effects.

## PHARMACOKINETICS Absorption: Readily from GI tract. **Onset:** 15–30 min. **Peak:** 1–2 h. **Duration:**

Common adverse effects in *italic;* life-threatening effects <u>underlined</u>; generic names in **bold;** classifications in SMALL CAPS; ♣ Canadian drug name; © Prototype drug

6–8 h. **Distribution:** Crosses placenta; distributed into breast milk. **Metabolism:** In liver via CYP3A4. **Elimination:** In urine. **Half-Life:** 2–3 h.

## NURSING IMPLICATIONS

### Assessment & Drug Effects

- Be aware that signs of developing tolerance or adaptation (with long-term use) include increased daytime anxiety, increased wakefulness during last one third of the night.
- Evaluate smoking habit. As with other benzodiazepines, smoking may decrease hypnotic effects.
- Monitor for symptoms of overdosage: Slurred speech, somnolence, confusion, impaired coordination, and coma.

### Patient & Family Education

- Do not drive or engage in potentially hazardous activities until response to drug is known.
- Avoid use of alcohol or other CNS depressants while on this drug; they may increase sedative effects.
- Do not stop taking drug suddenly, especially if you are subject to seizures. Withdrawal symptoms may occur and range from mild dysphoria to more serious symptoms (e.g., tremors, abdominal and muscle cramps, convulsions). Consult prescriber for schedule to discontinue therapy.
- Do not increase dose without prescriber's advice because of toxic potential of drug.

## TRIFLUOPERAZINE HYDROCHLORIDE

(trye-floo-oh-per'a-zeen)

**Classification:** ANTIPSYCHOTIC; PHENOTHIAZIDE
Therapeutic: ANTIPSYCHOTIC
**Prototype:** Chlorpromazine

**AVAILABILITY** Tablet

## ACTION & *THERAPEUTIC EFFECT*

Phenothiazine with antipsychotic effects thought to be related to blockade of postsynaptic dopamine receptors in the brain. *Effectiveness indicated by increase in mental and physical activity.*

**USES** Management of schizophrenia, short term for anxiety.

**CONTRAINDICATIONS** Hypersensitivity to phenothiazines or sulfites; comatose states; CNS depression; ethanol intoxication; blood dyscrasias; hematologic disease, bone marrow depression; dementia related psychosis in older adults; preexisting liver disease; lactation.

**CAUTIOUS USE** Previously detected breast cancer; history of QT prolongation; significant cardiac disease or pulmonary disease; compromised respiratory function; seizure disorders; impaired liver function; pregnancy (category C); children younger than 6 y.

## ROUTE & DOSAGE

### Schizophrenia

*Adult:* **PO** 2–5 mg once daily or b.i.d., may increase up to 15–20 mg/day
*Child (6–12 y):* **PO** 1 mg 1–2 × day, may increase up to 15 mg/day

### Anxiety

*Adult:* **PO** 1–2 mg 1–2 × day (max: 6 mg/day)

## ADMINISTRATION

### Oral

- Crush tablet and give with fluid or mix with food if patient will not or cannot swallow pill.

T

Common adverse effects in *italic;* life-threatening effects underlined; generic names in **bold;** classifications in SMALL CAPS; ✦ Canadian drug name; ✪ Prototype drug

1657

- Store in light-resistant container at 15°–30° C (59°–86° F) unless otherwise directed.

**ADVERSE EFFECTS (≥1%) CNS:** *Drowsiness,* insomnia, dizziness, agitation, *extrapyramidal effects,* neuroleptic malignant syndrome. **Special Senses:** Nasal congestion, *dry mouth,* blurred vision, pigmentary retinopathy. **Hematologic:** Agranulocytosis. **Skin:** Photosensitivity, skin rash, sweating. **GI:** Constipation. **CV:** Tachycardia, *hypotension.* **Respiratory:** Depressed cough reflex. **Endocrine:** Gynecomastia, galactorrhea.

**INTERACTIONS Drug: Alcohol** and other CNS DEPRESSANTS add to CNS depression. Do not use with agents that prolong QT interval (e.g., **bepridil, dofetilide, dronedarone, procaine, ziprasidone**). **Herbal: Kava** may increase risk and severity of dystonic reactions.

**PHARMACOKINETICS Absorption:** Well absorbed from GI tract. **Onset:** Rapid onset. **Peak:** 2–3 h. **Duration:** Up to 12 h. **Metabolism:** In liver. **Elimination:** In bile and feces.

## NURSING IMPLICATIONS

### Black Box Warning

*Trifluoperazine has been associated with increased risk of mortality in older adults with dementia-related psychosis.*

### Assessment & Drug Effects

- Monitor HR and BP. Hypotension is a common adverse effect.
- Hypotension and extrapyramidal effects (especially akathisia and dystonia) are most likely to occur in patients receiving high doses or in older adults. Withhold drug and notify prescriber if patient has dysphagia, neck muscle spasm, or if tongue protrusion occurs.

- Monitor I&O ratio and bowel elimination pattern. Check for abdominal distention and pain. Encourage adequate fluid intake as prophylaxis for constipation and xerostomia.
- Agitation, jitteriness, and sometimes insomnia may simulate original psychotic symptoms. These adverse effects may disappear spontaneously.
- Expect maximum therapeutic response within 2–3 wk after initiation of therapy.
- Monitor lab tests: Periodic CBC, serum electrolytes, lipid profile, and HbA1C.

### Patient & Family Education

- Take drug as prescribed; do not alter dosing regimen or stop medication without consulting prescriber.
- Consult prescriber about use of any OTC drugs during therapy.
- Do not take alcohol and other depressants during therapy.
- Avoid potentially hazardous activities such as driving or operating machinery, until response to drug is known.
- Cover as much skin surface as possible with clothing when you **must be** in direct sunlight. Use an SPF higher than 12 sunscreen on exposed skin.
- Urine may be discolored or reddish brown and this is harmless.

---

# TRIFLURIDINE
(trye-flure′i-deen)
Viroptic
**Classification:** ANTIVIRAL
Therapeutic: ANTIVIRAL

**AVAILABILITY** Ophthalmic solution

**ACTION & *THERAPEUTIC EFFECT***
Pyrimidine nucleoside that appears to inhibit viral DNA synthesis and viral replication. *Active against herpes simplex virus (HSV) types*

Common adverse effects in *italic;* life-threatening effects underlined; generic names in **bold;** classifications in SMALL CAPS; ♣ Canadian drug name; ℗ Prototype drug

1658

*1 and 2, vaccinia virus, and certain strains of adenovirus.*

**USES** Topically to eyes for treatment of primary keratoconjunctivitis and recurring epithelial keratitis caused by herpes simplex virus types 1 and 2. Also for other herpetic ophthalmic infections including stromal keratitis, uveitis, and for infections caused by vaccinia and *Adenovirus,* but clinical effectiveness has not been established.

**CONTRAINDICATIONS** Lactation.

**CAUTIOUS USE** Dry eye syndrome; pregnancy (category C); children younger than 6 y.

## ROUTE & DOSAGE

**Viral Infections of Eye**

*Adult:* **Ophthalmic** 1 drop 1% ophthalmic solution into affected eye q2h during waking hours until healing (reepithelialization) has occurred (max: 9 drops/day); when healing appears to be complete, dosage reduced to 1 drop q4h during waking hours for an additional 7 days (max: 5 drops/day); continuous administration beyond 21 days not recommended

## ADMINISTRATION

**Instillation**

- Wait several minutes between applications when used concurrently with other eye drops. Remove contact lenses prior to use.
- Store refrigerated at 2°–8° C (36°–46° F) unless otherwise directed.

**ADVERSE EFFECTS** (≥1%) **Special Senses:** Mild transient burning or stinging, mild irritation of conjunctiva or cornea, photophobia, edema of eyelids and cornea, punctal occlusion, superficial punctate keratopathy, epithelial keratopathy, stromal edema, keratitis sicca, hyperemia, increased intraocular pressure.

**PHARMACOKINETICS Absorption:** Following topical application to eye, trifluridine penetrates cornea and aqueous humor (inflammation enhances penetration). Systemic absorption does not appear to be significant.

## NURSING IMPLICATIONS

**Assessment & Drug Effects**

- Expect epithelial eye infections to respond to therapy within 2–7 days, with complete healing occurring in 1–2 wk.

**Patient & Family Education**

- Inform prescriber of progress and keep follow-up appointments. Herpetic eye infections have a tendency to recur and can lead to corneal damage if not adequately treated.

## TRIHEXYPHENIDYL HYDROCHLORIDE

(trye-hex-ee-fen'i-dill)

**Classifications:** CENTRALLY ACTING CHOLINERGIC RECEPTOR ANTAGONIST; ANTIPARKINSON; ANTISPASMODIC
**Therapeutic:** ANTIPARKINSON; ANTISPASMODIC
**Prototype:** Benztropine

**AVAILABILITY** Tablet; elixir

## ACTION & *THERAPEUTIC EFFECT*

Thought to act by blocking excess of acetylcholine at certain cerebral synaptic sites. Relaxes smooth muscle by direct effect and by atropinelike blocking action on the parasympathetic nervous system.

*Diminishes the characteristic tremor of Parkinson's disease.*

**USES** Symptomatic treatment of all forms of parkinsonism (arteriosclerotic, idiopathic, postencephalitic). Also to treat drug-induced extrapyramidal disorders.

**UNLABELED USES** Huntington's chorea, spasmodic torticollis.

**CONTRAINDICATIONS** Hypersensitivity to trihexyphenidyl; narrow angle glaucoma; tardive dyskinesia.

**CAUTIOUS USE** History of drug hypersensitivities; glaucoma; arteriosclerosis; hypertension; cardiac disease, kidney or liver disorders; MG; alcoholism; CNS diseases; obstructive diseases of GI or genitourinary tracts; BPH; older adults; pregnancy (category C); lactation. Safe use in children not established.

## ROUTE & DOSAGE

### Parkinsonism
*Adult:* **PO** 1 mg day 1, 2 mg day 2, then increase by 2 mg q3–5days up to 6–10 mg/day in 3 or more divided doses (max: 15 mg/day)

### Extrapyramidal Effects
*Adult:* **PO** 1 mg/day then increase as needed; usual dose 5–15 mg/day in 3–4 divided doses

## ADMINISTRATION

### Oral
▪ Give before or after meals, depending on how patient reacts. Older adults and patients prone to excessive salivation (e.g., postencephalitic parkinsonism) may prefer to take drug after meals. If drug causes excessive mouth dryness, it may be better given before meals, unless it causes nausea.
▪ Do not crush or chew sustained release capsules. These **must be** swallowed whole.
▪ Store at 15°–30° C (59°–86° F) in tight container unless otherwise directed.

**ADVERSE EFFECTS** (≥1%) **GI:** *Dry mouth, nausea,* constipation. **Special Senses:** *Blurred vision,* mydriasis, photophobia, angle-closure glaucoma. **Urogenital:** Urinary hesitancy or retention. **CNS:** *Dizziness, nervousness,* insomnia, drowsiness, confusion, agitation, delirium, psychotic manifestations, euphoria. **CV:** Tachycardia, palpitations, hypotension, orthostatic hypotension. **Body as a Whole:** Hypersensitivity reactions.

**INTERACTIONS Drug:** Reduces therapeutic effects of **chlorpromazine, haloperidol,** PHENOTHIAZINES; increases bioavailability of **digoxin;** MAO INHIBITORS potentiate actions of trihexyphenidyl. **Herbal: Betel nut** may increase risk of extrapyramidal symptoms.

**PHARMACOKINETICS Absorption:** Readily from GI tract. **Onset:** Within 1 h. **Peak:** 2–3 h. **Duration:** 6–12 h. **Elimination:** In urine.

## NURSING IMPLICATIONS

### Assessment & Drug Effects
▪ Be aware that incidence and severity of adverse effects are usually dose related and may be minimized by dosage reduction. Older adults appear more sensitive to usual adult doses.
▪ Monitor vital signs. Pulse is a particularly sensitive indicator of response to drug. Report tachycardia, palpitations, paradoxical bradycardia, or fall in BP.

- Assess for and report severe CNS stimulation (see ADVERSE EFFECTS) that occurs with high doses, and in patients with arteriosclerosis, or those with history of hypersensitivity to other drugs.
- In patients with severe rigidity, tremors may appear to be accentuated during therapy as rigidity diminishes.
- Monitor daily I&O if patient develops urinary hesitancy or retention. Voiding before taking drug may relieve problem.
- Check for abdominal distention and bowel sounds if constipation is a problem.

**Patient & Family Education**

- Learn measures to relieve drug-induced dry mouth; rinse mouth frequently with water and suck ice chips, sugarless gum, or hard candy. Maintain adequate total daily fluid intake.
- Avoid excessive heat because drug suppresses perspiration and, therefore, heat loss.
- Do not to engage in potentially hazardous activities requiring alertness and skill. Drug causes dizziness, drowsiness, and blurred vision. Help walking may be indicated.

# TRIMETHOBENZAMIDE HYDROCHLORIDE

(trye-meth-oh-ben′za-mide)

Tigan

**Classification:** ANTIEMETIC
Therapeutic: ANTIEMETIC
**Prototype:** Prochlorperazine

**AVAILABILITY** Capsule; rectal suppository; solution for injection

**ACTION & THERAPEUTIC EFFECT**
Primary locus of action is thought to be the chemoreceptor trigger zone (CTZ) in medulla. *Less effective than phenothiazine antiemetics but produces fewer adverse effects.*

**USES** Control of nausea and vomiting.

**CONTRAINDICATIONS** Uncomplicated vomiting in viral illness; parenteral use in children or infants; rectal administration in prematures and newborns; known sensitivity to benzocaine (in suppository) or to similar local anesthetics.

**CAUTIOUS USE** In presence of high fever, dehydration, electrolyte imbalance; pregnancy (category C); lactation; children.

**ROUTE & DOSAGE**

| **Nausea and Vomiting** |
| --- |
| *Adult:* **PO** 250–300 mg t i d. or q.i.d.; **IM** 200 mg t.i.d. or q.i.d. prn |

**ADMINISTRATION**

**Oral**
- Empty capsule and give with water or mix with food if patient cannot swallow capsule.

**Intramuscular**
- Give IM deep into upper outer quadrant of buttock.
- Minimize possibility of irritation and pain by avoiding escape of solution along needle track. Use Z-track technique. Rotate injection sites.
- Injection not for use in children or infants.

**ADVERSE EFFECTS** (≥1%) **Body as a Whole:** Hypersensitivity reactions (including allergic skin eruptions), muscle cramps, pain, stinging, burning, redness, irritation at IM site; local irritation following rectal administration. **CNS:** Pseudoparkinsonism. **CV:** Hypotension. **GI:** Diarrhea, exaggeration of nausea, acute hepatitis, jaundice.

**INTERACTIONS Drug:** Alcohol and other CNS DEPRESSANTS add to depressant activity; PHENOTHIAZINES may precipitate extrapyramidal syndrome. Do not use with **sodium oxybate.**

**PHARMACOKINETICS** **Onset:** 10–40 min PO; 15 min IM. **Duration:** 3–4 h PO; 2–3 h IM. **Elimination:** 30–50% of dose excreted unchanged in urine within 48–72 h.

## NURSING IMPLICATIONS

### Assessment & Drug Effects

- Monitor BP. Hypotension may occur particularly in surgical patients receiving drug parenterally.
- Report promptly and stop drug therapy if an acute febrile illness accompanies or begins during therapy.
- Antiemetic effect of drug may obscure diagnoses of GI or other pathologic conditions or signs of toxicity from other drugs.

### Patient & Family Education

- Report promptly to prescriber onset of rash or other signs of hypersensitivity (see Appendix F). Discontinue drug immediately.
- Do not drive or engage in potentially hazardous activities until response to drug is known.
- Do not drink alcohol or alcoholic beverages during therapy with this drug.

# TRIMETHOPRIM ℗
(trye-meth'oh-prim)
*Primsol*
**Classification:** URINARY TRACT ANTI-INFECTIVE

**Therapeutic:** URINARY TRACT ANTI-INFECTIVE

**AVAILABILITY** Tablet; oral solution

## ACTION & *THERAPEUTIC EFFECT*
Anti-infective and folic acid antagonist with slow bactericidal action. Binds and interferes with bacterial cell growth. *Effective against most common UTI pathogens. Most pathogens causing UTI are in normal vaginal and fecal flora. Effective in treatment of acute otitis media.*

**USES** Initial episodes of acute uncomplicated UTIs, acute otitis media in children.

**UNLABELED USES** Treatment and prophylaxis of chronic and recurrent UTI in both men and women; treatment in conjunction with dapsone of initial episodes of *Pneumocystis carinii* pneumonia; treatment of travelers' diarrhea; acne; otitis media.

**CONTRAINDICATIONS** Hypersensitivity to trimethoprim; megaloblastic anemia secondary to folate deficiency; creatinine clearance less than 15 mL/min, impaired kidney or liver function; possible folate deficiency; children with fragile X chromosome associated with mental retardation.

**CAUTIOUS USE** Possible folate deficiency; risk factors for hyperkalemia; renal disease; mild or moderate renal impairment; hepatic impairment; older adults; pregnancy (category C); lactation; children younger than 12 y.

## ROUTE & DOSAGE

**Urinary Tract Infection**
*Adult/Adolescent:* **PO** 100 mg b.i.d. or 200 mg once/day

Common adverse effects in *italic;* life-threatening effects <u>underlined</u>; generic names in **bold;** classifications in SMALL CAPS; ◆ Canadian drug name; ℗ Prototype drug

## ADMINISTRATION
### Oral
- Give with 240 mL (8 oz) of fluid if not contraindicated.
- Store at 15°–30° C (59°–86° F) in dry, light-protected place.

## ADVERSE EFFECTS (≥1%) GI: Epigastric discomfort, nausea, vomiting, glossitis, abnormal taste sensation. **Hematologic:** Neutropenia, *megaloblastic anemia*, methemoglobinemia, leukopenia, thrombocytopenia (rare). **Skin:** *Rash, pruritus*, exfoliative dermatitis, photosensitivity. **Body as a Whole:** Fever. **Metabolic:** Increased serum transaminases (ALT, AST), bilirubin, creatinine, BUN.

## DIAGNOSTIC TEST INTERFERENCE
Interferes with serum *methotrexate assays* that use a competitive binding protein technique with a bacterial dihydrofolate reductase as the binding protein. May cause falsely elevated *creatinine* values when *Jaffe reaction* is used.

## INTERACTIONS Drug: May inhibit **phenytoin** metabolism causing increased levels. Do not use with **dofetilide.**

## PHARMACOKINETICS Absorption: Almost completely from GI tract. **Peak:** 1–4 h. **Distribution:** Widely distributed, including lung, saliva, middle ear fluid, bile, bone, CSF; crosses placenta; appears in breast milk. **Metabolism:** In liver. **Elimination:** 80% in urine unchanged. **Half-Life:** 8–11 h.

## NURSING IMPLICATIONS
### Assessment & Drug Effects
- Reinforce necessity to adhere to established drug regimen. Recurrent infection after terminating

prophylactic treatment of UTI may occur even after 6 mo of therapy.
- Assess urinary pattern during treatment. Altered pattern (frequency, urgency, nocturia, retention, polyuria) may reflect emerging drug resistance, necessitating change of drug regimen. Periodically check for bladder distention.
- Be alert for toxic effects on bone marrow, particularly in older adults, malnourished, alcoholic, pregnant, or debilitated patients. Recognize and report signs of infection or anemia.
- Drug-induced rash, a common adverse effect, is usually maculopapular, pruritic, or morbilliform and appears 7–14 days after start of therapy with daily doses of 200 mg or less.
- Monitor lab tests. Baseline C&S.

### Patient & Family Education
- Drink fluids liberally (2000–3000 mL/day, if not contraindicated) to help flush out urinary bacteria.
- Report pain and hematuria to prescriber immediately.
- Do not postpone voiding even though increases in fluid intake may cause more frequent urination.
- Do not use douches or sprays during treatment periods; practice careful perineal hygiene to prevent reinfection.
- Report to prescriber promptly any symptoms of a blood disorder (fever, sore throat, pallor, purpura, ecchymosis).
- Consult prescriber if severe traveler's diarrhea does not respond to 3–5 days therapy (i.e., persistence of symptoms of severe nausea, abdominal pain, diarrhea with mucus or blood, and dehydration).
- Drug-induced rash, a common adverse effect, may appear 7–14 days after start of therapy. Report rash to prescriber for evaluation.

Common adverse effects in *italic;* life-threatening effects underlined; generic names in **bold;** classifications in SMALL CAPS; ♣ Canadian drug name; ⊘ Prototype drug

1663

## TRIMIPRAMINE MALEATE
(tri-mip′ra-meen)
Surmontil
**Classification:** TRICYCLIC ANTIDEPRESSANT
Therapeutic: TRICYCLIC ANTIDEPRESSANT (TCA)
**Prototype:** Imipramine

**AVAILABILITY** Capsule

**ACTION & THERAPEUTIC EFFECT**
Antidepressant effects are thought to result from postsynaptic sensitization to serotonin. *More effective in alleviation of endogenous depression than other depressive states.*

**USES** Treatment of depression.

**CONTRAINDICATIONS** Hypersensitivity to tricyclic antidepressants; prostatic hypertrophy; during recovery period after MI; AV block; QT prolongation; bundle-branch block; ileus; MAOI therapy; suicide ideation; concurrent use with linezolid or IV methylene blue.

**CAUTIOUS USE** Schizophrenia, electroshock therapy, psychosis; bipolar disease; Parkinson's disease; seizure disorders; increased intraocular pressure; history of urinary retention; history of narrow-angle glaucoma; hyperthyroidism; suicidal tendency; cardiovascular, liver, thyroid, kidney disease; pregnancy (category C); lactation. Safe use in children younger than 12 y not established.

**ROUTE & DOSAGE**

**Depression**
*Adult:* **PO** 25–50 mg daily in divided doses, may increase gradually up to 150 mg/day if needed (max dose: 300 mg/day)
*Geriatric/Adolescent:* **PO** 50 mg/day with gradual increases up to 100 mg/day

**Pharmacogenetic Dosage Adjustment**
*Poor CYP2D6 metabolizer:* Start with 30% of dose

**ADMINISTRATION**
**Oral**
- Give with food to decrease gastric distress. Administer maintenance doses as a single dose at bedtime.
- Store in tightly closed container at 15°–30° C (59°–86° F) unless otherwise specified.

**ADVERSE EFFECTS** (≥1%) **CNS:** Seizures, tremor, confusion, *sedation*, suicidality, dizziness, drowsiness, headache. **Special Senses:** Blurred vision. **CV:** Tachycardia, *orthostatic hypotension,* hypertension. **GI:** *Xerostomia, constipation,* paralytic ileus, appetite stimulation, dyspepsia. **Urogenital:** *Urinary retention,* ejaculation dysfunction. **Skin:** Photosensitivity, sweating.

**INTERACTIONS Drug:** CNS DEPRESSANTS, **alcohol,** HYPNOTICS, BARBITURATES, SEDATIVES potentiate CNS depression; may increase hypoprothrombinemic effect of ORAL ANTICOAGULANTS; **levodopa,** SYMPATHOMIMETICS (e.g., **epinephrine, norepinephrine**) increase possibility of sympathetic hyperactivity with hypertension and hyperpyrexia; do not use with MAO INHIBITORS; **methylphenidate** increases plasma TCA levels; **cimetidine** may increase plasma TCA levels. **Herbal: Ginkgo** may decrease seizure threshold; **St. John's wort** may cause **serotonin** syndrome.

Common adverse effects in *italic;* life-threatening effects underlined; generic names in **bold;** classifications in SMALL CAPS; ✦ Canadian drug name; ⊕ Prototype drug

## PHARMACOKINETICS **Absorption:** Rapidly absorbed from GI tract. **Peak:** 2 h. **Metabolism:** In liver (CYP2D6). **Elimination:** In urine and feces. **Half-Life:** 9.1 h.

## NURSING IMPLICATIONS

### Black Box Warning

*Trimipramine maleate has been associated with increased risk of suicidal thinking and behavior in children, adolescents, and young adults.*

### Assessment & Drug Effects
- Monitor for changes in behavior that may indicate increased incidence of suicidality.
- Assess vital signs (BP and pulse rate) during adjustment period of tricyclic antidepressant (TCA) therapy. If BP falls more than 20 mm Hg or if there is a sudden increase in pulse rate, withhold medication and notify prescriber.
- Orthostatic hypotension may be sufficiently severe to require protective assistance when patient is ambulating. Instruct patient to change position from recumbency to standing slowly and in stages.
- Report fine tremors, a distressing extrapyramidal adverse effect, to prescriber.
- Monitor bowel elimination pattern and I&O ratio. Severe constipation and urinary retention are potential problems, especially in older adults. Advise increased fluid intake to at least 1500 mL/day (if allowed).
- Inspect oral membranes daily with high-dose therapy. Urge outpatient to report symptoms of stomatitis or xerostomia.
- Regulate environmental temperature and patient's clothing carefully; drug may cause intolerance to heat or cold.

### Patient & Family Education
- Report immediately to prescriber signs of worsening mental status such as suicidal ideation, aggressiveness, agitation, anxiety, hostility, impulsivity, insomnia, irritability, panic attacks, and worsening of depression.
- Be aware that your ability to perform tasks requiring alertness and skill may be impaired.
- Do not use OTC drugs unless approved by prescriber.
- Understand that the actions of both alcohol and trimipramine are increased when used together during therapy and for up to 2 wk after the TCA is discontinued. Consult prescriber about safe amounts of alcohol, if any, that can be taken.
- Be aware that the effects of barbiturates and other CNS depressants may also be enhanced by trimipramine.

## TRIPTORELIN PAMOATE
(trip-tor'e-lyn)
Trelstar Depot, Trelstar LA, Triptodur
**Classification:** GONADOTROPIN-RELEASING HORMONE (GNRH) AGONIST ANALOG
Therapeutic: GNRH AGONIST ANALOG
**Prototype:** Leuprolide acetate

## AVAILABILITY Solution for injection

## ACTION & *THERAPEUTIC EFFECT*
An agonist analog of GnRH that causes suppression of ovarian and testicular hormone production due to decreased levels of LH and FSH with subsequent decrease in testosterone and estrogen levels. *In men, the level of serum testosterone is equivalent to a surgically castrated man.*

Common adverse effects in *italic;* life-threatening effects underlined; generic names in **bold;** classifications in SMALL CAPS; ♣ Canadian drug name; ☻ Prototype drug

1665

**USES** Palliative treatment of advanced prostate cancer; central percocious puberty.

**UNLABELED USES** Breast cancer hypersexuality, endometriosis, infertility, hirsutism.

**CONTRAINDICATIONS** Hypersensitivity to triptorelin, other LHRH agonists, or LHRH; dysfunctional uterine bleeding; pregnancy (category X); lactation.

**CAUTIOUS USE** Prostatic carcinoma; hepatic or renal dysfunction; patients with impending spinal cord compression or severe urogenital disorder; premenstrual syndrome; renal insufficiency. Safety and efficacy in children not established.

## ROUTE & DOSAGE

| Prostate Cancer |
| --- |
| *Adult:* **IM** 3.75 mg q4w OR 11.25 mg q12w or 22.5 mg q24w |
| **Central Percocious Puberty (Triptodur)** |
| *Adolescent/Child (older than 2 y):* **IM** 22.5 mg q24wk |

## ADMINISTRATION

**Intramuscular**
- Give deep into a large muscle.
- Alternate injection sites. Administer immediately after reconstitution.

**ADVERSE EFFECTS** (≥1%) **Body as a Whole:** *Hot flushes,* pain, leg pain, fatigue. **CV:** Hypertension, lower extremity edema. **GI:** Diarrhea, vomiting, nausea, anorexia. **Hematologic:** Anemia. **Musculoskeletal:** Musculoskeletal pain. **CNS:** Headache, dizziness, insomnia, impotence, emotional lability.

**Skin:** Pruritus, skin rash. **Urogenital:** Urinary retention, UTI. **Other:** Pain at injection site, hyperglycemia, increased serum testosterone, increased ALT/AST, increased BUN, decreased libido, gynecomastia.

## DIAGNOSTIC TEST INTERFERENCE
May interfere with tests for *pituitary-gonadal function.*

**INTERACTIONS Drug:** Do not use with **corifollitropin alfa.** Use with QT prolonging agents (e.g., **amiodarone, citalopram, dofetilide**) should be avoided.

**PHARMACOKINETICS Peak:** 1–3 h. **Duration:** 1 mo. **Metabolism:** Unknown. **Elimination:** Eliminated by liver and kidneys. **Half-Life:** 3 h.

## NURSING IMPLICATIONS

**Assessment & Drug Effects**
- Monitor for S&S of disease flare, especially during the first 1–2 wk of therapy: Increased bone pain, blood in urine, urinary obstruction, or symptoms of spinal compression.
- Monitor for S&S of emerging CV disease.
- Monitor lab tests: Periodic serum testosterone and HbA1C.

**Patient & Family Education**
- Disease flare (see ASSESSMENT & DRUG EFFECTS) is a common, temporary adverse effect of therapy; however, symptoms may become serious enough to report to the prescriber.
- Notify prescriber promptly of the following: S&S of an allergic reaction (itching, hives, swelling of face, arms, or legs; tingling in mouth or throat, tightness in chest or trouble breathing); weakness or loss of muscle control; rapid weight gain.

# TROPICAMIDE
(troe-pik′a-mide)
**See Appendix A-1**.

# TROSPIUM CHLORIDE
(tro-spi′um)
**Classifications:** ANTICHOLINERGIC; ANTIMUSCARINIC; ANTISPASMODIC
Therapeutic: URINARY SMOOTH MUSCLE RELAXANT
**Prototype:** Oxybutynin

**AVAILABILITY** Tablet; extended release capsule

**ACTION & *THERAPEUTIC EFFECT***
Antagonizes the effect of acetylcholine on muscarinic receptors in smooth muscle. Its parasympatholytic action reduces smooth muscle tone of the bladder. *Decreases urinary frequency, urgency, and urge incontinence in patients with overactive bladders.*

**USES** Treatment of overactive (neurogenic) bladder, urinary incontinence.

**CONTRAINDICATIONS** Hypersensitivity to trospium; patients with or at risk for urinary retention; uncontrolled narrow-angle glaucoma; gastroparesis; GI obstruction, ileus, pyloric stenosis, toxic megacolon, severe ulcerative colitis.

**CAUTIOUS USE** Significant bladder obstruction, closed-angle glaucoma; BPH; ulcerative colitis, GERD, intestinal atony; myasthenia gravis, autonomic neuropathy; moderate or severe hepatic dysfunction; severe renal insufficiency, renal failure; older adults; pregnancy (category C); lactation. Safety in children not established.

## ROUTE & DOSAGE

**Overactive Bladder**
*Adult:* **PO** 20 mg twice daily OR **Extended release** 60 mg daily
*Geriatric (75 y or older):* **PO** **Immediate release** 20 mg once daily

***Renal Impairment Dosage Adjustment***
*CrCl less than 30 mL/min:* **Immediate release** 20 mg once daily at bedtime

## ADMINISTRATION
**Oral**
▪ Give at least 1 h before meals or on an empty stomach.
▪ Store at 20°–25° C (66°–77° F).

**ADVERSE EFFECTS** (≥1%) **Body as a Whole:** Fatigue, dry skin. **CNS:** Headache. **GI:** *Dry mouth, constipation,* abdominal pain, dyspepsia, flatulence, vomiting. **Special Senses:** Dry eyes, blurred vision, skin rash. **Urogenital:** Urinary retention, urinary tract infection. **Cardiac:** Tachycardia. **Respiratory:** Nasopharyngitis, dry nose.

**INTERACTIONS Drug:** Increased anticholinergic adverse effects with ANTICHOLINERGIC AGENTS. Do not use with **potassium citrate** due to increased ulcerogenic effect.

**PHARMACOKINETICS Absorption:** Less than 10% absorbed orally. **Peak:** 5–6 h. **Metabolism:** In liver via CYP2D6. **Elimination:** Primarily in feces. **Half-Life:** 20 h.

## NURSING IMPLICATIONS
**Assessment & Drug Effects**
▪ Monitor bowel and bladder function. Report urinary hesitancy or significant constipation.

T

Common adverse effects in *italic;* life-threatening effects underlined; generic names in **bold;** classifications in SMALL CAPS; ♣ Canadian drug name; ✿ Prototype drug

1667

- Withhold drug and notify prescriber if urinary retention develops.
- Monitor for and report worsening of GI symptoms in those with GERD.

**Patient & Family Education**
- Report promptly any of the following: Signs of an allergic reaction (e.g., itching or hives), blurred vision or difficulty focusing, confusion, dizziness, difficulty passing urine.
- Moderate intake of tea, coffee, caffeinated sodas, and alcohol to minimize side effects of this drug.
- Avoid situations in which overheating is likely, as drug may impair sweating, which is a normal cooling mechanism.
- Do not engage in hazardous activities until response to the drug is known.

# ULIPRISTAL
(u-li-pris'tal)
Ella
**Classification:** PROGESTERONE AGONIST/ANTAGONIST; POSTCOITAL CONTRACEPTIVE
**Therapeutic:** POSTCOITAL CONTRACEPTIVE

**AVAILABILITY** Tablet

## ACTION & THERAPEUTIC EFFECT
A selective progesterone receptor modulator with antagonistic and partial agonistic effects. It binds to the progesterone receptor preventing the binding of progesterone. *If taken immediately before ovulation, it delays follicular rupture and inhibits ovulation. It may also alter the endometrium and interfere with implantation of a fertilized ovum.*

**USES** Postcoital contraception after unprotected intercourse or a known or suspected contraceptive failure.

**CONTRAINDICATIONS** Known or suspected pregnancy (category X); lactation.

## ROUTE & DOSAGE

**Postcoital Contraception**
*Adult:* **PO** 30 mg within 120 h of unprotected intercourse or known or suspected contraceptive failure; may repeat within 3 h if patient vomits initial dose

## ADMINISTRATION
**Oral**
- Give within 120 h of unprotected intercourse.
- Store at controlled room temperature 20°–25° C (68°–77° F).

**ADVERSE EFFECTS** (≥5%) **Body as a Whole:** *Abdominal and upper abdominal pain.* **CNS:** Fatigue, dizziness, *headache.* **GI:** *Nausea.* **Urogenital:** Dysmenorrhea.

**INTERACTIONS Drug:** Coadministration of CYP3A4 inducers (e.g., **carbamazepine, phenobarbital, phenytoin, rifampin, topiramate**) can decrease the levels of ulipristal. Coadministration of strong CYP3A4 INHIBITORS (e.g., **itraconazole, ketoconazole**) can increase the levels of ulipristal. **Food: Grapefruit juice** can increase the levels of ulipristal. **Herbal: St. John's wort** can decrease the levels of ulipristal.

**PHARMACOKINETICS Peak:** 1 h. **Distribution:** 94% plasma protein bound. **Metabolism:** Hepatic oxidation by CYP3A4 to active metabolite. **Half-Life:** 32.4 h.

## NURSING IMPLICATIONS
**Assessment & Drug Effects**
- Monitor for vomiting. Drug may be re-administered if patient vomits within 3 h of initial dose.

U

## Patient & Family Education

- Ulipristal is not intended for repeated use. It should not replace conventional means of contraception.
- Certain concurrently taken drugs may interfere with the contraceptive effects of ulipristal. Consult prescriber.
- Ulipristal may interfere with the length of the next menstrual cycle (i.e., cycle may occur sooner or later than expected).
- Ulipristal does not protect against sexually transmitted diseases.

# USTEKINUMAB
(us-te-kin'u-mab)
Stelara

**Classification:** IMMUNOMODULATOR; MONOCLONAL ANTIBODY; INTERLEUKIN-12 AND INTERLEUKIN-23 RECEPTOR ANTAGONIST
**Therapeutic:** IMMUNOSUPPRESSANT
**Prototype:** Basiliximab

**AVAILABILITY** Solution for injection

**ACTION & *THERAPEUTIC EFFECT***
A human monoclonal antibody that disrupts IL-12 and IL-23 mediated signaling and cytokine cascades. *Inhibits inflammatory and immune responses associated with plaque psoriasis thereby improving psoriasis.*

**USES** Treatment of moderate to severe plaque psoriasis; psoriatic arthritis.

**CONTRAINDICATIONS** Clinically significant hypersensitivity to ustekinumab; active infection (e.g., active TB); live vaccines; BCG vaccines within 1 y prior to, during, or 1 y following drug treatment; reversible posterior leukoencephalopathy syndrome (RPLS).

**CAUTIOUS USE** Chronic infection or history of recurrent infection (e.g.,

latent TB); prior malignancy; phototherapy; older adults; pregnancy (category B); lactation. Safety and efficacy in children younger than 18 y not established.

## ROUTE & DOSAGE

**Psoriasis**

*Adult 100 kg or less:* **Subcutaneous** 45 mg initially and 4 wk later, followed by 45 mg q12wk
*Adult over 100 kg:* **Subcutaneous** 90 mg initially and 4 wk later, followed by 90 mg q12wk

**Psoriatic Arthritis**

*Adult:* **Subcutaneous** 45 mg initially and 4 wk later then 45 mg q12w

## ADMINISTRATION

**Subcutaneous**

- Solution may contain a few small translucent or white particles. **Do not** shake.
- Note: Needle cover on prefilled syringe is natural rubber and should not be handled by latex-sensitive persons.
- When using a single-use vial, withdraw dose using a 27 gauge syringe with a one-half inch needle.
- Rotate injection sites and do not inject into an area that is tender, bruised, red, or irritated.
- Store unopened vials upright in refrigerator. Discard unused portions in single-use vials.

**ADVERSE EFFECTS** (≥1%) **CNS:** Depression, dizziness, fatigue, headache. **GI:** Diarrhea. **Musculoskeletal:** Back pain, myalgia. **Respiratory:** Nasopharyngitis, upper respiratory tract infection. **Skin:** Injection-site erythema, pruritus. **Body as Whole:** *Infection.*

**INTERACTIONS Drug:** LIVE VACCINES should not be administered

Common adverse effects in *italic*; life-threatening effects <u>underlined</u>; generic names in **bold**; classifications in SMALL CAPS; ♣ Canadian drug name; ✪ Prototype drug

1669

concurrently with ustekinumab therapy. Do not use with IMMUNOSUP-PRESANTS. Closely monitor use with narrow therapeutic index drugs (e.g., **warfarin**, **cyclosporine**).

## PHARMACOKINETICS **Peak:** 7–13.5 days. **Metabolism:** Degraded to smaller proteins. **Half-Life:** 14.9–45.6 days.

## NURSING IMPLICATIONS

### Assessment & Drug Effects

- Monitor for and promptly report S&S of TB or other infection.
- Monitor neurologic status and report promptly: Seizures, problems with vision, headaches, or confusion.
- Note: BCG vaccines should not be given during treatment, for one year prior to initiating treatment, or one year following discontinuation of treatment.
- Monitor lab tests: Prior to initiation of therapy, test for latent TB.

### Patient & Family Education

- Do not accept vaccinations with live vaccines while taking this drug. Note that non-live vaccines may not be effective if given during a course of ustekinumab.
- You should be tested for TB prior to taking this drug.
- Report promptly S&S of infection including: Chills, fever, cough, shortness of breath, diarrhea, stomach or abdominal pain, burning on urination, sores anywhere on your body, unexplained or excessive fatigue.
- Report immediately seizures, problems with vision, headaches, or confusion.

## VACCINIA IMMUNE GLOBULIN (VIG-IV)
(vac-cin′i-a)

**Classifications:** BIOLOGIC RESPONSE MODIFIER; IMMUNOGLOBULIN
**Therapeutic:** IMMUNOGLOBULIN
**Prototype:** Immune globulin

## AVAILABILITY Solution for injection

## ACTION & *THERAPEUTIC EFFECT*
Vaccinia immune globulin, VIG (VIG-IV) is a purified human immunoglobulin G (IgG). VIG (VIG-IV) contains high titers of anti-vaccinia antibodies. *VIG is effective in the treatment of smallpox vaccine adverse reactions secondary to continued vaccinia virus replication after vaccination.*

## USES Prevention of serious complications of smallpox vaccine; treatment of progressive vaccinia; severe generalized vaccinia; eczema vaccinatum; vaccinia infection in patients with skin conditions (e.g., burns, impetigo, varicella-zoster, poison ivy, or eczematous skin lesions); treatment or modification of aberrant infections induced by vaccinia virus.

## CONTRAINDICATIONS Predisposition to acute renal failure (i.e., preexisting renal insufficiency, DM, volume depletion, sepsis proteinemia, patients older than 65 y); AIDS; chronic skin conditions; bone marrow suppression; chemotherapy; radiation therapy; corticosteroid therapy, eczema; hematologic disease, thrombosis; hypotension; herpes infection; postvaccinal encephalitis; aseptic meningitis syndrome (AMS); pulmonary edema; lactation.

## CAUTIOUS USE Renal impairment; autoimmune disease; cardiomyopathy, impaired cardiac output, cardiac disease, history of hypercoagulation; pregnancy (category C). Safe use in children not established.

Common adverse effects in *italic;* life-threatening effects underlined; generic names in **bold;** classifications in SMALL CAPS; ♣ Canadian drug name; ⊙ Prototype drug

## ROUTE & DOSAGE

**Vaccinia**
*Adults:* **IV** 100–500 mg/kg
**Renal Impairment Dosage Adjustment**
Max dose: 400 mg/kg

## ADMINISTRATION

### Intravenous

*PREPARE:* **IV Infusion:** No dilution required. Use solution as supplied. Do not shake. Avoid foaming.

*ADMINISTER:* **IV Infusion:** Begin infusion within 6 h of entering the vial. Complete infusion within 12 h of entering the vial. ▪ Use inline filter (0.22 microns), infusion pump, and dedicated IV line [may infuse into a preexisting catheter if it contains NS, D2.5W, D5W, D10W, or D20W (or any combination of these)]. ▪ Infuse at 1 mL/kg/h the first 30 min, increase to 2 mL/kg/h the next 30 min, and then increase to 3 mL/kg/h until infused.

## ADVERSE EFFECTS (≥1%) **Body as a Whole:** Injection site reaction. **CNS:** Dizziness, *headache.* **GI:** Abdominal pain, nausea, vomiting. **Musculoskeletal:** Arthralgia, back pain. **Respiratory:** Upper respiratory infection. **Skin:** Erythema, flushing.

## INTERACTIONS **Drug:** May interfere with the immune response to LIVE VIRUS VACCINES. Vaccination with LIVE VIRUS VACCINES should be deferred until approximately 6 mo after administration of VIG-IV.

## PHARMACOKINETICS **Half-Life:** 22 days.

## NURSING IMPLICATIONS

### Black Box Warning

*Vaccinia immune globulin IV has been associated with serious renal dysfunction, acute renal failure, and death.*

### Assessment & Drug Effects

▪ Monitor vital signs continuously during infusion, especially after infusion rate changes.
▪ Slow infusion rate for any of the following: Flushing, chills, muscle cramps, back pain, fever, nausea, vomiting, arthralgia, and wheezing.
▪ Discontinue infusion, institute supportive measures, and notify prescriber for any of the following: Increase in heart rate, increase in respiratory rate, shortness of breath, rales or other signs of anaphylaxis.
▪ Have loop diuretic available for management of fluid overload.

### Patient & Family Education

▪ Promptly report any discomfort that develops while drug is being infused.

# VALACYCLOVIR HYDROCHLORIDE

(val-a-cy′clo-vir)

**Valtrex**

**Classification:** ANTIVIRAL; ANTIHERPES
**Therapeutic:** ANTIVIRAL; ANTIHERPES
**Prototype:** Acyclovir

## AVAILABILITY Tablet

## ACTION & *THERAPEUTIC EFFECT*

An antiviral agent hydrolyzed in the intestinal wall or liver to acyclovir, which interferes with viral DNA synthesis. *Active against herpes simplex virus types 1 (HSV-1) and 2 (HSV-2), varicella zoster virus, and cytomegalovirus. Inhibits viral replication.*

**V**

Common adverse effects in *italic;* life-threatening effects <u>underlined</u>; generic names in **bold**; classifications in SMALL CAPS; ♣ Canadian drug name; ⊙ Prototype drug

1671

**USES** Herpes zoster (shingles) in immunocompetent adults. Treatment and suppression of recurrent genital herpes; suppression of recurrent herpes in HIV-positive patients; treatment of cold sores; treatment of varicella infection.

**CONTRAINDICATIONS** Hypersensitivity to, or intolerance of valacyclovir or acyclovir.

**CAUTIOUS USE** Renal impairment, patients receiving nephrotoxic drugs, advanced HIV disease, allogeneic bone marrow transplant and renal transplant recipients, treatment of disseminated herpes zoster, immunocompromised patients, pregnancy (category B); lactation; children younger than 2 y for chicken pox.

## ROUTE & DOSAGE

**Herpes Zoster**

*Adult/Adolescent:* **PO** 1 g t.i.d. for 7 days, start within 48 h of onset of zoster rash

*Renal Impairment Dosage Adjustment*

*CrCl 30–49 mL/min:* 1 g q12h; *10–29 mL/min:* 1 g q24h; *less than 10 mL/min:* 500 mg q24h

**Treatment of Recurrent Genital Herpes**

*Adult/Adolescent:* **PO** 500 mg b.i.d. × 3 days

*Renal Impairment Dosage Adjustment*

*CrCl 29 mL/min or less:* 500 mg daily

**Suppression of Recurrent Genital Herpes**

*Adult:* **PO** 1 g daily; if patient has concurrent HIV infection 500 mg b.i.d.

**Treatment of Cold Sores**

*Adult/Adolescent:* **PO** 2 g 12 h × 2 doses

**Chickenpox**

*Adolescent/Child (2 y or older):* **PO** 20 mg/kg t.i.d. × 5 days (max: 1 g t.i.d.)

## ADMINISTRATION

**Oral**

- Start drug as soon as possible after diagnosis of herpes zoster, preferably within 48 h of onset of rash.
- Note: Dosage reduction is recommended for patients with renal impairment.
- Give valacyclovir after hemodialysis.
- Store at 15°–30° C (59°–86° F).

**ADVERSE EFFECTS** (≥1%) **CNS:** *Headache,* weakness, somnolence, dizziness, fatigue, lethargy, confusion. **GI:** *Nausea, vomiting, diarrhea,* abdominal pain, dyspepsia, flatulence, elevated hepatic enzymes. **Urogenital:** Glomerulonephritis, renal tubular damage, acute renal failure. **Skin:** Rash, urticaria, pruritus. **Respiratory:** Pharyngitis. **Body as a Whole:** Neutropenia.

**INTERACTIONS Drug: Probenecid, cimetidine** decrease valacyclovir elimination. **Zidovudine** may cause increased drowsiness and lethargy. Caution with **meperidine** due to elevated levels. Avoid LIVE VACCINES.

**PHARMACOKINETICS Absorption:** Rapidly absorbed from GI tract; 54% reaches systemic circulation as acyclovir. **Peak:** 1.5 h.

Common adverse effects in *italic;* life-threatening effects underlined; generic names in **bold;** classifications in SMALL CAPS; ♣ Canadian drug name; ◉ Prototype drug

**Distribution:** 13.5–17.9% bound to plasma proteins; distributes into plasma, cerebrospinal fluid, saliva, and major body organs; crosses placenta; excreted in breast milk. **Metabolism:** Rapidly converted to acyclovir during first pass through intestine and liver. **Elimination:** 40–50% in urine. **Half-Life:** 2.5–3.3 h.

## NURSING IMPLICATIONS

### Assessment & Drug Effects

- Monitor kidney function in patients with kidney impairment or those receiving potentially nephrotoxic drugs.
- Monitor for S&S of hypersensitivity; if present, withhold drug and notify prescriber. Monitor lab tests: LFTs.

### Patient & Family Education

- Be aware of potential adverse effects and do not discontinue drug until full course is completed.
- Note: Post-herpes pain is likely to be present for several months after completion of therapy.

## VALBENAZINE
(val-ben'a-zeen)

Ingrezza

**Classifications:** CENTRAL MONO-AMINE-DEPLETING AGENT; VMAT2-IN-HIBITOR

Therapeutic: CENTRAL NERVOUS SYSTEM AGENT

## AVAILABILITY Capsule

## ACTION & *THERAPEUTIC EFFECT*
Thought to reversibly inhibit the vesicular monoamine transporter 2 (VMAT2) transporter, affecting the uptake of monoamines to the synaptic vesicle from the cytoplasm. *Improves stiff and jerky involuntary musculoskeletal movement.*

## USES Treatment of tardive dyskinesia.

## CONTRAINDICATIONS Avoid in patients with congenital long QT syndrome or cardiac arrhythmias associated with prolonged QT interval; patients with severe renal impairment or renal failure; patients taking monoamine oxidase inhibitor therapy (MAOI therapy). Data regarding valbenazine use in human pregnancy is insufficient to provide information on drug-associated risks; lactation.

## CAUTIOUS USE History of hepatic disease. Safety in children not established.

## ROUTE & DOSAGE

### Tardive Dyskinesia

*Adult:* **PO** 40 mg daily; after 1 wk titrate to 80 mg daily
**Renal Impairment Dosage Adjustment**

*CrCL less than 30 mL/min:* Use is not recommended

**Hepatic Impairment Dosage Adjustment**

*Moderate to Severe impairment (Child-Pugh class B or C):* 40 mg daily

**Concomitant CYP3A4 Inhibitor/ Inducer**

*Strong CYP3A4 inducer:* Do not use
*Strong CYP3A4 inhibitor:* Max dose: 40 mg daily

## ADMINISTRATION

### Oral
- May be administered with or without food.
- Store at 20°–25° C (68°–77° F); excursions permitted to 15°–30° C (59°–86° F).

V

**ADVERSE EFFECTS** (≥2%) **CNS:** Drowsiness, sedation, dizziness, falling, drooling, insomnia. **Metabolic:** Hyperglycemia, weight gain. **GI:** Vomiting. **Neuromuscular:** Joint pain, involuntary movement. **Respiratory:** Infection.

**INTERACTIONS** CYP3A4 substrate; avoid use with strong CYP3A4 inducers (e.g., **carbamazepine**, **phenytoin**, **rifampin**); 40 mg daily max dose with CYP3A4 inhibitors (e.g., clarithromycin, itraconazole, ketoconazole) **Herbal: St. John's wort** should not be combined with valbenazine.

**PHARMACOKINETICS Absorption:** 49% bioavailability, AUC and $C_{max}$ decreased with high fat meals. **Distribution:** 99% protein bound. **Onset:** Peak effect in 0.5–1 h. **Metabolism:** Hepatic hydrolysis to an active metabolite, primarily by CYP3A4/5. **Elimination:** 30% in feces, 60% in urine. **Half-Life:** 15–22 h.

## NURSING7 IMPLICATIONS

### Assessment & Drug Effects
- Monitor for decrease in severity of tardive dyskinesia (abnormal involuntary movement) symptoms as indicative of efficacy.
- Monitor QT interval for patients at risk, prior to increasing the dose.
- EKG in patients at risk for QT prolongation.
- Monitor lab tests: Baseline LFTs.

### Patient & Family Education
- Notify all health care providers that you this drug is being taken. This includes prescribers, doctors, nurses, pharmacists, and dentists.
- Avoid driving or other tasks that require alertness until drug affects are known.
- Notify prescriber if taking digoxin. Blood work will need to be monitored more closely.

- Notify prescriber of pregnancy or plan to get pregnant.
- Do not breast-feed while taking this drug or at least 5 days after final dose. Milk should be pumped and dumped during this time.
- Notify prescriber right away with S&S of an allergic reaction: Rash, hives, itching, blistered skin, fever, wheezing, chest or throat tightness, trouble breathing, unusual hoarseness, swelling of the mouth, face, lips, tongue, or throat.
- Notify prescriber right away with difficulties in focusing, blurred vision, difficulty urinating, a fast heartbeat that does not feel normal, or fainting.

# VALGANCICLOVIR HYDROCHLORIDE
(val-gan-ci'clo-vir)
Valcyte
**Classification:** ANTIVIRAL
Therapeutic: ANTIVIRAL
**Prototype:** Acyclovir

**AVAILABILITY** Tablet; powder for oral solution

**ACTION & THERAPEUTIC EFFECT** Rapidly converted to ganciclovir by intestinal and hepatic enzymes. In cells infected with cytomegalovirus (CMV), ganciclovir is converted to ganciclovir triphosphate that inhibits viral DNA synthesis. *Effective antiviral that prevents replication of viral CMV DNA.*

**USES** Treatment or prevention of CMV retinitis; prevention of CMV disease in high-risk kidney, kidney-pancreas, and heart transplant patients (not effective in liver transplants).

**UNLABELED USES** Esophagitis, herpesvirus infection.

**CONTRAINDICATIONS** Hypersensitivity to valganciclovir, ganciclovir,

Common adverse effects in *italic*; life-threatening effects underlined; generic names in **bold**; classifications in SMALL CAPS; ◆ Canadian drug name; ● Prototype drug or acyclovir; dental work; antimicrobial resistance; neutropenia, thrombocytopenia; females of childbearing age; lactation.

**CAUTIOUS USE** Impaired kidney function; dental disease; anemia; leukopenia; bone marrow depression; irradiation; older adults; pregnancy (category C). Safe use in infants younger than 4 mo not established.

## ROUTE & DOSAGE

### Cytomegalovirus Prophylaxis

*Adult/Adolescent:* **PO** 900 mg once daily, starting within 10 days of transplantation until 100–200 days post-transplantation
*Child/Infant (older than 4 mo):* See package insert for dose calculation formula (max: 900 mg)

### Cytomegalovirus Retinitis Treatment

*Adult:* **PO** 900 mg b.i.d. × 21 days then 900 mg daily

### Renal Impairment Dosage Adjustment

*CrCl 40–59 mL/min:* 450 mg b.i.d. (induction) or daily (maintenance); *25–39 mL/min:* 450 mg daily (induction) or q2days (maintenance); *10–24 mL/min:* 450 mg q2days (induction) or twice weekly (maintenance)

## ADMINISTRATION

### Oral

- Exercise caution in handling tablets, powder for oral solution, and the oral solution. Do not crush or break tablets. Avoid direct contact of any form of the drug with skin or mucous membranes. Note that adults should receive tablets, not the oral solution.
- Give with food.

- Do not give to patients on hemodialysis.
- Store tablets at 25°–30° C (77°–86° F). Store oral solution at 2°–8° C (36°–46° F) for no longer than 49 days.

**ADVERSE EFFECTS** (≥1%) **Body as a Whole:** *Fever,* local and systemic infections, hypersensitivity reactions. **CNS:** *Headache, insomnia,* peripheral neuropathy, paresthesia, convulsions, psychosis, confusion, hallucinations, agitation. **GI:** *Diarrhea, nausea, vomiting, abdominal pain.* **Hematologic:** Neutropenia, anemia, thrombocytopenia, pancytopenia, bone marrow suppression, aplastic anemia. **Special Senses:** Retinal detachment.

**INTERACTIONS Drug:** ANTINEOPLASTIC AGENTS, **amphotericin B, didanosine, trimethoprimsulfamethoxazole (TMP-SMZ), dapsone, pentamidine, probenecid, zidovudine** may increase bone marrow suppression and other toxic effects of valganciclovir; may increase risk of nephrotoxicity from **cyclosporine;** ANTIRETROVIRAL AGENTS may decrease valganciclovir levels; valganciclovir may increase levels and toxicity of ANTIRETROVIRAL AGENTS; may increase risk of seizures due to **imipenem-cilastatin.**

**PHARMACOKINETICS Absorption:** 60% reaches systemic circulation as ganciclovir. **Onset:** 3–8 days. **Peak:** 1–3 h. **Duration:** Clinical relapse can occur 14 days to 3.5 mo after stopping therapy; positive blood and urine cultures recur 12–60 days after therapy. **Distribution:** Distributes throughout body including CSF, eye, lungs, liver, and kidneys; crosses placenta in animals; not known if distributed into breast milk. **Metabolism:** Metabolized in intestinal wall to

V

Common adverse effects in *italic;* life-threatening effects <u>underlined</u>; generic names in **bold;** classifications in SMALL CAPS; ✦ Canadian drug name; ⦿ Prototype drug

1675

ganciclovir, ganciclovir is not metabolized. **Elimination:** 94–99% of dose is excreted unchanged in urine. **Half-Life:** 4 h.

## NURSING IMPLICATIONS

### Black Box Warning

*Valganciclovir has been associated with granulocytopenia, anemia, and thrombocytopenia.*

### Assessment & Drug Effects
- Withhold drug and notify prescriber for any of the following: Absolute neutrophil count less than 500 cells/mm$^3$, platelet count less than 25,000/mm$^3$, hemoglobin less than 8 g/dL, declining creatinine clearance.
- Monitor for S&S of bronchospasm in asthma patients; notify prescriber immediately.
- Monitor lab tests: Baseline and frequent serum creatinine or creatinine clearance, CBC with differential, platelet count, Hct and Hgb.

### Patient & Family Education
- Schedule ophthalmologic follow-up examinations at least every 4–6 wk while being treated with valganciclovir.
- Keep all scheduled appointments for laboratory tests.
- Do not drive or engage in potentially hazardous activities until response to drug is known.
- Report any of the following immediately: Unexpected bleeding, infection.
- Use effective methods of contraception (barrier and other types) during and for at least 90 days following treatment.
- Discontinue drug and notify prescriber immediately in the event of pregnancy.

# VALPROIC ACID (DIVALPROEX SODIUM, SODIUM VALPROATE) ℞
(val-proe'ic)

Depacon, Depakene, Depakote, Depakote ER, Depakote Sprinkle, Epival ♦

**Classifications:** ANTICONVULSANT; GAMMA-AMINOBUTYRIC ACID (GABA) INHIBITOR

Therapeutic: ANTICONVULSANT

**AVAILABILITY** Capsule; sprinkle capsule; delayed release tablet; syrup; solution for injection

**ACTION & THERAPEUTIC EFFECT** The mechanisms of action is unknown. Its activity in epilepsy may be related to increased brain concentrations of gamma-aminobutyric acid (GABA). *Depresses abnormal neuron discharges in the CNS, thus decreasing seizure activity.*

**USES** Alone or with other anticonvulsants in management of absence (petit mal) and mixed seizures; mania; migraine headache prophylaxis.

**UNLABELED USES** Status epilepticus refractory to IV diazepam, petit mal variant seizures, febrile seizures in children, other types of seizures including psychomotor (temporal lobe), myoclonic, akinetic and tonic-clonic seizures, photosensitivity seizures, and those refractory to other anticonvulsants.

**CONTRAINDICATIONS** Hypersensitivity to valproate sodium; significant hepatic function impairment; known urea cycle disorders; hyperammonemia, encephalopathy; suicidal ideations; thrombocytopenia, patient with bleeding disorders or liver dysfunction or disease, drug induced pancreatitis; congenital metabolic disorders, mitochondrial disorders caused by mutations in mitochondrial DNA and children younger than 2 y who are suspected of having a mitochondial DNA polemerase related disorder; pancreatitis; pregnancy (category D); lactation.

**CAUTIOUS USE** History of suicidal tendencies; history of kidney disease, renal impairment or failure; history of mild or moderate liver impairment; congenital metabolic disorders, those with severe epilepsy; HIV; CMV-infected patients; hypoalbuminemia; organic brain syndrome or mental retardation; use as sore agent; older adults. Safe use in children with partial seizures younger than 10 y not established. Safe use for migraine use in children younger than 12 y not established.

## ROUTE & DOSAGE

Note: May need to increase dose when converting from immediate release to extended release products

**Management of Seizures**

*Adult/Child (10 y or older):* **PO/IV** 10–15 mg/kg/day in divided doses when total daily dose greater than 250 mg, increase at 1 wk intervals by 5–10 mg/kg/day until seizures are controlled or adverse effects develop (max: 60 mg/kg/day)

*Conversion of PO to IV:* Give normal dose in divided doses q6h

**Migraine Headache Prophylaxis**

*Adult:* **PO** 250 mg b.i.d. (max: 1000 mg/day) or **Depakote ER**

500 mg daily × 1 wk, may increase to 1000 mg daily

**Mania**

*Adult:* **PO** 750 mg/day administered in divided doses OR **Extended release** 25 mg/kg/day

**Hepatic Impairment Dosage Adjustment**

Dose reduction recommended

**Renal Impairment Dosage Adjustment**

Severe impairment may require close monitoring

## ADMINISTRATION

### Oral

- Give tablets and capsules whole; instruct patient to swallow whole and not to chew Instruct to swallow sprinkle capsules whole or sprinkle entire contents on teaspoonful of soft food, and instruct to not chew food.
- Avoid using a carbonated drink as diluent for the syrup because it will release drug from delivery vehicle, free drug painfully irritates oral and pharyngeal membranes.
- Reduce gastric irritation by administering drug with food.

### Intravenous

**PREPARE: IV Infusion:** Dilute each dose in 50 mL or more of D5W, NS, or LR.

**ADMINISTER: IV Infusion:** Give a single dose over at least 60 min (20 mg/min or less). ▪ Avoid rapid infusion.

**INCOMPATIBILITIES: Solution/additive:** Should avoid mixing with other drugs. **Y-site: Vancomycin.**

**ADVERSE EFFECTS** (≥1%) **CNS:** Breakthrough seizures, *sedation, drowsiness, headache, tremor, muscle*

**V**

Common adverse effects in *italic;* life-threatening effects underlined; generic names in **bold;** classifications in SMALL CAPS; ♣ Canadian drug name; ⊘ Prototype drug

1677

*weakness,* dizziness, increased alertness, hallucinations, emotional upset, aggression; <u>deep coma, death (with overdose)</u>. **GI:** *Nausea, vomiting, indigestion (transient),* hypersalivation, anorexia with weight loss, increased appetite with weight gain, abdominal cramps, diarrhea, constipation, <u>liver failure,</u> <u>pancreatitis</u>. **Hematologic:** *Prolonged bleeding time,* leukopenia, lymphocytosis, thrombocytopenia, hypofibrinogenemia, <u>bone marrow depression</u>, anemia. **Skin:** Skin rash, photosensitivity, transient hair loss, curliness or waviness of hair, alopecia. **Endocrine:** Irregular menses, secondary amenorrhea. **Metabolic:** Hyperammonemia (usually asymptomatic), hyperammonemic encephalopathy in patients with urea cycle disorders, <u>pancreatitis</u>. **Respiratory:** Pulmonary edema (with overdose).

## DIAGNOSTIC TEST INTERFERENCE
Valproic acid produces false-positive results for *urine ketones,* elevated *AST, ALT, LDH,* and *serum alkaline phosphatase,* prolonged *bleeding time,* altered *thyroid function tests.*

## INTERACTIONS **Drug:** Alcohol
and other CNS DEPRESSANTS potentiate depressant effects; other ANTICONVULSANTS, BARBITURATES increase or decrease anticonvulsant and BARBITURATE levels; **haloperidol, loxapine, maprotiline,** MAOIS, PHENOTHIAZINES, THIOXANTHENES, TRICYCLIC ANTIDEPRESSANTS can increase CNS depression or lower seizure threshold; **aspirin, dipyridamole, warfarin** increase risk of spontaneous bleeding; **clonazepam** may precipitate absence seizures; SALICYLATES, **cimetidine, isoniazid** may increase valproic acid levels and toxicity. **Mefloquine** can decrease valproic acid levels; **meropenem** may decrease valproic acid

levels; **cholestyramine** may decrease absorption. **Herbal: Ginkgo** may decrease anticonvulsant effectiveness.

## PHARMACOKINETICS **Absorption:** Readily from GI tract. **Peak:** 1–4 h valproic acid; 3–5 h divalproex. **Therapeutic Range:** 50–100 mcg/mL. **Distribution:** Crosses placenta; distributed into breast milk. **Metabolism:** In liver. **Elimination:** Primarily in urine; small amount in feces and expired air. **Half-Life:** 5–20 h.

## NURSING IMPLICATIONS

### Black Box Warning

*Valproic acid, sodium valproate, and divalproex sodium have been associated with severe hepatotoxicity, life-threatening pancreatitis, and fetal harm.*

### Assessment & Drug Effects
- Monitor patient alertness especially with multiple drug therapy for seizure control.
- Monitor patient carefully during dose adjustments and promptly report presence of adverse effects. Increased dosage is associated with frequency of adverse effects.
- Monitor for and report promptly S&S of pancreatitis (e.g., abdominal pain, nausea, vomiting, and/or anorexia).
- Multiple drugs for seizure control increase the risk of hyperammonemia, marked by lethargy, anorexia, asterixis, increased seizure frequency, and vomiting. Report such symptoms promptly to prescriber. If they persist with decreased dosage, the drug will be discontinued.
- Monitor lab tests: Baseline LFTs, platelet count, bleeding time, coagulation parameters, and serum ammonia; then repeat at least q2mo,

especially during the first 6 mo of therapy.

**Patient & Family Education**

- Women of childbearing age should be aware of the potential for birth defects should a pregnancy occur while taking this drug.
- Do not discontinue therapy abruptly; such action could result in loss of seizure control. Consult prescriber before you stop or alter dosage regimen.
- Notify prescriber promptly if spontaneous bleeding or bruising occurs (e.g., petechiae, ecchymotic areas, otorrhagia, epistaxis, melena).
- Withhold dose and notify prescriber for following symptoms: Visual disturbances, rash, jaundice, light-colored stools, protracted vomiting, diarrhea. Fatal liver failure has occurred in patients receiving this drug.
- Avoid alcohol and self-medication with other depressants during therapy.
- Consult prescriber before using any OTC drugs during anticonvulsant therapy, especially drugs containing aspirin or sedatives and medications for hay fever or other allergies.
- Do not drive or engage in potentially hazardous activities until response to drug is known.

# VALRUBICIN
(val-roo'bi-sin)
Valstar
**Classification:** ANTINEOPLASTIC; (ANTIBIOTIC) ANTHRACYCLINE
**Therapeutic:** ANTINEOPLASTIC
**Prototype:** Doxorubicin hydrochloride

**AVAILABILITY** Solution

## ACTION & *THERAPEUTIC EFFECT*
A cytotoxic agent that inhibits the incorporation of nucleosides in DNA

and RNA, resulting in extensive chromosomal damage. It arrests the cell cycle of the HIV virus in the G2 phase by interfering with normal DNA action of topoisomerase II, which is responsible for separating DNA strands and resealing them. *Valrubicin has higher antitumor efficacy and lower toxicity than doxorubicin.*

**USES** Intravesical therapy of BCG-refractory carcinoma *in situ* of the urinary bladder.

**CONTRAINDICATIONS** Hypersensitivity to valrubicin, doxorubicin, anthracyclines, or castor oil; patients with a perforated bladder, concurrent UTI, active infection; severe irritable bladder symptoms; severe myelosuppression; lactation.

**CAUTIOUS USE** Within 2 wk of a transureteral resection; compromised bladder mucosa; mild to moderate myelosuppression; history of bleeding disorders; GI disorders, renal impairment; pregnancy (category C).

## ROUTE & DOSAGE

**BCG-Refractory Bladder Carcinoma *in situ***
*Adult:* **Intravesically** 800 mg once/wk × 6 wk

## ADMINISTRATION

**Instillation**
Avoid skin reactions by using gloves during preparation/administration.

- Use only glass, polypropylene, or polyolefin containers and tubing.

***PREPARE:*** Slowly warm 4 vials (5 mL each) to room temperature. ■ When a precipitate is initially present, warm vials in hands until solution clears. ■ Add contents of 4 vials to 55 mL of 0.9% NaCl injection to yield 75 mL of diluted solution.

Common adverse effects in *italic;* life-threatening effects <u>underlined</u>; generic names in **bold;** classifications in SMALL CAPS; ♦ Canadian drug name; ⊘ Prototype drug

1679

*ADMINISTER:* Aseptically insert a urethral catheter and drain the bladder. ▪ Use gravity drainage to instill valrubicin slowly over several min. ▪ Withdraw catheter; instruct patient not to void for 2 h. ▪ Note: Do not leave a clamped catheter in place.

▪ Store vials in refrigerator. Do not freeze.

**ADVERSE EFFECTS** (≥1%) **Body as a Whole:** Abdominal pain, asthenia, back pain, fever, headache, malaise, myalgia. **CNS:** Dizziness. **CV:** Vasodilation. **GI:** Diarrhea, flatulence, nausea, vomiting. **Urogenital:** *Urinary frequency, urgency, dysuria, bladder spasm, hematuria, bladder pain, incontinence, cystitis, UTI,* nocturia, local burning, urethral pain, pelvic pain, gross hematuria, urinary retention. **Respiratory:** Pneumonia. **Skin:** Rash. **Other:** Anemia, hyperglycemia, peripheral edema.

**PHARMACOKINETICS Absorption:** Not absorbed. **Distribution:** Penetrates bladder wall. **Metabolism:** Not metabolized. **Elimination:** Almost completely excreted by voiding the instillate.

**NURSING IMPLICATIONS**

**Assessment & Drug Effects**
▪ Therapeutic effectiveness: Indicated by regression of the bladder tumor.
▪ Notify prescriber if bladder spasms with spontaneous discharge of valrubicin occur during/shortly after instillation.

**Patient & Family Education**
▪ Expect red-tinged urine during the first 24 h after administration.
▪ Report prolonged passage of red-colored urine or prolonged bladder irritation.
▪ Drink plenty of fluids during 48 h period following administration.
▪ Use reliable contraception during therapy period (approximately 6 wk).

# VALSARTAN
(val-sar'tan)
**Diovan**
**Classifications:** RENIN ANGIOTENSIN SYSTEM ANTAGONIST; ANTIHYPERTENSIVE
**Therapeutic:** ANTIHYPERTENSIVE; ANGIOTENSIN II RECEPTOR (AT₁) ANTAGONIST
**Prototype:** Losartan

**AVAILABILITY** Capsule

**ACTION & *THERAPEUTIC EFFECT***
An angiotensin II receptor antagonist that blocks the angiotensin converting enzyme (ACE). It inhibits the binding of angiotensin II to the AT₁ subtype receptors found in many tissues (e.g., vascular smooth muscle, adrenal glands). Angiotensin II is a potent vasoconstrictor and primary vasoactive hormone of the renin–angiotensin–aldosterone system (RAAS). *Blocking angiotensin II receptors results in vasodilation as well as decreasing the aldosterone-secreting effects of angiotensin II. These actions result in the antihypertensive effect of valsartan.*

**USES** Treatment of hypertension, heart failure; reduction of cardiovascular mortality in stable patients with left ventricular failure or left ventricular dysfunction (LVD) following acute myocardial infarction.

**CONTRAINDICATIONS** Hypersensitivity to valsartan or losartan; severe heart failure with compromised renal function; volume depletion; history of ACE inhibitor–induced angioedema concomitant use with aliskiren in patients with diabetes mellitus; children with CrCl of 30 mL/min/1.73 mm³; pregnancy (category D); lactation.

Common adverse effects in *italic;* life-threatening effects <u>underlined;</u> generic names in **bold;** classifications in SMALL CAPS; ♣ Canadian drug name; ⓟ Prototype drug

**CAUTIOUS USE** Severe renal impairment; hyperuricemia; hyperglycemia; increases in cholesterol and triglycerides; acute angle-closure glaucoma; SLE; history of allergy or bronchial asthma; mild to moderate hepatic impairment; biliary stenosis; renal artery stenosis; hypovolemia; hyperkalemia; transient hypotension; use prior to surgery; history of angioedema; congestive heart failure; older adults; children younger than 6 y.

## ROUTE & DOSAGE

**Hypertension**

*Adult:* **PO** 80 or 160 mg daily (max: 320 mg daily)
*Adolescent/Child (6–16 y):* **PO** 1.3 mg/kg (max: 40 mg/day)

**Heart Failure**

*Adult:* **PO** 40 mg b.i.d. and titrate up to 160 mg b.i.d.

**Left Ventricular Dysfunction Post MI**

*Adult:* **PO** 20 mg b.i.d. titrate to dose of 160 mg b.i.d. if tolerated

*Hemodialysis Dosage Adjustment*

Adjustment not needed

## ADMINISTRATION

**Oral**

- May be given with or without food.
- Reduce dosage with severe hepatic or renal impairment.
- Note: Daily dose may be titrated up to 320 mg.
- Store at 15°–30° C (59°–86° F).

**ADVERSE EFFECTS** (≥1%) **Body as a Whole:** Arthralgia, viral infection. **CNS:** Headache, dizziness, fatigue. **GI:** Diarrhea, nausea, abdominal pain. **Respiratory:** Cough, sinusitis. **Metabolic:** Hyperkalemia, neutropenia. **GU/Renal:** Increased BUN. **Cardiac:** Hypotension, syncope. **Musculoskeletal:** Arthralgia, back pain.

**INTERACTIONS** Do not use with **tranylcypromine.** Do not use within 12 h of **rituximab** administration. Use cautiously with **amifostine** due to increased risk of hypotension.

**PHARMACOKINETICS** **Absorption:** Rapidly from GI tract, 25% bioavailability. **Onset:** Blood pressure decreased in 2 wk. **Peak:** Plasma levels, 2–4 h; blood pressure effect 4 wk. **Distribution:** 99% protein bound. **Metabolism:** In the liver (CYP2C9). **Elimination:** Primarily in feces. **Half-Life:** 6 h.

## NURSING IMPLICATIONS

### Black Box Warning

*Valsartan has been associated with fetal toxicity.*

**Assessment & Drug Effects**

- Monitor BP periodically; take trough readings, just prior to the next scheduled dose, when possible.
- Monitor lab tests: Periodic renal function tests.

**Patient & Family Education**

- Inform prescriber immediately if you become pregnant.
- Note: Maximum pressure lowering effect is usually evident between 2 and 4 wk after initiation of therapy. Use precaution when changing positions.
- Notify prescriber of episodes of dizziness, especially those that occur when making position changes.
- Do not use potassium supplements or salt substitutes containing potassium without consulting the prescribing prescriber.

Common adverse effects in *italic*; life-threatening effects underlined; generic names in **bold**; classifications in SMALL CAPS; ♣ Canadian drug name; ◑ Prototype drug

1681

# VANCOMYCIN HYDROCHLORIDE ⊕

(van-koe-mye'sin)

**Vancocin**

**Classifications:** ANTIBIOTIC; GLYCOPEPTIDE

**Therapeutic:** ANTIBIOTIC

**AVAILABILITY** Capsule; solution for injection

**ACTION & THERAPEUTIC EFFECT**
Bactericidal action is due to inhibition of cell-wall biosynthesis and alteration of bacterial cell-membrane permeability and ribonucleic acid (RNA) synthesis. *Active against many gram-positive organisms.*

**USES** Parenterally for potentially life-threatening infections in patients allergic, nonsensitive, or resistant to other less toxic antimicrobial drugs. Used orally only in *Clostridium difficile* colitis and staphylococccal enterocolitis (not effective by oral route for treatment of systemic infections).

**UNLABELED USES** Rectal administration for complicated *C. difficile* infection.

**CONTRAINDICATIONS** Hypersensitivity to vancomycin.

**CAUTIOUS USE** Impaired kidney function, renal failure, renal impairment, hearing impairment; colitis, inflammatory disorders of the intestine; older adults; pregnancy (category B), children, neonates.

## ROUTE & DOSAGE

### Systemic Infections
*Adult/Adolescent:* **IV** 500 mg q6h or 1 g q12h or 15 mg/kg q12h

*Child/Infant (1 mo or older):* **IV** 30–40 mg/kg/day divided q6–8h
*Neonate:* **IV** 10–15 mg/kg q8–24h

### Clostridium difficile Colitis
*Adult:* **PO** 125 mg q.i.d. × 10 days
*Child:* **PO** 40 mg/kg/day divided q6h (max: 2 g/day)

### Staphylococcal Enterocolitis
*Adult:* **PO** 500 mg–2g in 3–4 divided doses × 7–10 days
*Child:* **PO** 40 mg/kg/day divided q6h (max: 2 g/day)

### Surgical Prophylaxis (in Patients Allergic to Beta-Lactams)
*Adult/Adolescent/Child (weight at least 27 kg):* **IV** 10–15 mg/kg starting 1 h before surgery
*Child (weight less than 27 kg):* **IV** 20 mg/kg starting 1 h before surgery

### Endocarditis
*Adult:* **IV** 500 mg q6h or 1 g q12h
*Infant older than 1 mo:* **IV** 10 mg/kg/dose q6h
*Neonate:* **IV** 15 mg/kg initial dose then 10 mg/kg q12h for first wk then q8h up to 1 mo old

### Renal Impairment Dosage Adjustment
*CrCl 40–60 mL/min:* Dose q24h; *less than 40 mL/min:* Extend interval based on monitoring levels

### Hemodialysis Dosage Adjustment
Not dialyzed

## ADMINISTRATION
### Oral
- May be given with or without food.

▪ Note: Some parenteral products may be administered orally; check manufacturer's package insert.

### Intravenous

*PREPARE:* **Intermittent:** Reconstitute 500 mg vial, 750 mg vial, or 1 g vial with 10 mL, 15 mL, or 20 mL, respectively, of sterile water for injection to yield 50 mg/mL. ▪ Further dilute each 500 mg with at least 100 mL, each 750 mg with at least 150 mL, and each 1 g with at least 200 mL of D5W, NS, or LR.

*ADMINISTER:* **Intermittent:** Give a single dose at a rate of 10 mg/min or over **not less** than 60 min (whichever is longer). ▪ Avoid rapid infusion, which may cause sudden hypotension. ▪ Monitor IV site closely; necrosis and tissue sloughing will result from extravasation.

*INCOMPATIBILITIES:* **Solution/additive: Aminophylline,** BARBITURATES, **aztreonam** (high concentration), **calcium chloride, chloramphenicol, chlorothiazide, ciprofloxacin, dexamethasone, heparin, methicillin, pentobarbital, phenobarbital, sodium bicarbonate, sodium fusidate, warfarin.** **Y-site: Albumin, aminophylline, amphotericin B cholesteryl, azathioprine, aztreonam, bivalirudin, cefazolin, cefepime, cefoperazone, cefotaxime, cefotetan, cefoxitin, ceftazidime, ceftriaxone, cefuroxime, chloramphenicol, clorazepate, dantrolene, daptomycin, defibrotide, diazepam, diazoxide, dimenhydrinate, drotrecogin epoetin, fluorouracil, foscarnet, furosemide, ganciclovir, gemtuzumab, heparin, ibuprofen, idarubicin, indomethacin, ketorolac, lansoprazole, leucovorin, mitomycin, moxifloxacin, nafcillin, omeprazole, phenytoin, piperacillin/tazobactam, rituximab, sargramostim, streptokinase, SMZ/TMP, temocillin, ticarcillin, ticarcillin/clavulanate, valproate sodium, warfarin.**

▪ Store oral and parenteral solutions in refrigerator for up to 14 days; after further dilution, parenteral solution is stable 24 h at room temperature.

## ADVERSE EFFECTS (≥1%) Special Senses: Ototoxicity (auditory portion of eighth cranial nerve). Urogenital: Nephrotoxicity leading to uremia. Body as a Whole: Hypersensitivity reactions (chills, fever, skin rash, urticaria, shock-like state), anaphylactoid reaction with vascular collapse, superinfections, severe pain, thrombophlebitis at injection site, generalized tingling following rapid IV infusion. Hematologic: Transient leukopenia, eosinophilia. GI: Nausea, warmth. Other: Injection reaction that includes *hypotension accompanied by flushing and erythematous rash on face and upper body* ("red-neck syndrome") following rapid IV infusion.

## INTERACTIONS Drug: Adds to toxicity of ototoxic and nephrotoxic drugs (AMINOGLYCOSIDES, **amphotericin B, colistin, capreomycin; cidofovir; cisplatin; cyclosporine; foscarnet; ganciclovir; IV pentamidine; polymyxin B; streptozocin; tacrolimus**). **Cholestyramine, colestipol** can decrease absorption of oral vancomycin; may increase risk of lactic acidosis with **metformin**.

## PHARMACOKINETICS Absorption: Not absorbed. Peak: 30 min

V

Common adverse effects in *italic;* life-threatening effects underlined; generic names in **bold;** classifications in SMALL CAPS; ♣ Canadian drug name; ⊙ Prototype drug

1683

after end of infusion. **Distribution:** Diffuses into pleural, ascitic, pericardial, and synovial fluids; small amount penetrates CSF if meninges are inflamed; crosses placenta. **Elimination:** 80–90% of IV dose in urine within 24 h; PO dose excreted in feces. **Half-Life:** 4–8 h.

## NURSING IMPLICATIONS

### Assessment & Drug Effects

- Monitor BP and heart rate continuously through period of drug administration.
- Assess hearing. Drug may cause damage to auditory branch (not vestibular branch) of eighth cranial nerve, with consequent deafness, which may be permanent.
- Be aware that serum levels of 60–80 mcg/mL are associated with ototoxicity. Tinnitus and high-tone hearing loss may precede deafness, which may progress even after drug is withdrawn. Older adults and those on high doses are especially susceptible.
- Monitor I&O: Report changes in I&O ratio and pattern. Oliguria or cloudy or pink urine may be a sign of nephrotoxicity (also manifested by transient elevations in BUN, albumin, and hyaline and granular casts in urine).
- Monitor lab tests: Periodic renal function tests, urinalysis, and WBC count; serial vancomycin blood levels (peak and trough) in patients with borderline kidney function, in infants and neonates, and in patients older than 60 y.

### Patient & Family Education

- Notify prescriber promptly of ringing in ears.
- Adhere to drug regimen (i.e., do not increase, decrease, or interrupt dosage. The full course of prescribed drug therapy **must be** completed).

# VARDENAFIL HYDROCHLORIDE

(var-den'a-fil hy-dro-chlo'ride)

Levitra, Staxyn

**Classifications:** IMPOTENCE AGENT; PHOSPHODIESTERASE (PDE) INHIBITOR; VASODILATOR

Therapeutic: IMPOTENCE; PDE TYPE 5 INHIBITOR

**Prototype:** Sildenafil

**AVAILABILITY** Tablet; orally disintegrating tablet

## ACTION & *THERAPEUTIC EFFECT*

Phosphodiesterases-5 (PDE5) is an enzyme that speeds up the degradation of cyclic guanosine monophosphate (cGMP), an enzyme needed to cause and maintain increased blood flow into the penis necessary for an erection. Vardenafil is a PDE5 inhibitor. *It enhances erectile function by increasing the amount of cGMP in the penis.*

**USES** Treatment of erectile dysfunction.

**CONTRAINDICATIONS** Hypersensitivity to vardenafil or sildenafil; coadministration of nitrates; QT prolongation, renal failure, severe renal impairment; retinitis pigmentosa. **Levitra:** Severe hepatic impairment (Child-Pugh class C); **Staxyn:** Moderate or severe hepatic impairment (Child-Pugh class B and C); lactation.

**CAUTIOUS USE** CAD, MI, or stroke within 6 mo; hypotension, or hypertension; risk factors for CVA; anatomic deformity of the penis; subaortic stenosis; sickle cell anemia, leukemia; multiple myeloma; leukemia; coagulopathy; active bleeding or a peptic ulcer; coagulopathy; GERD; hepatitis, cirrhosis; older adults; pregnancy (category B).

V

Common adverse effects in *italic;* life-threatening effects underlined; generic names in **bold;** classifications in SMALL CAPS; ✦ Canadian drug name; ⊙ Prototype drug

## ROUTE & DOSAGE

### Erectile Dysfunction

*Adult:* **PO** 10 mg approximately 60 min before sexual activity. May increase to max 20 mg/day (**Levitra** only) if needed.
*Geriatric:* **PO** Start with 5 mg 60 min before sexual activity (max: 20 mg/day)

### Hepatic Impairment Dosage Adjustment

*Moderate impairment:* For **Levitra** reduce dose to 5 mg (max: 10 mg/day). For **Staxyn** dosing do not use in patients with moderate or severe (class B or C) hepatic impairment.

### Drug Interaction Dosage Adjustment

If taking **Ritonavir,** max dose: 2.5 mg/72 h; if taking **erythromycin, indinavir, itraconazole, ketoconazole,** max dose: 2.5–5 mg/24 h

## ADMINISTRATION

### Oral

- Take approximately 1 h before expected intercourse, but preferably not after a heavy or high-fat meal.
- Store at 15°–30° C (59°–86° F).

## ADVERSE EFFECTS (≥1%) **Body as a Whole:** *Flushing,* flu-like syndrome, back pain, anaphylactoid reactions, asthenia, facial edema, pain, paresthesias. **CNS:** *Headache,* dizziness, insomnia, somnolence, vertigo. **CV:** Angina, hypertension, hypotension, MI, orthostatic hypotension, palpitations, syncope, sinus tachycardia. **GI:** Dyspepsia, nausea, vomiting, abdominal pain, abnormal liver function tests, diarrhea, dysphagia, esophagitis, gastritis, GERD, xerostomia. **Metabolic:** Increased creatine kinase. **Musculoskeletal:** Arthralgia, myalgia, hypertonia, hyperesthesia. **Respiratory:** Rhinitis, sinusitis, dyspnea, epistaxis, pharyngitis. **Skin:** Photosensitivity, rash, pruritus, sweating. **Special Senses:** Tinnitus, sudden vision loss, blurred vision, changes in color vision. **Urogenital:** Ejaculation dysfunction.

## INTERACTIONS **Drug:** May potentiate hypotensive effects of NITRATES, ALPHA-BLOCKERS, **alfuzosin, doxazosin, prazosin, tamsulosin, terazosin; amiodarone, dofetilide, procainamide, quinidine, sotalol** may increase $QT_c$ interval leading to arrhythmias; dosage adjustment required with potent CYP3A4 inhibitors (**atazanavir, erythromycin, idinavir, itraconazole, ketoconazole,** etc.). If taking ritonavir, max dose is 2.5 mg/72 h. If taking erythromycin, indinavir, itraconazole, ketoconazole, max dose is 2.5–5 mg/24 h.

## PHARMACOKINETICS **Absorption:** Rapidly absorbed, 15% reaches systemic circulation; 95% protein bound. **Onset:** Within 1 h. **Peak:** 0.5–2 h. **Metabolism:** In liver by CYP3A4, CYP3A5, and CYP2C. **Elimination:** Primarily in feces (90–95%). **Half-Life:** 4–5 h.

## NURSING IMPLICATIONS

### Assessment & Drug Effects

- Monitor CV status and report angina or other S&S of cardiac dysfunction.

### Patient & Family Education

- Do not take more than once a day and never take more than the prescribed dose.

Common adverse effects in *italic;* life-threatening effects underlined; generic names in **bold**; classifications in SMALL CAPS; ✤ Canadian drug name; ⊕ Prototype drug

1685

- Do not take this drug without consulting prescriber if you are taking drugs called "alpha-blockers" or "nitrates" or any other drugs for high blood pressure, chest pain, or enlarged prostate.
- Report promptly any of the following: Palpitations, chest pain, back pain, difficulty breathing, or shortness of breath; dizziness or fainting; changes in vision; dizziness; swollen eyelids; muscle aches; painful or prolonged erection (lasting longer than 4 h); skin rash, or itching.

# VARENICLINE
(var-en'i-cline)
Chantix
**Classifications:** SMOKING DETERRENT; NICOTINIC RECEPTOR AGONIST
Therapeutic: SMOKING CESSATION
**Prototype:** Nicotine

## AVAILABILITY Tablet

## ACTION & THERAPEUTIC EFFECT
Nicotine increases dopamine release in the brain and cravings for nicotine are stimulated by low levels of dopamine during periods of abstinence. Varenicline is a partial agonist at nicotinic acetylcholine receptors (nAChRs), the sites responsible for the dopamine effects of nicotine. It partially stimulates these receptors to produce a modest level of dopamine but blocks nicotine from binding to many of the nicotinic receptor sites. *By blocking nicotinic receptors, it reduces effects of nicotine in cases where patient relapses and uses tobacco.*

## USES Adjunct for smoking cessation in patients experiencing nicotine withdrawal.

**CONTRAINDICATIONS** Suicidal ideation; chronic depression; serious psychiatric disease; lactation.

**CAUTIOUS USE** History of suicidal tendencies, depression; renal impairment, older adults; pregnancy (category C). Safe use in children younger than 18 y not known.

## ROUTE & DOSAGE

### Smoking Cessation
*Adult:* **PO** Begin with 0.5 mg/day for 3 days, increase to 0.5 mg b.i.d. for 4 days, then increase to 1 mg b.i.d. on day 8. Treat for 12 wk and may repeat an additional 12 wk.
### Renal Impairment Dosage Adjustment
*CrCl 50 mL/min or less:* Titrate to 0.5 mg b.i.d. (max)

## ADMINISTRATION
### Oral
- Give after a meal with a full glass of water.
- Dose titration over 8 days (from 0.5 to 2 mg daily) is recommended to minimize adverse effects.
- Store at 15°–30° C (59°–86° F).

**ADVERSE EFFECTS** (≥1%) **Body as a Whole:** Fatigue, flushing, gingivitis, headache, influenza-like symptoms, lethargy, malaise, thirst. **CNS:** *Abnormal dreams,* anorexia, anxiety, asthenia, disturbance in attention, depression, dizziness, drowsiness, emotional lability, *insomnia,* irritability, *nightmares,* restlessness, sensory disturbance, *sleep disorder,* suicidality. **CV:** Chest pain, hypertension. **GI:** Abdominal pain, *constipation,* diarrhea, dyspepsia, *flatulence,* gastroesophageal

Common adverse effects in *italic;* life-threatening effects underlined; generic names in **bold;** classifications in SMALL CAPS; ◆ Canadian drug name; ● Prototype drug

V

reflux, *nausea, vomiting.* **Metabolic:** Abnormal liver function test, appetite stimulation, weight gain. **Musculoskeletal:** Arthralgia, back pain, muscle cramps, musculoskeletal pain, myalgia. **Respiratory:** Dyspnea, epistaxis, respiratory disorder, rhinorrhea. **Skin:** Hyperhidrosis, pruritus, rash. **Special Senses:** Dysgeusia, xerostomia. **Urogenital:** Menstrual irregularity, polyuria.

**INTERACTIONS Drug:** **Cimetidine** increases systemic exposure to varenicline by 29%.

**PHARMACOKINETICS Absorption:** Complete absorption from GI tract. **Peak:** 3–4 h. **Distribution:** Less than 20% protein bound. **Metabolism:** Minimal. **Elimination:** Primarily eliminated unchanged in the urine. **Half-Life:** 24 h.

**NURSING IMPLICATIONS**

**Black Box Warning**

*Varenicline has been associated with increased risk of depression, suicidal ideation, and suicide attempt.*

**Assessment & Drug Effects**
- Monitor smoking cessation behavior and adverse effects.
- Monitor BP for new-onset hypertension.
- Monitor diabetics for loss of glycemic control.
- Monitor for increased suicidality, or increase in agitation or aggression.

**Patient & Family Education**
- Report persistent nausea, vomiting, or insomnia to a health care provider.

- Report new-onset of depressed mood, suicidal ideation, or changes in emotion and behavior resulting from the use of varenicline.

**VARICELLA VACCINE**
(var-i-cel′la)
*Varivax*
**See Appendix J.**

**VASOPRESSIN INJECTION**
(vay-soe-press′in)
*Vasostrict*
**Classifications:** PITUITARY HORMONE; ANTIDIURETIC HORMONE (ADH)
**Therapeutic:** ADH REPLACEMENT

**AVAILABILITY** Solution for injection

**ACTION & *THERAPEUTIC EFFECT***
Produces concentrated urine by increasing tubular reabsorption of water (ADH activity), thus reabsorbing up to 90% of water in renal tubules. Causes contraction of smooth muscles of the GI tract as well as the vascular system, especially capillaries, arterioles, and venules. *Effective in reversing diuresis caused by diabetes insipidus. When given intravenously, it is effective as an adjunct in treating massive GI bleeding.*

**USES** Antidiuretic to treat diabetes insipidus, vasodilatory shock (Vasostrict only).

**UNLABELED USES** Test for differential diagnosis of nephrogenic, psychogenic, and neurohypophyseal diabetes insipidus; test to elevate ability of kidney to concentrate urine, and provocative test for pituitary release of corticotropin and growth hormone; emergency and adjunct pressor agent in the control of massive GI hemorrhage (e.g., esophageal varices).

**CONTRAINDICATIONS** Hypersensitivity to vasopression or any of the components in formulation; uncorrected nephritis accompanied by nitrogen retention; ischemic heart disease, PVCs, advanced arteriosclerosis; lactation.

**CAUTIOUS USE** Epilepsy; migraine; asthma; heart failure, angina pectoris; any state in which rapid addition to extracellular fluid may be hazardous; vascular disease; older adults; labor and delivery; pregnancy (category C); children.

## ROUTE & DOSAGE

### Diabetes Insipidus

*Adult:* **IM/Subcutaneous** 5–10 units aqueous solution 2–4 × day (5–60 units/day) or 1.25–2.5 units in oil q2–3days; **Intranasal** Apply to cotton pledget or intranasal spray
*Child:* **IM/Subcutaneous** 2.5–10 units aqueous solution 2–4 × day

### Vasodilatory Shock

*Adult:* **IV** 0.03 units/min can titrate up by 0.005 units/min at 10–15 min intervals (max: 0.1 unit/min)

### GI Hemorrhage

*Adult:* **IV** 20 units bolus then 0.2–0.4 units/min up to 0.9 units/min

### Septic Shock

*Adult:* **IV** 0.01 units/min then can titrate up by 0.005 units/min (max: 0.07 units/min)

## ADMINISTRATION

### Intramuscular/Subcutaneous

- Give 1–2 glasses of water with vasopressin to reduce adverse effects such as skin blanching, abdominal cramps and nausea.
- Give IM injection deeply into a large muscle.
- With subcutaneous injection, exercise caution not to inject intradermally.

### Intravenous

**PREPARE: Direct/IV Infusion:** Dilute with NS or D5W to a concentration of 0.1–1 units/mL.
**ADMINISTER: Direct:** Give rapid bolus dose. **IV Infusion:** Titrate dose and rate to patient's response.
- Ensure patency prior to injection or infusion as extravasation may cause severe vasoconstriction with tissue necrosis and gangrene.

**ADVERSE EFFECTS** (≥1%) **Skin:** Rash, urticaria. **Body as a Whole:** <u>Anaphylaxis</u>; *tremor,* sweating, bronchoconstriction, *circumoral and facial pallor,* angioneurotic edema, *pounding in head, water intoxication* (especially with tannate), gangrene at injection site with intraarterial infusion. **GI:** *Eructations, passage of gas, nausea, vomiting,* heartburn, abdominal cramps, increased bowel movements secondary to excessive use. **CV:** Angina (in patient with coronary vascular disease); <u>cardiac arrest</u>, hypertension, bradycardia, minor arrhythmias, premature atrial contraction, heart block, peripheral vascular collapse, coronary insufficiency, <u>MI</u>; cardiac arrhythmia, pulmonary edema, bradycardia (with intraarterial infusion). **Urogenital:** Uterine cramps. **Respiratory:** Congestion, rhinorrhea, irritation, mucosal ulceration and pruritus, postnasal drip. **Special Senses:** Conjunctivitis.

Common adverse effects in *italic;* life-threatening effects <u>underlined</u>; generic names in **bold;** classifications in SMALL CAPS; ✦ Canadian drug name; ⊙ Prototype drug

## DIAGNOSTIC TEST INTERFERENCE
Vasopressin increases *plasma cortisol* levels.

## INTERACTIONS Drug: Alcohol,
**demeclocycline, epinephrine, heparin, lithium, phenytoin** may decrease antidiuretic effects of vasopressin; **guanethidine, neostigmine** increase vasopressor actions; **chlorpropamide, clofibrate, carbamazepine,** THIAZIDE DIURETICS may increase antidiuretic activity.

## PHARMACOKINETICS Duration:
2–8 h in aqueous solution, 48–72 h in oil, 30–60 min IV infusion. **Distribution:** Extracellular fluid. **Metabolism:** In liver and kidneys. **Elimination:** In urine. **Half-Life:** 10–20 min.

## NURSING IMPLICATIONS
### Assessment & Drug Effects
- Monitor infants and children closely. They are more susceptible to volume disturbances (such as sudden reversal of polyuria) than adults.
- Establish baseline data of BP, weight, I&O pattern and ratio. Monitor BP and weight throughout therapy. (Dose used to stimulate diuresis has little effect on BP.) Report sudden changes in pattern to prescriber.
- Be alert to the fact that even small doses of vasopressin may precipitate MI or coronary insufficiency, especially in older adult patients. Keep emergency equipment and drugs (antiarrhythmics) readily available.
- Check patient's alertness and orientation frequently during therapy. Lethargy and confusion associated with headache may signal onset of water intoxication, which, although insidious in rate of development, can lead to convulsions and terminal coma.
- Monitor urine output, specific gravity, and serum osmolality while patient is hospitalized.
- Withhold vasopressin, restrict fluid intake, and notify prescriber if urine-specific gravity is less than 1.015.

### Patient & Family Education
- Be prepared for possibility of anginal attack and have coronary vasodilator available (e.g., nitroglycerin) if there is a history of coronary artery disease. Report to prescriber.
- With diabetes insipidus, measure and record data related to polydipsia and polyuria. Keep an accurate record of output. Understand that treatment should diminish intense thirst and restore undisturbed normal sleep.
- Avoid concentrated fluids (e.g., undiluted syrups), since these increase urine volume.

## VECURONIUM BROMIDE
(vek-yoo-roe'nee-um)
**Classifications:** NONDEPOLARIZING SKELETAL MUSCLE RELAXANT; ACETYLCHOLINE RECEPTOR ANTAGONIST
Therapeutic: SKELETAL MUSCLE RELAXANT
**Prototype:** Atracurium

## AVAILABILITY Intravenous solution

## ACTION & THERAPEUTIC EFFECT
Intermediate acting nondepolarizing skeletal muscle relaxant that inhibits neuromuscular transmission by competitively binding with acetylcholine at receptors located on motor endplate receptors. *Effective as a skeletal muscle relaxant.*

## USES Adjunct for general anesthesia to produce skeletal muscle relaxation during surgery.

Common adverse effects in *italic;* life-threatening effects underlined; generic names in **bold;** classifications in SMALL CAPS; ♣ Canadian drug name; ☺ Prototype drug

1689

**CONTRAINDICATIONS** Hypersensitivity to vecuronium.

**CAUTIOUS USE** Severe liver disease; impaired acid–base, fluid and electrolyte balance; long-term use; severe obesity; adrenal or neuromuscular disease (myasthenia gravis, Eaton-Lambert syndrome); patients with slow circulation time (cardiovascular disease, old age, edematous states); obesity, pregnancy (category C); lactation; children younger than 1 y and older than 7 wk.

## ROUTE & DOSAGE

**Skeletal Muscle Relaxation**

*Adult/Child (10 y or older):* **IV** 0.08–0.1 mg/kg initially, then after 25–40 min, 0.01–0.15 mg/kg q12–15min or 0.001 mg/kg/min by continuous infusion for prolonged procedures

*Child (1–10 y)/Infant:* **IV** Varies greatly; may require higher initial dose

**Obesity Dosage Adjustment**

Dose based on IBW

## ADMINISTRATION

Note: Vecuronium is administered only by qualified clinicians.

**Intravenous**

*PREPARE:* **Direct:** Reconstitute the 10 or 20 mg vial with 10 or 20 mL, respectively, of sterile water for injection (supplied). **Continuous:** Further dilute the reconstituted solution in up to 100 mL D5W, NS, or LR to yield 0.1–0.2 mg/mL. *ADMINISTER:* **Direct:** Give a bolus dose over 30 sec. **Continuous:** Give at the required rate.

*INCOMPATIBILITIES:* **Y-site:** Amphotericin B cholesteryl complex, diazepam, etomidate, furosemide.

• Refrigerate after reconstitution below 30° C (86° F), unless otherwise directed. Discard solution after 24 h.

**ADVERSE EFFECTS** (≥1%) **Body as a Whole:** Skeletal muscle weakness, malignant hyperthermia. **Respiratory:** Respiratory depression.

**INTERACTIONS Drug:** GENERAL ANESTHETICS increase neuromuscular blockade and duration of action; AMINOGLYCOSIDES, **bacitracin, polymyxin B, clindamycin, lidocaine, parenteral magnesium, quinidine, quinine, trimethaphan, verapamil** increase neuromuscular blockade; DIURETICS may increase or decrease neuromuscular blockade; **lithium** prolongs duration of neuromuscular blockade; NARCOTIC ANALGESICS increase possibility of additive respiratory depression; **succinylcholine** increases onset and depth of neuromuscular blockade; **phenytoin** may cause resistance to or reversal of neuromuscular blockade.

**PHARMACOKINETICS Onset:** Less than 1 min. **Peak:** 3–5 min. **Duration:** 25–40 min. **Distribution:** Well distributed to tissues and extracellular fluids; crosses placenta; distribution into breast milk unknown. **Metabolism:** Rapid nonenzymatic degradation in bloodstream. **Elimination:** 30–35% in urine, 30–35% in bile. **Half-Life:** 30–80 min.

## NURSING IMPLICATIONS

### Assessment & Drug Effects

• Use peripheral nerve stimulator during and following drug administration to avoid risk of overdosage and to identify residual paralysis during recovery period. This is especially indicated when cautious use of drug is specified.

V

- Monitor vital signs at least q15min until stable, then q30min for the next 2 h. Also monitor airway patency until assured that patient has fully recovered from drug effects. Note rate, depth, and pattern of respirations. Obese patients and patients with myasthenia gravis or other neuromuscular disease may have ventilation problems.
- Evaluate patients for recovery from neuromuscular blocking (curare-like) effects as evidenced by ability to breathe naturally or take deep breaths and cough, to keep eyes open, and to lift head keeping mouth closed and by adequacy of hand grip strength. Notify prescriber if recovery is delayed.
- Note: Recovery time may be delayed in patients with cardiovascular disease, edematous states, and in older adults.
- Monitor lab tests: Baseline serum electrolytes, acid–base balance, LFTs, and renal function tests.

## VEDOLIZUMAB

(ve dol'i-zu-mab)

Entyvio

**Classifications:** BIOLOGICAL RESPONSE MODIFIER; MONOCLONAL ANTIBODY; INTEGRIN INHIBITOR

Therapeutic: IMMUNOSUPPRESSANT

**Prototype:** Basiliximab

**AVAILABILITY** Lyophilized powder for reconstitution and injection

## ACTION & *THERAPEUTIC EFFECT*

Inhibits the migration of memory T-lymphocytes, which promote inflammation, across the endothelium into inflamed GI tissue. *Decreases inflammation and other responses*.

**USES** Treatment of moderate-to-severe ulcerative colitis (UC) and Crohn's disease (CD) in adults who have had inadequate response to a tumor necrosis factor (TNF) blocker or immunomodulator, or were unable to achieve corticosteroid-free remission.

**CONTRAINDICATIONS** Known serious or severe hypersensitivity to vedolizumab or any component of the formulation; dyspnea, bronchospasm; progressive multifocal leukoencephalopathy (PML); active serious infection; jaundice or liver injury due to vedolizumab.

**CAUTIOUS USE** History of recurrent mild or moderate infection; liver impairment. Safety and efficacy in children younger than 18 y not established.

## ROUTE & DOSAGE

### Ulcerative Colitis or Crohn's Disease

*Adult:* **IV** 300 mg infusion, again at wk 2 and wk 6, then 300 mg every 8 wk; discontinue if no benefit after wk 14

## ADMINISTRATION

### Intravenous

*PREPARE:* **IV Infusion:** Reconstitute vial with 4.8 mL of SW. Swirl gently for at least 15 sec but do not vigorously shake or invert. Allow vial sit up to 20 min at room temperature to allow foam to settle; vial can be swirled during this time. If not fully dissolved after 20 min, allow another 10 min for dissolution. Do not use the vial if the drug is not dissolved in 30 min. Prior to withdrawing the reconstituted solution from the vial for dilution, gently invert vial

V

Common adverse effects in *italic;* life-threatening effects <u>underlined</u>; generic names in **bold;** classifications in SMALL CAPS; ♣ Canadian drug name; ● Prototype drug

1691

3 times. Withdraw 5 mL (300 mg) of reconstituted solution and add to 250 mL of NS and gently mix the infusion bag. Use as soon as possible.
*ADMINISTER:* **IV Infusion:** Give over 30 min. **Do not** give IV push or bolus. Flush line after infusion with 30 mL of NS. Observe closely during infusion (until complete) and monitor for hypersensitivity reactions; stop infusion if a reaction occurs.
*INCOMPATIBILITIES:* Do not add any other drugs or solutions to the IV line.

- Store up to 4 h at 2°–8° C (36°–46° F). Do not freeze.

**ADVERSE EFFECTS** (≥3%) **Body as a Whole:** *Antibody development*, fever, influenza, infusion related reaction. **CNS:** *Headache*, fatigue. **GI:** Nausea. **Metabolic:** Elevated ALT and AST. **Musculoskeletal:** *Arthralgia*, back pain, pain in extremities. **Respiratory:** Bronchitis, cough, *nasopharyngitis*, oropharyngeal pain, upper respiratory tract infection. **Skin:** Pruritus, skin rash.

**INTERACTIONS Drug:** TUMOR NECROSIS FACTOR BLOCKERS may increase the risk of progressive multifocal leukoencephalopathy and other infections if given with vedolizumab. Concomitant use of vedolizumab with ANTINEOPLASTIC AGENTS, IMMUNOSUPPRESSIVES, IMMUNOMODULATING AGENTS, or **natalizumab** may enhance the risk of opportunistic infections.

**PHARMACOKINETICS Half-Life:** 25 d (300 mg dose).

## NURSING IMPLICATIONS

### Assessment & Drug Effects
- Monitor closely for S&S of a hypersensitivity reaction (see

Appendix F). Interrupt infusion and notify prescriber if hypersensitivity is suspected.
- Monitor for and report promptly S&S of an infection, especially in the upper respiratory tract.
- Monitor for signs of hepatotoxicity (see Appendix F).
- Monitor lab test: Baseline TB screening; periodic LFTs.

### Patient & Family Education
- Report immediately if you experience S&S of a hypersensitivity reaction (e.g., itching, rash, swelling about the mouth and face, difficulty breathing, dizziness, feeling hot, or palpitations).
- Needed immunizations should be brought up to date before beginning therapy with vedolizumab.
- Report promptly to prescriber S&S of an infection (e.g., sinus infection, fever, cough, bronchitis, flu-like symptoms).
- Report to prescriber if you develop S&S of liver damage (e.g., tiredness, loss of appetite, pain on the right side of abdomen, dark urine, or yellowing of the skin and eyes).
- If you are pregnant or plan to become pregnant, immediately consult prescriber.
- Do not breast-feed while taking this drug without consulting prescriber.

## VENLAFAXINE ℗

(ven-la-fax′een)
Effexor, Effexor XR

## DESVENLAFAXINE

Khedezla, Pristiq

**Classifications:** ANTIDEPRESSANT; SEROTONIN NOREPINEPHRINE REUPTAKE INHIBITOR (SNRI)
Therapeutic: ANTIDEPRESSANT; SNRI

**AVAILABILITY** Tablet; sustained release capsule; extended release tablet. **Desvenlafaxine:** Extended release tablet

## ACTION & *THERAPEUTIC EFFECT*
Potent inhibitor of neuronal serotonin and norepinephrine reuptake. *Antidepressant effect presumed to be due to potentiation of neurotransmitter activity in the CNS.*

**USES** Depression, generalized anxiety disorder; premenstrual dysphoric disorder; social anxiety disorder.

**UNLABELED USES** Diabetic neuropathy, migraine prevention, obsessive-compulsive disorder, hot flashes.

**CONTRAINDICATIONS** Hypersensitivity to venlafaxine, desvenlafaxine, or other SNRI drugs; concurrent administration with MAO inhibitors or within 14 days of last dose; initiation in patients receiving linezolid or IV methylene blue; abrupt discontinuation; treatment for bipolar depression; serotonin syndrome symptoms; hyponatremia; suicidal ideation; lactation.

**CAUTIOUS USE** Renal and hepatic impairment, renal failure; anorexia nervosa, history of mania or other psychiatric disorders, history of suicidal tendencies or increase in suicidality especially in individuals younger than 24 y; elevated intraocular pressure, acute closed-angle glaucoma; cardiac disorders, recent MI, heart failure; hypertension; hyperthyroidism; CNS depression; history of seizures or seizure disorders; volume depleted individuals; hypertriglycerides; risk factors for interstitial lung disease; older adults; pregnancy (category C). Safety in children younger than 18 y not established.

## ROUTE & DOSAGE

**Depression**

*Adult:* **PO Immediate release** 75 mg/day in 2–3 divided doses; **Extended release** 75 mg daily; **Desvenlafaxine:** 50 mg daily, may increase dose (max: 400 mg/day)

**Anxiety**

*Adult:* **PO Sustained release** Start with 75 mg daily and increase q4days (max: 225 mg/day)

**Social Anxiety Disorder**

*Adult:* **PO** 75 mg daily

***Renal Impairment Dosage Adjustment***

**Venlafaxine:** *CrCl 10–70 mL/min:* Reduce total daily dose by 25–50%, *less than 10 mL/min:* Reduce total daily dose by 50%; **Desvenlafaxine:** *CrCl 3–50 mL/min:* Max dose 50 mg/day; *less than 30 mL/min:* Max dose: 50 mg every other day

***Pharmacogenetic Dosage Adjustment***

*Poor CYP2D6 metabolizer:* Start with 70% of dose

## ADMINISTRATION
### Oral
- Give with food. Extended-release *capsules* **must be** swallowed whole or carefully opened and sprinkled on a spoonful of applesauce. The applesauce mixture should be swallowed without chewing and followed with a glass of water. Extended release *tablets* should be swallowed whole and not divided, crushed, or chewed.
- Dosage increments of up to 75 mg/day are usually made at 4 days or longer intervals.

---

Common adverse effects in *italic*; life-threatening effects underlined; generic names in **bold**; classifications in SMALL CAPS; ✦ Canadian drug name; ● Prototype drug

V

- Allow 14 days interval after discontinuing an MAO inhibitor before starting venlafaxine or desvenlafaxine.
- Do not abruptly withdraw drug after 1 wk or more of therapy.
- Store at room temperature, 15°–30° C (59°–86° F).

## ADVERSE EFFECTS (≥1%) CV: *Increased blood pressure and heart rate*, palpitations. CNS: *Dizziness*, fatigue, headache, anxiety, *insomnia, somnolence,* suicidality. Endocrine: Small but statistically significant increase in serum cholesterol, weight loss (approximately 3 lb). GI: *Nausea, vomiting, dry mouth,* constipation, anorexia. Urogenital: Sexual dysfunction, erectile failure, delayed orgasm, anorgasmia, impotence, abnormal ejaculation. Special Senses: Blurred vision. Body as a Whole: *Sweating,* asthenia, Stevens–Johnson syndrome.

## DIAGNOSTIC TEST INTERFERENCE

False positive *urine drug screen* may occur for amphetamine or phencyclidine; use alternative tests to confirm results.

## INTERACTIONS Drug: Cimetidine, MAO INHIBITORS, desipramine, haloperidol may increase levels and toxicity. Should not use in combination with MAO INHIBITORS: Do not start until greater than 14 days after stopping MAO INHIBITOR; do not start MAO INHIBITOR until 7 days after stopping venlafaxine/desvenlafaxine. Trazodone may lead to serotonin syndrome. Avoid use with agents that increase QT interval (e.g., dofetilide, dronedarone, posaconazole, voriconazole, ziprasidone). Herbal: St. John's wort, sour date nut may cause serotonin syndrome.

## PHARMACOKINETICS Absorption: Well absorbed from GI tract. Onset: 2 wk. Peak: Venlafaxine 1–2 h; metabolite 3–4 h. Duration: Extensively tissue bound. Metabolism: Undergoes substantial first-pass metabolism to its major active metabolite (CYP2D6, CYP3A4). Elimination: ~60% in urine as parent compound and metabolites. Half-Life: Venlafaxine 3–4 h, desvenlafaxine ~11 h.

## NURSING IMPLICATIONS

### Black Box Warning

*Venlafaxine has been associated with increased risk of suicidal thinking and behavior.*

### Assessment & Drug Effects

- Monitor for worsening of depression or emergence of suicidal ideation.
- Monitor cardiovascular status periodically with measurements of HR and BP.
- Monitor neurologic status and report excessive anxiety, nervousness, and insomnia.
- Monitor weight periodically and report excess weight loss.
- Assess safety, as dizziness and sedation are common.
- Monitor lab tests: Periodic lipid profile.

### Patient & Family Education

- Be aware of potential adverse effects and notify prescriber of those that are bothersome.
- Report promptly worsening mental status, especially thoughts of suicide.
- Do not drive or engage in potentially hazardous activities until response to drug is known.
- Avoid using alcohol while on venlafaxine.
- Do not use herbal medications without consulting prescriber.

V

Common adverse effects in *italic;* life-threatening effects <u>underlined;</u> generic names in **bold;** classifications in SMALL CAPS; ♣ Canadian drug name; ● Prototype drug

# VERAPAMIL HYDROCHLORIDE ⓟ

(ver-ap'a-mill)

Calan, Calan SR, Covera-HS, Isoptin SR, Verelan, Verelan PM

**Classifications:** CALCIUM CHANNEL BLOCKER; ANTIHYPERTENSIVE; CLASS IV ANTIARRHYTHMIC

Therapeutic: CLASS IV ANTIARRHYTHMIC; ANTIHYPERTENSIVE; ANTIANGINAL

**AVAILABILITY** Tablet; sustained release tablet; sustained release capsule; solution for injection

## ACTION & *THERAPEUTIC EFFECT*

Inhibits calcium ion influx through slow channels into cells of myocardial and arterial smooth muscle. Dilates coronary arteries and arterioles and inhibits coronary artery spasm. Decreases and slows SA and AV node conduction without affecting normal arterial action potential or intraventricular conduction. Dilates peripheral arterioles, causing decreased total peripheral resistance, and this results in lowering the BP. *Decreases angina attacks by dilating coronary arteries and inhibiting coronary vasospasms. Decreases nodal conduction, resulting in an antiarrhythmic effect. Decreased total peripheral vascular resistance; and therefore, reduction in BP.*

**USES** Supraventricular tachyarrhythmias; Prinzmetal's (variant) angina, chronic stable angina; unstable, crescendo or preinfarctive angina and essential hypertension.

**UNLABELED USES** Paroxysmal supraventricular tachycardia, atrial fibrillation; prophylaxis of migraine headache; and as alternate therapy in manic depression.

**CONTRAINDICATIONS** Severe hypotension (systolic less than 90 mm Hg), cardiogenic shock, cardiomegaly, digitalis toxicity, second- or third-degree AV block; Wolff–Parkinson–White syndrome including atrial flutter and fibrillation; accessory AV pathway, severe left ventricular dysfunction, severe CHF, sinus node disease, sick sinus syndrome (except in patients with functioning ventricular pacemaker); lactation.

**CAUTIOUS USE** Duchenne's muscular dystrophy; hepatic and renal impairment; mild to moderate left ventricular heart failure; MI followed by coronary occlusion, aortic stenosis; MG; Duchenne muscular dystrophy; GI obstruction, GERD, hiatal hernia, ileus; older adults; pregnancy (category C). **Extended release:** Safe use in children younger than 18 y not established.

## ROUTE & DOSAGE

### Angina

*Adult:* **PO** 80 mg q6–8h, may increase up to 320–480 mg/day in divided doses (Note: **Covera-HS must be** given once daily at bedtime)

### Hypertension

*Adult:* **PO Immediate release** 80 mg t.i.d.; **Sustained release tablet** 180 mg daily may increase to 240 mg daily (Note: Covera-HS **must be** given once daily at bedtime); **Sustained release capsule** 240 mg daily may adjust to response

### Supraventricular Tachycardia, Atrial Fibrillation

*Adult/Adolescent (15 y or older):* **IV** 5–10 mg after 30 min may give 10 mg (max total dose: 20 mg)

---

Common adverse effects in *italic;* life-threatening effects underlined; generic names in **bold;** classifications in SMALL CAPS; ♣ Canadian drug name; ⓟ Prototype drug

V

*Child/Adolescent (younger than 15 y):* **IV** 0.1–0.3 mg/kg (do not exceed 5 mg)
*Infant:* **IV** 0.1–0.2 mg/kg may repeat after 30 min

**Renal Impairment Dosage Adjustment**

*CrCl less than 10 mL/min:* Give 50–75% of dose

**Hemodialysis Dosage Adjustment**

Supplemental dose not necessary

**Hepatic Impairment Dosage Adjustment**

*Cirrhosis:* Use 20–50% of normal dose

## ADMINISTRATION

### Oral
- Give with food to reduce gastric irritation.
- Capsules can be opened and contents sprinkled on food. **Do not** dissolve or chew capsule contents.
- Do not withdraw abruptly; may increase and extend duration of pain in the angina patient.

### Intravenous

*PREPARE:* **IV Direct:** Given undiluted or diluted in 5 mL of sterile water for injection. ▪ Inspect parenteral drug preparation before administration. Make sure solution is clear and colorless.
*ADMINISTER:* **Direct:** Give a single dose over 2–3 min.
*INCOMPATIBILITIES:* **Solution/additive: Albumin, aminophylline, amphotericin B, hydralazine, trimethoprim/sulfamethoxazole. Y-site: Acyclovir, albumin, amphotericin B cholesteryl complex, ampicillin, azathioprine, cefperazone, ceftazidime, chloramphenicol, dantrolene, diazepam, diazoxide, ertapenem, fluorouracil, folic acid, foscarnet, ganciclovir, indomethacin, lansoprazole, nafcillin, oxacillin, pantoprazole, pentobarbital, phenobarbital, phenytoin, piperacillin/tazobactam, propofol, sodium bicarbonate, SMZ/TMP, thiotepa, tigecycline.**

▪ Store at 15°–30° C (59°–86° F) and protect from light.

## ADVERSE EFFECTS (≥1%)
**CNS:** Dizziness, vertigo, *headache,* fatigue, sleep disturbances, depression, syncope. **CV:** *Hypotension,* congestive heart failure, bradycardia, severe tachycardia, peripheral edema, <u>AV block</u>. **GI:** Nausea, abdominal discomfort, *constipation,* elevated liver enzymes. **Body as a Whole:** Flushing, <u>pulmonary edema</u>, muscle fatigue, diaphoresis. **Skin:** Pruritus. **Respiratory:** Pharyngitis, sinusitus.

## DIAGNOSTIC TEST INTERFERENCE
May cause false positive for ***urine screen*** detection of **methadone**.

## INTERACTIONS
**Drug:** BETA-BLOCKERS increase risk of CHF, bradycardia, or heart block; significantly increased levels of **digoxin** and **carbamazepine** and toxicity; potentiates hypotensive effects of HYPOTENSIVE AGENTS; levels of **lithium** and **cyclosporine** may be increased, increasing their toxicity; **calcium salts** (IV) may antagonize verapamil effects. **Food:** Grapefruit juice may increase verapamil levels. **Herbal:** Hawthorn may have additive hypotensive effects. **St. John's wort** may decrease efficacy.

## PHARMACOKINETICS
**Absorption:** 90% absorbed, but only 25–30% reaches systemic circulation (first pass metabolism). **Peak:** 1–2 h PO; 4–8 h sustained release; 5 min IV. **Distribution:** Widely distributed, including CNS; crosses placenta; present in breast milk. **Metabolism:** In

Common adverse effects in *italic;* life-threatening effects underlined; generic names in **bold;** classifications in SMALL CAPS; ♣ Canadian drug name; ⊙ Prototype drug

**V**

liver (CYP3A4). **Elimination:** 70% in urine; 16% in feces. **Half-Life:** 2–8 h.

## NURSING IMPLICATIONS

### Assessment & Drug Effects

- Establish baseline data and periodically monitor BP and pulse with oral administration.
- Following IV infusion, instruct patient to remain in recumbent position for at least 1 h after dose is given to diminish subjective effects of transient asymptomatic hypotension that may accompany infusion.
- Monitor for AV block or excessive bradycardia when IV infusion is given concurrently with digitalis.
- Monitor I&O ratio during IV and early oral maintenance therapy. Renal impairment prolongs duration of action, increasing potential for toxicity and incidence of adverse effects. Advise patient to report gradual weight gain and evidence of edema.
- Monitor ECG continuously during IV administration. Essential because drug action may be prolonged and incidence of adverse reactions is highest during IV administration in older adults, patients with impaired kidney function, and patients of small stature.
- Check BP shortly before administration of next dose to evaluate degree of control during early treatment for hypertension.
- Monitor lab tests: Baseline and periodic LFTs and renal function tests.

### Patient & Family Education

- Monitor radial pulse before each dose, notify prescriber of an irregular pulse or one slower than established guideline.
- Do not drive or engage in potentially hazardous activities until response to drug is known.
- Decrease intake of caffeine-containing beverage (i.e., coffee, tea, chocolate).

- Change positions slowly from lying down to standing to prevent falls because of drug-related vertigo until tolerance to reduced BP is established.
- Notify prescriber of easy bruising, petechiae, unexplained bleeding.
- Do not use OTC drugs, especially aspirin, unless they are specifically prescribed by prescriber.

## VILAZODONE

(vil-az'oh-done)

Vibryd

**Classifications:** SELECTIVE SEROTONIN REUPTAKE INHIBITOR (SSRI); PSYCHOTHERAPEUTIC AGENT; ANTIDEPRESSANT

Therapeutic: ANTIDEPRESSANT; SSRI

**Prototype:** Fluoxetine

### AVAILABILITY Tablet

### ACTION & THERAPEUTIC EFFECT

A selective serotonin reuptake inhibitor (SSRI). Antidepressant effect is presumed to be linked to inhibition of CNS neuronal uptake of the neurotransmitter, serotonin. *Improves mood in those with major depressive disorder.*

### USES Treatment of major depressive disorder.

### CONTRAINDICATIONS Concomitant use of MAOIs or MAOIs within the preceding 14 days; suicidal ideation.

### CAUTIOUS USE History of suicidal thoughts; potential precursors to suicidal impulses (e.g., anxiety, agitation, panic attacks, insomnia, irritability, hostility, aggressiveness, impulsivity, psychomotor restlessness, hypomania, mania); history of seizure disorder; concurrent use of NSAIDs, aspirin, or other drugs that affect coagulation or bleeding; pregnancy (category C);

V

Common adverse effects in *italic;* life-threatening effects <u>underlined</u>; generic names in **bold;** classifications in SMALL CAPS; ♣ Canadian drug name; ● Prototype drug

1697

lactation. Safety and efficacy in children younger than 18 y not established.

## ROUTE & DOSAGE

### Major Depressive Disorder

*Adult:* **PO** Initial dose of 10 mg once daily for 7 days, increase to 20 mg once daily for 7 days, then to 40 mg once daily

## ADMINISTRATION

### Oral

- Give with food to enhance absorption.
- Store at 15°–30° C (59°–86° F).

## ADVERSE EFFECTS (≥1%) **Body as a Whole:** Arthralgia, decreased appetite, feeling jittery, increased appetite. **CNS:** Abnormal dreams, akathisia, *dizziness*, fatigue, insomnia, libido decreased, migraine, abnormal orgasm, paresthesia, restless leg syndrome, restlessness, sedation, somnolence, tremor, <u>suicidality</u>. **CV:** Palpitations. **GI:** *Diarrhea*, dry mouth, dyspepsia, flatulence, gastroenteritis, *nausea*, vomiting. **Skin:** Hyperhidrosis, night sweats. **Special Senses:** Blurred vision, dry eye. **Urogenital:** Delayed ejaculation, erectile dysfunction.

## INTERACTIONS **Drug:** Inducers of CYP3A4 (e.g., **phenytoin**) may reduce the levels of vilazodone. Coadmination or moderate (e.g., **erythromycin**) and strong (e.g., **ketoconazole**) increase the levels of vilazodone and require a dosage reduction to 20 mg once daily. MONO-AMINE OXIDASE INHIBITORS increase the levels of vilazodone and should not be used in combination with vilazodone. Coadministration of serotonergic agents (e.g, **busipirone, tramadol, thyptophan,** SELECTIVE SEROTONIN REUPTAKE INHIBITORS, SEROTONIN–NOREPINEPHRINE REUPTAKE INHIBITORS, TRIPTANS) increase the risk of serotonin syndrome. Vilazodone can increase the risk of bleeding if used in combination with **aspirin** or NSAIDs. **Food:** Ingestion of food enhances the absorption of vilazodone.

## PHARMACOKINETICS **Absorption:** Bioavailability 72%. **Peak:** 4–5 h. **Distribution:** 96–99% plasma protein bound. **Metabolism:** Hepatic oxidative metabolism (CYP3A4). **Elimination:** Renal and fecal. **Half-Life:** 25 h.

## NURSING IMPLICATIONS

### Black Box Warning

*Vilazodone has been associated with increased risk of suicidal thinking and behavior.*

### Assessment & Drug Effects

- Monitor closely and report promptly any of the following: Worsening of clinical symptoms; emergence of suicidal ideation; agitation, irritability, or unusual changes in behavior; signs of serotonin syndrome or neuroleptic malignant syndrome (see Appendix F).
- Supervise patients closely who are high suicide risks; be especially vigilant for changes in behavior and suicidal ideation in children and adolescents.
- Monitor those at risk for volume depletion (e.g., diuretics use) for S&S of hyponatremia.
- Monitor lab tests: Periodic serum sodium.

### Patient & Family Education

- Report promptly worsening of condition, suicidal thoughts or thoughts of self-harm.
- Do not abruptly stop taking this drug without consulting prescriber.

V

- Notify prescriber if you become pregnant or intend to breast-feed.
- Do not drive or engage in other hazardous activities until response to drug is known.
- Consult prescriber prior to using nonsteroidal anti-inflammatory drugs (NSAIDs), aspirin, or other drugs that affect coagulation.

## VINBLASTINE SULFATE

(vin blast'cen)

**Classifications:** ANTINEOPLASTIC; MITOTIC INHIBITOR; VINCA ALKALOID
Therapeutic: ANTINEOPLASTIC
**Prototype:** Vincristine

**AVAILABILITY** Intravenous solution

**ACTION & *THERAPEUTIC EFFECT***
Cell cycle–specific drug that interferes with microtubules that form mitotic spindle fibers required to complete the process of mitosis. Has an effect on cell energy production needed for mitosis and interferes with nucleic acid synthesis. *Interrupts the cell cycle in metaphase, thus preventing cell replication and cancer cell proliferation.*

**USES** Palliative treatment of Hodgkin's disease and non-Hodgkin's lymphomas, choriocarcinoma, lymphosarcoma, neuroblastoma, mycosis fungoides, advanced testicular germinal cell cancer, histiocytosis, and other malignancies resistant to other chemotherapy. Used singly or in combination with other chemotherapeutic drugs.

**CONTRAINDICATIONS** Severe bone marrow suppression, significant granulocytopenia unless it is a result of the disease being treated; bacterial infection, adynamic ileus; older adult patients with cachexia or skin ulcers; men and women of childbearing potential; pregnancy (category D); lactation.

**CAUTIOUS USE** Malignant cell infiltration of bone marrow; leukopenia; obstructive jaundice, hepatic impairment; history of gout; use of small amount of drug for long periods; use in eyes; children.

## ROUTE & DOSAGE

**Antineoplastic**

*Adult:* IV 5.5 to 7.4 mg/m² weekly, dose varies based on protocol and may increase incrementally up to 18.5 mg/m² if tolerated
*Child:* IV 3–6 mg/m², dose varies based on protocol and may increase up to 12.5 mg/m² if tolerated

**Hepatic Impairment Dosage Adjustment**

*Bilirubin 1.5–3 mg/dL:* Reduce dose 50%; *bilirubin over 3 mg/dL:* Reduce dose 75%

## ADMINISTRATION

**Intravenous**

This drug is a cytotoxic agent and caution should be used to prevent any contact with the drug. Follow institutional or standard guidelines for preparation, handling, and disposal of cytotoxic agents.

***PREPARE:* Direct:** Add 10 mL NS to 10 mg of drug to yield 1 mg/mL. Do not use other diluents. ▪ Avoid contact with eyes. Severe irritation and persisting corneal changes may occur. Flush immediately and thoroughly with copious amounts of water. Wash both eyes; do not assume one eye escaped contamination.

V

Common adverse effects in *italic;* life-threatening effects <u>underlined</u>; generic names in **bold**; classifications in SMALL CAPS; ✤ Canadian drug name; ⊘ Prototype drug

1699

***ADMINISTER:* Direct:** Drug is usually injected into tubing of running IV infusion of NS or D5W over period of 1 min. ▪ Stop injection promptly if extravasation occurs. Use applications of moderate heat and local injection of hyaluronidase to help disperse extravasated drug. ▪ Observe injection site for sloughing. ▪ Restart infusion in another vein.

***INCOMPATIBILITIES:* Y-site: Amphotericin B, cefepime, dantrolene, diazepam, furosemide, gemtuzumab, lansoprazole, pantoprazole, phenytoin.**

▪Refrigerate reconstituted solution in tight, light-resistant containers up to 30 days without loss of potency.

## ADVERSE EFFECTS (≥1%) **Body as a Whole:** Fever, weight loss, muscular pains, weakness, parotid gland pain and tenderness, tumor site pain, Raynaud's phenomenon. **CNS:** Mental depression, peripheral neuritis, numbness and paresthesias of tongue and extremities, loss of deep tendon reflexes, headache, convulsions. **GI:** Vesiculation of mouth, stomatitis, pharyngitis, anorexia, *nausea, vomiting,* diarrhea, ileus, abdominal pain, constipation, rectal bleeding, hemorrhagic enterocolitis, bleeding of old peptic ulcer. **Hematologic:** Leukopenia, thrombocytopenia, and anemia. **Skin:** *Alopecia (reversible),* vesiculation, photosensitivity, phlebitis, cellulitis, and sloughing following extravasation (at injection site). **Urogenital:** Urinary retention, *hyperuricemia,* aspermia. **Respiratory:** Bronchospasm.

## INTERACTIONS **Drug: Mitomycin** may cause acute shortness of breath and severe bronchospasm; may decrease **phenytoin** levels; ALFA INTERFERONS, **erythromycin,** **itraconazole** may increase vinblastine toxicity.

## PHARMACOKINETICS **Distribution:** Concentrates in liver, platelets, and leukocytes; poor penetration of blood–brain barrier. **Metabolism:** Partially in liver. **Elimination:** In feces and urine. **Half-Life:** 24 h.

## NURSING IMPLICATIONS

### Black Box Warning

*Vinblastine extravasation has been associated with severe tissue irritation. Vinblastine is fatal if given intrathecally.*

### Assessment & Drug Effects
▪ Monitor for and report promptly unexplained bruising or bleeding.
▪ Adverse reactions seldom persist beyond 24 h with exception of leukopenia, and neurological adverse effects.
▪ Monitor GI adverse effects which may range from nausea and vomiting to severe constipation.
▪ Report promptly if oral mucosa tissue breakdown is noted.
▪ Monitor lab tests: Baseline and periodic CBC with differential and platelet count.

### Patient & Family Education
▪ Be aware that temporary mental depression sometimes occurs on second or third day after treatment begins.
▪ Avoid exposure to infection, injury to skin or mucous membranes, and excessive physical stress.
▪ Report immediately to prescriber development of sore mouth, sore throat, fever, or chills.
▪ Notify prescriber promptly about onset of symptoms of agranulocytosis (see Appendix F). Do not delay seeking appropriate treatment.

# VINCRISTINE SULFATE ⊙

(vin-kris'teen)

Vincasar PFS

**Classifications:** ANTINEOPLASTIC;
MITOTIC INHIBITOR; VINCA ALKALOID
Therapeutic: ANTINEOPLASTIC

**AVAILABILITY** Intravenous solution

**ACTION & *THERAPEUTIC EFFECT***
Cell cycle–specific vinca alkaloid
arrests mitosis at metaphase by inhibition of mitotic spindle function,
thereby inhibiting cell division. *Induction of metaphase arrest in 50%
of cells results in inhibition of cancer cell proliferation.*

**USES** Acute lymphoblastic and
other leukemias, Hodgkin's disease, lymphosarcoma, neuroblastoma, Wilms' tumor, lung and breast
cancers, reticular cell carcinoma,
and osteogenic and other sarcomas.

**UNLABELED USES** Idiopathic
thrombocytopenic purpura, alone
or adjunctively with other antineoplastics, breast cancer, colorectal
cancer, thymoma.

**CONTRAINDICATIONS** Obstructive jaundice; active infection; adynamic ileus; radiation of the liver;
patient with demyelinating form of
Charcot–Marie–Tooth syndrome; men
and women of childbearing potential;
pregnancy (category D); lactation.

**CAUTIOUS USE** Leukopenia;
preexisting neuromuscular or neurologic disease; hypertension; hepatic or biliary tract disease; older
adults; children.

## ROUTE & DOSAGE

### ALL
*Adult:* **IV** 1.4 mg/m² (max: 2 mg/
m²) at weekly intervals

*Child (weight greater than 10 kg):* **IV**
1.5–2 mg/m² at weekly intervals;
*weight less than 10 kg:* 0.05 mg/kg
initial weekly dose, then titrate

### Malignant Glioma/Hodgkin's Disease/non-Hodgkin's Lymphoma
*Adult/Adolescent/Child:* **IV**
1.4 mg/m² on days 1 and 8 every
28 days

### Neuroblastoma
*Child:* **IV** 1 mg/m²/day for
72 h

### Multiple Myeloma
*Adult/Adolescent/Child:* **IV**
0.4 mg/day × 4 days

### *Hepatic Impairment Dosage Adjustment*
*Bilirubin 1.5–3 mg/dL:* Use 50% of
dose; *3–5 mg/dL:* Use 25% of dose;
*greater than 5 mg/dL:* Skip dose

## ADMINISTRATION

### Intravenous

This drug is a cytotoxic agent and
caution should be used to prevent
any contact with the drug. Follow
institutional or standard guidelines for preparation, handling,
and disposal of cytotoxic agents.

**PREPARE: Direct:** No dilution is
required. Administer as supplied.
■ Avoid contact with eyes. Severe
irritation and persisting corneal
changes may occur. Flush immediately and thoroughly with copious amounts of water. Wash both
eyes; do not assume one eye escaped contamination.

**ADMINISTER: Direct:** Drug is usually injected into tubing of running
infusion over a 1 min period.
■ Stop injection promptly if extravasation occurs. Use applications

V

Common adverse effects in *italic*; life-threatening effects <u>underlined</u>; generic names
in **bold**; classifications in SMALL CAPS; ✤ Canadian drug name; ⊙ Prototype drug

1701

of moderate heat and local injection of hyaluronidase to help disperse extravasated drug. ▪ Restart infusion in another vein. Observe injection site for sloughing.

*INCOMPATIBILITIES:* **Y-site: Amphotericin B colloidal, cefepime, diazepam, furosemide, gemtuzumab, idarubicin, lansoprazole, nafcillin, pantoprazole, phenytoin, sodium bicarbonate.**

▪ Store solution in the refrigerator.

## ADVERSE EFFECTS (≥1%) CNS: *Peripheral neuropathy,* neuritic pain, *paresthesias, especially of hands and feet;* foot and hand drop, sensory loss, athetosis, ataxia, loss of deep tendon reflexes, muscle atrophy, dysphagia, weakness in larynx and extrinsic eye muscles, ptosis, diplopia, mental depression. **Special Senses:** Optic atrophy with blindness; transient cortical blindness, ptosis, diplopia, photophobia. **GI:** Stomatitis, pharyngitis, anorexia, nausea, vomiting, diarrhea, abdominal cramps, *severe constipation (upper-colon impaction), paralytic ileus (especially in children),* rectal bleeding; hepatotoxicity. **Urogenital:** Urinary retention, polyuria, dysuria, SIADH (high urinary sodium excretion, hyponatremia, dehydration, hypotension); uric acid nephropathy. **Skin:** Urticaria, rash, *alopecia,* cellulitis and phlebitis following extravasation (at injection site). **Body as a Whole:** Convulsions with hypertension, malaise, fever, headache, pain in parotid gland area, weight loss. **Metabolic:** Hyperuricemia, hyperkalemia. **CV:** Hypertension, hypotension. **Respiratory:** Bronchospasm.

## INTERACTIONS Drug: Mitomycin may cause acute shortness of breath and severe bronchospasm; may decrease **digoxin, phenytoin** levels.

## PHARMACOKINETICS Distribution: Concentrates in liver, platelets, and leukocytes; poor penetration of blood–brain barrier. **Metabolism:** Partially in liver (CYP3A4). **Elimination:** Primarily in feces. **Half-Life:** 10–155 h.

## NURSING IMPLICATIONS

### Black Box Warning

*Vincristine extravasation has been associated with severe tissue irritation. Vincristine is fatal if given intrathecally.*

### Assessment & Drug Effects
▪ Monitor I&O ratio and pattern, BP, and temperature daily.
▪ Monitor respiratory status. Report promptly shortness of breath (bronchospasms) which may occur within minutes or hours of drug infusion.
▪ Be aware that neuromuscular adverse effects, most apt to appear in the patient with preexisting neuromuscular disease, usually disappear after 6 wk of treatment. Children are especially susceptible to neuromuscular adverse effects.
▪ Assess for hand muscular weakness, and check deep tendon reflexes (depression of Achilles reflex is the earliest sign of neuropathy). Also observe for and report promptly: Mental depression, ptosis, double vision, hoarseness, paresthesias, neuritic pain, and motor difficulties.
▪ Provide special protection against infection or injury during leukopenic days.
▪ Avoid use of rectal thermometer or intrusive tubing to prevent injury to rectal mucosa.
▪ Monitor ability to ambulate and supply support as needed.
▪ Start a prophylactic regimen against constipation and paralytic ileus at beginning of treatment

(paralytic ileus is most likely to occur in young children).

- Monitor lab tests: Baseline and periodic CBC with differential; periodic LFTs, CBC with differential, and serum uric acid levels.

**Patient & Family Education**

- Notify prescriber promptly of stomach, bone, or joint pain, and swelling of lower legs and ankles.
- Report changes in bowel habit as soon as manifested.
- Report a steady gain or sudden weight change to prescriber.
- Women should use effective means of contraception during treatment.

# VINORELBINE TARTRATE

(vin-o-rel'been)

Navelbine

**Classifications:** ANTINEOPLASTIC; MITOTIC INHIBITOR; VINCA ALKALOID

Therapeutic: ANTINEOPLASTIC

**Prototype:** Vincristine

**AVAILABILITY** Intravenous solution

**ACTION & THERAPEUTIC EFFECT** A semisynthetic vinca alkaloid with antineoplastic activity. Inhibits polymerization of tubules into microtubules, which disrupts mitotic spindle formation. *Arrests mitosis at metaphase, thereby inhibiting cell division in cancer cells.*

**USES** Non–small-cell lung cancer.

**UNLABELED USES** Breast cancer, ovarian cancer, Hodgkin's disease.

**CONTRAINDICATIONS** Hypersensitivity to vinorelbine, infection; severe bone marrow suppression; granulocyte counts greater than or equal to 1000 cells/mm³; pulmonary toxicity to

drug; constipation, ileus; pregnancy (category D); lactation.

**CAUTIOUS USE** Hypersensitivity to vincristine or vinblastine; leukopenia or other indicator(s) of bone marrow suppression; chickenpox or herpes zoster infection; hepatic insufficiency, severe liver disease; pulmonary disease; preexisting neurologic or neuromuscular disorders; older adults. Safety and efficacy in children not established.

## ROUTE & DOSAGE

### Non–Small-Cell Lung Cancer

*Adult:* **IV** 25–30 mg/m² weekly; may require toxicity adjustment

*Hepatic Impairment Dosage Adjustment*

*Bilirubin 2.1–3 mg/dL:* Use 50% of dose; *greater than 3 mg/dL:* Use 25% of dose

## ADMINISTRATION

**Intravenous**

This drug is a cytotoxic agent and caution should be used to prevent any contact with the drug. Follow institutional or standard guidelines for preparation, handling, and disposal of cytotoxic agents.

**PREPARE: IV Infusion:** *Method One:* Dilute each 10 mg in a syringe with either 2 or 5 mL of D5W or NS to yield 3 mg/mL or 1.5 mg/L, respectively. *Method Two:* Dilute the required dose in an IV bag with D5W, NS, or LR to a final concentration of 0.5–2 mg/mL (e.g., 10 mg diluted in 19 mL yields 0.5 mg/mL).

**ADMINISTER: IV Infusion:** Give diluted solution over 6–10 min into the side port closest to an IV bag

Common adverse effects in *italic;* life-threatening effects underlined; generic names in **bold;** classifications in SMALL CAPS; ♣ Canadian drug name; ⊙ Prototype drug

1703

with free-flowing IV solution; follow by flushing with at least 75–125 mL of IV solution over 10 min. ■ Take every precaution to avoid extravasation. If suspected, discontinue IV immediately and begin in a different site. *INCOMPATIBILITIES:* **Solution/additive: Acyclovir, aminophylline, amphotericin B, ampicillin, cefazolin, cefoperazone, ceforanide, cefotaxime, cefotetan, ceftazidime, ceftriaxone, cefuroxime, fluorouracil, furosemide, ganciclovir, methylprednisolone, mitomycin, piperacillin, sodium bicarbonate, thiotepa.** **Y-site: Acyclovir, allopurinol, aminophylline, amphotericin B, amphotericin B cholesteryl complex, ampicillin, cefazolin, cefepime, cefoperazone, cefotetan, cefoxitin, ceftriaxone, cefuroxime, chloramphenicol, dantrolene, diazepam, fluorouracil, foscarnet, furosemide, ganciclovir, heparin, ketorolac, lansoprazole, methohexital, methylprednisolone, mitomycin, nitroprusside, pantoprazole, phenobarbital, phenytoin, piperacillin, sodium bicarbonate, SMZ/TMP, thiotepa.**

■ Store at 2°–8° C (36°–46° F).

## ADVERSE EFFECTS (≥1%) **CNS:** *Decreased deep tendon reflexes, paresthesia, fatigue, asthenia, peripheral neuropathy,* myalgia, jaw pain. **Hematologic:** *Anemia,* neutropenia, granulocytopenia, thrombocytopenia. **GI:** Paralytic ileus, *constipation, nausea, vomiting, diarrhea,* stomatitis, mucositis, hepatotoxicity *(elevated LFT).* **Body as a Whole:** *Pain on injection,* venous pain, thrombophlebitis, *alopecia,* myalgia, muscle weakness.

## INTERACTIONS **Drug:** Increased severity of granulocytopenia in combination with **cisplatin;** increased risk of acute pulmonary reactions in combination with **mitomycin; paclitaxel** may increase neuropathy.

## PHARMACOKINETICS **Distribution:** 60–80% bound to plasma proteins (including platelets and lymphocytes); sequestered in tissues, especially lung, spleen, liver, and kidney, and released slowly. **Metabolism:** In liver (CYP3A4). **Elimination:** Primarily in bile and feces (50%), 10% in urine. **Half-Life:** 42–45 h.

## NURSING IMPLICATIONS

### Black Box Warning

*Vinorelbine has been associated with severe granulocytopenia and increased risk of infection, and extravasation has been associated with severe local tissue necrosis.*

### Assessment & Drug Effects
■ Withhold drug and notify prescriber if the granulocyte count is less than 1000 cells/mm³.
■ Monitor for neurologic dysfunction including paresthesia, decreased deep tendon reflexes, weakness, constipation, and paralytic ileus.
■ Monitor for S&S of infection, especially during period of granulocyte nadir 7–10 days after dosing.
■ Vincristine lab tests: CBC with differential throughout therapy and on the day of treatment prior to each infusion. Periodic LFTs, kidney functions, and serum electrolytes.

### Patient & Family Education
■ Be aware of potential and inevitable adverse effects.

- Women should use reliable forms of contraception to prevent pregnancy.
- Notify prescriber of distressing adverse effects, especially symptoms of leukopenia (e.g., chills, fever, cough) and peripheral neuropathy (e.g., pain, numbness, tingling in extremities).
- Report changes in bowel habits as soon as manifested.

## VISMODEGIB ℞
(vis-mo-de′gib)
Erivedge
**Classification:** ANTINEOPLASTIC; BIOLOGICAL RESPONSE MODIFIER; SIGNAL TRANSDUCTION INHIBITOR; HEDGEHOG PATHWAY INHIBITOR
Therapeutic: ANTINEOPLASTIC

### AVAILABILITY Capsule

### ACTION & THERAPEUTIC EFFECT
Inhibits the Hedgehog pathway which is needed to produce angiogenic factors and decrease activity of apoptotic genes that allow for tumor expansion. *Slow basal cell tumor growth and development.*

### USES Treatment of adults with metastatic basal cell carcinoma, or locally advanced basal cell carcinoma.

### CONTRAINDICATIONS Pregnancy (category D); lactation.

### CAUTIOUS USE Renal and hepatic impairment; females of reproductive age. Safety and efficacy in children younger than 18 y not established.

### ROUTE & DOSAGE

| Basal Cell Carcinoma |
| --- |
| *Adult:* **PO** 150 mg once daily |

### ADMINISTRATION
**Oral**
- May be given without regard to food.
- Ensure that capsules are swallowed whole. They should not be opened or crushed.
- Store at 15°–30° C (59°–86° F).

### ADVERSE EFFECTS (≥10%) **Body as a Whole:** *Alopecia,* fatigue. **GI:** Ageusia, constipation, diarrhea, *dysgeusia, nausea,* vomiting. **Metabolic:** Azotemia, decreased appetite, hypokalemia, hyponatremia, *weight loss.* **Musculoskeletal:** Arthralgias, *muscle spasms.*

### INTERACTIONS **Drug:** Coadministration with drugs that inhibit P-glycoprotein (e.g., **clarithromycin, erythromycin, azithromycin**) may increase the levels of vismodegib. Drugs that alter the pH of the upper GI tract (e.g., PROTON PUMP INHIBITORS, H₂-RECEPTOR ANTAGONISTS, and ANTACIDS) may decrease the bioavailability of vismodegib.

### PHARMACOKINETICS **Absorption:** 32% bioavailability. **Distribution:** Greater than 99% plasma protein bound. **Metabolism:** In the liver. **Elimination:** Primarily fecal (82%). **Half-Life:** 4 days.

### NURSING IMPLICATIONS

| Black Box Warning |
| --- |
| *Vismodegib has been associated with embryo-fetal death and severe birth defects.* |

#### Assessment & Drug Effects
- Ensure that women and men understand the risks associated with fetal exposure to this drug during a pregnancy. Advise males of the potential risk of vismodegib exposure through semen.

V

Common adverse effects in *italic;* life-threatening effects underlined; generic names in **bold;** classifications in SMALL CAPS; ♣ Canadian drug name; ⊘ Prototype drug

1705

- Monitor lab tests: Baseline pregnancy test within 7 d before start of therapy; repeat pregnancy test anytime the possibility of a pregnancy arises.

**Patient & Family Education**
- If a dose is missed, skip the dose and wait for the next scheduled dose.
- Women should use a highly effective means of birth control during therapy and for at least 7 mo following completion of therapy. Contact your prescriber immediately if you become pregnant during treatment.
- Men (even those with a vasectomy) should always use a condom with a spermicide during sex with female partners during treatment and for 2 mo following completion of therapy. Report to prescriber immediately if your partner becomes pregnant or thinks she is pregnant while you are taking this drug.
- Do not breast-feed while receiving this drug.

---

# VITAMIN A
(vye′ta-min A)
Aquasol A, Del-Vi-A
**Classification:** VITAMIN SUPPLEMENT
Therapeutic: VITAMIN A REPLACEMENT

**AVAILABILITY** Tablet; capsule; solution for injection

**ACTION & *THERAPEUTIC* EFFECT**
Acts as a cofactor in mucopolysaccharide synthesis, cholesterol synthesis, and the metabolism of hydroxysteroids. *Essential for normal growth and development of bones and teeth, for integrity of epithelial and mucosal surfaces, and for synthesis of visual purple necessary for visual adaptation to the dark. Has antioxidant properties.*

**USES** Vitamin A deficiency and as dietary supplement during periods of increased requirements, such as pregnancy, lactation, infancy, and infections. Used during fat malabsorption diagnosis, ichthyosis, keratosis follicularis, measles.

**CONTRAINDICATIONS** History of sensitivity to vitamin A, hypervitaminosis A, oral administration to patients with malabsorption syndrome. Safe use in amounts exceeding 6000 international units during pregnancy (category X if greater than RDA) is not established.

**CAUTIOUS USE** Women on oral contraceptives, hepatic disease, hepatic dysfunction, hepatitis; renal disease; pregnancy (category A within RDA limit); lactation; children, low-birth weight infants.

## ROUTE & DOSAGE

**Severe Deficiency**
*Adult/Child (8 y or older):* **PO** 500,000 international units/day for 3 days followed by 50,000 international units/day for 2 wk, then 10,000–20,000 international units/day for 2 mo; **IM** 100,000 international units/day for 3 days followed by 50,000 international units/day for 2 wk
*Child (younger than 1 y):* **PO/IM** 7500–15,000 international units/day for 10 days; *1–8 y:* 17,000–35,000 international units/day for 2 wk

**Dietary Supplement**
*Child (younger than 4 y):* **PO** 300 mcg/day; *4–8 y:* 400 mcg/day

---

Common adverse effects in *italic;* life-threatening effects underlined; generic names in **bold;** classifications in SMALL CAPS; ♣ Canadian drug name; ⊙ Prototype drug

## ADMINISTRATION

### Oral

- Give on an empty stomach or following food or milk if GI upset occurs.
- Store in tight, light-resistant containers.

### Intramuscular

- Use IM route only if oral route not feasible.
- Inject deeply into a large muscle.

## ADVERSE EFFECTS (≥1%) CNS:
Irritability, headache, intracranial hypertension (pseudotumor cerebri), increased intracranial pressure, bulging fontanelles, papilledema, exophthalmos, miosis, nystagmus. **Metabolic:** Hypervitaminosis A syndrome (malaise, lethargy, abdominal discomfort, anorexia, vomiting), hypercalcemia. **Musculoskeletal:** Slow growth; deep, tender, hard lumps (subperiosteal thickening) over radius, tibia, occiput; migratory arthralgia; retarded growth; premature closure of epiphyses. **Skin:** Gingivitis, lip fissures, excessive sweating, drying or cracking of skin, pruritus, increase in skin pigmentation, massive desquamation, brittle nails, alopecia. **Urogenital:** Hypomenorrhea. **GI:** Hepatosplenomegaly, jaundice. **Endocrine:** Polydipsia, polyuria. **Hematologic:** Leukopenia, hypoplastic anemias, vitamin A plasma levels greater than 1200 international units/dL, elevations of sedimentation rate and prothrombin time. **Body as a Whole:** Anaphylaxis, death (after IV use).

## DIAGNOSTIC TEST INTERFERENCE
Vitamin A may falsely increase *serum cholesterol* determinations *(Zlatkis-Zak reaction);* may falsely elevate *bilirubin* determination (with *Ehrlich's reagent*).

## INTERACTIONS Drug: Mineral oil, cholestyramine, orlistat may decrease absorption of vitamin A.

## PHARMACOKINETICS Absorption: Readily from GI tract in presence of bile salts, pancreatic lipase, and dietary fat. **Distribution:** Stored mainly in liver; small amounts also found in kidney and body fat; distributed into breast milk. **Metabolism:** In liver. **Elimination:** In feces and urine.

## NURSING IMPLICATIONS

### Assessment & Drug Effects

- Take dietary and drug history (e.g., intake of fortified foods, dietary supplements, self-administration or prescription drug sources). Women taking oral contraceptives tend to have significantly higher plasma vitamin A levels.
- Monitor therapeutic effectiveness. Vitamin A deficiency is often associated with protein malnutrition as well as other vitamin deficiencies. It may manifest as night blindness, restriction of growth and development, epithelial alterations, susceptibility to infection, abnormal dryness of skin, mouth, and eyes (xerophthalmia) progressing to keratomalacia (ulceration and necrosis of cornea and conjunctiva), and urinary tract calculi.

### Patient & Family Education

- Avoid use of mineral oil while on vitamin A therapy.
- Notify prescriber of symptoms of overdosage (e.g., nausea, vomiting, anorexia, drying and cracking of skin or lips, headache, loss of hair).

## VITAMIN B₁
See Thiamine HCl.

## VITAMIN B₂
See Riboflavin.

Common adverse effects in *italic;* life-threatening effects underlined; generic names in **bold;** classifications in SMALL CAPS; ♣ Canadian drug name; ◉ Prototype drug

1707

## VITAMIN B₃
See Niacin.

## VITAMIN B₆
See Pyridoxine.

## VITAMIN B₉
See Folic acid.

## VITAMIN B₁₂
See Cyanocobalamin.

## VITAMIN B₁₂A
See Hydroxocobalamin.

## VITAMIN C
See Ascorbic acid.

## VITAMIN D
See Calcitriol, Ergocalciferol.

## VITAMIN E (TOCOPHEROL)
(vit′a-min E)

Aquasol E, Vita-Plus E, Vitec

**Classification:** VITAMIN SUPPLEMENT
Therapeutic: VITAMIN E
SUPPLEMENT

**AVAILABILITY** Tablet; capsule; liquid

**ACTION & *THERAPEUTIC EFFECT***
An antioxidant, it prevents peroxidation, a process that gives rise to free radicals (highly reactive chemical structures that damage cell membranes and alter nuclear proteins). *Prevents cell membrane and protein damage, protects against blood clot formation by decreasing platelet aggregation, enhances vitamin A utilization, and promotes normal growth, development, and tone of muscles.*

**USES** To treat and prevent hemolytic vitamin E deficiency; for the treatment of familial hypocholesterolemia. Also used topically for dry or chapped skin and minor skin disorders.

**UNLABELED USES** Muscular dystrophy and a number of other conditions with no conclusive evidence of value. A component of many multivitamin formulations and of topical deodorant preparations as an antioxidant.

**CONTRAINDICATIONS** Bleeding disorders; thrombocytopenia.

**CAUTIOUS USE** Large doses may exacerbate iron deficiency anemia; pregnancy (category A within RDA); children.

## ROUTE & DOSAGE

**Vitamin E Deficiency**
*Adult:* **PO** 60–75 international units/day
*Child:* **PO** 1 international unit/kg/day

**Prophylaxis for Vitamin E Deficiency**
*Adult:* **PO** 12–15 international units/day
*Child:* **PO** 7–10 international units/day
*Neonate:* **PO** 5 international units/day

**Familial Hypocholesterolemia**
*Child/Infant:* **PO** 50 international units/kg/day

## ADMINISTRATION
**Oral**
- Give on an empty stomach or following food or milk if GI upset occurs.
- Ensure that capsules are swallowed whole. They should not be crushed or chewed.

V

- Store in tight containers protected from light.

**ADVERSE EFFECTS** (≥1%) **Body as a Whole:** Skeletal muscle weakness, headache, fatigue (with excessive doses). **GI:** Nausea, diarrhea, intestinal cramps. **Urogenital:** Gonadal dysfunction. **Metabolic:** Increased serum creatine kinase, cholesterol, triglycerides; decreased serum thyroxine and triiodothyronine; increased urinary estrogens, androgens; creatinuria. **Skin:** Sterile abscess, thrombophlebitis, contact dermatitis. **Special Senses:** Blurred vision.

**INTERACTIONS Drug: Mineral oil, cholestyramine** may decrease absorption of vitamin E; may enhance anticoagulant activity of **warfarin.** Avoid use with **amprenavir, tipranavir** due to increased risk of bleeding.

**PHARMACOKINETICS Absorption:** 20–60% absorbed from GI tract if fat absorption is normal; enters blood via lymph. **Distribution:** Stored mainly in adipose tissue; crosses placenta. **Metabolism:** In liver. **Elimination:** Primarily in bile.

**NURSING IMPLICATIONS**

**Patient & Family Education**
- Natural sources of vitamin E are found in wheat germ (the richest source) as well as in vegetable oils (sunflower, corn, soybean, cottonseed), green leafy vegetables, nuts, dairy products, eggs, cereals, meat, and liver.

## VORAPAXAR
(vor-a-pax'ar)
Zontivity
**Classifications:** ANTIPLATELET; PROTEASE-ACTIVATED RECEPTOR-1 (PAR-1) ANTAGONIST

**Therapeutic:** PLATELET AGGREGATION INHIBITOR; ANTITHROMBOTIC

**AVAILABILITY** Tablets

**ACTION & *THERAPEUTIC EFFECT*** A reversible antagonist of the protease-activated receptor 1 (PAR-1) expressed on platelets; inhibits platelet aggregation induced by thrombin and thrombin receptor agonist peptide (TRAP). *Reduces the incidence of thrombus formation in those with preexisting risk factors*

**USES** Reduction of thrombotic cardiovascular events in patients with a history of myocardial infarction (MI) or with peripheral arterial disease (PAD).

**CONTRAINDICATIONS** History of stroke, TIA, or intracranial hemorrhage (ICH); active pathological bleeding (e.g., hemorrhage, peptic ulcer bleeding); severe hepatic impairment; lactation.

**CAUTIOUS USE** Any bleeding disorder; concomitant use of drugs that increase the risk for bleeding (e.g., anticoagulants, NSAIDs, SSRIs, SNRIs); depression; mild to moderate hepatic impairment; renal impairment; older adults; pregnancy (category B). Safety and efficacy in children younger than 18 y not established.

**ROUTE & DOSAGE**

| **Thromboembolism Prophylaxis** |
| --- |
| *Adult:* **PO** 2.08 mg once daily |

V

Common adverse effects in *italic;* life-threatening effects underlined; generic names in **bold;** classifications in SMALL CAPS; ♣ Canadian drug name; ⊘ Prototype drug

1709

## ADMINISTRATION

### Oral

- Give without regard to food.
- Store at 15°–30° C (59°–86° F) and protect from moisture.

## ADVERSE EFFECTS (≥1%) CNS:
Depression. **Hematological:** Anemia, hemorrhage. **Metabolic:** Iron deficiency. **Skin:** Eruptions, exanthemas, rash. **Special Senses:** Diplopia, oculomotor disturbances, retinopathy, retinal disorder.

## INTERACTIONS Drug: Strong
inhibitors of CYP3A (e.g., **boceprevir, clarithromycin, conivaptan, indinavir, itraconazole, ketoconazole, nefazodone, nelfinavir, posaconazole, ritonavir, saquinavir, telaprevir, telithromycin**) can increase the levels of vorapaxar and can increase the risk of bleeding if used in combination. Strong inducers of CYP3A (e.g., **carbamazepine, phenytoin, rifampin**) can decrease the levels of vorapaxar. **Herbal: St. John's wort** can decrease the levels of vorapaxar.

## PHARMACOKINETICS Absorption:
100% bioavailable. **Peak:** 1 h. **Distribution:** Greater than 99% plasma protein bound. **Metabolism:** In liver to active and inactive metabolites. **Elimination:** Fecal (58%) and renal (25%). **Half-Life:** 8 days (range 5–13 days).

## NURSING IMPLICATIONS

### Black Box Warning

*Vorapaxar has been associated with an increased risk of bleeding, including fatal bleeding events especially in those with a history of stroke, transient ischemic attack (TIA), or intracranial hemorrhage (ICH).*

### Assessment & Drug Effects

- Monitor for and report immediately S&S of bleeding. There is no antidote for vorapaxar-induced bleeding.
- Monitor closely those with risk factors for bleeding (e.g., older age, low body weight, reduced renal or hepatic function, history of bleeding disorders, and concomitant use of anticoagulants, NSAIDs, SSRIs, and SNRIs).
- Monitor lab test: Periodic Hct and Hgb.

### Patient & Family Education

- Immediately report to prescriber if you experience any of the following: Bleeding that is severe or that you cannot control; pink, red, or brown urine; vomiting blood or your vomit looks like coffee grounds; red or black tarry stools; coughing up blood or blood clots.
- Consult prescriber before taking any new prescription or OTC drugs to determine possible interaction the vorapaxar.

## VORICONAZOLE
(vor-i-con'a-zole)
**Vfend**
**Classifications:** ANTIBIOTIC; AZOLE ANTIFUNGAL
**Therapeutic:** ANTIFUNGAL
**Prototype:** Fluconazole

**AVAILABILITY** Solution for injection; oral suspension

## ACTION & THERAPEUTIC EFFECT
Inhibits fungal cytochrome P450 enzymes used for an essential step in fungal ergosterol biosynthesis. The subsequent loss of ergosterol in the fungal cell wall is thought to be responsible for the antifungal activity. *Voriconazole is active against Aspergillus and Candida.*

Common adverse effects in *italic;* life-threatening effects <u>underlined</u>; generic names in **bold**; classifications in SMALL CAPS; ♣ Canadian drug name; ☻ Prototype drug

**USES** Treatment of invasive aspergillosis, esophageal candidiasis, candidemia in nonneutropenic patients and disseminated skin infections, and abdomen, kidney, bladder wall, and wound infections due to *Candida*.

**CONTRAINDICATIONS** Known hypersensitivity to voriconazole; should be avoided in moderate or severe renal impairment (CrCl less than 50 mL/min) and severe Child-Pugh class C hepatic impairment; development of S&S of hepatic disease in response to voriconazole; history of galactose intolerance; Lapp lactase deficiency or glucose-galactose malabsorption; development of exfoliative cutaneous reaction; sunlight (UV) exposure; pregnancy (category D); lactation.

**CAUTIOUS USE** Mild to moderate hepatic cirrhosis, hepatitis, Child-Pugh class A and B hepatic disease; proarrhythmic conditions; renal disease; mild or moderate renal impairment; ocular disease; hypersensitivity to other azole antifungal agents such as fluconazole. Safety and efficacy in children younger than 12 y not established.

## ROUTE & DOSAGE

**Invasive Aspergillosis**

*Adult/Adolescent:* **IV** 6 mg/kg q12h x 2 doses then 4 mg/kg q12h. Treatment continues until 7–14 days after symptom resolution; *weight greater than 40 kg:* **PO** 200 mg q12h; *weight less than 40 kg:* **PO** 100 mg q12h

**Candidemia**

*Adult:* **IV** 6 mg/kg q12h x 2 doses then 3–4 mg/kg q12h; *weight greater than 40 kg:* **PO** 200 mg q12h may titrate dose; *weight less than 40 kg:*

100 mg q12h, may titrate dose

**Esophageal Candidiasis**

*Adult (weight greater than 40 kg):* **PO** 200 mg q12h for a minimum of 14 days and for at least 7 days after resolution of symptoms (max: 600 mg daily); *weight less than 40 kg:* 100 mg q12h for a minimum of 14 days and for at least 7 days after resolution of symptoms (max: 300 mg daily)

*Drug Interaction Dosage Adjustment*

Needed for concomitant CYP 450 enzyme inducers/substrates. See package insert for specific efavirenz and phenytoin adjustments.

*Renal Impairment Dosage Adjustment*

*CrCl less than 50 mL/min:* Switch to PO therapy after loading dose; hemodialysis does not require supplemental dose

*Hepatic Impairment Dosage Adjustment*

*Child-Pugh class A or B:* Reduce maintenance dose by 50%; *Child-Pugh class C:* Avoid drug use

## ADMINISTRATION

### Oral

- Give at least 1 h before or 1 h following a meal.
- Store tablets at 15°–30° C (59°–86° F).

### Intravenous

**PREPARE: Intermittent:** Use a 20-mL syringe to reconstitute each 200 mg powder vial with exactly 19 mL of sterile water for injection to yield 10 mg/mL.

V

Common adverse effects in *italic;* life-threatening effects underlined; generic names in **bold;** classifications in SMALL CAPS; ✦ Canadian drug name; ⊘ Prototype drug

1711

Discard vial if a vacuum does not pull the diluent into vial. Shake until completely dissolved. ▪ Calculate the required dose of voriconazole based on patient's weight. ▪ From an IV infusion bag of NS, D5W, D5/NS, D5/.45NS, LR or other suitable solution, withdraw and discard a volume of IV solution equal to the required dose. ▪ Inject the required dose of voriconazole into the IV bag. The IV solution should have a final voriconazole concentration of 0.5–5 mg/mL. ▪ Infuse immediately.

*ADMINISTER:* **Intermittent:** Infuse over 1–2 h at a maximum rate of 3 mg/kg/h. ▪ **Do not** give a bolus dose.

*INCOMPATIBILITIES:* **Solution/additive:** Do not dilute with **sodium bicarbonate;** do not mix with any other drugs. **Y-site:** Do not infuse with other drugs.

▪ Store unreconstituted vials at 15°–30° C (59°–86° F).

## ADVERSE EFFECTS (≥1%) **Body as a Whole:** Peripheral edema, *fever,* chills. **CNS:** Headache, *hallucinations,* dizziness, chills. **CV:** <u>Tachycardia</u>, hypotension, hypertension, vasodilation. **GI:** *Nausea,* vomiting, abdominal pain, abnormal LFTs, diarrhea, cholestatic jaundice, dry mouth. **Metabolic:** Increased alkaline phosphatase, AST, ALT, hypokalemia, hypomagnesemia, increased serum creatinine. **Skin:** *Rash,* pruritus. **Special Senses:** *Abnormal vision (enhanced brightness, blurred vision, or color vision changes),* photophobia.

## INTERACTIONS **Drug:** Due to significant increased toxicity or decreased activity, the following drugs are <u>contraindicated</u> with voriconazole: BARBITURATES, **carbamazepine, efavirenz,** ERGOT ALKALOIDS, **pimozide, quinidine, rifabutin, sirolimus; fosphenytoin, phenytoin, rifampin,** Avoid use with CYP3A4 inhibitors (e.g., **atazanavir, itraconazole, ketoconazole, ritonavir**). PROTEASE INHIBITORS (except **indinavir**) may increase voriconazole toxicity; voriconazole may increase the toxicity of BENZODIAZEPINES, **cyclosporine,** NONNUCLEOSIDE REVERSE TRANSCRIPTASE INHIBITORS, **omeprazole, tacrolimus, vinblastine, vincristine, warfarin, fentanyl, oxycodone,** NSAIDS; **Food:** Absorption reduced with high-fat meals. **Herbal: St. John's wort** may decrease efficacy.

## PHARMACOKINETICS **Absorption:** 96% absorbed. Has a nonlinear pharmacokinetic profile, a small change in dose may cause a large change in serum levels. Steady state not achieved until day 5–6 if no loading dose is given. **Peak:** 1–2 h. **Metabolism:** In liver by (and inhibits) CYP3A4, 2C9, and 2C19. **Elimination:** Primarily in urine. **Half-Life:** 6 h–6 days depending on dose.

## NURSING IMPLICATIONS
### Assessment & Drug Effects
▪ Visual acuity, visual field, and color perception should be monitored if treatment continues beyond 28 days.
▪ Withhold drug and notify prescriber if skin rash develops.
▪ Monitor cardiovascular status especially with preexisting CV disease.
▪ Concurrent drugs: Monitor PT/INR closely with warfarin as dose adjustments of warfarin may be needed. Monitor frequently blood glucose levels with sulfonylurea

drugs as reduction in the sulfonylurea dosage may be needed.
Monitor for and report any of the
following: S&S of rhabdomyolysis
in patient receiving a statin drug;
prolonged sedation in patient receiving a benzodiazepine; S&S of
heart block, bradycardia, or CHF
in patient receiving a calcium
channel blocker.
- Monitor lab tests: Baseline and
periodic LFTs; frequent renal function tests; trough serum drug concentrations on day 5 and weekly
thereafter for 4–6 wk; periodic CBC
with platelet count, Hct and Hgb,
serum electrolytes, blood glucose,
and lipid profile.

**Patient & Family Education**
- Use reliable means of birth control to prevent pregnancy. If you
suspect you are pregnant, contact
prescriber immediately.
- Do not drive at night while taking
voriconazole as the drug may
cause blurred vision and photophobia.
- Do not drive or engage in other
potentially hazardous activities
until reaction to drug is known.
- Avoid strong, direct sunlight
while taking voriconazole.

## VORTIOXETINE
(vor-ti-ox'e-teen)
Trintellix
**Classifications:** ANTIDEPRESSANT;
SEROTONIN MODULATOR
**Therapeutic:** ANTIDEPRESSANT

**AVAILABILITY** Tablet

**ACTION & THERAPEUTIC EFFECT**
Mechanism of action unknown but
thought to be through inhibition of
the reuptake of serotonin (5-HT),
5-HT3 receptor antagonism,
and 5-HT1A receptor agonism.

*Enhanced serotonergic activity in
the CNS is believed to produce an
antidepressant effect.*

**USES** Treatment of major depressive disorder (MDD).

**CONTRAINDICATIONS** Hypersensitivity to vortioxetine including angioedema; suicidal ideation;
MAOIs within 14 days of starting
vortioxetine or 21 days of stopping
vortioxetine; serotonin syndrome;
symptomatic hyponatremia; severe
hepatic impairment; lactation.

**CAUTIOUS USE** History of suicidal thoughts; history of or family
history of bipolar disorder, mania,
or hypomania; history of bleeding
disorders; history of GI bleeding;
mild to moderate hepatic impairment; older adults; pregnancy
(category C). Safety and efficacy in
children not established.

## ROUTE & DOSAGE

**Major Depressive Disorder**
*Adult.* PO 10 mg once daily; may
increase to 20 mg or decrease to
5 mg as needed or tolerated

*Metabolism Dosage Adjustment*
Use with a strong CYP2D6
inhibitor: Decrease dose by 50%
Use with a strong CYP2D6
inducer: Increase dose up to
3 × normal
Use in patients who are poor
CYP2D6 metabolizers: Maximum
dose is 10 mg once daily

## ADMINISTRATION
**Oral**
- May give without regard to food.
- To avoid adverse reactions, it is
recommended that doses of 15–20

Common adverse effects in *italic;* life-threatening effects underlined; generic names
in **bold;** classifications in SMALL CAPS; ◆ Canadian drug name; ● Prototype drug
1713

mg/day be decreased to 10 mg/day for 1 wk before discontinuation.
▪ Store at 15°–30° C (59°–86° F).

## ADVERSE EFFECTS (≥2%) CNS:
Abnormal abnormal dreams, *dizziness*. **GI:** Constipation, *diarrhea, dry mouth*, flatulence, *nausea*, vomiting. **Metabolic:** Hyponatremia. **Skin:** Pruritus. **Urogenital:** Sexual dysfunction.

## INTERACTIONS Drug:
Coadministration of other drugs that affect serotonin transmission (e.g., SSRIS, SNRIS, MAOIS, TRIPTANS, **buspirone, linezolid, tramadol**) may increase the risk of serotonin syndrome. Strong CYP2D6 inhibitors (e.g., **bupropion, fluoxetine, paroxetine, quinidine**) may increase the levels of vortioxetine. Strong CYP2D6 inducers (e.g., **carbamazepine, phenytoin, rifampin**) may decrease the levels of vortioxetine. **Food:** Tryptophan containing foods may increase the risk of serotonin syndrome.

## PHARMACOKINETICS Absorption:
75% bioavailable. **Peak:** 7–11 h. **Distribution:** 98% plasma protein bound. **Metabolism:** Hepatic oxidation via CYP2D6, CYP3A4/5, CYP2C19, CYP2C9, CYP2A6, CYP2C8, and CYP2B6. **Elimination:** Renal (59%) and fecal (26%). **Half-Life:** 66 h.

## NURSING IMPLICATIONS

### Black Box Warning

*Vortioxetine has been associated with suicidal thinking and behavior in children, adolescents, and young adults.*

### Assessment & Drug Effects
▪ Report immediately to prescriber signs of worsening mental status such as suicidal ideation, aggressiveness, agitation, anxiety, hostility, impulsivity, insomnia, irritability, panic attacks, and worsening of depression.
▪ Monitor for S&S of serotonin syndrome (see Appendix F). If serotonin syndrome is suspected withhold drug, notify prescriber and initiate supportive treatment.
▪ Monitor for and report promptly S&S of hyponatremia (see Appendix F) and any signs of abnormal bleeding.
▪ Monitor lab tests: Baseline LFTs and periodic serum sodium.

### Patient & Family Education
▪ Report promptly to prescribe suicidal ideation or behavior, aggressive or impulsive behavior, worsening depression or anxiety, mania or unusual changes in behavior or mood.
▪ Do not take OTC supplements such as tryptophan or St. John's wort without consulting prescriber.
▪ Inform prescriber if you are taking OTC nonsteroidal anti-inflammatory drugs (NSAIDs) or aspirin for pain relief.
▪ Report promptly any of the following: S&S of serotonin syndrome (see Appendix F); abnormal bleeding; S&S of low serum sodium (see hyponatremia Appendix F).
▪ Notify prescriber immediately if you are or suspect you are pregnant.
▪ Do not breast-feed while taking this drug.

# WARFARIN SODIUM
(war′far-in)

Coumadin, Jantoven, Warfilone ♦

**Classification:** ANTICOAGULANT
Therapeutic: ANTICOAGULANT

## AVAILABILITY Tablet

## ACTION & *THERAPEUTIC EFFECT*
Indirectly interferes with blood clotting by depressing hepatic synthesis of vitamin K-dependent coagulation factors: II, VII, IX, and X. *Deters further extension of existing thrombi and prevents new clots from forming.*

## USES Prophylaxis and treatment
of deep vein thrombosis and its extension, pulmonary embolism; treatment of atrial fibrillation with embolization. Also used as adjunct in treatment of coronary occlusion, cerebral transient ischemic attacks (TIAs), and as a prophylactic in patients with prosthetic cardiac valves; reduce the risk of death, recurrent MI, and thromboembolic events, post MI.

## CONTRAINDICATIONS Hem-
orrhagic tendencies, hemophilia, coagulation factor deficiencies, dyscrasias; active bleeding, open wounds, active peptic ulcer, visceral carcinoma, esophageal varices, malabsorption syndrome, uncontrolled hypertension, cerebral vascular disease; heparin-induced thrombocytopenia (HIT); pericarditis; severe hepatic or renal disease; continuous tube drainage of any orifice; subacute bacterial endocarditis; recent surgery of brain, spinal cord, or eye; regional or lumbar block anesthesia; threatened abortion; unreliable patients; pregnancy (category X).

## CAUTIOUS USE Alcoholism, al-
lergic disorders, during menstruation, senility, psychosis; debilitated patients; CVD; renal impairment; hepatic impairment. Endogenous factors that may increase prothrombin time response (enhance

anticoagulant effect): Carcinoma, CHF, collagen diseases, hepatic and renal insufficiency, diarrhea, fever, pancreatic disorders, malnutrition, vitamin K deficiency. Endogenous factors that may decrease prothrombin time response (decrease anticoagulant response): Edema, hypothyroidism, hyperlipidemia, hypercholesterolemia, chronic alcoholism, hereditary resistance to coumarin therapy; older adults; children.

## ROUTE & DOSAGE

### Anticoagulant
*Adult:* **PO** Usual dose 2–5 mg daily with dose adjusted to maintain a PT 1.2–2 × control or INR of 2–3 (target varies per disease state)

### *Pharmacogenetic Dosage Adjustment*
Variations in CYP2C9 or VKORC1 may require dose adjustments (see package insert for tables)

## ADMINISTRATION
Note: Antidote for bleeding—anticoagulant effect usually is reversed by omitting 1 or more doses of warfarin and by administration of specific antidote phytonadione (vitamin $K_1$) 2.5–10 mg orally. Prescriber may advise patient to carry vitamin $K_1$ at all times, but not to take it until after consultation. If bleeding persists or progresses to a severe level, vitamin K 10 mg IV is given, or a fresh whole blood transfusion may be necessary.

### Oral
- Give tablet whole or crushed with fluid of patient's choice.

## ADVERSE EFFECTS (≥1%) Body as a Whole: Major or minor hemor-

rhage from any tissue or organ; hypersensitivity (dermatitis, urticaria, pruritus, fever). **GI:** Anorexia, nausea, vomiting, abdominal cramps, diarrhea, steatorrhea, stomatitis. **Other:** Increased serum transaminase levels, hepatitis, jaundice, burning sensation of feet, transient hair loss. **Overdosage:** Internal or external bleeding, paralytic ileus; skin necrosis of toes (purple toes syndrome), tip of nose, buttocks, thighs, calves, female breast, abdomen, and other fat-rich areas.

## DIAGNOSTIC TEST INTERFERENCE

Warfarin (coumarins) may cause alkaline urine to be red-orange; may enhance **uric acid** excretion, cause elevation of **serum transaminases,** and may increase **lactic dehydrogenase** activity.

## INTERACTIONS **Drug:** In addition

to the drugs listed below, many other drugs have been reported to alter the expected response to warfarin; however, clinical importance of these reports has not been substantiated. The addition or withdrawal of any drug to an established drug regimen should be made cautiously, with more frequent **INR** determinations than usual and with careful observation of the patient and dose adjustment as indicated. The following may enhance the anticoagulant effects of warfarin: **Acetohexamide, acetaminophen,** ALKYLATING AGENTS, **allopurinol,** AMINOGLYCOSIDES, **aminosalicylic acid, amiodarone,** ANABOLIC STEROIDS, ANTIBIOTICS (ORAL), ANTIMETABOLITES, ANTIPLATELET DRUGS, **aspirin, asparaginase, capecitabine, celecoxib, chloramphenicol, chlorpropamide, chymotrypsin, cimetidine, clofibrate, cotrimoxazole, danazol, dextran, dextrothyroxine, diazoxide, disulfiram,** **erythromycin, ethacrynic acid, fluconazole, glucagons, guanethidine,** HEPATOTOXIC DRUGS, **influenza vaccine, isoniazid, itraconazole, ketoconazole,** MAO INHIBITORS, **meclofenamate, mefenamic acid, methyldopa, methylphenidate, metronidazole, miconazole, mineral oil, nalidixic acid, neomycin (oral),** NONSTEROIDAL ANTI-INFLAMMATORY DRUGS, **oxandrolone, plicamycin,** POTASSIUM PRODUCTS, **propoxyphene, propylthiouracil, quinidine, quinine, rofecoxib, salicylates, streptokinase, sulindac,** SULFONAMIDES, SULFONYLUREAS, TETRACYCLINES, THIAZIDES, THYROID DRUGS, **tolbutamide,** TRICYCLIC ANTIDEPRESSANTS, **urokinase, vitamin E, zileuton.** The following may increase or decrease the anticoagulant effects of warfarin: **Alcohol** (acute intoxication may increase, chronic alcoholism may decrease effects), DIURETICS. The following may decrease the anticoagulant effects of warfarin: BARBITURATES, **carbamazepine, cholestyramine,** CORTICOSTEROIDS, **corticotropin, glutethimide, griseofulvin,** LAXATIVES, **mercaptopurine,** ORAL CONTRACEPTIVES, **rifampin, spironolactone, vitamin C, vitamin K. Herbal:** Boldo, capsicum, celery, chamomile, chondroitin, clove, coenzyme Q10, danshen, devil's claw, dong quai, echinacea, evening primrose oil, fenugreek, feverfew, fish oil, garlic, ginger, ginkgo, glucosamine, horse chestnut, licorice root, passionflower herb, turmeric, willow bark may increase risk of bleeding; ginseng, green tea, seaweed, soy, St. John's wort may decrease effectiveness of warfarin. **Food:** Cranberry juice may increase **INR.** Green leafy vegetables may affect efficacy. **Avocado** may decrease effectiveness of warfarin.

## PHARMACOKINETICS Absorption: Well absorbed from GI tract. **Onset:** 2–7 days. **Peak:** 0.5–3 days. **Distribution:** 97% protein bound; crosses placenta. **Metabolism:** In liver (CYP2C9). **Elimination:** In urine and bile. **Half-Life:** 0.5–3 days.

## NURSING IMPLICATIONS

### Black Box Warning

*Warfarin has been associated with serious, sometimes fatal, bleeding events.*

### Assessment & Drug Effects

- Determine INP prior to initiation of therapy and then daily until maintenance dosage is established.
- Obtain a COMPLETE medication history prior to start of therapy and whenever altered responses to therapy require interpretation; extremely IMPORTANT since many drugs interfere with the activity of anticoagulant drugs (see INTERACTIONS).
- Dose is typically adjusted to maintain an INR of 2–4 depending on diagnosis.
- Note: Patients at greatest risk of hemorrhage include those whose INR is difficult to regulate, who have an aortic valve prosthesis, who are receiving long-term anticoagulant therapy, and older adult and debilitated patients.
- Monitor lab tests: INR prior to initiation of therapy and then daily until maintenance dosage is established. For maintenance dosage, INR determinations at 1–4-wk intervals depending on patient's response; periodic urinalyses, stool guaiac, and LFTs.

### Patient & Family Education

- Understand that bleeding can occur even though INR are within therapeutic range. Stop drug and notify prescriber immediately if bleeding or signs of bleeding appear: Blood in urine, bright red or black tarry stools, vomiting of blood, bleeding with tooth brushing, blue or purple spots on skin or mucous membrane, round pinpoint purplish red spots (often occur in ankle areas), nosebleed, bloody sputum; chest pain; abdominal or lumbar pain or swelling, profuse menstrual bleeding, pelvic pain; severe or continuous headache, faintness or dizziness; prolonged oozing from any minor injury (e.g., nicks from shaving).
- Stop drug and report immediately any symptoms of hepatitis (dark urine, itchy skin, jaundice, abdominal pain, light stools) or hypersensitivity reaction (see Appendix F).
- Take drug at same time each day, and **do not** alter dose.
- Risk of bleeding is increased for up to 1 mo after receiving the influenza vaccine.
- Fever, prolonged hot weather, malnutrition, and diarrhea lengthen INR (enhanced anticoagulant effect).
- A high-fat diet, sudden increase in vitamin K–rich foods (cabbage, cauliflower, broccoli, asparagus, lettuce, turnip greens, onions, spinach, kale, fish, liver), coffee or green tea (caffeine), or by tube feedings with high vitamin K content shorten INR.
- Avoid excess intake of alcohol.
- Use a soft toothbrush and floss teeth gently with waxed floss.
- Use barrier contraceptive measures; if you become pregnant

**W**

Common adverse effects in *italic*; life-threatening effects <u>underlined</u>; generic names in **bold**; classifications in SMALL CAPS; ♣ Canadian drug name; ⊕ Prototype drug

1717

while on anticoagulant therapy the fetus is at great potential risk of congenital malformations.
- Do not take any other prescription or OTC drug unless specifically approved by prescriber or pharmacist.

# XYLOMETAZOLINE HYDROCHLORIDE

(zye-loe-met-az'oh-leen)

Otrivin

**Classifications:** NASAL DECONGESTANT; VASOCONSTRICTOR

Therapeutic: NASAL DECONGESTANT

**Prototype:** Naphazoline

**AVAILABILITY** Nasal solution

## ACTION & *THERAPEUTIC EFFECT*

Markedly constricts dilated arterioles of nasal membrane. *Decreases fluid exudate and mucosal engorgement associated with rhinitis and may open up obstructed eustachian tubes.*

**USES** Temporary relief of nasal congestion associated with common cold, sinusitis, acute and chronic rhinitis, and hay fever and other allergies.

## CONTRAINDICATIONS

Sensitivity to adrenergic substances; angle-closure glaucoma; concurrent therapy with MAO inhibitors or tricyclic antidepressants; pregnancy (category C); lactation.

## CAUTIOUS USE

Hypertension; hyperthyroidism; heart disease, including angina; advanced arteriosclerosis, older adults, pregnancy (category C); children younger than 2 y and infants.

## ROUTE & DOSAGE

### Nasal Congestion

*Adult/Child (12 y or older):* **Nasal** 1–2 sprays or 1–2 drops of 0.1% solution in each nostril q8–10h (max: 3 doses/day)

*Child (2–12 y):* **Nasal** 1 spray or 2–3 drops of 0.05% solution in each nostril q8–10h (max: 3 doses/day)

## ADMINISTRATION

### Instillation

- Have patient clear each nostril gently before administering spray or drops.
- Store at 15°–30° C (59°–86° F) in a tight, light-resistant container.

## ADVERSE EFFECTS (≥1%) All:

Usually mild and infrequent; local stinging, burning, dryness and ulceration, sneezing, headache, insomnia, drowsiness. **With Excessive Use:** *Rebound nasal congestion* and vasodilation, tremulousness, hypertension, palpitations, tachycardia, arrhythmia, somnolence, sedation, <u>coma</u>.

## INTERACTIONS Drug:

May cause increase BP with **guanethidine, methyldopa,** MAO INHIBITORS; PHENOTHIAZINES may decrease effectiveness of nasal decongestant.

## PHARMACOKINETICS

**Onset:** 5–10 min. **Duration:** 5–6 h.

## NURSING IMPLICATIONS

### Assessment & Drug Effects

- Evaluate for development of rebound congestion (see ADVERSE EFFECTS).

### Patient & Family Education

- Prevent contamination of nasal solution and spread of infection by

Common adverse effects in *italic*; life-threatening effects <u>underlined</u>; generic names in **bold**; classifications in SMALL CAPS; ♣ Canadian drug name; ⊗ Prototype drug

X

rinsing dropper and tip of nasal spray in hot water after each use; restrict use to the individual patient.
▪ Note: Prolonged use can cause rebound congestion and chemical rhinitis. **Do not** exceed prescribed dosage and report to prescriber if drug fails to provide relief within 3–4 days.
▪ **Do not** self-medicate with OTC drugs, sprays, or drops without prescriber's approval.
▪ Note: Excessive use by a child may lead to CNS depression.

## ZAFIRLUKAST ℗
(za-fir-lu'kast)
Accolate
**Classifications:** RESPIRATORY SMOOTH MUSCLE RELAXANT; LEUKOTRIENE RECEPTOR ANTAGONIST (LTRA); BRONCHODILATOR
Therapeutic: BRONCHODILATOR; LTRA

### AVAILABILITY Tablet

### ACTION & *THERAPEUTIC EFFECT*
Selective leukotriene receptor antagonist (LTRA) that inhibits binding of leukotriene $D_4$ and $E_4$, thus inhibiting inflammation and bronchoconstriction. Leukotriene production and receptor affinity have been correlated with the pathogenesis of asthma. *Zafirlukast helps to prevent the signs and symptoms of asthma, including airway edema, smooth muscle constriction, and altered cellular activity due to inflammation.*

### USES Prophylaxis and chronic treatment of asthma in adults and children older than 5 y (not for acute bronchospasm).

### UNLABELED USES Chronic urticaria.

### CONTRAINDICATIONS Hypersensitivity to zafirlukast; acute asthma attacks, including status asthmaticus, acute bronchospasm; hepatic impairment including cirrhosis; lactation.

### CAUTIOUS USE Patients 65 y or older, pregnancy (category B); children younger than 5 y.

### ROUTE & DOSAGE

**Asthma**

*Adult/Child (12 y or older):* **PO** 20 mg b.i.d. 1 h before or 2 h after meals
*Child (5 y or older):* **PO** 10 mg b.i.d.

### ADMINISTRATION
**Oral**
▪ Give 1 h before or 2 h after meals.
▪ Store at 20°–25° C (68°–77° F); protect from light and moisture.

### ADVERSE EFFECTS (≥1%) **Body as a Whole:** Generalized pain, asthenia, myalgia, fever, back pain. **CNS:** *Headache,* dizziness. **GI:** Nausea, diarrhea, abdominal pain, vomiting, dyspepsia; liver dysfunction, increased liver function tests, <u>hepatic failure</u>. **Other:** <u>Churg-Strauss syndrome</u> (fever, muscle aches and pains, weight loss).

### INTERACTIONS **Drug:** May increase ***prothrombin time (PT)*** in patients on **warfarin. Erythromycin** decreases bioavailability of zafirlukast. Avoid use with CYP2C8 inhibitors and strong CYP2C9 inhibitors/inducers.

### PHARMACOKINETICS **Absorption:** Rapidly from GI tract, bioavailability

Common adverse effects in *italic;* life-threatening effects <u>underlined</u>; generic names in **bold**; classifications in SMALL CAPS; ♣ Canadian drug name; ℗ Prototype drug

1719  Z

significantly reduced by food. **Onset:** 1 wk. **Peak:** 3 h. **Distribution:** Greater than 99% protein bound; secreted into breast milk. **Metabolism:** In liver (CYP2C9). **Elimination:** 90% in feces, 10% in urine. **Half-Life:** 10 h.

## NURSING IMPLICATIONS

### Assessment & Drug Effects

- Assess respiratory status and airway function regularly.
- Monitor closely phenytoin level with concurrent phenytoin therapy.
- Monitor lab tests: Periodic LFTs, and INR with concurrent warfarin therapy.

### Patient & Family Education

- Taking medication regularly, even during symptom-free periods.
- Note: Drug is not intended to treat acute episodes of asthma.
- Report S&S of hepatic toxicity (see Appendix F) or flu-like symptoms to prescriber. Follow-up lab work is very important.
- Notify prescriber immediately if condition worsens while using prescribed doses of all antiasthmatic medications.

## ZALEPLON
(zal′ep-lon)
Sonata
**Classifications:** SEDATIVE-HYPNOTIC; NONBARBITUATE
**Therapeutic:** SEDATIVE-HYPNOTIC
**Prototype:** Zolpidem
**Controlled Substance:** Schedule IV

## AVAILABILITY Capsule

## ACTION & *THERAPEUTIC EFFECT*

Short-acting nonbenzodiazepine with sedative-hypnotic, muscle relaxant. *Reduces difficulty in initially falling asleep. Preserves deep sleep*

*(stages 3 through 4) at hypnotic dose with minimal-to-absent rebound insomnia when discontinued.*

## USES Short-term treatment of insomnia.

## CONTRAINDICATIONS Hypersensitivity to zaleplon, or tartrazine dye (Yellow 5); severe hepatic impairment; suicidal ideation.

## CAUTIOUS USE Hypersensitivity to salicylates; chronic depression; history of suicidal thoughts; history of drug abuse; COPD; respiratory insufficiency; hepatic impairment; pulmonary disease; older adults; pregnancy (category C); lactation. Safe use in children not established.

## ROUTE & DOSAGE

### Insomnia
*Adult:* **PO** 10 mg at bedtime (max: 20 mg at bedtime)
*Geriatric:* **PO** 5 mg at bedtime (max: 10 mg at bedtime)

## ADMINISTRATION

### Oral

- Give immediately before bedtime; not while patient is still ambulating.
- Ensure that extended release tablets are swallowed whole and are not crushed or chewed.
- Sublingual tablets should not be given with water and should not be swallowed.
- Oral spray container must be primed before first use. Ensure that a full dose (5 mg) is sprayed directly into the mouth over the tongue. For a 10 mg dose, administer a second spray.
- Store at 20°–25° C (68°–77° F).

## ADVERSE EFFECTS (≥1%) **Body as a Whole:** Asthenia, fever, *headache,* migraine, myalgia, back pain. **CNS:** Amnesia, dizziness, paresthesia,

Z

1720

Common adverse effects in *italic;* life-threatening effects <u>underlined;</u> generic names in **bold;** classifications in SMALL CAPS, ♣ Canadian drug name; ❼ Prototype drug somnolence, tremor, vertigo, depression, hypertonia, nervousness, difficulty concentrating. **GI:** Abdominal pain, dyspepsia, nausea, constipation, dry mouth. **Respiratory:** Bronchitis. **Skin:** Pruritus, rash. **Special Senses:** Eye pain, hyperacusis, conjunctivitis. **Urogenital:** Dysmenorrhea.

**INTERACTIONS Drug: Alcohol, imipramine, thioridazine, topiramate,** BARBITURATES, may cause additive CNS impairment; **rifampin** increases metabolism of **zaleplon**; **cimetidine** increases serum levels of **zaleplon**. Do not use with **sodium oxybate. Herbal: Valerian, melatonin** may produce additive sedative effects. **Food: High-fat meals** may delay absorption.

**PHARMACOKINETICS Absorption:** Rapidly and completely absorbed, 30% reaches systemic circulation. **Onset:** 15–20 min. **Peak:** 1 h. **Duration:** 3–4 h. **Distribution:** 60% protein bound. **Metabolism:** Extensively in liver (CYP3A4) to inactive metabolites. **Elimination:** 70% in urine, 17% in feces. **Half-Life:** 1 h.

**NURSING IMPLICATIONS**

**Assessment & Drug Effects**

- Monitor behavior and notify prescriber for significant changes. Use extra caution with preexisting clinical depression.
- Provide safe environment and monitor ambulation after drug is ingested.
- Monitor respiratory status with preexisting compromised pulmonary function.

**Patient & Family Education**

- Exercise caution when walking; avoid all hazardous activities after taking zaleplon.
- Do not take in combination with alcohol or any other sleep medication.

- Note: Exhibits altered effectiveness if taken with/immediately after high-fat meal.
- Do not use longer than 2–3 wk.
- Expect possible mild/brief rebound insomnia after discontinuing regimen.
- Report use of OTC medications to prescriber (e.g., cimetidine).
- Report pregnancy to prescriber immediately.

**ZANAMIVIR**

(zan′a-mi-vir)

Relenza

**Classification:** ANTIVIRAL; NEURAMINIDASE INHIBITOR

Therapeutic: ANTIINFLUENZA

**Prototype:** Oseltamivir

**AVAILABILITY** Blister for inhalation

**ACTION & THERAPEUTIC EFFECT** Inhibitor of influenza A and B viral enzyme; does not permit the release of newly formed viruses from the surface of the infected cells. *Prevents viral spread across the mucus lining of the respiratory tract, and inhibits the replication of influenza A and B virus. Relieves flu-like symptoms.*

**USES** Uncomplicated acute influenza in patients symptomatic less than 2 days; prophylaxis for influenza.

**CONTRAINDICATIONS** Hypersensitivity to zanamivir or milk protein; severe renal impairment, renal failure; COPD; severe asthma.

**CAUTIOUS USE** Renal impairment; cardiac disease; severe metabolic disease; older adults; preg-nancy (category C); lactation. **Acute influenza:** Safety and efficacy in children younger than 7 y not established. **Influenza prophylaxis:** Safe use in children younger than 5 y not established.

Common adverse effects in *italic;* life-threatening effects <u>underlined;</u> generic names in **bold;** classifications in SMALL CAPS; ♦ Canadian drug name; ⦿ Prototype drug

1721

Z

## ROUTE & DOSAGE

**Influenza Treatment**

*Adult/Child (7 y or older):*
**Inhaled** 2 inhalations (one 5 mg blister/inhalation) b.i.d. × 5 days

**Influenza Prophylaxis**

*Adult/Child (5 y or older):*
**Inhaled** 2 inhalations daily for 10 days (household prophylaxis) or for 28 days (community outbreak)

## ADMINISTRATION

**Inhalation**
- Most effective if initiated within 48 h of onset of flu-like symptoms.
- Give any scheduled inhaled bronchodilator before zanamivir.
- Store at 25° C (77° F).

## ADVERSE EFFECTS (≥1%) **Body as a Whole:** Headache, abnormal behavior. **CNS:** Dizziness. **GI:** Nausea, diarrhea, vomiting. **Respiratory:** Nasal symptoms, bronchitis, cough, sinusitis; ear, nose, throat infection.

## INTERACTIONS **Drug:** Do not use with LIVE VACCINES.

## PHARMACOKINETICS **Absorption:** 4–17% of inhaled dose is systemically absorbed. **Peak:** 1–2 h. **Distribution:** Less than 10% protein bound. **Metabolism:** Not metabolized. **Elimination:** In urine. **Half-Life:** 2.5–5.1 h.

## NURSING IMPLICATIONS

**Patient & Family Education**
- Start within 48 h of onset of flu-like symptoms for most effective response.
- Use any scheduled inhaled bronchodilator first; then use zanamivir.

## ZICONOTIDE
(zi-con′o-tide)
**Prialt**
**Classifications:** MISCELLANEOUS ANALGESIC; N-TYPE CALCIUM CHANNEL ANTAGONIST
**Therapeutic:** MISCELLANEOUS ANALGESIC

**AVAILABILITY** Solution for injection

## ACTION & *THERAPEUTIC EFFECT*
Ziconotide binds to N-type calcium channels located on the afferent nerves in the dorsal horn in the spinal cord. It is thought that these binding blocks of N-type calcium channels lead to a blockade of excitatory neurotransmitter release in the afferent nerve endings. *Ziconotide is effective in controlling severe chronic pain that is intractable to other analgesics.*

**USES** Management of severe chronic pain in patients for whom intrathecal (IT) therapy is warranted.

**UNLABELED USES** Spasticity associated with spinal cord trauma.

**CONTRAINDICATIONS** Hypersensitivity to ziconotide; preexisting history of psychosis; epidural or intravenous administration; sepsis; depression with suicidal ideation; cognitive impairment; bipolar disorder; schizophrenia; dementia; presence of infection at the injection site, uncontrolled bleeding, or spinal canal obstruction that impairs circulation of CSF; coagulopathy; seizures; lactation.

**CAUTIOUS USE** Renal, hepatic, and cardiac impairment; older adults; pregnancy (category C). Safe use in children and infants not established.

## ROUTE & DOSAGE

### Severe Chronic Pain

*Adult:* **Intrathecal** Initial 0.1 mcg/h; may titrate up 0.1 mcg/h q2–3days to 0.8 mcg/h (19.2 mcg/day)

## ADMINISTRATION

### Intrathecal

- May be administered undiluted (25 mcg/mL in 20 mL vial) or diluted using the 100 mcg/mL vials. Diluted ziconotide is prepared with NS without preservatives.
- Administer using an implanted variable-rate microinfusion device or an external microinfusion device and catheter.
- Note: Due to serious adverse events, 19.2 mcg/day (0.8 mcg/h) is the maximum recommended dose.
- Doses should normally be titrated upward by no more than 2.4 mcg/day (0.1 mcg/h) at intervals of 2–3 × wk.
- Refrigerate all ziconotide solutions after preparation and begin infusion within 24 h. Discard any unused portion left in a vial.

## ADVERSE EFFECTS (≥1%) **Body as a Whole:** Accidental injury, back pain, catheter complication, catheter-site pain, cellulitis, chest pain, chills, *fever,* flu syndrome, infection, malaise, neck pain, neck rigidity, *pain,* pump-site complication, pump-site mass, pump-site pain, viral infection. **CNS:** Abnormal dreams, *abnormal gait,* agitation, *anxiety, aphasia, asthenia, ataxia,* CSF abnormal, *confusion,* depression, difficulty concentrating, *dizziness,* dry mouth, *dysesthesia,* emotional lability, *headache,* hostility, hyperesthesia, *hypertonia,*

incoordination, insomnia, *memory impairment,* mental slowing, meningitis, *nervousness,* neuralgia, paranoid reaction, *paresthesia,* reflexes decreased, *somnolence, speech disorder,* stupor, abnormal thinking, tremor, twitching, *vertigo.* **CV:** Hypertension, hypotension, postural hypotension, syncope, tachycardia, vasodilation. **GI:** Abdominal pain, *anorexia,* constipation, *diarrhea,* dyspepsia, gastrointestinal disorder, *nausea, vomiting.* **Urogenital:** Dysuria, urinary incontinence, *urinary retention,* urinary tract infection, impaired urination. **Hematologic:** Anemia, ecchymosis. **Metabolic/ Nutritional:** Creatinine phosphokinase increased, dehydration, edema, hypokalemia, peripheral edema, weight loss. **Musculoskeletal:** Arthralgia, arthritis, leg cramps, myalgia, myasthenia. **Respiratory:** Bronchitis, cough increased, dyspnea, lung disorder, pharyngitis, pneumonia, rhinitis, sinusitis. **Skin:** Cutaneous surgical complication, dry skin, pruritus, rash, skin disorder, sweating. **Special Senses:** *Abnormal vision,* diplopia, *nystagmus,* photophobia, taste perversion, tinnitus.

## INTERACTIONS **Drug: Ethanol** and other CNS DEPRESSANTS may increase drowsiness, dizziness, and confusion.

## PHARMACOKINETICS **Distribution:** 50% protein bound. **Metabolism:** Hydrolyzed by peptidases. **Half-Life:** 4.6 h.

## NURSING IMPLICATIONS

### Black Box Warning

*Ziconotide has been associated with severe psychiatric symptoms and neurologic impairment.*

Common adverse effects in *italic;* life-threatening effects <u>underlined</u>; generic names in **bold**; classifications in SMALL CAPS; ♣ Canadian drug name; ⊘ Prototype drug

1723

Z

### Assessment & Drug Effects

- Monitor for and report S&S of meningitis, cognitive impairment, hallucinations, changes in mood or consciousness, or other psychiatric symptoms.

### Patient & Family Education

- Report any of the following to prescriber: Muscle pain, soreness, or weakness, confusion, unusual behavior, symptoms of depression or suicidal thoughts, fever, headache, stiff neck, nausea or vomiting, seizures.
- Note: Taking this drug with other depressants (e.g., alcohol, sedatives, tranquilizers) will increase the risk of side effects.

## ZIDOVUDINE (ZDV) (FORMERLY AZIDOTHYMIDINE, AZT)

(zye-doe'vyoo-deen)

Retrovir

**Classifications:** ANTIVIRAL; NUCLEOSIDE REVERSE TRANSCRIPTASE INHIBITOR

Therapeutic: ANTIVIRAL; NRTI
**Prototype:** Lamivudine

**AVAILABILITY** Tablet; capsule; syrup; solution for injection

## ACTION & THERAPEUTIC EFFECT

Appears to act by being incorporated into growing DNA chains by viral reverse transcriptase, thereby terminating viral replication. *Zidovudine has antiviral action against HIV, LAV (lymphadenopathy-associated virus), and ARV (AIDS-associated retrovirus).*

**USES** Treatment of HIV (along with other antiretroviral agents), prevention of perinatal transfer of HIV during pregnancy.

**UNLABELED USES** Postexposure chemoprophylaxis, thrombocytopenia.

**CONTRAINDICATIONS** Life-threatening allergic reactions to any of the components of the drug; drug induced lactic acidosis; pronounced hepatotoxicity; lactation.

**CAUTIOUS USE** Severe renal impairment; or impaired hepatic function, alcoholism; anemia; chemotherapy; radiation therapy; bone marrow depression; older adults; pregnancy (category C); children.

## ROUTE & DOSAGE

### HIV Infection

*Adult/Adolescent/Child (weight 30 kg or greater):* **PO** 300 mg b.i.d. OR 200 mg t.i.d.; **IV** 1 mg/kg given 5–6 × daily
*Adolescent/Child/Infant (older than 4 wk, weight less than 30 kg):* See package insert for weight based dosing

### Prevention of Maternal-Fetal Transmission

*Neonate (older than 34 wk):* **PO** 2 mg/kg q6h for 6 wk beginning within 12 h after birth; *Full term:* **IV** 1.5 mg/kg q6h × 6 wk
*Maternal:* **PO** 100 mg 5 × daily OR 300 mg b.i.d. from 14–34 wk gestation until delivery; **IV** During labor, 2 mg/kg loading dose, then 1 mg/kg/h until clamping umbilical cord

### Toxicity Dosage Adjustment

*Hemoglobin falls below 7.5 g/dL or falls 25% from baseline:* Interrupt therapy. *ANC falls below 750 cells/mm$^3$ or decreases 50% from baseline:* Interrupt therapy.

## ADMINISTRATION

### Oral

- May be given with or without food.

## Intravenous

*PREPARE:* **Intermittent:** Withdraw required dose from vial and dilute with D5W to a concentration not to exceed 4 mg/mL.
*ADMINISTER:* **Intermittent for HIV infection:** Give calculated dose at a constant rate over 60 min; avoid rapid infusion. **IV Infusions for Prevention of Maternal-Fetal Transmission:** Give maternal loading dose over 1 h, then continuous infusion at 1 mg/kg/h. **Intermittent Infusion for Prevention of Maternal Transmission of HIV to Neonate:** Give calculated dose at a constant rate over 30 min.
*INCOMPATIBILITIES:* Solution/additive: Meropenem. Y-site: Dexrazoxane, gemtuzumab, lansoprazole, meropenem.

- Store at 15°–25° C (59°–77° F) and protect from light. Store diluted IV solutions refrigerated for 24 h.

## ADVERSE EFFECTS (≥1%) **Body as a Whole:** *Fever,* dyspnea, *malaise, weakness, myalgia,* myopathy. **CNS:** *Headache,* insomnia, dizziness, paresthesias, mild confusion, anxiety, restlessness, agitation. **GI:** *Nausea, diarrhea, vomiting, anorexia,* GI pain. **Hematologic:** <u>Bone marrow depression, granulocytopenia, anemia.</u> **Respiratory:** *Cough, wheezing.* **Skin:** *Rash,* itching, diaphoresis. **Metabolic:** <u>Lactic acidosis.</u>

## INTERACTIONS **Drug:** **Acetaminophen ganciclovir, interferon-alfa** may enhance bone marrow suppression; **atovaquone, amphotericin B, aspirin, dapsone, doxorubicin, fluconazole, flucytosine, indomethacin, interferon alfa, methadone, pentamidine, vincristine, valproic acid** may increase risk of **AZT** toxicity; **probenecid** will decrease **AZT** elimination, resulting in increased serum levels and thus toxicity. **Nelfinavir, rifampin, ritonavir** may decrease zidovudine (**AZT**) concentrations; other ANTIRETROVIRAL AGENTS may cause lactic acidosis and severe hepatomegaly with steatosis; **stavudine, doxorubicin** may antagonize **AZT** effects.

## PHARMACOKINETICS **Absorption:** Readily from GI tract; 60–70% reaches systemic circulation (first-pass metabolism). **Peak:** 0.5–1.5 h. **Distribution:** Crosses blood–brain barrier and placenta. **Metabolism:** In liver. **Elimination:** 63–95% in urine. **Half-Life:** 1 h.

## NURSING IMPLICATIONS

### Black Box Warning

Zidovudine has been associated with hematologic toxicity (including neutropenia and severe anemia), myopathy, lactic acidosis, and severe hepatomegaly with steatosis.

### Assessment & Drug Effects

- Evaluate patient at least weekly during the first month of therapy.
- Myelosuppression results in anemia, which commonly occurs after 4–6 wk of therapy, and granulocytopenia in 6–8 wk.
- Monitor for common adverse effects, especially severe headache, nausea, insomnia, and myalgia.
- Monitor lab tests: Baseline and periodic CBC with differential; periodic LFTs.

### Patient & Family Education

- Contact prescriber promptly if health status worsens or any unusual symptoms develop.
- Report to prescriber any of the following: Muscle weakness, shortness of breath, symptoms of hepatitis or pancreatitis, or

Common adverse effects in *italic;* life-threatening effects <u>underlined</u>; generic names in **bold;** classifications in SMALL CAPS; ✦ Canadian drug name; ⊙ Prototype drug

1725

Z

any other unexpected adverse reaction.

- Understand that this drug is not a cure for HIV infection; you will continue to be at risk for opportunistic infections.
- Do not share drug with others; take drug exactly as prescribed.
- Drug does **not** reduce the risk of transmission of HIV infection through body fluids.

# ZILEUTON
(zi-leu'ton)
Zyflo, Zyflo CR
**Classifications:** RESPIRATORY SMOOTH MUSCLE RELAXANT; BRONCHODILATOR; LEUKOTRIENE RECEPTOR ANTAGONIST (LTRA)
Therapeutic: BRONCHODILATOR; LTRA
**Prototype:** Zafirlukast

**AVAILABILITY** Immediate release tablet; controlled release tablet

## ACTION & *THERAPEUTIC EFFECT*
Inhibits 5-lipoxygenase, the enzyme needed to start the conversion of arachidonic acid to leukotrienes, which are important inflammatory agents that induce bronchoconstriction and mucus production. *Zileuton helps to prevent the signs and symptoms of asthma including airway edema, smooth muscle constriction, and altered cellular activity due to inflammation.*

**USES** Prophylaxis and chronic treatment of asthma in adults and children older than 12 y.

## CONTRAINDICATIONS Hypersensitivity to zileuton or zafirlukast, active liver disease, status asthmaticus; QT prolongation; lactation.

**CAUTIOUS USE** Hepatic insufficiency; alcoholism; fever; infection; history of QT prolongation; older females; older adults; pregnancy (category C). Safety and efficacy in children younger than 12 y not established.

## ROUTE & DOSAGE

**Asthma**

*Adult/Child (12 y or older):* **PO Controlled release** 1200 mg b.i.d. OR **Immediate release** 600 mg q.i.d.

## ADMINISTRATION
**Oral**
- Ensure that controlled release tablets are swallowed whole. They should not be crushed or chewed.
- Store at room temperature, 15°–30° C (59°–86° F); protect from light.

**ADVERSE EFFECTS** (≥1%) **Body as a Whole:** Pain, asthenia, myalgia, arthralgia, fever, malaise, neck pain/rigidity. **CNS:** *Headache,* dizziness, insomnia, nervousness, somnolence. **CV:** Chest pain. **GI:** Abdominal pain, *dyspepsia,* nausea, constipation, flatulence, vomiting, elevated liver function tests, asymptomatic hepatitis. **Skin:** Pruritus. **Other:** Conjunctivitis, hypertonia, lymphadenopathy, vaginitis, UTI, leukopenia.

**INTERACTIONS Drug:** May double **theophylline** levels and increase toxicity. Increases hypoprothrombinemic effects of **warfarin.** May increase levels of BETA-BLOCKERS (especially **propranolol**), leading to hypotension and bradycardia.

**PHARMACOKINETICS Absorption:** Rapidly from GI tract. **Peak:**

1.7 h. **Duration:** 5–8 h. **Distribution:** 93% protein bound; secreted in the breast milk of rats. **Metabolism:** In liver primarily via glucuronide conjugation. **Elimination:** Primarily in urine (94%). **Half-Life:** 2.5 h.

## NURSING IMPLICATIONS

### Assessment & Drug Effects

- Assess respiratory status and airway function regularly.
- Monitor closely each of the following with concurrent drug therapy: With theophylline, theophylline levels; with warfarin, PT and INR; with phenytoin, phenytoin level; with propranolol, HR and BP for excessive beta blockade.
- Monitor lab tests: Baseline and periodic LFTs.

### Patient & Family Education

- Take medication regularly even during symptom-free periods.
- Drug is not intended to treat acute episodes of asthma.
- Report to prescriber promptly S&S of hepatic toxicity (see Appendix F) or flu-like symptoms. Follow-up lab work is very important.
- Notify prescriber if condition worsens while using prescribed doses of all antiasthmatic medications.

## ZIPRASIDONE HYDROCHLORIDE

(zip-ra-si'done)

Geodon

**Classification:** ATYPICAL ANTIPSYCHOTIC
**Therapeutic:** ANTIPSYCHOTIC
**Prototype:** Clozapine

**AVAILABILITY** Capsule; solution for injection

## ACTION & THERAPEUTIC EFFECT

Exerts antischizophrenic effects through dopamine ($D_2$) and serotonin ($5\text{-}HT_{2A}$) receptor antagonism. Exerts antidepressant effects through $5\text{-}HT_{1A}$ agonism, $5\text{-}HT_{1D}$ antagonism, and serotonin/norepinephrine reuptake inhibition. *Improves signs and symptoms of schizophrenia, schizoaffective disorder, and psychotic depression.*

**USES** Treatment of schizophrenia, acute bipolar mania, acute psychosis, agitation.

**UNLABELED USES** Tourette's syndrome.

**CONTRAINDICATIONS** Hypersensitivity to ziprasidone; history of QT prolongation including congenital long QT syndrome or with other drugs known to prolong the QT interval; recent MI or uncompensated heart failure; NMS; older adults with dementia-related psychosis; lactation.

**CAUTIOUS USE** History of seizures, CVA, dementia, Parkinson's disease, or Alzheimer disease; known cardiovascular disease, conduction abnormalities, cerebrovascular disease; hepatic impairment; seizure disorder, seizures; breast cancer; risk factors for elevated core body temperature; esophageal motility disorders and risk of aspiration pneumonia; schizophrenia; suicide potential; DM; pregnancy (category C); children older than 7 y for use in Tourette's syndrome only. Safety and efficacy in children or adolescents (except for treatment of Tourette's syndrome) not established.

## ROUTE & DOSAGE

### Schizophrenia

*Adult:* **PO** Start with 20 mg b.i.d. with food, may increase slowly as needed (normal dose 40–100 mg b.i.d.)

---

Common adverse effects in *italic;* life-threatening effects <u>underlined;</u> generic names in **bold;** classifications in SMALL CAPS; ✦ Canadian drug name; ◉ Prototype drug

1727

Z

**Acute Episodes of Agitation/
Acute Psychosis**
*Adult:* **IM** 10 mg q2h or 20 mg
q4h up to max of 40 mg/day

**Acute Mania/Bipolar Disorder**
*Adult:* **PO** Start with 40 mg b.i.d.
with food; may increase q2days
up to 80 mg b.i.d. if needed

## ADMINISTRATION

**Oral**
- Give with food.
- Make dosage adjustments at intervals of 2 days or more.

**Intramuscular**
- Give deep IM into a large muscle.
- Store at 15°–30° C (59°–86° F).

## ADVERSE EFFECTS (≥1%) **Body
as a Whole:** Asthenia, myalgia,
weight gain, flu-like syndrome, face
edema, chills, hypothermia. **CNS:**
*Somnolence,* akathisia, dizziness,
extrapyramidal effects, dystonia,
hypertonia, agitation, tremor, dyskinesias, hostility, paresthesia, confusion, vertigo, hypokinesia, hyperkinesias, abnormal gait, oculogyric
crisis, hypesthesia, ataxia, amnesia,
cogwheel rigidity, delirium, hypotonia, akinesia, dysarthria, withdrawal syndrome, buccoglossal
syndrome, choreoathetosis, diplopia, incoordination, neuropathy,
headache. **CV:** Tachycardia, postural
hypotension, prolonged $QT_c$ interval, hypertension. **GI:** *Nausea,* constipation, dyspepsia, diarrhea, dry
mouth, weight gain, abdominal pain,
vomiting. **Metabolic:** Hyperglycemia,
diabetes mellitus. **Respiratory:** Rhinitis, increased cough, dyspnea. **Skin:**
Rash, fungal dermatitis, photosensitivity, pain at injection site. **Special
Senses:** Abnormal vision.

## INTERACTIONS **Drug:** **Carba-
mazepine** may decrease **ziprasi-**
done levels; **ketoconazole** may
increase **ziprasidone** levels; may
enhance hypotensive effects of AN-
TIHYPERTENSIVE AGENTS; may antagonize effects of **levodopa;** increased
risk of arrhythmias and heart
block due to prolonged $QT_c$ interval with ANTIARRHYTHMIC AGENTS,
**amoxapine, arsenic trioxide,
chlorpromazine, clarithromycin, citalopram, daunorubicin, diltiazem, dolasetron,
doxorubicin, droperidol,
erythromycin, halofantrine,
indapamide, levomethadyl,**
LOCAL ANESTHETICS, **maprotiline,
mefloquine, mesoridazine,
octreotide, pentamidine,
pimozide, levofloxacin, moxifloxacin, sparfloxacin,** TRICY-
CLIC ANTIDEPRESSANTS, **tacrolimus,
thioridazine, troleandomycin;**
additive CNS depression with
SEDATIVE-HYPNOTICS, ANXIOLYTICS,
**ethanol,** OPIATE AGONISTS.

## PHARMACOKINETICS **Absorp-
tion:** Well absorbed with 60%
reaching systemic circulation.
**Peak:** 6–8 h. **Metabolism:** In liver
(CYP3A4). **Elimination:** Feces and
urine. **Half-Life:** 7 h.

## NURSING IMPLICATIONS

### Black Box Warning

*Ziprasidone has been associated
with increased mortality in older
adults with dementia-related psychosis.*

### Assessment & Drug Effects
- Monitor diabetics for loss of glycemic control.
- Monitor for S&S of torsade de
pointes (e.g., dizziness, palpitations,
syncope), tardive dyskinesia (see
Appendix F) especially in older

Common adverse effects in *italic;* life-threatening effects <u>underlined</u>; generic names
in **bold;** classifications in SMALL CAPS; ✦ Canadian drug name; ⊙ Prototype drug

adult women and with prolonged therapy, and the appearance of an unexplained rash. Withhold drug and report to prescriber immediately if any of these develop.

- Monitor for signs and symptoms of suicidality.
- Monitor I&O ratio and pattern: Notify prescriber if diarrhea, vomiting or any other conditions develops which may cause electrolyte imbalance.
- Monitor BP lying, sitting, and standing. Report orthostatic hypotension to prescriber.
- Monitor cognitive status and take appropriate precautions.
- Monitor for loss of seizure control, especially with a history of seizures or dementia.
- Monitor lab tests: Baseline and periodic serum potassium and serum magnesium, especially with concomitant diuretic therapy; periodic blood glucose.

### Patient & Family Education

- Carefully monitor blood glucose levels if diabetic.
- Be aware that therapeutic effect may not be evident for several weeks.
- Report any of the following to a health care provider immediately: Palpitations, faintness or loss of consciousness, rash, abnormal muscle movements, vomiting or diarrhea.
- Do not drive or engage in potentially hazardous activities until response to drug is known.
- Make position changes slowly and in stages to prevent dizziness upon arising.
- Avoid strenuous exercise, exposure to extreme heat, or other activities that may cause dehydration.

## ZIV-AFLIBERCEPT

(ziv-a-fli'ber-cept)

**Zaltrap**

**Classification:** BIOLOGICAL RESPONSE MODIFIER; GROWTH FACTOR INHIBITOR; SIGNAL TRANSDUCTION INHIBITOR; RECOMBINANT FUSION PROTEIN; ANTINEOPLASTIC
**Therapeutic:** ANTINEOPLASTIC

**AVAILABILITY** Solution

**ACTION & THERAPEUTIC EFFECT**
Binds to certain vascular growth factors thus inhibiting their binding to and activation of receptors that stimulate neovascularization (new blood vessel growth) and increased vascular permeability. *Decreased neovascularization in tumors slows growth of metastatic colorectal tumors.*

**USES** Treatment of metastatic colorectal cancer in combination chemotherapy with 5-flurouracil, leucovorin, and irinotecan in patients whose condition has progressed or is resistant to an oxaliplatin-containing combination

**CONTRAINDICATIONS** Severe hemorrhage, GI perforation; compromised wound healing; fistula development; 4 wk before or after elective surgery; hypertensive crisis or hypertensive encephalopathy; drug induced arterial thromboembolic event or nephrotic syndrome; reversible posterior leukoencephalopathy syndrome (RPLS); lactation.

**CAUTIOUS USE** Hypersensitivity to ziv-aflibercept; hemorrhage; history of GI perforation; poor wound healing; severe hypertension or hypertension; thromboembolic events; proteinuria; infection; diarrhea and dehydration; older adults; pregnancy (category C). Safety and efficacy in children younger than 18 y not established.

Common adverse effects in *italic*; life-threatening effects underlined; generic names in **bold**; classifications in SMALL CAPS; ✦ Canadian drug name; ● Prototype drug

1729

Z

## ROUTE & DOSAGE

### Colorectal Cancer

*Adult:* **IV** 4 mg/kg q2wk; administer prior to 5-flurouracil, leucovorin, and irinotecan

### Toxicity Dosage Adjustments

*Recurrent of severe hypertension:* Hold therapy until hypertension is controlled; permanently reduce dose to 2 mg/kg for subsequent cycles
*Proteinuria:* Hold therapy until proteinuria is less than 2 g/24 h; permanently reduce dose to 2 mg/kg for subsequent cycles

## ADMINISTRATION

### Intravenous

*PREPARE:* **IV Infusion:** Withdraw required dose of ziv-aflibercept and dilute to a final concentration of 0.6–8 mg/mL in NS or D5W (enter vial only once to withdraw dose). Dilute in PVC infusion bags containing bis (2-ethylhexyl) phthalate (DEHP) or polyolefin.
*ADMINISTER:* **IV Infusion:** Infuse over 1 h through a 0.2 micron polyethersulfone filter. Do not use filters made of polyvinylidene fluoride or nylon. **Do not** give IV push or as bolus dose. Use an infusion set made of PVC containing DEHP or one of the other materials approved by manufacturer.
*INCOMPATIBILITIES:* **Solution/additive:** Do not combine ziv-aflibercept with other drugs in the same IV solution. **Y-site:** Do not administer ziv-aflibercept in the same IV line with other drugs

• Store diluted solution at 2°–8° C (36°–46° F) for up to 4 h.

## ADVERSE EFFECTS (≥1%) **Body as a Whole:** Asthenia, *fatigue,* catheter site infection, hypersensitivity, injection site hemorrhage, injection site pain, pneumonia. **CNS:** Headache. **CV:** <u>Deep venous thrombosis, pulmonary embolism,</u> *hypertension.* **GI:** *Abdominal pain, diarrhea,* hemorrhoids, proctalgia, rectal hemorrhage, *stomatitis,* <u>GI perforation.</u> **Hematological:** <u>Leukopenia, neutropenia,</u> thrombocytopenia, <u>hemorrhage.</u> **Metabolic:** *Decreased appetite,* dehydration, *increased ALT and AST, weight decreased.* **Respiratory:** Dysphonia, dyspnea, epistaxis, nasopharyngitis, oropharyngeal pain, <u>pulmonary embolism,</u> rhinorrhea, upper respiratory tract infection. **Skin:** Palmar-plantar erythrodysesthesia syndrome, skin hyperpigmentation. **Special Senses:** Blurred vision, cataract, *conjunctival hemorrhage,* conjunctival hyperemia, corneal edema, corneal erosion, detachment of the retinal pigment epithelium, *eye pain,* eyelid edema, foreign body sensation in the eyes, increased intraocular pressure, increased lacrimation, retinal pigment epithelium tear, tooth infection, vitreous detachment, vitreous floaters. **Urogenital:** *Proteinuria, serum creatinine increased,* urinary tract infections.

## PHARMACOKINETICS **Peak:** 1–3 d. **Metabolism:** Via proteolysis. **Half-Life:** 5–6 d.

## NURSING IMPLICATIONS

### Black Box Warning

*Ziv-aflibercept has been associated with severe, sometimes fatal hemorrhage, GI perforation, and seriously compromised wound healing.*

## Assessment & Drug Effects

- Monitor vital signs, especially BP for exacerbation of hypertension.
- Monitor for and report immediately S&S of bleeding and GI perforation.
- Monitor for diarrhea and dehydration, especially in the older adult.
- Monitor lab tests: Baseline and prior to each cycle, CBC with differential; periodic LFTs, renal function tests, and urinalysis for proteinuria; 24 h urine when urinary protein creatinine ratio is greater than 1.

## Patient & Family Education

- Report promptly any of the following: S&S of bleeding including light-headedness; S&S of hypertension including severe headache, or dizziness; severe diarrhea, vomiting, or abdominal pain.
- Frequent monitoring of BP is advised. Contact prescriber if BP is elevated beyond usual parameters.
- Men and women should use effective means of birth control during therapy and for at least 3 mo following completion of therapy.
- Contact your prescriber immediately if you or your partner becomes pregnant during treatment with ziv-aflibercept.
- Do not breast-feed while receiving this drug without consultation with prescriber.

## ZOLEDRONIC ACID

(zo-le-dron'ic)

Aclasta ♦, Reclast, Zometa

**Classifications:** BISPHOSPHONATE; BONE METABOLISM REGULATOR

**Therapeutic:** BONE METABOLISM REGULATOR

**Prototype:** Etidronate disodium

**AVAILABILITY** Solution for injection

## ACTION & THERAPEUTIC EFFECT

Zoledronic acid inhibits various stimulatory factors of osteoclastic activity produced by bone tumors. It also induces osteoclast apoptosis. *Zoledronic acid blocks osteoclastic resorption of bone, thus reducing the amount of calcium released from bone.*

**USES** Treatment of hypercalcemia of malignancy, multiple myeloma, and bony metastases from solid tumors, Paget's disease (Reclast), postmenopausal or glucocorticoid-induced osteoporosis (Reclast).

**CONTRAINDICATIONS** Hypersensitivity to zoledronic acid preexisting hypocalcemia (**Reclast** only); serum creatinine less than 35 mL/min; pregnancy (category D); lactation.

**CAUTIOUS USE** Aspirin-sensitive asthma; cancer chemotherapy; renal and/or hepatic impairment, dental work; multiple myeloma; Paget disease; hypoparathyroidism, malabsorption syndrome; QT prolongation, cardiac arrhythmias; neurologic events; older adults. Safety and efficacy in children not established.

## ROUTE & DOSAGE

**Hypercalcemia of Malignancy (Zometa)**

*Adult:* **IV** 4 mg over a minimum of 15 min. May consider retreatment if serum calcium has not returned to normal, may repeat after 7 days

**Multiple Myeloma and Bone Metastases from Solid Tumors (Zometa)**

*Adult:* **IV** 4 mg over a minimum of 15 min q3–4wk

---

Common adverse effects in *italic*; life-threatening effects underlined; generic names in **bold**; classifications in SMALL CAPS; ♦ Canadian drug name; ☉ Prototype drug

Z

**Osteoporosis (Reclast)**
*Adult:* **IV** 5 mg infusion once/year

**Osteoporosis Prophylaxis in Postmenopausal Women (Reclast)**
*Adult:* **IV** 5 mg every other year

**Paget's Disease (Reclast)**
*Adult:* **IV** 5 mg dose, retreatment may be necessary

**Renal Impairment Dosage Adjustment (Zometa)**
*CrCl 50–60 mL/min:* 3.5 mg; *40–49 mL/min:* 3.3 mg; *30–39 mL/min:* 3 mg; *less than 30 mL/min:* Do not use

**Renal Impairment Dosage Adjustment (Reclast)**
*CrCl less than 35 mL/min:* Do not use

## ADMINISTRATION

**Intravenous**

Do not administer to anyone who is dehydrated or suspected of being dehydrated. Consult prescriber.

▪ Do not administer until serum creatinine values have been evaluated by the prescriber.

**PREPARE: IV Infusion:** *Reclast:* No further preparation is necessary. *Zometa concentrate:* Further dilute in 100 mL NS or D5W. *Powder for injection:* Reconstitute with 5 mL of sterile water for injection (provided) to yield 0.8 mg/mL. Further dilute in 100 mL NS or D5W prior to administration. ▪ If not used immediately, refrigerate. The total time between reconstitution and end of infusion must not exceed 24 h.

**ADMINISTER: IV Infusion:** Infuse a single dose over NO LESS than 15 min. Flush line with 10 mL NS following infusion.

**INCOMPATIBILITIES: Solution/additive and Y-site:** Do not mix or infuse with **calcium**-containing solutions (e.g., **lactated Ringer's**).

▪ Store at 2°–8° C (36°–46° F) following dilution. ▪ **Must be** completely infused within 24 h of reconstitution.

## ADVERSE EFFECTS (≥1%) **Body as a Whole:** *Fever,* flu-like syndrome, redness and swelling at injection site, asthenia, chest pain, leg edema, mucositis, rigors. **CNS:** *Insomnia, anxiety, confusion, agitation,* headache, somnolence, fatigue, dizziness, depression. **CV:** *Hypotension.* **GI:** *Nausea, vomiting, constipation, abdominal pain, anorexia,* dysphagia, candidiasis. **Hematologic:** *Anemia,* granulocytopenia, thrombocytopenia, pancytopenia. **Metabolic:** *Hypophosphatemia, hypokalemia, hypomagnesemia,* hypocalcemia, dehydration. **Musculoskeletal:** Skeletal pain, arthralgias, osteonecrosis of the jaw in cancer patients. **Respiratory:** *Dyspnea, cough,* pleural effusion. **Skin:** Alopecia, dermatitis. **Urogenital:** Renal insufficiency, UTI.

## INTERACTIONS **Drug:** NSAIDS may increase the risk of GI toxicity. **Thalidomide** and other NEPHROTOXIC DRUGS may increase risk of renal toxicity.

## PHARMACOKINETICS **Onset:** 4–10 days. **Duration:** 3–4 wk. **Metabolism:** Not metabolized. **Elimination:** In urine. **Half-Life:** 146 h.

## NURSING IMPLICATIONS

**Assessment & Drug Effects**

▪ Notify prescriber immediately of deteriorating renal function as indicated by rising serum creatinine levels over baseline value.

▪ Withhold zoledronic acid and notify prescriber if serum creatinine is not within 10% of the baseline value.

- Monitor closely patient's hydration status. Note that loop diuretics should be used with caution due to the risk of hypocalcemia.
- Monitor for S&S of *bronchospasm* in aspirin-sensitive asthma patients; notify prescriber immediately.
- Baseline dental exam prior to initiation of therapy for patients at risk for osteonecrosis including all cancer patients.
- Monitor lab tests: Baseline renal function tests prior to each dose and periodically thereafter; periodic ionized calcium or corrected serum calcium levels, serum phosphate and magnesium, electrolytes, CBC with differential, Hct and Hgb.

**Patient & Family Education**

- Maintain adequate daily fluid intake. Consult with prescriber for guidelines.
- Report unexplained weakness, tiredness, irritation, muscle pain, insomnia, or flu-like symptoms.
- Use reliable means of birth control to prevent pregnancy. If you suspect you are pregnant, contact prescriber immediately.

## ZOLMITRIPTAN
(zol-mi-trip'tan)

Zomig, Zomig ZMT, Zomig Nasal Spray

**Classifications:** SEROTONIN 5-HT₁ RECEPTOR AGONIST; ERGOT ALKALOID
**Therapeutic:** ANTIMIGRAINE
**Prototype:** Sumatriptan

**AVAILABILITY** Tablet; orally disintegrating tablet; nasal spray

## ACTION & *THERAPEUTIC EFFECT*
Selective serotonin (5-HT₁B/₁D) receptor agonist. The agonist effects at 5-HT₁B/₁D reverse the vasodilation of cranial blood vessels and inhibit release of pro-inflammatory neuropeptides. *Vasoconstricts dilated cranial blood vessels and decreased neuropeptide release relieve the pain of a migraine headache.*

**USES** Acute migraine headaches with or without aura.

**CONTRAINDICATIONS** Hypersensitivity to zolmitriptan; history of stroke or TIA; ischemic heart disease (angina, arteriosclerosis, ECG changes, history of MI or Prinzmetal's angina); cardiac arrhythmias associated with cardiac accessory conduction pathway disorders; symptomatic Wolff–Parkinson–White syndrome, uncontrolled hypertension; patients with other cardiac risk factors, such as diabetes, obesity, cigarette smoking, high cholesterol levels; hemiplegia or basilar migraine; concurrent administration of ergotamine or sumatriptan; concurrent use of MAOIs or within 14 days of use; vasospasm-related events, lactation.

**CAUTIOUS USE** Men older than 40 y; postmenopausal women; strong family history of CAD; GI disease, PVD, ischemic colitis, Raynaud's disease, hepatic impairment; adults older than 65 y; pregnancy (category C); children younger than 12 y.

## ROUTE & DOSAGE

| Acute Migraine |
|---|
| *Adult:* **PO** 1.25–2.5 mg, may repeat in 2 h if necessary (max: 10 mg/24 h) |
| *Adult/Adolescent:* **Nasal Spray** One spray into one nostril |

## ADMINISTRATION
**Oral**
- Give any time after symptoms of migraine appear. Give 2.5 mg or less by breaking a 5 mg tablet in

Common adverse effects in *italic;* life-threatening effects <u>underlined;</u> generic names in **bold;** classifications in SMALL CAPS; ♣ Canadian drug name; ● Prototype drug

1733

Z

half. If headache returns, may repeat q2h up to 10 mg in 24 h.

- **Do not** give zolmitriptan within 24 h of an ergot-containing drug or other 5-HT₁ agonist.
- Discard unused tablets that have been removed from the packaging.

**Intranasal**
- Unit-dose spray device delivers a 5 mg dose. Do not exceed the maximum dose of 10 mg in 24 h.
- Store at 2°–25° C (36°–77° F) and protect from light.

**ADVERSE EFFECTS** (≥1%) **Body as a Whole:** Asthenia, fatigue, malaise, pain, pressure sensation, paresthesia, throat pressure, warm/cold sensations, hypesthesia. **CNS:** Somnolence, dizziness, drowsiness, headache, hypesthesia, decreased mental acuity, euphoria, tremor. **CV:** Coronary artery vasospasm, transient myocardial ischemia, <u>MI</u>, ventricular tachycardia, ventricular fibrillation, chest pain/tightness/heaviness, palpitations. **GI:** Dry mouth, nausea, vomiting. **Respiratory:** Dyspnea. **Skin:** Flushing. **Other:** Hot flushes.

**INTERACTIONS Drug: Dihydroergotamine, methysergide,** other 5-HT₁ AGONISTS may cause prolonged vasospastic reactions; SSRIS have rarely caused weakness, hyperreflexia, and incoordination; MAOIS should not be used with 5-HT₁ AGONISTS; **cimetidine** increases half-life of zolmitriptan. **Herbal: St. John's wort** may increase TRIPTAN toxicity.

**PHARMACOKINETICS Absorption:** Rapidly absorbed, 40% bioavailability. **Peak:** 2–3 h. **Distribution:** 25% protein bound. **Metabolism:** In liver to active metabolite. **Elimination:** Primarily in urine (65%), 30% in feces. **Half-Life:** 3 h.

## NURSING IMPLICATIONS
### Assessment & Drug Effects
- Monitor for therapeutic effectiveness: Relief or reduction of migraine pain within 1–4 h.
- Monitor cardiovascular status carefully following first dose in patients at risk for CAD (e.g., postmenopausal women, men older than 40 y, persons with known CAD risk factors) or coronary artery vasospasms.
- Periodic cardiovascular evaluation is recommended with long-term use.
- Report to prescriber immediately chest pain, nausea, or tightness in chest or throat that is severe or does not quickly resolve.

### Patient & Family Education
- Carefully review patient information insert and guidelines for taking drug.
- **Do not** take zolmitriptan during the aura phase, but as early as possible after onset of migraine.
- Do not remove orally disintegrating tablet from blister until just prior to dosing.
- Concurrent oral contraceptive use may increase incidence of adverse effects.
- Contact prescriber immediately if any of the following occur after zolmitriptan use: Symptoms of angina (e.g., severe or persistent pain or tightness in chest or throat, sudden nausea), hypersensitivity (e.g., wheezing, facial swelling, skin rash, hives), fainting, or abdominal pain.
- Report any other adverse effects (e.g., tingling, flushing, dizziness) at next prescriber visit.

## ZOLPIDEM ℗
(zol'pi-dem)

Ambien, Ambien CR, Edluar, Intermezzo, Zolpimist
**Classifications:** SEDATIVE-HYPNOTIC, NONBARBITUATE
Therapeutic: SEDATIVE-HYPNOTIC
**Controlled Substance:** Schedule IV

**AVAILABILITY** Tablet; extended release tablet; sublingual tablet

## ACTION & *THERAPEUTIC EFFECT*
An agonist that binds the gamma aminobutyric acid (GABA)-A receptor chloride channel, thus inhibiting its action potential in the cortical region of the brain. *Effective as a sedative.*

**USES** Short-term treatment of insomnia.

**CONTRAINDICATIONS** Hypersensitivity of zolpidem including angioedema; suicidal ideation, worsening of depression; labor or obstetric delivery.

**CAUTIOUS USE** Depressed patients, psychiatric disorders; history of suical tendencies; hepatic/renal impairment, alcohol or drug abuse; patients with compromised respiratory status, COPD, sleep apnea; chronic depression; older adults; pregnancy (category C). Safe use in children younger than 18 y not established.

## ROUTE & DOSAGE

### Short-Term Treatment of Insomnia
*Adult:* **PO Immediate release/sublingual** 5–10 mg OR **Extended release** 12.5 mg at bedtime; **Spray** 1–2 sprays before bedtime

### Insomnia (Intermezzo Only)
*Adult:* **PO** 1.75 mg (women) or 3.5 mg (men) once/night if needed
*Geriatric:* **PO Immediate release/sublingual** 5 mg OR **Extended release** 6.25 mg at bedtime; **Spray** 1 spray before bedtime (max: 2 sprays)

### Hepatic Impairment Dosage Adjustment
**Immediate release** 5 mg OR **Extended release** 6.25 mg at bedtime

## ADMINISTRATION
### Oral
- Give immediately before bedtime; for more rapid sleep onset, **do not** give with or immediately after a meal.
- Ensure that sublingual tablets are not swallowed.
- Extended release tablets should be swallowed whole. Ensure that they are not crushed or chewed.
- Store at room temperature, 15°–30° C (59°–86° F).

**ADVERSE EFFECTS** (≥1%) **CNS:** *Headache on awakening, drowsiness, fatigue, lethargy,* drugged feeling, depression, anxiety, irritability, dizziness, double vision. Doses greater than 10 mg may be associated with anterograde amnesia or memory impairment. **GI:** Dyspepsia, nausea, vomiting, diarrhea. **Other:** Myalgia.

**INTERACTIONS Drug:** CNS DEPRESSANTS, **alcohol,** PHENOTHIAZINES by augmenting CNS depression. **Food:** Extent and rate of absorption of zolpidem are significantly decreased.

Common adverse effects in *italic;* life-threatening effects <u>underlined;</u> generic names in **bold;** classifications in SMALL CAPS; ♣ Canadian drug name; ✪ Prototype drug

1735

Z

## PHARMACOKINETICS Absorption:
Readily from GI tract. 70% reaches systemic circulation. **Onset:** 7–27 min. **Peak:** 0.5–2.3 h. **Duration:** 6–8 h. **Distribution:** Highly protein bound. Lowest concentrations in CNS, highest concentrations in glandular tissue and fat. Crosses placenta. **Metabolism:** In the liver to 3 inactive metabolites. **Elimination:** 79–96% in the bile, urine, and feces. **Half-Life:** 1.7–2.5 h.

## NURSING IMPLICATIONS

### Assessment & Drug Effects
- Assess respiratory function in patients with compromised respiratory status. Report immediately to prescriber significantly depressed respiratory rate (less than 12/min).
- Monitor patients for S&S of depression (see Appendix F); zolpidem may increase level of depression.
- Monitor closely older adult or debilitated patients for impaired cognitive or motor function and unusual sensitivity to the drug's effects.

### Patient & Family Education
- Avoid taking alcohol or other CNS depressants while on zolpidem.
- Do not drive or engage in other potentially hazardous activities until response to drug is known.
- Report vision changes to prescriber.
- Note: Onset of drug is more rapid when taken on an empty stomach.

## ZONISAMIDE ⒫
(zon-i'sa-mide)
Zonegran
**Classifications:** ANTICONVULSANT; SULFONAMIDE
Therapeutic: ANTICONVULSANT

## AVAILABILITY Capsule

## ACTION & *THERAPEUTIC EFFECT*
A broad-spectrum anticonvulsant that facilitates dopaminergic and serotonergic neurotransmission but does not potentiate the activity of gamma-aminobutyric acid (GABA) in the synapses of the CNS neurons. *Suppresses focal spike discharges and electroshock seizures. Effective against a variety of seizure types.*

## USES Adjunctive therapy for partial seizures.

## UNLABELED USES Antipsychotic-induced weight gain.

## CONTRAINDICATIONS Hypersensitivity to sulfonamides or zonisamide; suicidal ideation; worsening of depression; severe metabolic acidosis; abrupt discontinuation; lactation.

## CAUTIOUS USE Depressive individuals; CNS effects; history of suicidal tendencies; renal or hepatic insufficiency, dehydration, hypovolemia; renal impairment; older adults; pregnancy (category C). Safety and efficiacy in children younger than 16 y not established.

## ROUTE & DOSAGE

### Partial Seizures
*Adult/Child (16 y or older):* **PO** Start at 100 mg daily, may increase after 2 wk to 200 mg/day, may then increase q2wk, if necessary (max: 400 mg/day in 1–2 divided doses)

## ADMINISTRATION

### Oral
- Do not crush or break capsules; ensure capsules are swallowed whole with adequate fluid.

- Withdraw drug gradually when discontinued to minimize seizure potential.
- Store at 25° C (77° F); room temperature permitted. Protect from light and moisture.

**ADVERSE EFFECTS** (≥1%) **Body as a Whole:** Flu-like syndrome, weight loss. **CNS:** Agitation, irritability, anxiety, ataxia, confusion, depression, difficulty concentrating, difficulty with memory, *dizziness,* fatigue, *headache,* insomnia, mental slowing, nervousness, nystagmus, paresthesia, schizophrenic behavior, *somnolence,* tiredness, tremor, convulsion, abnormal gait, hyperesthesia, incoordination. **GI:** Abdominal pain, *anorexia,* constipation, diarrhea, dyspepsia, nausea, dry mouth, flatulence, gingivitis, gum hyperplasia, gastritis, stomatitis, cholelithiasis, glossitis, melena, rectal hemorrhage, ulcerative stomatitis, ulcer, dysphagia. **Metabolic:** Oligohidrosis, sometimes resulting in heat stroke and hyperthermia in children. **Respiratory:** Rhinitis, pharyngitis, cough. **Skin:** Ecchymosis, rash, pruritus. **Special Senses:** Difficulties in verbal expression, diplopia, speech abnormalities, taste perversion, amblyopia, tinnitus. **Urogenital:** Kidney stones.

**INTERACTIONS Drug: Phenytoin, carbamazepine, phenobarbital, valproic acid** may decrease half-life of zonisamide.

**PHARMACOKINETICS Peak:** 2–6 h. **Distribution:** 40% protein bound, extensively binds to erythrocytes. **Metabolism:** Acetylated in liver by CYP3A4. **Elimination:** Primarily in urine. **Half-Life:** 63–105 h.

## NURSING IMPLICATIONS
### Assessment & Drug Effects
- Withhold drug and notify prescriber if an unexplained rash or S&S of hypersensitivity appear (see Appendix F).
- Monitor for and report S&S of CNS impairment (somnolence, excessive fatigue, cognitive deficits, speech or language problems, incoordination, gait disturbances); oligohidrosis (lack of sweating) and hyperthermia in pediatric patients.
- Monitor lab tests: Periodic BUN and serum creatinine, and CBC with differential.

### Patient & Family Education
- Do not abruptly stop taking this medication.
- Increase daily fluid intake to minimize risk of renal stones. Notify prescriber immediately of S&S of renal stones: Sudden back or abdominal pain, and blood in urine.
- Report any of the following: Dizziness, excess drowsiness, frequent headaches, malaise, double vision, lack of coordination, persistent nausea, sore throat, fever, mouth ulcers, or easy bruising.
- Exercise special caution with concurrent use of alcohol or CNS depressants.
- Do not drive or engage in other potentially hazardous activities until response to drug is known.

## ZOSTER VACCINE ℗
(zos′ter)

Zostavax

**See Appendix J.**

Common adverse effects in *italic;* life-threatening effects <u>underlined</u>; generic names in **bold;** classifications in SMALL CAPS; ♣ Canadian drug name; ℗ Prototype drug

1737

Z

# APPENDICES

# ◆ APPENDIX A

(Generic names are in **bold**)

## APPENDIX A-1

### OCULAR MEDICATIONS

**BETA-ADRENERGIC BLOCKERS** **Prototype for classification: Propranolol HCl Use:** Intraocular hypertension and chronic open-angle glaucoma.

| | |
|---|---|
| **Betaxolol HCl**<br>Betoptic S,<br>0.25% suspension,<br>0.5% solution | *Adult:* **Topical** 1 drop in affected eye b.i.d. for 0.25% suspension; 1–2 drops in affected eye for 0.5% solution. |
| **Carteolol HCl**<br>Ocupress, 1% solution | *Adult:* **Topical** 1 drop b.i.d. |
| **Levobunolol**<br>Betagan,<br>0.25%, 0.5% solution | *Adult:* **Topical** 1–2 drops of 0.25% solution b.i.d. or 1–2 drops of 0.5% solution daily. |
| **Metipranolol HCl**<br>OptiPranolol,<br>0.3% solution | *Adult:* **Topical** 1 drop b.i.d. |
| **Timolol maleate**<br>Betimol, Istalol,<br>Timoptic, Timoptic XE,<br>0.25%, 0.5% solution | *Adult:* **Topical** 1 drop of 0.25–0.5% solution b.i.d.; may decrease to daily. Apply gel daily. Apply Istalol solution once daily. |

**ADVERSE EFFECTS/CLINICAL IMPLICATIONS** May cause *mild ocular stinging* and discomfort, tearing; may also have the adverse effects of systemic beta blockers. May precipitate thyroid storm in patients with hyperthyroidism. Patients with impaired cardiac function and the elderly should report to prescriber signs and symptoms of CHF (see Appendix G). Monitor BP for hypotension and heart rate for bradycardia.

**MIOTICS** **Prototype for classification: Pilocarpine HCl Use:** Open-angle and angle-closure glaucomas; to reduce IOP and to protect the lens during surgery and laser iridotomy; to counteract effects of mydriatics and cycloplegics following surgery or ophthalmoscopic examination.

| | |
|---|---|
| **Apraclonidine HCl**<br>Iopidine, 0.5%,<br>1% solution | **Intraoperative and Postsurgical Increase in IOP:** *Adult:* **Topical** 1 drop of 1% solution in affected eye 1 h before surgery and 1 drop in same eye immediately after surgery. **Open-Angle Glaucoma:** *Adult:* **Topical** 1 drop of 0.5% solution in affected eye q12h. |
| **Brimonidine tartrate**<br>Alphagan P,<br>0.1%, 0.15%,<br>0.2% solution | **Glaucoma:** *Adult:* **Topical** 1 drop in affected eye(s) t.i.d. approximately 8 h apart. *Child (2 y or older):* **Topical** 1 drop in affected eye t.i.d. approximatively 8 h apart. |

**Brinzolamide**
Azopt,
1% suspension

**Ocular Hypertension or Open-Angle Glaucoma:** *Adult:* **Topical** 1 drop in affected eye(s) t.i.d.

**Carbachol**
1.5%, 3% solution

**Glaucoma:** *Adult:* **Topical** 2 drops in affected eye(s) up to 3 × daily.

**Dorzolamide**
Trusopt,
2% solution

**Ocular Hypertension or Open-Angle Glaucoma:** *Adult, Child:* **Topical** 1 drop in affected eye(s) t.i.d.

**Pilocarpine HCl**
Isopto Carpine,
Pilopine HS,
1%, 2%, 4%
solution

**Acute Glaucoma:** *Adult:* **Topical** 1 drop of 1–2% solution in affected eye q5–10min for 3–6 doses, then 1 drop q1–3h until IOP is reduced. **Chronic Glaucoma:** *Adult:* **Topical** 1 drop of 0.5–4% solution in affected eye q4–12h or 1 ocular system (Ocusert) q7days. **Miotic:** *Adult:* **Topical** 1 drop of 1% solution in affected eye.

**ADVERSE EFFECTS/CLINICAL IMPLICATIONS Ocular:** Ciliary spasm with brow ache, twitching of eyelids, eye pain with change in eye focus, miosis, *diminished vision in poorly illuminated areas,* blurred vision, reduced visual acuity, sensitivity, contact allergy, lacrimation, follicular conjunctivitis, conjunctival irritation, cataract, retinal detachment. **CNS:** *Headache, drowsiness,* depression, syncope. **GI:** Abnormal taste, dry mouth. **Clinical Implications:** Wait 15 min after instillation before inserting soft contact lenses to avoid staining lenses. Use with MAO inhibitors may increase risk of hypertensive emergency. May increase the effects of beta-blockers and other antihypertensives on blood pressure and heart rate. TCAs may reduce the effects of **brimonidine. Brinzolamide** is a carbonic anhydrase inhibitor (prototype: Acetazolamide) and is a sulfonamide. It should not be used by patients with sulfa allergies. Reconstituted solutions of **echothiophate** remain stable for 1 mo at room temperature. Expiration date should appear on label. The length of time solutions remain stable under refrigeration varies with manufacturer. **Echothiophate** therapy is generally discontinued 2–6 wk before surgery. If necessary, alternate therapy is substituted. Medication should be given in the evening. Give at least 5 min apart from other topical ophthalmic drugs. The patient with brown or hazel eyes may require a stronger ophthalmic solution or more frequent instillation of **physostigmine** for desired effects than the patient with blue eyes.

**PROSTAGLANDINS Prototype for classification: Latanoprost**

**Use:** Open-angle glaucoma and intraocular hypertension.

**Bimatoprost**
Lumigan, 0.01%,
0.03% solution

*Adult:* **Topical** 1 drop in affected eye(s) once daily in the evening.

**Latanoprost**
Xalatan, 0.005%
solution

*Adult:* **Topical** 1 drop (1.5 mcg) in affected eye(s) once daily in the evening.

**Trafluprost**
Zioptan 0.015 mg/Ml

*Adult:* **Topical** 1 drop in the conjunctival sac of the affected eye(s) once daily in the evening.

**Travoprost**
Travatan, 0.004% solution

*Adult:* **Topical** 1 drop in affected eye(s) once daily in the evening.

**ADVERSE EFFECTS Ocular:** *Conjunctival hyperemia, growth of eyelashes, ocular pruritus,* ocular dryness, visual disturbance, ocular burning, foreign body sensation, eye pain, pigmentation of the periocular skin, blepharitis, cataract, superficial punctate keratitis, eyelid erythema, ocular irritation, eyelash darkening, eye discharge, tearing, photophobia, allergic conjunctivitis, increases in iris pigmentation (brown pigment), conjunctival edema. **Body as a Whole:** Headaches, abnormal liver function tests, asthenia, and hirsutism. **Clinical Implications:** Should instill in the evening. Wait 15 min after instillation before inserting soft contact lenses to avoid staining the lenses. Give at least 5 min apart from other topical ophthalmic drugs.

**MYDRIATIC Prototype for classification: Homatropine HBr**
**Use:** Mydriatic for ocular examination and as cycloplegic to measure errors of refraction. Also inflammatory conditions of uveal tract, ciliary spasm, as a cycloplegic and mydriatic in preoperative and postoperative conditions, and as an optical aid in select patients with axial lens opacities.

**Cyclopentolate HCl**
Cyclogyl, 0.5%, 1%, 2% solution

**Cycloplegic Refraction:** *Adult:* **Topical** 1 drop of 1% solution in eye 40–50 min before procedure, followed by 1 drop in 5 min; may need 2% solution in patients with darkly pigmented eyes. *Child:* **Topical** 1 drop of 0.5–1% solution in eye 40–50 min before procedure, followed by 1 drop in 5 min; may need 2% solution in patients with darkly pigmented eyes.

**Homatropine HBr**
Homatropaire, Isopto Homatropine, 2%, 5% solution

**Cycloplegic Refraction:** *Adult:* **Topical** 1–2 drops of 2% or 5% solution in eye repeated in 5–10 min if necessary. **Ocular Inflammation:** *Adult:* **Topical** 1–2 drops of 2% or 5% solution in eye up to q3–4h.

**Phenylephrine HCl**
AK-Dilate Ophthalmic, Mydfrin, 0.12%, 2.5%, 10% solution

**Ophthalmoscopy:** *Adult:* **Topical** 1 drop of 2.5% or 10% solution before examination. *Child:* **Topical** 1 drop of 2.5% solution before examination. **Vasoconstrictor:** *Adult:* **Topical** 2 drops of 0.12% solution q3–4h as necessary.

**Tropicamide**
Mydriacyl, Tropicacyl, 0.5%, 1% solution

**Refraction:** *Adult:* **Topical** 1–2 drops of 1% solution in each eye, repeat in 5 min; if patient is not seen within 20–30 min, an additional drop may be instilled. **Examination of Fundus:** *Adult:* **Topical** 1–2 drops of 0.5% solution in each eye 15–20 min prior to examination; may repeat q30min if necessary.

**CONTRAINDICATED IN** Primary (narrow-angle) glaucoma or predisposition to glaucoma; children younger than 6 y. **Cautious Use in:** Increased IOP, infants, children, pregnancy (category C), the elderly or debilitated; hypertension; hyperthyroidism; diabetes; cardiac disease. **Adverse Effects:** Increased IOP, *blurred vision, photophobia*. **Prolonged Use:** Local irritation, congestion, edema, eczema, follicular conjunctivitis. **Excessive Dosage/Systemic Absorption:** Symptoms of atropine poisoning (flushing, dry skin, mouth, nose; decreased sweating; fever, rash, rapid/irregular pulse; abdominal and bladder distention; hallucinations, confusion). **CNS:** Psychotic reaction, behavior disturbances, ataxia, incoherent speech, restlessness, hallucinations, somnolence, disorientation, failure to recognize people, grand mal seizures. **Clinical Implications:** Carefully monitor **cyclopentolate** patients with seizure disorders, since systemic absorption may precipitate a seizure. Photophobia associated with mydriasis may require patient to wear dark glasses. Since drug causes blurred vision, supervision of activity may be indicated.

**VASOCONSTRICTOR; DECONGESTANT** Prototype for classification: **Naphazoline HCl Use:** Ocular vasoconstrictor.

| | |
|---|---|
| **Naphazoline HCl** 0.012%, 0.02%, 0.1% solution | *Adult:* **Topical** 1–3 drops of 0.1% solution q3–4h prn or 1–2 drops of a 0.012–0.03% solution q4h prn. |
| **Tetrahydrozoline HCl** Opti-Clear, Visine Original, 0.05% solution | *Adult:* **Topical** 1–2 drops of 0.05% solution in eye b.i.d. or t.i.d. |

**CONTRAINDICATED IN** Narrow-angle glaucoma; concomitant use with MAO INHIBITORS or TRICYCLIC ANTIDEPRESSANTS **Cautious Use in:** Hypertension, cardiac irregularities, advanced arteriosclerosis; diabetes; hyperthyroidism; elderly patients. **Adverse Effects:** Pupillary dilation, increased intraocular pressure, rebound redness of the eye, headache, hypertension, nausea, weakness, sweating. **Overdosage:** Drowsiness, hypothermia, bradycardia, shocklike hypotension, coma.

**CORTICOSTEROID, ANTI-INFLAMMATORY** Prototype for classification: **Hydrocortisone Use:** Inflammation. **Unlabeled Use:** Anterior uveitis.

| | |
|---|---|
| **Difluprednate** Durezol, 0.05% suspension | *Adult:* **Topical** 1 drop in conjunctival sac q.i.d. for the first 24 h; q.i.d. for 2 wk; then b.i.d. for 2 wk. |
| **Fluorometholone** Flarex, FML Forte, FML Liquifilm, 0.1%, 0.25% suspension; 0.1% ointment | *Adult/Child (2 y or older):* **Topical** 1–2 drops of suspension in conjunctival sac q.h. for the first 24–48 h; then b.i.d. to q.i.d.; or a thin strip of ointment q4h for the first 24–48 h; then 1–3 × day. |

**Loteprednol etabonate**
Alrex, Lotemax, 0.2%, 0.5% suspension

*Adult:* **Topical** 1–2 drops in conjunctival sac q.i.d. during initial treatment, may increase to q1h if necessary.

**Prednisolone sodium phosphate**
Inflamase Mild, Pred Mild, Prednisol, Inflamase Forte, 0.11%, 0.12%, 0.9% suspension

*Adult:* **Topical** 1–2 drops in conjunctival sac q.h. during the day; then q2h at night; may decrease to 1 drop t.i.d. or q.i.d.

**Rimexolone**
Vexol, 1% solution

**Postoperative Ocular Inflammation:** *Adult:* **Topical** 1–2 drops q.i.d. beginning 24 h after surgery, continue through first 2 wk postoperatively. **Anterior Uveitis:** *Adult:* **Topical** 1–2 drops in affected eye every hour while awake for first wk, then q2h for second wk, then taper frequency until uveitis resolves.

**CONTRAINDICATED IN** Ocular fungal diseases, *herpes simplex* keratitis, ocular infections, ocular mycobacterial infections, viral disease of cornea or conjunctiva such as vaccinia, varicella. **Adverse Effects: Ocular:** Blurred vision, photophobia, conjunctival edema, corneal edema, erosion, eye discharge, dryness, irritation, pain. **Prolonged Use:** Glaucoma, ocular hypertension, damage to optic nerve, defects in visual acuity and visual fields, posterior subcapsular cataract formation, secondary ocular infections. **Other:** Headache, taste perversion. **Clinical Implications:** Shake all products well before use.

**OCULAR ANTIHISTAMINES Prototype for classification: Emedastine**
**Use:** Relief of signs and symptoms of allergic conjunctivitis

**Azelastine HCl**
OPTIVAR, 0.05% solution

*Adult/Child (3 y or older):* **Topical** 1 drop in affected eye(s) b.i.d.

**Bepotastine**
Bepreve, 1.5% solution

*Adult:* **Topical** 1 drop in affected eye(s) b.i.d.

**Cetirizine**
Zerviate, 0.24% solution

*Adult:* **Topical** 1 drop in each eye b.i.d.

**Cromolyn sodium**
Crolom, Opticrom, 4% solution

*Adult:* **Topical** 1–2 drops in each eye 4–6 × day.

**Emedastine difumarate**
Emadine, 0.05% solution

*Adult/Child (3 y or older):* **Topical** 1 drop in affected eye(s) up to q.i.d.

**Epinastine hydrochloride**
Elestat, 0.05% solution

*Adult/Child (3 y or older):* **Topical** 1 drop in affected eye(s) up to b.i.d.

| **Ketotifen fumarate** | *Adult:* **Topical** 1 drop in affected eye(s) |
| Zaditor, 0.025% solution | q8–12h. |
| **Lodoxamide** | *Adult/Child (2 mo or older):* **Topical** |
| Alomide, 0.1% solution | 1–2 drop in affected eye(s) q.i.d. for up to 3 mo. |
| **Nedocromil sodium** | *Adult/Child (3 y or older):* **Topical** |
| Alocril, 2% solution | 1–2 drops in affected eye(s) b.i.d. |
| **Olopatadine HCl** | *Adult/Child (3 y or older):* **Topical** |
| Patanol, 0.1% solution; Pata-day, 0.2% solution; Pazeo, 0.7% solution | 1–2 drops in affected eye(s) b.i.d. at least 6–8 h apart. |

**ADVERSE EFFECTS Ocular:** Allergic reactions, *burning, stinging,* discharge, dry eyes, eye pain, eyelid disorder, itching, keratitis, lacrimation disorder, mydriasis, photophobia, rash. **CNS:** Drowsiness, fatigue, headache. **Other:** Dry mouth, cold syndrome, pharyngitis, rhinitis, sinusitis, taste perversion. **Clinical Implications:** Wait 10 min after instilling **emedastine** before inserting soft contact lenses; do not use **olopatadine** with soft contact lenses.

## OCULAR NONSTEROIDAL ANTI-INFLAMMATORY DRUGS
**Prototype for classification: Ibuprofen Use:** Treatment of ocular pain and inflammation associated with cataract surgery.

| **Bromfenac** | *Adult:* **Topical** 1 drop into affected eye(s) b.i.d. |
| Xibrom, 0.09% solution | beginning 24 h after cataract surgery and continuing for 14 days. |
| **Diclofenac** | *Adult:* **Topical** 1–2 drops in affected eye(s) within |
| 0.1% solution | 1 h prior to surgery then 1–2 drops 15 min after surgery, then daily beginning 4–6 h after surgery, continue up to 3 days. |
| **Flurbiprofen** | *Adult:* **Topical** 1 drop q30min beginning 2 h |
| Ocufen, 0.03% solution | prior to surgery for total of 4 drops. |
| **Ketorolac** | *Adult:* **Topical** 1 drop to affected eye(s) 4 × day |
| Acular, Acular LS, Acuvail, 0.4% 0.45%, 0.5% solution | beginning 24 h after surgery and continuing for 14 days. |
| **Nepafenac** | *Adult/Child (10 y or older):* **Topical** 1 drop into |
| Nevanac, 0.1% suspension | affected eye(s) t.i.d. beginning 24 h after cataract surgery and continuing for 14 days. |

**ADVERSE EFFECTS Ocular:** Conjunctival hyperemia, ocular hypertension, foreign body sensation, decreased visual acuity, headache, iritis, ocular inflammation (e.g., edema, erythema), ocular irritation (burning/stinging), ocular pruritus, ocular pain, photophobia, lacrimation, abnormal sensation in the eye, delayed wound healing, keratitis, lid margin crusting, corneal erosion, corneal perforation, corneal thinning, and epithelial breakdown. Continued use can lead to ulceration or perforation. **Clinical Implications: Nepafenac** suspension **must be** shaken well prior to use.

## OCULAR ANTIBIOTIC, QUINOLONE

**Prototype for classification: Ciprofloxacin Use:** Treatment of ocular infection.

| | |
|---|---|
| **Besifloxacin**<br>Besivance, 0.6%<br>suspension | *Adult/Adolescent/Child (1 y or older):*<br>**Topical** 1 drop in affected eye(s) t.i.d. × 7 days |
| **Ciprofloxacin**<br>Ciloxin, 0.3% solution | *Adult/Adolescent/Child (1 y or older):*<br>**Topical** 1–2 drops in affected eye(s) q2h ×<br>2 days then q4h × 5 days. |
| **Levofloxacin**<br>0.5% solution | *Adult/Adolescent/Child (6 y or older):*<br>**Topical** 1–2 drops in affected eye(s) q2h<br>(up to 8 × day) on days 1 and 2 then q4h<br>(up to 4 × day) |
| **Moxifloxacin**<br>Vigamox, 0.5% solution<br>Moxeza, 0.5% solution | *Adult/Child (1 y or older):* **Topical** (Vigamox) 1<br>drop in affected eye(s) t.i.d. × 7 days. (Moxeza)<br>1 drop in affected eye(s) b.i.d. × 7 days |
| **Ofloxacin**<br>Ocuflox 0.3% solution | *Adult/Adolescent/Child:* **Ophthalmic** Instill<br>1–2 drops q2–4h for first 2 days, then q.i.d.<br>for up to 5 additional days |

**ADVERSE EFFECTS Ocular:** Conjunctival redness, blurred vision, irritation, pain, pruritus. **CNS:** Headache

## APPENDIX A-2

### LOW MOLECULAR WEIGHT HEPARINS

**ANTICOAGULANT, LOW MOLECULAR WEIGHT HEPARIN Prototype for classification: Enoxaparin Use:** Prevention and treatment of DVT following hip or knee replacement or abdominal surgery, unstable angina, acute coronary syndromes.

| | |
|---|---|
| **Dalteparin sodium**<br>Fragmin, 10,000<br>international units/mL,<br>25,000 international<br>units/mL | **DVT Prophylaxis, Abdominal Surgery:** *Adult:*<br>**Subcutaneous** 2500 international units daily<br>starting 1–2 h prior to surgery and continuing<br>for 5–10 days postoperatively. **DVT Prophylaxis,**<br>**Total Hip Arthroplasty:** *Adult:* **Subcutaneous**<br>2500–5000 international units daily starting<br>1–2 h prior to surgery and continuing for 5–14<br>days postoperatively. **Acute Thromboembolism:** |

*Adult:* **Subcutaneous** 120 international units/kg b.i.d. for at least 5 days. **Recurrent Thromboembolism:** *Adult:* **Subcutaneous** 5000 international units b.i.d. for 3–6 mo. **Unstable Angina/Non–Q-Wave MI:** *Adult:* **Subcutaneous** 120 international units/kg (max: 10,000 international units) q12h.

**DVT Prophylaxis with risk of PE:** *Adult:* **Subcutaneous** 5000 international units once daily for 12–14 days. **Extended Treatment of VTE or Proximal DVT:** *Adult:* **Subcutaneous** 200 international units/kg daily for 1 mo, then 150 international units/kg daily for 2–6 mo.

**Enoxaparin**
Lovenox,
100 mg/mL

**Prevention of DVT after Hip or Knee Surgery:** *Adult:* **Subcutaneous** 30 mg subcutaneously b.i.d. for 10–14 days starting 12–24 h post-surgery. **Prevention of DVT after Abdominal Surgery:** *Adult:* **Subcutaneous** 40 mg daily starting 2 h before surgery and continuing for 7–10 days (max: 12 days). **Treatment of DVT and Pulmonary Embolus:** *Adult:* **Subcutaneous** 1 mg/kg b.i.d.; monitor anti-Xa activity to determine appropriate dose. **Acute Coronary Syndrome:** *Adult:* **Subcutaneous** 1 mg/kg q12h × 2–8 days. Give concurrently with aspirin 100–325 mg/day.

**CONTRAINDICATED IN** Hypersensitivity to ardeparin, other low molecular weight heparins, pork products, or parabens; active major bleeding, thrombocytopenia that is positive for antiplatelet antibodies with ardeparin; uncontrolled hypertension; nursing mothers. **Tizaparin** contraindicated in patients over 90 years old with CrCl less than 60 mL/min. **Cautious Use in:** Hypersensitivity to heparin; history of heparin-induced thrombocytopenia; bacterial endocarditis; severe and uncontrolled hypertension, cerebral aneurysm or hemorrhagic stroke, bleeding disorders, recent GI bleeding or associated GI disorders (e.g., ulcerative colitis), thrombocytopenia, or platelet disorders; severe liver or renal disease, diabetic retinopathy, hypertensive retinopathy, invasive procedures; pregnancy (category C). **Adverse Effects: Body as a Whole:** Allergic reactions (rash, urticaria), arthralgia, pain and inflammation at injection site, peripheral edema, fever. **CNS:** *CVA*, dizziness, headache, insomnia. **CV:** Chest pain. **GI:** Nausea, vomiting. **Hematologic:** *Hemorrhage*, thrombocytopenia, ecchymoses, anemia. **Respiratory:** Dyspnea. **Skin:** Rash, pruritus. **Drug Interactions: Aspirin,** NSAIDS, **warfarin** can increase risk of hemorrhage **Clinical Implications:** Alternate injection sites using the abdomen, anterior thigh, or outer aspect of upper arms. **Lab Tests:** CBC with platelet count, urinalysis, and stool for occult blood should be tested throughout therapy. Routine coagulation tests are not required. Carefully monitor for and immediately report S&S of excessive anticoagulation (e.g., bleeding at venipuncture sites or surgical site) or hemorrhage (e.g., drop in BP or Hct). Patients on oral anticoagulants, platelet inhibitors, or with impaired renal function **must be** very carefully monitored for hemorrhage. Patient should be sitting or lying supine for injection. Inject deep subcutaneously with entire length of needle inserted into skin fold. Hold skin fold gently throughout injection and do not rub site after injection.

## APPENDIX A-3

### INHALED CORTICOSTEROIDS (ORAL AND NASAL INHALATIONS)

**CORTICOSTEROID, ANTIINFLAMMATORY Prototype for classification:
Hydrocortisone Use:** Oral inhalation to treat steroid-dependent asthma, nasal inhalation for the management of the symptoms of seasonal or perennial rhinitis.

| | |
|---|---|
| **Beclomethasone dipropionate** <br> Beconase AQ, Qnasl, QVAR | **Asthma:** *Adult:* **Oral Inhaler** 40–80 mcg b.i.d. may try to reduce systemic steroids after 1 wk of concomitant therapy; (max: 320 mcg/day). *Child (5–11 y):* **Oral Inhaler QVAR** 40 mcg b.i.d. (max: 160 mcg/day). *Child (4-5 y):* **Oral Inhaler Qvar Redihaler** 40 mcg b.i.d. **Allergic Rhinitis:** *Adult:* **Nasal Inhaler** 1 spray/nostril b.i.d. to q.i.d. Child (older than 6 y): 1–2 sprays daily. |
| **Budesonide** <br> Pulmicort, Rhinocort Aqua | **Asthma, Maintenance Therapy:** *Adult:* **Oral Inhalation** 360 mcg b.i.d. (max: 800 mcg b.i.d.). *Child (6 y or older):* **Oral Inhalation** 180 mcg b.i.d. (max: 400 mcg b.i.d.). *Child (12 mo–8 y):* **Nebulization** 0.5 mg/day in 1–2 divided doses. **Rhinitis:** *Adult/Child (6 y or older):* **Intranasal** 2 sprays/nostril in the morning and evening or 4 sprays/nostril in the morning. |
| **Ciclesonide** <br> Alvesco, Omnaris, Zetonna | **Rhinitis:** *Adult/Child (6 y or older):* **Intranasal** 1–2 sprays/nostril once daily (depends on product used) **Asthma:** *Adult/Child (12 y and older):* **Inhaled** 80 mcg b.i.d.; may increase to 160 mcg b.i.d. |
| **Flunisolide** <br> 0.025% solution | **Allergic Rhinitis:** *Adult:* **Intranasal** 2 sprays intranasally/nostril, b.i.d.; may increase to t.i.d., if needed. *Child:* **Intranasal** 6–14 y, 1 spray intranasally/nostril t.i.d. or 2 sprays b.i.d. |
| **Fluticasone** <br> ArmonAir RespiClick, Flonase, Flovent, Flovent HFA, 44 mcg, 110 mcg, 220 mcg aerosol, **Veramyst,** 27.5 mcg/actuation | **Seasonal Allergic Rhinitis:** *Adult:* **Intranasal** 100 mcg (1 inhalation)/nostril 1–2 × daily (max: 4 × daily). **Inhalation** 1–2 inhalations daily. *Child (4 y or older):* **Intranasal** 1 spray/nostril once daily. May increase to 2 sprays/nostril once daily if inadequate response, then decrease to 1 spray/nostril once daily. when control is achieved. *Adult/Adolescent/Child (12 y or older):* **Intranasal (Veramyst)** 2 sprays/nostril daily then reduce to 1 spray daily. *Child (2–11 y):* **Intranasal (Veramyst)** 1 spray/nostril daily, may increase to 2 sprays/nostril daily if necessary. *Adult/Adolescent:* **Inhaled (Advair)** 1–2 inhalations q12h. |

| | |
|---|---|
| **Fluticasone/ Vilanterol** Breo Ellipta, 100 mcg/25 mcg powder for inhalation | *Adult:* **Inhalation** 1 inhalation every 24 h. |
| **Mometasone furoate** Asmanex, Nasonex, 220 mcg/ inhalation, 50 mcg/ inhalation | **Allergic Rhinitis:** *Adult/Child (12 y or older):* **Intranasal** 2 sprays (50 mcg each) in each nostril once daily. *Child (2 y –11 y):* **Intranasal** 1 spray in each nostril once daily. *Adult/Child (12 y or older):* **Powder for Inhalation** 1 inhalation (220 mcg) once or twice daily (max: 1 inhalation b.i.d.). *Child (4–11 y):* **Powder for Inhalation** 200 mcg (may increase to 400 mcg) b.i.d. |
| **Triamcinolone acetonide** Nasacort, 100 mcg/inhalation | *Adult:* **Inhalation** 2 puffs 3–4 × day (max: 16 puffs/day) or 4 puffs b.i.d. **Nasal Spray** 2 sprays/ nostril once daily (max: 8 sprays/day). *Child (6–12 y):* **Inhalation** 1–2 sprays t.i.d. or q.i.d. (max: 12 sprays/day) or 2–4 sprays b.i.d. **Intranasal** 1 spray in each nostril daily. |

**CONTRAINDICATED IN** Nonasthmatic bronchitis, primary treatment of status asthmaticus, acute attack of asthma. **Cautious Use in:** Patients receiving systemic corticosteroids; use with extreme caution if at all in respiratory tuberculosis, untreated fungal, bacterial, or viral infections, and ocular herpes simplex; nasal inhalation therapy for nasal septal ulcers, nasal trauma, or surgery. **Adverse Effects: Oral Inhalation:** *Candidal infection of oropharynx* and occasionally larynx, hoarseness, dry mouth, sore throat, sore mouth. **Nasal (Inhaler):** *Transient nasal irritation, burning, sneezing,* epistaxis, bloody mucus, nasopharyngeal itching, dryness, crusting, and ulceration; headache, nausea, vomiting. **Other:** With excessive doses, symptoms of hypercorticism. Increased risk of adverse effects if Advair is used with other long-acting beta-agonists. **Clinical Implications:** Note that oral inhalation and nasal inhalation products are not to be used interchangeably. **Oral Inhaler:** Emphasize the following: (1) Shake inhaler well before using. (2) After exhaling fully, place mouthpiece well into mouth with lips closed firmly around it. (3) Inhale slowly through mouth while activating the inhaler. (4) Hold breath 5–10 sec, if possible, then exhale slowly. (5) Wait 1 min between puffs. Clean inhaler daily. Separate parts as directed in package insert, rinse them with warm water, and dry them thoroughly. Rinsing mouth and gargling with warm water after each oral inhalation removes residual medication from oropharyngeal area. Mouth care may also delay or prevent onset of oral dryness, hoarseness, and candidiasis. **Nasal Inhaler:** Directions for use of nasal inhaler provided by manufacturer should be carefully reviewed with patient. Emphasize the following points: (1) Gently blow nose to clear nostrils. (2) Shake inhaler well before using. (3) If 2 sprays in each nostril are prescribed, direct one spray toward upper, and the other toward lower part of nostril. (4) Wash cap and plastic nosepiece daily with warm water; dry thoroughly. Inhaled steroids do not provide immediate symptomatic relief and are not prescribed for this purpose.

## APPENDIX A-4

### TOPICAL CORTICOSTEROIDS

**CORTICOSTEROID, ANTI-INFLAMMATORY** **Prototype for classification: Hydrocortisone Use:** As a topical corticosteroid, the drug is used for the relief of the inflammatory and pruritic manifestations of corticosteroid-responsive dermatoses.

**Hydrocortisone**
Aeroseb-HC, Alphaderm, Cetacort, Cortaid, Cortenema, Dermolate, Hytone, Rectacort, Synacort, Caldecort, 0.5%, 1%, 2.5% cream, lotion, ointment, spray

*Adult:* **Topical** Apply a small amount to the affected area 1–4 × day. **PR** Insert 1% cream, 10% foam, 10–25 mg suppository, or 100 mg enema nightly.

**Hydrocortisone acetate**
Anusol HC, Carmol HC, Colifoam, Cortaid, Cort-Dome, Cortisaine, Cortifoam, Epifoam, 0.5%, 1% ointment, cream

**Alclometasone dipropionate**
Aclovate, 0.05% cream, ointment

*Adult:* **Topical** 0.05% cream or ointment applied sparingly b.i.d. or t.i.d.; may use occlusive dressing for resistant dermatoses.

**Amcinonide**
Cyclocort, 0.1% cream, lotion, ointment

*Adult:* **Topical** Apply thin film b.i.d. or t.i.d.

**Betamethasone dipropionate**
Diprolene, Diprolene AF, Diprosone, Maxivate, 0.05% cream, gel, lotion, ointment

*Adult:* **Topical** Apply thin film b.i.d.

**Betamethasone valerate**
Luxiq, Valisone, Psorion, Beta-Val, 0.1% cream, ointment, lotion; 0.12% aerosol foam

*Adult:* **Topical** Apply sparingly b.i.d.

**Clobetasol propionate**
Clobex, Cormax, Embeline, Olux, Temovate, 0.05% cream, gel, ointment, lotion, aerosol foam

*Adult:* **Topical** Apply sparingly b.i.d. (max: 50 g/wk), or b.i.d. 3 day/wk or 1–2 × wk for up to 6 mo.

**Clocortolone pivalate**
Cloderm, 0.1% cream

*Adult:* **Topical** Apply thin layer
1–4 × day.

**Desonide**
DesOwen, Tridesilon, 0.05%
cream, ointment, lotion

*Adult:* **Topical** Apply thin layer b.i.d.
to q.i.d.

**Desoximetasone**
Topicort, 0.05%, 0.25% cream,
ointment; 0.25% topical spray

*Adult:* **Topical** Apply thin layer b.i.d.

**Diclofenac**
Flector, Pennsaid, 1.3%
topical patch; 1% topical gel

*Adult:* **Topical** Up to 4 g 4 × day on
affected joint (max: 16 g).

**Diflorasone diacetate**
Florone, Florone E,
Maxiflor, Psorcon E,
Psorcon, 0.05% cream,
ointment

*Adult:* **Topical** Apply thin layer of
ointment 1–3 × day or cream 2–4 ×
day.

**Fluocinolone acetonide**
Fluoderm, Synalar, 0.025%
ointment, cream; 0.2%
cream; 0.01% cream,
solution, shampoo, oil;
0.59 mg ophthalmic insert

*Adult:* **Topical** Apply thin layer b.i.d.
to q.i.d.

**Fluocinonide**
Vanos, 0.05% cream,
ointment, solution,
gel; 0.1% cream

*Adult:* **Topical** Apply thin layer b.i.d.
to q.i.d.

**Flurandrenolide**
Cordran, Cordran SP,
0.05% cream, lotion; 4 mcg/
sq cm tape

*Adult:* **Topical** Apply thin layer b.i.d.
or t.i.d.; apply tape 1–2 × day at
12 h intervals. *Child:* **Topical** Apply
thin layer 1–2 × day; apply tape
once/day.

**Fluticasone**
Cutivate, 0.005%, 0.05%
cream; 0.005% ointment

*Adult/Child (3 mo or older):*
**Topical** Apply a thin film of cream
or ointment to affected area once or
twice daily.

**Halcinonide**
Halog, 0.1% cream,
ointment, solution

*Adult:* **Topical** Apply thin layer b.i.d.
or t.i.d. *Child:* **Topical** Apply thin
layer once/day.

**Halobetasol**
Ultravate, 0.05% cream,
ointment

*Adult:* **Topical** Apply sparingly b.i.d.

**Mometasone furoate**
Elocon, 0.1% cream,
lotion, ointment

*Adult:* **Topical** Apply a thin film of
cream or ointment or a few drops of
lotion to affected area once/day.

**Triamcinolone**
Kenalog, Triderm,
0.025%, 0.5%, 0.1%
cream, ointment; 0.025%,
0.1% lotion

*Adult:* **Topical** Apply sparingly b.i.d.
or t.i.d.

**CONTRAINDICATED IN** Topical steroids contraindicated in presence of varicella, vaccinia, on surfaces with compromised circulation, and in children younger than 2 y. **Cautious Use in:** Children; diabetes mellitus; stromal *herpes simplex;* glaucoma, tuberculosis of eye; osteoporosis; untreated fungal, bacterial, or viral infections **Adverse Effects: Skin:** Skin thinning and atrophy, *acne, impaired wound healing;* petechiae, ecchymosis, easy bruising; suppression of skin test reaction; hypopigmentation or hyperpigmentation, hirsutism, acneiform eruptions, subcutaneous fat atrophy; allergic dermatitis, urticaria, angioneurotic edema, increased sweating. **Clinical Implications:** Administer retention enema preferably after a bowel movement. The enema should be retained at least w1 h or all night if possible. If an occlusive dressing is to be used, apply medication sparingly, rub until it disappears, and then reapply, leaving a thin coat over lesion. Completely cover area with transparent plastic or other occlusive device or vehicle. Avoid covering a weeping or exudative lesion. Usually, occlusive dressings are not applied to face, scalp, scrotum, axilla, and groin. Inspect skin carefully between applications for ecchymotic, petechial, and purpuric signs, maceration, secondary infection, skin atrophy, striae or miliaria; if present, stop medication and notify prescriber. Warn patient not to self-dose with OTC topical preparations of a corticosteroid more than 7 days. They should not be used for children younger than 2 y. If symptoms do not abate, consult prescriber. Usually, topical preparations are applied after a shower or bath when skin is damp or wet. Cleansing and application of prescribed preparation should be done with extreme gentleness because of fragility, easy bruisability, and poor healing skin. Hazard of systemic toxicity is higher in small children because of the greater ratio of skin surface area to body weight. Apply sparingly. Urge patient on long-term therapy with topical corticosterone to check expiration date.

## APPENDIX A-5

### TOPICAL ANTIFUNGAL AGENTS

**USES** Treatment of fungal infections managed by topical agents. This could include: Tinea (pityriasis) versicolor due to *M. furfur* (formerly *P. orbiculare*), interdigital tinea pedis (athlete's foot), tinea corporis (ringworm) and tinea cruris (jock itch) due to *E. floccosum, T. mentagrophytes, T. rubrum,* and *T. tonsurans.* Shampoo for treatment of seborrheic dermatitis.

**Butenafine**
Lotrimin Ultra, Mentax, 1% cream

*Adult:* **Topical** Apply 1–2 × daily for
2–4 wk.

**Ciclopirox**
Ciclodan, CNL8 Nail, Loprox,
Pedipirox-4 Nail, Penlac,
8% solution, 1% shampoo,
0.77% gel

*Adult:* **Topical** Apply twice daily
(morning and evening). Nail lacquer
solution should be applied once daily.

**Econazole**
Ecoza, 1% cream, 1% foam

*Adult:* **Topical** Apply once daily ×
2–4 wk (depending on area).

**Efinaconazole**
Jublia, 10% solution

*Adult:* **Topical** Apply daily to affected
toenail × 48 wk.

**Luliconazole**
Luzu, 1% cream

*Adult:* **Topical** Apply to affected area
daily × 1–2 wk.

**Naftifine**
Naftin, 1%, 2% cream; 1%, 2% gel

*Adult:* **Topical** Apply cream once
daily or gel twice daily to affected
areas × 2–4 wk.

**Sertaconazole**
Eratczo, 2% cream

*Adult:* **Topical** Apply to affected area
b.i.d. × 4 wk.

**Tavaborole**
Kerydin 5% solution

*Adult:* **Topical** Apply to affected
toenails daily × 48 wk.

**Tolnaftate**
Fungi-Guard, Fongoid-D, Lamisil AF
Defense, Mycocide Clinical NS,
Podactin, Tinactin, Tinaspore,
1% solution, 1% powder, 1% cream,
1% aerosol, 1% aerosol powder

*Adult/Adolescent/Child (2 y or
older):* **Topical** Apply to affected area
1–2 times daily × 4 wk.

**CONTRAINDICATED IN** Patients with known or suspected sensitivity to
agent; administration via route other than oral.

**CAUTIOUS USE** Pregnancy or lactation, cautious use in children (except
tolnaftate), avoid use with occlusive dressing.

**ADVERSE EFFECTS** **Skin:** Stinging/burning at application site, contact dermatitis, erythema, irritation, itching. **Dermatologic:** Ingrown toenail.

**CLINICAL IMPLICATIONS** If symptoms not resolving within recommended
therapy duration patient needs to be re-evaluated. Patients using a nail
product should avoid pedicures, or use of nail polish during treatment.

# ◆ APPENDIX B  U.S. SCHEDULES OF CONTROLLED SUBSTANCES

## Schedule I

High potential for abuse and of no currently accepted medical use. Examples: heroin, LSD, ecstasy peyote. Not obtainable by prescription but may be legally procured for research, study, or instructional use.

## Schedule II

High abuse potential and high liability for severe psychological or physical dependence. Prescription required and cannot be renewed.[a] Includes opium derivatives, other opioids, and short-acting barbiturates. Examples: Amphetamine, cocaine, meperidine, morphine, fentanyl.

## Schedule III

Potential for abuse is less than that for drugs in Schedules I and II. Moderate to low physical dependence and high psychological dependence. Includes certain stimulants and depressants not included in the above schedules and preparations containing limited quantities of certain opioids. Examples: Ketamine, anabolic steroids, testosterone. Prescription required.[a,b]

## Schedule IV

Lower potential for abuse than Schedule III drugs. Examples: Certain psychotropics (tranquilizers), chlordiazepoxide, diazepam, meprobamate, phenobarbital. Prescription required.[a,b]

## Schedule V

Abuse potential less than that for Schedule IV drugs. Preparations contain limited quantities of certain narcotic drugs; generally intended for antitussive and antidiarrheal purposes and may be distributed without a prescription provided that:

1. Such distribution is made only by a pharmacist.
2. Not more than 240 mL or not more than 48 solid dosage units of any substance containing opium, nor more than 120 mL or not more than 24 solid dosage units of any other controlled substance may be distributed at retail to the same purchaser in any given 48-hour period without a valid prescription order.
3. The purchaser is at least 18 years old.

4. The pharmacist knows the purchaser or requests suitable identification.
5. The pharmacist keeps an official written record of: name and address of purchaser, name and quantity of controlled substance purchased, date of sale, initials of dispensing pharmacist. This record is to be made available for inspection and copying by U.S. officers authorized by the Attorney General.
6. Other federal, state, or local law does not require a prescription order.

Under jurisdiction of the Federal Controlled Substances Act:
[a] Except when dispensed directly by a practitioner, other than a pharmacist, to an ultimate user, no controlled substance in Schedule II may be dispensed without a *written* prescription, except that in emergency situations such drug may be dispensed upon oral prescription and a written prescription must be obtained within the time frame prescribed by law. No prescription for a controlled substance in Schedule II may be refilled.
[b] Refillable up to 5 × within 6 mo, but only if so indicated by prescriber.

In December 2014 the FDA released a final rule replacing the historic *letter categories* (listed below) with new detailed subsections describing the risk of medication exposure in the real-world context of caring for pregnant patients. The final rule requires the use of three subsections in the labeling titled, *Pregnancy, Lactation,* and *Females and Males of Reproductive Potential* that provide details about use of the drug or biological product. These changes will be implemented over the next several years; until that time the historic *letter categories* will still be in use and so are included below for reference. The categories described by the FDA are as follows:

### Category A

Controlled studies in women fail to demonstrate a risk to the fetus in the first trimester (and there is no evidence of risk in later trimesters), and the possibility of fetal harm appears remote.

### Category B

Either animal-reproduction studies have not demonstrated a fetal risk but there are no controlled studies in pregnant women, or animal-reproduction studies have shown an adverse effect (other than a decrease in fertility) that was not confirmed in controlled studies in women in the first trimester (and there is no evidence of a risk in later trimesters).

### Category C

Either studies in animals have revealed adverse effects on the fetus (teratogenic or embryocidal effects or other) and there are no controlled studies in women, or studies in women and animals are not available. Drugs should be given only if the potential benefit justifies the potential risk to the fetus.

### Category D

There is positive evidence of human fetal risk, but the benefits from use in pregnant women may be acceptable despite the risk (e.g., if the drug is needed in a life-threatening situation or for a serious disease for which safer drugs cannot be used or are ineffective). There will be an appropriate statement in the "warnings" section of the labeling.

### Category X

Studies in animals or human beings have demonstrated fetal abnormalities or there is evidence of fetal risk based on human experience, or both, and the risk of the use of the drug in pregnant women clearly outweighs any possible benefit. The drug is contraindicated in women who are or may become pregnant. There will be an appropriate statement in the "contraindications" section of the labeling.

Drugs approved after June 2015 will not have a *pregnancy category* but will instead include the categories of *Pregnancy, Lactation,* and *Females and Males of Reproductive Potential.*

## ◆ APPENDIX D   ORAL DOSAGE FORMS THAT SHOULD NOT BE CRUSHED

Some oral dosage forms should not be crushed or chewed. These dosage forms have been specially designed to release the drug slowly over several hours, to protect the drug from the low pH of the stomach, and/or to protect the stomach from the irritating effects of the drug.

Drugs may have an **enteric coating** which is designed to allow the drug to pass through the stomach intact with the drug being released in the intestines. This protects the stomach from the irritating effects of the drug, protects the drug from being destroyed by the acid pH of the stomach, and can delay the onset of action.

**Modified release** formulations are designed to release the drug over an extended period of time. These formulations can include multiple-layer compressed tablets where drug is released as each layer dissolves, mixed-release pellets that dissolve at different time intervals, and special tablets that are themselves inert but are designed to release drug slowly from the formulation. Some modified release dosage forms are scored and may be broken in half without affecting the release mechanism but still should not be crushed or chewed. Some mixed-release capsule formulations can be opened and the contents sprinkled on food. However, the pellets should not be crushed or chewed. Some modified release formulations can be identified by common abbreviations used in their brand names. These abbreviations include: CR (controlled release), CRT (controlled release tablet), LA (long acting), SR (sustained release), TR (time release), SA (sustained action), and ER or XL or XR (extended release).

Occasionally, drugs should not be crushed because they are oral mucosa irritants, are extremely bitter, or contain dyes that may stain teeth or mucosal tissue. Many medications that are combinations (containing multiple ingredients) should not be split.

The table contains a partial listing of drugs found in the Guide that should not be crushed or chewed. A liquid dosage form may be available for many of these drugs. However, the dose or frequency of administration may be different from the slow-release product. Check with your pharmacist for liquid availability and dosing conversions.

| | Generic Name | Comments |
|---|---|---|
| Absorica | isotretinoin | mucous membrane irritant |
| Accutane | isotretinoin | mucous membrane irritant |
| AcipHex | rabeprazole | slow release |
| Acticlate | doxycycline | film-coated |
| Actiq Oralet | fentanyl citrate | lozenge product |
| Actonel | risendronate | irritant |
| Adalat CC | nifedipine | slow release |
| Adderall XR | amphetamine | slow release |
| Advicor | niacin/lovastatin | slow release |

| | Generic Name | Comments |
|---|---|---|
| Afinitor | everolimus | mucous membrane irritant |
| Aggrenox | aspirin/dipyridamole | slow release; may be opened and contents taken without crushing |
| Allegra D | fexofenadine/pseudoephedrine | slow release |
| Alophen | bisacodyl | enteric coated |
| Altoprev | lovastatin | slow release |
| Amitiza | lubiprostone | slow release |
| Amrix | cyclobenzaprine | slow release |
| Apriso | mesalamine | extended release; pH range concerns |
| Aptivus | tipranavir | taste |
| Aricept | donepezil | crushing 25mg tablet significantly impacts absorption |
| Arthrotec | diclofenac/misoprostol | enteric coated |
| Asacol | mesalamine | slow release |
| Atelvia | risendronate | extended release |
| Augmentin XR | amoxicillin/clavulanic acid | slow release; may be scored and broken |
| Avinza | morphine | slow release; capsule may be opened |
| Avodart | dutasteride | skin contact may cause tumor production |
| Azor | amlodipine/olmesartan | combination product |
| Azulfidine En tabs | sulfasalazine | enteric coated |
| Bayer Extra Strength Enteric 500 | aspirin, enteric coated | enteric coated;  slow release |
| Bayer Low Adult 81 mg | aspirin, enteric coated | enteric coated |
| Bayer Caplet | aspirin, enteric coated | enteric coated |
| Biaxin XL | clarithromycin | slow release |
| Biltricide | praziquantel | taste |
| Bisacodyl | bisacodyl | enteric coated |
| Bisco-Lax | bisacodyl | enteric coated |
| Boniva | ibandronate | irritant |
| Briviact | brivaracetam | film-coated |

|  | Generic Name | Comments |
|---|---|---|
| Calan SR | verapamil | slow release; may break tablet |
| Cama Arthritis Strength | aspirin, magnesium ox- ide, aluminum hydroxide | special tablet formulation |
| Cardizem, Cardizem CD, Cardizem SR, Cardizem LA, Cartia XT | diltiazem | slow release; capsules may be opened and contents taken without chewing or crushing |
| Ceftin | cefuroxime | taste; use liquid formulation |
| Cellcept | mycophenolate | teratogenic potential |
| Chlor-Trimeton Repetab | chlorpheniramine | slow release |
| Choledyl SA | oxtriphylline | slow release |
| Cipro | ciprofloxacin | taste |
| Colace | docusate | taste |
| Colestid | colestipol | slow release |
| Commit | nicotine | lozenge form |
| Concerta | methylphenidate | slow release |
| Constant T | theophylline | slow release; capsules may be opened and contents taken without chewing or crushing |
| Coreg CR | carvedilol | extended release; may add capsule contents to chilled applesauce |
| Cotazym S | pancrelipase | enteric coated; capsules may be opened and contents taken without chewing or crushing |
| Covera-HS | verapamil | slow release |
| Creon | pancrelipase | slow release |
| Crixivan | indinavir | taste |
| Cymbalta | duloxetine | enteric coated |
| Cytovene | ganciclovir | skin irritant |
| Deconamine SR | chlorpheniramine, pseudoephedrine | slow release |
| Depakene | valproic acid | slow release; mucous membrane irritant |
| Depakote | valproate disodium | slow release |
| Desoxyn Gradumets | methamphetamine | slow release |

| | Generic Name | Comments |
|---|---|---|
| Detrol LA | tolterodine | slow release |
| Dexedrine Spansule | dextroamphetamine | slow release |
| Dexilant | dexlansoprazole | slow release |
| Diamox Sequels | acetazolamide | slow release |
| Dilacor XR | diltiazem | slow release |
| Dilatrate-SR | isosorbide dinitrate | slow release |
| Disophrol Chronotab | dexbrompheniramine, pseudoephedrine | slow release |
| Donnatal Extentab | atropine, scopolamine, hyoscyamine, phenobarbital | slow release |
| Donnazyme | pancreatin, pepsin, bile salts, atropine, scopolamine, hyoscyamine, phenobarbital | slow release |
| Drixoral | dexbrompheniramine, pseudoephedrine | slow release |
| Droxia | hydroxyurea | skin toxicity when exposed to powder |
| Dulcolax | bisacodyl | enteric coated |
| Easprin | aspirin | enteric coated |
| Ecotrin | aspirin | enteric coated |
| E.E.S. 400 | erythromycin ethylsuccinate | enteric coated |
| Effexor XR | venlafaxine | slow release |
| Embeda | morphine | slow release; do not give via NG tube |
| Enablex | darifenacin | slow release |
| E-Mycin | erythromycin | enteric coated |
| Ergomar | ergotamine | sublingual tablet |
| Erivedge | vismodegib | potential teratogen with skin contact |
| Ery-Tab | erythromycin | enteric coated |
| Erythrocin Stearate | erythromycin | enteric coated |
| Erythromycin Base | erythromycin | enteric coated |
| Evista | raloxifene | taste |

| | Generic Name | Comments |
|---|---|---|
| Exalgo | hydromorphone | extended release; could cause overdose |
| Extendryl JR | chlorpheniramine, methscopolamine, phenylephrine | slow release |
| Fedahist Timecaps | chlorpheniramine, pseudoephedrine | slow release |
| Feldene | piroxicam | mucous membrane irritant |
| Feosol | ferrous sulfate | enteric coated |
| Feosol Spansule | ferrous sulfate | slow release; capsules may be opened and contents taken without chewing or crushing |
| Fergon | ferrous gluconate | slow release; capsules may be opened and contents taken without chewing or crushing |
| Ferro-Sequels | ferrous fumarate, docusate | slow release |
| Flomax | tamsulosin | slow release |
| Fosamax | alendronate | mucous membrane irritant |
| Gleevec | imatinib | taste |
| Glucophage XR | metformin | slow release |
| Glucotrol XL | glipizide | slow release |
| Glumetza | metformin | slow release |
| Hydrea | hydroxyurea | powder may cause skin toxicities |
| Imdur | isosorbide mononitrate | slow release |
| Inderal LA | propranolol | slow release |
| Indocin SR | indomethacin | slow release; capsules may be opened and contents taken without chewing or crushing |
| Intelence | etravirine | may be dissolved in water |
| Iso-Bid | isosorbide dinitrate | slow release |
| Isoptin SR | verapamil | slow release |
| Isosorbide Dinitrate SR | isosorbide dinitrate | slow release |
| Janumet | sitagliptin/metformin | combination product |
| Jalyn | dutasteride/tamsulosin | pregnant patients should avoid crushed tablets |

| | Generic Name | Comments |
|---|---|---|
| Kadian | morphine | slow release |
| Kaon CL 10 | potassium chloride | slow release |
| Keppra | levetiracetam | taste |
| Klor-Con | potassium chloride | slow release |
| Klotrix | potassium chloride | slow release |
| K-Tab | potassium chloride | slow release |
| Levsinex Timecaps | hyoscyamine | slow release |
| Letairis | ambrisentan | slow release |
| Lithobid | lithium | slow release |
| Lovaza | fish oils | irritant |
| Meprospan | meprobamate | slow release; capsules may be opened and contents taken without chewing or crushing |
| Mestinon Timespan | pyridostigmine | slow release |
| Micro K | potassium chloride | slow release |
| Movantik | naloxegol | film coated |
| Moxatag | amoxicillin | slow release |
| MS Contin | morphine | slow release |
| Mucinex | guaifenesin | slow release |
| Nexium | esomeprazole | slow release |
| Nico 400 | niacin | slow release |
| Nicobid | niacin | slow release |
| Nitro Bid | nitroglycerin | slow release; capsules may be opened and contents taken without chewing or crushing |
| Nitroglyn | nitroglycerin | slow release; capsules may be opened and contents taken without chewing or crushing |
| Norflex | orphenadrine | slow release |
| Norpace CR | disopyramide | slow release |
| Norvir | ritonavir | decreases bioavailability |
| Novafed A | pseudoephedrine, chlorpheniramine | slow release |
| Oracea | doxycycline | slow release |
| Oramorph SR | morphine | slow release |

| | Generic Name | Comments |
|---|---|---|
| Pancrease | pancrelipase | enteric coated |
| Papaverine Sustained Action | papaverine | slow release |
| Perdiem | psyllium hydrophilic mucilloid | wax coated |
| Phazyme, Phazyme 95 | simethicone | slow release |
| Plendil | felodipine | slow release |
| Pradaxa | dabigatran | altered therapeutic effect |
| Prevacid | lansoprazole | slow release |
| Prilosec | omeprazole | slow release |
| Procainamide HCl SR | procainamide | slow release |
| Procan SR | procainamide | slow release |
| Protonix | pantoprazole | slow release |
| Procardia XL | nifedipine | slow release |
| Pronestyl SR | procainamide | slow release |
| Proventil Repetabs | albuterol | slow release |
| Ranexa | ranolazine | slow release |
| Rapamune | sirolimus | pharmacokinetics affected |
| Renagel | sevelamer | tablets expand if broken |
| Reyataz | atazanavir | use oral powder instead |
| Revlimid | lenalidomide | teratogenic potential |
| Ritalin SR | methylphenidate | slow release |
| Robimycin Robitab | erythromycin | enteric coated |
| Rondec TR | pseudoephedrine, carbinoxamine | slow release |
| Roxanol SR | morphine | slow release |
| Sinemet CR | levodopa, carbidopa | slow release; tablet is scored and may be broken in half |
| Slo-Bid Gyrocaps | theophylline | slow release; capsules may be opened and contents taken without chewing or crushing |
| Slo-Phyllin Gyrocaps | theophylline | slow release; capsules may be opened and contents taken without chewing or crushing |

| | Generic Name | Comments |
|---|---|---|
| Slow-Fe | ferrous sulfate | slow release |
| Slow-K | potassium chloride | slow release |
| Sorbitrate SA | isosorbide dinitrate | slow release |
| Strattera | atomoxetine | slow release |
| Sudafed 12 hour | pseudoephedrine | slow release |
| Tarka | trandolapril, verapamil | slow release |
| Tasigna | nilotinib | may increase toxicity risk |
| Tessalon Perles | benzonatate | slow release |
| Theo-24 | theophylline | slow release |
| Tiazac | diltiazem | slow release |
| Toprol XL | metoprolol | slow release |
| Tracleer | bosentan | teratogenic |
| Trental | pentoxifylline | slow release |
| Treximet | naproxen/sumatriptan | decreases efficacy |
| Uceris | budesonide | slow release |
| Uniphyl | theophylline | slow release |
| Valcyte | valganciclovir | irritant; teratogen |
| Verelan | verapamil | slow release; capsules may be opened and contents taken without chewing or crushing |
| Vortient | pazopanib | increase ADR risk |
| Wellbutrin SR, Wellbutrin XL | bupropion | slow release; mucous membrane irritant |
| Zolinza | vorinostat | irritant |
| ZORprin | aspirin | slow release |
| Zyban | bupropion | slow release |

Note: This listing is not comprehensive. Please check with your pharmacist for additional questions.

Information from The Institute for Safe Medication Practices available at: http://www.ismp.org/tools/DoNotCrush.pdf

**Acanya** (ANTIACNE) *gel:* benzoyl peroxide 2.5%/clindamycin (see p. 373) 1.2%.

**Accuretic** (ANTIHYPERTENSIVE) *tablet:* quinapril (see p. 1394) 10 mg/hydrochlorothiazide (see p. 782) 12.5 mg; 20 mg quinapril (see p. 1394)/12.5 mg hydrochlorothiazide; 20 mg quinapril/25 mg hydrochlorothiazide.

**Activella** (HORMONE REPLACEMENT THERAPY) *tablet:* estradiol (see p. 630) 1 mg/norethindrone acetate (see p. 1156) 0.5 mg.

**Actonel with Calcium** (BISPHOS-PHONATE) *tablet:* risedronate (see p. 1440) 35 mg/1250 calcium carbonate (see p. 246).

**ACTOplus Met** (ANTIDIABETIC) *tablet:* pioglitazone (see p. 1305) 15 mg/metformin (see p. 1018) 500 mg; pioglitazone 15 mg/metformin 850 mg.

**Advair Diskus** (BRONCHODILATOR) *Inhalation powder:* fluticasone propionate (see p. 715) 100 mcg/salmeterol (see p. 1466) 50 mcg; fluticasone propionate 250 mcg/salmeterol 50 mcg; fluticasone propionate 115 mcg/salmeterol 21 mcg; fluticasone propionate 230 mcg/salmeterol 21 mcg; fluticasone propionate 45 mcg/salmeterol 21 mcg.

**Advicor** (ANTILIPEMIC) *tablets, sustained release:* niacin (see p. 1128) 500 mg/lovastatin (see p. 969) 20 mg; niacin 1000 mg/lovastatin 20 mg.

**Aggrenox** (ANTIPLATELET) *extended release capsule:* dipyridamole (see p. 517) 200 mg/aspirin (see p. 122) 25 mg.

**AirDuo RespiClick** (BRONCHODILATOR) *inhalation powder:* fluticasone (see p. 715) 113 mcg/salmeterol (see p. 1466) 14 mcg; fluticasone 232 mcg/salmeterol 14 mcg; fluticasone 55 mcg/salmeterol 14 mcg.

**Aldactazide 25/25** (DIURETIC) *tablet:* spironolactone (see p. 1519) 25 mg/hydrochlorothiazide (see p. 782) 25 mg.

**Aldactazide 50/50** (DIURETIC) *tablet:* spironolactone (see p. 1519) 50 mg/hydrochlorothiazide (see p. 782) 50 mg.

**Allegra D 12 hour** (ANTIHISTAMINE, DECONGESTANT) *tablet, extended release:* fexofenadine (see p. 687) 60 mg/pseudoephedrine (see p. 1381) 120 mg.

**Allegra D 24 hour** (ANTIHISTAMINE, DECONGESTANT) *tablet, extended release:* fexofenadine (see p. 687) 180 mg/pseudoephedrine (see p. 1381) 240 mg.

**Anexsia** (NARCOTIC ANALGESIC [schedule III]) *tablet:* hydrocodone (see p. 784) 5 mg/acetaminophen (see p. 13) 500 mg.

**Anexsia 5/325** (NARCOTIC ANALGESIC [schedule III]) *tablet:* hydrocodone (see p. 784) 5 mg/acetaminophen (see p. 13) 325 mg.

**Anexsia 7.5/325** (NARCOTIC ANAL-GESIC [schedule III]) *tablet:* hydrocodone (see p. 784) 7.5 mg/acetaminophen (see p. 13) 325 mg.

**Anexsia 7.5/650** (NARCOTIC ANAL-GESIC [schedule III]) *tablet:* hydrocodone (see p. 784) 7.5 mg/acetaminophen (see p. 13) 650 mg.

**Angeliq** (HORMONE) *tablet:* drospirenone 0.5 mg/estradiol (see p. 630) 1 mg.

**Apresazide 25/25** (ANTIHYPERTEN-SIVE) *capsule:* hydralazine hydrochloride (see p. 780) 25 mg/

---

*For a complete list that includes nonprescription drugs, please see our companion website at www.prenhall.com

hydrochlorothiazide (see p. 782) 25 mg.

**Apresazide 50/50** (ANTIHYPERTENSIVE) *capsule:* hydralazine hydrochloride (see p. 780) 50 mg/hydrochlorothiazide (see p. 782) 50 mg.

**Apresodex** (ANTIHYPERTENSIVE) *tablet:* hydralazine hydrochloride (see p. 780) 25 mg/hydrochlorothiazide (see p. 782) 15 mg.

**Aralen Phosphate with Primaquine Phosphate** (ANTIMALARIAL) *tablet:* chloroquine phosphate (see p. 335) 500 mg (300 mg base)/primaquine phosphate (see p. 1348) 79 mg (45 mg base).

**Arthrotec 50** (NSAID) *tablet:* diclofenac sodium (see p. 488) 50 mg/misoprostol (see p. 1073) 200 mcg.

**Arthrotec 75** (NSAID) tablet: diclofenac sodium (see p. 488) 75 mg/misoprostol (see p. 1073) 200 mcg.

**Atacand HCT** (ANTIHYPERTENSIVE) *tablet:* candesartan (see p. 255) 32 mg/hydrochlorothiazide (see p. 782) 12.5 mg; candesartan 16 mg/hydrochlorothiazide 12.5 mg.

**Atripla** (ANTIRETROVIRAL) *tablet:* 600 mg efavirenz (see p. 569)/200 mg emtricitabine (see p. 574)/300 mg tenofovir (see p. 1568).

**Augmentin** (ANTIBIOTIC) *tablet:* amoxicillin (see p. 87) 250 mg/clavulanic acid 125 mg; amoxicillin 500 mg/clavulanic acid 125 mg; amoxicillin 875 mg/clavulanic acid 125 mg; amoxicillin 1000 mg/clavulanic acid 125 mg; *chewable tablet:* amoxicillin 125 mg/clavulanic acid 31.25 mg; amoxicillin 200 mg/clavulanic acid 28.5 mg; amoxicillin 250 mg/clavulanic acid 62.5 mg; amoxicillin 400 mg/clavulanic acid 57 mg; *suspension (per 5 mL):* amoxicillin 125 mg/clavulanic acid 31.25 mg; amoxicillin 200 mg/clavulanic acid 28.5 mg; amoxicillin 250 mg/clavulanic acid 62.5 mg; amoxicillin

400 mg/clavulanic acid 57 mg; amoxicillin 600 mg/clavulanic acid 42.9 mg.

**Auralgan Otic** (OTIC PREPARATION: DECONGESTANT, ANALGESIC) *solution:* acetic acid 0.1%, antipyrine 5.4%, benzocaine (see p. 175) 1.4%, u-polycosanol 410 0.01%.

**Avalide** (ANTIHYPERTENSIVE) *tablet:* irbesartan (see p. 860) 150 mg/hydrochlorothiazide (see p. 782) 12.5 mg; irbesartan 300 mg/hydrochlorothiazide 12.5 mg; irbesartan 300 mg/hydrochlorothiazide 25 mg.

**Avandamet** (HYPOGLYCEMIC AGENT) *tablet:* 1 mg rosiglitazone maleate (see p. 1459)/500 mg metformin HCl (see p. 1018); 2 mg rosiglitazone/500 mg metformin; 4 mg rosiglitazone/500 mg metformin; 2 mg rosiglitazone/1000 mg metformin; 4 mg rosiglitazone/1000 mg metformin.

**Avandaryl** (HYPOGLYCEMIC AGENT) *tablet:* rosiglitazone (see p. 1459) 4 mg/glimepiride (see p. 751) 1 mg; rosiglitazone 4 mg/glimepiride 2 mg; rosiglitazone 4 mg/glimepiride 4 mg.

**Azo Gantanol** (URINARY ANTI-INFECTIVE, ANALGESIC) *tablet:* sulfamethoxazole (see p. 1533) 500 mg, phenazopyridine hydrochloride (see p. 1280) 100 mg.

**Azo Gantrisin** (URINARY ANTI-INFECTIVE, ANALGESIC) *tablet:* sulfisoxazole (see p. 976) 500 mg/phenazopyridine hydrochloride (see p. 1280) 50 mg.

**Azor** (ANTIHYPERTENSIVE) *tablet:* amlodipine (see p. 82) 5 mg/olmesartan (see p. 1172) 20 mg; amlodipine 5 mg/olmesartan 40 mg; amlodipine 10 mg/olmesartan 20 mg; amlodipine 10 mg/olmesartan 40 mg.

**B-A-C** (ANALGESIC) acetaminophen (see p. 13) 650 mg/caffeine (see p. 240) 40 mg/butalbital 50 mg.

**Bacticort Ophthalmic** (ANTI-INFLAM-MATORY) suspension: hydrocortisone (see p. 785) 1%/neomycin sulfate (see p. 1120) 0.35%/polymyxin B (see p. 1318) 10,000 units.

**Bactrim** (URINARY TRACT AGENT) *tablet:* sulfamethoxazole (see p. 1533) 400 mg/trimethoprim (see p. 1662) 80 mg.

**Bactrim DS** (URINARY TRACT AGENT) *tablet:* sulfamethoxazole (see p. 1533) 800 mg/trimethoprim (see p. 1662) 160 mg.

**Benicar HCT** (ANTIHYPERTENSIVE) *tablet:* 20 mg olmesartan medoxomil (see p. 1172)/12.5 mg hydrochlorothiazide (see p. 782); 40 mg olmesartan medoxomil/12.5 mg hydrochlorothiazide; 40 mg olmesartan medoxomil/25 mg hydrochlorothiazide.

**Betoptic Pilo Suspension** (ANTIGLAUCOMA) *suspension:* betaxolol (see p. 182) 0.25%/pilocarpine (see p. 1297) 1.75%.

**Bevespi Aerosphere** (ANTICHO-LINERGIC/BETA AGONIST) *inhaler:* glycopyrrolate 9 mcg/formoterol fum 4.8 mcg.

**Beyaz** (ORAL CONTRACEPTIVE) *tablet:* drosperinone 3 mg/ethinyl estradiol 0.02 mg/levomefolate calcium 0.451 mg.

**BiDil** (ANTIHYPERTENSIVE) *tablet:* isosorbide dinitrate (see p. 876) 20 mg/hydralazine (see p. 780) 37.5 mg.

**Breo Ellipta** (BRONCHODIALATOR) *powder for inhalation:* fluticasone (see p. 715) 100 mcg/vilanterol 25 mcg.

**Blephamide** (OPHTHALMIC STEROID, SULFONAMIDE) *suspension:* prednisolone acetate (see p. 1343) 0.2%/sulfacetamide sodium (see p. 1530) 10%.

**Blephamide S.O.P.** (OPHTHALMIC STEROID, SULFONAMIDE) *ointment:* prednisolone acetate (see p. 1343) 0.2%/sulfacetamide sodium (see p. 1530) 10%.

**Brevicon** (MONOPHASIC ORAL CONTRACEPTIVE [ESTROGEN, PROGESTIN]) *tablet:* ethinyl estradiol 35 mcg/norethindrone (see p. 1156) 0.5 mg.

**Bromfed** (DECONGESTANT, ANTIHISTAMINE) *sustained release capsule:* pseudoephedrine hydrochloride (see p. 1381) 120 mg/brompheniramine maleate (see p. 217) 12 mg.

**Bromfed-PD** (DECONGESTANT, ANTIHISTAMINE) *sustained release capsule:* pseudoephedrine hydrochloride (see p. 1381) 60 mg/brompheniramine maleate (see p. 217) 6 mg.

**Bronchial Capsules** (ANTIASTHMATIC) *capsule:* theophylline (see p. 1588) 150 mg/guaifenesin (see p. 767) 90 mg.

**Byvalson** (ANTIHYPERTENSIVE) *tablet:* nebivolol 5 mg/valsartan 80 mg.

**Caduet** (ANTIHYPERTENSIVE/ANTILIPEMIC) *tablet:* 2.5 mg amlodipine (see p. 82)/10 mg atorvastatin (see p. 132); 2.5 mg amlodipine/20 mg atorvastatin; 2.5 mg amlodipine/40 mg atorvastatin; 5 mg amlodipine/10 mg atorvastatin; 10 mg amlodipine/10 mg atorvastatin; 5 mg amlodipine/20 mg atorvastatin; 10 mg amlodipine/20 mg atorvastatin; 5 mg amlodipine/40 mg atorvastatin; 10 mg amlodipine/40 mg atorvastatin; 5 mg amlodipine/80 mg atorvastatin; 10 mg amlodipine/80 mg atorvastatin.

**Cafergot Suppositories** (ANTIMIGRAINE) *suppository:* ergotamine tartrate (see p. 610) 2 mg/caffeine (see p. 240) 100 mg.

**Cam-ap-es** (ANTIHYPERTENSIVE) suspension, *tablet:* hydrochlorothiazide (see p. 782) 15 mg/reserpine (see p. 1420) 0.1 mg/hydralazine hydrochloride (see p. 780) 25 mg.

**Capital with Codeine** (NARCOTIC ANALGESIC [schedule V]) *suspension (per 5 mL):* codeine

phosphate (see p. 393) 12 mg/
acetaminophen (see p. 13) 120 mg.

**Carisoprodol Compound** (SKEL-
ETAL MUSCLE RELAXANT, ANALGESIC)
*tablet:* carisoprodol (see p. 277)
200 mg/aspirin (see p. 122) 325 mg.

**Carmol HC** (ANTI-INFLAMMATORY)
*cream:* hydrocortisone acetate
(see p. 785) 1%/urea 10%.

**Celestone-Soluspan** (GLUCOCORTI-
COID) *injection (suspension) (per
mL):* betamethasone acetate (see
p. 180) 3 mg/betamethasone
sodium phosphate (see p. 180)
3 mg.

**Cetacaine** (TOPICAL ANESTHETIC) *gel,
liquid, ointment, aerosol:* benzocaine (see p. 175) 14%/tetracaine
hydrochloride (see p. 1582) 2%/
butamben      2%/benzalkonium
chloride (see p. 174) 0.5%.

**Cheracol Syrup** (NARCOTIC ANTITUS-
SIVE, EXPECTORANT [schedule V])
*syrup (per 5 mL):* codeine
phosphate (see p. 393) 10 mg/
guaifenesin (see p. 767) 100 mg/
alcohol 4.75%.

**Cipro HC Otic** (ANTI-INFECTIVE/
ANTI-INFLAMMATORY) *topical:* ciprofloxacin (see p. 360) 2 mg/
dexamethasone (see p. 470)
10 mg otic suspension.

**Ciprodex Otic** (ANTI-INFECTIVE/
ANTI-INFLAMMATORY) *topical:* ciprofloxacin (see p. 360) 0.3%/dex-
amethasone (see p. 470) 0.1%
otic suspension.

**Claritin D** (ANTIHISTAMINE, DE-
CONGESTANT) loratadine (see
p. 963), 5 mg/pseudoephedrine
(see p. 1381) 120 mg; loratadine 10 mg/pseudoephedrine
240 mg.

**Clarinex D 24 hr** (ANTIHISTAMINE, DE-
CONGESTANT) *tablet:* desloratadine
(see p. 467) 5 mg/pseudoephed-
rine (see p. 1381) 240 mg.

**Climara Pro** (HORMONE REPLACEMENT
THERAPY) *transdermal patch:* estradiol (see p. 630) 0.045 mg/
levonorgestrel acetate 0.015 mg.

**Codiclear DH Syrup** (ANTITUSSIVE
[schedule III]) *syrup (per 5 mL):*
hydrocodone (see p. 784) 5 mg/
guaifenesin (see p. 767) 100 mg/
alcohol 10%.

**Codimal DH** (ANTITUSSIVE [sched-
ule III]) *syrup (per 5 mL):* phenylephrine hydrochloride (see
p. 1289) 5 mg/pyrilamine maleate
8.33 mg/hydrocodone bitartrate
(see p. 784) 1.66 mg.

**Codimal PH** (ANTITUSSIVE [schedule
III]) *syrup (per 5 mL):* codeine
(see p. 393) 10 mg/pyrilamine
maleate 8.33 mg/phenylephrine
(see p. 1289) 5 mg.

**Co-Gesic** (NARCOTIC ANALGESIC
[schedule V]) *tablet:* hydrocodone (see p. 784) 5 mg/acetami-
nophen (see p. 13) 500 mg.

**Coly-Mycin S Otic** (OTIC: STER-
OID, ANTIBIOTIC) *suspension
(per mL):* hydrocortisone acetate
(see p. 785) 1%/neomycin sulfate (see p. 1120) 3.3 mg/colis-
tin sulfate 3 mg/thonzonium
bromide 0.05%.

**Combigan** (GLAUCOMA) *ophthalmic
solution:* brimonidine (see p. 213)
0.2%/timolol (see p. 1609) 0.5%.

**CombiPatch** (HORMONE REPLACE-
MENT THERAPY) *transdermal
patch:* estradiol (see p. 630)
0.05 mg/norethindrone acetate
(see p. 1156) 0.14 mg; estradiol
0.05 mg/norethindrone acetate
0.25 mg.

**Combivent Respimat** (BETA-
AGONIST/ANTICHOLINERGIC BRON-
CHODILATOR) *inhalation solution:*
100 mcg albuterol sulfate/20 mcg
ipratropium

**Combivir** (ANTIVIRAL) *tablet:* zidovudine (see p. 1724) 300 mg/
lamivudine (see p. 903) 150 mg.

**Complera** (ANTIRETROVIRAL) *tablet:*
rilpivirine 25 mg/emtricitabine
200 mg/tenofovir 300 mg.

**Cortisporin** (OPHTHALMIC STER-
OID, ANTIBIOTIC) *suspension (per
mL):* hydrocortisone (see p. 785)

1%/neomycin sulfate (see p. 1120) (equivalent to 0.35% neomycin base)/polymyxin B sulfate (see p. 1318) 10,000 units.

**Cortisporin Ointment** (OPHTHAL-MIC STEROID, ANTIBIOTIC) *ointment:* hydrocortisone (see p. 785) 1%/ neomycin sulfate (see p. 1120) (equivalent to 0.35% neomycin base)/bacitracin zinc (see p. 157) 400 units, polymyxin B sulfate (see p. 1318) 10,000 units/g.

**Corzide** (ANTIHYPERTENSIVE) *tablet:* nadolol (see p. 1093) 40 mg/ben-droflumethiazide 5 mg; nadolol 80mg/bendoflumethiazide 5mg.

**Cosopt** (OPHTHALMIC, GLAUCOMA) *ophthalmic solution:* dorzola-mide (see p. 537) 2%/timolol (see p. 1609) 0.5%.

**Cyclomydril** (OPHTHALMIC DECON-GESTANT) *ophthalmic solution:* atropine hydrochloride 0.2%/ phenylephrine hydrochloride (see p. 1289) 1%.

**Decadron with Xylocaine** (GLU-COCORTICOID) *injection (per mL):* dexamethasone sodium phos-phate (see p. 470) 4 mg/lido-caine hydrochloride (see p. 937) 10 mg.

**Deconamine** (DECONGESTANT, AN-TIHISTAMINE) *syrup (per 5 mL):* pseudoephedrine hydrochloride (see p. 1381) 30 mg/chlorphe-niramine maleate (see p. 339) 2 mg; *tablet:* pseudoephedrine hydrochloride 60 mg/chlorphe-niramine maleate 4 mg.

**Deconamine SR** (DECONGESTANT, ANTIHISTAMINE) *sustained release capsule:* pseudoephedrine hydrochloride (see p. 1381) 120 mg/chlorpheniramine maleate (see p. 339) 8 mg.

**Depo-Testadiol** (ESTROGEN, ANDRO-GEN) *injection (per mL):* estradiol cypionate (see p. 630) 2 mg/ testosterone cypionate (see p. 1579) 50 mg.

**Descovy** (REVERSE TRANSCRIPTASE INHIBITOR) *tablet:* emtricitabine 200 mg/tenofovir alafenamide 25 mg.

**Diclegis** (ANTIEMETIC) *tablet:* doxy-lamine 10 mg/pyridoxine (see p. 1388) 10 mg.

**Dilaudid Cough Syrup** (NARCOTIC ANTITUSSIVE [schedule II]) *syrup:* hydromorphone (see p. 789) 1 mg/guaifenesin (see p. 767) 100 mg/alcohol 5%.

**Dilor G** (ANTIASTHMATIC) *liquid (per 5 mL):* dyphylline (see p. 561) 100 mg/guaifenesin (see p. 767) 100 mg.

**Diovan HCT** (ANTIHYPERTENSIVE) *tablet:* hydrochlorothiazide (see p. 782) 12.5 mg/valsartan (see p. 1680) 80 mg; hydrochlorothi-azide 12.5 mg/valsartan 160 mg; hydrochlorothiazide 25 mg/ valsartan 160 mg; hydrochlo-rothiazide 12.5 mg/valsartan 320 mg; hydrochlorothiazide 25 mg/valsartan 320 mg.

**Donnatal** (GASTROINTESTINAL AN-TICHOLINERGIC, SEDATIVE) *tab-let, elixir:* atropine sulfate (see p. 138) 0.0194 mg/scopolamine hydrobromide (see p. 1476) 0.0065 mg/hyoscyamine hydro-bromide or sulfate (see p. 800) 0.1037 mg/phenobarbital (see p. 1283) 16.2 mg. The elixir con-tains alcohol 23%/5 mL.

**Donnatal Extentab** (GASTROIN-TESTINAL ANTICHOLINERGIC, SEDA-TIVE) *tablet:* atropine sulfate (see p. 138) 0.0582 mg/scopolamine hydrobromide (see p. 1476) 0.0195 mg/hyoscyamine sulfate (see p. 800) 0.3111 mg/pheno-barbital (see p. 1283) 48.6 mg.

**Duac** (ANTIACNE) *gel:* clindamycin (see p. 373) 1%/benzoyl perox-ide 5%.

**Duavee** (HORMONE REPLACEMENT) tablet conjugated estrogen 0.45 mg/bazedoxifene 20 mg.

**Duetact** (ANTIDIABETIC) *tablet:* pioglitazone (see p. 1305) 30 mg/glimepiride (see p. 751) 2 mg; pioglitazone 30 mg/glimepiride 4 mg.

**Duexis** (ANTIULCERATIVE) *tablet:* ibuprofen 800 mg/famotidine 26.6 mg.

**Dulera** (CORTICOSTEROID/BETA-AGONIST) *inhaler:* mometasone 100 mcg/fomoterol 5 mcg; mometasone 200 mcg/fomoterol 5 mcg.

**DuoNeb** (BETA-AGONIST/ANTICHOLINERGIC BRONCHODILATOR) *inhalation solution:* 2.5 mg albuterol sulfate (see p. 38)/0.5 mg ipratropium bromide (see p. 859) per 3 mL.

**Duzallo** (ANTIGOUT) *tablet:* lesinurad (see p. 916) 200 mg/allopurinol (see p. 47) 200 mg; lesinurad 200 mg/allopurinol 300 mg.

**Dyazide** (DIURETIC) *capsule:* triamterene (see p. 1654) 37.5 mg/hydrochlorothiazide (see p. 782) 25 mg.

**Dymista** (ANTIHISTAMINE) *Nasal spray:* azelastine 137 mcg/fluticasone 50 mcg.

**Edarbyclor** (ANTIHYPERTENSIVE) *tablet:* azilsartan 40 mg/chlorthalidone 12.5 mg; azilsartan 40 mg/chlorthalidone 25 mg.

**Embeda** (ANALGESIC [schedule II]) *tablet:* morphine (see p. 1084) 20 mg/naltrexone (see p. 1103) 0.8 mg; morphine 30 mg/naltrexone 1.2 mg; morphine 50 mg/naltrexone 2 mg; morphine 60 mg/naltrexone 2.4 mg; morphine 80 mg/naltrexone 3.2 mg; morphine 100 mg/naltrexone 4 mg.

**Endocet** (NARCOTIC ANALGESIC [schedule II]) *tablet:* oxycodone (see p. 1206) 7.5 mg/acetaminophen (see p. 13) 325 mg; oxycodone 7.5 mg/acetaminophen 500 mg; oxycodone 10 mg/acetaminophen 325 mg; oxycodone 10 mg/acetaminophen 650 mg.

**Enlon Plus** (ANTICHOLINESTERASE) *solution:* edrophonium 10 mg/atropine 0.14 mg.

**Entresto** (NAPRILYSIN INHIBITOR/ANGIOTENSION II BLOCKER) *tablet:* sacubitril 24 mg/valsartan 26 mg; sacubitril 49 mg/valsartan 51 mg; sacubitril 97 mg/valsartan 103 mg.

**Epiduo** (ANTIACNE) *gel:* adapalene (see p. 28) 0.1%/benzoyl peroxide 2.5%.

**Epclusa** (ANTIVIRAL) *tablet:* sofosbuvir 400 mg/velpatasvir 100 mg.

**Epzicom** (ANTIRETROVIRAL AGENT) *tablet:* abacavir (see p. 1) 600 mg/lamivudine (see p. 903) 300 mg.

**Estratest** (ESTROGEN, ANDROGEN) *tablet:* esterified estrogens (see p. 638) 1.25 mg/methyltestosterone (see p. 1044) 2.5 mg.

**Estratest H.S.** (ESTROGEN, ANDROGEN) *tablet:* esterified estrogens (see p. 640) 0.625 mg/methyltestosterone (see p. 1044) 1.25 mg.

**Exforge** (ANTIHYPERTENSIVE) *tablet:* amlodipine (see p. 82) 5 mg/valsartan (see p. 1680) 160 mg; amlodipine 10 mg/valsartan 160 mg; amlodipine 5 mg/valsartan 320 mg; amlodipine 10 mg/valsartan 320 mg.

**Exforge HCT** (ANTIHYPERTENSIVE) *tablet:* amlodipine (see p. 82) 5 mg/valsartan (see p. 1680) 160 mg/hydrochlorothiazide (see p. 782) 12.5 mg; amlodipine 5 mg/valsartan 160 mg/hydrochlorothiazide 25 mg; amlodipine 10 mg/valsartan 160 mg/hydrochlorothiazide 12.5 mg; amlodipine 10 mg/valsartan 160 mg/hydrochlorothiazide 25 mg.

**Fioricet with Codeine** (NONNARCOTIC AGONIST ANALGESIC) *capsule:* acetaminophen (see p. 13) 300 mg/butalbital 50 mg/caffeine (see p. 240) 40 mg/codeine (30 mg).

**Fiorinal** (NONNARCOTIC AGONIST ANALGESIC [schedule III]) *capsule,* aspirin (see p. 122) 325 mg/butalbital 50 mg/caffeine (see p. 240) 40 mg.

**Fiorinal with Codeine** (NARCOTIC AGONIST ANALGESIC [schedule III]) *capsule:* codeine phosphate (see p. 394) 30 mg/aspirin (see p. 122) 325 mg/caffeine (see p. 240) 40 mg/butalbital 50 mg.

**Fosamax Plus D** (BISPHOSPHONATE) *tablet:* alendronate (see p. 40) 70 mg/vitamin D (see p. 1708) 2800 international units.

**Glucovance** (ANTIDIABETIC) *tablet:* glyburide (see p. 755) 1.25 mg/metformin (see p. 1018) 250 mg; glyburide 2.5 mg/metformin 500 mg; glyburide 5 mg/metformin 500 mg.

**Harvoni** (ANTIVIRAL) *tablet:* ledipasvir (see p. 912) 90 mg/sofosbuvir (see p. 912) 400 mg.

**Helidac** (ANTIULCER, ANTIBIOTIC) *tablet:* bismuth subsalicylate (see p. 193) 262.4 mg/metronidazole (see p. 1051) 250 mg/tetracycline (see p. 1584) 500 mg.

**Hycodan** (ANTITUSSIVE [schedule III]) *tablet, syrup:* hydrocodone bitartrate (see p. 784) 5 mg/homatropine methylbromide 1.5 mg.

**Hycotuss Expectorant** (ANTITUSSIVE [schedule III]) guaifenesin (see p. 767) 100 mg/hydrocodone (see p. 784) 5 mg.

**Hydrocet** (NARCOTIC ANALGESIC [schedule III]) *capsule:* hydrocodone (see p. 784) 5 mg/acetaminophen (see p. 13) 500 mg.

**Hyzaar** (ANTIHYPERTENSIVE) *tablet:* losartan (see p. 968) 50 mg/hydrochlorothiazide (see p. 782) 12.5 mg/losartan 100 mg/hydrochlorothiazide 12.5 mg/losartan 100 mg/hydrochlorothiazide 25 mg.

**Inderide 40/25** (ANTIHYPERTENSIVE) *tablet:* propranolol hydrochloride (see p. 1371) 40 mg/hydrochlorothiazide (see p. 782) 25 mg.

**Invokamet** (ANTIDIABETIC) *tablet:* canagliflozin (see p. 253) 150/metformin

(see p. 1018) 1000 mg; canagliflozin 50/metformin 500 mg.

**Jalyn** (BPH AGENT) *capsule:* dutasteride 0.5 mg/tamsulosin 0.4 mg.

**Janumet** (ANTIDIABETIC) *tablet:* sitagliptin (see p. 1500) 50 mg/metformin (see p. 1018) 500 mg; sitagliptin 50 mg/metformin 1000 mg.

**Janumet XR** (ANTIDIABETIC) *extended release tablet:* sitagliptin 100 mg/metformin 1000 mg; sitagliptin 50 mg/metformin 1000 mg; sitagliptin 50 mg/metformin 500 mg.

**Jentadueto** (ANTIDIABETIC) *tablet:* linagliptin 2.5 mg/metformin 1000 mg; linagliptin 2.5 mg/metformin 500; mglinagliptin 2.5 mg/metformin 850 mg.

**Jusvisync** (ANTIDIABETIC) *tablet:* sitagliptin 100 mg/simvastatin 10mg; sitagliptin 100 mg/simvastatin 20 mg; sitagliptin 100 mg/simvastatin 40 mg.

**Kazano** (ANTIDIABETIC) *tablet:* alogliptin (see p. 51) 12.5 mg/metformin (see p. 1018) 500 mg alogliptin 12.5 mg/metformin 1000 mg.

**Kisqali Femara** (ANTINEOPLASTIC) *tablet:* letrozole (see p. 919) 2.5 mg/ribociclib 200 mg; letrozole 2.5 mg/ribociclib 400 mg; letrozole 2.5 mg/ribociclib 600 mg.

**Kombiglyze XR** (ANTIDIABETIC) *extended release tablet:* saxagliptin 5 mg/metformin 500 mg; saxagliptin 2.5 mg/metformin 1000 mg; saxagliptin 5 mg/metformin 1000 mg.

**LidoSite** (LOCAL ANESTHETIC) *transdermal patch:* lidocaine (see p. 937) 100 mg/epinephrine (see p. 594) 1.05 mg.

**Limbitrol** (PSYCHOTHERAPEUTIC [schedule IV]) *tablet:* chlordiazepoxide (see p. 333) 5 mg/amitriptyline (see p. 80) 12.5 mg; chlordiazepoxide 10 mg/amitriptyline 25 mg.

**Limbitrol DS** (PSYCHOTHERA-PEUTIC [schedule IV]) *tablet:* chlordiazepoxide (see p. 333) 10 mg/amitriptyline (see p. 80) 25 mg.

**Liptruzet** (LIPID-LOWERING AGENT) *tablet:* atorvastatin (see p. 132) 10mg/ezetimibe (see p. 665) 10 mg atorvastatin 20mg/ezetimibe 10 mg atorvastatin 40mg/ezetimibe 10 mg atorvastatin 80mg/ezetimibe 10 mg.

**Loestrin 1/20** (ORAL CONTRACEP-TIVE) *tablet:* ethinyl estradiol 20 mcg/norethindrone acetate (see p. 1156) 1 mg.

**Loestrin 1/20 Fe** (ORAL CONTRA-CEPTIVE) *tablet:* ethinyl estradiol 20 mcg/norethindrone acetate (see p. 1156) 1 mg/ferrous fumarate 75 mg in last 7 tablets.

**Loestrin 1.5/30** (ORAL CONTRA-CEPTIVE) *tablet:* ethinyl estradiol 30 mcg/norethindrone acetate (see p. 1156) 1.5 mg.

**Loestrin 1.5/30 Fe** (ORAL CONTRA-CEPTIVE) *tablet:* ethinyl estradiol 30 mcg/norethindrone acetate (see p. 1156) 1.5 mg/ferrous fumarate 75 mg in last 7 tablets.

**Lomotil** (ANTIDIARRHEAL) *tablet:* diphenoxylate (see p. 516) 2.5 mg/atropine (see p. 138) 0.025 mg.

**Lo/Ovral 28** (ORAL CONTRACEPTIVE) tablet: ethinyl estradiol 30 mcg/norgestrel 0.3 mg.

**Lopressor HCT** (ANTIHYPERTENSIVE) *tablet:* metoprolol tartrate (see p. 1049) 50 mg/hydrochlorothiazide (see p. 782) 25 mg; metoprolol tartrate 100 mg/hydrochlorothiazide 25 mg; metoprolol tartrate 100 mg/hydrochlorothiazide 50 mg.

**Lorcet** (NARCOTIC ANALGESIC [schedule III]) *tablet:* hydrocodone (see p. 784) 5 mg/acetaminophen (see p. 13) 500 mg.

**Lorcet 10/650** (NARCOTIC ANALGESIC [schedule III]) *tablet:* hydrocodone (see p. 784) 10 mg/acetaminophen (see p. 13) 650 mg.

**Lorcet-HD** (NARCOTIC ANALGESIC [schedule III]) *tablet:* hydrocodone (see p. 784) 5 mg/acetaminophen (see p. 13) 500 mg.

**Lortab 5** (NARCOTIC ANALGESIC [schedule III]) *tablet:* hydrocodone (see p. 784) 5 mg/acetaminophen (see p. 13) 500 mg.

**Lortab 7.5/500** (NARCOTIC ANALGESIC [schedule III]) *tablet:* hydrocodone (see p. 784) 7.5 mg/acetaminophen (see p. 13) 500 mg.

**LoSeasonique** (ORAL CONTRACEP-TIVE) *tablet:* ethinyl estradiol 0.01 mg/ethinyl estradiol 0.02 mg/levonorgestrel (see p. 932) 0.1 mg.

**Lotensin HCT** (ANTIHYPERTENSIVE) *tablet:* hydrochlorothiazide (see p. 782) 25 mg/benazepril (see p. 171) 20 mg; hydrochlorothiazide 12.5/benazepril 20 mg; hydrochlorothiazide 12.5 mg/benazepril 10 mg.

**Lotrel** (ANTIHYPERTENSIVE) *tablet:* amlodipine (see p. 82) 2.5 mg/benazepril (see p. 171) 10 mg; amlodipine 5 mg/benazepril 10 mg; amlodipine 5 mg/benazepril 20 mg; amlodipine 10 mg/benazepril 20 mg; amlodipine 10mg/benazepril 40 mg.

**Lotrisone** (CORTICOSTEROID, ANTI-FUNGAL) *cream:* betamethasone (see p. 180) (as dipropionate) 0.05%/clotrimazole (see p. 390) 1%.

**Malarone** (ANTIMALARIAL) *tablet:* atovaquone (see p. 133) 250 mg/proguanil HCl (see p. 135) 100 mg; atovaquone 62.5 mg/proguanil HCl 25 mg.

**Maxitrol** (OPHTHALMIC STEROID, ANTIBIOTIC) *ophthalmic ointment, ophthalmic suspension:* dexamethasone (see p. 458) 0.1%/neomycin sulfate (see p. 1120) (equivalent to 0.35% neomycin base)/polymyxin B sulfate (see p. 1318) 10,000 units.

**Maxzide** (DIURETIC) *tablet:* triamterene (see p. 1654) 75 mg/hydrochlorothiazide (see p. 782) 50 mg.

**Maxzide 25** (DIURETIC) *tablet:* triamterene (see p. 1654) 37.5 mg/hydrochlorothiazide (see p. 782) 25 mg.

**Metaglip** (HYPOGLYCEMIC AGENT) *tablet:* glipizide (see p. 752) 2.5 mg/metformin HCl (see p. 1018) 250 mg; glipizide 2.5 mg/metformin 500 mg; glipizide 5 mg/metformin 500 mg.

**Micardis HCT** (ANTIHYPERTENSIVE) *tablet:* telmisartan (see p. 1561) 40 mg/hydrochlorothiazide (see p. 782) 12.5 mg; telmisartan 80 mg/hydrochlorothiazide 12.5 mg; telmisartan 80 mg/hydrochlorothiazide 25 mg.

**Minizide** (ANTIHYPERTENSIVE) *capsule:* polythiazide 0.5 mg/prazosin hydrochloride (see p. 1341) 1 mg; polythiazide 0.5 mg/prazosin hydrochloride 2 mg; polythiazide 0.5 mg/prazosin hydrochloride 5 mg.

**Modicon 28** (ORAL CONTRACEPTIVE) *tablet:* ethinyl estradiol 35 mcg/norethindrone (see p. 1156) 0.5 mg.

**Moduretic** (DIURETIC) *tablet:* amiloride hydrochloride (see p. 70) 5 mg/hydrochlorothiazide (see p. 782) 50 mg.

**Mycitracin** (OPHTHALMIC ANTIBIOTIC) *ophthalmic ointment:* polymyxin B sulfate (see p. 1318) 10,000 units/neomycin sulfate (see p. 1120) 3.5 mg/bacitracin (see p. 157) 500 units/g.

**Mycodone** (NARCOTIC ANALGESIC [schedule III]) *syrup (per 5 mL):* homatropine methylbromide 1.5 mg/hydrocodone (see p. 784) 5 mg.

**Mycolog II** (CORTICOSTEROID, ANTIFUNGAL) *cream, ointment:* triamcinolone acetonide (see p. 1652)

0.1%/nystatin (see p. 1161) 100,000 units/g.

**Mydayis** (ATTENTION DEFICIT DISORDER AGENT [schedule II]) *extended release capsule:* amphetamine aspartate 3.125 mg, amphetamine sulfate (see p. 91) 3.125 mg, dextroamphetamine saccharate 3.125 mg, dextroamphetamine sulfate (see p. 480) 3.125 mg.

**Neo-Cortef** (CORTICOSTEROID ANTIBIOTIC) *water-soluble cream, topical ointment:* hydrocortisone acetate (see p. 785) 1%/neomycin sulfate (see p. 1120) 0.5%.

**Neosporin** (OPHTHALMIC ANTIBIOTIC) *ophthalmic drops:* polymyxin B sulfate (see p. 1318) 10,000 units/neomycin sulfate (see p. 1120) 1.75 mg/gramicidin 0.025 mg/mL; *ophthalmic ointment:* polymyxin B sulfate 10,000 units/neomycin sulfate 3.5 mg/bacitracin zinc (see p. 157) 400 units/g.

**Neosporin G.U. Irrigant** (ANTIBIOTIC) *solution:* neomycin sulfate (see p. 1120) 40 mg/polymyxin B sulfate (see p. 1318) 200,000 units/mL.

**Neutra-Phos** (PHOSPHORUS REPLACEMENT) *capsule, powder:* phosphorus 250 mg/potassium (see p. 1325) 278 mg/sodium (see p. 1501) 164 mg/combination of monobasic, dibasic, sodium, and potassium phosphate.

**Norco** (NARCOTIC AGONIST ANALGESIC [schedule III]) *tablet:* hydrocodone bitartrate (see p. 784) 10 mg/acetaminophen (see p. 13) 325 mg; hydrocodone bitartrate 7.5 mg/acetaminophen 325 mg.

**Nordette 28** (ORAL CONTRACEPTIVE) *tablet:* ethinyl estradiol 30 mcg/levonorgestrel (see p. 932) 0.15 mg.

**Norgesic** (SKELETAL MUSCLE RELAXANT) *tablet:* orphenadrine citrate (see p. 1188) 25 mg/aspirin (see

p. 122) 385 mg/caffeine (see p. 240) 30 mg.

**Norgesic Forte** (SKELETAL MUSCLE RELAXANT, ANALGESIC) *tablet:* orphenadrine citrate (see p. 1188) 50 mg/aspirin (see p. 122) 770 mg/caffeine (see p. 240) 60 mg.

**Norinyl 1+35** (ORAL CONTRACEPTIVE) *tablet:* ethinyl estradiol 35 mcg/norethindrone (see p. 1156) 1 mg.

**Norinyl 1+50** (ORAL CONTRACEPTIVE) *tablet:* mestranol 50 mcg/norethindrone (see p. 1156) 1 mg.

**Odefsey** (NUCLEOSIDE REVERSE TRANSCRIPTASE INHIBITOR/NONNUCLEOSIDE REVERSE TRANSCRIPTASE INHIBITOR) *tablet:* emtricitabine 200 mg/rilpivirine 25 mg/tenofovir alafenamide 25 mg.

**Ortho Evra** (CONTRACEPTIVE) *transdermal patch:* norelgestromin 0.15 mg/ethinyl estradiol 0.02 mg.

**Oxycet** (NARCOTIC ANALGESIC [schedule II]) *tablet:* acetaminophen (see p. 13) 325 mg/ oxycodone (see p. 1206) 5 mg.

**Paremyd** (MYDRIATIC) ophthalmic *solution:* 1% hydroxyamphetamine hydrobromide, 0.25% tropicamide (see p. 1667).

**Percocet** (NARCOTIC ANALGESIC [schedule II]) *tablet:* oxycodone (see p. 1206) 2.5 mg/acetaminophen (see p. 13) 325 mg; oxycodone 7.5 mg/acetaminophen 325 mg; oxycodone 10 mg/acetaminophen 325 mg; oxycodone 10 mg/acetaminophen 650 mg.

**Percodan** (NARCOTIC ANALGESIC [schedule II]) *tablet:* oxycodone hydrochloride (see p. 1206) 4.5 mg/oxycodone terephthalate 0.38 mg/aspirin (see p. 122) 325 mg.

**Phrenilin** (NONNARCOTIC AGONIST ANALGESIC) *tablet:* acetaminophen (see p. 13) 325 mg/butalbital 50 mg.

**Phrenilin Forte** (NONNARCOTIC AGONIST ANALGESIC) *capsule:* acetaminophen (see p. 13) 650 mg/butalbital 50 mg.

**Polysporin Ointment** (ANTI-INFECTIVE [OPHTHALMIC]) *ophthalmic ointment:* polymyxin B sulfate (see p. 1318) 10,000 units/bacitracin zinc (see p. 157) 500 units/g.

**Prandimet** (HYPOGLYCEMIC AGENT) *tablet:* repaglinide (see p. 1419) 1 mg/metformin (see p. 1018) 500 mg; repaglinide 2 mg/metformin 500 mg.

**Pravigard Pac** (LIPID-LOWERING AGENT) *tablet:* pravastatin (see p. 1338) 20 mg/buffered aspirin (see p. 122) 81 mg; pravastatin 20 mg/buffered aspirin 325 mg; pravastatin 40 mg/aspirin 81 mg; pravastatin 40 mg/buffered aspirin 325 mg; pravastatin 80 mg/buffered aspirin 81 mg; pravastatin 80 mg/buffered aspirin 325 mg.

**Premarin with Methyltestosterone** (ESTROGEN, ANDROGEN) *tablet:* conjugated estrogens (see p. 638) 0.625 mg/methyltestosterone (see p. 1044) 5 mg.

**Premphase** (ESTROGEN, PROGESTERONE) *tablet:* conjugated estrogens (see p. 638) 0.625 mg/medroxyprogesterone acetate (see p. 993) 5 mg.

**Prempro** (ESTROGEN, PROGESTIN) *tablet:* conjugated estrogens (see p. 638) 0.3 mg/medroxyprogesterone (see p. 993) 1.5 mg; conjugated estrogen 0.45 mg/medroxyprogesterone 1.5 mg; conjugated estrogen 0.625 mg/medroxyprogesterone 2.5 mg; conjugated estrogen 0.625 mg/medroxyprogesterone 5 mg.

**Prestalia** (ACE INHIBITOR/CALCIUM CHANNEL BLOCKER) *tablets:* perindopril 14 mg/amlodipine besylate 10 mg; perindopril 3.5 mg/amlodipine besylate 2.5 mg; perindopril 7 mg/amlodipine besylate 5 mg.

**Prevacid NapraPAC** (PROTON PUMP INHIBITOR/ANTI-INFLAMMATORY) capsules and *tablets:* lansoprazole (see p. 907) 15 mg capsule/naproxen sodium (see p. 1105) 375 mg table; lansoprazole 15 mg capsule/naproxen sodium 500 mg tablet.

**Prevpac** (ANTIBIOTIC/ANTISECRETORY) capsules and *tablets:* amoxicillin (see p. 87) 500 mg capsules, clarithromycin (see p. 369) 500 mg tablets, lansoprazole (see p. 907) 30 mg capsules.

**Prinzide** (ANTIHYPERTENSIVE) *tablet:* hydrochlorothiazide (see p. 782) 12.5 mg/lisinopril (see p. 953) 10 mg; hydrochlorothiazide 12.5 mg/lisinopril 20 mg; hydrochlorothiazide 25 mg/lisinopril 20 mg.

**Probenecid and Colchicine** (ANTIGOUT) *tablet:* probenecid (see p. 1351) 500 mg/colchicine (see p. 395) 0.5 mg.

**Pyridium Plus** (ANALGESIC) *tablet:* phenazopyridine hydrochloride (see p. 1280) 150 mg/hyoscyamine hydrobromide (see p. 800) 0.3 mg/butalbital 15 mg.

**Qsymia** (ANTIOBESITY) *extended release capsule:* phentermine 3.75/topiramate 23 mg; phentermine 7.5/topiramate 46 mg; phentermine 11.25 mg/topiramate 69 mg phentermine 15 mg/topiramate 92 mg.

**Qtren** (ANTIDIABETIC) *tablet:* dapagliflozin (see p. 438) 10 mg/saxagliptin (see p. 1474) 5mg.

**Quartette** (ORAL CONTRACEPTIVE) *tablet:* various combinations of levonorgestrel and ethinyl estradiol.

**Rebetron** (INTERFERON, ANTIVIRAL) ribavirin (see p. 1427) tablet polythiazide 2 mg/reserpine (see p. 1420) 0.25 mg.

**Rifamate** (ANTITUBERCULOSIS) *capsule:* isoniazid (see p. 871) 150 mg/rifampin (see p. 1432) 300 mg.

**Rifater** (ANTITUBERCULOSIS) *tablet:* rifampin (see p. 1430) 120 mg/isoniazid (see p. 871) 50 mg/pyrazinamide (see p. 1384) 300 mg.

**Rimactane/INH Dual Pack** (ANTITUBERCULOSIS) *pack:* thirty isoniazid (see p. 871) 300 mg tablets, sixty rifampin (see p. 1432) 300 mg capsules.

**Rondec** (DECONGESTANT, ANTIHISTAMINE) *tablet:* pseudoephedrine hydrochloride (see p. 1381) 60 mg/carbinoxamine maleate 4 mg; *drops (per mL):* pseudoephedrine hydrochloride 25 mg/carbinoxamine maleate 2 mg; *syrup (per mL):* pseudoephedrine hydrochloride 60 mg/carbinoxamine maleate 4 mg.

**Roxicet** (NARCOTIC ANALGESIC [schedule II]) *tablet:* oxycodone (see p. 1206) 5 mg/acetaminophen (see p. 13) 325 mg; *syrup (per 5 mL):* oxycodone 5 mg/acetaminophen 325 mg.

**Ryzodeg 70/30** (INSULIN); *injection:* insulin degludec 70/insulin aspart 30.

**Simcor** (ANTILIPIDEMIC) extended release *tablet:* niacin (see p. 1128) 1000 mg/simvastatin (see p. 1495) 20 mg; niacin 1000 mg/simvastatin 40 mg, niacin 500 mg/simvastatin 20 mg; niacin 500 mg/simvastatin 40 mg, niacin 750 mg/simvastatin 20 mg.

**Soliqua** (ANTIDIATBETIC) *injection:* insulin glargine (see p. 841) 100 units/lixisenatide (see p. 957) 33 mg.

**Soma Compound** (SKELETAL MUSCLE RELAXANT) *tablet:* carisoprodol (see p. 277) 200 mg/aspirin (see p. 122) 325 mg.

**Soma Compound with Codeine** (SKELETAL MUSCLE RELAXANT [schedule III]) *tablet:* carisoprodol (see p. 277) 200 mg, aspirin (see p. 122) 325 mg/codeine phosphate 16 mg.

**Stalevo** (ANTIPARKINSON AGENT) *tablet:* carbidopa (see p. 266) 12.5 mg/levodopa (see p. 927) 50 mg/entacapone (see p. 589) 200 mg; carbidopa 18.75 mg/levodopa 75 mg/entacapone 200 mg; carbidopa 25 mg/levodopa 100 mg/entacapone 200 mg; carbidopa 31.25 mg/levodopa 125 mg/entacapone 200 mg; carbidopa 37.5 mg/levodopa 150 mg/entacapone 200 mg.

**Stiolto** (BRONCHODIALATOR) *powder for inhalation:* tiotropium 2.5 mcg/ olodaterol 2.5 mcg.

**Suboxone** (ANALGESIC) sublingual *tablet:* buprenorphine (see p. 223) 2 mg/naloxone (see p. 1101) 0.5 mg, buprenorphine 8 mg/naloxone 2 mg.

**Symbicort** (MINERALOCORTICOID/ BRONCHODILATOR) *inhaler:* budesonide (see p. 219) 0.08 mg/formoterol (see p. 721) 0.045 mg; budesonide 0.16 mg/formoterol 0.045 mg.

**Symbyax** (ATYPICAL ANTIPSYCHOTIC/ SSRI) *capsule:* olanzapine (see p. 1170) 6 mg/fluoxetine (see p. 706) 25 mg; olanzapine 6 mg/fluoxetine 50 mg; olanzapine 12 mg/fluoxetine 25 mg; olanzapine 12 mg/fluoxetine 50 mg.

**Synalgos-DC** (NARCOTIC AGONIST ANALGESIC [schedule III]) *capsule:* dihydrocodeine bitartrate 16 mg/aspirin (see p. 122) 356.4 mg/caffeine (see p. 240) 30 mg.

**Synera** (LOCAL ANESTHETIC) *transdermal patch:* lidocaine (see p. 937) 70 mg/tetracycline (see p. 1584) 70 mg.

**Syntest D.S.** (ESTROGEN, ANDROGEN) *tablet:* esterified estrogens (see p. 640) 1.25 mg/methyltestosterone (see p. 1044) 2.5 mg.

**Syntest H.S.** (ESTROGEN, ANDROGEN) *tablet:* esterified estrogens (see p. 640) 0.625 mg/methyltestosterone (see p. 1044) 1.25 mg.

**Taclonex Scalp** (NSAID) *topical suspension:* betamethasone (see p. 180) 0.064%/calcipotriene (see p. 242) 0.005%.

**Talacen** (NARCOTIC AGONIST-ANTAGONIST ANALGESIC [schedule IV]) *tablet:* pentazocine hydrochloride (see p. 1267) 25 mg/acetaminophen (see p. 13) 625 mg.

**Talwin NX** (NARCOTIC ANALGESIC [schedule IV]) *tablet:* pentazocine (see p. 1267) 50 mg/naloxone (see p. 1101) 0.5 mg.

**Tanafed DP** (DECONGESTANT, ANTIHISTAMINE) *suspension:* pseudoephedrine (see p. 1381) 75 mg/chlorpheniramine tannate 4.5 mg.

**Targiniq ER** (NARCOTIC ANALGESIC [schedule II]) tablet: oxycodone 10 mg/naloxone 5 mg, oxycodone 20 mg/naloxone 10 mg; oxycodone 40 mg/naloxone 20 mg.

**Tarka** (ANTIHYPERTENSIVE) *tablet:* trandolapril (see p. 1643) 2 mg/verapamil HCl (see p. 1695) 180 mg; trandolapril 4 mg/verapamil HCl 240 mg; trandolapril 1 mg/verapamil HCl 240 mg, trandolapril 2 mg/verapamil HCl 240 mg.

**Technivie** (ANTIVIRAL) *tablet:* ombitasvir 12.5 mg/paritaprevir 75 mg/ritonavir 50 mg.

**Tekamlo** (ANTIHYPERTENSIVE) *tablet:* aliskiren 150 mg/amlodipine 10 mg; aliskiren 150 mg/amlodipine 5 mg; aliskiren 300 mg/amlodipine 10 mg; aliskiren 300 mg/amlodipine 5 mg.

**Tekurna HCT** (ANTIHYPERTENSIVE) *tablet:* aliskiren (see p. 45) 150 mg/hydrochlorothiazide (see p. 762) 12.5 mg.

**Tenoretic 50** (ANTIHYPERTENSIVE) *tablet:* chlorthalidone (see p. 346) 25 mg/atenolol (see p. 128) 50 mg.

**Tenoretic 100** (ANTIHYPERTENSIVE) *tablet:* chlorthalidone (see p. 346) 25 mg/atenolol (see p. 128) 100 mg.

**Terra-Cortril Suspension** (OCULAR STEROID AND ANTIBIOTIC) *suspension:* hydrocortisone acetate (see p. 785) 1.5%/oxytetracycline 0.5%.

**Teveten HCT** (ANTIHYPERTENSIVE) *tablet:* eprosartan mesylate (see p. 605) 600 mg/hydrochlorothiazide (see p. 782) 12.5 mg; eprosartan 600 mg/hydrochlorothiazide 25 mg.

**Timolide** (ANTIHYPERTENSIVE) *tablet:* hydrochlorothiazide (see p. 782) 25 mg/timolol maleate (see p. 1609) 10 mg.

**Tobradex** (ANTI-INFECTIVE) *ophthalmic suspension:* dexamethasone (see p. 470) 0.1%/tobramycin (see p. 1618) 0.3%; ophthalmic ointment: dexamethasone 0.1%/tobramycin 0.3%.

**Treximet** (ANALGESIC) *tablet:* naproxen (see p. 1105) 500 mg/sumatriptan (see p. 1539) 85 mg.

**Triacin-C Cough Syrup** (ANTITUSSIVE [schedule V]) *syrup:* pseudoephedrine (see p. 1381) 30 mg/triprolidine 1.25 mg/codeine (see p. 394) 10 mg.

**Tribenzor** (ANTIHYPERTENSIVE) *tablet:* olmesartan 20 mg/amlodipine 5 mg/hydrochlorothiazide 12.5 mg; olmesartan 40 mg/amlodipine 10 mg/hydrochlorothiazide 12.5 mg; olmesartan 40 mg/amlodipine 10 mg/hydrochlorothiazide 25 mg; olmesartan 40 mg/amlodipine 5 mg/hydrochlorothiazide 12.5 mg; olmesartan 40 mg/amlodipine 5 mg/hydrochlorothiazide 25 mg.

**Tri-Hydroserpine** (ANTIHYPERTENSIVE) *tablet:* hydrochlorothiazide (see p. 782) 15 mg/reserpine (see p. 1420) 0.1 mg/hydralazine hydrochloride (see p. 780) 25 mg.

**Tri-Luma Cream** (STEROID) *cream:* 4% hydroquinone (see p. 791)/0.05% tretinoin (see p. 1650)/0.01% fluocinolone acetonide (see p. 703).

**Tri-Norinyl 28** (ORAL CONTRACEPTIVE) *tablet:* ethinyl estradiol (see p. 630) 35 mcg/norethindrone (see p. 1156) 0.5 mg × 7 d, ethinyl estradiol 35 mcg/norethindrone 1 mg × 9 d, ethinyl estradiol 35 mcg/norethindrone 0.5 mg × 5 d.

**Triple Antibiotic** (OPHTHALMIC ANTIBIOTIC) *ophthalmic ointment:* hydrocortisone (see p. 785) 1%/neomycin sulfate (see p. 1120) 0.5%/bacitracin zinc (see p. 157) 400 units/polymyxin B sulfate (see p. 1318) 10,000 units/g.

**Triumeq** (ANTIRETROVIRAL) *tablet:* abacavir (see p. 1) 600 mg/dolutegravir (see p. 530) 50 mg/lamivudine (see p. 903) 300 mg.

**Trizivir** (REVERSE TRANSCRIPTASE INHIBITOR) *tablet:* abacavir (see p. 1) 300 mg/lamivudine (see p. 903) 150 mg/zidovudine (see p. 1724) 300 mg.

**Truvada** (NUCLEOSIDE REVERSE TRANSCRIPTASE INHIBITOR) *tablet:* emtricitabine (see p. 580) 200 mg/tenofovir disoproxil fumarate (see p. 1568) 300 mg.

**Tussicap** (ANTITUSSIVE [schedule III]) *extended release capsule:* chlorpheniramine (see p. 339) 8 mg/hydrocodone (see p. 784) 10 mg.

**Tussigon** (ANTITUSSIVE [schedule III]) *tablet:* homatropine methylbromide 1.5 mg/hydrocodone (see p. 784) 5 mg.

**Tussionex** (ANTITUSSIVE [schedule III]) *tablet:* chlorpheniramine (see p. 339) 8 mg/hydrocodone (see p. 784) 10 mg.

**Twinrix** (VACCINE) *injection:* hepatitis A vaccine (see p. 777) 720 ELU/hepatitis B recombinant vaccine (see p. 777) 20 mcg per single dose vial.

**Twynsta** (ANTIHYPERTENSIVE) *tablet:* telmisartan 40 mg/amlodipine 5 mg; telmisartan 40 mg/amlodipine 10 mg; telmisartan 80 mg/

amlodipine 5 mg; telmisartan 80 mg/amlodipine 10 mg.

**Tylenol with Codeine No. 3** (NARCOTIC AGONIST ANALGESIC [schedule III]) *tablet:* acetaminophen (see p. 13) 300 mg/codeine phosphate 30 mg.

**Tylenol with Codeine No. 4** (NARCOTIC AGONIST ANALGESIC [schedule III]) *tablet:* acetaminophen (see p. 13) 300 mg/codeine phosphate 60 mg.

**Ultracet** (ANALGESIC/ANTIPYRETIC) *tablet:* tramadol (see p. 1640) 37.5 mg/acetaminophen (see p. 13) 325 mg.

**Uniretic** (ANTIHYPERTENSIVE) *tablet:* moexipril (see p. 1081) 7.5 mg/hydrochlorothiazide (see p. 782) 12.5 mg; moexipril 15 mg/hydrochlorothiazide 12.5 mg, moexipril 15 mg/hydrochlorothiazide 25 mg.

**Urised** (URINARY ANTI-INFECTIVE) *tablet:* methenamine (see p. 1024) 40.8 mg/phenyl salicylate 18.1 mg/atropine sulfate (see p. 138) 0.03 mg/hyoscyamine (see p. 800) 0.03 mg/benzoic acid 4.5 mg/methylene blue 5.4 mg.

**Vabomere** (ANTI-INFECTIVE) *solution for injection:* meropenem (see p. 1012) 1 g/vaborbactam 1g.

**Valturna** (ANTIHYPERTENSIVE) *tablet:* aliskiren (see p. 45) 150 mg/valsartan (see p. 1680) 160 mg; aliskiren 300 mg/valsartan 320 mg.

**Vaseretic** (ANTIHYPERTENSIVE) *tablet:* enalapril maleate (see p. 581) 10 mg/hydrochlorothiazide (see p. 782) 25 mg.

**Vasocidin** (OPHTHALMIC CORTICOSTEROID, ANTI-INFECTIVE) *ophthalmic solution:* prednisolone sodium phosphate (see p. 1343) 0.23%/sulfacetamide sodium (see p. 1530) 10%.

**Vasocon-A** (OPHTHALMIC DECONGESTANT) *ophthalmic solution:* naphazoline hydrochloride (see p. 1104) 0.05%/antazoline phosphate 0.5%.

**Veltin** (ANTIACNE) *gel:* clindamycin 1/2%/tretinoin 0.025%.

**Vicoprofen** (NARCOTIC AGONIST ANALGESIC [schedule III]) *tablet:* hydrocodone bitartrate (see p. 784) 7.5 mg/ibuprofen (see p. 804) 200 mg.

**Viekira XR** (ANTIVIRAL) *tablet:* ombitasvir 8.33 mg/paritaprevir 50 mg/ritonavir 33.33 mg/dasabuvir 200 mg.

**Vimovo** (ANALGESIC) *tablet:* naproxen 375 mg/esomeprazole 20 mg; naproxen 500 mg/esomeperazole 20 mg.

**Vosevi** (ANTIVIRAL) *tablet:* sofosbuvir (see p. 1505) 400 mg/velpatasvir 100 mg/voxilaprevir 100 mg.

**Vytorin** (ANTILIPEMIC AGENT) *tablet:* ezetimibe (see p. 665) 10 mg/simvastatin (see p. 1495) 10 mg; ezetimibe 10 mg/simvastatin 20 mg; ezetimibe 10 mg/simvastatin 40 mg; ezetimibe 10 mg/simvastatin 80 mg.

**Vyxeos** (ANTINEOPLASTIC) *powder for injection:* daunorubicin (see p. 451) 44 mg/cytarabine (see p. 420) 100 mg.

**Wygesic** (NARCOTIC AGONIST ANALGESIC [schedule IV]) *tablet:* 65 mg/acetaminophen (see p. 13) 650 mg.

**Xerese** (TOPICAL ANTIINFECTIVE) *cream:* acyclovir 5%/hydrocortisone 1%.

**Yasmin** (ORAL CONTRACEPTIVE) *tablet:* ethinyl estradiol 30 mcg/drospirenone 3 mg.

**Yosprala** (ANTIPLATELET/ANTIULCERATIVEE) *tablet:* aspirin 81 mg/omeprazole 40 mg; aspirin 325 mg/omeprazole 40 mg.

**Zepatier** (ANTIVIRAL/PROTEASE INHIBITOR) *tablet:* elbasvir 50 mg/grazoprevir 100 mg.

**Zestoretic** (ANTIHYPERTENSIVE) *tablet:* hydrochlorothiazide (see p. 782) 12.5 mg/lisinopril (see p. 953) 10 mg; hydrochlorothiazide 12.5 mg/lisinopril 20 mg; hydrochlorothiazide 25 mg/lisinopril 20 mg.

**Ziac** (ANTIHYPERTENSIVE) *tablet:* bisoprolol (see p. 194) 2.5 mg/ hydrochlorothiazide (see p. 782) 6.25 mg; bisoprolol 5 mg/hydrochlorothiazide 6.25 mg; bisoprolol 10 mg/hydrochlorothiazide 6.25 mg.

**Ziana** (ANTIACNE) *gel:* clindamycin 0.5%/tretinoin 0.025%.

**Zubsolv** (ANALGESIC) *sublingual tablet:* buprenorphine 1.4 mg/ naloxone 0.36 mg; buprenorphine 2.9 mg/naloxone 0.71 mg; buprenorphine 5.7 mg/naloxone 1.4 mg; buprenorphine 8.6 mg naloxone 2.1 mg; buprenorphine 11.4 mg/naloxone 2.9 mg.

**Zylet** (OPHTHALMIC ANTIBIOTIC) *solution:* loteprednol etabonate (see p. 969) 0.5%/tobramycin (see p. 1618) 0.3%.

**Zyrtec-D** (ANTIHISTAMINE/DECONGESTANT) *sustained release tablet:* cetirizine (see p. 323) 5 mg/ pseudoephedrine (see p. 1381) 120 mg.

**acute coronary syndrome** an acute ischemic event with or without marked ST segment elevation.

**acute dystonia** extrapyramidal symptom manifested by abnormal posturing, grimacing, spastic torticollis (neck torsion), and oculogyric (eyeball movement) crisis.

**adverse effect** unintended, unpredictable, and nontherapeutic response to drug action. Adverse effects occur at doses used therapeutically or for prophylaxis or diagnosis. They generally result from drug toxicity, idiosyncrasies, or hypersensitivity reactions caused by the drug itself or by ingredients added during manufacture (e.g., preservatives, dyes, or vehicles).

**afterload** resistance that ventricles must work against to eject blood into the aorta during systole.

**agranulocytosis** sudden drop in leukocyte count; often followed by a severe infection manifested by high fever, chills, prostration, and ulcerations of mucous membrane such as in the mouth, rectum, or vagina.

**akathisia** extrapyramidal symptom manifested by a compelling need to move or pace, without specific pattern, and an inability to be still.

**analeptic** restorative medication that enhances excitation of the CNS without affecting inhibitory impulses.

**anaphylactoid reaction** excessive allergic response manifested by wheezing, chills, generalized pruritic urticaria, diaphoresis, sense of uneasiness, agitation, flushing, palpitations, coughing, difficulty breathing, and cardiovascular collapse.

**anticholinergic actions** inhibition of parasympathetic response manifested by dry mouth, decreased peristalsis, constipation, blurred vision, and urinary retention.

**bioavailability** fraction of active drug that reaches its action sites after administration by any route. Following an IV dose, bioavailability is 100%; however, such factors as first-pass effect, enterohepatic cycling, and biotransformation reduce bioavailability of an orally administered drug.

**blood dyscrasia** pathological condition manifested by fever, sore mouth or throat, unexplained fatigue, easy bruising, or bleeding.

**cardiotoxicity** impairment of cardiac function manifested by one or more of the following: hypotension, arrhythmias, precordial pain, dyspnea, electrocardiogram (ECG) abnormalities, cardiac dilation, congestive failure.

**cholinergic response** stimulation of the parasympathetic response manifested by lacrimation, diaphoresis, salivation, abdominal cramps, diarrhea, nausea, and vomiting.

**circulatory overload** excessive vascular volume manifested by increased central venous pressure (CVP), elevated blood pressure, tachycardia, distended neck veins, peripheral edema, dyspnea, cough, and pulmonary rales.

**CNS stimulation** excitement of the CNS manifested by hyperactivity, excitement, nervousness, insomnia, and tachycardia.

**CNS toxicity** impairment of CNS function manifested by ataxia, tremor, incoordination, paresthesias, numbness, impairment of pain or touch sensation, drowsiness, confusion, headache, anxiety, tremors, and behavior changes.

**congestive heart failure (CHF)** impaired pumping ability of the heart manifested by paroxysmal nocturnal dyspnea, cough, fatigue or dyspnea on exertion, tachycardia, peripheral or pulmonary edema, and weight gain.

**Cushing's syndrome** fatty swellings in the interscapular area (buffalo hump) and in the facial area (moon face), distention of the abdomen, ecchymoses following even minor trauma, impotence, amenorrhea, high blood pressure, general weakness, loss of muscle mass, osteoporosis, and psychosis.

**dehydration** decreased intracellular or extracellular fluid manifested by elevated temperature, dry skin and mucous membranes, decreased tissue turgor, sunken eyes, furrowed tongue, low blood pressure, diminished or irregular pulse, muscle or abdominal cramps, thick secretions, hard feces and impaction, scant urinary output, urine specific gravity above 1.030, an elevated hemoglobin.

**disulfiram-type reaction** Antabuse-type reaction manifested by facial flushing, pounding headache, sweating, slurred speech, abdominal cramps, nausea, vomiting, tachycardia, fever, palpitations, drop in blood pressure, dyspnea, and sense of chest constriction. Symptoms may last up to 24 hours.

**enzyme induction** stimulation of microsomal enzymes by a drug resulting in its accelerated metabolism and decreased activity. If reactive intermediates are formed, drug-mediated toxicity may be exacerbated.

**first-pass effect** reduced bioavailability of an orally administered drug due to metabolism in GI epithelial cells and liver or to biliary excretion. Effect may be avoided by use of sublingual tablets or rectal suppositories.

**fixed drug eruption** drug-induced circumscribed skin lesion that persists or recurs in the same site. Residual pigmentation may remain following drug withdrawal.

**gamma-glutamyl transpeptidase** screening test for possible liver damage and/or suspected alcohol abuse.

**half-life ($t_{1/2}$)** time required for concentration of a drug in the body to decrease by 50%. Half-life also represents the time necessary to reach steady state or to decline from steady state after a change (i.e., starting or stopping) in the dosing regimen. Half-life may be affected by a disease state and age of the drug user.

**heart failure** left- and/or right-sided failure associated with systolic and/or diastolic dysfunction.

**heat stroke** a life-threatening condition manifested by absence of sweating; red, dry, hot skin; dilated pupils; dyspnea; full bounding pulse; temperature above 40° C (105° F); and mental confusion.

**hepatotoxicity** impairment of liver function manifested by jaundice, dark urine, pruritus, light-colored stools, eosinophilia, itchy skin or rash, and persistently high elevations of alanine amino-transferase (ALT) and aspartate aminotransferase (AST).

**hyperammonemia** elevated level of ammonia or ammonium in the blood manifested by lethargy, decreased appetite, vomiting, asterixis (flapping tremor), weak pulse, irritability, decreased responsiveness, and seizures.

**hypercalcemia** elevated serum calcium manifested by deep bone and flank pain, renal calculi, anorexia, nausea, vomiting, thirst, constipation, muscle hypotonicity, pathologic fracture, bradycardia, lethargy, and psychosis.

**hyperglycemia** elevated blood glucose manifested by flushed, dry skin, low blood pressure and elevated pulse, tachypnea, Kussmaul's respirations, polyuria, polydipsia; polyphagia, lethargy, and drowsiness.

**hyperkalemia** excessive potassium in blood, which may produce life-threatening cardiac arrhythmias, including bradycardia and heart block, unusual fatigue, weakness or heaviness of limbs, general muscle weakness, muscle cramps, paresthesias, flaccid paralysis of extremities, shortness of breath, nervousness, confusion, diarrhea, and GI distress.

**hypermagnesemia** excessive magnesium in blood, which may produce cathartic effect, profound thirst, flushing, sedation, confusion, depressed deep tendon reflexes (DTRs), muscle weakness, hypotension, and depressed respirations.

**hypernatremia** excessive sodium in blood, which may produce confusion, neuromuscular excitability, muscle weakness, seizures, thirst, dry and flushed skin, dry mucous membranes, pyrexia, agitation, and oliguria or anuria.

**hypersensitivity reactions** excessive and abnormal sensitivity to given agent manifested by urticaria, pruritus, wheezing, edema, redness, and anaphylaxis.

**hyperthyroidism** excessive secretion by the thyroid glands, which increases basal metabolic rate, resulting in warm, flushed, moist skin; tachycardia, exophthalmos; infrequent lid blinking; lid edema; weight loss despite increased appetite; frequent urination; menstrual irregularity; breathlessness; hypoventilation; congestive heart failure; excessive sweating.

**hyperuricemia** excessive uric acid in blood, resulting in pain in flank; stomach, or joints, and changes in intake and output ratio and pattern.

**hypocalcemia** abnormally low calcium level in blood, which may result in depression; psychosis; hyperreflexia; diarrhea; cardiac arrhythmias; hypotension; muscle spasms; paresthesias of feet, fingers, tongue; positive Chvostek's sign. Severe deficiency (tetany) may result in carpopedal spasms, spasms of face muscle, laryngospasm, and generalized convulsions.

**hypoglycemia** abnormally low glucose level in the blood, which may result in acute fatigue, restlessness, malaise, marked irritability and weakness, cold sweats, excessive hunger, headache, dizziness, confusion, slurred speech, loss of consciousness, and death.

**hypokalemia** abnormally low level of potassium in blood, which may result in malaise, fatigue, paresthesias, depressed reflexes, muscle weakness and cramps, rapid, irregular pulse, arrhythmias, hypotension, vomiting, paralytic ileus, mental confusion, depression, delayed thought process, abdominal distention, polyuria, shallow breathing, and shortness of breath.

**hypomagnesemia** abnormally low level of magnesium in blood, resulting in nausea, vomiting, cardiac arrhythmias, and neuromuscular symptoms (tetany, positive Chvostek's and Trousseau's signs, seizures, tremors, ataxia, vertigo, nystagmus, muscular fasciculations).

**hyponatremia** a decreased serum concentration (less than 125 mEq) of sodium that results in intracellular swelling. The resulting signs and symptoms include nausea, malaise, headache, lethargy, obtundation, seizures, and coma. There is significant variability in the symptomatology of hyponatremia manifested in patients.

**hypophosphatemia** abnormally low level of phosphates in blood, resulting in muscle weakness, anorexia, malaise, absent deep tendon reflexes, bone pain, paresthesias, tremors, negative calcium balance, osteomalacia, osteoporosis.

**hypothyroidism** condition caused by thyroid hormone deficiency that lowers basal metabolic rate and may result in periorbital edema, lethargy, puffy hands and feet, cool, pale skin, vertigo, nocturnal cramps, decreased GI motility, constipation, hypotension, slow pulse, depressed muscular activity, and enlarged thyroid gland.

**hypoxia** insufficient oxygenation in the blood manifested by dyspnea, tachypnea, headache, restlessness, cyanosis, tachycardia, dysrhythmias, confusion, decreased level of consciousness, and euphoria or delirium.

**immune reconstitution inflammatory syndrome (IRIS)** describes a collection of inflammatory disorders associated with worsening of preexisting infectious processes following initiation of highly active antiretroviral therapy in HIV-infected individuals. Usually the inflammatory reaction is self-limiting but long-term sequelae and fatal outcomes may occur, particularly when neurologic structures are involved.

**international normalizing ratio** measurement that normalizes for the differences obtained from various laboratory readings in the value for thromboplastin blood level.

**ischemic colitis** blood flow to part of the colon is reduced due to narrowing or blocked arteries resulting in insufficient oxygen to those cells. Signs and symptoms can include pain, tenderness, or cramping in the abdomen which can occur suddenly or gradually, bright red or maroon-colored blood in stool, or passage of blood alone from the rectum, a feeling of urgency to defecate, and diarrhea.

**lactic acidosis** is characterized by low pH (pH less than 7.35) in body tissues and blood (acidosis) accompanied by buildup of lactate. Lactate buildup results from metabolizing glucose anaerobically (low oxygen). Signs and symptoms include nausea, vomiting, hyperventilation, abdominal pain, lethargy, anxiety, hypotension, irregular heart rate, tachycardia, and severe anemia.

**leukopenia** abnormal decrease in number of white blood cells, usually below 5000 per cubic millimeter, resulting in fever, chills, sore mouth or throat, and unexplained fatigue.

**liver toxicity** manifested by anorexia, nausea, fatigue, lethargy, itching, jaundice, abdominal pain, dark-colored urine, and flu-like symptoms.

**metabolic acidosis** decrease in pH value of the extracellular fluid caused by either an increase in hydrogen ions or a decrease in bicarbonate ions. It may result in one or more of the following: lethargy, headache, weakness, abdominal pain, nausea, vomiting, dyspnea, hyperpnea progressing to Kussmaul breathing, dehydration, thirst, weakness, flushed face, full bounding pulse, progressive drowsiness, mental confusion, combativeness.

**metabolic alkalosis** increase in pH value of the extracellular fluid caused by either a loss of acid from the body (e.g., through vomiting) or an increased level of bicarbonate ions (e.g., through ingestion of sodium bicarbonate). It may result in muscle weakness, irritability, confusion, muscle twitching, slow and shallow respirations, and convulsive seizures.

**microsomal enzymes** drug-metabolizing enzymes located in the endoplasmic reticulum of the liver and other tissues chiefly responsible for oxidative drug metabolism (e.g., cytochrome P450).

**myopathy** any disease or abnormal condition of striated muscles manifested by muscle weakness, myalgia, diaphoresis, fever, and reddish-brown urine (myoglobinuria) or oliguria.

**nephrotoxicity** impairment of the nephrons of the kidney manifested by one or more of the following: oliguria, urinary frequency, hematuria, cloudy urine, rising BUN and serum creatinine, fever, graft tenderness or enlargement.

**neuroleptic malignant syndrome (NMS)** potentially fatal complication associated with antipsychotic drugs manifested by hyperpyrexia, altered mental status, muscle rigidity, irregular pulse, fluctuating BP, diaphoresis, and tachycardia.

**orphan drug** (as defined by the Orphan Drug Act, an amendment of the Federal Food, Drug, and Cosmetic Act which took effect in January 1983): drug or biological product used in the treatment, diagnosis, or prevention of a rare disease. A rare disease or condition is one that affects fewer than 200,000 persons in the United States, or affects more than 200,000 persons but for which there is no reasonable expectation that drug research and development costs can be recovered from sales within the United States.

**ototoxicity** impairment of the ear manifested by one or more of the following: headache, dizziness or vertigo, nausea and vomiting with motion, ataxia, nystagmus.

**pharmacogenetic** genetic variation affecting response to different drugs.

**post-transplant lymphoproliferative disorder (PTLD)** of B-cell proliferation that is a life-threatening complication after hematopoietic stem cell or organ transplant due to therapeutic immunosuppression after transplant. The majority of cases are associated with Epstein-Barr virus (EBV), while other causes are endogenous anti-T cell cytokine and anti-T cell antibodies, or production of interleukin-10. Some of the B cell mutations can result in lymphoma.

**prodrug** inactive drug form that becomes pharmacologically active through biotransformation.

**protein binding** reversible interaction between protein and drug resulting in a drug-protein complex (bound drug) which is in equilibrium with free (active) drug in plasma and tissues. Since only free drug can diffuse to action sites, factors that influence drug-binding (e.g., displacement of bound drug by another drug, or decreased albumin concentration) may potentiate pharmacologic effect.

**pseudomembranous enterocolitis** life-threatening superinfection characterized by severe diarrhea and fever.

**pseudoparkinsonism** extrapyramidal symptom manifested by slowing of volitional movement (akinesia), mask facies, rigidity and tremor at rest (especially of upper extremities); and pill rolling motion.

**pulmonary edema** excessive fluid in the lung tissue manifested by one or more of the following: shortness of breath, cyanosis, persistent productive cough (frothy sputum may be blood tinged), expiratory rales, restlessness, anxiety, increased heart rate, sense of chest pressure.

**QT prolongation** longer than normal time interval from the Q wave (QRS complex) to the end of the T wave; may be congenital or drug-induced.

**renal insufficiency** reduced capacity of the kidney to perform its functions as manifested by one or more of the following: dysuria, oliguria, hematuria, swelling of lower legs and feet.

**serotonin syndrome** may include several of the following: Confusion, agitation or restlessness, dilated pupils, headache, status changes, nausea and/or vomiting, diarrhea, rapid heart rate, tremor, loss of muscle coordination, twitching muscles, shivering, or diaphoresis.

**somogyi effect** rebound phenomenon clinically manifested by fasting hyperglycemia and worsening of diabetic control due to unnecessarily large p.m. insulin doses. Hormonal response to unrecognized hypoglycemia (i.e., release of epinephrine, glucagon, growth hormone, cortisol) causes insensitivity to insulin. Increasing the amount of insulin required to treat the hyperglycemia intensifies the hypoglycemia.

**superinfection** new infection by an organism different from the initial infection being treated by antimicrobial therapy manifested by one or more of the following: black, hairy tongue; glossitis, stomatitis; anal itching; loose, foul-smelling stools; vaginal itching or discharge; sudden fever; cough.

**tachyphylaxis** rapid decrease in response to a drug after administration of a few doses. Initial drug response cannot be restored by an increase in dose.

**tardive dyskinesia** extrapyramidal symptom manifested by involuntary rhythmic, bizarre movements of face, jaw, mouth, tongue, and sometimes extremities.

**torsade de pointes** a form of ventricular tachycardia nearly always due to drugs; characterized by a long QT interval.

**vasovagal symptoms** transient vascular and neurogenic reaction marked by pallor, nausea, vomiting, bradycardia, and rapid fall in arterial blood pressure.

**water intoxication (dilutional hyponatremia)** less than normal concentration of sodium in the blood resulting from excess extracellular and intracellular fluid and producing one or more of the following: lethargy, confusion, headache, decreased skin turgor, tremors, convulsions, coma, anorexia, nausea, vomiting, diarrhea, sternal fingerprinting, weight gain, edema, full bounding pulse, jugular vein distention, rales, signs and symptoms of pulmonary edema.

| | |
|---|---|
| **ABGs** | arterial blood gases |
| **ABW** | adjusted body weight |
| **a.c.** | before meals (*ante cibum*) |
| **ACD** | acid-citrate-dextrose |
| **ACE** | angiotensin-converting enzyme |
| **ACh** | acetylcholine |
| **ACIP** | Advisory Committee on Immunization Practices |
| **ACLS** | advanced cardiac life support |
| **ACS** | acute coronary syndrome |
| **ACT** | activated clotting time |
| **ACTH** | adrenocorticotropic hormone |
| **AD** | Alzheimer's disease |
| **ADCC** | antibody-dependent cell-mediated cytotoxicity |
| **ADD** | attention deficit disorder |
| **ADH** | antidiuretic hormone |
| **ADLs** | activities of daily living |
| **ad lib** | as desired (*ad libitum*) |
| **ADP** | adenosine diphosphate |
| **ADT** | alternate day drug (administration) |
| **AED** | antiepileptic drug |
| **AF** | atrial fibrillation |
| **AFL** | atrial flutter |
| **AIDS** | acquired immunodeficiency syndrome |
| **AIP** | acute intermittent porphyria |
| **alpha1-Pi** | alpha1-proteinase inhibitor |
| **ALS** | amyotrophic lateral sclerosis |
| **ALT** | alanine aminotransferase (formerly SGPT) |
| **AMI** | acute myocardial infarction |
| **AML** | acute myelogenous leukemia |
| **AMP** | adenosine monophosphate |
| **ANA** | antinuclear antibody(ies) |
| **ANC** | absolute neutrophil count |
| **ANG I** | angiotensin I |
| **ANG II** | angiotensin II |
| **ANH** | atrial natriuretic hormone |
| **ANLL** | acute nonlymphocytic leukemia |
| **AntiXa** | antifactor Xa |
| **APL** | acute promyelotic leukemia |
| **aPTT** | activated partial thromboplastin time |
| **ARC** | AIDS-related complex |
| **ARDS** | adult respiratory distress syndrome |
| **ASHD** | arteriosclerotic heart disease |
| **AST** | aspartate aminotransferase (formerly SGOT) |
| **ATIII** | antithrombin III |
| **AT$_1$** | angiotensin II receptor subtype I |
| **AT$_2$** | angiotensin II receptor subtype II |

| ATP | adenosine triphosphate |
|---|---|
| AUV | area under the curve |
| AV | atrioventricular |
| b.i.d. | two times a day |
| BMD | bone mineral density |
| BMI | body mass index |
| BMR | basal metabolic rate |
| BP | blood pressure |
| BPH | benign prostatic hypertrophy |
| bpm | beats per minute |
| BSA | body surface area |
| BSE | breast self-exam |
| BSP | bromsulphalein |
| BT | bleeding time |
| BUN | blood urea nitrogen |
| C | centigrade, Celsius |
| CAD | coronary artery disease |
| cAMP | cyclic adenosine monophosphate |
| CBC | complete blood count |
| CCR5 | cellular chemokine coreceptor-5 |
| CD | Crohn's disease |
| CDAD | clostridium difficile-associated diarrhea |
| CDC | Centers for Disease Control and Prevention |
| CDC | complement-dependent cytotoxicity |
| CF | cystic fibrosis |
| cGMP | cyclic guanosine monophosphate |
| CHC | chronic hepatitis C |
| CHF | congestive heart failure |
| CKD | chronic kidney disease |
| CLL | chronic lymphocytic leukemia |
| cm | centimeter |
| CML | chronic myeloid leukemia |
| CMV | cytomegalovirus-I |
| CNS | central nervous system |
| Coll | collyrium (eye wash) |
| COMT | catecholamine-O-methyl transferase |
| COPD | chronic obstructive pulmonary disease |
| COX-1 | cyclooxygenase-1 |
| COX-2 | cyclooxygenase-2 |
| CPK | creatinine phosphokinase |
| CPR | cardiopulmonary resuscitation |
| CRC | colorectal cancer |
| CrCl | creatinine clearance |
| CRF | chronic renal failure |
| CRFD | chronic renal failure disease |
| C&S | culture and sensitivity |
| CSF | cerebrospinal fluid |
| CSP | cellulose sodium phosphate |

| | |
|---|---|
| CSSSI | complicated skin and skin structure infections |
| CT | clotting time |
| CTZ | chemoreceptor trigger zone |
| CV | cardiovascular |
| CVA | cerebrovascular accident |
| CVP | central venous pressure |
| CYP | cytochrome P450 system of enzymes |
| CYP3A4 | cytochrome 3A4 |
| D5W | 5% dextrose in water |
| D&C | dilation and curettage |
| DIC | disseminated intravascular coagulation |
| DKA | diabetic ketoacidosis |
| dL | deciliter (100 mL or 0.1 liter) |
| DM | diabetes mellitus |
| DMARD | disease-modifying antirheumatic drug |
| DNA | deoxyribonucleic acid |
| DPD | dihydropyrimidine dehydrogenase |
| DTC | differentiated thyroid cancer |
| DTRs | deep tendon reflexes |
| DVT | deep venous thrombosis |
| ECG, EKG | electrocardiogram |
| ECT | electroconvulsive therapy |
| EEG | electroencephalogram |
| EENT | eye, ear, nose, throat |
| e.g. | for example (*exempli gratia*) |
| EGFR | epidermal growth factor receptor |
| eGFR | estimated glomerular filtration rate |
| EIB | exercise-induced bronchoconstriction |
| ENT | ear, nose, throat |
| EPS | extrapyramidal symptoms (or syndrome) |
| ER | estrogen receptor |
| ESRF | end-stage renal failure |
| F | Fahrenheit |
| FBS | fasting blood sugar |
| FDA | Food and Drug Administration |
| FSH | follicle-stimulating hormone |
| FTI | free thyroxine index |
| 5-FU | 5-fluorouracil |
| FUO | fever of unknown origin |
| g | gram |
| G6PD | glucose-6-phosphate dehydrogenase |
| GABA | gamma-aminobutyric acid |
| GERD | gastroesophageal reflux disease |
| GFR | glomerular filtration rate |
| GGT | gamma-glutamyl transferase |
| GGTP | gamma-glutamyl transpeptidase |
| GH | growth hormone |
| GI | gastrointestinal |

| | |
|---|---|
| GIST | gastrointestinal stomal tumor |
| GLP-1 | glucagon-like peptide-1 |
| GM-CSF | granulocyte-macrophage colony-stimulating factor |
| GnRH | gonadotropic releasing hormone |
| GPIIb/IIIa | glycoprotein IIb/IIIa |
| GTT | glucose tolerance test |
| GU | genitourinary |
| GVHD | graft-versus-host disease |
| h | hour |
| HACA | human antichimeric antibody |
| HbA1C | glycosylated hemoglobin |
| hBNP | human B-type natriuretic peptide |
| HBV | viral hepatitis B |
| HCG | human chorionic gonadotropin |
| Hct | hematocrit |
| HCV | hepatitis C virus |
| HDD-CKD | hemodialysis-dependent chronic kidney disease |
| HDL-C | high-density-lipoprotein cholesterol |
| HER | human epidermal growth factor |
| HF | heart failure |
| Hgb | hemoglobin |
| 5-HIAA | 5-hydroxyindoleacetic acid |
| HIT | heparin-induced thrombocytopenia |
| HIV | human immunodeficiency virus |
| HMG-CoA | 3-hydroxy-3-methyl-glutaryl coenzyme A |
| HPA | hypothalamic–pituitary–adrenocortical (axis) |
| HPV | human papillomavirus |
| HR | heart rate |
| HSV-1 | herpes simplex virus type 1 |
| HSV-2 | herpes simplex virus type 2 |
| 5-HT | 5-hydroxytryptamine (serotonin receptor) |
| IBD | inflammatory bowel disease |
| IBW | ideal body weight |
| IC | intracoronary |
| ICH | intracranial hemorrhage |
| ICP | intracranial pressure |
| ICU | intensive care unit |
| ID | intradermal |
| IFN | interferon |
| Ig | immunoglobulin |
| IGF-1 | insulin-like growth factor 1 |
| IL | interleukin |
| IM | intramuscular |
| INR | international normalized ratio |
| IOP | intraocular pressure |
| IPPB | intermittent positive pressure breathing |
| iPTH | idiopathic parathyroid hormone |
| IT | intrathecal |
| ITP | idiopathic thrombocytopenic purpura |

| | |
|---|---|
| IV | intravenous |
| JRA | juvenile rheumatoid arthritis |
| kg | kilogram |
| KGF | keratinocyte growth factor |
| 17-KGS | 17-ketogenic steroids |
| 17-KS | 17-ketosteroids |
| KVO | keep vein open |
| L | liter |
| LABA | long-acting beta-2 agonist |
| LDH | lactic dehydrogenase |
| LDL | low density lipoprotein |
| LDL-C | low-density-lipoprotein cholesterol |
| LE | lupus erythematosus |
| LFT | liver function test |
| LH | luteinizing hormone |
| LLN | lower limit of normal |
| LR | lactated Ringer's |
| LSD | lysergic acid diethylamide |
| LTRA | leukotriene receptor antagonist |
| LVEDP | left ventricular end diastolic pressure |
| LVEF | left ventricular ejection fraction |
| M | molar (strength of a solution) |
| m$^2$ | square meter (of body surface area) |
| MAC | mycobacterium avium complex |
| MAO | monoamine oxidase |
| MAOI | monoamine oxidase inhibitor |
| MBD | minimal brain dysfunction |
| MCH | mean corpuscular hemoglobin |
| MCHC | mean corpuscular hemoglobin concentration |
| mCi | millicurie |
| MCL | mantle cell lymphoma |
| mcg | microgram (1/1000 of a milligram) |
| MDD | major depressive disorder |
| MDI | metered dose inhaler |
| MDR | minimum daily requirements |
| MDS | muscular dystrophy syndrome |
| mEq | milliequivalent |
| mg | milligram |
| MI | myocardial infarction |
| MIC | minimum inhibitory concentration |
| min | minute |
| mL | milliliter (0.001 liter) |
| mm | millimeter |
| mo | month |
| MPS I | mucopolysaccharidosis I |
| MRSA | methicillin-resistant *Staphylococcus aureus* |
| MS | multiple sclerosis |
| MTC | medullary thyroid cancer |
| mTOR | mammalian target or rapamycin |

| | |
|---|---|
| mu-m | micrometer |
| N | normal (strength of a solution) |
| NADH | reduced form of nicotine adenine dinucleotide |
| NAPA | *N*-acetyl procainamide |
| nb | note well (*nota bene*) |
| NDD | non-hemodialysis dependent |
| NDD-CKD | non-hemodialysis-dependent chronic kidney disease |
| ng | nanogram (1/1000 of a microgram) |
| NMDA | N-methyl-D-aspartic acid |
| NMS | neuroleptic malignant syndrome |
| NNRTI | nonnucleoside reverse transcriptase inhibitor |
| NON-PVC | nonpolyvinyl chloride IV bag or tubing |
| NPN | nonprotein nitrogen |
| NPO | nothing by mouth |
| NRTI | nucleoside reverse transcriptase inhibitor |
| NS | normal saline |
| NS 3/4A | nonstructural protein (NS) 3/4A protease inhibitor |
| NSAID | nonsteroidal anti-inflammatory drug |
| NSCLC | non-small-cell lung cancer |
| NSR | normal sinus rhythm |
| NVAF | non-valvular atrial fibrillation |
| NYHA Class I, II, III, IV | New York Heart Association classes of heart failure |
| OA | osteoarthritis |
| OAB | overactive bladder |
| OATP | organic anion transporting polypeptide |
| OC | oral contraceptive |
| OCD | obsessive compulsive disorder |
| ODT | oral disintegrating tablet |
| 17-OHCS | 17-hydroxycorticosteroids |
| OTC | over the counter (nonprescription) |
| P450 | cytochrome P450 system of enzymes |
| PABA | *para*-aminobenzoic acid |
| PAR-1 | protease-activated receptor-1 |
| PAS | *para*-aminosalicylic acid |
| PAWP | pulmonary artery wedge pressure |
| PBI | protein-bound iodine |
| PBP | penicillin-binding protein |
| p.c. | after meals (*post cibum*) |
| PCI | percutaneous coronary intervention |
| PCP | *Pneumocystis carinii* pneumonia |
| PCWP | pulmonary capillary wedge pressure |
| PD-1 | programmed cell death receptors |
| PDD | peritoneal dialysis dependent |
| PDD-CKD | peritoneal dialysis-dependent chronic kidney disease |
| PDE | phosphodiesterase |
| PDE5 | phosphodiesterase type-5 |

| | |
|---|---|
| PE | pulmonary embolism |
| PERRLA | pupils equal, round, react to light and accommodation |
| P-gp | P-glycoprotein transporter |
| PG | prostaglandin |
| PGE$_2$ | prostaglandin E$_2$ |
| pH | hydrogen ion concentration |
| Ph | Philadelphia (chromosome) |
| PI | protease inhibitor |
| PID | pelvic inflammatory disease |
| PJP | *Pneumocystis jirovecii* pneumonia |
| PKU | phenylketonuria |
| PMDD | premenstrual dysphoric disorder |
| PML | progressive multifocal leukoencephalopathy |
| PND | paroxysmal nocturnal dyspnea |
| PNE | primary nocturnal enuresis |
| PO | by mouth or orally (*per os*) |
| PPES | Plantar Palmar Erythrodysesthesia |
| PPI | proton pump inhibitor |
| PPM | parts per million |
| PR | rectally (*per rectum*) |
| PRES | posterior reversible encephalopathy syndrome |
| prn | when required (*pro re nata*) |
| PSA | prostate-specific antigen |
| PSP | phenolsulfonphthalein |
| PSVT | paroxysmal supraventricular tachycardia |
| PT | prothrombin time |
| PTCL | peripheral T-cell lymphocyte |
| PTH | parathyroid hormone |
| PTLD | post-transplant lymphoproliferative disorder |
| PTSD | post-traumatic stress disorder |
| PTT | partial thromboplastin time |
| PUD | peptic ulcer disease |
| PVC | polyvinyl chloride IV bag or tubing |
| PVC | premature ventricular contraction |
| PVD | peripheral vascular disease |
| PZI | protamine zinc insulin |
| q.i.d. | four times daily |
| RA | rheumatoid arthritis |
| RAAS | renin angiotensin aldosterone system |
| RAI | radioactive iodine |
| RAR | retinoic acid receptor |
| RAST | radioallergosorbent test |
| RBC | red blood (cell) count |
| RDA | recommended (daily) dietary allowance |
| RDS | respiratory distress syndrome |
| REM | rapid eye movement |
| rem | radiation equivalent man |
| RES | reticuloendothelial system |

| | |
|---|---|
| RIA | radioimmunoassay |
| RNA | ribonucleic acid |
| ROM | range of motion |
| RSV | respiratory syncytial virus |
| RT | reverse transcriptase |
| RTK | receptor tyrosine kinase |
| $RT_3U$ | total serum thyroxine concentration |
| S&S | signs and symptoms |
| SA | sinoatrial |
| SARA | selective aldosterone receptor antagonist |
| SBE | subacute bacterial endocarditis |
| SC | subcutaneous |
| $S_{cr}$ | serum creatinine |
| SE | systemic embolism |
| sec | second |
| SERMs | selective estrogen receptor modulators |
| SGGT | serum gamma-glutamyl transferase |
| SGLT2 | sodium-glucose cotransporter 2 in proximal tubule of kidney |
| SGOT | serum glutamic–oxaloacetic transaminase (*see* AST) |
| SGPT | serum glutamic–pyruvic transaminase (*see* ALT) |
| SIADH | syndrome of inappropriate antidiuretic hormone |
| SI Units | International System of Units |
| SK | streptokinase |
| SL | sublingual |
| SLE | systemic lupus erythematosus |
| SLL | small lymphocytic lymphoma |
| SMA | sequential multiple analysis |
| SMZ/TMP | sulfamethoxazole/trimethoprim |
| SNRI | serotonin norepinephrine reuptake inhibitor |
| SOS | if necessary (*si opus cit*) |
| sp | species |
| SPF | sun protection factor |
| sq | square |
| SR | sedimentation rate |
| SRS-A | slow-reactive substance of anaphylaxis |
| SSRI | selective serotonin reuptake inhibitor |
| stat | immediately |
| STD | sexually transmitted disease |
| STEMI | ST elevated MI |
| SVT | supraventricular tachyarrhythmias |
| SW | sterile water |
| $t_{1/2}$ | half-life |
| $T_3$ | triiodothyronine |
| $T_4$ | thyroxine |
| TCA | tricyclic antidepressant |
| TG | total triglycerides |
| TIA | transient ischemic attack |

| | |
|---|---|
| t.i.d. | three times a day (*ter in die*) |
| TKI | tyrosine kinase inhibitor |
| TNF | tumor necrosis factor |
| tPA | tissue plasminogen activator |
| TPN | total parenteral nutrition |
| TPR | temperature, pulse, respirations |
| TSH | thyroid-stimulating hormone |
| TSS | toxic shock syndrome |
| TT | thrombin time |
| TTP | thrombotic cyclopenic purpura |
| UA | urinary analysis |
| UC | ulcerative colitis |
| ULN | upper limit of normal |
| URI | upper respiratory infection |
| USP | United States Pharmacopeia |
| USPHS | United States Public Health Service |
| UTI | urinary tract infection |
| UV-A, UVA | ultraviolet A wave |
| VDRL | Venereal Disease Research Laboratory |
| VEGF | vascular endothelial growth factor |
| VEGFR2 | vascular endothelial growth factor receptor 2 |
| VLDL | very low density lipoprotein |
| VMA | vanillylmandelic acid |
| VREF | vancomycin-resistant *Enterococcus faecium* |
| VRSA | vancomycin-resistant *Staphylococcus aureus* |
| VS | vital signs |
| wk | week |
| WBC | white blood (cell) count |
| WBCT | whole blood clotting time |
| y | year |

As patient interest in dietary supplements and other natural products increases, there is an increased need for information on this topic. These products are not standardized or stringently regulated by FDA guidelines; therefore, caution should be used when discussing these products. Consumers should note that since rigid quality control standards are not required for these products, substantial variability can occur in both potency and purity of a given product, especially between different commercial companies.

Many of these products have limited research on safety; thus, side effects and potential drug interactions are not well understood. Dietary supplements may either increase or decrease the level of a drug in the patient's body.

This table provides basic information on some of the most commonly sold dietary supplements. For additional information, a specialty resource on herbal and/or dietary supplements should be consulted.

| Name | Common Use | Significant Safety Concerns |
|------|-----------|----------------------------|
| Bilberry | Eye health | Long-term, high-dose use can cause liver problems |
| Black cohosh | Menopausal symptoms | Should be avoided in pregnant patients |
| Cranberry | Urinary tract infections | Considered safe at usual doses; high dose may increase bleeding risk |
| Echinacea | Infections | May cause allergic reactions; should be used only short-term |
| Eleuthera (Siberian ginseng) | Energy | Avoid use with digoxin |
| Evening primrose | Menopausal symptoms | May affect seizure threshold |
| Garcinia cambogia | Weight loss | Mild GI side effects |
| Flax | Cholesterol | Minor GI side effects |
| Garlic | Cholesterol | Significant drug interactions with drugs metabolized by CYP system |
| Ginger | Nausea | Overdoses may cause cardiac arrhythmias |

| Name | Common Use | Significant Safety Concerns |
|------|-----------|----------------------------|
| Ginkgo | Memory enhancement | Potential increased bleeding risk |
| Ginseng (American ginseng) | Energy | Should not be used with MAO inhibitors; may affect anticoagulants |
| Glucosamine | Osteoarthritis | Considered safe at usual doses; at higher doses, possible interaction with warfarin and other coumarin anticoagulants |
| Green tea | Energy, weight loss | High doses may cause cardiovascular side effects |
| Horny goat weed | Sexual function | Should be avoided in pregnant/lactating women |
| Horse chestnut | Congestive heart failure | Potential hepatotoxicity |
| Milk thistle | Liver function | May affect CYP metabolism and interact with drugs metabolized by this system |
| Saw palmetto | Benign prostatic hyperplasia | Adverse effects appear mild |
| Soy | Menopausal symptoms | GI-related side effects may be significant for some patients |
| St. John's wort | Depression | Significant drug interactions with several drugs metabolized by CYP system |
| Valerian | Sleep disorder | Potentially hepatotoxic |
| Yohimbe | Sexual function | Do not use with drugs affecting serotonin system |

# ◆ APPENDIX I LOOK-ALIKE, SOUND-ALIKE MEDICATIONS

There are a number of medications whose names look or sound similar when pronounced. The Institute of Safe Medication Practices, the Food and Drug Administration, the Joint Commission, and other patient safety groups have reported multiple medication errors related to these medications. The list below comes from the FDA approved list of established drug names that require use of Tall Man Letters (capitalized letters to more easily distinguish between similar medication names). More extensive lists of medications are available at http://www.ismp.org/tools/confuseddrugnames.pdf.

| | | |
|---|---|---|
| acetoHEXAMIDE | acetaZOLAMIDE | |
| ALPRAZolam | LORazepam | |
| aMILoride | amLODIPine | |
| ARIPiprazole | RABEprazole | |
| buPROPion | busPIRone | |
| chlorproMAZINE | chlorproPAMIDE | |
| clomiPHENE | clomiPRAMINE | |
| clonazePAM | cloNIDine cloZAPine cloBAZam | |
| cycloSPORINE | cycloSERINE | |
| DAUNOrubicin | DOXOrubicin | |
| dazePAM | diltiaZEM | |
| dimenhyDRINATE | diphenhydrAMINE | |
| DOBUTamine | DOPamine | |
| eriBULin | epiRUBicin | |
| glipiZIDE | glyBURIDE | |
| hydrALAZINE | hYDROmorphone | hydrOXYzine |
| LEVOleucovorin | leucovorin | |
| levOCARNitine | levETIRAceta | levoFLOXacin |
| hydroCHOROthiazie | hydrOXYzine | hydrALAZINE |
| medoxyPROGESTERone | methylPREDNISolone | methylTESTOSTERone |
| niCARdipine | NIFEdipine | |
| predniSONE | prednisoLONE | |
| risperiDONE | rOPINIRole | |
| sulfADIAZINE | sulfiSOXAZOLE | |
| TOLAZamide | TOLBUTamide | |
| vinBLAStine | vinCRIStine | |

ISMP's List of Confused Drug Names © ISMP 2015

The Centers for Disease Control and Prevention (CDC) contains detailed listings of what vaccinations are recommended for various age groups as well as patients with multiple concurrent disease states. The full recommendations are available at: http://www.cdc.gov/vaccines/recs/schedules/default.htm.

Dosing information is provided for some common vaccines. There are many other vaccines and vaccine formulations. Please consult the package insert for specific details regarding each of the following:

## BCG (BACILLUS CALMETTE-GUERIN) VACCINE
Tice, TheraCys

**USES** To protect groups with excessive rates of TB infection.

*Adult/Adolescent/Child (1 mo or older):* **Percutaneous** 0.2–0.3 mL of vaccine **Intradermal** 0.1 mL
*Child (younger than 1 mo):* **Percutaneous** Reduce adult dose by half, may need to reactivate at 1 y of age

**CONTRAINDICATIONS** Hypersensitivity to any vaccine component; active or past mycobacterial infection; immunosuppressed patients.

## DIPHTHERIA TOXOID/TETANUS TOXOID/ACELLULAR PERTUSSIS VACCINE, ADSORBED (DTaP/Tdap)
Adacel, Boostrix, Daptacel, Infanrix

**USES** Prevention of tetanus, diphtheria, and pertussis.

*Adult/Adolescent/Child (10 y or older):* **IM** 0.5 mL

**CONTRAINDICATIONS** Severe allergic reaction to any component of the formulation; encephalopathy within 7 days of a previous dose of pertussis antigen.

## HAEMOPHILUS B CONJUGATE VACCINE (HIB)
ActHIB, Hiberix, Liquid PedvaxHIB

**USES** To provide active immunity to *H. influenzae* type b (Hib) infection.

*Infant:* **IM** 0.5 mL at 2, 4, and 6 mo (ActHIB)
*Infant/Child:* **IM** 0.5 mL at 2 and 4 mo and again at 12 to 15 mo (Liquid PedvaxHIB)
*Child (15–59 mo):* **IM** 0.5 mL as booster (Hiberix)

**CONTRAINDICATIONS** Hypersensitivity to any vaccine components; fever of unknown etiology.

## HEPATITIS A VACCINE
Havrix, Vaqta

**USES** To provide active immunity to hepatitis A.

*Adult:* **IM** 1 mL dose then 1 mL 6–12 mo later
*Child (1–18 y):* **IM** 0.5 mL then 0.5 mL 1 mo later, then 0.5 mL booster dose 6–12 mo later

**CONTRAINDICATIONS** Hypersensitivity to any vaccine component; neomycin hypersensitivity.

## HEPATITIS B IMMUNE GLOBULIN
HepaGam B, HyperHep, Nabi-HB

**USES** To provide passive immunity to hepatitis B infections in individuals exposed to HBV or Hbs Ag-positive materials; to prevent hepatitis B recurrence in post-liver transplant (HepaGam B).

*Adult/Child:* **IM** 0.06 mL/kg as soon as possible post-exposure, then repeat 28–30 day post-exposure *Neonate:* **IM** 0.5 mL within 24 h of birth, then repeat at 3 and 6 mo *Adult:* **HepaGam B IV** 20,000 U/dose daily every 2 wk (2–12 wk) then monthly

**CONTRAINDICATIONS** Hypersensitivity to any vaccine component.

## HEPATITIS B VACCINE (RECOMBINANT)
Engerix-B, Recombivax HB

**USES** To provide active immunity to individuals at high risk for exposure.

*Adult (20 y or older):* **IM/Subcutaneous** 10 mcg then repeat at 1 and 6 mo (Recombivax); 20 mcg then repeat at 1 and 6 mo (Engerix-B) *Adult (younger than 20 y)/Adolescent/ Child/Infant:* **IM/Subcutaneous** 5 mcg then repeat at 1 and 6 mo (Recombivax) *Adult/Adolescent/Child (11 y or older):* **IM** 10–20 mcg then repeat at 1 and 6 mo (Engerix-B) *Neonate* **IM/Subcutaneous** 5 mcg within 12 h of birth then repeat at 1 and 6 mo (Recombivax); 10 mcg within 12 h of birth then repeat at 1 and 6 mo (Engerix-B)

**CONTRAINDICATIONS** Hypersensitivity to any vaccine component; yeast hypersensitivity.

## HUMAN PAPILLOMAVIRUS BIVALENT (RECOMBINANT)
Cervarix

**USES** To prevent disease associated with HPV exposure.

*Adult/Adolescent/Child (10 y or older):* **IM** 0.5 mL dose at 0, 1, and 6 mo

**CONTRAINDICATIONS** Hypersensitivity to any vaccine component; yeast hypersensitivity.

## HUMAN PAPILLOMAVIRUS QUADRIVALENT VACCINE (RECOMBINANT)
Gardasil

**USES** To prevent HPV-related disease; to prevent genital warts; to prevent anal cancer.

*Adult/Child (9 y or older):* **IM** 0.5 mL followed by doses at 2 and 6 mo

**CONTRAINDICATIONS** Hypersensitivity to any vaccine component; yeast hypersensitivity.

## HUMAN PAPILLOMAVIRUS 9-VALENT VACCINE
Gardasil 9

**USES** To prevent HPV-related disease; to prevent genital warts; to prevent anal cancer.

*Adult/Child (9–26 y):* **IM** 0.5 mL followed by doses at 2 and 6 mo

**CONTRAINDICATIONS** Hypersensitivity to any vaccine component; yeast hypersensitivity; previous use of other HPV vaccine.

## INFLUENZA VACCINE
Afluria, FLUAD, Fluarix, Flublok, FluLaval, Fluvirin, Fluzone, Flumist, FluMist Quadrivalent

**USES** To prevent influenza.

*Adult (younger than 49 y):* **Intranasal** 0.2 mL dose **IM** 0.5 mL *Geriatric:* FLUAD formulation **IM** 0.5mL
*Child (9 y or older):* **Intranasal** 0.1 mL per nostril
*Child (2–8 y):* **IM** 0.5 mL dose if it is the first vaccination, then repeat in 4 wk **Intranasal** 0.1 mL per nostril; dose may need to be repeated
*Infant/Child (6–35 mo):* **IM** 0.25 mL dose if it is the first vaccination, then repeat in 4 wk

**CONTRAINDICATIONS** Hypersensitivity to egg, kanamycin, neomycin or polymyxin.

## MENINGOCOCCAL DIPHTHERIA TOXOID CONJUGATE
Menveo, Menactra

**USES** To provide prophylaxis against meningococcal infection.

*Adult (younger than 56 y)/Adolescent/Child (2 y or older):* **IM** 0.5 mL injection
*Infant/Child (9 mo or older):* Menactra only: 0.5 mL injection (2 dose series)

**CONTRAINDICATIONS** Hypersensitivity to any vaccine component; history of Guillain-Barré syndrome, latex hypersensitivity.

## MEASLES, MUMPS AND RUBELLA VIRUS VACCINE
M-M-R II

**USES** Vaccination against measles, mumps, and rubella.

*Child (over 12 mo):* **Subcutaneous** 0.5 mL at ages 12–15 mo; second dose at ages 4–6 y

**CONTRAINDICATIONS** Hypersensitivity to any component of the vaccine, including gelatin Do not administer to patients who are pregnant, receiving immunosuppressive therapy.

## MENINGOCOCCAL GROUP B VACCINE
Bexsero, Trumenba

**USES** To provide prophylaxis against meningococcal infection.

*Adult/Adolescent/Child (ages 10–25 y):* **IM** 0.5 mL/dose as part of a 2 or 3 dose series

**CONTRAINDICATIONS** Hypersensitivity to the meningococcal group B vaccine or any component of the formulation.

## PNEUMOCOCCAL 13-VALENT VACCINE, DIPHTHERIA
Prevnar 13

**USES** To provide routine prophylaxis for infants and children as part of the primary childhood immunization schedule.

*Child/Adolescent (6–17 y):* **IM** 0.5 mL as single dose

*Child (2–6 y):* **IM** If no previous doses given, 0.5 mL single dose

*Child (12–23 mo):* **IM** If no previous doses given, 0.5 mL followed by a second dose after 8 wk (total of 2 doses)

*Infant (7–11 mo):* **IM** If no previous doses given, 0.5 mL followed by a second dose in 4 wk, then a third dose after the 1 y birthday (total of 3 doses)

*Infant (younger than 6 wk):* **IM** 0.5 mL dose repeated at 4–8 wk, then 4–8 wk after the second dose and again at 12–15 mo of age (total of 4 doses)

**CONTRAINDICATIONS** Hypersensitivity to any vaccine component.

## PNEUMOCOCCAL POLYSACCHARIDE VACCINE, 23-VALENT
Pneumovax 23

**USES** Pneumococcal disease prevention

*Adult/Adolescent/Child (2 y or older):* **Subcutaneous/IM** 0.5 mL; revaccination may be necessary in some patients with concurrent immunocompromised disease states.

**CONTRAINDICATIONS** Severe allergic reaction to pneumococcal vaccine or any component of the formulation.

## RABIES VACCINE
RabAvert, Imovax

**USES** Pre-exposure rabies prophylaxis

*Adult/Adolescent/Children/Infant:* **IM** Series of 3 injections 1 mL on days 0, 7, 21, or 28

**CONTRAINDICATIONS** Anaphylaxis to vaccine or vaccine component.

## ROTAVIRUS VACCINE
Rotarix, RotaTeq

**USES** To prevent gastroenteritis caused by rotavirus infection.

*Infant (6–32 wk) (RotaTeq only):* **PO** 2 mL at 2, 4, and 6 mo

*Infant (6–24 wk) (Rotarix only):* **PO** 1 mL at 6 wk; then second dose to follow at least 4 wk later

**CONTRAINDICATIONS** Hypersensitivity to any vaccine component, history of intussusception, or severe combined immunodeficiency.

## VARICELLA VACCINE
Varivax

**USES** To provide vaccination against varicella.

*Adult/Adolescent:* **Subcutaneous** 0.5 mL followed by a second dose 4–8 wk later

*Child (1–12 y):* **Subcutaneous** 0.5 mL single dose

**CONTRAINDICATIONS** Hypersensitivity to any vaccine component; AIDS; bone marrow suppression; concurrent chemotherapy or corticosteroid therapy; gelatin hypersensitivity; hypogammaglobulinemia; current leukemia or lymphoma; neomycin hypersensitivity; pregnancy; tuberculosis; concurrent radiation therapy.

# ZOSTER VACCINE LIVE
Zostavax

**USES** To prevent herpes zoster in people over 50 y old.

*Adult (50 y or older):* **Subcutaneous** Administer 0.65 mL as single dose.

**CONTRAINDICATIONS**  Hypersensitivity to any vaccine component; AIDS; gelatin hypersensitivity; immunosuppression; leukemia; lymphoma; neomycin hypersensitivity; pregnancy; people receiving antitumor necrosis factors.

# BIBLIOGRAPHY

*American Hospital Formulary Service (AHFS) Drug Information.* 2017. Bethesda, MD: American Society of Health-System Pharmacists.

*Clinical Pharmacology.* http://clinicalpharmacology.com. Elsevier/Gold Standard Media. 2017.

*Food and Drug Administration.* http://www.fda.gov. 2017.

Lacy CF, Armstrong LL, Goldman MP, Lance LL. *Drug Information Handbook.* 2017. http://online.lexi.com/.

National Institute of Health. *Daily Med.* http:/daily med.nlm.gov. 2016.

Trissel LA. *Handbook of Injectable Drugs.* 19th ed. Bethesda, MD: American Society of Health-System Pharmacists. 2016.

# INDEX

---

Drug categories are in SMALL CAPS. Prototypes are in **bold.**
Generic drug names are given in parentheses.

Drug categories are in SMALL CAPS. Prototypes are in **bold.**
Generic drug names are given in parentheses.

Drug categories are in SMALL CAPS. Prototypes are in **bold**.
Generic drug names are given in parentheses.

1805

Drug categories are in SMALL CAPS. Prototypes are in **bold.**
Generic drug names are given in parentheses.

Drug categories are in SMALL CAPS. Prototypes are in **bold**.
Generic drug names are given in parentheses.

1807

Drug categories are in SMALL CAPS. Prototypes are in **bold.**
Generic drug names are given in parentheses.

1809

Drug categories are in SMALL CAPS. Prototypes are in **bold.**
Generic drug names are given in parentheses.

Drug categories are in SMALL CAPS. Prototypes are in **bold**.
Generic drug names are given in parentheses.

1811

Drug categories are in SMALL CAPS. Prototypes are in **bold.**
Generic drug names are given in parentheses.

Drug categories are in SMALL CAPS. Prototypes are in **bold.**
Generic drug names are given in parentheses.

1813

Drug categories are in SMALL CAPS. Prototypes are in **bold.**
Generic drug names are given in parentheses.

Drug categories are in SMALL CAPS. Prototypes are in **bold**.
Generic drug names are given in parentheses.

Drug categories are in SMALL CAPS. Prototypes are in **bold.**
Generic drug names are given in parentheses.

Drug categories are in SMALL CAPS. Prototypes are in **bold**.
Generic drug names are given in parentheses.

1817

Drug categories are in SMALL CAPS. Prototypes are in **bold.**
Generic drug names are given in parentheses.

Drug categories are in SMALL CAPS. Prototypes are in **bold**.
Generic drug names are given in parentheses.

1819

Drug categories are in SMALL CAPS. Prototypes are in **bold.**
Generic drug names are given in parentheses.

Drug categories are in SMALL CAPS. Prototypes are in **bold.**
Generic drug names are given in parentheses.

1821

Drug categories are in SMALL CAPS. Prototypes are in **bold**.
Generic drug names are given in parentheses.

Drug categories are in SMALL CAPS. Prototypes are in **bold**.
Generic drug names are given in parentheses.

1823

Drug categories are in SMALL CAPS. Prototypes are in **bold**.
Generic drug names are given in parentheses.

1825

Drug categories are in SMALL CAPS. Prototypes are in **bold.** Generic drug names are given in parentheses.

Drug categories are in SMALL CAPS. Prototypes are in **bold.**
Generic drug names are given in parentheses.

Drug categories are in SMALL CAPS. Prototypes are in **bold.**
Generic drug names are given in parentheses.

1829

Drug categories are in SMALL CAPS. Prototypes are in **bold.**
Generic drug names are given in parentheses.

Drug categories are in SMALL CAPS. Prototypes are in **bold**.
Generic drug names are given in parentheses.
1831

Drug categories are in SMALL CAPS. Prototypes are in **bold.**
Generic drug names are given in parentheses.

Drug categories are in SMALL CAPS. Prototypes are in **bold.**
Generic drug names are given in parentheses.

1833

Drug categories are in SMALL CAPS. Prototypes are in **bold.**
Generic drug names are given in parentheses.

---

Drug categories are in SMALL CAPS. Prototypes are in **bold**.
Generic drug names are given in parentheses.

Drug categories are in SMALL CAPS. Prototypes are in **bold.**
Generic drug names are given in parentheses.

Drug categories are in SMALL CAPS. Prototypes are in **bold.**
Generic drug names are given in parentheses.

1837

Drug categories are in SMALL CAPS. Prototypes are in **bold.**
Generic drug names are given in parentheses.

Drug categories are in SMALL CAPS. Prototypes are in **bold.**
Generic drug names are given in parentheses.
1839

Drug categories are in SMALL CAPS. Prototypes are in **bold.**
Generic drug names are given in parentheses.

---

Drug categories are in SMALL CAPS. Prototypes are in **bold.**
Generic drug names are given in parentheses.

Drug categories are in SMALL CAPS. Prototypes are in **bold.**
Generic drug names are given in parentheses.

1843

Drug categories are in SMALL CAPS. Prototypes are in **bold**.
Generic drug names are given in parentheses.

Drug categories are in SMALL CAPS. Prototypes are in **bold**.
Generic drug names are given in parentheses.

1845

Drug categories are in SMALL CAPS. Prototypes are in **bold.**
Generic drug names are given in parentheses.

Drug categories are in SMALL CAPS. Prototypes are in **bold.**
Generic drug names are given in parentheses.
1847

Drug categories are in SMALL CAPS. Prototypes are in **bold.**
Generic drug names are given in parentheses.

Drug categories are in SMALL CAPS. Prototypes are in **bold.**
Generic drug names are given in parentheses.

1849

Drug categories are in SMALL CAPS. Prototypes are in **bold.**
Generic drug names are given in parentheses.

Drug categories are in SMALL CAPS. Prototypes are in **bold.**
Generic drug names are given in parentheses.

1851

Drug categories are in SMALL CAPS. Prototypes are in **bold.**
Generic drug names are given in parentheses.

Drug categories are in SMALL CAPS. Prototypes are in **bold.**
Generic drug names are given in parentheses.

1853

Drug categories are in SMALL CAPS. Prototypes are in **bold.**
Generic drug names are given in parentheses.

Drug categories are in SMALL CAPS. Prototypes are in **bold.**
Generic drug names are given in parentheses.

1855

Drug categories are in SMALL CAPS. Prototypes are in **bold.**
Generic drug names are given in parentheses.

Drug categories are in SMALL CAPS. Prototypes are in **bold.**
Generic drug names are given in parentheses.
1857

Drug categories are in SMALL CAPS. Prototypes are in **bold**.
Generic drug names are given in parentheses.

Drug categories are in SMALL CAPS. Prototypes are in **bold.**
Generic drug names are given in parentheses.

1859

Drug categories are in SMALL CAPS. Prototypes are in **bold.**
Generic drug names are given in parentheses.

Drug categories are in SMALL CAPS. Prototypes are in **bold.**
Generic drug names are given in parentheses.

1861

Drug categories are in SMALL CAPS. Prototypes are in **bold.**
Generic drug names are given in parentheses.

Drug categories are in SMALL CAPS. Prototypes are in **bold.**
Generic drug names are given in parentheses.

1863

Drug categories are in SMALL CAPS. Prototypes are in **bold.**
Generic drug names are given in parentheses.

## J

## K

Drug categories are in SMALL CAPS. Prototypes are in **bold.**
Generic drug names are given in parentheses.

Drug categories are in SMALL CAPS. Prototypes are in **bold.**
Generic drug names are given in parentheses.

Drug categories are in SMALL CAPS. Prototypes are in **bold.**
Generic drug names are given in parentheses.

1867

Drug categories are in SMALL CAPS. Prototypes are in **bold.**
Generic drug names are given in parentheses.

Drug categories are in SMALL CAPS. Prototypes are in **bold.**
Generic drug names are given in parentheses.

Drug categories are in SMALL CAPS. Prototypes are in **bold.**
Generic drug names are given in parentheses.

1871

Drug categories are in SMALL CAPS. Prototypes are in **bold.**
Generic drug names are given in parentheses.

Drug categories are in SMALL CAPS. Prototypes are in **bold.**
Generic drug names are given in parentheses.

1873

Drug categories are in SMALL CAPS. Prototypes are in **bold.**
Generic drug names are given in parentheses.

1875

Drug categories are in SMALL CAPS. Prototypes are in **bold.**
Generic drug names are given in parentheses.

Drug categories are in SMALL CAPS. Prototypes are in **bold.**
Generic drug names are given in parentheses.

1877

Drug categories are in SMALL CAPS. Prototypes are in **bold.** Generic drug names are given in parentheses.

Drug categories are in SMALL CAPS. Prototypes are in **bold.**
Generic drug names are given in parentheses.

1879

Drug categories are in SMALL CAPS. Prototypes are in **bold.**
Generic drug names are given in parentheses.

Drug categories are in SMALL CAPS. Prototypes are in **bold.**
Generic drug names are given in parentheses.

1881

Drug categories are in SMALL CAPS. Prototypes are in **bold.**
Generic drug names are given in parentheses.

---

Drug categories are in SMALL CAPS. Prototypes are in **bold.**
Generic drug names are given in parentheses.

Drug categories arc in SMALL CAPS. Prototypes are in **bold.**
Generic drug names are given in parentheses.

Drug categories are in SMALL CAPS. Prototypes are in **bold.**
Generic drug names are given in parentheses.

1885

Drug categories are in SMALL CAPS. Prototypes are in **bold.**
Generic drug names are given in parentheses.

Drug categories are in SMALL CAPS. Prototypes are in **bold.**
Generic drug names are given in parentheses.

1887

Drug categories are in SMALL CAPS. Prototypes are in **bold.**
Generic drug names are given in parentheses.

Drug categories are in SMALL CAPS. Prototypes are in **bold.**
Generic drug names are given in parentheses.

1889

Drug categories are in SMALL CAPS. Prototypes are in **bold**.
Generic drug names are given in parentheses.

Drug categories are in SMALL CAPS. Prototypes are in **bold.**
Generic drug names are given in parentheses.

1891

Drug categories are in SMALL CAPS. Prototypes are in **bold.**
Generic drug names are given in parentheses.

Drug categories are in SMALL CAPS. Prototypes are in **bold**.
Generic drug names are given in parentheses.

1893

Drug categories are in SMALL CAPS. Prototypes are in **bold.**
Generic drug names are given in parentheses.

Drug categories are in SMALL CAPS. Prototypes are in **bold.**
Generic drug names are given in parentheses.

1897

# INDEX

Drug categories are in SMALL CAPS. Prototypes are in **bold.**
Generic drug names are given in parentheses.

Drug categories are in SMALL CAPS. Prototypes are in **bold.**
Generic drug names are given in parentheses.
1899

Drug categories are in SMALL CAPS. Prototypes are in **bold.**
Generic drug names are given in parentheses.

Drug categories are in SMALL CAPS. Prototypes are in **bold.**
Generic drug names are given in parentheses.

1901

Drug categories are in SMALL CAPS. Prototypes are in **bold.**
Generic drug names are given in parentheses.

Drug categories are in SMALL CAPS. Prototypes are in **bold**.
Generic drug names are given in parentheses.
1903

Drug categories are in SMALL CAPS. Prototypes are in **bold.**
Generic drug names are given in parentheses.

Drug categories are in SMALL CAPS. Prototypes are in **bold.**
Generic drug names are given in parentheses.

1905

Drug categories are in SMALL CAPS. Prototypes are in **bold.**
Generic drug names are given in parentheses.

Drug categories are in SMALL CAPS. Prototypes are in **bold.**
Generic drug names are given in parentheses.

Drug categories are in SMALL CAPS. Prototypes are in **bold**.
Generic drug names are given in parentheses.

Drug categories are in SMALL CAPS. Prototypes are in **bold.**
Generic drug names are given in parentheses.

1909

Drug categories are in SMALL CAPS. Prototypes are in **bold.**
Generic drug names are given in parentheses.

Drug categories are in SMALL CAPS. Prototypes are in **bold.**
Generic drug names are given in parentheses.

1911